INTERNATIONAL TEXTBOOK OF MEDICINE

General Editors

A. H. SAMIY, M.D.

Professor of Clinical Medicine and Chief of
Division of Medicine, New York Hospital, Cornell Medical Center
New York, New York

LLOYD H. SMITH, JR., M.D.

Professor of Medicine; Associate Dean,
University of California, San Francisco, School of Medicine,
San Francisco, California

JAMES B. WYNGAARDEN, M.D.

Director, National Institutes of Health,
Bethesda, Maryland

VOLUME I
PATHOPHYSIOLOGY
The Biological Principles of Disease

VOLUME II
MEDICAL MICROBIOLOGY AND INFECTIOUS DISEASES

Volumes I and II of the International Textbook of Medicine
have been conceived and written to follow a logical pedagogical approach
and can readily be used in conjunction with the
CECIL TEXTBOOK OF MEDICINE.

Second Edition

PATHOPHYSIOLOGY
The Biological Principles of Disease

LLOYD H. SMITH, Jr., M.D.

Professor of Medicine; Associate Dean,
University of California, San Francisco, School of Medicine,
San Francisco, California

SAMUEL O. THIER, M.D.

Sterling Professor and Chairman, Department of Internal Medicine,
Yale University School of Medicine,
New Haven, Connecticut

1985

W. B. SAUNDERS COMPANY

Philadelphia, London, Toronto, Mexico City, Rio de Janeiro, Sydney, Tokyo, Hong Kong

W. B. Saunders Company: West Washington Square
Philadelphia, PA 19105

Library of Congress Cataloging in Publication Data

Main entry under title:

Pathophysiology: the biological principles of disease.

Includes bibliographies and index.

1. Physiology, Pathological.   I. Smith, Lloyd H., 1924–
   II. Thier, Samuel O., 1937–   .   [DNLM: 1. Disease.
   2. Pathology.   3. Physiology. QZ 140 P297]

RB113.P364 1985   616.07   85–2007

ISBN 0–7216–8411–4

Manuscript Editor: Donna Walker and Edna Dick
Indexer: Edna Dick
Production Manager: Frank Polizzano

Listed here is the latest translated edition of this book together
with the language of the translation and the publisher:

Spanish (*1st Edition*)—Editorial Medica Panamericana, Buenos Aires, Argentina

PATHOPHYSIOLOGY—The Biological Principles of Diseases   ISBN   0-7216-8411-4

Last digit is the print number: 9   8   7   6   5   4   3   2   1

Dedication

To medical students and physicians throughout the world,
who strive with dedication and hard work
to achieve better health for mankind.

CONTRIBUTORS

PETER S. ARONSON, M.D.

Associate Professor, Departments of Medicine and Physiology, Yale University School of Medicine, New Haven. Attending Physician, Yale-New Haven Hospital, New Haven, and Veterans Administration Hospital, West Haven, Connecticut.
The Kidney

LLOYD AXELROD, M.D.

Associate Professor of Medicine, Harvard Medical School. Associate Physician, Massachusetts General Hospital, and Chief of the Medical Unit, Massachusetts Eye and Ear Infirmary, Boston, Massachusetts.
Adrenal Cortex

C. RICHARD BOLAND, M.D.

Associate Professor of Medicine, University of Michigan School of Medicine. Chief of Gastroenterology, Veterans Administration Medical Center, Ann Arbor, Michigan.
The Colon

C. BUNCH, M.A., M.B., Ch.B., F.R.C.P.

Clinical Reader in Clinical Medicine, Nuffield Department of Clinical Medicine, University of Oxford. Honorary Consultant Physician, Oxfordshire Health Authority, England.
The Blood and Blood-Forming Organs

DAVID R. COX, M.D., Ph.D.

Associate Professor of Pediatrics, Biochemistry and Biophysics, University of California, San Francisco, School of Medicine, San Francisco, California.
Genetics

GILBERT H. DANIELS, M.D.

Associate Professor of Medicine, Harvard Medical School. Associate Physician and Director, Thyroid Clinic, Massachusetts General Hospital, Boston, Massachusetts.
Thyroid Pathophysiology

CLIFFORD W. DEVENEY, M.D.

Associate Professor of Surgery, University of California, San Francisco, School of Medicine. Surgeon, San Francisco Veterans Administration Medical Center, San Francisco, California.
The Stomach

MARILYN G. FARQUHAR, Ph.D.

Professor of Cell Biology, Yale University School of Medicine, New Haven, Connecticut.
Cell Biology

PHILIP FELIG, M.D.

President, Sandoz Research Institute, Sandoz, Inc., E. Hanover, New Jersey. Clinical Professor of Medicine, Yale University School of Medicine, New Haven, Connecticut.
Metabolism

THOMAS B. FITZPATRICK, M.D.

Wigglesworth Professor and Chairman, Department of Dermatology, Harvard Medical School. Chief of Dermatology Service, Massachusetts General Hospital, Boston, Massachusetts.
Pathophysiology of Skin

EDWARD J. GOETZEL, M.D.

Professor of Medicine and Microbiology and Director, Division of Allergy and Immunology, University of California, San Francisco, School of Medicine. Investigator, Howard Hughes Medical Institute, San Francisco, California.
Immunology

IRA S. GOLDMAN, M.D.

Assistant Professor of Medicine, Gastroenterology Division, University of California, San Francisco, School of Medicine, San Francisco, California.
Pathophysiology of the Esophagus

JAMES H. GRENDELL, M.D.

Assistant Professor of Medicine, Gastroenterology Division, University of California, San Francisco, School of Medicine, San Francisco, California.
The Pancreas

RICHARD J. HAVEL, M.D.

Professor of Medicine and Director, Cardiovascular Research Institute, University of California, San Francisco, School of Medicine. Attending Physician, Moffitt-Long Hospital, University of California Medical Center, San Francisco, California.
Metabolism

MARTIN F. HEYWORTH, M.D., M.R.C.P.

Assistant Professor of Medicine, University of California, San Francisco, School of Medicine. Staff Physician, San Francisco Veterans Administration Medical Center, San Francisco, California.
Pathophysiology of the Small Intestine

ANNE KLIBANSKI, M.D.

Assistant Professor of Medicine, Harvard Medical School. Assistant in Medicine, Massachusetts General Hospital, Boston, Massachusetts.
Reproductive Endocrinology

STEPHEN M. KRANE, M.D.

Professor of Medicine, Harvard Medical School. Physician and Chief, Arthritis Unit, Massachusetts General Hospital, Boston, Massachusetts.
Connective Tissue

JOHN F. MURRAY, M.D., D.Sc.(Hon.)

Professor of Medicine, University of California, San Francisco, School of Medicine. Chief, Chest Service, San Francisco General Hospital, and Member, Senior Staff, Cardiovascular Research Institute, University of California, San Francisco, California
Respiration

ROBERT M. NEER, M.D.

Associate Professor of Medicine, Harvard Medical School. Director, Mallinckrodt General Clinical Research Center, Massachusetts General Hospital, Boston, Massachusetts.

Connective Tissue

GEORGE E. PALADE, M.D.

Senior Research Scientist, Yale University School of Medicine, New Haven, Connecticut.

Cell Biology

FRED PLUM, M.D. (Cornell), M.D. (HC) (Karolinska Institute, Stockholm)

Anne Parrish Titzell Professor and Chairman, Department of Neurology, Cornell University Medical College, New York. Neurologist-in-Chief, New York Hospital, New York, New York.

Neurology

JEROME B. POSNER, M.D.

Professor of Neurology, Cornell University Medical College, New York. Chairman, Department of Neurology, Memorial Sloan-Kettering Cancer Center, New York, New York.

Neurology

RICHARD K. ROOT, M.D.

Professor and Chairman, Department of Medicine, University of California, San Francisco, School of Medicine, San Francisco, California.

Infectious Diseases: Pathogenetic Mechanisms and Host Responses

E. CHESTER RIDGWAY III, M.D.

Professor of Medicine and Head, Division of Endocrinology, University of Colorado Health Sciences Center, Denver, Colorado.

The Pituitary and Hypothalamus

MICHAEL ROSENBLATT, M.D.

Vice President for Biological Research, Merck Sharp & Dohme Research Laboratories, West Point, Pennsylvania.

Endocrinology; Hormonal Regulation of Calcium Metabolism

DANIEL RUDMAN, M.D.

Professor of Medicine and Director, Division of Geriatric Medicine, University of Health Sciences/Chicago Medical School. Chief of Geriatric Medicine, Veterans Administration Medical Center, North Chicago, Illinois.

Pathophysiologic Principles of Nutrition

MARVIN H. SLEISENGER, M.D., D.S.(Hon.)

Professor and Vice Chairman, Department of Medicine, University of California, San Francisco, School of Medicine. Chief, Medical Services, San Francisco Veterans Administration Medical Center, San Francisco, California.

Pathophysiology of the Gastrointestinal Tract

LLOYD H. SMITH, Jr., M.D.

Professor of Medicine and Associate Dean, University of California, San Francisco, School of Medicine, San Francisco, California.

Metabolism

NICHOLAS A. SOTER, M.D.

Professor of Dermatology, New York University School of Medicine. Attending Physician, University Hospital, New York University Medical Center, New York, New York.
Pathophysiology of Skin

JOHN D. STOBO, M.D.

Professor of Medicine, Investigator, Howard Hughes Medical Institute, San Francisco. Head, Section of Rheumatology/Clinical Immunology, University of California, San Francisco, School of Medicine, San Francisco, California.
Immunology

SAMUEL O. THIER, M.D.

Sterling Professor and Chairman, Department of Internal Medicine, Yale University School of Medicine, New Haven, Connecticut.
The Kidney

ANDREW G. WALLACE, M.D.

Professor of Medicine, Duke University School of Medicine. Attending Physician, Duke University Hospital, Durham, North Carolina.
Pathophysiology of Cardiovascular Disease

ROBERT A. WAUGH, M.D.

Associate Professor of Medicine, Duke University School of Medicine. Attending Physician, Duke University Hospital, Durham, North Carolina.
Pathophysiology of Cardiovascular Disease

D. J. WEATHERALL, F.R.C.P., F.R.S.

Nuffield Professor of Clinical Medicine, and Honorary Director, Medical Research Council Molecular Haematology Unit, University of Oxford. Honorary Consultant Physician, Oxford District and Regional Health Authority, John Radcliffe Hospital, Oxford, England.
The Blood and Blood-Forming Organs

PATRICIA JO WILLIAMS, M.M.Sc., R.D.

Clinical Faculty and Research Nutritionist, Clinical Research Facility, Emory University School of Medicine, Atlanta, Georgia.
Pathophysiologic Principles of Nutrition

DAVID ZAKIM, M.D.

Vincent Astor Distinguished Professor of Medicine, Cornell University Medical College. Professor of Cell Biology, Cornell University Graduate School of Medical Sciences. Attending Physician and Director, Division of Digestive Diseases, the New York Hospital, New York, New York.
Pathophysiology of Liver Disease

FOREWORD

The traditions of medicine are as old as recorded history and are interwoven into all civilizations, both past and present. Avicenna, Galen, Hippocrates, Maimonides, Harvey, Pasteur, Koch, and many others, celebrated and obscure, have created that tradition, which is still being modified in our time. Clearly, superstition in medicine is not yet expelled nor empiricism sufficiently narrowed. They remain to adulterate and diminish the science and humanism of medical practice.

The science of medicine is universal in its origins and in its relevance. In fact, universality in time and place is the bedrock of scientific observation. Human biology is basically the same in Sri Lanka as in Sweden. It is true that biological variation exists. Gene pools have been modified by mutation and natural selection. Balanced polymorphism, for example, seems to have created a high incidence of sickle cell disease only where the associated increased resistance to falciparum malaria constitutes a significant biological advantage. Such examples of differing gene pools in ethnic groups abound. Much more impressive, however, is the constancy of human biology, representing a high conservation of the human genome and therefore close homology of gene products. Out of infinite possibilities, the same molecular species transport oxygen, capture energy from carbohydrates, and transmit nerve impulses in all humans without regard for national borders. It would be astonishing if it were otherwise in view of the recentness of the "ascent of man" from a common ancestry. It is reasonable, therefore, to present Volume I of this textbook as "international." Its discussions of cell biology, genetics, immunology, hematology, metabolism, endocrinology, cardiology, respiration, nephrology, gastroenterology, neurology, connective tissue, and dermatology are universally relevant. They are the disciplines that underlie the practice of medicine in whatever setting that practice may occur.

Although human biology is relatively constant, the environments in which men exist are extraordinarily diverse. Differences in nutrition, culture, education, economics, climate, crowding, application of the technologies of public health and preventive medicine, and many other environmental influences dictate the occurrence of disease and the maintenance of health far more than do differences in genomic nucleotide sequences. Disease presents in different patterns, therefore, throughout the world (geographic medicine) and in subsets within a given society (epidemiology). Differences exist in the incidence of all kinds of diseases (cancer, cardiovascular disorders, rheumatic diseases); in fact, it is difficult to find any disorder with equal geographical prevalence. Nutritional disorders, the infectious and parasitic diseases, and their deadly interactions are without question the medical problems with the most sharply defined geographical and economic foci—largely in the developing countries of the world.

All living things protect themselves as vigorously from invasion by smaller living things as they do from engulfment by larger ones; for it is as bad to rot from within as to be eaten from without—at least it is as decisive. Poor nutrition causes that protection to falter in ways not yet fully explained. Inadequate sanitation, poverty, and crowding have their own epidemiology and assist the invasion by smaller living things. Furthermore, some infectious diseases, once comfortably remote from western countries, are now alarmingly close in a shrinking world marked by increasing commerce in goods and people. Lassa fever, although still confined to Africa, warrants attention; kuru may be an analog for slow virus diseases yet to be detected. Volume II, edited by Doctors Braude, Davis, and Fierer, is truly international in its description of the parasitic and infectious diseases. Fifty-eight participants from 27 countries outside the United States have contributed to its completion with the authority of direct personal observation. More than any single book now available, it describes the world experience with the parasitic and infectious diseases.

The first two volumes of the *International Textbook of Medicine* were designed to articulate with the *Cecil Textbook of Medicine,* which has had an international audience in internal medicine for more than half a century, to complete this "system of medicine." The practice of clinical medicine requires a frame of reference, which for this series is the western world with its assumption of the availability of high technology and its recommended therapeutic programs.

The *International Textbook of Medicine,* then, has created two new books designed to be used with a third, a well known classic textbook of medicine. All three of these textbooks are capable of standing alone and each will have its specific audience. What is the motivation for presenting them in such a series or system of medicine? More than three fourths of the earth's population live in the developing countries of the world. Achievement of better health is one of the highest aspirations of the people of these countries. "The health of all the people is really the foundation upon which all their happiness and all their powers as a state depend" (Disraeli). The prospects for better health in most of these countries, even in those that are wealthier and more fortunate, depend more directly upon the ultimate conquest of persistent poverty, malnutrition, illiteracy, and a multitude of other social problems than upon expansion of personal health services. These are problems that transcend the work of the physician, although the physician may be unusually influential in their alleviation. This is perhaps particularly true in countries where physicians constitute one of the few highly educated segments of society.

Despite the crushing burden of these external factors, most of which are beyond the traditional purview of medicine, the education of physicians and other health workers remains a top priority. The number of medical schools, medical students, and physicians continues to rise throughout the world. A severe limitation to both undergraduate and continuing medical education, however, has been a deficit of appropriate textbooks. Students living in the developing countries of Asia, Africa, or Latin America often have no easy access to libraries and can rarely afford to own the required textbooks. In most circumstances the student must rely on didactic lectures or notes distributed by teachers.

On the basis of these observations, as well as from many years of personal experience in medical education in developing countries, one of us (AHS) conceived this plan to publish a comprehensive textbook of medicine to meet the needs of students and physicians in the international medical community. Not unexpectedly, this turned out to be impossible to attain in a single volume. Volume I was therefore designed to give a comprehensive presentation of the most pertinent aspects of basic science and pathophysiology for medical practice. In view of the importance of infectious diseases as the leading cause of morbidity and mortality in the developing countries, it was considered essential to devote an entire volume to microbiology and to the clinical problems of infectious diseases. Of the many authoritative textbooks of clinical medicine, the *Cecil Textbook of Medicine* was judged to lend itself most readily to this series. At this time, the *International Textbook of Medicine* does not attempt to encompass all aspects of medical practice, such as pediatrics, surgery, or psychiatry. As such it is not totally comprehensive, but it is a start. It is also not a primer but rather presents medicine and its relevant pathophysiology at a level of rigor consistent with that taught at advanced medical schools throughout the world.

The practice of medicine is truly international in its scope. The editors hope that the *International Textbook of Medicine* will make a contribution to its common purposes.

ABDOL HOSSEIN SAMIY

LLOYD H. SMITH, JR.

JAMES B. WYNGAARDEN

PREFACE
TO THE SECOND EDITION

The first edition of *Pathophysiology, The Biological Principles of Disease,* defined as its goal the integration of science in a rational analysis of disease states. The text was meant to bridge the gap between the basic sciences as separate disciplines and the whole patient in whom knowledge of these disciplines can be integrated to explain clinical disorders. The reader is referred to the Preface to the First Edition, which elaborates upon the purposes for which this book was conceived. During the four years since the first edition appeared, the advance of knowledge in the basic biological sciences has, if anything, accelerated. The second edition attempts to keep pace with this new information and responds to many of the constructive criticisms that we have received. The text has been compressed and focused on human rather than on animal biology. Details have been limited as much as possible to those required to define broad concepts. Discussions of the clinical aspects and the natural history of diseases have been limited in this book, as being more appropriate for its companion, the *Cecil Textbook of Medicine.*

Cell biology and genetics remain a solid foundation for the understanding of other sections. A newly authored discussion of immunology is now followed by a new section on infectious diseases and host defense mechanisms, which provides a logical extension of the discussion of immunity and leads readily to a number of topics presented in the subsequent section on hematology. Metabolism and nutrition, a single section in the first edition, have been separated into independent sections. The sections on endocrinology and on neurology have been completely reorganized under new authorship. As part of this reorganization of the book, the sections on neoplasia and on clinical pharmacology have been omitted. It is believed that the concepts relevant to pathophysiology in those sections are adequately covered elsewhere in the book. All sections in this second edition have been updated to reflect recent advances and changing concepts.

Books do not simply congeal from submitted manuscripts. They require a considerable editorial effort. This effort varies from the development of a unified concept of scale, scope, and format to close attention to an enormous number of details necessary for accuracy and clarity of fact and of exposition. In all of these activities we have been greatly assisted by J. Dereck Jeffers at the W. B. Saunders Company and by the skilled editorial and production team that was assigned to this complex task: Lorraine Kilmer, Donna Walker, Edna Dick, and Frank Polizzano. The editors also depended heavily upon the invaluable contributions made by their editorial colleagues in San Francisco (Judith Serrell) and in New Haven (Jacqueline McKim). Without the coordinated effort of all of these individuals, this second edition would not have been possible.

If clinical medicine is to be understood in terms of our growing basic knowledge of biology, then pathophysiology must be a dynamic and changing field. We hope that this second edition of *Pathophysiology, The Biological Principles of Disease,* reflects that change and presents important knowledge to students and practicing physicians in a clear and usable form.

LLOYD H. SMITH, JR.

SAMUEL O. THIER

PREFACE
TO THE FIRST EDITION

By tradition, the practice of medicine is based on the personal qualities of the good physician. Each physician must discover these qualities for himself and within himself and each will attain and value them in different measure. Without compassion, dedication, equanimity, common sense, and the highest of ethical standards, no one can be a good physician. But these do not suffice. Compassion will not impede the logarithmic phase of bacterial growth; dedication will not diminish renal tubular reabsorption of sodium; equanimity is not sufficient as a response to cardiopulmonary arrest. The physician must apply, with skill and understanding, the most current medical science and technology of his time in the prevention, diagnosis, and treatment of disease. Medical science is merely a branch of applied biology, which is innately relevant, not antithetical, to the best in medical practice. The highest compassion may be that of making the right diagnosis. The complete physician is one who can synthesize both science and humanism within the traditions and ethical standards of the profession.

The biological sciences have grown enormously within the past generation. If the first half of the 20th century can be considered to have belonged to physics, the second half can equally be considered to belong to biology. New disciplines have evolved and have grown to maturity in this short time. In 1950, the structure of DNA was unknown and even its function was being debated despite the seminal work of Avery. Thirty years later, human genes are being sequenced, synthesized, and inserted into bacterial hosts by recombinant DNA technology. In 1950, the lymphocyte was a rather uninteresting small blue cell seen with Wright's stain of a blood smear, laboriously recorded in the differential count of leukocytes but otherwise relegated to obscurity. A generation later, the immune system has been revealed as an elaborate network for surveillance, communication, and defense, with circuits of specialized cells that secrete a variety of immune globulins and lymphokines. In endocrinology, the radioimmunoassay has allowed new orders of sensitivity and precision in measurement; the intricacies of hormone receptors, messengers, and cellular response have been considerably elucidated; new endocrine systems have been discovered (the prostaglandins, endorphins, the vitamin D system, calcitonin, somatomedins, and so on). Similar examples can readily be supplied within all of the biological sciences related to medical practice.

Each discipline is being investigated by scientists who have concentrated their scholarship on that particular sphere of biology. Intense scrutiny of a field is, of course, necessary for scientific progress. The science of medicine, however, has no such natural or contrived boundaries. It has a limitless scope that adds to its interest but makes more formidable the task of gaining and maintaining proficiency in it. Almost eight centuries ago, Alexander Neckam, Abbot of Cirencester, wrote an encyclopedia of current science entitled "The Nature of Things." He stated: "Science is acquired at great expense, by frequent vigils, by great expenditure of time, by sedulous diligence of labor, by vehement application of mind." This précis from a 13th century monastery is nowhere more pertinent than in the biological sciences applicable to medical practice. In the first two years in most medical schools in the United States, and with different packaging but similar effect in other countries, the student is assailed by scientific data that beat upon receptor mechanisms dangerously overloaded despite "sedulous diligence of labor." Within this brief period of time, the student is expected to master the scientific basis for a medical practice that may extend over four decades. Too often, also, the Henry Adams effect is at play: "Nothing in education is more pernicious than the amount of ignorance it accumulates in the form of inert facts."

Pathophysiology is a hybrid phrase that presumes a certain amount of hybrid vigor. It attempts to explain the biological basis of disease, making use of whatever scientific disciplines may be pertinent. Its goal is to integrate science in a rational analysis of a disease state. As such it can be broadly conceived as the ultimate scientific tool of the physician, who must see things whole rather than in separate compartments labeled anatomy, biochemistry, physiology, or pharmacology. This book attempts to integrate key aspects of the scientific basis of medical practice.

The editors asked Doctors George Palade and Marilyn Farquhar to introduce the book with a chapter on cell biology, a topic of basic importance in biology and one with which few physicians are now conversant. As the cell is composed of cytoplasm, organelles, supporting structures, and membranes, functional systems and organs are composed of specialized cells. Common to all nucleated cells is the transmission of genetic material and the potential for unregulated growth; these subjects are covered in chapters on genetics and oncology. Immunology encompasses one of the most rapidly expanding bodies of knowledge in medicine and has importance in pathologic processes affecting virtually every other organ system. Hematology, which overlaps with immunology, is then followed by chapters on most functional and organ systems—metabolism, endocrinology, connective tissue, nephrology, respiration, cardiovascular, neurology, gastroenterology, hepatology, and dermatology. We conclude with a chapter on clinical pharmacology, a subject critically dependent on an understanding of pathophysiology and one bridging the gap between mechanisms of disease and strategies of therapy. An understanding of basic disease mechanisms and clinical pharmacology, together with a knowledge of the clinical manifestations and natural history of disease, allows the development of a therapeutic strategy; the sum comprises the scientific basis of clinical medicine.

In each case the authors chosen are clinicians who both teach and utilize pathophysiology in medical practice. They were asked to describe within the space available the scientific basis of that system with which, in their opinion, the practicing physician should be conversant. For if, as John P. Peters said, "the disorders encountered in disease may be regarded as normal physiologic responses to unusual conditions," that scientific basis should be an essential need of the scholarly clinician.

LLOYD H. SMITH, JR.

SAMUEL O. THIER

CONTENTS

CELL BIOLOGY

GEORGE E. PALADE, M.D.,
and MARILYN G. FARQUHAR, PH.D.

Introduction _____

THE STUDY OF CELL BIOLOGY IN PREPARATION FOR A CAREER IN MEDICINE

The human organism consists of a very large number of cells, perhaps 1×10^{17}, that belong to a wide variety of cell types, each differentiated so as to perform a specific function with utmost efficiency. Each of these cell types is the result of the preferential expression of those genes (of the common genome* of all cells) that relate to its specialized function. Cells of one or more types—together with their products—form tissues. And tissues—integrated according to specific patterns—form organs. The next steps, toward still more elaborate organization, are tracts or systems that consist of organs performing complex, highly integrated functions. The final step is the human organism itself. The whole organism could be viewed as a vast aggregate of myriads of cells living together, performing their functions, and interacting with one another without detectable perturbations as long as the organism is healthy. Diseases, irrespective of the level at which they manifest themselves—the whole organism, a system, a certain organ, or a specific tissue—originate in cells or affect cells. Hence, diseases are basically the result of cumulative cell malfunction.

In the present state of development of the life sciences, it is possible to investigate and eventually to understand disease processes in terms of what is already known about normal cell function. Moreover, in many cases investigations can be carried out on human tissues or cells cultured in vitro as an extension of clinical research done (or being done) on human patients. Cellular pathology is increasingly becoming the natural basis of medicine. The trend is rapid enough to be expected to affect a good part (if not all) of medicine during the future professional career of today's students.

FUNDAMENTAL IMPORTANCE OF THE CELL IN BIOLOGY

The cell is the structural and functional unit of all living matter. This means that all living species are either single cells or orderly cell aggregates. Biologic

_____
Genome: totality of the genes (hereditary determinants) of a cell, organism, or species.

organization can be regarded as a hierarchy of progressively more complex levels of structure that starts with simple molecules and ends with whole organisms. Within this hierarchy, the cell is the simplest level at which emerges the most important characteristic of living matter: the capacity for self-reproduction. In fact, the whole organization of the cell can best be explained in terms of this dominant propensity. In order to reproduce itself, the cell must replicate its genome and must transcribe and translate the information encoded in it so as to generate the molecules and macromolecules needed for all the structures of its duplicate. These operations require a continuous supply of metabolic energy and a carefully controlled environment. Specialized cell organs (or subcellular components) carry out each of these operations and satisfy each of these requirements.

UNITY OF LIVING MATTER AT THE SUBCELLULAR AND CELLULAR LEVEL

Biochemistry has already established the general principle of unity of living matter at the molecular level. All living beings use essentially the same amino acids, the same nucleotides, and basically the same lipids and monosaccharides to build their specific macromolecules and to satisfy their metabolic needs. Their metabolic pathways follow the same steps or involve alternative reactions leading to similar products. Modern cell biology has taken the unity of living matter a few steps further. It has established the existence of two basic cell types, *prokaryotic* and *eukaryotic,* which (for the purpose of avoiding confusion) could be described as archetypes, and it has shown that the basic organization of all cells belonging to each archetype is essentially the same irrespective of taxonomy and cell differentiation. Since all cells possess the same kinds of macromolecular assemblies and subcellular components, the unity of living matter appears to extend—all the way up—to the cellular level of biologic organization.

THE ARCHETYPES

Bacteria and blue-green algae are prokaryotes; protozoa and the cells of all metazoa are eukaryotes, as are unicellular and multicellular plants. Eukaryotic cells are considerably larger than prokaryotes and generally have an elaborate system of intracellular membranes that defines a characteristic set of intracellular compartments. One of these compartments, *the nucleus,* is the residence of the genome, which is thus clearly separated from the rest of the cell—that is, *the cytoplasm*—through most of the cell's existence. The name eukaryote reflects this condition, since it means "properly nucleated." In prokaryotes the genome is not separated from the cytoplasm by any partition; thus these cells lack a distinct nucleus. Prokaryote means "prenucleated."

In medicine, prokaryotes are of importance primarily as pathogens. Our concern is this chapter is with the eukaryotic cells of the human organism. Given the unity of organization already mentioned, it should not be surprising that human cells are very similar to the cells of other mammals and vertebrates. Differences from one differentiated cell type to another within the same species are relatively large and easily recognizable; but differences from one species to another are generally small when the same types of differentiated cells are considered.

General Organization of the Eukaryotic Cell

SIZE AND SHAPE

Although ~1000 times larger than prokaryotes, eukaryotic cells are small objects, usually smaller than the limit of resolution of the human eye—that is, smaller than 0.1 mm, or 100 μm. In their vast majority, they have diameters—or sides—of 10 to 30 μm; this fact explains why research in cell biology depends heavily on magnifying instruments—that is, light and electron microscopes. There are, however, a few notable or even striking exceptions: the human oocyte is ~ 100 μm in diameter, and the main body of many nerve cells is of comparable size; moreover, some nerve cells have processes that extend over centimeters or meters.

The shape of the cells varies with their habitat: they are prismatic when closely packed; spherical or glob-

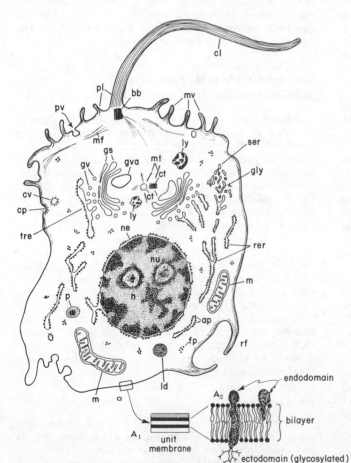

Figure 1. Diagram of a median section through an animal eukaryotic cell as seen at a magnification of ~10,000 ×.

n, nucleus; nu, nucleolus; ne, nuclear envelope; rer, rough endoplasmic reticulum; ser, smooth endoplasmic reticulum; tre, transitional element; gv, Golgi vesicles; gs, Golgi stacked cisternae; gva, Golgi vacuoles; ly, lysosome; fp, free polysome; ap, attached polysomes; ct, centriole; mt, microtubules; mf, microfilaments (in bundles); pl, plasmalemma; pv, plasmalemmal vesicle; cp, coated pit; cv, coated vesicle; rf, ruffle (lamellar pseudopodium); mv, microvilli; cl, cilium; bb, basal body; m, mitochondrion; p, peroxisome; ld, lipid droplet; gly, glycogen.

The rectangle marked a is further magnified (to ~100,000 ×) at A_1 to show the unit membrane structure of the plasmalemma. The diagram at A_2 gives the position of a transmembrane protein, of a protein buried half way in the bilayer, and of the head groups and fatty acyl chains of the phospholipids within the unit membrane at a magnification of ~500,000 ×.

ular when they live free in a fluid environment; and flattened, elongated, or fusiform when they adhere to a solid substrate.

COMPARTMENTATION

Each eukaryotic cell has a cell membrane or plasmalemma that separates it from the environment and a system of intracellular membranes that may exceed the plasmalemma by 1 or 2 decades in either mass or surface area. In animal eukaryotes, the intracellular membranes belong to ~ 10 different types of characteristic structure, biochemistry, and function, and each type is organized as a closed compartment. The final result is a highly compartmented system in which a variety of small compartments (that differ from one another in the nature of their membrane as well as their content) are enclosed in a relatively large, common, and continuous compartment called the *cytoplasmic matrix*.

The diagram in Figure 1 illustrates the main subcellular compartments and components so far identified in an average eukaryotic cell. It gives their names and portrays their characteristic structure, relative size, average density, and usual distribution. Note that the diagram is a two-dimensional representation of a three-dimensional object. It is, in fact, an idealized, two-dimensional electron microscope image given by a thin (~ 60 nm) "median" section through an idealized cell. Information collected from ~ 350 serial sections of this thickness would be needed to reconstruct a three-dimensional cell.

The next section will summarize our current knowledge on the structure, biochemistry, and function of these subcellular components, which are now recognized as specialized cell organs.

Cell Organs

Although rather diverse in their organization, *cell organs have a salient common feature: each of them is built to perform a special and unique function.* There are no obvious substitutes or alternatives; most of them are present, however, in multiple copies, which may represent evolution's formula for fail safe.

Some cell organs are macromolecular assemblies—that is, copolymers of a number of different large molecules (proteins or proteins and nucleic acids); most of them are located in the cytoplasmic matrix; a few are found in other intracellular compartments. Other, more elaborate cell organs are simple or complex membrane-bound compartments with a matrix of their own. Since membranes create and maintain chemical and electrochemical gradients between the compartments they separate, it can be assumed that the cell organs of the first type depend for their function on gradients maintained primarily by the plasmalemma, whereas the function of those of the second type requires special gradients produced by the cell organ's own membrane(s).

The distinction between the two classes of cell organs is quite clear, but the transition from large macromolecular assemblies identified as cell organs, to other less elaborate assemblies—usually described as multienzyme systems, filaments, or particles—is gradual. At this level, the distinction is often arbitrary.

PLASMALEMMA (OR CELL MEMBRANE)

The plasmalemma is the organ that mediates and controls the cell's interactions with all the components of the environment, be they small molecules, large molecules, or other cells.

STRUCTURE, BIOCHEMISTRY, AND FUNCTION

Unit Membrane. In the light microscope the cell membrane appears as an interface between the cell and its environment, but in electron micrographs of sectioned specimens it has a characteristic structure of its own, clearly visible when the section is normal to the plane of the membrane. It consists of two dense bands each ~ 2.5 nm in width separated by a light band ~ 3 nm wide. This layered structure is often referred to as the unit membrane (Fig. 2). In some cell types, the outer surface is covered by arrays of small particles (< 10 nm), and in practically all cells the inner surface is associated with a fine fibrillar meshwork.

Lipid Bilayer: The Diffusion Barrier. *The basic constituent of the plasmalemma is a bilayer of polar or amphipathic lipid molecules*—namely, phospholipids, glycolipids, and cholesterol—usually occurring in the ratio 70:5:25 (w:w:w). The bilayer functions as a diffusion barrier for water and hydrophilic solutes; lipid soluble molecules, including O_2 and CO_2, permeate it readily. *The bilayer is fluid at the temperature of the environment,* and cells make every effort to maintain it fluid when the ambient temperature changes. They control the viscosity of the bilayer by modifying the fatty acyls of its phospholipids. Short or highly unsaturated fatty acyls decrease the viscosity.

The light band in the unit membrane corresponds to the fatty acyl groups of the phospholipids of the bilayer, whereas the two dense bands represent their polar groups and (in part) their associated proteins.

Transport: Channels and Pumps. The inherently low permeability of the lipid bilayer for hydrophilic molecules is increased and rendered selective by protein molecules inserted across it. These proteins act as (1) channels (or pores) for various ions, (2) specific

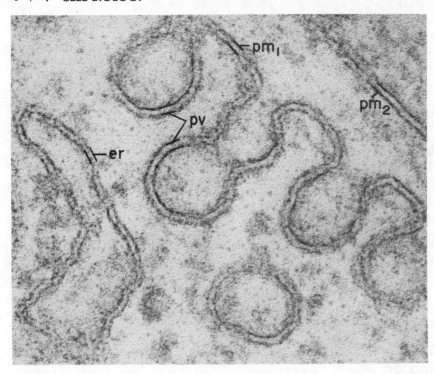

Figure 2. Unit membrane. The plasma-lemma (pm₁) of this endothelial cell (rat), the membranes of its plasmalemmal (pinocytic) vesicles (pv), and endoplasmic reticulum (er), as well as the plasmalemma of its neighboring pericyte (pm₂) have a typical stratified structure, described as "unit membrane." It is related to the presence of a lipid bilayer in all these membranes. The acyl chains of the bilayer's lipids are located in the middle, light band. 350,000 ×.

carriers or transporters for metabolites (amino acids, monosaccharides), and (3) "pumps" that preferentially concentrate certain ions (for example, K^+) in the cell sol, while keeping the concentration of other ions (for example, Na^+, Ca^{2+}) well below that of the environment. The pumps require metabolic energy, supplied as adenosine triphosphate (ATP) (see section on Cell Energetics) to transport ions against concentration gradients, in a process known as *active transport*. The most extensively studied pump is the Na^+ + K^+-dependent ATPase, also called *transport ATPase,* of mammalian cells. It works continuously against leaks (through pores, or channels), and by its activity it regulates the cell's volume, controls homeostasis, creates a resting potential that renders the cell excitable and its membrane conductive, and maintains the intracellular K^+ concentration at the level required for the activity of many enzymes, including those involved in protein synthesis.

The transport ATPase is a ubiquitous enzyme, but its concentration varies from one cell type to another. It is particularly high in cells specialized in large scale active transport of Na^+ and K^+ ions, like the cells of renal (nephron) epithelia, the source from which it has been recently isolated and purified. It is a large glycoprotein with two subunits of M_r (molecular weight) of ~ 100,000 and ~ 50,000, respectively. The Ca^{2+}-dependent ATPase is another important active-transport enzyme. It pumps Ca^{2+} continuously out of the cell to maintain its intracellular concentration at a low base level, $< 1 \times 10^{-6}M$. Above this level (up to 1 $\times 10^{-5}M$), Ca^{2+} acts as a *second messenger* for many cellular activities (contraction, secretion). At even higher concentrations, Ca^{2+} severely damages or kills the cells. The anion (chloride) channel of the human erythrocytic plasmalemma (also known as band 3 protein) has also been isolated; work on other channels

and pumps is being pursued actively in many laboratories.

Receptors and Second Messengers. In general, the plasmalemma is not permeable to hydrophilic molecules larger than 1 nm in diameter. Yet in humans and most other multicellular organisms, cells must respond to physiologic agents that integrate the activity of different cell populations with that of the whole organism. Some of these agents are relatively large, nonpermeant molecules. Integration is possible because the plasmalemma of the target cells is provided with specific receptor molecules that interact on its outer surface with physiologic ligands—for example, peptide hormones, neurotransmitters, immunoglobulins, lipoproteins, mitogens, and others. Some of these ligands (peptide hormones and neurotransmitters) are referred to as *first messengers*. Within the plasmalemma, the activated receptor interacts in turn with an enzyme system that generates a *second messenger,* usually cyclic adenosine monophosphate (cAMP) (or in some cases cyclic guanosine monophosphate [cGMP]), in the cytosol. This second messenger triggers a chain of intracellular reactions that eventually elicit the characteristic response of the target cell to its physiologic ligand. Very often these reactions involve the phosphorylation of effector enzymes by protein kinases. So far, only a few receptors have been isolated and characterized, notable among them being the acetylcholine receptor, the insulin receptor, the receptors for epidermal growth factor and platelet-derived growth factor, and the receptor for low density lipoproteins; but many more are under intensive investigation. Those so far studied are large glycoproteins. Many (but not all) receptors appear to be "internalized" (see below: *endocytosis*) together with their ligands. At present it is still uncertain whether this event is required for their activity or is part of the mechanisms that regulate receptor density in the plasmalemma. *A number of disorders appear to involve defective or damaged membrane receptors, such as the acetylcholine receptor in myasthenia gravis* and the lipoprotein receptor in familial hypercholesterolemia.** Not all hormone → receptor interactions generate cAMP or cGMP

---

*In myasthenia gravis, an autoimmune disease, the receptor is apparently inactivated by an autoantibody; in familial hypercholesterolemia, the low density lipoprotein receptors are defective or absent.

as secondary messengers. Some of them cause a depolarization of the plasmalemma followed by a rapid influx of Ca^{2+} into the cytoplasmic matrix, presumably as a result of the opening of the Ca^{2+} channels of the cell membrane. In such cases, Ca^{2+} behaves as the secondary messenger. Even when the interaction generates a cyclic nucleotide, intracellular Ca^{2+} concentration increases concomitantly by influx (as above) or by mobilization from storage sites within the cell (see sections on the Endoplasmic Reticulum and Mitochondria). The order of these fluctuations and the exact

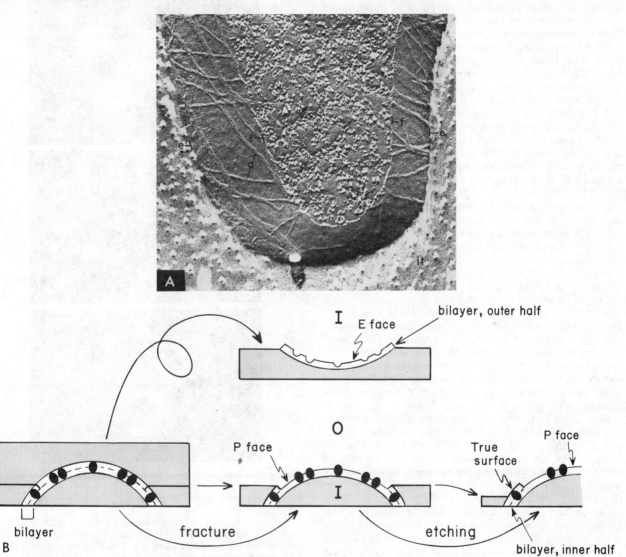

Figure 3. A, Replica of the freeze-fractured plasmalemma of a human erythrocyte. The P face, exposed from f to f, is marked by intramembranous particles (arrows), clustered because of the partial removal of the supporting infrastructure of the membrane. The true outer surface of the plasmalemma is exposed from f to e (by etching the ice table); it was decorated beforehand with actin filaments (a) to facilitate its identification. it, ice table. 123,000 ×. (Courtesy of Drs. T. W. Tillack and V. T. Marchesi: J Cell Biol 45:649, 1970.)

B, In this procedure, a frozen specimen is fractured in vacuum at −160° C. Metal is first evaporated at a low angle on the exposed surface to provide contrast. Then a surface replica is produced by evaporating carbon (at 90° C) on top of the metal. The metal shadowed replica is removed from the thawed specimen and examined in the electron microscope.

The fracture often cleaves cellular membranes along the middle plane of their lipid bilayers. The faces thereby exposed are called P face (inner half of the bilayer seen from outside) and E face (outer half of the bilayer seen from inside). P stands for protoplasm and E for external. The true surface of a membrane can be visualized only by etching the ice table before metalization and replication.

role of nucleotides and Ca^{2+} as intracellular messengers or mediators are still under investigation.

Membrane Architecture, Integral Versus Peripheral Membrane Proteins. As expected from their function, transporters and receptors are transmembrane proteins asymmetrically inserted into the lipid bilayer. This means that their ectodomain (the part of the molecule which protrudes into the external medium) is different from their endodomain (the part of the molecule located in the cytosol, or internal medium): each of them is built to interact with a different ion or molecule in a different environment. In sectioned specimens, the light band of the unit membrane (the lipid bilayer) appears continuous, although it must be locally interrupted by numerous transmembrane proteins. The latter are not detected because of lack of adequate contrast. The hydrophobic domains of the transmembrane proteins, like the fatty acyl groups of the phospholipids, cannot be "stained" by usual procedures. In freeze-fractured specimens (see legend for Fig. 3), however, membranes are often split along the middle plane of their lipid bilayers and the faces thus exposed show either particles ~8 nm in size or complementary pits. These *intramembranous particles* are assumed to represent clusters of transmembrane proteins (Fig. 3).

Transmembrane proteins belong to a group described as *integral* or *intrinsic* membrane proteins: they are retained in the plasmalemma primarily by hydrophobic interactions with the bilayer, and can be removed from the membrane only by detergents that solubilize the lipid. Other proteins, described as *peripheral* or *extrinsic,* are bound to the membrane by multiple weak hydrophilic interactions (ionic or stereospecific) and can be dissociated from it by agents that counteract such interactions (low or high ionic strength media, and denaturing or perturbing reagents). Peripheral membrane proteins are preferentially associated with the cytoplasmic aspect of the plasmalemma. They constitute the fibrillar meshworks already mentioned and appear to function as stabilizing or reinforcing infrastructures for the rest of the membrane.

Best known among peripheral membrane proteins are actin (M_r 45,000) and the high molecular weight spectrins ($M_r \sim 250,000$) of the erythrocyte plasmalemma. The presence of actin together with that of other contractile proteins—for example, α actinin, tropomyosin, and myosin—has been reported in situ in the immediate vicinity of the plasmalemma (or in plasmalemmal cell fractions) of other cells. These proteins appear to be involved in local movements of the cell's surface. The spectrins appear to be limited in their distribution to the plasmalemma of erythrocytes and a few other cells, but related proteins, called *fodrins,* are found associated with the plasmalemma of many other cell types.

Since the bilayer is fluid at the temperature of the ambient, lipid molecules as well as integral protein molecules are free to diffuse, in principle, in the plane of the membrane; experimental data indicate that they do move at relatively rapid rates (~ 1 μm $\cdot$ sec^{-1} for lipids and ~ 1 μm $\cdot$ min^{-1} for proteins) unless restrained by interactions with the infrastructure or by other means still unknown. For instance, interactions of the integral membrane proteins with an external, multifunctional ligand (for example, a lectin or an immunoglobulin) lead to their gradual aggregation. It begins by the formation of small patches within the plane of the membrane and it may end under extreme experimental conditions with the aggregation of the patches into a single large *cap* usually located over the tail of moving cells (Fig. 4). Patching or clustering of receptors may play a role in normal cell physiology, since many physiologic ligands are polyvalent. At present the general properties of the plasmalemma

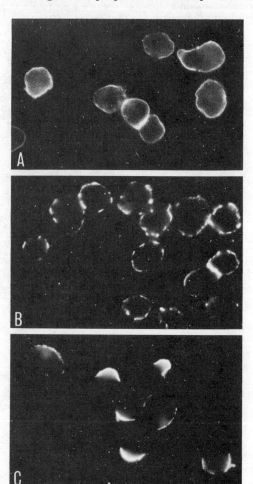

Figure 4. Changes in the distribution of a plasmalemmal integral protein (the histocompatibility antigen H2) upon interaction with multifunctional ligands (antibodies against H2 [anti H2]).

A, Fixed murine lymphocytes reacted first with anti H2 and then with an antibody against anti H2 (anti-anti H2) conjugated with a fluorescent dye. The fluorescent antibodies are evenly distributed over cell surfaces because the H2 antigens were immobilized beforehand by fixation in their original locations.

B, Unfixed murine lymphocytes reacted with antibodies as in A and then incubated at 0° C (for 60 min). The surface fluorescence has now a patchy distribution because the two layers of multifunctional ligands (anti H2 and anti-anti H2) have herded the H2 molecules into distinct patches.

C, As B, except that after antibody treatment the cells were incubated at 37° C (for 30 min). The fluorescent patches have been further herded into caps. Patching and capping of integral membrane proteins can be induced by multifunctional ligands because the lipid bilayers of the membranes are fluid (in this case even at 0° C). 1000 ×. (Courtesy of Dr. L. Bourguignon, University of Miami, Fla.)

(and all other cellular membranes) are rationalized in terms of a *fluid mosaic model* (advocated by S. J. Singer and G. Nicolson), according to which integral proteins, seen as the pieces or tesserae of a mosaic, float singly or as aggregates in a fluid lipid bilayer. *Membrane fluidity makes possible membrane expansion and membrane fusion without loss of permeability control.* These are processes that are critically required for cell growth and cell division, as well as many other cell activities (see below).

Structures Involved in Cell:Cell Interactions

The plasmalemma is also critically involved in cellular interactions. *Cell:cell recognition, preceding cell fusion or specific cell aggregation, is of crucial importance in gamete conjugation (fertilization) and in subsequent embryonic development. It is also important for the normal integration of cells into the tissues of the fully developed metazoon.* Relevant interactions are particularly striking in epithelia, in which cells must be retained in proper alignment with one another through attachment devices, and intercellular spaces must be sealed through occluding devices so as to restrict or control extracellular (or paracellular) traffic of ions and small hydrophilic solutes across the epithelium. These devices are local differentiations within the plasmalemma, each device being endowed with a characteristic structure. Occluding devices are belt-like structures called *tight junctions* or *occluding zon-*

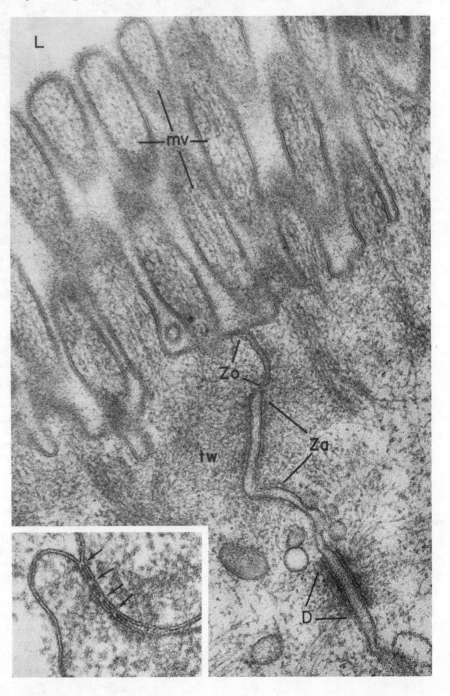

Figure 5. Junctional complex between two cells of the intestinal epithelium (rat). The complex consists of two belt-like devices, the occluding zonule (zonula occludens) (Zo) and the adhering zonule (zonula adherens) (Za), and a variable number of button-like devices called adhering maculae or desmosomes (D). The fibrils of the terminal web (tw) are anchored in the plasmalemma primarily at the level of the adhering zonule. L, lumen; mv, microvilli of the brush border (obliquely sectioned). 80,000 ×.

Inset: Occluding zonule between two pancreatic exocrine cells. The cell membranes are fused at a series of sites (arrows) that apparently correspond to the ridges seen in freeze-cleaved preparations (see Fig. 6). 160,000 ×. (From M. G. Farquhar and G. E. Palade: J Cell Biol 17:375, 1963.)

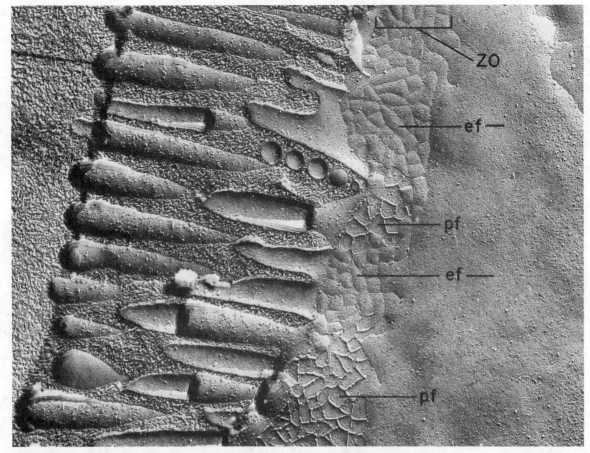

Figure 6. Occluding zonule in the intestinal epithelium (rat). Replica of a freeze-cleaved preparation. ZO, occluding zonule; ef, e face (see legend of Fig. 3); pf, p face. The occluding zonule appears as a network of protruding strands on the p face; the e face shows a complementary network of fine grooves. 70,000 ×. (Courtesy of Dr. N. B. Gilula, Baylor College of Medicine [from D. S. Friend and N. B. Gilula: J Cell Biol 52:758, 1973].)

ules* (Fig. 5). *At their level, the plasmalemma of a given cell appears to be fused with that of each of its neighbors.* In freeze-cleaved preparations (Fig. 6), the lines of potential fusion are seen as a series of interconnected ridges on the P face of the plasmalemma, with complementary grooves on the opposite E face. The number of successive ridges in an occluding zonule seems to correlate directly with the functional tightness of the junction. Besides occluding the intercellular spaces, the tight junctions attach each cell firmly to its neighbors. Other attachment devices are either belt-like structures, called *adhering zonules,* located abluminally to the occluding zonules, or button-like devices known as *adhering maculae*† or *desmosomes*.‡ The latter have a rather elaborate structure that involves both intra- and intercellular elements described in more detail in the legend of Figure 7. The size, complexity, and density of desmosomes increase roughly in proportion to the intensity of shearing forces acting on the epithelium. The stratified epithelia of the skin (epidermis), oral cavity, and esophagus provide impressive examples. *In certain epithelia, junctional ele-*

ments are characteristically grouped in junctional complexes in which the occluding zonule, located close to the luminal surface, is followed abluminally by an adhering zonule and by one or more desmosomes (Fig. 5).

In addition to adhering and occluding structures, the cells of multicellular organisms have evolved special *communicating junctions,* also called *gap junctions.* In freeze-cleaved preparations (Fig. 8), they appear as large, planar clusters or lattices of ~ 9 nm particles (on P faces). Each particle, called a *connexon,* appears to consist of subunits surrounding a central channel ~ 2 nm in diameter. *When in phase in the two interacting membranes, they are assumed to form intercellular channels through which ions and small molecules* ($M_r \leq 600$) *can diffuse directly from cell to cell (without leakage into the intercellular spaces), thus creating a common ionic environment and a common pool of small metabolites for large cell populations.* Communicating junctions occur not only in epithelia, but also in many other tissues. They are particularly prominent in the myocardium, in the intestinal and vascular smooth muscles of all mammals, and in the central nervous system of lower vertebrates. *Gap junctions make possible the propagation of impulses (membrane depolarization) from cell to cell and thus control the spreading*

Zonula: little belt (Latin).

†*Macula:* spot (Latin).

‡*Desmosome:* attachment body (Greek).

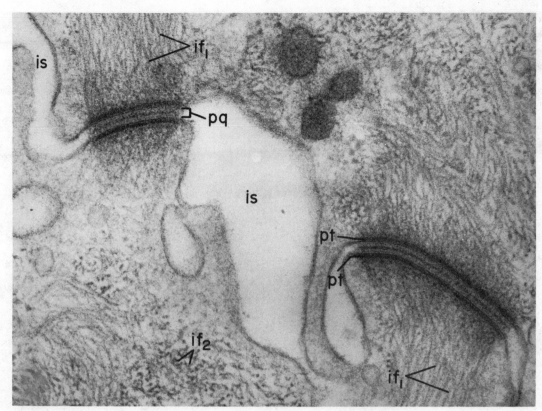

Figure 7. Desmosomes joining two adjacent epidermal cells (keratinocytes). Each desmosome consists of a dense, layered, intercellular plaque (pq) in phase with two dense intracellular plates (pt) located immediately under each plasmalemma. Bundles of intermediary filaments (~10 nm diameter) are anchored in these plates. In epidermal cells, the filaments consist of specific, polymerized proteins (cytokeratins). Such bundles appear in longitudinal section at if_1, and in cross section at if_2. is, intercellular space. The glycoproteins that form the intercellular plaque, the proteins (desmoplakins) that generate the intracellular plates, and a whole series of cell-specific cytokeratins, which form a large fraction of the intermediate filaments in epithelial cells, have been isolated and partially characterized. 115,000 ×. (From M. G. Farquhar and G. E. Palade: J Cell Biol 26:263, 1965.)

of contraction waves over long distances in visceral muscles, myocardium included. In electrophysiology, the presence of communicating junctions can be detected by measuring the resistance to electric current passed between electrodes implanted in adjacent cells. If gap junctions are present, the resistance is much lower than across the plasmalemma. The cells appear electrically coupled, a condition described as *low resistance coupling.* The function of the communicating junctions is critically dependent on Ca^{2+} concentration in their immediate environment. When the Ca^{2+} concentration increases in the cytosol or decreases in the extracellular medium, the junctions close, although their gross structure does not appear to be perturbed. They also close when the intracellular pH becomes acid. The closure of communicating junctions protects the immediate neighbors of a damaged or dying cell.

Differentiated Plasmalemmal Domains

Membrane molecules are expected to be evenly distributed over the plasmalemma on account of the fluidity of the bilayer. Yet domains of apparently stable biochemical composition are encountered at different dimensional levels, as a result of strong molecular interactions within or across the bilayer. Certain transmembrane proteins interact preferentially with certain lipids of the bilayer, which form around them a characteristic sleeve or annulus. Certain receptors are maintained in distinct clusters by interaction with a stabilizing infrastructure, the best-known example being that of the low density lipoprotein (LDL) receptors clustered into small (diam ~ 100 nm) invaginations of the plasmalemma called *coated pits* because their cytoplasmic aspect is covered by a characteristic coat. These pits detach from the plasmalemma to become *coated vesicles* (diam 80 to 100 nm) that function as carriers in receptor-mediated endocytosis (see below). The stabilizing coat consists of heavy and light chains of *clathrin* (M_r ~ 180,000 and ~ 30,000, respectively) which, together with other proteins, form (by self-assembly) structures reminiscent of geodetic cages. Connexons are probably maintained within the plaques of the communicating junctions by protein-protein interactions. Finally, in epithelia in which one side of the cells is exposed to an entirely different medium from that bathing the other sides, *the occluding zonules function as boundaries between plasmalemmal domains of very different composition and function.* A striking example is provided by the absorptive cells of the intestinal epithelium. The luminal domain of their plasmalemma, which faces the intestinal chyle, evolves into a highly characteristic structure, called the *brush border* (or cuticular border), specialized for

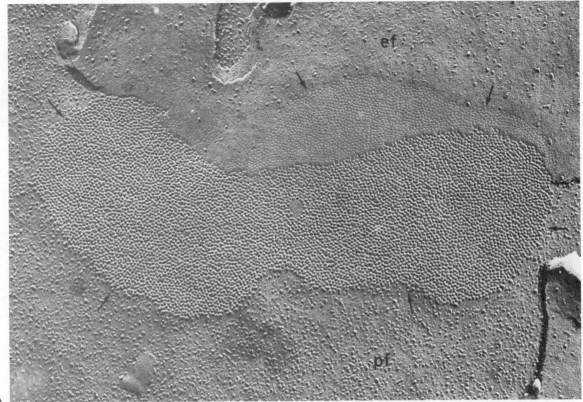

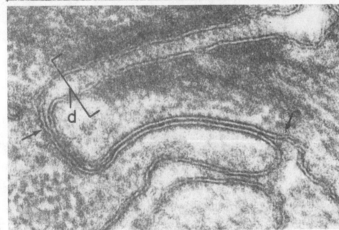

Figure 8. A, Gap (or communicating) junction between two hepatocytes (rat). Replica of a freeze-cleaved preparation. pf, p face; ef, e face. The limits of the junction are indicated by arrows. The connexons appear as clustered prominent particles on the p face. They have left small, complementary dimples on the e face. Note the difference in intramembranous particle density between the p and e faces. 96,000 ×. (Courtesy of Dr. N. B. Gilula, Baylor College of Medicine [from N. B. Gilula in Cell Communication. 1974, John Wiley and Sons].)

B, Cross section through a communicating junction between two keratinocytes in a thin section of rat skin. The limits of the junction are marked by arrows. d, desmosome. 170,000 ×.

terminal food digestion by integral membrane enzymes (disaccharidases, aminopeptidases), and for the inward transport of ions and metabolites (amino acids, monosaccharides, lipids). The surface area of the luminal domain is greatly amplified by the appearance of numerous, tightly packed, finger-like projections, called *microvilli*,* which together form the brush border. As expected for any well-designed piece of chemical equipment, the entire structure is provided with an elaborate system of stirrers made up of stiff bundles of actin (in the microvilli) mounted on a plate of contractile proteins (in the terminal web) (Figs. 5 and 9). The basolateral domains of the same cells face the interstitial fluid of the organism and are specialized for the outward transport (as far as the cell is concerned) of ions and metabolites. The existence of such differentiated domains makes possible the selective, vectorial (unidirectional) transport of a number of ions and molecules of evident usefulness for the entire organism. Comparable examples of luminal as opposed to basolateral differentiated domains are encountered in many other instances (the epithelia of the nephron, gallbladder, exocrine glands). Elaborate brush borders appear in the epithelium of the proximal tubule of the nephron, and microvilli in less orderly distribution are found on the surface of many other cell types.

Microvillus: fine hair (Greek-Latin hybrid).

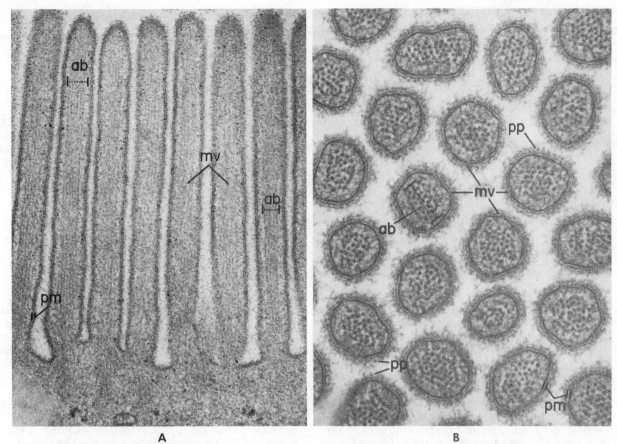

Figure 9. Uniform, regularly distributed microvilli of the type found in the brush border of the intestinal epithelial cells (enterocytes) (mouse). A, Longitudinal section and B, transverse section through the brush border. mv, microvilli; pm, plasmalemma; ab, actin bundles within individual microvilli; pp, particles protruding at the surface of the microvilli. Most of them are ectodomains of integral membrane proteins that function as digestive enzymes (aminopeptidases, disaccharidases). A: 82,000 ×; B: 160,000 ×.

NUCLEUS

After examining the structure and function of the plasmalemma, the interested student could enter the cell (figuratively speaking) and continue his or her exploratory journey from the cell's periphery to its center. This approach would not be particularly helpful because it lacks a unifying functional guide. It amounts to wandering rather than following a logical trail. The alternative we shall use will take us directly to the nucleus, which is usually located in the center of the cell. The nucleus plays a central role in the cell's life, and for this reason it can be used as the starting point for a functionally meaningful review of cellular organization.

The nucleus contains the cell's genome, which consists of a defined number of long DNA molecules, each of them having the characteristic double helix structure of DNA. In human cells the aggregate length of these molecules is 1.60 meters. The potential informational content of the genome is staggering: it amounts to ~ 9 × 10^{11} bits of information (a bit [short for binary digit] is the simplest unit of information), the equivalent of a library of ~ 180,000 volumes (if an average printed word were equated to ~ 36 bits and if there were ~ 150,000 words per volume). In addition, *the nucleus contains the equipment needed for the repair of the genome, for its replication (in anticipation of cell division), for its transcription (into RNA), and for the processing of the original RNA transcripts into mRNAs, tRNAs, and rRNAs (messenger, transport, and ribosomal RNAs, respectively). The assembly of ribosomal subunits (see below) also takes place within the nucleus concomitantly with the processing of rRNAs. Finally, at least part of the equipment involved in the regulation of gene replication and transcription is contained within the nucleus.*

Shape and Size. The nucleus of an average human cell is a spherical or oblate object, 3 to 5 μm in diameter. This gives a volume of ~ 100 μm³—that is, ≲ 10 per cent of the cell's total volume. Variations in size are numerous, and variations in shape even more extensive: they range from nearly perfect spheres to deeply indented and occasionally lobated or polymorphic bodies.

Nuclear Envelope. In a nondividing cell, the nucleus is a distinct intracellular compartment separated from the rest of the protoplasm* (that is, the cytoplasm)

Protoplasm: first formed (substance) (Greek) refers to the substance of the whole cells. It is resolved into *nucleoplasm* (substance of the nucleus) and *cytoplasm* (substance of the cell). *Cytos:* vesicle (in Greek) is used as a synonym for *cell*. *Cell (cella):* small room or cubicle (Latin). *Nucleus:* stone or pit (of a fruit) (Latin); the Greek equivalent is *karyon*.

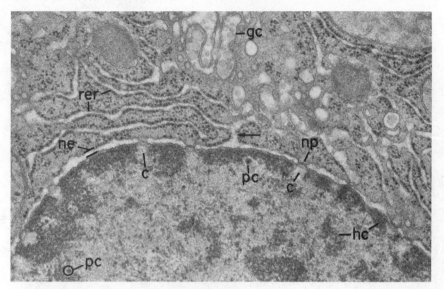

Figure 10. Partial view of the nucleus and adjacent cytoplasm in a hepatocyte (rat). Peripheral heterochromatin masses (hc) interrupted by channels (c) leading to nuclear pores (np) are seen in the nucleus. ne, nuclear envelope; pc, perichromatin granules. At the arrow, the nuclear envelope is continuous with an RER cisterna (rer) located at some distance in the cytoplasm. gc, Golgi complex. 18,000 ×.

by a characteristic membranous structure called the *nuclear envelope*. It consists of two successive membranes *(inner and outer nuclear membranes)* organized into a *perinuclear cisterna* (in fact, a tridimensional moat), which is part of the endoplasmic reticulum (see below) (Fig. 10). The envelope is extensively fenestrated and each fenestra, called a *nuclear pore,* measures ~ 80 nm in diameter and is provided with an elaborate structure—called *pore complex*—still poorly preserved by current preparation procedures. The surface density of nuclear pores appears to be connected with the rate of nucleocytoplasmic exchanges: in rapidly growing cells it may reach 10 units per μm^2. The pores are most probably the gates used by macromolecules and macromolecular assemblies (proteins, mRNAs, ribosomal subunits) to move out of, or into, the nucleus. Exchanges between the nucleus and the cisternal content of the nuclear envelope are probable, but little is known at present about them.

The outer membrane of the nuclear envelope is enzymologically similar to the membrane of the endoplasmic reticulum (see below) with which it is continuous (Fig. 10). Like the latter, it has attached polysomes involved in the production of secretory and lysosomal proteins, which can be shown (by appropriate cytochemical procedures) to be segregated into the perinuclear cisterna. The inner membrane is different: it rests on a laminar felt, called the *fibrous lamina,* on which the pore complexes are affixed, and it interacts through this lamina with the nuclear chromatin (see below).

In contradistinction with the limiting membranes of all other cell compartments, the nuclear envelope does not have a continuous existence: it is dismantled toward the end of each cell cycle—at the end of prophase—and it is reconstituted from its dispersed fragments toward the end of mitosis*—in telophase.

Cell Cycle—Chromosomes and Karyotype. At this point, a short description of the cell cycle (Fig. 11) is needed to understand not only the modulations of the nuclear envelope but also the general organization of the *nucleoplasm* and of the cell's genome.

Mitosis: filamentous state, or filamentization (Greek).

As the cell prepares itself for division, long filamentous bodies become progressively visible, by light microscopy, within the nucleoplasm. They have a high affinity for basic dyes and for this reason are called *chromosomes.** This process takes 1 hour, and at the end of the corresponding interval—called *prophase*—the nuclear envelope breaks down and peels off as small separate cisternae. During the next stage—called *metaphase*—each chromosome, now apparently immersed in the cytoplasm acquires a characteristic rod-like shape by progressive condensation. For this reason, *metaphase is the stage at which the general morphology of the entire chromosome set of the cell can be studied under the most favorable conditions.*

Swelling the cells by hypotonic treatment and then squashing them, and staining the squashes with appropriate dyes, spreads the chromosomes and reveals additional diagnostic details, since upon staining with certain dyes, each chromosome appears to have a characteristic banding pattern.

Chromosome: stained (or stainable) body (Greek).

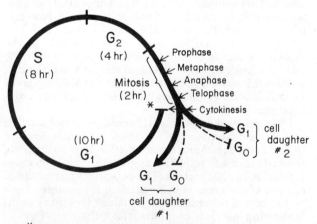

Figure 11. Diagram of the cell cycle for an assumed generation time of 24 hr. For shorter generation times, the interphase (that is G_1 + S + G_2) is correspondingly shorter.

Studies of the chromosome set—or *karyotype*—have led to the following conclusions.

1. The number of chromosomes is constant for all cells of a given species. For *Homo sapiens* the number is 46. The only exception is the male and female gametes, which in *Homo* have 23 chromosomes each.

2. In all cells, the chromosomes occur in pairs—23 in *Homo,* and in each pair the two components—called homologues—are morphologically identical. There is, however, an important exception: the human male (and the mammalian male, in general) has two unpaired chromosomes, designated X and Y, whereas the female has an XX pair. Since (with this exception) the chromosomes occur in duplicate, the karyotype can be described as *diploid** (see, however, page 17 and Section II for further details).

If cell divisions are traced back all the way to the fertilized egg, then one homologue can be shown to be inherited from the mother, through the female *haploid** gamete or oocyte, and the other from the father, through the male haploid gamete or sperm cell (recall that human gametes have only 23 chromosomes).

Careful observation reveals that each metaphase chromosome is split lengthwise into two symmetric halves, called *chromatids*† or *sister chromatids,* and that each chromatid is provided with a platelike structure, called *kinetochore,*‡ for the attachment of the *microtubule*§ (see below) of the mitotic spindle. The position of the kinetochore varies from one species to another; in *Homo* it is located near the center of most chromatids.

At the end of metaphase, the sister chromatids finally separate from each other and from now on each of them will be recognized as a distinct chromosome. During the next stage, called *anaphase,* microtubules attached to the kinetochores—working in concert with

---

Haploid, diploid: single(set) and double(set), respectively (Greek).

†*Chromatid*: descendant of chromosome or chromatin (Greek).

‡*Kinetochore*: movable plate (Greek).

§*Microtubule*: small tubule (Greek-Latin hybrid).

all the other components of the mitotic spindle (see below)—sort out two complete sets of 46 chromosomes, and move each set toward one of the two poles of the spindle. The end of the movement marks the beginning of a new stage, called *telophase,* during which the chromosomes cluster together, a nuclear envelope is reassembled around them, and the nucleus resumes its existence as a distinct compartment for the rest of the cell cycle. (A diagram of these phases is given in Fig. 12.)

The whole process that begins with chromosome condensation and ends with the formation of two progeny nuclei is called mitosis. It lasts for ~ 2 hours from late prophase to the end of telophase, and during the latter stage the body of the mother cell also divides by *cytokinesis.** Each of the daughter cells thus produced enters a relatively long *interphase* (~22 hours), during which it first synthesizes most of the macromolecules (RNAs, proteins, lipids, polysaccharides) needed for its own existence and for its future progeny. This active period, called G_1 (G stands for gap), takes ~10 hours and is followed by an ~8 hour interval, called S (for synthesis), during which the genome of the cell—that is, its nuclear DNA molecules—is replicated. S is followed by a short and relatively inactive stage, called G_2, at the end of which the cell enters into mitosis again. The first gap, G_1, is interposed between the end of mitosis and the beginning of S; the second, G_2, lasts from the end of S to the beginning of mitosis. In the process of cell differentiation, many cells leave the cycle and progress from G_1 to a stage described as G_0, which can last indefinitely without leading to S (Fig. 11). In the tissues of the human organism, the nuclei of the vast majority of the cells appear to be in interphase, because many differentiated cells are arrested in G_0 and because the mitosis of the cells that are still dividing is 10 times shorter than their interphase.

Mitotic Spindle

The mitotic spindle consists of a large number of microtubules that, in animal cells, are organized

---

Cytokinesis: cell movement (in fact, cell division) (Greek).

Mitosis

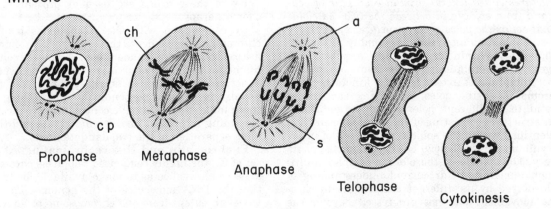

Figure 12. Mitosis. The diagram illustrates the most important steps and events in mitosis. To facilitate the understanding of the process, the number of chromosomes is reduced to four. Note that sister chromatids (that is, the two new replicas of an old chromosome) are still attached to each other at metaphase. They are completely separated at anaphase, when each of them is moving toward a different spindle pole. ch, chromosome; s, spindle; a, aster; cp, centriolar pair.

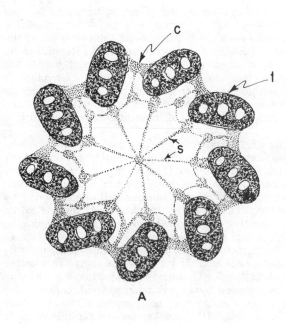

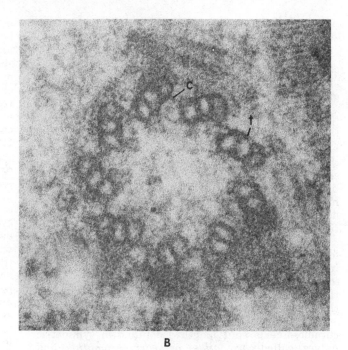

Figure 13. Centrioles and basal bodies.

A, Diagram of a cross section through an animal cell centriole (after E. de Harven). The centriole is a cylindrical body (length:350 nm, diam:150 nm) composed of nine dense, elongated elements, disposed like the blades of a turbine at the periphery of the cylinder. Each of these elements is a triplet (t) of fused microtubules. The triplets are linked to each other by peripheral connectors (c) and to an axial structure by a system of spokes (s). Small dense masses called centriolar satellites form a discontinuous ring around the centriole. Microtubules appear to be anchored in these satellites (see Fig. 28).

B, Cross section of the basal body of a flagellum in the green alga *Chlamydomonas reinhardtii.* t, triplet; c, peripheral connector.

The basic structure of the basal bodies of cilia and flagella is similar to that of centrioles. 280,000 ×.

around special cell organs called centrioles.* Details of their structure are given in the legend of Figure 13. During interphase, the cell appears to have a single pair of centrioles located in the vicinity of the nucleus often within the Golgi region (see below). Before the beginning of prophase, the centrioles are duplicated, and each of the two pairs migrates to opposite poles of the nucleus. *Microtubules produced by the polymerization of two soluble proteins, called tubulins* ($M_r \sim$ 55,000) *(see below for further details) form (a) radiating structures called asters† around each pair of centrioles and (b) a spindle in between the two centriolar pairs that act as the poles of the structure.* The spindle becomes visible soon after the disassembly of the nuclear envelope. Within its structure, a substantial contingent of microtubules stretches from pole to pole, but most microtubules extend from the kinetochores of the chromatids to the poles, connecting each sister chromatid to a different pole. Recently, additional fibrillar structures consisting of actin and myosin have been identified within the spindle and a shell of intermediary filaments (see below) has been detected at its periphery. The spindle is, therefore, a complex multicomponent apparatus. Our current understanding of the role played by its different components in chromosome movement has not progressed beyond the stage of conflicting hypotheses (for example, sliding of microtubules—as in cilia [see below]—versus shorten-

ing of pole-kinetochore microtubules coupled with lengthening of pole-pole microtubules (by depolymerization-polymerization of tubulins), versus movement effected by contractile proteins, with the microtubules serving only as guiding lines). It is known, however, that microtubules are required for chromosome translocation, since drugs that interfere with the polymerization of tubulins (for example, colchicine, vinblastine, vincristine) prevent the progress of mitosis beyond metaphase and lead eventually to extensive cell death. Some of these drugs are used at present in cancer chemotherapy.

By comparison with the mechanisms involved in chromosome movement, those at work in cytokinesis are reasonably well understood. A ring of contractile filaments consisting of actin, myosin, tropomyosin, and α actinin differentiates at the periphery of the cell usually in a plane perpendicular to the long axis of the spindle. Its progressive contraction produces at the beginning a *division furrow,* and at the end the complete separation of the two daughter cells.

Euchromatin and Heterochromatin.* At the onset of G_1, the highly condensed telophase chromosomes start to unravel so as to make available for transcription the DNA molecules of the genome. The process varies in extent from one chromosome to another and

---

*Centriole: little center (Latin).

†*Aster*: star (Greek).

---

*Chromatin: stainable substance; *euchromatin* and *heterochromatin*: true chromatin and different chromatin, respectively (Greek).

leads eventually to the following results. The morphologic identity of the chromosomes is lost, although their molecular identity is retained at least for their DNA and histones. *Chromosome segments under active transcription acquire a loose structure and are called, in their totality, euchromatin. Chromosome segments not involved in transcription decondense only partially; they appear as relatively large dense masses (heavily stained by basic dyes) called, in their totality, heterochromatin.* The size and distribution of the heterochromatin masses are expected to change with time, as different parts of the genome are made ready for transcription. Only exceptionally, chromosome segments or whole chromosomes are inactivated for the duration of the whole cycle. A typical example is one of the two X chromosomes of mammalian females. It persists throughout interphase as a permanent mass of heterochromatin attached to the nuclear envelope. It is known as *Barr's body* and it is extensively used to diagnose (when in doubt) the genotypic sex of the person whose cells are examined.

In the process of cell differentiation, many cells remain arrested in G_1 or G_0. As a result of their specialized biosynthetic activities, the transcription of their genome is restricted to specific genes, and the distribution of their heterochromatin acquires relatively characteristic patterns. A cell reentering the cycle from G_0 usually converts a large part of its heterochromatin to euchromatin, whereas in a sick or dying cell, in which transcription is coming to a standstill, most of the chromatin is condensed into large, confluent heterochromatin masses, a condition described as *pyknosis.** These various heterochromatin patterns are used extensively in pathology to identify cell types and to assess the general level of cell activity in the transcription and translation of its genetic information. In most cells, the heterochromatin forms a perforated shell located immediately under the nuclear envelope (Fig. 14). The perforations are channels leading to nuclear pores. Other shells of heterochromatin are usually found around nucleoli (see below).

Chromatin Fibrils and Nucleosomes. Irrespective of its status—loose, condensed (as in interphase nuclei), or hypercondensed (as in metaphase chromosomes)—chromatin can be resolved into a common unit structure, called *chromatin fibril,* of characteristic morphology (Fig. 15): it consists of a strand of considerable length, connecting a series of beads of ~10 nm diameter. Each bead is an octamer of 4 basic proteins, called histones, and the strand associated with it is a 200

Pyknosis: condensed state (Greek).

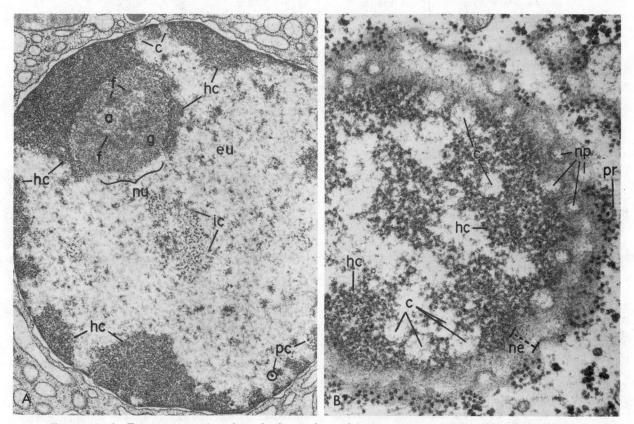

Figure 14. A, Transverse section through the nucleus of a pancreatic exocrine cell (guinea pig). hc, heterochromatin masses forming a shell around the nucleolus (nu) and around the periphery of the nucleus. The two shells are fused in part and the peripheral shell is interrupted by channels (c) leading to nuclear pores. g, f, and a: granular, fibrillar and amorphous parts of the nucleolus; pc, perichromatin granules; ic, cluster of interchromatin granules; eu, euchromatin. 36,000 ×.

B, Grazing section through the nucleus of a hepatocyte (rat), hc, peripheral heterochromatin masses; c, channels through the heterochromatin shell; np, nuclear pores; ne, oblique section through the nuclear envelope; pr, polysomes on the outer membrane of the nuclear envelope. 45,000 ×.

Chromatin fibril

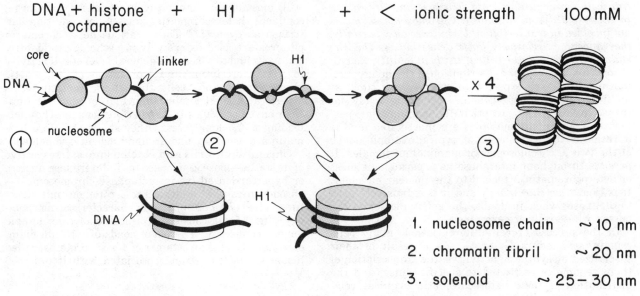

Figure 15. Nucleosomes and chromatin fibrils. The diagram illustrates the nucleosome, the packing unit of the genome, and the superstructures it forms.

Each nucleosome consists of a core and a linker. The core is a globular (more precisely, a disk-shaped) copolymer (octamer) of histones (H) built according to the formula $2 \cdot (H2a + H2b + H3 + H4)$ with a stretch of double-stranded DNA, ~140 base pair long, wrapped around it. The linker is the exposed stretch of DNA, ~60 base pair long, that connects two cores. This flexible chain of nucleosomes is the simplest chromatin fibril.

The addition of H1 to such fibrils (in vitro) extends the DNA wrapping around each core to two full turns, secures the exit of the DNA strand close to its entry, and thereby converts the loose chain of nucleosomes (10 nm maximum width) to a more compact, flat, ribbon-like fibril ~20 nm in width. If the ionic strength of the medium is progressively increased, the ribbon becomes a helical structure, 25 to 30 nm in diameter, with up to six nucleosomes per turn. It is assumed that similar conversions occur *in vivo*, presumably as a result of interactions with other nuclear proteins. (In part, after F. Thoma, Th. Koller, and A. Klug: J Cell Biol 83:403, 1979.)

base pair segment of a very long double helix DNA molecule. The latter is wrapped around each bead and extends from bead to bead as a 4 to 5 nm linker. One bead and one of its linkers constitute the repeat unit of the chromatin fibril which is called *nucleosome.** The addition of another histone (H1, M_r 21,000) to the linkers converts the beaded chain into a relatively tight coil of ~30 nm diameter. This reaction appears to be a key event in the conversion of euchromatin to heterochromatin. The histones, H2a, H2b, H3, and H4, are cationic, relatively small proteins, ranging in M_r from 12,000 to ~20,000, which have been highly conserved through evolution.

At present the nucleosome is considered the packing unit of the genome: a structural device that makes possible the accommodation of a whole genome—with an aggregate length of ~1.6 m in *Homo*—into a diminutive nuclear compartment less than 5 μm in diameter. Genes are transcribed without dismantling the nucleosomes, since the DNA molecules are accessible in shallow grooves at the surface of the beads. Access is facilitated, however, by special nonhistone proteins that bind preferentially to "activated nucleosomes."

---

*Nucleosome: nuclear body (Latin-Greek hybrid).

At present it is assumed that each chromosome contains, and is organized around, a single DNA molecule that, if stretched out, could be as long as 1 to 10 cm in *Homo*. Since the longest human chromosomes do not exceed 10 μm, it follows that premetaphase condensation produces a structure that is ~10^4 times shorter than the DNA molecule it contains. The first level of packing—via nucleosomes—gives a structure (the chromatin fibril) that is ~6 times shorter than its DNA. Hence, considerably more intrachromosome packing must take place during prophase and metaphase. The process is evidently well controlled, since each chromosome emerges with the same specific morphology at each metaphase.

Types of DNA Sequences. Within each DNA molecule, and within the entire genome, there are highly repetitive sequences that are replicated but not transcribed. In intact chromosomes, these sequences (referred to as *satellite DNA*) appear to be clustered in the vicinity of the kinetochore. They may play a structural rather than informational role. Most DNA sequences appear to be nonrepetitive, and are probably present in a single copy per haploid genome; these sequences are the carriers of genetic information. In between these extremes are moderately repetitive sequences that represent redundant genes (see below), and spacers or linkers in between usual genes.

DNA Replication

During S, DNA molecules are replicated bidirectionally, starting from a very large number (probably more than 1000) of initiation sites for an average length chromosome. The two strands of the double helix are locally unwound, and each strand serves as a template for a new DNA molecule produced by DNA-dependent DNA polymerases. The result of this semiconservative replication is two high fidelity copies of the original DNA molecule.

The information available on DNA replication and DNA polymerases in eukaryotic cells is still limited. Much more is known about the process in prokaryotes, in which three different DNA polymerases have been identified (in *Escherichia coli*). *All depend on a template (that is, a single DNA strand) for their activity, all need a "primer," a short complementary RNA sequence synthesized by a special polymerase called* primase, *and all of them function as nucleases and polymerases. This double function is important because it makes possible the elimination of damaged or mismatched bases and the complete repair of DNA molecules (hence, chromosomes) as long as the two DNA strands are not damaged at the same level.* In fact, one DNA polymerase (pol I) proofreads and edits the product of the other (pol III), thereby reducing the frequency of mistakes by 4 or 5 orders of magnitude. On one DNA strand (the lagging strand), DNA polymerases produce short sequences because they can proceed in one direction only (5′ to 3′) along the strands. As the replication fork advances and makes available for copying new stretches of single standed DNA, the polymerase on the lagging strand has to "jump back" repeatedly and start working anew each time close to the fork. The polymerase on the leading strand works without interruptions, since it always moves in its restricted direction: 5′ to 3′. The short sequences synthesized on the lagging strand and whatever interruptions may appear on the leading strand are subsequently linked to one another or repaired by other enzymes, called *DNA ligases*. Replication proceeds along similar lines in eukaryotic cells. DNA repair enzymes are deficient in the inborn human disease *xeroderma pigmentosum*, in which the skin of the afflicted person develops multiple malignant tumors as a result of its high sensitivity to sun and ultraviolet light (the latter is a common source of DNA damage).

Replication probably requires the dismantling of nucleosomes and the coordinated production and assembly of histones, so as to generate an additional chromatin fiber. Each DNA copy becomes the main component of a chromatid that will become progressively more visible as the cell approaches metaphase. From the end of S to the end of metaphase, the two sister chromatids remain attached to one another. Therefore, each prophase or metaphase chromosome contains genetic information in duplicate. Since each chromosome has a homologue, the genome is present in quadruplicate past the end of S. It will be reduced again to the duplicate level (diploid) at telophase.

A General View of Replication and Mitosis. One could consider the whole genome as a library containing all the information needed for the survival and replication of the corresponding cell. For the convenience of the processing of its informational content, the genome is divided into a number of chromosomes (the equivalents of a library's volumes). For safety's sake, each volume is present in duplicate: each chromosome has a homologue; therefore, the genome and the karyotype are diploid. During interphase, especially during G_1, the volumes are extensively unfolded—like giant Japanese silk books—and their information copied according to the cell's own program as adapted to the demands of the environment. During S each volume is replicated, but the two copies remain linked together through metaphase. For historical reasons, they are designated by a different name, chromatid (meaning descendants of chromatin), but for all purposes they are chromosomes with their full complement of genetic information. The library has now four copies of each volume. During prophase and metaphase the volumes are refolded, and at the end of metaphase the last links between replicate volumes are split. Strings are attached to each volume, and some well-controlled forces pull the strings to separate at anaphase and telophase a complete set of duplicate volumes for each daughter library, whose informational content is thus brought back to the diploid level. Finally, cytokinesis segregates each daughter library into a daughter cell. Mitosis appears, therefore, as a complex process by which, under normal conditions, an already replicated genome is precisely divided chromosome by chromosome and gene by gene between two daughter cells.

The Nucleolus*

The interphase nucleus contains two or more globular bodies of ~0.5 μm in diameter called nucleoli (Fig. 14). Their number is generally connected with the degree of ploidy of the nucleus (one nucleolus per haploid genome), and their size reflects the rate of ribosome production—hence, the overall rate of protein synthesis for either growth or secretion. This explains why nucleoli are prominent in rapidly growing cells, including tumor cells, as well as in cells with a large output of secretory proteins.

In electron micrographs, the nucleolus appears surrounded by a shell of heterochromatin that varies considerably in size from one cell type to another. In contradistinction to the vast majority of genes that are present in two copies per genome, genes coding for ribosomal RNAs (rRNAs) are redundant: the number of copies reaches ~400 in human somatic cells and exceeds 4000 in certain amphibian oocytes. In many cells, some of these redundant genes are not transcribed: they form a shell of *nucleolus-associated heterochromatin* around each nucleolus. The nucleolus proper can be resolved into two parts of different structure: one is finely fibrillar, the other granular. An "amorphous" part is also detected in some nucleoli. The geometry of these parts is complex and variable—the main structural characteristic appears to be a large area of contact between the fibrillar and the granular parts.

The organization of the nucleolus has been analyzed by a variety of procedures including biochemical assays of isolated nucleoli, enzyme digestion tests carried out in situ, and autoradiography after the incorporation of

---

Nucleolus: small pit (Latin).

radioactive RNA precursors. These studies have established that ribosomal genes under active transcription form euchromatin loops that penetrate into the fibrillar part, where they are transcribed by a special DNA-dependent RNA polymerase that is inhibited by the antibiotic actinomycin D. The primary transcript made by the polymerase is a single 45S rRNA molecule, which is extensively processed in the nucleolus by enzymic modification (base methylation) and cleavage, to give eventually a (23S + 5.8S) RNA and an 18S RNA for the large and the small ribosomal subunits respectively. Assembly of the rRNAs into ribosomal particles (by complex formation with proteins) proceeds in tandem with transcription. Two types of proteins, imported from the cytoplasm, are apparently used in the process: nucleolar proteins that appear to function as temporary scaffolding, and ribosomal proteins that become part of the final products. An additional small RNA molecule, 5S rRNA, the product of genes not associated with the nucleolus, is used for the large subunit. Ribosomal particles are assembled and temporarily stored in the granular part before being exported to the cytoplasm (most probably via nuclear pores). The small ribosomal subunits emerge into the cytoplasm more rapidly than the large ribosomal subunits.

Micrographs obtained by spreading detergent-treated nucleoli on an appropriate support (carbon film) reveal in remarkable detail the redundancy of ribosomal genes, their concurrent transcription by a large number of DNA-dependent RNA polymerases, and the assembly of rRNAs into ribosomal particles proceeding "in tandem" with transcription (Fig. 16). In prophase, the nucleolus decreases gradually in size, because the transcription of rDNAs is arrested and finally disappears (in most but not all cells) while the rDNAs* are

---

*rDNAs: genes coding for rRNAs.

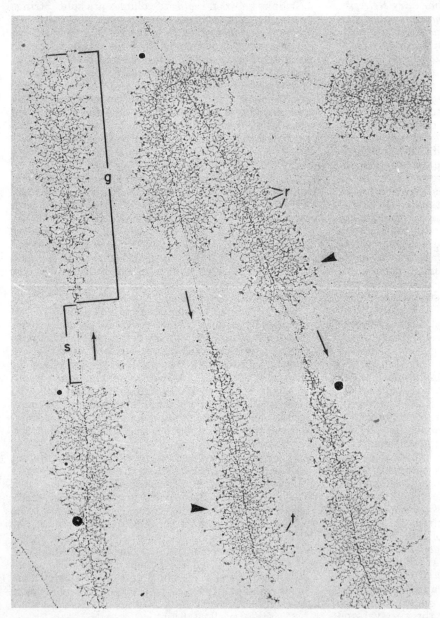

Figure 16. Genes (rDNA) for ribosomal RNAs visualized upon dispersing the nucleoli of an amphibian oocyte. Each of the "fernleaf"-figures in this micrograph is one of the oocyte's redundant rRNA genes under active transcription. The central vein of the "blade" is the gene itself (g), the connecting "stripes" are nontranscribed "spacers" (s). The dots on the genes are DNA-dependent RNA polymerases. The lateral veins of each leaf are the original transcripts (t). The particles at the end of these "veins" are ribosomal subunits (r) under assembly. Note that assembly proceeds in tandem with transcription. The direction of transcription is indicated by arrows; that of assembly by arrowheads. 35,000 ×. (Courtesy of Drs. O. L. Miller, Jr., and B. R. Beatty: Science 164:955, 1969.)

incorporated usually into a single pair of chromosomes. At the beginning of G_1, ribosomal production starts again from *nucleolus organizers*—that is, the parts of the chromosomes in which the redundant rDNAs are included.

hnRNAs and mRNAs

In euchromatin, gene transcription is carried out by other DNA-dependent RNA polymerases that are inhibited by α amanitin, the toxin of the mushroom *Amanita phalloides*. The primary transcripts are large and heterogeneous RNA molecules, designated hnRNAs (hn stands for heterogeneous, nuclear). It was already known that their intranuclear processing involves large RNA losses, but it was found only recently that *during this processing large internal sequences (called introns) of the original transcript are removed, the remaining sequences (called exons) being spliced together to produce functional mRNAs*. Splicing occurs at multiple sites and, with the exception of histone mRNAs, affects all primary transcripts so far investigated. This unexpected finding establishes a sharp discontinuity between prokaryotes and eukaryotes as far as gene transcription is concerned, since gene splicing occurs only in the latter. The meaning of this type of processing is still under discussion. It is assumed that it has accelerated evolution, but it is clear that it does have more immediate effects, since unedited transcripts are retained and degraded within the nucleus.

While still in the nucleus, mRNAs are provided with protective caps at their 5′ ends (the cap has a methylated guanosine and protects the 5′ end against phosphatases and nucleases), lengthened by adding polyA sequences at their 3′ end, complexed with a small number of specific proteins, and finally transferred to the cytoplasm as ribonucleoprotein particles.

tRNAs

Still another DNA-dependent RNA polymerase transcribes the genes for 5S rRNAs and tRNAs. The transcripts of the latter are extensively processed by chemical modifications of their bases, limited splicing, and short sequence additions before being ready for use in protein synthesis (see below).

Other Components of the Nucleoplasm

Besides heterochromatin, euchromatin, and nucleoli, other structural entities have been described in the nucleoplasm. They include perichromatin granules (diam ~30 nm) at the periphery of heterochromatin masses, and interchromatin granules (diam ~20 nm) that occur in clusters in the euchromatin. Neither is fully characterized chemically or functionally.

Nuclei contain, in addition to histones, a large number of proteins—more than 100 at the present level of electrophoretic resolution. Most of them are anionic. Upon nuclear fractionation, many of these proteins are recovered in chromatin fractions. Similar proteins are found in isolated chromosomes. The enzymes involved in DNA synthesis and repair, as well as those involved in RNA synthesis—that is, gene transcription—are among these nonhistone proteins. They are found associated with the DNA molecules of the genome during replication and transcription. But many other nonhistone proteins have no defined function. At present

it is assumed that some of them are involved in the processing of transcripts for each type of RNA (splitting, splicing, chemical modifications), and many more are expected to be part of the mechanisms that regulate replication, transcription, and packing of the genome. So far only a few regulatory proteins have been partially characterized. They bind steroid hormones and thyronines (thyroid hormones) and appear to be involved in the hormonal control (or modulation) of transcription.

CYTOPLASM

As already mentioned, the cytoplasm is extensively compartmented. It contains a series of ~10 distinct types of compartments, each of them outlined by its own membrane. These compartments vary in morphology, biochemistry (of their membranes and contents), function, and behavior, as will be shown in detail farther on. They are all enclosed in a common continuous space or compartment usually described as cytoplasmic matrix and sometimes referred to as the cytosol. The last term is misleading, since the matrix contains a large number of macromolecular assemblies that behave as solid structures, and since many of the matrix components can and do form reversible gels. The term cytosol should be reserved for the fluid phase of the cytoplasmic matrix.

A number of important cellular activities and the equipment or apparatus that supports them are located in the cytoplasmic matrix. They include the following:

1. Synthesis of essential biochemicals, such as amino acids, fatty acids, and monosaccharides
2. The intermediary metabolism in which these products are involved
3. The storage of metabolic reserves in the form of polysaccharides (primarily glycogen in animal eukaryotes) *and lipid droplets* (primarily triacylglycerols and cholesteryl esters)
4. The whole complex apparatus involved in protein synthesis or translation of the genome's transcripts

Included also in the cytoplasmic matrix is the locomotor apparatus of the cell, which consists of supportive or guiding assemblies (primarily microtubules and intermediary filaments) as well as contractile assemblies represented by actin and myosin filaments interacting with a large number of other proteins (α actinin, tropomyosin, troponins, calmodulin) involved in contraction and in its regulation. Actin is an unusually versatile protein. It exists in a number of isoforms specific for different groups of differentiated cells. It is used to construct contractile as well as supporting assemblies, and it interacts with a large number of actin-binding proteins that control the length of actin filaments, their mode of assembly (rigid rods versus compressible meshworks), and their attachment to membranes and other structures.

The enzymic equipment involved in the synthesis of amino acids, monosaccharides, and fatty acids, their metabolism, and their interconversion will not be discussed here. At present, all these enzymes are assumed to be soluble and their reactions are supposed to be governed by strict specificity and random collision with their substrates and modifiers. Even at this level, however, multienzyme systems have evolved; structurally they are macromolecular assemblies of enzymes working seriatim on a substrate and its successive metabolites. A well-documented case is the complex involved in fatty acid synthesis in a number of eukaryotic cells: it consists of seven enzymes and carries out a series of reactions that add a two-carbon segment at each cycle. The substrates remain bound to the complex until the final product, usually a 16C fatty acid, is released.

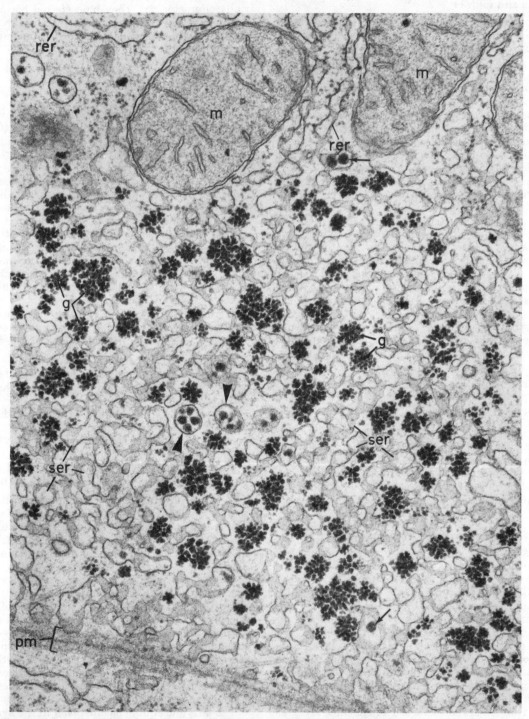

Figure 17. Smooth-surfaced endoplasmic reticulum. Rat hepatocyte. This part of the ER consists of a tightly meshed, tubular network (ser), in continuity (at the periphery of the field) with cisternal elements of the rough ER (rer). Glycogen particles (g) occur in the cytoplasmic matrix in close association with SER elements. Lipoprotein particles are seen in SER (arrows) and Golgi elements (arrowheads). m, mitochondria; pm, obliquely sectioned, overlapping plasmalemmata of two adjacent hepatocytes. 50,000 ×. (From G. Dallner, P. Siekevitz, and G. E. Pallade: J Cell Biol 30:73, 1966.)

Storage of Metabolic Reserves

Glycogen. In many cells, the cytoplasmic matrix contains glycogen particles that occur in a variety of sizes: a small compact particle of ~25 nm diameter is found in most cells, especially in muscle cells; a large particle (diam ~80 nm) which is an aggregate of the former occurs in hepatocytes (Fig. 17). Glycogen is a large, branched polyglucose molecule in which glucose residues are glycosidically linked α 1–4 in straight chains and α 1–6 at branching points. The enzymes that synthesize and degrade glycogen (glycogen synthetase and phosphorylase, respectively) as well as the enzymes (protein kinases) that regulate the synthetase and the phosphorylase are all soluble proteins, but some of these enzymes interact strongly enough with glycogen particles to separate with them upon cell fractionation.

Glycogen Synthesis and Degradation. A complex system that has been studied in detail in mammalian hepatocytes and striated muscle cells regulates the synthesis and degradation of glycogen. It depends on variations in glucose concentration in the blood plasma. A decrease in this concentration (hypoglycemia) activates the release of glucagon (from the α cells of pancreatic islands) and of epinephrine (from the adrenal medulla). The interaction of these hormones with specific receptor molecules in the plasmalemma activates an enzyme, adenylyl cyclase, which generates cyclic AMP (from ATP) in the cytoplasmic matrix. Cyclic AMP activates a protein kinase that phosphorylates the inactive form of phosphorylase (phosphorylase B), thereby converting it to active phosphorylase A. The activated enzyme begins to degrade (by phosphorolysis) the glycogen molecules of the cytoplasmic matrix. In hepatocytes, the final product of phosphorolysis (glucose-6-phosphate) is dephosphorylated by an integral enzyme of the ER membrane (glucose-6-phosphatase); the glucose thus produced leaves the cells and enters directly into the circulation to bring back into homeostatic range the concentration of glucose in the blood plasma. Concomitantly with the activation of phosphorylase, the protein kinase phosphorylates the glycogen synthetase. In this case, however, the phosphorylated enzyme is inactive, so that practically all the glucose generated by glycogen degradation can be used for export or intracellular consumption (glycolysis) with no competition from the synthetase. If glucose concentration increases beyond a certain range (hyperglycemia), glucagon and epinephrine release is curbed, and a converse series of intracellular events (inactivation of phosphorylase, activation of synthetase by specific protein phosphatases) leads to reaccumulation of glycogen. The system relies, therefore, on specific hormone receptors, a common link (adenylyl cyclase), a common secondary messenger (cAMP), specific kinases, and converse effects of enzyme phosphorylation and dephosphorylation on the catabolism vs anabolism of glycogen.

Lipids

Lipid droplets of various sizes (from 0.2 μm to 5 μm) are often found in the cytoplasmic matrix. They are particularly frequent in cells that rely on fatty acids for their energy needs as well as in cells that specialize in lipid (adipocytes) or steroid (cells producing steroid hormones) metabolism. In the former, the lipid droplets reach extreme dimensions (up to 80 μm); in the latter, the droplets contain large amounts of cholesteryl esters.

In the cells so far studied, the synthesis of triacylglycerols (from fatty acids and glycerol generated in the cytoplasmic matrix) is carried out by enzymes integral to the ER membrane. The product either appears in the cytoplasmic matrix (if the cells retain it as a metabolic reserve) or is segregated in the ER cisternae (if the product is destined for export as lipoprotein), as is the case in hepatocytes and enterocytes. The mechanisms involved in directing the product to one or the other compartment are unknown. The enzyme that transfers fatty acids from phosphatidylcholine to cholesterol to synthesize cholesteryl esters is a soluble component of the cytoplasmic matrix and of the blood plasma.

In the majority of cells the lipid droplets of the cytoplasmic matrix represent metabolic reserves to be used in ATP production via oxidative phosphorylation of fatty acids in mitochondria.

RIBOSOMES AND PROTEIN SYNTHESIS

Protein synthesis is undoubtedly the most important activity carried out in the cytoplasmic matrix of eukaryotic cells. It involves a large number of molecules and macromolecular assemblies of which the most conspicuous is the ribosome, a particle of ~20 to 25 nm diameter with a sedimentation coefficient of 80S.

Ribosomes are obligatory equipment for protein synthesis wherever it occurs. Hence, they are found in prokaryotic as well as eukaryotic cells; and in the latter, they occur in the cytoplasmic matrix but also in the matrix of those subcellular components, like mitochondria and chloroplasts, that have the ability to synthesize at least part of their proteins. Although organized along a common plan, prokaryotic ribosomes and different types of eukaryotic ribosomes differ in size and degree of biochemical complexity. In each case, the ribosome consists of a small and a large subunit that have been characterized in terms of general morphology, sedimentation coefficients, and component molecules, each subunit being a macromolecular assembly of RNA and protein molecules (designated rRNA and r proteins respectively). Prokaryotic ribosomes are smaller and simpler. They have been studied in considerably more detail than eukaryotic ribosomes. In fact, analytic studies of eukaryotic ribosomes have followed thus far leads obtained from the study of prokaryotic ribosomes. For this reason, it may be useful to present and compare current information on prokaryotic and eukaryotic ribosomes. The important data so far secured are given in Table 1.

PROKARYOTIC RIBOSOMES

Prokaryotic ribosomes consist of two unequal, asymmetric subunits, characterized by their morphology, sedimentation coefficient, and biochemical composition.

The *small subunit* is an oblong body (15 × 10 × 8 nm) marked by an asymmetric groove; it has a sedimentation coefficient of 30S, and thus is often referred

TABLE 1. RIBOSOMES: BASIC PARAMETERS

	S	DIMENSIONS *nm*	MASS *d*	rRNA *n*	*S*	r PROTEINS *n*
Prokaryotic	70S					
Small subunit	30S	$15 \times 10 \times 8$	0.9×10^6	1	16S	21
Large subunit	50S	$15 \times 15 \times 10$	1.6×10^6	2	23S	34
					5S	
Eukaryotic	80S					
Small subunit	40S	$23 \times 14 \times 11$	1.4×10^6	1	18S	~30
Large subunit	60S	$23 \times 22 \times 17$	2.9×10^6	3	23S	~50
					5.8S	
					5S	

S: sedimentation coefficient
d: daltons
n: number

to as the *30S subunit*. It consists of a single 16S rRNA molecule and of 21 r proteins. All these components have been isolated (from *Escherichia coli* 30S particles), purified, and sequenced. *Functional small subunits can be reconstituted in vitro starting from their isolated components; therefore, the structure of the latter contains all the information needed for self-assembly.* At present, the three-dimensional assembly diagram of the small subunit is under active investigation by a variety of means; the ultimate goal is to understand the position and function of each component and the way in which the entire assembly works during protein synthesis.

The *large subunit* has the shape of a skiff (15 × 15 × 10 nm) and a sedimentation coefficient of 50S, and is referred to as the *50S subunit*; it consists of two rRNA molecules (5S and 23S) and about 34 r proteins. Work on their characterization and three-dimensional assembly diagram is proceeding quickly along the lines already mentioned for the 30S subunit.

Protein Synthesis

In protein synthesis, the nucleotide sequences of mRNAs are translated by ribosomes into the amino acid sequences of proteins. Translation proceeds in the 5′ → 3′ direction on the mRNA while the cognate protein is synthesized from its N (amino) terminal to its C (carboxyl) terminal.

Translation is carried out in three sequential steps: initiation, elongation, and termination.

Initiation. The two ribosomal subunits associate reversibly in vitro at a Mg^{2+} concentration of ~5 mM. In vivo their association into functional ribosomes is controlled by a multiplicity of factors, all involved directly in protein synthesis. The most important among these factors is the processed mRNA of the protein to be synthesized: it forms a complex with a free 30S subunit and a special tRNA (tRNA$_f^{Met}$) charged with a modified (formylated) methionyl residue (fMet tRNA$_f$). This tRNA recognizes the initiation codon, AUG, located close to the 5′ end of the mRNA. Three soluble proteins called *initiation factors* and energy, supplied by splitting a GTP molecule, are required for the formation of this complex, which is now ready to associate with a 50S subunit into a functional ribosome. The events so far mentioned constitute the *initiation* step in protein synthesis. tRNA$_f^{Met}$ is used only once—for initiation—in the synthesis of any polypeptide on prokaryotic ribosomes, and for this reason it is called *initiation tRNA* (Fig. 18).

Elongation. When a functional ribosome is formed,

fMet tRNA$_f$ interacts with a special region of the 50S subunit, usually called *P site* (for peptidyl site). Next to it, on the same subunit, is another site, called *A site* (for aminoacyl site), that can bind any charged tRNA, but the one finally bound is the tRNA that recognizes the mRNA codon that follows immediately (in the 3′ direction) the initiation codon; in the newly formed 70S ribosomal complex, that codon is aligned with the A site. At this stage, when two charged tRNAs are bound to the ribosome, *a protein of the 50S subunit functioning as transpeptidase transfers the formylmethionyl residue from the initiation tRNA (in the P site) to the charged tRNA (in the A site).* The result of this operation is a dipeptidyl tRNA in the A site, and an uncharged tRNA$_f^{Met}$ in the P site. The latter is discharged promptly after losing its aminoacyl residue. *The next stage involves a complex operation called translocation, during which the mRNA-dipeptidyl tRNA complex and the ribosome move in opposite directions over the distance of a single codon;* this movement translocates the dipeptidyl tRNA to the P site and vacates the A site, which is now aligned with the codon specifying the third amino acid residue in the original polypeptide sequence. The specified charged tRNA binds to the A site, the transpeptidase makes another peptide band, translocation follows, the tripeptidyl tRNA is shifted to the P site, and the A site is made ready for a tRNA charged with the next amino acid in the sequence (Fig. 18). This entire series of reactions, called *elongation*, requires the participation of three soluble proteins (called elongation factors) and energy supplied by two GTP molecules; the first is used in binding the charged tRNA to the A site, and the second is needed to effect translocation.

Termination. The series of interactions involved in elongation is repeated n–1 times, n being the number of amino acid residues in the original translation product, until finally a special codon, UGA (or UAA), of the mRNA is aligned with the A site. These special codons, called *termination codons*, are not recognized by special tRNAs but by specific proteins called *termination factors*. In their presence, the transpeptidase splits the bond between the last tRNA and the polypeptide chain, the latter is discharged from the large subunit, the subunits dissociate from the mRNA and from one another and reenter the pool of free ribosomal subunits in the cytoplasmic matrix from where they can be recruited for the translation of another mRNA. This series of reactions constitutes the last step, called termination, in protein synthesis (Fig. 18).

Preparatory Steps. Complex and numerous as they

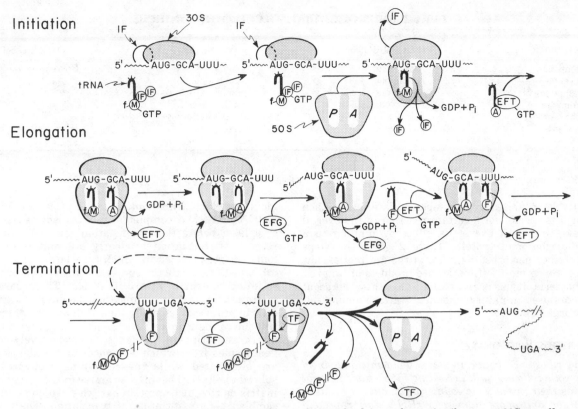

Figure 18. Protein synthesis. Phases and reactions so far resolved in prokaryotic ribosomes. 30S, small subunit; 50S, large subunit; IF, initiation factors; EFT and EFG, elongation factors; P, peptide site; A, aminoacyl site on the large ribosomal subunit; fM, formylmethionine; A, alanine; F, phenylalanine. Note that the first complex formed in initiation involves two initiation factors, the initiation tRNA, and GTP. The second complex includes the mRNA, the small ribosomal subunit, and an additional initiation factor.

appear from this summary description, the reactions involved in initiation, elongation, and termination cover only part of all the reactions needed for protein synthesis. For instance, prior to its binding to a cognate tRNA, each amino acid is activated by forming a mixed anhydride with adenylic acid. This is an endergonic reaction that consumes the equivalent of two high energy phosphate bonds. It follows that *cells invest the equivalent of four high energy phosphate bonds for each peptide bond formed during protein synthesis: two for the amino acid activation, one for binding the corresponding charged tRNA to the A site, and one for translocation. The energy of the first high energy bond invested is conserved in the aminoacyl adenylate and is used to generate the peptide bond.*

The equipment necessary to activate amino acids and generate charged tRNAs resides in its entirety in the cytoplasmic matrix. It includes about 60 different tRNAs (more than one for each amino acid) and a set of amino acid tRNA synthetases, large polymeric proteins that carry out in tandem the synthesis of amino acid adenylates and the charging of the cognate tRNAs.

Polysomes. *Usually, a mRNA is translated simultaneously by a number of ribosomes commensurate with the length of the mRNA, and hence with the molecular weight of the translated protein. This complex is called a polysome; it has a ribosome for ~30 codons of mRNA and therefore for each ~3300 daltons of translation product.*

The polysomes are seen as clusters of ribosomes of different sizes; after isolation, they appear as ribosome chains in which the ribosomal units are connected to one another by a fine strand (about 2 nm thick) presumed to be the mRNA. In the polysome assembly, the mRNA is located in between the two ribosomal subunits and most of the interactions with charged tRNAs apparently take place on the "shelf" of the 50S subunit adjacent but not covered by the 30S subunit. The exact position of the P and A sites is still unknown, but each of them appears to represent a cluster of interacting r proteins.

Free Versus Attached Polysomes. In prokaryotes, the vast majority of the ribosomes are present as polysomes. Most polysomes are free in the cytoplasmic matrix and are involved in the synthesis of soluble proteins or proteins for macromolecular assemblies. Before or soon after termination, the primary translate of free polysomes is modified by removing the first (and sometimes the second) amino acid residue from its N terminal. *A few polysomes are attached, however, to the plasmalemma; they produce secretory proteins (or periplasmic proteins), cell wall components, and integral membrane protein for the plasmalemma and the outer cell membrane (in gram-negative organisms).* In this case, the modifications incurred by the primary translate are more extensive than in the case of the products of free polysomes. These modifications will be discussed in more detail in conjunction with attached eukaryotic polysomes.

Protein synthesis in prokaryotes is strongly and

TABLE 2. ANTIBIOTICS THAT AFFECT PROTEIN SYNTHESIS

ANTIBIOTIC	TYPE OF RIBOSOME	TARGET (site or step)	OTHER EFFECTS
Streptomycin	Prokaryotic, 30S	Initiation	Code misreading
Tetracycline	Prokaryotic, 30S	A site (elongation)	
Chloramphenicol	Prokaryotic, 50S	Peptidyl transferase	
Erythromycin	Prokaryotic, 50S	Translocation	
Cycloheximide	Eukaryotic, 60S	Peptidyl transferase	
Puromycin*	Prokaryotic, 50S	A site	Premature termination
	Eukaryotic, 60S	A site	

*Puromycin acts as analog of aminoacyl tRNA; it binds to the A site and participates in peptide bond formation, but the peptidyl puromycin thus formed is discharged instead of being translocated.

Penicillin, one of the most widely used antibiotics, affects cell wall synthesis, not protein synthesis.

effectively inhibited by a number of antibiotics. Each of them is specific for a certain reaction in the overall process, and each exerts its effect by binding to a specific ribosomal protein. Table 2 gives the steps inhibited or perturbed by a few of the antibiotics now in use. Since most antibiotics are products of fungi or soil bacteria, it has been assumed that they represent reagents used in natural chemical warfare among soil microorganisms.

EUKARYOTIC RIBOSOMES

The ribosomes found in the cytoplasmic matrix of eukaryotic cells are built according to the same general plan as their prokaryotic counterparts, but they consist of larger and more numerous rRNA and r protein molecules; as a result, they are larger, more complex, and more difficult to analyze, yet *their general morphology is highly reminiscent of that seen in prokaryotic cells, and the way in which they function is basically the same.*

The small subunit measures $23 \times 14 \times 11$ nm, has a sedimentation coefficient of 40S, and consists of an 18S rRNA and ~30 r proteins. The sedimentation coefficient of the large subunit is 60S; this particle has three rRNA molecules (23S, 5.8S, and 5S) and ~50 r proteins, and measures $23 \times 22 \times 17$ nm.

Protein synthesis on eukaryotic ribosomes proceeds according to the same steps—that is, initiation, elongation, and termination—as in prokaryotes. The initiation codon is the same, AUG, but the initiation tRNA is different: its anticodon complements AUG, as in prokaryotes, but the aminoacyl residue it carries is an unmodified methionine.

Eukaryotic initiation, elongation, and termination factors are also different from their prokaryotic counterparts, but the reactions in which they are involved are similar. *Energy requirements are the same.* Eukaryotic elongation factors, however, can play a significant role in the control of translation. In erythroblasts, for instance, one of them (IF2) is phosphorylated and thereby inactivated by a protein kinase that is activated when the cells run out of heme. Erythroblasts synthesize primarily globins (for hemoglobin), but in the absence of heme continuous globin production would be useless. A similar inactivation of IF2 is induced by interferon, a glycoprotein secreted by virus-infected cells. Diphtheria toxin inactivates (by ADP-ribosylation) one of the eukaryotic elongation factors, the translocase. Protein synthesis is arrested with grave consequences for the cells and the patients.

Given the existence of a separate nuclear compart-ment in which transcription takes place, eukaryotic mRNAs must be completed and transported to the cytoplasm before their translation can start. In this respect, the situation is clearly different from that found in prokaryotes in which translation of a given mRNA starts at the 5' end of an mRNA while transcription continues toward its 3' end. The separation of transcription from translation enables eukaryotic cells to process extensively their mRNAs: in contradistinction to their prokaryotic counterparts, they are not direct transcripts of the genes, but extensively edited gene copies from which sequences of variable length are eliminated while the remaining sequences are spliced together. The mRNAs arrive in the cytoplasmic matrix as ribonucleoprotein particles, which are disassembled before initiation of translation. The poly A sequence they have at their 3' end (see page 19 and Section II) gets shorter with repeated rounds of translation, and for this reason it is supposed to control the turnover rate of mRNAs.

Although ribosomes can be considered as the epitome of truly basic and ubiquitous biologic machine tools, there is only limited homology between prokaryotic and eukaryotic ribosomal "parts" such as r proteins. Significantly, however, the few homologies so far established concern r proteins involved in critical reactions—for example, the binding of charged tRNAs. *This lack of evolutionary conservatism is of considerable practical importance in medicine. Most of the antibiotics that inhibit protein synthesis on prokaryotic ribosomes do not affect protein synthesis on eukaryotic cytoplasmic ribosomes and vice versa, and this is the basis for their efficiency and extensive use in treating infectious diseases* (see Table 2).

Eukaryotic Polysomes

As in prokaryotic cells, *the vast majority of eukaryotic ribosomal particles is found assembled in polysomes at any time; only a small fraction belongs to a pool of free dissociated subunits. Among polysomes, two distinct classes are easily recognizable: free polysomes, which appear to be randomly scattered in the cytoplasmic matrix, and bound or attached polysomes to the membrane of the endoplasmic reticulum* (see below), *this being the only type of eukaryotic cellular membrane to which ribosomes are apparently able to attach. So far, and in contradistinction to the situation found in prokaryotes, no binding of ribosomes to the plasmalemma has been recorded. It should be noted that, notwithstanding their attachment to the ER membrane, bound polysomes, like free polysomes, are immersed in the cytoplasmic matrix. All polysomes—free or at-*

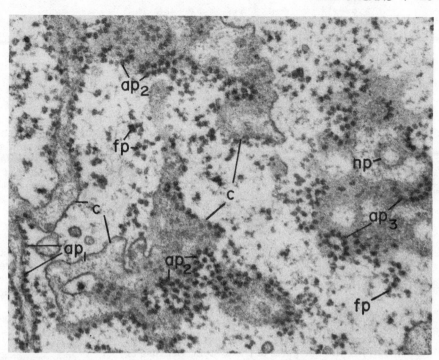

Figure 19. Polysomes in a rat hepatocyte. Free polysomes (fp) appear as ribosome clusters in the cytoplasmic matrix. Attached polysomes are seen in profile on normally sectioned ER membranes (ap_1), and in full-faced view on grazing sections of ER cisternae (ap_2) and the nuclear envelope (ap_3). np, nuclear pore; c, ER cisternae. 70,000 ×. (From G. E. Pallade: Science 189:347, 1975.)

tached—depend on a common cytosolic pool of amino acids, enzymes, tRNAs, and factors for their activity.

Attached polysomes form a small number of characteristic patterns on the cytoplasmic aspect of the ER membrane, the most common among them being loops, circles, rosettes, spirals, and double rows, in which variable numbers (from 5 to 20 or more) of ribosomes partake. In certain cell types, a single pattern predominates (for example, spirals in plasma cells or double rows in fibroblasts); in other cell types a varied mixture of polysomal patterns is found (Fig. 19).

The size of the total ribosomal population of a eukaryotic cell is directly related to its protein output. It can often exceed 1×10^6 units.

Free polysomes synthesize proteins destined to function intracellularly at a variety of sites. Among them are soluble proteins for the cytosol, monomeric units for the protein assemblies of the cell's locomotor apparatus, peripheral proteins for cellular membranes, and proteins destined for transport to certain intracellular compartments—for example, the nucleus, mitochondria, peroxisomes (and chloroplasts in plant cells), where they will become either membrane or matrix proteins. Free polysomes account for the majority of the ribosomal population in undifferentiated, rapidly growing cells, and in differentiated (or differentiating) cells whose function calls for a large amount of matrix proteins, such as myoblasts and erythrocyte precursors. In such cells, attached polysomes are a small minority of the total ribosomal population. Attached polysomes synthesize proteins for overt secretion—that is, for export to some extracellular compartment—as well as proteins for intracellular use, such as lysosomal enzymes (covert secretion, see below). They also synthesize integral membrane proteins. Since exportable proteins are usually produced in larger amounts and at a much faster rate than proteins for intracellular use, the fraction of attached polysomes in the total ribosomal population reflects primarily the cell's output of

secretory proteins. It reaches its highest values in exocrine or endocrine cells, outstanding examples being the hepatocytes, plasma cells, and acinar cells of the pancreas and salivary glands. All these cells have, however, a minority subpopulation of free polysomes, as expected because of the functions already enumerated for this type of polysome.

Ribosomal subunits are interchangeable, and all polysomes—free or attached—are assembled from free 40S and 60S subunits recruited from the pool located in the cytoplasmic matrix. Cells have the ability to shift their ribosomes from the free to the attached state or vice versa according to the demands put on them or according to their inherent developmental program. An exocrine cell, for instance, begins its differentiation process with a predominant population of free polysomes, needed to support its growth and replication and the assembly of the equipment required for its future activities. At the end of the process, when the cell is finally engaged in full scale production of secretory proteins, attached polysomes predominate.

The processing of polypeptides produced by free polysomes is limited, in most cases, to the removal of the methionyl residue from the original N terminal. Processing is much more extensive and elaborate in the case of attached polysomes, where it is connected with the complete or partial translocation of newly synthesized polypeptides across the ER membrane. The details of the process will be discussed in their proper context when the functions of the endoplasmic reticulum will be considered.

INTRACELLULAR MEMBRANE SYSTEMS

THE ENDOPLASMIC RETICULUM

General Morphology

As already stated, eukaryotic cells are highly compartmented systems. *Among their many intracellular compartments none is more complex geometrically and more diversified functionally than the endoplasmic reticulum, a network of membrane bounded channels or spaces that pervades the cytoplasm all the way from the nucleus to the plasmalemma.* It forms around the nucleus the perinuclear cisterna or nuclear envelope (already discussed), and it is restricted to the internal, more fluid, part of the cytoplasm called *endoplasm** (hence the name endoplasmic reticulum). It usually remains separated from the plasmalemma by a thin, relatively dense layer of fibrillar infrastructures (designated in the past as *exoplasm**). Contact and especially continuity of the ER membrane with the plasmalemma are extremely rare and, for the time being, can be considered as accidents of either nature or preparatory procedures.

The network is limited by a thin (about 6 nm) membrane that separates its contents from the cytoplasmic matrix. It consists of tubules, about 50 nm in diameter, often contorted and anastomosed, and of flattened sacks, called *cisternae†*, ~50 to 70 nm deep but as large as ~10 μm in the other two dimensions. When numerous, the cisternae tend to be disposed in parallel arrays, an arrangement that often obscures the existence of the network, which is in general more evident in the tubular parts of the system. Because of the frequent predominance of cisternal elements, the space enclosed by the ER membrane and the matter it contains are called *cisternal space* and *cisternal content*, respectively (see below, however, for the extension of these terms to other compartments). When the cisternal space is enlarged by extensive accumulation of cell products, the reticular geometry of the system becomes much more evident (in sectioned specimens). It is probable that the cisternal space is continuous throughout the entire ER, but the assumption is difficult to prove: it would require a three-dimensional reconstruction from a large number (for example, 300 to 400) of sections. The geometry of the system is labile: under a wide variety of abnormal conditions, including plasmalemmal damage, the tubules as well as the cisternae of the ER dilate and break down into a large collection of separate spherical vesicles 50 to 100 nm in diameter. Cell fractionation procedures take advantage of this phenomenon. ER vesicles are produced in situ when the plasmalemma is ruptured by shearing forces used for cell or tissue homogenization. These vesicles can be separated (from other subcellular components) as a distinct cell fraction, called the *microsomal fraction,* by a variety of centrifugal procedures. The vesicles of the fraction are called *microsomes.‡* The separation is, however, imperfect and incomplete, since not all microsomes represent ER-derived vesicles and not all ER-derived vesicles are recovered in the microsomal fraction.

Local Differentiations

A remarkable feature of the endoplasmic reticulum is its local association with other subcellular components or cell organs. It generates structurally and

functionally differentiated domains within the system; the best-studied of these domains are the following:

1. *The perinuclear cisterna or nuclear envelope,* surrounding the nucleus during interphase and controlling the traffic in and out of the nucleus through the nuclear pores.
2. *The rough-surfaced endoplasmic reticulum (RER),* characterized by its association with attached polysomes; it is the part of the network in which large cisternal elements predominate (Fig. 20).
3. *The smooth-surfaced endoplasmic reticulum (SER)* is the part of the system free of attached ribosomes. It consists of fine tubules organized in a tight meshwork; it is associated in some cell types with glycogen deposits, but this association is far from being as regular and as consistent as those mentioned above (Fig. 17).
4. In some cells, especially in invertebrates, part of the ER is differentiated into arrays of fenestrated cisternae reminiscent in their organization of the nuclear envelope but located in packages within the cytoplasm. They are called *annulate lamellae** and their functional significance is still unknown. Of potential interest is their frequent occurrence in mammalian, including human, tumor cells.
5. The transitional elements at the boundary between the ER and the Golgi complex will be described in a more appropriate context in relation to the Golgi apparatus.

These local differentiations occur, or can occur, in all animal eukaryotic cells. In addition, in certain cell types, special and functionally important modifications of the system have evolved, the most striking example being the sarcoplasmic reticulum, a highly elaborate structure associated with the sarcomeres of the myofibrils in striated (skeletal and cardiac) muscle.

As expected from the discussion on attached polysomes, the rough ER is highly developed in cells producing secretory proteins. The smooth ER is prominent in cells specialized in lipid, especially cholesterol, metabolism. It reaches its highest development in cells producing or catabolizing steroids and steroid hormones—for example, cells of the adrenal cortex, interstitial cells of the testis, cells of the corpus luteum, and hepatocytes.

Irrespective of the variety and degree of development of these differentiated domains, they are always in continuity with one another: they have a common, continuous membrane surrounding a common, continuous space as shown by·electron microscopy on favorable sections and by the distribution of physiologic tracers: proteins with an enzymatic activity detectable in situ by cytochemical procedures.

Biochemistry and Function

Microsomal Fractions. Microsomal fractions have been extensively used to collect information on the biochemistry and function of the endoplasmic reticulum. Most of this information has been obtained from (rat) liver fractions, a point worth remembering. Considerably more work is needed to find out to what extent the data obtained are of general applicability. The original microsomal fraction isolated by Claude

---

*Endoplasm and *exoplasm*: inner and outer cytoplasm respectively (Greek).

†*Cisterna*: reservoir or cistern (Latin).

‡*Microsome*: small body (Greek).

---

*Annulate lamellae: lamellae provided with rings (Latin).

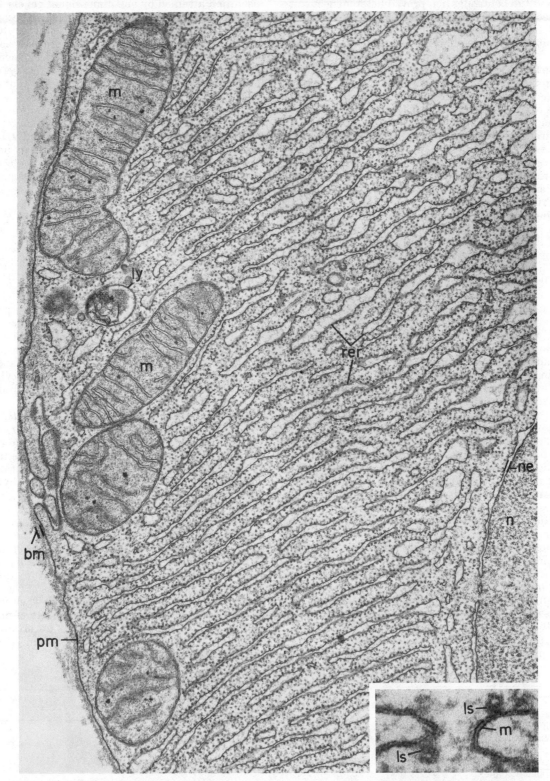

Figure 20. Rough-surfaced ER (rer) in a pancreatic exocrine (acinar) cell. The highly developed RER of this cell consists of numerous cisternal elements (rer) packed in parallel arrays. This organization is typical for all cells specialized in the massive production of secretory proteins. m, mitochondrion; ly, lysosome; n, nucleus; ne, nuclear envelope; pm, plasmalemma (basal domain); bm, basement membrane. 25,000 ×.

Inset: Part of two RER cisternae at high magnification to show the layered structure of the ER membrane (m) and the attachment of the large ribosomal subunit (ls) to the membrane. 240,000 ×. (From G. E. Pallade: Science 189:347, 1975.)

by differential centrifugation proved heterogeneous: it contained, in addition to vesicles of ER origin, vesicles derived from the Golgi complex, plasmalemma, and outer mitochondrial membranes. The demonstration of differentiated domains within the ER prompted attempts at their separation; more recently, cell fractionation protocols have been improved to yield a nuclear envelope fraction and Golgi fractions and to separate vesicles originating from the RER from those derived from the SER. Reasonably homogeneous rough microsomal fractions (derived from the RER) and Golgi fractions can be obtained at present by isopyknic or velocity sedimentation or flotation. The smooth microsomal fraction is still uncomfortably contaminated by plasmalemmal vesicles, Golgi elements, and outer mitochondrial membranes.

Biochemistry. *Lipids* in microsomal fractions are derived primarily from the polar lipids of the bilayer of the ER membrane. Some contamination by content lipids is, however, possible in hepatocytes and enterocytes. The fraction, presumably the ER membrane, is unusually rich in phosphatidylcholine (see Table 3) and in other phospholipids, and relatively poor in sphingomyelin and especially in cholesterol. However, the latter does not appear to be a contaminant contributed by non-ER membranes, since the terminal enzymes in cholesterol synthesis are located in the ER membrane and since their product is expected to partition, in part, into the latter's bilayer.

The fatty acyl groups of the phospholipids are medium-sized and highly unsaturated. Thus, lipid composition is compatible with a highly fluid and highly permeable membrane. In fact, as isolated, microsomal vesicles appear to be permeable to molecules as large as M_r ~5000, and their response to changes in medium osmolality is limited. They are impermeable, however, to proteins of M_r >20,000, and hence to most proteases.

Proteins. The proteins of the microsomal fractions can be resolved into content—and membrane proteins. In addition, a relatively large amount of soluble proteins is found relocated by adsorption on the outer surface of the microsomal vesicles, especially in rough microsomes.

The separation of content from membrane proteins is still imperfect. The former include secretory proteins, in different states of processing, as well as proteins that apparently remain in the cisternal space, where they act as posttranslocational modifiers of secretory proteins. Membrane proteins are numerous, varied in size, and diverse in function. At the level of

resolution attained by one-dimensional gel electrophoresis, more than 50 different bands can be recognized. The number of bands (and, hence, of separable proteins) is expected to increase with improved resolution.

Most of the information available on ER membrane proteins has been obtained by enzymic assays, which have identified a large number of resident (not exportable) activities. Some of the enzymes have been isolated and purified. In fact, the ER membrane is, at present, the cellular membrane with the largest number of well-characterized components. Finally, in some cases, information obtained by enzymic assay has been correlated with information obtained from electrophoretograms. As a result of this diversity of approaches, the following important biochemical processes have been localized in ER membranes:

Enzymes Involved in Lipid Metabolism

Synthesis of triacylglycerols (from fatty acids and glycerol produced in the cytoplasmic matrix) with glycerol phosphate and phosphatidic acid (PA) as intermediates. The products appear either in the cisternal space, where they become part of lipoprotein particles produced for export, or in the cytoplasmic matrix, where they are stored in lipid droplets as metabolic reserves. What controls the direction of discharge is still unknown. Production of lipids for metabolic reserves is a general process; production of triacylglycerols for export (as lipoproteins) appears to be limited to enterocytes and hepatocytes.

Synthesis of phospholipids from phosphatidic acid and activated choline, serine, ethanolamine or inositol. The cells have two options in this process: to proceed de novo all the way from phosphatidylserine to phosphatidylethanolamine (PE) (by decarboxylation) and phosphatidylcholine (PC) (by successive methylation), or to recover choline (from catabolized components), activate it (to phosphatidylcholine), and bind it to PA.

The enzymic equipment needed to produce these important components of all cellular membrane bilayers appears to be exclusively localized in the ER membrane. This virtual monopoly implies the existence of transport systems of phospholipids from the ER to all other membranes. Some potential components of the system have been identified and characterized. They function in vitro as exchange proteins for a variety of phospholipids; their activity in vivo is still uncertain. They could be part of a more elaborate system capable of effecting net transfer of phospholipids.

TABLE 3. LIPID COMPOSITION OF CELLULAR MEMBRANES

	ER MEMBRANES (%)	GOLGI MEMBRANES (%)	PLASMALEMMA (%)
Phospholipids			
Phosphoglycerides			
Phosphatidylcholine	45	30	20
Phosphatidylethanolamine	30	25	10–20
Phosphatidylserine	10	5	5
Phosphatidylinositol	5	5	5
Sphingolipids			
Sphingomyelin	5	15	20
Cholesterol	5	20	30–40

Figures given are (approximate) per cent of the total amount of polar lipids in each membrane fraction. Glycolipids are not included.

The degree of unsaturation of the fatty acyl groups of the phospholipids is ~45% for ER membranes, ~35% for Golgi membranes, and ~30% for the plasmalemma. These parameters describe the following gradient of bilayer fluidity: ER > Golgi complex > plasmalemma.

Synthesis of sphingolipids and partial synthesis of sphingoglycolipids.

Synthesis of cholesterol; in this case only a key "early" enzyme, 3-hydroxy-3-methylglutaryl CoA reductase (whose immediate product is mevalonate), and a chain of terminal enzymes responsible for converting squalene to lanosterol and the latter finally to cholesterol are located in the ER membrane. It should be noted that the monopoly of the ER applies to practically all polar lipids found in bilayers. Hence, transport systems must be in operation for all these lipids.

Modifying enzymes operating at different levels:

1. *transacylases that reshuffle the fatty acyl composition of the phospholipids and reacylate lysophosphatides;*

2. *enzymes that elongate fatty acids;*

3. *an enzyme system that desaturates fatty acids. This system is a chain of three enzymes, NADH-cyt b_5 reductase, cytochrome b_5, and desaturase, all of them integral membrane proteins.* The first two have been isolated, purified, and characterized. They have a large hydrophilic domain protruding into the cytoplasmic matrix and a smaller hydrophobic domain buried in the bilayer. The desaturase is more hydrophobic and hence more deeply buried in the bilayer. The system functions as an electron transport chain from NADH and fatty acids to O_2. It is inducible in the sense that the key enzyme (the desaturase) has a short half-life and the amount produced can be adjusted continuously to the cell's needs. As already stated, cells maintain fluid, at the temperature of the ambient, the lipid bilayers of their membranes: to achieve this goal, they adjust continuously the degree of unsaturation of the phospholipids of their bilayers.

Lipid-modifying enzymes are present in all cellular membranes, but for some of them (for example, those of the desaturating system) concentration and total amount are highest in the ER membrane.

Transport Enzymes

Biochemical assays and cytochemical tests have been used to localize a number of phosphatases in the ER or ER membrane. Among them are the following:

The Ca^{2+} ATPase present as majority protein component in the membrane of the sarcoplasmic reticulum. Comparable, but lower, activities have been recorded in neurons and other cells. The enzyme is part of a homeostatic system that maintains Ca^{2+} activity or ionic concentration at a low level in the cytosol ($\sim 10^{-6}M$) by pumping the Ca^{2+} into the cisternal space of the ER where the ion is sequestered by another protein. Muscle cells use variations in Ca^{2+} concentration to trigger contraction or achieve relaxation of their contractile assemblies. It may be assumed that a comparable system operates in all cells, since all cells have contractile assemblies (though of different types), but this issue is still unsettled.

As already mentioned, another Ca^{2+} ATPase, located in the plasmalemma, pumps Ca^{2+} from the cytosol into the extracellular medium, and thereby maintains a low basal intracellular Ca^{2+} concentration. That enzyme is the main active component of the Ca^{2+} homeostatic system.

Nucleoside mono-, di-, and triphosphatases have been found in the ER and microsomal fractions of many cell types. Their local function is still unknown. Some of the corresponding proteins may represent components for other membranes (plasmalemma) en route to their final destination or engaged in recycling.

Glucose-6-phosphatase is an integral membrane enzyme in the ER of hepatocytes, enterocytes, nephron epithelia, and possibly other cells. It dephosphorylates glucose-6-phosphate, the final product of glycogen phosphorolysis. The glucose thus produced is supposed to diffuse or be transported rapidly to the blood plasma (or interstitial fluid) through the plasmalemma. The phosphate appears in the cisternal space (or within microsomal vesicles), where it can be precipitated by Pb^{2+} or other trapping agents used in cytochemical reactions. The meaning of this sequestration is still obscure. Glucose-6-phosphatase has been considered in the past as a marker enzyme for the microsomal fraction (and hence for the ER) and has been used extensively to estimate the degree of contamination of other fractions by ER-derived vesicles. More recently, the enzyme was detected in other cellular membranes (for example, Golgi vesicles). Moreover, it is not expected to be a marker for the ER of all cells. Hence, its use for monitoring cell fractionation procedures requires caution and, if possible, independent supporting evidence.

Mixed Function Oxygenases

In certain cell types, the ER membrane contains an enzyme system that hydroxylates hydrophobic aromatic compounds imported from the environment or produced by the cells themselves. Hydroxylation renders such compounds more soluble in water and more easy to metabolize and eliminate. In mammals (*Homo* included) the system is present in the cells of the intestinal epithelium and is highly developed in hepatocytes. These are cells to which exogenous cyclic compounds (often found in food) have immediate or rapid access. The system consists of a flavoprotein that transfers electrons from NADPH to a specific member of a family of cytochromes (cyt P-450, P-448). The reaction of the reduced cyt P-450 with O_2 leads to the reduction of an O atom to water and to the introduction of the other O atom in the cyclic compound, which is thereby hydroxylated (Fig. 21). In hepatocytes, this system is involved in part in the hydroxylation of excess cholesterol. The products are bile acids, which are eventually excreted into the bile.

The Cyt P-450 Chain Functions as a Detoxifying System. Many drugs are cyclic compounds potentially toxic and relatively hydrophobic. A typical example is the barbiturates. Such drugs are processed by the cyt P-450 chain, which is often called (for this reason) the *detoxifying system.* It should be noted, however, that some of the intermediate metabolites in the detoxifying process (epoxides, for instance) can be more toxic or more carcinogenic than the original compounds.

The Detoxifying System Can Be Induced. When exposed to excess amounts of exogenous aromatic compounds, the cells are capable of accumulating large amounts of hydroxylating enzymes by stepping up their rate of synthesis while slowing down their degradation. The process, known as *induction,* can be readily triggered in experimental animals (and probably in humans) by administering aromatic drugs or steroid hormones. Induction causes a characteristic

Microsomal
Mixed function oxidase

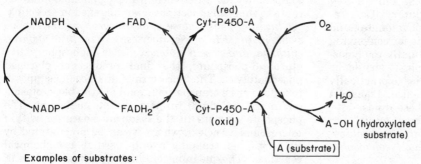

Examples of substrates:

    <u>drugs</u> : phenobarbital, morphine, codeine, amphetamine ;

    <u>carcinogens</u> : methylcholanthrene ;

    <u>metabolites</u> : sterols, steroids

Figure 21. The mixed function oxygenase is a short, multienzyme chain located in the membrane of the ER. Its components (NADPH-cyt P450) reductase (a flavoprotein) and a family of specific cytochromes (cyt P450-P448) are all integral membrane proteins.

proliferation of the ER, especially smooth ER, since the affected cells need more ER membrane to accommodate the increased amounts of detoxifying enzymes, which are all integral membrane proteins.

    Other Detoxifying Systems. Besides hydroxylation, cells use other enzymic reactions to increase the solubility and facilitate the elimination of either metabolites or drugs. These reactions include conjugation with glucuronate or amino acids; the corresponding enzymes are also associated with the ER membrane. Typical examples are the glucuronidation of bilirubin and the conjugation of bile acids with glycine or taurine.

Role of the ER in the Processing of Secretory Proteins

    Segregation: Signal Sequence. It has been known for some time that proteins destined for secretion are synthesized by attached polysomes and rapidly segregated into the cisternal space of the ER, but the means by which cells control protein traffic and achieve segregation of secretory products were only recently understood. The 5′ end of the mRNA of a secretory protein codes for a sequence of 15 to 30 amino acids, called signal sequence (or leader sequence) that begins with the initiating amino acid residue (or its neighbor). Translation of the mRNA into a secretory peptide starts in the cytoplasmic matrix, but upon the emergence of the nascent peptide from the large ribosomal subunit, the signal sequence recognizes (and it is recognized by) a relatively large ribonucleoprotein particle, called *signal recognition particle* (SRP), which consists of a small RNA molecule (7S) and a cluster of six proteins. SRP is recognized in turn by an integral ER membrane protein (SRP receptor or docking protein) and this interaction leads to the attachment of the ribosome (by the large subunit) to the ER membrane. SRP and the SRP receptor leave the ribosome and two ER membrane glycoproteins, called *ribophorins,* secure it in place. Upon ribosome attachment, the elongating polypeptide penetrates the membrane and is transferred across it cotranslationally—that is, as translation proceeds. The signal sequence is removed, also cotranslationally, by an endopeptidase on the

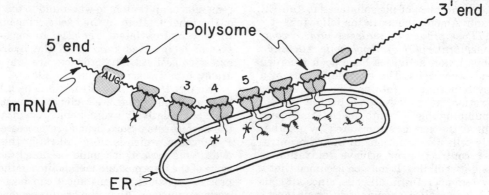

Figure 22. Signal sequence and traffic regulation of proteins within the cytoplasmic matrix. The initiation codon, AUG, of the mRNAs of secretory, lysosomal and some membrane proteins is followed by a sequence of 15 to 30 codons translated into a signal sequence that is recognized by a specific ribonucleoprotein particle (signal recognition particle) when it projects far enough from the large ribosomal subunit. The recognition is followed by ribosome attachment to the ER membrane and translocation of the newly synthesized polypeptide to the cisternal space of the ER. mRNA translation (for ER-directed proteins) begins therefore in the cytoplasmic matrix. Translocation occurs cotranslationally. The signal recognition particle is not included in this diagram.

cisternal side of the ER membrane. When translation is terminated and the transfer, or translocation, of the newly synthesized polypeptide to the cisternal space is completed, the ribosome detaches from the membrane, its subunits dissociate and reenter the pool of free ribosomal particles in the cytosol (Fig. 22). The molecules, the molecular mechanisms, and the forces involved in translocation are still unknown. If the mRNA of a secretory protein is translated in vitro in the absence of ER membranes (introduced as microsomal vesicles), the product is a larger relative of the protein found in the cisternal space, because its signal sequence is still present as an extension at its N terminal. This product, which is referred to as *preprotein* (and in some cases as *preproprotein,* see below), is not found in normal cells. In the absence of microsomal membranes (in *in vitro* experiments), and presumably in the absence of available translocation sites on the ER in intact cells, SRP blocks reversibly the elongation of nascent polypeptides and acts, therefore, as a controlling factor for the translation of ER-directed proteins.

The mRNAs of proteins synthesized for the various components of the cytoplasmic matrix have no signal sequences. The polysomes involved in their production remain free and the final product, discharged into the cytosol, is the same (or practically the same) as the original translate.

Further Modifications of Segregated Proteins. In the cisternal space, the segregated polypeptides are further processed by disulfide bridge formation, partial glycosylation (in the case of glycoproteins), and modification of certain amino acid residues (for example, hydroxylation of proline and lysine residues in collagens). As a result of these multiple modifications, the secretory proteins assume their final (or prefinal) tertiary structure while in the cisternal space. The modifying enzymes are either membrane or content proteins of the ER (Fig. 23). Most remarkable among them are those that carry out the synthesis and transfer in block of oligosaccharide chains for the glycosylation of proteins. Each chain consists of 14 hexose residues (2 *N*-acetyl-glucosamines, 9 mannoses, and 3 glucoses). Its transfer involves a special lipid carrier, namely a phosphate ester of a long isoprenoid chain called *dolichol*; the transferred oligosaccharide is N-linked cotranslationally to an asparagine residue.* The polymerization of polypeptide chains into heteropolymeric proteins like collagens and immunoglobulins occurs also within the cisternal space.

Recent evidence indicates that lysosomal enzymes are synthesized, segregated, and further processed in the same way as secretory proteins. It follows that the cisternal space accommodates within a common pool proteins for overt secretion, lysosomal enzymes, as well as resident ER proteins, like some of the modifying enzymes mentioned above. Cells evidently know how to sort out the different components of the pool and to direct them to their final destination, but the mechanisms at work are still unknown.

---

*Much less is known at present about the intracellular distribution of the enzymes involved in the O-glycosidic linkage of oligosaccharides to the serine and threonine residues of glycoproteins. These enzymes are probably Golgi-membrane proteins.

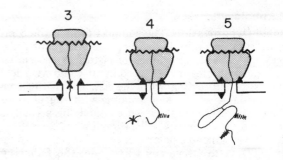

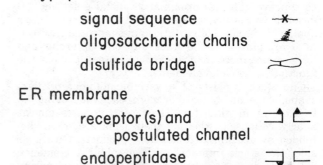

Polypeptide chain

   signal sequence

   oligosaccharide chains

   disulfide bridge

ER membrane

   receptor (s) and
       postulated channel

   endopeptidase

Figure 23. Cotranslational modifications of secretory (and membrane) proteins include (1) removal of the signal sequence by an endopeptidase, (2) proximal glycosylation, and (3) disulfide bridge formation. The processed translate assumes its tertiary structure as a result of these modifications. 3, 4, 5 refer to ribosomes 3, 4, 5 in the polysome in Figure 22.

Synthesis and Assembly of Transmembrane Proteins. The few plasmalemmal glycoproteins and the more numerous viral envelope glycoproteins so far investigated are synthesized and processed like secretory proteins, except that the transfer of the corresponding polypeptide (initiated by a signal sequence) is arrested halfway through the membrane so that the protein acquires a transmembrane topography with an endodomain still in the cytosol and an ectodomain in the cisternal space. Only the ectodomain is glycosylated.

THE GOLGI COMPLEX

The Golgi apparatus (or the Golgi complex) is a set of membrane-bound compartments interposed between the ER and the plasmalemma. Its constant and most characteristic structural component is a stack of smooth-surfaced cisternae.*

Its functions include posttranslational modifications of secretory proteins (primarily through terminal glycosylation and partial proteolysis); packaging of secretory products into membrane containers capable of exocytosis; sorting out of lysosomal enzymes for transport to lysosomes; terminal N-glycosylation, O-glycosylation; and sorting out of glycoproteins for Golgi subcompartment-, lysosome-, and secretion granule–membranes, and for the plasmalemma and each of its differentiated domains, when present.

---

*Golgi is the name of the discoverer of the apparatus, the Italian cytologist Camillo Golgi.

Morphology

Basic Organization. The simplest form of the complex is found in multiple distinct copies in plant cells. Each copy consists of a stack of cisternae associated with small vesicles (called peripheral Golgi vesicles) on the side interacting with the ER, and with large Golgi vacuoles on the side trading with the plasmalemma. The first side is called *cis*, and the second is designated *trans* (Fig. 24). The complex has, therefore, a clearly recognizable polarity.

In addition to cis versus trans side, the following pairs of synonyms are widely used in the literature to describe the polarity of the Golgi complex: (1) convex vs concave side, (2) proximal vs distal side, and (3) forming vs maturing side; (1) and (2) are not always applicable because of variations in shape and intracellular orientation of the stacks of Golgi cisternae, and (3) assumes more than we know at present about the function of cis Golgi elements.

The stack consists of a variable number of disk-shaped cisternae (3 to 10 or more) each measuring 0.5 to 1.0 μm in diameter. Their central parts appear nearly collapsed, whereas their rims are often distended by accumulated secretory products. On its cis side, the stack interacts with special ER elements, called *transitional elements*, because their limiting membrane has attached polysomes (like the ER) on one side, and is smooth (like Golgi vesicles) and often provided with small protrusions on the other side. The small (diam ~50 nm) peripheral Golgi vesicles, already mentioned, are clustered in between the transitional ER elements and the stacks as well as around the circumference of the stacks. The vacuoles on the trans side of the stacks measure 0.2 to 1.0 μm in diameter and, depending on the cell type, are distended to a varied extent by secretory products in different states of concentration. In such instances (see below), Golgi vacuoles are also called *condensing vacuoles*.

In many cells, the limiting membrane of Golgi elements is thin, ~6 nm (ER-like), on the cis side of the complex and noticeably thicker, ~10 nm (plasmalemma-like), on the trans side, the transition from one type of membrane to the other occurring at the level of the stacked cisternae.

Golgi Complex of Animal Cells. In animal cells, the basic organization of the complex is the same, but the piled cisternae are larger in size and more variable in shape than in plant cells. Moreover, the individuality of the complex is less evident and the arrangement of its elements less regular primarily because the Golgi area and its immediate vicinity are crowded by many other subcellular components, such as ER elements, coated vesicles, and lysosomes. In many animal cells, the Golgi complex is disposed around a pair of centrioles, which, with their associated satellites, microtubules, and fibrillar bundles, constitute the *centrosphere* (see Fig. 28).

On the trans side of many (but not all) Golgi stacks occurs a cisterna of characteristic morphology. It has a rigid appearance, a relatively constant thickness, and a dense, laminated content. Since acid phosphatase activity (reminiscent of lysosomes) can be detected therein, it has been postulated that this cisterna and its associated structures constitute a link between the *G*olgi (complex), the *ER*, and the *L*ysosomes; hence, the acronym GERL is used for its designation.

Functions

The functions of the Golgi complex have been less extensively investigated than those of the ER, primarily because satisfactory Golgi fractions became available only relatively recently. At present, the following conclusions emerge from biochemical assays on isolated Golgi fractions and from studies carried out in situ by cytochemical tests and autoradiographic procedures.

1. Golgi elements are heterogeneous: cytochemical reactions differentiate between cisternae in extreme cis and trans positions; the functional meaning of these differences is now being elucidated.

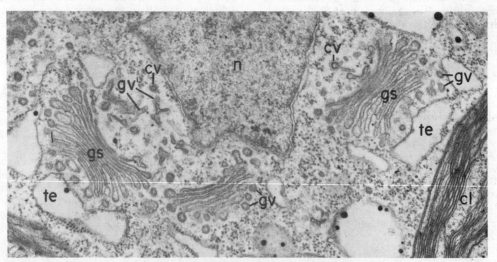

Figure 24. Three Golgi complexes in a unicellular plant, the alga *Chlamydomonas reinhardtii*. gs, stacks of Golgi cisternae; gv, small, peripheral Golgi vesicles; te, transitional elements of the rough ER; gv', Golgi vacuoles (collapsed in this case; see Figures 25 and 28 for dilated appearances); cv, coated vesicles; n, nucleus; cl, chloroplast. 38,000 ×. (From M. G. Farquhar and G. E. Palade: J Cell Biol 91:77s, 1981.)

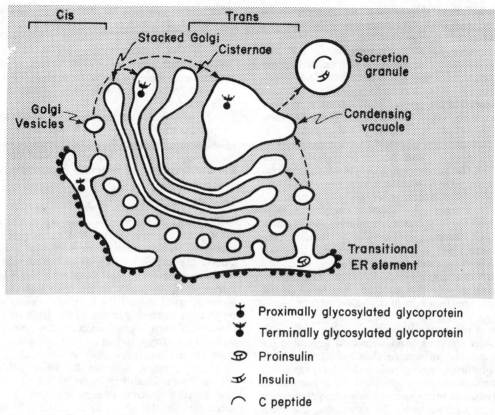

ꙮ Proximally glycosylated glycoprotein

ꙮ Terminally glycosylated glycoprotein

ꙮ Proinsulin

ꙮ Insulin

⌒ C peptide

Figure 25. Diagram of the organization of the Golgi complex. Posttranslational modifications incurred by secretory (and membrane) proteins within the Golgi complex include (1) terminal glycosylation, (2) proteolytic processing (as in the case of insulin and albumin), (3) phosphorylation (as in the case of caseins), and (4) sulfation (as in the case of proteoglycans). Only (1) and (2) are illustrated. Interrupted lines indicate the traffic pathways from ER to the Golgi complex and secretion granules. The return pathways (recycling) are not indicated.

2. The Golgi complex is involved in the transport, posttranslational modification, and packaging of secretory and other proteins received from the ER.

Transport. Secretory proteins are transported in small vesicular containers, or carriers, that are assumed to function as shuttles between the transitional elements of the ER and the distended rims of Golgi cisternae, or the Golgi vacuoles on the trans side of the complex (Fig. 25). The peripheral Golgi vesicles found on the cis side of the Golgi stacks are probably reserve vesicular carriers. In certain cell types, however, patent tubular connections have been described between ER and Golgi elements. The transport is vectorial and energy-dependent. The products are moved in one direction only (from the ER to the Golgi), and are blocked at the level of transitional ER elements if the cell cannot synthesize ATP.

Modifications. While in transit through the Golgi complex, some (but not all) secretory proteins are modified by partial proteolysis and/or by glycosylation (Fig. 25). One or more proteolysis steps remove(s) from the polypeptide chains short, terminal segments (as in the case of albumin in hepatocytes) or loops (as in the case of insulin in the β cells of the pancreatic islets). In other cell types (for example, cells of the pituitary gland) a large common precursor is converted into a series of distinct peptides. In such cases, the product received from the ER is called a proprotein (proalbumin, proinsulin, and so on), the usual name being

reserved for the product finally discharged by the cell. Recall that proinsulin is derived from a primary translate that is referred to as preproinsulin. The same series of pre and pro precursors is found for many other (but not all) secretory proteins.

Secretory glycoproteins arrive in the Golgi complex already partially glycosylated. Upon arrival, their oligosaccharides are partially trimmed, down to two N-acetylglucosaminyl and three mannosyl residues, by resident glycosidases. The remnant chains are further glycosylated by the stepwise addition of other monosaccharides—namely, N-acetylglucosamine, galactose, sialic acid (in this order), and, occasionally, fucose. The transferases that catalyze these reactions are Golgi membrane proteins, and one of them (the galactosyltransferase) is considered a marker enzyme for the Golgi complex.

Sulfation of glycoproteins and glycosaminoglycans (linked to proteoglycans) is also restricted to the Golgi complex, and the same apparently applies for the phosphorylation of secretory proteins—like the caseins, produced by mammary gland cells, for instance.

Packaging. In the Golgi complex, secretory proteins are packaged in membrane containers competent to interact with the plasmalemma and to deliver by exocytosis (see below) their content to the extracellular medium. These containers are called *secretion vacuoles* or *secretion granules*. Information available in a rapidly increasing number of cases indicates that the membrane proteins of these containers appear to be different from, and less numerous than, those of the plasmalemma and Golgi membranes.

Other Secretion-Related Functions. In addition to the operations described above, which occur in most (if not all) cells, certain glandular cells have the ability to concentrate secretory products in Golgi vacuoles that, by progressive filling and concentration of their content, become secretory granules. Concentration appears to be achieved by complex (or aggregate) formation, which leads to a reduction in osmotic activity within Golgi vacuoles and hence to passive water movement from the vacuoles to the cytosol. Concentration (and its corollary, secretion granule formation) appear in cells that store their secretory products intracellularly. Intracellular storage enables them to deliver in mass their secretory products upon stimulation by either neurotransmitters or hormones. Concentration takes place either in trans Golgi vacuoles (called for this reason *condensing vacuoles*) or in the distended rims of stacked Golgi cisternae. The proteolytic processing of secretory proteins, initiated in the Golgi complex, continues in many cases within secretion granules.

Secretory Pathway. Protein-secreting cells use their ER, Golgi complex, and secretion granules (or vacuoles) as a series of connectable compartments in which their products, segregated in the cisternal space of the ER, are successively modified (in a number of different ways), and often concentrated and temporarily stored prior to discharge. By extension, the term cisternal space is used for the content space of all these compartments, which are referred to collectively as the secretory pathway or (more appropriately) the ER→plasmalemma pathway. The pathway is reminiscent of an assembly line in which different production steps are logically separated in time and space.

Sorting of products and traffic patterns within the Golgi complex. Information obtained over the last few years has considerably advanced our understanding of the functional organization of the Golgi complex. Each cisterna (or small group of cisternae) of the Golgi stack appears to have its own set of resident membrane proteins with specific enzymatic or receptor activities; each cisterna, therefore, is equipped to perform a specific function. For instance, galactosyltransferase (the "marker enzyme" of the Golgi complex) has been localized by immunocytochemistry to a single cisterna (or pair of cisternae) on the trans side of the Golgi stack, together with a UDPase that degrades the nucleotide (UDP) involved in galactose activation. The mannose-6-phosphate receptor for lysosomal enzymes (see below) has been localized by immunocytochemistry to a single cisterna (or pair of cisternae) on the cis side of the stack. Other localizations by similar procedures may be forthcoming.

The substrates (secretory, lysosomal, and membrane proteins) for these resident Golgi enzymes and receptors are brought to the distended rims of the Golgi cisternae by vesicular carriers that move them in succession from one Golgi cisterna to the next until they are ready for transport—by other vesicular carriers—to their final destinations, e.g., secretion granules, lysosomes, or plasmalemma. Since all these carriers seem to recycle, the Golgi complex appears to function as the hub of the intracellular vesicular traffic.

Sorting of proteins for different destinations is probably effected at different levels along the Golgi stacks. Each protein probably leaves the main pathway at the level of the cisterna in which it has acquired its "mature form" and has encountered its receptor. Lysosomal enzymes, for instance, probably leave the main pathway from cisternae located on the cis side of the Golgi stacks.

Recently, vesicular transport between Golgi subcompartments has been demonstrated *in vitro* in reconstituted, subcellular systems. Experiments of this kind may uncover the molecular mechanisms involved in the traffic control of vesicular carriers.

Exocytosis*

Proteins, glycoproteins, and lipoproteins produced for export are moved in membrane-bound containers (called secretion vesicles or secretion granules) from the Golgi complex to the plasmalemma. The membrane of these containers can fuse with the plasmalemma either spontaneously or upon cell stimulation by a secretagogue† (usually a hormone, releasing factor, or neurotransmitter). Fission of the lipid bilayers within the area of membrane fusion creates an orifice through which secretory products can be discharged in mass from their containers. Exocytosis enables the cell to discharge macromolecules in mass while retaining intact its permeability barriers for small molecules. The process requires energy and Ca^{2+} mobilized from intracellular storage sites or coming from the extracellular medium.

The membrane of the containers is rapidly recovered as small vesicles (often coated vesicles) and is probably repeatedly used or recycled. In exocrine cells, competency for exocytosis is limited to the luminal domain of the plasmalemma.

LYSOSOMES‡

Lysosomes are sac-like structures that contain digestive enzymes and function as an intracellular digestive system.

Structure and Biochemistry

The important general properties of lysosomes are their content of digestive enzymes, their limiting membrane, and their structural heterogeneity. As far as their enzyme content is concerned, they contain over 40 digestive enzymes, at latest count, including proteases, nucleases, glycosidases, lipases, phospholipases, sulfatases, and phosphatases. With this enzyme complement, lysosomes are capable of digesting most constituents of cells and tissues—that is, proteins, nucleic acids, lipids, carbohydrates, and glycosaminoglycans—down to their basic building blocks (amino acids or dipeptides, sugars, and fatty acids). The vast majority of lysosomal enzymes are acid hydrolases (optimally active at pH 5.0 or below). Intralysosomal pH is maintained lower than that of the cytosol by an H^+-depend-

---

Exocytosis: discharge by cell (Greek); it refers, in fact, to discharge of matter in bulk.

†*Secretagogue*: substance that promotes secretion (Latin-Greek hybrid).

‡*Lysosome*: lytic body (Greek).

ent ATPase (a proton pump), which is an integral lysosomal membrane protein. Several enzymes have been used extensively as marker enzymes for the identification of lysosomes during cell fractionation (acid phosphatase, *N*-acetyl-β-glucosaminidase, cathepsin C) or in tissue sections (acid phosphatase and aryl sulfatase). The limiting membrane of the lysosome, which is a typical unit membrane of the plasmalemmal variety, acts as a shield between the digestive enzymes and the cytosol, preventing leakage of these potentially lethal hydrolases into the cytoplasmic matrix. The structural heterogeneity of the lysosomes is created by the fact that, in addition to acid hydrolases, lysosomes contain materials undergoing digestion that may be present in varying stages of degradation (Fig. 26). Often residues of partially digested extracellular or intracellular components (cell organs) can be recognized among the contents. This heterogeneity of form and content has rendered the identification of lysosomes in tissue sections and their isolation as a pure cell fraction difficult, since they do not have uniform morphologic or sedimentation characteristics. Hence, use of marker enzymes has played an essential role in the study and characterization of lysosomes by both cell fractionation and cytochemistry since their discovery.

The Lysosomal System

In reality lysosomes represent not a single entity but a whole system—sometimes referred to as the vacuolar or lysosomal system (diagrammed in Fig. 27), which functions as an intracellular digestive tract. This system has as its evolutionary forerunner the digestive vacuoles of amebae and other protozoa, which function in the nutrition of these organisms: foodstuffs are taken in bulk, digested in food vacuoles, and the products used for cell metabolism. Lysosomes are ubiquitous in animal cells (except for the mammalian red blood cell), and comparable organelles are found in plant cells from yeast to higher plants. However, in higher organisms the primitive activity of intracellular digestion has been adapted in a variety of ways to subserve the needs of the whole organism as will be described below.

Entry into Lysosomes

Substances that gain access to lysosomes can come either from outside the cell by *heterophagy** or by direct *permeation* or from inside the cell by *autophagy** or *crinophagy** (as described below).

Heterophagy consists of uptake of materials in bulk by invagination of the plasma membrane or *endocytosis*.† Incorporation can be in small, fluid-filled vesicles

---

**Heterophagy, autophagy,* and *crinophagy*: eating other (substance than its own), eating itself, and eating secretion, respectively (Greek).

†*Endocytosis*: incorporation by cells (Greek).

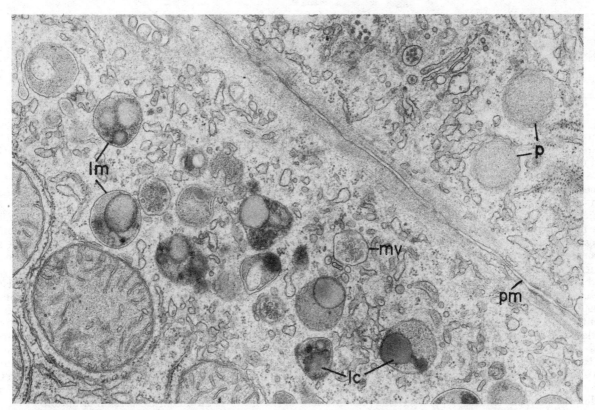

Figure 26. Cluster of secondary lysosomes (ly) in a hepatocyte (rat). Each lysosome is bounded by a single membrane (lm) and has a characteristically heterogeneous content (lc) that represents primarily digestion residues. Some of the simplest and earliest secondary lysosomes are filled with small vesicles and are called multivesicular bodies (mv). The plasmalemma (pm) of this part of the cell has an extensive fibrillar infrastructure; p, peroxisomes. 27,000 ×.

THE LYSOSOMAL OR VACUOLAR SYSTEM

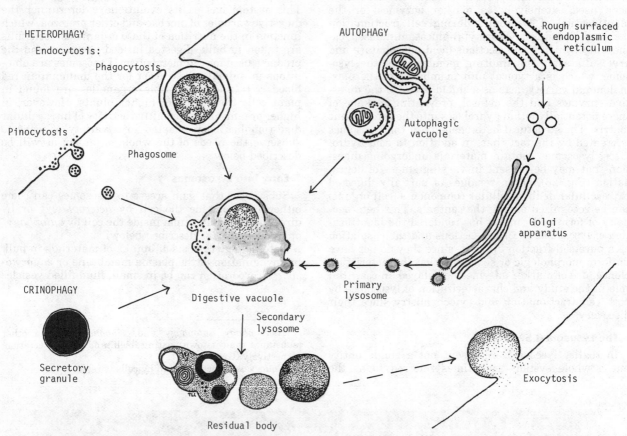

Figure 27. Input of substrates into the digestive vacuole (in the center of the diagram) comes primarily from the extracellular medium via endocytosis (pinocytosis and phagocytosis), and occasionally from intracellular sources via autophagic vacuoles (autophagy) and secretory granules (crinophagy). Input of digestive enzymes comes from the RER via the Golgi complex and primary lysosomes. An active digestive vacuole is called a secondary lysosome; as digestion proceeds, the residue-loaded vacuole becomes a residual body whose content is occasionally discharged by exocytosis. (Courtesy of Drs. T. Lentz and M. G. Farquhar, Yale University.)

containing small molecules or particles *(pinocytosis)** or in large pockets that accommodate microorganisms, cell debris, or even whole cells *(phagocytosis)*.* In the case of phagocytosis the membrane is usually tightly adherent to the entering particle, whereas in pinocytosis the incorporated molecules enter as part of the vesicle content *(fluid-phase pinocytosis)* or bound to the membrane *(adsorptive or receptor-mediated endocytosis)*. Endocytosed material does not reach the lysosomes directly; it is channeled instead through a series of vacuoles called *endosomes*. The watery content of the latter has a low pH (because their membranes have a proton pump), but no lysosomal enzymes. Many receptors lose their ligands in these low pH compartments and recycle to the cell surface undamaged. Endosomes are the ports of entry for many infections with enveloped (i.e., membrane bound) virus particles. In their acid environment, the glycoproteins of viral envelopes undergo changes that make them "fusogenic," i.e., capable of fusing their membrane with the endosome membrane. As a result of this membrane fusion, the undamaged viral genome can reach the cytoplasmic matrix wherein it can start its replication. In time, endosomes acquire lysosomal enzymes by fusion with primary or secondary lysosomes (see below).

A few substances gain access to endosomes and lysosomes by direct permeation or passive diffusion; owing to their small size and solubility in lipid bilayers, they can directly penetrate the cell membrane and the endosomal and lysosomal membranes. They enter these acid compartments in uncharged form, are converted into charged forms and thus are trapped and concentrated therein. Examples of substances of interest that are believed to be concentrated in this manner include weak bases, certain basic dyes (neutral red, acridine orange), drugs (chloroquine), and carcinogens (chlorinated hydrocarbons).

Cellular constituents can gain access to lysosomes by direct fusion—for example, of vesicles or secretory granules (referred to as *crinophagy*) or by *autophagy*. The latter is an elaborate version of uptake in bulk in which bits of cytoplasm, often containing recognizable cell organs, become surrounded by smooth-membrane–cisternae (derived from the Golgi or from the ER), and are eventually segregated from the surround-

---

*Pinocytosis and *phagocytosis*: cell drinking and cell eating, respectively (Greek).

ing cytoplasm. Autophagy is common in cell populations undergoing remodeling (as during embryogenesis and metamorphosis), when there is extensive cell involution, or when a cell suffers sublethal injury.

Fate of Ingested Materials

All of the ingested materials, whether incorporated by heterophagy, autophagy, or crinophagy, are collected together in lysosomes where they undergo a common fate—that is, advanced or complete digestion. The products (dipeptides, amino acids, sugars, and fatty acids) are small enough to diffuse readily across the lysosomal membrane, enter the free cytoplasmic pools, and be reutilized in biosynthesis. Normally, lysosomes undergo repeated cycles of incorporation and digestion, being continually recharged with a new complement of digestive enzymes by fusion with primary lysosomes (that is, granules or vesicles derived from the Golgi that are filled with newly synthesized lysosomal enzymes). Sometimes lysosomes become stuffed with indigestible residues, either locally produced (lipofuscin pigment) or accidentally introduced (silica, asbestos) from the environment. Residues of the latter type can cause defects in lysosomal function or lead to lysosomal rupture. Some cells can discharge such indigestible residues by exocytosis. For example, hepatocytes discharge their lysosomal residues into bile along the bile front of their plasmalemma.

The membrane used in the delivery of incorporated substances into endosomes and lysosomes is reutilized or recycled; that is, after fusion with an endosome or lysosome, the incoming membrane pinches off and is eventually returned to the plasmalemma, from where it can participate in another endocytosis cycle.

Source of Lysosomal Enzymes

Available evidence indicates that lysosomal enzymes are glycoproteins that are synthesized and processed in the same manner and along the same route as secretory proteins. They are sorted out therefrom in the Golgi complex and packaged into small vesicles (usually of the clathrin-coated variety) in most cells, or into distinct granules in special cases, as in granulocytes. The content of these vesicles or granules, known as *primary lysosomes,* is delivered to endosomes or to already enzymically active *secondary lysosomes* by membrane fusion. Endosomes are converted to lysosomes by fusion events of two types: endosome—primary lysosome, or endosome—secondary lysosome.

Soon after their entry into the Golgi complex, newly synthesized lysosomal enzymes are modified by a set of specific resident enzymes, which phosphorylate (in the 6 position) a few mannose residues of their mannose-rich oligosaccharide chains. The phosphorylated residues are the signal recognized by specific receptors (called *mannose-6-P receptors*) that bind the enzymes, remove them from the common pathway, and transport them to lysosomes or endosomes. The mannose-6-P receptor is an integral membrane protein found in the membranes of cis-Golgi cisternae and associated coated-vesicle carriers that recycle between the Golgi complex and lysosomes (or endosomes). Upon arriving in lysosomes, the newly arrived enzymes dissociate from their receptors (owing to the local acid pH) and are dephosphorylated and proteolytically processed to

forms able to function for a relatively long time in their new harsh environment. The receptors recycle back to the Golgi complex. In mutants that cannot synthesize the mannose-6-P signal, the lysosomal enzymes cannot be sorted out and segregated into lysosomes; instead they are discharged into the extracellular medium, just like secretory proteins.

Specialized Cell Functions Mediated by Lysosomes

As already indicated, the primitive digestive function that the lysosomal system has in protozoa has been adapted by multicellular organisms to subserve a remarkable variety of functions. For example, *defense* (phagocytosis of microorganisms by granulocytes and macrophages); *cell turnover* (removal of old erythrocytes, leukocytes, and platelets from the circulation by splenic macrophages); *protein absorption* (recovery of filtered plasma proteins by the cells of the proximal kidney tubule); *hormone secretion* (processing of thyroglobulin to T_3* and T_4* by the lysosomes of thyroid cells); *renewal of retinal rod outer segments* (the disks of the tips of the rod outer segments are phagocytized [and digested in lysosomes] by the pigment epithelium); and *glycoprotein catabolism* (removal of altered glycoproteins from the circulation by hepatocytes, followed by their degradation in lysosomes).

Receptor-Mediated Endocytosis

In addition, it has recently become evident that lysosomes are involved in even more elaborate regulatory mechanisms of the metabolism of animal cells. The best-studied case in point is the regulation of intracellular cholesterol metabolism in cells other than hepatocytes. The low density lipoproteins (LDL) (derived from very low density lipoproteins secreted by hepatocytes) are the predominant cholesterol-carrying particles of the blood. LDL bind to specific receptors located in *coated pits* in the plasmalemma of their target cells, and are internalized (as receptor-LDL complexes) in coated vesicles that subesquently fuse with endosomes. After fusion the receptor recycles back to the plasmalemma, whereas the LDL are transported to, and degraded within, lysosomes. The cholesterol released in the process diffuses into the cytosol, where it turns off cholesterol production by suppressing 3-hydroxy-3-methylglutaryl-CoA reductase, the rate-controlling enzyme of cholesterol synthesis. The increase in free cholesterol concentration in the cytoplasm leads also to the turning off of the synthesis of LDL receptors. (Familial hypercholesterolemia, an inborn disease that leads to early, fatal arteriosclerosis, is the result of defective LDL receptors.) Other examples of macromolecules, important in the regulation of cell metabolism, that are taken up by receptor-mediated endocytosis are peptide hormones (insulin, epidermal growth factor, β-melanocyte-stimulating hormone, gonadotropins), transcobalamin, transferrin, yolk proteins, polymeric immunoglobulin A, and maternal immunoglobulins. In these cases, the biologic consequences of uptake are less clear, but in many instances their effects on cellular metabolism involve

---

*T_3 and T_4: triiodo- and tetraiodothyronine, the active forms of thyroid hormones.

the participation of lysosomes. In a few cases (yolk proteins, polymeric immunoglobulin A, and maternal immunoglobulins) lysosomes appear to be bypassed. Immunoglobulins are transported unaltered by vesicular carriers (transcytosis*) across cells organized in epithelia, and yolk proteins are stored undegraded for later use in embryonic development. Since each of these problems is under extensive investigation, rapid progress in defining the biologic consequences of endocytosis and lysosomal digestion of receptors and cognate ligands (hormones, growth factors) can be anticipated.

Medical Implications: Cell Pathology

At present there is more known about the role of lysosomes in cell pathology than about that of any other cell organ. To begin with, owing to their monopoly on digestive functions, they are involved either directly or indirectly in every disease process in which there is cell death, cell involution, or cell injury. In addition, there is a large group of diseases—over 20 at latest count—known as lysosomal storage diseases, that are due to a genetic defect or deletion of one or more lysosomal enzymes. As a result, the substrate of the missing enzyme accumulates within lysosomes, and these organelles become large and numerous enough to interfere with normal cell function. Examples are Pompe's disease, which leads to accumulation of glycogen in lysosomes (owing to the absence or low activity of lysosomal α-glucosidase), and Tay-Sachs disease, in which a ganglioside (GM_2) accumulates in lysosomes (owing to absence or deficiency of lysosomal hexosaminidase A).

In other situations, such as in gout and silicosis, the underlying pathology is due to an accumulation of undigestible residues (uric acid and silica respectively) within lysosomes that damage the lysosomal membrane, causing leakage of lysosomal enzymes, thereby resulting in cell death and tissue injury.

We have pointed out that the normal functioning of the host defense to infectious diseases depends on the amplification of heterophagy and enhanced activity of the lysosomal system of granulocytes and macrophages during the inflammatory response. Some diseases, primarily granulomatous diseases, result from the fact that the causative organisms have learned how to interfere with normal heterophagy. For example, toxoplasmas, brucellae, listeriae, and tubercle bacilli are incorporated normally by phagocytosis, but they produce substances that interfere with fusion between phagosomes and primary lysosomes, and they thrive within phagosomes.† Another type of interference is found in leprosy; the organism responsible for this disease has a capsule that resists digestion by lysosomal enzymes, enabling it to thrive within phagolysosomes.‡ In still other cases, microorganisms are believed to produce membranolytic toxins that cause rupture of the phagolysosomal membrane after their ingestion; streptolysins produced by streptococci are believed to act in this manner.

THE LOCOMOTOR APPARATUS

General Types of Motility. Unicellular eukaryotes have developed a variety of locomotive mechanisms among which the most common and effective are based either on ciliary (or flagellar) beats or on movement of contractile assemblies within the cell body. The first mechanism is epitomized by ciliated or flagellated protozoa; the second by amebae.

In multicellular organisms, both types of locomotion are encountered, but, in addition, a number of highly differentiated modes of locomotion are found in different types of muscle cells.

Certain human cells live as free individuals in the fluid content of different body compartments (blood, lymph, interstitial fluid) and are capable of active movements, often directed by chemotactic responses. Granulocytes, lymphocytes, macrophages, and many others belong to this group. Other cells live in a relatively fixed location—as in the case of epithelial cells, secured in place by junctional complexes, but even such cells are potentially mobile. Besides, certain activities of all cells require movement of cell parts or subcellular components on a relatively large scale. Foremost among these activities are chromosome separation, cell division, intracellular transport, exocytosis, and endocytosis.

Other cells of multicellular organisms retain cilia or flagella. Those incorporated into epithelia generate waves by coordinated ciliary beats, and these waves move fluid (usually secreted mucus with adsorbed or embedded particles) over the exposed surface of the epithelium. This type of movement is of considerable importance in the physiology of the respiratory tract and of the female reproductive system. The only clear example of a free-swimming, flagellated cell in mammals is the male gamete (the sperm cell or the spermatozoon).

CYTOSKELETON

Movement requires contractile or motor devices as well as relatively rigid, but movable, components. The latter can be considered as the equivalent of an internal skeletal system, and for this reason they are often referred to as *cytoskeleton*. They consist of *microtubules* and bundles of *intermediary filaments*.

Microtubules

The microtubules are long, hollow, cylindric structures that measure ~25 nm in diameter; their wall consists of 13 parallel protofilaments, each formed by the polymerization of heterodimeric units produced by the copolymerization of two proteins (M_r ~55,000) called *tubulin a* and *tubulin b*. Microtubules depolymerize at high pressure or low temperature into heterodimers. Polymerization of the heterodimers into microtubules requires low Ca^{2+} concentrations and is facilitated by a number of other proteins, including some high molecular weight species called *microtubule-associated proteins* that copurify with the tubulins.

Transcytosis: transport across a cell (Latin-Greek hybrid).

†*Phagosome*: phagocytic body or vacuole (before fusing with a lysosome) (Greek).

‡*Phagolysosome*: body involved in uptake and lysis (or a transition form from phagosome to lysosome) (Greek).

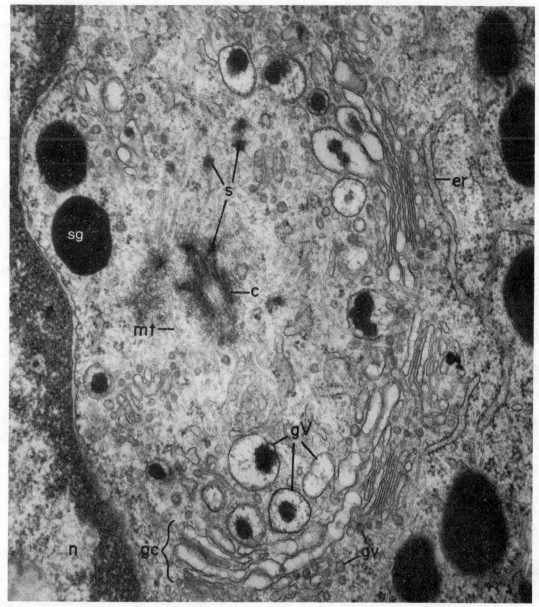

Figure 28. Centriole and Golgi complex in a neutrophilic promyelocyte (rabbit bone marrow). The Golgi complex consists of stacks of Golgi cisternae (gc) disposed in a semicircle. Some of these cisternae have distended rims in which secretory products are concentrated in dense masses. Small Golgi vesicles (gv) and RER elements (er) are seen on the cis side of the stacks, while large Golgi vacuoles (gV) occur on the trans side. The center of the Golgi area is occupied by a centriole (c) surrounded by centriolar satellites (s) on which microtubules (mt) converge. sg, mature secretion granules; n, nucleus. 50,000 ×. (From D. F. Bainton and M. G. Farquhar: J Cell Biol. 28:277, 1966.)

The cells use microtubules for a variety of purposes:

1. To achieve and maintain shapes other than globular; long cell processes such as the dendrites and axons of nerve cells exist only because they are internally reinforced by numerous microtubules.

2. To construct a system of guidelines or "monorails" along which various subcellular components are moved. This function is particularly obvious in melanocytes, in which pigment granules move from the cell's center to the cell's periphery (and back) along such lines. Besides form-enforcing, the microtubules of nerve axons perform a similar function in guiding the transport of various particulate components (synaptic vesicles, mitochondria) from the cell body to axonal endings.

3. To construct the mitotic spindle already described.

4. To produce the special microtubules of cilia and flagella (see below).

In many cells, microtubules radiate from a set of small, dense masses of unknown chemical nature located around the centrioles and called *centriole satellites* or *microtubule organizing centers* (Fig. 28). The way in which they end at the periphery is unknown for groups 1 and 2, but it is generally assumed that they interact at close range with the infrastructure of the plasmalemma.

Microtubules are in equilibrium with a pool of soluble heterodimers that lose the capacity to polymerize or repolymerize when reacted with certain alkaloids such as colchicine, vinblastine, and podophylotoxin. The result is progressive depolymerization of all cellular microtubules with a single exception, the microtubules of the cilia and flagella. The most obvious effect of these alkaloids is the disorganization of the mitotic spindle and the arrest of dividing cells in mitosis. For this reason the alkaloids mentioned are often referred to as mitotic poisons.

Intermediary Filaments

The other macromolecular assemblies that appear to function as cytoskeletal elements are microfilaments of ~10 nm in diameter. They are grouped in bundles and are called *intermediary filaments,* because they are finer than microtubules and thicker than actin filaments. These filaments are the result of the polymerization of 1, 2, or more proteins of M_r 50,000 to 60,000 that vary in nature from one group of cell types to another. In epithelial cells they belong to a family of *prekeratins* or *cytokeratins,* related to the keratins of hair and nails; in cells of mesodermal origin they appear to be antigenically different, and for this reason were given a different name: *vimentins.** Related proteins, capable of fibril formation by polymerization, have been detected in muscle cells.

In epithelial cells, the bundles of cytokeratin fibrils are anchored in desmosomal plates and crisscross the cytoplasm from one desmosome to another. The arrangement creates a system of intracellular bracing structures that connect intercellular adhering devices, thereby contributing to the ability of the cells and epithelia to withstand the pressure and shearing forces to which they are subjected during their existence. Vimentin bundles, like cytokeratin bundles, crisscross the cytoplasm, but their relations with other cell structures are poorly understood at present.

CILIA†

Structure. The cilium is a slender (diam ~0.2 μm) long structure that protrudes as much as 10 to 20 μm above the cell's surface. It consists of a complex assembly of microtubules, called the *axoneme,‡* which is ensheathed within a long extension of the plasmalemma and is affixed to a special structure called basal body located close to the cell's surface.

The axoneme consists in turn of nine peripheral pairs of microtubules disposed around a tenth central pair. This arrangement (referred to as the 9 + 1 pattern) is found in all ciliated cells and is clearly visible on cross-sectioned cilia (Fig. 29). In each peripheral pair, the microtubules are fused lengthwise to form a doublet, in which one of the microtubules is incomplete and the other is provided with perpendicularly and periodically attached arms long enough to reach the neighbor doublet. In contradistinction to the peripheral doublets, the central pair consists of two well-separated microtubules.

Vimentin (from vimentum): woven twigs (Latin).
†*Cilium*: eyelash (Latin).
‡*Axoneme*: axial filament (Greek).

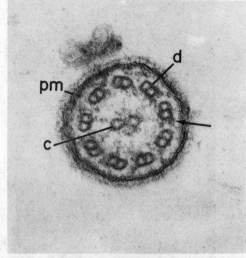

A

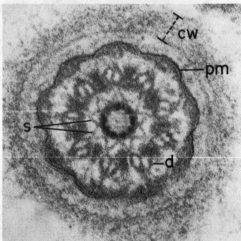

B

Figure 29. Flagellum. Cross sections of a flagellum of the green alga *Chlamydomonas reinhardtii* at the level of the flagellar shaft (A), and immediately distal to the corresponding basal body (B). In A, the nine peripheral doublets (d) of the axoneme are clearly visible; each of them consists of two parallel, partially fused microtubules. Dynein arms are marked by arrow. The central pair of separate microtubules (c) is clearly resolved, but structures (spokes) connecting them to the peripheral doublets are not. Such structures (s) are clearly seen in B. Note that at this level the central pair of microtubules is replaced by a special (cylindrical) structure. pm, plasmalemma; cw, cell wall. A: 130,000 ×; B: 140,000 ×.

Biochemistry. Ciliary microtubules, like other microtubules, are formed by polymerized tubulins. Their arms contain a large macromolecular assembly, a copolymer of many proteins, with ATPase activity, called *dynein.* The peripheral doublets are attached to the central pair and the plasmalemmal sheath by a large number of proteins that form a complex system of spokes and linkers. Their function is to keep together the various elements of the cilium during its movements.

Function. The basic mechanism of ciliary motion is reminiscent of striated muscle contraction. It involves the sliding of doublets against one another and proceeds by successive cycles of attachment and detachment of the dynein arms of one doublet to (and from) its next neighbor. Each cycle requires energy supplied as ATP. The integration of the sliding motions of all doublets so as to give a ciliary beat is still not fully understood.

The structure of the basal body is similar to that of the centriole. In certain cell types, the basal body is anchored within the cytoplasmic matrix by striated fibrillar structures called *rootlets*.

FLAGELLA*

Except for greater length and a number of associated supporting structures, the organization of flagella is comparable to that of cilia.

Mutations that affect dynein arms occur in many organisms, *Homo* included. The affected individuals are sterile (if males) and prone to repeated respiratory infections because they have defective, paralyzed flagella and cilia.

Contractile Assemblies

Until recently it was assumed that contractile proteins were present only in differentiated smooth or striated muscle cells, but during the last few years it was established that practically all cells so far investigated contain a complete or nearly complete set of muscle proteins that includes actin, myosin, α actinin, and tropomyosin. These proteins have the properties of usual muscle proteins, although they appear to be, in all cases, the products of different genes. Their filamentous assemblies function in the same way as in muscle, essentially by actin filaments sliding along myosin filaments, but the organization of the contractile assemblies is quite different.

Actin Filaments Involved in Movement. Actin microfilaments of ~6 nm in diameter often form ordered bundles anchored on the cytoplasmic aspect of the plasmalemma at the tip of microvilli, at the level of adhering zonules, or at other, less differentiated, sites. Some of these filaments interact with short myosin filaments and other contractile proteins to form motor units of varied sizes, conformations, and function. An elaborate example is the terminal web under the brush border of intestinal epithelial cells. The highly ordered, rod-like assemblies that occur in the core of microvilli function as passive stirrers "activated" by the muscle plate of the terminal web. The veil-like assemblies found in plasmalemmal folds (or "ruffles") move particles or fluid droplets into plasmalemmal pockets in phagocytosis or pinocytosis. The ring-like assemblies developed during cytokinesis constrict and finally break the body of a dividing cell into two parts. The large lamellar assemblies found in pseudopodia are involved in the movement of the cell body as a whole.

In many cells, these contractile assemblies are transient: they are dismantled in one location to be reassembled in another, whereas in differentiated muscle cells the contractile assemblies appear to have permanent locations. The concentration of myosin in nonmuscle cells is low, and for this reason the force generated during contraction is weak. However, be-cause of the transient character of their contractile assemblies, nonmuscle cells have the advantage of being able to change the site and the direction of the movement imparted to their parts. Differentiated muscle cells are more efficient but less versatile: they can contract only in a single, fixed direction.

Actin Filaments in Stabilizing Infrastructures. Actin also forms felt-like filamentous structures under the plasmalemma either alone or in association with other proteins (spectrins in erythrocytes or related proteins, like fodrins, in other cells). Its interaction with the cell membrane is so strong that actin is found in relatively large amounts in isolated plasmalemmal fractions and is considered a peripheral membrane protein in many cell types, including the mature erythrocyte. In these situations, actin is used by the cells to construct stabilizing infrastructures rather than contractile assemblies under the plasmalemma. Actin filaments can be cross-linked to one another by a number of large M_r proteins, which thereby convert the cytoplasmic matrix into a reversible gel. This is expected to affect many cell functions, including motility. Actin is therefore a multipurpose protein used by the cells to stabilize membranes and to move (or immobilize) various cell parts. A large and rapidly growing number of cytoplasmic proteins, generically called *actin-binding proteins*, control the size, the direction of growth, and the pattern of aggregation (bundles vs plates vs meshworks) of actin filaments.

Microtrabeculae.* Recently, a system of *microtrabeculae* connecting microfilaments, microtubules, and practically all other subcellular components was described in the cytoplasm of animal cells examined under a high voltage electron microscope. The fast electrons generated in this microscope can penetrate relatively thick specimens and can give a tridimensional image of layers of cytoplasm up to 1.0 or 1.5 μm in thickness. The microtrabeculae may be the expression of gelation phenomena like the one mentioned above, but their importance for the general physiology of the cell, locomotion included, is difficult to assess at present because of lack of sufficient information.

CELL ENERGETICS

To carry out the functions already described, and to produce and maintain the equipment that effects these functions, cells depend critically on a number of intracellular systems that generate and supply energy. These systems are, in fact, convertors rather than generators of energy.

Animal eukaryotes depend exclusively on chemical energy imported as organic nutrients from the environment, and for this reason are called *chemotrophs*† or *heterotrophs*.† Plant eukaryotes provided with chloroplasts convert solar energy into the chemical energy of a variety of organic compounds; accordingly, they do not have to import such compounds from their ambience, and for these reasons are called *phototrophs*† or *autotrophs*.† In both cell types, the chemical energy

---

Flagellum: whip (Latin).

**Microtrabeculae*: little beams (Greek-Latin hybrid).

†*Heterotrophs, chemotrophs, phototrophs, autotrophs*: organisms depending for their nutrition on others, on chemicals, on light, or on themselves respectively (Greek).

of imported or locally generated metabolites is converted to the chemical energy of the last two phosphate bonds of *adenosine triphosphate* (ATP). These bonds are called *high energy phosphate bonds* because they deliver when hydrolyzed a large amount of free energy (~7.5 kilocalories per bond per mole). The high energy phosphate bonds of ATP—or some immediate derivative such as GTP—are the form of chemical energy that can be readily used by all pieces of cell equipment involved in energy-requiring reactions. *ATP is therefore the common intracellular energetic currency of all cells, and intracellular energy-generating systems are essentially producers and distributors of ATP.*

ENERGETICS OF ANIMAL CELLS

Animal cells operate in tandem two ATP-generating systems: (1) *glycolysis* in the cytosol, and (2) *oxidative phosphorylation* in mitochondria.

Glycolysis

The cells of higher metazoa, *Homo* included, use glucose as primary fuel for energy generation. Glucose is imported from the blood or interstitial fluid; in addition it can be locally generated in some cell types from other metabolites (for example, lactic acid, deaminated residues of amino acids) in a process called *gluconeogenesis.*

Glycolysis is carried out by ten enzymes that operate a linear series of reactions called the *glycolytic pathway.* The first three enzymes phosphorylate glucose and convert it to fructose diphosphate. A fourth enzyme *(aldolase)* splits fructose diphosphate into two phosphorylated *trioses* (3 carbon sugars), which, in subsequent steps, acquire high energy phosphate bonds and are used as immediate chemical precursors for the synthesis of ATP. The final product of the glycolytic pathway is pyruvate. If enough oxygen is available, pyruvate becomes the primary substrate for oxidative phosphorylation; if not, it is converted to lactate, which in turn can be used to regenerate glucose by gluconeogenesis.

Glycolysis generates four molecules of ATP for each molecule of glucose processed but, since two ATP molecules must be used to prime the chain of reactions (by phosphorylating glucose and fructose), the yield is only two molecules of ATP per molecule of glucose. Two molecules of the coenzyme NAD^+ (nicotinamide adenine dinucleotide) are also reduced in the process to NADH, an efficient electron donor that can be used in reductive reactions. NADH is also a primary electron donor in mitochondrial oxidative phosphorylation (see below).

Glycolysis does not require oxygen; in fact, it can proceed in its absence and, on this account, it is the only source of ATP in the obligate anaerobes found among prokaryotic cells.

All the enzymes involved in glycolysis (and most of those involved in gluconeogenesis) are soluble proteins, assumed to function as independent units in the cytosol.

Glycolysis is a wasteful yet efficient process: it releases only ~5 per cent of the potential energy in glucose (the balance remains in pyruvate), but it converts nearly 40 per cent of the energy released into ATP, the rest being lost as heat. In bioenergetics, a 40 per cent energy recovery denotes high efficiency.

Oxidative Phosphorylation

Eukaryotic cells have developed early in biologic evolution another ATP-generating system that utilizes pyruvate as a primary substrate and hence appears to take off from where glycolysis ends. It is based, however, on different principles: energy is released from metabolites by stepwise oxidation and is converted to ATP by a tightly coupled oxidation-phosphorylation process called *oxidative phosphorylation.* This system improves energy recovery from glucose by more than one order of magnitude, and it is all assembled within a special cell organ, the *mitochondrion,*[*] present in more than one copy per cell. With the exception of the mature erythrocyte (which relies entirely on glycolysis), all human cells have mitochondria and depend on them for most of their energetic needs.

MITOCHONDRIA

Morphology

In general, mitochondria are either filamentous or granular bodies of large enough dimensions to be seen under the light microscope in either living or fixed-and-stained cells. Special optics or special preparation procedures are required, however, for their optimal visualization. They measure 0.3 to 0.5 μm in diameter and up to 10 μm in length. Observations on living cells show that neither the shape nor the number of mitochondria is stable; both are continuously changing. Mitochondria branch and fuse with one another to form extensive networks, and conversely they break down into isolated granular bodies under conditions that are not fully understood. It is known, however, that cell damage often leads to mitochondrial swelling and fragmentation. Mitochondrial counts have, therefore, limited meaning. Mitochondrial volume density and mass fraction are more informative parameters. Both are low (~5 per cent) in most cells, but reach high values in cells whose activities require a high ATP production (for example hepatocytes, ~20 per cent; muscle cells of the myocardium, ~30 per cent).

Irrespective of shape variations, all mitochondria have the same basic organization detectable only by electron microscopy (Fig. 30). They are limited by an outer mitochondrial membrane of simple geometry and have an extensively infolded inner mitochondrial membrane. The infoldings, called *mitochondrial cristae*[†] *(cristae mitochondriales),* are flat folds (~25 nm in thickness) in most cases; tubular or other forms of cristae are encountered, however, in certain cell types. Both mitochondrial membranes measure ~6 nm in thickness, and both have the usual unit membrane structure, which means that their polar lipids are organized in bilayers (Fig. 31). *The inner aspect of the inner membrane is covered by small particles (diam ~9 nm) attached to the membrane by a fine stalk.* These *inner membrane particles* can be visualized optimally in negatively stained specimens. The outer membrane

---

[*]*Mitochondrion*: filament-granule (Greek).
[†]*Crista*: ridge (Latin).

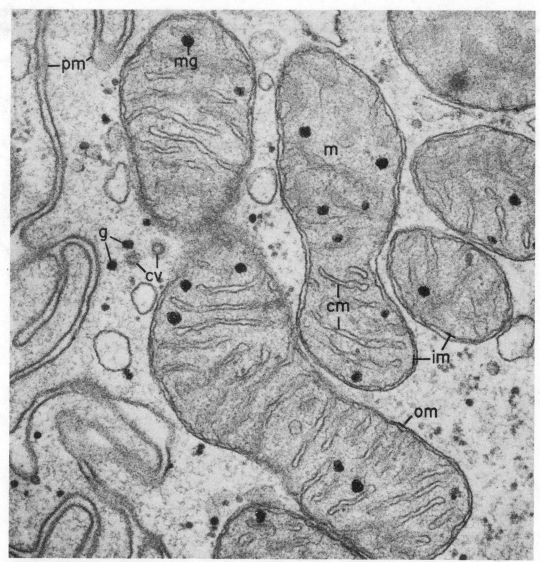

Figure 30. Mitochondria in an intestinal epithelial cell (rat). om, outer membrane; im, inner membrane; cm, cristae (seem clearly only when normally sectioned); m, mitochondrial matrix; mg, intramitochondrial granules; g, glycogen particles; pm, plasmalemma; cv, coated vesicles. 75,000 ×.

is separated from the inner membrane by an *outer mitochondrial chamber* that extends (as *intracristal space*) within each crista. The content of this chamber is of characteristically low density. The inner membrane forms the boundary of an *inner mitochondrial chamber* filled by an amorphous content of high density called *mitochondrial matrix* (Fig. 32). Embedded in this matrix are *intramitochondrial granules* (diam ~30 nm), *mitochondrial ribosomes* (diam ~15 nm) and the *mitochondrial genome,* a usually circular DNA molecule ~20 μm in length.

Mitochondrial Fractions and Mitochondrial Functions

Mitochondria were among the first cell organs isolated (as crude cell fractions) by cell fractionation procedures. Refined over the years, cell-fractionation procedures yield at present reasonably homogeneous mitochondrial fractions from a variety of sources (liver, kidney, or myocardium homogenates). Moreover, mitochondrial subfractions representing the inner or outer membrane are available and can be subfractionated in turn into enzyme complexes and finally into individual molecular components. Hence, a rather extensive inventory of mitochondrial components is available and the location of most components within the mitochondrial context is known. Yet, it took a long time to understand the basic working mechanisms of this ATP-generating unit.

Biochemistry of Mitochondrial Subfractions. Studies carried out on mitochondrial fractions and subfractions have established the following facts.

(1) *Enzymes involved in oxidative phosphorylation are present only in mitochondria.* (2) *The inner mitochondrial membrane and the mitochondrial matrix are the most important structural components of the system.* (3) *The matrix contains a series of enzymic sets that oxidize substrates and reduce them to a form required by the next set in line.*

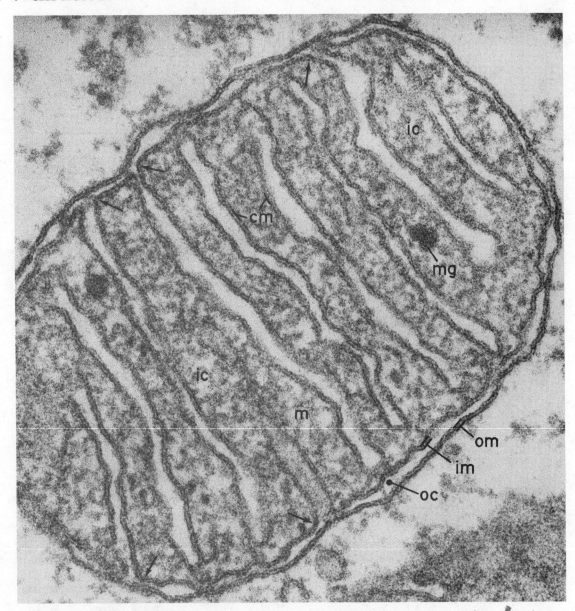

Figure 31. Mitochondrion in a pancreatic centroacinar cell (guinea pig). om, outer membrane; im, inner membrane (note that at this magnification the lipid bilayer is resolved in both membranes); oc, outer chamber; ic, inner chamber occupied by mitochondrial matrix (m) and intramitochondrial granules (mg); cm, cristae; points where the continuity of the cristae with the inner membrane is visible are marked by arrows. 200,000 ×.

The first set includes: a complex multienzyme system, called *pyruvate dehydrogenase,* that converts pyruvate to acetyl coenzyme A (Acetyl CoA), and reduces NAD⁺ to NADH; a series of enzymes involved in the stepwise oxidation of fatty acids (β oxidation) that generates also acetyl CoA; and an enzyme, glutamate dehydrogenase, that deaminates glutamate to produce α-ketoglutarate (an intermediate than can be used by the second enzymic set).

The second set of enzymes operates a cyclic series of reactions called the citric acid cycle (or the Krebs cycle) because it begins with the synthesis of citrate (6 carbon compound) from acetyl CoA (the 2 carbon product of the first set) and oxaloacetate (the 4 carbon product of

the cycle itself). Citrate is oxidized and decarboxylated in a series of steps to yield 5 carbon and 4 carbon intermediates and to generate two CO_2 molecules for each turn of the cycle (Fig. 33). The final product of the cycle, oxaloacetate, is used to resynthesize citric acid (as already mentioned), and with this reaction the cycle starts again. During each turn of the cycle, the dehydrogenases that oxidize its successive intermediates reduce three molecules of NAD⁺ to NADH and one molecule of FAD* to FADH₂; they also generate

---

*FAD: flavin adenine dinucleotide, the prosthetic group of succinate dehydrogenase; *FADH₂*: its reduced form.

one GTP molecule from a high energy chemical precursor (as in glycolysis). NADH and $FADH_2$ are the required substrates for the next set of mitochondrial oxidative enzymes.

All the enzymes that catalyze the citric acid cycle are soluble proteins of the mitochondrial matrix with one notable exception: succinate dehydrogenase, which is an integral membrane protein of the inner mitochondrial membrane. The functional implications of this difference in distribution are unknown.

The third set: the mitochondrial electron transport chain. The third set of mitochondrial enzymes involved in substrate oxidation is a chain of electron carriers that effect the transport of electrons from NADH and $FADH_2$ to molecular O_2. With one exception (namely, coenzyme Q, or ubiquinone, which is a lipid) all these carriers are proteins of the inner mitochondrial membrane. *The electron transport chain begins with NADH dehydrogenase, a complex flavoprotein that removes two electrons from NADH and transfers them to ubiquinone,* the second link in the chain. *From ubiquinone, the electrons flow (one at a time) through a series of 5 cytochromes (cyt b, cyt c_1, cyt c, cyt $a + a_3$) to oxygen and reduce it to H_2O* (Fig. 33). All the protein components of the chain are integral proteins of the inner mitochondrial membrane with the exception of cytochrome *c*, which is a peripheral protein attached to the outer aspect of the same membrane.

Proton Gradient and ATP Synthesis. The electron transport chain loops three times back and forth through the inner membrane. This arrangement facilitates the ejection of 6 protons (H^+) (2 at a time) for each pair of electrons that moves down the chain, and thus creates a proton gradient and an electrical potential (inside negative) across the inner membrane (Fig. 34). Together, *the proton gradient and the electrical potential represent a temporary energy storage that is used to generate ATP.* The protons run down the gradient back to the inner mitochondrial chamber through channels presumably located in the stalk of the inner membrane particles. The head of these particles is an ATP synthetase that binds ADP and inorganic phosphate. Its interaction with the incoming protons leads to ATP synthesis by mechanisms that remain to be elucidated. Three ATP molecules are synthesized for each pair of electrons moving down the entire length of the electron transport chain, but only two ATP molecules are produced per electron pair that

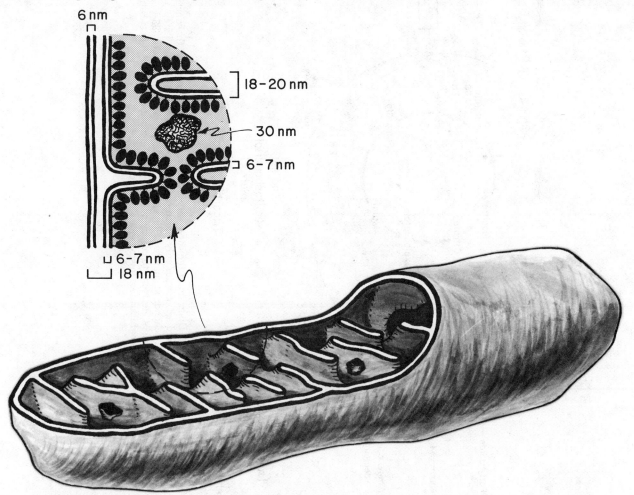

Figure 32. Tridimensional model of a mitochondrion. The inset shows in further detail the mitochondrial sector outlined by a semicircle. It illustrates the layered structure of the mitochondrial membranes, and the inner membrane particles attached to the inner aspect of the cristae and inner membrane. These particles are the ATP-synthesizing complex.

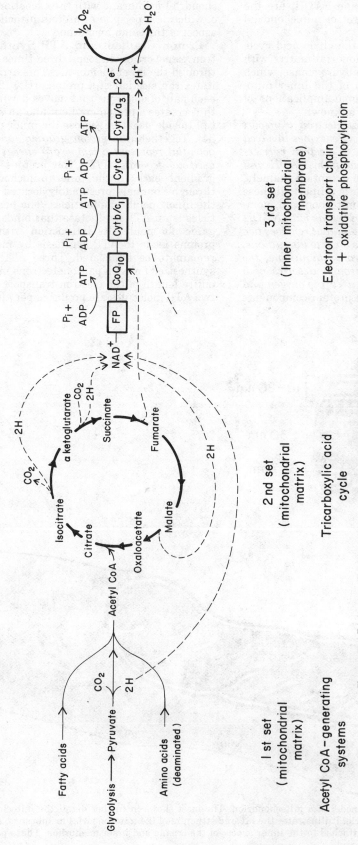

Figure 33. Diagram of the three sets of mitochondrial enzymes and their activities. The electron transport chain (third set) carries only electrons. The protons needed at the final step (reduction of O_2) come from the inner mitochondrial chamber. Not shown: (1) the glycerol 3-phosphate (G3-P) shuttle; the G3-P dehydrogenase transfers electrons to coenzyme Q_{10}; (2) the generation of GTP (via substrate level phosphorylation) by the α ketoglutarate dehydrogenase complex.

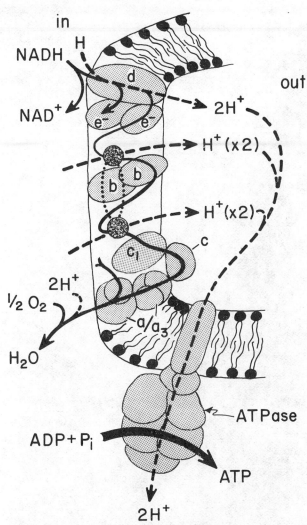

Figure 34. Diagram of the electron transport chain of the inner mitochondrial membrane. The components of the chain are: d, the NADH-dehydrogenase complex (a flavoprotein and two [or more] iron-sulfur proteins); •, coenzyme Q_{10} (ubiquinone); b, cytochrome b; c_1, cytochrome c_1; c, cytochrome c; a/a_3, the cytochrome oxidase complex.

→e^-, pathway followed by electrons; it loops three times across the membrane. Electrons are transported in pairs at the beginning of the chain and as single particles through the rest. Only one of the identical segments of the chain is shown (to simplify the diagram).

---→H^+, pathway followed by protons.

ATPase, ATP-synthesizing complex. The exact relationship of the complexes to the electron transport chain within the membrane is still unknown. in, inner mitochondrial chamber; out, outer mitochondrial chamber.

enters the chain at ubiquinone, as is the case for the $FADH_2$ of succinate dehydrogenase. The bulk of ATP generation in the mitochondrion does not depend on high energy chemical precursors (as is the case with substrate-level phosphorylation). It depends on the proton motive force generated by the proton gradient mentioned above. This relatively new concept, known as the *chemiosmotic hypothesis,* provides at present a reasonably satisfactory explanation of the complex process of oxidative phosphorylation.

Permeability of the Inner Mitochondrial Membranes: Transporters and Shuttles. As expected from its ability to maintain a proton gradient, the inner mitochondrial membrane has an unusually low permeability. Inflow of substrates (pyruvate, fatty acids, and amino acids) is carefully controlled and effected by specific transport systems. The outflow of ATP is coupled with the inflow of ADP and is mediated by a specific exchange system. It follows that ATP can be delivered by mitochondria to the rest of the cell only if ADP is available in the cytoplasm, which means only if the cell is using ATP. As a double insurance, ATP is synthesized in the mitochondria only if ADP is available in the mitochondrial matrix; and electron transport proceeds only if ATP can be synthesized. Respiration is therefore tightly coupled to phosphorylation, and the key factor in ATP synthesis is ADP availability, which is another way of saying that mitochondria synthesize ATP only if the cell needs ATP. Experimentally, respiration and phosphorylation can be uncoupled by a series of compounds, such as dinitrophenol, that run down the proton gradient by increasing the permeability of the inner membrane.

The inner membrane is impermeable to both NAD^+ and NADH. As glycolysis proceeds in the cytosol, NADH is generated and its concentration increases at the expense of NAD^+. This situation could create a problem, since NAD^+ is required for glycolysis to proceed. The cells have solved the problem by transporting electrons instead of NADH to the mitochondrial matrix. NADH reduces dehydroxyacetone 3-phosphate to glycerol 3-phosphate in the cytosol (and is thereby oxidized to NAD^+). Glycerol 3-phosphate is transported by a shuttle across the inner mitochondrial membrane. A membrane-bound glycerol 3-phosphate dehydrogenase oxidizes it to dehydroxyacetone 3-phosphate, which is returned to the cytosol by the same shuttle and is ready to oxidize another NADH molecule. The electrons removed from glycerol 3-phosphate reduce FAD, the prosthetic group of its dehydrogenase, to $FADH_2$ and enter the electron transport chain at ubiquinone. The glycerol 3-phosphate shuttle generates, therefore, only 2 ATP molecules per electron pair.

Energetic Balance Sheet. *The complete oxidation of a glucose molecule (to CO_2 and H_2O) generates 36 ATP molecules: 2 during glycolysis in the cytosol, and 34 in the mitochondria. The ratio 2:34 illustrates clearly the importance of mitochondria and oxidative phosphorylation in cellular energetics.*

Outer Mitochondrial Chamber. In contrast to the mitochondrial matrix, the outer mitochondrial chamber contains a few proteins at low concentration. Notable among them are nucleoside diphosphokinases (including adenylate kinase or myokinase), whose function is to make available ADP for the ATP-ADP exchange system.

Outer Mitochondrial Membrane. The outer membrane is different in many respects from the inner mitochondrial membrane. It does have a number of enzyme activities, but none of them is directly connected with ATP generation. The best studied among them is *monoamine oxidase,* an enzyme involved in the inactivation of catecholamines. The outer membrane is highly permeable and relatively rigid. It does not behave as a diffusion barrier for small molecules and it does not respond osmotically. Since the inner

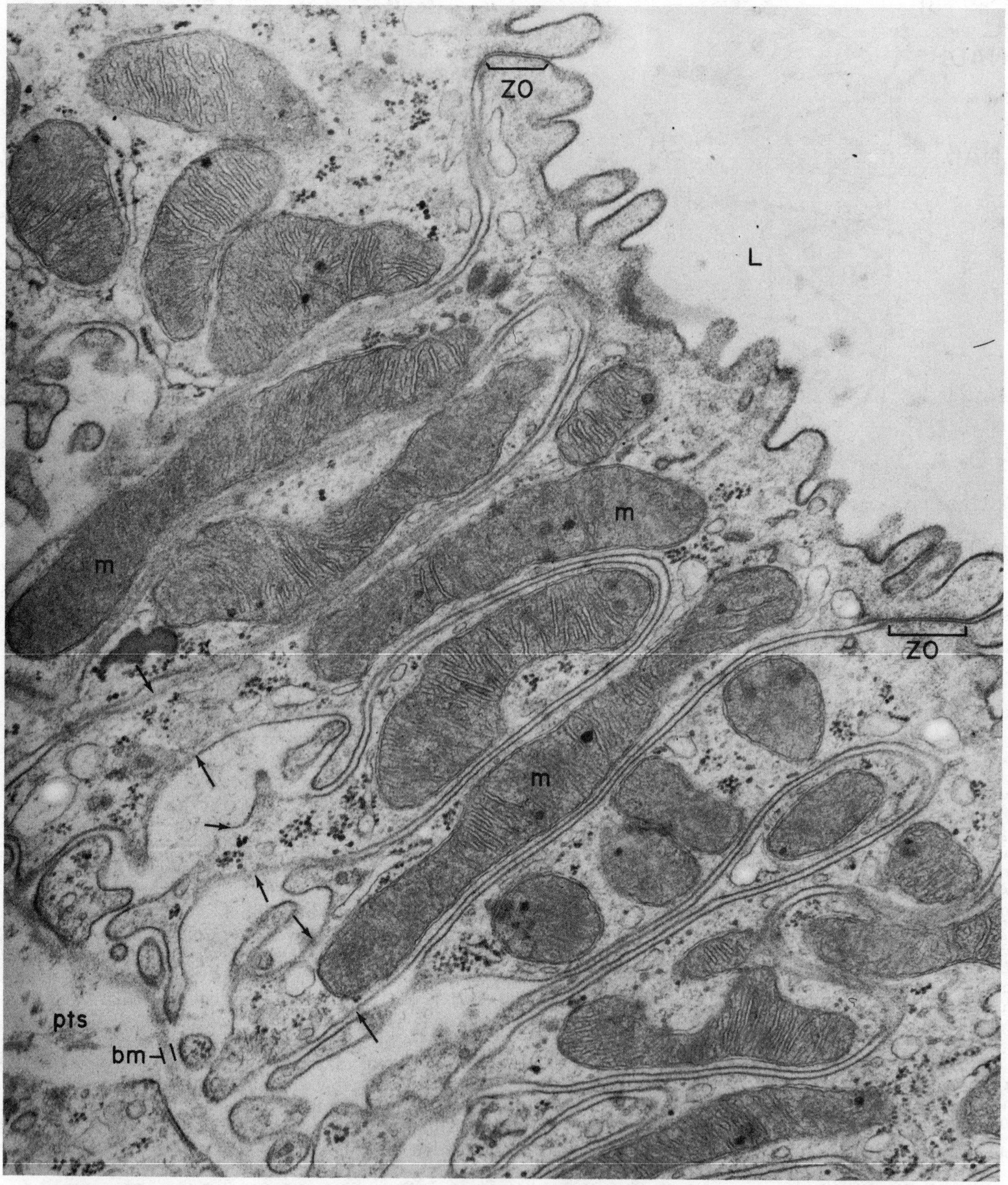

Figure 35. Association of mitochondria with plasmalemmal infoldings in the cells of the distal tubule of the nephron (rat). The infoldings belong to the basal-lateral domain of the plasmalemma in which the $Na^+ + K^+$ ATPase (transport ATPase) is highly concentrated.

Each deep infolding (in between arrows) usually contains a single mitochondrion, (m). This is an example of strategic distribution of ATP generators (mitochondria) in relation to ATP-dependent effectors (plasmalemmal transport ATPase). It amplifies their area of close relationship and reduces ATP diffusion paths. L, lumen; ZO, occluding zonules; bm, basement membranes; pts, peritubular spaces. 40,000 ×. (From M. G. Farquhar and G. E. Palade: J Cell Biol 17:375, 1963.)

membrane behaves like an osmometer, the relative volume of the two mitochondrial chambers and the regularity of the cristae are affected by the osmotic activity of the environment. At high osmotic activity the usual appearance of the mitochondria is replaced by a "condensed state."

Other Mitochondrial Functions. Ions accumulate in the mitochondrial matrix either by exchange (PO_4^{-3} exchanged for OH^-) or by active transport powered by ATP. Ca^{2+} and other bivalent cations are concentrated in the intramitochondrial granules already mentioned. On account of their ability to accumulate Ca^{2+}, mitochondria function in intracellular homeostasis and may release Ca^{2+} in the cytoplasm when needed for a variety of purposes (exocytosis, contraction).

Mitochondria also accumulate iron needed for the intramitochondrial synthesis of heme molecules, the prosthetic groups of cytochromes.

Functional Associations of Mitochondria. In the majority of cell types, mitochondria are distributed at random and appear to change their position continuously. In other types, however, persistent and characteristic associations occur and can be rationalized in terms of a reduction of distances over which either ATP must diffuse to various effectors, or substrates have to diffuse to mitochondria. Mitochondria are associated with elaborate infoldings of the plasmalemma in cells specialized in the active transport of ions, especially Na^+ and K^+ (Fig. 35). Active transport requires ATP and is effected by ion-dependent ATPases that—as already mentioned—are integral plasmalemmal proteins. Mitochondria are strategically disposed around the flagellum of sperm cells and around the myofibrils of red muscle fibers. They are also found wrapped around lipid droplets in cells obliged to depend primarily on fatty acid oxidation for their energetic needs.

Mitochondrial Biogenesis

Mitochondria are endowed with temporal continuity: they are inherited without discontinuity from cell generation to cell generation. They are not produced de novo. In anticipation of cell division, they grow by expansion of their preexisting membranes and by commensurate increase of their matrix components. *Mitochondria have their own "chromosome," a single, small DNA molecule, and a complete apparatus for the transcription and translation of the genetic information it contains.* The molecules needed for their growth come from two different sources. Mitochondria produce their own rRNAs, all their tRNAs, and a limited number of mRNAs as transcripts of their genes. Proteins synthesized locally by mitochondrial ribosomes, as translates of mitochondria mRNAs, are few in number but functionally critically important. They include part of the subunits of the ATPase and of the cytochromes c_1, b, and $a + a_3$. All the other mitochondrial proteins, including the enzymes and the structural components of the transcription-translation apparatus, the matrix, and the membranes (amounting to more than 90 per cent of the total mitochondrial protein), are produced by cytoplasmic free polysomes as translates of nuclear mRNAs and are transported for assembly into mitochondria across one or two membranes. The basic operation is the same as in the case of the ER: proteins are translocated across lipid bilayers, but the procedures are different. In the cases so far investigated, mitochondrial membranes or matrix proteins exist transiently as soluble precursors of larger M_r (by $\sim$ 3 to 4 K) in the cytosol. They are translocated posttranslationally (not cotranslationally as in the case of ER-directed proteins), and in the process they are proteolytically cleaved in one or two steps to their "mature" size.

This intricate pattern of biosynthetic relations reflects the extensive, mutual interdependence between the mitochondria and the rest of the cell. This unusual situation is currently rationalized by assuming that mitochondria were originally prokaryotic symbionts of early eukaryotic cells that, during evolution, have lost a large part of their genetic independence. A similar hypothesis, with photosynthetic prokaryotes as symbionts, has been advanced to explain the comparable situation of chloroplasts in plant cells.

PEROXISOMES

Certain oxidases oxidize their substrates by reducing O_2 to H_2O_2 (hydrogen peroxide), which is reduced at a subsequent step to H_2O by the enzyme catalase through either a peroxidatic or a catalytic mechanism. In animal cells, catalase and a variable number of H_2O_2–generating oxidases are packed together in special cell organs called peroxisomes, because within these bodies catalase is assumed to reduce H_2O_2 by the peroxidatic mechanism.

Morphology

Peroxisomes (or microbodies) were originally detected by electron microscopy in nephron epithelia and hepatocytes. In these cells they are relatively large globular bodies, 0.5 to 1.0 μm in diameter, limited by a single membrane and containing a dense, homogeneous matrix in which is embedded a crystal usually referred to as the *core* (Fig. 36). This crystal is not, however, a constant peroxisomal feature.

Biochemistry and Function

These large peroxisomes have been isolated in reasonably homogeneous cell fractions and their components have been partially characterized. The peroxisomal membrane, like the mitochondrial inner membrane, has a carnitine carrier that transports fatty acids from the cytoplasm to the peroxisomal matrix. Catalase is a constant and major component of the peroxisomal matrix, which contains, in addition, a D-amino acid oxidase, and an L-α hydroxyamino acid oxidase. The core is a urate oxidase crystal. All these oxidases generate H_2O_2. More recently, it was found that the peroxisomes can carry out the β-oxidation of fatty acyl-CoAs. They contain a set of fatty acid oxidizing enzymes comparable to that present in the mitochondrial matrix, except that the first enzyme of the peroxisomal set generates H_2O_2. The number of peroxisomes and their mass fraction increases markedly in the hepatocytes of animals treated with hypolipidemic agents—that is, drugs that reduce the concentration of lipids in the blood plasma. The peroxisomes produce acetyl-CoA and reduce NAD^+ to NADH; both products can be used in mitochondria to generate ATP. At present, the role of the peroxisomes

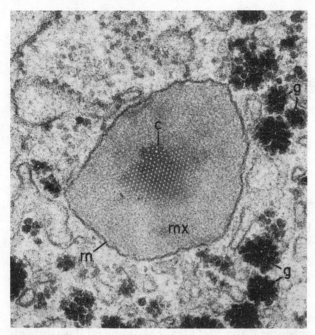

Figure 36. Peroxisome in a guinea pig hepatocyte. The globular (though rather irregular) body is limited by a single membrane (m) and contains a dense homogeneous matrix (mx) in which is embedded a crystalline core (c). The crystal consists of urate oxidase; the matrix contains H_2O_2-generating oxidases and catalase. g, glycogen particles. 110,000 ×.

in the energetics and lipid metabolism of normal cells is not yet fully understood. Plant cells have more complex and versatile peroxisomes that contain an additional enzyme system, known as the glyoxylate cycle, capable of converting fatty acids to glucose. For this reason they are called *glyoxisomes*.

Because of their catalase content, peroxisomes can be detected by histochemical reactions for peroxidatic activities. These reactions reveal the presence of a type of small (diam 0.1 to 0.2 μm) core-free peroxisomes (called *miniperoxisomes*) in practically all cell types so far examined. The function of these miniperoxisomes is still unknown.

Biogenesis. The enzymes of the peroxisomal matrix are synthesized by free cytosolic polysomes translating cognate nuclear mRNAs. The primary translates have apparently the same M_r as the mature peroxisomal proteins. They are translocated across the peroxisomal membrane posttranslationally without undergoing detectable proteolysis. The same seems to apply for peroxisomal membrane proteins.

EXTRACELLULAR MATRIX

In multicellular organisms, *Homo* included, the cells modify the content of certain compartments of their immediate environment (primarily the interstitial fluid and the blood plasma) by discharging therein a large amount of secretory proteins, glycoproteins, and proteoglycans. In the interstitia, these secretory products and the structures they form, together with associated small solutes, ions, and water, constitute the *extracellular matrix*.

The proteins of the blood plasma, secreted primarily by hepatocytes and plasma cells, function in osmotic regulation, metabolite transport, control of blood coagulation, and immune responses (among others). Because of the high permeability of the vascular endothelium, all these proteins are also present in the interstitial fluid and lymph.

Structure and Chemistry. A wide variety of cell types (mesenchymal as well as epithelial) secrete a variety of procollagen molecules into the interstitia of the tissues. In this case, posttranslational modifications continue after secretory discharge: partial proteolysis by procollagen proteases (produced apparently by the same cells that secrete procollagens) remove amino acid sequences from both the N- and C-terminal of the discharged molecules, thereby converting them to collagens. These proteolytic steps make possible the staggered lateral aggregation of collagens into long fibers of variable diameter and characteristic periodic banding patterns. Only certain collagens, i.e., collagen types I, II, and III, form fibers as described above. Protocollagen type IV is not proteolytically processed upon discharge; as a result, it does not form fibrils. Instead, it generates, by interaction with other glycoproteins (collagen V, fibronectin, laminin, entactin) and proteoglycans, laminated meshworks known as *basement membranes* or *basal laminae*. Basement membranes ensheath cells that are long-term nonmigrating residents of the interstitia, e.g., smooth and striated muscle cells, Schwann cells; they also form a continuous substrate under all endothelia and epithelia. In basement membranes, collagen IV is the molecular constituent that imparts tensile strength to the structure. Laminin, a heavy M_r glycoprotein, facilitates the attachment of epithelial cells to different substrates, basement membranes included. Fibronectin, a ~ 450 Kd glycoprotein, acts as a diversified linker: the molecule has distinct specific domains that recognize collagens, proteoglycans, and receptors on the plasmalemma of adjacent (epithelial and mesenchymal) cells. Integral membrane proteins interact with fibronectin outside the cell and with peripheral membrane proteins (or cytoskeletal proteins) inside the cell to create a mechanically continuous system.

Proteoglycans are large molecules with a large number of covalently linked glycosaminoglycan chains that are sulfated (to a variable degree) in the case of chondroitin-, heparan-, dermatan-, and keratan-sulfate, and nonsulfated in the case of hyaluronate. The proteoglycans associated with basement membranes provide them with fixed negative charges, that affect their permeability; in addition, they form clusters that seem to function as attachment sites for endothelial or epithelial cells.

Proteoglycans are present as soluble components in the interstitial fluid and as integral or adsorbed proteins on cellular membranes. In the interstitia, they control the degree of hydration of the extracellular matrix and the diffusion of large and small solutes, acting, in the last case, much like ion exchange columns.

Biosynthesis. All the molecules of the extracellular matrix are secretory glycoproteins produced by both epithelial and mesenchymal cells, in steps common to all secretory proteins. Elastin and elastic fibers are produced, as far as is known, only by mesenchymal cells, primarily by fibroblasts and smooth muscle cells. Among the proteins of the extracellular matrix, collagens represent a special case. They are the products of a relatively large family of genes. They are long ($\sim$ 320 nm) polypeptide chains that are extensively modified in the ER cisternal space by hydroxylation of their numerous proline residues. This modification makes possible the association of three polypeptide chains into a triple helical structure that is responsible for the characteristically high tensile strength of collagen fibrils. Again, in the ER cisternal space, some of their lysine residues are hydroxylated to be used later for intermolecular crosslinkage. In the biosynthesis of collagens, the intracellular stage produces triple helices and the extracellular stage generates fibrils.

Function. By its fibrillar components, the extracellular matrix creates a solid framework that is maintained under tension by the high degree of hydration of its proteoglycans and in which collagen fibrils are disposed along lines of propagation of the physical forces exerted on the system. Linkers, such as fibronectin and laminin, attach the cells to the framework, thereby creating a mechanically continuous system that can resist pressure, stress, and tension by distributing their impact throughout the entire system. The extracellular matrix is produced by cells that can alter its chemical composition in specific ways, depending on the local cell population. But once produced, it affects the cells that have created it: it controls their attachments, their mobility, their shape and—in subtle ways—their metabolism. Cells and extracellular matrix become extensively interdependent as structurally and functionally integrated parts at a higher level of biologic organization characteristic for tissues and organs in multicellular organisms.

EPILOGUE

Upon reading this chapter, the student may be impressed by the amount and depth of knowledge now available on the structure, biochemistry, and function of different cell organs. Yet he or she should realize that we are still very far from a complete understanding of the object of our interest—the eukaryotic cell. For many cell organs, the inventory of chemical components is still incomplete, and functional roles are still beyond clear, comprehensive understanding. *The most important deficiencies in our knowledge concern, however, the mechanisms that regulate the function of each cell organ, and especially the mechanisms that integrate effectively the specialized activities of a multitude of diverse subcellular components so as to achieve that ultimate goal, which is the survival and the regular reproduction of the entire cell.*

SECTION II

GENETICS

DAVID R. COX, M.D., PH.D.

All of the information required to direct development of a human organism from the single cell created by fusion of an egg and a sperm is encoded in the human genome. This genetic blueprint is made up of functional units, or genes, each of which directs the synthesis of one of the 100,000 different protein molecules found in every individual. Although each cell in the human body contains the complete human genome, it is the selective expression of only a specific fraction of these genes, and thus the selective synthesis of only a subset of the total proteins, that determines the specialized structures and functions of any particular cell. All of the chemical reactions in the cell, including those that lead to the formation of membranes and cellular organelles, are a consequence of the specific proteins contained in that cell.

Since all humans contain the same basic set of genes and, thus, the same proteins, the developmental and structural similarities between human beings are not surprising. More remarkable than these similarities, however, are the differences between individuals. Marked variations in size, facial features, hair texture, eye color, and personality are only a few of the differences that distinguish individuals from one another. Such variation is due in large part to minor differences in the form of individual proteins and thus of individual genes. It has been estimated that over 25 per cent of the proteins in any given person have structures or functions that vary slightly from the forms of those same proteins in the majority of human beings.

In certain cases, variation in a protein and the gene that codes for it is so marked that the protein can no longer carry out its specified function, resulting in cell malfunction and disease. Such conditions are referred to as genetic diseases. As a result of advances in medical care, which have reduced perinatal mortality and increased the lifespan of the average human being, genetic diseases now represent a significant proportion of those human disorders that physicians are called upon to diagnose and treat.

The goal of treatment of genetic disease is to modify the chemistry of malfunctioning cells so that they function normally, allowing an affected person to live a healthy life despite the presence of one or more abnormal genes. However, in order to achieve this goal, the pathogenesis of genetic disease must be understood. This involves an understanding of the molecular alterations that distinguish an abnormal gene from a normal one, an understanding of how abnormal genes lead to disturbances in the structure and function of particular proteins, and an understanding of how abnormalities of particular proteins lead to cell and tissue malfunction. Knowledge at each of these levels of organization is required for the development of logical treatment plans for genetic diseases.

THE GENETIC MATERIAL

DNA STRUCTURE

The polymeric molecule deoxyribonucleic acid, or DNA, is the chemical of heredity and contains all of

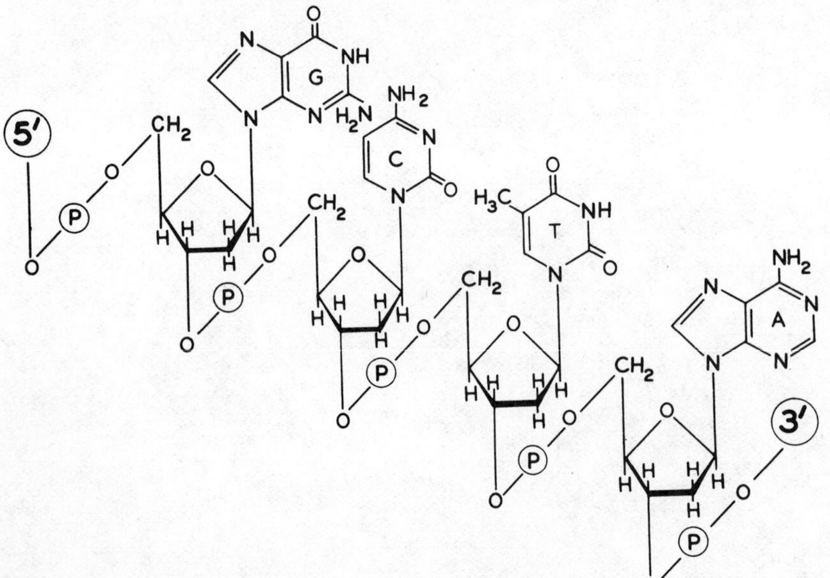

Figure 1. A segment of a structure of DNA molecule in which the purine and pyrimidine bases adenine (A), thymine (T), cytosine (C), and guanine (G) are held together by a phosphodiester backbone between 2′-deoxyribosyl moieties attached to the nucleobases by an N-glycosidic bond. Note that the backbone has a polarity (i.e., a direction). (From Harper, H. A., Rodwell, V. W., and Mayes, P. A.: Review of Physiological Chemistry. 17th ed. Los Altos, CA, Lange Medical Publications, 1979, p. 137.)

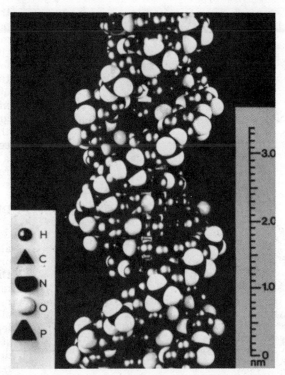

Figure 2. The Watson and Crick model of the double helical structure of DNA. *Left,* Diagrammatic representation of structure (modified). A = adenine, C = cytosine, G = guanine, T = thymine, P = phosphate, S = sugar (deoxyribose). *Right,* Space-filling model of DNA structure. (Photograph from James D. Watson, Molecular Biology of the Gene. 3rd ed. Copyright © 1976, 1970, 1965, by W. A. Benjamin, Inc., Menlo Park, CA. Drawing and photograph combination from Harper, H. A., Rodwell, V. W., and Mayes, P. A.: Review of Physiological Chemistry. 17th ed. Los Altos, CA, 1979, p. 137.)

the genetic information required to specify the human organism. Surprisingly, DNA is a relatively simple polymeric molecule, consisting of only four different types of monomeric units linked together to form a long chain. The monomers of DNA are the four different nucleobases adenine (A), thymine (T), guanine (G), and cytosine (C), each with a deoxyribose sugar molecule attached to it. These nucleobase-sugar moieties are strung together by phosphodiester bonds (Fig. 1) such that the resulting polymer possesses a polarity or direction, with a 5′ phosphate group at one end and a 3′ hydroxyl group at the other end of the strand.

DNA exists naturally as a double-stranded helical molecule, with the two strands held together by non-covalent hydrogen bonds between the nucleobases (Fig. 2). This pairing between nucleobases on opposite DNA strands is very specific and depends on the fact that adenine hydrogen bonds exclusively with thymine, while guanine bonds exclusively with cytosine (Fig. 3). This base pairing restriction in double-stranded DNA results in a molecular content of A equal to that of T, and a content of G equal to that of C. The two strands of the double-stranded DNA molecule are held together in such a way that the 3′ end of one strand is bonded to the 5′ end of the other strand (Fig. 4). This is somewhat analogous to two parallel streets, each one way but running in opposite directions.

Since the two strands of the DNA double helix are held together by noncovalent bonds between the nucleobases, the double-stranded structure can be "melted" or denatured into two single strands in solution by increasing the temperature or decreasing the

Figure 3. Schematic representation of base pairing and antiparallel orientation of polynucleotide strands in a double helix. (From Fristrom, J. W., and Spieth, P. T.: Principles of Genetics. New York, Chiron Press, Inc., 1980, p. 31.)

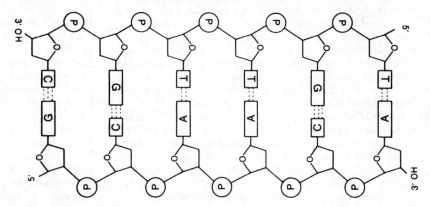

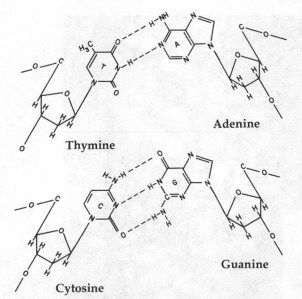

Figure 4. Base-pairing between adenine and thymine and between cytosine and guanine as proposed by Watson and Crick. The broken lines represent hydrogen bonds. (The phosphodiester bridges are not shown.) (From Harper, H. A., Rodwell, V. W., and Mayes, P. A.: Review of Physiological Chemistry. 17th ed. Los Altos, CA, Lange Medical Publications, 1979, p. 138.)

salt concentration, thereby disrupting the hydrogen bonds between the nucleobases on opposite strands. However, when the temperature is lowered or the salt increased, the two complementary DNA strands are able to renature spontaneously into the orginal double-stranded structure. This ability of a single-stranded piece of DNA to anneal specifically with another single strand of DNA that has a complementary sequence of nucleobases forms the basis for the DNA hybridization techniques described later in this chapter.

The genetic information in DNA resides in the specific sequence of nucleobases that make up the DNA molecule. Each DNA molecule can be functionally divided into units referred to as genes. Since human DNA molecules are very large, each such molecule contains many genes. In general, one gene specifies the structure of one polypeptide chain or protein molecule. All of the chemical reactions in the cell, such as the synthesis of carbohydrate, the synthesis of complex lipid, the formation of membranes, and the construction of cell organelles, occur as a consequence of the action of specific proteins. The human genome consists of approximately 3×10^9 base pairs of DNA, which is enough double-stranded DNA to code for about three million different average-size proteins. However, a variety of estimates indicates that only about 100,000 different proteins are made by all of the various cell types that comprise the human body. Although these estimates are crude, they nevertheless indicate that no more than 2 to 3 per cent of the human genome is composed of genes that code for proteins.

Some DNA sequences code for structural RNA molecules that are components of the machinery for protein synthesis. Unlike the protein-coding genes, each of which is usually present in only two copies per cell, the genes that code for structural RNA are present in multiple copies in every cell. Therefore, even though there are only a few different types of structural RNA,

the genes coding for these molecules make up about 1 per cent of the total cellular DNA. Even taken together, however, the genes coding for proteins and those coding for structural RNA molecules still account for less than 5 per cent of total human DNA. Although there has been much speculation concerning the role of the remaining DNA, the precise function of the vast majority of human DNA is essentially unknown. The amount of DNA per cell (i.e., twice the genome size) is the same in all human cells. This precise control of cellular DNA content implies that most of the DNA in a cell does play an important role, even though this role is poorly defined at present.

DNA Replication

The nucleus of every cell in the human body contains all of man's genetic information. Since the human organism contains a very large number of cells, the DNA initially present in the first cell of an individual must replicate many times during development in a process of high fidelity, for any change in the sequence of nucleobases would alter the genetic information, leading to mutations. The complementarity of the two strands of the double-stranded DNA molecule immediately suggests a mechanism whereby DNA can be replicated with the necessary fidelity. If each strand of the double-stranded molecule were to separate from its complement during replication, then each could serve as a template on which a new complementary strand could be synthesized (Fig. 5). The two newly formed double-stranded DNA molecules, each containing one of the original strands from the parental DNA molecule, could then be sorted between two daughter cells during division. The DNA molecule in each daughter cell would thus have the information or sequence identical to that of the parent. This semiconservative mode of DNA replication, first demonstrated in bacteria, appears to be the mechanism of DNA replication in all organisms. The replication of the double-stranded DNA molecule occurs on both strands simultaneously. However, since there is no enzyme capable of polymerizing DNA in the 3' to 5' direction, both of the newly replicated DNA strands cannot grow in the same direction simultaneously. Instead, a single enzyme replicates one strand continuously in the 5' toward the 3' direction, while it replicates the other strand discontinuously in short pieces 150 to 250 bases long, which are subsequently joined together into a continuous DNA strand (Fig. 6). DNA replicates simultaneously on both strands in both directions, at many different sites in a mammalian cell. In the process "replication bubbles" are generated (Fig. 7).

During the replication of the double-stranded helix of DNA, the molecule must unwind to allow the formation of the new DNA helices. This unwinding process appears to be catalyzed by specific proteins that stabilize the single-stranded portion of DNA at replication sites. Replication of DNA in mammalian cells occurs only at a specified time during the life cycle of the cell. This DNA synthetic or S phase is temporally separated from the mitotic phase when the cell divides by nonsynthetic periods referred to as gap1(G1) and gap2(G2), occurring before and after the S phase, respectively (see Section I, Fig. 11). The regulation of the entry of a cell into the S phase is highly complex

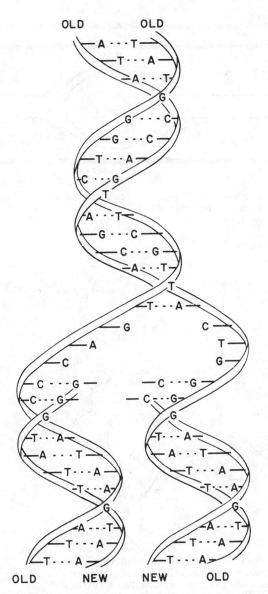

OLD · · · OLD

OLD · · NEW · · NEW · · OLD

Figure 5. The double-stranded structure of DNA and the template function of each old strand on which a new complementary strand is synthesized. (From Harper, H. A., Rodwell, V. W., and Mayes, P. A.: Review of Physiological Chemistry. 17th ed. Los Altos, CA, Lange Medical Publications, 1979, p. 460. Originally from James D. Watson, Molecular Biology of the Gene. 3rd ed. Copyright © 1976, 1970, 1965, by W. A. Benjamin, Inc., Menlo Park, CA.)

and poorly understood. However, it is clear that the regulation of DNA replication plays an important role in cell growth and division. These phenomena are further discussed in Section I, Cell Biology.

RNA STRUCTURE

Although all of the genetic information is contained in DNA, expression of this information requires ribonucleic acid or RNA. RNA is a polymer of nucleobases, each attached to a sugar molecule and held together by phosphodiester bonds, quite analogous to DNA (Fig. 8). However, there are important differences between RNA and DNA: (1) Although RNA is made up of the nucleobases adenine, guanine, and cytosine, it does not contain thymine. Instead, RNA contains the nucleobase uracil (U). (2) The sugar molecule that is attached to the nucleobases in RNA is ribose, as opposed to deoxyribose, which is present in DNA. (3) RNA exists natively as a single-stranded molecule and thus does not have the double-stranded helical structure of DNA.

As is the case with DNA, RNA harbors information in its sequence of polymerized nucleobases. This information in RNA is derived from DNA, with the sequence of nucleobases in the RNA molecule complementary to the sequence of nucleobases in one strand of the double-stranded DNA (Fig. 9). The DNA strand that serves as the template for RNA is referred to as the "sense" strand, while the other DNA strand is referred to as the "antisense" strand. For double-stranded DNA molecules that contain many different genes, the sense strand for each gene will not necessarily be the same strand of the DNA double helix. Thus, a given strand of a double-stranded DNA molecule will serve as the sense strand for some genes and the antisense strand for other genes (Fig. 10). The base pairing rules between the DNA sense strand of a gene and the RNA molecule for which it codes are similar to those for double-stranded DNA, except that the adenine of the DNA pairs with uracil in the RNA molecule, since RNA does not contain thymine.

There are three major classes of RNA molecules: messenger RNA (mRNA), transfer RNA (tRNA), and ribosomal RNA (rRNA). These classes differ from each other by size, function, and general stability. mRNA molecules are the most heterogeneous in size and stability and make up approximately 2 to 4 per cent of the RNA present in the cytoplasm of a cell. Each mRNA molecule serves as a template for the polymerization of amino acids in a defined sequence to form a specific protein molecule, the ultimate product of a

Figure 6. The process of semidiscontinuous, simultaneous replication of both strands of double-stranded DNA. (From Harper, H. A., Rodwell, V. W., and Mayes, P. A.: Review of Physiological Chemistry. 17th ed. Los Altos, CA, Lange Medical Publications, 1979, p. 468.)

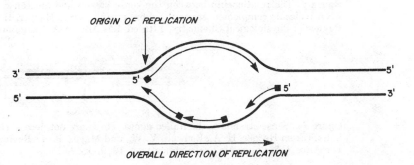

ORIGIN OF REPLICATION

3' — 5'
5' — 3'

OVERALL DIRECTION OF REPLICATION

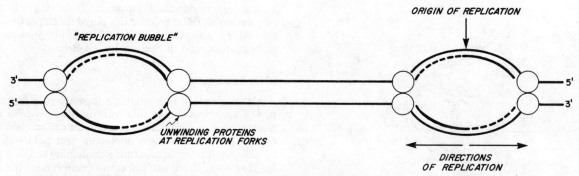

Figure 7. The generation of "replication bubbles" during the process of DNA synthesis. The bidirectional replication and the proposed positions of unwinding proteins at the replication forks are depicted. (From Harper, H. A., Rodwell, V. W., and Mayes, P. A.: Review of Physiological Chemistry. 17th ed. Los Altos, CA, Lange Medical Publications, 1979, p. 468.)

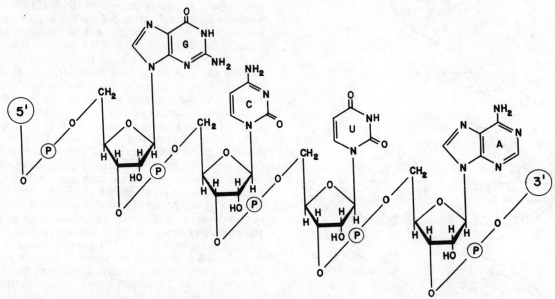

Figure 8. A segment of a ribonucleic acid (RNA) molecule in which the purine and pyrimidine bases—adenine (A), uracil (U), cytosine (C), and guanine (G)—are held together by phosphodiester bonds between ribosyl moieties attached to the nucleobases by N glycosidic bonds. Note that the polymer has a polarity. (From Harper, H. A., Rodwell, V. W., and Mayes, P. A.: Review of Physiological Chemistry. 17th ed. Los Altos, CA, Lange Medical Publications, 1979, p. 143.)

DNA STRANDS:

ANTISENSE → 5'-TGG AATTGTGAGCGGATAACA AT T TCACACAGGAAACAGCT ATG ACCATG-3'
SENSE ———→ 3'-ACCTTAACACTCGCCTATTGTTAAAGTGTGTCCTTTGTCGATACT GGTAC-5'

RNA TRANSCRIPT 5' pAUUGUGAGCGGAU AACA AUUUCAC ACAGGAAACAGCUAUGACCAUG 3'

Figure 9. The relationship between the sense strand and antisense strand in the DNA molecule and the RNA molecule complementary to the sense strand. (From Harper, H. A., Rodwell, V. W., and Mayes, P. A.: Review of Physiological Chemistry. 17th ed. Los Altos, CA, Lange Medical Publications, 1979, p. 474.)

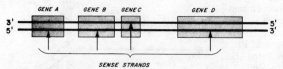

Figure 10. Sense strands of the linked genes. These are not necessarily the same strand of the DNA double helix. (From Harper, H. A., Rodwell, V. W., and Mayes, P. A.: Review of Physiological Chemistry. 17th ed. Los Altos, CA, Lange Medical Publications, 1979, p. 474.)

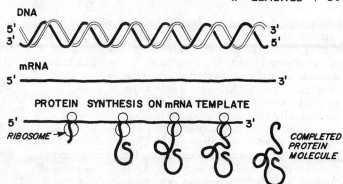

Figure 11. The expression of genetic information in DNA into the form of an mRNA transcript. This is subsequently translated by ribosomes into a specific protein molecule. (From Harper, H. A., Rodwell, V. W., and Mayes, P. A.: Review of Physiological Chemistry. 17th ed. Los Altos, CA, Lange Medical Publications, 1979, p. 144.)

protein coding gene (Fig. 11). Transfer RNA molecules are 75 to 80 bases long and serve as adaptors for the translation of an mRNA base sequence into a specific sequence of amino acids. There are at least 20 different types of tRNA molecules in every cell, with each type corresponding to a specific amino acid. Ribosomal RNA molecules form the skeleton of the ribosomes, those cytoplasmic nucleoprotein particles that contain the machinery necessary for the synthesis of proteins. Each human ribosome consists of two major subunits, the larger of which contains at least three different rRNA molecules, along with more than 50 specific protein molecules. The smaller subunit of a ribosome consists of a single rRNA molecule and approximately 30 different protein molecules. Thus, each cell contains at least four different types of ribosomal RNA molecules, which together make up the bulk of cellular cyto-

plasmic RNA. The structure and function of ribosomes are further described in Section I.

GENETIC EXPRESSION

GENE STRUCTURE

With the advent of recombinant DNA technology and the availability of techniques that allow one to determine rapidly the base sequence of a DNA molecule, the structures of a number of specific mammalian genes have now been determined. The majority of eukaryotic genes that code for proteins share certain constant features. For example, eukaryotic genes are constructed in pieces, such that the DNA sequences coding for a particular protein, the exons, are interrupted by one or more intervening sequences of DNA (introns) that do not code for protein (Fig. 12). Not all

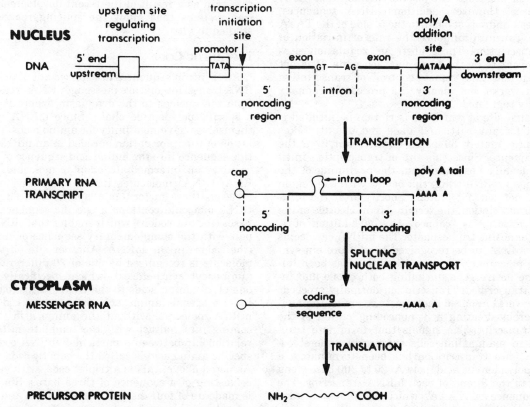

Figure 12. Eukaryotic gene structure and the steps involved in eukaryotic gene expression. (From Cox, D. R., and Epstein, C. J.: In Emery, A. E. H., and Rimoin, D. L. (eds.): Principles and Practice of Medical Genetics. Edinburgh, Churchill Livingstone, 1983, p. 7.)

genes contain the same number of introns, and both introns and exons can vary greatly in length. The average exon is about 200 bases long. Each exon in a gene appears to code for a specific structural-functional domain of its resultant protein. One is led to the conclusion that eukaryotic genes exist in pieces as a result of evolution, which has built functionally and structurally complex molecules from simpler ones.

A number of similarities in DNA sequence are shared by most mammalian genes. The sequence TATA is found 30 or more bases upstream from the 5' end of the first exon, while the sequence AATAAA is present several hundred nucleotides downstream from the 3' end of the last exon. Although each intron has a different DNA sequence, all of the introns studied to date share the base sequences GT and AG at their 5' and 3' ends, respectively. The significance of these interesting similarities is still being investigated.

GENE TRANSCRIPTION

The enzyme DNA-dependent RNA polymerase is responsible for the polymerization of RNA bases with a sequence complementary to the sense strand of the gene. Mammalian cells possess several different DNA-dependent RNA polymerases, each of which seems responsible for the transcription of different sets of genes. The TATA sequence found at the 5' end of eukaryotic genes appears to be essential for the initiation of transcription, since deletions or mutations in this DNA sequence dramatically reduce transcription initiation. This TATA sequence may represent a binding site for at least one of the mammalian RNA polymerases. However, additional DNA sequences, sometimes hundreds of bases to the 5' side of the TATA sequence, can also influence the rate of initiation of RNA transcription. These upstream regulation sites do not appear to be the same for each gene. It is not yet known how this "remote control" of transcription initiation works, but clearly the process is complex and highly regulated.

The actual site at which transcription is initiated is invariant for any particular gene and usually takes place approximately 30 bases downstream from the TATA sequence. Since this site of transcription initiation is usually upstream from the beginning of the first exon, an mRNA transcript begins with a 5' region that does not code for protein. Shortly after the initiation of transcription, the terminal 5' nucleotide of the mRNA transcript is "capped" by the addition of 7-methyl guanosine triphosphate. The mRNA cap seems to allow mRNA to be recognized by the protein-synthesizing machinery. Once transcription has been initiated, the entire gene, including both exons and introns, is transcribed. Transcription normally proceeds at least several hundred bases past the end of the final exon, thereby creating a 3' noncoding region of the mRNA transcript. The signals that terminate transcription in mammalian cells are poorly understood. However, once transcription has been terminated, a "tail" of polyadenylic acid (poly A) 20 to 300 bases long is added to the 3' end of each mRNA transcript. The DNA sequence AATAAA, which is almost always found 15 to 30 bases upstream from the poly A tail, serves as a signal for the proper site of poly A addition

to the mRNA molecule. This sequence does not appear to play a significant role, however, in determining the site of transcriptional termination per se. The function of the poly A tail remains unknown.

In summary, the primary transcription product of a typical protein-coding mammalian gene contains a capped 5' end, a 3' poly A tail, and includes exons and introns, as well as 5' and 3' noncoding regions (Fig. 12).

RNA PROCESSING

In order for the primary RNA transcript of a protein-coding gene to serve as a functional messenger RNA, the sequences corresponding to the introns must be removed and the sequences corresponding to the exons precisely spliced or joined together (Fig. 12). Some facts concerning RNA splicing are known: (1) The dinucleotides GT and AG at the 5' and 3' ends of introns, respectively, are critical for proper splicing. (2) When a primary RNA transcript contains several introns, these are spliced out in a preferred but not obligatory order that is not necessarily sequential. (3) Intron splicing is critical for proper transport of mRNA from the nucleus to the cytoplasm and for the production of stable mRNA. (4) The splicing mechanism seems to have been highly conserved during evolution, since any mammalian cell is able to splice correctly primary RNA transcripts derived from other species. It is likely that the secondary structure of the primary RNA transcript is involved in the splicing reaction. To date, no "splicing enzyme" has been identified in mammalian cells. Rapid progress will likely be made in this area as a result of the recent development of cell-free systems that allow the splicing reaction to be studied in vitro.

THE GENETIC CODE

After intron sequences are spliced out of the primary RNA transcript, mature messenger RNA is transported from the nucleus to the cytoplasm, where it codes for a specific polypeptide chain. Since mRNA molecules themselves have no affinity for amino acids, the translation of the information encoded in an mRNA nucleotide sequence into the amino acid sequence of a protein requires an intermediate adaptor molecule. Transfer RNA (tRNA) molecules in the cytoplasm of the cell serve as these molecular adaptors. One site on each tRNA molecule contains a specific sequence of three bases (the anticodon), which enables that tRNA to base pair with the complementary sequence of three bases (the codon) in the mRNA. Another site on the tRNA molecule is recognized by one of 20 different enzymes (aminoacyl synthetases), which specifically attaches one of 20 amino acids to the tRNA. Thus, each tRNA links a specific amino acid to a specific codon in the mRNA molecule, without the amino acid itself ever coming into contact with the template mRNA. This relationship between a particular mRNA codon and a specific amino acid is called the genetic code (Table 1). As noted above, this is a triplet code, with each codon consisting of a sequence of three bases. Since mRNA is made up of four distinct bases (A,U,G, and C), there are 64 possible triplets to provide for 20 amino acids. Almost all amino acids are represented by more than

TABLE 1. THE GENETIC CODE*

AAA AAG	} Phe	AGA AGG	}	ATA ATG	} Tyr	ACA ACG	} Cys
AAT AAC	} Leu	AGT AGC	} Ser	ATT ATC	} Stop	ACT ACC	Stop Trp
GAA GAG GAT GAC	} Leu	GGA GGG GGT GGC	} Pro	GTA GTG	} His	GCA GCG GCT GCC	} Arg
				GTT GTC	} Gln		
TAA TAG	} Ile	TGA TGG	}	TTA TTG	} Asn	TCA TCG	} Ser
TAT TAC	} Met	TGT TGC	} Thr	TTT TTC	} Lys	TCT TCC	} Arg
CAA CAG CAT CAC	} Val	CGA CGG CGT CGC	} Ala	CTA CTG	} Asp	CCA CCG CCT CCC	} Gly
				CTT CTC	} Glu		

*DNA codons specifying the twenty amino acids.

A = adenine; C = cytosine; G = guanine; T = thymine; Stop = termination codon. The amino acids are abbreviated as follows; Ala = alanine; Arg = arginine; Asp = aspartic acid; Asn = asparagine; Cys = cysteine; Gln = glutamine; Glu = glutamic acid; Gly = glycine; His = histidine; Ile = isoleucine; Leu = leucine; Lys = lysine; Met = methionine; Phe = phenylalanine; Pro = proline; Ser = serine; Thr = threonine; Trp = tryptophan; Tyr = tyrosine; Val = valine. (From Cox, D. R., and Epstein, C. J.: In Emery, A. E. H., and Rimoin, D. L. (eds.): Principles and Practice of Medical Genetics. Edinburgh, Churchill Livingstone, 1983, p. 9.)

a single codon, but codon use is nonrandom in that certain codons are used more frequently than others for specifying a given amino acid. Why one of several codons specifying a given amino acid should be repeatedly used in preference to the others is unknown. Since more than one codon specifies a particular amino acid, the genetic code is degenerate. For any specific codon, however, only a single amino acid is indicated. Thus, the genetic code is unambiguous, even though it is degenerate. This distinction between ambiguity and degeneracy is an important concept to be emphasized. Since a special tRNA that recognizes the codon AUG is required for polypeptide chain initiation on ribosomes, all polypeptides that do not undergo post-translational processing contain methionine as the amino terminal amino acid. Three codons are not recognized by any of the tRNA molecules; these "nonsense codons" serve as polypeptide chain terminators, causing the nascent polypeptide chain to be released from the tRNA-mRNA-ribosomal complex.

As noted previously, the ribosome is the cellular component on which tRNA, mRNA, and amino acids interact to assemble a functional protein. Since this process is outlined in detail in Section I, Cell Biology, it will not be repeated here. The reading of the genetic code during the process of protein synthesis does not involve any overlap of codons. Furthermore, once the reading is begun at a specific codon there is no punctuation between codons. The message is read in a continuing sequence of nucleotide triplets until a nonsense codon is reached. Although most nascent mammalian polypeptides do not differ significantly in their rates of elongation and termination, eukaryotic mRNAs do differ in the rates with which they form initiation complexes with the ribosome. These differences in the rate of initiation complex formation may well result from intrinsic differences in the base sequence and secondary structure of the various mRNA molecules.

REGULATION OF GENE EXPRESSION

Each cell in the human body contains the complete genome, but only a fraction of the protein-coding genes are expressed in any given cell. Each cell contains a subset of the total human proteins, which includes both "household" proteins and tissue-specific proteins. Household proteins are those gene products that are present in virtually every cell in the body, while tissue-specific proteins are restricted to a particular differentiated cell type or tissue. About 5,000 to 10,000 of the human protein-coding genes are thought to specify household proteins, while the rest code for tissue-specific proteins. How the expression of some genes but not others in a particular cell is regulated is poorly understood. This regulation of gene expression seems to occur at multiple levels, including mRNA transcription, mRNA processing, and mRNA translation.

Transcription of mRNA. In many cases, particular nuclear proteins interact with a gene to determine whether or not it will be transcribed. This interaction is thought to change the three-dimensional structure of the gene, thereby making it either more or less accessible for binding by RNA polymerase. In some cases, a covalent modification of DNA determines whether or not a gene will be transcribed.

METHYLATION OF CYTOSINE. A small proportion of the cytosine bases in human DNA have a methyl group added covalently at the 5 position, resulting in 5-methylcytosine. Those genes that are not expressed in a given cell generally contain a higher proportion of 5-methylcytosine residues as compared to actively transcribed genes, suggesting that DNA methylation inhibits gene transcription. Actively transcribed genes do contain some 5-methylcytosine residues, however, so the relationship between DNA methylation and gene transcription is a complicated one.

GENE REARRANGEMENT. In rare instances, the expression of a particular gene is secondary to a DNA rearrangement, and thus a primary change in the DNA sequence of the gene. Immunoglobulin gene expression is the best example of structural DNA rearrangement leading to gene transcription (see Section III, Immunology).

Processing of mRNA. In addition to the association of genes with particular nuclear proteins, DNA methylation, or changes in gene structure, all of which regulate gene transcription, gene expression can also be regulated at the level of mRNA processing. The expression of a gene coding for myosin, a major protein in muscle, is one such example. Although all muscle cells contain a form of myosin protein called myosin light chain, the amino acid sequence of myosin light chain in embryonic muscle is slightly different from that in adult muscle. Since these two polypeptides have different amino acid sequences, it seems that they must be coded for by two separate genes. However, we now know that both proteins are coded for by a single gene, whose primary mRNA transcript is processed differently in embryonic and adult muscle cells. A DNA sequence that is an intron in the myosin light chain gene and processed out of the primary mRNA transcript in embryonic muscle cells is not processed out of the transcript in adult muscle cells, thereby resulting in a larger mRNA. When this larger mRNA is translated in adult muscle cells, it produces a larger myosin light chain protein with a different amino acid sequence from that found in embryonic muscle cells. Only a few such examples of gene regulation at the level of mRNA processing are currently known.

Translation of mRNA. Gene expression is also regulated at the level of mRNA translation. An example is the hormonal regulation of ornithine amino transferase (OAT) gene expression in liver cells. OAT is a mitochondrial enzyme involved in the biosynthesis of the amino acid proline. Although OAT protein is increased more than 10-fold in liver cells treated with certain hormones as compared to untreated liver cells, the amount of OAT mRNA is essentially the same in treated and untreated liver. The increased amount of OAT protein in hormonally treated liver is due to an increased frequency of initiation of translation of OAT mRNA molecules in these cells. The overall rate of translation of individual OAT mRNA molecules once translation has been initiated does not differ between the treated and untreated liver cells, however. Thus, even though hormonally treated and untreated liver cells have the same number of OAT mRNA molecules per cell, many more of these molecules are being translated in the hormonally treated liver cells, leading to increased amounts of OAT protein in these cells.

The same hormones that increase the amount of OAT protein in liver cells also increase the level of OAT protein in the kidney. However, unlike the situation in liver, hormonally treated kidney cells contain 10 times the amount of OAT mRNA of untreated kidney cells and demonstrate no increase in the initiation of translation of OAT mRNA molecules. This example is most instructive, since it illustrates that regulation of the expression of a single gene (OAT) by a single effector molecule (hormone) leading to the same end result (increased OAT protein) can occur by very different mechanisms in different cell types.

Alterations in Degradation. So far, we have concentrated on those processes that alter the rate of synthesis of a specific mRNA molecule or of a specific protein. However, the final concentration of any molecule in the cell is determined by a balance between its rate of synthesis and its rate of degradation. Therefore, regulation of the rate of degradation of mRNA or protein molecules also plays a major role in the control of gene expression. Individual proteins and mRNA molecules show great variation in stability; very little is known about the factors responsible for these differences in protein and mRNA degradation in a particular cell. One example of gene regulation at the level of protein degradation involves the enzyme glutamine synthetase, which catalyzes the formation of glutamine from glutamate and ammonia. When rat hepatoma cells are grown in vitro, removal of glutamine from the culture medium results in a 15-fold decrease in the rate of degradation of the glutamine synthetase protein without altering the rate of synthesis of the enzyme, thereby increasing the steady-state cell concentration of the protein 15-fold. Adding excess glutamine to the culture medium increases the rate of degradation of glutamine synthetase protein without altering the rate of degradation of other cellular proteins. It is clear that glutamine somehow induces a specific function that is responsible for the selective, enhanced degradation of glutamine synthetase.

In summary, those factors that determine the subset of genes expressed in any given cell, as well as the concentration of individual gene products in the cell, operate at many different levels, including gene transcription, mRNA processing, mRNA translation, and processes that affect both the rates of synthesis and degradation of individual mRNA and protein molecules.

MUTAGENESIS AND REPAIR

A mutation is defined as a heritable change in the base sequence of a DNA molecule. By far the most common type of mutation found in humans is the replacement of a single base in a gene by a different base, resulting in a "point" mutation.

Missense Mutations. Most point mutations change the meaning of the codon that contains the altered base, so that a different amino acid is inserted into the protein at the position of the mutation. Such point mutations are called "missense" mutations. An example of a missense mutation is the alteration in the gene coding for the β chain of hemoglobin that results in sickle cell anemia. Normally the sixth codon of the β globin gene contains the triplet CTC, which specifies glutamic acid as the sixth amino acid in the protein. However, the mutation that causes sickle cell anemia changes the sixth codon to CAC, specifying valine instead of glutamic acid at position 6 in the protein. Owing to the degeneracy of the genetic code, not all point mutations are missense mutations. For instance, replacement of an AAT codon, which codes for leucine, by AAC would not alter the amino acid sequence of the protein, since AAC also specifies leucine.

Nonsense Mutations. When a point mutation changes a codon to either ATT, ATC, or ACT, the result is premature termination of the polypeptide chain, since none of these three DNA codons specifies an amino acid. Such point mutations are called "nonsense" mutations. Consider a gene normally coding for a protein 100 amino acids long with an AAT codon specifying leucine at the third position, which undergoes a mutation changing the third codon to ACT. Even though the mRNA molecules produced from the mutant and normal genes would be the same length, the mutant mRNA would result in a polypeptide only two rather than 100 amino acids long, owing to termination of polypeptide synthesis and release of the polypeptide from the ribosome when translation reached the mutant codon. As is evident from this example, nonsense mutations usually cause drastic changes in protein structure.

Frameshift Mutations. Another class of mutations is additions and deletions in which bases are added to or deleted from the sequence of a gene. Deletion and addition mutations most commonly result in what are known as "frameshift" mutations, since all the codons in the gene following the addition or deletion will be read out of phase, leading to numerous amino acid changes in the mutant protein. For example, the DNA sequence CAA TCT AAT AGA would code for valine-arginine-leucine-serine. However, deletion of the fourth base in this sequence would give CAA CTA ATA GA, which codes for valine-aspartic acid-tyrosine. Additions or deletions that are multiples of three bases do not result in frameshifts but instead simply add or delete amino acids in the protein coded for by the mutant gene. Frameshift mutations, like nonsense mutations, result in mutant proteins with markedly altered properties compared to their normal counterparts.

Spontaneous Mutations. Errors in DNA replication are thought to be a major source of many of the so-called spontaneous mutations in man. Such errors result from the introduction of an erroneous base at one position of a newly synthesized single DNA strand during DNA replication. Although the specific pairing of bases, A with T and G with C, normally determines the order of bases on the newly synthesized DNA strand, approximately one time in 100,000 an error in pairing results in the insertion of a "mutant" base into the new DNA strand. Fortunately, the cell has a backup mechanism that removes all such improperly paired bases in the newly formed strand, replacing them with correctly paired bases. Occasionally, even this DNA repair mechanism fails to replace an improperly paired base. In such a case, the "mutant" base is perpetuated in the next round of DNA replication by the normal base pairing mechanism, which results in a double-stranded DNA molecule with a mutant base on each strand (i.e., a mutant base pair). Thus, a single incorrectly paired base has been converted into a heritable change in the sequence of the DNA molecule. It is estimated that such a "spontaneous" mutational event occurs approximately 3×10^{-9} per base per cell division. This number must be multiplied by approximately 7 to arrive at the total mutability per codon as expressed in amino acids substitutions (i.e., each base of a codon can be replaced by three others and approximately 75 per cent of all base replacements lead to amino acid substitutions). This implies a total mutation rate of about 2×10^{-8} per codon. Since an average gene is made up of about 300 codons, this would give a mutation rate of 6×10^{-6} per gene per cell division, which is consistent with empirically derived estimates of spontaneous, single-gene mutations in man.

Mutagenic Agents. Mutations can also be caused by many different types of physical and chemical agents. The most common mutagenic physical agents include x-rays, ultraviolet irradiation, irradiation from radioactive elements, and heat. The chemical agents capable of generating mutations are very diverse, not only in their structure, but also in their mechanisms of mutagenesis. In general, however, both physical and chemical mutagens act by altering the structure of one or more bases in a DNA molecule, resulting in faulty pairing of the altered DNA bases during subsequent DNA replication, which in turn leads to mutations as described above. Most organisms, including humans, have developed sophisticated enzymatic processes that remove DNA bases that have been altered by physical or chemical mutagens and replace them with structurally normal bases, thereby preventing mutations that would otherwise have occurred during subsequent DNA replication. Some chemical compounds cause mutation indirectly by inhibiting various components of this DNA repair system.

The various components that make up the human DNA repair process are poorly defined. However, there are several human genetic diseases in which the primary defect is a failure of one or more of the components of this DNA repair system. In one such disease, xeroderma pigmentosum, patients have an increased sensitivity to ultraviolet light, resulting in skin atrophy and eventually skin cancer. Such individuals have a specific inability to repair those types of altered DNA bases that result from UV light exposure (see Section XVI for a further discussion of this disorder).

Somatic Mutations. Mutations can occur in any cell in the body, but it is important to distinguish between mutations that occur in somatic cells and those that occur in the germ cells. A somatic mutation will be transmitted to the daughter cells and all subsequent cells derived from the original cell carrying the mutation. However, all other cells in the body will be normal. Thus, a somatic mutation cannot be transmitted to one's offspring. In contrast, a mutation in a germ cell will be present in some of the eggs or sperm derived from that germ cell and therefore may be transmitted to one's progeny. Since there are many more somatic cells than germ cells in the human body, somatic mutations occur much more frequently than germinal mutations. However, it is germinal mutations that result in the majority of human genetic diseases.

THE GENETIC APPARATUS

CHROMATIN AND CHROMOSOMES

The DNA present in the nucleus of each cell exists as a complex with a nearly equal mass of small basic proteins, called histones, as well as with a smaller amount of nonhistone proteins. The DNA, together with these proteins, forms a structure called the chromatin fibril, which resembles a group of beads on a string (Fig. 13). Each bead, or nucleosome core, consists of 146 base pairs of DNA coiled around a central histone octamer containing two each of the histone proteins H2A, H2B, H3, and H4. These nucleosome cores are joined together by linker segments of DNA, which are continuous with the DNA surrounding the

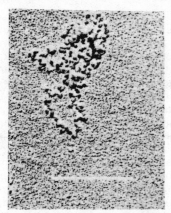

Figure 13. Electron micrograph of nucleosomes attached by strands of nucleic acid. (White bar represents 2.5 μm.) (From Harper, H. A., Rodwell, V. W., and Mayes, P. A.: Review of Physiological Chemistry. 17th ed. Los Altos, CA, Lange Medical Publications, 1979, p. 139. Originally from Chambon, P.: Cell 4:281, 1975.)

cores. The superpacking of nucleosomes in nuclei seems to depend on the interaction of another histone, H1, with the double-stranded DNA connecting the nucleosome cores (see page 61). Each gene is made up of many individual nucleosome cores with their connecting DNA linker segments. In addition to this simple repeating structure, there are complex local variations in the distribution of nonhistone proteins along the chromatin fibril. It is unclear what determines which segments of a gene are packaged into nucleosome cores as opposed to linkers, or what determines the spacing between nucleosome cores. However, the association of histones with double-stranded DNA to form nucleosomes does not depend on the sequence of nucleotides in the DNA molecule.

The chromatin of each human cell is divided into exactly 46 individual pieces called chromosomes, which vary in their state of packing, depending on the stage of the cell cycle. Individual chromosomes can be visualized only during mitosis, when they are in their most condensed state. Chromosomes occur in pairs; the two members of any particular chromosome pair (called homologues) are morphologically identical. Since the chromosomes occur in duplicate, the entire chromosome set is described as being *"diploid."* Eggs and sperm are exceptions, as they each contain only 23 unpaired chromosomes. These gametes are described as containing a *"haploid"* rather than a diploid set of chromosomes.

Each individual chromosome at mitosis is made up of two identical longitudinal halves, or chromatids, which are held together by a constriction known as the centromere (Fig. 14). The position of the centromere is characteristic for any given chromosome but varies for different chromosomes, dividing each chromosome into arms of equal or unequal length. In addition to a characteristic size and centromere position, each chromosome also has a unique "banding pattern" following exposure to trypsin and staining with Giemsa dye (Fig. 15). Thus, on the basis of size, centromere position, and banding pattern, each of the 23 pairs of human chromosomes can be uniquely identified.

The standard means of displaying the chromosomes

of a given mitotic cell is to prepare a *karyotype*—that is, to take a picture of the chromosomes of the cell, cut out the individual chromosomes from the picture, and arrange these individual chromosomes in pairs, according to size. By convention, the largest chromosome pair is designated chromosome 1 and the smallest chromosome 22. A typical karyotype is shown in Figure 16. Note that in this figure, it is difficult to identify the two chromatids of each individual chromosome because these chromatids are so close together. For one of the chromosome pairs, labeled X and Y, the two members of the pair are not of the same size, nor do they have the same banding pattern. These chromosomes are called the *sex chromosomes*, as opposed to the other 22 pairs of chromosomes, which are called *autosomal chromosomes*. The sex chromosomes are so named because they differ in male and female cells. Males contain one X and one Y chromosome, while females contain two X chromosomes and no Y. Thus, the standard nomenclature to describe a normal male karyotype is 46XY, while that for a normal female karyotype is 46XX.

Each chromatid of an individual metaphase chromosome consists of a single continuous chromatin fibril folded on itself many times with higher levels of organization. Thus, each chromatid represents a continuous piece of double-stranded DNA. Since chromosomes are visualized at mitosis, after the time when DNA replication has occurred, it is not surprising that each chromosome consists of two identical chromatids at this stage of the cell cycle. The two chromatids simply represent identical copies of a double-stranded DNA molecule that has been replicated in preparation for cell division. If an individual chromosome could be

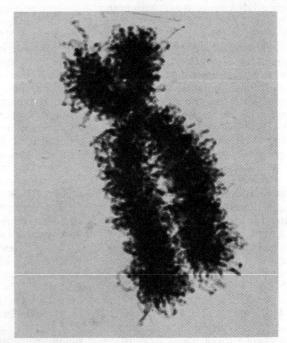

Figure 14. Human chromosome 12 (× 27,850). (From Harper, H. A., Rodwell, V. W., and Mayes, P. A.: Review of Physiological Chemistry. 17th ed. Los Altos, CA, Lange Medical Publications, 1979, p. 140. Originally from DuPraw, E. J.: DNA and Chromosomes. New York, Holt, Rinehart, & Winston, 1970.)

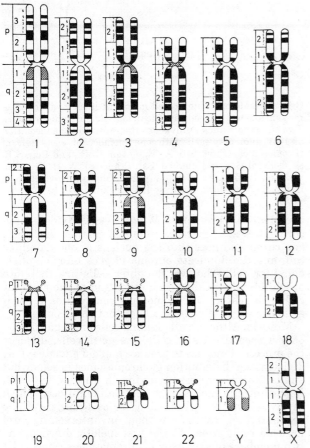

Figure 15. A depiction of the Giemsa-banding pattern of a haploid set of human chromosomes. (From Vogel, F., and Motulsky, A. G.: Human Genetics: Problems and Approaches. 2nd ed. Berlin, Springer-Verlag, 1982, p. 29. Originally from Paris Conference, 1971, Standardization in Human Cytogenetics. New York, National Foundation–March of Dimes, 1972.)

visualized at a stage of the cell cycle prior to DNA replication, it would consist of only a single chromatid. In the following discussion, we will use the term chromosome to mean a single chromatid prior to DNA replication. That is to say, each chromosome represents a different piece of double-stranded DNA, containing its own unique sequence of bases and thus its own genes. The position of any particular gene on the DNA molecule that makes up a chromosome is called the genetic locus. Each gene resides at a specified genetic locus on one particular chromosome. Since chromosomes exist as pairs, every cell contains two copies of each gene prior to DNA replication. However, this is not necessarily true for genes that are located on the sex chromosomes, X and Y. As noted previously, these chromosomes are different morphologically, and they do not contain the same genes. Female cells, which contain two X chromosomes, contain two copies of each X chromosome–specific gene, while male cells, which contain a single X chromosome, contain only one copy of each X chromosome gene. Furthermore, female cells contain none of the Y chromosome–specific genes that are present in males. With the exception of these genes on the X and Y chromosomes, the genetic makeup of males and females is identical.

ALLELIC VARIATION

Each individual contains the same set of genes coding for the proteins that make up the human organism. However, more than 25 per cent of these proteins, and thus of their corresponding genes, exist in a form that differs slightly from the one present in the majority of the population. Such individual variation in a particular gene frequently consists of a single base change that slightly alters the structure of the protein coded for by the gene without dramatically changing its function. This remarkable degree of genetic variability or polymorphism that characterizes "normal" human beings accounts for much of the

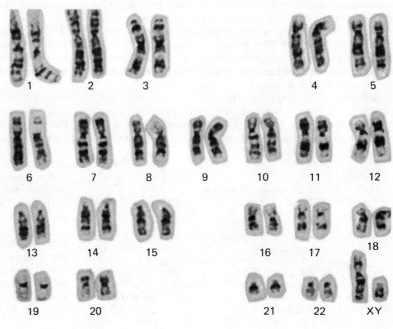

Figure 16. A human karyotype (of a man with a normal 46 XY constitution), in which the chromosomes have been stained by the Giemsa method and aligned according to the Paris Convention. (From Harper, H. A., Rodwell, V. W., and Mayes, P. A.: Review of Physiological Chemistry. 17th ed. Los Altos, CA, Lange Medical Publications, 1979, p. 141. Appeared in Harper et al. by courtesy of Helen Lawce and Dr. Felix Conte, Department of Pediatrics, University of California School of Medicine, San Francisco.)

naturally occurring variation in body traits such as facial features, eye color, and height. The alternate forms of a particular gene in a population are known as "alleles" of that gene. A gene may have only a single allele or as many as 10 alleles. However, since any given individual in the population contains only two copies of a particular gene, one individual can contain no more than two different alleles of any one gene. When the two copies of a single gene in an individual are the same allele, the individual is said to be *homozygous* for that allele. If the two copies of the gene represent two different alleles, the individual is *heterozygous* for each allele.

Each chromosome of a particular chromosome pair contains the same genetic loci as its chromosome partner; the homologues of the two members of a chromosome pair are therefore equivalent. This statement is not strictly correct, however, since an allele at a particular genetic locus on one chromosome is frequently different from the allele at the same genetic locus on the other member of the chromosome pair. This allelic variation between genetic loci on homologous chromosomes, coupled with the fact that either member of a chromosome pair can be included in any particular gamete, results in an enormous genetic diversity among the gametes generated by each individual. Since there are 23 chromosome pairs, each of which includes either one of its two members into any particular gamete, there are 2^{23} or approximately eight million different possible combinations of chromosomes that can result. Thus, there is one chance in eight million that two gametes from a single individual will contain the same combination of chromosomes and, therefore, the same array of genetic alleles.

MITOSIS AND MEIOSIS

Every human cell has the same complement of chromosomes. How is this regularity of the human chromosome complement maintained? How is the regular diploid complement of chromosomes kept constant through the successive nuclear divisions that take place during development of the organism from a single fertilized egg? How are haploid gametes, each with one member of each pair of chromosomes, generated from diploid germ cells? The process responsible for the regularity of the diploid chromosome complement in somatic cells is called mitosis, while the process leading to haploid gametes is called meiosis.

Mitosis. The essential characteristics of mitosis, which have been described in detail in Section I, are very simple (Fig. 17). Each chromosome duplicates itself so that at the time of cell division, it consists of

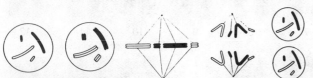

Figure 17. Mitosis. Identical copies of each chromosome separate as the nucleus divides, so that the daughter nuclei are identical in chromosomal constitution. (From Srb, A. M., Owen, R. D., and Edgar, R. S.: General Genetics. 2nd ed. San Francisco, W. H. Freeman and Co., 1965, p. 72. Originally from Sharp: Introduction to Cytology. New York, McGraw-Hill Book Co., 1934.)

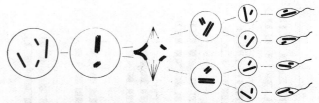

Figure 18. Meiosis. Duplicated members of each pair of chromosomes come to lie side by side in four-strand configurations. Two successive nuclear divisions then result in the formation of four gametes, each with one member of each pair of chromosomes. (From Srb, A. M., Owen, R. D., and Edgar, R. S.: General Genetics. 2nd ed. San Francisco, W. H. Freeman and Co., 1965, p. 81. Originally from Sharp: Introduction to Cytology. New York, McGraw-Hill Book Co., 1934.)

two identical chromatids. When the cell divides, these chromatids are separated from one another, such that one chromatid goes into the nucleus of one daughter cell, and the duplicate chromatid goes into the other daughter cell. The two daughter cells are therefore absolutely identical to each other and to their parent cell with respect to chromosome constitution as well as to the array of genetic alleles that they contain.

Meiosis. Although all dividing cells undergo mitosis, only a special class of cells, the germ cells, undergo the process of meiosis to produce haploid gametes. This division and distribution of chromosomes is somewhat similar to the process occurring in mitosis, but with important differences (Fig. 18). Unlike mitosis, which involves a single cell division, meiosis consists of two sequential cell divisions, without any intervening chromosome replication. At the first meiotic division, the two members of each pair of chromosomes come to lie side by side in the nucleus. Each chromosome of the pair has replicated at this stage and consists of two identical chromatids, so that a total of four different chromatids are associated to form a tetrad. Note that no such tetrad formation occurs during mitosis, since the two homologues of a chromosome pair do not associate during mitosis. Spindles attached to the centromeres of each chromosome then separate one member of each chromosome pair into a daughter cell, so that each daughter cell now contains 23 chromosomes rather than 23 pairs of chromosomes. Note that the two chromatids of individual chromosomes do not separate from one another during this first meiotic division. Without any replication, the 23 chromosomes in each of the cells derived from the first meiotic division align themselves in the center of the cell and undergo the second meiotic division. At this stage the chromatids of the individual chromosomes separate from one another, as in mitosis, with one chromatid from each chromosome going into daughter cells resulting from the second meiotic division. The resulting nuclei are haploid, with each nucleus containing one member of each pair of chromosomes. Thus, meiosis of a diploid germ cell results in four haploid gametes.

The process of meiosis is the same in males and females, but there is one important difference in male and female gamete formation. In the male, four functional sperm are formed from each meiotic event, while in the female, each meiosis results in only one functional egg. Three of the four products of each meiotic event in females are small abortive cells called polar bodies, which contain little cytoplasm and which bud off from the egg as meiosis proceeds. While the first meiotic division in the human eggs is complete at the time the eggs are ovulated, the second meiotic division occurs only after the ovulated eggs have been fertilized and a sperm has entered the egg.

GENETIC LINKAGE

Although each chromosome pair segregates independently during meiosis, those genes that are located on any particular chromosome will be transmitted together. As a result, such genes are said to be "linked." One consequence of genetic linkage is that the combination of alleles on a particular chromosome remains unchanged by the events of meiosis. For example, the genetic locus specifying the Rh blood group antigen and the locus specifying the enzyme phosphoglucomutase (PGM) are located in close proximity on chromosome 1. Thus, if the R^1 allele of the Rh locus, and the PGM^a allele of the PGM locus are present on one copy of chromosome 1, while the $R \cdot$ allele of the Rh gene and the PGM^b allele of the PGM gene are located on the other chromosome 1 in a particular individual, then offspring who receive the R^1 allele at the Rh locus will always inherit the PGM^a allele at the PGM locus. Conversely, offspring who receive the $R \cdot$ RH allele will always receive the PGM^b allele.

In other words, the inheritance of a particular allele at one genetic locus predicts which allele has been inherited at a second linked genetic locus. If an allele at the second locus is one that leads to disease, then the linked allele at the first locus becomes a "marker" for the disease and can be used to predict whether or not the offspring of an affected individual will develop the disease. For instance, the genetic locus on human chromosome 1 that specifies the Duffy blood group antigen is closely linked to another genetic locus, one allele of which, CMT1, results in a late-onset neurological disease in adults. If an individual heterozygous for the CMT1 allele is also heterozygous for two alleles, D1 and D2, at the Duffy locus, and if the D1 allele is present on the same chromosome as CMT1, those offspring who inherit the D1 allele and who express the corresponding Duffy antigen on their blood cells can be predicted to have inherited the CMT1 allele and will develop neurological disease in their later years. Those offspring who inherit the D2 allele will not have inherited CMT1 and will be normal. The concept of genetic linkage implies only an association between two genetic loci and does not imply a consistent association between a particular Duffy allele and the CMT1 allele in different families. Although the allele leading to neurological disease will be linked to one particular Duffy allele in any given family, the particular Duffy allele associated with CMT1 will differ from family to family. Linkage analysis is currently useful for the diagnosis of only a small number of human genetic disorders. With the isolation of large numbers of polymorphic DNA probes over the next several years, linkage will almost certainly become a major means of diagnosing genetic disease in man.

RECOMBINATION

The array of alleles on a particular chromosome remains unchanged by the events of meiosis. This statement is only true, however, for genetic loci that are in very close proximity to one another on a chromosome. The allelic relationships of loci more distant from one another on a chromosome are frequently altered by a process known as *genetic recombination*. This process takes place in meiosis prior to the first meiotic division, during the period when the two members of a chromosome pair are associated with one another. Remember that each chromosome has replicated its DNA by this stage of meiosis and thus consists of two sister chromatids. Genetic recombination involves the physical breakage of one chromatid from each chromosome followed by reunion, to yield an exchange or crossover of genetic material between homologous chromosomes (Fig. 19). Since the breakpoint is identical on the two chromatids involved in the recombination event, no genetic material is gained or lost. However, the array of alleles on the recombinant chromatids is altered from that of either of the two original chromosomes. Thus, if two genetic loci on a chromosome are separated by a recombination event, the presence of a particular allele at one locus no longer precisely predicts which allele will be inherited at the second locus. The farther apart two genetic loci are on the same chromosome, the more likely a recombination event will occur in a region of the chromosome

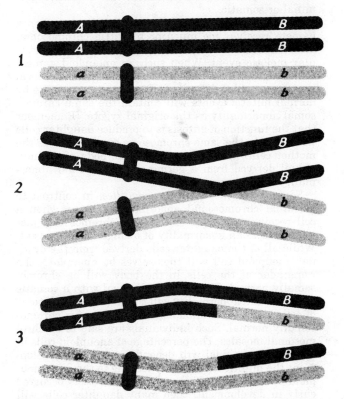

Figure 19. Schematic diagram of genetic recombination. (1) The two members of a chromosome pair, each consisting of two identical chromatids, form a tetrad prior to the first meiotic division. One chromosome carries alleles A and B at two different genetic loci, while the other chromosome carries alleles a and b. (2) Two chromatids break at corresponding places and exchange fragments. (3) Two recombinant chromatids are created following rejoining of the exchanged fragments, one of which carries alleles A and b and the other alleles a and B. (From Stent, G. S.: Molecular Genetics. San Francisco, W. H. Freeman and Co., 1971, p. 20.)

between them, disrupting the linkage relationship of the alleles at the two loci. During any particular meiosis, each chromosome pair usually is involved in at least one recombination event, which can occur at any point along the chromosome. Thus, genetic recombination is frequent. In view of this fact, a genetic disease can be effectively diagnosed by linkage analysis only when the genetic locus causing disease is in such close proximity to a marker locus on the same chromosome that recombination between the two loci almost never occurs.

HUMAN DISEASE DUE TO CHROMOSOMAL ABNORMALITIES

GERMINAL VERSUS SOMATIC ABNORMALITIES

In spite of the elegance and precision of mitosis and meiosis, these processes sometimes fail to deliver a diploid complement of chromosomes to a daughter cell or a haploid number of chromosomes to a gamete, resulting in what is called an unbalanced chromosomal abnormality. Any cell or gamete that contains other than the normal diploid or haploid amount of chromosomal material, respectively, is said to be aneuploid. Such chromosomal abnormalities can be either germinal or somatic.

Germinal chromosomal abnormalities occur when a gamete receives too much or too little chromosomal material as a result of an abnormality during a particular meiotic event. When such an aneuploid gamete combines with a chromosomally normal gamete to form a zygote, each of the cells derived from that zygote by normal mitotic events will contain the same chromosomal abnormality as the original zygote. (Remember that the function of mitosis is to produce daughter cells with exactly the same chromosome constitution as the mother cell.) Thus, every cell in the body of an individual derived from a germinal chromosomal abnormality will be aneuploid.

Somatic chromosomal abnormalities, in contrast to germinal chromosomal abnormalities, occur when a cell receives too much or too little chromosomal material due to an abnormality of a single mitotic event. While all of the daughter cells derived from the original aneuploid cell will themselves be aneuploid, the remainder of the cells in the body will be chromosomally normal. Thus, each individual with a somatic chromosomal abnormality will contain two populations of cells, one that is aneuploid and one that is chromosomally normal. Such individuals are said to be chromosomal mosaics. The percentage of aneuploid cells in a mosaic individual will depend on when in development the mitotic abnormality leading to the first aneuploid cell occurred. If the abnormal mitosis occurred early in development, then many daughter cells will result from the original aneuploid cell, and the percentage of aneuploid cells in the body will be large. On the other hand, if the abnormal mitotic event occurred very late in development, in a single lymphocyte for instance, then the percentage of aneuploid cells in the body will be small.

The clinical effect of both germinal and somatic chromosomal abnormalities, whether they consist of too much or too little chromosomal material, is to produce a broad spectrum of developmental abnormalities, including mental retardation. Although many different unbalanced chromosomal abnormalities result in a similar spectrum of developmental defects, each particular unbalanced chromosomal abnormality results in its own specific pattern of developmental anomalies. In other words, clinical defects associated with a particular chromosomal abnormality depend on the "quality" as well as the quantity of chromosomal material that is either extra or missing. Given that each chromosome contains a specific array of genes, it is not too surprising to find this association between specific chromosomal abnormalities and specific patterns of developmental abnormality.

TYPES OF CHROMOSOMAL ABNORMALITIES

Chromosome abnormalities can be grouped into two major classes: (1) abnormalities of chromosome number, and (2) abnormalities of chromosome structure.

Abnormalities of Chromosome Number. The most common abnormalities of chromosome number are those situations in which a single specific chromosome is either added to or missing from the normal diploid chromosome complement. *Trisomy* refers to the presence of a single additional chromosome in the cell, while *monosomy* refers to the absence of a single chromosome. Thus, trisomic cells contain 47 rather than 46 chromosomes, while monosomic cells contain only 45 chromosomes. The karyotype of a male cell trisomic for chromosome 21 is written 47XY, +21, while a female cell trisomic for chromosome 13 would be designated 47XX, +13. Similarly, a male cell monosomic for chromosome 21 would be designated as 45XY, −21. In addition to trisomy and monosomy, other rarer types of numerical chromosome abnormalities include triploidy (3n), in which each cell contains three copies of every chromosome or 69 total chromosomes, and tetraploidy (4n), in which each cell contains four copies of every chromosome or 92 total chromosomes.

Abnormalities of Chromosome Structure. These abnormalities result from breakage and rearrangement of specific chromosomes and can be either balanced or unbalanced. *Balanced reciprocal translocations,* the most common type of structural chromosomal abnormality, result from two separate chromosome breaks, one break on each of two different chromosomes, followed by rejoining of broken fragments (Fig. 20). This chromosomal abnormality is "balanced" because no chromosomal material is added or deleted; the two chromosomes involved in the translocation are simply rearranged. Individuals who carry a balanced reciprocal translocation are usually clinically normal. However, they are at significant risk for producing aneuploid gametes, as will be discussed below. The most common type of balanced reciprocal translocation is called a *Robertsonian translocation,* which involves rearrangement between any two chromosomes from pairs 13, 14, 15, 21, and 22. These are the human acrocentric chromosomes, so named because the centromere is located very near one end of the chromosome. A Robertsonian translocation generally results from a chromosome break on one acrocentric chromosome just below the centromere, and a second break on a second acrocentric chromosome just above the

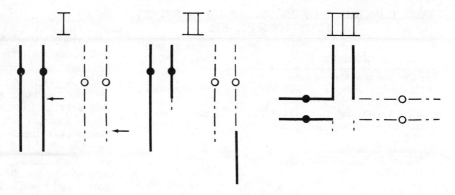

Figure 20. Reciprocal translocation. Origin of a reciprocal translocation by breakage of two nonhomologous chromosomes (I) followed by restitution with the broken ends interchanged (II). At meiosis I, the two normal chromosomes and their reciprocally translocated partners may form a cross-shaped figure (III). (From Thompson, J. S., and Thompson, M. W.: Genetics in Medicine. 3rd ed. Philadelphia, W. B. Saunders Co., 1980, p. 147.)

centromere, followed by rejoining (Fig. 21). The net effect is to remove the centromere from one acrocentric chromosome and to join that chromosome to the centromere of a second acrocentric chromosome. The reciprocal product, which consists of the centromere from the first chromosome and a very small amount of chromosomal material from the second chromosome, is generally lost from the cell. Thus, strictly speaking, Robertsonian translocations are not completely balanced. However, since the reciprocal product that is lost is extremely small, individuals with Robertsonian translocations are phenotypically normal.

Inversions, a second type of balanced structural chromosome abnormality, occur less commonly than reciprocal translocations. Inversions result from two chromosomal breaks occurring on a single chromosome with rejoining of the broken ends (Fig. 22). As in the case of balanced translocations, individuals who carry an inversion are phenotypically normal but at increased risk for generating aneuploid gametes.

The *unbalanced translocation* involves both a duplication and a deficiency of chromosomal material, resulting in a significant alteration in the total amount of chromosomal material present in the cell. Unbalanced translocations, the most common type of unbalanced structural chromosomal abnormality, most commonly result from aneuploid gametes that themselves are derived from individuals who carry balanced translocations (see below). Unbalanced translocations result in significant clinical abnormalities, which vary depending on which chromosomal material is duplicated and which is deficient.

Chromosomal deletions represent a second type of unbalanced structural chromosomal abnormality and result from breakage of a single chromosome with subsequent loss of some material from that chromo-

some. Deletions almost always lead to clinical abnormalities.

INCIDENCE OF CHROMOSOMAL ABNORMALITIES

Incidence in Live Births. Chromosomal abnormalities are a common cause of human genetic disease. Approximately one in 200 liveborn babies has a detectable chromosomal aberration. Of these, about one third are trisomic for either chromosome 21, chromosome 18, or chromosome 13 (Table 2). Trisomy 21 or Down's syndrome, the most common chromosomal abnormality in humans, is characterized clinically by a regular pattern of dysmorphic facial features (Fig. 23), hypotonia, mental retardation, congenital heart disease, an increased incidence of infection and leukemia, and an increased incidence of presenile dementia and premature aging in older individuals. Trisomy 18, which is at least 10 times less frequent than Down's syndrome, is characterized by severe failure to thrive and mental retardation, a prominent occiput, micrognathia, congenital heart disease, and multiple additional malformations. Trisomy 13, which is also rare

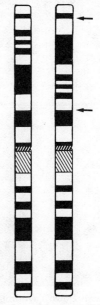

Figure 22. An inversion of human chromosome 1, with a normal chromosome on the left and an inverted chromosome on the right. The two breakpoints of the inversion are indicated by the arrows.

Robertsonian Translocation

Nonhomologous acrocentric chromosomes

Translocation chromosome

Figure 21. The formation of a Robertsonian translocation chromosome from the fusion of two nonhomologous acrocentric chromosomes.

TABLE 2. INCIDENCE OF CHROMOSOMAL DISORDERS AMONG LIVEBORN INFANTS

DISORDER		APPROXIMATE INCIDENCE
Sex Chromosome Abnormalities		
Klinefelter's syndrome	(47XXY)	1 in 1000 males
XYY syndrome	(47XYY)	1 in 1000 males
Triple X syndrome	(47XXX)	1 in 1000 females
Turner's syndrome	(45X)	1 in 2500 females
Autosomal Trisomies		
Trisomy 21 (Down's syndrome)		1 in 800
Trisomy 18		1 in 5000
Trisomy 13		1 in 10,000
Structural Rearrangements		
Balanced		1 in 500
Unbalanced		1 in 2000

in comparison to Down's syndrome, is characterized by severe mental retardation and failure to thrive, abnormal development of the eyes, cleft lip and palate, extra digits, and congenital heart disease. Although Down's syndrome is frequently compatible with life into adulthood, the vast majority of children with trisomy 18 or trisomy 13 die by one year of age.

Another one third of the babies born with chromosome aberrations have numerical abnormalities of the sex chromosomes, the most common of which are 47XXY (Klinefelter's syndrome), 47XYY, 47XXX (triple X syndrome), and 45X (Turner's syndrome). Males with Klinefelter's syndrome are usually tall, with testicular atrophy and infertility and a slightly feminized body habitus, and occasionally have behavioral problems and/or a mildly impaired intelligence. Males with the XYY syndrome are also frequently quite tall and occasionally have behavioral abnormalities, but are generally normal and fertile. Females with the triple X syndrome occasionally have mild mental retardation and/or learning disabilities as well as abnormal ovarian function, but are otherwise normal. Finally, females with Turner's syndrome have short stature, ovarian dysgenesis, failure of secondary sexual development, and occasional difficulties with spatial-perceptual tasks. They are not mentally retarded. Approximately 20 per cent have coarctation of the aorta, and renal anomalies are also fairly common.

The remaining one third of newborns with chromosomal abnormalities have structural rearrangements of the chromosomes, most of which are balanced reciprocal translocations and which do not lead to clinical abnormalities.

Incidence in Spontaneous Abortuses. The incidence of chromosomal abnormalities in spontaneous abortuses is remarkably higher than that in live births. Over 50 per cent of all clinically recognizable spontaneous abortions in humans are associated with and presumably result from a chromosomal abnormality. Since 15 to 20 per cent of all human conceptions end in spontaneous abortion, no less than 10 per cent of all clinically recognizable conceptions are chromosomally abnormal. Over half of these abnormal abortions are trisomic for an autosomal chromosome, while about 10 per cent have Turner's syndrome (45X). Another 10 per cent of the abnormal abortuses are either triploid (3n) or tetraploid (4n). The remainder have either structural rearrangements or are chromosomal mosaics (Table 3). Many different autosomal trisomies, in addition to trisomy 21, trisomy 13, and trisomy 18, are represented in the abortus material. Thus, it seems that the reason we find only trisomies 21, 13, and 18 in the liveborn is not because these particular chromosomes have an increased propensity for abnormality, but rather because these are the only autosomal trisomies that are compatible with life. Even these three trisomic conditions are associated with significant mortality. For every child with Down's syndrome born alive, some three to four are spontaneously aborted. Even a greater percentage of trisomy 18 and trisomy 13 conceptions end as spontaneous abortions. Probably most surprising, only one out of 300 conceptions with Turner's syndrome survives to birth. The sex chromosome trisomies 47XXY, 47XYY, and 47XXX are not seen in the abortus material, indicating that these conditions are not associated with significant mortality. Why the sex chromosome trisomies should be so much less deleterious than the autosomal trisomies will be considered later in this section.

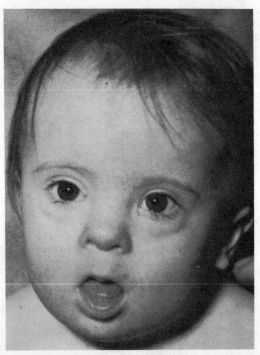

Figure 23. A child with Down's syndrome. (From Thompson, J. S., and Thompson, M. W.: Genetics in Medicine. 3rd ed. Philadelphia, W. B. Saunders Co., 1980, p. 158. Originally from Smith, D. W.: Recognizable Patterns of Human Malformation. 2nd ed. Philadelphia, W. B. Saunders Co., 1976.)

TABLE 3. INCIDENCE OF CHROMOSOMAL DISORDERS AMONG SPONTANEOUS ABORTIONS

DISORDER	APPROXIMATE INCIDENCE
Autosomal trisomy (all types)	1 in 4
Turner's syndrome (45X)	1 in 10
Triploidy (3n)	1 in 10
Tetraploidy (4n)	1 in 30
Structural abnormalities	1 in 50

Etiology of Numerical Chromosomal Abnormalities

Effect of Age. The only etiological factor that has unequivocally been linked with trisomy in man is advanced maternal age. Older women are at a significantly greater risk than are younger women for having trisomic offspring. Figure 24 illustrates the relative frequency of live births with trisomy 21 in women of different ages as compared to the population average. Thus, a 40-year-old woman has approximately a one in 100 chance of having a child with trisomy 21 with each pregnancy, a figure that is about 10 times that found for 30-year-old women (Table 4). This increased risk of trisomic livebirths in older women is not just for trisomy 21, however, but for other trisomic condi-

TABLE 4. BIRTH INCIDENCE OF DOWN'S SYNDROME BY MATERNAL AGE GROUP*

MATERNAL AGE	INCIDENCE OF DOWN'S SYNDROME/1000 BIRTHS	
–19	0.43	(1/2300)
20–24	0.62	(1/1600)
25–29	0.82	(1/1200)
30–34	1.13	(1/880)
35–39	3.45	(1/290)
40–44	10.00	(1/100)
45–	21.76	(1/46)

*From Collman and Stoller: Am J Publ Health 52:813, 1962.

tions as well, including trisomy 13, trisomy 18, 47XXY (Klinefelter's syndrome), and 47XXX (triple X syndrome) (Fig. 25). Thus, the overall chance that a 35-year-old woman will give birth to a trisomic infant in any given pregnancy is about 1 per cent. In contrast to advanced maternal age, advanced paternal age does not seem to increase the risk of numerical chromosomal abnormalities in offspring.

It has been suggested that the increased incidence of trisomic liveborns found in older mothers is due to a selective decrease in the rate of spontaneous abortion of trisomic fetuses as compared to normal fetuses in older versus younger women. However, this is unlikely to be the case, since the frequency of trisomy 21 in spontaneous abortuses of 40-year-old women is 10 times as high as for 30-year-old women. Although such comparisons are complicated by the fact that the overall frequency of spontaneous abortion is different in younger versus older women, it nevertheless appears that the increased incidence of trisomic liveborns in older women is due to an absolute increase in the number of trisomic conceptions in older women.

Even though the maternal age effect on trisomic births is quite dramatic, younger mothers do produce trisomic babies. In fact, since the overall number of babies born to younger mothers is much greater than the number of babies born to older mothers, the ma-

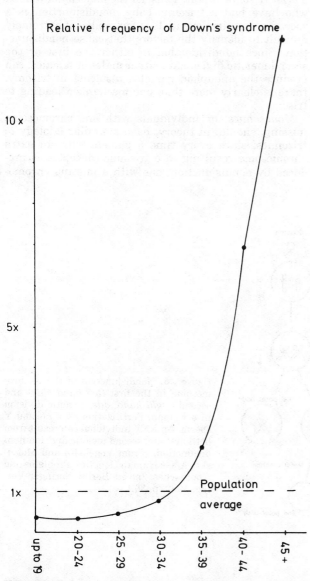

Figure 24. Relative incidence of Down's syndrome, compared with the average risk of the female population in relation to maternal age. (From Vogel, F., and Motulsky, A. G.: Human Genetics: Problems and Approaches. 2nd ed. Berlin, Springer-Verlag, 1982, p. 284.)

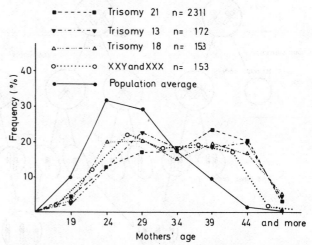

Figure 25. Maternal age distribution of trisomies 21, 13, 18, and a combined sample of XXY, XXX compared with the population average. (From Vogel, F., and Motulsky, A. G.: Human Genetics: Problems and Approaches. 2nd ed. Berlin, Springer-Verlag, 1982, p. 285.)

jority of trisomic infants have younger as opposed to older mothers.

Irradiation. In addition to maternal age, maternal (but not paternal) irradiation may possibly play a role in the etiology of trisomy 21. Some but not all studies have shown such a correlation with an increased frequency of trisomy 21, especially in older mothers. The doses of x-irradiation involved are very low, and the data suggest that the radiation effects may accumulate over many years, with the maximal effect produced by irradiation occurring 10 years or more prior to conception.

Parental Origin of Extra Chromosome. In theory, the production of an aneuploid gamete, which would result in a trisomic zygote when combined with a normal gamete, could occur in either the male or the female parent. The evidence for a strong maternal age effect, and lack of evidence of a paternal age effect, might suggest that the aneuploid gametes resulting in trisomic zygotes are produced only in females. However, in approximately one third of cases of Down's syndrome, the extra chromosome 21 is derived from the father, not the mother. Thus, the abnormal event that produces an aneuploid gamete resulting in a trisomy 21 can occur in either the father or the mother, although in the majority of cases such aneuploid gametes are produced during female gametogenesis.

Nondisjunction. The meiotic abnormality leading to the production of aneuploid gametes with two copies rather than one copy of a specific chromosome is called *nondisjunction* and can occur in either the first or the second meiotic division (Fig. 26). This example illustrates nondisjunction of the X chromosome in a female. The final result, an egg with two X chromosomes instead of a single X chromosome, is the same whether the abnormal event leading to nondisjunction occurs at the first or the second meiotic division. However, there are ways to determine at which step in meiosis a particular nondisjunction event has occurred. Nondisjunction in humans almost always occurs during the first meiotic division, but it can occur rarely during the second meiotic division. In summary, a nondisjunction event in the first meiotic division during female gamete formation is the most common origin of the aneuploid gametes that result in trisomic babies.

Almost nothing is known about what causes such nondisjunction events to occur. Women who have had one trisomic infant appear to have only a slightly increased risk for having a second trisomic baby, as compared to women of a similar age who have not had a prior trisomic infant. Thus, for the majority of women who have had a trisomic baby, nondisjunction is a sporadic, one-time event. This fact makes it extremely difficult to identify the factors that cause nondisjunction. Since nondisjunction in either the first or the second meiotic division, in either males or females, can produce the aneuploid gametes resulting in trisomy, there is clearly more than one mechanism leading to trisomy.

Monosomics, or individuals with one chromosome missing, should, in theory, have a similar etiology to trisomics, since every time a gamete with an extra chromosome resulting in a trisomic conceptus is produced by nondisjunction, one with a missing chromo-

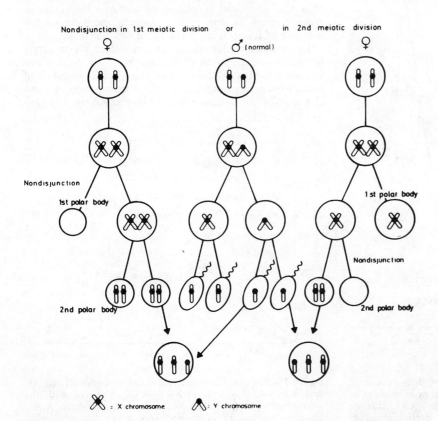

Figure 26. Nondisjunction of the X chromosome in the first *(left-hand side)* and second *(right-hand side)* meiotic division in a woman. Fertilization by a normal Y sperm. An XXY individual can result from both first and second meiotic division nondisjunction. (From Vogel, F., and Motulsky, A. G.: Human Genetics: Problems and Approaches. 2nd ed. Berlin, Springer-Verlag, 1982, p. 39.)

some resulting in a monosomic conceptus should also be produced (Fig. 26). If this is the case, the vast majority of monosomic conceptuses must be lost prior to developing into a clinically recognizable pregnancy, because with one exception, 45X or Turner's syndrome, virtually no monosomics are found among liveborn humans or among spontaneous abortuses. In fact, monosomics die very early in development, usually prior to implantation of the zygote, as noted in animal studies.

Turner's syndrome (45X) is rare and no etiological agent has been associated with the production of 45X conceptuses in man. Specifically, 45X is not associated with increased maternal age or with a history of maternal irradiation. Approximately 75 per cent of 45X conceptuses have a maternal X chromosome and thus are deficient for a paternal sex chromosome. This suggests that the majority of 45X conceptuses result from either the fertilization of a normal egg by a sperm that has 22 autosomal chromosomes and no sex chromosomes, or by the loss of the paternal sex chromosome during the first mitotic division of the zygote. The first of these possibilities would be caused by a meiotic error during male gametogenesis (i.e., nondisjunction of the sex chromosomes during either the first or second meiotic division). The second possibility would result from a mitotic error during the first cell division of the zygote, such that the paternally derived sex chromosome would be lost on the mitotic spindle and not included in either of the daughter cells. Each daughter cell would thus receive a single chromatid from the maternal X chromosome and would be 45X (Fig. 27). The available evidence argues in favor of a mitotic rather than a meiotic origin for the majority of 45X conceptuses, consistent with the fact that many individuals with Turner's syndrome are 45X/46XX or 45X/46XY mosaics, containing two different populations of cells. Such an individual would result if loss of the paternally derived sex chromosome occurred in only one of the two daughter cells at the first mitotic division (Fig. 27). In summary, the primary mechanism responsible for the majority of 45X conceptuses is mitotic loss of the paternally derived sex chromosome

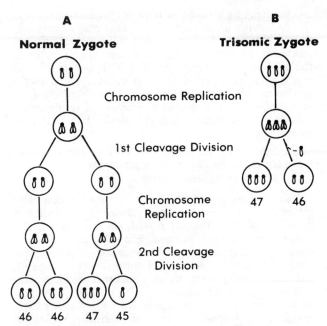

Figure 28. Mosaic Down's syndrome due to mitotic errors. *A*, Mitotic nondisjunction of chromosome 21 at the second cleavage division of a normal zygote. The monosomy 21 cell line is frequently lost due to poor growth, resulting in a 46XX/47XX + 21 mosaic. *B*, Mitotic loss of one copy of chromosone 21 at the first cleavage division of a trisomy 21 zygote, resulting in a 46XX/47XX + 21 mosaic.

during an early mitotic division of the zygote, a mechanism very different from that which generates trisomic conceptuses.

Mosaics. About 2 per cent of all individuals with Down's syndrome are found to be mosaics containing normal diploid cells as well as aneuploid trisomy 21 cells. As would be expected, the clinical features of such mosaic individuals vary markedly, depending on the percentage of trisomy 21 cells in any particular organ. As in the case of 45X/46XX or 45X/46XY mosaics, trisomy 21 mosaics are generated by a mitotic error in an early cell division of the zygote. This could either be by mitotic nondisjunction of chromosome 21 in a chromosomally normal zygote or, more likely, by mitotic loss of a chromosome 21 in a trisomy 21 zygote (Fig. 28). Such conceptuses are thus the result of both a meiotic error and a separate mitotic error of chromosome segregation.

Polyploidy. Polyploid fetuses have either three haploid or four haploid sets of chromosomes per cell, rather than the usual two. As discussed above, triploid fetuses (with three haploid sets and 69 chromosomes per cell) and tetraploid fetuses (with four haploid sets and 92 chromosomes per cell) make up about 10 per cent of all spontaneous human abortions. Both triploidy and tetraploidy are lethal, although on rare occasions a fetus of either type may come to term. There are multiple possible mechanisms that could generate triploid embryos, but the two most probable are (1) failure of either the first or the second meiotic division to occur during a particular meiosis, resulting in a diploid gamete, which, when combined with a normal haploid gamete, would yield a triploid zygote, or (2) fertilization of a normal haploid egg by two haploid spermatozoa. There are examples documenting each of these

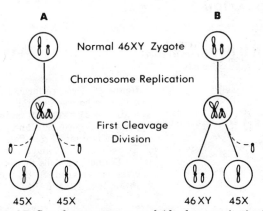

Figure 27. Sex chromosome aneuploidy due to mitotic chromosome loss. *A*, Both copies of the paternally derived Y chromosome are lost due to anaphase lagging at the first cleavage division, resulting in Turner's syndrome, 45X. *B*, Only one copy of the Y chromosome is lost at the first cleavage division, resulting in sex chromosome mosaicism 45X/46XY.

mechanisms as a cause of triploidy in humans. As is the case with all numerical chromosomal abnormalities in humans, the factors that cause polyploidy are unknown. Maternal age is not an etiological factor in the production of polyploids. Both high estrogen levels and a prolonged period between ovulation and fertilization may be associated with an increased frequency of polyploidy, but a definitive etiological relationship between these factors and polyploidy has not been established.

CONSEQUENCES OF BALANCED STRUCTURAL CHROMOSOMAL ABNORMALITIES

Balanced reciprocal translocations are the most frequent structural chromosomal abnormalities found in man and of these the balanced Robertsonian translocations are the most common. Since balanced Robertsonian translocations are not associated with significant additions or deletions of chromosomal material, individuals who carry these structural chromosomal rearrangements are phenotypically normal. However, such individuals are at significant risk of generating aneuploid gametes and thus of producing offspring with unbalanced chromosomal abnormalities and the developmental defects that accompany them. Figure 29 outlines the types of gametes that arise during meiosis in an individual carrying a balanced Robertsonian translocation between a number 14 chromosome and a number 21 chromosome. Every cell of this translocation carrier will have one normal 14 chromosome, one normal 21 chromosome, and one (14;21) translocation chromosome. Since each of the other chromosome pairs will be normal and will segregate normally during meiosis, they do not need to be considered further. During the first meiotic division in a normal germ cell, each of the chromosomal pairs forms its own tetrad. Thus, there would be one tetrad representing the number 14 pair of chromosomes and one tetrad representing the number 21 pair of chromosomes. However, in the first meiotic division of a germ cell from a balanced (14;21) translocation carrier, the (14;21) translocation chromosome, the normal 14 chromosome, and the normal 21 chromosome, each composed of two identical chromatids, all pair together to form one tetrad instead of the normal two. When the chromosomes from this "super tetrad" segregate into daughter cells following the first meiotic division, one of the following three different types of segregation can occur.

1. The normal number 14 and the normal number 21 can go into one daughter cell and the (14;21) translocation chromosome can go into the other. This is called *alternate segregation* and produces two types of gametes following the second meiotic division, each of which is chromosomally balanced. One type of gamete will carry the (14;21) translocation chromosome, resulting in offspring who, like their parent, will carry the balanced Robertsonian translocation. The other type of gamete will contain a normal number 14 and normal number 21 and thus be perfectly normal, resulting in a chromosomally normal child.

2. The normal number 21 and the (14;21) translocation chromosome can segregate to one daughter cell while the normal number 14 chromosome segregates to the other daughter cell. Following the second meiotic division, this will result in two classes of gametes, one with a normal number 21 and the (14;21) translocation, which will produce trisomy 21 when combined with a normal gamete from the other parent, and one with a normal chromosome 14 and no chromosome 21, which will produce an embryo monosomic for chromosome 21, a lethal condition. Thus, segregation of this second type at the first meiotic division produces only aneuploid gametes.

3. The normal chromosome 14 and the (14;21) translocation segregate to one daughter cell, while the normal chromosome 21 segregates to the other daughter cell, resulting in gametes following the second meiotic division that produce trisomy 14 zygotes or monosomy 14 zygotes, respectively. Thus, this third type of segregation at the first meiotic division also produces only aneuploid gametes.

In any given meiosis, only one of the three possible types of chromosome segregation can occur at the first meiotic division. If these occur with equal frequency,

TRANSMISSION OF A 14/21 TRANSLOCATION

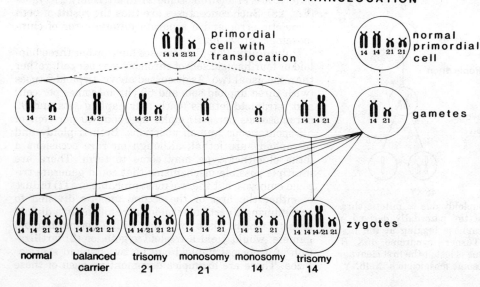

Figure 29. Zygotes formed from a mating between an individual with a 14/21 translocation in the primordial germ cells and a normal individual. (From Potts, W. E., Schroer, R. S., and Taylor, H. A.: Counseling Aids for Geneticists. Greenwood, S. C., Jacobs Press, Inc., 1984, p. 14.)

we would expect one sixth of the offspring of a balanced (14;21) translocation carrier to be balanced carriers like the parent, one sixth to be chromosomally normal, one sixth to carry the translocation chromosome and be trisomic for chromosome 21, one sixth not to carry the translocation chromosome but to be monosomic for chromosome 21, one sixth to carry the translocation chromosome and be trisomic for chromosome 14, and one sixth not to carry the translocation chromosome but to be monosomic for chromosome 14 (Fig. 29). Since monosomy 21, monosomy 14, and trisomy 14 are lethal conditions, one third of the liveborn infants would be chromosomally normal, one third would be balanced translocation carriers like the parent, and one third would carry the (14;21) translocation chromosome as well as two normal 21 chromosomes and thus would be trisomic for chromosome 21.

In practice, the three types of segregation possible at the first meiotic division in a balanced (14;21) translocation do not occur with equal frequency, and the probability that aneuploid gametes will result depends on whether it is the mother or the father who is the balanced translocation carrier. Thus, if the father is a balanced (14;21) translocation carrier, only 3 to 8 per cent of his offspring will have trisomy 21, while if the mother is the balanced (14;21) translocation carrier, 10 to 15 per cent of her offspring will have trisomy 21. These figures are derived empirically and are considerably lower than one would predict based on random chromosome segregation as outlined above. It is not known why female translocation carriers have a higher frequency of aneuploid offspring than do male translocation carriers. What is clear, however, is that the proportion of aneuploid offspring varies with each different reciprocal translocation, and thus, empirical recurrence risks must be determined separately for each particular type of translocation. In practice, the recurrence risks are very similar for the more common Robertsonian translocations [i.e., (13;14), (14;21), (13;15), and (15;21)] with the exception of (21;21) balanced translocation carriers, who always produce aneuploid gametes and thus can never have normal children. [Prove to yourself that this is the case by following the reasoning outlined above for the (14;21) example.]

Approximately 3 per cent of all children with Down's syndrome carry a Robertsonian translocation involving chromosome 21 as well as two normal 21 chromosomes. Thus, they are unbalanced Robertsonian translocation carriers. These individuals with "translocation Down's syndrome" are phenotypically indistinguishable from those children with regular trisomy 21. As outlined above, individuals with translocation Down's syndrome can be produced by parents who are balanced carriers of translocations involving chromosome 21. However, not all infants with translocation Down's syndrome have a parent who is a translocation carrier. About 50 per cent of children with translocation Down's syndrome represent new structural chromosomal rearrangements that occurred in a single germ cell during meiosis, and such individuals have parents with completely normal chromosomes.

Like balanced reciprocal translocation carriers, individuals who carry a chromosomal inversion are at risk for producing aneuploid gametes. However, such aneuploid gametes are produced by inversion carriers only if a recombination event takes place during meiosis in the region of the inverted chromosome that lies between the inversion breakpoints. If no such recombination event takes place, then chromosomally balanced gametes are produced. For further details regarding these events in carriers of chromosomal inversions, the reader should refer to one of the standard human genetics texts listed at the end of this chapter.

The causes of the chromosome breakage leading to reciprocal translocations and inversions in human germ cells are obscure. X-irradiation and γ-irradiation of germ cells can certainly produce structural chromosomal rearrangements in experimental animals as well as in humans, but it is not known if radiation is the major etiological agent generating the "spontaneous" structural chromosomal rearrangements found in man.

PATHOGENESIS OF THE DEVELOPMENTAL DEFECTS CAUSED BY ANEUPLOIDY

Almost nothing is known concerning the mechanisms by which trisomy for chromosome 21 causes the structural and functional abnormalities of development that characterize Down's syndrome. Trisomy for only the distal third of chromosome 21 is sufficient to cause the dysmorphic features, the mental retardation, and the congenital heart disease of the Down's syndrome, while trisomy for the proximal two thirds of chromosome 21 does not result in these features. Thus, there is a specific association between the Down's syndrome phenotype and the presence of three rather than two copies of those genes located on the distal third of chromosome 21.

Gene Dosage Effect. Several hundred genes are estimated to be present on this segment of chromosome 21, but only three have been identified. The protein products of each of these genes are present in trisomy 21 cells in amounts that are 150 per cent of those found in normal diploid cells. Thus, the steady-state level of those chromosome 21 gene products studied to date is directly proportional to the gene copy number in a cell (i.e., a gene dosage effect). It is postulated, but not proven, that the majority of the genes on chromosome 21 will show a gene dosage effect in trisomy 21, but how a 50 per cent increase in the expression of several hundred chromosome 21 genes can cause the developmental defects of Down's syndrome is moot.

Effect on Gene Expression. In addition to the gene dosage effects discussed above, it is also possible that trisomy 21 results in abnormal development by altering the expression of genes that are located on chromosomes other than chromosome 21. Trisomy 21 does not result in massive qualitative or quantitative changes in total cellular proteins, but there are several examples in which the expression of nonchromosome 21 genes is increased in trisomy 21 cells. One attractive, but as yet untested hypothesis, is that trisomy 21 "shuts off" certain normally expressed genes. It is much easier to envision how failure of a group of genes to be expressed could result in developmental abnormalities than it is to explain how a 150 per cent increase in several hundred gene products could lead to developmental defects. Another untested hypothesis is that trisomy 21 results in developmental defects by causing genes to be expressed at the wrong time in development or in the wrong tissues.

Monosomic Lethality. Why does monosomy arrest development so much earlier than does trisomy? At present no one knows. It has been suggested that monosomy "uncovers" recessive lethal mutations on the monosomic chromosome that would normally not cause a problem in a diploid cell. However, this explanation is unlikely to be the cause of early monosomic lethality, since monosomic embryos generated from extensively inbred mouse strains that do not carry any such recessive lethal genes still die much earlier than trisomic mouse embryos.

Trisomic Sex Chromosomes. Why is trisomy for the sex chromosomes 47XXY, 47XXX and 47XYY so much less deleterious than trisomy for autosomal chromosomes? The answer in large part is due to the phenomenon of X chromosome inactivation, discussed in Section I and later in this section. In brief, in any cell with more than one X chromosome, the genes from only a single X chromosome are expressed, while the genes on the other X chromosome(s) are inactive. Thus, as a result of X chromosome inactivation, gene expression in 47XXY and 47XXX cells is very similar to that in diploid cells, in contrast to cells trisomic for an autosomal chromosome, in which expression of genes on the trisomic chromosome is not suppressed. 47XYY is thought not to cause major developmental abnormalities because the Y chromosome contains very few expressed genes, even in normal diploid male cells.

HUMAN DISEASE DUE TO GENE MUTATION

SINGLE GENE DISORDERS

Mutation at any one of the many genetic loci that make up the human genome can lead to human disease by resulting in functional abnormality of the protein encoded by the mutant gene. Such single gene mutations are a major cause of human genetic disease. The mutant gene products responsible for most single gene disorders are unknown, as are the corresponding molecular alterations at the DNA level. These diseases are therefore recognized and classified clinically according to the alterations of cell and tissue function that each individual mutation produces. In other words, single gene disorders are diagnosed indirectly by their specific disease "phenotypes" rather than by

direct identification of their mutant "genotypes." Based on characteristic patterns of inheritance of these disease phenotypes, single gene disorders can be distinguished from other types of human disease and grouped into three main classes: autosomal dominant disease, autosomal recessive disease and sex-linked or X-linked disease.

Autosomal Dominant Disease. When mutation of only one of the two alleles at a particular autosomal genetic locus is sufficient to result in a characteristic disease, that disease is called an autosomal dominant disorder. Fifty per cent of gametes produced by an individual with an autosomal dominant disease will contain the mutant allele and result in offspring with the same disease as the affected parent, while the remaining 50 per cent of gametes will contain a functionally normal allele at the locus in question, resulting in clinically normal offspring. Thus, on the average, 50 per cent of the offspring of a person with an autosomal dominant disease married to a normal individual will have the same disease as their affected parent, while 50 per cent of the offspring will be normal and not carry the mutant allele. The affected offspring when married to normal mates, will themselves have an average of 50 per cent affected children and 50 per cent normal children. The normal offspring, when married to normal mates, will have only normal children. Since the mutant allele is on an autosomal chromosome, both males and females will be affected in equal numbers, and the disease will be transmitted by both males and females. These patterns of inheritance that characterize autosomal dominant disease result in family trees or "pedigrees" such as that shown in Figure 30. (Figure 31 defines some of the symbols commonly used in pedigree charts.)

Autosomal Recessive Disease. When mutation of both alleles at a particular autosomal genetic locus is required to result in a disease, while the same mutation at only one allele leads to no clinical abnormality, the disease is called an autosomal recessive disorder. Simultaneous mutation at both alleles of a single genetic locus is an extremely rare event. Patients with autosomal recessive disease almost always result therefore from the mating of two phenotypically normal individuals, each of whom carries one nonfunctional mutant allele at the locus in question. Since each of these heterozygous "carrier" parents will produce 50 per cent gametes with the mutant allele and 50 per cent gametes with the normal allele, one in four of their offspring will receive a normal allele from each

AUTOSOMAL DOMINANT INHERITANCE

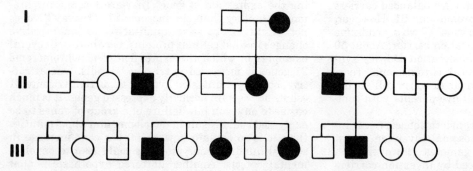

Figure 30. Pedigree of an autosomal dominant disease. Note the "vertical" pattern of transmission. (From Potts, W. E., Schroer, R. S., and Taylor, H. A.: Counseling Aids for Geneticists. Greenwood, S. C., Jacobs Press, Inc., 1984, p. 24.)

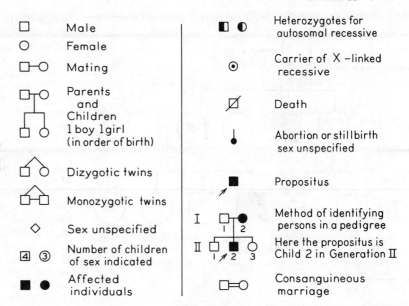

Figure 31. Symbols commonly used in pedigree charts. (From Thompson, J. S., and Thompson, M. W.: Genetics in Medicine. 3rd ed. Philadelphia, W. B. Saunders Co., 1980, p. 55.)

parent and will be clinically normal; one half of offspring will contain a mutant allele from one parent and a normal allele from the other and will be clinically normal; and one in four of the offspring will receive a mutant allele from each parent and develop the genetic disease. Thus, individuals with autosomal recessive disease usually have clinically normal parents but on the average have 25 per cent of brothers and sisters who are similarly affected, resulting in a pedigree as shown in Figure 32.

Offspring of an individual with an autosomal recessive disease and a normal mate who carries no mutant alleles at the locus in question will all be phenotypically normal, although each will be a "carrier," having inherited one mutant allele from the affected parent. Again, since the mutant allele is located on an autosomal chromosome, the number of males and females affected with any given autosomal recessive disease will be equal.

Sex-linked Disease. The final class of single gene disorder, sex-linked disease, is due to mutation at a

locus on the X chromosome that leads to disease. Sex-linked or X-linked disease can be either recessive or dominant. Mutation at a locus on the X chromosome that leads to disease in males who carry the mutation on their single X chromosome, but not in heterozygous females who carry the mutant allele on one X chromosome and a functionally normal allele on the other, is called *X-linked recessive disease*. Males with an X-linked recessive disease will produce only normal male offspring, since these sons must receive a Y chromosome from their affected father, and not the X chromosome containing the mutant allele. All daughters of males with an X-linked recessive disease will be clinically normal, although they will all be heterozygous "carriers" for the same disease as their father, since each daughter will receive from her father the single X chromosome that contains the mutant gene. Female carriers of an X-linked recessive disease will produce 50 per cent sons who receive the X chromosome with the mutant allele and who develop disease and 50 per cent normal sons. In addition, 50 per cent of

AUTOSOMAL RECESSIVE INHERITANCE

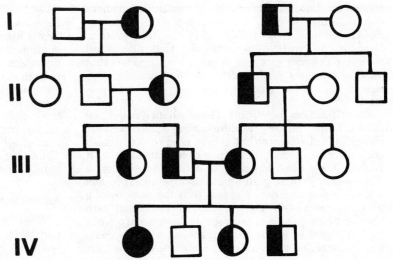

Figure 32. Pedigree of an autosomal recessive disease. (From Potts, W. E., Schroer, R. S., and Taylor, H. A.: Counseling Aids for Geneticists. Greenwood, S. C., Jacobs Press, Inc., 1984, p. 26.)

X-LINKED INHERITANCE

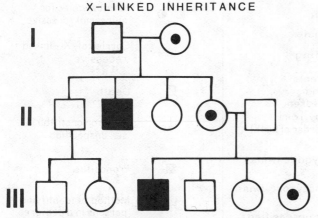

Figure 33. Pedigree of an X-linked recessive disease. (From Potts, W. E., Schroer, R. S., and Taylor, H. A.: Counseling Aids for Geneticists. Greenwood, S. C., Jacobs Press, Inc., 1984, p. 29.)

their daughters will be phenotypically normal carriers of the mutant gene, while 50 per cent of daughters will be both phenotypically and genotypically normal. Thus, X-linked recessive disease is characterized by affected males, normal females, and no male-to-male transmission of disease, generating pedigrees as shown in Figure 33.

Mutation at a locus on the X chromosome such that one copy of the mutant allele causes disease in females as well as males results in an *X-linked dominant disorder*. The hallmark of an X-linked dominant disease is that all daughters of an affected male will have the same disease as their father, while all sons will be normal. Women who have an X-linked dominant disease will have an average of 50 per cent offspring with the disease and 50 per cent normal offspring, irrespective of the sex of the offspring. Almost all human diseases resulting from mutation of a single gene on the X chromosome are X-linked recessive rather than X-linked dominant.

The distinction between dominant and recessive disease is based solely on whether heterozygotes or homozygotes for a given mutation develop disease. Thus, knowledge that a given disease is dominant or recessive does not necessarily provide any information about the molecular basis of the mutation leading to the disease, or about the nature of the mutant protein. However, in practice, it turns out that almost all recessive disorders are due to mutations in genes that code for enzymes, while many dominant disorders are due to mutations in genes coding for structural proteins.

Identification of Single Gene Disorders. Each class of human single gene disorder has a characteristic pattern of inheritance that can be used to distinguish such disorders from other types of human disease. It is not always easy, however, to determine whether a disease that is present in a particular family is in fact a single gene disorder. The fact that the pattern of a particular disease in a given family is consistent with that of single gene disease does not necessarily mean that the disease is due to mutation at a single gene. For instance, consider a family of twelve children, six

boys and six girls, in which three of the boys and three of the girls, as well as their father, have tuberculosis. Although the pattern of disease in this family is consistent with an autosomal dominant disorder, we would be wrong if we concluded that tuberculosis was due to a single gene mutation. In general, before one can conclude that a particular disease is a single gene disorder, that disease must follow the rules of single gene inheritance in a number of different families.

Even when a disease has been shown to follow the rules of single gene inheritance in a number of families, it is still not easy to be sure that the disease in any particular family is due to a single gene mutation. This is because a variety of different mechanisms can result in a single human disorder. Deafness is a good example. Although a significant proportion of all cases of profound childhood deafness are due to a single gene mutation resulting in autosomal recessive inheritance of deafness, over half of all cases of severe childhood deafness are due to infection or some other environmental insult and do not involve gene mutation. Even though the mechanisms leading to deafness are very different, the final disease is identical clinically. Thus, when a couple with normal hearing and no family history of deafness has a severely deaf child, it is frequently impossible to determine whether or not this represents a single gene disorder.

Correct identification of single gene disorders is further complicated by the fact that mutation at different genetic loci can often result in the same disease. This is called genetic heterogeneity. Again, deafness is a good example. It has been estimated that mutation in any one of more than 10 different human genetic loci can result in childhood deafness, which can be inherited as either an autosomal dominant, an autosomal recessive, or a sex-linked disorder. Only in those families in which there is sufficient information to exclude all but one of these modes of inheritance is it possible to determine accurately the recurrence risk for deafness.

Prevalence of Single Gene Disorders. In spite of the difficulties outlined above that are frequently associated with the diagnosis of human single gene disorders, there are a large number of human diseases that are quite distinctive and have unique modes of inheritance due to mutation at a single genetic locus. Over 1600 different human single gene disorders have been identified in which the mode of inheritance is firmly established. Of these 57 per cent are autosomal dominant diseases, 36 per cent are autosomal recessive disorders, and 7 per cent are X-linked diseases. Although each such disorder is quite rare, in the aggregate, single gene disorders are fairly common. One of every 100 babies is born with a single gene disorder. Such diseases account for approximately 5 per cent of all pediatric hospital admissions, and for about 1 per cent of all adult hospital admissions. Tables 5, 6, and 7 list those disorders that make up the bulk of single gene disease in man.

AUTOSOMAL DOMINANT DISEASE

What are the mechanisms by which mutation of only one of the two alleles at a particular genetic locus leads to human disease? On first consideration, it

TABLE 5. HUMAN AUTOSOMAL DOMINANT DISORDERS

DISEASE	CLINICAL MANIFESTATION	MUTANT PROTEIN
Familial hypercholesterolemia	Hypercholesterolemia; atherosclerotic cardiovascular disease	Cell surface receptor for low density lipoprotein (LDL)
Adult onset polycystic kidney disease	Multiple renal cysts; progressive renal failure	Unknown
Multiple exostoses	Bony growths at metaphyses; asymmetry of long bones; mechanical difficulties at affected joints	Unknown
Hereditary spherocytosis (several types)	Hemolysis; splenic sequestration of spherocytic red cells	Red cell membrane protein
Neurofibromatosis	Subcutaneous neurofibromas; hyperpigmented skin lesions (i.e., café au lait spots); mental retardation	Unknown
Hereditary polyposis (several types)	Intestinal polyps that become malignant	Unknown
Tuberous sclerosis	Hypopigmented skin lesions; angiofibromas; seizures; mental retardation	Unknown
Myotonic dystrophy	Skeletal muscle dystrophy; myotonia; cataracts; mental retardation	Unknown
Huntington's chorea	Late onset progressive chorea; dementia; psychiatric symptoms	Unknown
Osteogenesis imperfecta (several types)	Multiple fractures; thin bones; blue sclera	α_1 Collagen (in some cases)
Achondroplasia	Disproportionate short-limbed dwarfism	Unknown
Marfan syndrome	Thin habitus; long limbs; dislocated lenses; aortic aneurysm	α_2 Collagen (in some cases)
Ehlers-Danlos syndrome (several types)	Hyperextensible skin; joint hypermobility and dislocations; skin fragility; easy bruisability	Unknown
Acute intermittent porphyria	Abdominal pain; peripheral motor neuropathy; psychiatric symptoms	Porphobilinogen deaminase
Deafness (several types)		Unknown
Blindness (several types)		Unknown

seems perplexing that dominant disease exists at all, since the nonmutant allele should produce a normal protein product even though the mutant allele results in a functionally abnormal protein. In those few cases in which the pathophysiology of autosomal dominant disease has been worked out, the answer appears to be that the functionally abnormal mutant protein interacts with the product of the normal allele so as to alter the function of the normal gene product, thereby resulting in disease. The classes of proteins most often involved in autosomal dominant disease are multimeric structural proteins and those proteins that function as the rate-limiting step of a complex metabolic pathway. Several examples will be described briefly.

Autosomal dominant hemolytic anemia due to an unstable hemoglobin molecule is a good example of how mutation altering one component of a multimeric protein can lead to dominant single gene disease. Each functional adult human hemoglobin molecule consists of four polypeptide chains, two identical α chains, and two identical β chains. A single genetic locus on human chromosome 11 codes for the β chains, while a different locus on chromosome 16 codes for the α chains. A proper spatial relationship between the four subunits in the hemoglobin molecule is essential for the normal functioning of the molecule. Individuals with a mutation at only one allele of the β chain locus will produce both mutant and normal β chain proteins. However, the majority of their hemoglobin molecules will be abnormal, consisting of one mutant β chain, one normal β chain, and two normal α chains. Such abnormal hemoglobin molecules are commonly unstable due to an altered spatial relationship between the four subunits, resulting in precipitation of the hemoglobin in the red cell, which in turn results in increased red cell destruction and hemolytic anemia. Over 70 different unstable human hemoglobins have been described that result in autosomal dominant hemolytic anemia. The majority of these are due to missense mutations at different positions in gene coding for the β chain of hemoglobin.

Autosomal dominant osteogenesis imperfecta, a dis-

TABLE 6. HUMAN AUTOSOMAL RECESSIVE DISORDERS

DISEASE	CLINICAL MANIFESTATION	MUTANT PROTEIN
Amino Acid Metabolism		
Phenylketonuria	Abnormal brain development; mental retardation	Phenylalanine hydroxylase
Methylmalonic acidemia	Metabolic ketoacidosis; developmental retardation	Methylmalonyl CoA mutase
Oculocutaneous albinism	Deficient skin pigmentation; nystagmus; decreased visual acuity	Tyrosinase
Carbohydrate Metabolism		
Galactosemia	Mental retardation; cataracts; liver and kidney dysfunction	Galactose-1 phosphate uridyl transferase
Lipid Metabolism		
Dysbetalipoproteinemia	Hyperlipidemia and atherosclerosis	Apoprotein E^D
Steroid Metabolism		
Congenital adrenal hyperplasia	Deficient cortisol; virilization	21-Hydroxylase
Metal Metabolism		
Hemochromatosis	Liver, heart, and pancreas dysfunction due to iron accumulation	Unknown
Wilson's disease	Copper accumulation in liver and basal ganglia; cirrhosis; psychiatric symptoms	Unknown
Connective Tissue		
α_1-Antitrypsin deficiency	Cirrhosis; lung disease	α_1 Antitrypsin
Blood		
Sickle cell anemia	Hemolysis; tissue ischemia; infarction	β Globin
β Thalassemia	Microcytosis; hemolysis; ineffective erythropoiesis	β Globin
α Thalassemia	Microcytosis; hemolysis; ineffective erythropoiesis	α Globin
Transport		
Cystinuria	Urinary tract calculi	Unknown
Cystic fibrosis	Pancreatic insufficiency; pulmonary infections	Unknown
Lysosomal Storage		
Tay-Sachs disease	Neurologic degeneration	Hexosaminidase A
Gaucher's disease, type I	Splenomegaly; hepatomegaly; bone pain	Glucocerebrosidase
Deafness		
(Several loci)		Unknown
Blindness		
(Several loci)		Unknown
Isolated Mental Retardation		
(Several loci)		Unknown

ease characterized by frequent fractures of the long bones, is another example in which mutation of one component of a multisubunit structural protein leads to autosomal dominant disease. In this case, it is mutation in a gene coding for one of the subunits of type I collagen that results in an unstable type I collagen molecule. The unstable collagen precipitates intracellularly, leading to a reduction in collagen secretion and therefore a reduction in the collagen available for bone formation, resulting in thin weak bones. Osteogenesis imperfecta is discussed further in Section IX.

Acute intermittent porphyria (AIP) is an example of an autosomal dominant disorder resulting from altered activity of a rate-limiting enzyme in a complex metabolic pathway. Patients with AIP have markedly increased activity of δ-aminolevulinic acid (ALA) synthase, the first and normally the rate-limiting enzyme in the heme biosynthetic pathway (Fig. 34). Increased ALA synthase activity results in overproduction of ALA as well as porphobilinogen (PBG), the product of the second enzyme in heme biosynthesis. The elevated level of ALA and PBG secondarily cause a number of neurovisceral symptoms, including abdominal pain,

TABLE 7. HUMAN X-LINKED RECESSIVE DISORDERS

DISEASE	CLINICAL MANIFESTATION	MUTANT PROTEIN
Hemophilia A	Impaired coagulation; bleeding	Factor VIII
Hemophilia B	Impaired coagulation; bleeding	Factor IX
Duchenne's muscular dystrophy	Progressive dystrophy of skeletal muscles	Unknown
Glucose-6-phosphate dehydrogenase (G6PD) deficiency	Hemolytic anemia	G6PD
Fabry's disease	Renal failure; cerebral vascular disease	α-Galactosidase A
Ocular albinism	Reduction in skin and iris pigment; nystagmus; decreased visual acuity	Unknown
Testicular feminization	Androgen resistance; feminization	Androgen receptor protein
Steroid sulfatase deficiency	Ichthyosis	Steroid sulfatase
X-linked mental retardation (several forms)		Unknown

peripheral motor neuropathy, and psychiatric disturbances. The increased activity of ALA synthase in patients with AIP is not due to a mutation in the gene coding for ALA synthase, but rather to a mutation in PBG deaminase, the enzyme catalyzing the third step in heme biosynthesis (Fig. 34). Patients with AIP contain one mutant allele of the PBG deaminase gene, which results in a nonfunctional protein. Thus, such individuals contain only 50 per cent of the normal amount of PBG deaminase activity. This 50 per cent decrease in PBG deaminase activity does not significantly affect the rate of heme biosynthesis under normal conditions. However, under conditions that require an increased rate of heme biosynthesis, the reduction in PBG deaminase activity makes this the rate-limiting step in the pathway. Normally, an increased de-

mand for heme is met by an increase in ALA synthase activity, since ALA synthase is under feedback repression by heme. However, as the demand for heme increases in individuals with AIP, the level of ALA synthase and thus the steady-state levels of ALA and PBG must be increased much more than in normal individuals in order to overcome the partial block in the heme biosynthetic pathway caused by the reduction in PBG deaminase activity. The markedly elevated steady-state levels of ALA and PBG in patients with AIP lead to disease. AIP is a particularly interesting genetic dsease, since affected patients exhibit symptoms only intermittently, when increased demand for heme leads to increased rates of heme biosynthesis.

Familial hypercholesterolemia (FHC) is another example of an autosomal dominant disorder in which

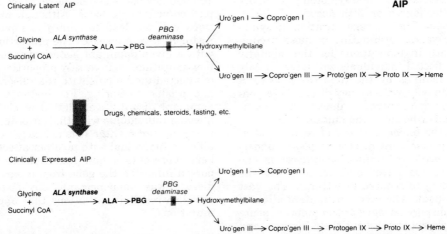

Figure 34. The enzymatic defect in AIP is a partial (~ 50 per cent) deficiency of PBG deaminase activity. The extent of the enzyme deficiency is the same in clinically latent *(top)* and clinically expressed AIP *(bottom)* subjects. Full clinical expression of the AIP gene defect occurs with exposure to agents such as hormones, drugs, etc., which appear to activate the disease primarily by inducing ALA synthase *(bold letters)* in the liver. Activation of the disease is associated with excess production and excretion of ALA and PBG *(bold letters)*. A similar transition from clinically latent to clinically expressed disease characterizes hereditary coproporphyria (HCP) and variegate porphyria (VP). ALA, δ-aminolevulinic acid; PBG, porphobilinogen; Uro'gen, uroporphyrinogen; Copro'gen, coproporphyrinogen; Proto'gen, protoporphyrinogen; Proto, protoporphyrin. (From Kappas, A., Sassa, S., and Anderson, K. E.: The porphyrias. In Stanbury, J. B., Wyngaarden, J. B., Fredrickson, D. S., et al.: The Metabolic Basis of Inherited Disease. 5th ed. New York, McGraw-Hill Book Co., 1983, p. 1348.)

mutation indirectly alters the activity of a rate-limiting enzyme leading to disease. This disorder is described in considerable detail in Section VI.

The above examples illustrate how mutation of genes that code for multimeric stuctural proteins or rate-limiting proteins in metabolic pathways can lead to autosomal dominant disease. The nature of the mutant gene product is unknown, however, for the vast majority of human autosomal dominant diseases.

Two characteristics of many autosomal dominant diseases are *reduced penetrance* and *variable expressivity*. Penetrance refers to the proportion of individuals carrying a mutant gene who display some clinical features of disease, while expressivity refers to the severity of the disease in an affected individual. Expressivity can be discussed only when a condition is penetrant.

Reduced Penetrance. In many autosomal dominant conditions, the disease becomes penetrant only late in life, after the reproductive age of affected individuals. Such age-dependent penetrance frequently makes it impossible to determine whether or not a young individual has inherited a particular mutant gene from an affected parent. Adult polycystic kidney disease and Huntington's chorea are the two most common autosomal dominant diseases that display age-dependent penetrance. *Polycystic kidney disease* is characterized by multiple renal cysts that expand with time to fill the kidneys. Since the cysts themselves have no normal renal function, and since they compress the surrounding normal nephrons, decreasing their function, individuals with this disorder experience progressive renal failure. Penetrance for this disorder is nearly complete by the middle of the sixth decade in individuals who carry the mutant allele.

Huntington's chorea is an autosomal dominant neurological disorder that includes severe emotional disturbance, choreic movements, seizures, and progressive dementia that is frequently accompanied by violent and paranoid behavior. These symptoms gradually appear late in the fourth or fifth decade of life in affected individuals. The average duration of symptoms is 13 to 15 years, terminating in most circumstances with death in institutions for the mentally disabled. Many affected individuals will have already completed their families by the time the disease is suspected. As with polycystic kidney disease, the penetrance for Huntington's chorea is almost 100 per cent in older individuals who carry the mutant gene.

In most cases, the biological basis of reduced penetrance in a given dominant disease is poorly understood. However, *acute intermittent porphyria* is one example in which we have some insight into the mechanisms leading to reduced penetrance. The vast majority of individuals who carry one mutant allele of PBG deaminase display no signs or symptoms of acute intermittent porphyria throughout their lifetime, and thus, the penetrance in this disorder is very low. Individuals who carry the PBG deaminase mutation who are exposed to drugs, such as barbiturates, or certain hormones that induce the synthesis of cytochrome P450 and thus stimulate heme biosynthesis, do develop symptoms of acute intermittent porphyria owing to elevations of ALA and PBG as described above. Thus, the low penetrance of acute intermittent porphyria in individuals who carry the mutant gene

can be explained by the fact that most such individuals are never placed in a situation in which they need to synthesize greater than normal amounts of heme. Clearly, the interaction of the mutant gene product with a number of environmental factors determines the penetrance in acute intermittent porphyria and probably a number of other dominant diseases as well.

Variable Expressivity. In addition to reduced penetrance, many autosomal dominant disorders display marked variability in the severity of symptoms, even among the affected individuals in a single family. Since each affected individual in a particular family has inherited the identical mutant allele, the variability in symptoms must be due to the interaction of the mutant gene product with products of other genetic loci or with environmental factors that differ between the affected family members. As a result of such interactions, it is common for a person who is mildly affected by a dominant disorder to have a severely affected child, or visa versa.

New Mutation. One final aspect of autosomal dominant disease is the concept of new mutation. Although half of the offspring of an individual with an autosomal dominant disorder will inherit the mutant allele and develop the same disease as their affected parent, it is not necessarily true that each affected person must have an affected parent. This is because a certain proportion of affected individuals owe their disorder to a new mutation in either the egg or sperm from which they were derived. The parent in whose germ cell the mutation arose would be clinically normal. Since the mutation arose in a single germ cell, the siblings of the affected individual would also be normal. Thus, only the affected individual would be at risk for having affected offspring. As discussed above in the section dealing with mutation, the average mutation rate in man is about 6×10^{-6} per gene per generation. Since a dominant disease requires mutation at only one of the pair of alleles at a locus, approximately 1 in 100,000 newborns should have a new mutation at any particular genetic locus. Although many such mutations will not lead to clinical symptoms, others will result in severe disease. The proportion of individuals with a given dominant genetic disease who represent new mutations is inversely proportional to the ability of affected individuals with that disorder to reproduce and produce offspring. For instance, if a particular dominant disorder were lethal in childhood, then all affected individuals with that disorder must represent new mutations. Often it is not easy to determine if an affected individual with no other affected family members represents a new mutation, or if that affected person inherited the gene from a parent in whom the disease was nonpenetrant. Obviously, nonpaternity can also result in situations that appear to be "new mutations."

AUTOSOMAL RECESSIVE DISEASES

In general, autosomal recessive diseases exhibit complete penetrance and much less variability than do most autosomal dominant disorders. For most autosomal dominant diseases the mutant proteins leading to disease have yet to be discovered. In contrast, defective gene products have been identified in a number of different autosomal recessive disorders, providing insight into the pathogenesis of these diseases. Most autosomal recessive diseases are due to mutations in genes coding for enzymes and result from proteins with absent or severely reduced catalytic activity. Enzymes do not function in isolation, but rather catalyze one or more steps in a metabolic pathway. The net effect of a mutation causing a catalytically inactive enzyme is to alter the flux and concentration of metabolic intermediates in the metabolic pathway that contains the mutant enzyme. Individuals who are heterozygous for such a mutation (i.e., carry one mutant allele and one normal allele at the locus in question) do not develop disease, for even though they generally have only 50 per cent of the normal amount of the enzymatic activity as a result of the mutation, this is sufficient catalytic activity to allow the metabolic pathway to function normally. On the other hand, patients homozygous for the mutation have a marked reduction or complete absence of enzyme activity, resulting in deficiency of the products as well as accumulation of the substrates of the defective enzyme. While the basic defect has been elucidated in many human autosomal recessive disorders, there are still a large number of autosomal recessive disorders for which the primary mutant protein is unknown. Cystic fibrosis, one of the most common autosomal recessive diseases in Caucasians, is such a disorder. Autosomal recessive diseases produce their phenotypical abnormalities through several mechanisms, which will be described and illustrated briefly.

Accumulation of Toxic Substrates. When a mutation produces a block in a catabolic pathway, it is generally the accumulation of toxic compounds proximal to the defective enzyme that causes disease.

Phenylketonuria (PKU), the most common autosomal recessive disorder of amino acid metabolism, is one such example. The primary defect in PKU is a mutation in the gene coding for phenylalanine hydroxylase, the enzyme that converts phenylalanine to tyrosine (Fig. 35). As a result of decreased phenylalanine hydroxylase activity, patients with PKU have elevated tissue, plasma, and urine concentrations of phenylalanine, which in turn lead to mental retardation, the most important and consistent clinical feature of this disorder. Elevated phenylalanine is thought to compete with other amino acids for transport into brain neurons, creating an amino acid imbalance within these cells, which inhibits protein synthesis and synapse formation. Reduction of hyperphenylalanemia in PKU patients by dietary therapy can prevent the mental retardation that is otherwise inevitable in these individuals.

Tay-Sachs disease is another example of an autosomal recessive disorder due to mutation of a catabolic enzyme, resulting in accumulation of substrates leading to disease. Tay-Sachs disease is a degenerative neurological disorder characterized by motor weakness beginning at three to six months of age, followed by rapid mental and motor deterioration after one year of age. By 18 months, progressive deafness, blindness, convulsions, and spasticity appear. Most patients die from pneumonia by three years of age. The primary defect in Tay-Sachs disease is a mutation in the gene coding for the lysosomal enzyme hexosaminidase A, an enzyme involved in the catabolism of gangliosides. Although these glycosphingolipids are normally present in highest concentration in the brain, where they are localized primarily in nerve ending membranes, gangliosides are present in most cells in the body. Hexosaminidase A deficiency in patients with Tay-Sachs disease leads to massive accumulation of the substrate GM_2 ganglioside in neuronal lysosomes, resulting in neuronal dysfunction by causing axonal degeneration and secondary central demyelination. Tay-Sachs disease is only one of many autosomal recessive lysosomal storage diseases in which deficiency of a lysosomal enzyme involved in a catabolic pathway results in massive substrate accumulation in the lysosomes, causing cellular dysfunction.

Deficiency of a Product. In contrast to the situation in catabolic pathways where accumulation of substrates proximal to an enzymatic defect results in disease, the deficiency of products distal to the defective enzyme most commonly causes disease when a mutation produces a block in an anabolic pathway. *Oculocutaneous albinism* due to mutation in the gene coding for tyrosinase is such an example. Tyrosinase is a key enzyme in the metabolic pathway that produces mel-

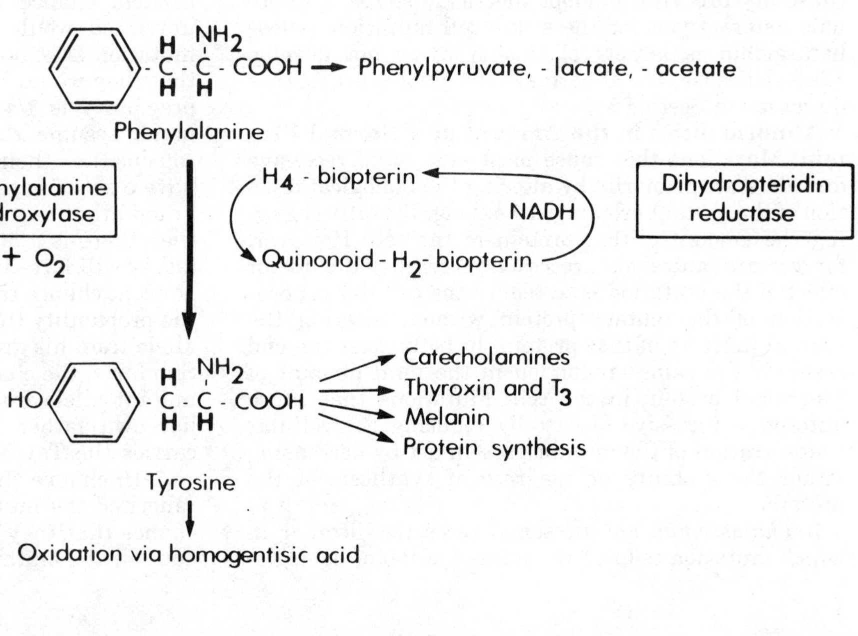

Figure 35. Pathways of phenylalanine and tyrosine metabolism. (From Smith, L. H., Jr.: The hyperphenylalaninemias. In Wyngaarden, J. B., and Smith, L. H., Jr. (eds.): Cecil Textbook of Medicine. 17th ed. Philadelphia, W. B. Saunders Co., 1985, p. 1126.)

anin, the major molecule contributing to skin and eye pigmentation. Tyrosinase deficiency leads to absence of melanin production, resulting in reduced skin pigmentation and secondarily leading to increased susceptibility of the skin to ultraviolet radiation–induced damage and cancer. Patients with oculocutaneous albinism also have nystagmus, decreased visual acuity, and abnormal optic neuronal pathways, all postulated to be due to absence of pigment in the developing optic cup. (See Section XVI for a more extensive discussion of melanin metabolism and albinism.)

Transport Defects. Although many autosomal recessive disorders are due to enzyme deficiency, mutation in genes that code for nonenzymatic proteins can also result in autosomal recessive disease. *Cystinuria* is an example of an autosomal recessive disease due to defective transepithelial transport of specific amino acids in renal tubules and the gastrointestinal tract. Individuals homozygous for this mutation have impaired transport of the basic amino acids cystine, lysine, arginine, and ornithine, resulting in increased concentrations of these amino acids in the urine. Owing to insolubility of cystine, it precipitates to form calculi in the urinary tract, often leading to obstruction and infection, and sometimes resulting in renal insufficiency. This disease is discussed further in Section X as it relates to kidney stone diathesis.

Abnormalities of Structural Characteristics. In addition to mutations that cause enzyme deficiency or alter transport across cell membranes, mutation in genes coding for cellular proteins that carry out other specialized functions can also result in autosomal recessive disease. *Sickle cell anemia* caused by a missense mutation in the gene coding for the β chain of hemoglobin is probably the best example. Hemoglobin molecules that contain two mutant β chains combined with two normal α chains are unstable and aggregate in the erythrocyte, causing the cell to assume a characteristic "sickle" shape. Such sickled cells clog small blood vessels, causing local ischemia and pain. In addition, "sickled" cells are rapidly cleared by the spleen, leading to anemia. Since a hemoglobin molecule consisting of one β chain with the sickle mutation, one normal β chain, and two normal α chains does not cause erythrocytes to adopt the sickle shape, individuals heterozygous for the sickle cell mutation, whose hemoglobin is largely of this type, do not develop clinical disease. The abnormal hemoglobins are further discussed in Section V.

Abnormalities in the Amount of a Normal Protein. Mutations that cause most autosomal recessive disorders act primarily by altering the biological function of the mutant protein, without significantly changing the amount of that protein in the cell. However, for certain autosomal recessive diseases, the major effect of the mutation is to reduce the cellular concentration of the mutant protein without altering the normal function of that protein. In both cases the end result is the same—reduction in the total amount of functional protein in the cell. Mutations that cause autosomal recessive disease by reducing the cellular concentration of the mutant protein act by decreasing either the stability or the rate of synthesis of the protein.

β *Thalassemia*, an autosomal recessive disorder in which mutation reduces the concentration of hemoglobin β chains in the red cell, results in excess uncombined α-globin chains, which disrupt red cell maturation and function, causing microcytosis, ineffective erythrocytosis, and hemolysis. β Thalassemia is a particularly instructive disorder, since it illustrates how a number of distinct mutations in the β chain gene can produce the same final result by totally different mechanisms.

The majority of patients with β thalassemia are homozygous for a mutation in the β chain gene that reduces the rate of synthesis of β chains. This is most commonly a nonsense mutation at codon 39. Individuals homozygous for this mutation produce normal amounts of β chain mRNA but fail to translate any full length β chain molecules owing to the stop codon in the middle of the message. Other patients with β thalassemia have a reduction in the rate of β chain synthesis due to mutations that reduce the amount of β chain mRNA in the cell. Most of these are either point mutations that interfere with the proper splicing of β chain mRNA or large deletions of the β chain gene itself. Rare patients with β thalassemia have a point mutation in the promoter region of the β chain gene such that RNA polymerase cannot bind properly, leading to reduced transcription of the gene. Thus, a variety of different mutations results in β thalassemia by reducing the rate of β chain synthesis. In addition, several mutations in the β chain gene dramatically reduce the stability of the β chain protein, resulting in a decreased steady-state concentration of the protein in erythrocytes.

Role of Consanguinity. A characteristic associated with autosomal recessive disease but not with dominant disorders is consanguinity; that is, the heterozygous parents of a child with an autosomal recessive disorder often have an ancestor in common. Autosomal recessive disease requires that both parents of an affected individual carry a rare mutant allele at the same genetic locus, and the likelihood of this event is increased if both parents are descended from a common ancestor who is a heterozygous carrier of the rare mutant allele. For instance, about 1 in 200 individuals in the general population carry the mutant allele that results in Tay-Sachs disease when homozygous. The random chance that a husband and wife who are unrelated would both be carriers of the Tay-Sachs mutation is $1/200 \times 1/200 = 1/40,000$, and the chance that they would have an affected child with any given pregnancy is 1/4 of this, or 1/160,000. On the other hand, assume that the husband and wife are first cousins (i.e., their fathers are brothers) and thus, they have a set of grandparents in common. If the common grandfather is a carrier for the Tay-Sachs mutation, then there is a 50 per cent chance that the husband's father will have inherited this mutant allele, and a 50 per cent chance that he transmitted it to his son. Thus, the probability that the husband inherited the mutant allele from his grandfather, through his father, is 1/4. Similarly, the chance that the wife inherited the same mutant allele from the common grandfather through her own father is 1/4. If the common grandfather carries the Tay-Sachs mutation, there is a $1/4 \times 1/4 = 1/16$ chance that both husband and wife will have inherited the mutant allele, and a $1/16 \times 1/4 = 1/64$ chance that they will produce a child who is homozygous for the mutant allele and therefore has Tay-Sachs disease. Since the random chance that the common grandfather would carry the Tay-Sachs mutation is 1/200, the probability that such a couple would have a child with Tay-Sachs disease by inheritance of a mutant allele through the common grandfather is 1/200 × 1/64 = 1/12,800. However, remember that such a couple also shares a common grandmother who could be a Tay-Sachs carrier, and from whom they could each inherit a mutant Tay-Sachs allele. Thus, the overall probability that a husband and wife who are first cousins will both be carriers for a Tay-Sachs mutation and have an affected child will be 1/12,800 + 1/12,800 = 1/6,400, a risk that is 25-fold greater than if this couple were not related to each other. The rarer the mutant allele in the general population, the greater the probability that the parents of an affected individual will be consanguineous.

Segregation in Ethnic Groups. A final characteristic of autosomal recessive disorders is the tendency for certain recessive diseases to occur in particular ethnic groups. For instance, Tay-Sachs disease is very common in Ashkenazi Jews; sickle cell anemia is common in blacks; and cystic fibrosis occus most frequently in Caucasians. Since individuals in a given ethnic group tend to mate within their own group, if a rare mutation occurs in one such individual, the chance that the mutant allele will be inherited by others in that small ethnic group is high, resulting in a higher frequency of heterozygous carriers in the ethnic group as compared to the general population. It has been estimated that 1 in 38 Ashkenazi Jews carries the Tay-Sachs mutation, as compared to 1 in 350 non-Jewish individuals. Even though many autosomal recessive diseases exhibit ethnic clustering as a result of selective mating within, as opposed to between, ethnic groups, a given recessive disease can occur in individuals of any ethnic background.

X-LINKED DISEASE

X-linked disease is due to mutation of genes that are located on the X chromosome. Since many more genes are present on the autosomal chromosomes, most dominant and recessive diseases are autosomal rather than X-linked.

A single mutant allele at an X chromosome locus will produce X-linked disease in males. Affected males can therefore acquire the mutant allele (1) by inheritance from a carrier mother, or (2) by new mutation, as described for autosomal dominant disease. If only a single male is affected in a given family, it is important to distinguish between these possibilities, since the recurrence risk of disease is very different in each case. Consider a situation in which a male is born with hemophilia A due to a mutation in the X-linked gene coding for clotting factor VIII, resulting in abnormal hemostasis. If the mother is a carrier for this mutant gene, half of her subsequent male children, on the average, will have hemophilia A and half her subsequent daughters will carry the mutant gene (even though they are clinically normal). On the other hand, if the affected male represents a new mutation in the gene coding for factor VIII (which occurred in a single germ cell during maternal gametogenesis), then neither his mother nor any of his sibs will carry the mutant allele, and they will not develop hemophilia or transmit it to their offspring.

In practice, even if the mutant protein resulting in a given X-linked disease has been identified, as in the case of hemophilia A, it is not always easy to determine whether or not the mother of an isolated affected male is a carrier of the mutant gene. Unlike the situation for autosomal genes, where both alleles at a given locus are expressed in each cell, only one of the two alleles of an X chromosome gene is expressed in any given female somatic cell. Since females have two X chromosomes while males have only one, and since the Y chromosome in males does not contain X chromosome genes, mechanisms of *"dosage compensation"* have evolved to make the production of proteins coded for by X chromosome genes equal in the two sexes.

X Chromosome Inactivation. Dosage compensation is achieved in humans by inactivation of all of the alleles on one of the two X chromosomes in each somatic cell of the female, resulting in only one functional X chromosome per cell. The following properties characterize the X chromosome inactivation process: (1) X chromosome inactivation occurs at a specific stage early in embryonic development, at about the time of implantation of the embryo. Prior to this stage, both of the X chromosomes in a female embryo are genetically functional. (2) Once X chromosome inactivation has occurred in a somatic cell, it is irreversible in that cell and all its progeny. Thus all daughter cells derived from an original inactivated cell will have the same active X chromosome. (3) X chromosome inactivation is random. Therefore, when the inactivation process occurs, on the average half of the somatic cells of the embryo will have an active X chromosome that is maternally derived, and half will have a paternally derived active X chromosome. (4) The inactive X chromosome is highly condensed throughout the cell cycle, giving rise to the "sex chromatin body" or "Barr body," which is cytologically detectable in the nucleus of female somatic cells. (5) When female germ cells begin the process of meiosis, the inactive X chromosome in the germ cell is reactivated, resulting in two functional X chromosomes. Such reactivation never occurs in somatic cells. (6) Because of X chromosome inactivation, each human female contains two genetically different types of cells, one in which only the paternally derived X chromosome is active, and one in which the maternally derived X is active. Thus, females are genetic mosaics.

Female Mosaicism. Females heterozygous for an X-linked mutation will have two populations of cells, one in which the X chromosome containing the mutant allele is genetically active, and one in which the X chromosome containing the normal allele is active. The former population of cells will be mutant and functionally equivalent to cells from a male carrying the same X-linked mutation, while the latter population of cells will be completely normal. Females heterozygous for an X-linked mutation are therefore quite different from individuals heterozygous for an autosomal mutation, who contain a single population of cells, with each cell expressing both the normal and the mutant allele at the genetic locus in question.

Since the X chromosome inactivation process is statistically random, the proportion of normal and mutant cells is not necessarily equal in any particular female carrier of an X-linked mutation. Thus, some females heterozygous for an X-linked mutation will contain mostly cells that are phenotypically entirely normal. Without a direct analysis at the DNA level, it is virtually impossible to identify such women as carriers of an X-linked mutation. On the other hand, some females heterozygous for an X-linked mutation will have more abnormal than normal cells, and such women may exhibit mild symptoms of the X-linked disorder which are usually observed only in males. Female carriers of the X-linked mutation that causes Duchenne's muscular dystrophy (DMD) illustrate this point. DMD is a common X-linked recessive condition almost completely penetrant by five years of age in males who carry the mutation. The affected boys have very weak but paradoxically prominent muscles of the lower extremities. The muscle weakness is progressive and eventually becomes quite generalized, affecting both skeletal and cardiac muscle. Affected males are often confined to a wheelchair by 10 years of age and usually die in the second decade owing to cardiac and/or respiratory complications. The primary defect resulting in this disease is unknown. While females are generally not affected by the DMD mutation, some mothers of boys with this disorder do show mild calf muscle hypertrophy and limb girdle muscle weakness, presumably due to skewing of the X-chromosome inactivation process leading to higher proportion of mutant muscle cells in such women.

As discussed above, in many cases it is difficult to determine whether or not the mother of an isolated male with an X-linked disorder is a carrier of the mutant gene. However, if the disease is lethal in males prior to the reproductive years, as is the case for DMD, and if the spontaneous mutation rate is assumed to be equal in males and females, then approximately one third of isolated affected males should be due to new mutations, while two thirds of isolated affected males will have mothers who are heterozygous carriers of the mutant allele. For X-linked recessive disorders such as hemophilia A, in which affected males survive to reproduce, the proportion of isolated cases in which the mother is a carrier of the mutation will be even higher.

MULTIFACTORIAL GENETIC DISEASE

Many inherited diseases do not result from the effects of a single defective gene but are due to the interaction between alleles at many different genetic loci. Such disorders are called polygenic as opposed to single gene diseases. When environmental factors also play a major role, such disorders are termed "multifactorial." Most common birth defects, including congenital heart disease, cleft lip and palate, and spina bifida, as well as many common chronic diseases, such as diabetes mellitus and atherosclerotic heart disease, are multifactorial disorders.

The genetic influences in multifactorial disease are best documented by twin studies. In general, if one member of a pair of identical twins has a multifactorial disorder, such as congenital heart disease, then in 30 to 50 per cent of cases, the other twin will have the same disorder. In contrast, when one member of a pair of nonidentical twins, which share only half of their genes in common, has such a disease, the concordance rate is only 1 to 5 per cent in the other twin. Although such studies demonstrate the importance of genetic factors in these diseases, the fact that identical twins are not always concordant for a multifactorial disorder, even though they have the same genetic endowment, illustrates that environmental factors as well as genetic factors play an important role in multifactorial disease.

Multifactorial diseases are determined by the interaction of many different genetic alleles with each other and with the environment. The inheritance pattern of these disorders is therefore complex. The precise number of genes involved in any given multifactorial disorder is unknown; this makes it impossible to determine accurately the recurrence risk as is done for single gene disorders. As a result, recurrence risks for multifactorial disorders are derived from empirical data, rather than from a theoretical treatment of gene segregation. Such empirical data demonstrate a number of basic principles:

1. The more genes an individual shares in common with a family member who has a given multifactorial disease, the higher the probability that the individual will develop the same disease. Since the parents, offspring, and sibs of an affected individual are all first degree relatives, sharing one half of their genes in common, each of these relatives has a similar empirical risk for developing the disease. Second degree relatives, who include grandparents, aunts, and uncles, will share only one fourth of their genes with the affected individual, and thus will have a much lower chance of having the disease. For most multifactorial disorders, first degree relatives of an affected individual have a 5 to 10 per cent risk for developing the disorder.

2. The more first degree relatives who are affected with a given disorder, the higher is the recurrence risk for the individual in question. For instance, while the recurrence risk for spina bifida is approximately 4 per cent for individuals who have one affected sib, this risk rises to 10 to 12 per cent if two sibs are affected.

3. For many multifactorial disorders, differences in severity, sex, and ethnicity influence the recurrence risk. When an affected individual is a member of the sex or ethnic group that is less commonly affected by a specific disorder, he or she is more likely to possess a larger number of alleles that contribute to the multifactorial disorder and will be more likely to transmit the disorder to offspring. Similarly, those individuals more severely affected with a particular disorder are more likely to have relatives with a similar disease than are mildly affected individuals.

Although multifactorial diseases clearly have a genetic component, the genetic information that exists is not very helpful either for diagnosing or for understanding the mechanisms that lead to these diseases.

DIAGNOSIS AND TREATMENT OF GENETIC DISEASE

GENETIC COUNSELING

Genetic counseling is that aspect of medical practice dealing with the human problems associated with the occurrence, or the risk of occurrence, of a genetic disorder in an individual or a family. The principles of genetic counseling, which are essentially those used in any medical decision making process, include diagnosis, communication, and delineation of the available options. The process of genetic counseling involves an attempt to help the family (1) to comprehend the medical facts, including the diagnosis, the probable course of the disorder, and the available management; (2) to appreciate the way in which heredity contributes to the disorder and the risk of recurrence in specific relatives; (3) to understand the options for dealing with the risk of recurrence; (4) to choose the course of action that seems appropriate to them in view of their risk and their family goals and act in accordance with that decision; and (5) to make the best possible adjustment to the disorder in an affected family member and/or the risk of recurrence of that disorder. The goal of genetic counseling is not necessarily the prevention of genetic disease, although this frequently turns out to be the desire of the individual who comes for counseling. The role of the genetic counselor should be that of a provider of information. One of the reasons for this nondirective approach is that many of the decisions that need to be made are based on moral, philosophical, or religious rather than medical issues.

The single most important step in the process of genetic counseling is to obtain a correct diagnosis. Because of the notorious heterogeneity of genetic diseases, this is often not an easy task. The counselor must obtain a complete medical history, physical examination, and laboratory evaluation of the affected individuals as well as those at risk. There are some genetic disorders that have such characteristic and specific symptoms that the diagnosis is unequivocal and the mode of inheritance can be inferred from previous knowledge about the disease in other families. In many cases, however, an unambiguous diagnosis can be made only after both the phenotype and the mode of inheritance of the disorder have been determined in the particular family being counseled.

Once a diagnosis and a mode of inheritance have been documented for a disorder within the family in question, the next step is to determine the genotype of the individual who has come for counseling (i.e., the consultand). This genotype is usually inferred from the diagnosis, when the consultand is affected with the disorder, or from the family history, as when the father of the consultand has an X-linked recessive disorder. For some genetic diseases, laboratory data such as a karyotype or enzyme level on cultured skin fibroblasts may provide sufficient information as to the genotype of the consultand. Despite these several sources of information, however, the genotype of the consultand cannot always be determined with certainty. If the genotype of the consultand can be determined, the counselor then outlines the recurrence risks for the consultand and/or for specific relatives of the consultand, and delineates the options available for dealing with these risks. For instance, consider a couple who comes for counseling because they had a child with Tay-Sachs disease. Based on this diagnosis and family history, both parents are carriers of the Tay-Sachs mutation and have a 25 per cent chance, with each subsequent pregnancy, of having a child with Tay-Sachs disease. This disorder can be diagnosed prenatally (see below), but at present no effective treatment for Tay-Sachs disease is available. Since this couple wants to have further children, but only if they can be certain they will not have another child with Tay-Sachs disease, the options open to them are (1) prenatal diagnosis, with termination of the pregnancy if the fetus is affected with Tay-Sachs disease, (2) artificial insemination, and (3) adoption. The option that is most appropriate will depend on the particular family being counseled.

PRENATAL DIAGNOSIS

Prenatal diagnosis of genetic disorders and other birth defects has developed into one of the most powerful tools of the medical geneticist. Beginning with the diagnosis of chromosomal abnormalities and a limited number of enzyme deficiencies, the scope of prenatal diagnosis has now grown to include over 100 inborn errors of metabolism, over 30 other single gene disorders, and a rapidly increasing number of structural abnormalities with multifactorial etiologies. In this discussion emphasis will be given to new methods that are being developed, beyond those of chromosomal karyotyping and specific enzyme assays.

Amniocentesis. Amniotic fluid can be aspirated transabdominally from the uterus at 16 weeks of gestation. This provides a safe technique that can be used to diagnose a number of genetic disorders at a stage of gestation early enough to terminate the pregnancy if the fetus is found to be affected. The risk of spontaneous abortion due to amniocentesis is considerably less than 1 per cent. Nevertheless, this procedure is generally not performed unless the information gained from the study will be critical to any decision that the potential parents make concerning the continuation or termination of that pregnancy. Both the amniotic fluid itself and cultured cells derived from the fluid are useful for prenatal diagnosis, the latter most frequently. Since these cells are derived from the fetus, they accurately reflect the genetic constitution of the fetus and can be used to determine whether or not a fetus at risk for a given genetic disease has inherited that disease.

It is usually a straightforward matter to determine if a fetus has a chromosomal abnormality by simply karyotyping the amniotic fluid cells. However, it is frequently not so easy to determine if a fetus at risk for a genetic disorder caused by gene mutation has inherited that disease. Prenatal diagnosis by analyzing the cells for the presence of the mutant gene product depends upon two variables: (1) the basic defect of the disease in question must be known, and (2) the gene must be normally expressed in amniotic fluid cells. Using such an approach, many genetic inborn errors of metabolism can be detected by assaying for specific enzyme activities.

Direct Analysis of Abnormal Gene Structure. Unfortunately, not all genes are expressed in amniotic fluid cells. For instance, the gene coding for phenylalanine hydroxylase, the defective enzyme in PKU, is expressed only in liver, while the genes coding for the α and β chains of hemoglobin are expressed only in erythroid cells. Thus, even though the basic defects leading to PKU and thalassemia are known, it is not possible to diagnose these disorders by assaying for the mutant gene products in amniotic fluid cells. The advent of the techniques of modern molecular biology, however, make it possible to detect alterations in gene structure directly at the level of DNA. It is now possible to use DNA from amniotic fluid cells to diagnose genetic disorders even when the mutant gene products are not expressed in amniotic cells. In this technique restriction enzymes that cleave DNA at specific nucleotide sequences are used as well as a gel electrophoresis blotting technique called "Southern blotting." It further requires the availability of a radioactive piece of DNA or "probe" with a base sequence like that of the gene to be analyzed. Each restriction enzyme recognizes a specific sequence of four or six bases in double-stranded DNA and cleaves the DNA at those positions where the specific recognition sequence is present. There are hundreds of different restriction enzymes, and each has its own recognition sequence. These enzymes are therefore extremely useful reagents for cutting the large DNA molecules that make up the human genome into thousands of smaller reproducible pieces that vary in size. One of the more commonly used restriction enzymes is designated Eco RI. If the gene of interest, for example the gene coding for the β chain of hemoglobin, does not contain any recognition sites for Eco RI, then when total genomic human DNA is cut with Eco RI, the β globin gene will be present on a single DNA fragment whose length is defined by the position of the Eco RI recognition sites that flank the gene.

In order to distinguish the DNA fragment that contains the β globin gene from all the other fragments of genomic DNA, one uses the Southern blotting procedure. This technique involves the separation of genomic DNA fragments according to size by electrophoresis on an agarose gel. Since the gel is difficult to work with, the fragments are transferred or "blotted" to a sheet of nitrocellulose filter paper, retaining the same array that they had in the gel, with the largest fragments at the top and the smallest fragments at the bottom. The specific fragment containing the β globin gene is then identified using a radioactive probe with a complementary nucleotide sequence to a portion of the β globin gene, taking advantage of the fact that a single strand of denatured DNA will renature with another single strand to form a double-stranded molecule only if the second strand has a complementary base sequence to the first (see the discussion of DNA structure). The double-stranded DNA fragments in the gel are denatured into single strands (without changing their position in the gel) prior to transfer to the nitrocellulose filter. Therefore, when the denatured, single-stranded radioactive probe is placed on the filter under conditions that allow single-stranded DNA to renature into double-stranded molecules, the probe will bind only to the particular DNA fragment on the filter that contains the β globin gene. Following such "hybridization," the filter is washed, dried, and exposed to x-ray film, which reveals a band at the position on the filter where the radioactive probe hybridized to the β globin gene DNA fragment (Fig. 36).

Direct analysis of abnormal gene structure was first used to diagnose disorders resulting from gene deletion. Certain lethal forms of thalassemia, which are inherited in an autosomal recessive fashion, are due to deletion of all copies of the gene coding for the α chain of hemoglobin. Therefore, prenatal diagnosis of

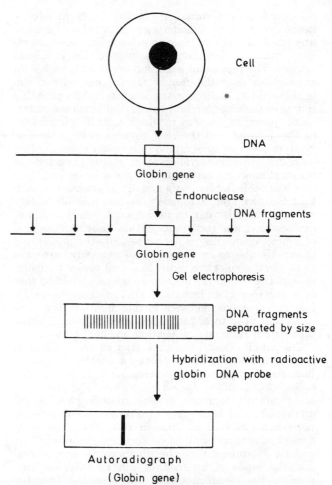

Figure 36. Visualization of globin genes. DNA from any cell nucleus is chemically prepared. This DNA will contain the globin genes. Various restriction endonucleases will break up the DNA into many fragments. Different endonucleases recognize different sequences of nucleotides. The DNA fragments are separated on gel electrophoresis by size. A specific radioactive DNA probe for globin is prepared and reacted with the DNA fragments. Hybridization of the radioactive globin probe occurs with a globin gene and can be visualized following radioautography. (From Vogel, F., and Motulsky, A. G.: Human Genetics: Problems and Approaches. 2nd ed. Berlin, Springer-Verlag, 1982, p. 251.)

a fetus at risk for this type of α thalassemia can be performed by simply analyzing Eco RI–digested fetal DNA prepared from amniotic fluid cells for the presence of α gene–specific DNA fragments as described above. If no such fragments are found, then the fetus is homozygous for the α gene deletion and will have the disease.

Prior to the development of this direct analysis of α globin genes, the prenatal diagnosis of α thalassemia required the study of α globin protein synthesis in fetal blood samples obtained by a procedure called fetoscopy (see below). Given the limited availability of fetoscopy and the 5 per cent risk of fetal loss associated with this technique even in experienced centers, the ability to diagnose α thalassemia using fetal DNA prepared from amniotic fluid cells represents a significant technical advance. Not only is amniocentesis a safer and more reliable procedure than fetoscopy, but the analysis of α-specific DNA fragments in fetal DNA is much simpler than the measurement of α globin chain synthesis in fetal blood.

The majority of human β globin genetic diseases, including sickle cell anemia, are presumably due to point mutations rather than deletions. An assay more specific than that just described is required for the prenatal diagnosis of these disorders. Such an assay using fetal DNA and restriction endonuclease analysis is now available which allows for the prenatal diagnosis of virtually all cases of sickle cell anemia. This assay is based on the use of the restriction enzyme Mst II, which cleaves DNA at the sequence CCTNAGG (i.e., N indicates that the base at this position in the sequence can be any of the four bases present in DNA). In the normal β globin gene (β^A), this sequence occurs in the region coding for amino acids 5, 6, and 7 (CCT-GAG-GAG: Pro Glu Glu) as well as at positions 1.15 Kb 5' and 0.2 Kb 3' from that site (i.e., 1 Kb = 1000 bases). The sickle mutation converts the DNA sequence in the region coding for amino acids 5, 6, and 7 to CCTGTGGAG, thereby replacing valine for glutamic acid at position 6 of the β globin protein and at the same time abolishing the Mst II recognition site in this region of the gene. Whereas Mst II digestion of the normal β globin gene will result in two DNA fragments 1.15 Kb and 0.2 Kb in length, similar digestion of a mutated sickle gene (β^S) produces only a single fragment 1.35 Kb in length. Thus, using the 1.15 Kb Mst II β globin gene fragment as a radioactive probe with Southern blot analysis, Mst II–digested DNA from individuals with two normal β^A genes will contain a single 1.15 Kb DNA fragment that reacts with the probe. DNA from individuals with two β^S genes will contain a single 1.35 Kb DNA fragment, and DNA from heterozygotes for the sickle mutation will contain both the 1.15 Kb and the 1.35 Kb fragments. In the short time that this assay has been available, it has proven to be a rapid, sensitive, and accurate technique for the prenatal diagnosis of sickle cell anemia.

Development of the Mst II assay has been a major breakthrough in the prenatal diagnosis of sickle cell anemia, but the probability that similar assays will be developed for other genetic disorders resulting from point mutations is low. Not only must the point mutation alter a restriction endonuclease recognition site, but the fragments produced must differ in size and be large enough to be detected. In light of these considerations, an additional assay for the prenatal diagnosis of sickle cell disease has been developed that provides a general method for the diagnosis of any genetic disease involving a point mutation, provided that the change in the DNA sequence caused by the mutation is known. This alternate approach involves the synthesis of two oligonucleotides, each 19 bases long, one complementary to the normal β^A gene and one complementary to the β^S gene. The site of the sickle mutation is placed near the center of the sequences in order to maximize thermal instability of mismatch hybridization. Although differing by only a single base, these oligonucleotides, when radioactively labeled and used as probes, can distinguish the normal β globin gene from the sickle cell gene. The advantage of this general approach is that oligonucleotide sequences can be designed and synthesized precisely according to need, eliminating dependence on a restriction enzyme recognition site alteration, as in the case of the Mst II assay. This oligonucleotide approach has already been used to synthesize probes that can detect the single base change that causes α_1 antitrypsin deficiency, and these probes have been used successfully to diagnose α_1 antitrypsin deficiency prenatally by direct analysis of fetal DNA.

Restriction Fragment Length Polymorphisms. Direct analysis of abnormal gene structure has led to remarkable advances in the prenatal diagnosis of a few human genetic diseases. This approach, however, requires knowledge of primary genetic defects at the nucleotide level. Unfortunately, for many human genetic diseases, such as cystic fibrosis or Duchenne muscular dystrophy, we do not yet know the primary gene product, let alone the precise molecular basis of the mutation. Thus, a different approach must be used for the prenatal diagnosis of the vast majority of human genetic diseases. With the discovery that 1 to 2 per cent of the nucleotides in regions of human DNA not coding for protein are polymorphic, resulting in individual variation in the location of recognition sites for restriction endonucleases, it has been proposed that random, single-copy human DNA sequences could be used as probes to detect restriction fragment length polymorphisms (RFLPs) tightly linked to genes that result in human disease. Such RFLPs could then serve as genetic markers for the prenatal diagnosis of linked genetic diseases. The most attractive feature of such an approach is that it would enable one to use fetal DNA obtained from amniotic fluid cells to diagnose any single gene disorder prenatally, without requiring knowledge of the basic genetic defect. However, the disadvantage of prenatal diagnosis by linkage analysis is that it will be incomplete and complicated due to such factors as genetic recombination (see discussion of linkage analysis). In order for prenatal diagnosis by RFLP linkage analysis to become generally useful, a large number of polymorphic RFLPs, distributed so as to saturate the entire human genome, must be isolated. Although this will be a formidable task, strategies for efficiently detecting and characterizing RFLPs have already been devised. It is encouraging that over a very short time, numerous human RFLPs have been identified, one of which is tightly linked to the Huntington's chorea locus and two which flank the Duchenne muscular dystrophy locus. In the very near future, prenatal diagnosis of these disorders by linkage analysis may become available.

Visualization of the Fetus. Linkage analysis using RFLPs should allow the prenatal diagnosis of a large number of human single gene disorders even when the basic genetic defect is unknown, but this approach is not useful for the prenatal diagnosis of multifactorial diseases. Other techniques, such as *ultrasonography*, that allow direct visualization of the fetus are already being used for the prenatal diagnosis of neural tube defects and, in some instances, of congenital heart disease. Measurement of α-fetoprotein levels in amniotic fluid, combined with a careful ultrasonographic examination of the fetus provides a safe, sensitive, and specific technique for the prenatal diagnosis of both spina bifida and anencephaly. *Fetoscopy*, the technique of direct fetal visualization using a fiberoptic endoscope, has already proven useful for fetal blood sampling, fetal skin biopsy, and fetal surface examination. The 5 per cent risk of spontaneous abortion associated with this technique, coupled with the fact that it can be used only to visualize surface structures, has generally made ultrasonography the technique of choice for fetal visualization.

Fetal Chorionic Biopsy. Amniocentesis has to be performed in the second trimester; the technique of fetal chorionic biopsy now being developed allows one to obtain fetal tissue samples in the first trimester of pregnancy. This technique would be of great benefit in terms of both a reduced waiting period for results and a safer method of abortion, if that proves to be necessary. In chorionic biopsy a small catheter is passed into the uterine cavity, under sonographic control, at 8 to 12 weeks of gestation to aspirate a sample of villi from the chorion under the decidua capsularis. Since these villi are normally lost by 14 to 15 weeks of pregnancy, their removal should theoretically cause no harm to the fetus. This technique holds great promise, particularly for those diseases diagnosable by DNA analysis, but experience is currently too limited to evaluate its safety or reliability.

TREATMENT OF GENETIC DISEASE

Mutant genes can lead to disease by a large number of different mechanisms, as illustrated in the preceding pages. Thus, any logical approach to treatment of a particular genetic disease requires some knowledge of the pathophysiology of that disorder. Five general approaches have been used to treat patients with genetic disease: (1) replacement of a mutant protein with the normal gene product, (2) alteration of a mutant protein to restore its function, (3) removal or reduction of a toxic compound accumulated as a result of a mutant gene product, (4) replacement of a deficient end product, and (5) replacement of a defective organ. A few examples of these approaches will be described below.

Replacement of a Mutant Protein. The replacement of a defective gene product with a normal product has proved successful for several inherited diseases. In hemophilia A, the deficiency of functional clotting factor VIII can be overcome by the administration of fresh plasma or cryoprecipitate containing normal factor VIII.

In adenosine deaminase deficiency, normal adenosine deaminase (ADA) can be given to individuals with an inherited deficiency of that enzyme by transfusions with normal, irradiated erythrocytes. Deoxyadenosine accumulates in ADA-deficient patients and is toxic to lymphocytes, resulting in immunodeficiency. However, following transfusion of such patients with normal erythrocytes, the deoxyadenosine enters the infused erythrocytes containing normal ADA, where it is deaminated and therefore detoxified by the normal enzyme. Although this approach to replacing the defective enzyme is only temporary, the immunocompetency of a number of patients with ADA deficiency has been regained at least for a year or two by monthly infusions. ADA deficiency is discussed more extensively in Section III.

Restoration of Biological Activity of a Mutant Protein. In general, attempts to treat enzyme deficiency diseases by infusions of normal enzyme have met with limited success. More effective treatment has resulted from attempts to increase the residual biological activity of the mutant enzyme. Some defective enzymes exhibit reduced affinity for a cofactor required for normal catalytic activity and thus function poorly at normal cofactor concentrations. By increasing the cofactor concentration, one can overcome the reduced affinity of the enzyme and restore normal biological activity. A classic example is the control of seizures by the administration of high doses of pyridoxine to infants with an inherited deficiency of the enzyme glutamate decarboxylase. Pyridoxal phosphate is an essential cofactor in the enzymatic conversion of glutamic acid to the inhibitory neurotransmitter γ-aminobutyric acid (GABA). Patients with a deficiency of glutamate decarboxylase activity due to a reduced affinity of the enzyme for pyridoxal phosphate have a deficiency of GABA, which is thought to predispose the brain to hyperirritability and seizures. Treatment with high doses of pyridoxine restores glutamate decarboxylase activity as well as brain GABA concentrations, controlling the seizures. A number of other so-called vitamin-dependency syndromes have been described in which very large amounts of a vitamin are necessary for normal enzymatic activity.

Removal or Reduction of a Toxic Compound. Dietary treatment has been effectively used in a number of genetic diseases to reduce toxic compounds that accumulate as a result of mutant gene products. Treatment of patients with phenylketonuria with diets deficient in phenylalanine reduces the hyperphenylalaninemia and prevents the mental retardation that otherwise results from the elevated phenylalanine levels. Toxic compounds can also be reduced by the administration of specific drugs, as in the case of patients with cystinuria. Administration of penicillamine to such patients results in the formation of complexes between penicillamine and the excess cystine in the urine. Since these complexes are much more soluble than cystine itself, the tendency to form cystine stones is reduced.

Replacement of a Deficient End Product. An example lies in the standard means of treating patients with congenital adrenal hyperplasia resulting from an enzymatic deficiency of adrenal steroidogenesis. As a result of the inherited enzyme deficiency, the level of cortisol, the end product of the metabolic pathway, is decreased in patients with congenital adrenal hyperplasia. This results in a secondary overproduction of ACTH, which leads to excessive synthesis of steroid precursors proximal to the enzyme defect, as well as to accumulation of the products of those adrenal hormones whose synthesis is not blocked by the enzymatic defect. Ambiguous genitalia at birth due to overproduction of adrenal steroids is a prominent clinical feature of the disorder. All of these metabolic abnormalities can be corrected simply by supplying cortisol, the deficient end product. As another example, hereditary orotic aciduria can be successfully treated by the oral administration of uridine, supplying a source of pyrimidine nucleotides beyond the site of the block in synthesis.

Replacement of a Defective Organ. This approach has been used to treat a number of genetic diseases.

The transplantation of normal kidneys into patients with polycystic kidney disease has been carried out with considerable success, prolonging life and alleviating signs and symptoms of the disease. In addition, organs of the immune system, such as the thymus, have been transplanted into individuals with inherited immunodeficiency diseases with successful reconstitution of immune competency.

To date, no human genetic disease has been successfully treated by replacement or repair of a defective gene. However, the potential for such treatment exists through future advances in molecular genetics.

REFERENCES

Cavalli-Sforza, L. L., and Bodmer, W. F.: The Genetics of Human Populations. San Francisco, W. H. Freeman and Co., 1971.

de Grouchy, J., and Turleau, C.: Clinical Atlas of Human Chromosomes. 2nd ed. New York, John Wiley and Sons, 1984.

Emery, A. E. H., and Rimoin, D. L. (eds.): Principles and Practice of Medical Genetics. Edinburgh, Churchill Livingstone, 1983.

Epstein, C. J., Cox, D. R., Schonberg, S. A., et al.: Recent developments in the prenatal diagnosis of genetic diseases and birth defects. Annu Rev Genet 17:48, 1983.

McKusick, V. A.: Heritable Disorders of Connective Tissue. 5th ed. St. Louis, The C. V. Mosby Co., 1978.

McKusick, V. A.: Mendelian Inheritance in Man. Catalogs of Autosomal Dominant, Autosomal Recessive, and X-linked Phenotypes. 6th ed. Baltimore, The Johns Hopkins University Press, 1983.

Murphy, E. A., and Chase, G. A.: Principles of Genetic Counseling. Chicago, Year Book Medical Publishers, 1975.

Smith, D. W.: Recognizable Patterns of Human Malformation: Genetic, Embryologic, and Clinical Aspects. 3rd ed. Philadelphia, W. B. Saunders Co., 1982.

Stanbury, J. B., Wyngaarden, J. B., Fredrickson, D. S., et al.: The Metabolic Basis of Inherited Disease. 5th ed. New York, McGraw-Hill Book Co., 1983.

Vogel, F., and Motulsky, A. G.: Human Genetics: Problems and Approaches. Berlin, Springer-Verlag, 1982.

SECTION III

IMMUNOLOGY

EDWARD J. GOETZL, M.D.,
and JOHN D. STOBO, M.D.

A. Introduction

The human immune system encompasses the principal pathways by which individuals respond adaptively to foreign and endogenous challenges. The proteins of the immune system comprise 20 to 25 per cent of the total concentration of plasma proteins, and the cells that participate in the system constitute approximately 15 per cent of body cells. The types of immune responses generally are considered in terms of *immunity,* which is a beneficial reaction of the host to foreign or non-self elements and a mechanism for the eradication of abnormal host cells, and *hypersensitivity,* which is a detrimental manifestation of immunity and may be directed to components of the host as a consequence of the similarity of host and non-self elements. An understanding of immune responses, as well as inherited and acquired disorders of these responses, requires attention to both the recognition mechanisms, typified by sites for antigen binding on antibodies and lymphocytes, and the effector pathways, such as complement proteins and cytotoxic lymphocytes, which are recruited to deal with the perceived threats to the host. The time course of immune responses is also a basis for classification. The immediate hypersensitivity reaction to proteins of pollens or stinging insect venoms begins within seconds of the challenge, whereas the delayed hypersensitivity to *Mycobacterium tuberculosis* or poison ivy is manifested only after 24 to 48 hours. The effectiveness of immune responses of host defense is in part attributable to cooperative interactions with the simpler and less adaptable natural defenses, such as mucosal barriers, the reticuloendothelial system, and the alternative pathway of complement. For example, both microbial organisms and damaged host erythrocytes are recognized with great sensitivity and removed with higher efficiency by the reticuloendothelial system when they are coated with antibodies that accelerate cell contact and facilitate endocytosis.

The components of the immune system are presented in this chapter in the order of involvement in immune responses. First T lymphocytes or T cells, which detect soluble and cell-associated antigens, then antibody proteins, and B cells, which produce antibodies under the regulatory influence of T cells, are described. These primary cellular and molecular constituents of immune recognition have the capacity to initiate a specific response. Then the effector mechanisms recruited by antibodies such as the chemical mediators of mast cells and basophils, complement, and immune complexes are presented, and finally involvement of T cells in hypersensitivity and cytotoxicity is discussed. Examples of diseases mediated by the immune system or that develop as a result of immune deficiencies will be included in each section to emphasize the major points.

The enormous expansion of immunology as a basic biologic and clinical discipline in the past two decades is evident both from the scope of this chapter and the immunologic content of other chapters. The applications of the diverse technologies of molecular and cellular genetics, cell biology, and biochemistry have contributed to and benefited from the explosion of knowledge in immunology. The intent of the authors is to provide both the essential tools and a framework for the growth of understanding of immunology for students of human biology and medicine. The chapter does not attempt an exhaustive compilation of comprehensive details, but should allow readers a general survey of current developments in immunology.

90

B.   Cells and Molecules of the Immune System

T Lymphocytes

ONTOGENY OF T CELLS (THYMUS-DERIVED LYMPHOCYTES)

Role of the Thymus

In the formation of T cells, stem cells from the bone marrow enter the thymic cortex and within the thymic microenvironment are induced to differentiate into relatively mature cells prior to their emigration into the peripheral lymphoid tissue. This stepwise differentiation, which takes approximately three days, occurs as thymocytes traverse the thymus from cortex to the medulla and is marked by changes in specific cell surface molecules (Table 1) as well as by changes in function (Fig. 1). Within the cortex, thymocytes exist as a single line of cells bearing the T markers T11, T10, T8, T6, T4, and T1. The migration from cortex to medulla is accompanied by three important changes: (1) The lineage splits into two different lines, one of which displays T4 surface molecules but not T8 molecules (T4 positive, T8 negative), while the other displays T8 molecules but not T4 molecules (T4 negative, T8 positive). (2) Both lines of cells express a molecule, T3, not expressed on the majority of cortical thymocytes. (3) The T3-positive medullary thymocytes first exhibit functions characteristic of thymus-derived lymphocytes, suggesting that expression of T3 may be important for T cell activation. After undergoing further differentiation within the medulla, thymocytes emigrate to the peripheral lymphoid tissue where they can be generally divided into two broad populations, again based on the differential expression of the T4 and T8 markers. As indicated in Figure 1, both peripheral T cell populations share the T11, T3, and T1 molecules. One population (approximately 65 per cent of peripheral T cells) is T4 positive and T8 negative, while another (approximately 35 per cent of peripheral T cells) is T4 negative and T8 positive.

The thymic stromal cells (also referred to as thymic macrophages, or thymic nurse cells) play a critical role in T cell differentiation in at least two ways: (1) They release thymic hormones, which are required for full T cell maturation accompanied by the expression of new cell surface antigens and for the development of T cell function. (2) They imprint the ability to recognize products of genes in the major histocompatibility complex (MHC). As will be discussed subsequently, activation of peripheral T cells by antigens requires that they "see" not only the antigen itself but also products of genes in the MHC. In other words, activation of peripheral T cells requires at least two signals. One of

TABLE 1. SURFACE ANTIGENS USEFUL FOR EXPLORING HUMAN T CELL DIFFERENTIATION AND FUNCTION

ANTIGENS	MOLECULAR* WEIGHT	MONOCLONAL† ANTIBODY	% POSITIVE Thymocytes	Periph. T	COMMENTS
T11	55,000	OKT11 LEU-5	95	100	Assoc. with SRBC rosette receptor
T10	37,000	OKT10	95	5	Present on early stem cells, some B cells, activated periph. T cells
T9	190,000	OKT9	10	0	Transferrin receptor, present on activated T
T8	32,000 43,000	OKT8 LEU-2a LEU-2b	80	35	Present on cytotoxic/suppressor cells
T6	44,000	OKT6 LEU-6	70	0	Equivalent to murine TL antigen
T4	60,000	OKT4 LEU-3	75	65	Present on helper/inducer T cells
T3	20,000 23,000 26,000	OKT3 LEU-4	20	100	Assoc. with T cell receptor for antigen
T1	67,000	OKT1 LEU-1	95	100	Equivalent to murine Lyt-1 antigen

*All molecular weights are determined under nonreducing conditions, except T8, which is determined under reducing conditions.
†OK refers to monoclonal antibodies produced by Ortho Diagnostics Systems Inc., Raritan, NJ, and LEU to monoclonal antibodies produced by Becton-Dickinson FACS Systems, Sunnyvale, CA.

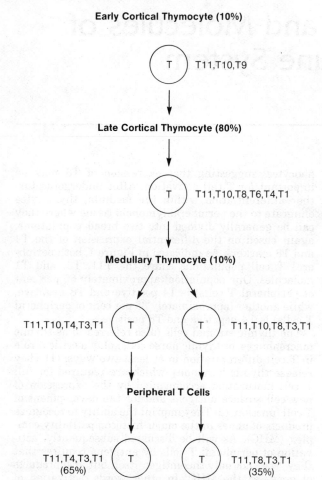

Early Cortical Thymocyte (10%)

T T11,T10,T9

Late Cortical Thymocyte (80%)

T T11,T10,T8,T6,T4,T1

Medullary Thymocyte (10%)

T11,T10,T4,T3,T1 T | T T11,T10,T8,T3,T1

Peripheral T Cells

T11,T4,T3,T1 T | T T11,T8,T3,T1
(65%) (35%)

Figure 1. T cell differentiation and expression of cell surface molecules. The display of the various T molecules (see Table 1) by cortical thymocytes, medullary thymocytes, and peripheral T cells is shown. The figures in parenthesis indicate the frequency of thymocytes or peripheral T cells at each stage of differentiation.

the signals is represented by antigen and the other is represented by MHC gene products (these products are referred to as class I or class II molecules). Recognition of either signal alone is not sufficient for T cell activation.

The ability of T cells to recognize self MHC molecules is acquired during their maturation within the thymus. The following illustration serves to emphasize this point. If animals of strain X are infected with virus Y, cytotoxic T cells are generated that demonstrate specificity for the virus seen in conjunction with the self MHC molecules. These cytotoxic T cells will not lyse cells from a different animal strain (e.g., Z) infected with the same virus. If, however, the thymus of strain X is removed and replaced with a thymus from strain Z animals, then virus-specific cytotoxic T cells appearing in the periphery will have specificity for the virus (Y) seen in conjunction with the strain Z and not the strain X MHC molecules. The MHC molecules that T cells view in conjunction with the antigen are those that are displayed on the surface of the stromal cells present in the thymic environment during differentiation. The thymic mechanism by which T cells are

taught to recognize self MHC gene products is still unclear.

Specificity of Peripheral Location

After emigration from the thymus the T cells move into the peripheral circulation and then into secondary lymphoid tissues such as the peripheral lymph nodes, spleen, and Peyer's patches. This migration into the secondary lymphoid tissue is mediated by specific interactions occurring between molecules on the surface of the lymphocytes and molecules on the surface of endothelial cells lining postcapillary, high endothelial venules (HEV) and is highly directed rather than random. For example, if lymphocytes from a peripheral lymph node are injected back into the circulation of an animal, they preferentially localize to the peripheral lymph nodes and not to the spleen or Peyer's patches. A comparable, preferential homing pattern of Peyer's patch lymphocytes to Peyer's patches and not to peripheral lymph nodes or spleen can be demonstrated. Treatment of the lymphocytes with enzymes that remove cell surface molecules destroys the specificity of their homing so that it is no longer directed but is random. A specific surface molecule is involved in the preferential homing of lymphocytes to peripheral lymph nodes, but is not present on the surface of Peyer's patch lymphocytes. A monoclonal antibody with specificity for this 80,000-dalton molecule blocks binding of lymphocytes to lymph node HEV but not to Peyer's patch HEV. Coating of the lymphocytes with antibody followed by injection into an animal inhibits the homing of lymphocytes to peripheral lymph nodes but not to Peyer's patches. These studies clearly support the notion that the recirculation patterns of lymphocytes in the periphery are mediated via cell surface recognition structures present on the surface of the lymphocytes and endothelial cells of HEV.

PHENOTYPIC AND FUNCTIONAL HETEROGENEITY AMONG PERIPHERAL T CELLS

Peripheral T cells participate in both effector and regulatory functions. Effector functions include such reactivities as delayed hypersensitivity and cytotoxicity, while regulatory functions include the ability of T cells to either help or suppress immune reactivities, including the differentiation of B cells into immunoglobulin-secreting plasma cells. These different functions do not represent the capabilities of a single clone of pluripotential T cells. Instead, discrete populations of T cells exist, each of which mediates a single or limited number of effector or regulatory functions. Moreover, these discrete functions correlate with the differential expression of the T molecules. Peripheral blood T cells can be broadly divided into two populations (Table 2 and Fig. 1): (1) Cells positive for T1, T3, T4, and T11 represent approximately 65 per cent of T cells, and (2) cells positive for T1, T3, T8, and T11 represent approximately 35 per cent of peripheral blood T cells.

These two populations can be further distinguished by differences in their effector and regulatory functions:

(1) The *T4-positive T cells*. This population contains

TABLE 2. PHENOTYPIC AND FUNCTIONAL HETEROGENEITY AMONG PERIPHERAL BLOOD T CELLS

	T CELL PHENOTYPE	
	$T1^+, T3^+, T4^+, T11^+$	$T1^+, T3^+, T8^+, T11^+$
FUNCTION	(65%)	(35%)
Effector cells for delayed hypersensitivity	+	−
Effector cells for cytotoxicity	−	+
Help for Ig synthesis	+	−
Help for cytotoxicity	+	−
Suppressor for Ig synthesis and delayed hypersensitivity	−	+
Inducer of suppressor	+	−

the effector cells required to initiate delayed hypersensitivity, T cells capable of helping B cells develop into immunoglobulin-secreting plasma cells, and T cells capable of inducing active suppressor cells that in turn inhibit immunoglobulin production. Functional subpopulations within the T4-positive cells differ in their display of other cell surface molecules. Approximately 80 per cent of the T4-positive population displays a molecule easily detectable by a circulating antibody present in the serum of some patients with active juvenile rheumatoid arthritis as well as a molecule reactive with the monoclonal antibody, OKTQ1. The remaining 20 per cent of the T4-positive T cells lack the marker depicted by the antibody present in the serum from patients with active juvenile rheumatoid arthritis and lack the TQ1 marker. Although both subpopulations of T4-positive cells contain helper cells for immunoglobulin synthesis, only the former and not the latter subpopulation contains T cells capable of inducing the generation of active suppressor cells.

(2) The *T8-positive T cells*. This population, in contrast, contains cytotoxic T cells as well as suppressor cells capable of directly inhibiting the differentiation of B cells into immunoglobulin-secreting plasma cells. The T8-positive population of T cells is also functionally and phenotypically heterogeneous. A portion of these cells can be induced to express a differentiation marker reactive with the monoclonal antibody, OKT20. This population contains cytotoxic cells. The T8-positive cells that lack the OKT20 marker do not contain the cytotoxic effector cells but do contain active suppressor cells.

THE MAJOR HISTOCOMPATIBILITY COMPLEX (MHC)

The genes of the major histocompatibility complex and their products play a critical role in both the initiation and subsequent regulation of immunity. The MHC contains genes whose products are transplantation antigens, which are displayed on the surface of nucleated cells, including cells involved in immune reactivity. These products are important in controlling immune reactivity. This link between transplantation antigens and immune reactivity can be understood better from a historical perspective. In the 1940s the

genetic locus in mice (H-2 locus of chromosome 17) that contained genes for transplantation antigens was identified. A few years later similar transplantation antigens were described in humans, coded for by genes in the HLA region of chromosome 6. In the 1960s Benacerraf demonstrated that the ability of an individual strain of rodents to produce either cell-mediated or antibody responses following immunization with simple, synthetic antigens was under genetic control. These immune response (Ir) genes were subsequently demonstrated to reside in the same genetic region that contained transplantation genes and to code for transplantation antigens. In the early 1970s it was found that killer T cells induced by virus infection can only lyse virally infected cells that share transplantation antigens with the killer T cells, i.e., the killer T cells must recognize two sets of determinants for them to exert their effect. One set of determinants is represented by the virus and the other set by transplantation antigens displayed on the surface of the virally infected cell. The primary function of transplantation antigens, therefore, is not to mediate graft rejection and frustrate transplantation surgeons. Instead they serve as a signpost that guides cellular interactions necessary for immunologic homeostasis. Indeed, this concept has been overriding in modern immunology.

The human MHC, termed the HLA locus, occupies a 3-centimorgan length of DNA on the short arm of chromosome 6 (Fig. 2). Based on differences in their structure and tissue distribution, the products of these genes can be divided into two major groups:

(1) *Class I molecules*. These molecules, coded for by genes in the HLA-A, B, and C loci, are 45,000-dalton glycoproteins that exist on the surface of all nucleated cells in association with a 13,000-molecular weight protein, beta$_2$ microglobulin. Only the 45,000-molecular weight chain of this bimolecular complex is encoded for by genes in the MHC. Beta$_2$ microglobulin is coded for by genes residing on chromosome 15.

Each of the three well-defined loci that code for the 45,000-molecular weight class I molecule contains many alleles in the general population: approximately 20 different forms of HLA-A genes, 30 different forms of HLA-B genes, and 8 different forms of HLA-C genes. A single individual can have a maximum of only two alleles for each gene. Differences in HLA-A, B, and C molecules, as well as differences in the product of different alleles of an individual locus, are reflected by differences in the amino acid sequence of the 45,000-dalton chain. Two individuals who have different HLA-A, B, and C alleles will have differences in the amino acid sequence of the HLA-A, B, and C molecules. In contrast, the amino acid sequence of beta$_2$ microglobulin is invariant in HLA-A, B, and C molecules from the same or even from different individuals. The differences in amino acid sequence in the heavy chain can be detected by using the sera from multiparous women, which contain antibodies to paternal class I molecules generated in response to repeated sensitization by fetal cells during pregnancy. Based on the reactivity of cells with these typing reagents it is possible to assign a numerical designation to specific HLA-A, B, and C molecules, i.e., HLA-A3, HLA-B5, HLA-C6. Class I molecules are inherited in a codominant fashion. Therefore, in any heterozygous individual six class I HLA molecules will be displayed on the

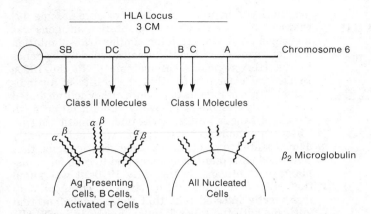

Figure 2. The human major histocompatibility complex. The human major histocompatibility complex, termed the HLA region, occupies a 3-centimorgan (*CM*) region of DNA on the short arm of chromosome 6. The HLA-A, B, and C loci contain genes coding for class I molecules, while the HLA-D, DC, and SB loci contain genes coding for class II molecules. B_2 microglobulin, which is associated on the cell surface with Class I molecules, is coded for by genes on chromosome 15.

surface of nucleated cells. Tissue typing in a heterozygote could reveal a profile such as HLA-A1, HLA-A2, HLA-B3, HLA-B5, HLA-C6, HLA-C7.

As noted previously, the specificity of cytotoxic effector T cells for virus-infected cells is not only for viral determinants but also for the host's own class I molecules. Interaction between the effector T cell and virus alone or between the effector T cell and cells bearing class I molecules alone is not sufficient to activate the cytolytic mechanism. The T cell must recognize both sets of determinants, i.e., virus plus class I, for cytotoxicity to ensue. The cytotoxic T cell receptor could theoretically consist of two distinct components, one of which recognizes virus and the other of which recognizes class I, or it could be a single component that recognizes a new determinant generated by interactions between virus and self class I molecules. This requirement for dual recognition perhaps prevents cytotoxic T cells from being inactivated by circulating free virus and ensures that the cytolytic mechanism will concentrate at the site of viral replication. The high degree of structural polymorphism of class I molecules, which are displayed on all nucleated cells, may afford protection against a large number of viruses. These molecules may direct the immune reaction against pathogens that can have tropism for a great number of different types of cells.

(2) *Class II molecules.* These molecules are coded for by genes in the HLA-D, HLA-DC, and HLA-SB loci. They also exist on the surface of cells as a bimolecular complex consisting of an alpha chain of 34,000 molecular weight and a beta chain of 29,000 molecular weight. In contrast to class I molecules, both chains of this bimolecular complex are coded for by genes in the MHC. Class II molecules are not present on every nucleated cell. They are displayed only on the surface of cells that participate in immune reactivity, including antigen-presenting cells (i.e., macrophages, dendritic cells), B lymphocytes, and activated T cells.

Class II molecules are coded for by genes in regions that are distinct from those coding for class I molecules. Each of three well-defined regions encodes for a distinct family of class II molecules, the HLA-DR, the HLA-DC, and the HLA-SB molecules, respectively. In a single individual, differences that distinguish each of the class II molecules from one another are reflected by differences in the amino acid sequence of the alpha and the beta chain. For example, the amino acid sequence of HLA-DC alpha and beta chains is different

from the amino acid sequence of HLA-DR alpha and beta chains. Differences that distinguish the class II molecules from one individual from the same class II molecules of another individual are reflected predominantly by differences in the amino acid sequence of the beta chain, although differences in the amino acid sequence of the alpha chain also exist.

The number of different alleles in the general population for class II genes appears to be less than that demonstrated for class I genes. To date there are ten different HLA-D alleles, approximately six HLA-DC alleles, and six HLA-SB alleles. The products of these alleles, reflected by differences in the amino acid sequence of the beta chain, can be depicted by antibodies present in the sera of multiparous women. For example, the ten serologically distinct HLA-DR molecules are designated by the numerals HLA-DR1 through HLA-DR10. Monoclonal antibodies are capable of depicting the products of different alleles in the HLA-DC locus and HLA-SB locus. As with class I genes, class II genes are inherited in a codominant fashion. Thus in a heterozygous individual, antigen-presenting cells, B cells, and activated T cells will display on their surface two different HLA-D, two different HLA-DC, and two different HLA-SB molecules.

Class II molecules have a structure and tissue distribution quite distinct from those of class I molecules, consistent with their distinct function of dictating interactions among immunocompetent cells. These are necessary both for the initiation and subsequent regulation of immunity rather than for controlling cytotoxicity. The class II molecules appear to be the products of the Ir genes, and therefore they are also called immune response-associated or Ia molecules. For example, a monoclonal antibody with specificity for class II molecules can inhibit immune reactivity, and slight changes in the amino acid sequence of the beta chain of class II molecules can drastically alter the immune response.

The mechanism by which Ir genes and class II molecules control immune reactivity is not known. Three hypotheses have been suggested:

(1) The Ia molecules control which antigen-reactive T cells appear in the periphery. Direct interactions between thymic epithelial cells bearing surface class II molecules and thymocytes play a crucial role in T cell maturation. This interaction may dictate which clones of antigen-reactive cells undergo intrathymic death and which undergo further maturation leading

to export into peripheral lymphoid tissue. The immune response of an animal can be altered by changing the class II molecules displayed in the thymic environment. Transplantation of the thymus from a strain of mice that is a responder to antigen X into a nonresponder strain results in peripheral T cells that react to antigen X. These T cells are derived from stem cells present in the bone marrow of the nonresponder recipient but that have developed in the environment of the donor responder thymus.

(2) Class II molecules influence immune reactivity by controlling the way antigen is presented to T cells. Antigen activation of T cells, such as effector T cells and helper T cells, requires recognition not only of the antigen but also of class II molecules displayed on the surface of the antigen-presenting cells. If an animal is a genetic nonresponder to antigen X, the class II molecules of the animal may not interact with antigen X in such a way as to be appropriately perceived by T cells. T cells from a nonresponder to antigen X can be activated by X when it is "seen" in conjunction with antigen-presenting cells from a responder strain of mice. Conversely, T cells from an X-responder animal are not activated when X is presented by antigen-presenting cells from an X-nonresponder animal.

(3) Class II molecules dictate the relative degree to which helper and suppressor cells are activated, rather than affecting the initiation of immunity. It is clear that net immune reactivity not only reflects the intrinsic capabilities of effector cells but also the balance between helper and suppressor influences capable of regulating that reactivity. In some situations immune unresponsiveness controlled by Ir genes reflects a predominance in suppressor influences rather than a failure to activate helper cells.

There are experimental data to support each of the three hypotheses for the mechanism by which Ir genes and their products, class II molecules, control immune reactivity. It is possible that the class II molecules exert their effect at each of the three levels suggested, i.e., development of antigen-reactive T cells, antigen presentation, and activation of regulatory cells, and that these effects may differ from antigen to antigen. Class II molecules are normally found only on cells that participate directly in immune reactivity, consistent with a primary function in both the initiation and the subsequent expression of immunity.

MHC GENES AND THE EXPRESSION OF DISEASE

Human response genes and their products have significant associations with specific clinical disorders. First studied were class I products of alleles in the HLA-A, B, and C molecules, which control cytotoxic cells and are not products of human Ir genes. Specific human class I molecules might be expected to be associated with certain viral infections but not with diseases dependent on a specific immune response. Indeed this appears to be the case. For example, during influenza infection effector T cells can be demonstrated whose cytotoxicity requires recognition of virus in conjunction with HLA-A and HLA-B determinants. Individuals in whom these cytotoxic T cells can be demonstrated appear to clear virus more effectively than individuals lacking these cytotoxic T cells.

The association between HLA-B27 and ankylosing spondylitis is the most striking association yet found between a human class I molecule and a disease. Neither the HLA-B27 molecule nor ankylosing spondylitis is found in Australian aborigines or African blacks. In contrast, 51 per cent of the Haida Indians in British Columbia are HLA-B27 positive, and 10 per cent of the adult Haida males have sacroiliitis. In Caucasians, approximately 8 per cent of the general population is HLA-B27 positive, whereas the frequency of HLA-B27 in Caucasians with ankylosing spondylitis is 90 per cent. This means that the relative risk of developing ankylosing spondylitis in Caucasians who are HLA-B27 positive is approximately 104. The relative risk is defined as the risk of developing a disease in an individual possessing a particular HLA antigen compared to the risk of developing the disease in an individual lacking the antigen. This is calculated using the following formula: per cent of patients with the antigen multiplied by the per cent of controls without the antigen/per cent of controls with the antigen multiplied by the per cent of patients without the antigen. The significance of this strong association between HLA-B27 and ankylosing spondylitis is unknown. Since spondylitis can be preceded by infection with enteric organisms it has been suggested that the B27 molecule is in some way important in the immune response to certain gram-negative organisms. This is unlikely, since class I molecules are involved in restricting cytotoxic T cell responses to viruses but not to bacteria. Hemochromatosis is the only other disorder so far found to have a significant association with a specific class I molecule (HLA-A3). While 18 to 31 per cent of control populations are HLA-A3 positive, 70 to 100 per cent of unrelated patients with idiopathic hemochromatosis have this same HLA phenotype. Why this genetic disorder of iron absorption exhibits this linkage is not known.

Class II molecules, the products of Ir genes, have been found to have a more significant association with specific clinical disorders than have class I molecules. Some of the most striking associations are outlined in Table 3. These findings suggest that genes linked to those coding for the associated HLA-DR molecule control immune reactivity to a specific antigen that is important in the expression of the disease. Thus the association between Goodpasture's disease and HLA-DR2 might indicate that genes linked to those coding for HLA-DR2 control reactivity to antigens present in glomerular and pulmonary basement membrane. While this is an attractive hypothesis it has not been proven for any of the diseases listed in Table 3.

Several different "autoimmune" disorders are associated with the HLA-DR3 phenotype, each of which is characterized by an immune response to a different self antigen (Table 3). This observation suggests that genes linked to those coding for HLA-DR3 may, in some way, code for immunologic hyperreactivity, i.e., increase the baseline immunologic reactivity to a level necessary for the generation of immunity to a self antigen, the specificity of which is dictated by some other factor. Normal HLA-DR3–positive individuals demonstrate enhanced cell-mediated and humoral im-

TABLE 3. ASSOCIATION BETWEEN HLA-DR TYPES AND DISEASE

DISEASE	DR PHENOTYPE	CONTROLS*%	% DR TYPE IN PATIENTS	RELATIVE RISK†
Goodpasture's syndrome	2	32	88	16
Buerger's disease	2	22	60	5
Multiple sclerosis	2	29	50	5
Myasthenia gravis	3	19	36	3
Graves' disease	3	21	54	5
Addison's disease	3	21	70	9
Chronic active hepatitis	3	19	78	14
Sjögren's syndrome	3	10	69	19
Systemic lupus erythematosus	3	22	54	5
Rheumatoid arthritis	4	20	60	5

*Different control series have shown moderate differences in the incidence of various DR phenotypes.

†The relative risk indicates the chance of developing the disease in an individual with the specific HLA-DR phenotype vs. the risk of developing the disease in an individual lacking the specific HLA-DR phenotype. See text for explanation.

munity when compared to HLA-DR3–negative individuals. Three observations suggest how this might occur: (1) Normal HLA-DR3–positive individuals lack a population of mitogen-induced suppressor cells capable of inhibiting immunoglobulin production. This suggests that genes linked to those coding for HLA-DR3 in some way prevent normal activation of suppressor cells. (2) Macrophages from HLA-DR3–positive individuals degrade antigens more slowly than do macrophages from HLA-DR3–negative subjects, suggesting that antigen may remain accessible to the immune system longer in HLA-DR3–positive subjects when compared to HLA-DR3–negative subjects. (3) Red cells coated with anti–red cell antibody are cleared less rapidly from the blood of normal HLA-DR3–positive individuals than from the blood of normal HLA-DR3–negative individuals. This observation suggests that the defect in HLA-DR3–positive individuals may be related to a relative inability to clear products of autoimmune responses.

Many diseases do not show a significant association with a specific HLA-DR phenotype. Possibly specific Ir genes, and therefore specific immune responses, do not influence the expression of the disease. On the other hand, Ir genes and specific immune responses may be associated with the disease but not depicted by a single, identifiable, HLA-DR reagent. In addition to the HLA-D locus the HLA-DC and HLA-SB loci also code for molecules that have the tissue distribution and structure of Ir gene products (Fig. 2). Serologic reagents capable of depicting distinct HLA-DC and HLA-SB molecules are not readily available.

The techniques of molecular biology have provided a useful way to examine the influence of Ir genes, specifically those in the HLA-SB and the HLA-DC regions, in the expression of diseases. cDNA probes capable of hybridizing with DR, DC, and SB alpha and beta chain genes have been developed and used to examine directly the structure of these Ir genes, utilizing a technique termed restriction mapping. In insulin-dependent diabetes an association between the disease and a specific restriction map has been noted. This technique has also been useful in delineating genetic polymorphisms associated with thalassemia, sickle cell anemia, and phenylketonuria, and will almost certainly be useful in delineating further associations between Ir genes and disease.

More than one Ir gene may be required for the

expression of disease; examples include insulin-dependent diabetes and herpes gestationis. Each disease shows a relatively low risk with either HLA-DR3 or HLA-DR4 alone. For example, the relative risk for developing insulin-dependent diabetes in individuals who are HLA-DR3 positive is 3.3 and in individuals who are HLA-DR4 positive is 4.4. When both the HLA-DR3 and the HLA-DR4 molecules are present, however, the relative risk of developing insulin-dependent diabetes increases dramatically to 34. Similarly, with herpes gestationis the risk of developing the disease is 5.5 in individuals who are HLA-DR3 positive, 1.1 in individuals who are HLA-DR4 positive, and 24.4 when both molecules are present. Therefore the expression of either disease is influenced most by having genes that are linked to those coding for both HLA-DR3 and HLA-DR4 as compared to having either gene alone.

T CELL ACTIVATION

T cell activation by antigen requires recognition of that antigen by receptors on the surface of the T cell. The structure of these T cell receptors is incompletely known; current data can be summarized as follows (Fig. 3): (1) The receptor is a heterodimer consisting of a 46,000 to 51,000 and a 40,000 to 43,000 chain linked by disulfide bonds on the T cell surface. This basic structure pertains to receptors isolated from either T4-positive helper or T8-positive cytotoxic T cell clones. (2) The alpha and beta chains of these receptors resemble immunoglobulin in having both variable and shared constant regions. (3) The receptor is coded for by genes distinct from those that code for immunoglobulins and MHC. (4) The receptor is noncovalently associated on the cell surface with the T3 molecule (Fig. 3). Indeed it appears that this association is important and necessary for T cell activation to occur. The role that the T3 molecule plays in activation is not known.

The T4 and T8 molecules may also participate in the antigen-induced activation of helper and suppressor/cytotoxic T cells, respectively. During primary immune responses, T4 and T8 increase the avidity with which the T cell can interact with the MHC molecules displayed by accessory or virally infected cells. During secondary responses the antigen receptor heterodimer itself is sufficient to cause high-avidity interactions, and the T4 and T8 complex are not necessary for T cell activation to proceed.

Activation of antigen-reactive T cells requires two signals. The first signal is the interactions between the T cell receptor and antigen plus MHC determinants (Fig. 4). The second signal is mediated by soluble materials. Accessory cells can provide both these signals. Examples of the accessory cells that can function in antigen processing and presentation include macrophages, dendritic cells, Langerhan cells of the skin, Kupffer cells of the liver, B cells, activated T cells, and, in some cases, endothelial cells.

Accessory cells can process and present antigen in conjunction with surface MHC determinants in a manner sufficient for this complex to be recognized by the T cell antigen receptor. This requires that the accessory cells display a sufficient density of Ia molecules on that surface. How antigens are "processed" by accessory cells has not been clarified. Some metabolic degradation may be required for processing large complex antigens, but does not seem to be required for small, simple antigens. Whether antigen presentation actually involves a physical association between surface Ia molecules and antigen determinants is also not known.

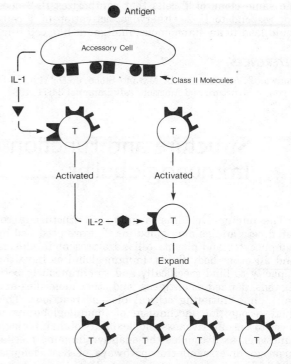

Figure 4. Events involved in the activation of T cells by soluble antigen. Activation of T cells by antigen requires recognition of antigen in conjunction with class II molecules as well as soluble materials such as interleukin-1 *(IL-1)* and interleukin-2 *(IL-2)*. (From Stobo, J. D.: Lymphocytes: Structure and function. *In* McCarty, D. J. (ed.): Arthritis and Allied Conditions: A Textbook of Rheumatology, 10th ed. Philadelphia, Lea & Febiger. In press: Reproduced with permission.)

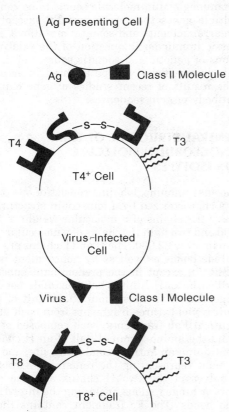

Figure 3. Molecules involved in T cell activation. The receptor for antigen plus class II or class I molecules displayed by T4- and T8-positive cells is a disulfide-linked heterodimer. The T3 complex, which consists of three molecules, is noncovalently associated with this receptor. The T4 and T8 molecules can participate in the recognition of class II and class I MHC molecules, respectively, and may be important in increasing the avidity of interaction between T cells and MHC-bearing cells.

Accessory cells also secrete soluble materials necessary for T cell activation. This secretion, which does not require expression of MHC molecules, includes the synthesis of interleukin-1 (IL-1), a 15,000-molecular weight polypeptide. IL-1 by itself cannot induce T cells to proliferate and to become activated; it must act in conjunction with another signal, that mediated by antigen plus MHC molecules. IL-1 may enhance T cell activation by (1) affecting the fluidity of the T cell membrane and thus increasing the accessibility of the antigen-binding receptor to the antigen-MHC complex, or (2) inducing synthesis of a second soluble material, interleukin-2 (IL-2), which enhances and expands T cell proliferation (Fig. 4). Formerly called T cell growth factor, IL-2 has a molecular weight of 17,000, and when added to T cells that express IL-2 receptors can initiate proliferation in the absence of any other signal. The activation of antigen-reactive T cells by antigen can be summarized as follows (Fig. 4): An antigen–class II molecule complex presented by accessory cells in conjunction with IL-1 initiates T cell activation. These activated cells then synthesize and secrete IL-2. This IL-2 acts on another clone of T cells of similar antigen specificity that has been induced by interactions with antigen and MHC determinants to display surface IL-2 receptors. The IL-2 then promotes expansion of this clone, which can manifest effector and regulatory functions. It is necessary to postulate that the same clone of T cells that synthesizes IL-2 does not respond to IL-2. Otherwise, activation of T cells could lead to an autonomous, malignant-like cell line.

REFERENCES

Gonwa, T. A., Peterlin, B. M., and Stobo, J. D.: Human Ir genes: Structure and function. Adv Immunol 34:71, 1983.

Reinherz, E. L., Meuer, S. L., and Schlossman, S. F.: The human T cell receptor: Analysis with cytotoxic T cell clones. Immunol Rev 74:83, 1983.

Reinherz, E. L., and Schlossman, S. F.: The differentiation and function of human T lymphocytes. Cell 19:821, 1980.

Thomas, Y., Rogozinski, L., and Chess, L.: Relationship between human T cell functional heterogeneity and human T cell surface molecules. Immunol Rev 74:113, 1983.

Structure and Function of Human Immunoglobulins

The immunoglobulins, a group of structurally related beta and gamma globulins that are produced by lymphocytes and plasma cells, are present in plasma and all other body fluids. Immunoglobulins have the capacity to bind specifically and simultaneously both ligands, defined as antigens, and other molecules and cells, thus initiating critical biologic reactions. This dual recognition mechanism of immunoglobulins is basic to the effectiveness and flexibility of their biologic functions, as it couples the adaptive immune mechanism to diverse effector pathways of host defense. Antibodies are immunoglobulins elicited in response to a definable antigenic challenge. Myeloma proteins and macroglobulinemia proteins are completely homogeneous immunoglobulins, termed monoclonal immunoglobulins, that are produced by abnormally proliferating clones of plasma cells or lymphocytes without apparent stimulation by antigen. The structure and functions of these monoclonal immunoglobulins, including an ability in some cases to bind antigen, are analogous to those of elicited antibodies. The recent development of techniques to fuse antibody-producing lymphocytes with myeloma plasma cells or other monoclonal immunoglobulin-producing cells in vitro has permitted the establishment of long term cultures of fused cells that produce monoclonal antibodies capable of recognizing the original antigen and others bearing the same determinant.

Immunoglobulins exhibit an unprecedented degree of molecular heterogeneity. They thus have become a model for the study of mechanisms of evolution of proteins and of the interplay of genetic and somatic factors in the determination of the diversity of proteins in any individual. It has been possible to begin to unravel the myriad structural variations that are fundamental to the observed differences in compartmental distribution, rates of turnover, antigenic specificities, and biologic activities of antibodies. The normal modulation of these critical functions of antibodies underlies their ability to contribute to host defense. Any disorders affecting antibody production or function may lead not only to failures in the humoral phases of defense, as in some immunodeficiency states, but also to production of inappropriate antibodies, as in some autoimmune diseases.

This section will focus on human immunoglobulin structure and function, both in normal humans and in relation to certain diseases, and will cite data from other species only when relevant human information is not available. General aspects of structure that apply to all immunoglobulins will be considered initially, followed by analysis of the bases for the definition of classes, subclasses, and several levels of genetic variation of immunoglobulins. The fine structure of the antigen-combining site common to all immunoglobulins will be presented. Biologic functions shared by all classes of immunoglobulins and those unique to a given class of immunoglobulins will be discussed in relation to differences in antibody structure. The synthesis of each immunoglobulin molecule seems to be controlled by multiple genes that are especially susceptible to DNA rearrangements and somatic mutations. Finally the classic immunologic question of the relative contributions of genetic and somatic sources of diversity of antibody specificity will be updated in accordance with the results of recent studies of gene expression and antibody protein sequences.

THE GENERAL STRUCTURE OF THE IMMUNOGLOBULIN MOLECULE AND ITS ISOTYPES

All normal immunoglobulins consist of one or more subunits characterized by a four-chain structure with two heavy (H) chains of a molecular weight of 50,000 to 70,000 and two light (L) chains of a molecular weight of approximately 22,000. The H and L chains are linked by disulfide bonds as well as by noncovalent interactions (Fig. 5), except in the predominant subclass of IgA_2, which lacks H-L interchain disulfide bonds. Papain digestion of the basic four-chain unit of immunoglobulins yields three fragments from each unit: (1) two identical Fab fragments, each composed of one L chain and the amino-terminal half of an H chain and each containing an antigen combining site, and (2) an Fc fragment representing the remaining carboxy-terminal halves of the two H chains and the joining segments or hinge regions, including the inter-H chain disulfide bonds. The Fc fragment contains the sites responsible for the mediation of most biologic functions. The exposure of immunoglobulins to pepsin at an acidic pH cleaves the basic immunoglobulin unit at a point distal to the hinge region and thus liberates a portion of the carboxy-terminal region that is smaller than the papain Fc fragment, and a bivalent section comparable to two papain-derived Fab fragments, which is termed the $F(ab')_2$. The successful cleavage

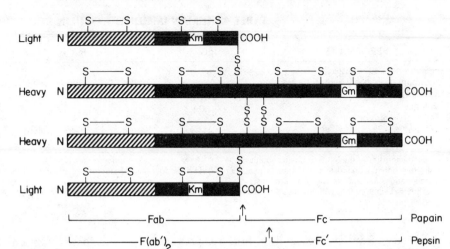

Figure 5. Linear representation of human κ IgG₁.

N = Amino-terminal end of polypeptide chain

COOH = Carboxy-terminal end of polypeptide chain

S—S = Disulfide bond

Km and *Gm* are genetic markers for κ and γ chains, respectively.

by papain of immunoglobulin units into one Fc and two Fab fragments in part reflects the conformational arrangement of these fragments as three compact regions of the native molecule connected by the flexible and exposed peptide segments of the hinge regions of the H chains.

There are two apparent subdivisions of L chains and four in H chains (Fig. 5), each such subdivision containing one intrachain disulfide bond that is highly conserved among the otherwise heterogeneous structures of immunoglobulins. The domain hypothesis of the structure of IgG, formulated by Edelman, proposes that the chains of the IgG molecule are composed of linear series of compact globular subdivisions, termed domains, which contain approximately 100 amino acids and are linked to each other by more loosely folded stretches of peptide chain. This model of immunoglobulin structure has been confirmed by x-ray crystallographic analyses (Fig. 6). The amino-terminal domain of the H chain and the amino-terminal domain of the L chain are homologous. Both amino-terminal domains exhibit several regions of extreme variability of sequence from one immunoglobulin to another, suggesting that they contain the contact amino acid residues of the antigen combining site of each Fab fragment. The term *variable region* has been applied to these domains of the heavy chain (V_H) and light chain (V_L) of IgG and other immunoglobulins. In contrast, the amino acid sequences of the carboxy-terminal domain of the light chains and the three or, in some immunoglobulins, four carboxy-terminal domains of the heavy chains exhibit far less variability among related immunoglobulins and thus have been termed the constant regions. The accepted domain nomenclature designates the constant region of the L chains as C_L and the contiguous domains in the constant region of the IgG H chains as $C\gamma_1$, $C\gamma_2$, and $C\gamma_3$, numbering from the variable region to the carboxy-terminus of the Fc fragment.

The x-ray crystallographic model of IgG (Fig. 6) supports the domain structural hypothesis in that it consists of two rounded cylindric Fab portions that are approximately four times the volume of the smaller cylindric $C\gamma_2$ domain to which each Fab is connected by the peptide chain of a flexible hinge piece. The hinge pieces of the two H chains are linked by disulfide

bonds, which vary for each subclass of immunoglobulin, as will be discussed. The glycosylated $C\gamma_2$ domains do not interact, but the $C\gamma_3$ domains interact strongly in a manner that stabilizes the structure of IgG. The details of the structure of the antigen combining site and of the localization within other domains of the many functions of immunoglobulins will be covered in subsequent sections. Importantly, the integrity of the structure of each domain appears to have evolved to perform certain specific and usually exclusive functions. This intramolecular differentiation represents the structural and evolutionary basis for the bifunctional potential of immunoglobulins, which links the

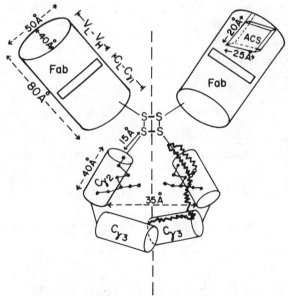

Figure 6. X-ray crystallographic model of the functional domains of human IgG₁.

S—S = Inter-heavy chain disulfide bond

⊙●⊙ = Intra-domain disulfide bond

ᗡᗡᗡ = Peptide chains outside the main globular domains

•—•—• = Carbohydrate chain

ACS = Antigen combining site

V = Variable region

C = Constant region

TABLE 4. HUMAN IMMUNOGLOBULIN STRUCTURE

PROPERTIES	CLASSES				
	IgG	IgA	IgM	IgD	IgE
Heavy chain subclasses	$\gamma_1, \gamma_2, \gamma_3, \gamma_4$	α_1, α_2	μ_1, μ_2	δ	ϵ
Sedimentation coefficient (S20, w)	7	7* (9, 11 . . .19)†	19	7	8
Molecular weight	150,000	160,000*	900,000	160,000	200,000
Valence	2	2*	10(5)	2	2
Secretory component	—	SIgA‡	—	—	—
J chain	—	Serum and secretory polymers	+	—	—
Carbohydrate content (% by weight)	2.5–3	7–10	10–12	10–13	10–11

*Characteristics of the IgA four-chain subunit.

†Serum polymers consisting of dimers to pentamers of the basic four-chain monomeric subunit exist at low concentrations in normal IgA and at higher concentrations in some IgA myeloma proteins.

‡SIgA = Secretory IgA, which consists of two monomeric units, a J chain, and a secretory component.

+ = present; − = absent.

specificity of antigen recognition to the expression of diverse effector functions constituting host defense.

The five major classes of human immunoglobulins, designated IgG, IgA, IgM, IgD, and IgE, differ in their antigenic, chemical, and physical properties (Table 4). The two H chains in an individual immunoglobulin subunit are identical and can be antigenically classified as γ, α, μ, δ, or ϵ. Likewise, each four-chain unit contains two identical L chains, which are antigenically of either the κ or λ serologic type. Therefore the molecular formulas of the monomeric units of the immunoglobulin classes are as follows: $\gamma_2\kappa_2$ or $\gamma_2\lambda_2$, $\alpha_2\kappa_2$ or $\alpha_2\lambda_2$, $\mu_2\kappa_2$ or $\mu_2\lambda_2$, $\delta_2\kappa_2$ or $\delta_2\lambda_2$, and $\epsilon_2\kappa_2$ or $\epsilon_2\lambda_2$. About 60 per cent of normal immunoglobulins possess κ chains and 30 to 40 per cent possess λ chains, whereas the distribution of H chains reflects the relative concentrations of each class in serum. There is some heterogeneity among the classes of H chains. Four subclasses of γ chains, two subclasses each of α and μ chains, and possibly two subclasses of δ and ϵ chains have been found. As the members of each subclass of H chain and each type of L chain are represented in all normal humans, the subclasses of immunoglobulins are termed isotypes and the antigenic determinants that distinguish them are designated isotypic determinants.

Immunoglobulins of the IgG subclasses, designated IgG_1, IgG_2, IgG_3, and IgG_4, consist of two L chains and two H chains; each H chain contains one variable and three constant region domains. The hinge region is rich in proline, and contains the cysteine residues that are involved in the disulfide bridges that link the two H chains (Figs. 5 and 6). In IgG_1, but not in the other subclasses of IgG, disulfide linkages in the hinge region also connect the H and L chains (Fig. 5). The γ subclasses are identical with respect to over 95 per cent of the amino acid sequences of the domains, and the major subclass-related differences are in the hinge piece.

Both IgA and IgM generally exist in a polymeric state. The serum IgA polymers consist of a continuous spectrum with from two to five four-chain subunits, while serum IgM contains five four-chain subunits arranged in a cyclic pentamer and exhibits occasional higher degrees of aggregation of the pentamers. Both IgA and IgM polymers contain a J chain, which is a unique constituent of polymeric immunoglobulins (Fig. 7). The J chain has an apparent molecular weight of 15,000 and is structurally different from all other immunoglobulin polypeptides. It is rich in cysteine residues, forms a loop that is stabilized by disulfide bridges, and is linked by disulfide bonds to IgA and IgM subunits in a molar ratio of one J chain per polymer irrespective of the size of the polymer (Fig. 7). Except in some disease states, serum IgA is largely monomeric and contains only a small proportion of decreasing concentrations of linear dimers, trimers, tetramers, and pentamers, which are composed of disulfide-linked monomeric units. Secretory IgA (SIgA), a special form of IgA found predominantly in the respiratory and gastrointestinal secretions, consists of two monomeric IgA subunits and a secretory component or transport piece of molecular weight approximately 70,000 that is attached by disulfide bonds to the immunoglobulin units. The special properties and functions of SIgA will be considered later in the chap-

Secretory IgA

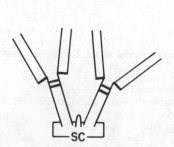

IgM Pentamer

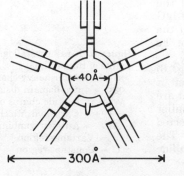

Figure 7. Immunoglobulin polymers.
∩ = J chain
SC = Secretory component

ter. The IgM molecule that predominates in human serum is a rigid cyclic pentamer composed of five identical four-chain subunits and one J chain linked by disulfide bonds. The variations in the physical forms of the immunoglobulins of the five major classes explain the differences in their antigen-binding valences (Table 4). While IgG, IgD, IgE, and monomeric IgA can bind up to two antigens per molecule, polymeric IgA binds up to four antigenic determinants per dimer and six per trimer at saturation. The maximum apparent valence of IgM is not realized with all antigens. While the valence of the IgM pentamer is ten for small antigens, it may not exceed five for larger antigens, possibly as a consequence of steric inhibition of binding.

IMMUNOGLOBULIN HETEROGENEITY UNRELATED TO THE ANTIGEN COMBINING SITE

In addition to the isotypes that make up the major classes and subclasses of immunoglobulins, numerous other levels of structural heterogeneity bear no apparent relationship to the specificity of the combining site. The genetic polymorphisms that distinguish individuals of a species are termed allotypes. Allotypes are detected by intraspecies antisera, as might be obtained in humans after inadvertent immunization by the transfusion of whole blood. Allotypes appear to be the product of a single autosomal codominant gene. In some instances, allotypic differences in immunoglobulins are responsible for major structural differences in the entire four-chain subunit. The Am2+ allotype, which is the predominant fraction of the human IgA_2 subclass, lacks a cysteine residue at position 130. This deletion results in the absence of the H-L chain interchain disulfide bonds characteristic of all other subclasses of immunoglobulins, including the Am2− allotype of human IgA_2. In general, the amino acid sequence differences that have been attributable to allotypic variation involve interchanges at one or two contiguous positions that are not critical to the overall structure or function of the immunoglobulin molecule. Thus, allotypic markers have served predominantly as genetic markers and as probes in studies of the mechanisms of immunoglobulin synthesis.

Several complex systems of genetic markers exist in the constant region of human H chains; these have been designated Gm on γ chains (for γ marker, Fig. 5), of which over 20 have been identified, Am_2 on α_2 chains, and Mm on μ chains. Comparable allotypic markers exist in the constant region of L chains, as exemplified by the Km system (Fig. 5). The genetic information obtained from analyses of human immunoglobulin allotypes in the constant and variable regions, in conjunction with amino acid sequence data, led to the current understanding of the polygenic control of the synthesis of individual H and L chains. Antiallotypic sera have also been used to analyze the ontogeny of immune responses and to study the structure of the antigen combining site. The administration of specific antiallotype antiserum to rabbits both selectively suppresses the production of antibodies of that allotype and preferentially depletes lymphocytes bearing membrane-associated IgM with the same allotypic marker.

The return of the allotypically defined lymphocyte subpopulation in greater than normal numbers before the reappearance of allotypically identical serum IgG provides corroborating evidence that lymphocyte-associated IgM immunoglobulins precede fluid-phase IgG in the development of an antibody response. Antiallotypic sera may prove to be valuable practical tools as well, as allotypic suppression of specific immune responses in rabbits prevents allograft rejection in some instances. Finally, simultaneous analyses of V_H and V_L region allotypes and combining site–specific idiotypes have begun to lead to an understanding of the structural basis for the specificity of the antigen combining site and have provided definitive insights into its evolution.

Idiotypes are markers for antibody combining sites and represent those portions of the variable regions that are directly responsible for the antigen-binding capacity of antibodies with identical specificity. The binding of anti-idiotypic antisera to the combining site is frequently prevented by the simultaneous presence of the homologous antigen. Some V_H and V_L allotypes are markers for the framework residues of the variable regions that determine the shape of the combining site, while idiotypes correlate with the hypervariable sequences that constitute the binding surfaces of the site that are complementary to the antigen. Analyses of subclasses of V_H regions have revealed a greater stability in the allotypic markers as compared with the idiotypic markers, which presumably reflects an evolutionary requirement for strict conservation of the overall shape and the common features of the fine structure of the antigen combining site. There is also generally a close linkage between a given idiotype and one set of V region allotypes. A few exceptions to this rule exist, however, thereby suggesting the possibility that more than one gene may control the V region of each chain so that multiple genes may influence the combining site.

THE ANTIGEN COMBINING SITE

Antigen binding is solely a function of the Fab portion of antibodies. Both H and L chains are required for optimal binding. H chains isolated by disaggregation of both antibodies and myeloma proteins with binding activity bind antigen with less than half the affinity of the intact molecule. Reassociation of the H chains with heterologous L chains increases the binding of antigen, but it is only fully restored by the addition of homologous L chains. The role for both chains is further emphasized by the necessity for the presence of specific antigen to achieve optimal recombination of homologous H and L chains, a process that is more random in the absence of antigen. The reaction of antibodies with anti-idiotypic sera, which exhibit specificity for the intact binding site, is frequently reduced by dissociation of the H and L chains. Analyses of amino acid sequences of many myeloma proteins in each subclass revealed the existence of hypervariable regions in H and L chains. In addition, affinity labeling of presumed contact residues in the combining site—by means of antigen analogues containing substituents capable of forming covalent bonds with specific amino acids and subsequent assessment of the distribution of label on isolated chains—implicated both chains in the recognition portion of the site. When amino acid residues critical for antigen binding in a number of myeloma proteins and conventional antibodies were affinity labeled by such reagents, binding affinity for the antigen was substantially reduced and the label was found in the hypervariable regions of both H and L chains. The final proof of the critical involvement of H and L chains in the combining site came from x-ray crystallography of complexes of myeloma proteins and defined specific antigens in which structural determinants known to be critical for the specific binding of the antigen were closely apposed to residues of the hypervariable regions of both chains.

Myeloma proteins represent acceptable models for antibody structural analyses, as some of these proteins bind antigens with an affinity comparable to that of conventional antibodies of the same specificity and also react with anti-idiotypic sera in a manner identical to elicited antibodies. For example, several independently generated mouse myelomas that bind phosphorylcholine antigens not only have similar variable region amino acid sequences and idiotypic specificities within the myeloma series, but also share these properties with elicited mouse antiphosphorylcholine antibodies. The finding in multiple species of similar and frequently identical amino acid sequences in the hypervariable regions of H and L chains of immunoglobulins of the same antigen-binding specificity unequivocally established the relationship of these small portions of the amino acid sequence to combining site specificity. Light chains of human and mouse myeloma proteins and of homogeneous rabbit antistreptococcal and antipneumococcal polysaccharide antibodies share some hypervariable regions, and each exhibits one or more unique segments of hypervariable sequence. Less information is available for the H chains of these immunoglobulins, but the regions so far presumed to be involved in expressing antigen-binding complementarity demonstrate both amino acid sequence and segment length variability comparable to the L chain hypervariable regions. The remainder of the amino acid sequences of the V_L and V_H domains are far less variable than the few small segments implicated in antigen contact. These so-called framework portions of the variable regions are controlled by clear genetic patterns, contain several allotypic markers, and are involved in maintaining the shape of the combining site so that the spatial arrangement of the complementarity-determining residues of the hypervariable regions provides maximal specificity and binding affinity. The framework regions not only have a less variable amino acid sequence, but do not participate in the deletions, insertions, and short-sequence base change events that are documented for the complementarity-determining sequences of the hypervariable regions. The framework residues most highly conserved in the V_L regions were frequently found to be identical for the immunoglobulins studied in several species. That the hypervariable and framework regions may be under separate genetic controls has been alluded to and will be discussed in more detail in a subsequent section.

X-ray crystallographic studies of Fab fragments of myeloma proteins with antigen-binding activity have provided strong confirmation of the nature and structural bases of the combining site (Fig. 6). The V_L and V_H domains are in spatial proximity at one end of the Fab fragment and create a 20Å × 25Å groove of variable width that is lined by the complementarity-determining residues of the hypervariable regions of both domains (Fig. 6). Binding depends on small differences in molecular structure in numerous series of analogues of small antigens as well as antigens with defined repeating subunits. The antigen appears to fit precisely into the homologous combining site and is held in place by multiple, weak noncovalent interactions. Each such interaction has a binding energy of less than 10 Kcal/mole, and the individual reactions possess extremely rapid kinetics. Nonetheless, the aggregate binding affinity of many such bonds may yield association constants in excess of 10^{10} M^{-1}. The combining site delineated structurally provides for all of these characteristics. The shape of the combining site is rigidly conserved by the framework amino acid sequences of the V_H and V_L domains and the overall conformation maintained by their interaction. The contact residues of the hypervariable region are displayed on the inner surfaces of the narrow groove that comprises the combining site in a pattern that maximizes the number of specifically complementary noncovalent bonds with the determinants of the antigen.

DISTRIBUTION AND FUNCTIONAL ROLES OF IMMUNOGLOBULINS

Although the details of the evolution of the five classes and numerous subclasses of immunoglobulins have not been fully elucidated, sufficient critical information exists concerning differences in their distribution and functional properties to allow an understanding of their biologic roles (Table 5). IgG not only is the quantitatively predominant immunoglobulin in adult serum, but also is the only class of antibody that crosses the placental barrier. This passive protection is just a part of the humoral immunologic defense system of the fetus and newborn infant, since IgM and some IgG antibodies can be endogenously synthesized during the third trimester and the neonatal period. IgA and probably IgE are absent until the third or fourth month of life and reach adult levels in serum far more slowly than IgM and IgG.

In the immune responses of adults, numerous antigens lead to the rapid development of antibodies of the IgM class, which persist only as long as antigen remains. In contrast, IgG antibodies appear early but reach peak levels later, persist longer, and predominate in secondary responses that follow additional challenges with the same antigen. In addition to differences in their appearance with maturation and after antigenic stimulation, human immunoglobulins exhibit class-specific patterns of distribution and catabolism that greatly influence the site of their antibody activities. IgG, IgE, and monomeric IgA are approximately equally distributed between the intravascular and other extracellular compartments. In contrast, more than 75 per cent of IgD and polymeric IgM is in the intravascular space, while monomeric IgM and IgD are the predominant immunoglobulins intrinsic to the surface of lymphocytes. The major immunoglobulin class represented in external secretions of the respiratory, gastrointestinal, and other systems is IgA,

TABLE 5. DISTRIBUTION AND SOME IMMUNOLOGIC FUNCTIONS OF HUMAN IMMUNOGLOBULINS

	CLASSES				
	IgG	IgA	IgM	IgD	IgE
Serum concentration (mean, mg/ml)	12	3	1	0.03	0.0001
Plasma survival (T½, days)	16–23	6	5	3	1–2
Distribution (approximate %)					
Intravascular	50	50	>75	>75	50
Extravascular	50	50	<25	<25	50
Present in secretions	+	SIgA	+	?	+
Transferred across placenta	+	−	−	−	−
Surface localization on unstimulated B lymphocytes	−	−	monomer	+	−
Sensitization of mast cells and basophils	(IgG$_4$*)	−	−	−	+
Initiation of complement pathways					
Classic	+	−	+	?	−
Alternative	−	+	−	?	±

+ = present or capable of a function; − = absent or incapable of a function.
*Transient preparation only.

which appears largely as secretory IgA. External secretions also contain IgE, IgM, and some IgG. The degradation of immunoglobulins, regardless of their location, is a function of class-specific determinants on the Fc fragment and thus is subject to controls separate from those that regulate synthesis and antigenic specificity. IgG possesses the lowest fractional catabolic rate (6.5 per cent per day), which is linearly related to its serum concentration, and thus IgG persists at substantial levels for more than a month, even after passive systemic administration. IgA, IgM, and IgD are degraded more rapidly than IgG. The catabolic rates are unrelated to the serum levels of IgA and IgM and possibly inversely related to the concentration of IgD. On the other extreme of the catabolic spectrum is IgE, which is replaced totally every 36 to 48 hours and has an intravascular fractional catabolic rate of nearly 90 per cent per day.

The immunoglobulin classes also differ profoundly with respect to their abilities to participate in cellular immunologic pathways and to activate immunologic effector systems (Table 5). Human B lymphocytes bear endogenous IgD and monomeric IgM, which can coexist on the membrane of the same cell, in contrast to the generally exclusive presence of a single type of immunoglobulin in the cytoplasm of a plasma cell. The surface IgD appears and achieves a maximum density after surface IgM in the development of each lymphocyte, and this transition process is both antigen and T lymphocyte independent. In contrast to the adsorbed IgG on the surface membranes of human null or K cells, the B lymphocyte IgM and IgD are maintained in culture, are subject to continuous turnover with a half-life of 20 to 80 hours in unstimulated cells, and are rapidly reexpressed if stripped off by exposure to anti-immunoglobulin antisera. Further, more than 80 per cent of the immunoglobulins made by unstimulated B lymphocytes are retained on the membranes. These and other properties have implicated lymphocyte surface IgM and IgD as the specific antigen recognition receptors that initiate lymphocyte proliferation and differentiation after the binding of the homologous antigen. The recruitment of immediate hypersensitivity pathways, which will be discussed in detail later, is a unique function of the IgE class of antibodies. Under some circumstances, human IgG antibodies,

especially those of the IgG$_4$ subclass, can transiently prepare primate mast cells and basophils for antigenic activation. However, only IgE antibodies can sensitize these target cells for a duration consistent with a significant role in the in vivo expression of immediate hypersensitivity reactions.

The classic complement pathway is most efficiently activated by IgM and IgG antibodies, with IgG$_4$ exhibiting essentially no activity relative to the other three subclasses of IgG. Initiation of the alternative, or properdin, pathway of complement can be accomplished by human immune complexes or aggregated immunoglobulins of the subclasses IgA$_1$ and IgA$_2$ and by secretory IgA, with less activity for IgE complexes and none for the other classes. Activation of the alternative complement pathway by human IgA and IgE is a function of class-specific determinants on the Fc fragment.

THE SECRETORY IgA SYSTEM

Secretory IgA (SIgA) is a copolymer of two IgA molecules and one J chain, derived from plasma cells, and a secretory component or transport piece with a molecular weight of 70,000 (Fig. 7), which is synthesized by the epithelial cells of the glands that secrete the IgA polymer. SIgA, which constitutes 80 to 90 per cent of the IgA and most of the immunoglobulins in all secretions, is uniquely capable of surviving diverse secretory conditions. There are high concentrations of SIgA in all secretions, but the ratio of IgA to other immunoglobulins typically exhibits segmental variations and is higher in saliva than in the jejunum or colon. The concentrations of SIgA in most glandular fluids reach adult levels by age one year, when serum IgA is at only 20 per cent of its adult concentration. Further, more than 85 per cent of the plasma cells in the intestinal lamina propria are dedicated to the elaboration of IgA, most of which is assembled into SIgA. IgA-producing plasma cells are the product of a complex lymphoid cycle that is separate from any involved in the elaboration of other immunoglobulins. Finally, secretory IgA is predominantly responsive to antigenic challenge at the body surfaces, and a maximal level of SIgA antibody is stimulated only by such local antigenic challenge. SIgA represents a critical first line of defense against some pathogens and other noxious elements in the environment.

In addition to those functions it shares with serum IgA, such as viral neutralization and complement activation by the alternative pathway, a variety of special properties have been attributed to SIgA. SIgA appears more resistant than serum IgA to proteolytic digestion by numerous enzymes. Perhaps of importance in the normal homeostasis of the gastrointestinal tract, SIgA specifically prevents bacterial adherence to the intestinal mucosal surface and inhibits uptake of protein and other macromolecular antigens by the gut and other absorptive surfaces. Only a small fraction of the IgA in plasma administered to patients with agammaglobulinemia reaches the saliva, and none of the maternal colostral SIgA is detectable in the infant's blood. These observations provide confirmation of the compartmental restriction of the antibodies in a normally elicited SIgA response. While oral immunization has little impact in terms of a systemic antibody response in the IgA or other classes, it stimulates high levels of SIgA antibodies. The oral introduction of polio viruses led to a specific local secretory IgA response, which was even segmentally constrained. Thus application of polio virus in a colostomy gave detectable levels of SIgA antibodies in the colonic secretions but not in the saliva. Such results are also of great practical significance, as orally administered polio vaccines are more effective than systemic vaccines, which fail to stimulate the production of SIgA anti-polio virus antibodies.

The lymphocytes capable of producing IgA are subject to a series of controls that ensure their maturation and accumulation below mucosal surfaces, especially in the gastrointestinal tract. The highly regulated distribution of IgA-producing cells was initially suggested by lymphocyte seeding experiments in irradiated rabbits. Reconstitution of the lymphoid systems of such rabbits with lymphocytes derived from Peyer's patches led to the development of plasma cells and the synthesis of IgA in the intestinal lamina propria. In contrast, the administration of lymphocytes derived from the spleen and lymph nodes preferentially repopulated organs other than the gastrointestinal and respiratory tracts and restored the synthesis of IgG but not IgA. The development of IgA production, as well as of IgG and IgE synthesis and elaboration, was demonstrated to be thymus dependent. IgA concentrations were even more severely depressed than those of IgG and IgE in thymus-deficient states. This information and these analyses of the migration and fate of radiolabeled precursors of IgA-producing plasma cells led to the current concepts of the synthesis and assembly of SIgA.

Precursor lymphocytes bearing surface IgM without IgA migrate from the secretory organs to regional lymphatic nodes. From there, the lymphocytes enter the thoracic duct, are carried into the peripheral circulation, and return by way of local capillary beds to the lamina propria of the intestines and other secretory organs, guided by unknown homing mechanisms to complete the antigen-independent cycle. After local antigenic stimulation, the conditioned lymphocytes develop into plasma cells and secrete dimeric IgA antibodies, which are prevented from entering the intestinal lumen directly by virtue of the interepithelial

tight junctions. The secretory components synthesized by the epithelial cells combine with the IgA antibodies and facilitate the entrance of the now complete SIgA units into the intracellular space, from where they are secreted into the intestinal lumen. The mechanisms by which secretory components accomplish the translocation of IgA antibodies, first into the epithelial cells and then into the intestinal fluid, may involve a membrane receptor function for the secretory components. The complexity of the SIgA system and the dependence of its full capacity on the status of the secretory organs is highlighted by the effects of malnutrition. Although cellular immunity is more consistently compromised by protein-calorie malnutrition than is humoral immunity, the levels of SIgA are selectively decreased relative to those of other immunoglobulins as intestinal mucosal alterations supervene, even though the serum IgA concentration is generally elevated.

SPECIFIC BIOLOGIC ACTIVITIES OF HUMAN IMMUNOGLOBULINS

The critical and specific roles of antibodies in host defense, acting both directly and by way of activation of humoral and cellular effector pathways, are amply demonstrated by the natural illustrations of inborn and acquired immunoglobulin deficiencies. Depression or absence of the IgG antibody response alone leaves the host more susceptible to gram-positive bacterial infections, while deficiencies in responses of other classes may reduce resistance to other microbial pathogens. Although varying in relative efficiency, both IgG and IgM antibodies agglutinate bacteria, prepare them with the aid of complement for phagocytosis by circulating polymorphonuclear and mononuclear leukocytes, and neutralize microbial toxins (Table 6). IgG antibodies alone are capable of opsonizing bacteria for phagocytosis and bactericidal destruction by tissue macrophages and other leukocytes in the absence of the complement proteins of plasma, whereas IgE can sensitize some nematodes for the parasiticidal action of macrophages. IgA is more restricted in its antibacterial effects, exhibiting only a capacity for toxin neutralization. However, IgA antibodies can provide specific microbicidal potential by virtue of their uniquely efficient activation of the alternative complement pathway, while IgG and IgM antimicrobial antibodies initiate the complement cascade by way of the classic pathway (Table 5). As with many functions of IgG antibodies, a subclass-specific pattern of distribution for microbicidal activities is evident (Table 6). Bacterial agglutination and opsonization in the presence of serum are functions of all subclasses, although IgG_4, which lacks substantial complement-activating activity, is a weak opsonin. In contrast, direct opsonization in the absence of complement is efficiently mediated only by the IgG_1 and IgG_3 subclasses, and IgG_1 is specially suited to the neutralization of microbial toxins. Antibody-dependent cytotoxicity, which is largely a property of K lymphocytes, is a component of host defense predominantly directed against foreign cells and abnormal clones of host cells. K lymphocyte cytotoxicity is mediated solely by antibodies of the IgG_1, IgG_2, and IgG_3 subclasses in humans. The IgE-depend-

TABLE 6. BIOLOGIC ACTIVITIES OF HUMAN IMMUNOGLOBULINS

| | CLASSES | | | | | | | |
| | IgG | | | | IgA | IgM | IgD | IgE |
	IgG_1	IgG_2	IgG_3	IgG_4				
HOST DEFENSE								
Microbial toxin neutralization	+	±	±	−	+	+	−	−
Bacterial agglutination	+	+	+	+	−	+	−	−
Opsonization of particles in serum	+	+	+	±	−	+	−	−
Neutrophil attachment	+	+	+	+	+	−	−	−
Monocyte-macrophage preparation	+	−	+	±	−	−	−	+
K lymphocyte cytotoxicity*	+	+	+	−	−	−	−	−
Local vascular permeability alterations and eosinophilia	−	−	−	±	−	−	−	+
TISSUE INJURY								
Anti–factor VIII	−	−	−	+	−	−	−	−
Anti-Rh	+	−	±	−	−	−	−	−
Antithyroglobulin	+	±	±	−	−	−	−	−
Cystic fibrosis factor	+	+	−	−	−	−	−	−
Serum sickness	+	+	+	±	−	±	−	#
Immune complex nephritis	+	+	+	±	−	±	−	#
Anti-DNA	+	+	−	−	−	−	−	−
Rheumatoid factor	−	±	±	−	±	+	−	−
Local and systemic anaphylaxis	−	−	−	±	−	−	−	+

*Antibody-dependent cytotoxicity mediated by K lymphocytes.
#Facilitates immune complex deposition in some tissues.

ent activation of mast cells and basophils is another special component of host defense pathways that will be considered in a subsequent section. The ability of immediate hypersensitivity reactions to rapidly provide local concentrations of protective antibodies, complement components, and inflammatory cells is almost certainly the exclusive province of IgE antibodies.

An additional dimension of immunoglobulin function is the deviation of antibody activities to the deleterious inhibition of important normal humoral and cellular pathways or to host tissue injury (Table 6). Antibodies directed to factor VIII, which may lead to an acquired hemorrhagic diathesis, are predominantly of subclass IgG_4, while the anti-Rh antibodies that mediate erythroblastosis fetalis and the antithyroglobulin antibodies in autoimmune thyroiditis are predominantly of subclass IgG_1. The controversial cystic fibrosis–associated serum factor, which immobilizes cilia in respiratory tract models, is restricted to subclasses IgG_1 and IgG_2. The distribution of antibodies that mediate immune complex diseases may reflect the nature of the basic disorder. Acute serum sickness and immune complex nephritis are typified by broad responses in the IgG subclasses with a minor contribution from IgM antibodies. In contrast, the anti-DNA antibodies in systemic lupus erythematosus are restricted largely to subclasses IgG_1 and IgG_2. The anti-IgG, which is detected as rheumatoid factor in nodular rheumatoid arthritis, is a similarly restricted response of the IgM class. Anti-IgG antibodies of other classes that may predominate in rheumatic diseases other than seropositive rheumatoid arthritis are not detected to any extent by the latex or bentonite flocculation tests, which are far more sensitive to a comparable level of pentavalent IgM anti-IgG. IgE antibodies not only mediate urticaria and systemic anaphylaxis, but may influence both the distribution of deposition and the

quantity of immune complexes deposited by selective alterations in vascular permeability induced by chemical mediators of the mast cells.

The concept of a molecular division of the functions of immunoglobulins based on their structural organization into domains was implicit in Edelman's original hypothesis. Fragments can be prepared corresponding to single domains, and the ability of such fragments to perform specific effector functions can be quantitatively assessed to provide direct evidence for the localization of the biologic activities of immunoglobulins. Several of the functional capabilities of IgG are solely attributable to a single domain of the Fc fragment. Initiation of the classic pathway of complement by the interaction of IgG and C1q, the binding substituent of the first component of complement, is an activity independently expressed by the $C\gamma_2$ domain alone and appears to involve an exposed hydrophobic center at the indole ring of tryptophan 277, which is associated with several positively charged side chains. The catabolic rate of unbound IgG is an exclusive function of the Fc fragment. Studies with labeled fragments and isolated domains of rabbit IgG showed the same rate of clearance from the rabbit circulation for IgG, Fc, and $C\gamma_2$, while $C\gamma_3$ and Fab were eliminated at four to five times the rate of intact IgG. As binding of $C\gamma_2$ to other proteins was specifically excluded, the site of control of the catabolic rate of the entire IgG molecule appears to reside in the $C\gamma_2$ domain. The ability of homologous IgG to bind to human monocytes and guinea pig macrophages was substantially blocked by the presence of equimolar $C\gamma_3$ and was totally inhibited by excess $C\gamma_3$. The binding of isolated radiolabeled $C\gamma_3$ was equal to that of intact IgG, thus establishing that the major macrophage-monocyte receptor is located solely in the $C\gamma_3$ domain. Some binding activity was also demonstrated for the $C\gamma_2$ domain in other studies, but it apparently is not expressed in the interaction of native IgG with these cell types. Many of the genetic determinants are also located in the $C\gamma_3$ domain, including the Gm allotypes (Fig. 5).

In contrast to those biologic activities of IgG that are localized exclusively in one domain, the Fc receptor recognition units for neutrophils and K lymphocytes appear to require an intact Fc fragment. Neither isolated $C\gamma_2$ nor $C\gamma_3$ monomers inhibited the respective binding of Fc fragments. Suggested interpretations include a localization of the cell receptor in one domain but a requirement for modulation by either the other domain of the Fc fragment or the dimeric partner and a joint structural site requiring both domains. There is, however, little evidence either for cooperative effects requiring multiple domains in the Fc fragments or for the transmission of functionally significant energy from the Fab to the Fc fragments. Antigen binding to the antibody combining site provides some stabilization of chain structure, leads to spreading of the inter-Fab angle, shields some charged amino acid side chains, and may induce other minor conformational changes. No substantial allosteric alterations or exposure of biologically active sites have been documented to result from the simple occupancy by antigen of the combining site. The major mechanisms by which antigen initiates the biologic functions of antibodies are fluid-phase aggregation, which creates multi-component sites with new activities, and bridging of cell-bound antibodies, which results in membrane perturbation and cellular activation. This explains the frequent requirement for multivalent antigen, which improves both the aggregating and bridging efficiency of the antigen.

REGULATION OF ANTIBODY SYNTHESIS—ORIGINS OF DIVERSITY

The existence of multiple classes and subclasses of immunoglobulins, each characterized by the structure of its heavy chain, was established by immunochemical analyses of isotypic determinants with antisera prepared against monoclonal immunoglobulins. Further insights into the genetic bases of regulation of immunoglobulin synthesis required additional studies of allotypic polymorphism and careful evaluation of accumulated amino acid sequences of both monoclonal immunoglobulins and homogeneous elicited antibodies. The distribution of human constant region allotypic markers within subclasses of γ chains (Gm), one subclass of α chains (Am2), and κ chains (Km) was defined in the immunoglobulins of a few population groups and in some series of monoclonal immunoglobulins. Both the structural and genetic lines of information suggested the existence of a series of closely linked autosomal genes responsible for controlling the synthesis of the constant domains of human H chains. A few γ chains appeared to represent products of apparent cross-over events, and thus analyses of their allotypes and those of parental γ chains permitted a preliminary assignment of the order for the subclass genes as γ_4, γ_2, γ_3, and γ_1. The presence of closely linked genes regulating the synthesis of a group of homologous polypeptide chains pointed to the possibility of gene duplications in the course of evolution from a

common primitive H chain constant region gene. The two genes controlling the synthesis of the constant regions of κ and λ L chains appeared not to be linked to each other or to the cluster of H chain genes.

The second fundamental concept to emerge from the analyses of amino acid sequences and allotypes of monoclonal immunoglobulins is revolutionary and of great biologic significance. Those portions of the V_H and V_L domains not characterized by sufficient hypervariability of amino acid sequence to be implicated in the antigen contact regions of the combining site clearly fall into a few general subclasses: four subclasses for all H chains, three for κ chains, and five for λ chains. The basic V region structure thus appears to be conserved as rigidly as the C regions during the evolution of immunoglobulins. Each V_H subclass is associated with all of the C_H classes, and each V_L subclass is linked to C_L regions with differing allotypic determinants. The synthesis of immunoglobulin chains, unlike that of any other known proteins, can therefore be presumed to be controlled by more than one gene. One gene carries the information critical to the general conformation of the antigen combining site, which is common to all classes of antibodies. The other genes contain the coding for the biologic activities of antibodies, which are class specific and must be linked to the combining site. Additional characteristics of immunoglobulin genes should account for the differential initiation of production of H and L chains, the transition from membrane-bound to secreted antibodies, and both allelic and isotypic exclusion.

MOLECULAR CHARACTERISTICS OF HUMAN IMMUNOGLOBULIN GENES

The recent application of techniques of molecular genetics to analyses of the genes of human normal and malignant B lymphocytes (B cells) has led to a greater understanding of the mechanisms of generation of antibody diversity. Extreme flexibility in somatic recombination and a high rate of somatic mutation both serve to maximize the number of unique antibody molecules, termed idiotypes, that can be generated from a limited number of germline gene subsegments. The apparent disadvantages of somatic processing of gene subsegments are the high rate of errors that lead to ineffective genes, and the likelihood of translocation of genes from other chromosomes to the loci of immunoglobulin genes. One deleterious outcome of the latter process is the combination of oncogenes with immunoglobulin genes that leads to some human malignant B cells. This section will describe the components of genes for immunoglobulin chains, the features of different forms of rearrangement of the gene components, and the controls that seem to ensure that the numerous genetic sources of antibody diversity do not interfere with the restriction of immunoglobulin production by each mature B cell to a single isotype.

The human κ light chain gene is located at band 2p13 of the short arm of chromosome 2 and consists of subsegments coding for diverse variable regions, one constant region, and five joining segments that are displayed sequentially and are connected to the 5' end of the constant region (Fig. 8). Although similar in fundamental structure to the κ light chain gene, the λ

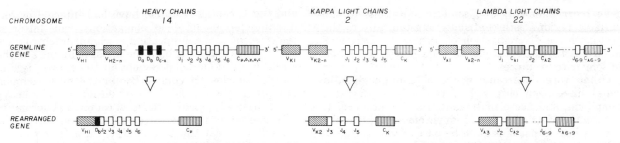

Figure 8. Human gene loci for heavy chains and κ and λ light chains on three different chromosomes. J = joining and D = diversity segments

light chain gene has between six and nine constant regions, each of which is preceded by a distinct joining segment. The variability in the total number of constant regions is attributable to differences in the amplification of the second and third constant regions, which may include additional nucleic acid sequences coding for up to a total of five separate regions. The heavy chain gene is analogous to the κ light chain gene, but has six joining segments and also contains a region that codes for at least three different families of diversity segments, which are displayed sequentially between the variable and joining regions (Fig. 8). The diversity segments code for a portion of the third hypervariable region. The gene subsegments or recombinations that account for the first and second hypervariable regions have not been recognized as yet.

Studies of heavy chain and light chain gene rearrangements in the monoclonal expansions of human B cell precursors of different stages, which are found in some types of acute lymphocytic leukemia, have elucidated partially the serial stages of rearrangements of the genes. The rearrangement of immunoglobulin genes precedes sequentially from heavy chains to κ light chains and then to λ light chains (Fig. 8). Thus the earliest definable B cells, termed pre-B cells, undergo μ chain gene rearrangement and express μ heavy chains without light chains, as will be discussed in the next section. In heavy chain genes, it appears that recombinations of D and J subsegments are accomplished prior to the joining of D and V regions. The recombination of a gene subsegment coding for a light chain V region with one J subsegment linked to

a light chain C region is similarly specific. The observed precedence of κ before λ gene rearrangement may be attributable to a difference in the relative rates of recombination of the two genes or to the effect of a regulatory element associated with one or both genes. Although the mechanisms responsible for the orderly rearrangement of immunoglobulin genes into effective synthetic units are not clear, the sequential nature of the events on different chromosomes would increase the diversity of antibody products.

The maturation of B cells, which will be described in detail subsequently, involves the development of a capacity to generate IgG, IgA, and IgE from the primitive activity of producing only IgM or IgM and IgD. The simultaneous production of IgM and IgD is based on the proximity of the two genes. Since the switch from the production of IgM/IgD to that of other immunoglobulins transfers previously established combining site specificities, a second type of heavy chain gene rearrangement was postulated (Fig. 9). This type of rearrangement was shown to be mediated by switch regions, which are composed of repetitive elements of five base pairs and are located on the 5′ side of each constant region. The respective S sites for the other immunoglobulin isotypes interact with that of IgM (S_μ) to substitute a new constant region for C_μ. The switch does not change the VDJ section, which determines the specificity of the antibody combining site, but effectively recombines the previously formed VDJ with a new constant region. The latter rearrangements serve to couple multiple effector functions to one antigen combining site. The two types of immunoglobulin

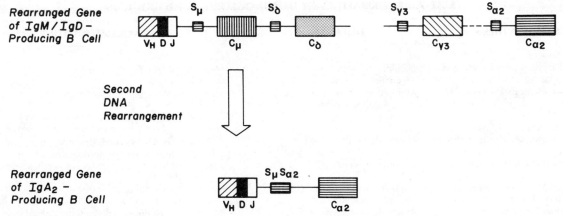

Figure 9. Gene rearrangements in B cell precursors that lead to production of a mature range of isotypes of immunoglobulins.
S = switch region

gene rearrangements and somatic mutations in the variable regions both contribute substantially to the post-germline diversification of antibodies. Deletions in mRNA may also account for the C_μ to C_γ transition in some circumstances.

Other rarer rearrangements of immunoglobulin genes have been observed in the cells of Burkitt's lymphoma and acute malignant transformation of B cells, some of which result from chromosomal translocations but do not appear to be part of the normal B cell maturation process. One such reciprocal translocation of chromosome 14q32 and chromosome 8q24 is of fundamental interest because of the location of oncogene c-Myc at 8q24. An enhancer sequence within the heavy chain gene is capable of augmenting the production of extraneous genes, and thus may increase the production of the translocated c-Myc gene. Speculation about the significance of the translocation of an oncogene to the locus of the heavy chain gene has included a role for c-Myc in malignant transformation of B cells.

ABNORMALITIES OF IMMUNOGLOBULIN PRODUCTION

A variety of disorders of immunoglobulin synthesis has been described. Detailed analyses of these disorders have provided not only additional insight into normal and abnormal immunoglobulin synthesis, but also have been the basis for the development of an objective classification of these disorders. Immunoglobulin deficiency states are discussed in Section IV, Host Defenses. The two basic categories of pathologic production of immunoglobulins include quantitative excesses of a single immunoglobulin or L chain and qualitative abnormalities of H or L chains that appear alone or as part of an immunoglobulin molecule (Table 7). The myeloma and macroglobulinemia proteins consist of normal intact immunoglobulins, and the Bence Jones proteins are normal L chains found in association with myeloma proteins or occasionally alone. Rarely, abnormal chain structures have been identified in myeloma proteins. For example, the γ chains of one monoclonal immunoglobulin lacked a hinge region,

and the L chains of others have had internal or terminal deletions or even elongations. The latter is reminiscent of the duplication mechanism felt to have led to the evolution of both the major domains and the multiple disulfide bond regions in the hinge piece of some γ subclass H chains. By far the most common group of H chain defects is that designated the heavy chain diseases, in which the most common abnormality is a deletion of C_{H1} and a variable portion of V_H. It is most likely that the defect in synthesis is either an error in DNA joining or the result of a nonsense codon leading to inappropriate termination of the synthesis of a polypeptide segment. The nature of the deletional abnormalities constitutes additional support for the speculation that H chain synthesis may be under the control of a complex series of genes rather than simply a V_H and a C_H gene. In contrast to the H chain disease proteins, the abnormal L chain fragments that represent one component of some forms of amyloid are most likely postsynthetic degradative products of normal L chains.

REGULATION OF ANTIBODY PRODUCTION BY LYMPHOCYTE SURFACE MEMBRANE IMMUNOGLOBULINS: IMMUNOLOGIC NETWORKS

The evolving body of knowledge relevant to the specific binding of antigens by antibodies, the biologic activities of various classes of antibodies, and the activation of effector pathways by antigen-antibody reactions far exceeds the current understanding of the mechanisms by which antibodies modulate the immune response. Some observations have suggested the existence of a complex immunoregulatory network in which several populations of lymphocytes exert selective stimulatory or inhibitory effects on a given set of antibody-producing lymphocytes by virtue of the unique antigenic determinants of the antibodies elaborated. The essentially monoclonal antibody response to Balb/c mice to phosphorylcholine antigens is accompanied by the simultaneous production of anti-idiotype antibodies directed to the phosphorylcholine combining

TABLE 7. ABNORMALITIES OF IMMUNOGLOBULIN PRODUCTION

CHAIN SYNTHESIS	DISEASE	ABNORMAL PROTEINS
Normal Structure		
H and L chain production equal	Multiple myeloma	Monoclonal IgG, IgA, IgD, or IgE
	Macroglobulinemia	Monoclonal IgM
Excess L chain production	Multiple myeloma and macroglobulinemia	Monoclonal Ig + Bence Jones protein*
Structurally Abnormal Chains		
Production of abnormal H chain only	Heavy chain disease	γ, α, or μ chains with deletion of V_H, C_{H1}, and/or the hinge region in various combinations
Abnormal H chain in intact Ig	Multiple myeloma	γ without a hinge region in IgG molecules; even rarer α or μ defects
Abnormal L chain in intact Ig	Multiple myeloma	Internal or terminal deletions or elongations of L chains
Combined defect	Multiple myeloma	Monoclonal IgG and γ heavy chain disease protein
Abnormal L chains	Amyloidosis (primary and that of lymphoid malignancies)	Portions of L chains (? postsynthetic degradation)

*Bence Jones proteins are only rarely found in macroglobulinemia but are common in multiple myeloma.

site. Further, T and B lymphocytes capable of reacting with idiotypic determinants on autologous immunoglobulins have been demonstrated in several species after immunization. Finally the administration of exogenous anti-idiotype antisera inhibits or stimulates B and T lymphocytes displaying that idiotype, which anti-idiotypic T lymphocytes selectively suppress the production of antibodies with the same idiotype. The coexistence and concomitant stimulation of antibody-producing lymphocytes bearing homologous idiotypes and complementary anti-idiotypic lymphocytes and antibodies represent the experimental basis for the network theory of Jerne (Fig. 10). The lymphocyte clone that produces antibodies and retains some antigen-binding immunoglobulin on the cytoplasmic membrane (Fig. 10*A*) is regulated by at least three other sets of lymphocytes with cross-reactive surface receptors. It is postulated that a set of inhibitory lymphocytes has specific anti-idiotypic receptors (Fig. 10*B*), a set exhibiting stimulatory effects has surface immunoglobulin of an idiotype that cross-reacts with the eliciting antigen (Fig. 10*C*), and another set or sets have immunoglobulin receptors with a cross-reacting idiotype (Fig. 10*D*) or anti-idiotype (Fig. 10*E*). It has not been demonstrated that autologous anti-idiotype reactions occur in conventional immune responses in humans or possess a modulating capacity if they do occur. However, the accumulating data favor such a mechanism, and some evidence also suggests that allotypic, as well as idiotypic, networks may exert control over antibody responses. The ability to inhibit, stimulate, and alter qualitatively an antibody response by selectively manipulating regulatory lymphocytes and anti-idiotypic antibodies is an extremely basic and flexible tool with potential applications to the treatment of immune deficiency and autoimmune diseases as well as allograft rejection.

REFERENCES

Korsmeyer, S. J., Bakhshi, A., Arnold, A., et al.: Genetic rearrangements of human immunoglobulin genes. In

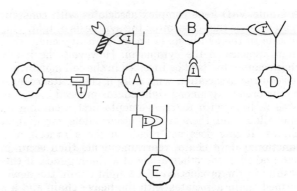

Figure 10. Regulation of antibody production by lymphocyte surface immunoglobulin interactions.

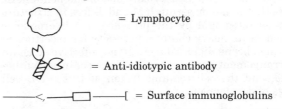

= Lymphocyte

= Anti-idiotypic antibody

= Surface immunoglobulins

I = Homologous idiotypic determinant
I' = Cross-reacting idiotypic determinant
——□ = Surface antigenic determinant

Greene, M. I., and Nisonoff, A. (eds.): Biology of Idiotypes. New York, Plenum Publishing Corp. 1984, pp. 75–95.

Leder, P., Max, E. E., Seidman, J. G., et al.: Recombination events that activate, diversify, and delete immunoglobulin genes. Cold Spring Harbor Symp Quant Biol 45:859, 1981.

Schechter, I., Wolf, O., Zemell, R., et al.: Structure and function of immunoglobin genes and precursors. Fed Proc 38:1839, 1979.

Wall, R., and Kuehl, M.: Biosynthesis and regulation of immunoglobulins. Annu Rev Immunol 1:393, 1983.

B Lymphocytes

ONTOGENY OF B CELLS

In birds the differentiation steps required for the development of stem cells into B lymphocytes occurs in a portion of the hindgut termed the bursa of Fabricius. Removal of the bursa results in a B cell-deficient, agammaglobulinemic chicken. In mammals there is no homologue of this bursa. During fetal life human B cell differentiation occurs in the liver; in adult life it occurs in the bone marrow.

B lymphocytes function in the humoral immune arm through their production of antibody. The differentiation steps occurring among the B cell lineage that culminate in the production of antibody can be divided into three major stages represented by pre-B cells, B cells, and plasma cells. Pre-B cells contain immunoglobulins in their cytoplasm, but neither express immunoglobulin molecules on their surface nor secrete

immunoglobulins into the circulation. B lymphocytes contain easily detectable immunoglobulin molecules on their surface, but do not secrete immunoglobulin molecules into the environment. Plasma cells do not express immunoglobulin molecules on their surface, but do secrete large amounts of immunoglobulin. This differentiation and maturation occurring among the B cell lineage may be best understood by recounting the events involved in the organization of immunoglobulin genes.

Pre-B Cell

At the level of the stem cell there is no rearrangement among genes encoding for the synthesis of either heavy or light chains of immunoglobulin. These genes therefore are said to be in the germ line configuration. The first event in B cell differentiation is reflected by rearrangements occurring among heavy chain genes.

A single VJD gene complex associates with constant region genes that determine the synthesis of IgM. This results in the synthesis of an intact heavy chain that then appears in the cytoplasm. However, the heavy chain cannot by itself be inserted in the cell membrane; it requires association with a light chain. Rearrangements occurring among light chains proceed in a stepwise fashion with rearrangements first occurring on one allele and then on the other allele for κ light chains. If this does not result in the synthesis of a functional light chain, rearrangements then occur in one and then the other allele of λ chain genes. If this results in the production of a λ light chain, the newly formed chain associates with the heavy chain and a λ IgM molecule appears on the cell membrane. This IgM molecule is represented by only one of the pentameric units that make up serum IgM and differs in structure from secreted IgM by the presence of a hydrophobic region in its heavy chain: a necessity for insertion in the membrane lipid bilayer. If no effective λ chain rearrangement occurs, then no light chain is synthesized, and the cell remains frozen at this pre-B cell stage of development.

B Cells and Plasma Cells

When the lymphocyte displays membrane immunoglobulin it is identifiable as a B cell. In the early stages of differentiation B cells express only IgM, but subsequently they synthesize and express IgD molecules. At the gene level this is represented by the association of a single VDJ heavy chain complex with constant μ and constant φ genes. Display of both IgM and IgD appears to be an important event in B cell activation, as B cells expressing only IgM are difficult to activate and appear particularly susceptible to the development of tolerance. The appearance of surface IgD allows the B cells to move forward into distinct differentiation pathways where they display IgG only, IgE only, or IgA. At this stage of B cell development, all immunoglobulin gene rearrangements have been completed, and the cell synthesizes large amounts of immunoglobulin containing a single antigenic specificity and a single immunoglobulin class and subclass. Generally B cells displaying a specific immunoglobulin class give rise to plasma cells secreting the same class of immunoglobulin. For example, IgG–bearing B cells develop into IgG–secreting plasma cells, and the same holds true for other immunoglobulin classes.

This ordered sequence of immunoglobulin gene expression that occurs during B cell development (IgM→IgG→IgA) is mirrored by the appearance of serum immunoglobulin during fetal and neonatal development. Synthesis of IgM begins at 10 to 11 weeks, IgG at 12 weeks, and IgA after 30 weeks of fetal development. Adult levels of IgM occur by one year of age, IgG by five years of age, and IgA by early teens.

REGULATION OF B CELL DIFFERENTIATION AND IMMUNOGLOBULIN PRODUCTION

B cells displaying IgM and plasma cells secreting IgM can occur in the absence of T cells, but differentiation of B cells into plasma cells synthesizing other immunoglobulin classes requires the presence of T cells. Indeed, T cells play a crucial role in B cell differentiation, acting both to help and suppress this process. Interactions between T cells and B cells involved in enhancing the immunoglobulin production appear to involve direct contact between T and B cells as well as the liberation of soluble materials by T cells and perhaps by other cells such as macrophages. These interactions can be best understood by examining a relatively well defined system of murine B cell differentiation (Fig. 11). Murine splenic B cells can be divided into two broad populations based on the expression of a differentiation antigen termed Lyb 5. Approximately 50 per cent of splenic B cells are Lyb 5 positive while the other 50 per cent are Lyb 5 negative. These two major populations, both of which display immunoglobulin molecules on their surface, differ in terms of the nature of interactions required for their differentiation into immunoglobulin-secreting plasma cells.

Lyb 5-positive cells can be activated by cross-linking surface IgM receptors with either anti-IgM antibodies or multivalent antigens. Increased RNA synthesis results, and the cell moves from resting (G_0) into an early activation (G_1) phase. Further movement from G_1 through the phase of DNA synthesis (S) requires interactions with two soluble materials: (1) B cell growth factors (BCGF) derived from T cells (BCGF binds only to activated Lyb 5-positive cells, not to resting cells.) and (2) a macrophage-derived factor that may be IL-1. The combination of these signals, multivalent antigen, BCGF, and IL-1 is sufficient to induce B cell proliferation. However, it is not sufficient to induce a differentiation of B lymphocytes into immunoglobulin-secreting plasma cells. (It is important to note that proliferation among B cells cannot be equated with their differentiation into plasma cells.) The development of activated B cells into immunoglobulin-secreting plasma cells requires another T cell-derived factor termed T cell-replacing factor (TRF).

Lyb 5-negative cells require interaction among the B cells, antigen, and T lymphocytes for their activation. This interaction with T cells appears to require direct cell-to-cell contact between T and B cells bearing homologous class II molecules and cannot be substituted for by T cell-derived soluble materials. This combination of interactions can push the differentiation of Lyb 5-negative cells forward into proliferation but not to plasma cell development. As noted for Lyb 5-positive cells, differentiation of activated Lyb 5-negative cells into plasma cells requires the action of TRF.

In summary, different populations of B cells appear to differ in their requirements for activation. One population of B cells requires interactions between antigen and soluble materials derived from T cells and macrophages to proliferate. Another distinct population of B cells cannot be induced to proliferate by soluble materials, but requires more intimate interactions between antigen and T cells. The final pathway of differentiation of both populations of B cells into plasma cells is similar and is mediated by a soluble material liberated by T cells.

T cells can also influence the development of B cells displaying specific immunoglobulin classes and the development of plasma cells secreting specific immunoglobulin isotypes. For example, a population of T cells specifically promotes the development of IgA-bearing B cells from IgM-bearing B cells, and another

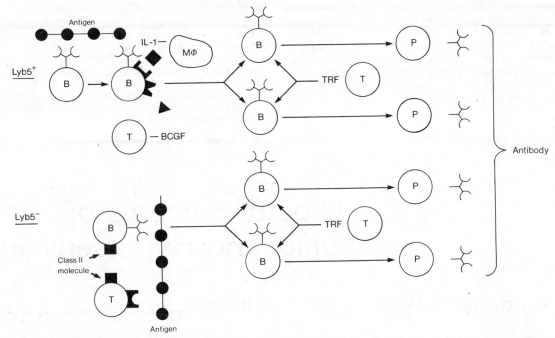

Figure 11. Differentiation of B cells. In mice, two distinct populations of B cells can be delineated, based on differences in their expression of the Lyb 5 molecule. For each, early events involved in their differentiation are different (see text).
BCGF = B cell growth factor
IL-1 = interleukin-1
TRF = T cell-replacing factor
(From Stobo, J. D.: Lymphocytes: Structure and function. *In* McCarty, D. J. (ed.): Arthritis and Allied Conditions: A Textbook of Rheumatology, 10th ed. Philadelphia, Lea & Febiger. In press. Reproduced with permission.)

population of T cells is specifically required for the differentiation of these IgA-bearing B cells into IgA-secreting plasma cells. To date, such isotype specific helper T cells have been demonstrated for IgG, IgA, and IgE.

In keeping with the concept of ordered immunologic reactivity, mechanisms exist for damping B cell differentiation, mediated by suppressor T cells that are phenotypically distinct from the helper T cell population. Activated or effector suppressor T cells bear the T8 phenotype, and T cells capable of activating these effector cells reside among a subpopulation of T4-positive cells. The mechanism by which these T cells damp B cell development has not been determined. Although soluble materials capable of mediating suppression of B cell development have been described, they are poorly characterized.

Both cell-mediated and humoral immunity can be regulated in an antigen-specific fashion. For example, immunization with antigen X can result in the activation of helper and suppressor influences that modulate only the response to X and not to Y. A "network theory" proposed to explain this specificity postulates that recognition of self idiotypes constitutes the basis of an immunoregulatory network. (Idiotypes are antigen determinants represented by the unique amino acid sequences in the antigen combining region of antibodies. Antibodies with different antigenic speci-

ficites will have different idiotypes.) According to the model, immunization with antigen X results in the production of antibody 1 (Ab1) with a specific idiotype (Id1). This in turn stimulates the production of an anti-idiotype antibody (Ab2) that has a unique idiotype (Id2). This then triggers the production of an anti-anti-idiotype (Ab3) bearing Id3, and so on. The effect is like dropping a rock into a pond. The initial splash results in the generation of large waves that become progressively damped as they move from the center and finally disappear. There is substantial evidence to support the idiotype network. For example, infusion of an animal with anti-idiotype antibodies can either augment or enhance antibody reactivity to a specific antigen. The ultimate effect on immune reactivity depends on the amount and affinity of the anti-idiotype antibody infused. Anti-idiotypes can be detected during the normal response following challenge with antigen, supporting a role for the idiotype network in immunologic homeostasis.

The demonstration of immunoregulatory influences has important implications for both understanding and correcting immune-mediated disorders. Disorders of hypoimmune and hyperimmune reactivity reflect not only intrinsic abnormalities in effector T and B cells but also imbalances in helper and suppressor influences. However, caution should be exercised in thinking that all immune-mediated defects represent immunoregulatory abnormalities. Clearly, abnormalities in immunoglobulin gene transcription and translation within B cells are as important in immunoglobulin deficiency as a deficiency of helper or a preponderance of suppressor T cells. Similarly the modulation of immunoregulatory influences to correct immune-mediated diseases, although a potential mechanism of therapy, is still experimental.

REFERENCES

DeFranco, A. L., Kung, J. T., and Paul, W. E.: Regulation of growth and proliferation in B cell subpopulations. Immunol Rev 64:161, 1982.

Fauci, A. S., Lane, C., and Volkman, D.: Activation and regulation of human immune responses: Implications in normal and disease states. Ann Intern Med 99:61, 1983.

Ishizaka, K., Yodoi, J., Suemura, M., et al.: Isotype-specific regulation of the IgE response by IgE-binding factors. Immunol Today 4:192, 1983.

C.   Effector Systems of Immunity and Hypersensitivity

Immediate-Type Hypersensitivity

ALLERGY, ATOPY, AND ANAPHYLAXIS

Anaphylaxis, the capacity of repeated injections of a toxic substance to elicit an adverse reaction rather than a protected state, was recognized by Porter and Richet in 1902 and so designated in contradistinction to prophylaxis. At that time severe immediate reactions to horse and other heterologous antisera, to diphtheria toxin, and to other bacteria or bacterial products dominated the clinical experience in humans. An understanding of the immunologic and cellular mechanisms of immediate hypersensitivity is directly relevant to the diagnosis and treatment of the reactions to drugs, insect stings, and other common environmental challenges. Immediate adverse reactions to penicillin became the most common form of human anaphylaxis in the mid 1940s, and the mortality from penicillin anaphylaxis in the United States continues to be estimated at 100 to 500 per year. The diverse group of haptens eliciting the typical clinical sequence is continually expanding with the introduction of new diagnostic and therapeutic chemicals. Anaphylaxis resulting from stings by insects of the Hymenoptera order is a persistent problem; serious systemic reactions have been estimated to occur in 0.4 per cent of the population. Anaphylaxis or anaphylactic shock may obstruct the upper airway because of laryngeal edema, or obstruct the distal bronchioles with secondary vascular collapse, or result in primary circulatory failure without antecedent respiratory difficulty, with a fatal outcome. The anaphylactic reaction is the most severe syndrome at one extreme of the spectrum of diseases of immediate hypersensitivity.

Allergy, a term originally used by von Pirquet in 1906, encompasses the less severe respiratory, cutaneous, and other manifestations of immediate hypersensitivity, which are attributable to the same basic mechanisms as anaphylaxis. IgE antibodies, which are bound to mast cells and basophils of a previously sensitized individual, initiate allergic reactions when they interact with a sufficient quantity of a bivalent antigen. The chemical factors released from the activated mast cells and basophils mediate diverse vascular, smooth muscle, and inflammatory responses that constitute local or systemic allergic reactions or both. Whether such a reaction is local or systemic and mild or severe depends on the intensity and distribution of antigen challenge, the degree of sensitization and resultant concentration of IgE antibody, and the effectiveness of an array of control mechanisms.

The association of allergic rhinitis and asthma in the same patient, often with a familial background, and the presence in the serum of IgE antibody to the clinically relevant antigen(s) led initially to use of the term *atopy* to imply a propensity to develop an altered state of reactivity without undue or unusual prior exposure to the antigens. As presently used, *atopic allergy* implies a familial tendency to manifest alone or in combination such clinical conditions as bronchial asthma, rhinitis, urticaria, and eczematous dermatitis (atopic dermatitis). The actual symptoms and signs expressed depend on the allocation of specific immune response genes, the primary determinants of total IgE, the tissue distribution of IgE-producing B lymphocytes and plasma cells, and the affinities of IgE for antigen and mast cell receptors, respectively. When contemplating the full spectrum of diseases of immediate hypersensitivity, it is also pertinent to consider the regulation of mediator generation and release in response to specific immunologic activation and the extracellular controls of mediator function.

Some reactions appear to be allergic on clinical grounds but have no demonstrable IgE antibodies as part of their pathogenesis. Examples of such disorders include the adverse reactions to aspirin, sodium sulfite, and radiographic contrast media. This suggests that non-IgE mechanisms can also activate mast cells and basophils. Indeed, many natural peptides and proteins can release the full range of mediators of allergic reactions in the absence of IgE.

The category of immediate-type hypersensitivity diseases adequately encompasses the anaphylactic syndrome, many forms of urticaria, and allergic rhinitis. It does not, however, explain the chronic irritability of the asthmatic airway during asymptomatic periods or the cutaneous lesions of atopic dermatitis. Mast cells and basophils may have such capabilities on the basis of their constituent mediators. Both early and late pulmonary and cutaneous responses to aerosol and intracutaneous administration of *Aspergillus* and avian materials have been demonstrated. Similar late or dual responses in sensitive subjects have been observed in skin with *Bacillus subtilis* enzyme preparations and in both skin and airways with grass pollen. Normal subjects also respond to intradermal crystalline *B. subtilis* alpha amylase after passive transfer of IgE antibodies and to the F(ab')$_2$ fragment of sheep antihuman IgE. These latter studies reveal that IgE–dependent mast cell activation is sufficient to achieve a secondary local inflammatory response with clinical erythema, swelling, and discomfort, characterized histologically by mast cell degranulation and subsequent infiltration of polymorphonuclear and mononuclear leukocytes.

BASOPHILS AND TISSUE MAST CELLS: CELLULAR CHARACTERISTICS AND THE IgE RECEPTOR

Mast cells are thought to derive from fixed, undifferentiated, mesenchymal cells, although this has not been clearly established. Mast cells are found in organs rich in connective tissue, such as mammary gland, lung parenchyma, the respiratory and digestive tracts, skin, and serous membranes in general. Normal human skin contains between 7225 and 12,100 mast cells per cu mm. Mast cells can replicate and migrate in tissues and increase in number at sites of chronic mast cell stimulation.

Mast cell granules, bounded by a membrane, vary in their structure. Two subgranular components are common to all human mast cell granules: dense lamellar or scroll structures and fine granular material. In addition, human skin mast cells are distinguished by long villous extensions of the plasma membrane, granules that contain crystalline lattices, and prominent microfilaments. By transmission electron microscopy the degranulation process is classic exocytosis with maintenance of cellular integrity and exposure of the membrane-free granule to the microenvironment. An initial fusion between the cell membrane and the membranes of the most peripherally located granules proceeds to involve more centrally located granules through fusion of adjacent granule membranes. This sequential recruitment of more internally located granules, resulting in the formation of cavities, is referred to as compound exocytosis.

The basophilic leukocyte is a polymorphonuclear granulocyte derived from the bone marrow and distinct from the tissue mast cell. Although readily identified in peripheral blood smears stained with Wright's stain, basophils are difficult to preserve properly and there-fore are infrequently visualized in tissue sections. Basophils and mast cells have similar cytoplasmic granules and membrane receptors for IgE, and probably functionally supplement each other in many circumstances. Circulating in the blood, basophils may be quickly mobilized to a site of immediate or delayed hypersensitivity. By contrast, new mast cells must arise by a slower process of replication and differentiation that requires a period of days or weeks.

Basophil granules are round-to-oval, membrane-bound structures that contain dense particles. Basophil granules appear to release their contents by two mechanisms: (1) Adjacent granule membranes may fuse to form chains or clusters of granules enveloped by a single limiting membrane. These commonly join with the plasma membrane, leading to continuity between granules and the cell exterior. (2) Vesicles or vacuoles may form a chain-like arrangement that, in some instances, extends from granules deep in the cell cytoplasm to the cell surface. These changes may provide a transport mechanism by which small quantities of basophil granule material may be extruded from the cell over an extended period.

IgE is unique in its capacity to bind firmly to a surface receptor on mast cells and basophils. The binding is not known to produce any perturbation of the cell until the cell is exposed to a divalent or multivalent antigen that interacts with and bridges two or more IgE molecules. The binding of human IgE to human mast cells requires the Fc portion of the immunoglobulin and probably is dependent on the integrity of the heat-labile $C_{\epsilon 3}$ and $C_{\epsilon 4}$ domains together.

Digestion of human lung tissue and isolation of lung mast cells has allowed direct demonstration of IgE binding to tissue mast cells, and the capacity of antigen and anti-IgE to generate and release mediators. The location of mast cells in the perivenular areas of connective tissues, as well as intraepithelially in the portio vaginalis uteri, tonsils-adenoids, pulmonary airways, and nasal tissues, affords their membrane-bound IgE ready access to potential antigens.

A normal rodent mast cell binds 500,000 ± 300,000 molecules of IgE when the cell is incubated with radioactive IgE. Cells from parasite-infected animals show an expected reduction in the number of unsaturated sites owing to their endogenous exposure to the higher serum IgE levels. Human lung mast cells have 20,000 to 100,000 high-affinity receptors per mast cell, of which only approximately 5000 per mast cell are free of endogenous IgE.

The basophil receptor for IgE is highly specific, and the binding of IgE is not affected by a 1000-fold to 10,000-fold excess of immunoglobulins of other isotypes or of heterologous IgE. The binding of IgE to high-affinity cellular receptors is rapidly reversible and is governed by a simple bimolecular forward reaction and first order dissociation. The high-affinity IgE receptors are univalent, are mobile in the plasma membrane, and are susceptible to aggregation by bridging of bound IgE with antigen or anti-IgE and with antireceptor antibodies. The IgE receptor appears to be an integral membrane protein that is largely embedded in the membrane with one portion exposed to the extracellular medium and another to the cellular cytoplasm.

The IgE receptor solubilized from cultured rat basophilic leukemia cells (RBL-1 cells) contains multiple different glycoprotein subunits that constitute the major functional receptor of approximate molecular weight 100,000. One type of subunit on the plasma membrane, which recognizes and binds IgE with high affinity, is connected by an intramembranous subunit to a third subunit, which is in communication with the cytoplasm and presumably transduces the signal for basophil/mast cell activation. In the IgE-mast cell system it appears that the signal is generated by a cross-linking of the surface IgE.

BIOCHEMICAL EVENTS IN MAST CELL ACTIVATION AND SECRETION

Once the mast cell is perturbed, a cascade of steps occurs, including calcium ion influx, the uncovering of a serine esterase, an energy-requiring phase, a second calcium-dependent event involving contractile cellular proteins, and a change in the level of intracellular cyclic $3',5'$-adenosine monophosphate (cyclic AMP) (Fig. 12). The initial perturbation may be by IgE-dependent mechanisms or by IgE-independent stimuli, such as the anaphylatoxin fragments of complement proteins C5a and C3a, platelet factor 4 (PF4), or lymphocyte-derived basophil- and mast cell-activating factors (BAF/MAF). This cellular activation and coupled secretory reactions culminate in the release from the exposed granule of preformed mediators in a fully active form, such as histamine and the tetrapeptides known as eosinophil chemotactic factor of anaphylaxis (ECF-A), and of granule-associated putative mediators such as heparin and chymotrypsin-like protease or chymase, which require further release to express full activity (Table 8). Activation, in addition, leads to the generation and release of unstored factors, such as the leukotrienes of slow-reacting substance of anaphylaxis (SRS-A), and phospholipid platelet-activating factors (PAFs). This array of mediators may then alter the microenvironment to allow for host defense or tissue injury.

Stimulation of both human basophilic leukocytes and rat mast cells requires a bivalent or multivalent antigen or antireceptor/anti-IgE antibody compatible with a requirement for ligand bridging of the IgE receptor to accomplish the relevant membrane perturbation. Clustering or capping of receptor-bound IgE is not required for activation of the basophil or the isolated rat peritoneal mast cell where the maximum size of a stimulatory cluster is less than 10 IgE molecules. Soon after an antigen challenge of mast cells or mast cell–rich tissue fragments, an extracellular calcium ion–dependent serine esterase with chymotrypsin-like properties is uncovered (Fig. 12). An energy-requiring step, either glycolysis or oxidative phosphorylation, is necessary to maintain the sequence leading to noncytotoxic mediator release from mast cells. A second calcium-dependent step in the activation cascade of human lung fragments and mast cells occurs after and separately from the early extracellular calcium ion–dependent step and after the energy-dependent step. A requirement for intracellular calcium is compatible with the activation of contractile protein that is inhibited through phosphorylation by a cyclic AMP-dependent kinase. Mast cells appear to contain contractile filaments in degranulating cells. The basophil release reaction is influenced by agents that act on microtubules; augmented by heavy water (D_2O) and inhibited by colchicine for example. These observations support the theory of a cyclic nucleotide–regulated secretory process (Fig. 12).

Two distinct mechanisms have been described for release of functional mediators to the microenvironment:

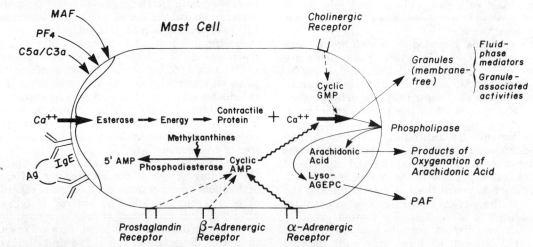

Figure 12. Biochemical mechanisms and pharmacologic modulation of the activation of mast cells.
$\longrightarrow$ = Action, release, or conversion
$\dashrightarrow$ = Stimulation
$\rightsquigarrow$ = Inhibition
$Ca++$ = Calcium ion
PF_4 = Platelet factor 4
MAF = Mast cell-activating factor
Ag = Antigen
$\succ\!=$ = IgE antibody

TABLE 8. MEDIATORS OF IMMEDIATE HYPERSENSITIVITY

CATEGORY	MEDIATOR	STRUCTURE	MAJOR EFFECTS	INACTIVATION
Preformed	Histamine	β-imidazolylethylamine	Contracts smooth muscle; increases vascular permeability	Histaminase, histamine methyltransferase
	Serotonin	5-HT*	Increases vascular permeability	5-HT deaminase
	ECF-A†	Hydrophobic acidic tetrapeptides (m.w. 360–390)	Chemotactic for eosinophils and neutrophils; enhances eosinophil cytotoxicity	Peptidases
	Intermediate m.w. ECF	Peptides (m.w. 1500–3000)	Chemotactic for eosinophils and neutrophils	Peptidases
	NCF-A‡	Protein (m.w. $\simeq$ 750,000)	Chemotactic for neutrophils	—
	Heparin	Acidic proteoglycan (m.w. $\simeq$ 60,000)	Anticoagulant; antagonizes complement and platelet factor 4	—
	Hydrolases	Chymase (m.w. 25,000)	Proteolysis	—
		N-acetyl β-glucosaminidase (m.w. 150,000)	—	—
		Arylsulfatase A (m.w. 115,000)	—	—
Newly generated	Leukotriene B$_4$	5(S), 12(R)-dihydroxy-eicosa-6,14 cis-8,10 transtetraenoic acid	Chemotactic for eosinophils and neutrophils; stimulates pulmonary airway secretion	Oxidation
	Leukotrienes C$_4$, D$_4$, and E$_4$ (SRS-A§)	5(S)-hydroxy-6-S-tripeptide, dipeptide, or cysteine-eicosa-7, 9 trans-11,14 cis-tetraenoic acid	Contract smooth muscle; stimulate pulmonary airway secretion; dilate microvasculature	Oxidation, peptidolysis
	Prostaglandin D$_2$		Increases vascular permeability	—
	PAF‖	1-0-hexadecyl-octadecyl-2-acetyl-sn-glyceryl-3-phosphoryl-choline (AGEPC, PAFacether)	Stimulates platelet aggregation and secretion; contracts smooth muscle	Deacetylation, phospholipases

*5-Hydroxytryptamine.
†Eosinophil chemotactic factor of anaphylaxis.
‡Neutrophil chemotactic factor.
‖Platelet-activating factor.
§Slow-reacting substance of anaphylaxis.

(1) The initial exposure of the granule to extracellular fluid releases those mediators bound by low-affinity charge interaction, such as histamine, 5-hydroxytryptamine, and ECF-A. Physiologic degranulation involves both ready exchange of mediators from the granule and actual extrusion of the discharged granule matrix from the confines of the cell. The fate of the extruded granule matrix and its major components—heparin, chymase, and acetyl-β-D-glucosaminidase—is not well defined. The granule may be phagocytosed by eosinophils and fibroblasts, but solubilization under physiologic conditions has not been shown.

(2) Mast cells and basophils, when appropriately stimulated, newly synthesize and release certain specific lipid agents (Fig. 12, Table 8). Isolated purified human and rat basophils and mast cells generate both oxygenation products of arachidonic acid, such as prostaglandin D$_2$, prostaglandin E$_2$, leukotrienes, and phospholipid platelet-activating factors (PAFs), which are released with the same time course as histamine and peptide mediators.

STRUCTURAL AND FUNCTIONAL CHARACTERISTICS OF THE MEDIATORS OF IMMEDIATE HYPERSENSITIVITY

The preformed mediators of immediate hypersensitivity are considered to be any granule-associated, biologically active substances that may come into contact with the extracellular environment. Some diffuse readily from the granule in physiologic buffer; others are more tightly granule associated and thus require a step beyond granule exocytosis for full expression of their functions (Fig. 12, Table 8). In reality, this distinction represents a spectrum: Histamine, 5-hydroxytryptamine, the tetrapeptides of eosinophil chemotactic factor of anaphylaxis (ECF-A), the oligopeptides with ECF activity, and arylsulfatase A are readily diffusible from the discharged granule in physiologic ionic medium; acetyl-β-D-glucosaminidase is partially released from the discharged or isolated granule; and macromolecular heparin and chymase are not released from the rat mast cell granule until it undergoes dissolution.

The newly generated mediators represent more than one type of lipid. The source of many of these substances is membrane phospholipids, broken down by specific phospholipases, that yield arachidonic acid and precursors of PAF.

Chemical Mediators Stored in Mast Cell/Basophil Granules

Histamine. Histamine, which is widely but variably distributed in mammalian tissue, is associated with the granules of the mast cell. The histamine content per mast cell is reasonably constant in normal tissue; human lung mast cells contain 1.0 to 5.5 pg of histamine per cell for example, an amount equal to or greater than that of the human basophil. Histamine also is found in blood platelets and in the mucosa of the parietal region of the stomach in adults, as well as in fetal liver cells. Histamine is formed by decarboxylation of L-histidine and degraded either by oxidative deamination or by methylation and oxidative deamination, so that the principal excretion products are imidazoleacetic acid-riboside and 1-methyl imidazoleacetic acid, respectively. An increase in histidine decarboxylase activity occurs in tissue not normally rich in mast cells, in response to a variety of nonspecific stimuli, and the alleged product of this adaptive enzyme activity has been referred to as induced histamine to distinguish it from that stored in mast cells.

Histamine (Table 8) increases permeability of venules, which is attributed to partial disconnection of the endothelial cells from each other, and may contract smooth muscle both directly and reflexly. Intravenously administered histamine increases pulmonary resistance or decreases specific conductance and compliance in the human lung by direct and reflex mechanisms. Biologic activities of histamine are mediated through at least two different histamine receptors: (1) H_1 tissue effects include venular dilatation and bronchial and intestinal smooth muscle contraction, which are inhibited by standard antihistamines. (2) H_2 action increases gastric acid secretion and inhibits certain leukocyte functions, including human lymphocyte-mediated cytotoxicity, suppressor T cell function affecting the production of macrophage inhibition factor (MIF) by guinea pig lymphocytes, and the IgE-mediated release of histamine from rat mast cells and human basophils. These H_2 receptor-mediated effects of histamine on the function of lymphocytes and mast cells/basophils in delayed and immediate hypersensitivity reactions also extend to eosinophil and neutrophil migration and other functions. The apparent capacity of histamine to facilitate via H_1 and dampen via H_2 receptors the responses of leukocytes of several classes forms an integral part of the thesis for the role of immediate-type hypersensitivity in the regulation of subacute and chronic processes. The H_2 receptor is blocked competitively by the thiourea derivatives burimamide, metiamide, and cimetidine.

Serotonin. In mammalian tissue, serotonin (5-hydroxytryptamine) is localized in the mucosal layer of the gastrointestinal tract and, to a lesser extent, in brain tissue and platelets. In the gastrointestinal tract, serotonin is presumably in the enterochromaffin cells. Serotonin is not present in human mast cells in contrast to those of the rat and mouse, but is in the platelets of most species, including man. Normally, human blood contains 0.1 to 0.2 µg of serotonin per milliliter, of which virtually all is in platelets. Immediate-type hypersensitivity reactions elaborate PAFs that release platelet amines, including serotonin. Serotonin is derived from the amino acid tryptophan by the introduction of a hydroxyl group into the 5 position and decarboxylation. Detoxification by deamination to 5-hydroxyindoleacetic acid is accomplished by amine oxidase, an enzyme present in many tissues.

Serotonin contracts smooth muscle and produces leaking venules by partial disconnection of the endothelial cells from each other. In humans, however, its primary role is probably as a neurotransmitter. In human hypersensitivity reactions it is classified as a preformed tertiary mediator derived from the action of PAFs on platelets.

Eosinophil Chemotactic Factors of Anaphylaxis. The prominence of the eosinophil in clinical and experimental in vivo allergic reactions led to the discovery in 1971 of a new mast cell capability—namely, the release of preformed granule–associated eosinophil chemotactic activity (Table 8). The mast cell-derived activity stimulates the directed migration of human eosinophils along a concentration gradient of the mediator, a phenomenon termed chemotaxis.

The eosinophil chemotactic activity results from at least two distinct acidic peptides that have amino acid sequences of Val-Gly-Ser-Glu and Ala-Gly-Ser-Glu. The maximal chemotactic activity of the peptides, alone or in combination, is observed at concentrations of 3×10^{-8} M to 3×10^{-7} M. The preferential in vitro eosinophil activity of ECF-A was initially surmised from studies of its chemotactic and deactivating activities for eosinophils, neutrophils, and mononuclear leukocytes in parallel with other defined stimuli over wide ranges of concentrations. At concentrations of each stimulant that elicited equivalent neutrophil chemotactic responses, purified native ECF-A and synthetic tetrapeptides attracted greater numbers of eosinophils than kallikrein or C5a but had only marginal effects on mononuclear leukocyte migration. The synthetic tetrapeptides also attracted eosinophils into human skin in vivo, with maximum activity at concentrations of 10^{-3} M to 10^{-4} M. The ECF-A tetrapeptides also have the capacity to increase the apparent number of C3b and, to a lesser extent, IgG and IgE-Fc receptors on eosinophils. This function augments the immune adherence–dependent functions of the eosinophil attracted to a site of hypersensitivity, including cytotoxicity for helminthic parasites.

Intermediate Molecular Weight Eosinophil Chemotactic Factors. At least three preformed intermediate molecular weight peptide chemotactic factors that preferentially attract eosinophils have been isolated from rat mast cells and human lung tissue fragments. The marked overall heterogeneity in terms of size, charge, and hydrophobicity of mast cell-derived, granule-associated, eosinophilotactic principles of low and intermediate molecular weight released after mast cell activation would create multiple gradients to which the eosinophil could respond for sustained intervals, and may mediate diverse other functions of eosinophils in host defense.

Neutrophil Chemotactic Activity. The eosinophilotactic mast cell–derived factors have secondary specificity for neutrophilic polymorphonuclear leukocytes, and thus also may attract the cardinal cell of an acute/subacute inflammatory response. In addition, there is evidence for the presence of a factor with preferred specificity for the neutrophilic polymorphonuclear leukocyte. This high molecular weight neutrophil chemotactic factor of anaphylaxis (NCF-A) has been found to be released, along with histamine and ECF-A, into the venous effluent of a cold-immersed extremity of patients with idiopathic cold urticaria and into the blood of asthmatics in whom attacks of bronchospasm were induced by exercise or aerosol antigen challenge. The NCF-A, which has a molecular weight of approximately 600,000 to 750,000, has a marked chemotactic preference for human neutrophils relative to eosinophils and monocytes and requires a concentration gradient for expression of this function. Although the specific mast cell origin and preformed state of the mediator have not been established, the time course of NCF-A release with histamine and ECF-A in IgE-mediated reactions of patients justifies its tentative inclusion as a preformed mast cell/basophil-derived mediator.

Heparin. Proteoglycans are composed of glycosaminoglycan chains covalently linked to a protein core; the composition of the glycosaminoglycan determines the classification of the proteoglycan (see subsequent discussion in Section IX). Heparin and heparan sulfate differ from the chondroitin sulfates, dermatan sulfate, and keratan sulfate in having alternating $\alpha 1,4$- and $\beta 1,4$-glycosidic linkages instead of alternating $\beta 1,3$ and $\beta 1,4$. Instead of having predominantly glucuronic or iduronic acid, both heparin and heparan sulfate have a mixture of the two. Heparin is also distinguished by having N-sulfate groups instead of N-acetyl groups on a large proportion of the glucosamine residues, in contrast to chondroitin sulfate, dermatan sulfate, keratan sulfate, and hyaluronic acid. Heparan sulfate contains a mixture of N-acetylated and N-sulfated glucosamine units and thus contain less sulfate per disaccharide unit than heparin. The presence of sulfate or carboxyl groups or both on each disaccharide unit makes the glycosaminoglycan chains strong polyanions with corresponding physical properties.

Human mast cell heparin proteoglycan has an average molecular weight of 60,000 by gel filtration and releases glycosaminoglycan chains of approximately 20,000 molecular weight when degraded by alkali. The small human heparin proteoglycan exhibits metachromasia, characteristic biochemical properties, and anticoagulant activity. [^{35}S]Heparin, labeled in vivo or in vitro, is released from purified rat peritoneal mast cells by guinea pig antirat IgE or rabbit antirat F(ab')$_2$ and by a calcium ionophore. The released [^{35}S]heparin correlates in linear fashion with net per cent histamine release. This is further evidence that mast cell activation by immunologic means (or by a calcium ionophore) results in secretion of the whole granule.

Whether intracellular proteoglycans merely have a matrix or carrier function when present in secretory granules or are truly primary mediators with important extracellular actions is not established. Human lung heparin glycosaminoglycan, like commercial heparin, contains a subfraction with antithrombin III binding and marked anticoagulant activity. Rat heparin proteoglycan and commercial heparin glycosaminoglycan are active in preventing formation of the amplification convertase (C3b,Bb) of the human alternative complement pathway. Additional inhibitory effects of heparin have been observed on the interactions of the early components of the classic complement system. The major unresolved issues concerning the intracellular proteoglycans of mast cells and basophils include the class and molecular weight, the possible relationships of proteoglycan class or size to the associated biologically active principles transported with the granule or released from it, and the nature of the nonstorage, nontransport functions of the proteoglycans.

Hydrolases. A chymotrypsin-like enzyme, termed chymase, can be demonstrated histochemically in mast cell granules or by the capacity of mast cell and granule extracts to cleave synthetic substrates of pancreatic alpha-chymotrypsin. Rat mast cell chymase is a single cationic protein composed of a single polypeptide chain of 25,000 molecular weight. The extracellular action of this neutral protease could include degradation of proteoglycans.

The lysosomal arylsulfatase A is the only arylsulfatase that can rightly be considered a primary mast cell/basophil mediator because of its release upon immunologic activation of rat peritoneal mast cells. Rat mast cells contain both arylsulfatases A and B, but secrete only arylsulfatase A when activated by calcium ionophores or rabbit antirat F (ab')$_2$.

N-acetyl β-glucosaminidase activity is present in the granules of rat peritoneal mast cells and is released by immunologic challenge in a linear relationship to histamine release, thereby confirming its existence in the secretory granule. Hexosaminidases, which contain two major isoenzymes (A and B), are present in rat mast cells as is the lysosomal form of glucuronidase. Release by rabbit antirat F(ab')$_2$ of both enzymes is time and dose dependent and coincident with release of histamine. Hexosaminidase A accounts for 85 per cent of the cell content and appears to be selectively released. A kallikrein-like protease, capable of liberating bradykinin from kininogen, is also released from preformed stores in basophils.

Newly Generated Mediators

The newly generated mediators of mast cells and basophils, as well as those from the monocyte/ macrophage populations of chronic hypersensitivity reactions, are produced from substrates made available by the cleavage of membrane phospholipids. The selection of mediators to be mentioned in the context of immediate hypersensitivity will be limited to the small group specifically identified as major products of mast cells and basophils (Table 8) and considered to make a functional contribution to the overall reaction.

Leukotriene B$_4$, the C-6 Peptide Leukotrienes C$_4$, D$_4$, and E$_4$, and Prostaglandin D$_2$ (Fig. 13). The arachidonic acid liberated from membrane phospholipids is converted by cyclo-oxygenation principally to prostaglandin (PG) D$_2$ in mast cells and to PGE$_2$ in basophils, and by 5-lipoxygenation and further metabolism to leukotriene (LT) B$_4$, C$_4$, and D$_4$ in both types of cells (Table 8). LTC$_4$, LTD$_4$, PGE$_2$, and PGD$_2$ act on blood vessels, smooth muscle, and glands, while LTB$_4$ has major functional effects on polymorphonuclear leukocytes and T lymphocytes. Mast cells, basophils, and macrophages generate large quantities of lipid mediators for export to the extracellular fluid. For each of these sources, the 5-lipoxygenation of arachidonic acid yields 5-hydroperoxy-eicosatetraenoic acid (5-OOHETE), which is converted to either 5-hydroxy-eicosatetraenoic acid (5-HETE) or to 5,6-epoxy-eicosatetraenoic acid that is designated LTA$_4$. LTA$_4$ is coupled to glutathione to form 5-hydroxy-6-S-glutathionyl-eicosatetraenoic acid (LTC$_4$) or is transformed by enzymatic hydration to 5(S),12(R)-di-hydroxy-eicosa-6,14 cis-8,10 trans-tetraenoic acid (LTB$_4$) and nonenzymatically to several other 5,12-di-HETE isomers. LTC$_4$ is subjected to sequential peptidolysis to yield 5-hydroxy-6-S-cysteinyl-glycyl-eicosatetraenoic acid (LTD$_4$) and 5-hydroxy-6-S-cysteinyl-eicosatetraenoic acid (LTE$_4$). The same cells also generate different

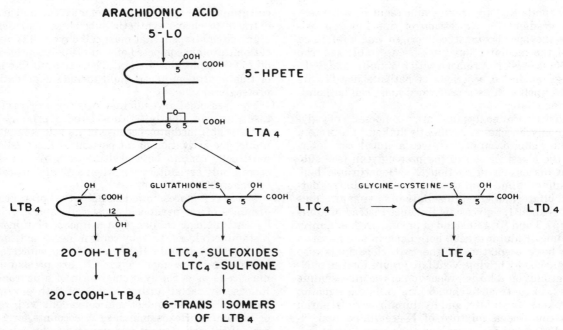

Figure 13. The 5-lipoxygenation of arachidonic acid as a source of mediators.
5-LO = 5-Lipoxygenase
LT = Leukotriene
HPETE = Hydroperoxyeicosatetraenoic acid
Although the individual double-bonds are not depicted, the characteristics of the basic shape of each molecule indicate the differences between the double bond geometry of 5-HPETE, LTB₄, and the peptide leukotrienes, as well as the similarity of LTA₄, LTC₄, LTD₄, and LTE₄. (From Goetzl E. J.: Leukocyte recognition and metabolism of leukotrienes. Fed Proc 42:3128, 1983. Reproduced with permission.)

amounts of mono-HETEs and di-HETEs from the 15-lipoxygenase and other lipoxygenase pathways.

Extracellular lipoxygenase products appear rapidly, and the quantity of each is a function of both the specific cells and stimulus. Macrophages and mast cells, for example, generate predominantly LTC₄ and LTB₄ of the complex mediators, whereas basophils generate largely LTD₄ and LTB₄.

Purified natural and synthetic LTC₄, LTD₄, and LTE₄, the constituents of slow-reacting substance of anaphylaxis (SRS-A), and PGD₂ are potent mediators of smooth muscle contraction. The leukotrienes contract guinea pig ileum and other smooth muscle with the characteristically slow onset and relaxation times that serve to differentiate "slow-reacting" substances from histamine, bradykinin, PGF₂α, and some other contractile factors. LTD₄ is 5 to 20 times more potent than LTC₄ and LTE₄ and approximately 50 to 500 times more potent than histamine in contracting the smooth muscle of guinea pig ileum.

The leukotrienes of SRS-A seem to play an important role in the homeostatic regulation and disease-associated abnormalities of airway tone. Intravenous administration of partially purified SRS-A and synthetic LTC₄ or LTD₄ markedly decreases the dynamic compliance of peripheral airways in guinea pigs, while smaller decreases occur in the conductance of the large central airways. In contrast, the ratio of the decrease in pulmonary compliance to the decrease in airway conductance is significantly smaller and of shorter duration for histamine than for SRS-A, indicating a greater activity of histamine on large airways. These in vivo results have been borne out by in vitro studies

of the effects of SRS-A, the leukotrienes and histamine on the contraction of parenchymal strips of guinea pig lung, a model for small airways, and the constriction of guinea pig trachea, a model for large airways. LTC₄ and LTD₄, respectively, are approximately 200-fold and 20,000-fold more potent than histamine in contracting parenchymal strips of guinea pig lung. LTB₄ exhibited a potency 1/10,000 to 1/1000 that of LTD₄ in the same assay system. LTC₄ and LTD₄ are only 30-fold to 100-fold more potent than histamine in constricting segments of guinea pig trachea, which confirms the generally greater effect of leukotrienes on small airways than on larger airways.

Purified SRS-A, the synthetic leukotrienes, PGE₂, and PGD₂ also alter vascular tone and vasopermeability (Table 8). LTD₄ is slightly more potent than LTC₄ and purified natural SRS-A in evoking a transient decrease in arterial blood pressure when intravenously administered to guinea pigs. Native SRS-A, synthetic LTD₄, LTE₄, and, to a lesser extent, LTC₄ similarly alter the permeability of the cutaneous microvasculature in guinea pigs and some other animals, which results in the leakage of intravascular fluid and proteins into the tissue. LTE₄ and LTD₄ are each 100 times more potent than histamine in inducing an increase in vasopermeability in guinea pig skin. The decrease in arterial blood pressure induced in guinea pigs by LTD₄ and LTC₄ implies that these mediators may dilate arterioles as well as other blood vessels. In fact, LTC₄ and LTD₄ can be shown to dilate small cutaneous vessels, sometimes following a transient vasoconstriction, in some cutaneous models in experimental animals and man. LTC₄ and LTD₄ vasoconstrict large arteries in some organs, especially in the heart and lungs of several species. Histamine, some prostaglandins, 12-HETE, LTB_4 and especially LTC_4 and LTD_4 all stimulate the secretion of mucous glycoproteins by airway tissues of the lungs.

LTC_4, LTD_4, and LTE_4 have potent vasoactive and smooth muscle contractile functions, but lack activity for leukocytes, while LTB_4 is a potent chemotactic factor for polymorphonuclear (PMN) leukocytes and eosinophils. In addition to exhibiting chemotactic activity, LTB_4 also increases adherence, stimulates aggregation, augments the expression of C3b receptors, and initiates limited degranulation of PMN leukocytes and eosinophils. The only effect of LTC_4 and other C-6 peptide leukotrienes on PMN leukocytes is increased adherence, as assessed in vitro, while PGD_2 and PGE_2 decrease adherence slightly and stimulate random migration but not chemotaxis. The effects of LTC_4 and LTD_4 on adherence are largely prevented by indomethacin and are associated with increased production of thromboxane B_2. The latter findings suggest that the effect of LTC_4 and LTD_4, but not of LTB_4, on PMN leukocytes is mediated by stimulation of the cyclooxygenation of arachidonic acid and the generation of thromboxane A_2, which is known to increase PMN leukocyte adherence.

LTB_4 suppresses human T-lymphocyte proliferative and synthetic responses to mitogens through several complex mechanisms. LTB_4 inhibits T helper cell proliferation and stimulates T suppressor cell proliferation, resulting in bidirectional modulation of the principal functional subsets of T lymphocytes. LTB_4 can also augment the expression of natural cytotoxic cell activity by a thromboxane-dependent mechanism.

Platelet-Activating Factors

PAF activity, which stimulates platelets to release their secretory granules, is generated by IgE-mediated reactions in human and rabbit basophils and human lung mast cells. The predominant PAF activity in most instances is attributable to 1-0-hexadecyl-/octadecyl-2-acetyl-sn-glyceryl-3-phosphorylcholine (AGEPC or PAFacether). The precursor 2-lyso-PAFacether is released from membrane lipids of the respective cell sources in a phospholipase-dependent reaction and PAFacether is generated by 2-acetylation. PAFacether aggregates rabbit and human platelets and induces the noncytotoxic release of serotonin, platelet factor 4, and other granule constituents at concentrations as low as 10^{-11}M. The systemic and local administration of PAFacether to rabbits evokes not only thrombocytopenia, but also bronchospasm, leukopenia, and hypotension, the latter of which is mediated in part by platelet-independent mechanisms. Partially purified rat PAF, rabbit basophil PAFacether, and synthetic PAFacether are substantially inactivated by phospholipase D from eosinophils but not by proteolytic enzymes, arylsulfatase B, or phospholipases A and B.

MODULATION OF MEDIATOR GENERATION AND RELEASE BY THERAPEUTIC AGENTS

Agents capable of stimulating adenylate cyclase, such as beta-adrenergic agents and prostaglandins of the E series, decrease IgE-dependent mediator release

(Fig. 12). Phosphodiesterase inhibitors, such as aminophylline, also block mediator release and demonstrate synergistic effects with the beta-adrenergic agonists. Consistent with these observations, purified populations of rat peritoneal and human lung mast cells exhibit inhibition of immunologic release of histamine when intracellular cyclic 3′:5′-adenosine monophosphate (cyclic AMP) levels are increased.

Mediator release from human lung fragments is also modulated by alpha-adrenergic and cholinergic prototype receptors (Fig. 12). Alpha-adrenergic agonists, alone or with beta blockers such as propranolol, reduce lung fragment levels of cyclic AMP and augment IgE-dependent mediator release. This observation may have relevance to the clinical finding that an underlying bronchospastic condition may be unmasked or aggravated in some patients receiving beta blockers for cardiovascular problems. Cholinergic stimulation of human lung fragments with acetylcholine or carbamylcholine increases tissue levels of cyclic 3′5′-guanosine monophosphate (cyclic GMP) and enhances IgE-dependent mediator release, as well as cellular generation and release of leukotrienes and PAF. The effect is blocked by atropine pretreatment, thereby identifying the muscarinic nature of the prototype cholinergic receptor. The precise relationship of the in vitro findings with isolated lung mast cells to their function in lung tissue is uncertain, as is suggested by the failure of corticosteroids to inhibit the release of $PGF_{2\alpha}$ from mast cells at concentrations that inhibit fully the release of $PGF_{2\alpha}$ from lung tissue fragments.

The view that mediator release contributes to a disease such as bronchial asthma is supported by the therapeutic efficacy of disodium cromoglycate (DSCG). DSCG is unique in suppressing mediator release selectively from mast cells by a mechanism independent of the cellular level of cyclic nucleotides, possibly by trapping calcium ions at the mast cell surface and thereby preventing activation. DSCG has little or no direct bronchodilatory action on airway smooth muscle; its usefulness in the management of allergic and nonallergic forms of asthma implies that the mechanism involves inhibition of the release of smooth muscle contractile mediators from mast cells. The beta-adrenergic agents and phosphodiesterase inhibitors could well be acting both by decreasing mediator generation and release from the target mast cell and by direct antispasmodic effects on the airway smooth muscle.

ENDOGENOUS REGULATION OF MEDIATOR AVAILABILITY AND FUNCTION

The composite events that follow antigen bridging of mast cell receptor–fixed IgE include the following: (1) the biochemical concomitants of membrane perturbation, designated *activation*; (2) the biochemical events essential for *granule exocytosis and solubilization*; (3) the *generation of unstored mediators* from membrane phospholipids; (4) the *target cell effects* of preformed mediators, dissociated from granules or granule bound, and newly generated mediators; and (5) the *degradation* of the mediators. Some of the regulatory events appear to involve eosinophils, which serve not only as target cells for mast cell–derived mediators but exert bidirectional effects on mast cell

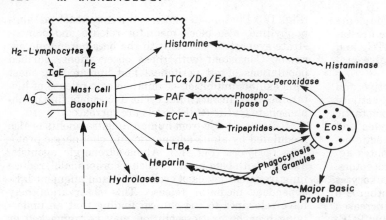

Figure 14. Natural regulation of mediator availability and activity.

$\longrightarrow$ = Action, release, uptake, or conversion

$---\rightarrow$ = Stimulation

$\sim\!\sim\!\rightarrow$ = Inhibition or inactivation

Ag = Antigen

$\succ\!\!=$ = IgE antibody

H_2 = H_2 receptor for histamine

H_2-*Lymphocytes* = Histamine-sensitive lymphocytes

activation and degrade several mast cell mediators (Fig. 14).

Activation. The membrane perturbation that results in activation requires the proximity of pairs of specific IgE for effective bridging. A number of variables affect activation, including immune response genes, effects of histamine and LTB$_4$ to suppress lymphocyte function, affinity of specific IgE for both antigen and the IgE receptor, the differences in numbers of IgE cell receptors at different times in the life cycle of mast cells and basophils, and the competition of nonspecific IgE or even poorly binding subclasses of IgG for the receptors. Noncytotoxic activation by other principles, such as the anaphylatoxin fragments C3a and C5a of the complement system, platelet factor 4, 15-HETE, or lymphokine-like principles, requires generation of those principles. Variables in the functional response to a fixed activating stimulus have been noted, but there is as yet no basis for determining whether the differences observed are in the biochemical events of activation or granule secretion. Eosinophils attracted to the site of mast cell activation by ECF-A and LTB$_4$ release the major basic protein, which can activate other mast cells early or as part of a late response.

Granule exocytosis and solubilization. Exogenous agents that elevate cyclic AMP suppress mediator release. Primary mediators such as histamine exert an endogenous feedback control through H$_2$ receptors linked to adenylate cyclase of human basophils or rat mast cells. Newly generated mediators, such as the prostaglandins, can dampen or augment mediator release owing to the opposing actions of different classes on the levels of cyclic AMP and cyclic GMP. Some of the mediators do not fully express all their activities while granule bound. For example, "second activation" by solubilization of the granule is required to reveal completely the metachromatic and limited anticoagulant activities of native heparin, since the bound protein partially masks the biologically active sulfate groups of the proteoglycan. In contrast, the inhibition of alternative pathway amplification convertase C3b,Bb formation is well expressed by the granules, which suppress generation of C3a and C5a. Likewise the granule-bound chymase, although it may have the capacity to act on small peptides such as bradykinin, is apparently sterically blocked from protein substrates such as casein.

Generation of unstored mediators. Many mediators are synthesized de novo after stimulation. This syn-

thesis is modulated by many of the principles that alter the release of stored mediators, as described previously.

Target cell action. The endogenous regulation of cell types and humoral systems influenced by the release of mediators can be illustrated by the eosinophil. Inhibitory tripeptides derived from ECF-A by peptidolysis of the tetrapeptides in eosinophils compete with the ECF-A tetrapeptides for membrane sites. Histamine can either enhance the eosinophil response to ECF-A or, at higher concentrations, suppress it. Another example of target tissue interaction of mediators is the ability of PGE$_1$ and PGE$_2$ to augment the response of the same smooth muscle to LTC$_4$ and LTD$_4$.

Degradation of mast cell-derived mediators. Both heparin and hydrolases, at least in their granular forms, are phagocytosed and apparently digested by the eosinophil. Eosinophils contain a histaminase capable of oxidative deamination of histamine, a peroxidase that can degrade the C-6 peptide leukotrienes of SRS-A, and a phospholipase D with the capacity to inactivate PAF. These enzymes inactivate the mediators in a time- and dose-dependent manner.

THE MOLECULAR BASIS OF IMMEDIATE TYPE HYPERSENSITIVITY REACTIONS IN HEALTH AND DISEASE

Mast cells and basophils are the only cell types normally possessing specific IgE recognition units for noxious foreign substances that are coupled to a capacity to generate and secrete large quantities of diverse potent mediators of cell function (Fig. 15). It is tempting to speculate that the physiologic role of mast cells and basophils in host defense is to recruit proteins, including immunoglobulins and complement, and to stimulate the ingress of phagocytic leukocytes to the reaction site. Once specific antibody and complement, followed in hours by eosinophils and other leukocytes, have arrived at the reaction site, the essential ingredients of the *humoral* and *cellular phases* of host defense are established locally. The initial or humoral phase of the host response would be mediated by the factors capable of altering local vascular permeability, such as histamine, LTC$_4$, PGD$_2$, and PAF (by its ability to elicit the release of platelet serotonin and other vasoactive principles). The cellular phase would be evoked by mediators, such as the tetrapeptides of ECF-

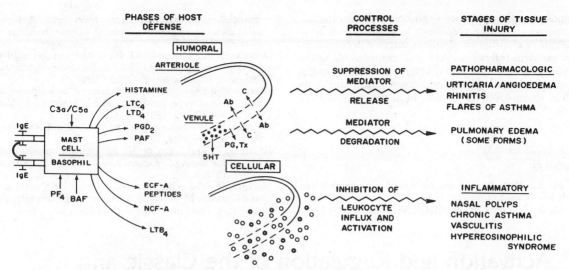

Figure 15. Contributions of immediate hypersensitivity to host defense and tissue injury. Effects of the mediators are depicted in relation to an arteriolar-venular loop.

$\longrightarrow$ = Action or release
$\rightsquigarrow$ = Penetration of control processes
Ag = Antigen
$\equiv$ = IgE antibody
C = Complement
Ab = Antibody
PG = Prostaglandin
Tx = Thromboxane
$5HT$ = Serotonin

A, the intermediate molecular weight ECF(s), NCF-A and LTB$_4$ (Fig. 15). The wide spectrum of molecular sizes and chemical composition of the leukocyte chemotactic factors would tend to stabilize the overall gradient, because the principles of smaller size or greater aqueous solubility would diffuse more rapidly and the stimuli of larger size or lower solubility more slowly.

The manner in which the immediate-type hypersensitivity response can facilitate host defense can be considered in terms of helminth infestations. Immediate-type hypersensitivity is present in patients experiencing metazoan parasite infections, as revealed by specific immediate-type skin tests and the release of histamine and ECF-A from peripheral leukocytes interacted with specific helminth antigen. The clinical course may include signs compatible with immediate-type hypersensitivity reactions and is characteristically marked by profound elevations in IgE, of which only a fraction is specific. In an intriguing study, which suggested an advantage in being atopic, serum IgE and peripheral blood eosinophil levels were found to be more elevated and fecal egg counts of *Necator americanus* were substantially reduced in atopic as compared with nonatopic native inhabitants of a hookworm-infected region of New Guinea.

The capacity of the tissue mast cell to recruit blood protein and cellular elements in its response to specific antigen or to a parasitic degranulating factor might be particularly pertinent to the control of the skin-penetrating or gut-attaching phase of a helminth cycle. In schistosomiasis, killing of the schistosomula and the encysted egg in vitro by human and peripheral blood leukocytes is an IgG antibody- and complement-dependent function of eosinophils and macrophages.

This special cellular protective function of eosinophils has been confirmed in in vivo studies of both schistosomula and *Trichinella* infections in mice. In such a circumstance the eosinophil would play a dual role in host defense: IgG- and complement-dependent cytotoxicity for the invading parasite and inactivation of many of the mast cell-derived mediators released directly by parasite-specific factors or by parasite antigen. Whereas the neutrophil influx is the critical factor in local host defense against bacteria, the eosinophil would still be useful as a regulatory element of an appropriately contained response. Parasites such as schistosomula and *T. cruzi* directly activate the alternative complement pathway and accumulate surface bound C3b with secondary mast cell involvement via the anaphylatoxins C3a and C5a. This reveals a mechanism of local host defense that involves the interplay of complement and mast cells in the nonimmune subject.

Failure to limit the mast cell response through an excessive reaction or a failure of local control processes, as in any other type of immunologic reaction, leads to disease (Fig. 15). In the case of immediate-type hypersensitivity, the mediators altering vascular permeability and smooth muscle tone are most likely responsible for the pathopharmacologic reactions of systemic anaphylaxis, urticaria, some instances of pulmonary edema, and acute exacerbations of asthma and rhinitis. The more chronic diseases of the atopic class are associated with cellular infiltration—that is, inflammation—but, in addition, the contributions of the hydrolases also must be considered. The result might be nasal polyps, persistent asthma, vasculitis, or an invasive hypereosinophilic syndrome. Numerous other defects have been described that may, in some cases, predispose to allergy rather than host defense, including abnormal cellular responses to endogenous beta-adrenergic or cholinergic agonists, enzyme deficiencies, or chronic viral infections. As for all components of the immune system, immediate reactions occur frequently, as part of normal physiologic responses, and only manifest themselves as disease in a minority of individuals.

REFERENCES

Bach, M. K.: Mediators of anaphylaxis and inflammation. Annu Rev Microbiol 36:371, 1982.

Caulfield, J. P., Lewis, R. A., Hein, A., et al.: Secretion in dissociated human pulmonary mast cells: Evidence for solubilization of granule contents before discharge. J Cell Biol 85:299, 1980.

Dvorak, A. M., Dickersin, G. R., Connell, A., et al.: Degranulation mechanisms in human leukemic basophils. Clin Immunol Immunopathol 5:235, 1976.

Goetzl, E. J.: Oxygenation products of arachidonic acid as mediators of hypersensitivity and inflammation. Med Clin North Am 65:809, 1981.

Ishizaka, K.: Cellular events in the IgE antibody response. Adv Immunol 23:1, 1976.

Ishizaka, T., and Ishizaka, K.: Biology of immunoglobulin E: Molecular basis of reaginic hypersensitivity. Prog Allergy 19:60, 1975.

Metzger, H.: The cellular receptor for IgE. In Cuatrecasas, P., and Greaves, M. F. (eds.): Receptors and Recognition, Series A, Vol. 4. London, Chapman and Hall, 1977, p. 75.

Activation and Regulation of the Classic and Alternative Complement Pathways

Complement is the major serum effector system for host defense against microbial infections and mediates many subacute and chronic inflammatory reactions. The two principal pathways of complement provide both adaptive protection through specific antibodies in the classic sequence and ready natural defense through broad recognition of microbial surfaces by the alternative sequence. Many general features of protein-protein and protein-cell/particle interactions are represented in the complex reactions of the diverse proteins of the complement system. The activation of the classic and alternative pathways of complement consists of the sequential interaction of at least 18 different proteins, which are macromolecules present in serum at substantial concentrations (Table 9). The noncovalent and occasional covalent associations of complement proteins that occur during activation of both sequences are followed by autocatalytic proteolysis, as for C1r, or proteolysis by an associated component, as for C1s or B. Cleavage of each component and conformational alterations in the major fragment generate intermediates that are unstable and decay in the fluid phase, but are stabilized by attachment to the developing complex of complement proteins. Many

TABLE 9. EFFECTOR AND REGULATORY COMPONENTS OF THE COMPLEMENT PATHWAYS

DESIGNATION	SIZE (daltons)	STRUCTURAL CHARACTERISTICS	HUMAN SERUM CONCENTRATION, MEAN (μg/ml)
C1q	400,000	Hexamer of globular heads attached to a central collagen-like stem	70
C1r	95,000	C1r and C1s both have two polypeptide chains, with serine protease activity in the light chain	35
C1s	85,000		35
C4	180,000	Glycoprotein composed of α, β, and γ chain	400
C2	117,000	Single-chain glycoprotein	25
C3 (factor A)	185,000	β globulin composed of α and β chain	1500
C5	200,000	β globulin composed of α and β chain	85
C6	128,000	Single-chain β globulin	75
C7	121,000	Single-chain β globulin	55
C8	153,000	γ globulin composed of α, β, and γ chain	55
C9	80,000	Single-chain α globulin	200
B (C3 proactivator)	95,000	Single-chain β globulin	250
D (C3 proactivator convertase)	25,000	Single-chain α globulin	2
P	149,000	Tetramer γ globulin	25
C1INH	105,000	Single-chain α globulin	180
C4-bp	540,000-590,000	Multiple identical subunits of approximately 70,000 m.w.	250
H	150,000	Single-chain β globulin	400
I (C3b/C4b inactivator)	90,000	β globulin composed of α and β chain	50

*C1INH = inhibitor of the activated first component of complement
C4-bp = serum-binding protein of C4
P = properdin
H = factor H or β1H
I = C3bINA or inactivator of C3b and C4b

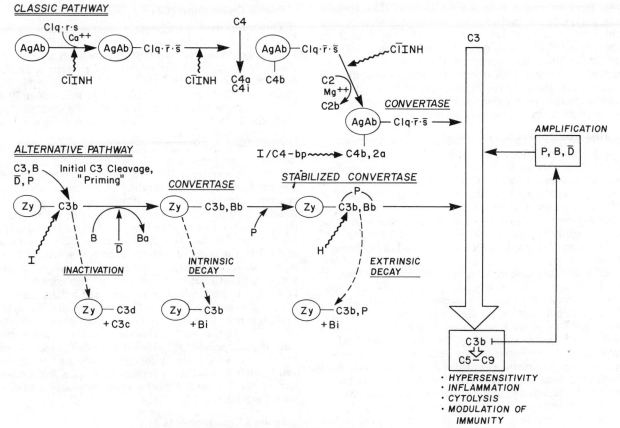

Figure 16. Major functional pathways of the complement system.
Zy = Zymosan particle
$AgAb$ = Antigen-antibody complex
P = Properdin
Mg^{++} = Magnesium ion
Ca^{++} = Calcium ion
⟶ = Reaction or conversion
⤳ = Inhibition or inactivation
----⟶ = Decay

of the low molecular weight cleavage fragments of complement proteins are potent fluid-phase mediators of hypersensitivity and inflammation that account for much of the noncytotoxic activity of complement. The activation and activities of complement are regulated at multiple levels, including the enzymes required for the development of the protein complexes, the established C3 and C5 convertases, the major cleavage fragments of complement proteins that can be displaced from the complexes, and both the major and minor fragments that are inactivated by further proteolysis.

Proteins of the classic pathway of C3 activation and of the effector pathway are designated by the capital letter C and an arabic number: C1, C4, C2, C3, C5 to C9, while the constituent proteins of the alternative pathway are denoted by capital letters: B,D,P,H,I (Table 9 and Fig. 16). C3 is involved in both pathways of initiation of complement activation and thus also may be referred to as factor A. Cleavage fragments of complement proteins are designated by lower case suffixes, as for C3a, C3b, Ba, Bb, while the letter i signifies inactive components, as in C2ai and Bbi. The bars over some numbers or letters signify the enzymatically active form of that complement protein.

PROTEIN CHEMISTRY AND BIOCHEMISTRY OF COMPLEMENT AND COMPLEMENT ACTIVATION

The most critical step in the generation of the biologic activities of complement is the cleavage of C3 and the liberation of the major fragment, termed C3b (Fig. 16). The functional subdivisions of the complement system include two pathways, the classic and alternative, for the formation of two different convertases capable of cleaving C3, an amplification limb of the alternative pathway that uses the initial C3b formed to augment C3 cleavage, and a final common effector pathway that C3b uses to recruit the terminal complement proteins C5 to C9 for cytolysis (Fig. 16).

THE CLASSIC PATHWAY OF COMPLEMENT COMPONENT ACTIVATION FOR C3 CLEAVAGE

If antibody that is aggregated by binding to polyvalent antigen or by physical cross-linking in the absence of antigen is added to serum, the first component (C1) is bound and converted into an active protease that catalyzes the activation of the fourth (C4) and second (C2) components (Fig. 16). Activated components in the form of major fragments C4b and C2a form a complex, C4b,2a, that also has proteolytic activity and catalyzes the cleavage and activation of the third component (C3). C3, as noted in detail below, may also be activated by an alternative pathway, which is initiated by contact with microbial surfaces and altered tissue membranes in the absence of antibodies. In both pathways the specific cleavage of C3 leads to sequential activation of the subsequent components.

First Component (C1)

C1 is formed from three subcomponents, C1q, C1r, and C1s (Table 9). In serum with a normal concentration of calcium, C1r and C1s are in a tight equimolar complex, but their interaction with C1q is weak. The C1r-C1s complex does not bind to IgG at all, unless C1q is present. C1q binds weakly to monomeric IgG, but strongly to aggregated IgG. Hence, interaction of C1 with antibody aggregates is presumed to be through C1q.

C1q contains nine dimers, of which six are composed of two different, A and B, polypeptide chains and three consist of two similar, C, polypeptide chains. The A, B, and C polypeptide chains have a similar but not identical amino acid sequence, and each contains a stretch of amino acids near the N-terminal that is typical of the collagen amino acid sequence. This sequence has glycine in every third position, and contains hydroxyproline and hydroxylysine residues, the latter being glycosylated in many cases with the disaccharide glucosylgalactose. The 18 peptide chains of C1q are bound together in a hexamer structure, joined in six fibrils formed from the collagen-like sections, and with globular heads. Interaction between C1q and aggregated antibody probably occurs through the second constant domain of the heavy chains of the antibody and the noncollagenous heads of the C1q hexamer structure.

C1r and C1s have similar structures of a single polypeptide chain of about 83,000 molecular weight. On activation, both C1r and C1s are split to produce active proteases formed from two peptide chains of about 56,000 and 27,000 molecular weight linked by disulfide bonds (Table 9). C1r and C1s are proteolytically inactive precursors of the serine esterases C$\overline{1}$r and C$\overline{1}$s and are activated on binding to antibody aggregates through C1q. They have a number of structural homologies with other serine esterase types of proteins. Zymosan-bound C1r is not activated by C$\overline{1}$r, and zymosan-bound C1s is not activated by C$\overline{1}$s, so that neither step is an autocatalytic event. Further, C$\overline{1}$s does not alter the state of C1r; yet activation of C1r to C$\overline{1}$r requires the presence of C1s, presumably to function in an activation complex but not as a protease. The kinetics of C1r activation in the C1 complex by an immune complex suggest an initial maximal rate upon binding without an autocatalytic element. The binding of a C1r-C1s complex to C1q, which has attached to aggregated immunoglobulin, probably causes a conformational change in C1r with uncovering of a catalytic site followed by an internal cleavage to present C$\overline{1}$r. C$\overline{1}$r then cleaves a peptide bond in C1s to yield C$\overline{1}$s; C$\overline{1}$s is then involved in the cleavage of C4 and C2 to form the classic C3 convertase, C4b,2a.

Fourth Component (C4)

This component is a glycoprotein of molecular weight 209,000 that is composed of three polypeptide chains linked by strong noncovalent interaction as well as disulfide bonds. The size of the alpha chain is 93,000 daltons, the beta chain 78,000, and the smaller gamma chain 33,000. Cleavage of C4 by C$\overline{1}$s releases a 7000 to 11,000 molecular weight fragment, designated C4a, from the N-terminus of the alpha chain; the residual major fragment is C4b.

C4b serves five functions: (1) irreversible binding to immune complexes and cell membranes via a nascent site that otherwise undergoes rapid decay to nonbinding fluid-phase C4i; (2) binding to immune adherence receptors present on a variety of cells via a stable binding site on C4b; (3) interaction with C$\overline{1}$ to allow more efficient cleavage of C2; (4) binding to activated C2 to form C4b,2a, the classic pathway C3 convertase; and (5) in the state of C4b,2a, interaction with C3b to form C4b,2a,3b, which is the classic pathway C5 convertase. Fluid-phase C4i retains all the capacities of C4b except the binding to membranes by the nascent site, and these functions of C4i and C4b are lost after cleavage into C4c and C4d. The mechanism for the effect of C4b/C4i on C2 cleavage by C$\overline{1}$ is unknown, but might include an allosteric modification of the active site of C$\overline{1}$, an allosteric modification of the substrate C2, or the provision of a site for deposition of the product, C2a, to allow interaction of C$\overline{1}$s with additional C2.

Second Component (C2)

C2 is a single-chain glycoprotein of 117,000 molecular weight that is cleaved by C$\overline{1}$s into C2a and C2b. The C2a fragment of 85,000 molecular weight is catalytically active, whereas the C2b fragment of 35,000 molecular weight serves as an activation peptide with a linkage function. C2a, like C$\overline{1}$r and C$\overline{1}$s, is a serine esterase. C2a must be associated with C4b or C4i in a magnesium ion–dependent binding to express C3-cleaving activity. Thus C2 has two interdependent sites uncovered by the action of C$\overline{1}$s: an enzymic site on C2a and a binding site for C4b on the smaller C2b fragment. C4b,2a undergoes temperature-dependent decay with a half-life at 37° C of five to ten minutes because of release of the bound C2a fragment, which is designated C2i as it lacks the binding site of C2b required for convertase function. The residual C4b is capable of reforming new C4b,2a convertase upon cleavage of additional C2 by C$\overline{1}$s, indicating that decay of the convertase is secondary to loss of C2a and that native C2 displaces any residual C2b on the C4b site. Since C4b,2a may activate the effector sequence of complement C3-C9, its formation completes the classic pathway of complement activation.

THE ALTERNATIVE AMPLIFYING AND ACTIVATION PATHWAYS FOR C3 CLEAVAGE

The alternative pathway was originally separated from the classic pathway on the basis of the independence of the sequence of proteins leading to utilization of C3 and the absence of a requirement for antibody aggregates to initiate activation. It is now clear, however, that the alternative pathway proteins amplify both antibody-dependent and antibody-independent C3 cleavage. The amplifying function is essential to any regulated expression of alternative pathway activation and augments antibody-dependent classic complement activation (Fig. 16); thus it serves both the nonimmune and immune host. The proteins of the amplification pathway are the same as those of the alternative initiating pathway—namely, properdin, B, D, and C3, with the only distinction being the requirement for the C3b state to shift their interaction to the amplified state. Since their sequential interaction in the amplified state is well known, it will be presented in a discussion of structural and functional relationships, followed by a description of the complex molecular events that initiate the alternative pathway of complement.

Third Component (C3)

C3, originally recognized as the substrate for classic C3 convertase, is now also known to be factor A of the original alternative or properdin pathway. C3, a beta globulin of 190,000 molecular weight, is composed of two polypeptide chains, alpha of 120,000 molecular weight and beta of 70,000 molecular weight, linked by disulfide bonds. Cleavage of C3 during the initiation of the alternative pathway, by the amplification C3 convertase, or by the classic C3 convertase (Fig. 16) yields a 6000 to 8000 molecular weight fragment, C3a, from the N-terminus of the alpha chain and a residual C3b fragment (Fig. 17). This fragment, like C4b of the classic C3 convertase, serves as the receptor for another protein, which then provides the C3-cleaving site.

B

B is a 100,000 molecular weight beta globulin consisting of a single polypeptide chain. When in a magnesium ion–dependent reversible association with C3b, B expresses some C3-cleaving activity, which is markedly increased upon cleavage by $\overline{D}$ to yield Bb, an 80,000 molecular weight fragment, and a 20,000 molecular weight activation fragment Ba. The Bb fragment is released in an inactive form, Bi, following which the residual C3b is capable of re-forming new C3b,Bb convertase upon association with additional B and attendant $\overline{D}$ cleavage.

$\overline{D}$

$\overline{D}$, a single polypeptide chain alpha globulin serine esterase of about 23,500 molecular weight, cleaves B in the presence of C3b to uncover fully the C3 convertase activity of the bimolecular complex, C3b,Bb. The analogies of the amplification pathway to the classic initiating pathway include: (1) formation of a magnesium ion–dependent bimolecular complex, C4b,2 and C3b,B, respectively; (2) action of a serine esterase, C1 and $\overline{D}$, to uncover the full C3-cleaving activity of the fragments 2a and Bb in the respective convertases, C4b,2a and C3b,Bb; and (3) decay of convertase function through release of the nonbinding C2i and Bi (Fig. 16). The differences are in the order of the molecular events. In the classic system the fixation of antibody to antigen determines the site of C1 activation to $\overline{C1}$ and the point of deposition of C4b,2a, the classic C3 convertase. In the alternative pathway, the association of C3b,B on the initiating surface facilitates the generation by $\overline{D}$ of C3b,Bb, and the amplification C3 convertase at that site. Since the substrate specificity of $\overline{D}$ for B is not expressed until formation of the bimolecular complex, there is control of the capability of $\overline{D}$ without invoking a zymogen, D.

Properdin

Properdin, a non-immunoglobulin gamma globulin of 220,000 molecular weight, adsorbs to the surface of particles during initiation of the alternative pathway. Properdin exists in two functional forms: native, as defined by reversible binding to C3b; and fully activated, as characterized by irreversible binding to C3b and unmasking of the capacity to permit assembly of the fluid-phase amplification convertase upon addition to normal serum in the absence of an activating particle. The two forms of properdin exhibit identical subunits of 56,000 molecular weight, noncovalently linked to form a tetramer. Properdin binds to and effects a nonenzymatic conformational change in C3b, and in this manner stabilizes the amplification convertase, C3b,Bb, by retarding the decay-dissociation of Bb as Bi.

Initiation

Since $\overline{D}$ is normally present in serum and plasma, there is presumably continuous but low-grade action

Figure 17. The effector sequence of the complement system and the biologically active fragments and complexes that are generated during cleavage of C3 and C5 by the classic and amplification C3 and C5 convertases, respectively. (Modified from Fearon, D. T., and Austen, K. F. *In* McCarty, D. J., and Hollander, J. L. (eds.): Arthritis and Allied Conditions. 9th ed. Philadelphia, Lea and Febiger, 1979. Reproduced with permission of the authors and publisher.)

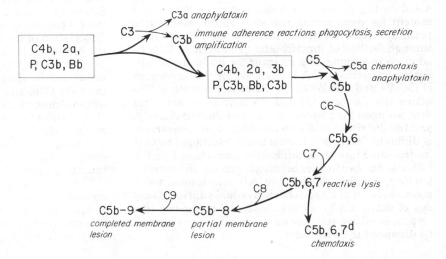

of $\overline{D}$ on B that has been complexed to C3. The resultant C3Bb would cleave C3 in plasma to continuously generate small quantities of the C3b fragment, which is central to the formation of the amplification convertase as described above. This initial fluid-phase C3 cleavage by the alternative pathway proteins may be facilitated by properdin stabilization of the less efficient C3 convertases, such as C3Bb, or even with inadequate amounts of D, C3b,B. Nonetheless, under the usual circumstances, the fluid-phase interactions of C3, B, D, and P would be prevented from amplifying by the action of the regulatory proteins. Microbial and mammalian cell surfaces that activate the alternative pathway in the absence of specific antibody nonspecifically bind the small "priming" quantities of C3b generated in continuous low-grade fashion by the regulated fluid-phase interaction. Although the initial C3b uptake by such surfaces is no greater than for nonactivating principles, the amplification effect is limited to activating surfaces. Such surfaces protect C3b from inactivation by C3b inactivator (I) in the presence of H and protect C3b,Bb,P from being dissociated by H, which can displace Bb with attendant decay of convertase function (Fig. 16). The intense deposition of C3b on such surfaces facilitates further activation of the convertase on the particle in a manner analogous to acceleration of the activation of the classic convertase by accumulation of specific antibody on surface determinants. Indeed, were specific antibody to be present to permit classic initiation, the benefits of amplification would be further appreciated. In any event, the alternative pathway may be viewed as a two-phase system: continuous, low-grade C3 cleavage with complete regulation of the putative actions of C3b, and amplified cleavage of C3 by a C3b-dependent convertase protected from the regulatory mechanisms largely by the nature of the surface taking up C3b from the fluid phase.

THE EFFECTOR COMPLEMENT COMPONENT SEQUENCE

The classic and amplifying C3 convertases recruit the effector proteins of the complement system, C3, C5, C6, C7, C8, and C9 (Figs. 16 and 17).

Third Component (C3)

The structural characteristics of native C3 were noted during its previous consideration as the central protein for determining the shift of the alternative pathway from low-grade turnover to amplification through facilitated function and generation of C3b. In addition to serving as a receptor for Bb in the amplification convertase, C3b is essential for the conversion of C4b,2a and C3b,Bb to the C5 convertase state. The active site for both C3 and C5 convertase activities depends upon the presence of C2a and Bb, respectively, and the distribution of C3b involved in the conversion is different from and quantitatively additional to that incorporated into the amplification convertase, C3b,Bb. C3b also has two further binding functions: irreversible binding, possibly covalent, to cell membranes via a nascent site of marked lability available during cleavage of native C3 by a convertase; and adherence to a trypsin-sensitive receptor on many cells types, as will be discussed in detail later.

Components 5, 6, 7, 8, and 9 (C5–C9)

C5 and C8 are multichain globulins, while C6, C7, and C9 are proteins of a single polypeptide chain (Table 9). Cleavage of C5 by either classic or amplification C5 convertase releases a peptide of about 11,000 molecular weight, C5a, from the alpha chain, leaving the major fragment, C5b.

C5b may bind directly to membranes bearing the convertase, complex with C6 in the fluid phase to form C5b,6, or remain in the fluid phase as C5i owing to irreversible decay of the membrane binding site. Membrane-bound C5b is labile, being subject to decay to C5i unless it complexes with C6. The membrane binding site on fluid-phase C5b,6 is not available until complexed with C7 to form C5b,6,7, which is capable of transiently binding to unsensitized membranes, a mechanism known as reactive lysis, which extends the cytolytic effects of complement to innocent bystander cells. If C5b,6,7 does not encounter an appropriate membrane, the binding site of C5b decays, and the complex becomes C5i,6,7, a cytolytically inactive but chemotactically active unit.

Formation of membrane-bound C5b,6,7 permits binding of C8 to the C5b fragment to create a partial membrane lesion, resulting in slow lysis. Although C8 possesses as many as six binding sites for C9, formation of a complex containing only one C9 accelerates the lytic reaction. These final steps in the complement sequence do not involve cleavage of C6-C9, but represent noncovalent assembly and conformational alterations of the components of the C5-C9 multimolecular complex. An additional serum protein, distinct from known complement components, has been found in C5-C9 complexes formed in the fluid phase. The function of this additional protein is now believed to be regulatory and to interfere with the insertion of the terminal pentamolecular complex and thus with formation of the membrane lesion leading to cytolysis.

REGULATORY PROTEINS OF THE COMPLEMENT SEQUENCES

Regulation of the reactions of the complement components occurs because of the intrinsic lability of certain essential binding steps and through the action of extrinsic control proteins. Inherent control is exemplified by the rapid decay under physiologic conditions of the C3 convertases, C4b,2a, C3,Bb, and C3b,Bb due to dissociation of the proteins bearing the catalytic activity, but which have lost a critical binding site. Another example of this type of control is the lability of the membrane binding sites appearing with generation of the C4b, C3b, and C5b fragments such that failure to achieve immediate membrane fixation results in loss of that potentiality. The implication of this lability of binding sites involved in protein-protein interactions and protein-membrane interactions is that, to be efficient, cleavage activation must occur at or near the initiating principle.

The extrinsic control proteins of the reaction sequence include the inhibitor of the activated first component (C$\overline{1}$INH) and the C4-binding protein (C4-bp), which regulate the classic activation pathway, and the inactivator of C3b (I) and H, which together regulate activation of the alternative pathway and amplification of either pathway. An additional type of control is represented by the anaphylatoxin inactivator, which inactivates a class of biologically active reaction by-products rather than the sequence itself.

C1INH

C1INH consists of a single polypeptide chain alpha globulin of 105,000 molecular weight, which has an unusually high carbohydrate content of approximately 35 per cent. C1INH controls assembly of C4b,2a by binding to the light chain of C1s, which bears the serine esteric site, thereby irreversibly inhibiting its capacity to cleave C4 and C2 (Fig. 16). The complex formation between C1INH and C1s is firm so the inhibitor is removed, although it is not broken down by its reaction with the enzyme. C1INH also blocks the esterolytic activity of C1r, thereby regulating both activation of C1 and expression of its function. C1INH also functions as a control protein for the Hageman factor–initiated pathways, since it inhibits the capacity of activated Hageman factor to activate prekallikrein and Factor XI of the clotting system and suppresses the kinin-generating and chemotactic activities of kallikrein. Inherited deficiency of this control protein results in hereditary angioedema, the disease that is characterized by recurrent nonpitting, noninflammatory swellings of the cutaneous and mucosal upper respiratory and gastrointestinal surfaces. The mucosal lesions can be obstructive, thus leading to respiratory distress and recurrent abdominal pain. The condition is associated with chronically depressed serum levels of C4 and C2 because of their cleavage by uninhibited C1 that is spontaneously generated. C3 serum levels are not correspondingly depressed, attesting to the relative inefficiency of forming and expressing the classic C3 convertase in the fluid phase.

C4-bp

C4-bp is a plasma protein, existing in two genetically distinct forms of 540,000 and 590,000 molecular weight, that is composed of identical subunits of 70,000 molecular weight and that, like C1INH, inhibits only the classic pathway. The binding of C4-bp to C4b results in three different inhibitory effects, including prevention of uptake of C2 by C4b, accelerated dissociation and decay of the C2a already bound to C4b, and greater susceptibility of C4b to cleavage inactivation by I.

I(C3b/C4b INA)

I is a beta-globulin of 93,000 molecular weight that is composed of two polypeptide chains, an alpha chain of 55,000 and a beta chain of 42,000 molecular weight, linked by disulfide bonds.

I cleaves the alpha' chain of C3b without fragmentation, resulting in the loss of such functions as formation of the amplification convertase, conversion of C3b,Bb and C4b,2a to C5 convertases, and immune adherence. Inactivation is followed by further cleavages to yield C3c and the smaller 25,000 molecular weight fragment C3d, providing that trace amounts of a noncomplement tryptic protease such as plasmin are present. Whereas this inactivation cleavage of the alpha' chain of C3b by I is well expressed when the substrate is surface fixed, a cofactor, H, appears to be particularly important when the C3b is in the fluid phase. Fluid-phase C4b also appears to be inactivated by cleavage of the alpha' chain without fragmentation in the presence of a cofactor protein, suggesting that I may have a regulatory role to play in the diminishing regeneration of both the classic and amplification convertases. I cannot inactivate C3b in the bimolecular C3 convertase, C3b,Bb, although it will inactivate the additional C3b, which converts the C3b,Bb convertase to a C5 convertase.

H(Beta-1H)

H is a beta globulin of 150,000 molecular weight that is composed of a single polypeptide chain. It functions, as noted above, to facilitate inactivation of C3b by I, especially in the fluid phase, and to dissociate Bb from the complex C3b,Bb. Neither H alone nor I alone is sufficient to prevent the interaction of C3, B, D, and P from progressing to amplification, and patients genetically lacking I are depleted of C3 and B by their amplified utilization. The secondary C3 deficiency leads to impaired host defense with recurrent infection by pyogenic microorganisms. The three levels of control of the amplification convertase are complementary and necessary, especially in the presence of properdin stabilization. Intrinsic and H-mediated extrinsic decay release Bb from C3b,Bb. The loss of Bb is only partially effective in preventing continuous activation of C3, since the C3b may re-form new convertase with B and D, unless C3b is inactivated by I. I acts only on C3b that is unassociated with Bb, and this reaction is augmented by H independent of its capacity to displace Bb and C3b,Bb.

Anaphylatoxin Inactivator (AI)

AI, which inactivates C3a and C5a, is an alpha$_2$ globulin with a molecular weight of 310,000, which consists of eight apparently identical noncovalently bound subunits of molecular weight 36,000. AI cleaves the C-terminal arginine from C3a and C5a and from bradykinin. The active site of AI is inhibited by high concentrations of epsilon-aminocaproic acid.

Two serum proteins, termed chemotactic factor inactivators, are capable of abolishing the chemotactic activities of C3- and C5-derived fragments. These inactivators are aminopeptidases and are not inhibited by metal ion chelators, thereby distinguishing them from the metal-dependent AI.

BIOLOGIC EFFECTS OF THE COMPLEMENT PATHWAYS

The biologic activities of complement activation in host defense and tissue injury stem both from the assembly of the pentamolecular terminal complex of C5b-C9 and from the cleavage of C3 and C5. The terminal complex is directly cytolytic for the host cell or for the organism that provided the surface for complement activation. Two general classes of mediators that are not directly cytolytic are also generated during complement activation. The first is composed of the surface-bound bifunctional fragments of complement proteins that are attached specifically to the targets of complement activation and then interact

TABLE 10. RECEPTORS FOR COMPLEMENT ON LEUKOCYTES AND OTHER CELLS

RECEPTOR	SPECIFICITY	CELLS	EFFECTS ON CELLS
		Cell or Particle-Bound Complement Proteins	
Clq	Clq	Neutrophils	Enhanced respiration
		Monocytes	
		B lymphocytes	
		T lymphocytes (subpopulation)	Augmented ADCC
		Null lymphocytes	
CRI	C3b	Neutrophils	Enhanced endocytosis and phagocytic
		Monocytes	recognition
		Eosinophils	
		B lymphocytes	
		T lymphocytes (subpopulation)	
		Glomerular cells	
		Mast cells	
		Erythrocytes	Binding (clearance) of immune complexes
			Facilitation of cleavage of C3B
CR2	C3d	B lymphocytes	
		Other lymphocytes	Enhanced proliferation and ADCC
CR3	C3d,g	Neutrophils	Enhanced secretion
		Macrophages	Enhanced phagocytosis
		Natural killer cells	Facilitation of cytotoxicity
		B lymphocytes (subpopulation)	
		Low Molecular Weight Complement Protein Fragments	
C3e	C3e	Neutrophils	Increased mobilization
C3a	C3a >>C4a	Mast cells	Mediator secretion
		Basophils	
		Platelets	Enhanced secretion and aggregation
		Helper T lymphocytes	Suppressed function
C5a	C5a	Mast cells	Mediator secretion
		Basophils	
		Neutrophils	Chemotaxis and other functions
		Eosinophils	
		Monocytes	Chemotaxis and protein production
		Lymphocytes	Augmented function

with effector cells that bear receptors for the fragments (Table 10). An example of this class is C3b attached to a bacterium, which promotes the phagocytosis of the bacterium by neutrophils and macrophages. The second class of noncytolytic complement mediators consists of low molecular weight cleavage fragments of complement proteins, which act locally to modify normal cellular functions or to incite or modulate inflammatory responses (Table 10, Fig. 17). An example of this class is C5a, which stimulates mast cell and platelet secretion, neutrophil and monocyte chemotaxis, and smooth muscle contraction.

Cytolysis

The formation of the multimolecular complex C5b-C9 on a cell membrane impairs osmotic regulation, which may cause cytolysis. A single membrane-bound C5b-C9 complex per cell may be sufficient for lysis. Both the classic and alternative activating pathways and fluid-phase C5b,6,7 alone have the capacity to prepare cells for lysis upon addition of C8 and C9. There appears to be no requirement for membrane-associated protein, since liposomes, which are free of protein, are similarly susceptible to the lytic action of the C5b-C9 complex.

Electron microscopy of erythrocytes that have been lysed by human complement has revealed characteristic doughnut-shaped lesions on the outer leaflet that have a dark central portion with a diameter of 10 to 11 nm surrounded by a lighter ring. The dark central area may be a depression in the membrane or a hydrophilic region, whereas the outer ring may be a relatively raised or hydrophobic region. These lesions are thought to represent alterations in the outer leaflet of the lipid layer of the membrane created by insertion of the nascent C5b,6,7 complex, assembled on or near a cell, into the phospholipid bilayer. The subsequent sequential interaction of C8 and C9 promotes further penetration of the final pentamolecular complex so as to create a transmembrane channel that impairs osmotic regulation and leads to cytolysis.

Anaphylatoxins

Anaphylatoxin is the trivial name for the low molecular weight peptides C3a and C5a. Human C3a and C5a contract isolated guinea pig ileum at concentrations of $10^{-8}M$ and $10^{-9}M$, respectively, and cause degranulation of human skin mast cells with wheal and flare reactions at $10^{-12}M$ and $10^{-15}M$, respectively. These actions are blocked by antihistamines. C3a and C5a do not exhibit cross tachyphylaxis on the guinea pig ileum, indicating the presence of different subsets of receptors for the two peptides. In addition, direct smooth muscle contractile activity that is independent of histamine release is attributable to C3a and C5a. Both types of activities of C3a and C5a are abolished rapidly by anaphylatoxin inactivator, which removes the C-terminal arginine from the peptides. Although unable to release histamine, the des-arginine derivative of C3a binds to mast cells and partially inhibits histamine release by active C3a. This mode of receptor blockage may represent another control mechanism for limiting the biologic activity of anaphylatoxins.

Chemotactic Activities

The anaphylatoxin C5a, the hemolytically inactive C5b,6,7 complex, and C3b,Bb presented as the bimolecular convertase have chemotactic activity for leukocytes, with different specificities. Generation of these chemotactic principles may occur not only by sequential activation of either the classic or alternative pathways, but also by the action of other proteolytic enzymes. For example, trypsin and a neutral protease present in lysosomal granules generate chemotactically active fragments from C5. Exposure of neutrophils to one chemotactic principle usually renders them unresponsive to the original as well as to others in reactions termed deactivation and cross-deactivation, respectively. Deactivation prevents further directed migration and may serve either to hold cells at an inflammatory focus, so that other functions can be expressed, or to exclude them so as to permit an alteration in the cellular composition of the infiltrate. Deactivation is linked to chemotactic activation in specificity; thus the capacity of the amplification convertase, C3b,Bb, to render human neutrophils unresponsive to the chemotactic action of C5a suggests a chemotactic capacity for the convertase or its Bb-associated fragment.

Leukocyte-Mobilizing Factor

A fragment released from C3 by the classic convertase, C4b,2a, has been found to release mature polymorphonuclear leukocytes from perfused isolated bone. This polypeptide of approximately 10,000 molecular weight, termed C3e, is derived from the remaining alpha′ chain of C3c. Administration of this fragment to rabbits by the intravenous route produced minimal leukopenia followed by marked leukocytosis. Although structurally and functionally distinct from the anaphylatoxic fragment C3a, C3e resembles C3a in also augmenting vascular permeability at cutaneous sites. C3e has no chemotactic or chemokinetic activity.

THE SPECIFICITY OF NONCYTOLYTIC INTERACTIONS OF COMPLEMENT WITH CELLS: CHARACTERISTICS OF COMPLEMENT RECEPTORS

There are at least four noncytolytic activities of activated components of complement and small fragments of complement proteins that are expressed in normal subjects but may not be in individuals with specific deficiencies of complement components:

(1) Clearance of immune complexes from the circulation. The recognition by leukocytes of C1q and C3b on immune complexes and the binding by erythrocytes of immune complex–associated C3b both appear to be examples of mechanisms for removing such complexes from the circulation.

(2) The production, distribution, and function of phagocytic leukocytes. Such effects include the enhancement of bone marrow generation of polymorphonuclear leukocytes by C3e, and the chemotactic

attraction and sequestration in lung tissue of polymorphonuclear leukocytes by C5a.

(3) The classic humoral functions of complement. Examples include smooth muscle contraction and enhanced microvascular permeability mediated by C3a and C5a.

(4) The modulation of immunity by complement. The ability of C3d to enhance antibody-dependent cellular cytotoxicity of some lymphocytes and the suppression of helper T lymphocyte functions by C3a are examples of this class of functions.

Three proteins attach to the target of complement activation, namely, C1q, H, and C3b and its further degradation products. The cellular receptor for C3b will be described in some detail, followed by briefer descriptions of other complement receptors (Table 10).

The immune adherence (IA) reaction occurs between C3b-coated complexes and certain cells that bear specialized membrane-associated receptors (IA receptors) for C3b. Human cells possessing the IA receptor are erythrocytes, mast cells, neutrophils, eosinophils, macrophages, monocytes, B lymphocytes, and some T lymphocytes. The presence or absence of other complement components does not influence adherence; C3b passively absorbed to tannic acid–treated erythrocytes supports the reaction. IA does not require divalent cations or energy metabolism, but is temperature dependent, presumably because aggregation of IA receptors is inhibited by the relative rigidity of the membrane at reduced temperatures. Treatment of particle-bound C3b with I abolishes its adherence to human erythrocytes, indicating the presence on this cell type of receptors only for intact C3b. The IA receptor is trypsin sensitive and contains sulfhydryl bonds, which contribute to the integrity of the site. The biologic consequences of IA depend upon the cell type, and binding to the membrane IA receptor acts as a signal for which the cell response has been programmed.

Although complexes sensitized with IgG are subject to phagocytosis after binding to the membrane receptors for the Fc fragment of IgG, prior interaction of the immune complex with complement greatly increases the rate and extent of phagocytosis. The components required for enhanced phagocytosis are precisely those needed for IA. The two events can be dissociated, however, since phagocytosis of immune complexes by polymorphonuclear leukocytes, monocytes, and macrophages is depressed by metabolic inhibitors, organophosphorus compounds, and chelation of divalent cations, while IA is unaffected. Further, particles coated with IgM do not adhere to monocytes, whereas such particles bearing, in addition, C3b manifest IA without subsequent phagocytosis unless the monocyte is independently activated. The importance of the activity of C3b in host defense is exemplified by patients with genetic or acquired deficiency of C3 who experience repeated bacterial infections. In the case of genetic deficiency, restoration of the C3 content with purified C3 corrects the in vitro opsonic defects. The C3b receptor, also designated CR1, is only one of three cellular recognition sites for C3 (Table 10). The CR1 receptor for C3b is a 250,000 molecular weight glycoprotein that is detectable by reaction with specific antireceptor antibodies in all of the cells that bind C3b.

The receptor for C3d, designated CR2, is a 72,000-

molecular weight glycoprotein found on B lymphocytes and possibly some subsets of large granular lymphocytes. The C3d receptor seems to be coupled to mixed lymphocyte- and mitogen-induced lymphocyte proliferation and lymphocyte-mediated antibody-dependent cellular cytotoxicity (ADCC). The C3 receptor named CR3 appears to bind C3d,g selectively and is located on monocytes, some B lymphocytes, and neutrophils. The use of lymphocyte subset–specific monoclonal antibodies to alter the binding properties of CR3 resulted in the tentative conclusion that murine natural killer cells bear CR3 and that it facilitates cytotoxicity. Although some lymphocytes and other leukocytes recognize factor H, it is unclear whether the complement-activating target displays H alone or after binding to C3b. The functional effects of H also require further investigation.

After $\overline{C1}$INH binds to and induces the dissociation of $\overline{C1}$r and $\overline{C1}$s, C1q becomes available for binding to neutrophils, monocytes, B lymphocytes, and subsets of T lymphocytes and null lymphocytes. C1q receptors facilitate the binding of C1q-containing immune complexes and opsonized particles to phagocytic leukocytes and enhance lymphocyte-mediated ADCC.

Mast cells, basophils, platelets, and some subsets of helper T lymphocytes have receptors for C3a. Binding of C3a to receptors on the various types of cells both stimulates and inhibits cell functions. C3a initiates the secretion of mediators by mast cells and basophils through a mechanism distinct from that of IgE-directed activation. C3a inhibits helper T lymphocyte function by C3a by suppressing both lymphokine generation and helper cell function for B lymphocytes.

C5a is the most potent and functionally diverse of the low molecular weight complement fragment mediators. C5a, like C3a, induces the release of histamine and other preformed constituents of granules from mast cells and basophils. Although leukotrienes are secreted from lung tissue fragments exposed to C5a, the mast cell is probably not the source. C5a, unlike C3a, is chemotactic for neutrophils, eosinophils, monocytes, and basophils. In addition, C5a increases neutrophil adherence to endothelial cells and other surfaces, enhances the expression of C3b receptors, and initiates both the oxidative burst and the release of lysosomal enzymes. That lower concentrations of C5a stimulate chemotaxis and increased adherence than the cytotoxic effector functions suggests that the C5a promotes neutrophil localization at sites of complement activation prior to the expression of the bactericidal potential of the neutrophils. C5a, in contrast to C3a, appears to exert immunostimulatory effects, including increases in production of interleukin 1 by macrophages and lymphocyte proliferative responses to antigen.

INTERACTIONS OF THE COMPLEMENT SEQUENCE WITH OTHER EFFECTOR PATHWAYS

The ability of $\overline{C1}$INH to inhibit the activated Hageman factor and its fragments illustrates how the utilization of $\overline{C1}$INH by $\overline{C1}$ would favor initiation of fibrinolysis, coagulation, and kinin generation by active Hageman factor. Additional interactions of $\overline{C1}$INH with kallikrein limit the proteolytic kinin-generating

and chemotactic activity of the active site. Plasmin can activate C1 to $\overline{C1}$ and cleave C3 to yield C3b, thus initiating classic and amplifying complement function. An antigenic relationship exists between the D factor of the alternative complement pathway and prothrombin and an autocatalyzed fragment of thrombin, possibly representing an essential link between two sequences with effector functions independent of a specific immune response. The modulation between the Hageman factor–dependent sequences and the classic and alternative complement pathways could profoundly influence the intensity and chronicity of an inflammatory host response.

The interplay of the complement system with immune complexes is highlighted by the activation of the classic pathway. However, antibody directed against a microorganism that itself has the surface properties necessary for initiating the alternative pathway would have an augmented effect—that is, recruitment and stabilization of the amplification pathway with a synergistic interplay of the IgG(Fc) and C3b receptors in phagocytosis or cytotoxicity.

The implications of cellular immunity for complement function are only in the early stages of definition. The production of C2 by human monocytes is stimulated with lymphokine-rich supernates. The recent finding of bidirectional modulation of lymphocyte function by C3a and C5a may presage the revelation of other important links between the generation and action of complement and the diverse functions of lymphocytes.

Finally, although the capacity of the anaphylatoxins to activate tissue mast cells for the release of the mediators of immediate hypersensitivity has long been recognized, the capacity of the mast cell products to modulate complement function is only now being appreciated. Commercial heparin has numerous anticomplementary effects on the classic complement pathway. Commercial heparin directly inhibits binding of C1q to immune complexes, interaction of $\overline{C1}$s with C4 and C2, and binding of C2 to C4b, and thus suppresses generation of the classic convertase, C4b,2a. This effect is enhanced in the presence of $\overline{C1}$INH because heparin acts as a cofactor to increase its inhibitory activity against $\overline{C1}$. In the effector sequence, heparin inhibits formation of the C5b,6,7 complex as assessed by expression of the chemotactic activity of that trimolecular macromolecule. Commercial heparin in concentrations exhibiting anticoagulant and antithrombin III cofactor activity suppresses generation of the amplification convertase, C3b,Bb. More importantly, native 750,000 molecular weight rat and mouse mast cell heparin proteoglycan is as active an inhibitor as commercial heparin when both materials are compared on the basis of uronic acid content. Since numerous microorganisms directly recruit the amplification pathway to their surface, the mast cell with its mucosal, cutaneous, and perivenular locations could be an important modulating cell of nonimmune host defense.

BIOSYNTHESIS AND METABOLISM OF COMPLEMENT PROTEINS

The metabolic behavior of highly purified and radiolabeled human complement components C4, C3, C5, and B reveals a fractional catabolic rate for all four proteins in the same relatively high range. This fractional catabolic rate of about 2 per cent of the plasma pool per hour or 50 per cent of the plasma pool per day indicates that these proteins are among the most rapidly metabolized human plasma proteins. Although fractional catabolic rates among normal subjects are independent of serum levels of the protein, synthetic rates for each of these complement proteins correlated well with plasma levels. Thus, in normal persons the rate of complement component synthesis is the major determinant of the plasma concentration.

Even in patients with inflammatory diseases, the synthetic rates remain well correlated with the plasma concentration, reflecting the acute phase response of the constituents of this effector system. Hypercatabolism in diseases with an immunologic element, such as systemic lupus erythematosus or rheumatoid arthritis, is accompanied by compensatory hypersynthesis. In certain abnormal circumstances, as in membranoproliferative glomerulonephritis and IgG-IgM cryoglobulinemia, C3 and C4, respectively, are hyposynthesized with or without evidence of hypercatabolism. The pathobiologic mechanism of depressed component synthesis is not known, and in most acquired diseases reduced plasma concentrations reflect increased catabolism to a degree that overcomes compensatory hypersynthesis.

The macrophage appears to be a source of proteins involved in convertase formation. Thus, such cells have been shown in culture to synthesize C4 and C2 of the classic convertase and B, $\bar{D}$, C3, and P of the alternative and amplification convertases. Although such a source would represent a significant link of these acute phase effector proteins to cells involved in host defense and activated by both T and B cell-derived mediators and complement fragments, other cell types are also involved routinely. C1 and thus its three subunits are synthesized by epithelial cell cultures, although C1q may, in addition, be macrophage derived. The major source of the effector proteins of the terminal sequence appears to be the hepatocyte, which has been demonstrated as a source for C3, C5, and C9. Liver transplantation changes the C3 and C6 polymorphic type from that of the recipient to that of the donor. The regulatory protein C$\bar{1}$INH is also synthesized in the liver, but no data exist at present regarding the sites of I and H synthesis.

Polysomes from guinea pig liver homogenates synthesize C4 as a single polypeptide chain of 200,000 molecular weight, designated pro-C4. C4 secreted from the intact cells is composed of the three chains, alpha, beta, and gamma, linked by disulfide bridges. C4 protein derived from human plasma is about 1 to 3 per cent in the single-chain pro-C4 state, whereas the remainder exhibits the three-chain structure characteristic of the postsynthetic modification apparently related to its secretion.

THE MOLECULAR BASIS OF THE ROLE OF THE CLASSIC AND ALTERNATIVE PATHWAYS IN HEALTH AND DISEASE

Many insights have been gained concerning the role of complement in host defense from the study of patients with inborn errors. The expectation that deficiencies would lead to defects in host resistance and increased susceptibility to infection has been validated only for patients with homozygous C3 deficiency, in whom the recurrent bacterial infections are reminiscent of agammaglobulinemia. Since such patients do mount a specific antibody response, their susceptibility is attributed to absence of C3b-mediated amplification of classic pathway complement function and lack of C3b-mediated immune adherence enhancement of phagocytosis. A susceptibility of such patients to their initial encounter with a particular microorganism would have been predicted from the role of the alternative initiation and amplification pathway in coating bacteria with C3b in the nonimmune host. However, the susceptibility to recurrent infections without age-related amelioration indicates that the synergistic action of the IgG(Fc) and C3b receptors is critical to full defense of immune hosts against pyogenic microorganisms controlled by phagocytosis.

Although individuals with deficiencies in the terminal complement components have been recognized with single or recurrent gonococcal or meningococcal infections, it is difficult to state that the frequency or susceptibility differs from normal. Recurrent pyogenic infections are not an issue in this group, attesting to the central role of their normal concentrations of C3. The bactericidal reaction is lacking in such sera, and it seems logical to speculate that this lack might predispose to prolonged bacteremia with organisms generally susceptible to lysis by this mechanism.

The studies of genetic defects in regulation have been particularly informative since the clinical concomitants were not predictable at the time the deficiencies were recognized. The definition of C$\bar{1}$INH permitted the development of clinical assays and the molecular definition of the disease termed hereditary angioedema. Kindreds with hereditary angioedema generally have no antigenic protein but in a minority of instances produce a nonfunctioning variant protein. The uninhibited action of C$\bar{1}$ on its natural substrates C4 and C2 generates a fragment that, upon further cleavage by plasmin, has the capacity to alter vascular permeability directly. As the C$\bar{1}$INH controls both C$\bar{1}$ activation and function and the ability of activated Hageman factor and its fragments to utilize cofactors that activate plasminogen, the lack of C$\bar{1}$INH could permit a significant interaction between these systems. Of the conventional forms of treatment, the efficacy of the antifibrinolytic agents, epsilon-aminocaproic acid and 4-aminomethyl cyclohexane carboxylic acid, is attributed to their inhibition of plasmin generation, thus preventing plasmin from cleaving the pathogenetic peptide from the fragment of C2. Effective prophylaxis with antifibrinolytic agents is not associated with a correction in the chronically reduced levels of C4 and C2 or a decrease in activated and uninhibited C$\bar{1}$. The efficacy of methyltestosterone and attenuated androgens is associated with a rise in the levels of C4 into the normal range and even a restoration with the attenuated androgens of the plasma levels of C$\bar{1}$INH. The attenuated androgens are used in a relatively greater anabolic dose than the methyltestosterone and correct the biochemical defect more strikingly but without greater clinical efficacy. Since the disease is inherited as an autosomal dominant characteristic, the heterozygous patients could manifest about half the normal level of C̄1INH rather than the usual value of one-fifth or less. The excessive reduction in C̄1INH is acquired by its interaction with C̄1, and thus the low level of this protein in hereditary angioedema results from a combination of reduced synthesis and increased utilization. The regular and attenuated androgens are presumed to stimulate the product of the functioning gene so as to generate enough C̄1INH to control C̄1 action, which is revealed by the rise in the plasma level of the C̄1 substrate, C4.

Two regulatory defects of the amplification pathway, an inborn deficiency of I and acquired development of the C3 nephritic factor (C3Nef), have also afforded important mechanistic insights. The I deficiency permits C3b, from the interaction of C3, B, D, and P, to lead to uncontrolled formation of the amplification convertase C3b,Bb with consequent C3 and B deficiency. The secondary C3 deficiency presents clinical problems comparable to inborn deficiency in terms of recurrent infections. Restoration of I by plasma infusion permits transient restoration of C3 and B levels. C3Nef, an activity originally described in the serum of patients with membranoproliferative glomerulonephritis, is now generally recognized to be an oligoclonal immunoglobulin directed against the amplification convertase, C3b,Bb. The interaction of this autoantibody with the convertase creates a highly stable equimolar complex of C3b,Bb,C3Nef, which does not undergo inherent decay or H-mediated extrinsic decay dissociation. Thus the I cannot inactivate C3b protected in the complex, and the Bb active site of the convertase profoundly depletes C3. The same factor appears to be present in some patients with partial lipodystrophy. Physiologic amplification, as already discussed, is surface initiated and surface directed, by circumvention of regulatory mechanisms normally applied to the fluid-phase reaction and to nonactivating surfaces. The amplification of C3, B, and D interaction by I deficiency or the presence of C3Nef illustrates fluid-phase circumvention of regulatory mechanisms.

Perhaps the most unexpected consequence of complement deficiency is the association of diseases such as systemic lupus erythematosus, hypersensitivity angiitis, and polymyositis with homozygous deficiency of C1r, C4, and C2. Indeed, systemic lupus erythematosus–like disease has even been noted in several kindreds with C̄1INH deficiency, presumably in rela-

tion to persistent depletion of C4. Since C1 and C4 have been demonstrated to increase the efficiency of antibody-dependent neutralization of certain viruses, it could be argued that some obscure viral agent is responsible for the disease, especially in the form of a persistent immune complex. The deficiency in the classic pathway components would contribute both to poor neutralization of the virus and perhaps, more importantly, to inadequate clearance or solubilization of immune complexes. Although components of the alternative pathway are critical to the complement-dependent solubilization of immune complexes formed with protein antigens, the classic system increases the rate of the solubilization process. The linkage of silent or null genes for certain complement components (namely, C4, C2, and B) to alleles of genes within the histocompatibility complex on chromosome 6 that may control immune responsiveness is one hypothesis for the association of complement deficiencies with rheumatic diseases. Since C1q, C1r, C1s, and C̄1INH are not encoded in the major histocompatibility region, but deficiencies of these components are also associated with rheumatic diseases, some deficiencies may also have a primary role in pathogenesis. This role may relate to disordered regulation of lymphocyte function or to impaired clearance of immune complexes.

REFERENCES

Colten, H. R.: Complement synthesis. In Day, N. K., and Good, R. A. (eds.): Biological Amplification Systems in Immunology. New York, Plenum Medical Book Co., 1977, p. 47.

Fearon, D. T., and Wong, W. W.: Complement ligand-receptor interactions that mediate biological responses. Annu Rev Immunol 1:243, 1983.

Glass, D. N., Fearon, D. T., and Austen, K. F.: Inherited abnormalities of the complement system. In Stanbury, J. B., Wyngaarden, J. B., Fredrickson, D. S., et al. (eds.): The Metabolic Basis of Inherited Disease, 5th ed. New York, McGraw-Hill Book Co., 1983, p. 1934.

Mayer, M. M.: Complement, past and present. Harvey Lect 72:139, 1976-1977.

Müller-Eberhard, H. J., and Schreiber, R. D.: Molecular biology and chemistry of the alternative pathway of complement. Adv Immunol 29:1, 1980.

Porter, R. R.: Structure and activation of the early components of complement. Fed Proc 36:2191, 1977.

The Immunopathogenic Involvement of Immune Complexes in Human Disease States

The production of specific antibodies is one of the fundamental elements of host defense against pathogens. Localized concentrations of such antibodies react with microbial antigens and both activate humoral cytotoxic pathways and facilitate recognition and destruction of the pathogens by phagocytes. Appropriate antibody responses also augment the elimination of other foreign particulate and soluble materials, dimin-

ish the absorption of noxious substances through mucosal surfaces of the respiratory and gastrointestinal tracts, and increase the efficiency of immunologic surveillance for autologous cell clones with malignant potential. The combination of antibodies with diverse antigens also forms antigen-antibody complexes, termed immune complexes, in the circulation and in some tissues. Whether such complexes will be sequestered and degraded uneventfully or will prove injurious to the host is, in part, related to the quantities and characteristics of the antigens and subclasses of antibodies that make up the immune complexes, but is also influenced by the size and the antigen:antibody ratio of the complexes. The latter qualities of the immune complexes determine the pattern of their deposition in organs and the specific immunopathogenic consequences of their tissue localization. In most animal models of tissue inflammation and damage induced by immune complexes, the most potent complexes are those formed in antigen excess. An exuberant antibody response, yielding complexes in antibody excess, may herald the subsidence of the tissue reaction. This subsidence may be a function of both altered tissue distribution and lack of relevant immunologic and inflammatory activity of the immune complexes that are formed in antibody excess. However, in some tissues, immune complexes in antibody excess may exhibit unique pathogenetic capabilities. For example, the intracutaneous injection of immune complexes preformed in antibody excess produces granulomatous lesions in guinea pig skin, a reaction not elicited by complexes in antigen excess. Although immune complexes have been demonstrated in the circulation and tissues in many human diseases by indirect assays, a detailed characterization, including the identification of the relevant antigen, has been provided only in a few conditions. Antibodies of many classes may participate in immune complex formation, but most analyses have focused in IgG complexes, since they predominate quantitatively in the vast majority of immune complex states.

THE STRUCTURE AND FUNCTION OF IMMUNE COMPLEXES

The addition of increasing quantities of a homogeneous antigen to a given amount of specific antibody generally results in progressively increasing precipitation of the antibody up to the point of maximal precipitation, termed the equivalence point (Fig. 18). At the equivalence point, the resultant series of antigen-antibody complexes further associate to form an extensive lattice structure in the precipitate, and no free antigen or free antibody can be detected in the supernatant. Total precipitation of the antibody is rarely achieved at the equivalence point, and soluble immune complexes account for the remaining portion of antibody. The concentrations of such soluble complexes are greater on either side of the equivalence point and up to the regions of moderate excess of antibody or antigen. The size, solubility, and biologic activities of the supernatant complexes are a function of multiple factors that include the characteristics of the antigen, the subclass and binding affinity of the antibody, and the antigen:antibody ratio. On one extreme of the scale of antigens, those that are univalent exhibit a simple and nonprecipitating binding relationship with antibodies. Complexes composed of bivalent antigens are either small or limited to linear polymerization, and thus not only are unlikely to precipitate at equivalence but may be highly soluble in only moderate antigen excess. In contrast, multivalent antigens usually form extensive interconnecting lattices exhibiting nearly total precipitation. The interaction of bivalent or multivalent antigens with antibodies not only is more complex than the interaction with univalent antigens but is significantly influenced by the spacing between antigenic determinants. The very special spacing of antigenic determinants, which permits one antigen molecule to occupy both combining sites of an antibody, leads to the saturation of combining sites in complexes of the formula Ag_1Ab_1 for bivalent antigens, Ag_1Ab_2 for tetravalent antigens, and so forth.

The heterogeneous soluble complexes formed by the reaction of antibodies of the IgG class and multivalent antigens encompass a wide spectrum of structures and immunologic activities (Fig. 18). Those with antibody-predominant formulas that are formed in the region of antibody excess vary considerably in size. The complexes found at equivalence contain equal molar

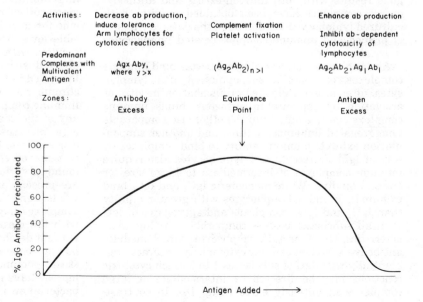

Figure 18. Relationship of antigen:antibody ratio to the immunologic and biologic activities of immune complexes.
Ag = Antigen
Ab = Antibody

amounts of antigen and antibody, while immune complexes formed in the regions of antigen excess comprise a series of decreasing size down to those of formula Ag_1Ab_1. The limit complex expected in vast antigen excess, which is depicted by the formula Ab_1Ag_2, has not been found in multivalent systems. Although the bivalency of IgG antibodies is usually realized in the formation of immune complexes, a low antibody-binding affinity may lead to a decrease in the effective valence of IgG at equilibrium. Thus a substantial proportion of low-affinity antibodies in any mixture of antibodies would favor the formation of complexes with small lattice structures and increased concentrations of soluble complexes at all ratios of antigen to antibody. Bivalent antibodies of high affinity also may appear univalent owing to the steric properties of antigens contained within a surface, as is the case for the reaction of "incomplete" anti-D antibodies with the surface of erythrocytes. The incomplete anti-D antibodies bind with high affinity to the erythrocytes but fail to agglutinate them, as the surface distribution of D antigens favors the saturation of antibody sites by D antigen on individual erythrocytes and opposes bridging between cells.

The ratio of antigen to antibody is a critical determinant of the immunobiologic effects of immune complexes (Fig. 18). The administration of immune complexes prepared in antigen excess leads to enhanced numbers of germinal centers in animals and a striking stimulation of the production of homologous antibodies without a comparable effect on cell-mediated immunity. The antibody response that antigen-excess complexes evoke in unprimed animals is kinetically and quantitatively similar to a secondary immune response rather than to the primary response that would be seen with a comparable initial dose of antigen alone. In contrast, the injection into animals of immune complexes in antibody excess elicits either no response or a diminished response relative to antigen alone. Such immune complexes in antibody excess may also suppress for prolonged periods the production of specific antibody in response to subsequent antigen challenge, without decreasing delayed hypersensitivity. Analogous results with both antigen-excess and antibody-excess complexes have been obtained in vitro with cultured lymphocytes as well as in the passive transfer of primed and immune complex–treated lymphocytes to irradiated hosts.

Although many classes of lymphocytes bind immune complexes, one specific subpopulation of T lymphocytes, after either prolonged preincubation in vitro or activation by exposure to mitogens, binds immune complexes more avidly than the otherwise comparable unaggregated immunoglobulins, and another subpopulation exhibits a unique ability to bind complexes by way of IgM Fc receptors. T lymphocytes also require immune complexes of intermediate to large size for optimal binding. While monomeric IgG_1 and IgG_3 bind to human B and T lymphocytes with greater affinity than IgG_2 and IgG_4, complexes and aggregates of IgG from all subclasses possess comparable binding characteristics. The K, or null, lymphocytes, which mediate antibody-dependent cellular cytotoxicity, interact preferentially with IgG of subclasses 1 to 3. Such cytotoxic reactions may be directed by intermediate or large complexes in antibody excess (Fig. 18). In contrast, immune complexes formed in antigen excess block antibody-dependent cytotoxicity of K lymphocytes, and may represent one portion of the blocking factor activity associated with some tumors and allografts. Immune complexes also interact with and activate other leukocytes and platelets, and thereby contribute to the expression of diverse effector pathways.

DETECTION AND QUANTITATION OF CIRCULATING IMMUNE COMPLEXES IN HUMAN DISEASES

The implication of immune complexes in human diseases is often initially based on the clinical presentation and the findings of cryoglobulins and a depressed level of serum hemolytic complement (CH_{50}). The diagnosis of immune complex disease may be further established by the demonstration of immune reactants in sections of involved tissues, as well as by assays of circulating immune complexes. These latter assays also provide a quantitative means of following the course of the disease and the results of treatment. The diversity of structures and biologic activities of immune complexes is reflected in the numerous assays that have been developed for the measurement of various subpopulations of complexes. Each indirect assay measures only a small proportion of the many subpopulations of immune complexes. This must be taken into account in the standardization of the method and the interpretation of results, and is borne out by the application of the assays to human disease states. Circulating immune complexes have been detected in myriad human diseases by such indirect assays, but in only a relatively few conditions have the complexes been characterized in detail and implicated etiologically in the basic disease or its complications.

Elevated levels of immune complexes exist in the circulation of patients with numerous chronic and acute neurologic diseases, including subacute sclerosing panencephalitis, amyotrophic lateral sclerosis, and Landry-Guillain-Barré syndrome. In these diseases, both IgG and C3 can be detected in electron microscopy and immunofluorescent analysis in deposits in the glomeruli of renal biopsies. Although antibodies specific for measles virus, the agent purportedly responsible for subacute sclerosing panencephalitis, are associated with the circulating complexes from patients affected with this disease, no specific antigen has been identified in the immune complexes in this or the other chronic neurologic states. Further, the presence of immune complexes has not been definitively related to any of the characteristic manifestations of the neurologic diseases, and the patients generally lack any expression of immune complex diseases. High concentrations of circulating immune complexes also are found in various forms of interstitial pneumonitis and are present as well in the interstitial regions of involved lung. Those patients with circulating immune complexes have active exudative lesions as compared with the chronic fibrosis in lung biopsies of patients without demonstrable complexes. The relevant antigen has not been demonstrated in the complexes of interstitial pneumonitis. On the other hand, patients with leprosy have circulating complexes containing specific bacterial antigens, but the complexes do not deposit in tissues to any significant extent and do not contribute to any known feature of the disease.

The failure of some immune complexes to deposit in tissues may explain the paradoxic findings in some chronic liver diseases. Immune complexes are present in high concentrations in the circulation of more than 90 per cent of patients with primary biliary cirrhosis, as assessed by indirect assays, and can be isolated in cryoprecipitates. Patients with this form of biliary cirrhosis rarely exhibit extrahepatic manifestations characteristic of hypersensitivity diseases, although there may be evidence for in vivo activation of the complement pathways. Patients with acute or chronic active hepatitis, who frequently develop signs reminiscent of autoimmune diseases, have a lower incidence of circulating immune complexes than patients with biliary cirrhosis. Nonetheless the concentration of immune complexes measured in indirect assays correlates with the occurrence of immune complications in several forms of active hepatitis. Thus the assays currently employed do not generally distinguish among immune complexes with respect to their immunopathogenetic potential.

In several human diseases, immune complexes with defined antibodies and antigens are pathogenically significant in terms of the basic disease or a prominent complication (Table 11). Glomerulonephritis is the predominant pathologic manifestation of the presence of circulating immune complexes in numerous infectious diseases and some malignant diseases. The course of the glomerulonephritis varies for each cause, but may lead to acute or chronic renal failure in some cases. Specific target organs other than the kidney may be selectively or preferentially involved, as in thyroiditis, where the specificity of the antibodies and localization of the thyroglobulin antigens are determining factors. The usual compartmentalization of rheumatoid arthritis is largely attributable to the fact that the immune response to altered IgG or viral antigens is primarily mounted locally in the affected joints. Even patients with systemic complications of rheumatoid arthritis, which may be attributable to the local production of immune complexes in other tissues, do not manifest glomerulonephritis unless they develop a high level of circulating complexes, which is generally detectable as cryoglobulinemia.

The prototype multisystem immune complex disease is systemic lupus erythematosus (SLE), in which

TABLE 11. VARIOUS HUMAN DISEASES WITH IMMUNE COMPLEX INVOLVEMENT

	DISEASE	TARGET ORGANS	SOURCE OF ANTIGENS	COURSE
Glomerulonephritis as the sole or predominant manifestation	β-hemolytic streptococcal infections		Plasma membranes of streptococci	Acute or subacute
	Syphilis		Treponema	Subacute to chronic
	Typhoid fever		Salmonella (Vi)	Subacute
	Toxoplasmosis		Toxoplasma	Acute to chronic
	Quartan malaria		Plasmodium malariae	Subacute to chronic
	Schistosomiasis		Schistosoma mansoni	Chronic
	Renal tubule hypersensitivity		Renal tubular antigen	Subacute
	Colonic carcinoma		Specific tumor product or carcinoembryonic antigen	Subacute to chronic
	Bronchogenic carcinoma		Specific tumor product	Subacute
	Renal cell carcinoma		Proximal tubule brush border	Subacute
Predominant manifestation in nonrenal target organs	Thyroiditis in thyroid carcinoma	Thyroid	Thyroglobulin	Subacute to chronic
	Rheumatoid arthritis	Joints; occasional involvement of skin, lungs, heart, nerves, or eyes	Altered IgG; viral products in some cases	Chronic with exacerbations
Multiple organ involvement with variable patterns	Bacterial endocarditis	Kidneys, skin, eyes, heart, nervous system	Bacteria	Acute to subacute
	Serum hepatitis	Skin, joints, nerves	Hepatitis B antigen	Subacute
	Mixed cryoglobulinemia	Skin, joints, nerves, kidneys, gastrointestinal tract	Altered IgG	Subacute to chronic
	Serum sickness	Skin, joints, nerves, kidneys	Heterologous proteins, hormones, drugs	Acute to subacute
	Systemic lupus erythematosus	Skin, joints, mucous membranes, serosal surfaces, kidneys, gastrointestinal tract, nervous system	DNA, nucleoproteins, C-type virus particles	Chronic with exacerbations

DNA–anti-DNA complexes may be found in the circulation and in relation to inflammatory lesions in virtually any organ. Fluctuations in the circulating levels of anti-DNA, DNA, and other antigens usually precede flares of disease activity, while the serum level of hemolytic complement (CH_{50}) and the serum concentrations of some complement components fall concomitantly. Indirect assays of immune complexes also reflect the changes in levels of circulating complexes associated with clinical exacerbations and the response to treatment. The nephritis of SLE exhibits great heterogeneity with respect to the histologic pattern, distribution of immune complex deposits, degree of proteinuria, urinary sediment abnormalities, and presence and rate of progression of renal failure. Irrespective of such differences, a high percentage of the patients with diffuse glomerulonephritis have decreased serum CH_{50} levels and abnormally low serum concentrations of C3 in association with circulating immune complexes and elevated levels of antinative DNA and other immune reactants. The morphology of the renal lesion in the diffuse glomerulonephritides of SLE is related to the frequency of proteinuria and the abnormalities detectable in the urinary sediment. Of the patients with early diffuse glomerulonephritis and normal renal function, those with the membranous form of glomerulonephritis all have proteinuria and one-half have sediment abnormalities, while up to one-third of those with the proliferative form of glomeru-lonephritis may lack proteinuria and over three-fourths may have normal urinalyses. In view of the ominous prognosis of diffuse glomerulonephritis in SLE, especially in the proliferative form, the demonstration of circulating immune reactants and glomerular immune complex deposits can provide valuable evidence of potentially progressive renal impairment early in the course for those patients with clinically silent glomerulonephritis and may allow earlier treatment. Thus measurements of levels of circulating immune complexes and immune reactants may indicate that patients with SLE should be subjected to renal biopsy for the more definitive demonstration of glomerular immune complex deposits by transmission electron microscopy and immunofluorescence. Despite the technical problems inherent in assays of immune complexes, the performance of several such assays based on different principles can both predict clinically significant glomerulonephritis in SLE early in the course and provide an awareness of exacerbations of glomerulonephritis before they are clinically apparent. The possible applicability of this approach to the diagnosis and management of other diseases mediated by immune complexes will be appreciated only when other well-controlled correlative studies are completed.

REFERENCE

Theofilopoulos, A. N., and Dixon, F. J.: The biology and detection of immune complexes. Adv Immunol 28:89, 1979.

T Cell Functions

DELAYED HYPERSENSITIVITY

Delayed hypersensitivity is the prototype of T cell effector function and is involved in host defense to viruses, microbacteria, and fungi. Macrophages operate at both the afferent and efferent limbs of this response. Activation of T cells for a specific antigen involves the accessory cell (e.g., macrophage)–dependent pathways discussed in the preceding section; antigen presentation and synthesis of soluble materials such as interleukin-1 (IL-1). Examples of antigen presenting cells that function in this regard and that play an important role in initial events required for host defense include Langerhan cells of the skin and the alveolar macrophages in the lung. The number of T cells specific for a given antigen is relatively small (1 to 10 of every 10,000 T cells). Therefore the system of delayed hypersensitivity has been developed so that once this small number of T cells is activated their reactivity is magnified. This occurs through the synthesis and secretion of soluble materials generically referred to as lymphokines. Examples of these include macrophage-activating factor, leukocyte inhibition factor, macrophage inhibition factor, and a variety of other not fully characterized materials whose net effect is to attract and accumulate other cell types into the area and arm them for destroying the invading pathogen. The morphologic correlate of delayed hypersensitivity is the accumulation of mononuclear cells and in some cases the formation of granuloma.

In humans, effector cells required for the initiation of delayed hypersensitivity reside among the T4-positive population. T cells capable of inhibiting this effector function reside among the T8-positive population. The relationship between effector cells and suppressor cells involved in the expression of delayed hypersensitivity is exemplified by the immune reactivity seen in response to infection with *Mycobacterium leprae*. Infection with *M. leprae* can result in one of two polar forms of the disease. Tuberculoid leprosy is characterized by well-circumscribed and limited lesions that contain very few, if any, viable organisms. Lepromatous leprosy is characterized by numerous and diffuse lesions containing large numbers of viable organisms. In the former type of disease there is adequate cell-mediated immunity and delayed hypersensitivity to *M. leprae* mediated by T4-positive cells. This results in killing and clearing of the organisms. In lepromatous leprosy there is specific in vivo and in vitro unresponsiveness to *M. leprae,* thus allowing the maintenance and proliferation of viable organisms. This unresponsiveness to *M. leprae* in lepromatous leprosy may reflect absence of antigen-specific T4-positive cells. Alternatively, such cells might exist but with their activity inhibited by T8-positive suppressor cells. Several observations support this latter possibility. Examination of the relative frequency of T4- and T8-positive cells demonstrates a predominance of T4-positive over T8-positive cells in tuberculoid but a predominance of T8-positive cells in lepromatous lesions. Depletion of T8-positive cells in the peripheral blood of individuals with lepromatous leprosy results in the appearance of in vitro reactivity to *M. leprae* in some patients. Addition of exogenous IL-2 to in vitro cultures of cells from patients with lepromatous leprosy restores in part their reactivity to *M. leprae*. These observations indicate that the absence of cell-mediated immunity to *M. leprae* in individuals with lepromatous leprosy represents immunosuppression by T8-positive cells. A portion of this immunosuppression may involve inhibition of IL-2 secretion or of its activity. Similar interactions between effector and regulatory cells are most likely involved in the net expression of delayed hypersensitivity seen in reactivity to other antigens and organisms.

T cell proliferation and the synthesis of new DNA is not required for delayed-hypersensitivity effector cells to mediate their reactivity. Therefore, in vitro T cell proliferation occurring in response to stimulation with a specific antigen is not a good correlate for in vivo delayed hypersensitivity. The best in vitro correlate of in vivo delayed hypersensitivity is to measure antigen-induced synthesis of lymphokines such as macrophage inhibition factor. The best in vivo correlate of delayed hypersensitivity is the delayed-hypersensitivity skin test.

CYTOTOXICITY

Cytotoxicity by T cells plays an important role not only in host defense against infection with organisms that replicate intracellularly but also in immunosurveillance of malignant cells. The specificity and function of cytotoxic T cells was first explored in systems that analyzed T cell reactivity to foreign transplantation antigens. These studies demonstrated that mixing of lymphocytes from different strains of animals or unrelated individuals resulted in the proliferation of T cells, similar to that seen when cells were stimulated with soluble antigens. This proliferation, termed a mixed lymphocyte reaction, represents activity among a T4-positive population of cells in response to recognition of foreign class II molecules. A consequence of this proliferation is the development of T cells capable of killing the allogeneic stimulator cells. This cytotoxicity represents the reactivity of a T8-positive population of cells. These cytotoxic T cells demonstrate specificity not for class II but for foreign class I molecules. An important step in the generation of these cytotoxic T cells is the liberation of IL-2. These reactivities are schematically outlined in Figure 19. T4-positive cells are activated by recognition of foreign class II molecules, and in conjunction with soluble materials such as IL-1 these cells proliferate. This represents the mixed lymphocyte component of the reactivity and is accompanied by the synthesis and secretion of IL-2. In the presence of IL-2, T8-positive cells specific for foreign class I molecules can be activated and induced to proliferate, and give rise to an expanded number of cytotoxic cells capable of lysing cells bearing the foreign class I molecules.

As indicated previously, infection of mice with a virus results in the generation of T cells whose cytotoxicity is specific for virally infected cells bearing self class I molecules. These cells are contained within a T

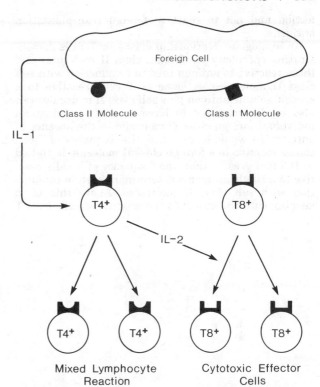

Figure 19. Events involved in the activation of T cells by alloantigens. In response to foreign class II molecules plus soluble materials such as interleukin-1 *(IL-1)*, T4-positive cells proliferative and liberate interleukin-2 *(IL-2)*. In conjunction with IL-2 and recognition of class I molecules, T8-positive cells can give rise to cytotoxic T cells. (From Stobo, J. D.: Lymphocytes: Structure and function. *In* McCarty, D. J. (ed.): Arthritis and Allied Conditions: A Textbook of Rheumatology, 10th ed. Philadelphia, Lea & Febiger. In press. Reproduced with permission.)

cell population that is analogous to human T8-positive cells. Their specificity is somewhat different from that noted for T8-positive T cells reactive to foreign class I molecules. In the former situation the effector cells recognize viral determinants in conjunction with self class I molecules, while in the latter they recognize foreign class I molecules alone. To determine the relationship between these two specificities the following experiment was performed: A clone of cytotoxic T cells specific for virus plus self class I molecules was assayed for its cytolytic activity against a panel of foreign cells, each of which displayed a different, foreign class I molecule in the absence of any definable virus. The results of this experiment showed that the T cell clone could lyse one of the foreign targets. This suggests that reactivity of T cells to a foreign class I molecule represents cross-reactivity by a cell whose original specificity is for a virus seen in association with self class I molecules. The frequency of T cell clones reactive to a single foreign class I molecule (1 of 100) is greater than that noted for T cells reactive to an individual virus plus self class I molecules (1 of 1000). Therefore the total reactivity for foreign class I molecules must represent the sum of reactivities occurring among several different T cell clones, each of which has specificity for a different viral determinant plus self class I. This is in keeping with the notion that the immune system was initially designed to prevent infection and not to react to foreign transplantation antigens.

An analogous relationship exists for T cells demonstrating specificity for foreign class II molecules and those reactive to antigen seen in conjunction with self class II molecules. A clone of T cells reactive to a specific soluble antigen plus self class II molecules can also be demonstrated to have reactivity against an individual foreign class II molecule in the absence of antigen. As would be expected, the frequency of T cell clones reactive to a foreign class II molecule is 10-fold to 100-fold greater than the frequency of T cells reactive to a single antigenic determinant seen in conjunction with self class II molecules. Again this is in keeping with the idea that the original specificity of T cells is for foreign antigens in conjunction with self class II molecules rather than for foreign class II molecules alone.

REFERENCES

Askenase, P. W., and Van Lovern, H.: Delayed-type hypersensitivity: Activation of mast cells by antigen-specific T-cell factors initiates the cascade of cellular interactions. Immunol Today 4:259, 1983.

Brunner, K. T., Weiss, A., MacDonald, H. R., et al.: Cytotoxic T lymphocyte clones recognizing murine sarcoma virus-induced tumor antigens. In Fathman, C. G., and Fitch, F. W. (eds.): Isolation, Characterization and Utilization of T Lymphocyte Clones. New York, Academic Press, 1982, p. 297.

INFECTIOUS DISEASES: PATHOGENETIC MECHANISMS AND HOST RESPONSES

RICHARD K. ROOT, M.D.

Introduction

Fever, a cardinal response to infection, has been known and feared as a sign of disease since antiquity. It was not until approximately 100 years ago, however, that the disorders we now know as infectious diseases were defined and the insight gained into the essential elements of infectious agents and corresponding host defense systems. This chapter will provide a conceptual framework for understanding the pathophysiology of various infectious diseases, stressing common host responses to acute infections. Typical host responses are central to alerting the clinician to the possibility of an infection, and thereby lead to attempts at specific diagnosis and therapy.

Infectious diseases occur as the result of invasion of the body by microorganisms or the action of their products or both. Their clinical manifestations can be ascribed to injury, dysfunction, or destruction of host cells and organs, events that are usually accompanied by alterations in homeostatic mechanisms. The initial injury or alteration may be mediated directly by the microbes or their products or indirectly by host defense mechanisms. Figure 1 outlines the critical phases in the infectious process: the interrelationships between host defense mechanisms, clinical manifestations, and outcome.

Clinically apparent infections begin only after new organisms colonize the host, after previously acquired organisms are no longer held in check by host defense mechanisms (reactivation of latent infections), or when colonizing organisms acquire new characteristics that make them more virulent. Microbiology as it relates to infectious diseases defines those properties of microorganisms that allow them to grow and replicate in vitro when isolated from infectious sites. It is also concerned with those factors that endow the organisms with virulence—the capacity to cause disease. Using clinical manifestations or other markers as points of reference, the epidemiology of infectious disease concerns the means by which organisms spread from one susceptible individual or population to another and the relationships of disease to immunity. The clinician must integrate an understanding of microbiology and epidemiology with the clinical expression of the disease in order to establish a diagnosis and to treat.

This discussion will focus on the several integrated host responses to acute infection. These include the actions of various host defense mechanisms against infectious agents, the pathophysiology of the febrile response, and the events that occur during bacterial or fungal invasion of the bloodstream. The key events that initiate infection will be reviewed, as will properties of some virulence factors of microorganisms. Features of several prototypic infections will be presented to highlight interactions between microbes and the host and to emphasize basic points in the pathophysiology of infectious disease.

MICROBIAL FACTORS IN THE PATHOGENESIS OF INFECTIOUS DISEASE

To cause infections, organisms must be acquired by the host from some source, survive, and must replicate effectively in competition with other flora (colonization). The capacity to cause *disease* is usually a function of virulence factors that permit survival in the face of host defense mechanisms as well as factors that cause cellular and organ injury or dysfunction. The latter may be a consequence of direct invasion of cells and tissues by the infecting organisms, actions of toxins elaborated during microbial growth, or interaction of microbial components with host mediation systems.

As indicated in Figure 1, the defense mechanisms of the host can be brought to bear against the organisms at a number of different points and usually involve well-regulated stages. Some organisms may cause clinically inapparent infection sufficient to initiate a specific immune response. This discussion will review the major phases of the infectious process as well as virulence factors of some organisms. For ease of discussion, the phases of microbial occupation of the host can be subdivided into colonization and local proliferation, invasion and dissemination.

DOCUMENTATION OF INFECTION

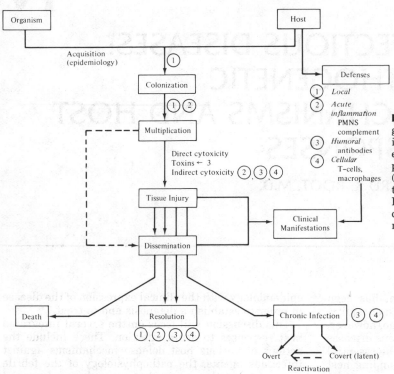

Figure 1. Idealized interplay between microorganisms and host factors that lead to infection, infectious disease, and resolution. These processes may be interrupted at any stage in the prevention or therapy of infectious disease. (From Root, R. K., and Heirholzer, W. L.: Infectious Diseases. In Melmon, K. L., and Morelli, H. F. (eds.): Clinical Pharmacology: Basic Principles in Therapeutics. 2nd ed. New York, Macmillan Company, 1978, p. 725.)

COLONIZATION

The human fetus lives in an environment that is usually sterile. Under optimal conditions the acquisition of organisms begins only at birth, and a normal flora is gradually established in the immediate postnatal period and during infancy. The fact that the host can coexist with the literally billions of microorganisms that colonize the skin, as well as the mucous membranes of the airway and gastrointestinal tract, without displaying any manifestations of disease is a tribute to the balance between active host defense mechanisms and microbial virulence factors.

Colonization must be preceded by acquisition of an organism (Table 1). Acquisition can occur through direct contact (droplets or touch from other colonized persons or animate or inanimate objects), air-borne spread, ingestion of contaminated food or water (vehi-

cles), or action of biting insects (arthropod-borne). The portal of entry of colonizing organisms can play a major role in dictating the site of a subsequent infection. It is not surprising that organisms transmitted by sexual contact cause lesions on the contact mucous membranes and skin, that inhaled organisms cause pneumonia, that ingested organisms produce enteric infections and hepatitis, and that anthropod-borne infections are usually systemic with a blood-borne phase. Thus, the setting in which the disease has developed and the epidemiologic contacts must be strongly considered in the evaluation of patients with repeated infectious diseases. In some infectious diseases the epidemiologic history coupled with clinical manifestations may be so characteristic that a solid working diagnosis can be made before definitive data are available.

Not every acquired organism can successfully colo-

TABLE 1. MECHANISMS OF ACQUISITION OF INFECTIOUS AGENTS

MECHANISM	MODE	REPRESENTATIVE ORGANISMS
Contact		
Direct	Skin to skin, mucous membranes	Gram-negative rods, *N. gonorrhoeae, T. pallidum*
Indirect	Droplets, secretions	Group A streptococcus, *N. meningitidis,* rhinoviruses
Vehicle-borne	Fomites	*Staphylococcus aureus*
	Food or water	Salmonella, Shigella, Hepatitis A
	Drugs, intravenous fluids	Gram-negative rods
Air-borne	Ventilation	Tuberculosis, varicella, mycoses
Vector-borne	Arthropods	*Yersinia pestis*, Malaria plasmodia, rickettsioses, encephalitis viruses
	Animals	Rabies, Brucella

TABLE 2. SOME BACTERIAL ADHESINS AND RECEPTORS*

BACTERIA	ADHESIN	RECEPTOR	CELLS
Streptococcus pyogenes	Lipotechoic acid M protein, fibrillae	Albumin-like protein, fibronectin	Oral and pharyngeal epithelium
Enterobacteriaceae	Type I, fimbriae	D-mannose	Alimentary tract epithelium
E. coli, uropathogenic	Fimbriae	Globotetraosyl ceramide	Periuretheral epithelium, intestinal brush border
E. coli, enteropathogenic	Fimbriae	GM_2 ganglioside	Small intestinal epithelium
Vibrio cholerae	Fimbriae	GM_2 ganglioside	
Mycoplasma	Membrane protein	Sialic acid glycophorin	Respiratory epithelium
Neisseria gonorrhoeae	Fimbriae, peptides, outer membrane proteins	GM_2 ganglioside	Vaginal epithelium, PMNs
Viridans streptococci	Dextran, fimbriae	?	Dental plaque, heart valve endothelium

*Modified from Beachey, E. L.: Bacterial adherence: Adhesin-receptor interactions mediating the attachment of bacteria to mucosal surfaces. J Inf Dis 143:325, 1981.

nize and proliferate within the host. Several conditions must be present to foster colonization. These can include: (1) a sufficiently large inoculum of organisms, (2) the ability of colonizing organisms to adhere to site-specific mucosal cells, (3) a favorable local environment, (4) an adequate nutritional supply to support new microbial growth, (5) a paucity of other flora that can compete successfully for limited nutrients or that may manufacture inhibitory substances (for example, bacteriocins) and (6) the avoidance of recognition and destruction by normal host defense mechanisms at the colonizing site.

Of the mechanisms involved in the initial stages of colonization, much attention has been paid to the ability of organisms, particularly bacteria, to adhere to mucosal cells of the alimentary canal and the genitourinary and the respiratory tract. So-called *adhesins* on the cell surface of organisms link to specific cellular receptors (Table 2). The availability, distribution, and turnover of receptors in different locations appear to play a major role in regulating the character of the local microbial flora.

Adhesins are usually located in hair-like structures that project from the microbial surface (fimbria, pili, or fibrillae) (Fig. 2). The nature of these structures varies with the organism, as shown in Table 2. Cellular receptors include simple proteins and sugars (for example, α D-mannose), more complex sialic acid containing surface carbohydrates linked to lipids (gangliosides), or glycoproteins.

The expression of receptors on different cell types regulates the site-specific adherence of different organisms. Furthermore, the expression of specific adhesins can be closely linked to virulence in some organisms. For example, enteropathogenic *E. coli* express adhesins that specifically link them to intestinal brush-border gangliosides, whereas uropathogenic *E. coli* have adhesins for periuretheral epithelial cell receptors.

The availability of cellular receptors may be altered competitively by other bacteria or by receptor analogues. For example, sugars such as α-D-methyl mannoside can block adherence of some enteropathogenic *E. coli*, and free gangliosides may inhibit attachment of other *E. coli* (Table 2). The expression of cellular receptors may be modified by disease states, including prior infection with viruses. Cells infected by influenza virus show increased adherence of streptococci. Gram-negative bacteria adhere more avidly to oropharyngeal

epithelial cells from seriously ill patients than from normal persons.

Conversely, bacterial adhesins may be altered or lost by antimicrobial treatment or by the binding of specific antibodies. Considerable effort is being expended to develop vaccines using adhesin-containing antigens (pili) from gonorrhea and intestinal pathogens. Antimicrobial prophylaxis against group A streptococcal infection may work by releasing adherent lipotechoic acids from the bacterial surface. Similarly, beyond the colonization stage antimicrobial prophylaxis for endocarditis may operate principally by blocking adherence to heart valves rather than by killing the infecting organisms.

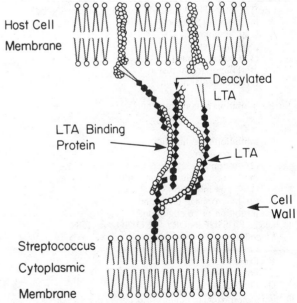

Figure 2. Hypothetical model of the interaction between lipoteichoic acid (LTA) and M protein on the surface of *Streptococcus pyogenes* cells (bottom). The interaction of LTA and deacylated LTA with several M protein molecules would result in a fibrillar network of LTA and protein and would permit exposure of the lipid ends of firmly anchored LTA molecules to interact with receptors in host cell membranes (top). (From Beachey, E. H., et al.: Attachment of streptococcus pyogenes to mammalian cells. Rev Inf Dis 5:S670, 1983.)

Information in this developing field holds considerable promise for enhanced understanding of microbial pathogenetic mechanisms as well as site-specific host responses and their modification by antibiotics or protective antibodies.

LOCAL PROLIFERATION

Once an organism has obtained a foothold in the host, the production of disease usually depends on the ability to proliferate locally. The interplay between local environmental factors, the established resident flora, the action of host defense mechanisms, and the protective virulence factors of the colonizing organism (Table 3) determines the outcome of this event. Local environmental factors that affect colonization and proliferation include the pH, the presence or absence of microbicidal fatty acids or other inhibitory substances such as lactoferrin elaborated by the host, as well as the availability of nutrients in competition with the established resident flora. The local host defense factors will be discussed in more detail in a later section.

Microbial factors that may limit or promote colonization and proliferation are complex. Resident organisms may serve as a mechanical impediment to further colonization, may block cellular receptors for other microbial adhesins, may compete for nutrients, or may produce substances that inhibit or kill other organisms. Perhaps the most dramatic example of this phenomenon was observed by Alexander Fleming, who isolated and characterized the active component from Penicillium mold that inhibits the growth of a wide variety of bacteria. On the other hand, within the human host the characterization of those factors produced by organisms to regulate colonization and local proliferation has received much less attention. A variety of bacteriocins have been isolated from certain species or strains of bacteria that inhibit or kill other organisms. The enhanced capacity of newly colonizing organisms to occupy sites within the host and to express disease following antibiotic treatment has been attributed in part to the depletion of these factors. Conversely, some organisms such as *Entamoeba histolytica* depend strongly on establishing a symbiotic axenic relationship with resident bacterial flora to successfully colonize and invade the mucosa in the colon. The ability of new organisms to colonize the host and cause disease following manipulation of the resident flora with antimicrobial treatment has become an increasingly important issue for clinicians. It can affect both the choice and duration of therapy with various antimicrobials.

The third major determinant of local microbial survival is the ability to withstand elimination by normal host defense mechanisms. The nature of these host defense mechanisms as they apply to microbial eradication will be discussed more fully later. Suffice it to say that many microbial virulence factors fall into the "protection from host defense mechanisms" category (Table 3).

Nowhere is this better demonstrated than when one considers the fate of rough (unencapsulated) pneumococci as opposed to those that are fully encapsulated when they are inoculated into a susceptible host such as a mouse. The rough organisms are rapidly engulfed

TABLE 3. MICROBIAL VIRULENCE FACTORS

I. PROTECTION FROM HOST DEFENSE MECHANISMS	
A. Inhibition of phagocytic cells	Examples
(1) Chemotaxis	Capnocytophagia, *B. pertussis*
(2) Phagocytosis	Organisms with capsules, M-protein, pili
(3) Oxidative burst	*Salmonellae*
(4) Phagolysomal fusion	*Toxoplasma gondii, Mycobacterium tuberculosis*, Legionellae
(5) Leukocidal action	*S. aureus*, Clostridia, group A streptococcus, *Entamoeba histolytica*
B. Inhibition of complement	Thick peptidoglycan cell wall (gram-positive bacteria), serum-resistant gram-negative bacteria, antigen-antibody complexes
C. Inhibition of antibodies	
(1) Formation	AIDS agent?
(2) Action	IgA proteases, protein A (IgG)
D. Inhibition of cellular immunity	
(1) T cell inhibition	AIDS agent, Ebstein-Barr virus, herpesviruses, others
(2) Macrophage inhibition	*Toxoplasma*, Mycobacteria
E. Inhibition of "recognition"	Schistosomes
II. DIRECT TISSUE INJURY OR DYSFUNCTION	
Mechanism	*Examples*
A. Cellular invasion with cytolysis	*Neisseria*, Shigellae, Salmonellae, most viruses
B. Exotoxins	Diphtheria toxin, clostridial toxins
C. Enterotoxins	*E. coli, Vibrio cholera, S. aureus*
D. Endotoxins	Gram-negative bacteria
III. INDIRECT TISSUE INJURY OR DYSFUNCTION	
Mechanism	*Examples*
A. Activation of acute inflammation	Pyogenic bacteria
B. Activation of host humoral mediator systems (e.g., complement, coagulation, kinins, arachidonic acid metabolites)	Endotoxins, bacterial peptidoglycan, teichoic acids
C. Disruption of vascular supply or hemostasis	Platelet activation, vascular occlusion or injury
D. Antibody/complement dependent cellular cytoxicity	Herpesviruses
E. T cell cytotoxicity	Hepatitis viruses

and killed by phagocytic cells. In the absence of opsonizing antibodies the encapsulated (smooth) organisms multiply rapidly and overwhelm the animal, eventually killing it. The same events presumably take place in the human lung when smooth pneumococci are aspirated into the alveolar space. In the absence of protective antibodies the encapsulated organisms proliferate, generate a brisk but initially ineffective inflammatory response, and cause pneumonia. Conversely, the rough organisms are ingested and killed and cause no disease.

Other microbial virulence factors can include those that inhibit the locomoting function of polymorphonuclear leukocytes (PMNs). Some organisms induce high intracellular levels of cyclic adenosine monophosphate (cholera toxin, Bordetella toxins) that inhibit leukocyte motility. Others destroy PMNs directly through the action of leukocidins. Both staphylococcal and streptococcal leukocidins appear to act by promoting intracellular lysosomal dissolution. Release of potent hydrolytic enzymes into the cellular cytoplasm rather than into the sanctuary of a phagocytic vacuole causes death of the cell. Organisms may survive within phagocytic cells for many reasons: e.g., they are resistant to the microbicidal products of these cells, they actually decrease the magnitude of cellular production of toxic oxygen products, or they block phagolysosomal fusion. The adaptability of Legionellae to survive in the intracellular location in human monocytes or macrophages is so striking that organisms grow much better after engulfment than before.

On mucosal surfaces certain pathogens can cleave secretory IgA$_2$ near the hinge region through the action of specific IgA proteases. Cleavage of IgA markedly reduces its ability to block adherence to mucosal surfaces. Nonpathogenic Neisseria do not contain these proteases; thus their capacity to cause invasive disease appears to be reduced. A variety of other pathogenic organisms that colonize mucosal surfaces do contain IgA$_2$ proteases; however, the relationship of these enzymes to pathogenicity is less clear.

Gram-positive cocci have thick and heavily cross-linked peptidoglycan cell walls—these form an impenetrable barrier to the deposition of complement proteins on the bacterial cell membrane. Gram-negative organisms, on the other hand, have an outer envelope rich in lipids, polysaccharides, proteins, and complex molecules that contain both a lipid and polysaccharide portion. These lipopolysaccharides or endotoxins can activate the complement system directly by the alternative pathway. When the terminal components are deposited, a lytic action is generated that leads to destruction of the gram-negative outer envelope and changes its permeability characteristics, causing lysis of the entire organism.

The majority of gram-negative organisms that live as relatively harmless commensals are highly susceptible to the lytic action of complement. Those causing bacteremic infection are often resistant to lysis. When protective antibodies develop against these latter organisms, they may induce lysis by enhancing complement deposition or by promoting opsonization and destruction by phagocytic cells. Conversely, IgA antibodies may paradoxically block the deposition of IgG or IgM complement-fixing antibodies on the microbial surface and promote bacteremic infection by this mechanism. When the IgA antibodies cross-react with other gram-negative organisms, host defense against these bacteria may be correspondingly altered.

The possession of one or more protective virulence factors of the type described above allows pathogenic organisms to survive at the local site. In addition, they may act to protect microorganisms from the immediate defenses of the acute inflammatory response or the complement system once the local site has been breached.

INVASION AND DISSEMINATION

Many organisms produce their clinical manifestations by first invading host tissues locally, then disseminating more widely. Information is just beginning to emerge on how organisms such as Neisseria and Shigellae invade mucosal cells. In a process analogous to phagocytosis, nonciliated cells are induced to take up these organisms, thereby transporting them to an intracellular site where cytolytic infection begins. Chlamydia also have the capacity to induce endocytosis by normally nonphagocytic cells and reach an intracellular location at their sites of infection.

Viruses must achieve an intracellular location to replicate. A variety of cellular receptors have been characterized as points of attachment for different viruses. For example, influenza viruses have a hemagglutinating (H) surface protein that binds to N-acetylneuraminic residues on mammalian mucosal cells as well as erythrocytes and leukocytes. Through the action of an adjacent protein (N), which is a neuraminidase, the cell membrane is penetrated and the uncoated organisms reach the cellular cytoplasm, where they replicate and eventually induce cytolysis. This frees newly produced organisms to attach to other cells and to repeat the cycle. Major pandemics of influenza occur when mutation leads to the production of new H proteins; minor epidemics develop as the result of new N protein synthesis without alterations in the H protein.

Many organisms do not produce disease by invading cells, but rather by remaining in the extracellular location. The pneumococcus is a good example of an obligate extracellular parasite. Its capsule inhibits phagocytosis. In infected sites in the lung three zones can be characterized histochemically: a central cell-free zone containing many extracellular bacteria, a middle zone where PMNs are found together with bacteria, and an outer zone rich in PMNs with few organisms. If the PMN defenses are overwhelmed, multiplying pneumococci can escape into lymphatics and travel to local lymph nodes and then eventually to the bloodstream. The mechanisms by which the pneumococci traverse the intact alveoli in this process are not known. Activation of the acute inflammatory response—in particular, PMNs and complement—produces many of the clinical manifestations of pneumococcal infection.

Still other organisms elaborate toxins that may have systemic effects far beyond the local site of infection. *Corynebacterium diphtheriae* are gram-positive bacilli that become capable of producing an exotoxin—a toxin released from the bacterial cells—when they are infected with a lysogenic bacteriophage virus. This toxin is an acidic globular protein; one portion (B subunit) promotes binding to mammalian cells and once bound, the other (A subunit) enters cells and disrupts protein synthesis by inhibiting peptide chain elongation. The result is cellular dysfunction and death. When diphtheritic pharyngeal infection occurs in nonimmune subjects, local destruction of mucosal cells coupled with generation of an acute inflammatory response leads to formation of a thick, gray membrane. This can be so large as to cause airway obstruction. Absorption of the toxin systemically has particularly devastating effects on the myocardium. In nonimmune individuals with extensive pharyngeal-laryngeal diphtheria, the incidence of myocarditis is about 10 per cent, with fatalities seen in up to 20 per cent of affected patients. Antibodies against diphtheria toxin are protective against all phases of the disease without altering colonization or eradicating the organisms.

Other striking examples of toxigenic infections are those caused by clostridial species. *Clostridium perfringens* causes marked cellular and myonecrosis (gas gangrene); other species (*C. botulinum, C. tetani*) cause botulism and tetanus. Again, antitoxic antibodies are protective and can be administered therapeutically or can be developed by immunization with toxoids (inactivated toxins). *Toxic shock syndrome* (fever, rash, diarrhea, hypotension) is a recently recognized complication of local infection with strains of *S. aureus* that produce a systemically absorbed toxin.

Enterotoxins are microbially produced proteins specifically directed at gastrointestinal mucosal cells. *Vibrio cholerae* is a bacterium that is incapable of invading or destroying the small intestinal mucosa and does not produce disseminated infection. Instead, it produces an 84,000-dalton protein that binds specifically to so-called GM_1-type gangliosides on intestinal mucosal cells. Binding is followed by induction of cellular adenyl cyclase activity and a marked increase in net active secretion of isotonic fluids from the small intestine. The resulting profound diarrhea (in severe cases in adults, stool volumes may average one liter per hour) and its attendant metabolic acidosis cause circulatory collapse and death unless corrective fluid therapy is administered. The disease is self-limited if death does not intervene. Considerable effort is being expended to develop a successful vaccine against the cholera toxin.

Other enterotoxins have been isolated from strains of *E. coli* that cause "traveler's diarrhea," as well as from other enteric pathogens (Shigellae and Salmonellae). The exact role of toxins in disease pathogenesis is difficult to separate from the cellular invasive properties of Salmonellae and Shigellae.

Finally, explosive epidemics of a short-lived illness characterized by nausea, vomiting, diarrhea, and fever have been traced to the ingestion of foods (often carbohydrate-rich) contaminated with enterotoxin-producing *S. aureus*. Toxin production is not a feature of all staphylococci but only of those bearing plasmid DNA coding for the formation of one of five polypeptide toxins. In contrast to staphylococcal infections elsewhere, which are characterized by necrosis and pus formation, enterotoxic staphylococcal infection has no associated tissue damage. Most of the staphylococcal enterotoxins, rather than acting directly on intestinal cells, appear to cause a vagally mediated emesis and hyperosmolarity of intestinal secretions.

Bacterial endotoxins differ from exotoxins and enterotoxins in that they are integral components of the outer envelope of virtually all gram-negative organisms. They are complex lipopolysaccharides rather than proteins. In the cell envelope location or when released during bacterial growth or destruction, they can have a wide variety of effects on both humoral and cellular host mediator systems as well as causing direct toxicity to some cells (for example, vascular endothelium). Since gram-negative bacteria comprise a huge component of the normal flora of the gastrointestinal tract, it is not surprising that oral ingestion of endotoxins produces none of the untoward effects seen during active gram-negative infections of tissues or the bloodstream. More will be said about the structure-function relationships of gram-negative endotoxins and host responses and immunity in the discussion of septicemia.

In summary, while many organisms are capable of tissue invasion and wide dissemination following their proliferation at a local site, pathogenetic mechanisms vary considerably, even among strains of a given species. An understanding of the virulence factors of organisms and a definition of the pathogenetic mechanisms have been instrumental in developing specific immunotherapies to be used prophylactically (vaccines) or therapeutically (immune serum) during acute infection. Furthermore, to the extent that host responses contribute to the tissue injury or dysfunction seen in acute infection, careful manipulation of these responses may also have potential benefit. This concept has yet to be applied safely to many infectious diseases but is worthy of further consideration as we take up the discussion of normal host defense mechanisms and the pathogenesis of fever.

Host Defense Mechanisms Against Infection

After understanding the conditions and mechanisms by which pathogenic microorganisms may establish themselves and initiate the infectious process in the human host, it is appropriate to consider how the host deals with these invaders. The discussion of immunology provided detailed information on the biology and pathophysiology of the specific immune response and its relationship to nonspecific effector systems mediated by phagocytic cells and the complement system. This discussion views these mechanisms as they relate to infection.

The host defenses can be divided into four major limbs (Table 4): local, phagocytic, humoral, and cellular immune. The phagocytic and complement systems are available to be activated immediately by appropriate stimuli to deal with colonizing or invading micro-

TABLE 4. HOST DEFENSES: DEFECTS, CONSEQUENCES, EVALUATION, AND CORRECTION*†

HOST DEFENSE SYSTEM	PREDOMINANT ORGANISMS CAUSING INFECTION‡	CIRCUMSTANCES THAT MAY IMPAIR HOST DEFENSES	METHODS OF IDENTIFYING DEFECTS	CORRECTIVE MEASURES
Local	Bacteria > fungi	Dermatitis, mucosal ulceration, catheters, foreign bodies, bronchiectasis, urinary stones or strictures, cystic fibrosis	Physical examination, radiographics, measures, sweat test	Remove foreign bodies, drainage
Phagocytic	Bacteria, opportunistic fungi, Nocardia	Neutropenias, GP 150 deficiency, hyper-IgE, chronic granulomatous disease, Chédiak-Higashi syndrome, MPO deficiency, diabetes, cirrhosis, uremia, acidosis	Leukocyte count, skin window, NBT test, leukocyte chemotaxis, phagocytosis, killing, metabolism	Leukocyte transfusion, ? ascorbate therapy, ? marrow transplant
Humoral				
Complement	Encapsulated bacteria Neisseria sp.	C3, C5-C9 deficiencies, SLE, immune complex disorders, cirrhosis	Complement components, functional assays	Vaccines, plasma
Antibodies	Encapsulated bacteria, some viruses, *Giardia lamblia*	Congenital or acquired hypogamma-globulinemia, multiple myeloma, lymphoma, lymphocytic leukemia, nephrotic syndrome, burns, steroid or cyto-toxic therapy	Serum protein electropho-resis, quantitative immu-noglobulins, antibody levels, B cell counts, lymphocyte mitogenesis	Immune serum globu-lin, plasma
Cellular	Intracellular bacteria, mucocutaneous Candida, invasive fungi, DNA viruses, protozoans, parasites	DiGeorge's syndrome, SCID, Wiskott-Aldrich syndrome, steroid therapy, uremia, sarcoidosis, Hodgkin's disease, burns, malnutrition, carcinomatosis, cytotoxic therapy	Delayed hypersensitivity skin tests, T cell counts, lymphocyte mitogenesis	γ-Interferon, interleukin II, transfer factor, treat underlying condition

*MPO = myeloperoxidase; NBT = nitroblue tetrazolium; SLE = systemic lupus erythematosus; GP = granulocyte protein; SCID = severe combined immune deficiency.
†Modified from American College of Physicians: MKSAP V Syllabus, 1979.
‡When the host defense system is defective.

organisms. The responses of the specific immune system (antibodies and cellular immunity) require a longer time to develop and serve to amplify and focus the more primitive inflammatory mechanisms.

Organisms can—in general—be characterized by which systems are most responsible for their eradication. Thus, pyogenic bacteria are usually eradicated by the combined action of phagocytes and opsonins. The latter are provided by the complement and humoral immune systems. Antibody and complement are critical to the effective elimination of obligate extracellular organisms, such as encapsulated pneumococci. Lysis by complement is a major defense against gram-negative organisms such as the *Neisseria*—a process that is enhanced by the development of complement-fixing antibodies against these organisms. Cellular immune mechanisms are particularly important in dealing with organisms normally resistant to the effects of phagocytosis. These include tubercle bacilli, *Legionellae*, fungi, protozoans (such as *Toxoplasma gondii* and *Leishmania, Pneumocystis carinii*), and DNA viruses—in particular, those of the herpesvirus group. Specific deletions in one or more of the limbs of host defense can give rise to repeated or unusually severe infections with organisms that reflect the limb involved. The nature of the infection often provides a clue to the nature of the impairment. The study of patients with various genetic host defense defects has provided insights into the specific mechanisms used by normal subjects in anti-infective defense as well as their alteration by disease states.

LOCAL DEFENSES

Local defense mechanisms operate at body surfaces, including the skin and mucosal linings: they constitute the first line of defense against most microorganisms. Keratin production by squamous epithelium provides a thick, relatively impenetrable protective layer against most skin bacteria, viruses, and fungi. Alterations in keratin production—as in various types of dermatitis—or penetration of this barrier by trauma or burns is a necessary prelude to most cutaneous infections. In addition to keratin, sebaceous glands in the skin form and secrete fatty acids (which may be bacteriostatic or cidal). Obstruction of these glands or sweat ducts permits their secondary infection by surface bacteria, of which *S. aureus* is a particularly prevalent pathogen.

On mucosal surfaces, cellular integrity provides a mechanical barrier; other factors intervene to limit microbial growth. These include the secretion of hydrolytic enzymes such as lysozyme or oxidizing enzymes such as lactoperoxidase. Using peroxide generated by colonizing bacteria, lactoperoxidase can form oxidants that kill susceptible organisms. Lysozyme may attack and destroy the cell walls of some grampositive cocci. Acid secretion is another mucosal bactericidal mechanism, most striking in the stomach where organism counts may be reduced by ten to 100-thousand fold from those found in the oropharynx and esophagus. Achlorhydria can markedly increase susceptibility to infection by enteric pathogens such as Salmonella. Neutralization of the normally acid pH of cervical and vaginal secretions by blood flow during the menses may be a factor in augmenting susceptibility to gonorrheal infection. In the urinary tract the acid pH of the urine and acidic bladder mucosal secretions serve to restrict growth of some bacterial species.

Mechanical cleansing of mucosal surfaces is also an important antimicrobial defense. In the airway this is provided by the cough reflex for large particles and by the flow of the mucociliary blanket for particles 3—10 μm in diameter. Impaired cough results in aspiration pneumonias in alcoholic or neurologically impaired patients. Bronchitis, bronchopneumonias, and destruction of bronchioles (bronchiectasis) can be the consequences of abnormal mucociliary flow as is seen in influenza infections, heavy smoking, and in some asthmatics and patients with certain genetic disorders (cystic fibrosis and the immotile cilia syndrome). Diarrhea may serve as an attempt to expel organisms in enteric infections or intestinal parasitism. Diuresis lowers bacterial counts in the urine by as much as several hundredfold during infection. Conversely, urinary obstruction—or obstruction of other drainage tracts (lungs, biliary tree, salivary glands)—predisposes to bacterial infection proximal to the obstructive site.

Foreign bodies constitute a special problem in that they may obstruct normal drainage tracts, injure mucosal or squamous epithelial cells, and protect bacteria against the action of host phagocytes. When the presence of a foreign body leads to infection, proper management usually demands its removal.

When local defenses are impaired, pyogenic bacterial infections are the usual consequence (Table 4). The organisms are most frequently the normal flora at the site or proximal to it. Repeated urinary tract infections—particularly of the relapsing variety (same strain of organism)—demand an investigation of urinary tract anatomy. Recurring obstruction of the apocrine sweat glands that can develop during puberty leads to the syndrome known as *chronic hidradenitis suppurativa*. The most common causes of recurrent pneumonias are not inadequate phagocytic, humoral, or cellular immune defenses, but are diseases that affect the airways.

PHAGOCYTIC DEFENSES

The principal phagocytic cells are polymorphonuclear leukocytes (PMNs) and macrophages. Of these two "professional" phagocyte populations, the most is known about the microbicidal mechanisms of PMNs. PMNs are highly mobile cells no longer capable of dividing after leaving their site of production in the bone marrow. They are capable of rapid entry into an infectious site and swift ingesting and destruction of a large variety of bacteria and fungi. Organisms too large to be ingested may be killed by PMNs that attach to their surface. The PMNs that form the pus of pyogenic infections have a brief life span once engulfment is completed. Old PMNs are rapidly replaced by new cells released from the marrow; daily production rates for normal adults may reach the 100 billion range.

In contrast to PMNs, macrophages provide the host with a more stable long-lived phagocytic population. Macrophages derived from monocyte precursors in the bone marrow and circulation represent the first defense against bacteria that reach the alveolar spaces. Macrophages in the venous sinusoids of the liver (Kupffer cells) and spleen play a key role in removing infectious agents from the bloodstream. Splenectomy leaves some patients susceptible to life-threatening bacteremic infections with pneumococci and other streptococci because of the loss of this clearance function. Macrophages in the dermis and other organs are also firstline defenders until the influx of the more rapidly acting PMNs reaches the site of microbial invasion.

The microbicidal power of macrophages can be modulated by the action of specific lymphokines; thus they are important effectors of cellular immunity. Besides this effector role macrophages operate with helper T cells in the afferent limb of the specific immune response in antigen processing. The generation of the T lymphocyte activating factor, interleukin 1, by macrophages is a key initial event in the development of specific immunity.

Eosinophils are also capable of phagocytosis, but to a lesser degree than PMNs and macrophages. While their precise role in host defense is not totally known, they participate importantly in the eradication of some metazoan parasites. Their functions as secretory cells in immunologically mediated events are described earlier in this text.

PMN KINETICS AND INFECTION

For this discussion the important points relate to PMN transit in various compartments and the production and characteristics of these cells during active bacterial infection. Under normal conditions (Fig. 3), PMNs spend about 14 days in the bone marrow undergoing proliferation and maturation from directed precursor stem cells. These two phases are divided into about equal seven-day periods. At the promyelocyte stage the major products of protein synthesis are single membrane–bound organelles (lysosomes) that contain hydrolytic enzymes, antibacterial cationic proteins, and the oxidizing enzyme myeloperoxidase (Table 5). These lysosomes (called *azurophilic granules* because of their staining characteristics) are divided among several daughter cells and their production ceases. At the myelocyte stage protein synthesis is directed primarily toward generating the contents of a second group of single membrane–bound organelles known as the specific granules. These, too, are distributed into

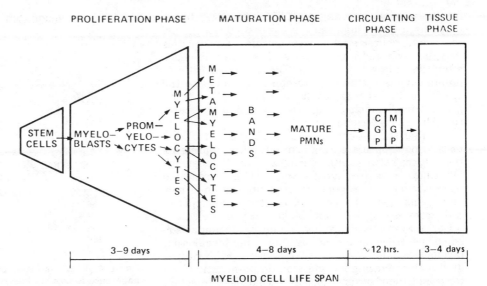

Figure 3. The phases of development circulation and disposition of polymorphonuclear leukocytes in humans. The relative size of the blocks correlates with size of the pool at each phase. CGP, circulating granulocyte pool; MGP, marginated granulocyte pool.

daughter metamyelocytes during the last divisional stage of myeloid proliferation. In the normal mature PMN the number of specific granules outnumbers azurophilic granules by about three to one and is responsible for the pink appearance of those cells with Wright's or Giemsa stains. Specific granules also contain some hydrolytic enzymes (lysozyme), as well as the iron-binding antimicrobial protein lactoferrin and B_{12}-binding protein. By the time PMNs reach morphologic maturity, the Golgi apparatus has regressed and the cells are filled with their secretory granules. Protein synthesis by mature PMNs is minimal. Mitochondria are scarce and glycogen stores abundant. The shape of the nucleus and the high degree of deformability allow PMNs to squeeze through small interstices between cells as well as in tissue spaces.

PMNs in the circulation are in transit from the bone marrow to potential sites of infection or inflammation. The average time normally spent in the circulation before exit is about 12 hours. About one half of the cells circulate freely in the central axial stream. The remainder are in a so-called "marginated pool" that does not circulate freely but can exchange readily with the circulating cells. Splenic and pulmonary vascular PMNs constitute a significant proportion of the marginated pool. Other PMNs marginate as a prelude to

leaving the circulation during the acute inflammatory response. The percentage of PMNs that marginate can be increased by factors that induce fusion of some of the specific granules into the plasma membrane, with extracellular discharge of their contents. A relative shift of cells into or out of the marginated pool may induce neutropenia or neutrophilic leukocytosis, respectively, without actually changing the number of cells in the circulation.

During acute bacterial infection, a number of changes take place in PMN kinetics. These may include the prompt and accelerated release of cells from the maturation or storage pool in the marrow. A cleavage product of complement known as C3e appears to play an active role in promoting marrow release. This release causes not only a neutrophilic leukocytosis but also the appearance of proportionally more immature cells in the circulation, an event known as a "shift to the left." The time in the circulation is reduced by as much as 50 to 90 per cent as cells marginate and exit more swiftly. Within several days the enhanced production and action of myelopoietic factors in the marrow causes an expansion in the total myeloid series. Marrow proliferation and maturation can be shortened to as little as five to seven days. This capacity for expansion and decreased time of retention

TABLE 5. CONTENTS OF LEUKOCYTE LYSOSOMES

POLYMORPHONUCLEAR LEUKOCYTES	MACROPHAGES	EOSINOPHILS
Azurophilic granules	**Primary and Secondary Lysosomes**	**Primary Granules**
Acid hydrolases	Acid hydrolases	Eosinophil Peroxidase
Myeloperoxidase	Lysozyme	Aryl sulfatase
Neutral proteases	Neutral proteases	Acid hydrolases
Collagenases	Collagenases	**Secondary**
Elastase	Elastase	**(Specific) Granules**
Cationic antimicrobial proteins	Plasminogen activator	Eosinophil peroxidase
Lysozyme	Angiotensin-converting enzyme	Eosinophil cationic protein
Specific Granules	Cationic antimicrobial proteins	Major basic protein
Lysozyme	Arginase	Acid hydrolases
Lactoferrin		Neutral proteases
B_{12}-binding proteins		**Specific**
		Microgranules
		?

in the marrow may augment PMN turnover by as much as five to tenfold above basal conditions. Furthermore, characteristic morphologic immaturities may be seen reflecting decreased cellular divisions after the promyelocyte stage. The increased ratio of prominent, dark staining azurophilic granules to the specific granules that results has been called "toxic granulation," emphasizing the inflammatory states that lead to its occurrence.

Whether the patient develops neutrophilic leukocytosis or neutropenia during acute infection represents the balance between production, exit from the marrow, margination vs free circulation, and exit from the intravascular space. When marrow production is normal, demand usually does not outstrip the supply of cells from myelopoiesis, and leukocytosis is the rule.

Certain organisms are notable for producing a paradoxic neutropenia during infection either by affecting myelopoiesis (for example, DNA viruses of the Herpes group) or enhancing margination (gram-negative bacteria and their surface lipopolysaccharides). Infection by the Herpes group of viruses appears to induce a suppressor cell population that actively inhibits the production of colony-stimulating factor (CSF) by marrow macrophages. Lipopolysaccharides activate the complement system and injure endothelium; both serve to cause neutrophil aggregation and enhance adherence in the microvasculature.

When neutropenia is the result of marrow failure, susceptibility to infection with a variety of bacteria and fungi is markedly enhanced. Neutropenia contributes importantly to the morbidity and mortality from infection experienced by patients on cytotoxic chemotherapy or with acute leukemia. A fall in circulating neutrophils below 1000/μl sharply reduces the participation of these cells in the inflammatory process and provides a rationale for the use of adjunctive neutrophil transfusions for some patients with infection. The decision to transfuse depends upon the nature of the infecting organism, the response to antimicrobial therapy, and the projected duration of the neutropenia or marrow failure.

The kinetics of macrophages and eosinophils have not been as extensively studied. Blood monocytes are derived from promonocyte precursors in the marrow. There is no storage pool in the marrow for monocytes comparable to that for PMNs. Monocytes spend several days in the circulation before departing and undergoing further maturation in the tissues to become fixed or wandering macrophages. Eosinophils develop from an independent myeloid cell line. Mature eosinophils circulate for about 12 to 24 hours before exiting into tissues. Conditions that induce eosinophilia expand eosinophil production and prolong time in the circulation.

ADHERENCE

Enhanced adherence of circulating PMNs to endothelial cells constitutes a major initial step in a tissue inflammatory response. Postcapillary venules are the usual site of exit of PMNs from the vasculature (Fig. 4). This increase in adherence is accompanied by changes in the PMN cell membrane related to specific granule fusion, reduction in the net negative surface charge, and increased deformability as well as by

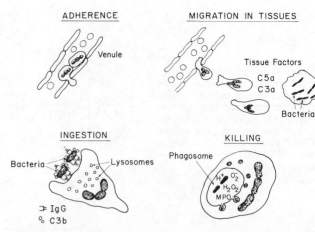

Figure 4. The four major phases in neutrophil function are adherence to postcapillary venules, migration into tissues in response to chemotactic factors, ingestion of organisms opsonized by IgG and C3B, and, finally, killing of organisms in phagocytic vacuoles by the combined action of lysosomal enzymes (myeloperoxidase), superoxide, H_2O_2, and acidity (H^+). (From Root, R. K.: Host defense factors in infectious diseases. American College of Physicians Medical Knowledge Self Assessment Program V, 1979, p. 31.)

aggregation of cells. The initial event appears as a secretory one that has the dual effect of coating the cell surface with the positively charged iron-binding protein lactoferrin, as well as inserting reactive sites into the cell membrane. Specific receptors for a cleavage product of the third component of complement, C3bi, are integral parts of these sites and appear to participate in adherence and aggregation, as well as phagocytosis. Monoclonal antibodies directed against these receptors inhibit PMN adherence and aggregation. In addition, patients who lack plasma membrane glycoproteins that incorporate the C3bi receptor have a circulating leukocytosis, fail to form pus normally, and suffer from serious recurrent bacterial infection in the lungs and a variety of soft tissue sites (see Table 4). In vitro, their cells show (1) markedly reduced adherence/aggregation properties to a variety of surfaces, (2) diminished surface-dependent chemotaxis, and (3) altered C3bi-dependent receptor function. Monocytes and macrophages also bear surface receptors for C3bi, which presumably play a similar role in these cells as in PMNs.

Humoral factors can serve to activate or modulate the adherence process. Stimuli that trigger specific granule fusion and secretion include the complement cleavage product C5a, formylated peptides analogous to those produced by bacteria, and arachidonic acid metabolites (for example, leukotriene B4 [LTB4]). High doses of glucocorticoids or alcohol induce a plasma factor that inhibits PMN adherence, as do agents that increase the ratio of intracellular cyclic adenosine monophosphate (cAMP) to cyclic guanosine monophosphate (cGMP). Bacterial infections that complicate high-dose steroid therapy or acute alcohol intoxication may complicate this blockade of the inflammatory process at the adherence step. Conversely, reduction of PMN adherence by glucocorticoids appears to be central to their anti-inflammatory action in tissues and may protect endothelial cells from injury during conditions of augmented adherence and triggering, such as sepsis complicated by shock (see below). The critical role that adherence plays in the participation of PMNs in the inflammatory response in vivo is highlighted by the infectious complications that may develop when it is impaired.

While not as extensively studied, monocytes respond to factors that augment or reduce adherence to surfaces—including endothelial cells—by mechanisms similar to PMNs.

CHEMOTAXIS

The ability of a cell to move in a tightly regulated fashion into and along an increasing concentration gradient of a motility stimulating factor is known as chemotaxis. This contrasts with the enhanced random motility exhibited by cells in the presence of a chemotactic factor without the establishment of a gradient. PMNs that leave the vasculature do so by squeezing between intact endothelial cells of the postcapillary venule in response to chemotactic factors. Localization of PMNs at a site of infection or inflammation follows migration along an increasing chemotactic factor gradient to its source. Receptors for a variety of chemotactic factors on the cell surface have been defined and play a key role in initiating motility responses. A failure of exit, migration, and localization can thus be a consequence of altered cellular properties (such as poor deformability, reduced receptor-mediated signaling, or altered locomotion) or a failure of synthesis of chemotactic factor. Examples of both types of defects have been found by the systematic study of patients with recurrent pyogenic bacterial infections.

A variety of chemotactic factors have been defined. Among the best studied are the complement cleavage product C5a, and the formylated tripeptides (for example, *N*-formyl-methionine-leucyl-phenylalanine [FMLP]). These latter compounds share structural homologies with those produced and released by bacteria. Denatured collagen, kallikrein, and 5-lipoxygenase arachidonic acid metabolites (LTB$_4$) and certain derivatives of 5-hydroxyeicosotetraenoic acid (5-HETE) are also potent chemotaxins. When peptides with chemotactic activity insert into their specific receptor, a number of events are triggered that initiate and direct cellular motility. These include an immediate transmembrane flux of sodium and calcium ions, membrane depolarization with a change in cellular surface charge, and calcium-dependent binding of the contractile protein actin to another protein, gelsolin. Gelsolin promotes actin binding to a second contractile protein, myosin—following which occurs a change in the gelsol state of these proteins. Movement is initiated at the sites adjacent to the chemotactic factor binding by the formation of a broad, organelle-free pseudopod that advances and adheres to the surface in front of the cell (Fig. 5). The continued forward thrust of the cytoplasm over the adherent membrane maintains motion in much the same fashion as the treads of a tank progress forward. The integrity of the microtubular network that constitutes the cytoskeleton of the cell appears to be importantly involved in maintaining direction. When this network is altered by drugs (for example, colchicine) or congenital defects such as the immotile cilia syndrome, the directional responses to chemotactic signals are impaired.

When cells are moving along an increasing gradient of chemotactic factor, speed and direction are maintained as progressively more receptors and presumably lower affinity receptors are engaged with increasing chemotactic factor concentrations. Cells may make short, angled turns or even reverse their directions if the gradient is altered accordingly. In the absence of a concentration gradient of chemotactic factor, movement occurs by much the same mechanisms, although it is random in nature. The percentage of cells engaged in random motility is increased if chemotactic factors are added to the medium without establishing a gradient.

Functional regulation of chemotactic receptor activity is achieved by a variety of mechanisms. When receptors are occupied by their specific chemotactic factor protein or peptide, they are blocked for receipt of new signals (so-called "down regulation"). This reg-

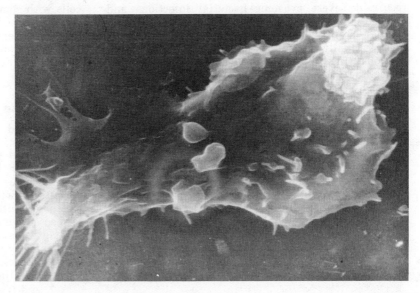

Figure 5. Scanning electron micrograph of a motile human PMN. The front of the cell is at the left.

ulation appears to be factor specific so that cells down-regulated for FMLP responses respond well to C5a and vice versa. It is not clear whether receptor-factor complexes are then internalized or remain on the cell membrane in all situations. New receptor activity can be generated by separation of the factor-receptor ligand, or by the insertion or uncovering of new receptor proteins in the plasma membrane. Neutrophil specific granules appear to be the major intracellular source of new receptors for complement and formylated peptides in these cells. As the concentration of chemotactic factors is increased, fusion of specific granules with the cell-membrane occurs, resulting in the appearance of new receptor activity. In this way, the cells become endowed with new or renewed functional capacity as they near the site of an infection or an inflammatory stimulus. Movement stops when all chemotactic receptors are occupied or when chemotactic receptors are inactivated. For example, myeloperoxidase, using H_2O_2 as a substrate, can oxidize the sulfhydryl groups on FMLP, thereby inactivating it.

A number of disorders of the chemotactic process contribute to the pathogenesis of pyogenic infections in certain acquired or congenital diseases. Both cellular abnormalities and humoral inhibitors of cellular function have been described. Patients with uremia, diabetes mellitus, rheumatoid arthritis, and cirrhosis have all had deficiencies in PMN chemotaxis reported (see Table 4). Evanescent cellular abnormalities have been reported in diabetes that do not relate strictly to diabetic control. Some patients with cirrhosis may have circulating inhibitors of chemotaxis. Uremia can inhibit the ability of normal PMNs to respond to chemotactic stimuli. Cells that are immature not only exhibit poor motility but are relatively rigid and do not adhere well to surfaces. This immaturity undoubtedly contributes to the cause of infections in untreated myelocytic leukemias or in other myeloid dysplastic states.

The study of patients with congenital disorders of chemotaxis has also provided important information about normal cellular mechanisms. For example, the importance of contractile proteins in the function of human PMNs was demonstrated in an infant with recurrent severe pyogenic bacterial infections and marked leukocytosis. In addition to markedly reduced cellular motility, his cells were unable to ingest particles normally and to form phagosomes. Polymerization of actin in his PMNs was abnormal and caused the cellular defects.

Patients with the Chédiak-Higashi syndrome have abnormally high turnover rates of microtubular proteins, accompanied by impaired chemotaxis and lysosomal degranulation. Their phagocytic cells also have unusually high intracellular levels of cAMP. Administration of ascorbate to some patients with the Chédiak-Higashi syndrome has reduced intracellular cAMP and restored normal microtubule-dependent functions.

In the immotile cilia syndrome (ICS), various microtubule-associated proteins are missing (dynein arms or radial spokes). Cytoskeletal functions related to these structures are lost or modified. While the chemotactic abnormalities in the ICS may be relatively unimportant in the pathogenesis of their infections, they have provided information about the participation of microtubules in cell orientation during movement.

Patients with recurrent staphylococcal soft tissue abscesses, an eczematous dermatitis, eosinophilia, and markedly elevated levels of immunoglobulin E have a disorder referred to as "Job's syndrome." The features of this syndrome mimic the Biblical trials of Job, who had recurrent boils and carbuncles. The patients have a T cell immunoregulatory abnormality that indirectly affects PMNs. Perhaps triggered by cutaneous staphylococcal infections, the diminished actions of a T-suppressor cell population fail to regulate IgE production (which may contain antistaphylococcal antibody) as well as fail to inhibit the elaboration of a lymphokine that normally reduces leukocyte motility (leukocyte inhibitory factor or LIF). The discovery of LIF and its relationship to this syndrome has emphasized the interconnected role played by specific cellular immune mechanisms and regulation of the acute inflammatory response. There is no effective therapy for this syndrome.

Some children who have unusually severe periodontitis have chemotactic deficiencies caused by a circulating inhibitor(s). While the nature of these inhibitors has not been defined for the majority of patients, in one group, the organism Capnocytophaga elaborates a potent inhibitor of neutrophil chemotaxis in vitro. In at least one case, therapy with the appropriate antibiotic in vivo led to a reversal of the defect.

These latter studies have helped to define a new dimension in host-parasite interactions in which microbial virulence factors modulate normal host defense mechanisms. While of less certain importance clinically, both cholera toxin (an inducer of host-cell adenylcyclase activity) and Bordetella pertussis toxin (which itself is a potent adenylcyclase) inhibit PMN chemotaxis. Infections with these agents lack pus—which may reflect this inhibitory activity. The in vitro studies with these toxins have helped to define an intracellular regulatory role for cyclic nucleotides in cell movement.

The chemotaxis of monocytes, macrophages, and eosinophils has also been studied. Mechanisms similar to those described for PMNs are shared with these cells with some modifications. Eosinophils, for example, appear to be regulated in their movement in vivo by specific peptides contained in mast cell granules as well as by products of the lipoxygenase pathway of arachidonic acid metabolism (see discussion of immunology).

PHAGOCYTOSIS

Interpreted broadly, phagocytosis refers to all of those events involving the attachment and uptake of large, usually particulate, molecules by cells and their incorporation into single membrane–bound intracellular vacuoles. The vacuolar membrane contains components of both the plasma membrane and those of lysosomes with which it has fused; the vacuole is termed a *phagolysosome.*

Phagocytosis involves cooperation between cellular mechanisms and humoral factors that affect the phagocytic particle. The cellular mechanisms include changes in the gel-sol state of contractile proteins, which lead to the formation of a pseudopod at the leading edge of the cell. Once contact is made and a particle has bound to appropriate sites on the cell membrane, ingestion occurs by a process of progressive engulfment of the particle. Lysosomal fusion at the site of engulfment occurs promptly, leading to formation of the phagolysosome. The interior of the phagolysosome contains the contents of the fused lysosomes—as well as other constituents—including some from the extracellular medium.

Whether or not a particle can be ingested by a phagocyte is a function of both its size and its surface characteristics. Particles in excess of 5 μm in diameter are usually too large to be ingested. Negatively charged particles or those with a neutral surface charge are more likely to be ingested than those that are positively charged. Ingestibility can also be correlated with the lipophilic characteristics of the particle. Hydrophilic particles are not usually ingested until their surface characteristics have been changed to make them more lipophilic. In the case of many pathogenic microorganisms or other cells, this change is accomplished by the process known as opsonization.*

Opsonins include immunoglobulins of the IgG$_1$ and IgG$_3$ subclasses that can bind directly to phagocytic cell receptors specific for the Fc portions of these molecules. When bound to an antigen, IgM and IgG antibodies act as opsonins indirectly by activating the complement cascade via the classical pathway. Cleavage products of C3, specifically C3b, and the product of its limited proteolysis, C3bi, also bind to specific cellular receptors termed CR1 and CR3, respectively. Thus when opsonins coat a phagocytic particle, they not only alter surface charge but also can form a receptor-specific ligand with the phagocytic cell that is involved in triggering the ingestion process. With macrophages, phagocytosis is more likely to occur when Fc receptors are engaged than when binding to cells occurs by complement receptors only. With these cells the complement receptors appear to be more involved in particle adherence to cells than ingestion per se. Receptor-mediated phagocytosis appears to occur by a progressive engagement of phagocytic receptors in a so-called "zipper" effect (Fig. 6). Fibronectin, a glycoprotein found in the blood and distributed widely in the extracellular spaces of most tissues, promotes phagocytosis of *S. aureus* and perhaps gram-negative bacterial endotoxins, apparently through nonreceptor-mediated mechanisms.

As phagocytes, PMNs are more effective and rapidly acting than mononuclear cells. Eosinophils are least effective in particle ingestion. Macrophages can increase their phagocytic activity when "activated" by lymphokines. Gamma-interferon released by immunologically activated T lymphocytes appears to play a major role in this process.

The capacity for phagocytosis occurs rather late in PMN development; immature cells exhibit reduced phagocytic activity. Both cellular motility and phagocytic activity are impaired by hyperosmolarity, as may occur in uncontrolled diabetes mellitus. Several genetic defects in phagocytic activity of PMNs have been described, including in a patient who lacked actin-

Opsonos: to prepare to eat (Greek).

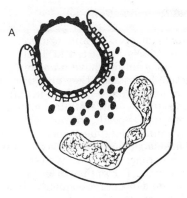

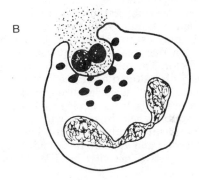

A. "Zipper" model of phagocytosis

B. "Regurgitation through feeding"

Figure 6. Two phases in PMN function: *A*, phagocytosis. (Modified from Silverstein, S. C., Steinman, R. M., and Cohn, Z.: Endocytosis. Annu Rev Biochem 46:669, 1977.) *B*, lysosomal degranulation during bacterial ingestion. (Modified from Weissman, G.: Lysosomal mechanisms of tissue injury in arthritis. N Engl J Med 286:141, 1972.)

binding proteins in his PMNs, and in patients whose PMNs lack membrane glycoproteins encompassing the C3bi receptor. Finally, when antibody-forming capacity or the ability to deposit C3b on the particle surface is impaired (either by C3 deficiency or reduced complement activation), phagocytic activity will be reduced in vivo. Interest is now centered on finding compounds that stimulate phagocytosis in vivo or that provide increased opsonic activity through active or passive vaccination.

Cellular Events Accompanying Phagocytosis

Phagocytosis is accompanied by lysosomal degranulation and triggering of a burst in cellular oxidative metabolism. Both are centrally involved in the killing and digesting of microorganisms or conversely in promoting inflammation. In addition, macrophages can process antigens and activate T lymphocytes through the elaboration of the monokine interleukin-1. PMNs or eosinophils that have ingested particles or have been triggered by other stimuli to degranulate and increase respiratory activity ultimately die within hours. Their role in antigen-processing appears to be a peripheral or secondary one at best.

Lysosomal Degranulation

The contents of specific and azurophilic granules (lysosomes) of PMNs are listed in Table 5. In PMNs only azurophilic granules have an acidic pH and contain acid-active hydrolases; they are "true" lysosomes. Specific granules are more involved in PMN secretory activity than in the intracellular microbicidal and digestive functions. Specific granule discharge can be provoked by minimal stimuli such as adherence of PMNs to various surfaces, and may be important in regulating adherence itself as well as responses to chemotactic factors. During particle ingestion specific granule fusion and discharge sequentially precede that of azurophilic granules.

The most important antimicrobial protein identified within specific granules is lactoferrin. This iron-binding protein may be microbiostatic or microbicidal depending upon the organism's requirement for iron as a growth factor. The presence of lactoferrin on the cell surface may also alter the surface charge. The hydrolytic enzyme lysozyme is localized predominately to the specific granules. Its action is restricted to cleaving N-acetyl muramic acid linkages with N-acetylglucosamine in bacterial peptidoglycan. It is bactericidal only for a few species and appears to be mainly involved in microbial digestive activity by PMNs and macrophages.

Azurophilic granules contain several classes of proteins involved importantly in microbial killing and digestion as well as inflammation. Myeloperoxidase is a heme protein that utilizes H_2O_2 as a substrate to promote a number of oxidizing reactions that may kill microorganisms or injure mammalian cells. Cationic proteins, some having tryptic activity, can modify the permeability characteristics of the outer membrane of gram-negative organisms and (by other mechanisms) cause their rapid death. Others kill fungi and gram-positive bacteria. Hydrolases, which have their optimal activity at an acid pH, can degrade proteins, DNA, and complex carbohydrates. Other metalloproteases have their optimal action at a neutral pH and show substrate specificity for elastin and collagen. While elastase and neutral tryptic proteases have mild antimicrobial properties, their primary action appears to be directed at host tissues. Some proteases can cleave the complement factors C3 and C5 directly, leading to the generation of biologically active C3a and C5a. Others can activate or inactivate the kinin system. The release of these proteins outside the cell before vacuole closure is complete ("regurgitation during feeding") (Fig. 6) can contribute to acute inflammation and its accompanying tissue injury.

As in the events that precede changes in cellular motility, fluxes in divalent (calcium) and monovalent (Na^+ and K^+) cations accompany degranulation. Furthermore, compounds called *ionophores,* which transport these ions across the plasma membrane or from one membrane-bound pool to another, may trigger degranulation. Rapid decreases in lysosomal osmolarity may also contribute to the degranulation mechanism. Once the phagolysosome is formed, it characteristically enlarges, as osmotically active molecules trap more solute-free fluid, and may fuse with other phagolysosomes in the cell. The assembly of microtubules also regulates lysosomal degranulation. When assembly is impaired—for example, by exposure to the drug colchicine—degranulation is reduced.

Relatively few naturally occurring examples of lysosomal abnormalities have been defined. A patient with missing specific granules has had problems with recurrent but not severe pyogenic infections. Upon stimulation his cells do not increase expression of receptors for chemotactic peptides or surface CR3 receptors. Cells from patients with the Chédiak-Higashi syndrome have abnormal single membrane–bound organelles. In PMNs this is expressed as giant lysosomes that contain proteins of both specific and azurophilic granules. The microbicidal activity of Chédiak-Higashi PMNs and monocytes is delayed due to faulty fusion of the giant lysosomes with phagosomes. Abnormal microtubule assembly may also play a role in this phenomenon.

Lysosomes in macrophages are of two types, primary structures formed by the Golgi apparatus (which contain a variety of acid hydrolases), and secondary lysosomes (which are actually phagolysosomes). The latter bring high molecular weight and particulate materials into these cells for further processing; their formation is increased when macrophages are activated by lymphokines. In contrast to PMNs, monocytes lose myeloperoxidase activity as the cells mature to become macrophages. Relatively little is known of other antimicrobial factors in macrophage lysosomes, although they contain cationic proteins that have actions similar to those found in PMNs; they also contain lysozyme. Other lysosomal enzymes allow macrophages to interact with the coagulation and renin-angiotensin systems, as well as to participate importantly in inflammatory processes.

Mature eosinophils possess two structurally distinct types of large granules; both contain peroxidase activity. A smaller dumbbell-shaped granule of uncertain function has also been found. The large granules are probably different developmental stages of the same lysosomes formed by eosinophilic promyelocytes. The majority of the large granules are marked by the presence of a discrete central bar that is less dense than the surrounding matrix. Termed *crystalloids,* these bars may accumulate in secretions rich in eosinophils and form Charcot-Leyden crystals. Peroxidase and other acid hydrolase activity is found in the matrix of the granules. Hydrolase activity includes arylsulfatase. This enzyme is unique to the eosinophil and inactivates specific leukotrienes involved in bronchial smooth muscle contraction (see discussion of immunology).

The eosinophil granule crystalloid is composed of an 11,000 dalton M_r basic protein that has broad cytotoxic activity against eukaryotic cells, including parasites and host endothelial cells. Compared to myeloperoxidase, eosinophil peroxidase is not as potent a bactericidal enzyme and is structurally and chemically distinct. A cationic protein has been described in eosinophils that has no microbicidal activity but that can interact with the coagulation and kallikrein systems, promoting both coagulation via the intrinsic pathway as well as activation of fibrinolysis. Eosinophil granules appear to be involved more in secretory functions of these cells as they interact with foreign surface antigens than in intracellular microbicidal and digestive actions. Besides their antimicrobial functions, eosinophils are important participants in the dampening of immediate hypersensitivity reactions as outlined in the discussion on immunology.

Metabolic Changes Accompanying Phagocytosis

All phagocytic cells undergo a striking burst in respiratory activity during particle ingestion or when the cell membrane is altered by other stimuli. The stimuli can be quite diverse and can include binding of cells to inert surfaces, insertion of chemotactic factors into their membrane receptors, exposure to structurally unique organic (phorbol) esters of myristic acid, arachidonic acid metabolites, or the action of calcium ionophores. All of these stimuli are capable of triggering the activation of a membrane-bound oxidase through apparently separate pathways that lead to a final common event. The mechanisms that trigger oxidase activation are thus tied closely to others that affect PMN surface properties—namely, cellular adherence, motility, degranulation, and phagocytosis itself. As with these other responses, oxidase activation is preceded by depolarization of the PMN plasma membrane followed by rapid hyperpolarization. Cationic fluxes—particularly those involving calcium—have been proposed to play a mechanistic role in oxidase activation.

The events known collectively as the *respiratory burst* are listed in Table 6; Figure 7 depicts their interrelationships. This respiratory activity is not tied to energy metabolism, but rather to oxygen utilization by a separate pathway. Mature PMNs have relatively few mitochondria and utilize anaerobic glycolysis for energy. Since PMNs are not dependent upon oxidative metabolism for motility, adherence, or phagocytosis, they can function well in areas of low oxygen tension such as the interior of abscesses and foci of chronic bone infection. In macrophages the number of mitochondria and dependence upon aerobic metabolism as an energy source vary considerably with the location of the usual site of operation of these cells. Macrophages in the alveolar spaces of the lung are rich in mitochondria, whereas those in the peritoneal cavity depend more upon anaerobic glycolysis for energy.

The oxidative pathways of the respiratory burst and their interrelationships have been defined and the central role of a superoxide-forming oxidase clarified. Superoxide is the one electron reduction product of oxygen. It is a common intermediate in biologic oxidation-reduction reactions that involve the eventual reduction of oxygen to water. In phagocytic cells the superoxide-forming oxidase is a complex enzyme with at least two major components (Fig. 8). A flavoprotein oxidase removes electrons from cytoplasmic pyridine nucleotide donors (NADPH is the primary donor) and transfers them to a terminal oxygen reductase, a B-type cytochrome. The localization of the cytochrome to the plasma membrane at the site of particle ingestion

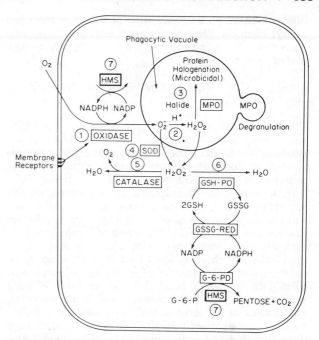

Figure 7. Events that occur during oxidative killing. Abbreviations: HMS, hexose monophosphate shunt; MPO, myeloperoxidase; SOD, superoxide dismutase; GSH-PO, glutathione peroxidase; GSH, reduced glutathione; GSSG, oxidized glutathione; G-6-PD, glucose-6-phosphate dehydrogenase; G-6-P, glucose-6-phosphate. (From Root, R. K.: The microbicidal mechanisms of human neutrophils and eosinophils. Rev Inf Dis 3:565, 1981.)

allows the formation of O_2^- directly in the phagosome or on cell surfaces.

O_2^- is a labile molecule that can undergo further reaction with itself—that is, "dismutation"—to form the two-electron oxygen reduction product peroxide or that can react with other electron-rich sites such as unsaturated carbon bonds in lipids and nucleic acids.

TABLE 6. THE LEUKOCYTE RESPIRATORY BURST

1. ↑ O_2 consumption	5. ↑ Glucose oxidation
2. ↑ O_2 generation	6. ↑ Chemiluminescence
3. ↑ H_2O_2 production	7. ↑ NBT reduction
4. ↑ Iodination	

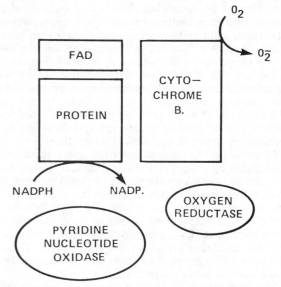

Figure 8. Proposed structure of the superoxide-forming oxidase. FAD: flavin adenine dinucleotide; NADPH, NADP: nicotinamide adenine dinucleotide phosphate, reduced and oxidized forms.

Superoxide may also react with peroxide to form hydroxyl radicals (OH·) and singlet oxygen ($^1O_2$)—both also powerful oxidants—by what is known as the Haber-Weiss reaction:

$$O_2^- + H_2O_2 \rightarrow OH^- + OH^· + {}^1O_2$$

This reaction is catalyzed by iron, which, in the PMN, can be supplied by lactoferrin. In this way the oxidizing potential of O_2^- is further enhanced. It may be accompanied by the generation of chemical light (chemiluminescence) as $^1O_2$ decays to ground state triplet O_2.

H_2O_2 formed by dismutation of O_2^- serves as the substrate for both myeloperoxidase and eosinophil peroxidase. In the presence of halide cofactors, myeloperoxidase can catalyze the formation of hyphalous ions such as hypochlorous acid. Hypochlorous acid can in turn catalyze chlorination of amines forming toxic chloramines. This transfer of oxidizing potential can culminate in peptide bond cleavage, creation of lipid peroxides, oxidation of iron centers of heme enzymes, and breaks in the structure of DNA and RNA. Iodination of proteins by hypoiodous acid may also disrupt their function and contribute to the microbicidal and cytocidal activity of the myeloperoxidase-H_2O_2-halide complex.

The above series of reactions describe what has come to be understood as a vital oxygen-dependent killing system in PMNs. The increase in the activity of the cytoplasmic pentose shunt can be related to the metabolism of H_2O_2 through reduced glutathione-dependent pathways; these result in formation of NADP, which is the rate-limiting substrate for the pentose shunt. This system functions to detoxify H_2O_2 in the cytoplasmic location in concert with the heme enzyme catalase. O_2^-, which enters the cytoplasm, is rapidly dismuted to H_2O_2 by the action of the metalloenzyme superoxide dismutase (SOD). SOD-promoted dismutation prevents O_2^- from reacting with competing electron donors or recipients. These can include H_2O_2, thereby blocking hydroxyl radical and singlet oxygen formation. Similar to catalase and glutathione peroxidase, SOD is a "protective" enzyme in aerobic cells and is ubiquitously distributed in all aerobic species.

The activity of the superoxide-forming oxidase can be assessed quickly in stimulated cells by the use of the electron scavenger dye nitroblue tetrazolium (NBT). This dye—yellow in its oxidized state—is turned into a black insoluble precipitate when it is reduced. A rapid histochemical assay that measures NBT reduction by cells adherent to glass surfaces or stimulated by phagocytosis, endotoxin, or phorbol esters has been employed to screen for deficiencies of the superoxide-forming oxidase. Direct measurements of oxygen consumption, superoxide and H_2O_2 formation, chemiluminescence, pentose shunt oxidation myeloperoxidase activity, and myeloperoxidase-mediated protein iodination are also relatively simple. Thus it is a relatively easy matter to evaluate the integrity of these various oxidative pathways.

The importance of oxygen-dependent microbicidal and cytocidal activity is highlighted by their impairment when cells are placed in an anaerobic environment. Similarly, genetic defects in oxidase activity have serious consequences for the host. The most common of these, *chronic granulomatous disease* (CGD), is inherited as an X-linked trait and results in a deletion of cytochrome B. In these patients intracellular bacteria and fungi must be killed by nonoxidative mechanisms and cellular immunity assumes an important role in the eradication of catalase-positive organisms such as *S. aureus, S. marcescens, Candida,* and *Aspergillus* species. The result is a mixture of granuloma and pus formation. The disease usually becomes apparent in childhood; it can be readily diagnosed by the NBT test, which will show no reduction by resting or stimulated cells. Catalase-negative bacteria are killed normally by CGD cells, since they suicidally supply a small amount of H_2O_2 to be used in myeloperoxidase-mediated bactericidal activity. A number of variants of CGD exist, involving changes in NADPH oxidase affinity or functions, impaired NADPH supply, and coexisting abnormalities in glutathione peroxidase metabolism.

Of much less serious consequence is a genetic deletion in the formation of myeloperoxidase. Whereas CGD occurs in the low frequency of one/million population, the frequency of myeloperoxidase deficiency is about one/ten thousand. Myeloperoxidase-deficient cells have a markedly reduced ability to kill *Candida albicans* and other fungi while preserving almost normal microbicidal activity against bacteria. Myeloperoxidase deficiency is not usually complicated by infection unless other impairments (particularly diabetes mellitus) are present. Diabetic patients with myeloperoxidase deficiency are prone to visceral candidiasis.

Thus formation of O_2^- and H_2O_2 is essential for normal killing of most catalase positive bacteria; myeloperoxidase activity is needed for optimal killing of eukaryotic cells and accelerates H_2O_2-dependent killing of bacteria. Nonoxidative killing mechanisms of PMNs include the acidification of vacuolar pH, the action of lactoferrin, the function of cationic proteins, and the weak activity of lysosomal hydrolases and proteases. Monocytes and macrophages also utilize both oxidative and nonoxidative killing systems. Myeloperoxidase, however, is not normally involved in oxidative killing by macrophages, unless it is somehow supplied to these cells. Macrophage "activation" by lymphokines results in an augmentation of their capacity to form H_2O_2 and O_2^-; this may contribute to their enhanced cidal activities.

Eosinophils generally exhibit exaggerated oxidative metabolism at rest and with stimulation. Eosinophil peroxidase does not utilize chloride as a cofactor and is a relatively weak microbicidal enzyme. Major basic protein represents the principal nonoxidative microbicidal factor that has been characterized for eosinophils.

A second metabolic pathway of phagocytic cells, which becomes activated by phagocytosis or the other stimuli, appears to have little to do with direct microbicidal activity but is important in acute inflammation. Activation of a calcium-dependent membrane-bound phospholipase A_2 cleaves bound arachidonic acid from membrane phospholipids. Platelet-activating factor is released by the same mechanism. PMNs, macrophages, and eosinophils contain both cyclooxygenases and lipoxygenases, which oxidize arachidonic acid at different sites (see discussion on immunology). The role of these metabolites in the inflammatory process and the pathogenesis of some of the features of septic shock are discussed below.

HUMORAL DEFENSES

The complement and antibody systems comprise the humoral host defenses. They are similar in that they are both composed of soluble proteins that are found in the blood, in interstitial fluid, and on mucosal surfaces in various quantities and activities. They differ functionally in that the complement system is available for immediate activation when appropriately triggered and is relatively nonselective in many of its actions, whereas antibody development is highly specific in its response to antigens and may take days to weeks to become important in host defense.

THE COMPLEMENT SYSTEM

The complement system plays a crucial role in dealing with organisms that invade the bloodstream. It is also centrally involved in the generation of an effective acute inflammatory response. Complement proteins can link the actions of specific antibodies to those of phagocytes or cause lytic destruction of organs or infected cells themselves. Furthermore, alternative pathway activation may be triggered by microbial products directly without the need for antibody. This property places the complement system with PMNs and macrophages as the key host defenses before the development of specific immunity. The details of the complement activation sequences and their mechanisms have been covered in the discussion of immunology. This discussion will emphasize interactions between microorganisms and the complement system as it operates in host defense mechanisms and inflammation.

COMPLEMENT ACTIVATION BY MICROBIAL PRODUCTS

Surface properties of microorganisms play a key role in initiating complement activation. They may do so by serving as antigens for the development of complement-fixing antibodies or they may bind to the initiating proteins directly. For example, classical pathway activation may be triggered by IgG_1 or IgG_3 or IgM antibodies bound to surface antigens of microbes. In the absence of antibody, the lipid A core of the envelope lipopolysaccharides of gram-negative rods may fix and assemble the first component of complement; protein A of staphylococci can initiate the same sequence.

The alternative pathway of complement activation is triggered when C3b, bound to a microbial surface component, is protected from inactivation by the proteolytic action of factor H (C3b inactivator). Factor I promotes the binding of factor H to its substrate, C3b. The polysaccharide portion of gram-negative lipopolysaccharides inhibits the binding of factors H and I to intact organisms or fragments of gram-negative cell walls while not affecting that of C3b. Thus, the integrity of bound C3b is maintained, permitting in turn the binding and cleavage of properdin factors B and D as well as factor P. A C3 convertase is assembled that

proteolytically attacks and cleaves C3, depositing more C3b on the cell surface and accelerating the sequence in a positive feedback system.

Other microbial substances that may promote complement activation by the alternative pathway include the peptidoglycan and teichoic acid moieties of gram-positive organisms such as group B streptococci, as well as polysaccharide components of fungi. Conversely, organisms or cells rich in surface sialic acids actively *promote* binding of factors H and I to C3b, thereby inactivating it and protecting these organisms from the actions of the complement system. Removal of the sialic acid residues has the reverse effect, thereby triggering alternative complement pathway activation. In this way surface sialic acids can serve as virulence factors by preventing the survival of C3b on the microbial surfaces. Antibody directed against the sialic acid residues can promote opsonization by either the classical or alternative pathway and thereby be protective.

The binding of C3b to organisms can aid in their eventual destruction by promoting either opsonization or the assembly of the terminal lytic membrane attack sequence. The importance of the alternative complement pathway as a major defense mechanism against intravascular invasion by bacteria before antibody is developed is highlighted by the ability of humans to live in apparent symbiosis with the huge number of gram-negative organisms that constitute the normal flora. Major bacteremic infections occur in patients who lack alternative complement pathway components. This stands in striking contrast to patients missing components of the classical activation pathway (C1, C4, C2) who have no increased propensity to infection unless there is coexisting immunoglobulin deficiency. The function of an intact alternative complement pathway in these subjects is apparently sufficient to protect them from major infectious complications.

EFFECTOR ACTIONS OF COMPLEMENT IN MICROBIAL ERADICATION

Fixation of C4b to some viruses promotes their uptake and inactivation by macrophages. The major biologic activities of the complement system are generated, however, following the deposition of products of C3 on antigen-antibody complexes or cellular surfaces (Table 7). Cleavage of C3 into bound (C3b) and soluble (C3a) components initiates systems that can irradicate invading microorganisms either by augmenting the activities and action of the acute inflammatory response or by a direct lytic destructive attack.

The membrane attack sequence of complement consists of the components C5b, 6, 7, 8, and 9. The last enzymatic step in complement activation is carried out by bound C3b and is the limited proteolytic cleavage of factor 5 leading to the formation of bound (C5b) and soluble (C5a) fragments. C5b promotes the sequential binding of factors 6, 7, 8, and 9. The binding of C9 accelerates the detergent-like action of factor 8 in concert with the other proteins by creating ionic channels in the cell membrane. This results in a net flow of water ions and the disruption of the osmotic integrity of the cell. The membrane attack sequence is highly effective against gram-negative organisms and results

TABLE 7. MAJOR BIOLOGIC FUNCTIONS OF COMPLEMENT IMPORTANT IN HOST DEFENSES*

FACTORS	FUNCTION
Alternative (properdin) pathway	Activation by endotoxin, or polysaccharides of organisms to cleave C3.
Classical pathway	Activation by specific antibodies (IgG1, IgG3, IgM) combining with antigenic sites on organisms or lipid A (gram-negative rods), protein A (*S. aureus*) to cleave C3. C4b opsonic for some viruses.
C3	Cleavage into bound (C3b) and soluble (C3a) subcomponents leads to cleavage of C5 (C3b), opsonization (C3b, C3bi) and vasodilatation, and increased capillary permeability. C3e promotes release of marrow PMNs.
C5	Cleavage by C3b leads to formation of soluble C5a (chemotactic, vasodilatory, neutrophil-activating, histamine-releasing) and bound C5b.
C5b6789	Fixation (binding) leads to cell-free lysis of susceptible organisms or cells.

*Modified from American College of Physicians: MKSAP V Syllabus, 1979.

in rapid destruction of the lipopolysaccharide-rich outer envelope. Similar events may lead to destruction of intact eukaryotic cells, including those of the host, if the sequence is successfully completed. The lytic activity of complement is not effective against gram-positive organisms because their thick cell wall protects the bacterial cell membrane from lytic attack.

Against gram-positive organisms and other bacteria, or microbes resistant to the lytic action of the membrane attack complex, the major protective function of complement relates to the operation of C3b as an opsonin. C3b deposited on the microbial surface and the product of its limited proteolytic cleavage, C3bi, can interact with appropriate receptors on phagocytic cells and trigger their ingestion as described above.

The complement proteins C3 and C5 also are vital in promoting the acute inflammatory response. The C3a cleavage product of C3 can augment capillary permeability and promote vasodilation (C3a anaphylatoxin). The soluble cleavage product of C5, C5a, is also an anaphylatoxin. These actions increase blood flow to a site of inflammation and promote the entry of complement proteins and immunoglobulins into the site. The role of C3- and C5-derived protein opsonization and PMN adherence, marrow release, chemotaxis, oxidase activation, and degranulation has been discussed.

The participation of C3 and C5 cleavage products in normal inflammatory mechanisms can be a two-edged sword; it contributes to the injury of host tissues during sepsis. Thus, PMNs attached to sites such as the meninges, joint spaces, and lungs can injure these tissues through the release of toxic oxygen metabolites and proteolytic and other hydrolytic enzymes. The anaphylatoxins can cause local swelling or generalized pulmonary edema. C5a—through its multiple effects on activating PMNs and altering vessels—may play a contributory role in the hypotension of septic shock as well as PMN-mediated pulmonary capillary and alveolar injury.

Deficiencies in the production or action of certain complement components may have major consequences to normal host defense (Table 8). Deletions of components of the classical complement pathway or its regulators have little impact on host defense because of the reserve activity of the alternative complement pathway. On the other hand, patients who lack alternative complement components such as factor B are subject to life-threatening bacteremias. The same is true of patients who are deficient in complement factor 3, either as a result of its genetic deletion or of its

unregulated activation (factor H deficiency). Both of these very rare disorders are marked by severe infections with encapsulated bacteria, involving the lung or bloodstream of affected patients. Recurrent episodes of systemic infection with Neisserial species characterize subjects who lack components of the terminal membrane attack complex (C5–C9). The relatively high frequency of complement-deficient states in meningococcemia or meningococcal meningitis indicates the need to measure hemolytic complement titers and individual components in patients who develop these infections.

The integrity of either the classical or the alternative complement pathway can be measured functionally with hemolytic assays. Such assays usually employ sheep erythrocytes coated with either IgM heterophil antibody (classical pathway) or C3b and properdin factor B (alternative pathway). The individual components may also be measured using specific immunoassays.

ANTIBODIES

The development of antibodies in response to the challenge of various antigens constitutes one of the two major limbs of the specific immune response. All antibodies are complex glycoproteins known as *immunoglobulins*. The mechanisms by which they are produced and details of their structure and function are summarized in the discussion on immunology. Of the five major classes or isotypes of immunoglobulins, those belonging to the G, M, A, and E subclasses have been defined as playing a major role in the effector arm of host defense. Immunoglobulins of the IgG isotype comprise 75 per cent of the total in serum; IgA 15 per cent, IgM 10 per cent, IgG 0.2 per cent, and IgE only 0.004 per cent, respectively. Approximately 50 per cent of IgG, IgA, and IgE is intravascular as compared to 75 per cent of IgM and IgD. IgG is the most prominent immunoglobulin in lymphatic fluid and is the only one to be actively transported across the placenta. IgA, particularly that of the dimeric subclass IgA$_2$, is the predominant immunoglobulin on mucosal surfaces and in various secretions such as saliva, tears, and colostrum. IgM exists in the circulation as a pentamer and is the first immunoglobulin to be formed in response to new antigens. Through its complement-fixing properties it appears to play a particularly prominent role in early defense against blood-borne infection.

TABLE 8. DEFECTS OF THE COMPLEMENT SYSTEM AND THEIR CONSEQUENCES TO HOST DEFENSE AGAINST INFECTION*

COMPONENT	ASSOCIATED DISEASES	EFFECTS ON HOST DEFENSES[a]
C1		
C1q	Combined immunodeficiency, SLE	Major[b]
C1r	SLE, glomerulonephritis	Minor[b]
C1s	SLE	Minor[b]
C1 inhibitor	HAE (hereditary angioedema)	None
C4	SLE (systemic lupus erythematosus)	Minor[b]
C2	None, discoid LE, SLE, polymyositis, encapsulated bacterial infections	None through Major[b, c]
C3	Hereditary deficiency, cirrhosis, SLE, nephritis, immune complex disorders	Major[b, c]
C3b inactivator (I)	Encapsulated bacterial infections	Major[c]
C5	Neisserial infections, SLE	Major[c]
C5 "dysfunction"	Bacterial infections, diarrhea, eczema (Leiner's syndrome)	Major[c]
C6	Neisserial infections, none	Moderate[b, c]
C7	Neisserial infections, none, Raynaud's	Moderate[b, c]
C8	Neisserial infections, SLE, none	Moderate[b, c]
C9	None	None
Alternate pathway	Sickle cell disease, splenectomy?	Major[b, c]
Factor B	Associated with C2 deficiency	Major[c]

*Reprinted with permission from Root, R. K.: Humoral Immunity. In Mandell, G., Douglas, G., and Bennett, J. (eds.): Principles and Practice of Infectious Diseases. 2nd ed. New York, John Wiley and Sons, in press.
[a]Major effects on host defenses are manifested by severe, recurrent bacterial infections, whereas minor effects are marked by infrequent infections.
[b]Effects on host defense appear to be mediated as much or more by the associated disease rather than by the complement deficiency per se.
[c]Effects on host defense are mediated primarily by the complement deficiency.

Immunoglobulins are bifunctional molecules: one function is to bind to specific antigens; the other is to elicit the biologic response. The majority of these responses involves the action of either phagocytes or the complement system.

Binding of antibody initiates the actions of phagocytosis or the fixation of complement via the classical pathway. Immunoglobulins of the IgA and IgE isotypes do not activate the complement system and do not bind to phagocytic cells.

The differing distribution, the biological properties, and the developmental sequences of individual immunoglobulin isotypes account for their activity at different sites in the body as well as different times in response to newly infecting agents. There is no evidence that antibodies are capable of penetrating intact cells to affect intracellular organisms. Thus, their action against invading microbes is restricted to the extracellular location. Finally, with chronic antigenic stimulation, specific antibodies or immune complexes may play a pathogenetic role in the manifestations of some infections.

FUNCTION OF ANTIBODIES IN HOST DEFENSE

Antibodies may eradicate or limit infecting organisms by several mechanisms. The actions of different antibodies and the major isotypes involved are outlined in Table 9. Antibodies may function as opsonins by forming a ligand directly between an organism and Fc receptors of the phagocytic cells. These actions are limited to antibodies of the IgG isotypes with IgG_1 and IgG_3 as the major subclasses involved. IgM (as well as IgG) has opsonic activity by virtue of its ability to activate the classical complement pathway and to generate bound C3b on the surface of the organism.

When the host lacks the capacity to develop opsonizing antibodies, recurrent and severe infections with encapsulated bacteria ensue.

Antibodies of the IgG and IgM subclass can also activate complement-derived lytic activity against susceptible organisms. Patients who lack bactericidal antibodies against Hemophilus influenzae are prone to recurrent septicemic infection with this organism. The administration of vaccines containing polysaccharides of Neisseria meningitidis or Hemophilus influenzae leads to the development of bactericidal or opsonizing antibodies that operate through the complement system. Lytic antibodies may also be directed against infected cells. In this case the cellular lysis is accomplished by the complement system rather than an antibody dependent cellular mechanism. Some virus-infected cells are killed by this mechanism.

Antibodies of the IgG and IgM subclasses may bind to protein toxins produced by organisms and neutralize their action. Vaccines developed against diphtheria and tetanus are basically antitoxic in their action. The IgG antibodies that develop in vaccine recipients have

TABLE 9. ROLE OF ANTIBODIES IN HOST DEFENSE

1. Inhibit adherence	(IgA, IgG)
2. Opsonization	(IgG)

3. Activate complement
   Opsonization
   Bacteriolysis
	(IgG, IgM)

4. Neutralize toxins	(IgG)
5. Neutralize viruses	(IgM, IgG, IgA)
6. Antibody-dependent-cellular cytotoxicity	(IgG)
7. Basophil and mast cell granule discharge	(IgE)

no significant activity against the organisms themselves but block the binding of potent exotoxins to cells, thereby neutralizing them. More recently, antibodies of the IgM subclass developed in recipients of a rough, mutant strain of *E. coli* have been used to reduce the morbidity and mortality of gram-negative sepsis in hospitalized patients. These antibodies appear to act by inhibiting the toxic properties of the lipopolysaccharides of multiple gram-negative bacteria.

The capacity of bacteria to colonize the mucosal surfaces of human and other mammalian hosts depends in part upon their ability to adhere to epithelial cells. IgA antibodies inhibit adherence at various colonizing sites. Some patients who lack the capacity to form mucosal IgA are prone to chronic and severe infections with intestinal parasites such as *Giardia lamblia*. Such patients may also develop malabsorption, presumably related to superinfection with bacteria. The malabsorption state is accompanied by atrophy of the intestinal villi and may respond to antimicrobal treatment.

Viral neutralizing antibodies may include IgG, IgM, and IgA isotypes. Viruses can be neutralized by antibody-dependent inhibition of their ability to bind to or penetrate target cells, or coating with complement components—in particular with C4b—to aid in their ingestion. The development of neutralizing antibodies limits the capacity of viruses to spread from an extracellular location, as on a mucosal surface or by a hematogenous route. The production of neutralizing antibody is synonymous with immunity against infection with viruses causing the common childhood exanthems or poliomyelitis. Conversely, viruses that are spread directly from one cell to another may not be amenable to the action of neutralizing antibodies. In this case cellular immune mechanisms predominate in host defense.

Certain viruses may modify the molecular structure of infected target cell surfaces, resulting in an antibody response directed against the infected cell. Lysis of the altered target cell may be achieved by the combined action of antibody and complement or by the binding of effector "killer" lymphocytes, neutrophils, or macrophages via their Fc regions. This antibody-dependent cellular cytotoxicity (ADCC) may be responsible for some of the tissue injury that occurs during viral infections. Lysis of the infected cell can be accomplished by oxidative or nonoxidative mechanisms of the phagocytic cells.

The action of IgE to trigger granule release from mast cells and basophils has been described earlier. Smooth muscle contraction induced in the gastrointestinal tract by the action of IgE may serve to expel parasites. IgE bound to the surface of schistosome larvae can be microbicidal, either through activation of the complement system or through the binding of effector eosinophils to the surface of the organisms. Killing under these conditions is achieved through the combined action of the major basic protein of eosinophil lysosomal granules, eosinophil peroxidase, and eosinophil oxidative products.

ANTIBODY DEFICIENCY STATES

Antibody deficiency states vary in their associated clinical symptoms. IgA deficiency affects one in 600 to 800 of the United States population, yet relatively few people are symptomatic. Those patients with IgA deficiency who have clinical symptoms are prone to (1) sinopulmonary infections; (2) atopy; (3) gastrointestinal tract disease; (4) autoimmune disorders such as systemic lupus erythematosus, rheumatoid arthritis, and pernicious anemia; and (5) certain malignancies (diffuse histiocytic lymphoma or gastrointestinal carcinoma). The absence of protective IgA on mucosal surfaces may allow access of antigens normally limited to these surfaces to submucosal or other tissue sites, thereby inciting an aberrant immune response. Affected patients have markedly reduced levels of IgA in both serum and secretions, and normal or increased values of other immunoglobulins. Some patients with IgA deficiency have associated reductions of IgG_2; they are likely to have problems with bacterial infection.

Deficiency of IgG and its subclasses is much more rare than IgA deficiency, but more likely to have clinical consequences. IgG levels below 400 mg/dl are associated with defective microbial opsonization and lead to recurrent infections with pyogenic encapsulated bacteria. Conditions that are associated with IgG deficiency may be "physiologic" and include the transient hypogammaglobulinemia of infancy, occurring between the ages of 6–10 months before normal endogenous production of IgG takes place. Other patients have defective B cell production. The sex-linked disorder known as Bruton's agammaglobulinemia is characterized by absent mature B cells in the blood and lymphoid organs, a complete lack in the formation of mature plasma cells, and impaired production of antibodies of all subclasses. Another disorder associated with deficiencies in IgG production as well as other immunoglobulins is the so-called common variable or "acquired" hypogammaglobulinemia. This appears to be a heterogeneous disorder first affecting adolescents or young adults. An immunoregulatory defect involving either a lack of T cell helper or exaggerated suppressor cell activity is responsible for the development of this disorder in different patients. Finally, some patients have combined deficiencies of both cellular and humoral immunity. The development of lymphoid and thymic tissue is usually minimal or absent. Affected subjects are prone to infections with encapsulated bacteria as well as a variety of intracellular organisms.

Patients who have serum IgG concentrations <200 mg/dl are candidates for replacement therapy with IgG. To date, the other immunoglobulin isotypes cannot be prepared in sufficient purity and quantity for therapeutic administration. IgG is available both for intramuscular as well as intravenous use. The latter material employs modified IgG that is not likely to form aggregates in the circulation. Formation of aggregates can lead to activation of the complement system and the occurrence of anaphylactic reactions. Treatment of deficient patients with IgG is usually given at regular intervals to maintain blood levels above 400 mg/dl of IgG and to restore near normal opsonization. The duration of the effect is usually about one month and is related to the half-life of the administered IgG.

ROLE OF ANTIBODIES IN TISSUE INJURY DURING INFECTION

The development of the specific humoral immune response may play a role in some of the manifestations of infections. For example, circulating immune complexes produced during chronic antigenic stimulation in bacterial endocarditis may cause glomerulonephritis or Arthus-like cutaneous lesions and arthritis. The hemorrhagic manifestations of some patients with dengue fever can be ascribed to circulating immune complexes, vascular injury, and activation of the coagulation system. Finally, antibody-dependent cytotoxicity reactions may cause tissue injury.

CELLULAR IMMUNITY

Cellular immunity is the coordinated operation of T lymphocytes and macrophages in the eradication of microorganisms that are normally resistant to destruction by phagocytosis or lysis by complement. In a primary response it takes about three weeks to become operative. Cellular immunity provides the paramount protection against intracellular parasites. It also plays a crucial role in protection against neoplasia as well as engraftment of foreign tissues. The functional correlate of this system in vivo is delayed type hypersensitivity (DTH) reactions to intradermally administered antigens. Characteristically, these reactions do not appear until 24 to 72 hours after antigen inoculation, and they are infiltrated with mononuclear cells. DTH reactions to antigens derived from microorganisms have been used to assess in vivo cellular immunity against different agents—for example, the tubercle bacillus. The mechanisms and function of T lymphocytes and macrophages in the afferent limb of the immune response have been described in detail earlier. The effector mechanisms of this system as they relate to defense against infection will be briefly reviewed here.

The cytotoxic mechanisms of an effective cellular immune response can involve the direct action of lymphocytes or the indirect lymphocyte-mediated activation of macrophages. Lymphocyte cytotoxicity can be directed against eukaryotic cells marked by different histocompatibility antigens or those altered in their surface antigenic properties by neoplasia or by viral infection. The cytotoxic activity of natural killer (NK) cells is directed predominantly against tumor cells or HLA-incompatible cells but may also be active against viral-infected cells in vitro and, presumably, in vivo. Cytotoxic T cells undergo clonal proliferation in response to foreign antigens. They are highly immunologically specific in their actions. Intimate cell contact by viable effector T lymphocytes is essential for cytotoxicity to occur. The exact nature of the cytotoxic reaction remains to be defined but differs from cytotoxicity mediated by soluble substances known as lymphotoxins produced by T lymphocytes under mitogenic stimulation. The specific role for lymphotoxins as opposed to other cell-mediated cytotoxic reactions in antimicrobial host defense remains to be established.

LYMPHOKINES AND ANTI-INFECTIOUS HOST DEFENSE

T lymphocytes operate broadly in augmenting and modulating host defenses through the production of glycoproteins (lymphokines), which affect other cells. Various lymphokines affect other T cells (for example, interleukin-2), B lymphocytes (B cell growth factor), macrophages (migration inhibitory factor, migration activation factor, chemotactic factors, gamma-interferon), polymorphonuclear leukocytes (chemotactic factors and inhibitors, activating factors), or eosinophils (chemotactic factor). In the eradication of infecting organisms, the clearest role for lymphokines is augmenting macrophage function. They may serve as chemotactic factors or increase the capacity of these cells to ingest and kill intracellular organisms. The major macrophage activating lymphokine is gamma-interferon. Under the influence of this compound, macrophages increase in size, in their capacity to spread and adhere to surfaces, in their content of lysosomal enzymes, in their oxidative metabolism resulting in the production of toxic oxygen metabolites, and in the display and function of surface receptors for phagocytosis.

Activated macrophages acquire the ability to kill resistant intracellular organisms such as the tubercle bacillus or *T. gondii*. Both of these organisms resist killing by nonactivated macrophages, apparently by inhibiting lysosomal degranulation. Other intracellular parasites such as the amastigotes of leishmania resist killing by nonactivated macrophages through their capacity to scavenge oxygen products. The activated macrophage produces these products in amounts too large for these organisms to resist.

Besides the array of lymphokines mentioned above, both alpha-interferon and gamma-interferon are produced by T lymphocytes during viral infection or by mitogenic stimulation. Alpha-interferon has some action on immune effector mechanisms but functions primarily to limit intracellular replication of viruses at several steps. These include inhibition of the initiation of viral protein synthesis, degradation of single-stranded RNA by activation of an endoribonuclease, and inhibition of the synthesis of viral envelope proteins. Gamma-interferon is not as active as alpha-interferon against viral replication mechanisms but has the properties of promoting macrophage activation and augmenting both NK cell activity and T cell cytotoxicity.

IMPAIRED CELLULAR IMMUNITY AND INFECTION

Cellular immunity may be impaired by mechanisms ranging from a genetic failure of the thymus or thymus-regulated lymphoid tissue to develop, through immunoregulatory abnormalities involving deficient helper or exaggerated suppressor cell activities, to defects in macrophage function. High doses of glucocorticosteroids blunt the acute inflammatory response and impair the traffic of T lymphocytes, with profound effects on cellular immunity. Advanced protein-calorie malnutrition has its major impact on the cellular immune limb of host defense. Both are common conditions in which cellular immunity is impaired.

Patients who have defective cellular immunity develop a characteristic spectrum of infectious complications (see Table 4). Patients with overwhelming miliary tuberculosis usually exhibit anergy against this organism. Conversely, treatment with high doses of steroids or the development of malnutrition are common ways of activating latent tuberculosis. Legionellosis and systemic infection with *Listeria monocytogenes* are two intracellular bacterial infections that are complications of reduced cellular immunity, and mucocutaneous candidiasis or progressive systemic infection by the primary mycoses are fungal complications. Persistent or overwhelming infections with DNA viruses of the Herpes group (cytomegalovirus, EB virus, *Herpes zoster,* and *Herpes simplex*) are major causes of morbidity and mortality in patients whose cellular immune mechanisms are depressed. Such patients are also prone to overwhelming infection with parasites and protozoans, including *T. gondii, P. carinii,* and *Strongyloides stercoralis.*

Infection of T lymphocytes by retroviruses may lead to their cytolysis or to leukemic transformation. Blood-borne retrovirus infection is responsible for the development of the acquired immune deficiency syndrome—which has occurred in male homosexuals, Haitians, heroin addicts, and hemophiliacs. The array of infections with organisms of normally low virulence in these subjects is a direct consequence of marked depressions in cellular immunity.

Patients with primary deficiencies of the cellular immune system are subject to the same types of infections as those with acquired immunodeficiency. The extent and severity of the infections parallel those of the immunodeficiency disorder. DiGeorge's syndrome (Table 10) describes patients with an embryonic failure in the development of the third and fourth pharyngeal pouches. Affected infants have thymic and parathyroid aplasia and consequent hypocalcemia. Cardiac malformations may also be present. The presence of ectopic thymic tissue in some patients ameliorates their immunodeficiency; T cell number and immune depression range from profoundly decreased to near normal. B cells and humoral immunity are normal. The cellular immune deficiency tends to abate with age as the population of normal T cells slowly increases. Immune reconstitution has been accomplished with thymic transplantation or extracts.

Combined immunodeficiency involves abnormalities of both cellular and humoral immunity. A number of specific subgroups of patients with severe combined immunodeficiency (SCID) have been recognized (Table 10). Exhibiting either sex-linked or autosomal inheritance, almost all patients with SCID develop complicating infections within the first few months of life. Infants with classic SCID may have a persistent morbilliform rash that becomes hyperpigmented. This is thought to be due to an abortive graft vs host reaction mediated by transplacentally acquired maternal T cells. Progressive mucocutaneous moniliasis, intractable diarrhea, and interstitial pneumonia caused by *Pneumocystis carinii* is a characteristic triad in SCID. Most have profound lymphopenia (less than 1000 lymphocytes/μl), but variant patients with SCID have B cells (Swiss) or immature T cells present in the circulation. Eosinophilia is common, but a rare subgroup have associated myelosuppression ("reticular dysgenesis"). The failure of T cells to express HLA A or B antigens in some patients has been called the "bare lymphocyte syndrome." A pathognomonic finding in SCID is the failure of Hassall's corpuscles to develop in the thymus; thymic biopsy is sometimes employed to make the diagnosis.

Approximately 50 per cent of patients with autosomal recessive inheritance of SCID will have a genetic deficiency of the enzyme adenosine deaminase. The natural substrates of this enzyme are adenosine and deoxyadenosine; adenosine triphosphate (ATP) and deoxyadenosine triphosphate (deoxy ATP) accumulate when the enzyme is deficient. Preferential metabolism of deoxyadenosine to deoxyadenosine monophosphate by an active kinase found in lymphoblasts leads to toxic accumulation of deoxy ATP in lymphocytes; deoxy ATP inhibits ribonucleotide reductase, thereby aborting DNA synthesis. Adenosine deaminase deficiency can be treated with transfusion of normal erythrocytes, which contain the enzyme to metabolize the excess nucleotides.

Another example of toxic accumulation of metabolites that is destructive to lymphocytes is seen in the very rare disorder purine nucleoside deficiency. In contrast to adenosine deaminase deficiency, deoxyguanosine triphosphate accumulation—which is the consequence of purine nucleoside phosphorylase deficiency—is selectively toxic to T cells, particularly suppressor T cells. B cells and immunoglobulin production are normal: treatment can be accomplished with infusions of the enzyme using either irradiated red cells or plasma from normal subjects.

The Wiskott-Aldrich syndrome, an X-linked disorder, consists of a unique combination of severe eczema, thrombocytopenia, and susceptibility to infection with encapsulated bacteria or viruses. Affected males also exhibit a high incidence of lymphoreticular malignancies. The immune disorder is attributed to three factors: (1) a progressive decline with age in T cell number and function, (2) reticuloendothelial hyperplasia with increased fractional turnover rate of immunoglobulins, and (3) a selective impairment in the ability to make antibodies to polysaccharide antigens. Impaired antigen processing by macrophages has also been described; however, a unifying mechanism for this disorder has not been provided. Allogenic bone marrow transplantation has reversed the immune deficiencies and the skin disorder but not the thrombocytopenia.

Patients with ataxia telangiectasia manifest cerebellar dysfunction early in life. They develop telangiectasias of the skin and conjunctivae and have

TABLE 10. PRIMARY CELLULAR IMMUNODEFICIENCIES

A. "Pure" defects
  DiGeorge's syndrome
  Purine nucleoside phosphorylase deficiency
B. Associated with antibody deficiency
  Severe combined immunodeficiency (SCID)
    Low T and B cell numbers
    Low T cell, normal B cell numbers (Swiss)
    Reticular dysgenesis
    "Bare lymphocyte syndrome"
    Adenosine deaminase deficiency
  Wiskott-Aldrich syndrome
  Ataxia telangiectasia

repeated sinopulmonary infections culminating in bronchiectasis. The thymus retains a fetal appearance and helper T cell function is impaired. The primary impact of the immune deficiency is on immunoglobulin production, particularly IgA (80 per cent of affected subjects deficient), IgE, and IgG. An abnormality in DNA repair has been seen in the cells of patients with ataxia telangiectasia. No satisfactory treatment exists.

EVALUATION OF CELLULAR IMMUNITY

The integrity of cellular immunity may be tested at several levels. Application of skin test antigens derived from microorganisms or other sources has been employed for years to examine the expression of cellular immunity in vivo. A positive DTH response to intradermal injection of protein antigens from the tubercle bacillus indicates prior infection with this organism, but it is not synonymous with active disease. Fungal skin tests are used to evaluate previous experience with specific mycoses as well as to examine the cellular immune response against these organisms in case of suspected infection.

A variety of monoclonal antibodies have been used to enumerate and characterize T cell subsets in vitro. Functional assays that correlate with in vivo expression of cellular immunity include mitogenic stimulation with plant lectins such as phytohemagglutinin and the mixed lymphocyte reaction. With a combination of in vivo skin testing, cellular enumeration, and functional assays, a complete profile of the integrity of the cellular immune response can be quickly generated. In addition, assays of macrophage function—including chemotactic responses, phagocytic capacity, metabolic activities, and killing functions—can be carried out.

THERAPY OF CELLULAR IMMUNE DEFICIENCY

Treatment of patients with deficient cellular immunity varies with the cause. Reduction in dosage of glucocorticosteroids and restoration of proper protein and caloric intake will reverse the defects induced with these acquired causes. Infusion of missing enzymes has improved the immunodeficiency state in patients who lack adenosine deaminase or purine nucleoside phosphorylase. Bone marrow transplantation has resulted in immune reconstitution in patients with SCID and the Wiskott-Aldrich syndrome. Thymic implants or extracts reverse the defects in DiGeorge's syndrome and have been attempted in the acquired immune deficiency syndrome. Interleukin-2 and gamma-interferon are also being employed to augment macrophage and helper cell function in this disorder.

Pathogenesis of Fever

Fever is a common manifestation of many acute and chronic infections, inflammatory disorders, and some neoplasms. Only recently has the pathophysiology of fever been understood and insights gained into its purpose in dealing with infection and in aiding host immune mechanisms.

THERMOREGULATORY MECHANISMS AND BODY TEMPERATURE

The body temperature is maintained by a carefully regulated balance between heat production and loss (Fig. 9). The action of thyroid hormone is responsible for generating the calories that give rise to the basal body temperature. This action is directed primarily at the regulation of the sodium-potassium ATPase in cell membranes. With cleavage of adenosine triphosphate (ATP) during active pumping out of intracellular sodium, heat is generated. Other major processes that contribute to heat generation through cleavage of ATP include muscle contraction and active transport of amino acids, carbohydrates, and lipids in the gastrointestinal tract. Thus, core body temperature tends to rise after vigorous exercise or following a meal.

Heat loss occurs primarily by radiation and convection under basal conditions when environmental temperature is cooler than the body surface. Evaporation of water from the respiratory passages also contributes to heat loss. Following an increase in the generation of core body heat as in vigorous exercise or after entry into a hot (35° C) environment, evaporative losses by sweating become the primary means to dissipate heat. Heat loss through radiation and convection is directly affected by cutaneous blood flow as well as by environmental temperature; vasodilatation or vasoconstriction of cutaneous blood vessels exerts a fine control over this process. When the ambient temperature falls, heat conservation mechanisms are activated, including the generation of more heat through shivering and a reduction of loss through cutaneous vasoconstriction. In

Figure 9. Schematic picture of relationships between heat production and loss mechanisms and role of the hypothalamic "thermostat" in maintaining thermoregulatory controls.

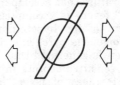

"Thermostat"

PRE—OPTIC HYPOTHALAMUS

HEAT PRODUCTION

1. Basal metabolism
2. Muscle contraction
3. Digestion

HEAT LOSS

1. Environmental Temperature
2. Cutaneous blood flow
3. Sweating

hairy mammals, contraction of muscles around hair follicles causes piloerection with the creation of an insulating layer of relatively warm, trapped air adjacent to the skin. In humans this is characterized by the development of so-called "goose flesh."

Coordination of heat regulatory mechanisms involves the interaction between thermal information received from peripheral and central receptors and neural centers in the hypothalamus. These centers function as a thermostat to allow a tight regulation of the core body temperature. During the day there is a normal cyclic variation in temperature of up to 2 to 3° Fahrenheit around a mean of 98.6° even in extremely hot and cold environments. The lowest temperatures usually occur at about 4 A.M. to 6 A.M. and the peak temperatures between 8 P.M. and 11 P.M.

The preoptic area of the hypothalamus contains two populations of thermally sensitive neurons that are responsive to either cold or warm stimuli. They generate thermoregulatory signals in response to information received from peripheral receptors on the skin surface or central receptors in the brain, spinal cord, viscera, and blood vessels, as well as the local temperature of the hypothalamus itself. The action of the two hypothalamic neuronal populations is reciprocal so that an increased rate of discharge from heat-sensitive neurons is accompanied by a decrease in the rate of discharge from the cold receptors. When the heat-sensitive neurons increase their discharge rate, cutaneous vasodilatation and sweating occur. Conversely, when cold-sensitive neurons increase their discharge rate, shivering, cutaneous vasoconstriction, and piloerection ensue. Sympathetic nerve fibers are responsible for carrying impulses involved in heat generation; parasympathetic nerves mediate heat loss responses. Thus drugs that affect the sympathetic or parasympathetic nervous system may have secondary effects on body temperature.

Core temperature increases when heat generation exceeds heat loss. During vigorous exercise temperatures may exceed 104° F until activity slows and heat is dissipated by sweating and cutaneous vasodilation. Similar accumulation of core heat may occur following prolonged motor seizure activity. Conditions such as hyperthyroidism may be accompanied by a sustained elevation in core temperature. Patients who are unable to regulate cutaneous blood flow precisely or to sweat normally because of disease or medication are particularly prone to develop dangerous increases in core temperature when in a hot environment. Heat stroke is an example of a failure of central heat loss mechanisms to dissipate heat; it usually occurs in the setting of prolonged exercise in extremely hot ambient temperatures. Elevated core temperatures may also be the result of impaired hypothalamic function induced by injury or by drugs.

THERMOREGULATORY MECHANISMS IN FEVER

The increase in body temperature that accompanies inflammation—that is, "true" fever—is accomplished by a change in the set point of the hypothalamic thermostat. In response to exogenous pyrogenic compounds an endogenous pyrogen is generated that has a direct action on thermally sensitive centers in the hypothalamus. In the initial stages of fever, heat generation and conservation mechanisms may both be activated, resulting in shivering and vasoconstriction. The body temperature rises abruptly to a new level at which point heat generation and heat loss again become equivalent, although at a higher rate as governed by an elevation of basal metabolism. Defervescence takes place through activation of the heat loss mechanisms—vasodilatation and sweating.

A variety of chemical mediators play a role in transmission of thermally induced information in the hypothalamus. Thus, endogenous pyrogen appears not to act directly upon thermally sensitive neurons but rather to affect the release or relocation of such intermediates as monoamines, sodium or calcium ions, prostaglandins, and cyclic nucleotides. Serotonin and norepinephrine both function as hypothalamic neurotransmitters; norepinephrine and related catechols participate in augmenting heat production responses, and seritonergic fibers appear to play a role in augmenting heat loss. Changes in the central partitioning of cations occur in experimental animals during fever.

Arachidonic acid metabolites—in particular, the classical prostaglandin PGE_1—appear to participate actively in mediating central responses to endogenous pyrogen. Intraventricular administration of PGE_1 causes fever in experimental animals; spinal fluid PGE_1 levels rise during fever induced by exogenous pyrogens. Aspirin, a compound that inhibits prostaglandin synthesis, attenuates fever and reduces the formation of PGE_1 in the spinal fluid of pyrogen-treated experimental animals. However, in experimental animals some specific antagonists of PGE_1 will not prevent fever after injection of endogenous pyrogen or after injection of arachidonic acid into the cerebral ventricles. Thus, metabolites of arachidonic acid other than PGE_1 could be participating as mediators of febrile responses. Nevertheless, the concept that antipyretics which inhibit prostaglandin synthesis act through a central mechanism remains an attractive one.

Cyclic nucleotides also participate in thermoregulatory responses, following in sequence the action of prostaglandins. Cyclic adenosine monophosphate (cAMP) levels are increased in the cerebral spinal fluid of animals given various pyrogens or PGE_1. Direct intracerebral injection of dibutyryl cAMP increases body temperature in experimental animals. Inhibition of the catabolism of cAMP by theophylline may augment febrile responses.

A proposed model for fever production involves the sequential activation of PGE_1 synthesis, caused by endogenous pyrogen (Fig. 10). PGE_1 induces norepinephrine release. As an alpha-adrenergic agonist, norepinephrine directly increases the production of cAMP, which then increases the rate of firing of heat conservation and heat generation neurons.

PYROGENS: EXOGENOUS AND ENDOGENOUS

Elevations of body temperature that are not caused by primary thermoregulatory changes result from the action of an endogenous pyrogen released from macrophages upon stimulation by a number of exogenous pyrogenic substances. The action of exogenous pyrogens has been defined in two ways: by their ability to cause temperature elevations when injected into humans or experimental animals, and to induce the

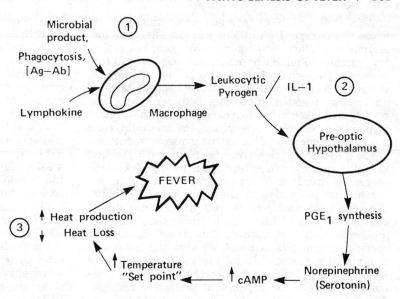

Figure 10. Proposed sequences in the pathogenesis of fever in mammals: (1) production of leukocytic pyrogen/interleukin 1 by stimulated macrophages; (2) site and sequences of action of leukocytic pyrogen; (3) thermoregulatory changes resulting in fever. Abbreviations: Ag-Ab, antigen-antibody complex; PGE, prostaglandin E. (Modified from Bernheim, H. A., Block, L. H., and Atkins, E.: Fever: Pathogenesis, pathophysiology and purpose. Ann Intern Med 91:261, 1979.)

release of endogenous pyrogen from macrophages. A variety of exogenous pyrogens from both microbial and nonmicrobial sources have been characterized (Table 10).

The best studied of the exogenous pyrogens are the lipopolysaccharides of gram-negative bacteria—that is, endotoxins. Intravenous administration of endotoxins produces a dose-dependent fever that begins in 15 to 30 minutes and usually reaches a peak between 90 to 120 minutes. The biologically active component of the lipopolysaccharide that causes fever has been shown to reside in the lipid A portion of the molecule. This portion is also involved in the pathogenesis of inflammatory events during gram-negative bacterial infection. These are discussed in the next section on septicemia and septic shock.

Shortly after the development of fever induced by the intravenous administration of endotoxins, a separate or "endogenous" pyrogen can be demonstrated in the circulation. Similarly, when endotoxins are incubated with phagocytic cells in vitro, pyrogenic activity appears in the medium that is separate from that of the endotoxin itself. In fact, subpyrogenic doses of endotoxins will induce pyrogen release from phagocytes. Similar experimental approaches have been used to demonstrate the pyrogenic activity and apparent mechanism of action of the other substances listed in Table 11.

Fevers may accompany inflammatory states of nonmicrobial origin. Pyrogenic substances can be produced during the immune response; for example, previously immunized animals develop fever when challenged intravenously with protein antigens. Passive transfer of immune complexes to normal recipients induces fever that is mediated by endogenous pyrogen; the immune complexes appear to trigger pyrogen production. Human lymphocytes incubated with mitogenic factors such as concanavalin A release a factor that causes monocytes to form and release endogenous pyrogen. When human lymphocytes from different donors are incubated together—producing what is known as the mixed lymphocyte reaction—formation and release of a pyrogen-inducing factor also occurs. The source of the pyrogen-inducing factor or lymphokine is T cells responding to specific antigenic stimulation. Administration of old tuberculin to BCG-sensitized animals causes fever through a lymphokine-mediated mechanism. Thus, microbes may cause fever through the direct action of pyrogenic substances in their structure or indirectly by induction of the immune response. Both humoral and cellular immunity may participate in this latter process.

Other substances of nonmicrobial origin that cause fever can also act directly on phagocytic cells. This mechanism may be responsible for fever complicating treatment with certain drugs or administration of adjuvants that stimulate the immune response.

The pyrogen released by phagocytic cells has been purified and characterized and the molecular mechanisms of its formation defined. While early studies suggested that the polymorphonuclear leukocyte was the source of endogenous pyrogen, it is now clear that monocytes and macrophages are the only cells capable of its production. Endogenous or leukocytic pyrogen is a protein of 15,000 dalton M_r. Its activity is destroyed by digestion with proteases, by heating, or by oxidation of free sulfhydryl groups. Higher molecular weight compounds demonstrated in vitro and circulating in vivo appear to be aggregates of the primary pyrogen.

The release of leukocytic pyrogen from monocytes requires a several-hour period of contact with the stimulus—the "activation" period. Leukocytic pyrogen is synthesized de novo during activation. Inhibitors of

TABLE 11. EXOGENOUS PYROGENS

MICROBIAL ORIGIN	NON-MICROBIAL ORIGIN
Gram-negative bacteria	Immune complexes
Lipopolysaccharide	Lymphokine-induced
Gram-positive bacteria	Pyrogenic steroids
Peptidoglycan	Polynucleotides
Exotoxins	Bleomycin
Fungi	Synthetic adjuvants
Polysaccharides	Urate crystals
Viruses	
Mycobacteria	
Spirochetes	

protein synthesis block pyrogen production and release. Cyclooxygenase inhibitors do not affect the formation and release of leukocytic pyrogen, but rather act centrally to inhibit hypothalamic responses to this molecule. Glucocorticoids are also potent anti-inflammatory and antipyretic agents. They appear to have dual sites of action, inhibiting both formation and release of leukocytic pyrogen as well as the central responses to this molecule. Estrogens are antipyretic compounds that inhibit leukocytic pyrogen production.

The structure of the active site of leukocytic pyrogen is highly conserved in nature. Cells from such diverse species as lizards and humans produce leukocytic pyrogens that are active in producing fever in rabbits. Whereas antibodies to leukocytic pyrogen from different species are highly specific, indicating that the antigenic sites are distinct, data from the crossed species experiments demonstrate that the molecular configuration responsible for the pyrogenic action is shared widely. This underscores the fundamental importance of fever as a potential protective response during infection in the animal kingdom.

PROTECTIVE ROLE OF FEVER IN INFECTION: RELATIONSHIPS OF LEUKOCYTIC PYROGEN TO INTERLEUKIN 1 AND LEUKOCYTE ENDOGENOUS MEDIATOR

Clinicians and investigators who tried for generations to explain the protective role of fever during infection have only recently been successful. Similarities between the molecular weight and chemical properties of the lymphocyte activating factor produced by macrophages and known as interleukin 1 and endogenous (or leukocytic) pyrogen led investigators to postulate that they might be identical. Interleukin 1 is a 15,000 dalton glycopeptide that is released by macrophages during phagocytosis or upon exposure to endotoxins. It acts on helper T cells to induce the production of the T cell growth factor, interleukin 2. In mitogenic assays that depend upon the action of interleukin 1 for cellular responses, highly purified leukocytic pyrogen will substitute. Conversely, intravenous administration of interleukin 1 to rabbits causes fever, confirming similarities between the biologic properties as well as structure of the two molecules. Since interleukin 1 is also a B cell activating factor, the opportunity for the interleukin 1/leukocyte pyrogen molecule to participate broadly in both limbs of the humoral immune response is evident. The answer to the question of whether leukocytic pyrogen and interleukin 1 are in fact identical awaits amino acid sequence analysis; nevertheless, they appear to share critical active sites.

Further insight into the role of fever in the specific immune process has been gained by the demonstration that lectin-induced mitogenesis of helper T lymphocytes as well as lymphokine production are both increased at febrile temperatures. Both interleukin 1-induced T cell proliferation (mediated by interleukin 2) and antibody production in vitro increase by up to 20-fold when cells are cultured at 39° C as opposed to 37° C. This exciting observation has provided the first meaningful insight into the potential protective role of the febrile response to augment specific immune responses during infection.

The material that circulates in animals administered gram-negative lipopolysaccharides or in the plasma of febrile human subjects and known as leukocyte endogenous mediator (LEM) may also be identical to leukocytic pyrogen/interleukin 1. LEM is a 15,000 dalton glycopeptide that induces myelopoiesis and the release of neutrophils from the bone marrow. The actions of LEM provide for enhanced inflammatory responses and nutritional alterations during infection. When purified leukocytic pyrogen is incubated with neutrophils in vitro it induces activation of these cells as measured by the release of specific granule enzymes, enhancement of chemotactic responsiveness, and the production of superoxide.

Finally, the accelerated catabolism of skeletal muscle proteins that accompanies severe trauma or infection may be caused by the action of a serum glycopeptide that appears to be leukocytic pyrogen. Mobilization of these proteins is presumably necessary to provide amino acids and energy for the development of protective responses or to supply metabolic needs that increase during these conditions. Incubation of muscle preparations with serum from febrile subjects or highly purified leukocytic pyrogen promotes proteolysis through the action of muscle lysosomal proteases, known as *cathepsins*. The effect of both the serum glycopeptide and leukocytic pyrogen is mediated through the generation of prostaglandin E_1 in the muscle tissue, and is blocked by the action of cyclooxygenase inhibitors or glucocorticoids. In this way, peripheral responses to leukocytic pyrogen mimic those in the hypothalamus, with the prostaglandins acting as important second messenger molecules.

Thus fever is not only a cardinal manifestation of infectious disease but the molecular mechanisms involved in its pathogenesis may have a wide role in augmenting the nutritional, acute inflammatory, and specific immune responses necessary to limit or eradicate the organisms responsible for infection.

Septicemia and Septic Shock

When microorganisms, in particular bacteria or their products, escape local portals of entry and invade the bloodstream, there develops a dramatic and often devastating constellation of clinical symptoms and signs. Known clinically as septicemia and complicated by hypotension and shock in a significant percentage of cases, the syndrome may have a fatal outcome even when it is recognized and appropriate treatment administered. While shock most frequently complicates gram-negative bacteremia, it may also develop with bloodstream infection caused by gram-positive bacteria, fungi, mycobacteria or rarely viruses. Bacteremia with septic shock is an unfortunate complication of infection in hospitalized patients often related to in-lying intravenous catheters or urinary bladder catheters, endotracheal tubes, tubes in other drainage sites, or surgical wounds.

Fewer septicemias and episodes of septic shock develop in the outpatient setting, complicating infections of the skin or soft tissues, urinary tract, lungs, intraabdominal sites, and less commonly the heart valves. While advances have been made in the prompt diagnosis and management of this syndrome, it continues to have a high mortality rate and its prevention remains one of the major challenges to modern medicine.

CLINICAL AND LABORATORY FEATURES

While bacteremia without symptoms may complicate such innocent procedures as brushing the teeth and may be prolonged and symptomatic in patients who have infections of the heart valves or typhoid fever, the term septicemia is usually reserved for conditions accompanied by the abrupt onset of symptoms and signs. Fever and chills are seen in almost all patients, although those at age extremes or with severe liver or renal disease or extensive burns have altered thermoregulatory mechanisms and may declare their septicemia with a paradoxic precipitous fall in body temperature. In the initial phases of septicemia, cardiac output is increased, predominately by an increase in cardiac rate. Hypotension occurs in about 40 per cent of sustained gram-negative bacteremias, but may be seen with other organisms as well (for example, about 5 per cent of gram-positive bacteremias). Most patients have increases in ventilation rate and about half alterations in mentation—including obtundation, confusion, agitation, and hallucinations. Disturbances of gastrointestinal motility occur in about a third of patients, marked by nausea and vomiting, diarrhea, or ileus. As the blood pressure falls, the shock syndrome can develop. This can be defined as progressive tissue hypoxia, microvascular injury, and ultimately organ failure. Finally, some patients may exhibit skin lesions ranging from petechiae to characteristic painful erythematous nodules or hemorrhagic vesicle-pustules known as ecthyma gangrenosum.

Laboratory abnormalities (Table 12) reflect triggering of the inflammatory response in the intravascular location and the consequences of reduced perfusion of tissues and organ failure.

A reasonably coherent picture is emerging of the pathophysiology of the syndromes of septicemia and

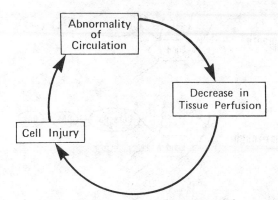

Figure 11. The "vicious circle" of shock.

septic shock. A critical interplay between factors that are unique to invading microbes and host mediator systems is responsible for the development of the clinical symptoms and signs of septicemia and the laboratory changes. From the standpoint of vascular perfusion and organ function, a vicious circle is established that results in progressive injury to the capillary endothelium and tissues as depicted schematically in Figure 11. Unless this circle is interrupted in the fully developed shock state, death results in the vast majority of patients.

MICROBIAL FACTORS IN PATHOGENESIS

Of the various microbial factors that may trigger the clinical and laboratory features of sepsis, none has received more attention than the endotoxins of gram-negative bacteria. These organisms when in the bloodstream have a high propensity to cause the shock syndrome, and many features of this syndrome can be reproduced by administration of fragments of these organisms or purified preparations of the lipopolysaccharide component of their endotoxins. Gram-negative lipopolysaccharides contain three major components (Fig. 12): an outer or terminal hydrophilic chain of repeating oligosaccharide units antigenically unique to each strain and serotype of organism, a central polysaccharide core consisting of four to five units that are shared among different gram-negative strains and species and a proximal nonpolar lipid component buried in the phospholipid layer of the outer envelope and chemically consistent among all strains and species. This lipid component—known as lipid A—is linked to the polysaccharide core via the sugar ketodeoxyoctulosonate. It is responsible for many of the toxic actions of lipopolysaccharide that result in cellular, tissue, and organ injury and ultimately death of the host. Acetylation or binding of the antibiotic polymyxin B to lipid A blocks most of its biologic properties as well as those of the intact LPS.

Composed of α 1, 6-linked D-glucosamine disaccharide further linked by acylation to toxic fatty acids such as myristic acid, lipid A can directly injure endothelial cells as well as induce synthesis of prostacyclin (Fig. 13A). It can activate macrophages to produce and release leukocytic pyrogen/interleukin 1, arachidonic acid metabolites, plasminogen activator, and lysosomal enzymes. It also causes release of clotting factors from platelets, resulting in their aggregation and destruc-

TABLE 12. SEPTICEMIA: LABORATORY FEATURES

PMNs: Increased or decreased, left shift
Platelets: Decreased
Coagulation: Decreased factor XII, V, VIII, fibrinogen; increased
  fibrin degradation products
Decreased arterial pO_2, pCO_2
Lactic acidosis
Increased blood urea nitrogen
Increased hepatic enzymes
Alterations in blood glucose

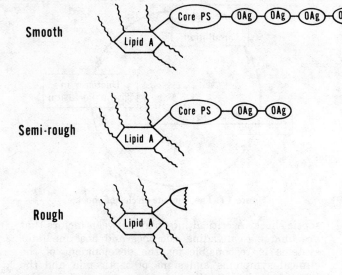

Figure 12. Schematic structure of three forms of bacterial lipopolysaccharides. (Reprinted with permission from Morrison, D. C., and Ulevitch, R. J.: The effects of bacterial endotoxins on host mediation systems. Am J Pathol 93:528, 1979.)

tion. The major interaction of lipopolysaccharides with neutrophils and mast cells is indirect and mediated by C5a.

Lipopolysaccharides interact with humoral mediator systems (Fig. 13*B*) and can trigger activation of the complement system by both the classical and alterna-

tive pathways. Classical pathway activation can be achieved following binding of IgM antibodies to the terminal polysaccharide portion of lipopolysaccharides or by lipid A itself. In the absence of antibody, alternative pathway activation can be triggered by the core and terminal polysaccharides. Lipid A activates the

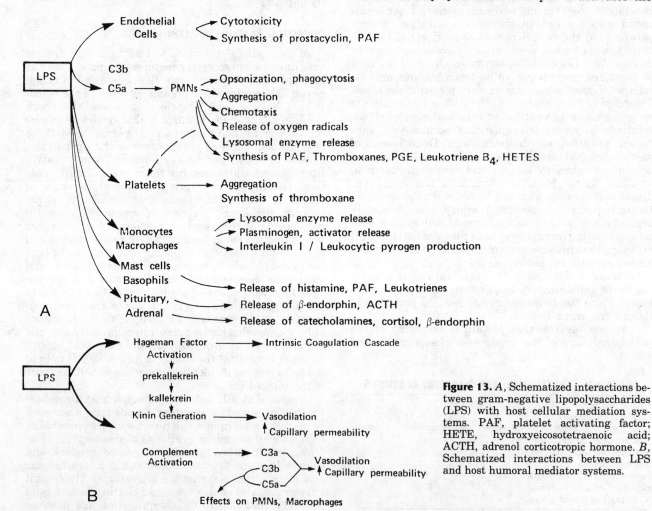

Figure 13. *A*, Schematized interactions between gram-negative lipopolysaccharides (LPS) with host cellular mediation systems. PAF, platelet activating factor; HETE, hydroxyeicosotetraenoic acid; ACTH, adrenol corticotropic hormone. *B*, Schematized interactions between LPS and host humoral mediator systems.

intrinsic clotting system through direct binding to, and activation of, factor XII (Hageman factor). Finally, lipid A triggers formation of kinins from kininogen precursors.

Other components of gram-negative organisms, gram-positive cocci, and fungi may trigger activation of the same mediator systems or injure vascular endothelium and tissues directly. They include the peptidoglycan moiety of bacterial cell walls as well as techoic acids and capsular polysaccharides, the cell wall polysaccharides of fungi and extracellularly released enzymes and toxins such as streptokinase of groups A, C, and G streptococci, and the pyrogenic enterotoxins of staphylococci. The formation of circulating antigen antibody complexes in some patients may serve as an additional factor that activates the complement system or that coats platelets, inducing aggregation and thrombocytopenia. This interplay between microbial factors and host mediator systems is a dramatic example of how the normally protective inflammatory mechanisms may contribute directly to vascular and tissue injury when unleashed in the wrong location.

HOST MEDIATOR SYSTEMS IN PATHOGENESIS

The cellular elements involved in generating the manifestations of sepsis contact microbial products within the vasculature or at the initiating site of the infection (Table 13). They include endothelial cells in the microvasculature, platelets, circulating polymorphonuclear leukocytes, monocytes and macrophages, basophils, and mast cells. The predominant humoral mediator systems include the circulating proteins and peptides of the complement, kinin, and coagulation systems. Although properly considered as mediators released by cells, the arachidonic acid metabolites and beta-endorphins are listed in Table 13 as humoral mediators in the sepsis syndrome for the purpose of our discussion because of their widespread cardiovascular effects.

The interactions of gram-negative lipopolysaccharides with the various mediator systems has been studied the most (Figs. 13*A, B*). Many of the effects of lipopolysaccharides can be mimicked by products of gram-positive bacteria and fungi as noted. Furthermore, the relative contributions and importance of these various factors in the pathogenesis of the sepsis syndrome remain to be established.

Intravascular Coagulation

During sepsis with gram-negative organisms or following intravenous injection of endotoxin into experimental animals, evidence for accelerated consumption of clotting factors and intravascular coagulation can

be documented. Turnover rates of factors XII, VIII, V, and fibrinogen increase and levels may fall if production cannot keep up with consumption. Plasmin is activated, both by activated Hageman factor (XII) and plasminogen activator released from macrophages; fibrin split products increase in the circulation. In the presence of abnormal liver function or massive intravascular coagulation, fibrin degradation products may increase sufficiently in the plasma to inhibit fibrin formation and contribute further to a secondary bleeding tendency. Coagulation is further accelerated by activation of platelets as noted below. Intravascular coagulation and secondary bleeding is a particularly prominent manifestation of septicemia caused by the meningococcus.

Administration of heparin to inhibit thrombin formation and replenishment of coagulation factors using fresh frozen plasma can reduce or reverse the intravascular coagulation and secondary bleeding. However, this treatment has not been shown to improve survival in the sepsis syndrome. Furthermore, many patients may develop severe and profound septic shock without evidence of disseminated intravascular coagulation. Thus, while these coagulation abnormalities may be important in the pathogenesis of some of the features of septic shock, they are not central in causing progressive tissue injury or death in this syndrome.

The Kinin System

Through the activation of Hageman factor, prekallikrein is activated and converted to kallikrein by limited proteolysis. Kallikrein, a neutral protease, can cleave bradykinin from kininogens. Bradykinin and related kinins are potent vasodilators and when injected locally, markedly increase the permeability of capillaries and postcapillary venules. They also stimulate pain fibers causing local painful swelling and tenderness. In patients with gram-negative bacteremia, prekallikrein is consumed and low levels of free circulating kinins generated. Through their vascular actions, the kinins may reduce systemic vascular resistance and alter capillary permeability, both characteristic of sepsis. Attempts to inhibit the formation or action of kinins in gram-negative bacteremia or endotoxemia have not been successful.

The Complement System

Activation of the complement system—principally by the alternative pathway—occurs in many patients with gram-negative bacteremia. The consumption of properdin factor B and C3 is accelerated and the levels of these components may fall below normal in patients with profound septic shock. Low C3 levels have correlated with a fatal outcome. Generation of the anaphylatoxins C3a and C5a may add to the effects of the kinins in causing systemic vasodilation and increased capillary permeability. Functioning as an opsonin, C3b can trigger phagocytosis of microorganisms in the bloodstream. During phagocytosis, both lysosomal enzymes and potentially toxic oxygen reduction products may escape phagocytic cells and contribute to vascular injury.

During bacterial sepsis, free C5a and its related product C5a-des-Arg appear in the circulation and may contribute in a major way to the peripheral margination and intravascular activation of PMNs. Thus, C5a

TABLE 13. HOST MEDIATOR SYSTEMS IN SEPTICEMIA AND SEPTIC SHOCK

CELLULAR	HUMORAL
Endothelial cells	Complement system
Platelets	Kinin system
Polymorphonuclear leukocytes	Coagulation system
Monocytes and macrophages	Phospholipid metabolites
Basophils and mast cells	β-endorphins

is of potentially great importance in the pathogenesis of the septic shock syndrome through its ability to recruit cellular mediators that contribute to tissue injury—in particular, that of the lung. However, a close relationship between circulating levels of C5a and clinical manifestations—including development of the acute respiratory distress syndrome during sepsis—has not been documented.

Phospholipid Products

As described in the discussion on immunology, almost all mammalian cells contain the long chain 20 carbon polyunsaturated hydrocarbon arachidonic acid (5, 8, 11, 14 eicosotetraenoic acid) bound in the phospholipids of the plasma membrane bilayer. In addition, another membrane phospholipid with considerable biologic activity, 1-0-alkyl-2-acetyl-sn-glyceryl-3-phosphoryl choline (abbreviated as AcGEPC and known as platelet activating factor [PAF]), is made by certain cells following stimulation. When appropriately triggered, arachidonic acid and PAF can be released from the cell membrane through the actions of phospholipases (Fig. 14).

Free arachidonate can be oxygenated at various sites by distinct oxygenase enzymes known as cyclooxygenase and lipoxygenases, forming prostaglandins or leukotrienes. Within the context of the septicemia and septic shock syndrome, major concerns must be focused on the relative ability of prostaglandins and leukotrienes to cause systemic vasodilation or local vasoconstriction, alterations in capillary permeability, aggregation of platelets, and aggregation and activation of neutrophils. Information as it relates to these properties of PAF and the major oxygenation products of arachidonic acid is summarized in Table 14. Much of this information has been obtained from studies with experimental animals and requires confirmation in humans—particularly during naturally occurring sepsis.

PAF. In the vasculature, neutrophils, platelets, basophils, macrophages, and endothelial cells contain the enzymatic machinery for PAF formation. PAF given intravenously to experimental animals causes hypotension resulting from a fall in vascular resistance and augments capillary permeability in the lung; given intradermally it causes a wheal. PAF causes platelets and neutrophils to aggregate and neutrophils to generate oxygen metabolites and to release lysosomal enzymes. PAF has a very short half-life (< 30 sec); elevated levels of free circulating PAF in septicemia have yet to be documented.

Cyclooxygenase Products. When arachidonic acid is oxygenated at carbon-11 by cyclooxygenase, a common intermediate, PGH_2, is formed. PGH_2 undergoes further modification by several different pathways to form either the classic prostaglandins (by isomerase enzymes), the thromboxanes (by the enzyme thromboxane synthetase), or prostacyclin (by the enzyme prostacyclin synthetase).

Formed mainly by platelets and PMNs, the thromboxanes are potent platelet aggregating agents and may cause vasoconstriction locally or systemically. The half-life of the most active compound—thromboxane A_2 (TX A_2)—is quite brief. Elevated levels of its more stable metabolite, TX B_2, have been documented in the circulation of some patients dying of gram-negative sepsis. In shock syndromes, TX A_2 may participate in platelet aggregation and localized vasoconstriction in the microvasculature. Pulmonary hypertension is common in experimental models of septic shock and contrasts with the fall in systemic vascular resistance. The use of specific inhibitors of thromboxane synthetase has reduced the pulmonary vascular changes that accompany endotoxin injection into experimental animals.

The "classic" prostaglandins, PGE_2 and PGD_2, decrease systemic vascular resistance and produce hypotension when administered in large doses. Both PGD_2 and PGE_2 inhibit platelet aggregation and may also inhibit some neutrophil functions through activating the synthesis of cyclic AMP. In animals with experimental septicemia, PGE_2 levels are elevated and may contribute to the fall in systemic vascular resis-

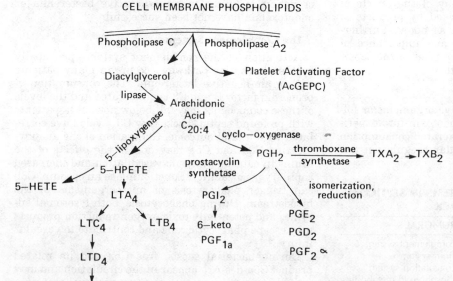

CELL MEMBRANE PHOSPHOLIPIDS

Figure 14. Schematic pathways for membrane phospholipid release by phospholipases and the synthesis of platelet activating factor [AcGEPC = (1-0-alkyl-2-acetyl-sn-glyceryl) (3-phosphoryl-choline)] and oxygenation products of arachidonic acid. PGH_2: prostaglandin H_2; TXA_2: thromboxane A_2; TXB_2: thromboxane B_2; PGE_2, PGD_2, PGF_2: prostaglandins E_2, D_2, $F_{2\alpha}$; PGI_2: prostacyclin; 6-keto-$PGF_{1\alpha}$: 6-ketoprostaglandin $F_{1\alpha}$ (stable metabolite of PGI_2); 5-HPETE: 5-hydroperoxyeicosotetraenoic acid; 5-HETE: 5-hydroxyeicosotetraenoic acid; LTA_4, LTB_4, LTC_4, LTD_4, LTE_4: leukotrienes A_4-E_4.

TABLE 14. EFFECTS OF CELLULAR PHOSPHOLIPID PRODUCTS ON VASCULAR FUNCTIONS, PLATELETS, AND PMNs

PRODUCT	SYSTEMIC VASCULAR RESISTANCE	MICROVASCULAR PERMEABILITY	EFFECTS ON PLATELETS	EFFECTS ON PMNs
Platelet activating factor (PAF)	Decrease	Increase	Aggregation	Aggregation, activation
Cyclooxygenase products				
TXA$_2$	Increase	±	Aggregation	
PGF$_{2\alpha}$	Increase	±		
PGE$_2$	Decrease	Augment	Dose-dependent inhibition of aggregation	Minor inhibition
PGD$_2$	Decrease	Augment	Inhibit aggregation	
PGI$_2$	Decrease	Augment	Inhibit aggregation	
Lipoxygenase products				
LTB$_4$	±	±	−	Chemotactic, activation, aggregation
LTC$_4$	Increase	Increase	−	−
LTD$_4$	Increase	Increase	−	−
LTE$_4$	Increase	Increase	−	−
5-HETE derivatives	−	−		Chemotactic, activation

tance and altered capillary permeability. Administration of PGE$_2$ increases contraction of smooth muscle in the gastrointestinal tract with nausea, vomiting, and diarrhea. Some of the gastrointestinal manifestions of clinical sepsis may be related to the action of this compound together with bradykinin and histamine.

Vascular endothelial cells and smooth muscle utilize PGH$_2$ preferentially to synthesize prostacyclin (PGI$_2$). Prostacyclin is a potent vasodilator, an inhibitor of platelet aggregation, and also augments vascular permeability. In animal models of septicemia, prostacyclin levels are elevated. Since its action may antagonize the effects of thromboxane at many sites, the net outcome will be determined by the relative concentrations of these compounds at local sites or in the circulation at large.

A precise role for each and all the products of PGH$_2$ metabolism in the pathogenesis of many features of the septicemia and septic shock syndromes remains to be established. It is of interest that inhibition of cyclooxygenase by administration of aspirin—or other nonsteroidal antiinflammatory drugs such as indomethacin—can reduce or ablate hypotension and mortality secondary to intravenously administered endotoxin or gram-negative bacteria. Furthermore, the salutary effects of large doses of glucocorticoids in experimental endotoxin or gram-negative bacterial shock have been ascribed to the inhibition of phospholipase A$_2$ and blockade of all subsequent pathways of phospholipid metabolism.

LIPOXYGENASE PRODUCTS

The metabolism and role of the various leukotrienes in the pathogenesis of immediate hypersensitivity reactions has been discussed earlier in detail. With respect to the acute inflammatory process and features of the septic shock syndrome, LTB$_4$ is of greatest interest because of its ability to cause activation and aggregation of neutrophils and to function as a chemotactic factor. This compound is synthesized in relatively large amounts by neutrophils and macrophages. When administered intravenously to experimental animals, LTB$_4$ acutely causes neutropenia by increased PMN margination. LTC$_4$ and LTD$_4$ can both increase

systemic vascular resistance and augment microvascular permeability and are major products of arachidonate metabolism in mast cells and eosinophils. The actions of LTC$_4$ and LTD$_4$ on capillary permeability may thus be additive to those of the kinins, C3a and C5a, other arachidonic acid metabolites, and histamine.

5-HPETE, the product of arachidonic and oxygenation by 5-lipoxygenase, can also undergo simple reduction to 5-HETE. Although not as striking, 5-HETE has effects on neutrophils that may mimic those of LTB$_4$. Because of its short half-life, little is known about the role of 5-HETE in experimental or clinical sepsis.

Endorphins

Small peptides of 500 to 15,000 dalton M$_r$ that may function both as neurotransmitters centrally and hormones peripherally have been characterized as endogenous opiates. The beta-endorphin (from "endogenous morphine-like") compound is one of the best characterized from the standpoint of its chemistry, tissue localization, and suggested actions. In the anterior and intermediate lobes of the pituitary gland beta-endorphin is formed from beta lipotropin, which in turn is derived from a precursor molecule, pro-opiomelanocortin. In response to such diverse events as acute trauma, intravenous administration of endotoxins, and hypoglycemia, pro-opiomelanocortin is cleaved into the various active components (including adrenocorticotropin) that are released into the bloodstream. Other opiatelike peptides are synthesized and released from the adrenal medulla by stimuli that activate the sympathetic nervous system.

Described in detail elsewhere, the opiate peptides have profound effects on central nervous system functions including mood alteration and pain relief, as well as cardiovascular effects. With respect to shock syndromes, beta-endorphin has received the most attention. Injection of beta-endorphin slows gastrointestinal motility and may cause ileus, an occasional complication of sepsis. Beta-endorphin reduces cardiac output directly by negative inotropic effects and indirectly by augmentation of vagus nerve activity (negative chronotropic effect), causing a fall in blood pressure. Use of the specific opiate antagonist naloxone has reversed experimental hypotension caused by blood loss, spinal shock, or administration of intravenous endotoxin. Naloxone appears to act on both central and peripheral opiate receptors to produce this effect.

With respect to endotoxin-induced shock, naloxone is most effective when administered with or soon after the lipopolysaccharide. Initial results with the use of naloxone in the therapy of septic shock were promising and have led to a number of clinical trials with this compound. While it is too early to determine the precise role of opiate antagonists in the management of septic or other shock syndromes, it is apparent that their administration late in the development of shock is without benefit.

Endothelial Cells

Autopsy studies of patients dying of sepsis or animals administered lipopolysaccharide have shown widespread degenerative changes in the microvasculature of virtually all organs. These changes range from vacuolation of the cytoplasm to frank destruction and active vasculitis, particularly at sites of organism deposition. These cells apparently serve as a primary target for the action of many of the humoral mediators described above as well as the action of products released by PMNs, platelets, macrophages, and basophils. Endothelial cells synthesize prostacyclin and also release activators of the extrinsic coagulation pathway when damaged. Extensive injury favors local activation of coagulation and contributes to plugging of the microvasculature by platelet and fibrin thrombi. Microthrombosis and localized vasoconstriction contribute actively to tissue hypoxia and secondary organ failure. A primary goal of treatment of profound shock states, including septic shock, is to prevent the development of an irreversible phase that is manifested by widespread endothelial injury.

Polymorphonuclear Leukocytes

During sepsis PMNs may be induced to aggregate, to engage in phagocytosis, and to form and release potentially toxic oxygen products as well as lysosomal enzymes. When this occurs in the vasculature, as opposed to the normal extravascular sites of inflammation, endothelial and vascular injury occurs. Characteristic changes in both the number and morphology of neutrophils occur during septicemia. For example, administration of lipopolysaccharide to experimental animals or humans induces neutropenia followed by a neutrophilic leukocytosis. The neutropenia is caused predominantly by an increase in margination of these cells in the microvasculature of the lungs and is accompanied by generation of a plasma factor(s) that mediates increases in their adherence and aggregating properties. One of the active plasma factors is C5a; LTB_4 may also play a role in PMN aggregation in vivo. In one study, the degree of plasma-mediated leukocyte adherence to surfaces in vitro correlated directly with the development of shock complicating bacteremia.

Whether a patient with bacterial septicemia has neutrophilic leukocytosis or a reduction in the circulating count is a function of the balance between supply and demand as well as the extent of margination of cells. It is not unusual for some patients with mild to moderate marrow suppression (through chronic alcohol ingestion, for example) to respond to bacteremia with a fall in circulating neutrophils. A "left shift"—that is, an increase in percentage of myelocyte and band forms in the circulation—is characteristic of sepsis, as is evidence of intravascular activation of cells. The relative percentage of azurophils to specific granules ("toxic granulation") is increased because of a reduced number of divisions after the promyelocyte stage, thereby shortening marrow transit time. Activation leads to the formation of vacuoles or may be marked by the presence of intracellular bacteria. When nitroblue tetrazolium is added to measure the activation state of neutrophils, the percentage of cells spontaneously reducing this dye increases markedly in most patients with sepsis.

Products of oxygen metabolism or lysosomal enzymes released from activated cells can injure adjacent tissues, including the endothelium and basement membrane and activate coagulation. Furthermore, through their production of PAF, thromboxane, and LTB_4, neutrophils may not only cause platelet aggregation and vascular spasm in areas in which they collect, but they may recruit more neutrophils into the region and secondarily cause their activation as well. Leukocyte thrombi in the lungs may contribute to obstruction of the microvasculature and pulmonary injury. One model of the acute respiratory distress syndrome that complicates sepsis invokes a central role for polymorphonuclear leukocytes in the pathogenesis of its altered capillary permeability and alveolar injury. Depletion of neutrophils has prevented the development of pulmonary injury following the intravenous administration of gram-negative lipopolysaccharides. C5a can be demonstrated to play a central role in the lipopolysaccharide-mediated activation of these cells.

The administration of high doses of glucocorticosteroids can inhibit the response of neutrophils to activating stimuli as well as reduce synthesis of arachidonic acid metabolites. These properties of glucocorticoids have been invoked to support the empiric use of these compounds in the therapy of bacterial sepsis.

Evidence of the role neutrophils play in the vascular and tissue injury of human septicemia is conflicting, and highlights the dual action of these cells in protection from infection as well as in the pathogenesis of inflammation. For example, severely neutropenic subjects are more prone to develop septicemia from bacteria or fungi because of the loss of this protective mechanism. Septic shock may develop in these patients despite a lack of circulating neutrophils. On the other hand, patients who are severely neutropenic may be less likely to develop profound shock complicating septicemia than are those with normal neutrophil supplies. Thus, neutrophils undoubtedly contribute to many of the pathogenetic features of the septic shock syndrome. However, their presence is not an essential requirement for this syndrome to develop and their absence may in fact promote it as a direct consequence of reduced antimicrobial defense.

Platelets

Thrombocytopenia of mild degrees is seen in up to 80 per cent of patients with bacterial septicemia. Platelet halftime is shortened in vivo and immature platelets are observed in the circulation. Platelets derived from patients with sepsis show increased aggregation in vitro and may be coated with IgG. Platelets activated in vivo by mediators such as PAF and thromboxane may aggregate and cause thrombi that further reduce blood flow and oxygen delivery from the microvasculature. The synthesis and release of thromboxane and serotonin from activated platelets can aggregate other platelets in the region and further promote thrombosis. Platelet-fibrin plugs in the microvasculature are characteristic findings in some patients dying with gram-negative bacteremia. In one investigation the degree of thrombocytopenia that complicated bacteremia correlated directly with lung injury as represented by the acute respiratory distress syndrome.

Monocytes and Macrophages

Exposure of monocytes and macrophages to lipopolysaccharides or other microbial products can have profound local effects and be responsible for fever, one of the cardinal manifestations of sepsis. The role of interleukin 1/leukocytic pyrogen in causing fever and its effects on immunity have been discussed extensively above. Besides release of interleukin 1, release of lysosomal enzymes and plasminogen activator is induced by these factors. Proteases released from macrophages lining the circulation may play a role in local organ injury in the lung, liver, spleen, and perhaps even the kidneys.

Mast Cells and Basophils

As described in the discussion on immunology, triggering of mast cells and basophils causes release of histamine, serotonin, and a variety of oxygenation products of arachidonic acid. Histamine is a vasodilator that is not as potent as bradykinin. It also augments capillary permeability, adding to the action of other similarly acting factors in sepsis. Serotonin is a platelet aggregating agent and with histamine and bradykinin can augment gastrointestinal motility. Release of leukotrienes E4 and D4 from pulmonary mast cells may contribute to augmented capillary permeability as well as induce bronchospasm in some patients who have sepsis.

SUMMARY OF PATHOGENETIC MECHANISMS IN SEPSIS

The entry of aerobic gram-negative bacteria, pneumococci, group A, B, C, or G streptococci, *S. aureus,* certain anaerobic bacteria, opportunistic fungi and rarely other bacteria, mycobacteria, or viruses into the bloodstream can trigger the abrupt onset of a septicemic and shock syndrome. This has profound consequences for cardiovascular function, the integrity and perfusion of the microvasculature, and tissue oxygenation. Major changes occur in cellular and humoral systems in the blood. Unless corrected, the net result is multiple organ failure with the liver, kidney, and lungs being major shock organs in sepsis. Each event that compromises the circulation or injures vascular endothelium can worsen tissue oxygenation and lead to cellular, tissue, and organ injury (Fig. 11). The septic shock syndrome differs from cardiogenic or hypovolemic shock in that the primary event is not a circulatory abnormality but rather cell injury induced directly by microbial products or indirectly by host

mediators. It can be thought of conceptually as the inflammatory process unleashed in a poorly regulated intravascular location rather than in the appropriate better-regulated extravascular sites. This results in circulatory abnormalities that decrease tissue perfusion and further contribute to cell injury and eventually organ system failure.

The cardiovascular features of septicemia and septic shock are distinguished by an early fall in systemic vascular resistance, mediated presumably by the integrated or additive action of kinins, prostaglandins, prostacyclins, C3a, C5a, histamine, and PAF. There is a compensatory rise in cardiac output accomplished predominantly through an increase in heart rate, and mediated in part through the action of beta-adrenergic catecholamines and the sympathetic nervous system. Hypotension results when cardiac output cannot be appropriately sustained. This may be a consequence of reductions in "preload" from intravascular volume redistribution and the negative inotropic effects of circulating beta-endorphin. In the initial stages of sepsis, patients are usually warm and apparently well perfused; when hypotension is added to this setting this has been termed the "warm shock" phase. In the later stages as cardiac output falls, systemic vascular resistance increases through the action of counterregulatory hormones—including norepinephrine and angiotensin—and a "cold shock" phase may ensue. Eventual prognosis has been related to the initial cardiac output or to the degree of reduction of systemic vascular resistance and inversely to the cardiac ejection fraction.

As in other forms of shock, lactate production increases in septic shock due to tissue hypoxemia and reduced metabolism of lactate by the liver. Systemic acidosis usually becomes quite severe in the late stages of septic shock and carries an ominous prognosis. Other than a marked propensity to develop the acute respiratory distress syndrome and the rare occurrence of bilateral renal corticalnecrosis in some patients, such as pregnant women or those with meningococcemia, there is nothing that particularly distinguishes septic from other forms of shock in the pattern of manifestations of progressive organ failure.

Patients with sepsis hyperventilate both in response to the effects of lactate on the respiratory center and as a consequence of stimulation of Hering-Breuer reflexes in the lung during incipient or overt pulmonary edema. Ventilation-perfusion imbalance in the lung gives rise to hypoxemia that may serve as an additional respiratory stimulus and further contributes to systemic hypoxia.

The obtundation and mental confusion that are features of sepsis may be rapidly reversed in some patients by the administration of opiate antagonists suggesting a role for beta-endorphin and other opiate peptides in this process. In others, hypoperfusion appears to play the critical role in producing these symptoms.

Azotemia in sepsis is a consequence of renal hypoperfusion in the majority of patients and less commonly due to acute renal failure or renal corticalnecrosis. Cardiac failure in the late stages of septic shock may be accompanied by evidence of myofibril degeneration at autopsy. The precise mechanism for these changes is not known, but similar alterations have been induced by prolonged infusion of catecholamines.

TREATMENT

Treatment of septicemia and septic shock is directed primarily toward establishing a specific microbial diagnosis and an entry site for the responsible microorganisms. The cornerstone of therapy is the proper selection of antibiotics and necessary surgical intervention to drain abscesses or to remove infected foreign bodies. While important in the general management of patients with sepsis, the administration of oxygen, intravenous fluids to expand circulating blood volume, bicarbonate to treat metabolic acidosis, and restoration of depleted clotting factors all play a secondary role. While some have claimed striking therapeutic success with the administration of large doses of glucocorticoids intravenously, these observations are by no means universal. Similarly, treatment with specific inhibitors of cyclooxygenase or thromboxane synthetase remains experimental.

As with most disorders that involve multiple major organ system failure, prevention remains the most important therapeutic goal for the future. Recently, encouraging results have been observed with the use of an immune serum raised in normal subjects against a common core antigen of LPS composed of lipid A, ketodeoxyoctulosonate, and attached common oligosaccharides. J-5 (rough) *E. coli* lack the outer specific polysaccharides in their lipopolysaccharides and provide an appropriate immunogenic stimulus when killed (see Fig. 12). Immunization with J-5 antiserum leads to the development of IgM antibodies, which are capable of detoxifying the endotoxins from a variety of gram-negative bacteria. Administration of J-5 antiserum to patients with gram-negative bacteremia has reduced mortality in a large controlled study.

REFERENCES

Texts

Braude, A. I.: Medical Microbiology and Infectious Diseases. Philadelphia, W. B. Saunders Co., 1981.

Mandell, G., Douglas, G., and Bennett, J.: Principles and Practice of Infectious Diseases, 2nd ed. New York, John Wiley & Sons, 1985.

Root, R. K., and Sande, M. A.: Septic Shock: New Concepts in Pathophysiology and Treatment. New York, Churchill-Livingstone, 1985.

Williams, W. J., Beutler, E., Erslev, E. J., and Lichtman, M. A.: Hematology, 3rd ed. New York, McGraw-Hill Book Co., 1983.

Articles and Reviews

Anderson, D. C., Schmalstieg, F. C., Arnaout, M. A., et al.: Abnormalities of polymorphonuclear leukocyte function associated with a heritable deficiency of high molecular weight surface glycoproteins (GP138): Common relationship to diminished cell adherence. J Clin Invest 74:536, 1984.

Bernheim, H. A., Block, L. H., and Atkins, E.: Fever: Pathogenesis, pathophysiology and purpose. Ann Intern Med 91:261, 1979.

Dinarello, C. A., and Wolff, S. M.: Molecular basis of fever in humans. Am J Med 72:799, 1982.

Fearon, D. T., and Austen, K. F.: The alternative pathway of complement: A system for host resistance to microbial infection. N Engl J Med 303:259, 1980.

Gallin, J. I.: Human neutrophil heterogeneity exists, but is it meaningful? Blood 63:977, 1984.

Goetzl, E. J.: Oxygenation products of arachidonic acid as mediators of hypersensitivity and inflammation. Med Clin North Am 65:809, 1981.

Holaday, J. W.: Cardiovascular effects of endogenous opiate systems. Ann Rev Pharmacol Toxicol 23:541, 1983.

McCabe, W. R., Treadwell, T. L., and DeMaera, A.: Pathophysiology of bacteremia. Am J Med 75:7, 1983.

Morrison, D. C., and Ulevitch, R. J.: The effects of bacterial endotoxins on host mediation systems. Am J Pathol 93:528, 1979.

Root, R. K., and Cohen, M. S.: The microbicidal mechanisms of human neutrophils and eosinophils. Rev Inf Dis 3:565, 1981.

Rosen, F. S., Cooper, M. D., and Wedgwood, R. J. P.: The primary immunodeficiencies (2 parts). N Engl J Med 311:235, 300, 1984.

Samuelsson, B.: Leukotrienes: Mediators of immediate hypersensitivity reactions and inflammation. Science 220:568, 1983.

Sheagren, J. N.: Septic shock and corticosteroids. N Engl J Med 305:456, 1981.

Silverstein, S. C., Steinman, R. M., and Cohn, Z.: Endocytosis. Annu Rev Biochem 46:669, 1977.

Swanson, J. P., Sparling, P. F., and Puziss, M.: Bacterial virulence and pathogenicity. Rev Inf Dis Supplement, Sept.-Oct., 1983.

Tauber, A. I., Borregard, N., Simons, E., and Wright, J.: Chronic granulomatous disease: A syndrome of phagocyte oxidase deficiencies. Medicine 62:286, 1983.

Wilson, J. J., Neame, P. B., and Kelton, J. G.: Infection-induced thrombocytopenia. Sem Thrombos Hemostas 8:217, 1982.

Ziegler, E. J., McCutchan, J. A., Fierer, J., et al.: Treatment of gram-negative bacteremia and shock with human antiserum to a mutant *E. coli*. N Engl J Med 303:1225, 1982.

THE BLOOD AND BLOOD-FORMING ORGANS

D. J. WEATHERALL, F.R.C.P., F.R.S., *and* C. BUNCH, F.R.C.P.

The pathophysiology of the blood and blood-forming organs is a subject of particular fascination in clinical medicine. Because of the central importance of blood in body metabolism there are few serious diseases that do not cause changes in the blood at some time during their course. Similarly, the primary hematologic disorders may have secondary effects on almost any organ system. Knowledge of the pathophysiology of blood diseases has increased dramatically over the last 20 years. This is one of the few branches of clinical science in which it is possible to define at least a few disease processes at the molecular level; this is because the easy accessibility of the blood and cells of the blood-forming organs, and their specialized nature, have made it possible to examine several blood diseases using the tools of molecular biology. Hence, study of the pathophysiology of these disorders is of particular value, not only for understanding blood diseases, but also for a better appreciation of pathophysiologic mechanisms in general.

General Description of the Blood _____

THE CONSTITUENTS OF NORMAL BLOOD

Blood consists of several different types of cells suspended in a nutrient fluid medium called *plasma*. If a blood sample is treated so that it does not clot it will be found that after standing or gentle centrifugation the cells make up approximately 45 per cent and the plasma about 55 per cent of the total volume. If blood is allowed to clot the fluid component is called *serum*. The absence of the clottable proteins, particularly fibrinogen, in serum differentiates it from plasma.

The formed elements of the blood consist of the *red cells, white cells,* and *platelets*. The red cells, or *erythrocytes,* are biconcave disks measuring approximately 7 to 8 μm in diameter. Erythrocytes consist of a highly organized membrane and contain water, the respiratory pigment hemoglobin, and a variety of other proteins, salts, and vitamins. They are of relatively uniform shape and size and contain similar amounts of hemoglobin. In health, the red cells in the peripheral blood do not contain a nucleus. However, on supravital staining approximately 1 per cent of them have a reticular appearance. This is an artifact produced by the dye acting on residual ribosomes, mitochondria, and other organelles. These are newly released red cells and because of their staining characteristics are called *reticulocytes*.

The white cell series can be divided by morphologic appearance into the *granulocytes* (polymorphonuclear leukocytes), *monocytes,* and *lymphocytes*. The granulocytes and monocytes are phagocytic cells, while the lymphocytes are involved in a variety of immune mechanisms. In the peripheral blood the granulocyte series includes a relatively small number of newly produced cells in which the nucleus is horseshoe-shaped but still single. These are called *band cells* or *juvenile polymorphonuclear leukocytes*. The majority of the granulocytes have matured beyond this stage, and their nuclei consist of two or more lobes separated by thin filamentous chromatin strands. They are about 12 to 15 μm in diameter. The granulocyte series is further classified according to the staining characteristics of the granules into *neutrophils, eosinophils,* and *basophils*. Neutrophil granules are numerous and stain violet pink, eosinophilic granules stain pale red, and basophilic granules stain a dense blue or black and are larger than the other two. While the neutrophil nucleus has from two to five lobes, the eosinophils and basophils usually have bilobed nuclei. The monocytes are also about 12 to 15 μm in diameter. The nuclei are oval, not horseshoe shaped, with a light, purple-pink-staining chromatin. Their cytoplasm is slate-colored with some lilac-colored granules. In normal blood two forms of lymphocyte can be seen: the large lymphocyte with a diameter of 8 to 16 μm and a smaller form measuring 7 to 9 μm. They are round cells with a round nucleus and light blue cytoplasm. In the large lymphocytes the nucleus fills approximately half of the cell, whereas in the small lymphocytes it almost completely fills the cell. This morphologic heterogeneity of the peripheral blood lymphocytes is not related to differences in function. Small and large lymphocytes are not distinct classes in the sense of being either T or B cells (see later discussion). Rather, their size appears to reflect their state of activity and stage of differentiation.

The platelets are disk-shaped cells approximately 2 to 3 μm in diameter. In normal blood they are relatively homogeneous in structure; little of their fine structure can be distinguished by conventional light microscopy.

A detailed description of the fine structures of the blood cells and their precursors appears later in this section.

EXAMINATION OF THE BLOOD

THE NORMAL BLOOD COUNT AND ITS PHYSIOLOGIC VARIATIONS

A great deal of useful information can be obtained by a relatively small number of simple studies of the peripheral blood. From a 5 ml anticoagulated blood sample it is possible to prepare a stained blood film and to examine the morphology of the formed elements. On the same sample the relative volume of packed red cells and white cells, the hemoglobin level, and the red cell, white cell, and platelet counts can be determined. By a series of calculations relating the volume of packed red cells, hemoglobin level, and red cell count, it is possible to derive useful information about both the size and the hemoglobinization of the red cells. Finally, the relative numbers of reticulocytes and the erythrocyte sedimentation rate can be determined.

THE STAINED BLOOD FILM

A careful examination of a stained blood film is the most important investigation in clinical hematology. Each of the formed elements is studied separately.

The red cells are examined for their degree of hemoglobinization and shape; if both are normal the film is described as normochromic and normocytic. Disorders of the red cell are frequently associated with changes in their morphology. The latter includes variation in size of the cells, or anisocytosis; cells that are larger than normal are called *macrocytes*; cells smaller than normal are called *microcytes*. Variation in red cell shape is called *poikilocytosis*. Pale staining of the cells indicates underhemoglobinization and is termed *hypochromia*. Variation in the degree of staining from cell to cell is known as *polychromasia*. In addition to these changes there may be more specific alterations in morphology of the red cells. These include target forms, which are thin flat cells with a centrally stained area that gives the cell its name. This deformity is thought to reflect a large "floppy" cell that has "folded" as the film has been made, hence giving the cell the appearance of having a thickened center. *Spherocytes* are spherical cells that appear to be densely hemoglobinized on the blood film. *Elliptocytes* are, as their name implies, elliptic or oval red cells. *Stomatocytes* are red cells that have a thin central slit rather fancifully thought to resemble a mouth. In addition, there are a variety of forms of irregularly contracted cells, including triangular-shaped fragments, elongated forms or *schistocytes*, helmet-shaped cells, cells with conspicuous spines called burr cells, and cells with a sickled conformation. *Acanthocytes* are crenated cells with surface projections. In addition to these changes in shape or size of the red cells abnormal inclusions may be seen on the peripheral blood film. These are described in detail on pages 242 to 243 and in Table 1. Nucleated red cells appear in the blood during periods of rapid regeneration or in association with a wide variety of disorders of the marrow. The clinical significance of these red cell changes is summarized in Table 1 and is described in detail later. Illustrative blood films are shown in Figure 1.

The white cells may be abnormal in number or morphology. An increased white cell count is called *leukocytosis*. If this involves the polymorphonuclear series it is called polymorphonuclear leukocytosis or *granulocytosis*. An elevated eosinophil, basophil, monocyte, or lymphocyte count is called *eosinophilia, basophila, monocytosis,* or *lymphocytosis,* respectively. A reduced white cell count is called *neutropenia* or *lymphopenia,* depending on the cell type involved. An absence of granulocytes in the blood is called *agranulocytosis*. As with the red cells, much can be learned by morphologic examination of the polymorphonuclear cells. The white blood cells are said to show a "shift to the left" if there are relatively more young polymorphonuclear leukocytes present than is normal. This is

TABLE 1. SIGNIFICANCE OF MORPHOLOGIC CHANGES OF THE RED CELL

RED CELL CHANGE	CLINICAL SIGNIFICANCE
Hypochromia	Defective hemoglobinization; usually iron deficiency or a defect in hemoglobin synthesis.
Microcytosis	Same as for hypochromia.
Macrocytosis	Dyserythropoiesis or premature release. May indicate megaloblastic erythropoiesis, hemolysis, or myelodysplasia.
Anisochromia	Variability of hemoglobinization or presence of young red cell populations—e.g., in hemolysis.
Spherocytes	Usually indicates damage to membrane. May occur as a genetic defect or an acquired abnormality often due to antibody damage.
Target cells	Large "floppy" cells that occur with deficient hemoglobinization or in liver disease. Also occur in hyposplenism.
Elliptocytes	Usually a genetic defect in the red cell membrane.
Poikilocytes: include burr cells, helmet cells, schistocytes, fragmented forms, etc.	Usually indicates damage to red cells in microcirculation—microangiopathy. A variable degree of poikilocytosis occurs in the megaloblastic anemias and other dyserythropoietic anemias. "Teardrop" cells are particularly characteristic of myelosclerosis.
Sickle cells	Occur in the sickling disorders.
Acanthocytes	Occur in genetic disorders of lipid metabolism.
Inclusions: Iron granules (siderocytes), Howell-Jolly bodies, and Cabot's rings (nuclear remnants), basophilic stippling and Heinz bodies	Iron granules and nuclear remnants are often seen after splenectomy. Basophilic stippling indicates defective hemoglobin synthesis—e.g., lead poisoning. Heinz bodies are precipitated hemoglobin or globin subunits.

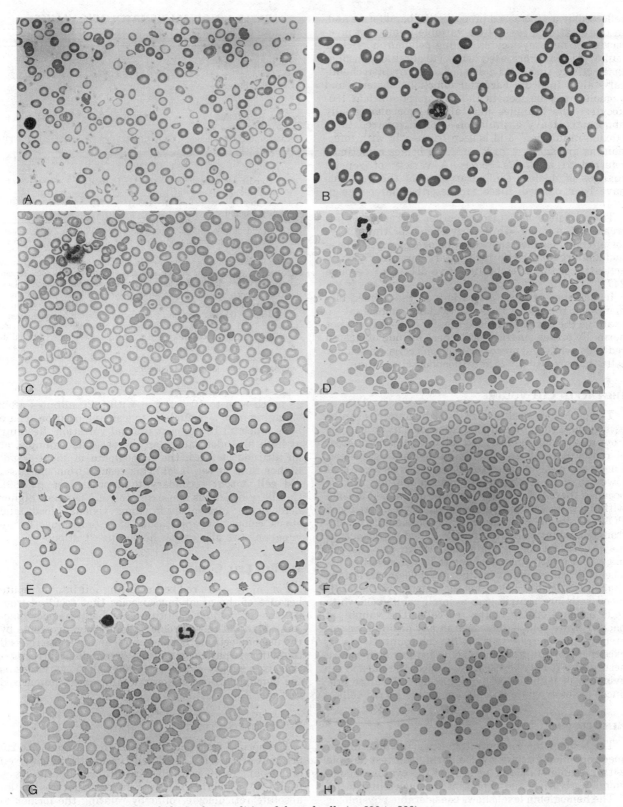

Figure 1. Morphologic abnormalities of the red cells (× 600 to 800).

(A) Hypochromia and microcytosis.
(B) Macrocytosis and poikilocytosis. This film is from a patient with pernicious anemia and shows a hyperlobulated polymorphonuclear leukocyte.
(C) Target cells.

(D) Spherocytes.
(E) Poikilocytosis with schistocytes.
(F) Ovalocytes.
(G) Acanthocytes.
(H) Heinz bodies.

reflected by an increased proportion of band forms and, in more extreme cases, by a variable number of myelocytes or metamyelocytes. Young polymorphonuclear leukocytes have increased leukocyte alkaline phosphatase activity that can be demonstrated by histochemical stains. In acute bacterial infections bacteria and vacuoles may be seen in the polymorphonuclear leukocytes. The granules may also be morphologically abnormal. Heavy granulation is often referred to as "toxic granulation" and is seen frequently with infection, as are small (1 to 2 μm) oval bodies sometimes referred to as *Döhle bodies*. A variety of genetic changes of nuclear configuration or of the granules have been defined; these are described later (see p. 264).

The platelets may also be either decreased or increased in number—thrombocytopenia or thrombocytosis. They also may show morphologic changes. These include large bizarre forms that are particularly characteristic of the myeloproliferative diseases (see page 247).

In addition to these alterations in the formed elements of the blood it is particularly important to examine the peripheral blood film for cells that are not normally present in the blood. These include nucleated red cells, while cell precursors, plasma cells, and tumor cells that are usually of reticuloendothelial origin.

THE PACKED CELL VOLUME

The packed cell volume (PCV, or hematocrit) can be estimated either by centrifugation or can be derived from measurement of the red cell volume and number of red cells using an electronic cell-counting system. The latter method yields results as much as 3 per cent lower than those obtained by centrifugation. This is because there is a variable amount of trapped plasma within a column of centrifuged erythrocytes. A reduced PCV usually indicates anemia but occasionally results from hemodilution. A raised PCV, called *polycythemia*, may represent an absolute increase in the red cell mass or a relative increase due to hemoconcentration. The PCV shows many of the physiologic variations that are described below for the hemoglobin level. If blood cells are centrifuged, a small column of white cells appears on top of the red cells. The volume of packed white cells is increased in any disorder associated with an increase in the white cell count. However, except in certain leukemias, it is too low to measure accurately. It may be useful to inspect the plasma for evidence of jaundice or hyperlipemia; the latter produces a cloudy white flocculation above the red cells.

HEMOGLOBIN

The hemoglobin concentration is usually determined spectrophotometrically by comparing the test sample with a stable standard, usually of the cyanmethemoglobin derivative, and is presented as g/deciliter (dl).

The hemoglobin level shows considerable physiologic variation. The normal range related to sex and age is given in Tables 2 and 3, and Gaussian distribution curves from which data of this kind can be derived are shown in Figure 2. The hemoglobin level is also related to physical exercise, posture, and environment. The level rises after muscular exercise and may change by

TABLE 2. NORMAL HEMATOLOGIC VALUES*†

	MEN	WOMEN
White cell count, × 10³ μl blood	7.25 (3.9–10.6)	7.28 (3.5–11.0)
Red cell count, × 10⁶ μl blood	5.11 (4.4–5.9)	4.51 (3.8–5.2)
Hemoglobin, g/100 ml blood	15.5 (13.3–17.7)	13.7 (11.7–15.7)
Volume packed RBC, ml/100 ml blood	46.0 (39.8–52.2)	40.9 (34.9–46.9)
Mean corpuscular volume, μm³/red cell	90.1 (80.5–99.7)	90.4 (80.8–100.0)
Mean corpuscular hemoglobin, pg/red cell	30.2 (26.6–33.8)	30.2 (26.4–34.0)
Mean corpuscular hemoglobin concentration, g/100 ml RBC	33.9 (31.5–36.3)	33.6 (31.4–35.8)
Platelet count, × 10³/μl blood	295 (150–440)	295 (150–440)

*From Williams, W. J., and Schneider, A. S.: In Williams, W. J., Beutler, E., Erslev, A. J. and Lichtman, M.A. (eds.): Hematology. 3rd ed. New York, McGraw-Hill, 1983.

†The nomenclature and units used in this table are still in use in many laboratories. However, it should be noted that new terminology is being introduced to describe the absolute values. "Corpuscular" is being replaced by "cell" (mean cell volume, mean cell hemoglobin, etc.). Furthermore, the Système International d'Unités (SI) is gradually being introduced for blood values. Thus red cell and white cell counts are being reported in units of 10¹²/l and 10⁹/l respectively and hemoglobin values in g/dl (deciliter). The mean cell volume is expressed in femtoliters (fl) and the mean cell hemoglobin concentration in g/dl in this system. The platelet count is expressed as 100s × 10⁹/l. The use of SI units in hematology is summarized in the Journal of Clinical Pathology 27:950, 1974.

as much as 5 to 10 per cent within 20 minutes after changing from a recumbent to a sitting position. There is as much as 15 per cent diurnal variation. Residing at high altitudes causes an increase; for example, at an altitude of 2 km the hemoglobin is about 1 g/dl higher than at sea level. This results from increased red cell output secondary to hypoxia (see p. 189). Capillary blood has approximately a 5 per cent higher hemoglobin concentration than venous blood, and stasis caused by application of a tourniquet before venepuncture also causes hemoconcentration.

THE RED CELL COUNT

For many years red cell counting fell into disrepute because of the great inaccuracies that resulted from the use of manual counting chambers (hemocytometers). Many of these problems have been overcome by the use of electronic cell counters, and now the red cell count forms part of a routine hematologic investigation. It is subject to the same physiologic variables as the hemoglobin level. Normal values are summarized in Table 2.

RETICULOCYTE COUNT

The normal reticulocyte count ranges from 0.2 to 2.0 per cent of total red blood cells in adults and children and from 2 to 6 per cent in full-term infants. It is useful to convert the per cent reticulocytes to an absolute reticulocyte count by relating the former to the red cell count.

ABSOLUTE INDICES

The red cell indices are derived from a series of calculations using the packed cell volume, hemoglobin

TABLE 3. NORMAL HEMATOLOGIC VALUES AT VARIOUS AGES*†

AGE	LEUKOCYTES (total)	NEUTROPHILS Total	Band	Segmented	EOSINOPHILS	BASOPHILS	LYMPHO-CYTES	MONOCYTES	HEMOGLOBIN (g/100 ml blood)
12 mo	11.4 (6.0–17.5)	3.5 (1.5–8.5) *31*	0.35 *3.1*	3.2 *28*	0.30 (0.05–0.70) *2.6*	0.05 (0–20) *0.4*	7.0 (4.0–10.5) *61*	0.55 (0.05–1.1) *4.8*	11.6 (9.0–14.6)
4 yr	9.1 (5.5–15.5)	3.8 (1.5–8.5) *42*	0.27 (0–1.0) *3.0*	3.5 (1.5–7.5) *39*	0.25 (0.02–0.65) *2.8*	0.05 (0–0.20) *0.6*	4.5 (2.0–8.0) *50*	0.45 (0–0.8) *5.0*	12.6 (9.6–15.5)
6 yr	8.5 (5.0–14.5)	4.3 (1.5–8.0) *51*	0.25 (0–1.0) *3.0*	4.0 (1.5–7.0) *48*	0.23 (0–0.65) *2.7*	0.05 (0–0.20) *0.6*	3.5 (1.5–7.0) *42*	0.40 (0–0.8) *4.7*	12.7 (10.0–15.5)
10 yr	8.1 (4.5–13.5)	4.4 (1.8–8.0) *54*	0.24 (0–1.0) *3.0*	4.2 (1.8–7.0) *51*	0.20 (0–0.60) *2.4*	0.04 (0–0.20) *0.5*	3.1 (1.5–6.5) *38*	0.35 (0–0.8) *4.3*	13.0 (10.7–15.5)
21 yr	7.4 (4.5–11.0)	4.4 (1.8–7.7) *59*	0.22 (0–0.7) *3.0*	4.2 (1.8–7.0) *56*	0.20 (0–0.45) *2.7*	0.04 (0–0.20) *0.5*	2.5 (1.0–4.8) *34*	0.30 (0–0.8) *4.0*	♂15.8 (14.0–18.0) ♀13.9 (11.5–16.0)

*From Williams, W. J., and Schneider, A. S.: In Williams, W. J., Beutler, E., Erslev, A. J., and Lichtman, M. A. (eds.): Hematology. 3rd ed. New York, McGraw-Hill, 1983.
†Values are expressed as "cells × 10³/μl." The numbers in italic type are percentages.

level, and the red cell count (Table 4). The mean cell volume (MCV), calculated in femtoliters (fl), gives an indication of the size of the erythrocytes; it is derived from the erythrocyte count and the packed cell volume, which measures the proportion of the blood occupied by erythrocytes expressed as volume rather than per cent. The mean cell hemoglobin (MCH), expressed in picograms (pg), is an indication of the amount of hemoglobin per cell and is derived from the hemoglobin value and red cell count. The mean cell hemoglobin concentration (MCHC) represents the concentration of hemoglobin in g/dl (100 ml) of erythrocytes. The red cell indices are *average* values and do not take into account the heterogeneity of cell populations. Their values are remarkably constant in health. The normal ranges are summarized in Tables 2 and 5.

The red cell indices may be used together with an examination of the stained blood film to classify various forms of anemia. Reduced values for the MCH and MCV indicate poorly hemoglobinized blood cells and usually accompany a hypochromic anemia. The MCHC falls only with a gross degree of hypochromic anemia and is therefore a relatively insensitive indicator of the degree of hemoglobinization of the red cells. The MCV is elevated in all forms of macrocytic anemia and usually accompanies a reticulocytosis when it reflects the larger size of relatively young red cells.

THE TOTAL AND DIFFERENTIAL LEUKOCYTE COUNT

The total number of leukocytes in the circulating blood can be determined either with a counting chamber or electronically. The total leukocyte count shows considerable physiologic variation. The normal range at different ages is summarized in Table 3. There is also a sex difference, which becomes greater in older age groups (that is, after the age of 50 years when the count becomes lower in women than in men). There are rhythmic variations during the menstrual cycle and a diurnal cycle with minimum counts in the morning with the subject at rest. Light activity may increase the count slightly, while strenuous exercise causes an increase of up to 30 × 10⁹ per l. There may

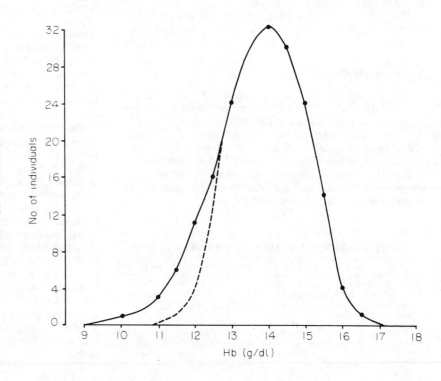

Figure 2. A frequency curve for hemoglobin levels in a population of normal women at sea level. The interrupted line represents a normalized Gaussian distribution. The acuteness of the original distribution curve indicates that the community was not entirely healthy. The 95 per cent (2 standard deviations) limits are 11.8 to 16.2 g/dl. (From Lewis, S. M.: *Blood and Its Disorders.* 2nd ed. Hardisty, R. M., and Weatherall, D. J. (eds.). Oxford, Blackwell Scientific Publications, 1982.)

TABLE 4. THE ABSOLUTE VALUES (OR INDICES)

Mean cell volume (MCV) $= \dfrac{\text{volume of packed erythrocytes/1000 ml}}{\text{red cell count, millions/mm}^3}$

expressed in femtoliters (fl)

Mean cell hemoglobin (MCH) $= \dfrac{\text{hemoglobin in grams/1000 ml}}{\text{red cell count, millions/mm}^3}$

expressed in picograms (pg)

Mean cell hemoglobin concentration (MCHC) $= \dfrac{\text{hemoglobin in grams/100 ml} \times 100}{\text{packed cell volume \%}}$

expressed in grams/100 ml (dl) of red cells

be a slight increase in the count during emotional stress and after food. A moderate leukocytosis is common during pregnancy with the peak about eight weeks before parturition; the count returns to normal about one week after delivery.

The differential white cell count also shows striking physiologic variation. The changes with age are summarized in Table 3. In the sex difference with age, mentioned above, the neutrophil count falls parallel with the total white count in postmenopausal females. In pregnancy the neutrophil count rises parallel with the total white cell count, whereas the lymphocyte count remains relatively constant, apart from a slightly lower mean count in the first trimester. The eosinophils are especially prone to diurnal variation with differences of as much as 100 per cent between the lowest counts, which occur in the day, and the highest counts, which occur at night. This remarkable variability is controlled to some extent by the activity of the adrenal cortex; the changes parallel and vary inversely with diurnal glucocorticoid fluctuations.

The total and differential white cell count shows many alterations in disease. These are described later (p. 262).

THE PLATELET COUNT

The normal platelet count varies with the method used. With currently standardized methods the range in health is approximately 150×10^9 to 400×10^9 per l. There have been no sex differences described and there appears to be no diurnal variation. A slight fall in platelet count has been described in females at about the time of menstruation and there is some evidence of a cycle with a 21- to 35-day rhythm. There are no obvious changes related to age.

TABLE 5. ABSOLUTE VALUES AT DIFFERENT AGES*

	3 MOS	1 YR	10–12 YRS	ADULTS
Mean cell volume (fl)	83–110	77–101	77–95	76–96
Mean cell hemoglobin (pg)	24–34	23–31	24–30	27–32
Mean cell hemoglobin concentration (g/dl)	27–34	28–33	30–33	30–35

*Based on Lewis, S. M.: In Hardisty, R. M., and Weatherall, D. J. (eds.): Blood and Its Disorders. 2nd ed. Oxford, Blackwell Scientific Publications, 1982.

THE BLOOD VOLUME, RED CELL MASS, AND PLASMA VOLUME

The measurement of the peripheral-blood hematocrit or hemoglobin level gives only an approximate indication of the true red cell mass. In general, with hematocrit values between 20 and 50 per cent but not outside this range there is a fairly close correlation between the hematocrit and circulating red cell mass. Furthermore, as discussed below, the peripheral-blood hematocrit is not a true measure of the total body hematocrit. Hence it is not possible to derive total blood volume from the red cell volume and blood hematocrit, and to obtain an accurate estimate of the blood volume it is necessary to measure it directly. This is usually done by measuring the red cell volume (RCV) and the plasma volume (PV) by radioisotope dilution.

The RCV is measured by radiolabeling red cells, usually with ^{51}Cr. For measuring PV the use of dyes, including Evans blue, has been largely superseded by the use of isotope-labeled albumin. The most frequently used label is ^{125}I. The RCV is calculated by comparing the radioactivity of 1 ml of labeled packed red cells with the radioactivity of 1 ml of a postinjection sample of packed red cells drawn after a period of equilibration. There may be a delay in the mixing time when there is sequestration of red cells, such as occurs in patients with massive splenomegaly or in patients in shock. The plasma volume is calculated in a similar way but with the use of 1 ml of labeled protein and with a comparison of its radioactivity with 1 ml of a postinjection sample of plasma again drawn after a period of postinjection equilibration.

Although in theory it should be possible to obtain an accurate measurement of the blood volume from the RCV plus the venous hematocrit, this is not the case. This inaccuracy results because the whole body hematocrit is not the same as the venous hematocrit, owing to the lower hematocrit of blood in the visceral capillaries as compared with the larger vessels. In normal persons the ratio of whole body to venous hematocrit is approximately 0.9, but this does not apply when there is sequestration of blood in organs such as the spleen. Furthermore, the whole body hematocrit is lower than normal in patients with liver disease, nephritis, or cardiac failure, and is increased in pregnancy. It varies greatly in normal subjects and is increased particularly in residents at high altitudes. Therefore, although it may sometimes be possible to obtain the blood volume from an estimate of the RCV and peripheral hematocrit, there are many situations in clinical practice in which a total blood volume has to be determined by measuring both the PV and RCV.

The blood volume of normal subjects varies considerably in relation to their height and weight. Furthermore, because adipose tissue is relatively avascular, relating blood volume to total body weight can also introduce inaccuracies. Total blood volume can be expressed in ml/kg of total body weight, in ml/kg of lean body weight, in relation to height and weight, or as a total volume together with predicted volume for a normal subject of the same height, weight, and age. That so many corrections have been applied to the estimated blood volume suggests that none of them is ideal.

TABLE 6. NORMAL RED CELL AND PLASMA VOLUMES*

	MALES	FEMALES
Red cell volume	30 ± 5 ml/kilo	25 ± 5 ml/kilo
Plasma volume	40–50 ml/kilo	40–50 ml/kilo
Total blood volume	60–80 ml/kilo	60–80 ml/kilo

*Based on Lewis, S. M.: In Hardisty, R. M., and Weatherall, D. J. (eds.): Blood and Its Disorders. 2nd ed. Oxford, Blackwell Scientific Publications, 1982.

In clinical practice it is usual to simply calculate the RCV or PV as ml/kg. The wide range of normal values is shown in Table 6. There is considerable physiologic variation. At birth the total blood volume is about 300 ml, and it fluctuates over the first year of life. It gradually increases until puberty and then increases more rapidly in males than in females. In pregnancy both plasma and total blood volume increase; the plasma volume increases especially in the first trimester, although the greatest increase in total blood volume occurs during the middle third of pregnancy. These changes take about one to two weeks to revert to normal after delivery. Prolonged immobility is associated with a reduction in blood volume due to contraction of the plasma volume.

THE ERYTHROCYTE SEDIMENTATION RATE

The erythrocyte sedimentation rate (ESR), sometimes called the blood sedimentation rate (BSR), is a measure of the suspension stability of red cells in blood. Various techniques have been devised for its measurement, and the results depend on the method used and particularly on the care with which the ESR tubes are set up. A numeric value in mm is obtained by measuring the distance from the surface meniscus to the upper limit of the red cell layer in the column of blood after 60 minutes. The ESR depends on the difference in specific gravity between the red cells and plasma but is also influenced by many other factors, particularly the rate at which the red cells clump or form rouleaux, because large clumps are heavier and therefore sediment more rapidly than in single cells. Other factors affecting the sedimentation rate include anemia, any tilt of the tube from the horizontal, the dimensions of the tube, and the nature of the anticoagulant used. Rouleaux formation is related to the concentration of fibrinogen, other acute phase proteins, and immunoglobulins in the plasma.

Because of the technical difficulties of standardizing the ESR estimation, normal values must be related to the method used, and even then they range widely.

The ESR is still widely used in clinical medicine as a nonspecific index of organic disease. It is elevated in many acute or chronic infections, neoplastic disease, collagen disease, renal insufficiency, and any disorder associated with a change in the plasma proteins. Anemia may cause increased sedimentation; although many attempts have been made to apply formulae to correct for this, none are very satisfactory. It is important to note that the ESR may vary in certain physiologic states, particularly pregnancy and increasing age. In men and women over the age of 60 a modestly elevated ESR (up to 25 to 35 mm/hour) may be found without any obvious cause.

The Formation of Blood

In this section the general principles that govern the formation of blood will be considered. A detailed account of the different precursors of the red cells, white cells, and platelets is given in appropriate sections later in this chapter.

HEMOPOIESIS DURING DEVELOPMENT

The earliest blood formation occurs in the primitive yolk sac. At about 19 days gestation blood islands appear in the yolk sac and differentiate in two directions. The cells at the periphery of the islands form the walls of the first blood vessels, while those in the center become the primitive blood cells, or *hemocytoblasts*. Similar blood islands soon appear throughout the mesodermal tissues of the body stalk. Hemopoiesis declines during this mesodermal stage of development from about the sixth week of gestation. By the fifth to sixth gestational week hemopoiesis is established in the liver, which serves as the major site of blood production until about the sixth fetal month and probably continues to produce some red cells until about term. The hemopoietic cells of the liver are almost exclusively erythropoietic in contrast to the mixed population of cell precursors produced by the marrow.

Hemopoiesis in the latter site commences about the fourth to fifth fetal month, and the marrow becomes the major organ of hemopoiesis from the sixth month onward. The spleen also becomes a hemopoietic organ from approximately the second to seventh month of gestation.

In the embryo two populations of erythrocytes are present. The large nucleated megaloblastic forms are the derivatives of the primitive mesoderm and these are replaced by smaller nonnucleated cells that are presumably produced by the liver. A fascinating question, which has not been completely resolved, is whether the cells from the primitive mesoderm migrate and populate the liver and then form the precursors of the next developmental stage of red cells. Alternatively, there may be two distinct cell lines, one derived from the primitive yolk sac and the other arising de novo from the fetal liver. The yolk-sac-derived cells carry specific embryonic hemoglobins, while the liver-derived population produce mainly fetal and small amounts of adult hemoglobins (see p. 202). During the later months of gestation, when hemopoiesis moves from the liver to the bone marrow, there is a switch from fetal to adult hemoglobin production. There is no evidence that a particular hemoglobin is produced in any one hemopoietic site, and the switch from fetal to

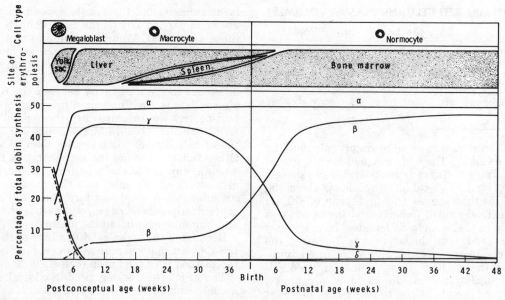

Figure 3. Changes in hemoglobin constitution, erythropoiesis, and the sites of hemopoiesis during fetal development. (From Wood, W. G.: British Medical Bulletin 32:282, 1977.)

adult hemoglobin production occurs synchronously throughout the organs of the developing fetus. These relationships are summarized in Figure 3.

During the early months of gestation a few granulocytes can be found in the peripheral circulation. In contrast, lymphocyte counts are higher in the first half of gestation and fall subsequently. Megakaryocytes are present in the yolk sac by the sixth gestational week and at this time they also appear in the liver, where they can be seen up to term. From about the third gestational month onward megakaryocytes are also present in the bone marrow.

The many differences between the peripheral blood at birth and in adult life are summarized in Tables 3 and 5, which show the sequential changes in the hemoglobin level, red cell count and indices, and in the white cell count. The red cells of newborn infants show many biochemical and antigenic differences from those of adults. Some of the most important are summarized in Table 7. The morphology of the red cells of newborn infants, partly those born prematurely, may reflect the immaturity of the neonatal spleen—that is,

they are those of hyposplenism (see p. 253). Immediately after birth the rate of erythropoiesis declines markedly, and for the first few months red cell production occurs at a very low level. The rate of erythropoiesis gradually increases from about the second to third month. These changes are reflected by the associated reticulocyte counts. In addition the red cell indices show striking changes during this period; the cells are relatively large at birth but are replaced by a smaller population in the first few weeks (Table 5).

During the first few years of life cellular bone marrow extends throughout the long bones, ribs, sternum, skull, pelvis, and vertebrae. From about the age of four years, however, growth of the bone cavities outstrips that of the blood cell precursors, and the fatty reserve of the bone cell precursors, and the fatty replacement occurs first in the diaphyses of the peripheral long bones and then extends centrifugally until by the age of about 18 years hemopoietically active bone marrow is found only in the vertebrae, ribs, sternum, skull, and proximal epiphyses of the long bones. If for any reason there is a drive to increased erythropoiesis in adult life this fatty marrow may be replaced by active erythropoietic tissue. Extramedullary hemopoiesis in the spleen or liver as a response to anemia is unusual after the early years of life.

THE BONE MARROW

An understanding of the morphology and functions of the bone marrow is an essential basis for studies of the blood in health and disease. In this section the structure and general morphologic appearances of the normal bone marrow and the various ways in which it can be examined are considered. A more detailed description of the different developmental stages of the hemopoietic precursor cells that are found in the marrow appear later in the chapter under individual sections dealing with the red cells, white cells, and platelets, respectively.

TABLE 7. SOME CHARACTERISTICS OF FETAL ERYTHROPOIESIS

Red cells larger than in adult life.
Red cell survival shorter than that of adult cells.
Red cells contain mainly Hb F ($\alpha_2\gamma_2$).
Hbs A and A_2 present at low levels.
Ratio of $^G\gamma:^A\gamma$ chains is about 3:1 in Hb F* and changes to about 2:3 in Hb F in normal adults.
Embryonic hemoglobins (Gower and Portland) present up to 8 weeks gestation.
Red cells have high oxygen affinity.
Carbonic anhydrase isozymes B and C much reduced as compared with adult cells.
High levels of i and low levels of I reactivity.
Erythropoiesis controlled by erythropoietin produced in liver.

*Human fetal hemoglobin is a mixture of molecules with the formulae $\alpha_2\gamma_2^{136gly}$ and $\alpha_2\gamma_2^{136ala}$. The γ chains of the former are called $^G\gamma$, and the later $^A\gamma$. They are the products of separate genes.

Structure

Bone marrow is made up of a delicate network of vessels and nerves, reticuloendothelial cells, and progenitor cells at various stages of maturation, together with fatty tissue, which acts as a "filler" (Fig. 4). The blood supply is derived from the nutrient arteries of the bones. These enter through the nutrient foramina and branch several times before terminating in capillaries that enter the haversian system of the bone or sinusoids of the marrow. The arterioles derived from these vessels empty into a complex sinusoidal venous system (Fig. 5), which drains into a central collecting vein. Hemopoiesis occurs outside the sinusoidal system, and newly produced cells have to pass through narrow openings in the endothelial vascular lining in order to enter the circulation. This fine, sieve-like barrier probably plays a role in erythroblastic nuclear extrusion and in removing various intracellular inclusions both in health and in disease. The sinuses are lined with endothelial cells. Flattened reticular cells extend from the fat cells to the sinusoids and serve as centers of hemopoietic cells or "blood islands." Plasma

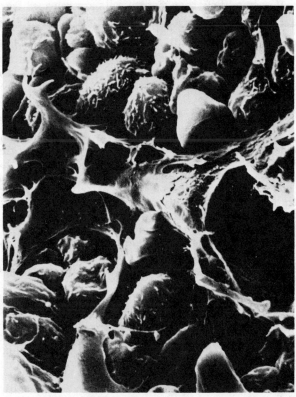

Figure 5. A vascular sinus of the bone marrow. The broad structure in the center of the field is a cytoplasmic expanse of adventitial reticular cell that covers much of the outside surface of the vascular sinus and branches richly, far out into the hemopoietic compartment. Its process is passed between the hemopoietic cells, and at one place reticular cell cytoplasm almost completely envelops a myelocyte. Several cells bearing microvilli lie close against the adventitial surface of the sinus at its upper aspect. These microvilli may well have developed preparatory to transmural passage of these cells. It should be noted that many hemopoietic cells have been removed in this preparation by the loosening effects of perfusion. Those that remain are separated from one another. (From Erslev, A. J., and Weiss, L.: In *Hematology*. 3rd ed. Williams, W. J., Beutler, E., Erslev, A. J., and Lichtman, M. A. (eds.). New York, McGraw-Hill, 1983.)

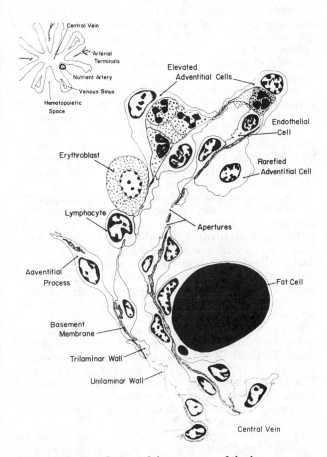

Figure 4. A general view of the anatomy of the bone marrow. The figure in the upper left-hand corner depicts a cross section of the marrow with spokelike sinusoids draining into a central longitudinal vein. The main diagram depicts sinusoidal basement membrane covered on one side by reticular cells acting as phagocytes, as "nurse" cells to hemopoietic elements, and as guards of the fenestrations in the basement membrane. (Weiss, L.: In *Regulation of Hematopoiesis*. Vol. 1. Gordon, A. S. (ed.). New York, Appleton-Century-Crofts, 1970.)

cells are in close contact with the sinusoidal wall and become stretched along the sinusoidal membrane.

The scanty connective tissue of hemopoietic marrow is found largely in association with sinuses and vessels. In the former it forms an incomplete basement membrane. The extracellular connective tissue can be stained with silver and by the periodic acid–Schiff (PAS) technique. In health it contains only small amounts of reticulin fibers.

There is an extensive nerve supply to the marrow. Some of the nerves lie close to the hemopoietic islands, and it is possible that they sense pressure changes caused by cellular proliferation. It has been suggested that such signals are transmitted by local reflex arcs to vessel walls. In this way an autoregulatory system may exist, capable of adjusting blood flow to permit proliferation and maturation before the cells are released into the circulation. In situations in which there is increased hemopoietic activity the total blood flow to the marrow may increase enormously.

It seems likely that mature cells are released from the marrow once they have become sufficiently "plastic" to negotiate the walls of the sinusoids. Alternatively, the sinus capillaries may open intermittently, although this seems less likely. Many diseases of the bone marrow are characterized by premature release of red and white cell precursors into the blood.

EXAMINATION OF THE BONE MARROW

Bone marrow may be examined by needle aspiration, needle biopsy, or open surgical biopsy. In adults the sites most readily available are the sternum and the anterior or posterior iliac crests, although the latter tend to become rather fatty in elderly subjects. In children less than a year old the anterior medial surface of the tibia is the site of choice; in older children the iliac crests or occasionally the lumbar vertebral spines are suitable. After aspiration of marrow, films are made and stained with a Romanowsky stain. Needle or surgical biopsy samples are fixed and sectioned by standard methods.

The bone marrow films are examined initially under "low power" to assess the cellularity and the relative amounts of fat and hemopoietic cells and for the presence of any abnormal cells. It is sometimes useful to obtain a differential count—that is, the relative numbers of each of the precursors of the different cell lines (Table 8). From this the myeloid:erythroid (M:E) ratio can be determined. This is approximately 3:1 in health, although when there is increased erythroid activity this ratio may reach unity or less.

Once the overall cellularity and the M:E ratio have been determined, the morphology of the individual cells is examined. In particular, the maturation pattern of the red cell, white cell, and megakaryocyte series is assessed. Finally, the marrow is examined for the presence of any abnormal cells, such as tumor cells, and storage or related abnormal forms.

TABLE 8. THE DIFFERENTIAL COUNT ON NORMAL BONE MARROW*

	PER CENT
Reticulum cells	0.1–2
Hemocytoblasts	0.1–1
Myeloblasts	0.1–3.5
Promyelocytes	0.5–5
Myelocytes	
Neutrophil	5–20
Eosinophil	0.1–3
Basophil	0–0.5
Metamyelocytes	10–30
Polymorphonuclears	
Neutrophil	7–25
Eosinophil	0.2–3
Basophil	0–0.5
Lymphocytes	5–20
Monocytes	0–0.2
Megakaryocytes	0.1–0.5
Plasma cells	0.1–3.5
Pronormoblasts	0.5–5
Basophilic and polychromatic normoblasts	2–20
Pyknotic normoblasts	2–10

*Based on Lewis, S. M.: In Hardisty, R. M., and Weatherall, D. J. (eds.): Blood and Its Disorders. 2nd ed. Oxford, Blackwell Scientific Publications, 1982.

The biopsy specimen is of value for looking at the overall cellularity of the bone marrow and relating the amount of hemopoiesis to the fatty tissue. It is of particular value when the marrow is replaced by fibrous or tumor tissue that may not aspirate readily. Using appropriate stains it is possible to estimate the amount of reticulin present, and hence to determine whether there is any degree of myelosclerosis (see p. 247), and to determine the quantity and distribution of iron.

More specialized techniques of marrow examination, including special histochemical methods, are considered in later sections.

ASSESSMENT OF BONE MARROW ACTIVITY AND FUNCTION

Some indication of bone marrow function is obtained from examination of the peripheral blood and from the morphologic appearances of the bone marrow. However, it may also be helpful to measure the rates of production and turnover of the red cell series using radioactive iron (see p. 194). Using isotopes, it is also possible (1) to take scintigrams that show the distribution of erythropoietic or reticuloendothelial marrow throughout the body; (2) to determine the overall size and hemopoietic and red cell sequestering function of the marrow; and (3) to determine iron storage in the spleen and liver. In addition, bone blood flow, which may be abnormal in hematologic disorders, can be assessed.

Erythropoietic bone marrow can be best assessed using the short-lived positron-emitting isotope ^{52}Fe. Pictures taken with a positron scintillation camera show normal adult erythropoietic marrow in the ribs, spine, pelvis, scapula, and clavicle. There is considerable individual variation in the amount of marrow in the skull and in the degree to which it extends down the shafts of the long bones.

The reticuloendothelial portion of the marrow can be labeled with any radiocolloid of an appropriate particle size, but the most effective is ^{99M}Tc–sulfur colloid. One disadvantage of the use of colloids of this type for visualization of the marrow is that a great deal of the dose goes to the liver and spleen, making it difficult to visualize the marrow in the spine behind these organs. Scanning of this type is useful for determining overall marrow function and for demonstrating invasive lesions such as tumors.

It is possible to examine blood flow in bone marrow using the short-lived positron-emitting isotope of fluorine, ^{18}F. There is remarkable similarity between the distribution of flow and the distribution of marrow. The close relationship between perfusion rate and marrow growth suggests that growth of hemopoietic marrow induces a high blood perfusion rate in the surrounding bone.

Imaging techniques are of use in a variety of hematologic problems. They are capable of giving an overall indication of the amount of active bone marrow and demonstrating sites of extramedullary hemopoiesis. In addition, it is possible to determine whether bone marrow failure is due to tumor infiltration or to ineffective erythropoiesis and to assess the extent of involvement of the marrow in such conditions as Hodgkin's disease (see p. 278).

THE EARLY STAGES OF HEMOPOIESIS

The origins and control of the early hemopoietic cells have been of interest to hematologists for many years. Much of what is currently known is derived from experimental work on small animals. Hence part of the information presented in this section depends on the mouse model; although this may provide a general picture of what is happening in larger animals, it must be read with the reservation that it is a big evolutionary jump from mouse to man!

In considering the cellular kinetics of hemopoiesis, certain concepts have to be mastered. Cells are often described as existing in "compartments." Clearly no such anatomic structures exist! The cell biologist uses this term to define cells that are in particular phases of differentiation; for example, the erythroid compartment "contains" those cells that have become genetically programmed to develop into red cells. Alternatively, some cell populations may still have the ability to differentiate into more than one form of mature blood cell; they would then be described as occupying an "uncommitted" compartment. In addition, cells can be categorized in terms of their particular cycle state—that is, whether they are actively synthesizing DNA, in the process of mitosis, out of cycle, and so on. The standard nomenclature for the different phases of the cell cycle is shown in Figure 6.

In considering the early stages of hemopoiesis it is necessary to define what is meant by hemopoietic stem cells, summarize what is known about their kinetics and regulation, and then consider our limited knowledge of the early differentiation steps in the pathway to mature blood cells. Each of these topics has an important bearing on an understanding of abnormal marrow function.

HEMOPOIETIC STEM CELLS

Stem cells can maintain their own numbers in spite of physiologic removal of cells into the populations to which they give rise. "Maintain their own numbers" implies that this is achieved by proliferation within the population and not by entry of cells from another population. Hence this definition is applicable not only to hemopoietic stem cells but to all cell populations capable of maintaining their numbers throughout healthy life by turnover or regeneration through their own proliferative capacity.

There has been considerable diversity of opinion about the origin and identity of stem cells. However, in the last few years experimental work in the mouse and humans has provided unequivocal evidence that hemopoietic stem cells are pluripotential.

EVIDENCE FOR A PLURIPOTENTIAL STEM CELL

First evidence for the existence of a pluripotential stem cell in the mouse was derived from studies in which it was shown that a single chromosomally marked cell clone can repopulate the entire hemopoietic system of lethally irradiated and subsequently bone-marrow–grafted mice. This evidence was confirmed by studies showing that injections of bone marrow cells into lethally irradiated mice form macroscopically visible nodules in the spleen. Furthermore, each of these nodules constitutes a clone or colony originating from a single cell that is capable of giving rise to erythroid, myeloid, and megakaryocytic lines. The term "Colony Forming Unit" was used to describe those cells in the donor marrow that are capable of forming such hemopoietic colonies. These cells are usually called CFU-S, where S stands for spleen.

The fact that CFU-S containing a specific chromosome marker can give rise to colonies that go on to make red cells, white cells, and platelets, each containing the same marker, indicates that they are a pluripotential population. Obviously a point of great interest is whether this stem cell population also gives rise to lymphocytes. Experiments in the mouse, again using chromosomal markers, indicate that lymphocytes are derived from the same population as the other hemopoietic cells. Evidence for a common lineage of lymphocytes and the other hemopoietic cells in humans is scanty. One patient with acquired sideroblastic anemia (see p. 217) has been reported in whom glucose-6-phosphate dehydrogenase isozyme studies indicated that all the hemopoietic cells and B and T lymphocytes were derived from a single cell line. On the other hand, in patients with chronic myeloid leukemia (see p. 276) the specific chromosome marker of the disease involves the red cell, white cell, and platelet lines but is not found in the lymphocyte population. However, even in the mouse, lymphopoiesis and granulopoiesis are functionally divorced. For example, there is a specific genetic strain of anemic mice, named W/W^v, in which there is a greatly reduced capacity for CFU-S to form granulocytic and erythropoietic colonies. However, these animals are immunologically competent; that is, they produce lymphocytes normally. An attempted resolution of these apparent discrepancies suggests that the differentiation event that separates CFU-S from lymphoid progenitors may occur prior to loss of capacity for self-renewal, and hence the lymphoid component may behave quite differently from the myeloid component although originally they were derived from the same cell line. This complicated concept of diver-

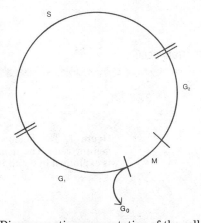

Figure 6. Diagrammatic representation of the cell cycle. The following symbols are used: M is the phase of mitosis, which lasts about ½ to 1 hour; G_1 is the postmitotic, or presynthetic, phase, which lasts about 10 hours; S is the phase of DNA synthesis, which lasts about 9 hours; and G_2 is the postsynthetic, or premitotic, phase, of about 4 hours. The total generation time of normally proliferating bone marrow is about 24 hours. A resting or nonproliferating cell is described as being in G_0.

gence of cell lineage early in stem cell differentiation is illustrated in Figure 7.

Quite recently, clonal assay systems for the detection of human pluripotent progenitor cells have been described. These progenitors give rise to mixed colonies in methyl cellulose in 5 per cent of medium conditioned with leukocytes, in the presence of phytohemagglutinin and erythropoietin. The cellular composition of these colonies varies greatly and may include neutrophil and eosinophil granulocytes, erythroblasts, megakaryocytes, and macrophages. In addition, approximately 20 per cent of them contain cells that give rise to different types of secondary hemopoietic colonies when replated as a single cell suspension. This finding indicates that they contain early progenitors for red cells or white cells. The clonal nature of the mixed colonies has been confirmed by the finding of a linear relationship between the number of cells plated and the number of colonies and the presence or absence of Y-chromatin in co-culture experiments with male and female cells.

If conditions can be found that allow the reproducible growth of these pluripotential progenitors, it should soon be possible to produce clonal assays for human pluripotential progenitor cells and to apply them to the study of disorders of bone marrow function. However, it is not yet absolutely certain that the cells that are being assayed in these in vitro colony systems are identical to the CFU-S as defined in the mouse spleen assay system.

The Kinetics and Regulation of CFU-S

The cell kinetics of the CFU-S have been examined by several techniques. Perhaps the most useful is the "thymidine suicide"–labeling approach. In experiments of this type high doses of ^{3}H thymidine are given in vitro or in vivo and it is found that only about 10 per cent of the CFU-S are killed. This indicates that the majority of this population was not synthesizing DNA and hence is out of cycle (or in G_0 as represented in Fig. 6). The CFU-S killed increases up to greater than 50 per cent during induced states of proliferation. These findings suggest that the pluripotential hemopoietic stem cell population is primarily a noncycling population that can be triggered into cycle on demand for proliferation. The doubling time for the CFU-S is about 20 to 24 hours.

There is relatively little information about the regulation of the CFU-S. Proliferative capacity, while clearly controlled by demand, is also under genetic control. There are genetically anemic strains of mice in which CFU-S are almost undetectable and no colony formation is detected when marrow from these mice is inoculated into irradiated normal animals. This indicates that the genetic defect lies in the CFU-S and not in the environment. On the other hand, there is another genetic strain of mice in which the opposite situation exists; that is, when the marrow of such mice is grafted into irradiated normal mice it can form colonies, suggesting that the defect in this case is in the marrow environment rather than in the CFU-S. The implications of these models to the problems of human marrow failure become apparent later in this chapter.

Unfortunately, the general regulatory mechanisms involved in the proliferation of CFU-S are ill-understood. What, for example, is the stimulus for the CFU-S to differentiate down any particular pathway? Various models have been proposed. One is based on the observation that if spleen colonies in the irradiated mouse are examined, development is usually restricted to a single cell type at early times after inoculation of the bone marrow but at later times cells of other types appear. This suggests that there may be specific environmental domains that have been called hemopoietic inductive microenvironments, or HIM. In other words, restriction to a single differentiation pathway early in

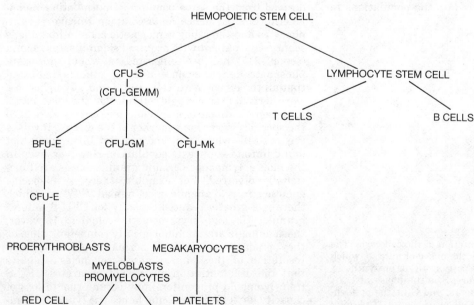

Figure 7. The hemopoietic progenitor cells. The nomenclature is explained in detail in the text.

colony growth might be attributed to the specific area of the spleen in which the CFU-S lodged. However, the validity of this model has been questioned because it is thought that the restriction to a single cell type at early times after inoculation of the bone marrow in the irradiated mouse may be due to seeding by primitive progenitors that are already programmed (see later discussion). Another model suggests that stem cell regulation is achieved by cellular interaction rather than interaction between CFU-S and the local environment. It has also been suggested that the first steps in differentiation result from the appearance of receptors for specific target hormones—for example, erythropoietin. This plethora of models and lack of experimental data underlies our current state of ignorance about these early differentiation steps and about how the stem cell population is controlled with regard to meeting the particular demands of hemopoiesis.

COMMITTED PRECURSOR CELLS

Nothing is known about the critical step that commits a stem cell to differentiation down one particular pathway during hemopoiesis. Presumably after a cell division, at least in the steady state, one daughter cell remains in the stem cell compartment while the other becomes "committed" to a differentiation pathway—otherwise, the stem cell compartment would be depleted. There are increasing data that suggest that there are intermediate stages of differentiation in the committed precursor compartments before recognizable erythroid or granulocyte precursors appear. A brief description of these precursor cells and what little is known about their kinetics follows.

THE ERYTHROPOIETIN-RESPONSIVE CELL

The CFU-S is not responsive to erythropoietin, the hormone that controls erythropoiesis (see p. 189). Using the ^{3}H thymidine "suicide technique," it has been shown that in a steady state the CFU-S is a slowly turning-over population, while the erythropoietin-responsive cell (ERC) is part of a fast-cycling population even in the absence of erythropoietic demand. There seems little doubt that there is a population of erythroid precursor cells that are derived from pluripotent stem cells and that precede the cells that synthesize hemoglobin. This compartment seems to act as an amplifier; that is, it is involved with regulating the numbers of erythroid precursors. It has been suggested that the ERC has cell-age–related compartments, and kinetic experiments indicate that there is a pre- or early ERC population that is interpolated between the pluripotential stem cells and the population that is fully responsive to erythropoietin. Although the pre-ERC's are committed to erythroid differentiation, they cannot respond to erythropoietin by differentiation into recognizable erythroid cells without first having matured during their extensive proliferation. Thus these cells are only susceptible to higher concentrations of erythropoietin than those later ERC precursor cells and respond by increasing the number of proliferative cycles—that is, by amplification of the compartment rather than by differentiation.

Most of the ideas outlined above have been derived from experiments in vivo. Recently it has become possible to define different populations of erythroid precursors that are probably part of the early committed erythroid population. Using either plasma clots or methylcellulose as supporting media it has been possible to grow colonies of these erythroid precursors and erythrocytes after incubation of mouse fetal liver or marrow cells, and, more recently, cells from human fetal or adult bone marrow. The first colonies to appear are small and consist of about 8 to 16 cells; these are usually fully developed after a few days of incubation. After a longer period in culture and at relatively high erythropoietin levels, larger colonies or "bursts" appear that contain up to several thousand cells. The small colonies are called erythropoietin-dependent colony-forming units, or CFU-E (colony-forming units, erythroid), and the progenitors of the bursts are called erythropoietin-dependent burst-forming units, or BFU-E. It seems very likely that the CFU-E are the more differentiated of the two and probably close to proerythroblasts in the differentiation pathway. On the other hand, the BFU-E are probably a much earlier population and may approximate to the pre-ERC compartment as defined above (Fig. 8).

As yet nothing is known about the stimulus for the differentiation of early BFU-E from pluripotential stem cells (CFU-S). Early BFU-E require a factor (or factors) termed burst-promoting activity (BPA) for in vitro growth (Fig. 8). Furthermore, at least under some experimental conditions they require the presence of T cells for their growth in culture. The requirement for BPA, in contrast to erythropoietin, seems to decrease with maturation from early to late BFU-E. To date, BPA activity has not been clearly separated from other factors that promote growth of granulocyte or lymphocyte colonies (see below). There are also doubts about the relevance of agents that enhance the cloning efficiency of CFU-E, such as β-adrenergic agonists, thyroid hormones, growth hormone, and androgenic and nonandrogenic steroids. It is possible that these substances modulate the rate of erythropoiesis, but none of them is capable of replacing erythropoietin in the in vitro colony systems.

THE COMMITTED PROGENITORS OF WHITE CELLS AND PLATELETS

Studies of the development of the granulopoietic pathway were greatly advanced by the finding that murine bone marrow cells maintained in semisolid or viscous media were capable of yielding granulocytic colonies. These "colony-forming units of cells in culture" (CFU-C or CFC-C) have also been found in human bone marrow and peripheral blood. For colony growth of this type a colony-stimulating activity or factor (CSA or CSF) must be incorporated into the culture medium. CSA can be obtained from human urine and in media conditioned by human leukocytes. A variety of studies have shown that CFU-C are different from CFU-S and have confirmed their lineage one from the other.

Evidence is accumulating that a spectrum of in vitro colony-forming cells and colony-stimulating factors may exist (see Fig. 7). This new information has brought with it an increasingly complex nomenclature. Currently, in defining specific progenitors and the

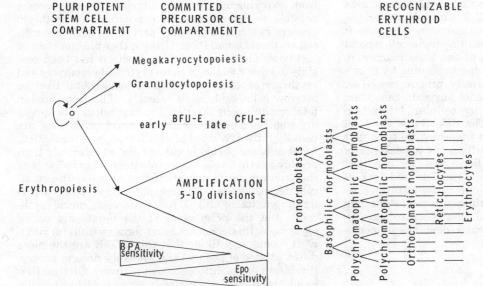

Figure 8. The various precursor populations of erythroid cells. BPA = burst-promoting activity; Epo = erythropoietin.

assay systems used, the abbreviations for colony-forming cell (FC) or unit (FU) are used in conjunction with an abbreviation such as C for in vitro culture and D for diffusion chamber. Furthermore, if possible, the nature of the cell produced in these colonies must also be defined. For example, GM is used to define a granulocyte/macrophage colony (CFU-GM), and the prefix N (for neutrophil) or Eo (eosinophil) can be used if more specific information is available concerning the differentiation potential of the progenitor. Additional abbreviations that have been adopted in this field include Mg or Mk (megakaryocyte), M (macrophage), Mo (monocyte), BL or TL (B or T lymphocyte), MIX or GEMM (mixed morphology), and F (fibroblast).

Very little is known about the humoral regulation of CFU-C. Even in the case of the reasonably well-defined committed precursor of granulocyte/monocyte colonies, the CFU-GM, it is not clear how its particular colony-stimulating factor (GM-CSF) operates—whether it simply increases the numbers and/or speed of cell cycle in the population or whether it increases the rate of differentiation of the pluripotent CFU-S into CFU-C. The concentration of GM-CSF increases in the serum during infection and in response to antigenic stimulation, and when injected in vitro it causes an increase of CFU-C and also a monocytosis and increased granulopoiesis. Unfortunately, many of these observations have been made using CSF preparations from different sources and of varying purity. Recently, a variety of purified preparations of what are apparently different CSF's have been described, but their roles and cell-line specificities remain to be explored further.

There are complex feedback loops in the humoral regulation of granulopoiesis. The monocyte/macrophage population not only produces CSF but also a diffusible inhibitor of CSF action that may be prostaglandin E (PGE). It has been suggested that the monocyte/macrophage populations are functionally heterogeneous with respect to obligatory CSF producers, inducible CSF producers, and PGE producers. These

feedback loops may be further modified by factors produced by mature granulocytes. For example, a glycoprotein, possibly lactoferrin, effectively inhibits CSF production by macrophages.

It appears, therefore, that we are just beginning to sense the complexities of the regulation of hemopoiesis. Recently it has been possible to isolate progenitors for eosinophils, lymphocytes, and megakaryocytes and to demonstrate the existence of pluripotent progenitors (CFU-GEMM, CFU-MIX). Furthermore, it has been possible to make a start at defining at least some of the growth factors that are responsible for the differentiation of various progenitor cells and to obtain pure proteins by recombinant DNA technology. At least four different factors have now been defined: *GM-CSF, interleukin-3 (IL-3), G-CSF,* and *M-CSF.* It appears that IL-3 is indifferent to cell lineage and promotes growth and development of all the different myeloid progenitor cells. In addition, it facilitates self-renewal of pluripotent stem cells and multipotent stem cells. GM-CSF is more restricted, stimulating both proliferation and development of only granulocyte, macrophage, and eosinophil colony-forming cells and the proliferation (but not the subsequent development) of the CFC-MIX. The growth factors G-CSF and M-CSF are more restricted in their activities. With the ability to clone the genes for these different regulatory proteins, and to obtain pure proteins for analysis in cell culture, it should gradually be possible to define the hierarchy of growth factors and other regulatory proteins involved in the different steps of differentiation of the hemopoietic cells.

SUMMARY OF THE EARLY STAGES OF HEMOPOIESIS

In this short section, which has dealt with what is called "hematology without the microscope," it has been seen how limited our knowledge is regarding the properties of stem cells and the populations that are produced in the early stages of the differentiation pathways toward recognizable cell types. Considerable progress has been made in the operational identification of intermediate populations in the early stages of these pathways, although their significance in clinical medicine is not yet clear. What is certain, however, is that the recognizable precursors of the cellular elements of the blood constitute a population that is in the final stages of differentiation and amplification. In other words, hemopoiesis can be looked upon as a two-stage differentiation system, from the pluripotent cells to the committed precursors and from the committed to the recognizable precursors. Each step is followed by maturation as well as by proliferation.

The Pathophysiology of the Red Cell

In the next sections we shall consider the development, structure, and functions of the red cell and the way in which they are altered in disease states. It is possible to understand modern ideas about the pathology of the red cell only if its physiology is fully appreciated.

In describing the physiology of the red cell it is impossible to separate the mature red cells of the peripheral blood from their precursor forms in the bone marrow. For this reason the total circulating red cell mass and its bone marrow precursors are called the "erythron." This term emphasizes the functional unity between all of the red cells, whether fixed in the bone marrow or circulating in the peripheral blood.

ERYTHROPOIESIS

The term "erythropoiesis" is applied to the formation of the erythrocyte population. In considering erythropoiesis in health it is necessary to describe briefly the morphologic and biochemical development of the red cell, how red cell production is controlled, the actions of the factors required for red cell proliferation and maturation, and the normal life-span and mode of destruction of red blood cells.

MORPHOLOGIC AND BIOCHEMICAL DEVELOPMENT OF THE RED CELL

During the early part of this century it was possible to describe the development of the red cell only in terms of the morphologic changes that occur as its precursors mature. More recently, however, some of the biochemical changes that accompany these maturation steps have been characterized. It is important to understand how these morphologic and biochemical maturation steps are related if the abnormalities of red cell maturation are to be fully appreciated.

The nucleated erythroid precursors are derived from the bone-marrow stem-cell pool. In the previous section the early stages of erythropoiesis were described up to the CFU-E. The process is now analyzed at the level of the identifiable red cell precursors in the marrow. The total maturation time of these precursors is approximately five days (Fig. 9). The first two days are spent in cell division; approximately 16 daughter cells are produced from each primitive red cell precursor. During the remaining three days, devoted almost entirely to cellular maturation and hemoglobin synthesis, the nucleus is extruded. After this phase of maturation the red cell precursor, which is called a reticulocyte, remains in the bone marrow for a further 24 hours

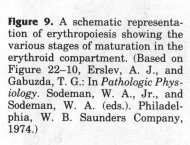

Figure 9. A schematic representation of erythropoiesis showing the various stages of maturation in the erythroid compartment. (Based on Figure 22–10, Erslev, A. J., and Gabuzda, T. G.: In *Pathologic Physiology.* Sodeman, W. A., Jr., and Sodeman, W. A. (eds.). Philadelphia, W. B. Saunders Company, 1974.)

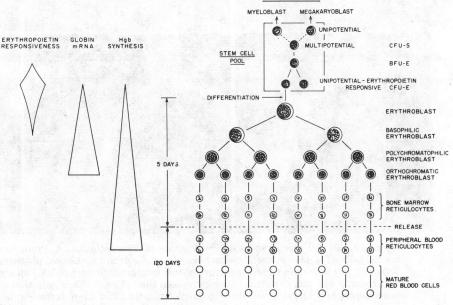

and then is delivered into the peripheral circulation, where it matures to an adult red blood cell in one day. Approximately 1 per cent of the total red cell mass is destroyed during each 24-hour period; therefore, in normal individuals there are a comparable number of reticulocytes delivered daily into the circulation. Thus, approximately 1 per cent of circulating red cells are reticulocytes.

The morphologic appearances of the red cell precursors at different stages of development are summarized in Figure 10. Probably the earliest recognizable form is the basophilic pronormoblast. This is a large cell with a diameter of about 23 μm. The deep-blue staining cytoplasm with Romanowsky stains indicates that there is as yet no hemoglobin present in the cytoplasm. The nuclear chromatin is loosely arranged in fine aggregates and there is a well-marked nucleolus. The next maturation step is the polychromatophilic normoblast, which has an orange-pink cytoplasm, indicating that hemoglobin synthesis has commenced. The nucleus is smaller than the pronormoblast and the chromatin is already starting to clump. By the fourth maturation division the cells are all morphologically at the orthochromatic normoblast phase, in which the cytoplasm is uniformly pink and the nuclear chromatin is becoming highly compressed. The nucleus is then lost from the cell by a process called pyknosis. The next stage of development is the reticulocyte. This cell

contains polyribosomes and some mitochondria. It is just larger than the mature red cell and has a slight diffuse basophilia. On exposure to supravital stains, such as brilliant cresyl blue or methylene blue, the cytoplasmic organelles clump artifactually into a blue-staining reticulum that can be easily recognized by light microscopy. The reticulocyte probably remains in the marrow pool for about 24 hours and then is released into the circulation. During its life span in the marrow and blood it loses its mitochondria and ribosomes and hence its capacity for hemoglobin synthesis. The reticulocytes enter the blood by physical extrusion through gaps in the wall of the marrow sinusoids. As already mentioned, the normal reticulocyte count is approximately 1 per cent of the total circulating red cells and can be expressed either as a percentage or as an absolute value when related to the red cell count.

The orderly maturation cycle described above does not occur without a certain amount of cell loss. It has been estimated that about 10 per cent of the red cell precursors die during their passage through the bone marrow. The reason for this "cellular infant mortality" is not known. This type of failure of maturation of red cell precursors is called "ineffective erythropoiesis." As will be seen later, in certain disorders of red cell maturation the degree of ineffective erythropoiesis is considerably elevated above the normal baseline of 10 per cent.

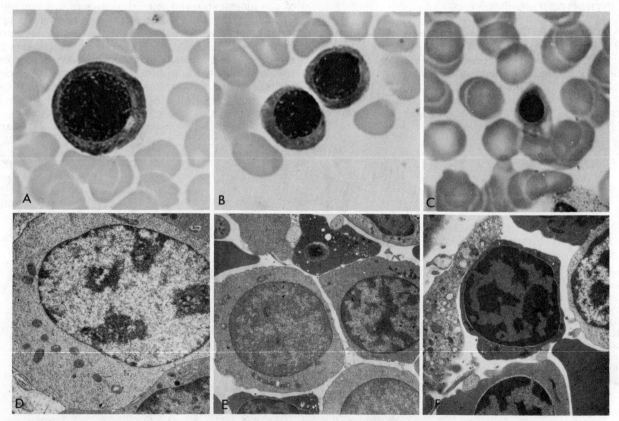

Figure 10. Red cell precursors at different stages of differentiation. *A,* Pronormoblast; *B,* two intermediate normoblasts; *C,* a late pyknotic normoblast; *D,* an electron microscopic photograph of a pronormoblast (× 7500); *E,* an electron microscopic picture of two intermediate normoblasts showing increased condensation of chromatin and more electron dense cytoplasm than *D* (× 5000); *F,* electron microscopic photograph of a later normoblast showing advanced hemoglobinization and even further condensation of chromatin (× 7500).

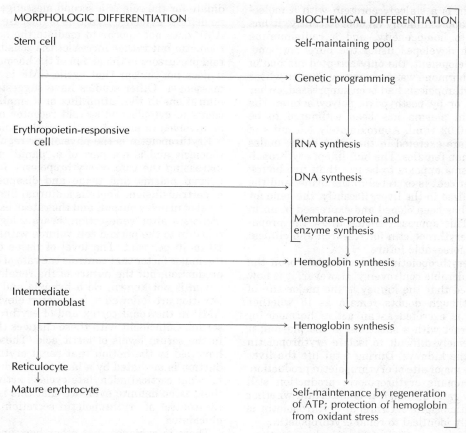

MORPHOLOGIC DIFFERENTIATION

Stem cell

Erythropoietin-responsive
cell

Intermediate
normoblast

Reticulocyte

Mature erythrocyte

BIOCHEMICAL DIFFERENTIATION

Self-maintaining pool

Genetic programming

RNA synthesis

DNA synthesis

Membrane-protein and
enzyme synthesis

Hemoglobin synthesis

Hemoglobin synthesis

Self-maintenance by regeneration
of ATP; protection of hemoglobin
from oxidant stress

Figure 11. Schematic representation of the relationship between morphologic and biochemical differentiation in erythropoiesis.

The well-characterized morphologic changes of red cell maturation are accompanied by important changes in the chemistry of the red cell precursors (Fig. 11). The precursors have well-formed Golgi apparatus and mitochondria. They are capable of DNA, RNA, and protein synthesis together with oxidative metabolism. At approximately the polychromatophilic normoblast stage, DNA and RNA synthesis ceases. By this time nearly all nonhemoglobin protein synthesis is complete, and thus the red cells are fully equipped with their various enzyme systems and surface antigens. Since RNA synthesis has ceased, all subsequent protein synthesis must use preformed messenger RNA, and the amount of protein produced depends on the stability of these messenger molecules. The later stages of development are given over almost entirely to hemoglobin synthesis. When the nucleus is extruded, the reticulocyte, which still contains polysomes and mitochondria, can synthesize protein and heme and has some oxidative capacity. After further maturation the mitochondria and RNA are lost and the cell is then able to metabolize glucose only through the Embden-Meyerhof pathway and hexose-monophosphate shunt. Although this seems to be an extremely simple and unsophisticated biochemistry with which to go out into the rough world of the peripheral circulation, as discussed later, it is beautifully suited to the needs of the circulating red cell.

It is clear, therefore, that there is a well-defined relationship between morphologic and biochemical changes during the erythroid maturation cycle.

THE REGULATION OF ERYTHROPOIESIS

The rate of erythropoiesis in health is regulated so that the loss of 1 per cent of red cells per day is made up by a comparable production of reticulocytes. Clearly there must be a highly adaptable regulatory mechanism so that there is the possibility of increasing or decreasing the output of red cells, depending on the oxygen requirements of the tissues.

The rate of erythropoiesis is governed by the rate of oxygen transport to the tissues. Tissue oxygenation depends on many factors, including the oxyhemoglobin concentration of the blood, the cardiac output, and the ease with which the blood gives up its oxygen to the tissues. These complicated interactions are considered in the later discussion of anemia. Here it is important to concentrate on the fundamental question of what is the effector that "informs" the bone marrow to modify its rate of erythropoiesis, depending on the state of oxygenation of the tissues.

The idea that there might be a humoral intermediary for the hypoxic stimulus to erythropoiesis was proved to be correct by Reismann. He took a pair of parabiotic rats—that is, animals in which a common circulation had been produced surgically—and showed that if one of the pair was maintained in a hypoxic atmosphere both animals showed stimulation of erythropoiesis. This indicated that a hormone produced in the hypoxic animal had crossed the joined circulation and stimulated the bone marrow of its partner. This hormone was later called erythropoietin or erythropoiesis-stimulating factor (ESF).

Erythropoietin is a sialoglycoprotein with a molecular weight of approximately 33,000. Recently, it has been purified to homogeneity, and a radioimmune assay has been developed using the pure hormone. Before this development, the only accepted method of measuring the hormone was by bioassay in mice whose endogenous erythropoiesis had been suppressed, either by transfusion or by posthypoxic polycythemia. The concentration in plasma has been estimated to be approximately 0.02 U/ml. Approximately 4.0 units of erythropoietin are excreted in the urine daily; males excrete more than females. The half-life of erythropoietin in the plasma appears to be less than five hours; less than 10 per cent is excreted in the urine, and the bulk is metabolized in the liver. Recently, the gene for erythropoietin has been cloned and expressed in an in vitro system. This approach should allow the preparation of pure erythropoietin for research and clinical use within the forseeable future.

The site of erythropoietin production has been the subject of considerable controversy. However, it is now generally agreed that the kidney is the major site of production, although doubts remain as to whether erythropoietin is excreted as an active hormone or must first interact with a substrate in the plasma; it has been extremely difficult to isolate erythropoietin directly from the kidneys. During fetal life the liver seems to be the major site of erythropoietin production. In anephric humans erythropoietin production still occurs at a low rate, although it is uncertain whether this is of hepatic origin. Extrarenal erythropoietin is immunologically identical to renal erythropoietin.

How does erythropoietin act to stimulate erythropoiesis? Erythropoietin does not act on the stem cell population but on the committed red cell compartment. There appears to be an increasing sensitivity to erythropoietin during the maturation of the red cell progenitor populations, BFU-E and CFU-E. Whether this reflects the appearance of specific receptors during maturation of these populations has not yet been determined. Many actions of the hormone have been demonstrated, including an increased rate of hemoglobin synthesis in developing erythroblasts, stimulation of nonhemoglobin protein synthesis, and an increased rate of transit of the red cell precursors through their maturation cycle and release into the peripheral blood. In red cell precursors exposed to erythropoietin, RNA synthesis increases within 15 minutes. Initially, this increase is in a very large (150S) RNA species, which may represent messenger RNA precursors. Subsequently, increases in ribosomal, transfer, and globin messenger RNA can be demonstrated. These changes are accompanied by a sequential elevation of RNA polymerases II and I and by an increased rate of nonhistone protein synthesis. Although increased DNA synthesis also occurs, it usually follows the stimulation of RNA synthesis. Furthermore, inhibition of DNA synthesis does not block erythropoietin-induced stimulation of RNA production. On the other hand, inhibition of RNA synthesis blocks erythropoietin-dependent increase in DNA formation. Thus it appears that the primary action of the hormone is to stimulate RNA synthesis. It could act either by entering the cell or indirectly through an intermediate intracellular messenger. Available evidence suggests that the second model is more likely. Cyclic AMP is an obvious candidate for the role of a second messenger, but there is no definite evidence that this is the case. In fact, cyclic AMP does not appear to mediate the action of erythropoietin but rather increases the sensitivity of erythroid precursors to the action of the hormone. Similarly, it does not appear that cyclic GMP is the secondary messenger. Other studies have suggested that either alterations in the cation flux or a small protein analogous to cytoplasmic steroid receptor molecules may be involved in mediating the erythropoietin response.

Erythropoietin is the physiologic regulator of erythropoiesis and is not part of a "panic" mechanism for increasing the rate of erythropoiesis. It is present in normal plasma and urine and disappears following hypertransfusion. There is a diurnal fluctuation in the level of urinary output, and the rate of excretion, which increases after venesection, bears a logarithmic relationship to the packed cell volume within the range of 20 to 40 per cent. The level of tissue oxygenation is the major factor that controls the rate of erythropoietin production, but the nature of the renal sensing mechanism is not known. Both hypoxia and cobalt administration are followed by sequential elevations of cyclic AMP in the renal cortex and of erythropoietin in the serum. Coincident with these changes there are peaks in the serum levels of lactic acid. These observations have led to the notion that renal erythropoietin production is mediated by a lactic acid-induced alteration in renal cortical adenylate cyclase activity. However, there is no definite evidence that this is the case, and the control of erythropoietin secretion remains to be elucidated.

There is evidence that other hormones and related agents affect red cell production. It has been possible to study the effect of these agents on the plating efficiency and growth of erythroid progenitor colonies in vitro. Corticosteroids, androgens, growth hormone, thyroid hormone, β adrenergic agonists, cyclic AMP, and certain prostaglandins all have a stimulatory effect on erythroid colony production. The existence of receptors for these agents on red cell progenitors suggests a mechanism whereby modulation of response of the erythroid cells to erythropoietin may be mediated. These observations suggest a possible mechanism for the hematologic changes seen in a disorder such as hyperthyroidism.

It is clear, therefore, that despite the many gaps in our knowledge about the mode of action of erythropoietin and other hormones involved in the control of erythropoiesis, a general picture of how the erythron works can be put together (Fig. 12). The oxygen content of arterial blood is the primary determinant of erythropoietin production. This is seen quite clearly from the response obtained when a normal individual receives a transfusion to a high hemoglobin level; erythropoietin production falls below a measurable level. On the other hand, after repeated phlebotomy urinary erythropoietin levels increase exponentially. Similarly, when arterial-blood oxygen saturation is decreased by ascent to high altitudes, erythropoietin production increases and a predictable increase in red cell production occurs. It appears, therefore, that there are renal sensors that in the face of a fall in oxygen content of arterial blood increase erythropoietin output and stimulate red cell production until the arterial oxygen content reaches normal levels. This beautifully bal-

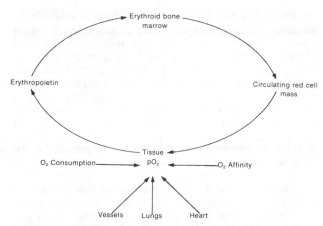

Figure 12. The factors involved in the regulation of erythropoiesis.

anced mechanism also may be modified by many factors that alter the oxygen content of the arterial blood and the availability of oxygen to the tissues. These include such central factors as cardiac output and pulmonary function as well as the rate of dissociation of oxygen from the hemoglobin of red cells (Fig. 12).

Erythropoietin stimulation of erythropoiesis produces certain well-defined cellular changes. Because of the shortened marrow transit time, and hence the skipping of late maturation divisions, polychromatic macrocytes appear in the peripheral blood and there is an accompanying reticulocytosis. The dense-staining macrocytes are called "shift," or "stress," cells. The bone marrow shows evidence of increased proliferation and differentiation of erythroid precursors with a shift of the myeloid:erythroid ratio, normally 3:1, toward unity. A third effect of increased proliferation is expansion of erythroid bone marrow tissue down the shafts of the long bones—a reversion to the fetal sites of erythropoiesis. All of these changes are seen in disease states in which there is an increased rate of red cell production.

FACTORS REQUIRED FOR NORMAL ERYTHROPOIESIS

The main factors required for normal erythropoiesis are summarized in Table 9. Before describing the pathophysiology of anemias caused by deficiencies of these substances, it is necessary to describe briefly their mechanisms of absorption and metabolism and actions in red cell production.

Iron. Iron is a vital nutritional requirement for normal erythropoiesis. It is required for hemoglobin synthesis but also seems to directly affect the rate of erythroid proliferation. In a normal adult, of the approximately 25 mg of iron used daily for erythropoiesis about 95 per cent is derived from hemoglobin degradation, and the remainder is iron absorbed from the gastrointestinal tract and from the body iron stores.

The total body iron content of a normal adult varies between 2 and 6 g, depending on body size and hemoglobin level. Approximately 2½ g of iron are present in the circulating hemoglobin and 1 g is present in the iron stores. The rest is distributed among the iron-containing tissue enzymes, the plasma, and myoglobin (Table 10). The two iron storage compounds, ferritin and hemosiderin, are found mainly in the reticuloendothelial cells of the liver, spleen, and bone marrow, where iron is released after hemoglobin breakdown. The storage compounds form a reserve of iron that can be mobilized when body requirements are increased. They are also found in liver parenchymal cells, which provide the main buffer from any excess iron in the body and hold the bulk of ferritin iron present in the liver.

Ferritin is a large molecule consisting of a protein shell that encloses an iron core. The ferritin apoprotein has a molecular weight of 450,000 and is composed of 24 identical subunits, each with a molecular weight of about 18,500. The latter form an almost spherical shell, which encloses a central core that contains up to 4500 iron atoms in the form of iron hydroxyphosphate. Isoelectric focussing studies of ferritin indicate that there is heterogeneity between tissues. Human liver and spleen have a range of isoferritins with isoelectric points between 5.3 and 5.8; heart isoferritin is in the range of 4.8 to 5.2. Ferritin synthesis in red cell precursors and reticuloendothelial storage cells is stimulated by increasing iron concentrations, and degradation occurs when no iron is incorporated. Hemosiderin appears to be a degraded form of ferritin in which the protein shells have partly disintegrated, thus allowing the iron cores to aggregate.

Before examining the factors that control the delicate balance between iron intake and loss in health it is necessary to examine briefly the various steps of

TABLE 9. FACTORS REQUIRED FOR HEMOPOIESIS*

Iron	Riboflavin
Vitamin B$_{12}$	Vitamin E
Folate	Amino acids and protein
Pyridoxine (vitamin B$_6$)	Trace metals Cu, Mn, Co, Zn
Ascorbic acid	

*In clinical practice, anemia is usually associated with iron-, vitamin B$_{12}$- or folate deficiency. The consequences of pyridoxine-, ascorbic acid- or vitamin E deficiency are considered in the text. Anemia due to trace metal deficiency must be exceedingly rare in man. In gross malnutrition—for example, kwashiorkor—protein deficiency may contribute to the anemia. Occasional cases of anemia responsive to other B vitamins, such as pantothenic acid and niacin, have been reported.

TABLE 10. DISTRIBUTION OF IRON IN A 70-kg MAN*

PROTEIN	TISSUE	TOTAL IRON (mg)
Hemoglobin	Red cells	2600
Myoglobin	Muscle	400
Mitochondrial cytochromes	All tissues	17
Microsomal cytochromes	Liver	2–4
Catalase	Liver and red cells	5
Transferrin	Plasma	8
Nonheme iron (ferritin and hemosiderin)	Liver	410
	Spleen	48
	Kidney	11
	Muscle	730
	Marrow	300
	Brain	60

*Modified from Jacobs, A.: In Hardisty, R. M., and Weatherall, D. J. (eds.): Blood and Its Disorders. 2nd ed. Oxford, Blackwell Scientific Publications, 1982.

iron metabolism. These can be divided into absorption, transport, utilization, and storage.

ABSORPTION. Dietary iron can be divided into two main groups consisting of heme iron compounds and inorganic iron. Although iron can be absorbed from any part of the gut, the process is most efficient in the duodenum and becomes progressively less so further down the alimentary canal (Fig. 13).

Heme iron, derived mainly from animal foods, is relatively efficiently absorbed, being taken up directly by mucosal cells. Within the cells the iron is released by the action of the enzyme heme oxygenase. By contrast, the availability of nonheme iron, which constitutes a much greater proportion of food iron in most diets, is greatly affected by other dietary constituents and by gastrointestinal secretions. In the alkaline medium of the upper small bowel iron precipitates as ferric hydroxide complexes and is unavailable for absorption unless kept in solution as a complex with proteins or organic acids. Among the lumenal factors that influence nonheme iron absorption, hydrochloric acid in gastric secretions is most important for solubilizing nonheme iron. Patients with iron deficiency anemia and normal acid secretion absorb more ferric iron from a test dose than those with achlorhydria, and in subjects with complete achlorhydria absorption is greater when iron is administered with hydrochloric acid. A variety of other inhibitory and enhancing substances are present in different foods. For example, phytates and phosphates form complexes with iron and retard absorption, while reducing substances such as ascorbate, lactate, pyruvate, and cysteine help to keep iron in the more soluble ferrous form and hence available for absorption. Alcohol enhances absorption, though the mechanism is unknown. Since foods of animal origin both contain more heme iron and on digestion yield products that enhance the solubility and availability of nonheme iron components of the diet, iron is much more efficiently absorbed from diets that contain meat than from vegetarian diets. These considerations are particularly important when considering iron balance in the developing countries.

Besides the intraluminal factors affecting iron absorption, the intestinal mucosal cell plays a major role in iron balance. These are specific receptors for iron on the brush border of the mucosal cell, though the form in which the iron is presented to them is unclear. In addition, it is suggested that a mechanism exists whereby the mucosal cells trap iron when the iron stores are replete and allow iron through into the circulation in the states of iron depletion. Radio-iron labeling studies suggest that iron remaining in the mucosal cell is incorporated into ferritin. The shedding of iron-loaded endothelial cells may be a mechanism whereby inappropriate iron absorption is prevented in the presence of adequate body iron supplies. There may be an intracellular iron carrier in mucosal cells, although the relationship of this protein to the regulation of iron absorption is not clear. Similar uncertainties exist about the mechanism of the delivery of iron from the mucosal cell to transferrin in the plasma. Iron release from isolated perfused epithelial cells is enhanced by the addition of apotransferrin to the medium. However, even in the absence of transferrin, rapid transfer of iron from isolated duodenal loops to the perfusion medium occurs. Transfer from the intestinal lumen to plasma may require the formation of low molecular weight iron chelates whose progress across the cell depends on interactions with intracellular ligands or macromolecules.

A variety of other factors influence iron absorption. It is increased by hypoxia, anemia, depletion of iron stores, and increased erythropoiesis and is reduced by hypertransfusion.

TRANSPORT. Having crossed the intestinal mucosa, iron is bound in the ferric form to a specific iron-binding protein called transferrin, a β-globulin with a molecular weight of 80,000. Transferrin has two iron-binding sites; the functional significance of these sites is still not clear. Transferrin synthesis occurs mainly in the liver, although it is produced in low amounts in many tissues. The mechanisms regulating the level of circulating transferrin are not known. Transferrin levels increase in iron deficiency and in pregnancy, while low levels are found in states of iron overload and acute and chronic inflammation. The normal concentration of iron in plasma is about 100 μg/100 ml. Normally, transferrin can bind about 300 μg/100 ml. This is called the iron binding capacity of plasma. Thus, transferrin is usually about 30 per cent saturated.

Although only about 4 mg of iron is present in the plasma at any time, the daily turnover is about 30 mg.

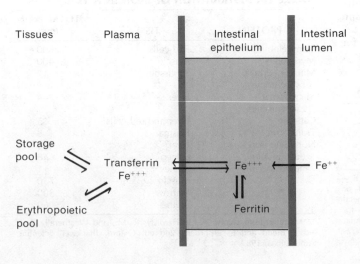

Figure 13. Iron absorption.

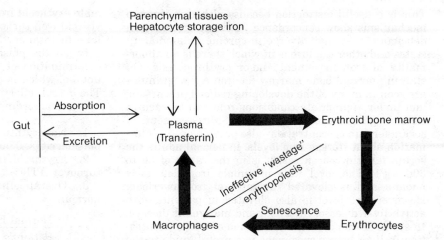

Figure 14. The various iron compartments and pools.

Most of the iron entering the plasma is released from reticuloendothelial cells following the breakdown of time-expired red cells. Smaller amounts enter the plasma from intestinal absorption, from mobilization of storage iron, and from parenchymal iron pools (Fig. 14). Iron is removed from the circulation mainly by the erythron, but, as shown in Figure 14, some is taken up by the parenchymal tissues in an amount that depends on the transferrin saturation; as the saturation rises so does the amount of iron entering the parenchymal iron stores. This mechanism has important implications in states of iron overload.

It is apparent, therefore, that transport iron represents a tiny fraction of the total body iron and that it is in a dynamic state, its concentration varying rapidly according to particular requirements. Its level also shows a significant diurnal variation.

UTILIZATION. Since about 1 per cent of the circulating red cells are broken down each day, approximately 20 to 25 mg of iron is liberated from hemoglobin catabolism. This is almost the amount of iron required for hemoglobin synthesis in normal circumstances. It is transported to the developing red cell precursors attached to transferrin. Transferrin binds to specific receptors on the red cell-precursor membranes. The structure of the transferrin receptor is now known. The protein is approximately 180,000 molecular weight and is composed of two equal subunits. Recent studies suggest that iron movement into cells involves the internalization of transferrin and its receptor by means of membrane vesicles in which iron is released and rapidly incorporated into cytosolic ferritin. After iron is released, apotransferrin present in the vesicle is recycled to the exterior of the cell. Iron release within the vesicles seems to be pH dependent. Iron that is not utilized for hemoglobin synthesis is incorporated into ferritin and hence into hemosiderin, which can be seen as small cytoplasmic aggregates in normal red cell precursors; cells of this type are called *sideroblasts*. Iron in this form remains in the red cell precursors during their maturation cycle. Once these cells lose their nucleus they are called *siderocytes*. At least some of the iron granules appear to be removed from the red cells during their passage through the spleen; siderocytes appear in the peripheral blood only in splenectomized individuals.

IRON BALANCE. Clearly iron hemostasis is delicately balanced (Table 11). In health only 1 to 2 mg of iron is absorbed each day, and this amount can be doubled in iron deficient states or in the presence of increased rates of erythropoiesis. In males, approximately 1 mg of iron is lost each day through the skin and mucous membranes. Females lose on average an additional 1 mg per day through menstruation, and in pregnancy require an additional 2 mg per day for the needs of the fetus and placenta. Normally about 5 to 10 per cent of dietary iron is absorbed. If the daily average iron content of a Western diet is about 13.5 mg, it should not be difficult for a male with normal iron losses to stay in iron balance. Clearly, the situation in females is much more precarious. These simple calculations explain much about the pathophysiology of iron metabolism. There is a delicate balance between intake and output, and if there are increased requirements, if the diet is deficient in iron, or if there is an increased rate of loss of iron through bleeding, a state of negative iron balance may easily follow. On the other hand, the body has no means of removing excess iron. Therefore, in individuals who are receiving blood transfusions or who have increased gastrointestinal iron absorption there is a gradual accumulation of iron in the body. The significance of these observations in various clinical disorders becomes apparent later in this chapter.

ASSESSMENT OF IRON STATUS. In assessing iron status it is useful to make the distinction between supply, which is assessed by the plasma iron level and transferrin saturation, and the iron stores, which can be estimated by staining the bone marrow for iron or indirectly by determining the plasma ferritin level.

TABLE 11. IRON BALANCE*

INTAKE	LOSSES
10–30 mg in diet	1 mg (stool, skin, hair, etc.)
1–3 mg absorbed	1 mg/day average over month for menstrual losses in females

*From these figures it is clear that, assuming a 10% absorption, an average daily intake of 10 mg of iron is required by the adult male and 20 mg by a menstruating female. A normal pregnancy uses about 900 mg iron. During this time, about 280 mg of iron is conserved owing to cessation of menses, leaving a debit of about 600 mg iron or an additional requirement of 2 mg iron per day throughout pregnancy. Many pregnant women cannot maintain an intake of 3 mg of iron from diet alone and require iron supplements.

These figures indicate that normal iron balance is precarious and that even small, regular blood loss or excessive menstrual loss will lead to a negative iron balance.

This is a useful distinction because although the two mechanisms show concordance in states of true iron deficiency, they may diverge in chronic inflammatory states and other conditions in which there is an abnormality of iron movement and/or erythropoiesis. On staining normal bone marrow for iron a few granules are seen in many of the developing red cell precursors, and under appropriate conditions iron can be seen in the storage elements of the marrow. Measurements of serum ferritin concentrations also provide useful information about storage iron levels. In normal adults the serum ferritin concentration is in the range of 50 to 300 μg/1. The level falls in simple iron deficiency anemia and is elevated in states of iron overload. However, the level is also elevated in patients with active liver disease, infection, and malignant disease. In states of iron overload estimation of iron concentration in liver biopsy specimens is a useful guide to the response of therapy. The practical value of these measurements is considered later in the chapter.

FERROKINETICS. The measurement of iron kinetics as an indicator of iron utilization and the level of erythropoiesis is useful as a research tool and occasionally for the assessment of marrow function in clinical disorders (Fig. 15).

As shown in Figure 14, internal iron exchange is normally dominated by the cycle between plasma transferrin, erythroid marrow, and the breakdown of senescent red cells in the macrophages that release their iron to plasma transferrin. This means that if transferrin-bound radioiron is injected the plasma iron turnover in normal subjects mainly reflects the activity of the erythroid marrow. The iron turnover per unit of whole blood can be derived from the initial clearance of transferrin-bound ^{59}Fe (assumed to be a single exponential), the plasma iron level, and the hematocrit. Thus, PIT is

$$\frac{\text{Plasma iron} \times (1 - \text{Hct} \times 0.9)}{\text{T}^{1/2}\,^{59}\text{Fe}}$$

mg iron/dl whole blood/24 hours.

In early studies the 14-day utilization by red cells of ^{59}Fe was used to calculate the fraction of the total plasma iron turnover that was contributing to erythroid iron turnover—in normal people about 80 per cent of the plasma iron turnover. This approach has proved inadequate, particularly in pathologic red cell production, since not all the radioiron taken up by the erythron during the initial clearance of the labeled transferrin is released as circulating hemoglobin within red cells. This is because even in normal people there is some degree of ineffective erythropoiesis, which short-circuits the radioiron directly to macrophages (see Fig. 14). The major unresolved problem in ferrokinetics is quantification of the degree of this reflux and hence the relative level of effective and ineffective erythropoiesis. One approach to this question involves a detailed computer analysis of plasma radioiron levels over 14 days. The difficulty with this method is that there is no way of knowing how much radioiron, generated by ineffective erythropoiesis and taken up by macrophages, remains in these cells rather than being released to circulating transferrin in which it can be detected. Thus this approach may underesti-

mate erythroid iron turnover and overestimate nonerythroid iron turnover. A simpler approach is to calculate the total erythroid iron turnover as the difference between the plasma iron turnover and an empirical determination of the parenchymal nonerythroid iron uptake, which is dependent on the plasma iron level. The overall effectiveness of erythropoiesis can then be assessed according to the following formulas:

1. Nonerythroid iron turnover = plasma iron × plasmacrit × 0.0035
2. Erythroid iron turnover (EIT) = plasma iron turnover (PIT) − non-EIT
3. Overall efficiency of erythropoiesis (fraction of normal) =

$$\frac{\text{Normal EIT*}}{\text{Patient's EIT}} \times \frac{\text{Patient's hematocrit}}{45}$$

Vitamin B$_{12}$. In 1926, Minot and Murphy observed that it was possible to treat pernicious anemia by feeding raw liver. In 1929, Castle discovered that the intestinal absorption of the anti–pernicious-anemia principle of liver, which he called extrinsic factor (vitamin B$_{12}$), depended on its first being bound to a factor secreted by the gastric mucosa, which he called intrinsic factor. Further developments included the identification of the chemical structure of vitamin B$_{12}$ and the elucidation of its mechanism of action.

Vitamin B$_{12}$ is synthesized only in certain microorganisms. Animals depend on microbial synthesis for their vitamin B$_{12}$ supply. Human foods that contain the vitamin are of animal origin (meat, liver, fish, eggs, and milk). The average daily diet in Western countries contains 5 to 30 μg of vitamin B$_{12}$, of which 1 to 5 μg is absorbed. The total body stores of the vitamin in adults range from 2 to 5 mg, of which approximately 1 mg is found in the liver. The daily dietary requirement is about 2 to 3 μg. Hence, after stopping intake of vitamin B$_{12}$, or after total gastrectomy, it takes several years to deplete the body stores and for the symptoms of vitamin B$_{12}$ deficiency to develop.

The structure of vitamin B$_{12}$, or cyanocobalamin, was elucidated in 1955 by the x-ray crystallographic analysis of Dorothy Hodgkin. The vitamin B$_{12}$ molecule (Fig. 16) consists of two main parts: (1) a planar group, a ring structure surrounding the cobalt atom, that resembles the porphyrin ring of heme except for a bond linking two pyrrole rings directly together instead of through a bridging carbon atom—this structure is called a corrin ring; and (2) a nucleotide group containing the base 5,6 dimethylbenzimidazolyl and phosphorylated ribose esterified with 1 amino, 2 propranol. Finally, a cyanide group is carried by the trivalent cobalt atom, which is also linked to the benzimidazole base. The term vitamin B$_{12}$ may be used to describe cyanocobalamin, although it is often used to include other forms of the vitamin in which the –CN is replaced by another side group. In nature, vitamin B$_{12}$ exists largely as the two forms, methylcobalamin and 5′deoxyadenosylcobalamin. These are labile and are converted to a fourth form of vitamin B$_{12}$, hydroxycobalamin. Both cyanocobalamin and hydroxycobalamin are used therapeutically.

---

*0.5 mg/dl blood/24 hours.

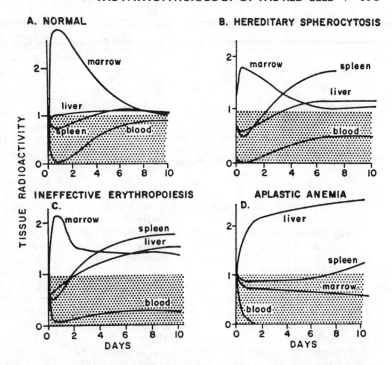

A. NORMAL

B. HEREDITARY SPHEROCYTOSIS

INEFFECTIVE ERYTHROPOIESIS

APLASTIC ANEMIA

Figure 15. Ferrokinetic studies in health and disease. The abscissa value of 1 represents the level of radioactivity immediately after injection of ^{59}Fe. The blood curve reflects the reappearance of incorporated isotope in circulating red cells. If red cell iron utilization reached 100 per cent, the curve would reach the 1 level again. *A,* Normal pattern; rapid uptake of iron into the marrow and appearance of isotope in hemoglobin. *B,* The pattern in hemolytic anemia; rapid uptake into the marrow and redelivery of isotope but less than 60 per cent of injected iron appears in the red cells because of splenic destruction of newly formed cells. *C,* Ineffective erythropoiesis; rapid marrow uptake but poor delivery with less than 40 per cent iron utilization because of death of red cell precursors in the bone marrow. The other curves suggest splenic uptake of newly produced cells and liver uptake of isotope because of high serum iron. *D,* Aplastic anemia; no marrow uptake with no utilization in hemoglobin synthesis. The isotope is deposited in liver cells. (From Finch, C. A., et al.: Medicine 49:17, 1970.)

Dietary vitamin B_{12} is released from protein and peptide complexes in the stomach, where it attaches to both intrinsic factor and a second vitamin B_{12} binding protein called R-binder. Intrinsic factor is a glycoprotein that contains 15 per cent carbohydrate and is

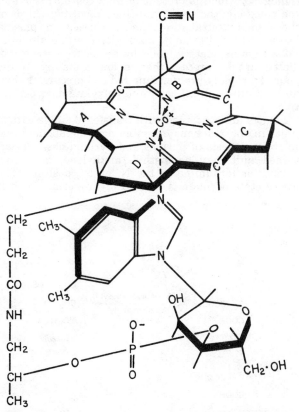

Figure 16. The structure of vitamin B_{12}. (From Hoffbrand, A.V.: In Hardisty, R. M., and Weatherall, D. J. (eds.): Blood and Its Disorders. Oxford, Blackwell Scientific Publications, 1974.)

secreted by the parietal cells of the body and the fundus of the stomach. One molecule of intrinsic factor binds to one molecule of vitamin B_{12} in the region of the edge of the corrin ring. The R-protein is degraded by pancreatic secretions and the vitamin B_{12} released binds to further intrinsic factor. This step is impaired in patients with pancreatic disease, leading to reduced vitamin B_{12} absorption. The normal site of absorption appears to be the distal ileum. It is possible to absorb up to 1.5 μg of vitamin B_{12} from a single oral dose of intrinsic factor–vitamin B_{12} complex. Following absorption, the ileum is refractory to further vitamin B_{12} absorption for several hours. At a neutral pH and in the presence of calcium ions, intrinsic factor–vitamin B_{12} complex passively attaches to receptor sites on the brush borders of the ileal mucosa. It then enters the mucosal cell, where it is found in the cytosol. After exit from the ileal enterocyte, vitamin B_{12} is attached to a second major vitamin B_{12} transport protein (transcobalamin II, see below) which is synthesized in the ileal cells. Thereafter, the vitamin is transferred to the portal blood, the peak blood level being reached only 8 to 12 hours after an oral dose. Intrinsic factor does not enter the portal blood and its fate is not absolutely clear. Only about 1 per cent of an oral dose of the order of 30 to 300 μg of vitamin B_{12} is absorbed in the absence of intrinsic factor. This form of absorption occurs throughout the gut by simple passive means.

Vitamin B_{12} is transported on specific binding proteins called *transcobalamins (TC),* of which three forms, TCI, II, and III, have been isolated. TCII is the main delivery protein that transports cobalamins to tissues such as marrow and in the nervous system. It is synthesized by a variety of cells, including macrophages, ileal enterocytes, and the liver. The TCII-vitamin B_{12} complex attaches to a receptor site on the surface of various target cells and is internalized by pinocytosis. TCII is essential for vitamin uptake by cells, and in its absence a severe vitamin B_{12} deficiency state develops. The functions of TC's I and III, which

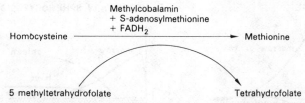

Figure 17. The role of vitamin B_{12} in homocysteine and methionine metabolism. (From Hoffbrand, A. V.: In *Blood and its Disorders*. Hardisty, R. M., and Weatherall, D. J. (eds.). Oxford, Blackwell Scientific Publications, 1974.)

are probably produced by leukocytes, are unknown. The TC levels vary in a variety of disease states. As might be expected, TCI levels rise markedly in various forms of granulocytic leukemia and other myeloproliferative diseases and also during the leukocytosis of infection. Increased TCII levels are observed in liver disease and pregnancy.

The metabolic functions of vitamin B_{12} are only understood in three well-defined reactions. One is the conversion of homocysteine to methionine, as shown in Figure 17. The enzyme involved is homocysteine-methionine methyl transferase, and the reaction requires 5-methyl tetrahydrofolate as a methyl donor, S-adenosylmethionine, and the reducing agent (FADH2) as well as methyl-B_{12} as a coenzyme. Vitamin B_{12}-dependent methionine synthesis is important in the regeneration of tetrahydrofolate from methyltetrahydrofolate. The second reaction involving vitamin B_{12}, as deoxyadenosylcobalamin, is the conversion of propionate to succinate, as shown in Figure 18. This reaction is part of the route by which cholesterol and odd-chain fatty acids as well as a number of amino acids and thymine are used for energy requirements via the Krebs cycle. Patients with vitamin B_{12} deficiency may excrete excess methylmalonic acid. Finally, vitamin B_{12} is involved in the isomerization of β-leucine to α-leucine; in vitamin B_{12} deficiency β-leucine accumulates while α-leucine is decreased. The interrelationships between vitamin B_{12} and folate metabolism in the synthesis of DNA are considered later—it is this function of vitamin B_{12} that undoubtedly accounts for the megaloblastic erythropoiesis and related phenomenon of abnormal DNA synthesis found in

vitamin B_{12} deficiency states. Vitamin B_{12} is also essential for the function of metabolic pathways in the central nervous system.

Folate. Folic acid, or pteroylmonoglutamic acid, is the parent compound of a large family of compounds known collectively as the folates. The molecule consists of three parts: (1) a pteridine derivative, (2) a para-amino benzoic acid residue, and (3) a L-glutamic acid residue (Fig. 19A). Folic acid occurs naturally as conjugates in which multiple glutamic acid residues are attached by gamma peptide linkages to the glutamic acid. Pteroylmonoglutamate is usually referred to as pteroylglutamate. Higher conjugates are termed pteroyl-diglutamate, pteroyl-triglutamate, and so on, or pteroyl-polyglutamates.

Folates are present in virtually all foods, the highest concentrations being found in liver, green vegetables, chocolate, and nuts. They are easily destroyed by cooking. Adults require about 100 μg of folate daily. The total body stores are from 6 to 20 mg and are found mainly in the liver. This store is sufficient for only a few months and clinical folate deficiency occurs in about four months on a diet completely lacking in folate.

Folate absorption occurs mainly through the duodenum and jejunum. All folates enter the portal blood as a single compound, 5-methyltetrahydrofolate. At least three reactions are required to convert the natural forms of folate in foods to this compound: (1) deconjugation, (2) reduction, and (3) methylation. Deconjugation is brought about by an enzyme folate conjugase, which is present in high concentrations in the mucosa of the small intestine. About two-thirds of the 5-methyltetrahydrofolate is carried in plasma loosely attached to an α_2 macroglobulin and albumin. Folate enters marrow cells by an active carrier-mediated uptake process that is found mainly in the younger, rapidly proliferating red cell precursors. Folate is built up in all cells into polyglutamate derivatives.

Folates are concerned with transfer of single carbon units in the reactions of amino acid metabolism and in the synthesis of purines and pyrimidines. The attached unit may be methyl, methylene, methenyl, formyl, or formimino at the N_5 or N_{10} position. The active state of folate is the tetrahydro-form, which is

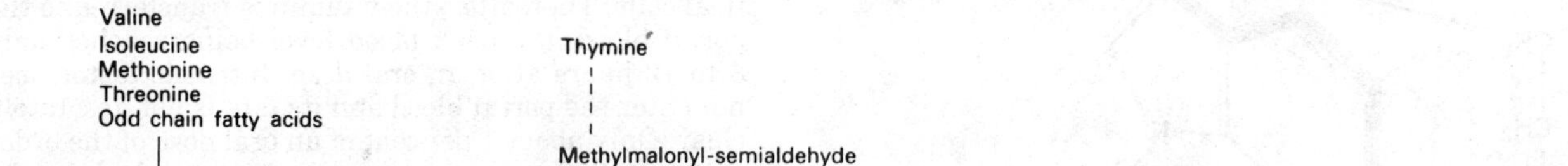

Figure 18. The metabolic interactions of propionyl CoA and succinyl CoA and the role of vitamin B_{12}. (From Hoffbrand, A. V.: In *Blood and Its Disorders*. Hardisty, R. M., and Weatherall, D. J. (eds.). Oxford, Blackwell Scientific Publications, 1974.)

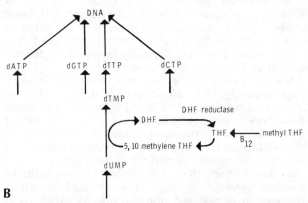

Folic acid (pteroylglutamic acid)

Figure 19. *A,* The structure of folic acid; *B,* the metabolic interrelationships between folate and vitamin B_{12} and their role in DNA synthesis. Folate coenzymes are also needed for two steps in purine synthesis (not illustrated). dATP = deoxyadenosine triphosphate; dGTP = deoxyguanosine triphosphate; dTTP = deoxythymidine triphosphate; dCTP = deoxycytidine triphosphate; dTMP = deoxythymidine monophosphate; dUMP = deoxyuridine monophosphate; dU = deoxyuridine (not a natural precursor); DHF = dihydrofolate; THF = tetrahydrofolate. (From Hoffbrand, A. V.: In *Blood and Its Disorders.* Hardisty, R. M., and Weatherall, D. J. (eds.). Oxford, Blackwell Scientific Publications, 1974.)

maintained by the enzyme dihydrofolate reductase. This reduces dihydrofolic acid (formed during thymidylate synthesis) to its active tetrahydrofolate state. The biochemical reactions of folates in mammalian cells are summarized in Table 12. They are involved in purine and pyrimidine synthesis and amino acid interconversions. Of the latter, the three most important are those involved in histidine, serine-glycine, and methionine metabolism. One of the pathways of histidine metabolism involves its degradation to glutamic acid. The first step in this conversion is that of histidine to urocanic acid. This is then converted to formiminoglutamic acid (FIGLU). Folate is required for the subsequent removal of the formimino group, which is transferred to tetrahydrofolate. In the absence of folate, FIGLU accumulates and is excreted in the urine, forming the basis for a test of folate deficiency.

The interactions of folate and vitamin B_{12} in the synthesis of RNA and DNA are summarized in Figure 19*B*. Because of their interrelationships in one-carbon metabolism, a theory has been proposed to account for the impairment of DNA synthesis in vitamin B_{12} deficiency as well as in folate deficiency. This theory has been called the "methyltetrahydrofolate trap" hypothesis. It is clear from Figure 19*B* that 5,10 methylene tetrahydrofolate is vital for the methylation of deoxy-

uridine monophosphate (dUMP) to thymidine monophosphate (dTMP) mediated by the enzyme thymidylate synthetase. By this mechanism folate deficiency could result in abnormal DNA synthesis. It is also clear that vitamin B_{12} is essential for the conversion of methyl tetrahydrofolate (entering cells from plasma) to tetrahydrofolate and so to 5,10 methylene tetrahydrofolate. It is suggested, therefore, that folate is "trapped" as methyltetrahydrofolate in the absence of vitamin B_{12}, and the cell becomes functionally folate depleted.

Attractive though this hypothesis is, it may not be the whole story. Accumulation of methyl folate in vitamin B_{12} deficiency has never been demonstrated in either humans or animals. Indeed, it is now clear that levels of folate in cells fall when there is a lack of vitamin B_{12}. Furthermore, in vitamin B_{12} deficiency tetrahydrofolate itself is not properly utilized. The anesthetic gas nitrous oxide has the remarkable effect of being cleaved in the presence of vitamin B_{12}, in vivo and in vitro, and of simultaneously oxidizing and inactivating the vitamin. Exposure to nitrous oxide thus produces a vitamin B_{12}-deficient animal. Such animals cannot utilize tetrahydrofolate, but they can use 10,formyltetrahydrofolate, for example, for making folate-polyglutamate coenzyme. Not only does formyl folate overcome vitamin B_{12} inactivation, but methionine is equally active. Indeed, methionine appears to give rise to formyl tetrahydrofolate through a pathway involving S-adenosylmethionine. Thus, in vitamin B_{12} deficiency there is a lack of single carbon units at the formate level of oxidation; this has been called the "formate starvation" hypothesis.

Whichever of these mechanisms is responsible, the basis for the abnormal DNA metabolism and megaloblastic changes associated with vitamin B_{12} or folate deficiency is still not clear. It has not been possible to demonstrate a reduced supply of any of the deoxyribonucleoside triphosphates which might, during the S phase of the cell cycle, impair the cell's ability to elongate newly initiated DNA fragments. Indeed, the levels of all four nucleotides are significantly elevated in vitamin B_{12} deficiency.

TABLE 12. BIOCHEMICAL REACTIONS OF FOLATES*

1. **Formate Fixation**
   Conversion of formate to 10-formyltetrahydrofolate

2. **Purine Synthesis**
   (a) Formylation of glycinamide ribotide to formyl glycinamide ribotide
   (b) Formylation of aminoimidazole carboxamide ribotide (AICAR) to FICAR

3. **Pyrimidine Synthesis**
   Methylation of deoxyuridine monophosphate to thymidylate monophosphate

4. **Amino-acid Interconversion**
   (a) Removal of formimino group from formiminoglutamic acid (FIGLU) to form glutamic acid
   (b) Glycine-serine interconversion
   (c) Methylation of homocysteine to methionine

*Based on Hoffbrand, A. V.: In Hardisty, R. M., and Weatherall, D. J. (eds.): Blood and Its Disorders. 2nd ed. Oxford, Blackwell Scientific Publications, 1982.

Ascorbic Acid. This is important in several aspects of erythropoiesis. Its action as a reducing agent for facilitating iron absorption has been mentioned. It may also be involved in releasing iron from the reticuloendothelial tissues, and this has been shown to be important in iron-loading states. There is no evidence that ascorbic acid has any direct effect on erythroid maturation.

Pyridoxine. Pyridoxal phosphate is an important coenzyme in the heme synthetic pathway; its action on heme synthesis will be considered in a later section.

Riboflavin. It is not clear what role riboflavin plays in normal erythropoiesis. Depression of red cell production has been described in states of riboflavin deficiency and can be produced experimentally in man with diets deficient in riboflavin. Whether it plays a part in normal erythropoiesis is unclear.

Vitamin E. This vitamin probably is essential for normal erythrocyte membrane metabolism, but there is no evidence that it is involved in red cell development.

Amino Acids and Protein. Amino acids and protein are essential for normal erythropoiesis as precursors for a variety of red cell constituents. Severe protein deprivation reduces the rate of erythropoiesis, and selective erythroid hypoplasia has been observed in children with malignant malnutrition.

THE LIFESPAN AND DESTRUCTION OF RED CELLS

Normal red cells survive for between 100 and 130 days. As they age there is a general "running down" of the red cell enzyme pathways, and the red cells are finally destroyed in the reticuloendothelial system. The precise mechanism that determines the age at which a red cell is destroyed is unknown.

LIFESPAN OF RED CELLS

The lifespan of red cells may be assessed by several methods: the use of antigenically recognizable cells (the Ashby technique); cohort-labeling of newly produced erythrocytes with radioactive glycine, selenomethionine, iron, or other markers; labeling of a sample of circulating erythrocytes with ^{51}Cr or DF^{32}P; or by calculations derived from estimation of the rate of production of bilirubin. In clinical practice ^{51}Cr-labeling of samples of circulating erythrocytes is the most convenient technique. Elution of label from erythrocytes in the circulation causes an exponential decay of activity. Correction for elution may be made, but the more usual method is to express the result in terms of half-life (T½) of the label in the circulation. The normal T½ for ^{51}Cr-labeled red cells is 25 to 36 days, depending on the technique employed.

Red Cell Destruction and the Fate of Hemoglobin (Fig. 20). In health, erythrocytes are phagocytosed by the reticuloendothelial cells of the spleen, liver, and elsewhere, and the liberated hemoglobin is degraded. The first stage is the splitting up of heme and globin. Then heme is converted to biliverdin by the enzyme heme oxygenase. One molecule of carbon monoxide is produced with each biliverdin molecule. Subsequent degradation of biliverdin is achieved by the action of

biliverdin reductase with the production of bilirubin. This pigment, which is not soluble, is released from the reticuloendothelial system and travels in the blood bound to albumin, in which form it is not excreted by the kidney. It is taken up by the liver and conjugated by several microsomal enzyme systems, principally glucuronyl transferase. The conjugated bilirubin is excreted via the bile into the intestine, where it is converted into a group of compounds known collectively as *stercobilinogen,* or *fecal urobilinogen.* This last conversion depends on the microorganisms in the gut and may be defective in patients who are receiving broad-spectrum antibiotics. There is some reabsorption of urobilinogen, most of which is reexcreted through the bile, but a small amount appears in the urine as urinary urobilin. On exposure to air urobilinogen forms a dark brown pigment. Normally, about 50 to 250 mg of fecal urobilinogen is excreted per day.

Not all bilirubin is derived from senescent red cells. Approximately 10 to 20 per cent of normal bilirubin production may be derived from the loss of normoblasts during erythroid maturation—that is, from ineffective erythropoiesis. Furthermore, some bilirubin is probably not derived from any of these erythroid sources but from nonhemoglobin porphyrin in the liver.

In health, very little hemoglobin escapes into the plasma. However, in cases of accelerated hemolysis hemoglobin is released into the plasma, where it is bound to haptoglobin, an α_2 globulin that preferentially binds the α chains of hemoglobin. Hemoglobin-haptoglobin complex is rapidly cleared by the reticuloendothelial system. Since the rate of removal of bound haptoglobin may exceed that of new haptoglobin production, its level decreases in the serum and is an extremely sensitive sign of accelerated red cell destruction. The physiologic role of haptoglobin is not clear, although these proteins may have evolved as a mechanism for iron conservation, since, presumably, small amounts of hemoglobin are continually escaping from the RE system during hemoglobin catabolism. In the absence of haptoglobin, free hemoglobin in the plasma is dissociated into heme and globin, and the iron of the heme is oxidized to ferriheme or hematin. The latter becomes loosely attached to albumin to form methemalbumin, which is therefore an indicator of intravascular hemolysis (see p. 229). Normal plasma also contains a β_1 globulin, called hemopexin, which firmly binds heme in equimolar amounts. Its physiologic role is unknown. However, it should be emphasized that haptoglobin and hemopexin binding of hemoglobin can be demonstrated only in states of pathologically increased red cell destruction.

THE ASSESSMENT OF ERYTHROPOIESIS

Erythropoiesis is usually assessed by simple clinical and hematologic studies. However, occasionally it is necessary to try to determine the relative rate and degree of effectiveness of erythropoiesis, together with the rate of red cell destruction, by more sophisticated means.

To assess erythropoiesis, the balance between red cell production and red cell destruction must be considered. The absolute reticulocyte count is one indicator of marrow function. A further guide to the activity

EXTRAVASCULAR

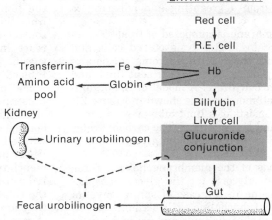

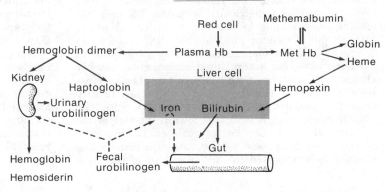

Figure 20. The metabolic pathways of hemoglobin breakdown.

INTRAVASCULAR

of the erythron can be obtained from the M:E ratio of the bone marrow. Additional information can be obtained by ferrokinetic measurements as described on page 194. In assessing the rate of destruction of red cells, determination of red cell survival is very helpful. Estimations of bile pigment production are less useful. Fecal urobilinogen excretion is modified by many factors, including the state of the bacteria of the gut and the amount of bile pigment being derived from ineffective erythropoiesis. Urinary urobilinogen estimations suffer from the same disadvantages, although a gross increase in urinary urobilinogen is usually indicative of hemolysis. For research purposes, it is possible to estimate the amount of pigment being produced by ineffective erythropoiesis by using labeled glycine to study heme metabolism.

The Structure and Functions of the Red Cell

We have now seen how the red cell is produced and that it survives for approximately 120 days in the circulation before it is destroyed in the reticuloendothelial system. The fact that it survives at all is quite remarkable. During its life-time it travels somewhere in the region of 100 miles. It is pumped out of the heart with considerable force, dragged through the microvasculature, and jammed together with its fellows in the osmotic backwaters of the spleen. Throughout this time it is bombarded with oxidants that continually tend to oxidize hemoglobin to a state in which it is useless as an oxygen carrier. From these considerations it is apparent that the red cell must carry out two major functions—maintain its own integrity and keep its hemoglobin in a suitable state for oxygen transport.

STRUCTURE OF THE RED CELL

The mature red cell is a biconcave disc, 8.5 μm in diameter, 2.5 μm thick at the periphery, and 1 μm thick at the center. Its volume is 85 to 90 fl and its surface area is approximately 140 μ^2. A sphere of this volume would have a diameter of approximately 5.5 μm and a surface area of 95 μ^2. The excess surface area allows the red cell to assume a discocytic shape, a conformation that offers maximal surface area for respiratory exchange. The cell is composed of about 70 per cent water, the remainder consisting of hemoglobin and small amounts of lipid, sugar, and enzyme proteins. The red cell membrane allows the cells to control their internal environment of anions, cations, and water, and the negatively charged outer phase provides the necessary electrostatic repulsion forces required to prevent the cells from aggregating and adhering to endothelium.

The red cell membrane is composed of lipids, carbohydrates, and proteins. After lysis of red cells and exhaustive washing, the resulting stroma consists of 40 to 50 per cent protein, 35 to 45 per cent lipid, and 5 to 15 per cent carbohydrate. A model of the organization of the red cell membrane is shown in Figure 21. Essentially, this consists of a lipid bilayer with intercollated proteins and glycoproteins. The carbohydrates are present mainly in the form of glycolipids and glycoprotein.

The phospholipids of the membrane have a three carbon background, glycerol for the glycerophospholipids and sphingosine in the case of sphingomyelin. Lecithin or phosphatidylcholine (PC) accounts for 28 per cent of the total phospholipids and sphingomyelin (SM) for 25 per cent. The amino phospholipids are phosphatidyl serine (PS, 13 per cent) and phosphatidyl ethanolamine (PE, 26 per cent). These phospholipids are arranged asymmetrically with the PC and SM choline phospholipids localized to the outer half of the bilayer and the amino phospholipids, PE and PS, on the inner half. The mature red cell does not synthesize lipids do novo, but several lipid components, notably cholesterol, exchange with lipids in the plasma. Cholesterol is able to cross the bilayer with greater facility than phospholipid and exchanges totally with the plasma cholesterol. It is located toward the core of the bilayer, where it may be intercalated between the phospholipid fatty acid side chains. The membrane glycolipids are located in the outer half of the lipid

bilayer. Their structure consists of a sphingosine as the lipid portion, with a series of sugars extending from the carbon-1 of the backbone. Specific enzymes control the addition of sugars, and these glycolipids react in turn with glycoproteins to determine the specific blood group antigens of the ABO, Lewis, and P blood group systems (see later section).

The major proteins of the red cell membrane are illustrated in Figure 22. They are defined by their electrophoretic properties after separation by sodium dodecyl sulfate (SDS) gel electrophoresis and detection with either a protein stain or the periodic acid–Schiff (PAS) base carbohydrate stain. The conventional nomenclature for the protein staining bands of the human red cell membrane is shown in Figure 22. However, as the roles of these different proteins are characterized, they are referred to by functional names. Two classes of membrane protein are identified in this way. Easily extracted and relatively poor water-soluble proteins are found at the cytosol face or internal surface and are called the *peripheral proteins*. The second group, the *integral membrane proteins,* require more stringent techniques for extraction, presumably because of their close association with the membrane lipids.

The peripheral or extrinsic membrane proteins are involved in the formation of an extensive submembranous reticulum, which is usually called the red cell *cytoskeleton.* The major components of this network are bands 1 and 2 (spectrin), band 2.1 (ankyrin), band 4.1, and band 5 (actin). This cytoskeleton controls the shape, integrity, and flexibility of the membrane. Its removal causes the membranes to fragment into small vesicles. On the other hand, treatment of the mem-

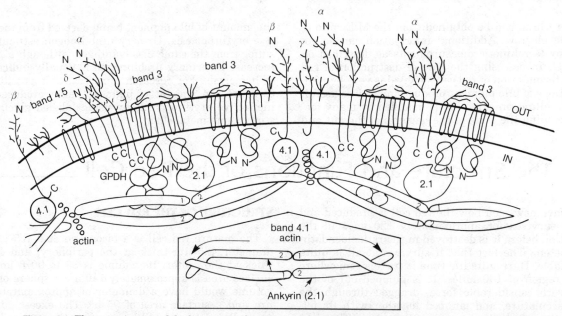

Figure 21. The organization of the human erythrocyte membrane. Schematic diagram of interactions between the components of the human erythrocyte membrane. There is evidence that the anion transport protein (band 3) is present in dimeric and possibly more highly aggregated oligomers and that the sialoglycoproteins (alpha and possibly delta) are associated with these oligomers. The anion transport protein-sialoglycoprotein aggregates probably form the intramembranous particles visualized by freeze-fracture electron microscopy. The glycoprotein oligosaccharides are shown as treelike structures extending from the peptide chains. The small treelike structures directly attached to the outer surface of the membrane represent glycolipids. The inset shows the sites of interaction of other components with the spectrin tetramer. (With kind permission of Dr. Michael Tanner.)

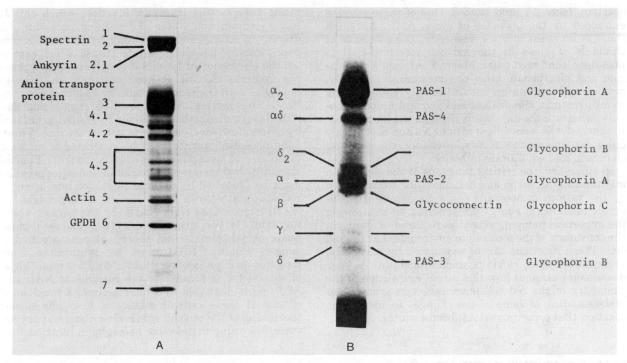

Figure 22. Proteins of the human erythrocyte membrane. *(A)* Sodium dodecyl sulfate (SDS) gel electrophoresis of erythrocyte membrane proteins stained with Coomassie blue. *(B)* SDS gel electrophoresis stained with periodic acid–Schiff stain. The nomenclature of the bands is shown. (By kind permission of Dr. Michael Tanner.)

branes with nonionic detergent that solubilizes the lipid layer and the integral membrane proteins leaves a structure containing the cytoskeleton protein, which retains the discoid shape of the cell. The spectrin bands 1 and 2 are both fibrous molecules that are associated with each other at one end to form a heterodimer. The open ends of two dimers associate tail to tail to give the spectrin tetramer, which seems to be the building block of the cytoskeleton. Band 4.1 associates with the ends of the tetramer, while band 2.1 binds to the band 2 chain near to the center of the tetramer. The association between spectrin tetramers to form a two-dimensional network involves both band 4.1 and short-actin protofilaments. This meshwork is connected to the lipid bilayer by the association of band 2.1 with the N terminal region of the anion transport protein and perhaps also by the association of band 4.1 with the C terminal cytoplasmic portion of sialoglycoprotein β (glycoconnectin) (see below).

The integral membrane proteins consist of band 3, or the anion transport protein, proteins in the band 4.5 region, which include the glucose transport protein, and the sialoglycoproteins, glycophorins A (α), B (δ), and C (β).

The anion transport protein (band 3) is the predominant integral protein of the membrane and makes up 25 per cent of the membrane protein, which is equivalent to 1.2×10^6 copies per red cell. It is involved in the transport of HCO_3^- and Cl^-. This protein is made up of two domains. The N terminus consists of a 40,000 molecular weight (M_r) portion located within the cytoplasm and is associated with many peripheral proteins, including glycolytic enzymes and hemoglobin. This domain also binds band 4.2 and forms part of the linkage between the membrane and the red cell cytoskeleton by association with ankyrin (band 2.1). The C terminal portion of the band 3 protein (M_r of approximately 55,000) carries out anion exchange and is membrane-bound. The band 3 protein carries a single N-linked oligosaccharide, which is heterogeneous in size and contains a variable number of repeating N-acety-lactosamine units. These are involved in the Ii blood group antigen determination.

The major red cell sialoglycoprotein, A (α), consists of a 23-residue hydrophobic segment that traverses the membrane and an extracellular N-terminal domain, which is densely glycosylated and contains 15 O-linked sialotetrasaccharides. The blood group M,N antigens are located on glycophorin A. The N-terminal sequence of sialoglycoprotein C (β) differs from that of α. This protein has been called glycoconnectin, since there is evidence that it may be associated with the erythrocyte cytoskeleton network by attachment to band 4.1.

The red cell membrane has a variety of transport systems, including Na⁺, K⁺-ATPase which is involved in the transportation of Na⁺ out of and K⁺ into the cell, Ca⁺⁺, Mg⁺⁺-ATPase, and acetylcholinesterase. The membrane pumps are of critical importance for maintaining electrolyte hemostasis in the red cell. Sodium is actively pumped from the cell against a concentration gradient of 10 mEq/l inside the cell to 145 mEq/l in the plasma. Potassium, on the other hand, is pumped into the cell against a concentration gradient of about 4.5 mEq/l in the plasma to 100 mEq/l in the cell. The calcium-magnesium pump requires phospholipid for full activation and mediates Ca⁺⁺ efflux against a 50- to 100-fold concentration gradient, converting one molecule of ATP to ADP for each two molecules of Ca⁺⁺ extruded. The entry of Ca⁺⁺ into the red cell causes the activator protein, calmodulin, to move from cytosol to membrane. The membrane also has several protein kinases that can phosphorylate spectrin, band 2.1, and band 3. One of these may be enhanced by the presence of cyclic AMP. Although there is no morphologic evidence for the existence of channels or pores in the red cell membrane, it is presumed that such exist. Monovalent ions like chloride and bicarbonate cross the membrane passively, more slowly than water, but still rapidly, equilibrating in milliseconds. Monovalent and divalent anions probably penetrate the membrane through the band 3 site. In contrast, the monovalent cations Na and K passively cross the membrane slowly, probably via separate channels, and equilibrate in hours.

In summary, the critical functions of the red cell in maintaining its shape and deformability are mediated by the various components of its membrane. Considerable amounts of energy are required for subserving the important pumping activities required to maintain the constancy of the electrolyte environment of the red cell. These functions can be modulated by hormones, cyclic nucleotides, calcium, and calmodulin. A later discussion examines how this recent knowledge of the chemistry of the red cell membrane can promote an understanding of some of the changes in membrane function that occur in various disease states.

ENERGY PATHWAYS IN THE RED CELL

The red cell loses its mitochondria and hence its capacity for oxidative energy production during its maturation cycle. It is delivered into the circulation with relatively simple "pay as you go" energy pathways. It needs to produce the high energy phosphate bonds of ATP to maintain its membrane pumps. In addition it requires energy to perform biochemical reduction to protect its hemoglobin and membrane from oxidative damage. There are two main reducing systems. One uses NADH and maintains the iron atoms of hemoglobin in the reduced state. The other is responsible for maintaining the cell's thiol groups and hence for protecting the membrane and hemoglobin. This latter pathway is mediated through NADPH, which works by maintaining glutathione in the reduced state.

Glucose, the only source of energy in the mature red cell, is metabolized mainly through the anaerobic Embden-Meyerhof pathway with the production of lactate as the end product (Fig. 23). There is a net production of 2 mol of ATP and the reduction of 2 mol of NAD to NADH per mole of glucose via this anaerobic pathway. The other energy pathway is the hexose monophosphate (HMP) shunt, or pentose phosphate pathway, in which there is reduction of 2 mol of NADP to NADPH per mole of glucose. This pathway is stimulated by certain redox compounds and oxidants. There is a "metabolic siding" in the EM pathway called the Rapoport-Luebering shunt (Fig. 23), controlled by diphosphoglycerate mutase, which generates 2,3-diphosphoglycerate (2,3-DPG). This is the most abundant intracellular phosphate in human erythrocytes, and it plays an important role in controlling oxygen uptake and release by hemoglobin.

The metabolic functions of the red cell can be summarized as follows. First, the red cell must maintain its osmotic stability through the activity of its membrane pumps. This transport function, which entails losing sodium and water and gaining potassium, is driven by ATP generated mainly by the membrane-bound enzyme phosphoglycerate kinase, which catalyzes the conversion of 1,3-diphosphoglycerate to 3-phosphoglycerate. Second, it must maintain the iron of hemoglobin in the reduced state, by reducing Fe^{+++} to Fe^{++}. The enzyme system involved, methemoglobin reductase or diaphorase, is driven by NADH generated by glyceraldehyde-3-phosphate dehydrogenase. Third, 2,3-diphosphoglycerate must be generated to act as a modulator of hemoglobin function (see below). Fourth, the sulfhydryl groups of hemoglobin and other proteins must be protected by maintaining adequate levels of reduced glutathione. This system is dependent on NADPH generated from NADP by the pentose pathway and its two principle enzymes, glucose-6-phosphate dehydrogenase and phosphogluconate dehydrogenase. Finally, NAD must be synthesized from nicotinic acid, glutamine, glucose, and inorganic phosphate. NADP is formed by the reaction of NAD and ADP. As is discussed in a later section, a breakdown of any of these critical metabolic functions causes shortening of the red cell survival or abnormal oxygen transport owing to defective hemoglobin function.

THE STRUCTURE, FUNCTION, AND SYNTHESIS OF HEMOGLOBIN

Probably more is known about the structure and function of hemoglobin than any other mammalian protein. It is essential to have a simple understanding of the way in which this protein functions and how its structure is genetically determined to form a basis for the description of its disorders, which are considered in a later section.

STRUCTURE

All human hemoglobins have a similar basic structure. They consist of two different pairs of peptide chains, each chain having one heme molecule attached to it. Normal adults have two hemoglobin fractions, a major component, Hb A, and a minor component, Hb A_2. Hb A has two α chains and two β chains and is written $\alpha_2\beta_2$; Hb A_2 has the structure $\alpha_2\delta_2$. The main hemoglobin of fetal life is Hb F, which has α chains combined with γ chains ($\alpha_2\gamma_2$). At a very early stage of development there are specific embryonic hemoglobins, but their synthesis ceases by the eighth gestational week. The structures of all the human hemoglobins are summarized in Table 13.

In addition to the hemoglobins described, the structures of which are genetically determined, certain postsynthetic modifications of the human hemoglobins occur. There are several hemoglobins that result from this type of process. One of particular clinical interest, hemoglobin A_{1C}, has the same structure as hemoglobin A except that the amino terminal residue of the β chain is linked to glucose by a Schiff base. The relative amount of hemoglobin A_{1C} is elevated in patients with diabetes mellitus and its level correlates well with the severity of the glucose intolerance.

The α chains of hemoglobin are made up of 141 amino acids (or residues) and the β chains consist of

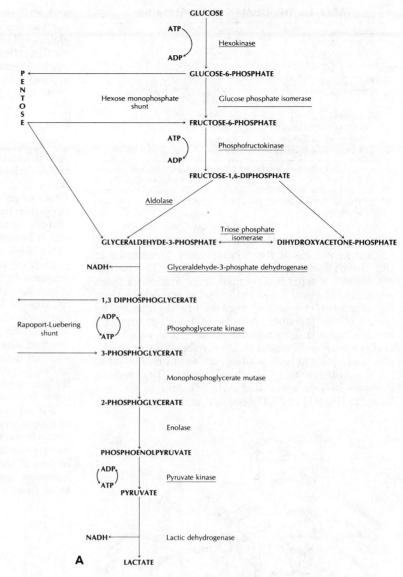

Figure 23. The major metabolic pathways of the red cell. *A,* The Embden-Meyerhof pathway. The relationships to the HMP and Rapoport-Luebering pathways are indicated. *B,* The hexose monophosphate shunt. This diagram shows schematically the relationship between glucose-6-phosphate dehydrogenase and the maintenance of reduced glutathione (GSH). *C,* The Rapoport-Luebering pathway for the synthesis of 2,3-diphosphoglycerate. The diagram indicates the relationship to the Embden-Meyerhof pathway as shown in *A.*

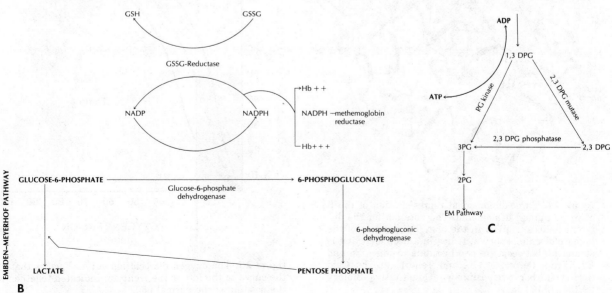

TABLE 13. THE HUMAN HEMOGLOBINS

Adult

Hemoglobin A	$\alpha_2\beta_2$
Hemoglobin A$_2$	$\alpha_2\delta_2$

Fetal*

Hemoglobin F	$\alpha_2\gamma_2(\alpha_2\gamma_2^{136gly}\ \alpha_2\gamma_2^{136ala})$

Embryonic

Hemoglobin Gower 1	$\xi_3\epsilon_2$
Hemoglobin Gower 2	$\alpha_2\epsilon_2$
Hemoglobin Portland	$\xi_2\gamma_2$

*Hemoglobin F contains two distinct types of γ chains, one with glycine at position 136 ($^G\gamma$) and the other with alanine at this position ($^A\gamma$). The $^G\gamma$ and $^A\gamma$ chains are the products of distinct gene loci. The ratio $^G\gamma{:}^A\gamma$ changes during maturation and in various conditions with persistence or reactivation of Hb F production.

146 residues. The order (or sequence) of these amino acids is known as the *primary structure*. Some areas of the chains form a helical configuration. The helical segments are separated by nonhelical areas and there are also nonhelical areas at the end of each chain (Fig. 24). Each of the helical regions are designated by letters of the alphabet (A to H) and each amino acid residue has a specific number. Hence, it is possible to designate an amino acid by its number—for example, β^{99}—and by its helical position; β^{99} would be H3—that is, the third residue in the H helix. The regions between helices are called AB, BC, and so on, and those at the NH and CO terminal ends are called NA

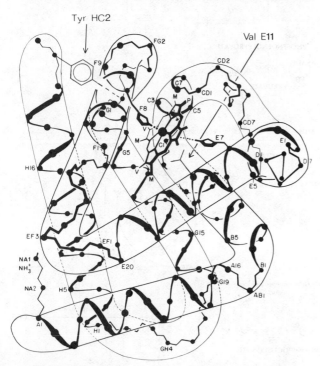

Figure 24. Three-dimensional representation of the β chain of human hemoglobin. The notation for the different helices is given in the text. The position of the heme molecule is shown; it lies in a deep cleft and is strung up between the two histidine residues F8 and E7. (From Perutz, M. F., and Teneyck, L. F.: Cold Spring Harbor Symposium on Quantitative Biology 29:197, 1964.)

and HC, respectively. Because of the interactions of the various amino acid side chains that make up the globin subunits they fold up into a complex tertiary configuration. Finally, the four subunits, two α and two β, fit together into a snug quaternary configuration to form a finished molecule with heme groups in deep clefts in its surface (Fig. 24).

FUNCTION

Why is the hemoglobin molecule so complex and how does it function as an oxygen carrier? The oxygenation of hemoglobin, as depicted by the oxygen dissociation curve (Fig. 25), has the well-known sigmoid shape. This curve relates the per cent saturation with the oxygen tension. A convenient index of the oxygen affinity is the p50, or partial pressure of oxygen at which hemoglobin is half saturated. The shape of this curve is beautifully adapted to the oxygen-transporting properties of hemoglobin. At relatively high oxygen tensions in the lungs oxygen is rapidly taken up, and it can be released readily at tensions encountered in the tissues. Myoglobin, which consists of a single globin chain with heme attached to it, has a hyperbolic oxygen dissociation curve. The older schools of physiologists realized that the transition from a hyperbolic to a sigmoid curve must indicate some form of interaction or "cooperativity" within the hemoglobin molecule. It is now possible to describe the molecular basis for these interactions.

The sigmoid oxygen dissociation curve is the result of cooperativity between the subunits, which is called heme-heme interaction. When one heme group takes on oxygen the affinity for oxygen of the remaining hemes of the tetramer increases markedly. This phenomenon is explained by the fact that hemoglobin can exist in two configurations, deoxy (T) and oxy (R). (T

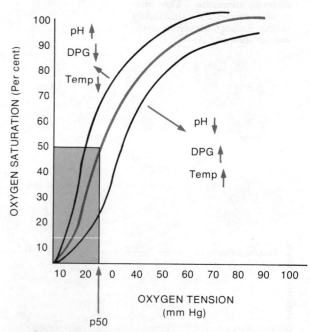

Figure 25. The oxygen dissociation curve. Factors that shift the curve to the left or the right are indicated together with the position of the normal p50.

and R stand for tight and relaxed states, respectively.) The T form has a lower affinity for ligands such as O_2 and CO than has the R form. At some point during the sequential addition of oxygen to the four hemes a transition from the T to R configuration occurs and at this point the oxygen affinity of the partial liganded molecule increases markedly. This remarkable change in oxygen affinity involves a series of interactions between the iron of the heme groups and various bonds within the molecule that cause subtle spatial alterations with the giving up and taking on of oxygen. This mechanism has interesting clinical implications because, if genetic variants of the hemoglobin molecules alter the shape at areas where these critical spatial interactions occur, heme-heme interaction is diminished and hemoglobin does not give up its oxygen as readily as normally.

The other important functional property of hemoglobin is the Bohr effect—that is, the decrease in oxygen affinity that occurs with increasing CO_2 tensions. This phenomenon is largely pH dependent. The mechanism of the Bohr effect is illustrated in Figure 26. It offers the physiologic advantage of facilitating oxygen unloading at tissue level, where a drop in pH due to CO_2 influx lowers oxygen affinity, thereby enhancing oxygen release. In contrast, in the lungs efflux of CO_2 and increase in intracellular pH increase oxygen affinity and hence uptake. Carbon dioxide influences hemoglobin in two ways. First, diffusion of CO_2 into the red cells, where carbonic anhydrase produces carbonic acid, decreases the pH, lowering oxygen affinity via the Bohr effect. Second, by combining with terminal amino groups forming carbamino compounds (Fig. 27), CO_2 further lowers oxygen affinity. Since deoxyhemoglobin forms carbamino complexes more readily than does oxyhemoglobin, increasing the relative amounts of carbamino hemoglobin tends to reduce oxygen affinity.

The position of the oxygen dissociation curve—that is, the p50—can be shifted to the right or left in a variety of ways. How pH and CO_2 can produce this effect has already been discussed. Another important constituent of the red cell that can modify oxygen transport is 2,3-diphosphoglycerate (2,3-DPG). Increasing concentrations of 2,3-DPG shift the oxygen dissociation curve to the right (that is, cause a state of reduced oxygen affinity), while diminishing concentrations shift the curve to the left—that is, produce a high oxygen affinity state. 2,3-DPG fits into the gap between the two β chains of hemoglobin when this becomes

$$Hb (H) + 4 O_2 \rightleftharpoons Hb (O_2)_4 + 2.4 H^+$$

Figure 26. The principle of the Bohr effect. Because CO_2 moves into red cells in the capillary circulation, there is an increase in intracellular H^+ and HCO_3^- concentrations. The binding of protons to hemoglobin represents the most important buffer system for maintaining intracellular pH. Oxyhemoglobin is a stronger acid than deoxyhemoglobin. Deoxyhemoglobin has a higher affinity for protons than has oxyhemoglobin. Perutz and his colleagues have constructed models that form a stereochemical basis to account for most of the alkaline Bohr effect; these models identify four specific acid groups of hemoglobin that are more readily protonated in the deoxy form. Thus there is a mechanism that favors the deoxy configuration in the tissues and the oxy configuration in the higher pH environment of the lungs.

$$H-HbNH_2 + CO_2 \rightleftharpoons H-HbNHCOOH$$

Figure 27. The binding of carbon dioxide to hemoglobin to form carbaminohemoglobin. This reaction depends on the existence of free amino groups in the protein. If the amino group is protonated, the reaction will not occur. The N-terminal amino group of each polypeptide chain and the ε amino group of lysine are the main binding groups. The latter group has a pK of about 9, and at neutral pH they are 99 per cent protonated and unable to bind CO_2. In contrast, the pK of the N-terminal amino groups is close to 7. Hence the carbamino reaction is pH-dependent, and, furthermore, deoxyhemoglobin binds CO_2 much more readily than does oxyhemoglobin.

widened during deoxygenation, and interacts with several specific binding sites in the central cavity of the molecule. However, in the oxy conformation the gap between the two β chains narrows and 2,3-DPG cannot be accommodated. In more simple terms, the β chains can be imagined as a pair of nutcrackers with the nut, 2,3-DPG, held between them. In the oxy configuration, the nut slides out as the nutcrackers move together! It follows, therefore, that with increasing concentrations of 2,3-DPG more molecules are held in the deoxy configuration, and the oxygen dissociation curve is shifted to the right. This interaction has important clinical implications.

METHEMOGLOBIN AND CARBOXYHEMOGLOBIN

Oxidation of the iron of hemoglobin from Fe^{++} to Fe^{+++} results in the formation of methemoglobin. Methemoglobinemia exceeding 1.5 g/dl results in clinical cyanosis and may occur either as a genetically determined disorder or by exposure of normal cells to severe oxidant stress. The congenital form is due either to a deficiency of the NADH-dependent methemoglobin reductase or to an inherited amino acid substitution in either the α or β chain near the heme attachment site (see p. 207). The latter hemoglobin variants are all called hemoglobin M and further identified by their place of discovery or particular substitution. The acquired form follows exposure to such oxidants as nitrites, nitrates, certain drugs, and aniline derivatives.

Carboxyhemoglobin results from exposure to CO. The affinity of heme for CO is over 200 times that for oxygen. After severe exposure, patients assume a "cherry red" color rather than a cyanotic hue. Exposure may result from self-poisoning or from exposure to industrial pollution or tobacco tar.

The defect in hemoglobin function is similar in the two conditions. A certain proportion of heme molecules are unable to bind oxygen. Because of the mechanism of heme-heme interaction (see p. 207), the hemoglobin molecules carrying the affected heme molecules become fixed in the oxy configuration—that is, there is a marked left shift in the oxygen dissociation curve. The presence of a 30 per cent methemoglobin or carboxyhemoglobin is much more serious than a drop of 30 per cent in the hematocrit, because each hemoglobin tetramer with a single oxidized or liganded heme is rendered physiologically useless. The end result is severe tissue hypoxia.

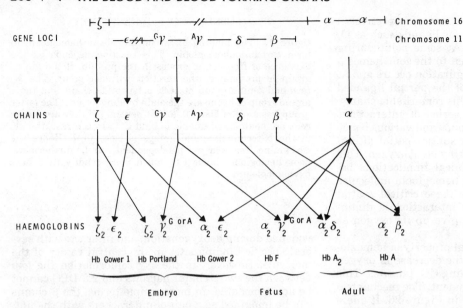

Figure 28. The genetic control of human hemoglobin production at various stages of development.

GENETIC CONTROL OF HEMOGLOBIN SYNTHESIS

The structure of the different hemoglobins is determined by specific structural gene clusters. The α globin gene cluster is on chromosome 16 and the non-α gene cluster is on chromosome 11 (Fig. 28). Parts of these regions of the genome have been cloned in bacteriophage, and their structure has been analyzed in detail (Fig. 29). The non-α globin gene cluster on chromosome 11 is contained in approximately 60 kilobases (kb; a thousand nucleotide bases). The genes in this cluster are arranged in the order 5'-ϵ-$^{G}\gamma$-$^{A}\gamma$-$\psi\beta$1-δ-β-3'. The $\psi\beta$1 locus is a so-called pseudogene, which is a locus that has structural similarities to the β locus but that has mutations that prevent its normal transcription. Pseudogenes of this type, which are found in many mammalian gene clusters, may be "burnt-out" evolutionary remnants of previously active gene loci. The α globin genes lie in a smaller cluster on chromosome 16 in the order 5'-ζ2-$\psi\zeta$1-$\psi\alpha$-α2-α1-3'. The $\psi\zeta$1 and $\psi\alpha$ genes are pseudogenes. All the globin genes have a similar basic structure. They consist of coding regions (exons) separated by noncoding intervening sequences (introns). The non-α genes each contain two introns of 122 to 130 and 850 to 900 base pairs between codons 30 and 31 and 104 and 105, respectively. At the 5' (upstream) side of the genes there are blocks of sequence homology, which are similar in many mammalian structural genes. These regions are thought to be involved in the initiation of transcription, that is, they probably represent promotor sequences.

The primary transcripts of the globin genes are large messenger RNA precursor molecules that contain both introns and exons. Before passing into the cytoplasm the introns are removed, and the exons are spliced together to form the definitive globin messenger RNA's (Fig. 30). Once in the cytoplasm of the red cell precursors, the various globin messenger RNA's act as templates for globin chain synthesis. Each chain combines with one heme molecule, synthesized by a separate pathway (Fig. 31). Finally, the various subunits combine to form definitive hemoglobin molecules. Very little is known about the regulation of the globin genes, although it is thought that, while there may be some fine adjustment at the translational level, control is mediated mainly by varying the rates of transcription.

CHANGES DURING DEVELOPMENT

During normal human development there is sequential activation of the embryonic, fetal, and adult globin genes (Fig. 28). Embryonic globin chain synthesis ceases by about the eighth week of development. Fetal hemoglobin production continues until a few weeks before term, after which adult hemoglobin production takes over, and by the end of the first year of life only traces of hemoglobin F are produced. Adult β chain synthesis occurs at a low level from early in intrauterine life and makes up about 10 per cent of non-α globin chain synthesis in the early stages of fetal development. This observation has important implications for prenatal diagnosis of hemoglobin disorders.

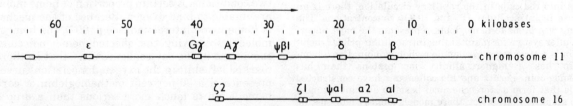

Figure 29. The arrangement of the α and β-like globin genes on chromosomes 16 and 11. The genes designated ψ are pseudogenes, that is, they have sequence similarities to functional genes but have mutations that would prevent their normal functioning. They are thought to be evolutionary remnants of once active genes. Kb = kilobase or 1000 nucleotide bases.

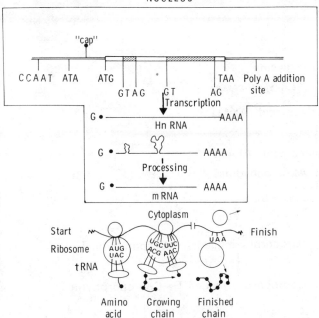

NUCLEUS

Figure 30. A schematic representation of the steps involved in the transcription of a human hemoglobin gene and the various processing mechanisms involved in producing a definitive globin messenger RNA. The globin gene is represented as a box between the start codon (ATG) and the stop codon (TAA). The unshaded regions represent the exons and the hatched regions the introns. The primary transcript (HnRNA) contains both intron and exons. While they are in the nucleus the introns are removed and the three exons are spliced together. The definitive messenger RNA is capped (C) and has a string of adenylic acid residues added to it (AAAA). It then moves into the cell cytoplasm to form a template for globin chain synthesis.

Hemoglobin F shows very little interaction with 2,3-DPG, and hence the oxygen affinity of fetal blood is higher than that of adult blood. This may be an important adaptive function for oxygenation of the fetus. The mechanism that regulates the beautifully coordinated switches from embryonic to fetal and from fetal to adult hemoglobin is completely unknown. It is not organ-specific; that is, during the switch from fetal to adult hemoglobin production the changeover occurs at the same rate in both fetal-liver and bone-marrow erythropoietic tissue. There is a family of genetic variants with the general title hereditary persistence of fetal hemoglobin. Many of these conditions result from deletions of the adult globin genes, but although it has been suggested that these deletions also remove regions of the non-α globin gene cluster that are involved in the regulation of the switch from fetal to adult hemoglobin production, so far it has not been possible to define such regions with precision.

MUTATIONS OF THE HEMOGLOBIN GENE LOCI

Many different mutations of the globin gene loci have been characterized, and in some instances the molecular basis for these lesions has been defined. These mutations give rise to two main classes of clinical disorders. First, there are the structural hemoglobin variants, which usually result from single base changes in one of the globin gene loci. The second group is made up of a series of disorders characterized by a reduced rate of production of one or more of the globin chains. These latter lesions give rise to the clinical phenotype of thalassemia. So far, over 200 structural hemoglobin variants have been discovered. In many cases they are harmless, but if the amino acid replacement is at a critical part of the molecule it may alter its function or stability and give rise to a clinical disorder. Later sections of this chapter examine how these changes produce different disease states and the many different types of mutation that give rise to a reduced output of globin chains, which causes the clinical phenotype of thalassemia.

THE RED CELL AND ADAPTATION TO HYPOXIA

The term hypoxia means a state of reduced oxygen tension in the tissues. It can result from a variety of causes, including a reduced oxygen tension in the inspired air, decreased cardiac output, diminished gaseous exchange in the lungs, a diminished ability of hemoglobin to give up its oxygen to the tissues, a reduced oxygen carrying capacity of the blood due to a paucity of red cells and/or hemoglobin, or from increased metabolic requirements by the tissues.

The unloading of oxygen to the tissues is controlled by three independent variables, which can be expressed by the Fick equation:

$$VO_2 = 1.39 \times Hb \times Q(Sat_A - Sat_V)$$

where VO_2 is the amount of oxygen released (1/min), 1.39 is the amount of O_2 in ml bound by 1 g of fully saturated hemoglobin, Q is blood flow (l/min), and Sat_A and Sat_V are arterial and mixed venous oxygen saturations (per cent). During hypoxic stress a patient may increase VO_2 by altering any one or more of three variables: (1) increase the cardiac output, (2) increase the red cell mass, (3) decrease the whole blood oxygen affinity. In many hypoxic states there is a shift to the right in the oxygen dissociation curve mediated through increased synthesis of red cell 2,3-DPG. How does hypoxia increase the rate of production of 2,3-DPG? Unfortunately, the answer to this question is far from clear, but one major contributing factor may be an increase in intracellular pH. Hypoxic patients often have a respiratory alkalosis; furthermore, there may be an increase in intracellular pH because of the Bohr effect. Alkalosis stimulates glycolysis in general and, more specifically, may increase 2,3-DPG formation and catabolism by the Rapoport-Lueberling shunt (see pp. 202 to 205 for further discussion of this mechanism). Whatever the mechanism, increased 2,3-DPG production shifts the oxygen dissociation curve to the right. This allows the liberation of relatively more oxygen from blood perfusing the tissues. This mechanism occurs in a variety of conditions that are summarized in Table 14. Its importance is examined in the adaptation to anemia in the next section, but here it should be noted that it is part of the process of adaptation to high altitude, pulmonary hypoxia, congestive cardiac failure, thyrotoxicosis, and the hyperphosphatemia of the immediate newborn period.

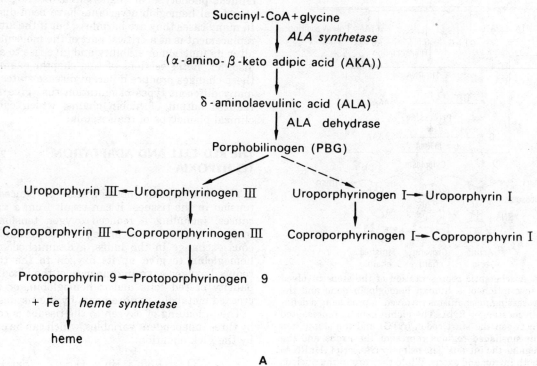

Figure 31. *A*, The biosynthetic pathways for heme production in red cell precursors. *B*, The structure of heme.

The converse situation to that described above—that is, a shift to the left in the oxygen dissociation curve with a relatively high oxygen affinity—can also occur in a variety of pathologic states. 2,3-DPG production is reduced in states of acidosis (Fig. 25). 2,3-DPG levels also decline in stored blood; hence a left shift in the oxygen dissociation curve may occur after blood transfusion. Other conditions in which this happens are summarized in Table 14.

Unfortunately, it is still not known how important the relative oxygen affinity is in any particular disease state in which many other complicating factors may occur. One excellent example of how complicated the situation can become in a state of severe metabolic upset is illustrated from what happens in diabetic coma. In this disorder there is usually severe acidosis. This tends to reduce 2,3-DPG production, which shifts the oxygen dissociation curve to the left. However, the direct effect of intracellular acidosis is to shift the oxygen dissociation curve to the right through the Bohr effect, and therefore the p50 may be relatively normal in patients with severe diabetic acidosis. However, some physicians (perhaps unwisely) tend to correct the acidosis rapidly with bicarbonate. The danger of rapid correction is that it immediately overcomes the Bohr effect. However, it takes several hours to generate 2,3-DPG, and so the bicarbonate causes a sudden shift in the oxygen dissociation curve to the left with a high affinity state. It remains to be proved that this is the mechanism for the deleterious effects of overrapid correction of acidosis in diabetic coma.

TABLE 14. CHANGES IN RED CELL 2,3-DIPHOSPHOGLYCERATE

Increased Levels
  Anemia
  Alkalosis
  Hyperphosphatemia
  Renal failure
  Altitude hypoxia
  Chronic pulmonary disease
  Pregnancy
  Cyanotic congenital heart disease
  Hepatic cirrhosis
  Thyrotoxicosis
  Some red cell enzyme deficiencies—e.g., PK deficiency

Decreased Levels
  Acidosis
  Cardiogenic or septicemic shock
  Hypophosphatemia
  Hyperparathyroidism
  Hypopituitarism
  Hypothyroidism
  Following replacement with stored blood

It is clear from the description of the adaptive functions of the red cell that the p50 can be varied widely according to particular environmental changes. How these compensatory mechanisms are related to the pathophysiology of anemia is examined in the next section.

Anemia

DEFINITIONS AND PATHOPHYSIOLOGY

There are several ways of defining anemia. In clinical practice it is usual to define it as a reduction in the circulating hemoglobin concentration or red cell count below that which would be normal for an individual's age and sex. There is a wide range of individual variation in the hematocrit, hemoglobin, and red cell count, and this should be borne in mind when making a diagnosis of anemia. Furthermore, a fall in the hematocrit can result from a reduction in the circulating red cell mass or from an increase in the plasma volume. Thus it is important to distinguish between *true* anemia and relative anemia due to hemodilution.

Although extremely valuable in day-to-day clinical practice, the definition of anemia by the hematocrit or hemoglobin concentration has many limitations from the point of view of function and pathophysiology. Since the job of the red cells is to transport oxygen to the tissues, the best functional definition of anemia is that state in which the volume of the circulating red cell mass is insufficient to meet the oxygen demands of the tissues. This definition takes into account that there are many ways in which the body can compensate for anemia and that in any individual patient it is important to assess not only the hematocrit level but also the compensatory mechanisms that may be at work to overcome the deleterious effects of the reduced red cell mass.

ADAPTATION TO ANEMIA

What are the effects of anemia and how does compensation occur? The red cell mass has to provide the tissues with about 250 ml oxygen per minute. The oxygen-carrying capacity of normal blood is 15 × 1.39 ml or 20 ml/100 ml of blood. With a cardiac output of 5000 ml per minute, 1000 ml of oxygen per minute is made available to the tissues. Extraction of one fourth of this reduces the oxygen tension from 100 mm Hg in the arterial end of the capillary to 40 mm Hg in the venous end. In anemia the extraction of the same amount of oxygen would lead to a greater hemoglobin desaturation and a lower oxygen tension at the venous end of the capillary. Since this would ultimately lead to cellular hypoxia, or anoxia, compensatory mechanisms are required to supply blood and oxygen to the tissues and hence to maintain an adequate oxygen gradient.

Some of the compensatory mechanisms that occur in anemia are summarized in Table 15. These can occur both centrally and peripherally. The most important central mechanism is an increased cardiac output. The latter remains constant until the hemoglobin level falls

TABLE 15. COMPENSATION FOR ANEMIA

Central Mechanisms
  Increased cardiac output

Peripheral Mechanisms
  Decreased blood viscosity
  Decreased peripheral resistance
  Redistribution of flow

Red Cell Mechanisms
  Increased production of 2,3-DPG
  Increased p50 and reduced oxygen affinity of Hb

Tissue Changes
  Changes in respiratory enzymes (?)

to about 7 to 8 g/dl. The output then increases in proportion to the hemoglobin decrease and may reach four to five times normal. The pulse rate/volume and circulation rate increase, and because of anemia the viscosity of the peripheral blood is reduced. The systolic blood pressure is well maintained but the diastolic pressure is usually decreased, and hence the workload on the right and left ventricles is only slightly increased. Blood in the coronary sinus is already extremely unsaturated at rest, and any increase in oxygen delivery to the myocardium must result from increased flow rather than from increased oxygen extraction. This is why, particularly in the presence of associated coronary artery disease, severe anemia sometimes produces angina.

Despite a great deal of study, the mechanism for the increased stroke volume in chronic anemic states has not been worked out. An increase in ventricular filling pressure or in total blood volume is not essential for the increase in cardiac output. Furthermore, it has been found recently that an intact β-adrenergic receptor system is not essential for the cardiac response to chronic anemia. It seems likely that the major mechanism is a decrease in afterload secondary to decreased peripheral resistance and/or blood viscosity.

The total blood volume is extremely variable in patients with chronic anemia. It may be normal or slightly reduced in cases of severe deficiency anemia. On the other hand, if there is associated hypersplenism or massive hypertrophy of the bone marrow, as occurs in dyserythropoietic states such as thalassemia and some of the other dyserythropoietic anemias, there may be a marked increase in the total blood volume as a result of expansion of the plasma volume.

Compensation for anemia also occurs at the tissue and cellular levels. There is early redistribution of blood from tissues with relatively low oxygen requirements and a high blood supply, such as skin and kidneys, to oxygen-dependent tissues, such as brain and myocardium. This redistribution is manifest by cutaneous vasoconstriction. However, the effect on renal excretory function is relatively minor, since the decrease in blood supply is offset by an increase in the plasmacrit of the perfusing anemic blood. At a cellular level the most striking change is a shift in the oxygen dissociation curve to the right, permitting the extraction of increased amounts of oxygen without a decrease in oxygen pressure. This shift is due mainly to an increased production of 2,3-DPG. It seems likely that with an increased concentration of deoxygenated

hemoglobin, more 2,3-DPG is bound, and this releases glucose metabolism from feedback inhibition of DPG on diphosphoglycerate mutase so that more 2,3-DPG is formed. This DPG becomes available to interact with and decrease the oxygen affinity of hemoglobin. This type of compensatory mechanism has its limitations, however. For example, certain hemoglobins, such as fetal hemoglobin, do not interact with 2,3-DPG. Therefore, the DPG mechanism cannot compensate for severe anemia in fetal life. Similarly, in certain red cell enzyme defects there is reduced synthesis of 2,3-DPG. In others, however, such as pyruvate kinase deficiency, 2,3-DPG levels are increased, and compensation for anemia is extremely efficient. Certain structural hemoglobin variants like sickle hemoglobin have relatively low oxygen affinities as compared with normal adult hemoglobin, and hence affected patients compensate well for anemia.

Therefore, when considering any individual patient the effects of anemia must be examined in terms of the state of the myocardium and lungs and the adequacy of compensation at the cellular level.

EFFECTS OF ANEMIA

If the various aspects of the pathophysiology of anemia outlined above are understood, the general effects of anemia are easy to work out. They are summarized in Table 16. Anemic patients are pale, partly because of peripheral vasoconstriction and partly because of low hemoglobin content of perfusing blood. Cardiorespiratory symptoms and signs usually appear with a relatively severe degree of anemia. They include exertional dyspnea, tachycardia, palpitations, angina of effort, claudication, and night cramps. There may also be increased arterial pulsation, capillary pulsations, bruits over the vessels, and cardiac enlargement. Some patients with severe chronic anemia and no underlying heart disease develop clinical features that are usually associated with congestive cardiac failure such as elevated systemic venous pressure with distended neck veins, hepatomegaly, and peripheral edema. However, these patients have several hemodynamic differences from those with congestive cardiac failure caused by other types of heart disease. They have an elevated resting cardiac output and can in-

TABLE 16. GENERAL EFFECTS OF ANEMIA

Cardiorespiratory	Gastrointestinal
Dyspnea; air hunger	Anorexia; nausea
Palpitations; arterial pulsation	Constipation or diarrhea
Angina	
Tachycardia	**Skin**
Cardiac enlargement	Pallor
Flow murmurs	
High output cardiac failure	**Genitourinary**
Increased respiratory rate	Menstrual irregularity
	Loss of libido
Neuromuscular	Frequency of micturition
Headache; faintness	
Tinnitus	**Metabolic**
Cold sensitivity	Fever
Easy fatigability	Raised BMR
Lack of concentration	
Fundal hemorrhages	

crease their output in response to exercise. Digoxin is ineffective in lowering the systemic venous pressure. Although the basis for this state of "high output" failure is not known, it appears that at very low hemoglobin levels compensatory mechanisms may not be able to overcome myocardial hypoxia, and hence myocardial failure may occur. These observations indicate that blood transfusion in patients with severe chronic anemia may be extremely hazardous. Because of the relative anoxia of the nervous system a variety of neurologic effects are seen. These include headache, vertigo, tinnitus, roaring in the ears, subjective sensitivity to cold, lack of mental concentration and, in states of severe anemia, hemorrhages in the optic fundi. Gastrointestinal symptoms, including anorexia, nausea, and bowel disturbance are common although their pathophysiology is not understood. Similarly, there may be menstrual irregularity, urinary frequency, and loss of libido. All these symptoms and signs may be associated with general disturbances, such as weight loss, an increased basal metabolism rate, and low-grade fever.

CLASSIFICATION OF ANEMIA

Most pathologic phenomena result from complex interactions that make classification difficult—anemia is no exception.

When presented with an anemic patient it is possible to approach the problem in a simple and methodical way. Anemia may occur if blood is being lost more rapidly than it is being produced or if there is a primary defect in the production of red cells. Blood may be lost either in the circulation or in the reticuloendothelial system, or because of bleeding. Deficient production of blood may be either because the critical building blocks for red cell production are missing, because there is a defect in cellular maturation, or because there is a failure at the factory for red cell production—that is, disease of the bone marrow. This very simple clinical approach to anemia is summarized in Table 17.

A classification of anemia based on pathophysiologic considerations is shown in Table 18. It is derived from the descriptions of the way in which red cells are produced, mature, and survive in the peripheral circulation. Thus the anemias can be divided into those that result from defective red cell maturation, defective proliferation, or combined defects of maturation and proliferation. A further group can be defined as being

TABLE 17. CLINICAL CLASSIFICATION OF ANEMIA*

Excessive Blood Loss
  Hemorrhage
  Hemolysis

Defective Blood Formation
  Deficiency of factors essential for hemopoiesis
  Defective maturation of hemopoietic precursors with normal
    levels of hemopoietic factors
  Bone marrow failure

Reduced Tissue Requirements for Oxygen

*In practice it is common for more than one mechanism to be responsible for anemia.

TABLE 18. PATHOPHYSIOLOGIC CLASSIFICATION OF ANEMIA

Excessive Blood Loss
  Hemorrhage
  Hemolysis—genetic or acquired

Defective Blood Formation
  Ineffective erythropoiesis
    Impaired hemoglobin synthesis—genetic or acquired
    Impaired DNA synthesis—genetic or acquired
    Iron loading of red cell precursors
  Defective proliferation of red cell precursors
    Hypoplasia—genetic or acquired
    Secondary to infiltrative disease of bone marrow

Combination of Above

caused by a reduced red cell survival or excessive blood loss. Finally, in any classification of anemia those states must be considered in which there is a relative decrease in the red cell mass because of an expansion of the plasma volume.

ANEMIA DUE TO DEFECTIVE RED CELL MATURATION

IRON DEFICIENCY ANEMIA

Iron deficiency is the most frequent cause of anemia and is one of the world's commonest disorders. It has been estimated that 10 to 30 per cent of the world population is deficient in iron; this is a major public health problem in underdeveloped countries.

Etiology. The precarious balance between iron intake and loss was described earlier in this section (pp. 191 to 193). Iron deficiency has different causes at different stages of development. It is relatively common in the newborn period, particularly in premature infants, since the majority of the iron is taken on during the last trimester of pregnancy. During the first year of life a full-term infant requires 160 mg of iron and a premature infant requires 240 mg. About 50 mg is provided by red cell destruction that occurs during the first few weeks of life. The remainder must come from the diet. Particularly in the underdeveloped countries, prolonged breast feeding is a major cause of iron deficiency, and there is much current interest in the use of widespread fortification of infant foods with iron. Another danger period is in early adolescence after the growth spurt. In adult females the usual cause of iron deficiency is a poor diet associated with multiple pregnancies or excessive menstrual loss. Diets poor in animal products and rich in carbohydrates or tea are especially likely to cause iron deficiency. In males iron deficiency is usually due to blood loss, often from the gastrointestinal tract. Common sites include hiatus hernia, esophageal varices, peptic ulcers, neoplasia of the stomach or large bowel, and hemorrhoids. Intestinal parasites—in particular the various forms of hookworm—are a major cause of blood loss iron deficiency in the third world. Patients who have had partial gastrectomy may develop iron deficiency. Hydrochloric acid in the stomach plays an important role in iron absorption; reduced absorption of both inorganic iron and heme iron has been demonstrated after gastrectomy. There may be intermittent blood loss from the anastomosis, which results in a state of negative iron balance. Furthermore, many of these patients go into surgery with depleted iron stores that are never adequately replenished after surgery. Occasionally, malabsorption of iron due to small bowel disease may result in iron deficiency. This is particularly common in celiac disease in childhood.

Evolution of Iron Deficiency. It is very important to understand the evolution of iron deficiency once a state of negative iron balance is entered (Fig. 32). At first, iron is removed from the body stores. Once the stores are depleted, the plasma iron level starts to fall and the total iron-binding capacity of the plasma increases. At this stage the hemoglobin level starts to fall, but the red cell morphology and indices may still be relatively normal. Hence, the anemia may be initially normochromic, but once severe iron deficiency is established the cells become pale-staining (hypochromic) and smaller than normal (microcytic) (Fig. 33). These changes are reflected in the red cell indices; they show low mean corpuscular hemoglobin concentration and mean corpuscular volume values. A stained peripheral blood film shows hypochromia, microcytosis, and a variable degree of anisopoikilocytosis. Finally, when there is a state of severe iron deficiency there is, in addition to anemia, epithelial damage presumably caused by depletion of iron-containing enzymes in the tissues. This leads to a variety of tissue changes. Besides the low serum iron and increased total iron-

binding capacity, other changes of iron deficiency include absence of sideroblasts and storage iron in the bone marrow, and a reduced plasma ferritin level. In addition, a glance at Figure 31 explains why free protoporphyrin accumulates in the red cells.

Effects of Iron Deficiency. The symptoms and signs of iron deficiency anemia are those of any form of anemia. Because iron is vital for the enzyme systems of many other tissues, a variety of additional systemic effects are observed. There may be brittleness of the fingernails, which can become spoon-shaped (koilonychia). Dysphagia may occur owing to the formation of a web in the upper esophagus, a premalignant condition. Glossitis is common, and the tongue becomes smooth and depapillated. The full picture of glossitis, dysphagia, and koilonychia is often known by the eponymous title of *Plummer-Vinson,* or *Foster-Kelly-Patterson, syndrome.* It is unusual today to see the full syndrome in developed countries because severe chronic iron deficiency is not usually allowed to reach this advanced state. Iron deficiency is often associated with mild depression and other psychologic changes, but the whole relationship between iron metabolism and the central nervous system is still controversial.

Diagnostic Problems. Iron deficiency is not the only cause of hypochromic anemia, and it is important to remember the common disorders that may be confused with iron deficiency. These are listed in Table 19.

Response to Iron. When iron deficiency is treated

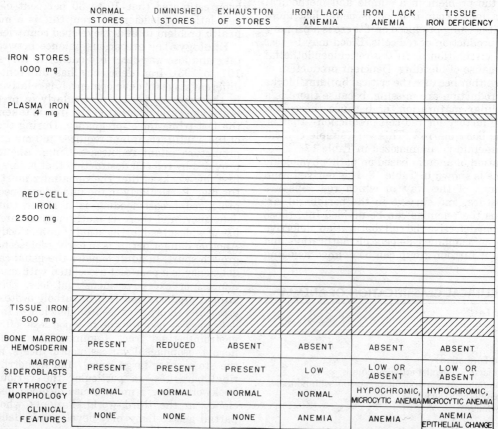

Figure 32. The evolution of iron deficiency. (From Harris, J. W., and Kellermeyer, R. W.: *The Red Cell.* Boston, Harvard University Press, 1970.)

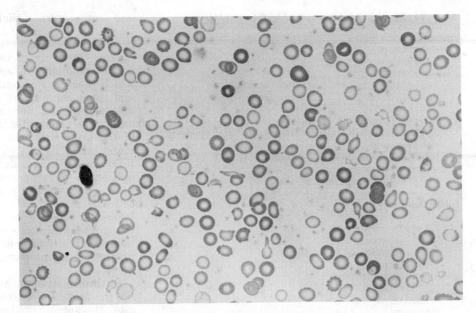

Figure 33. The blood film appearance in iron deficiency anemia (× 800).

with adequate doses of oral iron there is a slow rise in hemoglobin at a rate of approximately 1 g/dl per week. This is associated with a reticulocytosis on about the fifth to seventh day after iron has been administered. However, the reticulocyte count rarely rises above 10 per cent, not at all like the remarkable response that occurs after treatment of megaloblastic anemia, in which the count may rise to 30 to 50 per cent or more. This is probably because iron deficiency produces a defect in cellular proliferation as well as maturation and because the marrow in iron deficiency is somewhat hypoplastic rather than hyperplastic, as it is in megaloblastic anemia. Thus there is a gradual increase in the rate of erythropoiesis, which is reflected by only a modest reticulocytosis. In the megaloblastic anemias, in which the marrow is grossly hyperplastic, the administration of a factor that allows normal maturation produces a remarkable burst of reticulocytes about a week after the start of therapy. The methods available for assessing iron stores and for confirming the diagnosis of iron deficiencies are summarized on page 194.

Iron Overload. Iron overload occurs in several well-defined situations. It occurs in primary hemochromatosis in which there is a genetically determined increase in iron absorption, despite there being normal or increased iron stores. The second group of iron-loading states are those secondary to repeated blood transfusion or increased gastrointestinal iron absorption associated with hemolysis or dyserythropoiesis. Iron may be deposited in reticuloendothelial cells or, if iron loading progresses, in parenchymal cells.

The distribution of iron in iron-loading states accounts for the associated clinical disorders. It is laid down in the liver, spleen, endocrine glands, skin, gonads, and myocardium. Tissue damage to these organs may lead to cirrhosis; a variety of endocrine deficiency states, including diabetes mellitus and hypogonadism; and cardiac death due to progressive heart failure or arrhythmia. How iron produces tissue damage and fibrosis is not clear. Two well-documented effects that may be important are disruption of lysosomes and stimulation of collagen synthesis. Iron may also cause free radical generation with subsequent cell damage. Iron loading is discussed further in the sections on sideroblastic anemia and thalassemia.

THE MEGALOBLASTIC ANEMIAS

The megaloblastic anemias are usually caused by either vitamin B_{12} or folate deficiency. The main causes are summarized in Table 20. The metabolic functions of these vitamins were summarized earlier in this chapter (see pp. 194 to 196). Their deficiency gives rise to a primary defect in DNA metabolism and hence in cellular proliferation and maturation. As might be expected, this effect is mediated mainly in rapidly dividing cell populations, particularly those of the bone marrow, epithelia, and gonads. The main result of deficiency of these vitamins on the hemopoietic system is an abnormal form of red cell production called *megaloblastic erythropoiesis,* which in turn leads to a type of anemia in which the red cells are larger than normal and are therefore called *macrocytes.* The underlying abnormality of DNA metabolism is also reflected by abnormalities in the maturation of the white cell series and platelets.

Megaloblastic Erythropoiesis. The pathophysiology of megaloblastic erythropoiesis is still not entirely understood. There is a defect in maturation of the red

TABLE 19. THE HYPOCHROMIC ANEMIAS

Iron Deficiency
    Reduced intake
    Excessive demands or loss
    Reduced absorption
    Defective utilization (chronic disorders)
    Genetic defects in iron transport

Defective Hemoglobin Synthesis
    Globin synthesis—thalassemia
    Heme synthesis*—congenital and acquired sideroblastic
      anemia
    Hemoglobin instability. Some unstable hemoglobin disorders

*It is still not established that all these anemias are due to a primary defect in heme synthesis.

TABLE 20. THE MEGALOBLASTIC ANEMIAS

Vitamin B$_{12}$ Deficiency
Reduced intake
　Veganism
Reduced absorption
　Intrinsic factor deficiency (acquired or congenital)
　Postgastrectomy
　Ileal resection
　Disease of ileum—e.g., Crohn's disease, tropical sprue
　Stagnant-loop syndrome (blind loop, jejunal diverticula, etc.)
　Fish tapeworm
　Selective malabsorption with proteinuria
Abnormal transport
　Congenital transcobalamin deficiency

Folate Deficiency
Reduced intake
　Dietary insufficiency
Reduced absorption
　Adult and childhood celiac disease
　Tropical sprue
　Dermatitis herpetiformis
　Jejunal resection
Increased demands
　Pregnancy
　Hemolysis
　Myeloproliferative disorders
　Hemodialysis
Drugs
　Dihydrofolate reductase inhibitors—e.g., methotrexate
　By unknown mechanisms—anticonvulsants, alcohol
Metabolic
　Homocystinuria

Not Due to Vitamin B$_{12}$ or Folate Deficiency
Acquired
　Erythroleukemia
　Cytotoxic drugs
Congenital
　A variety of rare metabolic disorders, including orotic-
　　aciduria, Lesch-Nyhan syndrome, and others

and open pattern of their nuclear chromatin (Fig. 34). Curiously, despite the defect in nucleic acid synthesis, protein synthesis may occur normally, and hemoglobin appears in many of these large immature erythroblasts, producing a rather striking appearance in which there is apparent asynchrony between nuclear and cytoplasmic maturation. All developing red cells are larger than normal, and the mature red cells emerge as macrocytes. However, presumably because of the gross defect in maturation, these cells show many other distinctive changes, including poikilocytosis and striking anisocytosis with huge macrocytes and small misshapen cells mixed on the film. The macrocytes typically are oval. Maturation of the white cell and platelet series is also abnormal. The total leukocyte count is often reduced, as is the platelet count. The white cells are larger than normal and the neutrophils show five or more lobes—that is, hypersegmentation. Giant metamyelocytes are frequently observed.

Pathophysiology. Megaloblastic anemia is probably the best-studied example of ineffective erythropoiesis. The anemia produces a striking drive to erythropoiesis through the erythropoietin pathway, and there is marked hypertrophy of the bone marrow with extension down the shafts of the long bones. This is the typical picture of ineffective erythropoiesis: the marrow is extremely hyperplastic and yet the patient is anemic! Erythrokinetic studies indicate that there is a major breakdown of erythroid precursors in the bone marrow and that this is the main cause of anemia. There is some peripheral hemolysis, presumably due to the abnormal shape and size of the red cells, but the main cause of the anemia is the abnormal maturation and intramedullary destruction of the red cell precursors. Indeed, erythrokinetic data obtained from untreated patients with pernicious anemia provide an extraordinary picture of ineffective erythropoiesis. They show that total marrow erythropoiesis is increased up to about three times normal but that effective red cell production is less than normal. Since the erythrocytes that are delivered into the peripheral blood do not survive long, an equilibrium is reached at a severe degree of anemia. Total erythropoiesis is somewhat less, and effective erythropoiesis much less,

cell series that is reflected by the presence of many more primitive red cell precursors than normal in the bone marrow. There is marrow hyperplasia with intramedullary death of cells late in the maturation pathway. Nucleated red cell precursors show an arrest in nuclear maturation as reflected by the finely divided

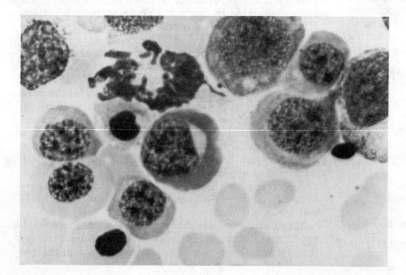

Figure 34. The bone marrow appearance in megaloblastic anemia. The megaloblasts show wide open chromatin in their nuclei and premature hemoglobinization of the cytoplasm. A single mitotic figure is seen (× 1200).

than would be expected of a normal marrow under comparable and sustained hypoxic stimulus.

With appropriate vitamin B_{12} or folic acid treatment there is a remarkably rapid return to normoblastic erythropoiesis. If the bone marrow is examined even within 24 to 48 hours of the start of treatment, red cell maturation is more normal in appearance, although there is still marked erythroid hyperplasia. Within three to five days the reticulocyte count in the peripheral blood starts to rise and reaches a peak at 7 to 10 days, at which time levels of up to 50 per cent reticulocytes may occur. There is a steady rise in the hemoglobin level, and the anemia is usually fully corrected by three months.

The findings outlined above are common to both vitamin B_{12} deficiency and folate deficiency, both of which produce abnormal DNA synthesis. These deficiency states must now be considered separately.

Vitamin B_{12} Deficiency

Pathogenesis. The most common cause of vitamin B_{12} deficiency is a deficiency of gastric intrinsic factor, which causes the clinical picture of pernicious anemia. A more complete classification of the causes of vitamin B_{12} deficiency is shown in Table 20. Like most vitamin deficiency states, they can be classified into those caused by defective intake, defective absorption, and defective utilization.

Inadequate dietary intake of vitamin B_{12} is rare, except in populations that for religious or other reasons adhere to a very strict vegetarian diet. It may also occur in total vegetarians, called vegans. The commonest cause of intrinsic factor deficiency is gastric atrophy, which is the basic underlying pathology of pernicious anemia. There is a rare congenital form of pernicious anemia that behaves as an autosomal recessive in which there is failure of intrinsic factor production. Total gastrectomy predictably leads to megaloblastic anemia after about two to six years, but vitamin B_{12} deficiency occurs only rarely after partial gastrectomy, unless there has been an extensive resection of the intrinsic-factor producing area. Since vitamin B_{12} is absorbed in the ileum, disease of this area causes vitamin B_{12} deficiency. Examples include surgical resection or involvement with regional ileitis, lymphoma, or tuberculosis of the ileum. Extensive disease of the small bowel, as occurs with tropical sprue or adult celiac disease, may occasionally cause vitamin B_{12} deficiency. There is a rare abnormality of the terminal ileum that causes a megaloblastic anemia in childhood and is usually associated with proteinuria; this is known as *Imerslund's syndrome*. Certain structural disorders of the small bowel reduce the availability of vitamin B_{12}. Any anatomic lesion that causes stasis and pooling of the lumenal contents with proliferation of bacteria may cause a situation in which vitamin B_{12} is taken up in the stagnant area and utilized by the bacteria. Such "blind loop" syndromes are caused by strictures of the small bowel, fistulas, and large diverticulae. A similar mechanism explains the megaloblastic anemia associated with the fish tapeworm (*Diphyllobothrium latum*).

Acquired intrinsic factor deficiency is by far the commonest cause of vitamin B_{12} deficiency, and the associated clinical disorder is known as *pernicious anemia*. It was first described in 1885 at Guy's Hospital, London, by Thomas Addison, and is sometimes known as *Addisonian pernicious anemia*. The basic defect is atrophy of the gastric mucosa, which results in an intrinsic factor deficiency. The etiology of the gastric atrophy is still far from certain. It seems likely that both genetic and autoimmune factors are involved. A genetic basis is suggested by the high incidence in certain races, such as Scandinavians, and by its association with blood group A. Furthermore, there is an increased incidence of the disorder among sibships and a markedly increased incidence of latent pernicious anemia within families. Latent pernicious anemia is characterized by lack of gastric acidity and decreased vitamin B_{12} absorption without the full hematologic features of pernicious anemia.

The atrophic gastritis of pernicious anemia is characterized by lack of normal gastric mucosa with a striking lymphocytic infiltration and an absence of gastric acid and pepsin production even after full stimulation with histamine or with pentagastrin. The serum gastrin level is raised. An autoimmune basis for this pathology has been suggested by the finding of autoantibodies against the cytoplasm of the gastric parietal cell in the serum of 90 per cent of patients with pernicious anemia. It should be noted, however, that individuals who do not have the disorder may have the same antibody. This includes 60 per cent of all individuals with atrophic gastritis, 30 per cent of relatives of patients with pernicious anemia, and about 10 per cent of the normal adult population. Patients with pernicious anemia frequently have antibodies directed against parenchymal tissue of endocrine glands, most commonly the acinar glands of the thyroid. On the other hand, patients with primary myxedema, or Hashimoto's thyroiditis, have a 30 per cent incidence of parietal cell antibodies and a 12 per cent incidence of coexisting pernicious anemia. Of more direct interest, however, is the finding that in about 57 per cent of patients with pernicious anemia there are anti-intrinsic factor antibodies in the serum, saliva, and gastric juice. These antibodies are polyclonal and may be IgG or IgA. It appears that they react to two different sites on the intrinsic factor molecule; there are blocking antibodies preventing the binding of vitamin B_{12} to intrinsic factor and binding antibodies that do not interfere with the attachment but impede absorption in the ileum. Intrinsic factor antibodies are found much less frequently than parietal cell antibodies in the general population and seem to be more specifically associated with pernicious anemia.

It appears, therefore, that individuals with a genetic predisposition toward pernicious anemia may develop autoimmune damage to the gastric mucosa and antibodies to intrinsic factor. It is unclear, however, whether the production of autoantibodies is a primary event or is secondary to whatever causes damage to the gastric mucosa.

Tissue and Neurologic Changes. There is a specific neurologic syndrome of vitamin B_{12} deficiency that is called subacute combined degeneration of the spinal cord. The pathologic changes are characterized by degenerative lesions in the dorsal and lateral columns. Early changes include swelling of individual myelinated nerve fibers and these lesions later coalesce into large foci involving many fiber systems. Similarly patchy degeneration occurs in the white matter of the brain. This produces a variety of clinical pictures, including cerebral manifestations ("megaloblastic madness"), perversions of taste and smell, defects in vision with central scotomata and optic atrophy, ataxia due to reduced dorsal column function, peripheral neuropathy, and, in some cases, a spastic paraplegia or quadriplegia when the lateral columns are involved.

In addition to the symptoms and signs of anemia and neurologic damage, patients with pernicious anemia have a lemon-yellow color due to slightly elevated unconjugated bilirubin, and about a third of them have palpable enlarged spleens.

Diagnosis of Vitamin B_{12} Deficiency. The laboratory investigation of vitamin B_{12} deficiency is based on an understanding of its pathophysiology. The finding of a macrocytic peripheral blood picture with a megaloblastic bone marrow usually indicates either vitamin B_{12} deficiency or folate deficiency. With vitamin B_{12} deficiency, the serum vitamin B_{12} level, as assayed microbiologically with *Lactobacillus leishmanii* or *Euglena gracilis,* or by isotope dilution, is reduced. In true pernicious anemia there is a histamine or pentagastrin-fast achlorhydria. Radioactive vitamin B_{12} absorption can be assayed by the Schilling test, in which a dose of ^{58}Co- or ^{57}Co-labeled cyanocobalamin is given by mouth at the same time as an intramuscular "flushing" dose of nonradioactive cyanocobalamin, and the amount of radioactivity in the urine is measured. The reason for giving the intramuscular dose of vitamin B_{12} is that normally when the vitamin is taken by mouth, it enters the liver, and only after a large dose given by injection to preload the liver does sufficient orally administered B_{12} appear in the urine to be easily measured. In the absence of intrinsic factor reduced amounts of radioactivity appear in the urine. The second part of the Schilling test consists of giving radioactive vitamin B_{12} together with intrinsic factor, after which a considerable portion of the radioactivity appears in the urine if the patient has genuine intrinsic factor deficiency. If vitamin B_{12} is due to small bowel disease, absorption is not corrected by intrinsic factor. Absorption can also be measured by monitoring the patient in a whole-body counter. In cases in which a blind loop is suspected, vitamin B_{12} absorption can be measured before and after giving a course of broad-spectrum antibiotics, which destroy the bacteria in the stagnant loop. Structural disease of the small bowel requires radiologic investigation and jejunal biopsy. Another test for vitamin B_{12} deficiency is the measurement of methylmalonic acid in the urine, which is elevated if there is a vitamin B_{12} deficiency (see pp. 194 to 195).

FOLATE DEFICIENCY

Pathogenesis. The causes of folic acid deficiency are summarized in Table 20. They include insufficient intake, defective absorption or utilization, and excessive demand.

Insufficient intake of folate may result from a diet poor in fruit and vegetables and is relatively common in the sick or malnourished and in alcoholics. Infants fed on goat's milk, which is poor in folate, are also prone to deficiency. Defective absorption of folate occurs most commonly with small bowel disease involving the jejunum. It occurs in celiac disease and in the other malabsorption syndromes and is particularly common in tropical sprue. Increased requirements for folate occur in pregnancy and also in patients with increased bone marrow activity, particularly with chronic hemolytic anemias and in the myeloproliferative disorders. Certain drugs interfere with folate metabolism, notably methotrexate and related antifolates. The anti-convulsant drugs, particularly the hydantoinates, produce folate deficiency quite frequently, although the precise mechanism is unknown. They may interfere with intestinal absorption.

Effects of Folate Depletion. Folate deficiency produces a macrocytic anemia with megaloblastic hemopoiesis identical to that which occurs with vitamin B_{12} deficiency. Similarly, the effects on the gastrointestinal mucosa and skin are the same in the two deficiency states. However, folate deficiency rarely produces neurologic symptoms.

Diagnosis of Folate Deficiency. Folate deficiency results in a low serum folate level, which is usually assayed using a microbiologic procedure with *Lactobacillus casei.* The serum folate level may be low long before megaloblastic changes occur, and assay of red cell folate probably gives a better assessment of the level of folate coenzymes in tissues. Red cell folate levels in patients with vitamin B_{12} deficiency are often low, whereas serum folate levels in "pure" vitamin B_{12} deficiency are usually elevated. There are no readily available tests of folate absorption, and when in doubt the results of a therapeutic trial of physiologic doses of folic acid—that is, 50 to 100 μg daily—may be used to distinguish folate from vitamin B_{12} deficiency. The estimation of formimino glutamic acid (FIGLU) excretion after histidine loading is occasionally used as a test for folate deficiency, but it is less reliable than red cell folate values. Recently, the deoxyuridine (du) suppression test has been developed to distinguish vitamin B_{12} deficiency from folate deficiency. This is illustrated in Figure 35.

OTHER CAUSES OF MEGALOBLASTIC ANEMIA

There are some rare inborn errors of metabolism that result in megaloblastic anemia. These are of interest largely because of the light they throw on the normal metabolic pathways for vitamin B_{12} and folate. They are summarized in Table 20. Drugs interfering directly with DNA synthesis—for example, hydroxyurea, cytosine arabinoside, and 6-mercaptopurine—may also cause megaloblastic anemia.

OTHER ACQUIRED DEFECTS OF ERYTHROID MATURATION

There are other, but less common, groups of acquired disorders of erythroid maturation in which there is no evidence of iron deficiency or vitamin B_{12} deficiency and in which the underlying basis for the maturation abnormality is not understood. These disorders have gone under the general term of "refractory anemia with hyperplastic bone marrow" but more recently it has become possible to classify them into several subgroups, depending on the morphologic appearance of the red cell precursors. By far the commonest are the sideroblastic anemias.

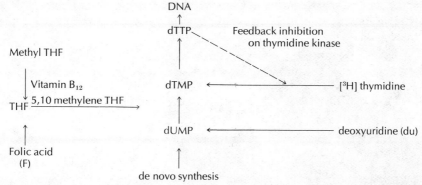

Figure 35. The principle of the deoxyuridine monophosphate (dUMP) test for vitamin B_{12} deficiency. The test measures the incorporation of [^{3}H] thymidine into DNA. In megaloblastic anemia due to vitamin B_{12} deficiency or folate deficiency deoxyuridine (dU) does not suppress incorporation of labeled thymidine into DNA to the same degree as it does in normal marrow. This is thought to be due to a block in conversion of dUMP (formed from dU) to thymidine monophosphate (dTMP) and so to a failure of feedback inhibition on thymidine uptake in the cells. In vitamin B_{12} deficiency this can be corrected in vitro by vitamin B_{12} and folic acid but not by methyltetrahydrofolate. In folate deficiency the defect can be corrected by folic acid and methyltetrahydrofolate but not by vitamin B_{12}.

Sideroblastic Anemia. In an earlier section it was pointed out that many normal red cell precursors contain iron granules scattered throughout their cytoplasm. These cells are called *sideroblasts*. However, there are some anemias in which there is pathologic accumulation of iron in the red cell precursors that is distributed in a ring, or "collar," around the nucleus. These erythroblasts are called *ring sideroblasts*. Their presence is the characteristic feature of a heterogeneous group of disorders known as the sideroblastic anemias. Electron microscopic analysis of the bone marrow shows that the iron is present in the mitochondria, which show marked disruption and loss of normal structure (Fig. 36). It is presumed that this pathologic process causes the abnormal red cell maturation and ineffective erythropoiesis that characterizes these conditions.

A classification of the different types of sideroblastic anemia is shown in Table 21. The congenital forms are very rare. Usually the condition occurs in middle or late life and no obvious cause is found. In some cases there is a history of exposure to drugs, particularly chloramphenicol or isoniazid, or toxins such as lead and alcohol, while in others the sideroblastic anemia may be the first indication of a disorder that may evolve into leukemia or other myeloproliferative states. Although some cases may respond partially to

pyridoxine therapy, there is no evidence that genuine pyridoxine deficiency can produce sideroblastic anemia, except very rarely in patients with malabsorption syndromes. The fact that there are frequently two erythroid populations present in patients with idiopathic sideroblastic anemia—one normochromic and the other hypochromic—suggests that the condition may result from a somatic mutation with the production of a cell line with a metabolic defect in iron handling, which results in iron loading of the mitochondria and ineffective erythropoiesis. Although it has been suggested that the basic lesion in this disorder is an acquired defect in heme synthesis, no specific enzyme deficiency in the heme synthetic pathway has been demonstrated.

The hematologic findings are common to all the forms of sideroblastic anemia. There is usually a moderate degree of anemia with a dimorphic blood picture—that is, both hypochromic and normochromic populations. The marrow is hyperplastic and there is a maturation abnormality in the erythroid precursors with many large forms that have some megaloblastic features. Iron staining shows gross iron loading of the red cell precursors, a high proportion of which show the typical "ring" sideroblast appearance (Fig. 36). The serum iron level is usually normal or elevated and there may be increased iron absorption and deposition of iron in the reticuloendothelial cells, particularly in the liver. Ferrokinetic studies indicate a marked degree of ineffective erythropoiesis. Other features of the sideroblastic anemias and a comparison of the acquired form with the congenital form of the disorder are summarized in Table 22. The congenital form is described further on p. 226.

Refractory Anemia with Hyperplastic Bone Marrow. Finally, in any account of the disorders of cellular maturation a heterogeneous group must be included in which there is anemia together with a hyperplastic bone marrow that does not show an increase in ring sideroblasts. This condition is often associated with a marked degree of ineffective erythropoiesis and the presence of increased levels of fetal hemoglobin and fetal antigens on the red cell surface.

TABLE 21. THE SIDEROBLASTIC ANEMIAS

Congenital
  X-linked
  Others
Acquired
  Primary or idiopathic
  Secondary
    Drugs—INH, chloramphenicol
    Alcohol
    Lead
    Malabsorption
    Myeloproliferative disorders
    Leukemia
    Secondary carcinoma

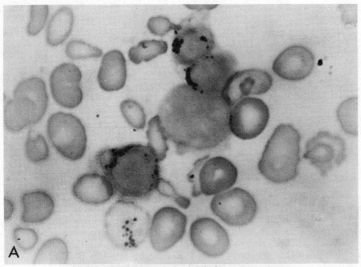

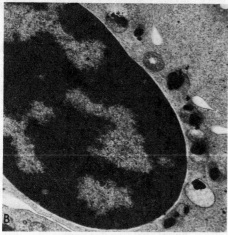

Figure 36. Sideroblastic anemia. *A,* Ring sideroblasts demonstrated by iron staining of bone marrow sample using Pearls reagent. *B,* Electron microscopic appearance of a ring sideroblast showing iron loading of the mitochondria. (Prepared by Professor S. Wickremasingh.)

It may remain as a simple refractory anemia for many years or evolve into a myeloproliferative disorder, such as acute leukemia.

Recently, these disorders have been grouped together under the general heading of the *myelodysplastic syndrome.* Attempts are being made to subclassify these conditions according to cytogenetic and surface markers to permit definition of subgroups of the syndrome according to their prognostic characteristics.

GENETIC DISORDERS OF RED CELL MATURATION

Genetic disorders of red cell maturation involve either the synthesis of globin (the thalassemias) or the synthesis of heme (the congenital sideroblastic anemias). In addition, there is a rare group of anemias characterized by a primary defect in red cell maturation and division of unknown etiology that bear the term "congenital dyserythropoietic anemias (CDA)."

THALASSEMIA

Thalassemia was first described by Thomas Cooley in 1925. Its name is derived from the Greek "thalassa," the sea, because the early cases reported in the United States were all of Mediterranean background. It is now realized that there are many forms of thalassemia and that these conditions have a worldwide distribution. Indeed, they are the commonest single gene disorders in the world population. The reason for this extraordinarily high gene frequency is still uncertain but there is some evidence that heterozygous carriers are, or have been, at an advantage in areas where malaria is, or was, endemic.

The new techniques of recombinant DNA technology have provided a great deal of evidence about the molecular pathology of the thalassemias. Indeed, more is known about the molecular basis of these disorders than about any other groups of human diseases, and their study is providing a great deal of information about human genetics in general.

Definition and Pathogenesis. The thalassemias are defined as a group of genetic disorders of hemoglobin synthesis in which there is a reduced rate of production of one or more of the globin chains of hemoglobin (Tables 23, 24, and 25). According to which chain is affected, they can be divided into the α, β, $\delta\beta$, $\gamma\delta\beta$, and δ-thalassemias, respectively. The α- and β-thalassemias are by far the most common and important forms of the condition. Both α- and β-thalassemia can be further subdivided into α^0- or β^0-thalassemia, in which no α or β chains are produced, and α^+- and

TABLE 22. CLINICAL AND HEMATOLOGIC FEATURES OF SIDEROBLASTIC ANEMIA

CONGENITAL	ACQUIRED
Mainly males	Both sexes
Mild splenomegaly	Splenomegaly unusual, unless part of a myeloproliferative disorder
Dimorphic blood picture with an extremely hypochromic population	Dimorphic blood picture; usually a population of moderately hypochromic cells
Reduced overall MCH and MCV	Overall MCV often normal or increased and MCH normal or slightly reduced
Marrow hyperplasia with large percentage of ring sideroblasts	Marrow hyperplastic, normal cellularity or hypoplastic; variable number of ring sideroblasts
Platelets and white cells normal	White cells usually normal; platelets reduced in 30% of cases
Red cell protoporphyrin reduced	Red cell protoporphyrin elevated
Hb A_2 reduced; Hb F normal	Hb A_2 reduced or normal; Hb F normal

TABLE 23. THE β-THALASSEMIAS

TYPE	HOMOZYGOTE	HETEROZYGOTE	MOLECULAR LESION
β°	Transfusion dependent Hbs F and A_2 No Hb A	Mild anemia Low MCH and MCV Raised Hb A_2	Partial deletion of β globin gene Premature stop codon Frameshift mutation Splice junction mutation
β⁺	Transfusion dependent Hbs F, A, and A_2	Same as above	Mutation causing cryptic splice site Promotor sequence mutation

TABLE 24. THE α-THALASSEMIAS

TYPE	HOMOZYGOTE	HETEROZYGOTE	MOLECULAR LESION
α°	Hb Bart's hydrops Hbs Bart's + Portland No Hb F	Mild anemia Low MCH and MCV Normal Hb A_2 5–10% Hb Bart's at birth	Deletion of both α globin genes Four different sized deletions identified
α⁺ (deletion)	Mild anemia Low MCH and MCV Normal Hb A_2 5–10% Hb Bart's at birth	Normal Slightly reduced MCH and MCV in some cases 1–2% Hb Bart's at birth in some cases	Deletion of one of the pair of linked α globin genes Two different sized deletions identified
α⁺ (nondeletion)	In some cases not yet defined. The Saudi Arabian form causes Hb H disease Hb Constant Spring produces a mild hemolytic anemia and splenomegaly	As for α⁺ (deletion) Hb Constant Spring carriers have about 1% of the variant	Very heterogeneous. Some forms result from the synthesis of very unstable hemoglobin variants. Hb Constant Spring results from a chain termination mutation, UAA→CAA. The Saudi Arabian form results from different mutations in the α1 and α2 genes

*Each type is very heterogeneous. Hemoglobin H disease results from the compound heterozygous state for α⁺- and α°-thalassemia or the homozygous state for the Saudi Arabian form of α⁺-thalassemia.

TABLE 25. THE DIVERSITY OF δβ-THALASSEMIA*

TYPE	HOMOZYGOTE	HETEROZYGOTE	MOLECULAR LESION
(δβ)° Lepore thalassemia	Thalassemia major Hbs F and Lepore	Thalassemia minor ~ 10% Hb Lepore	Unequal crossing over with the product of a δβ fusion gene
^{G}γ^{A}γ(δβ)°-thalassemia	Thalassemia intermedia 100% Hb F	Thalassemia minor ~ 15% Hb F	Deletion of δ and β globin genes†
^{G}γ(δβ)°-thalassemia	Thalassemia intermedia 100% Hb F	Thalassemia minor ~ 15% Hb F	Deletion of δ, β, and part of ^{A}γ genes†
(γδβ)°-thalassemia	Not viable	Thalassemia minor Normal Hb A_2	Deletion of ^{G}γ, ^{A}γ, and δ globin genes†
^{G}γ^{A}γ(δβ)° HPFH	Thalassemia minor 100% Hb F	Normal hematology 25% Hb F	Deletion of δ and β globin genes†

*The diversity of δβ-thalassemia illustrates the phenotypes produced by gene deletions as shown in Figure 42. In hereditary persistence of fetal hemoglobin (HPFH) the output of γ chains almost completely compensates for the absence of δ and β chains; this is not the case in the different forms of δβ-thalassemia.
†It is presumed that differences in the extent of the deletions are responsible for the different phenotypes.

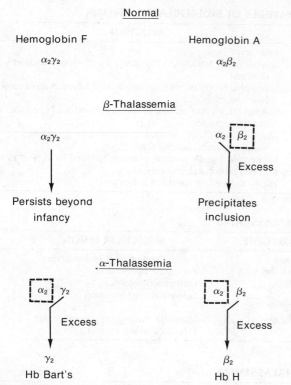

Figure 37. The pathophysiology and main subdivisions of the thalassemias.

β^+-thalassemia, in which some α or β chain synthesis occurs but at a reduced rate.

A general plan of the pathogenesis of the α- and β-thalassemias is shown in Figure 37. The β-thalassemias only affect the production of adult hemoglobin; fetal hemoglobin synthesis is normal, and therefore the disease only appears after birth when adult hemoglobin synthesis is established. The excess α chains that are produced in β-thalassemia are unable to form a tetramer and precipitate in the red cell precursors. On the other hand, α-thalassemia affects both fetal and adult hemoglobin synthesis, since α chains are shared by both types of hemoglobin. Unlike β-thalassemia, the excess non-α chains that are produced in α-thalassemia are capable of forming a hemoglobin tetramer. In fetal life, excess γ chains form γ_4 tetramers, or hemoglobin Bart's. In adult life, excess β chains form β_4 molecules that are called hemoglobin H.

Molecular Genetics. The precise molecular defect that causes some types of thalassemia has now been established. In some cases it has been possible to achieve this by simple restriction enzyme mapping of the globin genes. In cases in which the molecular lesion is more subtle and is not associated with a major gene rearrangement or deletion, it has been necessary to clone the appropriate genes in bacteriophage and to sequence them. A picture of remarkable molecular diversity has emerged from these sophisticated studies.

Over 30 different mutations have been found to underlie the β-thalassemias (Fig. 38). Several forms of β-thalassemia result from either the insertion or loss of one or more nucleotide bases, which causes a shift in the reading frame of the genetic code. Because genetic information is stored as a triplet code, the insertion or loss of one, two, or four bases throws the reading frame completely out of sequence. Messenger RNA transcribed from genes affected in this way can only be translated normally up to the point of the frame shift; beyond that point the sequence changes completely, or translation ceases. In either case it is not possible to synthesize a viable globin chain. Other forms of β-thalassemia result from so-called nonsense or premature chain termination mutations. In this case a single base change produces a new termination

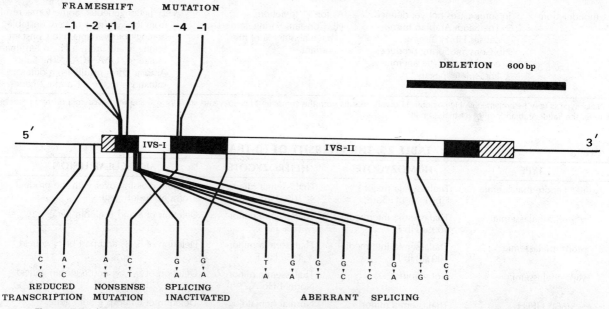

Figure 38. A summary of some of the mutations responsible for β-thalassemia. The β-globin gene is represented as a box with two introns (IVS-1 and IVS-2) and three exons in dark shading. The hatched regions represent the parts of the gene that code for the nontranslated regions of the globin messenger RNA. bp = base pairs.

codon; instead of an amino acid being inserted when the message is translated, premature chain termination occurs and a nonviable globin chain is produced. Another group of β-thalassemias result from single base mutations that interfere with processing of the messenger RNA precursors. These mutations may occur at exon-intron junctions (see p. 206) and hence interfere with the normal splicing of the exons after the excision of the introns. These mutations prevent any normal messenger RNA being produced and thus are associated with the phenotype of β⁰-thalassemia. More subtle base changes may produce so-called cryptic splice mutations. In this case a new splice site is produced such that part of the intron is incorporated into the messenger RNA, and hence it cannot be used as a template for normal β globin synthesis. In these cases the normal splice sites are not affected. There may be both normal and abnormal β messenger RNA produced, giving rise to the phenotype of β⁺-thalassemia. This type of mechanism is illustrated in Figure 39. Yet another group of β-thalassemias results from single base changes in the regulatory regions upstream from the 5′ end of the β globin gene. These interfere

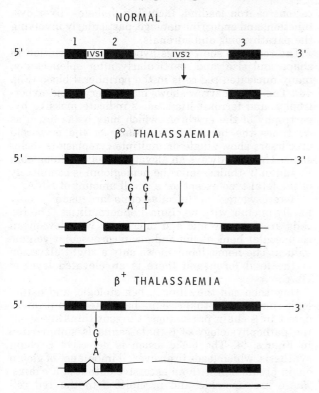

Figure 39. Splicing defects in β-thalassemia. The top figure shows how normally IVS-1 and IVS-2 are removed and the three exons are joined together. In the form of β⁰-thalassemia shown here there is a defect at the splice junction between the second exon and the second intron. In addition, there is a G → T substitution within the first intron, which produces a new splicing site. Splicing is completely defective because of the G → A substitution at the intron-exon junction. Two abnormal messenger RNA molecules are produced. In the β⁺-thalassemia defect there is a G → A substitution in the first intron, which produces a new splice site. The majority of messenger RNA produced is abnormal because it contains some of the first intron sequences, but a small amount of normal messenger RNA is also synthesized.

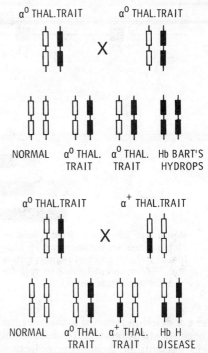

Figure 40. The genetics of α-thalassemia. Normal α genes are shown by open boxes and defective α genes by shaded boxes. The α⁰-thalassemia haplotype is characterized by defective production by both the linked α genes; α⁺-thalassemia trait results from α chain production by only one of the linked pairs of α genes.

with the transcription of β globin messenger RNA. Finally, one form of β⁰-thalassemia results from a 600 base deletion involving the 3′ end of the β globin gene.

The molecular pathology of the common forms of α thalassemia is different from that of β-thalassemia (Fig. 40). As mentioned earlier (see p. 206), there are two α globin genes per haploid genome. The common forms of α-thalassemia result from a series of gene deletions that involve either one or both of the linked α globin genes. The α⁺-thalassemias are caused by the loss of one α globin gene, thus leaving one functional α globin gene per haploid genome. The α⁰-thalassemias result from different length deletions, which involve both linked α globin genes and hence leave only the embryonic ζ globin genes intact on chromosome 16 (Fig. 41). The situation is not quite as simple as this, however. It is becoming apparent that there are some nondeletion forms of α-thalassemia. The commonest is a chain termination mutation called *hemoglobin Constant Spring*. This variant occurs in up to 5 per cent of some populations in Southeast Asia. It results from a single base change in the α chain termination codon, UAA→CAA. CAA codes for glutamine, so that instead of terminating at the usual position glutamine is inserted and then α globin messenger RNA at the 3′ end that is not normally translated is translated for a further 90 nucleotides until another stop codon is reached. This results in the production of an elongated α chain with 31 extra amino acid residues at the C terminal end. For some reason the translation of this extra messenger RNA renders it unstable, and hence these elongated α chains are made in very low amounts and are associated with the phenotype of α⁺-thalasse-

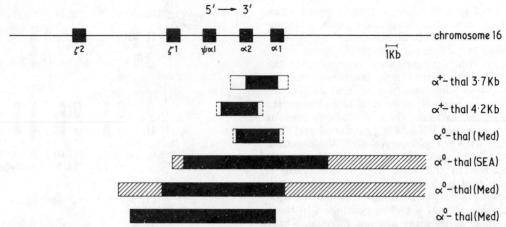

Figure 41. The various gene deletions responsible for α-thalassemia. The arrangement of the α globin genes on chromosome 16 is as depicted in Figure 29. The different deletions are shown in black, and the hatched regions represent uncertainty about their full extent. The designations Med and SEA represent lesions seen in the Mediterranean region and Southeast Asia, respectively. 1Kb = 1000 nucleotide bases.

mia. Other nondeletion forms of α-thalassemia are due to single base substitutions that produce highly unstable α chain variants or to splicing defects of a type similar to some forms of the β-thalassemia described earlier.

The δβ-thalassemias are also very heterogeneous at the molecular level (Fig. 42). In some cases they result from long deletions that remove the δ and β globin genes. Another form of δβ-thalassemia is due to the production of hemoglobin in which normal α chains are combined with non-α chains that consist of part δ and part β chain. This δβ fusion chain is directed by a δβ fusion gene, which has arisen by an accident of meiosis in which the chromosomes carrying the δ and β chain genes have become misaligned, and there has been unequal crossing over with the production of a δβ fusion gene. This novel hemoglobin is called *hemoglobin Lepore* (after the family name of the first recorded case). There are several different forms of this variant, depending on the point of abnormal crossing over between the δ and β chain genes.

β-Thalassemia. In the homozygous state for the different forms of β-thalassemia there is usually severe anemia from about the third month of life. Affected children are usually maintained on regular blood transfusion and survive until about the second decade. As they develop, they become pigmented and have increasing hepatosplenomegaly. Their bones are brittle and they develop thickening of the long bones and of the skull. The skull assumes a curious shape with frontal bossing and overdevelopment of the zygomata. The eyes are wide set, and the whole facial appearance comes to resemble that seen in the Mongoloid races. As these children develop, and particularly if they are not adequately transfused, they become stunted in growth and hypermetabolic, with a raised BMR, fever, and wasting. They have increased folate requirements and may develop megaloblastic anemia. The major cause of death is iron loading. Nearly all of them die a cardiac death related to the effects of cardiac siderosis. Very few β-thalassemia homozygotes go into normal puberty, and they develop a variety of compli-

cations of iron loading, including diabetes, liver dysfunction, and endocrine damage, particularly involving the parathyroids and adrenals.

The red cells show gross hypochromia, variation in shape and size, and, particularly after splenectomy, many nucleated red cells in the peripheral blood (Fig. 43). The bone marrow shows marked erythroid hypertrophy, and ferrokinetic studies indicate massive hypertrophy of the erythron, which may be as much as 40 times the normal mass. Many of the erythroid precursors show single or multiple cytoplasmic inclusions. There is always an elevated level of hemoglobin F, and in β⁰-thalassemia the hemoglobin is completely of the fetal type except for a small amount of Hb A₂.

Heterozygotes for β-thalassemia are usually only mildly anemic with no clinical abnormalities. The red cells are hypochromic and microcytic with low mean corpuscular hemoglobin and mean corpuscular volume values. The hemoglobin shows only a slight elevation of the fetal form, and there is an elevated level of HbA₂.

How then can the clinical, hematologic, and pathologic changes of β-thalassemia be related to a primary defect in β chain production? Current thinking about the pathophysiology of β-thalassemia is summarized in Figure 44. The basic lesion is defective β chain synthesis, which leads to an overall imbalance of globin chain production with an excessive output of α chains. These are unstable and precipitate in the red cell precursors to form large ragged inclusions. It is these inclusions that cause grossly abnormal red cell maturation and massive intramedullary destruction of red cell precursors. The precipitated α chains may cause damage by rendering the cells more rigid or by interfering with cell division, or both. Cells that do reach the peripheral blood contain inclusions, and these produce a rigid cell that is prematurely destroyed in the spleen and other parts of the reticuloendothelial system. Thus the anemia of β-thalassemia is due to a combination of infective erythropoiesis (due to abnormal red cell maturation) and hemolysis.

Some β-thalassemic red cell precursors retain the

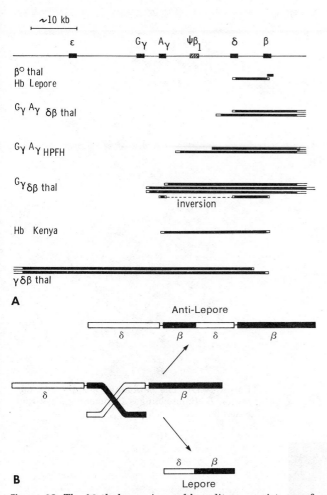

~10 kb

ε $^G\gamma$ $^A\gamma$ $\psi\beta_1$ δ   β

β° thal
Hb Lepore

$^G\gamma$ $^A\gamma$ δβ thal

$^G\gamma$ $^A\gamma$ HPFH

$^G\gamma$ δβ thal

inversion

Hb Kenya

γδβ thal

A

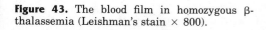

Anti-Lepore

δ   β   δ   β

δ   β

δ   β

B   Lepore

Figure 42. The δβ-thalassemias and hereditary persistence of fetal hemoglobin (HPFH). *A,* The various deletions responsible for these conditions. The β globin gene cluster is as depicted in Figure 29. The deletions are shown in black, and the open ends represent uncertainty about their full extent. The small deletion responsible for β°-thalassemia is shown for comparison. *B,* The production of hemoglobin Lepore and its mirror image, anti-Lepore, by chromosomal misalignment and unequal crossing over at the closely linked δ and β chain loci.

ability to make fetal γ chains and hence bind α chains to produce Hb F. This occurs only in a limited number of precursors, and the Hb F–producing population in β-thalassemia is better hemoglobinized and survives longer because its precursors contain relatively fewer α chain inclusions. Hb F–containing cells have a higher oxygen affinity than cells that contain adult hemoglobin, and this, together with the severe degree of anemia, produces a tremendous drive to erythropoietin production. This in turn causes massive hypertrophy of the erythroid bone marrow, which spreads down the long bones and between the diploë of the skull and into extramedullary sites, such as the spleen, liver, and even into the chest or spinal canal. However, in this massively expanded erythroid marrow, most of the erythropoiesis is ineffective and therefore of little use to the affected child. It is this massively expanded and rapidly turning over erythropoietic marrow that produces the hypermetabolic state, fever, and wasting of β-thalassemia. These patients need regular blood transfusions. Each unit of blood contributes 200 mg of iron, so that by the time they reach the middle of the second decade many of these patients have accumulated as much as 60 to 80 g of iron. Furthermore, with the massively expanded erythron there is increased iron absorption. It is easy to see why these unfortunate children become massively iron loaded. The iron has a particular predilection for the endocrine system, liver, and myocardium. How it damages and causes fibrosis of these organs is not clear, but it is deposited in the lysosomes and causes their disruption, with the release of enzymes leading to tissue damage (see p. 213).

α-Thalassemia. There are two main α-thalassemia determinants, α°-thalassemia and α⁺-thalassemia. Although these are heterogeneous at the molecular level, the important clinical forms of α-thalassemia result from the interaction of these two main classes of determinants (Fig. 40 and Table 24). The homozygous state for α°-thalassemia, in which no α globin chains are synthesized, results in the hemoglobin Bart's hydrops syndrome. The compound heterozygous state for α°- and α⁺-thalassemia, in which there is only one functional α globin gene, causes hemoglobin H disease. As mentioned earlier, there is at least one common

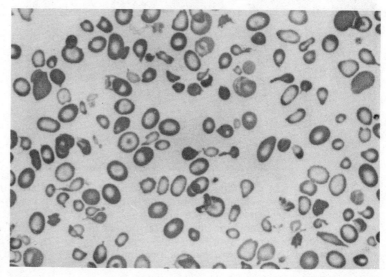

Figure 43. The blood film in homozygous β-thalassemia (Leishman's stain × 800).

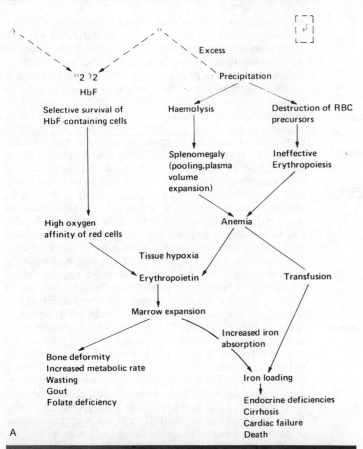

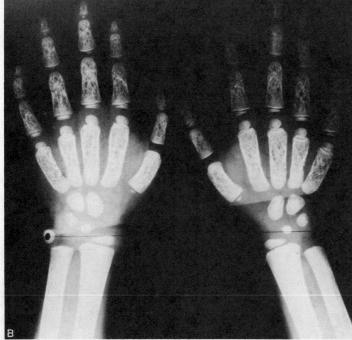

Figure 44. *A*, The pathophysiology of β-thalassemia. *B*, Bone changes in homozygous β-thalassemia.

nondeletion form of α^+-thalassemia that is characterized by the synthesis of hemoglobin Constant Spring. The compound heterozygous state for α^0-thalassemia and the hemoglobin Constant Spring determinant also produce a form of hemoglobin H disease.

The Hb Bart's hydrops syndrome is a common cause of stillbirth throughout Southeast Asia. Affected infants have no α chain genes and make no α chains. Thus their hemoglobin consists of hemoglobin Bart's (γ_4) and a small amount of Hb H (β_4). Since oxygen transport depends on normal heme-heme interaction, which in turn requires interaction between α and non-α subunits, these hemoglobins are physiologically useless. These babies have a gross defect in hemoglobin synthesis, and the hemoglobin that they do produce has the properties of myoglobin; that is, it does not give up its oxygen at physiologic tensions. Hence, they are usually stillborn at about 34 weeks, although occasionally they survive to term and are liveborn but die within a few hours of birth. Considering their hemoglobin physiology it is remarkable that they survive at all. The stillborn infants show gross edema—that is, hydrops fetalis, and pallor. There is massive hepatosplenomegaly and extramedullary erythropoiesis. All the organs are edematous, and there is ascites with pleural effusions. The reason for this severe edema is not fully understood, although these infants are probably hypoalbuminemic, possibly because of the effect of intrauterine anemia on albumin synthesis, and also from diversion of albumin precursors into the expanded erythron. There is severe anemia with the typical thalassemic blood picture and many circulating normoblasts. The marrow shows gross erythroid hyperplasia. It seems likely that these infants are anemic because hemoglobin Bart's is relatively unstable, so that there is a marked hemolytic component; furthermore, because the red cells contain a hemoglobin that does not give up its oxygen at physiologic tensions, the infants are profoundly hypoxic. The fact that hemoglobin Bart's has a very high oxygen affinity is a nice confirmation of the fact that normal heme-heme interaction requires both α and β chains—that is, the interaction of unlike subunits. Similarly, hemoglobin H is equally useless as an oxygen carrier.

Hemoglobin H disease is characterized by a variable degree of anemia and splenomegaly. The red cells show marked hypochromia and variation in shape and size. If they are mixed with a redox agent, such as brilliant cresyl blue, they generate large numbers of inclusion bodies owing to precipitation of Hb H by the dye. After splenectomy, large preformed single inclusions are found in the red cells. The pathophysiology of the anemia is well understood. There is less ineffective erythropoiesis than in β-thalassemia because the excess β chains form soluble tetramers (β_4). However, these tetramers are relatively unstable and form inclusion bodies as red cells age, and these cause the cells to be damaged in their passage through the spleen and other parts of the reticuloendothelial system, the result being a marked hemolytic anemia. Interestingly, hemoglobin H disease is not associated with much iron loading. Although there is increased iron absorption from the gastrointestinal tract these patients are not usually transfusion dependent. Furthermore, since hemoglobin binds to haptoglobin through its α chains, Hb H, which contains no α chains, does not bind to haptoglobin, and this allows increased urinary iron loss to compensate for the increased rate of iron absorption.

The heterozygous carrier states for α^0-thalassemia and α^+-thalassemia are characterized by mild abnormalities of red cell morphology and hemoglobinization. There are no associated changes in hemoglobin pattern except at birth, when increased levels of Hb Bart's are present.

δβ-**Thalassemia.** The δβ-thalassemias (Table 25) are milder than the β-thalassemias or severe forms of α-thalassemia. Homozygotes have a mild anemia and splenomegaly, thalassemic red cell changes, together with 100 per cent hemoglobin F. It appears that when the δ and β globin genes are completely deleted, γ chain synthesis more efficiently compensates for the lack of β chain production than is the case in β-thalassemia. The hemoglobin Lepore thalassemias are more severe and in the homozygous states more closely resemble the severe forms of β-thalassemia. For some reason, γ chain production is less efficient if there is a δβ fusion gene than if the δ and β globin genes are deleted.

There is a group of conditions related to δβ thalassemia called hereditary persistence of fetal hemoglobin (HPFH) (Table 25). Although these conditions are of no clinical significance, they provide an important group of models for studying the genetic regulation of the control of fetal and adult hemoglobin during development. They are characterized by defective or absent δ and β globin chain synthesis, but this is almost completely compensated for by persistent γ chain production. As is the case in the different forms of δβ-thalassemia, the conditions may be associated with persistent $^G\gamma$ and $^A\gamma$ synthesis or by the production of only $^G\gamma$ chains. These observations provide the basis for the nomenclature of the δβ-thalassemias and HPFH, that is, allows them to be divided into $^G\gamma$ or $^G\gamma^A\gamma$ types (Table 25).

Other Thalassemic Disorders. The thalassemic disorders described above are those in which the genetics are most clearly understood. However, there are many other thalassemia-like states in which the genetics have not been fully worked out. There are several forms of β-thalassemia of a severity intermediate to that of the homozygous and heterozygous states; these conditions are called "β-thalassemia intermedia." Although in some cases the reason for this mild expression of the β-thalassemia genes is unknown, in others it appears that the patients are homozygous for β-thalassemia genes but have also inherited an α-thalassemia gene. The latter reduces the amount of globin chain imbalance and hence causes a milder disorder. This elegant "experiment of nature" provides excellent proof that β-thalassemic children are anemic largely because of imbalanced globin chain production. Another important group of thalassemic disorders are those due to the inheritance of both thalassemia and a structural hemoglobin variant. The commonest are those that result from the inheritance of a gene for β-thalassemia with that for either Hb S, C, or E. The resulting conditions, Hb S thalassemia, Hb C thalassemia, and Hb E thalassemia are widespread in Africa and Southeast Asia. Hemoglobin S thalassemia is associated with a clinical disorder similar to sickle cell anemia, although in some cases it is milder. Hemoglobin E thalassemia is widespread throughout Southeast Asia, and the clinical disorder is similar to homozygous β-thalassemia intermedia. Hemoglobin E is a β chain variant that is inefficiently synthesized and hence is associated with the clinical phenotype of a mild form of β-thalassemia. It appears that the base change responsible for the hemoglobin E mutation results in a cryptic splice site similar to those that underlie some of the milder forms of β^+ thalassemia (see p. 222).

CONGENITAL SIDEROBLASTIC ANEMIA

The congenital sideroblastic anemias are rare disorders with a clinical picture similar to that of the acquired sideroblastic anemias. The hematologic changes are summarized in Table 22. There is anemia from early life, and the peripheral blood shows a dimorphic picture with well-filled red cells mixed with grossly hypochromic forms. The bone marrow shows erythroid hyperplasia with many ring sideroblasts. This disease is seen most often in males and may have a sex-linked mode of inheritance. Female carriers show a small population of hypochromic cells. The genetics is not always as simple as this, and several families have been reported in which the genetic transmission does not follow a clear-cut sex-linked pattern.

CONGENITAL DYSERYTHROPOIETIC ANEMIA (CDA)

This is another rare group of congenital disorders in which there is normochromic anemia associated with a hyperplastic bone marrow and evidence of a defect in red cell maturation and division. The striking feature of this group of anemias is the multinuclearity of the red cell precursors, which have well-marked internuclear bridges. There are several forms of CDA defined by the associated serologic findings and the morphology of the bone marrow. Their etiology is completely unknown.

ANEMIAS DUE TO DEFECTIVE PROLIFERATION OF RED CELL PRECURSORS

The hypoplastic anemias may be classified in several ways (Table 26). First, they may be divided into idiopathic and secondary, depending on whether there is any obvious etiologic factor involved. Second, they may be subdivided into those in which there is selective red cell asplasia with normal production of white cells and platelets and those in which the defective red cell formation is associated with a defect in the formation of the other formed elements of the blood. Finally,

TABLE 26. THE APLASTIC AND HYPOPLASTIC ANEMIAS

As Part of a Generalized Bone Marrow Failure
Congenital aplastic anemia (Fanconi's anemia)
Acquired aplastic anemia
  Primary (or idiopathic)
  Secondary
    Drugs
    Chemicals
    Ionizing radiation
    Virus infection
    Part of PNH syndrome

Selective Red Cell Aplasia or Hypoplasia
Congenital (Diamond-Blackfan anemia)
Acquired red cell aplasia
  Primary (or idiopathic; acute transient or chronic)
  Secondary
    Thymic tumor
    Infection (usually with hemolytic anemia)
    Renal disease
    Carcinoma
    Lymphoma
    Riboflavin deficiency

defective proliferation of red cell precursors may occur in a bone marrow that is infiltrated with malignant cells; this group includes the leukemias, myeloproliferative disorders, and other neoplastic infiltrations.

APLASTIC ANEMIA

The aplastic and hypoplastic anemias are a group of conditions characterized by a reduced output of all the formed elements of the blood. They may be idiopathic or secondary to a variety of agents that damage the bone marrow. There is a further group that presents early in life and probably represents a congenital form of the condition.

Acquired Aplastic Anemia. The varieties of acquired aplastic anemia are summarized in Table 26. In the so-called idiopathic form, no history of exposure to drugs, chemicals, or other agents can be obtained. There is considerable interest in the possibility that some forms of idiopathic aplastic anemia have an immune basis. Some patients who have had bone marrow transplantation and in whom the graft has not taken have gone into a spontaneous remission that is possibly mediated by the immunosuppressive preparation for the transplant. In addition, there have been reports of apparent improvement in patients with aplastic anemia treated with antithymocyte globulin. These observations suggest that a form of immune-mediated suppression of hemopoiesis may be the basis for some forms of aplastic anemia. Further evidence in support of this notion has come from in vitro colony studies that have shown that peripheral blood mononuclear cells from patients with aplastic anemia are capable of inhibiting colony formation. However, the evidence for there being a subgroup of aplastic anemias related to an active suppressor mechanism must be reviewed critically. For example, marrow culture studies, even when undertaken with HLA-matched target marrow, may demonstrate colony inhibition caused by transfusion sensitization of the patient to minor histocompatibility differences. Thus, although there is circumstantial evidence that some cases of aplastic anemia have an immune basis, the natural tendency for spontaneous remission and the inherent difficulties of standardizing the in vitro assay systems make it difficult to evaluate the place of immune mechanisms in the pathogenesis of the condition.

Many agents can produce a secondary aplastic anemia; some of these are listed in Table 27. The commonest are drugs, particularly anti-inflammatory agents, some antibiotics, and the antithyroid drugs. In some cases there appears to be individual hypersensitivity to the drug because marrow aplasia occurs after small doses; in others there is always marrow damage if enough of the drug is given. Chloramphenicol may cause marrow damage by both of these mechanisms. The role of infection in producing hypoplastic anemia is uncertain. Hypoplastic anemia may be a complication of virus infection. This is certainly true of infectious hepatitis, and there have been occasional reports of hypoplasia following EB virus infection. The transient marrow aplasia that occurs in patients with hemolytic anemia may, in some cases, be caused by a parvovirus infection. In vitro colony studies have shown that this virus is capable of reducing the numbers of CFU-E and BFU-E, although it has less effect

TABLE 27. DRUGS AND CHEMICALS THAT MAY CAUSE APLASTIC ANEMIA*

	DEFINITE ASSOCIATION	POSSIBLE ASSOCIATION
Antibiotics	Chloramphenicol	Thiamphenicol
	Sulfonamides	Streptomycin
		Penicillin
		Methicillin
		Tetracycline
		Nitrofurantoin
		Para-aminosalicylic acid
		Isoniazid
Anti-inflammatory agents	Phenylbutazone	Indomethacin
	Oxyphenbutazone	Penicillamine
	Amidopyrine	Colchicine
	Gold salts	
Anti-epileptic drugs	Phenytoin	
	Methoin	
	Troxidone	
Oral hypoglycemic agents	Tolbutamine	
	Chlorpropamide	
Drugs used for parasite infections	Mepacrine	Amodiaquine
	Organic arsenicals	Pyrimethamine
Antithyroid drugs	Potassium perchlorate	Carbimazole
		Thiouracil
Antihistamines		Chlorpheniramine
		Tripelennamine
Psychoactive drugs		Phenothiazines
		Chlordiazepoxide
		Meprobamate
Diuretics		Acetazolamide
		Chlorthiazide
		Hydroflumethiazide
Others		Quinidine bisulfate
		Gamma benzene hexachloride
		Naphthalene

*Modified from Lewis, S. M., and Gordon-Smith, E. C.: In Hardisty, R. M., and Weatherall, D. J. (eds.): Blood and Its Disorders. 2nd ed. Oxford, Blackwell Scientific Publications, 1982.

on the growth of CFU-C. Viruses also may be responsible for destruction of hemopoietic precursors in the bone marrow, particularly in immunosuppressed patients. The name *virus hemophagocytic syndrome* has been given to a condition in which there is intense erythrophagocytosis in the marrow associated with fever, rapidly progressive pancytopenia, and a severe systemic illness. The pathophysiology of this condition, which may be associated with several different viral infections, remains to be determined.

Ionizing radiation is a well-defined cause of bone marrow suppression. Radiation energy is capable of breaking molecular bonds in critical intracellular macromolecules. Its effects are particularly marked on rapidly turning over populations, such as the bone marrow precursor cells. Acute exposure to high-energy radiation may produce extensive destruction of the bone marrow and early death, while exposure to lower doses may produce a chronic aplastic anemia. Other important marrow-depressing agents include benzene and its derivatives and some heavy metals.

The pathophysiology of both primary and secondary aplastic anemia is similar. There is a variable degree of anemia with normochromic red cells. In addition there is granulocytopenia and thrombocytopenia. It is now clear that the prognosis can be related to the initial granulocyte and platelet counts. Absolute granulocyte counts lower than $200/\mu l$ or platelet counts lower than $10,000/\mu l$ indicate a poor prognosis. A bone marrow aspiration is hypocellular and a trephine biopsy shows an extremely hypocellular fragment consisting mainly of fat spaces. There may be moderate lymphocyte infiltration with increased numbers of plasma cells. The marrow appearances are very variable in this condition, however, and it is possible to find hyperplastic fragments with evidence of dyserythropoiesis. Radioactive iron uptake is markedly reduced, and there is diminished activity when external scanners are applied to the sacrum or vertebrae. Further evidence of diminished marrow activity is the reticulocytopenia, which is almost invariably present in these patients.

The clinical manifestations of aplastic anemia are related directly to the pathophysiology. These include symptoms of anemia and a hemorrhagic tendency due to the associated thrombocytopenia. There is a high frequency of bacterial infections due to the granulocytopenia. Death usually results from bleeding or infection.

It is not uncommon to find an acid-sensitive red cell line similar to that found in paroxysmal nocturnal hemoglobinuria in patients with a hypoplastic bone marrow. This association is considered in a later section (p. 241).

Constitutional or Congenital Hypoplastic Anemia. This condition, also known as *Fanconi's anemia,* is a rare but extremely interesting form of aplastic anemia. Although it appears to be due to an inborn defect in cellular proliferation, it may not become manifest until early childhood. It is characterized by a pancytopenia associated with congenital abnormalities, such as skin pigmentation; renal hypoplasia; bone defects, including an absent radius; and microcephaly. That this disorder results from a primary defect in cellular proliferation is suggested by the finding of multiple abnormalities of the chromosomes, with tendency for frequent breaks. The basic defect in this disorder is in DNA repair. There is an increased incidence among sibships and some epidemiologic evidence that affected families have a higher incidence of other cancers and leukemia than is normal. For unknown reasons, some children with Fanconi's anemia respond to androgen therapy.

There has been successful bone marrow transplantation in both congenital and acquired aplastic anemia. The results of these transplants suggest that many aplastic anemias are primarily disorders of stem cells rather than the marrow environment, since the transplanted stem cells seem to proliferate normally.

SELECTIVE RED CELL APLASIA

Acquired Red Cell Aplasia. Pure red cell aplasia is a rare disorder. It may occur acutely, usually following a viral infection, in patients with hemolytic anemia (see earlier discussion). A transient erythroblastopenia may occur in early childhood; the cause is unknown. A more chronic form occurs sometimes in association with tumors of the thymus or sometimes without any associated disorder. It has also been reported in patients with systemic lupus erythematosus or as a side effect of drugs. In some cases antibodies directed against erythroid bone marrow red cell precursors can be found in the serum. The existence of antibodies directed against erythropoietin has also been recorded. Why these should occur in patients with thymic tumors is not clear, but remission has been reported after thymectomy, which suggests a true causal relationship.

Congenital Red Cell Aplasia. This rare condition was first described by Blackfan and Diamond and is known as *Blackfan-Diamond anemia.* Affected children are anemic from birth, and bone marrow examination reveals a complete absence or marked diminution of red cell precursors. White cell and platelet production is normal. Many of these patients require blood transfusion for survival, but some of them respond to corticosteroids and androgens and may in fact go into remission with the use of these drugs. This is a heterogeneous disorder, and some cases may have an immunologic basis similar to acquired red cell aplasia.

ANEMIAS DUE TO ABNORMAL MATURATION AND PROLIFERATION

THE ANEMIA OF CHRONIC DISORDERS

A mild anemia that is refractory to hematinics occurs in association with inflammation, collagen vascular disease, any form of neoplasia, and renal disease. A particularly good example is the anemia that accompanies the syndrome of polymyalgia rheumatica and temporal arteritis. This extremely common type of anemia has several distinguishing features (Table 28). The anemia is mild and the red cells are normochromic or only slightly hypochromic. The serum iron level is usually reduced in the range of 30 to 60 µg/dl, and the total iron binding capacity is moderately depressed between 100 and 300 µg/100 ml with a saturation of about 20 per cent. The bone marrow shows normal or slightly reduced numbers of red cell precursors that contain reduced amounts of iron in their cytoplasm. However, iron is present in normal or increased amounts in the reticuloendothelial storage cells of the bone marrow.

The pathophysiology of this form of anemia is poorly understood. There appears to be a decrease in the iron supply for hemoglobin synthesis due to a block in the release and utilization of iron from the reticuloendothelial cells. This is mirrored by an increase in reticuloendothelial iron, decreased plasma iron, and per cent transferrin saturation and a decrease in the number of sideroblasts in the marrow. There is an increase

in red cell protoporphyrin and occasionally a mild defect in hemoglobin synthesis as shown by the hypochromic red cells. In addition, however, there is a failure of erythropoietin response and hence a proliferation and maturation defect, and also a slightly reduced red cell lifespan. All of these changes are corrected when the underlying disorder is treated.

CHRONIC RENAL FAILURE

Anemia may be a major problem in patients with chronic renal failure. Its pathophysiology and hematologic features have much in common with the anemia of chronic disorders. However, additional factors seem to occur in renal disease. The hemolytic element is often quite marked and the red cell defect is extracorpuscular, since the patient's red cells survive normally when injected into healthy recipients. There is an almost linear relationship between the blood urea and red cell survival. Furthermore, the red cell survival improves after dialysis. The agent responsible for this extracorpuscular hemolytic effect of uremic plasma is unknown. In addition, there is some degree of ineffective erythropoiesis and lack of full response to erythropoietin. Also, there may be a failure of erythropoietin production that presumably is caused by damage to the erythropoietin-producing areas of the kidney. Anemia may be exacerbated by iron deficiency due to gastrointestinal blood loss because of an increased bleeding tendency. Folic acid deficiency occurs, particularly in patients undergoing intensive dialysis, since this agent is dialyzable.

The pathogenesis of the anemia of renal failure may be even more complicated. For example, patients maintained on continuous ambulatory peritoneal dialysis (CAPD) are less anemic than those maintained on hemodialysis. Since the clearance of some middle molecular weight substances is greater with CAPD than with hemodialysis, this suggests that these substances may have a role in suppressing erythropoiesis. Individuals whose hemoglobin level responds to CAPD seem to be capable of increasing their erythropoietin output; particularly good responses occur in patients with cystic disease of the kidney. It has also been suggested that secondary hyperparathyroidism plays a role in producing a poor erythropoietic response to erythropoietin in patients with chronic renal failure. This is particularly interesting in view of the occurrence of refractory anemia in primary hyperparathyroidism, possibly due to marrow fibrosis (see later discussion).

Complicated compensatory mechanisms may modify the effects of the anemia of renal failure. For example, phosphate retention may cause a "right shift" in the oxygen dissociation curve. This effect may be augmented by acidosis. However, the latter tends to reduce the level of 2,3-DPG, which increases oxygen affinity.

ANEMIAS ASSOCIATED WITH ENDOCRINE DISORDERS

A mild normochromic anemia is found commonly in patients with hypopituitarism or hypothyroidism. It was thought that the thyroid hormones have a direct stimulatory effect on erythropoiesis and that this effect is reduced in states of hypopituitarism or hypothyroid-

---

TABLE 28. THE ANEMIA OF CHRONIC DISORDERS

Mild hypochromic or normochromic anemia
MCH and MCV normal or slightly reduced
Serum iron reduced
Total iron binding capacity reduced
Transferrin saturation normal or slightly reduced
Sideroblasts in marrow reduced
Reticuloendothelial iron in marrow increased
Plasma copper increased
Red cell protoporphyrin increased

ism. It has been suggested, however, that anemia is an appropriate response to a decreased cellular demand for oxygen. In other words, such patients are not functionally anemic. However, patients with hypothyroidism frequently have menorrhagia and may be iron deficient, and there is a strong association between hypothyroidism and pernicious anemia; therefore, there may be a true vitamin B_{12} deficiency. It is interesting that patients with hyperthyroidism who have increased oxygen requirements are not polycythemic. This may be because the thyroid hormones cause increased cardiac output and tissue perfusion, and therefore an increased red cell mass is not required to increase the rate of oxygen delivery to the tissues. Furthermore, there is an increase in erythrocyte 2,3-DPG in thyrotoxicosis which, by shifting the oxygen dissociation curve to the right, may increase the rate of release of oxygen to the tissues. Patients with hyperthyroidism may have a very mild anemia with a slightly reduced mean corpuscular volume; these changes revert to normal after treatment. Overall, patients with hypothyroidism tend to have a slightly elevated mean corpuscular volume.

About 5 per cent of patients with primary hyperparathyroidism have a normochromic normocytic anemia that cannot be related to blood loss or associated renal failure. While bone marrow biopsy may show a considerable degree of myelosclerosis, this condition is not associated with hepatosplenomegaly or any of the peripheral blood changes usually found in patients with myelofibrosis. Correction of the hyperparathyroidism is followed by improvement of the anemia.

HEMOLYTIC ANEMIA

When the red cell lifespan is shortened, there is a reduction in the circulating red cell mass. This leads to relative tissue hypoxia, which results in an increased output of erythropoietin. This stimulates erythropoiesis, and the red cell mass may be restored to normal. Therefore, if the survival time is not too short and the bone marrow is healthy, a normal red cell mass can be maintained. The condition is then called a compensated hemolytic state. However, when the rate of red cell destruction is in excess of eight times normal (that is, the red cell survival is less than 15 days), even a normal bone marrow cannot compensate, and a hemolytic anemia results. If the bone marrow is abnormal or if there is an inadequate supply of iron or other substances required for hemopoiesis, anemia may occur when the red cell survival is considerably greater than 15 days.

PATHOPHYSIOLOGY OF HEMOLYSIS

Sites of Red Cell Destruction. The destruction of red cells may take place either intravascularly or extravascularly, or, as occurs more commonly, in both sites. The site of destruction depends on the type and degree of damage to the red cells. For example, complement-damaged cells have large holes in the membrane and are destroyed intravascularly, whereas IgG-coated cells are removed in the reticuloendothelial system.

Breakdown of Hemoglobin. Approximately 80 per cent of the heme liberated by the breakdown of hemoglobin is converted to bilirubin. Since the opening of the heme ring is associated with the production of carbon monoxide, this can be used as a measure of the degree of hemolysis. The fate of bilirubin was considered earlier in this chapter. In hemolytic states there is an increased rate of production of bilirubin and also an increased production of urinary and fecal urobilinogen. Fecal and urinary urobilinogen levels are unreliable as a precise measure of the rate of hemolysis, however, because bilirubin may be derived from ineffective erythropoiesis and because the level of fecal urobilinogen also depends on the activity of microorganisms in the gut. The level of circulating bilirubin present in patients with hemolysis depends on the rate of hemolysis and on the ability of the liver to conjugate and excrete bilirubin. For example, in the neonatal period immaturity of the fetal liver may lead to very high levels of bilirubin with relatively low-grade hemolysis. Unconjugated bilirubin does not appear in the urine, and therefore the hyperbilirubinemia of hemolysis is sometimes described as acholuric jaundice.

Metabolism of Hemoglobin in the Circulation and Kidneys. When hemoglobin is liberated into the circulation it is bound to haptoglobin. The haptoglobins are a group of α globulins that are synthesized in the liver. Several molecular varieties have been identified by their electrophoretic migration, and their structure is determined by two allelic systems. Three phenotypes are recognized: 1-1, 2-2, and 2-1. They are made up of similar subunits but differ with respect to molecular weight, hemoglobin-binding capacity, and clearance rates. Normally, sufficient haptoglobin is present to bind 100 to 140 mg of hemoglobin/100 ml of plasma. Hemoglobin-haptoglobin complex is not excreted by the kidney but is cleared from the plasma by the reticuloendothelial system at a rate of approximately 15 mg of hemoglobin/100 ml per hour. Thus, the most sensitive guide to intravascular hemolysis is a reduction in the serum haptoglobin level. This occurs even when the hemolysis is primarily extravascular, presumably because there is some "leak" of free hemoglobin into the circulation. If the binding capacity of haptoglobin is exceeded, hemoglobin appears in the plasma, where it is degraded and the liberated heme binds to hemopexin. Hemopexin is a β glycoprotein that consists of two components, I and II. I is a monomer, and II, which contains four electrophoretic bands, is a polymeric form. Its normal concentration is approximately 80 mg/100 ml of plasma. Hemopexin-heme complexes are removed from the circulation by the liver. When this is saturated, heme may bind to albumin, forming methemalbumin, and with severe intravascular hemolysis the plasma may assume a dirty brown color owing to the presence of this metabolite.

When there is marked intravascular hemolysis, hemoglobin may appear in the urine. Tetrameric hemoglobin freely dissociates into α and β dimers with a molecular weight of 32,000, which is small enough to permit glomerular filtration. With plasma hemoglobin levels of 13 mg/ml or less, no hemoglobin appears in the urine because it is reabsorbed in the proximal renal tubules. At levels in excess of this, free hemoglobin appears in the urine. In states of low-grade intravascular hemolysis there may be no detectable hemoglobin in the urine but because there is repeated absorption of hemoglobin in the renal tubules, where it is subsequently degraded, hemosiderin forms in the tubular cells. These cells are cast off and appear in the urine, and the presence of hemosiderin in a spun-down urinary sediment is by far the most reliable indication of a state of chronic intravascular hemolysis. The iron granules may be demonstrated in the urine sediment by the Prussian blue reaction.

Compensatory Mechanisms. The anemia of hemolysis results in increased erythropoietin production and the stimulation of erythropoiesis. This leads to an increased number of red cell precursors in the bone marrow with a change in the myeloid:erythroid ratio toward unity or less. With further stimulation there is expansion of the marrow down the long bones. Hence, if there is chronic hemolysis from early childhood there may be expansion of the marrow cavities of the skull, vertebrae, and long bones, resulting in marked skeletal deformity. Another result of erythropoietin stimulation is to shorten the transit time of red cell precursors through the marrow with the production of large deep-staining macrocytes (shift cells) together with a variable reticulocytosis. The increased rate of erythropoiesis results in increased requirements for folic acid, and for maximal proliferative response the serum iron level must be in excess of 70 μg/dl. The erythroid hyperplasia results in increased absorption of iron, and hence chronic hemolysis may be associated with iron loading of the tissues.

The degree of compensation in any hemolytic process is modified by the oxygen affinity of the red cells. How this can occur with different structural hemoglobin variants and with changes in the level of intracellular phosphate, particularly 2,3-DPG, has already been discussed. Some hemoglobin variants that produce hemolytic anemia, like sickle cell hemoglobin, have a low oxygen affinity, and therefore the anemia is well compensated. Similarly, in some genetic defects of the glycolytic pathway, the level of 2,3-DPG is elevated and this also causes a right shift in the oxygen dissociation curve with increased delivery to the tissues. Congenital pyruvate kinase deficiency is an excellent example of the latter circumstance.

MECHANISMS OF PREMATURE RED CELL DESTRUCTION

Premature destruction of red cells occurs for the following reasons: (1) the membrane is abnormal in structure and/or function; (2) the red cells are exposed to excessive physical trauma in the circulation; and (3) the red cells are unusually rigid owing to the precipitation or abnormal molecular configuration of hemoglobin (Table 29).

Abnormalities of the Red Cell Membrane. If a red cell is to survive in the circulation it must be able to maintain a normal shape and permeability and undergo plastic deformation as it traverses the microcirculation. The plasticity of the cell depends mainly on its surface:volume ratio, which in turn depends on the integrity of its membrane. Normal membrane function relies on the production of energy for active transport of sodium and potassium out of and into the cell and the maintenance of the protein sulfhydryl

TABLE 29. MECHANISMS OF HEMOLYSIS

MECHANISM	EXAMPLES
Abnormalities of the Red Cell Membrane	
Genetic abnormality of membrane structure	Hereditary spherocytosis, elliptocytosis
Alteration in lipid constitution	"Spur cell" anemia
Altered sulfhydryl activity	Oxidant drugs
Altered properties resulting from interaction with complement or immunoglobulins	Immune hemolytic anemia
Increased permeability, reduced plasticity	Glycolytic enzyme defects
Increased Rigidity Causing Abnormal Flow	
Aggregation of hemoglobin molecules	Sickle-cell anemia
Decreased solubility of hemoglobin	Hemoglobin C disease
Inclusion (Heinz) body formation	Thalassemia, unstable hemoglobins, oxidant drugs
Direct Physical Trauma	
Direct external trauma	March and karate hemoglobinuria
Turbulent flow	Cardiac hemolytic anemia
Cleavage by fibrin strands	Microangiopathic hemolytic anemia

groups in a reduced state. It also depends on the existence of a system for the renewal of membrane lipids to preserve a normal lipid composition. Abnormalities of any of these functions tend to produce a spherical cell that has a small surface area for a given volume and hence is not easily deformed. The resultant loss of plasticity leads to selective sequestration of the affected cells in the spleen and other parts of the reticuloendothelial system. This process occurs in any condition in which the membrane is structurally abnormal, so that there is an increased influx of sodium. Thus it is observed in hereditary spherocytosis, in situations in which there is a reduced amount of energy produced in the cell because of genetic deficiencies of its glycolytic enzymes, in other forms of enzyme deficiency that render the cell sensitive to oxidant stress or cause oxidation of the membrane sulfhydryl groups, and in disorders associated with abnormal lipid metabolism. Membrane damage may also result from the interaction of antibodies on the cell surface with macrophages of the reticuloendothelial system and by the direct effects of trauma, chemicals, bacteria, or parasites. Severe destruction of the membrane may follow when complement is activated on the cell surface. Finally, inherited structural alterations in the protein components of the red cell membrane may provide a basis for some forms of congenital hemolytic anemia.

Trauma. The red cell may undergo excessive trauma in a variety of ways. It may be involved in excessive turbulence created by cardiac valve prosthesis. It may be damaged as it becomes caught up in fibrin strands in any condition in which there is intravascular deposition of fibrin. Finally, it may be damaged by excessive pressure on external body surfaces.

Increased Red Cell Rigidity Due to Abnormalities of Hemoglobin. Red cells that contain abnormally aggregated or precipitated hemoglobin molecules are less deformable and are destroyed in the marrow, spleen, or microcirculation. This type of process occurs in the sickling disorders, in which there is aggregation of hemoglobin molecules causing cellular deformity, or in conditions in which there is precipitation of hemoglobin with the production of a rigid Heinz body. The latter mechanism is observed in the thalassemias, disorders with unstable hemoglobin and in cells unusually sensitive to oxidant damage, particularly those deficient in glucose-6-phosphate dehydrogenase. It may occur in normal red cells, provided that the degree of oxidant damage is of sufficient magnitude.

THE DIAGNOSIS OF HEMOLYSIS

The diagnosis of hemolysis depends on an understanding of its pathophysiology (Table 30). It relies on the following: (1) recognition that there is an increased rate of red cell destruction; (2) finding of concomitant evidence of increased red cell production; and (3) confirmation by measurement of the red cell survival time.

Increased Red Cell Destruction. If the rate of red cell destruction exceeds the liver's capacity to conjugate and excrete bilirubin, the level of plasma bilirubin will increase. This bilirubin is unconjugated and because of its low water solubility is not excreted by the kidney, giving the clinical picture of acholuric jaundice. The excretion of fecal and urinary urobilinogen is increased, but for reasons outlined earlier the levels of these metabolites are only an approximate guide to the rate of hemolysis. Even in the presence of extravascular hemolysis there is usually a decreased level of haptoglobin, and in the presence of severe hemolysis haptoglobins disappear from the serum. If intravascular hemolysis is suspected, the most useful investigations are the plasma hemoglobin level, Schumm's test for methemalbumin and an examination of the urine for hemoglobin, and, in cases of chronic hemolysis, hemosiderin. The level of lactic dehydrogenase (LDH) in the serum is often elevated, owing to its release from damaged red cells.

Evidence of Increased Red Cell Production. The stained blood film usually shows anisochromia with deep-staining macrocytes. There is a variable increase in the reticulocyte count. The marrow shows erythroid hyperplasia with an alteration in the myeloid: erythroid ratio toward unity or less.

Direct Measurement of Red Cell Survival. It is not necessary to assess the red cell survival in cases in which there is obvious hemolysis. However, where mild hemolysis is suspected or where there is associated marrow disease so that the contribution of the hemolytic component to the overall degree of anemia is uncertain, direct measurements of red cell survival are useful. Furthermore, when splenectomy is being considered, it is helpful to combine the red cell survival studies with external scanning to determine the site of maximal red cell destruction.

After injection of labeled red cells, survival curves can be plotted (see p. 198) and, by comparing the radioactivity over the precordium, liver, and spleen, some indication of the site of destruction can be obtained. The slope of elimination of ^{51}Cr-labeled cells, when plotted on arithmetic graph paper, is usually curvilinear. In clinical practice the $T\frac{1}{2}$ ^{51}Cr (number of days when 50 per cent of the ^{51}Cr has been eliminated) is an adequate indication of the red cell survival. The normal range of $T\frac{1}{2}$ is between 25 and 33 days. Red cell survival data are invalidated if there is bleeding from any source.

CLASSIFICATION OF THE HEMOLYTIC ANEMIAS

The causes of an increased rate of red cell destruction are often multifactorial and no classification is completely satisfactory. A useful approach is to divide them into (1) those that result from genetic disorders of either the red cell membrane, energy-producing pathways, or hemoglobin and (2) those that result from acquired abnormalities of the red cell membrane or metabolism. This classification has the disadvantage that some of the congenital abnormalities of the red cell, particularly those due to enzyme or hemoglobin variants, require the presence of an environmental factor such as a drug to produce a hemolytic response.

The Congenital Hemolytic Anemias

The genetically determined hemolytic anemias fall into three groups (Table 31): (1) enzyme deficiencies that result in abnormal energy metabolism; (2) hemoglobinopathies; and (3) disorders of the red cell membrane.

TABLE 30. DIAGNOSIS OF HEMOLYSIS

Evidence of Increased Rate of Red Cell Destruction
Intravascular
  Decreased haptoglobins
  Increased plasma hemoglobin
  Methemalbumin increased in plasma
  Hemoglobinuria
  Hemosiderinuria (in chronic intravascular hemolysis)
Extravascular
  Increased bilirubin production, jaundice
  Increased urinary urobilinogen
  Increased fecal urobilinogen
  Increased carbon monoxide (CO) production
Evidence of Increased Rate of Red Cell Production
  Reticulocytosis, normoblasts in peripheral blood
  Red cell polychromasia, "shift cells" on blood film
  Erythroid hyperplasia of bone marrow
  Skeletal deformities caused by marrow expansion
Direct Evidence of Decreased Red Cell Survival Time
  Shortened chromiun isotope half-life (^{51}Cr T$\frac{1}{2}$)
Associated Effects of a Hemolytic State
  "Work hypertrophy" of the spleen
  Increased folic acid requirements
  Increased uric acid production
  Sequestration of cells in spleen and reticuloendothelial system

---

TABLE 31. CONGENITAL HEMOLYTIC ANEMIA

The Red Cell Membrane
  Hereditary spherocytosis
  Elliptocytosis
  Stomatocytosis
  Acanthocytosis in abetalipoproteinemia
  Pyropoikilocytosis
Hemoglobin (Hemoglobinopathies)
  Structural hemoglobin variants
  Thalassemia syndromes
Energy Pathways
  Enzyme deficiencies in the EM (Embden-Meyerhof) pathway
  Enzyme deficiencies in the hexose monophosphate (HMP) shunt
  Other enzyme deficiencies

Genetic disorders of the red cell enzyme systems may involve either the hexose monophosphate or Embden-Meyerhof pathways. Genetic defects in these pathways can result in unusual susceptibility to the hemolytic properties of certain drugs or a continuous hemolytic process called *congenital nonspherocytic hemolytic anemia (CNSHA)*. The abnormal hemoglobin disorders that cause hemolysis are those associated with hemoglobins S, C, and E, or the unstable hemoglobins. Finally, there are conditions that are thought to be due to primary defects in the metabolism or structure of the red cell membrane.

Red Cell Enzyme Deficiency

Glucose-6-phosphate Dehydrogenase Deficiency. G-6-PD deficiency is an extremely common X-linked disorder. It has been estimated that it affects about 100 million individuals in the world population. G-6-PD activity is essential for normal HMP function, and hence deficiency of the enzyme leaves the red cell poorly protected against oxidant damage (see p. 202).

Analysis of the red cells of G-6-PD–deficient individuals indicates that the disorder is extremely heterogeneous. Affected Negroes have 10 to 15 per cent of normal enzyme activity in their red cells. There are two electrophoretic types of G-6-PD, designated A and B, in the Negro population. Type A is confined to Negroes and the AB phenotype is found only in females, while Negro males may have either A or B type but never both. Enzyme deficiency in the Negro is nearly always due to an unstable variant of the A enzyme called the A⁻ variant. Reticulocytes of individuals with the A⁻ variant have normal enzyme activity but this declines more rapidly than normal as the red cells age. Hence a hemolytic reaction in a Negro G-6-PD–deficient subject is self-limiting, since the young cell population with newly synthesized A⁻ enzyme appears in the blood, and these cells are resistant to the drug that has provoked the hemolysis. Furthermore, an enzyme-deficient Negro may appear to have normal enzyme activity if a blood sample has been obtained during reticulocytosis.

G-6-PD deficiency of the non-Negro variety is widespread in the Mediterranean, Middle East, and Orient. Affected males have low or absent activity in their red cells. The electrophoretic mobility of G-6-PD in these individuals is the same as the normal B enzyme, but studies of several functional parameters, such as heat stability, pH optima, and Michaelis constants indicate that some of the variant enzymes are structurally abnormal. Using these techniques, over 50 G-6-PD variants have now been isolated and characterized, but only some of them are associated with reduced enzyme activity. The A type of G-6-PD differs from the B type by a single amino acid substitution, asparagine to aspartic acid. G-6-PD Hectoen also has a single amino acid substitution, in this case histidine to tyrosine. Recently, the G-6-PD gene has been cloned. By developing suitable molecular probes it should be possible to analyze the molecular pathology that underlies many of the G-6-PD variants.

The precise mechanism of hemolysis in G-6-PD deficiency is not yet understood. It is possible that the drugs cause generation of hydrogen peroxide, oxidation of glutathione, and precipitation of hemoglobin following the formation of mixed disulfides with the cysteine residues of the β chain.

The hemolysis associated with G-6-PD deficiency is predominantly intravascular. The precipitating hemoglobin produces intracellular inclusions, or Heinz bodies, and these cause damage to the red cell in the microcirculation. Hence there is intravascular hemolysis often associated with hemoglobinuria. Because of the nature of the A⁻ enzyme the hemolysis is usually self-limiting in Negroes but may be life-threatening in the non-Negro varieties of the disorder.

The clinical manifestations of G-6-PD deficiency are summarized in Table 32. They include hemolysis after administration of oxidant drugs, such as sulfonamides, primaquine, nitrofurantoin, and phenacetin. The enzyme deficiency is also associated with neonatal jaundice in some populations and with favism, a reaction to the bean *Vicia fava*, which causes an acute episode of intravascular hemolysis. There is some evidence that hemolysis may occur in G-6-PD–deficient individuals with intercurrent infections, diabetic coma, and liver disease. Occasionally, G-6-PD deficiency results in chronic continuous hemolysis, which is not precipitated by drugs—that is, it is one cause of congenital nonspherocytic hemolytic anemia.

Enzyme Deficiencies in the Embden-Meyerhof Pathway. Investigation of patients with congenital nonspherocytic hemolytic anemia has shown that this condition can result from a variety of enzyme deficiencies in the Embden-Meyerhof (EM) pathway (Table 33). Most of these are rare, and the only one that has been seen commonly and is well characterized is pyruvate kinase (PK) deficiency.

PYRUVATE KINASE (PK) DEFICIENCY. PK deficiency is inherited as an autosomal recessive trait. Homozygotes have markedly reduced or absent enzyme activity in their red cells, while heterozygous carriers may have significantly reduced levels. PK deficiency results in an extremely inefficient generation of ATP by the mature erythrocyte. It seems likely that patients with this disorder survive because they have an unusually high reticulocyte count; reticulocytes retain the functions of oxidative phosphorylation for maintenance of ATP. Incubation of PK-deficient blood with cyanide, which inhibits oxidative phosphorylation, produces a striking and rapid decrease in red cell ATP content, whereas normal reticulocytes do not show this effect. PK-deficient erythrocytes have a marked increase in oxygen consumption as compared with normal. Furthermore, if such cells are maintained in a hypoxic environment there is a marked reduction in ATP production. It is likely that this is one of the major causes of shortened red cell survival in this condition, particularly when the cells are packed together in the spleen. An ATP-depleted red cell loses its membrane-pumping properties, and potassium loss tends to exceed

TABLE 32. CLINICAL MANIFESTATIONS OF G-6-PD DEFICIENCY

Drug-induced hemolytic anemia
Favism
Neonatal jaundice
Congenital nonspherocytic hemolytic anemia
Hemolysis during intercurrent acute illness

sodium gain. The resultant loss of cations is accompanied by an osmotic loss of water and a reduction in cell volume. The cells become shrunken and spiculated. Such dehydrated red cells, which have been called "dessicytes," are presumably destroyed prematurely in the spleen and probably in other parts of the reticuloendothelial system.

Because PK occurs relatively late in the EM pathway, there is an increased concentration of intermediates behind the block. Of particular importance is the increased level of 2,3-DPG, which tends to push the oxygen dissociation curve to the right; hence PK-deficient patients can compensate well for a marked degree of anemia. A unique feature of this disorder is that although there may be an improvement in the hemoglobin level after splenectomy, the reticulocyte count may rise and remain extraordinarily high after the operation.

As might be expected, PK deficiency is characterized by a chronic hemolytic anemia, which often appears in the neonatal period. There is splenomegaly, and in severe cases there may be expansion of the long bones and skull.

Other Red Cell Enzyme Deficiencies. A large number of enzyme deficiencies have been reported in individual cases or in a few families. Some are summarized in Table 33. In most of these disorders there is a variable degree of hemolytic anemia without other systemic features. However, in the case of triose-phosphate-isomerase deficiency there are associated neurologic complications, including impaired motor development, muscle weakness, and flaccidity, and death in early infancy is common. Pyrimidine 5-nucleotidase deficiency is being recognized quite frequently. The condition causes a mild hemolytic anemia, and the blood film is notable for the presence of marked basophilic stippling that is rather similar to that seen in lead poisoning. The red cells contain high concentrations of cytidine and uridine nucleotides and there is an associated, but unexplained, increase in GSH concentration and a partial deficiency of ribose phosphate pyrophosphokinase. The hemolytic anemia associated with increased adenosine deaminase levels is of particular interest because this is the only disorder described so far in which there seems to be a shortened red cell survival associated with the marked elevation of an enzyme.

Hemolytic Anemia Due to Genetic Disorders of Hemoglobin

The genetic disorders of hemoglobin have been mentioned several times in this chapter. They are summarized in Table 34.

Hemolysis may occur in patients homozygous for Hbs, S, C, D, and E and in individuals heterozygous for a variety of unstable hemoglobin variants. In addition, there is a hemolytic component in the thalassemia syndromes. A classification of the abnormal hemoglobin disorders is shown in Table 34. Their molecular basis was considered on page 206.

The Sickling Disorders. By far the most important of the abnormal hemoglobin disorders are the sickle cell syndromes. These consist of the heterozygous state for Hb S or the sickle cell trait (A-S), the homozygous state or sickle cell disease (S-S), and the compound heterozygous state for Hb S together with Hbs C, D, E, or other structural variants. In addition, there are several disorders resulting from the inheritance of the sickle cell gene together with different forms of thalassemia.

Hemoglobin S differs from Hb A by the substitution of valine for glutamic acid in position 6 in the β chain. It is still not precisely known how this amino acid substitution causes the sickling phenomenon. Sickling appears to be due to the unusual solubility characteristics of Hb S, which undergoes liquid crystal or tactoid formation as it becomes deoxygenated (Fig. 45). In the deoxygenated state, aggregates of sickled hemoglobin molecules are arranged in parallel rod-like structures with a diameter of 160 Å. The molecules of the strands are in a helical configuration with low pitch, six mol-

---

TABLE 33. ERYTHROCYTE ENZYME DEFICIENCIES ASSOCIATED WITH HEMOLYTIC ANEMIA

Clearly associated with hemolytic anemia
A. Enzymes of Embden-Meyerhof pathway
    Hexokinase (HK)
    Glucose phosphate isomerase (GPI)
    Phosphofructokinase (PFK)
    Aldolase (ALD)
    Triosephosphate isomerase (TPI)
    Diphosphoglycerate mutase (DPGM)
    Phosphoglycerate kinase (PGK)
    Pyruvate kinase (PK)
B. Enzymes of the hexose monophosphate (HMP) shunt and of glutathione metabolism
    Glucose-6-phosphate dehydrogenase (G-6-PD)
    Glutathione peroxidase (GSH-Px)
    GSH deficiency secondary to deficiency of
      γ-glutamyl cysteine synthetase
    GSH synthetase
    Glutathione reductase (GSSG-R)
C. Enzymes of nucleotide metabolism
    Adenylate kinase
    Pyrimidine 5'-nucleotidase
Association with hemolytic anemia uncertain
A. Enzymes relating to HMP shunt, nucleotide metabolism, or glycolysis
    6-Phosphogluconate dehydrogenase (6-PGD)
    Adenosinetriphosphatase (ATPase)
    Glutathione reductase (GSSG-R), partial
    The "high ATP" syndromes
    Lactate dehydrogenase (LDH)

TABLE 34. THE SPECTRUM OF CLINICAL DISORDERS CAUSED BY STRUCTURAL HEMOGLOBIN VARIANTS

Hemolytic Anemia
    Hemoglobin S
    Hemoglobin C
    Hemoglobin E
    Unstable hemoglobins—Zürich, Köln, Hammersmith
Methemoglobinemia
    Hemoglobin M
Polycythemia
    Hemoglobin Chesapeake
    Hemoglobin Radcliffe
    Others
Hypochromic Anemia
    Hemoglobin E
    Hemoglobin Lepore
    Hemoglobin Constant Spring

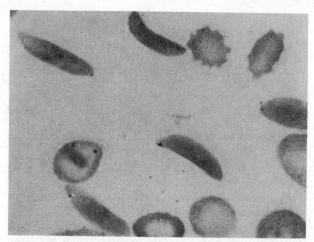

Figure 45. Sickle cells. Peripheral blood film from a patient with sickle-cell thalassemia shows a number of sickle red cells (× 600).

ecules occupying the space that makes up one turn. It seems likely that there is a tendency for hemoglobin molecules to become lined up in normal red cells when the hemoglobin is in the deoxy configuration, and in sickle cells the β6 valine substitution somehow stabilizes these molecular stacks. As mentioned earlier (pp. 204 to 205), conformational changes in hemoglobin molecules occur between the deoxy- and oxy- states. The key to sickling seems to be the behavior of a hydrophobic acceptor pocket between the E and F helices that is present in deoxyhemoglobin but absent in oxyhemoglobin. When residue 6 in the β chain is changed from glutamic acid to valine, its side chain can rest snugly in this pocket in the deoxy configuration; that is, only in this conformation (the T state, see pp. 204 to 205) is the acceptor pocket shaped in a way that promotes interaction with hydrophobic side chains from donor molecules. This probably accounts for the

fact that sickling only occurs in the deoxy configuration.

There is great variation in the degree to which different hemoglobins are able to participate in the sickling process with Hb S. This almost certainly accounts for the clinical variability of the sickling conditions; for example, Hb F is almost completely excluded from the sickling phenomena, and therefore increasing concentrations of Hb F in the red cell tend to reduce the degree of sickling.

Red cells go through a series of cycles of sickling and unsickling, but finally, owing to loss of membrane and increased membrane permeability, the cells become irreversibly sickled. Sickling of red cells has two main effects. First, the sickled erythrocytes have an increased mechanical fragility and a shortened red cell survival. Hence the disorder is characterized by chronic hemolysis. Second, because of aggregation of sickled erythrocytes, particularly in the microvasculature, the viscosity of the blood increases with slowing of the flow, resulting in further sickling and in extreme cases complete blockage of the small vessels with damage to the tissues beyond the block. Hence the other major complication of sickle cell anemia is tissue infarction. This occurs particularly in areas that are relatively poorly vascularized or rely on a few small vessels for their blood supply. Hence the heads of the femur and humerus are particularly prone to infarction with subsequent aseptic necrosis (Fig. 46). Bone infarcts tend to become secondarily infected, leading to chronic osteomyelitis; the typhoid bacillus is a common causative organism. Infarction of the superficial skin vessels may be responsible for the chronic leg ulcers of this disorder. Infarction also occurs in the kidney, lungs, liver, and central nervous system.

The vascular occlusive episodes of sickle cell anemia usually occur as part of acute exacerbations of the illness, called crises. They take many forms, but the commonest is the "painful crisis" that often follows

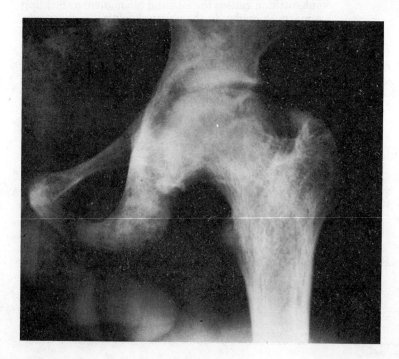

Figure 46. Aseptic necrosis of the femoral head in a case of sickle cell anemia.

infection. It is presumed that pain is due to the infarction of organs, and bone pain has been shown to result from extensive infarction of the bone marrow. Infarction due to acute blockage of blood supply is reflected in several clinical syndromes. These include painful dactylitis in childhood ("hand-foot" syndrome); cerebrovascular accidents; the "lung" syndrome, which is associated with the clinical picture of a pulmonary infarction; and recurrent priapism. Massive bone marrow infarction may result in bone marrow emboli and acute right heart failure.

In addition to painful crises there are several types of "hematologic" crises. There may be an increased rate of hemolysis during intercurrent infection, but more serious is the so-called aplastic crisis, in which red cell precursors almost disappear from the bone marrow. As a result of marrow shutdown, and because there is a very short red cell survival, patients may become profoundly anemic over a period of a few hours. These episodes frequently result from intercurrent virus infections, and at least in some cases the parvovirus has been implicated. Another important but fortunately rare type of hematologic crisis is the so-called sequestration crisis. In this condition, large numbers of sickled erythrocytes become trapped in the spleen or liver, both of which may become extremely large over a period of a few hours. Postmortem examination of patients who have died of this condition shows massive red cell sequestration in these organs, which may contain a high proportion of the circulating red cell mass.

The long-term complications of sickle cell anemia, which may be crippling, can be easily understood on the basis of the pathophysiology of the sickled erythrocyte. Because of repeated infarction of the spleen there is usually splenic atrophy by the time a homozygote has reached the second decade. There may be chronic damage to the vessels of the retina, with a proliferating retinitis. Infarction of areas of the brain may lead to chronic neurologic disability. Repeated infarction of the lung may lead to pulmonary hypertension and right heart failure. Repeated bone infarction may cause severe deformity, particularly of the hip joints. Infarcts involving the dorsal vein of the penis may cause recurrent priapism and lead to severe fibrosis with permanent deformity. Because of repeated infarction of the renal papilla there is a gradual diminution of the power to concentrate urine. In some cases a frank nephrotic syndrome may occur.

The blood picture is characterized by chronic hemolysis with a hemoglobin concentration in the 7 to 9 g/dl range. There is persistent reticulocytosis in the 10 to 20 per cent range. The red cells are well hemoglobinized, but there is usually anisocytosis, and sickled forms are seen on the peripheral film. All the biochemical abnormalities of chronic hemolysis described earlier in this chapter are found in this condition. The hemoglobin consists of Hb S with variable amounts of Hb F (Fig. 47).

The clinical manifestations of sickling depend on the amount of Hb S in the red cell. The heterozygous state usually has about 30 per cent Hb S (Fig. 47); this is symptomless except in conditions of severe oxygen deprivation, such as in the case of a badly-given anesthetic or when flying in unpressurized aircraft at high altitude. The clinical manifestations of disorders

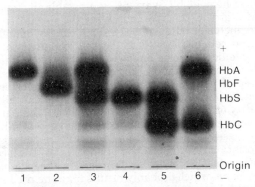

Figure 47. Hemoglobin electrophoresis shows the following from left to right: (1) normal adult hemoglobin, (2) umbilical cord blood containing mainly hemoglobin F, (3) sickle cell trait (AS), (4) SS disease, (5) hemoglobin SC disease (SC), and (6) hemoglobin C trait (AC).

in which the sickle cell gene is inherited together with another hemoglobin variant depend on the amount of interaction that occurs between the particular hemoglobin variant and Hb S.

Hemoglobin SC disease is a much milder disorder than sickle cell anemia, but there is a significant incidence of vascular occlusive episodes. Ocular complications including a severe proliferation of retinal vessels are common and may lead to blindness. This is also observed in some patients with Hb SD disease. Sickle cell thalassemia is a disorder of variable severity, depending on the type of thalassemia gene that is inherited. Sickle cell β^0-thalassemia may be as severe as sickle cell anemia, while sickle cell β^+-thalassemia is usually milder because of the presence of Hb A in the red cells. Individuals heterozygous for both Hb S and hereditary persistence of fetal hemoglobin usually have few clinical problems because the large amount of Hb F protects them against sickling.

Other Hemoglobin Variants (Table 34). Hemoglobin C differs from Hb A by the substitution of lysine for glutamic acid at position 6 in the β chain. Hemoglobin C is less soluble than Hb A and the red cells containing this variant are less deformable than normally. It is thought that this is the reason they have a slightly shortened survival time. The homozygous state for Hb C is characterized by a very mild hemolytic anemia and splenomegaly. The blood film shows large numbers of target cells and Hb C often crystallizes on the smear, giving the red cells a characteristic appearance with oblong hemoglobin precipitates across their centers. Hemoglobin E is extremely common in Southeast Asia, and the homozygous state is characterized by mild hemolytic anemia. Hemoglobin E is slightly unstable and appears to be synthesized less efficiently than Hb A (see p. 225). Hence there is a mild hemolytic anemia with target cells and mild hypochromia. Hemoglobin S, C, and E thalassemia were considered earlier (p. 225).

The unstable hemoglobin disorders are all rare. They result from amino acid substitutions in the region of the heme pocket, in the heme binding sites, or at critical areas that cause distortion of the globin chains. In some cases these hemoglobin variants result from deletions of one or more amino acids, which produces an unstable globin chain.

If a hemoglobin variant is unstable it tends to precipitate in the red cells with the formation of a rigid inclusion (Heinz) body. This causes damage to the red cell membrane as the cell is pulled through the splenic sinusoids or microvasculature of other organs. Thus the degree of hemolysis depends on the degree of instability of the hemoglobin molecule, accounting for the marked variability of the clinical severity of these conditions. Furthermore, some unstable hemoglobins have an abnormal oxygen affinity; in some cases this causes a right shift in the oxygen dissociation, and hence the anemia is well tolerated. Another feature of these disorders is the passage of dark urine, which probably results from the production of breakdown products of heme liberated from the precipitated globin chains in the red cells.

Because at least some of the unstable hemoglobins result from amino acid substitutions that do not alter the charge of the hemoglobin molecule, these conditions cannot be diagnosed by hemoglobin electrophoresis. However, nearly all the unstable hemoglobin variants are heat precipitable and can be demonstrated by warming a solution of hemoglobin to about 50° C.

Genetic Disorders of the Red Cell Membrane

Hereditary Spherocytosis (HS). This is a relatively common disorder that is inherited as an autosomal dominant trait. A genetic defect in the membrane results in spherical red cells that are prematurely destroyed in the spleen. Although the basic molecular defect in this disorder is still unknown, several well-defined metabolic abnormalities have been demonstrated. There is an increased permeability to sodium, which leads to an increased rate of glycolysis to provide energy for pumping excess sodium out of the cell. In addition, there is deficiency of the normal membrane lipid composition required to reduce the surface area of the cells. These metabolic changes, although not of great significance when the cells are in the circulation, interact to produce premature destruction of the cells when packed together in the osmotically unfavorable environment of the spleen. There is a specific molecular alteration in the red cell membrane skeleton in some but not all families with hereditary spherocytosis. There appears to be an alteration in spectrin-protein-4.1 interaction because of a defective spectrin molecule. This defect leads to a weakened spectrin-protein-4.1 complex, which in turn may lead to the friable membrane skeleton and the membrane instability characteristic of this disorder. One of the classic features of hereditary spherocytosis is that the red cells are more sensitive to lysis in hypotonic solutions than are normal red cells. In a hypotonic medium a normal red cell behaves as an almost perfect osmometer. On exposure to solutions of decreasing ionic strength its shape changes from its normal biconcave configuration until it has reached a spherical form. At this stage, the greatest volume is contained within the minimal surface area—that is, the surface area equal to that of the formerly biconcave disk. Once the red cell has reached this stage, the membrane becomes rigid and any further osmotic stress results in lysis. Thus the susceptibility to hemolysis in hypotonic solutions is thought to be a function of the ability of a red cell to swell before it reaches a critical spherical shape. Hence the decreased resistance to osmotic lysis in the cells of patients with hereditary spherocytosis is consistent with the finding that many of the cells in this condition are spherical or nearly spherical in the circulation. The decreased osmotic fragility in mild cases of hereditary spherocytosis can be demonstrated by incubation of red cells under sterile conditions for 24 hours before the osmotic fragility test is carried out. The flat underhemoglobinized cells of iron deficiency or thalassemia show the opposite pattern to that seen in hereditary spherocytosis; that is, they exhibit decreased osmotic fragility. Furthermore, since these cells tend to lose potassium and water during periods of sterile incubation, the decreased osmotic fragility is even more marked after a period of incubation under these conditions.

The condition has a variable clinical course characterized by a hemolytic anemia associated with intermittent jaundice and splenomegaly. The most important complications are hemolytic or aplastic crises usually related to infection, gallstone formation, the development of hemochromatosis due to increased iron absorption, and chronic leg ulceration. If obstructive jaundice develops, the spherocytosis becomes less marked and the red cell fragility may revert to normal.

Elliptocytosis. This condition is transmitted as an autosomal dominant trait and is characterized by the presence of a variable proportion of elliptic or oval cells in the peripheral blood. In many cases it is of no clinical importance and does not cause any increase in the rate of hemolysis. Occasionally, however, it may be associated with a severe hemolytic disorder and splenomegaly. There are two distinct genetic varieties of the condition, one linked to the Rh blood group locus, the other not. The latter form is associated with severe hemolysis and usually responds well to splenectomy. At least some forms of hereditary elliptocytosis result from a deficiency of a protein related to band 4.1 on electrophoresis of the red cell membrane proteins (see pp. 200 to 201).

Acanthocytosis. The presence of cells with spikes and horny excrescences is associated with the absence of β lipoprotein in the serum. The full syndrome is characterized by malabsorption, diffuse involvement of the central nervous system, and retinitis pigmentosa. Acanthocytosis has also been described in association with bizarre neurologic disorders in the absence of β lipoprotein deficiency. Although changes in red cell membrane lipid composition have been demonstrated in acanthocytes, the reason for the particular shape of the cells is unknown.

Stomatocytosis. Stomatocytosis is the name for any condition in which the red cells have a curious staining appearance in which there is a linear gap in the middle of the cell (see page 174). This type of cell has been observed in association with a hereditary hemolytic anemia in which the cells have an unusually high content of sodium and low levels of potassium together with increased intracellular water; the osmotic fragility is increased. Although the basic defect in this condition remains to be determined, recent studies point toward an abnormality of membrane protein. For example, one study has shown diminution in band 7. Furthermore, incubation of stomatocytic red cells with a bifunctional cross-linking reagent corrects the morphologic abnormality and is accompanied by a marked improvement in cation composition.

Stomatocytes are also observed in many acquired conditions, such as liver disease, alcoholism, lead poisoning, and malignant disease. They may also represent smear artifacts!

Hereditary Pyropoikilocytosis. This condition is characterized by a congenital hemolytic anemia accompanied by striking microspherocytosis and cells with blunted projections that are triangular. The diagnostic feature is that the red cells undergo fragmentation at a temperature of 45° C, whereas normal cells do not show these changes below 49° C. This condition may result from a structural change in the α subunit of spectrin. This finding is particularly interesting, since the 80K region of the α subunit appears to be involved in spectrin-spectrin interactions, which are responsible for oligomer formation.

The Acquired Hemolytic Anemias

The main types of acquired hemolytic disorders are summarized in Table 35. They fall into two main groups, according to whether or not the hemolysis is associated with a demonstrable antibody.

Immune Hemolytic Anemias

Immune hemolytic anemias are characterized by premature destruction of the red cells by one or more components of the immune system. There are two main groups, isoimmune and autoimmune. The antibodies that cause red cell destruction are of two main classes, warm and cold.

Mechanism of Red Cell Destruction. The mechanism of red cell destruction by the two main classes of antibodies has a different pathophysiology.

Warm antibodies are 7S IgG molecules that are

TABLE 35. ACQUIRED HEMOLYTIC ANEMIA

Associated with Antibodies to the Red Cell
Isoantibodies
  Hemolytic disease of the newborn
Transfusion reactions
Autoimmune hemolytic anemia
  Warm antibody type
  Drug-induced
  Cryopathic hemolytic syndromes
Not Associated with Antibody Formation
Acquired membrane defects
  Paroxysmal nocturnal hemoglobinuria (PNH)
  Liver disease
  Uremia
  Vitamin E deficiency
Trauma
  Microangiopathic hemolytic anemia
  Cardiac hemolysis
  March hemoglobinuria
Chemical and physical agents
Infection
  Parasitic
  Bacterial
Multifactoral
  Anemia of chronic disorders
  Hypersplenism
  Malignancy
  Renal failure

maximally active at 37° C. They do not agglutinate red cells and usually do not fix or activate complement. They are classified, therefore, as incomplete antibodies. (For a further consideration of incomplete antibodies see p. 257). They cause no morphologic or metabolic alteration of the red cells and usually lack specificity for the ABO blood group antigens but may have specificity for the Rh antigens. These antibodies cause destruction of the red cells in the spleen and other parts of the reticuloendothelial system and often produce a marked spherocytosis. The mechanism of cell destruction is complicated and probably multifactorial. Antibody-coated cells adhere to splenic macrophages and while doing so may lose part of their membrane, in a process that leads to spherocyte formation. Such macrophages have receptors highly specific for IgG subclasses IgG1 and IgG3. It is also possible that the incomplete antibodies, by altering the zeta potential (electrostatic charges that cause red cells to repel each other), allow closer interaction of the cells, particularly in the spleen. This may be a secondary cause of premature red cell destruction. Destruction of red cells can occur with very small numbers of IgG molecules on their surface. For example, destruction has been observed with as few as 10 molecules of anti-D per cell, and autoimmune hemolytic anemia has been observed with as few as 70 molecules per cell. This is well below the number of bound IgG molecules demonstrated by the standard antiglobulin test.

In some cases of autoimmune hemolytic anemia associated with IgG autoantibody, complement deposition occurs on the red cell surface by a mechanism that is not yet clear. Red cells are removed from the circulation by the binding of the active form of C3, C3b, by macrophages. Attachment to macrophages only occurs during the initial stages of complement deposition because C3b is rapidly split to C3c and C3d; although C3d remains on the cell surface, it does not bind to macrophage receptors.

Cold antibodies usually are 19S IgM molecules with a temperature optimum at or near 4° C. The thermal range of these antibodies is considerable, and occasionally they may be active almost up to body temperature. The cold antibody is complete; that is, it causes macroscopic and microscopic agglutination (see p. 257). These antibodies activate complement, and the red cells may become coated with the major complement component, C_3. C_3-sensitized red cells may be sequestered by the reticuloendothelial system, particularly in the liver. Rarely, if the IgM is a vigorous complement-binding antibody and the number of cell-bound C_3 molecules is high enough, more extensive complement-mediated hemolysis may occur. Complement fixation begins with the activation of the sequence by antigen-antibody complex. The classic pathway is usually triggered through C_1, C_4, and C_2. Lysis of the red cells occurs when the entire complement system has been activated through to C_9, producing holes in the membrane that can be seen by the electron microscope. These holes are 80 to 100 Å in diameter and thus are large enough to allow hemoglobin through and to cause intravascular hemolysis. It is interesting that the complement activation sequence is often interrupted at C_3, although the reason for this is not known. For a detailed discussion of the complement system, see Section III on Immunology.

Detection of Antibodies on Red Cells. A technique called the Coombs test is used to demonstrate the presence of various fractions of the plasma proteins on red cell membranes (see p. 257). In its simplest form (direct Coombs test) it is performed by adding a heterologous antiserum against human serum protein (Coombs reagent) to washed red cells. Cells coated with incomplete antibody are visibly agglutinated by this method. The antisera can be made more specific and to interact only with IgG, IgG plus complement (C), or complement alone. In addition to detecting antibody, the Coombs test can be used to detect red cell antibodies in the serum (indirect Coombs test). Cells from normal donors are incubated with test serum and then treated with the Coombs reagent as described above. If serum antibodies become attached to the normal red cells, the cells are agglutinated. Normal cells that have been pretreated with certain proteolytic enzymes, such as papain, show increased susceptibility to agglutination by incomplete antibodies. Agglutination may also occur on exposure to such antibodies without the use of Coombs sera by suspending the cells in agents that alter the zeta potential, such as albumin, dextran, and polyvinylpyrrolidone.

The Coombs test as practiced routinely in clinical laboratories is relatively crude and is only capable of demonstrating relatively large numbers of bound antibodies, probably in excess of a thousand or more. Recently, more sensitive radioimmune techniques have been developed that are capable of measuring less than 100 antibodies on the red cell surface.

Isoimmune Hemolytic Disease

The term "isoimmune hemolytic disease of the newborn" describes a group of conditions that result from the transplacental passage of maternal blood group antibodies that destroy the infant's red cells in utero.

Serology. The antibodies are usually of the Rh or ABO blood group systems. Rh isoimmune disease follows an immunizing event, usually the transplacental passage of fetal red cells into the maternal circulation when an Rh-positive infant is carried by an Rh-negative mother. Isoimmune hemolysis may then occur during subsequent pregnancies (see p. 256). Transfusion of Rh-positive blood to an Rh-negative woman may result in isoimmunization and hemolytic disease of the newborn in any subsequent pregnancy. One pregnancy with a full-term ABO-compatible infant immunizes about 17 per cent of Rh-negative women; antibodies appear immediately in about half and appear during subsequent Rh-positive pregnancies in the remainder. If no immunization has occurred after two pregnancies, the chances of carrying an affected infant in future are reduced. It is not certain whether the transplacental passage of red cells in pregnancies that end in abortion is a frequent cause of rhesus immunization, although this seems unlikely, especially in spontaneous abortions. Only IgG isoantibodies are transported across the placenta. Within the ABO blood group system, either spontaneously occurring or postimmunization, isoantibodies may be present that have some major components in the IgG (7S) immunoglobulin class. ABO incompatibility accounts for about half of all cases of neonatal hemolytic disease and Rh incompatibility for most of the remainder. Occasional cases result from the minor blood groups, such as Kell

(see pp. 256 to 257). In terms of severity, however, Rh incompatibility is by far the most important; ABO incompatibility rarely causes dangerous neonatal hemolysis.

Pathophysiology. The transfer of maternal antibodies and their reaction with incompatible erythrocytes causes hemolysis and raised levels of unconjugated bilirubin. Compensatory hemopoiesis results in normoblastemia and extramedullary erythropoiesis. Severe intrauterine anemia may lead to fetal death with massive edema and hypertrophy of the placenta. This picture, called *hydrops fetalis,* is probably due to fetal cardiac failure and hypoalbuminemia, possibly due to diminished albumin synthesis. In milder cases there is anemia and neonatal jaundice (icterus neonatorum). The fetus has a limited capacity for conjugating bilirubin. Unconjugated bilirubin penetrates and directly injures the nerve cells in the basal nuclei, leading to kernicterus. Since bilirubin can be moved into the maternal circulation via the placenta, this occurs only after delivery. The cord blood bilirubin level is closely related to the severity of the disease; values above 4 mg/100 ml suggest severe disease. Peak levels are usually reached by the fourth day after delivery.

The main hematologic changes in Rh hemolytic disease are anemia, normoblastemia, and reticulocytosis. The normal hemoglobin value at birth is 19.0 ± 2.2 g/dl. Values of 14 g/dl for cord blood hemoglobin are significantly reduced and in the fully developed hydrops picture levels as low as 3 to 5 g/dl may be encountered. The direct Coombs test is positive and antibodies may be demonstrated in the serum. The mechanism of red cell destruction is that described for warm antibodies in the previous section.

In ABO incompatibility there are usually spherocytes on the blood film. The degree of anemia is milder than in Rh incompatibility and the direct Coombs test may not be positive; special serologic techniques may be required to demonstrate the antibodies.

Autoimmune Hemolytic Anemia

Autoimmune hemolytic anemia (AHA) can be classified in terms of the type of autoantibody present and on the presence or absence of an underlying disorder. Using the former approach, AHA can be divided into the "warm" and "cold" antibody types, and both groups can be subdivided further into either primary or secondary (Table 35).

Warm Antibody Hemolytic Anemia. In the majority of patients with warm AHA the autoantibodies are of the IgG class. In the minority of cases these antibodies have specificity for a particular blood group antigen, usually anti-C or anti-E of the Rh system (see p. 256). About a third of the antibodies that lack apparent specificity have some specificity, because they fail to react with Rh-null red cells, that is, cells with no detectable Rh antigens (see p. 256). This observation suggests that these antibodies react with a "core" structural component common to the Rh antigens. Warm antibodies are identified on the cells by the use of the direct Coombs test (see previous section and p. 257). IgG is detected on the cell surface in about 80 per cent of cases, while in about 50 per cent components of the complement system, principally C_3 and C_4, are detected with anticomplement-specific antisera. About 10 per cent of affected patients show positive reaction only with anti-C. It is thus important to use a "broad-spectrum" antiglobulin reagent that will detect both IgG and C-coating of the cells for the direct Coombs test. Hemolysis may occur in any of these patterns of red cell sensitization—that is, IgG alone, C alone, or both. However, while hemolysis nearly always occurs when the cells are coated with IgG only, about half of the patients with C alone show definite hemolysis. In many cases, free antibody can be detected in the serum by the use of the indirect Coombs test and enzyme-treated red cells (see p. 257).

About 50 per cent of cases of warm antibody AHA have demonstrable underlying disorders. These include lymphomas, chronic lymphatic leukemia, systemic lupus erythematosus (SLE), other collagen vascular disorders, and ovarian malignancies. There is no correlation between the serologic findings and the presence or absence of an underlying disorder, although patients with SLE may have both IgG and complement on their red cells.

The disorder is characterized by icterus, splenomegaly, anemia, and a reticulocytosis. The blood film shows polychromasia with spherocytosis and anisocytosis, and there are often nucleated red cells in the peripheral blood. The hemolysis is primarily extravascular, although in severe cases intravascular hemolysis and hemoglobinuria can occur. The diagnosis can be confirmed by the presence of a positive direct Coombs test with the serologic characteristics already mentioned.

"Cold" Autoimmune Disease (the cryopathic hemolytic syndromes). There are two disorders in which increased red cell destruction occurs at below normal body temperature; these are cold agglutinin disease and paroxysmal cold hemoglobinuria.

A marked elevation of cold agglutinins may occur either as a transient phenomenon in association with infections, particularly those caused by *Mycoplasma pneumoniae,* or may be more persistent as part of the idiopathic cold agglutinin disorder of old age or in association with neoplasia, particularly the reticuloses. The cold agglutinins are IgM antibodies that, if present in high titers, interact with complement in the cooler parts of the body to produce intravascular hemolysis. In addition, intravascular agglutination of red cells may result in blockage of vessels, causing Raynaud's phenomenon or physical damage to the cells.

In the condition associated with *M. pneumoniae* infection there is usually a brisk hemolytic episode often with hemoglobinuria, which occurs two to three weeks after a short respiratory illness. In the chronic idiopathic form of the disease, which occurs usually in old people, the symptoms are mainly those of anemia with Raynaud's phenomenon and diffuse mottling of the skin after cooling. In more severe cases hemoglobinuria may occur.

The peripheral blood picture shows changes typical of hemolysis with a variable degree of anemia, reticulocytosis, and some spherocytosis. The red cells show autoagglutination after cooling to 4° C; this is dispersed at 37° C. The cold agglutinin titer is markedly elevated and with high titers of antibodies there may be a substantial activity up to 30° C or higher. The direct Coombs test is usually positive because of the ability of the cold antibody to fix C_3 and C_4 components of complement; it has specificity against the inactive form of C_3 in most patients. Electrophoresis of the plasma proteins usually shows a "monoclonal" band; the serum IgM is in the 500 to 1500 mg/100 ml range. Most cold agglutinins of the IgM type react with I antigen, although with hemolysis associated with infectious mononucleosis the antibodies may have anti-i specificity.

Paroxysmal cold hemoglobinuria is a rare form of acquired hemolytic anemia characterized by intermittent attacks of intravascular hemolysis and hemoglobinuria due to an antibody system that is cold-dependent. This disorder was formerly seen frequently in association with syphilis, particularly the congenital form, but now it is rare and usually occurs as a single acute episode following a viral illness such as measles or mumps. The causative autoantibody (termed the *Donath-Landsteiner (DL) antibody)* is able to fix complement in the cold. When the cells are warmed to 37° C the complement sequence is completed and lysis results. The DL antibody is an IgG immunoglobulin that usually has specificity for the red cell antigen P in both idiopathic and syphilitic forms. The condition is associated with attacks of hemoglobinuria with backache and cramps; additional features are a Raynaud-like phenomenon and cold urticaria. The blood picture shows a typical picture of hemolytic anemia, often associated with leukopenia.

Immune Hemolytic Anemia Associated with Drugs

Although it has been known for many years that hemolytic anemia may be associated with direct injury to the red cells by drugs, it has become clear only recently that many of the hemolytic anemias associated with drug therapy have an immune basis. Other ways in which drugs may damage red cells have been mentioned in previous sections and are summarized in Table 36. There is now a long list of drugs capable of producing immune hemolysis, and at least three distinct immune mechanisms have been worked out in the pathogenesis of these anemias.

Hapten. In this type of disorder, the drug, presumably acting as hapten, evokes the production of antibodies, usually of the IgG class. On subsequent exposure to the drug the antibody interacts with erythrocytes that are coated with the drug. Antibody can be demonstrated on the red cells by the direct Coombs test. The commonest cause of this type of hemolytic reaction is the administration of massive

TABLE 36. DRUG-INDUCED HEMOLYTIC ANEMIA

Oxidant Damage
Genetically susceptible red cells
    G-6-PD deficiency
    Other enzyme deficiencies
    Hb H disease
    Other unstable hemoglobins
Normal red cells
    Any severe oxidant stress—e.g., phenacetin

Immune Damage
    Hapten
    "Innocent bystander"
    Autoimmune

Unknown Mechanism
    Sulfonamides

doses of penicillin. Thus, in addition to acting as an immunologic stimulus, the drug becomes tightly bound to the red cell membrane, in vitro or in vivo. It is possible to prepare penicillin-sensitized cells for demonstrating the presence of an IgG penicillin antibody. The hemolytic reaction is usually of slow onset with a gradual fall in hemoglobin level and minimal intravascular hemolysis.

Innocent Bystander Mechanism. Another way in which drugs cause hemolysis has been called the "innocent bystander" mechanism (a name that is more ornamental than scientifically accurate). In this type of disorder, the drug evokes an immune response with the production of an antibody of the IgM class. It has been suggested that, when the drug is given again, drug-antibody complexes are formed that are capable of interacting with the red cell membrane with the attachment of complement components. The drug-antibody complex dissociates and leaves the cell with a positive (anticomplement) Coombs test, but the cells do not react with anti-IgM reagents. Typical examples of this type are the immune anemias associated with quinidine, quinine, and stibophen. The hemolytic reaction can be dramatic, with intravascular hemolysis and hemoglobinuria following a second exposure to the drug.

Autoimmune Mechanism. Drugs may cause true autoimmune hemolytic anemia; this has been worked out for the antihypertensive agent methyldopa. Approximately 25 per cent of patients receiving this drug develop a positive Coombs test after three to six months of treatment. The antibodies have serologic properties identical to those of the warm antibody autoimmune hemolytic anemias, and many of them show Rh specificity. Only a minority of patients with the positive Coombs test develop hemolytic anemia. Some affected patients develop antinuclear antibodies and a small proportion also have thrombocytopenia. The Coombs test may remain positive for some months after the drug has been withdrawn.

The Coombs test may become positive in the absence of hemolysis in patients on drugs other than methyldopa. For example, a positive direct Coombs test may be found after the administration of large doses of cephalothin or cephaloridine. There are no drug-dependent antibodies present in the serum or eluate. Patients receiving large doses of rifampicin may develop a positive Coombs test; in this case there are drug-dependent antibodies, although hemolysis is rare. The positive Coombs test of patients taking carbromal is thought to have the same basis as that of the penicillin-induced hemolytic anemia.

The Nonimmune Acquired Hemolytic Anemias

The red cell may be prematurely destroyed through the action of increased mechanical stress, chemical agents, infections, or acquired defects of red cell membrane.

Hemolytic Anemia Due to Trauma to the Red Cells

There are three mechanisms whereby red cells may be damaged by trauma: (1) increased rigidity of vessel walls associated with turbulence or other abnormalities of flow; (2) diseases of the small blood vessels that interfere with the microcirculation; and (3) direct trauma to the red cells in exposed areas, such as the feet.

Cardiac Hemolytic Anemia. Abnormal turbulence set up by diseased or artificial cardiac valves can produce intravascular hemolysis by direct trauma to the red cells. There is often a low-grade hemolytic process associated with valvular abnormalities, particularly aortic stenosis. The degree of hemolysis is not usually enough to cause anemia. Severe hemolytic anemia has followed several different forms of repair or replacement operations for aortic or mitral valve disease. It has been reported after Teflon-patch repair of septal defects, aortic valve replacement with a variety of prostheses, in particular the Starr-Edwards valve, and also after mitral valve replacement. These anemias have a complex origin that is probably related mainly to abnormal flow dynamics, particularly regurgitation of blood through or around a prosthesis, to fibrin deposition on the artificial valves, and to the action of regurgitant jets of blood impinging on a foreign (unendothelialized) patch. This type of red cell trauma causes a moderate to severe intravascular hemolysis with hemoglobinuria and hemosiderinuria in the postoperative period. This goes on to a state of chronic intravascular hemolysis and the blood film shows marked fragmentation of the red cells (Fig. 48). The magnitude of iron loss through the kidneys may be sufficient to cause iron deficiency anemia, which reduces the marrow response to the hemolytic anemia.

Microangiopathic Hemolytic Anemia. The microangiopathies are a group of disorders in which there is intravascular hemolysis and fragmentation of the red blood cells secondary to disease of the small vessels. The actual pathologic basis of the small vessel disease varies, and there may be arteritis, fibrinoid necrosis, or invasion of the capillaries by malignant cells. Furthermore, the disorders that produce disseminated intravascular coagulation (DIC) may be associated with a microangiopathy. These observations suggest that small thrombi are the cause of hemolysis and that the red cells are fragmented as they pass through fibrin meshes. Some examples of microangiopathic hemolysis follow.

Hemolytic uremic syndrome (HUS) is the term used to describe the association of an acute hemolytic anemia with renal failure in infancy or early childhood. This condition often follows an acute febrile illness and is characterized by a variable degree of hemolytic anemia with nephritis. There may be a very rapid fall in the hemoglobin level with marked hemoglobinuria. The condition is also characterized by severe systemic upset, including fever and abdominal pain, and the renal failure may go on to complete anuria. There is often purpura and drowsiness leading to coma in some cases. The peripheral blood picture shows the typical microangiopathic appearance with fragmentation and distortion of the red cells, small spherocytes, and marked polychromasia. There is a variable degree of thrombocytopenia and a leukocytosis. Studies for evidence of disseminated intravascular coagulation have given equivocal results, possibly because such changes occur only early in the evolution of the illness. There is an elevated blood urea, and urinalysis provides evidence of nephritis.

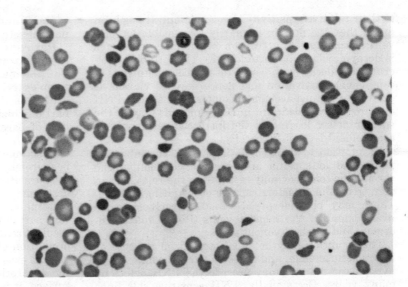

Figure 48. The peripheral blood film of a patient with microangiopathic hemolytic anemia. The film shows the typical small fragmented cells. (Leishman's stain × 600.)

Thrombotic thrombocytopenic purpura (TTP) is an acute disorder of unknown origin characterized by hemolytic anemia together with neurologic and renal disease. It is predominantly a disease of young adults and is characterized by a sudden onset of fever, renal failure, and neurologic signs characterized by paralysis, psychiatric disturbances, and coma. In addition, there is generalized purpura and anemia with hemoglobinuria. The hematologic changes are those of a microangiopathy with thrombocytopenia. In most cases there is no evidence of disseminated intravascular coagulation. Current theories regarding the etiology of HUS and TTP are discussed below.

Microangiopathic hemolytic anemia may occur in association with disseminated mucus-secreting carcinoma, particularly of the stomach. The precise etiology of the microangiopathic process is unknown, but it may result from the direct invasion of small vessels by tumor with subsequent tumor emboli or may follow the liberation of thromboplastic material from the mucus-secreting tumor.

Microangiopathic hemolytic anemia may also be seen in a variety of other conditions, including collagen vascular disorders, toxemia of pregnancy, septicemia, purpura fulminans, malignant hypertension, and in association with cavernous hemangiomata.

March Hemoglobinuria. This is characterized by attacks of hemoglobinuria following strenuous physical exercise, such as running, particularly on hard surfaces. The condition results from mechanical trauma to red cells in the soles of the feet. A similar mechanism probably accounts for the hemoglobinuria that follows karate and other strenuous activity associated with direct trauma to body surfaces.

Acquired Defects of the Red Cell Membrane

Liver Disease. Although there may be some shortening of red cell survival in patients with infectious hepatitis and cirrhosis or biliary obstruction, the degree of hemolysis is usually mild. However, there are two conditions in which liver disease may be associated with a more severe hemolytic process. In *Zieve's syndrome,* acute hemolytic episodes associated with abdominal pain occur, usually in alcoholics with liver disease, following a bout of drinking. There is associated hyperlipidemia and jaundice. The pathophysiology of the shortened red cell survival is not understood. Another group of patients whose liver disease may be complicated by severe hemolysis are those with the so-called *spur-cell syndrome.* This condition is usually associated with severe hepatocellular disease and is characterized by the appearance of markedly deformed red cells, resembling acanthocytes, in the peripheral blood; there is usually a marked hemolytic anemia. The nature of the defect in the red cell membrane is unknown although it may result from increased accumulation of cholesterol in the red cell membrane.

Paroxysmal Nocturnal Hemoglobinuria (PNH). This is a rare condition of unknown etiology that is characterized by chronic intravascular hemolysis, exacerbations associated with hemoglobinuria, and a marked thrombotic tendency. The hemoglobinuria tends to occur at night but may be continuous.

The basic defect in PNH is in the erythrocyte membrane, which is sensitive to lysis by acidified serum. This is because the PNH cell is much more sensitive than normal to lysis by complement, and complement lysis is particularly active in the lower pH range. This property of the PNH cell forms the basis for the acidified serum lysis test for the disorder, first described by Ham. The cells are also unusually sensitive to low ionic strength solutions, such as sucrose, which is a further characteristic of complement sensitivity. Following exposure to complement, large holes appear in the PNH red cell membrane similar to those that occur in normal cells after complement lysis. However, the PNH cell is lysed at much lower serum complement levels than is a normal red cell. The PNH cell is believed to be the product of an abnormal erythroid clone arising de novo or in the setting of a previously damaged marrow—for example, in aplastic anemia. The PNH cell also shows a marked sensitivity to anti-i (see p. 256), the basis for the cold antibody lysis test. This anti-i sensitivity is also due to increased sensitivity to complement, since the degree of antibody binding is not greatly enhanced. As well as normal red cells, several different populations have been identified in PNH that have been classified types I to III according to their relative sensitivity to complement. It has been found that the protein primarily responsible for preventing complement activation on human erythrocytes is decay-accelerating factor (DAF). This protein accelerates the decay of C_3 convertase of both pathways of complement activation and hence may be viewed as protective against accidental complement attack. PNH erythrocytes are deficient in DAF, and this may be the specific defect leading to the increased sensitivity to complement lysis of PNH cells.

In addition to the hemolytic process, thrombocytopenia and leukopenia are observed commonly. The thrombotic tendency may result from the release from damaged cells of factors capable of initiating clotting. There may be widespread venous thrombosis with involvement of the hepatic veins (Budd-Chiari syndrome) and cerebral venous sinuses.

The condition may be superimposed on aplastic or hypoplastic anemia, and indeed a pancytopenia with a hypoplastic marrow may precede the PNH defect by many years. Occasionally, PNH sensitive cell lines occur in the myeloproliferative disorders, including acute leukemia. Thus, the PNH abnormality may occur in a broad spectrum of clinical settings; at one end is the typical severe hemolytic anemia with nocturnal hemoglobinuria and at the other the presence of small clones of complement-sensitive cells in patients with a wide variety of disorders of the bone marrow.

Other Disorders of the Red Cell Membrane. The burr cells of renal failure result from the presence of a heat-labile factor in uremic serum. The degree of hemolysis is not usually severe in renal failure. Because membrane lipids are subject to peroxidation, deficiency of vitamin E, which is an antioxidant, might be expected to cause hemolysis. This may occur in newborn infants and in later life in patients with thalassemia major. The degree to which vitamin E deficiency contributes to the hemolysis of the latter condition is uncertain.

Hemolytic Anemia Due to Infection

Hemolytic anemias that accompany infection result from a variety of mechanisms. In bacterial infection the cells may be destroyed by the direct action of bacterial toxins on the red cell, by immune interaction between bacteria and the red cell, or by DIC precipitated by the infection (see p. 312), leading to a microangiopathic hemolytic anemia. In addition, the red cell may be damaged directly by parasites.

Septicemia. The hemolytic anemia that occurs in some patients with septicemia may well be due to DIC, leading to a microangiopathic hemolytic anemia. However, in some cases, particularly those of infection with *Clostridium perfringens* (also called *C. welchii*), the organism produces a lecithinase that acts on the red cell lipoproteins, causing their destruction. In such conditions there is fragmentation of the red cells and clear evidence of DIC. In some bacteremias there may be absorption of bacterial polysaccharides onto the red cells, which are then agglutinated by the action of antibodies directed against the coated cells. Rarely, there may be unmasking of T-type antigens by the bacteria, which makes the cell polyagglutinable. All human red cells carry the T antigen, which can be activated by bacterial enzymes. Since normal serum contains anti-T, such cells become agglutinable by any normal sera.

Parasitic Disorders. Globally, parasitic disorders are an extremely important cause of hemolytic anemia. The anemia of *Plasmodium falciparum* malaria has a complex etiology, which is not fully understood. In acute infections there is a major hemolytic component, part of which undoubtedly results from the sequestration of parasitized red cells in the spleen and other parts of the reticuloendothelial system. However, hemolysis may continue after the parasitized cells have been removed from the circulation, suggesting that nonparasitized erythrocytes may also be prematurely destroyed in this condition. Although the picture may be complicated by acute renal failure, it seems likely that part of the hemolytic component of this condition results from a nonspecific macrophage activation. A proportion of patients with *P. falciparum* malaria develop a positive Coombs test, probably as a result of the absorption of malarial antigen onto the red cell surface. It is not clear whether this contributes to the shortened red cell survival. Finally, patients with acute malaria do not respond adequately to hemolysis, and there is a component of dyserythropoiesis. This seems to be more marked in individuals with recurrent *P. falciparum* infections in whom the pathogenesis of the anemia may be further complicated by hypersplenism secondary to massive splenomegaly.

The hemolytic component in infections with *Bartonella bacilliformis* seems to be due to direct involvement of the red cells by the parasite. On the other hand, the acute hemolytic anemia of childhood *leishmaniasis* appears to be caused by macrophage activation throughout the reticuloendothelial system. Hemolysis may also occur as a result of the effect of drugs used in the treatment of parasitic illnesses. This is particularly important in the case of malaria in G-6-PD–deficient individuals.

Virus Infection. The relationship between viral illness and hemolysis is complex. In disorders such as infectious mononucleosis there may be a clear-cut immune hemolytic anemia. Cytomegalovirus infection, particularly in the newborn, may be associated with marked hemolysis; the mechanism is unknown. Hemolysis may also be a factor in the virus hemophagocytosis syndrome described earlier in this chapter (see p. 227).

Hemolytic Anemia Due to Direct Damage by Drugs, Chemicals, and Other Toxins, and Physical Agents

The production of hemolytic anemia by the action of drugs on red cells with an intrinsic enzyme defect and by an immune basis were considered earlier in this chapter. However, certain drugs in a high enough concentration damage normal red cells. For example, phenacetin can cause a Heinz body anemia, presumably by its oxidant properties. The acute hemolytic reaction to certain sulfonamides has never been adequately explained. Red cell damage can be produced by some of the heavy metals, arsenic in particular. Inhalation of arsine gas can produce anemia, jaundice, and severe hemoglobinuria. *Lead poisoning* produces a moderate degree of anemia with an extremely complex origin. There is a hemolytic component, possibly owing to the effect of lead on the membrane sulfhydryl groups; in addition, there is a defect in hemoglobin synthesis due to the effect of lead on both heme and globin production. Copper in large doses may also produce a hemolytic process. Some patients with *Wilson's disease* have severe hemolytic episodes. Sodium or potassium chlorate may produce methemoglobinemia, Heinz bodies, and hemolytic anemia. Exposure to certain physical agents can produce a hemolytic proc-

ess. One of the most interesting of these involves the breathing of 100 per cent oxygen by astronauts, in which the mechanism for hemolysis is unknown. The stings from a variety of insects, including bees and spiders, may occasionally cause hemolytic anemias. Despite the fact that snake venom causes hemolysis in vitro by converting lecithin to isolecithin, hemolysis does not occur often in vivo. Severe hemolysis may accompany extensive burns and other thermal injuries.

Polycythemia

The term "polycythemia" is used to describe an increased red cell count. In fact, it can be applied to any condition in which there is a significant increase above normal of the number of red cells or the hematocrit or hemoglobin levels. There are two classes: (1) relative, in which there is a reduction in the plasma volume with a normal red cell mass, and (2) true, in which there is an actual increase in red cell mass. These major subdivisions of polycythemia are still used today, although they are usually called relative polycythemia and absolute polycythemia, respectively.

A simple clinical classification of the different forms of polycythemia is shown in Table 37. The major divisions are relative and absolute polycythemia, and the latter group is further subdivided into primary polycythemia, or polycythemia vera, and the secondary polycythemias. This is a useful classification because in clinical practice it is first important to decide whether there is an absolute or relative polycythemia and, if the former is the case, to determine whether the polycythemia is due to an abnormal proliferation of red cell precursors or is secondary to any of the large number of conditions that can produce an increased red cell mass.

A more pathophysiologic approach to the classification of polycythemia is shown in Table 38. As discussed earlier, the rate of proliferation of red cell precursors is regulated by the level of erythropoietin. Polycythemia could occur if the red cell precursors were to proliferate independently of erythropoietin. It could also occur as a response to increased erythropoietin production mediated by an appropriate response such as hypoxia. Another potential mechanism would be

the production of increased amounts of erythropoietin in situations in which the normal feedback suppression by an adequate oxygen content of the circulating red cells was lost. Such inappropriate production of erythropoietin might result from its secretion by tumors; there are many examples of the inappropriate production of hormones in this way, which are examined in the sections that follow.

ABSOLUTE POLYCYTHEMIA

An absolute polycythemia is defined as a state in which the red cell mass is significantly elevated. It may result from an abnormal proliferation of red cell precursors of unknown origin or from a variety of conditions that are associated with an increased output of erythropoietin.

POLYCYTHEMIA VERA

Polycythemia vera results from abnormal proliferation of the red cell precursors and often of the other formed elements of the blood. It is one of a family of diseases called the myeloproliferative disorders, which are characterized by an abnormal proliferation of the formed elements of the blood; the red cells, white cells, and platelets may be affected in any combination. The disorders encompass a broad spectrum of conditions, ranging from polycythemia vera through essential thrombocythemia to chronic myeloid leukemia and

TABLE 37. CLINICAL CLASSIFICATION OF POLYCYTHEMIA

Relative or pseudopolycythemia ("stress" polycythemia)
Absolute polycythemia
  Primary—polycythemia vera
  Secondary
    Altitude
    Chronic lung disease
    Cyanotic congenital heart disease
    Renal disease—tumors, cysts, hydronephrosis, posttransplant
    Nonrenal tumors—hepatoma, cerebellar hemangioma
    Endocrine—Cushing's disease, pheochromocytoma
    Genetic—abnormal hemoglobin
       —abnormal erythropoietin metabolism
    Obesity—Pickwickian syndrome

TABLE 38. PATHOPHYSIOLOGIC CLASSIFICATION OF POLYCYTHEMIA

Relative
  Reduced plasma volume
Absolute
  Normal or low erythropoietin levels. Abnormal proliferation
    Polycythemia vera
  Increased erythropoietin levels
    Appropriate
      Lung disease, cyanotic heart disease, altitude, abnormal hemoglobin, obesity
    Inappropriate
      Renal tumor, other rare genetic defects of erythropoietin regulation, erythropoietin-secreting tumors, post renal transplant
  Mechanism unknown
    Endocrine disease, Cushing's disease, pheochromocytoma

myelosclerosis. "Myeloproliferative" is useful only as a descriptive term in that it includes a series of disorders that are unlikely to have a common etiology.

Etiology. Polycythemia vera results from abnormal proliferation of red cell precursors derived from a single clone and probably from a single stem cell. The reason for the abnormal proliferation of this line is completely unknown. Evidence that the line is derived from a single stem cell has been obtained from studies of the red cell enzymes of Negro females with polycythemia vera. Because of inactivation (Lyonization) of one X chromosome per cell at an early stage of embryonic development, women heterozygous for the G-6-PD types A and B (see p. 232) should have two distinct types of somatic cells—that is, one containing the B enzyme and one containing the A enzyme. This is certainly the case in their red cells. Several persons of this type have been found who also have polycythemia vera. In these patients more than 90 per cent of the peripheral blood red cells have been found to carry one form of G-6-PD (that is, they contain either the A or the B enzyme), whereas in other tissues a more or less equal number of cells containing either A or B type enzyme are found. These observations indicate that the majority of their red cells are the progeny of a single stem cell. Presumably the basic defect in this disease is a change in the genetic constitution of this cell, such that its progeny proliferate independently of the normal control mechanisms involved in erythropoiesis. The increased number of white cells and platelets that are often found in this disorder suggests that this abnormal proliferation is not confined to the erythroid line.

The general concept of the etiology of polycythemia vera outlined above is strengthened by studies of the control of erythropoiesis in this condition. Erythropoietin levels are extremely low in the blood and urine, but there is an appropriate rise after venesection. In in vitro culture the red cell precursors obtained from patients with polycythemia vera show increased and prolonged unstimulated erythropoiesis as well as responsiveness to added erythropoietin. These studies suggest that there is not a primary defect in erythropoietin metabolism and that the normal feedback mechanisms for reducing erythropoietin output are intact (see pp. 109 to 191). Rather, they suggest that the disorder results from the emergence of a clone of red cell precursors whose proliferative capacity is not erythropoietin-dependent and hence continues to proliferate despite low erythropoietin levels. Since the red cell precursors are responsive to erythropoietin in an in vitro culture system, it seems unlikely that the abnormal proliferation is due to an altered receptor state for erythropoietin on the red cell surface, although this possibility requires further study.

During the course of the presumed neoplastic proliferation of the abnormal clone in patients with polycythemia vera, abnormal proliferation of white cells and platelets may occur and both lines may show abnormalities of function. Ultimately, there may be a marked fibrotic reaction in the marrow with progression to myelosclerosis, or the condition may terminate in acute myeloblastic leukemia. Hence, the natural history of polycythemia vera bears at least a superficial resemblance to that of chronic myeloid leukemia (p. 276).

Pathophysiology. When measured in capillary tubes, viscosity of blood increases exponentially with increases in hematocrit. When the rate of blood flow is measured (that is, as the reciprocal of viscosity) at varying hematocrit levels, it is seen to decrease as an essentially linear function of the increasing hematocrit (Fig. 49). If the flow rate is multiplied by oxygen content the product provides an indication of the rate of oxygen transport at different hematocrit values. As shown in Figure 50, optimum oxygen transport occurs at intermediate hematocrit values of about 40 to 50 per cent. If no compensatory mechanisms occurred, there would be a reduced rate of oxygen transport with a slight increase in hematocrit. In fact, tissue oxygen tension in hypervolemic animals remains relatively normal. This degree of compensation is achieved because there is an increase in the total blood volume, particularly the plasma volume, and an increased cardiac output. In addition, the peripheral vascular bed enlarges, leading to a fall in peripheral resistance. Indeed, at a hematocrit of 60 per cent these changes produce an increase in oxygen transport (Fig. 50). Castle has summarized the situation as follows: "homeostasis of hemoglobin level and oxygen transport depend on the independent and opposite influences of blood viscosity and blood volume." Hypervolemia per se increases oxygen transport because the increased blood oxygen content and cardiac output more than compensate for the increased viscosity of the blood. However, polycythemia vera is a disease of middle and old age, and if there are associated cardiovascular disorders, such as hypertension or coronary artery disease, these compensating mechanisms may break down. This will be particularly likely at very high hematocrit levels when there may be a marked increase in workload for both the left and right sides of the heart because of the high blood viscosity in the systemic and pulmonary circulations. Indeed, at hematocrits in excess of 60 per cent, net oxygen transport is reduced.

The complications of polycythemia vera can be related to the hemodynamic changes and abnormal function of the aberrant cell line. Thrombotic episodes probably result from reduced flow of thick viscous blood, the high platelet counts that commonly accom-

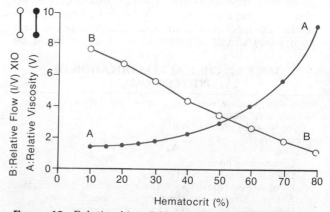

Figure 49. Relationship of blood viscosity (curve A) and relative blood flow through a capillary tube (curve B) of human blood at various hematocrits. (From Castle, W. B., and Jandl, J. H.: Seminars in Hematology 3:193, 1966.)

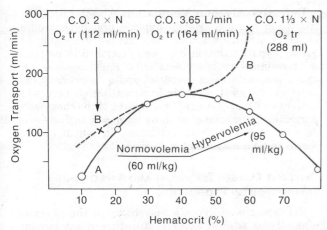

Figure 50. Relative oxygen transport by blood of various hematocrits in vitro and in vivo. Curve A was constructed by multiplying the values for relative blood flow at various hematocrits in curve B of Figure 49 by their corresponding hematocrits. Curve B shows the relative transport of oxygen in vivo calculated for blood with hematocrits of 15, 42, and 60 per cent, respectively. Note the large increase in the last as a result of the increased cardiac output of blood with increased oxygen content. (From Castle, W. B.: In *Pathologic Physiology: Mechanisms of Disease*. 4th ed. Sodeman, W. A., and Sodeman, W. A., Jr. (eds.). Philadelphia, W. B. Saunders Company, 1967.)

pany the disorder, and the associated abnormalities of platelet function (see p. 295). Such episodes may involve cerebral vessels on the arterial or venous sides and have a particular predilection for the portal and hepatic venous systems. Damage to the intestinal mucosa following a thrombotic episode may account for the high incidence of mucosal ulceration. The hemorrhagic tendency is not well understood. There are no consistent defects in the clotting factors, but platelet function is often abnormal; in particular, abnormalities of aggregation and interaction with epinephrine and collagen have been demonstrated. The bleeding or thrombotic manifestations of the condition together with cardiovascular complications due to the increased cardiac work are the commonest causes of morbidity or death.

Because of the increased hemopoietic activity and turnover of red cell precursors, many patients with polycythemia vera have hyperuricemia and secondary gout. For the same reason, folic acid deficiency may occur; the patient may become anemic only to become polycythemic again after folate therapy! The pruritus, which is a common accompaniment, is unexplained, although it has been suggested that hyperhistaminemia may be involved.

Clinical Features. The clinical features are easily understood if the pathophysiology has been appreciated. Affected patients have a ruddy complexion and complain of headache, dizziness, vertigo, visual disturbances, cardiovascular symptoms, and the effects of arterial or venous thromboses or hemorrhages. Pruritus is a very common presenting symptom. The physical findings include plethora; dilated superficial vessels, particularly over the face and neck; and splenomegaly. The pathophysiology of the latter is not understood; there is no evidence that it results from extramedullary hemopoiesis.

Blood Findings. There is a variable increase in the hemoglobin, hematocrit, and red cell count. There is an absolute increase in the circulating red cell mass and very frequently an elevation in the white cell and/or platelet count, although some patients with genuine polycythemia vera may go for many years with normal granulocyte and platelet counts. Early in the course of the illness the morphology of the formed elements of the blood is usually normal; although, as the disease progresses, complications such as myelosclerosis or leukemic transformation may occur, and the peripheral blood may become markedly abnormal. The bone marrow shows proliferation of the erythroid, myeloid, and megakaryocytic series with extension down the long bones and the extremities. Marrow biopsy shows replacement of the fat spaces with highly cellular marrow in which all the formed elements are present. The amount of stainable iron is usually reduced. This may reflect associated bleeding and the fact that iron stores are shifted into the intravascular compartment as a result of the increased red cell mass. Even early in the course of the illness special staining may show an increase in reticulin; as the disease progresses this may become more extensive when the appearances become typical of myelosclerosis. Other findings include hyperuricemia, an increased leukocyte alkaline phosphatase and an increased level of the vitamin B_{12} binding protein transcobalamin I. There may be a slight decrease in the arterial oxygen saturation. Pulmonary function tests have not provided an adequate explanation for this phenomenon. Studies of the chromosomes have given conflicting results, partly because many of them have been carried out on patients who have been treated with radioactive phosphorus or cytotoxic therapy. However, about 10 per cent of patients have an extra C group chromosome.

Course. The course of polycythemia vera is extremely variable and the condition may go on relatively unchanged for many years or cause early death owing to cardiovascular, thrombotic, or hemorrhagic complications. Ultimately, the blood picture gradually changes to one of myelosclerosis with anemia and massive splenomegaly (see p. 252). At this stage the bone marrow becomes difficult to aspirate and biopsy shows a marked increase in reticulin. Alternatively, the condition may suddenly deteriorate and the blood picture changes to that of acute myeloblastic leukemia. The risk of leukemic transformation is increased if patients are treated with alkylating agents such as chlorambucil, although cases treated by venesection alone also occasionally terminate in acute leukemia.

SECONDARY ABSOLUTE POLYCYTHEMIA

The secondary polycythemias are shown in Table 37. Secondary polycythemia can occur when the tissues are hypoxic, and hence there is a compensatory elaboration of erythropoietin, or where tissue oxygenation is normal but there is an inappropriate production of erythropoietin.

COMPENSATORY ERYTHROPOIETIN PRODUCTION

Altitude. The low PO_2 at high altitudes decreases arterial oxygen saturation. After a rapid rise to a high altitude, there is an increase in cardiac output and ventilation that results in a reduction in the oxygen gradient between atmospheric and alveolar air but also causes some degree of alkalosis. The effect of this alkalosis is to shift the oxygen dissociation curve to the left. However, within 24 hours of ascent there is an increase in the concentration of 2,3-diphosphoglycerate and ATP in the red cells that shifts the oxygen dissociation curve to the right and hence facilitates the delivery of oxygen to the tissues. Within a few days there is a reticulocytosis and then a steady rise in the hematocrit. This is associated with an increase in the total blood volume, which enables the increased red cell mass to improve oxygen transport. These changes are associated with less well-understood adaptive alterations in the tissue enzymes and in regional distribution of blood flow. The overall result is that an acclimatized individual exposed to air at two-thirds to one-half atmospheric pressure experiences no greater degree of tissue hypoxia than that needed to mobilize and maintain the mechanisms of acclimatization.

Cardiopulmonary Disease. Chronic lung disease may be associated with cyanosis and arterial oxygen desaturation, and there may be a marked increase in hematocrit. However, there is considerable variability of erythropoietic response in chronic chest disease, and the relationship between the degree of arterial oxygen desaturation and the red cell mass is far from consistent. This may be partly due to an increased production of 2,3-diphosphoglycerate with a consequent shift to the right of the oxygen dissociation curve, but this is of no greater magnitude than the shift observed at high altitudes. A further factor may be decreased erythropoiesis secondary to chronic infection, which is frequently present in patients with chronic lung disease. While both these factors undoubtedly play a part, it is far from clear why the erythropoietic response is so variable in patients with lung disease. Sometimes patients with respiratory failure have an extremely high hematocrit level and this may add to the cardiac workload, particularly of the right ventricle, which is already increased owing to lung disease and to pulmonary hypertension secondary to hypoxia. The value of reducing the hematocrit in such patients remains controversial.

Right to Left Shunting. Infants with congenital heart disease may have profound arterial oxygen desaturation with marked cyanosis and extreme polycythemia. Indeed, the hematocrit levels in such infants may be higher than in any other condition. This phenomenon is often associated with venous thrombosis, particularly during periods of intercurrent illness and dehydration. These infants often have thrombocytopenia and an associated defect in coagulation, possibly resulting from a relative deficiency in fibrinogen associated with the extremely high hematocrit levels. The value of venesection in correcting both viscosity and hypocoagulability is controversial. In acquired heart disease and congestive cardiac failure there may be a slight degree of polycythemia, although this is often exaggerated by a relative polycythemia that occurs owing to dehydration by diuretic therapy. The mild polycythemia of liver disease probably results from the presence of acquired pulmonary arteriovenous shunting between the portal and pulmonary systems. A similar syndrome has been described in patients with pulmonary arteriovenous aneurysms.

Defective Alveolar Ventilation. Alveolar hypoventilation can cause arterial hypoxia and hypercapnia, cyanosis, somnolence, and secondary polycythemia. Alveolar hypoventilation has been described in patients with cerebral vascular accidents, Parkinsonism, encephalitis, with drug overdose, and as a primary disorder. Peripheral alveolar hypoventilation occurs in patients with mechanical impairment of the chest wall, particularly associated with neuromuscular disease or as part of Pickwickian syndrome, in which obesity seems to be a major factor.

DEFECTIVE OXYGEN TRANSPORT AND APPROPRIATE ERYTHROPOIETIN PRODUCTION

Relative tissue hypoxia may occur in the presence of a normal arterial oxygen saturation in any circumstance that impairs the binding or release of oxygen by hemoglobin. Chronic exposure to carbon monoxide results in increased concentrations of carboxyhemoglobin, which shifts the oxygen dissociation curve to the left (see p. 205). This is the basis for the mild polycythemia of some heavy cigarette smokers. Several different abnormal hemoglobins are responsible for the genetic, or familial, polycythemias. In each case the increased oxygen affinity results from a single amino acid substitution at a critical part of the hemoglobin molecule, which interferes with subunit interaction or 2,3-diphosphoglycerate binding (see pp. 204 to 205). In all these cases the arterial oxygen saturation is normal and the diagnosis is suggested by the finding of a reduced p50—that is, increased oxygen affinity—of the hemoglobin.

Hemoglobin fails to transport oxygen when its iron is in the oxidized (Fe^{+++}) state. The congenital and acquired methemoglobinemias are described on page 205. Affected patients are rarely polycythemic, but in those that are, the increased red cell mass probably results from a left shift in the oxygen dissociation curve rather than from arterial oxygen desaturation.

Finally, tissue hypoxia may result from substances that cause tissue damage. A good example is cobalt, which binds SH groups and interferes with tissue oxygen utilization. Sublethal concentrations of cyanide have a similar effect because of the action of cyanide on the cytochrome system.

INAPPROPRIATE ERYTHROPOIETIN PRODUCTION

Increased erythropoietin production, inappropriate to the arterial oxygen saturation of the peripheral blood, is an occasional cause of polycythemia. Since the major source of erythropoietin in adult life is the kidney, this is most commonly found with renal lesions, including cysts, hypernephroma, hydronephrosis, and after renal transplantation. It has also been found in association with certain extrarenal tumors, such as hepatoma, cerebellar hemangioma, and uterine myoma. There is considerable controversy about whether the association with the latter tumor results from impairment of renal function due to back pressure on the ureters resulting from the large tumor mass in the pelvis or whether these tumors actually secrete erythropoietin. The latter mechanism is probably the most important. Occasionally polycythemia has been reported in patients with pheochromocytomas, aldosterone-producing adenomas, or as part of Cushing's syndrome. The mechanism for the polycythemia in these conditions is not clear. It also occurs in patients who have received large doses of androgens for malignant disease or in association with androgen-secreting tumors.

Finally, there are reports of polycythemia in families or in individuals in whom obvious inherited causes such as abnormal hemoglobins have been excluded. Studies of these patients, including erythropoietin assays and in vitro colony assays, have suggested a variety of mechanisms for increased red cell production. These include a primary overproduction of erythropoietin, suggesting that the feedback mechanism whereby oxygenation reduces erythropoietin output is abnormal. Other cases seem to result from proliferative abnormalities of the red cell precursors, that is, an abnormal response to erythropoietin.

RELATIVE POLYCYTHEMIA

Relative polycythemia is defined as a state in which the red cell mass is normal but in which there is a contraction of the plasma volume. It can result from any cause of dehydration and is frequently observed in patients who have been overtreated with diuretics.

There is an extremely interesting and common form of relative polycythemia called "stress polycythemia," which makes up over half of all referrals to hematology departments with the diagnosis of "polycythemia." Affected individuals have a red cell mass that is normal, or at the upper limit of normal, with a decreased plasma volume. There is considerable variation

in the hematocrit from day to day, and no definite abnormality of body fluid hemostasis has been demonstrated. Studies of aldosterone metabolism and distribution of body fluids have all given equivocal results, and the reason for the contraction of plasma volume remains unsolved.

This type of hematologic abnormality is often found in anxious, overweight, and mildly hypertensive middle-aged males. There seems to be an increased incidence of angina and claudication in this group of patients. There has been some criticism about the validity of the association between stress polycythemia and these disorders.

There are no abnormal hematologic findings except the apparent polycythemia, and there is no evidence that the high hematocrit per se is dangerous. A condition that has been known in the medical literature for many years as the *Gaisböck syndrome* describes the association of polycythemia and hypertension and is almost certainly a form of stress polycythemia.

There is considerable interest in determining the significance of relative polycythemias or high-normal red cell mass values. This problem has been highlighted by epidemiologic studies that have shown that a high-normal hemoglobin level appears to be a factor in determining the incidence of stroke. Furthermore, in patients with polycythemia vera there is an increased risk of occlusive vascular disease even in what would be considered to be a high-normal hematocrit range (45 to 50 per cent). The question that has not been answered is whether otherwise normal individuals who have high normal hematocrit or hemoglobin values are at increased risk for occlusive vascular disease and, if so, whether reducing the hematocrit has any therapeutic value.

Other Myeloproliferative Disorders _____

The myeloproliferative disorders have been defined as a group of conditions characterized by the abnormal proliferation of one or more of the formed elements of the blood. The abnormal proliferation of red cell precursors as the basis for polycythemia vera has already been described. In this condition there is often an associated proliferation of white cell and platelet precursors. A spectrum of myeloproliferative disorders exists in which there is usually a predominance of one formed element. In polycythemia vera this is the red cell, in primary thrombocythemia the platelet, in chronic myeloid leukemia the neutrophil, and in myelofibrosis the supportive elements of the bone marrow. At least two of these conditions, polycythemia vera and chronic myeloid leukemia, are clonal disorders resulting from the proliferation of an abnormal stem cell population; the same may be true of the other conditions in this group, although this remains to be proved. The inclusion of these conditions under the heading of "myeloproliferative states" is clinically useful because there is much overlap between them as regards the abnormal proliferation of the formed elements of the blood. In polycythemia vera there may be

high platelet and white cell counts, and in primary thrombocythemia there may be slightly elevated red cell or white cell counts. In chronic myeloid leukemia it is not uncommon for there to be a high platelet count or even mild polycythemia at some time during the illness (see p. 276). Furthermore, polycythemia vera and chronic myeloid leukemia often go on to a stage of marrow fibrosis resembling primary myelosclerosis. However, while the concept of myeloproliferative disorder is useful clinically, it should be remembered that these conditions may have completely different etiologies and that fibrosed bone marrow may be the end point of a variety of different pathophysiologic mechanisms. Thrombocythemia is dealt with on page 301 and chronic myeloid leukemia on page 276. Here the pathophysiology of myelosclerosis is briefly described.

MYELOSCLEROSIS

Progressive fibrosis of the bone marrow occurs either as one of the myeloproliferative disorders, primary myelosclerosis, or secondary to bone marrow damage from a variety of causes.

PRIMARY MYELOSCLEROSIS

Primary myelosclerosis is a myeloproliferative disorder characterized by anemia and abnormal proliferation of hemopoietic precursors, associated with a variable degree of fibrosis of the bone marrow and myeloid metaplasia of the spleen, liver, and other organs. This last characteristic is the reason for the variety of alternate names for the condition, which include myeloid metaplasia, agnogenic myeloid metaplasia, and megakaryocytic splenomegaly! Myelofibrosis is a disorder of unknown etiology. Although it was once thought that the abnormal fibrous tissue proliferation in the marrow in this condition might reflect the product of an abnormal cell line, G-6-PD isozyme studies have not confirmed that this is the case. The cardinal feature of the bone marrow in this condition is abnormal fibroblast proliferation and collagen deposition associated with the presence of large numbers of morphologically abnormal megakaryocytes. It has been suggested that the process leading to excessive deposition of marrow collagen is initiated by the abnormal presence in marrow intercellular spaces of megakaryocytic-derived constituents, particularly megakaryocyte-derived growth factor and factor 4 (see p. 293). High concentrations of megakaryocyte-derived growth factor stimulate fibroblast proliferation and collagen secretion.

Although it was originally thought that myeloid metaplasia in the spleen, liver, and lymph nodes was a compensatory mechanism for bone marrow failure secondary to fibrosis, it is now believed that myeloid activity in these organs is part of a neoplastic proliferation by abnormal myeloid precursors.

Pathophysiology. There are two major pathologic processes that appear to be going on simultaneously in myelosclerosis—that is, progressive fibrosis of the bone marrow (Fig. 51) and myeloid metaplasia in the liver, spleen, and lymph nodes. The fibrosis of the bone marrow is extraordinarily patchy, and there may be areas of hyperplasia that can cause diagnostic difficulties. The hyperplasia involves all the formed elements, particularly the megakaryocytes. Indeed, megakaryocytic proliferation is a major feature of the disorder. Despite the apparent hyperplastic areas of the marrow, red cell production is generally diminished, and while in early stages of the illness there may be raised white cell and platelet counts, these tend to fall with progressive fibrosis of the bone marrow. Hence, one major factor in producing the clinical picture of the disease is progressive bone marrow failure. The second factor is hypersplenism caused by progressive enlargement of the spleen (see p. 251). Splenic enlargement and associated hepatic enlargement seem to be largely due to myeloid metaplasia. This extramedullary hemopoiesis probably represents part of a neoplastic proliferation but may also play a variable part in compensation for the bone marrow failure. The mechanism by which the massive spleen causes worsening of the anemia, thrombocytopenia, and neutropenia are described in a later section (see p. 251).

The clinical and hematologic features of myelosclerosis are the result of the two pathophysiologic mechanisms outlined above. There is a slowly progressive anemia that is characteristically leukoerythroblastic; that is, there are both red cell and white cell precursors in the peripheral blood. The latter are usually myelo-

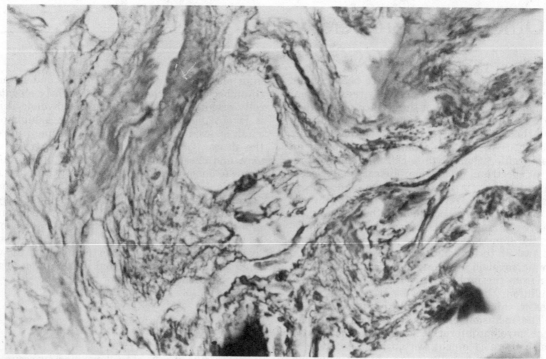

Figure 51. The bone marrow in myelosclerosis. This trephine sample has been stained with a silver stain and shows the marked increase in reticulin that is characteristic of the disorder.

cytes and metamyelocytes, although blast cells may be present in small numbers. Though originally the leukoerythroblastic picture was thought to result from extramedullary hemopoiesis in the spleen, this is probably not the case and more likely reflects the premature release of immature red and white cell precursors from the diseased bone marrow. Indeed, after splenectomy there may be large numbers of nucleated red and white cell precursors together with increased numbers of abnormal platelets and megakaryocytic fragments in the peripheral blood. Presumably, many of these immature cells are filtered out of the blood when the spleen is intact. The abnormal proliferation of red cell precursors is probably responsible for the extraordinary morphologic abnormalities observed in myelosclerosis. These are characterized by anisopoikilocytosis and many bizarre-shaped red cells, including characteristic "tear drop" forms.

There is often a marked bleeding or bruising tendency in myelosclerosis, probably because abnormal platelet function and a variety of defects in platelet aggregation (see p. 295) have been demonstrated. Chronic gastrointestinal blood loss may lead to a secondary iron deficiency anemia.

The metabolic abnormalities in myelosclerosis are similar to those in the other myeloproliferative disorders. They result from increased turnover of abnormal precursors. There is secondary hyperuricemia occasionally leading to gout; folate deficiency, which may result in a megaloblastic anemia; and a raised serum alkaline phosphatase, which may be secondary to the bone involvement that occurs in about a third of patients with this condition.

With progressive enlargement of the liver and spleen, together with bone marrow failure, death may occur owing to anemia, infection, or bleeding. In addition to contributing to the anemia caused by hypersplenism, the massive spleen may infarct or rupture. If the spleen is removed, there is a marked thrombotic tendency associated with a massive thrombocytosis. Splenectomy late in the disease may be followed by marked hepatic enlargement with extensive myeloid metaplasia in the liver, which may ultimately lead to intrahepatic obstructive jaundice.

Clinical and Hematologic Features. The clinical picture of this disorder is easily understood from its pathophysiology, as outlined above. There is progressive anemia and splenomegaly with complicating features of blood loss, infection, bleeding, episodes of splenic pain, secondary gout, and progressive weight loss. The course is very variable, and some patients may go for years with the condition in a static state. The blood picture is as described above, and a characteristic finding is a "dry tap," when attempting a bone marrow aspiration. A few hypocellular fragments consisting mainly of megakaryocytes may be withdrawn. The diagnosis is confirmed by a bone marrow biopsy that shows increased reticulin interspersed with hyperplastic areas containing numerous megakaryocytes (Fig. 51). Needle biopsy of the liver or spleen shows extramedullary hemopoiesis. The red cell survival is usually shortened, and there is nearly always an increased blood volume and evidence of pooling of red cells in the spleen (see p. 251). Injected ^{59}Fe is slowly cleared and appears at a reduced rate in the red cells. External counting may indicate a decreased uptake over the marrow with a high uptake over the spleen and liver. Whether the latter phenomenon indicates effective erythropoiesis in these organs is uncertain.

The prognosis for patients with myelosclerosis is variable, with survival from 1 or 2 to 15 years or more. Death usually results from anemia related to marrow failure. Occasionally, the condition terminates in acute myeloblastic leukemia.

A very acute form of myelosclerosis has been described. It is characterized by fever, weight loss, leukoerythroblastic anemia, and dense myelosclerosis; splenomegaly is a variable finding.

SECONDARY MYELOFIBROSIS

Secondary myelofibrosis may be a reaction to a variety of agents that damage the bone marrow. It occurs late in the course of polycythemia vera or chronic myeloid leukemia. It is a variable feature of invasion of the marrow by neoplastic cells, either carcinoma or reticulosis.

The Spleen and Reticuloendothelial System _____

The term "reticuloendothelial system" (RES) is used to describe a heterogeneous group of organs, tissues, and cells that are involved with a wide variety of functions, including immune response, phagocytosis, filtration of blood and extravascular fluids, and hemopoiesis. The existence of this system was first demonstrated by Ehrlich and his associates, who injected dyes into animals and found supravital staining mainly in the endothelium of organs, such as liver, lymph nodes, and spleen. The term "reticuloendothelial system" was first used by Aschoff, who divided the system into four broad structures: (1) splenic phagocytes and blood histiocytes; (2) reticulum cells of the pulp cords of the spleen and cortical nodules and pulp cords of lymph nodes and other lymphatic tissues; (3)

histiocytes of connective tissue; and (4) reticuloendothelium of lymph sinuses, splenic sinuses, capillaries of the liver, bone marrow, adrenal cortex, and anterior lobe of the pituitary.

More recently, the validity of the RES concept has been questioned. Thus, although macrophages, endothelial cells, and fibroblasts are anatomically and functionally related, these cell types are not developmentally related. As we shall see later, macrophages are derived from marrow hemopoietic progenitors, whereas endothelial cells and fibroblasts are derived from the endoderm and mesenchyme, respectively. However, because of the functional interrelationships that were so well defined by the original workers in this field, the term continues to be widely used in clinical practice. Here, the pathophysiology of the spleen, which is central to our understanding of many hematologic disorders, is examined.

THE HEMATOLOGIC FUNCTIONS OF THE SPLEEN

The normal spleen has the shape of an irregular lens. Its convex surface is in contact with the left hemidiaphragm, and its anteromedial and concave surface is molded to the stomach, colon, and kidney. The anterior border is notched. In health it weighs between 120 and 200 g and cannot be palpated. It becomes palpable when it is enlarged to approximately three times its normal size. The enlarging spleen extends downward and medially toward the right iliac fossa and in extreme cases may enter the pelvis and be palpable per rectum.

The spleen consists of a capsule and trabeculae enclosing a pulp. The latter is divided into three zones: white pulp, a marginal zone, and red pulp. The capsule and trabeculae consist of dense fibrous tissue and carry the main afferent and efferent blood and lymphatic vessels and nerves. The fibrous trabeculae of the human spleen contain a small amount of elastic tissue, but not enough to make it a contractile organ.

The functional anatomy of the spleen is best appreciated by an understanding of its vasculature. The splenic artery arises from the celiac axis and divides at the hilum into five or six branches, each of which gives rise to several lesser divisions that make up the trabecular arteries. These progressively divide without forming significant interconnections, so that the organ is vulnerable to infarction after arterial occlusion. After several subdivisions the small arteries enter the pulp and here acquire periarterial lymphatic sheaths that collectively form the white pulp (Fig. 52). The periarterial lymphatic sheaths are populated mainly by small T lymphocytes embedded in loose connective tissue. Numerous lateral branches of these arteries penetrate the white pulp to reach the surrounding marginal zone. The latter is a specialized extension of the red pulp. The acute angle at which these branches leave their mainstreams is believed to "skim" plasma from the arterial stream as it enters the narrow arteries of the red pulp. A few of these arteries form direct connections with the first elements of the efferent vasculature known as the splenic sinuses. Others end in the open meshwork "cords" of the pulp between the sinuses and thereby subject blood to a complex filtration process through macrophage-rich channels before it re-enters the vasculature through the sinus walls (Fig. 52). The fine pathways at this level are some of the smallest orifices in the body through which blood cells have to pass.

The functions of the spleen are not fully understood. Its removal in adult life is not followed by any clinical

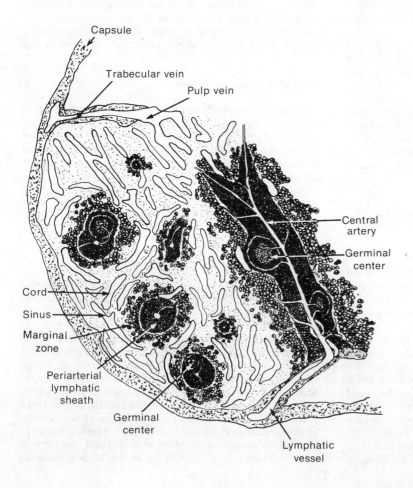

Figure 52. The structure of the spleen. The white pulp is composed of the periarterial lymphatic sheath (PLS) and the germinal centers. One PLS is shown sectioned longitudinally. The red pulp is the area of splenic cords and sinuses. The marginal zone is shown. In the human spleen the penicilliary arteries loop back and supply the germinal follicles. The short branch from the central artery to the follicle shown in the diagram is characteristic of other mammalian spleens. (From Weiss, L., and Tavassoli, M.: Seminars in Hematology 7:372, 1970.)

effects except a slightly increased susceptibility to infection. Removal during the first five years of life is associated with an increased incidence of overwhelming infection.

Several hematologic functions have been defined. The spleen filters abnormal cells and both intracellular and extracellular particulate matter from the circulating blood. This can be looked on as fine quality control, particularly of the erythrocyte populations. After splenectomy, morphologically abnormal red cells and platelets are present in the peripheral blood. The red cell abnormalities include target forms and small irregularly contracted cells. In addition, the red cells contain inclusions that are not seen if the spleen is intact. These include single inclusions that stain with Romanowsky stains, called Howell-Jolly bodies, and small granular bodies that stain for iron. When the latter take up Romanowsky stains they are called Pappenheimer bodies. It is believed that Howell-Jolly bodies are nuclear remnants that are normally removed in the spleen and that the small siderotic granules are derived from excess iron—which combines with apoferritin to form ferritin during erythroid maturation—and are removed from mature erythrocytes in the same way (see p. 193). Transfused red cells containing iron granules lose these granules in the normal spleen without the cells themselves being destroyed; this is called the "pitting" function of the spleen. It is very likely that reticulocytes spend some time in the spleen maturing and losing their residual RNA; similarly, the few nucleated red cells that escape from the bone marrow in health lose their nuclei in the spleen. Thus the spleen appears to scrutinize the circulating cells and removes those that are abnormal in shape or contain intracellular inclusions, in a mechanism that is called *culling*. The spleen is undoubtedly involved in a certain amount of remodeling of the red cell surface. During the first few days of its extramedullary existence the red cell becomes smaller in volume and in surface area. In the absence of the spleen the mean surface area of mature red cells may be larger than normal, while the volume still remains normal. All these processes are normal physiologic functions of the spleen. The spleen is also active in removing abnormal red cells; this mechanism is considered later. The hematologic results of splenectomy are summarized in Table 39.

Hemopoiesis occurs in the spleen only in fetal life. Postnatally, only lymphopoiesis occurs, mainly in response to immune stimuli; the basal rate in the absence of antigen challenge is low. Extramedullary hemopoiesis occurs in the spleen in adult life in certain pathologic circumstances, occasionally as a compensatory mechanism but usually as part of the neoplastic process of myeloid metaplasia. There is evidence that the spleen both contributes to antibody formation and produces cells that mediate immune responses.

Other, less-well defined functions have been ascribed to the spleen. A role in the regulation of hemopoiesis has been suggested, but there is very little experimental evidence for this. Since the human spleen contains only about 50 ml of blood, it does not have a significant storage function, unlike the spleen of some animals. However, it does store platelets, iron, and some proteins, including Factor VIII.

PATHOPHYSIOLOGY

The most important pathophysiologic mechanism of the spleen is the destruction or pooling of the formed elements of the blood. This may happen in two ways. First, if the spleen enlarges for any reason it may trap and/or destroy formed elements of the blood even if they are normal. Second, because of its peculiar vasculature and rich phagocytic cell population, it is particularly well designed to destroy red cells, white cells, or platelets that are intrinsically abnormal.

Hypersplenism. Hypersplenism is a syndrome that consists of splenomegaly associated with anemia, leukopenia (particularly neutropenia), and thrombocytopenia.

The spleen can produce anemia, neutropenia, or thrombocytopenia in two ways. First, because of its peculiar vascular and phagocytic properties, it may be the site of destruction of abnormal cells. The constant exposure of the spleen to such cells, particularly red cells, produces splenic enlargement, a phenomenon called "work hypertrophy" (see p. 252). Second, splenic enlargement due to primary disease of the reticuloendothelial system or other pathology may result in reduction in number of one or more of the formed elements of the blood even when the latter are normal in structure and function. It is to this second group of disorders that the term hypersplenism is usually applied. A working definition of hypersplenism is, therefore, a state characterized by splenomegaly caused by a wide variety of causes associated with the following: anemia, leukopenia, thrombocytopenia, or any combination of the three; a bone marrow that, if diseased at all, is capable of maintaining a higher output of the formed elements of the blood than is apparent from their numbers in the circulation and in which the cytopenia is corrected by splenectomy.

The intriguing question raised by this definition is how does an enlarged spleen produce anemia, neutropenia, and thrombocytopenia? Probably the most important mechanism, and one for which there is excellent experimental evidence, is pooling of formed elements of the blood. There is a significant degree of red cell pooling in most enlarged spleens. This is evident from a comparison of the venous hematocrit with the whole body hematocrit. Red cells accumulate in a splenic erythrocyte pool that increases significantly with increasing splenomegaly and that may constitute up to 50 per cent of the total red cell mass. In effect, then, at any particular time a significant proportion of the total red cell mass is sequestered

TABLE 39. HEMATOLOGIC CHANGES OF HYPOSPLENISM

Nucleated red cells in peripheral blood
Target cells
Burr cells
Red cell inclusions
    Siderocytes
    Howell-Jolly bodies
    Pappenheimer bodies
Thrombocytosis
Large platelets

"outside" the circulation; hence, the discrepancy between the peripheral venous hematocrit and the total body hematocrit as obtained by isotope dilution techniques. Similarly, it is possible to demonstrate that there is significant pooling of platelets in enlarged spleen. In health, approximately 10 per cent of the circulating platelets are in the spleen at any time; with significant splenomegaly, pooling increases progressively and may involve up to 90 per cent of the total peripheral blood platelet mass. There is also considerable pooling of granulocytes in enlarged spleens. The overall effect of cell pooling depends on the hemopoietic capability of the bone marrow; that is, the degree of anemia, neutropenia, and thrombocytopenia reflects a fine balance between the magnitude of pooling and the ability of the marrow to compensate. In disorders such as myelosclerosis or chronic myeloid leukemia, in which there may be a diminished bone marrow response, splenic pooling may cause a severe degree of anemia, thrombocytopenia, or neutropenia. This cytopenia may occur to a lesser extent or not at all if the marrow is healthy.

Another feature of splenomegaly is hypervolemia. In diseases that limit red cell production, the expanded volume is provided mainly by plasma. The result is a dilutional anemia that tends to add to the effect of splenic pooling of red cells. The favored mechanism is the development of a hyperkinetic portal circulation produced by the high blood flow through the enlarged spleen with expansion of the splanchnic vasculature upstream from the portal vein. How this actually produces an increased plasma volume is far from clear. As well as causing some degree of hemodilution, the high plasma volume renders patients with hypersplenism particularly difficult to treat with transfusions without circulatory overloading.

In addition to trapping a large proportion of the red cell mass in large spleens, there is good evidence that the survival of normal red cells may be reduced. This may result from various "metabolic stresses" applied to the red cells as they are packed together in the enlarged organ. These include glucose deprivation, lactate accumulation, and a fall in pH. It seems likely that repetitious exposure to conditions of this type causes a reduction in red cell survival. In general, however, the hemolytic component of this type of hypersplenism is mild. The evidence that thrombocytopenia and neutropenia are caused by a similar mechanism is less solid. There are no good data to suggest that the transit time of granulocytes in the circulation is reduced in patients with large spleens. Similarly, there is no definite evidence that otherwise normal platelets are destroyed prematurely in large spleens. Rather, the thrombocytopenia of hypersplenism seems to be almost entirely due to platelet pooling. If the bone marrow is incapable of compensating for the large splenic platelet pool, thrombocytopenia results.

SPECIFIC DESTRUCTION OF THE FORMED ELEMENTS OF THE BLOOD BY THE SPLEEN

Abnormal red cells may be destroyed in the spleen. The cells of patients with hereditary spherocytosis are particularly prone to be destroyed in this way, presumably because of their inherent metabolic abnormalities. Heinz bodies may be "pitted" out of cells with subsequent membrane damage. Similarly, in warm antibody autoimmune hemolytic disease, red cells coated with IgG, because of the peculiar anatomy of the spleen, come into close proximity with macrophages with specific receptors for these molecules. It is very likely that a similar general mechanism is responsible for the destruction of platelets in idiopathic thrombocytopenic purpura. Similarly, the neutropenia of Felty's syndrome (rheumatoid arthritis with splenomegaly) has an immune basis. Thus, studies quantitating IgG on the surface of the neutrophil have provided strong evidence that the neutropenia of Felty's syndrome is due to the presence of white cell antibodies. Clearly, the hypersplenism of these immune disorders of the red cells, white cells, and platelets is a reflection of the ability of the macrophages of the spleen to identify cells coated with specific antibodies.

CAUSES OF SPLENOMEGALY

The causes of splenomegaly are summarized in Table 40. The spleen may enlarge transiently in a variety of acute infections. The most common are the acute viral illnesses. The spleen may be enlarged in chronic infection, such as brucellosis and tuberculosis, and in subacute bacterial endocarditis. Massive splenomegaly may result from several tropical disorders, including malaria, kala-azar, and schistosomiasis. Enlargement may accompany any cause of portal hypertension.

Splenomegaly is a feature of a variety of disorders of the red cell. The fact that splenomegaly occurs in most chronic hemolytic anemias suggests that spleen growth may be stimulated by an increase in its workload (work hypertrophy). This concept suggests that when the spleen is being constantly bombarded with abnormal red cells it increases in size to allow a larger

TABLE 40. SOME CAUSES OF ENLARGEMENT OF THE SPLEEN

Acute bacterial, viral, and other infections
Chronic bacterial infections: TB and brucellosis
Chronic parasitic infections: malaria, kala-azar, schistosomiasis
Idiopathic nontropical splenomegaly
Tropical splenomegaly
"Congestive"; portal hypertension
Genetic hemolytic anemia
    Hereditary spherocytosis (HS)
    Symptomatic elliptocytosis
    Structural hemoglobinopathy
    Thalassemia
    Red cell enzyme defects
Acquired hemolytic anemia
    Warm antibody hemolytic anemia
    Cryopathic hemolytic syndrome
Primary blood dyscrasia
    Acute leukemia
    Chronic myeloid leukemia
    Chronic lymphatic leukemia
    Polycythemia vera
    Myelosclerosis
Reticulosis
    Hodgkin's disease
    Other reticulosis
Miscellaneous
    Amyloid, sarcoidosis, tumor of the spleen, storage diseases
Connective tissue disorders
    SLE
    Felty's syndrome

area for red cell destruction, creating a vicious circle of increasing red cell destruction. Indeed, there is experimental evidence for this mechanism. Small pieces of splenic tissue grow and function when auto-transplanted into the subcutaneous tissues of rats. If the rats are splenectomized, the transplanted slices of spleen grow to a greater size than in animals with intact spleens. These small transplanted spleens are able to trap labeled red cells that have been coated with incomplete antibody, and they show considerable stimulation of growth if the animal is treated with phenylhydrazine, which produces a chronic hemolytic state; that is, the transplanted spleens are continually perfused with abnormal red cells. This experimental system bears close resemblance to the clinical observation of hypertrophy of splenunculi or accessory spleens after splenectomy in patients with hemolytic disease.

Splenomegaly occurs in the myeloproliferative disorders. Although this has been explained by the process of myeloid metaplasia in myelosclerosis, histologic examination of the spleen in polycythemia vera does not show extramedullary erythropoiesis, certainly not in the early stages of the illness. The explanation for the splenomegaly of polycythemia vera is far from clear. The spleen may also enlarge in any form of leukemia or lymphoma; here the splenomegaly is the direct result of infiltration of the organ with abnormal cells. A similar mechanism is the basis for the splenomegaly of the various storage diseases. However, the enlarged spleens found in association with Hodgkin's disease or lymphoma do not always show histologic evidence of the tumor. The spleen may enlarge considerably and still show a normal architecture. An extreme example of this phenomena is *idiopathic nontropical splenomegaly*, in which massive splenomegaly, with relatively normal histology, may precede the clinical appearance of a lymphoma by months or even years.

The spleen may also enlarge because of infiltration with abnormal cells—other than neoplastic hemopoietic or RE cells—as occurs in the rare storage diseases, which are summarized in Table 41. The organ may also enlarge in sarcoidosis or, rarely, in amyloid disease. Occasionally, primary tumors or cysts may cause splenomegaly.

HYPOSPLENISM

The features of hyposplenism are summarized in Table 39. These are found invariably after splenectomy. Many of the red cell changes of hyposplenism

are also present in newborn infants owing to splenic immaturity. Congenital absence of the spleen is a rare anomaly sometimes associated with complex congenital cardiac abnormalities that make survival unlikely. Splenic hypoplasia may be part of the syndrome of Fanconi's anemia (see page 227). Acquired atrophy of the spleen is now a well-recognized accompaniment of celiac disease. It is also found occasionally in patients with essential thrombocythemia or in systemic lupus erythematosus and in most adults with sickle cell anemia, in which it results from repeated infarction.

Hyposplenism, or the absence of the spleen, may be suspected from the morphologic appearances of the red cells. The cells contain Howell-Jolly bodies and siderotic granules, and there may be a number of nucleated red cells and target cells on the peripheral blood film. In patients with reduced splenic function the red cells show small surface pits, and the number of cells affected in this way is a reliable guide to the degree of splenic hypofunction. Absence of the spleen can be confirmed by various scanning techniques using labeled colloids.

SPLENIC INFARCTION

Because of the peculiar vasculature of the spleen, infarction of an enlarged spleen is not uncommon. It occurs particularly in patients with myelosclerosis or chronic myeloid leukemia but can occur with almost any cause of splenomegaly. It results in an inflammatory reaction on the serous surface; if this occurs over the area of contact with the left dome of the diaphragm, it may be responsible for left basal pleurisy and pain referred to the left shoulder.

SPLENIC RUPTURE

Splenic rupture is a rare but important medical emergency. The commonest cause is direct trauma, but spontaneous rupture has been reported in a variety of pathologic spleens. Rupture may be into the peritoneal cavity or subcapsular, with the formation of a perisplenic hematoma. In some spleens involved with neoplasia there may be massive infarction of the organ as it enlarges, with rupture within the capsule.

INVESTIGATION OF THE SPLEEN

Assessment of splenic size is best carried out by palpation or by straight x-ray examination of the

TABLE 41. SOME LIPID STORAGE DISEASES

NAME	INHERITANCE	DEFECT	CLINICAL FEATURES
Gaucher's	Autosomal recessive	Heterogeneous with 3 defined types; absence of glucocerebrosidase with accumulation of glucocerebroside in histiocytes of RE system	Splenomegaly; anemia; hypersplenism; hepatomegaly; bone changes; Gaucher cells in marrow
Niemann-Pick	Autosomal recessive	Heterogeneous; 5 defined types; defect in sphingomyelin metabolism, which accumulates in RE cells; abnormal sphingomyelinase activity	Infiltration of organs with "foamy" macrophages; mental retardation; splenomegaly; hepatomegaly; bone changes; CNS changes
Gangliosidosis	Autosomal recessive	β galactoside deficiency; ganglioside accumulation in tissues	Mental retardation; CNS changes; splenomegaly; foamy cells in marrow
Tay-Sachs	Autosomal recessive	β hexosaminidase deficiency; ganglioside deposited in tissues	CNS changes; mental retardation; cherry spots in retina; no splenomegaly—disease in CNS only

abdomen. Radioisotope spleen scanning with a scintillation camera or a rectilinear scanner also detects enlargement of the organ. In addition, these techniques may indicate focal lesions, infarcts, splenic rupture, accessory spleens, and absence or hypoplasia of the spleen. Scanning can also be carried out by using heat-treated chromium-labeled red cells or by using a variety of radioactively labeled colloids.

In assessing hypersplenism a direct estimate of the total red cell mass isotopically compared with the venous hematocrit is a useful indication of the degree of pooling in the spleen. In most cases of severe hypersplenism, the plasma volume is markedly increased. ^{51}Cr labeling of the red cells with external scanning allows the red cell survival and degree of sequestration within the organ to be assessed. Further information can be gained by injecting labeled red cells and meas-

uring the time they take to achieve equilibration in the circulation; in the presence of pooling this time is markedly lengthened. In cases of myelosclerosis in which splenectomy is considered, it is important to first assess the degree of bone marrow activity by measuring the per cent incorporation of ^{59}Fe and the radioactivity over the marrow sites and spleen by external scanning techniques. Recently, techniques have been developed for measuring the splenic red cell pool size using cells labeled with ^{51}Cr. In addition, by determining the patterns of uptake and disappearance of injected ^{59}Fe by surface counting it is possible to obtain an approximate estimate of the degree of effective erythropoiesis in the spleen in various myeloproliferative disorders. This may be of practical importance in assessing the likelihood of success of splenectomy in myelosclerosis.

The Blood Groups

The discovery of the human blood groups by Landsteiner at the beginning of this century was a major landmark in clinical medicine. It led to the routine use of blood transfusion and opened up exciting new areas of study for geneticists and anthropologists. In this short section only those aspects of the subject are reviewed that are directly related to clinical hematology. The blood group systems cannot be appreciated without some elementary understanding of immune reactions, particularly the structure and interactions of antigens and antibodies. The latter topics are dealt with elsewhere in this book and the reader is advised to become familiar with these concepts before reading the following section.

THE ABO BLOOD GROUP SYSTEM

The ABO system was the first human blood group system to be discovered and is still the most important in clinical practice. It is characterized by four main blood groups, A, B, O, and AB (although subgroups of A can occur, vide infra) that are determined by the presence or absence of two antigens A and B, formerly called agglutinogens, on the erythrocyte membrane. There are corresponding antibodies, anti-A and anti-B, present in the serum in accordance with the rule that the corresponding antigens and antibodies do not coexist in the blood of the same person. Anti-A and anti-B are known as naturally occurring antibodies, since there is no obvious antigenic stimulation, although substances with chemical structures closely related to A and B are ubiquitous in nature and may be the stimulus for antibody development in early life. Under certain circumstances, such as in AB-incompatible pregnancies, immune anti-A and anti-B can be superimposed on the naturally occurring antibodies. The common antigens and antibodies of the ABO system are shown in Table 42. Also shown are the principal divisions of the A antigen into A_1 and A_2. Anti-A_1 is found in approximately 1 per cent of A_2 and 25 per cent of A_2B persons. Rarer subgroups of the A antigen also exist, such as A_3, A_4, and Am.

PROPERTIES AND GENETIC CONTROL OF THE ABO ANTIGENS

The A and B antigens are not confined to erythrocytes but are also present on white cells, platelets, tissue cells, and in most body fluids. The presence of blood group substances is controlled by the secretor (Se) genes that segregate independently from those that determine the blood groups. However, the Se genes are closely associated with these latter genes, since it is known that H substance, present in most erythrocytes and related to A and B substances, cannot be formed unless Se and H genes are present; thus the Se gene is regarded as a regulator gene. Secretor status of an individual is usually determined by the ability of saliva to neutralize anti-A, anti-B, or anti-H. The significance of secretor status is considered on p. 258.

H substance is an important constituent of the ABO system and is found in association with the major groups of this system in the following descending order of concentration: O, A_2, A_2B, B, A_1, and A_1B. H is inherited independently from A and B, and the two genotypes HH and Hh are H-positive while hh is H-negative. Occurrence of the latter leads to the rare Bombay, or O_h, blood group. The erythrocytes of such persons are not agglutinated with anti-A, anti-B, or anti-H, and their blood contains all three antibodies.

It is clear, therefore, that what appears to be a relatively straightforward blood group system has hidden complexities. With respect to the A and B genes, however, there is a simple mendelian inheritance. A

TABLE 42. MAJOR GROUPS AND ANTIBODIES OF THE ABO SYSTEM

GROUP	ANTIBODIES
A_1B	
A_2B	(anti-A_1)
A_1	anti-B
A_2	anti-B (anti-A_1)
B	anti-A
O	anti-A, anti-B

TABLE 43. INHERITANCE OF THE ABO GROUPS

GENES FROM PARENTS		GENOTYPE	PHENOTYPE
A	B	AB	AB
A	A	AA	A
A	O	AO	A
B	B	BB	B
B	O	BO	B
O	O	OO	O

and B genes are codominant, and the O gene is an amorph, that is, it has no demonstrable product. The genotypes and phenotypes in the ABO system are summarized in Table 43.

To understand how the primary blood group genes determine the presence of A and B antigens, it is necessary to understand the basis of the chemistry of these blood groups. The AB and H blood group substances on red cells are found principally on glycoproteins but also on glycolipids and on polyglycosyl ceramides. In plasma they occur as glycosphingolipids, and in body fluids they are glycoproteins. Antigenic specificity is determined by sugars at the nonreducing ends of the carbohydrate component.

The chemical backbone of the A, B, and H substances consists of two chains ending in galactosyl residues, thus:

Type I β-Gal-(1-3)-GNAc

Type II β-Gal-(1-4)-GNAc

where Gal = galactose and GNAc = N-acetyl-D-glucosamine. While both of the precursors can be acted upon by the products of the A, B, and H genes, type I structures are not synthesized by red cell precursors, while those of type II are. Thus A, B, and H substances in plasma have a basic type I structure, whereas those on red cells are of type II.

The first gene to be involved in development of these blood group antigens is H, which produces a 2-L-fucosyl-transferase that, in the presence of the regulator Se genes, adds L-fucose to the basic glycosyl residue in a 1-2 linkage. Thus, using the type II chain as the example:

$$\beta\text{-Gal-(1-4)-GNAc} \longrightarrow \beta\text{-Gal-(1-4)-GNAc}$$
$$| \; 1.2$$
$$\alpha\text{-Fucose}$$

This terminal structure is the H antigen, and it serves as the basic substrate for the glycosyltransferases that are the products of the A and B genes. The A gene produces a transferase that adds N-acetyl-D-galactosamine to the H substance, and the B gene causes the addition of D-galactose to confer A and B specificity, respectively. Thus:

$$\beta\text{ Gal-(1-4)-GNAc} \xrightarrow{A \text{ gene}} \alpha\text{-Gal NAc(1-3)-}\beta\text{-Gal-(1-4) GNAc}$$
$$| \; 1.2 \qquad\qquad\qquad\qquad\qquad | \; 1.2$$
$$\alpha\text{-Fucose} \qquad\qquad\qquad\qquad\qquad \alpha\text{-Fucose}$$
$$\xrightarrow{B \text{ gene}} \alpha\text{-Gal-(1-3)-}\beta\text{-Gal-(1-4)-GNAc}$$
$$| \; 1.2$$
$$\alpha\text{-Fucose}$$

It can be deduced from this process that since the O gene is amorphic, there is no conversion of the basic H substance under its influence, and therefore, the O blood group is rich in H substance. Also, A and B transferases do not convert all the H substance to A and B, and therefore, H can coexist with A and B although in different concentrations, as indicated above. The most noticeable differences exist between A_1 and A_2, and it is thought that the A_1 transferase is more efficient in converting H substance than is the A_2 transferase; thus the difference between A_1 and A_2 antigens is principally quantitative.

Closely related to the chemical structures of the A and B antigens are those of the P Lewis and Ii blood group systems. Of these, the Lewis system is the most closely associated being dependent upon interaction between Se and Le genes and using H substance as a substrate.

THE RHESUS BLOOD GROUP SYSTEM

In 1940, Landsteiner and Wiener reported that the injection of Rhesus monkey red cells into rabbits or guinea pigs led to the production of antibodies that agglutinated the red cells of about 85 per cent of white persons in the United States. The antibody was called anti-Rh and the antigen it detected, the Rh antigen. This antibody appeared to be identical to that found by Levine and Stetson in the blood of a pregnant group O woman who had not received previous transfusions and who received a transfusion of blood from her husband, had a reaction, and subsequently gave birth to a macerated fetus. The authors postulated that she had produced an antibody to a fetal erythrocyte antigen inherited from her husband, and the name anti-Rh was accepted for the human antibody. It was found later that there were differences between the human and animal antibodies. The human antibody has continued to be designated as anti-Rh, while the animal antibody was called anti-LW in honor of Landsteiner and Wiener.

While much has been learned about the Rh blood groups since that time, including the definition of over 40 different antigens, the basic division between Rh-positive and Rh-negative is still the most important from a clinical point of view. The importance of the Rh blood group systems as a cause of hemolytic disease of the newborn is described on page 238.

Inheritance. There has been much argument and confusion over the notation of the Rhesus antigens. Fisher and Race postulated that there are three closely linked loci in the production of the Rhesus antigens and that each gene, with one exception, produces an antigen that is given the same notation as the gene. The gene pairs are Cc, Dd, Ee, which give rise to the antigens C, c, D, E, e. The d gene has no product. The D antigen is the most potent immunogen in the system, and anti-D is the commonest antibody. The commonly used term "Rh-positive" refers to persons whose cells are agglutinated by anti-D. The commonly found gene complexes and their corresponding antigens based on the Fisher-Race nomenclature are given in Table 44. The shortened form is often used in laboratory work.

Table 44 also illustrates a nomenclature proposed by Wiener that is based on his different concept of Rh

TABLE 44. NOTATIONS FOR RHESUS BLOOD GROUPS

	FISHER-RACE (CDE)			WIENER (Rh-Hr)			
	Gene Complex	Antigens	Short Form	Allele	Agglutinogen	Factors	Rosenfield
RH Positive	CDe	C,D,e	R_1	R^1	Rh_1	Rho,rh',hr''	1,2,5
	CDE	C,D,E	R_2	R^2	Rh_2	Rho,hr',rh'	1,3,4
	cDe	c,D,e	R^o	R^o	Rh_o	Rho, hr',hr''	1,4,5
	CDE	C,D,E	R_z	R^z	Rh_z	Rho,rh',rh''	1,2,3
Rh Negative	cde	c,e	r	r	rh	hr',hr''	4,5
	Cde	c,e	r'	r'	rh'	rh',hr''	2,5
	cdE	c,E	r''	r''	rh''	hr',rh''	3,4
	CdE	C,E	r^y	r^y	rh^y	rh',rh''	2,3

inheritance, which he considered to be determined by a number of allelic genes situated at a single locus. Thus he considered the inheritance of CDe (Fisher-Race) to be controlled by a single gene, R^1, which could produce an agglutinogen, which in the example given above would be referred to as Rh_1. This agglutinogen in turn has several factors that are separately reacting parts of the antigenic structure.

While Wiener's theory of inheritance may be correct, his terminology is not as widely used as that of Fisher and Race and is not as explicit. As a compromise, Rosenfield proposed a numerical system for the Rh nomenclature (Table 44), and with the introduction of electronic data processing into blood group serology and blood transfusion the use of a numerical system is likely to gain wider acceptance in the future.

Rhesus Antibodies. Although Rhesus antibodies can be naturally occurring, they are more commonly immune in origin, arising as a result of incompatible transfusion or pregnancy. Anti-D is the commonest antibody, although many others have been encountered, including anti-C (rare as a single antibody), anti-E, anti-c, and anti-e. Many antibody complexes also are found, such as anti-C + D, which may be really anti-G, an antibody to a separate antigen found on all C-positive and most D-positive red cells, anti-Ce, and anti-cE. When Rh antibodies occur as autoantibodies, anti-e is the commonest specificity found.

Other Rh Variants. The commonest variant is the D^u antigen, which has the frequency of about 0.6 per cent but it is more common in Blacks. D^u may arise simply from the development of fewer antigen sites per cell than in the normal D-positive erythrocyte and can be inherited as such. Other instances of D^u arise from the suppressive effect of the Cde and CdE chromosomes in the transposition to a chromosome carrying the D antigen. Certain cells lack some or all of the Rh antigens, for example, -D-, CWD-, cD- and ---, in which all the antigens are missing. The latter are called Rh-null; such cells have a reduced survival time and presumably have a basic membrane structural defect. These cells may be useful in the study of autoimmune hemolytic anemia.

OTHER BLOOD GROUP SYSTEMS

There are many blood group systems, some of which are summarized in Table 45, with an indication of their clinical importance. After the ABO and Rh sys-

TABLE 45. SOME BLOOD GROUP SYSTEMS OF CLINICAL IMPORTANCE

SYSTEM	ANTIGENS	IMMUNOGLOBULIN CLASS	CLINICAL SIGNIFICANCE
ABO	A_1, A_2, B, H, A_3, A_m, Ax	IgM, IgG, IgA	Severe hemolytic reaction. Hemolytic disease of newborn.
MNSs	M, N, S, s, U, M^g, Mi^a, Hu, He, V^w, M^c	IgM, IgG	Occasional transfusion reaction. Hemolytic disease of newborn.
Rh	D, C, E, c, e, C^w, E^w, ce, Ce, G, CE, cE, D^u, C^u, LW	IgM, IgG, IgA	Hemolytic disease of newborn. Some autoimmune hemolytic diseases have antibodies specific for Rh system.
P	P_1, p^k, P_2 (Tj^a)	IgM	Anti-P found in paroxysmal cold hemoglobinuria (Donath-Landsteiner antibody).
Lutheran	Lu^a, Lu^b	IgM, IgG, IgA	—
Kell	K, k, Kp^a, Kp^b, Js^a, Js^b	IgG	Transfusion reaction or hemolytic disease of newborn.
Lewis	Le^a, Le^b, Le^c, Le^d	IgM	Hemolytic reactions after complement fixation are possible.
Duffy	Fy^a, Fy^b	IgG	Transfusion reaction or hemolytic disease of newborn.
Kidd	Jk^a, Jk^b	IgM, IgG	Transfusion reaction or hemolytic disease of newborn.
Diego	Di^a, Di^b	IgG	Rare transfusion reaction.
Yt	Yt^a, Yt^b	IgG	Rare transfusion reaction.
Xg	Xg^a	IgG	Sex linked; useful genetic marker of X chromosome.
Dombrock	Do^a	IgG	—

tems, the Kell, Duffy, and Kidd systems are the most important in transfusion therapy; they are systems of immune antibodies usually produced as a result of blood transfusion and less frequently by heterospecific pregnancy. The most frequently encountered antibodies are those that react in the cold and that, like the ABO antibodies, appear to be naturally occurring. Most of these antibodies are of little clinical significance, such as anti-P_1, and anti-A_1, although some, such as anti-Le^a and Le^b, may fix complement and react at 37° C. Some examples have been reported to cause hemolysis after incompatible blood transfusion. Also, the Lewis group differs from other systems in that its members are adsorbed onto the red cell from the plasma. In addition, there are developmental antigen systems, such as Ii. The two antigens I and i are found in reverse proportions in cord cells (i > I) and adult cells (I < i). The clinical importance of these antibodies in cold acquired hemolytic anemia has been summarized on page 239.

THE BLOOD GROUP ANTIGEN/ANTIBODY REACTION

Blood group antigens can be defined and the specificity of antibodies determined by a reaction that leads to an observable result. This is usually agglutination of the red cells or, less frequently, hemolysis.

Antibodies to blood group antigens are immunoglobulins and may comprise either IgM, IgG, and IgA classes, or a single antibody may exist as a combination of these classes. The nature of the reaction between an antibody and its corresponding antigen may depend on the class of immunoglobulin to which it belongs. Thus, in general, IgM antibodies usually agglutinate red cells when suspended in 0.15 mol NaCl, whereas most, but not all, IgG antibodies fail to do so. Such antibodies, however, coat or sensitize red cells in saline suspension, and agglutination may be effected by either increasing the protein concentration of the suspending medium, by the use of antiglobulin test, or by enzyme treatment of the red cells.

To understand the mechanism of agglutination it is necessary to consider some of the factors that are concerned with the union of the antibody with its antigen and the second stage of agglutination, which consists of bringing the red cells close enough so that an antibody molecule can bridge the gap between adjacent cells.

The combination of an antibody-binding site on an immunoglobulin molecule to the antigen depends on various factors, including the *equilibrium constant,* which represents the goodness of fit of the antibody to the antigen. In general, the higher the equilibrium constant the less readily will the antibody/antigen bond be broken. Other factors are the *ionic strength* of the medium, which affects the rate of association, and the number of *antigen sites.* Agglutination of antibody-coated red cells also depends on a number of factors. Red cells carry a negative charge and repel each other. When red cells are suspended in saline solution, the Na and Cl ions form an electrical double layer around each cell, with the positively charged Na ions forming the inner layer. The electric potential that develops between the cells' negative charge and the ionic layers

is known as the zeta potential, and this must be overcome before agglutination can occur. IgM antibodies, because of their size and multiple antibody binding sites, can effect agglutination of saline-suspended red cells. The smaller IgG molecule usually cannot, but those that are able to do so, such as anti-A and anti-B, probably effect agglutination as a result of the large number of antigen sites on the red cell's surface. The negative charge of the red cell is caused by the carboxyl groups of sialic acid, and therefore reduction of this charge can lower zeta potential, allowing the cells to approach each other more closely. The most efficient enzyme to reduce charge is neuraminidase, but this is not as effective in allowing IgG antibodies to agglutinate red cells in saline suspension as are the proteolytic enzymes, papain, ficin, and bromelain. Thus, although the zeta potential may be one factor in the agglutination reaction, it is probably not the only one, and the removal of peptide chains may further expose antigen sites and may also increase the mobility of antigens so that multiple bridges may form between clusters of antigens. Thus the treatment effectively increases localized antigen site density.

Another factor that may affect agglutination is the increase in the dielectric constant as a result of the addition of colloids, such as albumin, which also has the effect of lowering the zeta potential. Finally, the position of the antigen in relation to the outer surface of the erythrocyte membrane may be an important factor.

It can be seen that whether an antibody agglutinates red cells in saline suspension depends on many factors. It was formerly convenient to consider the saline agglutinins as complete and others as incomplete antibodies. These are misleading terms, since there is nothing "incomplete" about those IgG antibodies that fail to agglutinate saline-suspended erythrocytes.

Most IgG, IgM, and IgA antibodies can be detected by the antiglobulin test. Antiglobulin serum is raised in animals injected with human immunoglobulins and complement components, although monoclonal antiglobulin reagents are now becoming available. Therefore, the antiglobulin reagent comprises anti-IgG, -IgM, -IgA and antibodies to various complement components. After sensitizing the red cells with blood group antibody and washing to remove surplus proteins, the cells are incubated with antiglobulin reagent. The reagent allows the combination of blood group antibody on adjacent red cells with the antibodies to immunoglobulins in the antiglobulin reagent, the formation of intercellular bridges, and consequent agglutination. The test is most commonly used to detect IgG (or occasionally IgA) antibodies on red cells, since, as stated above, most IgM antibodies agglutinate the red cells in saline suspension; however, subagglutinating doses of IgM antibodies may fix C_3 and C_4 components of complement and can be detected by the presence of anti-C_3 and anti-C_4 in the antiglobulin reagent.

THE DISTRIBUTION OF BLOOD GROUPS

The incidence of blood group antigens varies from race to race. The most extensive data are those from the ABO system. The distribution of ABO groups in

TABLE 46. DISTRIBUTION OF ABO BLOOD GROUPS

	O	A	B	AB
United Kingdom	47	42	8	3
European gypsies	31	27	35	7
Asiatic Indians	33	24	24	9
Japanese	30	39	22	9
Maoris (Polynesians)	40	56	3	1
Some South American tribes	100	0	0	0

some populations is summarized in Table 46. There is also a striking difference in the distribution of the Rh genes. In the Negroid and Mongoloid races there is a high incidence of Rh positivity, while the Basques have an unusually high incidence of the Rh-negative state. The reason for these differences is not clear but may be related to the diseases to which different races have been exposed during evolution.

BLOOD GROUPS AND DISEASE

There are some extremely interesting examples of the association of blood groups with human diseases. For example, group A persons are more likely than those of groups B or O to develop carcinoma of the stomach or pernicious anemia, while nonsecretors of blood group O are more likely to develop duodenal ulcer. The cellular basis for these observations is not clear. Although there has been much speculation about the relative susceptibility of persons with different blood groups to common infectious diseases as a basis for the distribution of blood groups among different populations, evidence that would support this fascinating hypothesis is not yet available.

BLOOD TRANSFUSION

It is possible here to describe only in the barest outline the principles of blood transfusion. The trend over recent years has been to use, whenever possible, component therapy so that the patient can receive the benefit from transfusion of a particular component of blood in which he or she is deficient. However, several million units of red cells, as whole blood or red cell concentrates, are transfused each year, and it is important to consider the principles involved and the possible ill effects of such transfusions.

Blood donations are collected aseptically into a container, usually some form of plastic pack, with an anticoagulant. There has been a tendency during recent years to use citrate-phosphate-dextrose (CPD), often supplemented with adenine (CPD-A) instead of acid citrate dextrose (ACD), which was employed for many years. CPD has the advantage that 2,3-diphosphoglycerate (2,3-DPG) is maintained at a higher level during storage of the red cells at 4° C, a temperature chosen to minimize glycolysis and bacterial growth. Red cells depleted of 2,3-DPG have a high oxygen affinity, and therefore transfusion of large quantities of such red cells has immediate disadvantages in terms of oxygen transport because it takes approximately 12 hours for the 2,3-DPG to be restored after transfusion. The further addition of adenine allows an extended

storage period of up to 35 days by maintaining higher adenosine triphosphate levels. ACD-anticoagulated blood also has the disadvantage of adding to the acidosis, which may already affect severely injured patients, while such problems are reduced when CPD blood is used for massive transfusion.

Whenever possible, donor blood of the same ABO and Rh(D) groups as those of the patient should be selected for transfusion. Subgroups of A and AB are not usually important unless the recipient has anti-A_1 or anti-B reacting at temperature greater than 30° C. In an emergency group O blood can be used for transfusion of patients of other blood groups, but such transfusions should be kept to a minimum and preferably should be of red cell concentrates. The donor plasma should be free of high titer anti-A or anti-B antibodies. Donor blood for Rh recipients should be Rh-negative (cde/cde). Prior to transfusion of red cells, they should be cross-matched with the patient's serum at room temperature (18 to 22° C) and at 37° C by techniques to detect the presence of antibodies, either IgG, IgM or IgA, in the patient's serum that may result in destruction of the donor red cells at transfusion. The principles for these tests are outlined above. The tests would normally include agglutination tests in saline solution and albumin and the antiglobulin test.

There are several important complications of blood transfusion. The most serious is the acute hemolytic reaction that follows the combination of antibody with red cells possessing the corresponding antigen. The most severe cases are caused by anti-A, anti-B, anti-D, anti-c, and anti-Kell reacting in the recipient's plasma with the corresponding antigen on the red cells of the transfused blood. These reactions can largely be avoided by extreme care in cross matching the donor's cells with the recipient's plasma and by scrupulous care in making sure that the name on the blood bottles is correct and that the patient receives the right blood. If a transfusion reaction of this type occurs, it is usually heralded by rigor and pain in the lumbar region. There is also constricting pain in the chest that may be caused by blocking of pulmonary vessels by agglutinates of red cells. Acute intravascular hemolysis may set off intravascular coagulation. The pathophysiology of acute intravascular hemolysis was considered on page 230. With the massive breakdown of cells in the circulation, haptoglobin binding is saturated, and free hemoglobin appears in the urine. This is often accompanied by acute renal failure, the exact mechanism of which is not clear. Delayed hemolytic reactions may occur as a result of previous sensitization with resulting antibody that is below detectable levels when cross matching is performed. Antigenic stimulation leads to a rapid rise in antibody concentration and destruction of the donor red cells three to seven days after the transfusion.

Other important complications of blood transfusion include bacteremic shock from infected blood, reactions to various other antigens on transfused cells, air embolism, and circulatory overload in patients with high blood volume or cardiac failure. There are a variety of infections, in particular hepatitis, syphilis, and acquired immune deficiency syndrome (AIDS), that can be transmitted with blood, and in tropical countries it is particularly important to screen donors for malaria. It is current practice in most countries to screen blood

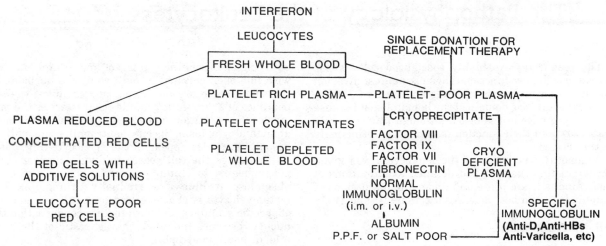

Figure 53. A flow diagram showing the processing of whole blood to obtain various blood components. (Courtesy of Dr. H. H. Gunson.)

donors for B virus hepatitis antigen. Cytomegalovirus in blood and some blood products has an important effect on certain groups of patients. This applies particularly to those who are immunodeficient, such as newborn infants, patients having transplantations, and children having treatment for acute leukemia. A proportion of donations, the number depending on the country of origin, may contain cytomegalovirus in the leukocytes. Freshly collected blood carries a higher risk, but stored blood may not always be safe. Procedures for assisting patients at risk can be the screening of donations for the absence of antibody to cytomegalovirus, the use of frozen blood, or passive immunization with specific immunoglobulin.

Blood Products. These can be divided into the components that can be separated from donations of whole blood, such as platelets, frozen cryoprecipitate, and fractionated blood products obtained from freshly collected plasma. Figure 53 illustrates the major components that can be obtained from whole blood, although it would not be realistic to obtain leukocytes from donations of whole blood, since they can be obtained more efficiently by the use of automated cell separators.

Blood transfusion centers separate plasma from up to 60 per cent of whole blood donations to obtain a sufficient quantity of fractionated products. This results in a depletion of whole blood donations, and a rationale for their use has to be determined. Any patient with anemia should receive red cell concentrates; indeed, the reduction in volume of the transfusion could be an advantage. In hemorrhagic states there is sufficient evidence to support the use of red cell concentrates, in conjunction with crystalloid solutions, when the loss is less than 30 per cent of the blood volume. Thereafter protein replacement is usu-

ally necessary, and it is sensible after the transfusion of two to four units of red cell concentrates to continue therapy, if required, with transfusion of whole blood. In an emergency, plasma protein fraction (PPF) can be used as a plasma volume expander. PPF, whose protein concentration is 5 g/dl, consists principally of albumin and can be pasteurized at 60° F for 10 hours to destroy the hepatitis and cytomegaloviruses. Excessive administration of this product should be avoided, since it causes a mobilization of extracellular fluids that may accumulate in the lungs.

Platelet concentrates can be obtained by differential centrifugation of the donation of whole blood. If stored at 4° C, their viability is significantly reduced, although they retain their hemostatic activity for up to 72 hours. More commonly, platelets are stored at 22° C when their recovery after 72-hour storage is between 40 and 70 per cent and their half-life is approximately three to four days. These platelet concentrates require a few hours after infusion to develop maximal hemostatic activity. The use of newer plastic containers will allow platelets to be stored at 22° C for up to five days. Since platelets carry the human leukocyte antigen (HLA) and specific antigens, the presence of antibodies to these antigens in the patient's blood causes their destruction and reduces their hemostatic function. It would be desirable, but not practical, to administer HLA-identical platelets (and white cells) to patients requiring repeated transfusions. When specific antibodies can be identified, it is desirable to carry out prior matching of platelets and leukocytes before transfusion.

The use of pooled blood products increases the risk of transmitting disease. For example, the acquired immune deficiency syndrome has been associated with frequent administration of factor VIII concentrates.

The Pathophysiology of the Leukocytes _____

The leukocytes are highly specialized cells whose principal collective function is defense against invasion and infection by microorganisms and viruses. Leukocytes come into the domain of the hematologist because of their presence in the blood, although this is merely transitory and their function is discharged principally in the tissues.

A general description of the leukocytes was given earlier in this chapter, and detailed examinations of their functions are presented under the discussions of immunology and host defenses (Sections III and IV).

THE NEUTROPHILS

MORPHOLOGY AND DEVELOPMENT (Fig. 54)

The earliest morphologically recognizable granulocyte precursor is the myeloblast, which is identical (at least morphologically) for neurotrophil, eosinophil, and basophil lines (Fig. 54B). In Romanowsky-stained smears it is of variable size (15 to 20 μm diameter)

with scanty basophilic cytoplasm and a large nucleus with fine open chromatin and two to five nucleoli. At this stage there are no cytoplasmic granules: the appearance of azurophilic granules characterizes the promyelocyte—a larger cell (20 to 25 μm) with more abundant cytoplasm. Specific neutrophil, eosinophil, or basophil granules appear in the myelocyte (Fig. 54C). At this stage the cell ceases to divide, nuclear chromatin begins to clump progressively, and the cytoplasm loses its blue color, gradually turning pink. The metamyelocyte is characterized by a full complement of specific granules, and with further condensation the nucleus becomes indented, characteristic of the juvenile, or band, neutrophil.

Mature neutrophils are 10 to 20 μm in diameter and have a segmented nucleus of two to five lobes. In females a nuclear appendage resembling a drumstick is found in approximately 3 per cent of cells and contains the inactivated X chromosome (Fig. 54D). There are about 600 cytoplasmic granules of two different types: azurophilic granules comprise 10 to 20

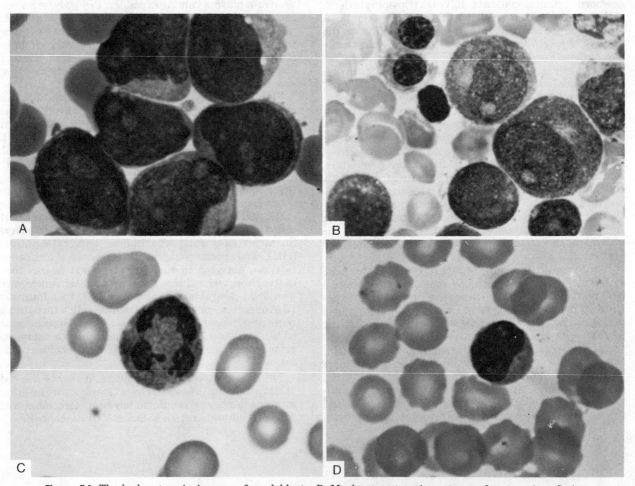

Figure 54. The leukocytes. *A*, A group of myeloblasts; *B*, Myelocytes at various stages of maturation; *C*, A mature neutrophil with a typical "drumstick" appendage; *D*, A lymphocyte.

per cent, and specific granules comprise the remainder. Azurophilic granules first appear in the promyelocyte, although in the mature cell they are indistinct by light microscopy. Electron microscopy shows them as dense bodies of 0.5 μm diameter with a limiting membrane. They appear to be typical lysosomes and contain myeloperoxidase, cathepsin G, elastase, lysozyme (muramidase) and a variety of acid hydrolytic enzymes, including acid phosphatase and other bactericidal cationic proteins. The specific granules are smaller (0.2 μm) and stain faintly pink. They contain principally lysozyme and lactoferrin, a heme-containing protein that is found also in milk. Lactoferrin has similar iron-binding properties to transferrins. Its function is unknown, but it is bacteriostatic, possibly because of its avidity for iron. It may also have some regulatory function and has been shown to inhibit in vitro granulocyte-colony–stimulating activity. Alkaline phosphatase is another enzyme that is found abundantly in neutrophils; it can be readily quantitated histochemically, and this is useful in distinguishing between leukemia and other cases of leukocytosis.

PRODUCTION

In common with erythroblasts, megakaryocytes, and possibly lymphocytes, granulocytes derive from a common pluripotent hematopoietic stem cell compartment (Fig. 55). This is a compartment of predominantly resting cells with an essentially limitless capacity for self-renewal, which, under the influence of as yet uncharacterized stimuli, undergo differentiation into one or another of the hematopoietic pathways. The early progenitor of the white cells was described earlier. There is growing evidence that both local and humoral influences play a role in the differentiation, maturation, and release of granulocytes. As mentioned earlier, at least four growth factors have now been defined that are involved in the regulation of the differentiation and maturation of the white cell series: interleukin-3, GM-CSF, G-CSF, and M-CSF. It appears that the capacity for stimulation of growth and differentiation by these different regulatory proteins varies considerably. For example, interleukin-3 is indifferent to cell lineage and promotes growth and development of all the different myeloid progenitor cells. In addition, it seems to facilitate self-renewal of stem cells and the progenitors of various mixed colonies. On the other hand, GM-CSF is more restricted in its activities and only stimulates proliferation and development of the granulocyte, macrophage, and eosinophil colony-forming cells. G-CSF and M-CSF seem to be even more restricted in their activities. It is also clear that granulopoiesis also requires the interaction of stromal cells, at least in vitro, presumably through the activity of diffusible molecules, although so far the nature of the latter has not been determined.

Humoral substances may also be involved in the control of granulocyte release from the marrow. Evidence for this comes from animal experiments in which plasma obtained shortly after administration of endotoxin causes rapid leukocytosis if it is later reinfused. Endotoxin itself induces leukopenia as a result of increased margination, so this would suggest that some other mediator that was responsible for the stimulation of granulocyte release had appeared after endotoxin administration.

The early committed granulocyte precursors undergo one or more amplifying divisions while differentiating into recognizable myeloblasts, which compose only 1 to 5 per cent of nucleated cells in the marrow. From the myeloblast to the myelocyte stage, there are four or five further divisions, each myeloblast thus giving rise to at least 16 myelocytes. The average time for a cell to traverse this proliferating compartment (stem cell to myelocyte) is estimated at five days. However, some four fifths of the myeloid cells in the marrow make up a postmitotic population undergoing final maturation (the maturation-storage compartment), and the time taken to traverse this second compartment is five to seven days.

After release from the marrow the neutrophils spend a short time in the bloodstream before randomly migrating to the tissues. A half-time of four to eight hours has been estimated for disappearance of neutrophils from the blood following reinjection of radiolabeled autologous neutrophils (Fig. 56). Furthermore, only about half the neutrophils can be accounted for after reinjection, as circulating neutrophils are in rapid equilibrium with a similar-sized pool of cells marginating along the walls of small blood vessels. The factors regulating the production and distribution of neutrophils are discussed with host defense.

It has been possible to estimate the relative size and kinetics of the various neutrophil pools and compartments. The circulating and marginating pools each

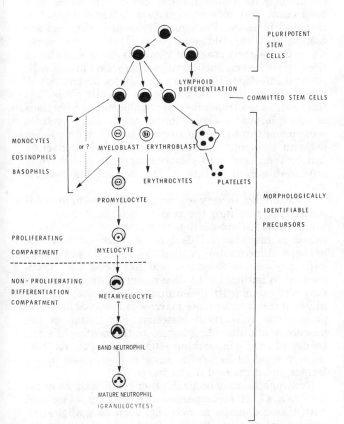

Figure 55. Schematic representation of the development of the leukocyte series.

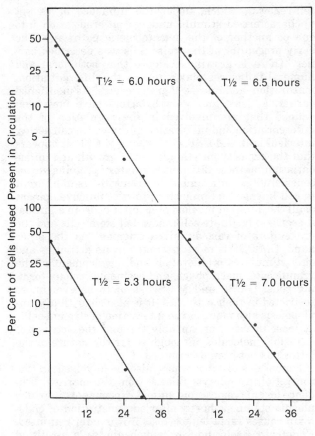

Figure 56. Disappearance of autologous ³²DFP-labeled granulocytes after reinjection in four normal subjects. (From Mauer, et al.: Journal of Clinical Investigation 39:1481, 1960.)

contain about 1.0 to 6.0 × 10⁸ cells/kg body weight. The average number of neutrophils released from the marrow each day is approximately 1.6 × 10⁹ cells/kg; the postmitotic maturation and storage compartment contains about 7.5 to 10 × 10⁹ cells/kg and the proliferating compartment about 2.5 × 10⁹ cells/kg.

NEUTROPHIL FUNCTION

Neutrophils are phagocytic cells whose prime function is to engulf and destroy bacteria that gain access to the body's tissues. The role of neutrophils in defense of the host as well as detailed coverage of neutrophil metabolism is provided in the discussion of host defenses (Section IV).

NEUTROPHIL DISORDERS

Neutrophils may be abnormal in number, structure, and function. The physiologic variations in the neutrophil count are summarized on page 177. Alterations in the circulating neutrophil numbers generally reflect changes in the rate of production, although alterations in utilization or in the distribution between marginating and circulating pools also are reflected in variations of the granulocyte count. A classification of the quantitative neutrophil disorders is given in Table 47.

TABLE 47. A CLASSIFICATION OF QUANTITATIVE GRANULOCYTE DISORDERS

Increased Production
  Appropriate: infection, tissue damage, etc.
  Inappropriate:
    Benign: leukemoid reactions
    Malignant: leukemia, myeloproliferative disorders

Decreased Production
  Reduced proliferation
    Primary: marrow failure (congenital or acquired)
    Secondary: drugs, toxins, irradiation, infiltration
  Ineffective myelopoiesis: megaloblastic anemia, drugs, alcohol

Increased Destruction or Utilization
  Infection, hypersplenism, antibodies, drug/antibody

Disturbance of Circulating/Marginating Pool Equilibrium
  Reduced margination: corticosteroids, exercise, epinephrine
  Increased margination: endotoxin, dialysis, racial

Neutrophilia

An increase in the circulating neutrophil count is called a neutrophilia or a neutrophil leukocytosis and is most commonly caused by increased neutrophil production in the face of tissue infection or injury. It is usually entirely appropriate to the body's needs and in general parallels the severity of the underlying condition. The circulating total leukocyte count is typically elevated into the 10,000 to 30,000/μl range but may occasionally be higher. The leukocytes are predominantly neutrophils; some less mature forms may be present and reflect premature marrow release in response to stress. Paradoxically, some infections are associated with mild leukopenia. This is seen sometimes in the early stages of viral infections and also in the enteric fevers, bacillary dysentery, and brucellosis. In viral infections there may be a direct destruction of leukocytes by the virus during the viremic phase, but the cause of neutropenia in certain bacterial infections is unexplained. Overwhelming sepsis may produce leukopenia through exhaustion of supply, with sudden demand stripping the storage pool before production can be increased, and this is exaggerated if there is any concomitant failure of the normal marrow response.

Occasionally, in very severe infections the neutrophil count may rise into the region of 50,000/μl or even higher, and differentiation from chronic myeloid leukemia is important. This type of reaction, which is, perhaps unfortunately, called "leukemoid," may occur with any severe infection and has been well documented in patients with disseminated tuberculosis. It may also occur with disseminated malignancy, particularly if the liver or bone marrow is involved or in the presence of concurrent infection. Estimation of the amount of alkaline phosphatase in the neutrophils can be useful in distinguishing leukemoid reactions from chronic myeloid leukemia, since it is elevated in the former and decreased in the latter.

Neutrophilia may occur in other conditions, as noted in Table 47. It accompanies any disorder associated with tissue damage or necrosis, such as malignancy, myocardial or other tissue infarction, and some collagen-vascular disorders. A neutrophilia following drug therapy can occur in several ways, such as demargination associated with glucocorticoid therapy, mobilization of the storage pool with etiocholanolone, and actual stimulation of granulopoiesis, such as may occur with lithium therapy.

Neutropenia

Neutropenia is defined as a circulating neutrophil count below 1500/μl, and most commonly occurs from reduced proliferation of myeloid precursors but may also result from ineffective myelopoiesis, increased utilization or destruction, or increased vascular margination. A complete absence of circulating neutrophils is termed *agranulocytosis*.

The clinical consequence of neutropenia is an increased susceptibility to bacterial infection. The risk is small with neutrophil counts over 1000/μl but becomes progressively greater with lower counts, and it is almost a certainty with agranulocytosis of more than a few days' duration. Infection occurs most commonly with organisms that normally colonize the skin and gastrointestinal tract, although this flora can be quickly augmented after admission to hospital by resistant hospital organisms that are often traceable to hospital food.

Neutropenia is most severe in conditions associated with marrow failure. It is most commonly associated with acute leukemia (both the disease and its treatment), the administration of drugs, and/or radiation for the treatment of other malignancies, or less commonly with idiopathic aplastic anemia. In these conditions there is usually failure of all marrow cell lines. Isolated neutropenia due to production failure may be produced by virtually any drug; the more common offenders are listed in Table 48. In most instances the effect is probably idiosyncratic, and it is obviously unwise for such a patient to be prescribed the same drug again. However, there is a group of drugs and other agents that predictably produce marrow depression, generally in a dose-related fashion. It includes, of course, the cytotoxic drugs and the list is similar to that producing general marrow aplasia (Table 27). Ineffective granulopoiesis with intramedullary destruction due to defective maturation occurs in megaloblastic states and may also be caused by drugs. A

TABLE 48. DRUG-INDUCED AGRANULOCYTOSIS

Defective Production
  a) Predictable
     Cytotoxic drugs
     Chloramphenicol
  b) Idiosyncratic
     Phenothiazine
     Thiouracil
     Phenylbutazone
     Many others
  c) Ineffective Granulopoiesis
     Hydantoin
     Primidone
     Others
Immune Destruction (Drug-Hapten-Antibody Interaction)
    Aminopyrine
    Many examples of single reports
Combination of 1 and 2
    Suspected for many drugs but not proved

mild to moderate pancytopenia may complicate conditions associated with splenomegaly, owing to increased trapping and/or destruction of cells by the spleen (Table 27). Infection is sometimes troublesome, but the main clinical problems are usually the result of anemia, thrombocytopenia, or the physical size of the spleen.

Immune destruction of neutrophils can occur for a variety of reasons, but it is not common. Transient neonatal isoimmune destruction results from placental transfer of maternal cytotoxic antibodies, in a manner similar to rhesus hemolytic disease of the newborn. Certain drugs may produce immune neutropenia (Table 48), and this is usually more rapid in onset than drug-induced marrow failure. Notable offenders are phenylbutazone (which may also produce general marrow aplasia), aminopyrine, and methylthiouracil. They are thought to act as haptens that combine with an unknown leukocyte antigen to induce antibody formation to the drug-antigen complex. Rapid leukoagglutination occurs following drug administration, but the antibody is ineffective in the absence of the hapten. Neutrophil autoantibodies have also been implicated in the neutropenia of rheumatoid arthritis, systemic lupus erythematosus, and Felty's syndrome (rheumatoid arthritis with splenomegaly), although in the latter the splenomegaly may contribute to the neutropenia. Occasionally, autoimmune neutropenia may be an isolated finding.

Blood neutrophil counts are physiologically lower in black populations than in white. This is thought to be due to an increase in the proportion of marginating cells. A quite dramatic but transient neutropenia follows the circulation of blood over an artificial surface such as a hemodialysis membrane or the nylon wool filters used to collect granulocytes for transfusion. The exact mechanism is not clear, but there is evidence that in some way complement is activated by blood flow over the artificial surface—probably by the alternate pathway. Leukocyte aggregation mediated by C_{5a} results in pulmonary sequestration and occasionally in hypoxia.

Certain neutropenias occur in early life. Although rare, they are of considerable interest because of the light they shed on genetic factors involved in granulocyte production. One of the earliest to be recognized was *Kostman's infantile genetic agranulocytosis*. This is characterized by a moderate to severe neutropenia that is present from the time of birth and that is associated with a marked tendency to infection. There is apparently a defect in granulocyte maturation, as normal or increased numbers of granulocyte precursors are found in the marrow. Another well-defined condition is *reticular dysgenesis with congenital aleukocytosis*. In this condition there is a striking granulocytopenia from birth that is associated with absent immunoglobulin production. A form of chronic neutropenia in childhood is described associated with various constitutional defects in the manner of Fanconi's familial pancytopenia (p. 227). Another association is that of neutropenia with congenital pancreatic insufficiency, although the mechanism is unknown. An autosomal dominant form of neutropenia is recognized in which persistently low neutrophil counts are found without any particularly severe liability to infection. These patients appear to have a reduced proliferating pool size. Finally, there is an extremely interesting form of genetic neutropenia that shows cyclic variations in the neutrophil count. This condition is also transmitted as an autosomal dominant trait but is probably underdiagnosed, since its cyclic nature may not always be suspected. Affected patients have a history of infection, often going back to early childhood, and the neutropenia is found to follow cycles lasting 14 to 21 days. There is often mild splenomegaly, and during the periods of neutropenia the marrow shows myeloid hyperplasia or an apparent arrest at the myelocyte stage. It is interesting that the condition may become milder with age and has disappeared entirely in several cases. A similar syndrome is seen in gray collie dogs and appears to be a stem cell disorder, in that cyclical fluctuations in red cell and platelet production have also been noted. Furthermore, it can be cured by transplantation of normal marrow and is transmitted by transplantation of affected marrow into normal dogs.

DISORDERS OF GRANULOCYTE FUNCTION
(Table 49)

Many systemic conditions are associated with an increased susceptibility to infection, including diabetes mellitus, ethanol ingestion, uremia, general debilitation, and corticosteroid therapy, but despite much research, no consistent defect in granulocyte function has been recorded in these disorders. There are, however, a few relatively well-defined congenital syndromes in which recurrent infections occur in the presence of normal granulocyte production. Some of these are severe and may be fatal. Certain syndromes are associated with defects in humoral immunity with defective chemotaxis and opsonization, but other disorders result from defective bacterial killing despite normal phagocytosis. These disorders are discussed in detail in the discussion of the kidney.

STRUCTURAL NEUTROPHIL ABNORMALITIES

A number of abnormalities of nuclear segmentation have been described, although none appear to be of functional significance. Although the development of nuclear segmentation occurs during cell maturation, it is no longer thought that the total number of lobes correlates with the age of the cell. An increase in the proportion of cells with more than five lobes is termed *hypersegmentation* and is characteristic of the megaloblastic anemias (p. 213). Hypersegmentation may also be inherited as an autosomal dominant trait; in some forms of this condition the cells themselves may

be twice the normal size but function quite normally. Failure of nuclear segmentation is characteristic of the *Pelger-Huët anomaly*. This is usually inherited as a dominant trait but may be acquired in certain hematologic disorders, such as leukemia, and in severe infection. The nucleus is round or dumbbell-shaped, but this appears to be of no functional significance.

Döhle bodies are small, bright blue, elliptic cytoplasmic inclusions that represent persisting rough endoplasmic reticulum. They are found in the neutrophils of some patients with severe infections. They have also been described in pregnancy, cancer, trauma, and following cytotoxic drug administration. In the rare *May-Hegglin anomaly* Döhle bodies are found in association with mild neutropenia, thrombocytopenia, and bizarre giant platelets. The disorder is inherited but surprisingly is not usually associated with clinical problems other than a mild hemorrhagic tendency in some individuals.

Auer rods are deep red-blue rodlike inclusions found in the cytoplasm of the myeloblasts and promyelocytes in many cases of acute myelogenous leukemia. They stain heavily with Sudan black and are an important feature in the differentiation of myelogenous from lymphoblastic leukemia. They result from an undefined abnormality of granule formation and probably represent abnormal lysosomes.

Other structural abnormalities, particularly those associated with infection or altered host defense, are examined under the discussion of host defense.

THE CLINICAL EVALUATION OF NEUTROPHIL KINETICS AND FUNCTION

In clinical practice the total peripheral blood leukocyte count and the absolute neutrophil count are the most commonly used guides to the status of neutrophil production. Because the peripheral blood population is transitory and represents only a small proportion of the total body neutrophil mass, this kind of static estimation does not always give a true indication of neutrophil production or destruction, the status of marrow reserve, or the distribution of neutrophils between different pools. Myelopoiesis can be assessed by examination of a stained marrow smear, although this suffers from the limitations of sampling errors and has relatively poor correlation with kinetics as estimated by other methods. For example, a marrow that shows an excess of early myeloid precursors is sometimes assumed to show "maturation arrest," although such an appearance does not distinguish between a true defect in cellular maturation and a

TABLE 49. DISORDERS OF GRANULOCYTE FUNCTION

DEFECT	CAUSES	CLINICAL PICTURE
Chemotaxis: Opsonization	Various antibody deficiency states; complement deficiencies; inhibition of activation.	Recurrent pyogenic infections
Migration: Phagocytosis	Actin dysfunction (rare); a variety of systemic illnesses, including immune complex diseases, burns, diabetes mellitus, drugs (ethanol, corticosteroids)	Recurrent infection failure of pus formation or may be subclinical
Bacterial killing	Deficiency of G-6-PD, pyruvate kinase, NADH oxidase, glutathione peroxidase	Chronic granulomatous disease
	Myeloperoxidase	Negligible

rapid mobilization from and depletion of the postmitotic storage pool. Despite these limitations, however, a careful examination of peripheral blood and marrow granulocyte populations provides sufficient information to resolve most clinical problems. If the absolute neutrophil count is <1000/μl and serial marrow aspirations are hypocellular, then the patient nearly always has impaired neutrophil production. The reverse may not always be true, however, since a cellular marrow and a normal blood count do not necessarily imply that production is normal.

A variety of other investigations have been developed to obtain a more precise picture of neutrophil kinetics. Relatively accurate assessments of leukocyte proliferation and distribution can be obtained by radioactive tracer techniques using diisopropylfluoro-^{32}phosphate, tritiated thymidine, or sodium-^{51}chromate, but concordance between results obtained with different labels is not absolute. Marrow neutrophil reserve can be assessed following endotoxin administration, since this stimulates neutrophil release from the storage pool; interpretation is complicated by an initial neutropenia resulting from increased cellular margination. A better agent is etiocholanolone, which stimulates release without increasing margination. Epinephrine administration on the other hand produces a shift from marginating to circulating pools and can be used to assess the relative distribution of neutrophils between these two pools.

Like the tests just described, neutrophil function tests have been useful in research but have little place in routine clinical practice. A variety of tests have been devised to study neutrophil locomotion. The best known is the Rebuck skin window technique, in which a sterile coverslip is applied to a dermal abrasion so that neutrophils migrating into the injured site adhere to the glass and can be subsequently enumerated. Phagocytosis has been studied in a variety of ways. The simplest is to perform a visual count of particles ingested after incubation with neutrophils, but this is unsatisfactory, since it is difficult to distinguish ingested particles from those simply adherent to the cell surface. Bacteria can be radioactively labeled and their ingestion estimated by scintillation counting of the neutrophils. Phagocytosis can also be indirectly monitored by measuring oxygen uptake during the burst of oxidative metabolism that accompanies phagocytosis or by detecting the associated chemiluminescence. The most popular of many tests of neutrophil metabolism is the nitroblue tetrazolium test: this colorless reagent is reduced to an insoluble blue-black formazan compound by the superoxide ion produced following phagocytosis. A histochemical technique is used and the test is of particular value in the diagnosis of chronic granulomatous disease. Several assays of bactericidal function have been developed that can assess the overall bactericidal activities of neutrophils, and abnormal results may be obtained in many congenital and acquired disease states.

It is rarely necessary to perform neutrophil function tests in clinical practice, but when a genetic disorder of neutrophil function is suspected, one of the ingestion assays, a screen for abnormal metabolism, including the nitroblue tetrazolium test, and one of the several assays of bactericidal activity should be performed (see the discussion of host defense).

THE MONOCYTES AND MACROPHAGES

THE MONOCYTES

The phagocytic capacity provided by the granulocytes is greatly enhanced by the monocyte-macrophage system. The peripheral blood monocytes number about 200 to 800/μl and are fairly large cells (10 to 18 μm), possessing a large indented nucleus with a fine open chromatin structure. The cytoplasm contains a number of distinct azurophilic granules that, like those of the granulocyte, contain typical lysosomal enzymes.

Monocytes are produced in the bone marrow and may be derived from the same precursor cells as granulocytes, as suggested by the finding of both monocytes and granulocytes in in vitro agar colonies grown from individual CFU and the frequent finding of a monocytic component in acute leukemias of myeloid origin. The monoblast has no unique morphologic characteristics to distinguish it from the myeloblast; the two may be one and the same cell, and it is not clear at which stage of differentiation the cell is programmed to become a monocyte. The promonocyte is slightly larger than the monocyte and has a higher nuclear-cytoplasm ratio with fewer cytoplasmic granules. Like the neutrophil, the monocyte spends a short time in the peripheral blood, where there are both circulating and marginating populations. The daily monocyte turnover has been estimated at 1.7×10^7 cells/kg/day, with a half-life in the blood of about eight hours. In contrast to the neutrophil, the monocyte retains the capacity for further division and differentiation in the tissues.

THE MACROPHAGES

The tissue macrophages, or histiocytes, are directly descended from the blood monocytes. Macrophages are widely distributed throughout the tissues, with a predilection for lymph nodes, liver, spleen, and bone marrow. Some are "fixed," or at least semipermanently attached, to endothelial structures lining the sinusoids of these organs. The term "reticuloendothelial system" has been applied to this widespread phagocytic function, although the macrophages are neither endothelial in origin nor the producers of reticulin fibers, as was once thought. Other macrophages are free to roam the tissues and can be readily recovered from the serous cavities and alveoli of the lungs. The term "macrophage" implies not only a capacious appetite but also a large cell, typically 20 to 80 μm, with abundant cytoplasm and plentiful lysosomes. Macrophages have an important role in the immune response in addition to their phagocytic function and may also be concerned in the regulation of hemopoiesis. Monocytes and macrophages are mobile cells and exhibit chemotaxis. They have receptors for IgG and C_3 and are able to consume a wide variety of particulate matter. They are particularly concerned in the defense against intracellular parasites, such as the organisms of tuberculosis, leprosy, and malaria. An important additional function of the fixed macrophages of the reticuloendothelial system is the capacity to remove from the circulation and digest effete blood cells.

The lifespans of the monocyte and the macrophage are more difficult to estimate but probably extend to many months. As monocytes differentiate into macrophages, the capacity for self-replication is retained, and alveolar macrophages recovered from patients with prolonged periods of marrow aplasia and profound blood monocytopenia still show good in vitro colony-forming ability.

The transition from monocyte to macrophage is accompanied by an increase in size and in the number of lysosomal granules. There is an increase in the amount of acid phosphatase, glucuronidase, lysozyme, aryl sulfatase, and other lysosomal enzymes but a decrease in myeloperoxidase. Energy metabolism involves both glycolytic and oxidative mechanisms, but the unique location of alveolar macrophages allows them to subsist on the latter. Bacterial killing relies heavily on glycolysis, and macrophages can work well in the anaerobic conditions of an abscess cavity, although function is improved in the presence of oxygen. The mechanism of phagocytosis and killing is similar to that of the neutrophil, but myeloperoxidase is probably of minor importance, as it is absent from the mature macrophage.

Interactions with the Immune Response

(The reader may also refer to the discussion of immunology, Section III).

Macrophages are involved in both the afferent (sensitizing) and efferent (effector) limbs of the immune response. Following phagocytosis of particulate antigen, the macrophage retains a small amount, possibly altering it in some way to enhance its immunogenicity. As a result of such "priming" with antigen, the macrophage is able to induce the transformation of virgin T lymphocytes into specifically sensitized cells. Indeed, lymphocyte transformation in vitro in response to antigenic stimulation is poor unless some macrophages or monocytes are also present. How the macrophage induces this specific transformation is not fully understood, but it is an energy-consuming process involving close physical contact between lymphocyte and macrophage, which must be genetically identical at some part of the main histocompatibility complex. Antigen-specific T cell responses are blocked by anti-HLA antisera, and the Ia molecule on the macrophage surface is essential for successful stimulation of T lymphocytes.

In response to phagocytosis and various other stimuli, the mononuclear phagocytes produce *interleukin-1* (IL-1), a single or closely related series of polypeptides with central and far-reaching effects on the acute-phase response to infection and inflammation. Release of IL-1 into the circulation produces fever (by a prostaglandin E_2-mediated effect on the hypothalamic thermo-regulatory center) and also stimulates the release and activation of marrow neutrophils and the synthesis of hepatic acute-phase proteins. Furthermore, IL-1 has an important role in the immune response, by activating both T and B lymphocytes. Activated T cells produce a series of mediators known as lymphokines; one of these, interleukin-2, induces clonal expansion of helper, suppressor, and cytotoxic T cell subsets. Other lymphokines, released by antigen-sensitized lymphocytes, activate macrophages to a state of enhanced phagocytic capability. Certain intracellular parasites, such as malaria, mycobacteria, and *Listeria,* are able to survive ingestion by the unactivated macrophages of the nonimmune host. Following an immune response, however, macrophages are activated and the organisms can be eliminated. It should be clear that, while macrophage activation is the result of interaction between macrophage and lymphocytes sensitized to a specific antigen, the increase in phagocytic potential is nonspecific.

Macrophages and Hemopoiesis

Macrophages may be involved in hemopoiesis. Islands of developing hemopoietic tissue in bone marrow sections can often be seen surrounding a macrophage, and some cell-cell interaction is thus possible. Furthermore, macrophages contain a heme-oxidase enzyme that breaks down hemoglobin following erythrophagocytosis and an active ferritin transport mechanism that may be involved in feeding iron to developing erythroblasts. It is also of interest that macrophages are a prime source of colony-stimulating factor required for growth of bone marrow colonies in vitro, and it is tempting to think that they may elaborate substances in vivo that are involved in the control of granulopoiesis.

MONOCYTE ABNORMALITIES

Because of their common origin, there is considerable overlap between production and function abnormalities of the monocyte and those of the granulocyte. Furthermore, the small number of circulating monocytes is not only difficult to enumerate accurately but represents a very small proportion of the total monocyte-macrophage system. Nevertheless, various associations between changes in the circulating monocyte count and certain disease states have been noted.

Decreased production of monocytes is most commonly seen following the administration of cytotoxic drugs and/or ionizing radiation in the treatment of malignant disease. Because mature macrophages are relatively insensitive to these agents and have a prolonged lifespan, problems directly ascribable to monocytopenia are less common and hard to separate from those related to the concomitant neutropenia. Patients who have received prolonged cytotoxic therapy, however, are more prone to deep-seated infections, often of fungal or protozoal origin, and a defective monocyte-macrophage system may be contributory.

Increases in peripheral blood monocyte numbers correlate reasonably well with increased monocyte turnover and are seen in a variety of conditions, in particular malignant disease (both hematologic and nonhematologic), infections such as tuberculosis and subacute bacterial endocarditis, and chronic inflammatory conditions such as collagen-vascular disorders and inflammatory bowel disease. Malignant disorders of the monocyte/macrophage series are discussed below.

Disorders of monocyte and macrophage function in the face of normal production are broadly similar to the neutrophil functional disorders outlined above. In particular, the defect in chronic granulomatous disease is present also in monocytes and macrophages, and this fact no doubt contributes to the severity of the clinical picture in this condition.

THE EOSINOPHILS

The eosinophil granulocytes have granules that stain deep red with eosin. They constitute less than 5 per cent of the total circulating leukocytes, or 40 to 440/μl. This level shows some diurnal fluctuation that is inversely correlated with adrenocortical activity. An increase in the eosinophil count has long been recognized in various allergic conditions and as an accompaniment of a variety of parasitic infestations. A reduction is seen with physiologic or pathologic increases in adrenocortical activity or after the administration of ACTH or adrenocortical steroids. Such observations are not new, but despite intensive research in recent years, the primary function of this cell is unclear.

The eosinophil resembles the neutrophil granulocyte except it has approximately 20 large refractile cytoplasmic granules that stain bright red with eosin. The cell is about 12 to 17 μm in diameter and has a bi- or trilobed nucleus with a condensed chromatin structure. With the electron microscope the specific granules are seen to be surrounded by a double membrane and to contain amorphous material with a dense crystalline core and a less dense matrix.

The contents of the eosinophil granules are of particular interest. About half the total protein is a strongly basic substance of molecular weight 11,000 called *major basic protein (MBP)*. Its purpose is unknown; it does not have antibacterial activity but it neutralizes heparin, as might any strongly basic substance. A peroxidase distinct from myeloperoxidase is also present, as are other enzymes, such as acid and alkaline phosphatases, aryl sulfatase, β-glucuronidase, and ribonuclease; apart from MBP, the eosinophil granules resemble typical lysosomes.

Eosinophils are thought to derive from the same stem cells as other myeloid cells, but eosinophilic development is not distinguishable until the myelocyte stage. The kinetics of production are less well documented than for the neutrophil. Postmitotic maturation in man occurs in the marrow with a postmitotic transit time of 2.5 days. Peripheral blood kinetics are complex and there is evidence for recirculation with an initial half-life in man of about four hours but with subsequent reappearance of all cells between 6 to 24 hours followed by a second period of slower disappearance over four days.

EOSINOPHIL FUNCTION

Eosinophils share some properties with neutrophils. They respond equally well to complement-mediated or other chemotactic stimuli, but this does not explain their selective migration to sites of parasitic infestation or allergic reaction. Several substances have been shown to attract eosinophils, including antigen-antibody complexes (perhaps by complement activation) and certain lymphokines. A substance specifically chemotactic for eosinophils is present in the cytoplasmic granules of the basophil and is released during basophil degranulation in response to the interaction of antigen and basophil-bound IgE (immediate hypersensitivity). This substance is called *eosinophil-chemotactic factor of anaphylaxis, ECFA*.

Eosinophils have some capacity for phagocytosis but are less efficient than neutrophils. They are capable of consuming zymosan particles, antigen-antibody complexes, mast cell granules, mycoplasma, and inert particles, as well as bacteria. Following ingestion, a limited degranulation occurs with discharge of the contents of adjacent granules into the phagosome. The eosinophil is also capable of discharging the contents of its granules to the exterior, and it has been shown that helminth larvae can be destroyed in this fashion without the need for phagocytosis. This may well be one of the major functions of this cell, although their accumulation at other sites of immediate hypersensitivity reactions suggests an important role in mechanisms of this type. They may simply be involved in the containment and modulation of such reactions by their ability to phagocytose some of the reaction products and by possessing in quantity a protein capable of neutralizing heparin, one of the potentially more hazardous substances released from basophils.

No patients have been described with a pure absence of eosinophils, so there are few clues as to how essential they are. A few patients have been described with hypogammaglobulinemia, eosinopenia, and thymoma; these patients, however, had normal cellular immunity, and no problems were observed that could be ascribed to the lack of eosinophils. A patient with absent eosinophils and basophils and reduced levels of IgA and IgE has been described who had repeated infections, rhinitis, and asthma, but the other deficiencies obviously complicate any interpretation of the effect of the eosinopenia.

EOSINOPHILS IN DISEASE

Increased eosinophil production with blood and tissue eosinophilia is a prominent feature of a wide variety of disorders with an immune basis (Table 50). It is seen in virtually every invasive metazoan infestation, although it is less predictable when infestation

TABLE 50. CAUSES OF EOSINOPHILIA AND EOSINOPENIA

Eosinophilia
  Parasitic infestations
  Allergic disorders
    Asthma
    Hay fever
    Drug and other hypersensitivity reactions
  Skin disorders
    Eczema
    Urticaria
    Pemphigus
    Dermatitis herpetiformis
  Pulmonary disorders
    Asthma
    Parasitic infestations
    Polyarteritis nodosa
  Malignancy
    Lymphoma
    Carcinoma
  Other
    Hypereosinophilic syndrome
    Sarcoidosis
    Hypoadrenalism
Eosinopenia
  Hypercorticoid states
    Cushing's disease
    Glucocorticoid administration
    Stress
  Epinephrine
  Congenital (rare)

is confined to the gastrointestinal tract or when larval forms become encysted, as does *Taenia solium*. Allergic disorders associated with eosinophilia include bronchial asthma, allergic rhinitis, certain drug allergies, and skin allergies, such as eczema, contact dermatitis, and urticaria. Various pulmonary conditions are associated with eosinophilia: the presence of metazoan larvae in the lungs is a regular cause, but eosinophilia may also occur with hypersensitivity to inhaled organic dusts and in pulmonary involvement with polyarteritis nodosa. Less frequently, eosinophilia may be seen in patients with malignant disease or with inflammatory conditions, such as collagen-vascular disease or with inflammatory bowel disease. The mechanism of eosinophilia in malignant disease is obscure, but in some instances of lung cancer with marked eosinophilia a humoral factor has been found with chemotactic properties for eosinophils.

Peripheral blood eosinophils are particularly sensitive to adrenocortical activity, and their numbers may thus be greatly reduced or absent in periods of stress, in patients with Cushing's disease, or in those on corticosteroid treatment. The mechanism is complex; initially, there is a peripheral sequestration or margination and impaired marrow release, but after prolonged exposure to excess steroid the picture is complicated by a decrease in marrow production. In contrast, mild eosinophilia is characteristic in patients with adrenocortical failure.

Because of common ancestry with other myeloid cells, an acute eosinophilic leukemia is not seen. Some patients have been described with a syndrome characterized by a progressive massive blood and tissue eosinophilia with splenomegaly and endomyocardial and pulmonary fibrosis. This has been termed the *hypereosinophilic syndrome*. Its origin is unknown: it seems that the tissue damage is a consequence of the eosinophilia, which in most cases is thought to be a reaction to an unidentified stimulus, although on occasions a true leukemic transformation is possible.

THE BASOPHILS

MORPHOLOGY AND PRODUCTION

The basophils are the least numerous of the leukocytes and number between 0 to 80/µl in the peripheral blood. They are about 10 to 14 µm in diameter and have abundant deeply basophilic cytoplasmic granules that largely obscure the bilobed or indented nucleus. The granules contain a variety of substances, including histamine, heparin, the eosinophil-chemotactic substance of anaphylaxis (p. 267), and a substance that promotes platelet aggregation and degranulation. They do not appear to contain proteolytic enzymes as do those of other granulocytes. Basophils have many similarities with, but are not identical to, the tissue mast cells, and their exact relationship is not clear. Blood basophils are produced in the marrow; the earliest recognizable precursor is the basophil myelocyte, but little is known of the kinetics of their production.

FUNCTION

The importance of basophils lies in their possession of membrane receptors for the Fc portion of IgE and their participation in immediate hypersensitivity reactions. IgE is the least abundant of the immunoglobulins; interaction of basophil-bound IgE with specific antigen produces basophil degranulation with release of granule contents into the surrounding tissues. Only very small amounts of antigen are required, sufficient to bridge two IgE molecules. The clinical effect of such interactions is dramatic and immediate and is manifested locally as urticaria, bronchial asthma, or rhinitis, or systemically as anaphylactic shock if antigen is administered or gains access to sensitized individuals. This type of reaction is not seen in everybody, but some individuals have an allergic or atopic tendency that may have a genetic component. These patients have more IgE bound to their basophils than do normal persons, and this may explain the severity of their reactions. The role of basophils in health remains to be defined.

Basophils in Disease

An increase in blood basophils occurs frequently in the myeloproliferative disorders, particularly myelosclerosis (p. 247) and chronic myeloid leukemia (p. 276). A marked increase in both tissue and blood basophils is seen in the rare disorders that constitute the syndrome of systemic mastocytosis, which is characterized by skin lesions, hepatosplenomegaly, skeletal changes, and many features of leukemia.

THE LYMPHOCYTES

For many years after their presence in the blood was noted, the lymphocytes were largely ignored because their function was unknown. During the past three decades, however, it has become clear that these apparently mundane cells have a fundamental role in the immune response and that their morphologic uniformity belies an impressive degree of functional heterogeneity. Extensive discussion of the structure of primary and secondary lymphatic organs as well as of the role of the lymphocyte in the immune response was presented in the discussion on immunology. Here aspects of the pathophysiology of lymphocytes of particular interest to the hematologist are examined.

Lymphocytes are round cells measuring 8 to 12 µm. They constitute 20 to 50 per cent of peripheral blood leukocytes (p. 173) and when stained with Romanowsky dyes have scanty pale blue cytoplasm containing occasional vacuoles and up to 15 very faint azurophilic lysosomal granules. The nucleus occupies most of the cell volume; it is round or slightly indented and stains darkly with densely packed chromatin. A small nucleolus is often visible but is more readily apparent by electron microscopy, which also demonstrates abundant condensed heterochromatin and typical cytoplasmic organelles—mitochondria, free ribosomes, and strands of rough endoplasmic reticulum. The scanning electron microscope shows a spherical cell with variable numbers of prominent short microvilli on the surface.

PRODUCTION

Lymphocytes descend from pluripotent stem cells, which they may have in common with other hematopoietic cells. During fetal life the thymus gland develops as an epithelial outgrowth of the third and fourth branchial pouches and becomes populated by stem cells that have circulated from primitive hematopoietic sites in the yolk sac, liver, and marrow. In birds, a second similar epithelial outgrowth in the region of the cloaca, called the bursa of Fabricius, is likewise populated with circulating stem cells. Intense proliferation and differentiation of lymphocytes is seen in both the thymus and the bursa, although much of it is ineffective. Differentiated lymphocytes from these organs are known as T cells and B cells, respectively. They are morphologically similar but differ markedly in function: B cells are concerned with humoral (antibody-mediated) immune processes and are, in fact, the precursors of antibody-secreting plasma cells; T cells, on the other hand, are concerned with a number of different processes collectively known as cell-mediated immune responses. Certain T cells have a direct cytotoxic, or "killer," capability against foreign cells, while others modulate B cell responses in a "helper" or "suppressor" capacity. In mammals there is no obvious counterpart to the avian bursa, and some other structure assumes the role of B cell induction. Its true identity remains unknown, although such a role has been suggested for the marrow, gut-associated lymphatic tissue, and the fetal liver.

The bursa (or the equivalent) and thymus are concerned with primary lymphocyte differentiation from stem cells and are thus known as primary lymphoid organs. Other lymphoid structures—the spleen, lymph nodes, and gut and bronchial-associated lymphatic tissues—are known as secondary lymphatic organs. They are mesenchymal in origin, develop later in fetal life, and are populated with differentiated T and B lymphocytes that circulate from the thymus and bursa or its analog. At this stage lymphocytes are "virgin," since they have not yet had contact with antigen, and they proliferate within secondary lymphatic structures only after antigenic stimulation.

Production of differentiated lymphocytes by the thymus and bursa-equivalent is most active in early life. In man, the thymus reaches its maximal size in adolescence and subsequently involutes. Its removal at this point does not result in any obvious defect in immune function, but evidence from animals does suggest that some delayed reduction in T cell number and function may result. On the other hand, neonatal thymectomy in mice is followed by a severe wasting disease, with a marked reduction in T cell numbers and in cell-mediated immunity, together with associated increased liability to infection.

The secondary organs are concerned directly with the immune response and are able to respond to antigen close to its point of entry into the body. The spleen is particularly well placed to clear antigenic particles from the bloodstream, and lymph nodes are strategically situated along lymphatic channels that convey tissue fluid (lymph) from the tissues to the bloodstream.

LYMPHOCYTE SUBPOPULATIONS AND DIFFERENTIATION MARKERS

Despite a uniform appearance, lymphocytes comprise a number of subpopulations that differ in various immunologic, biochemical, and functional respects.

The development of T and B lymphocytes has already been described, and the diverse functional characteristics of these cells are fully discussed under immunology (Section III). Lymphocyte subpopulations are also distinguished by *cell markers,* which reflect biological differences between different cell types at different stages of maturation. Such markers include surface antigens and intracellular enzymes and are invaluable in the study of lymphoproliferative disorders. Traditionally the detection of surface antigens has relied on immunofluorescent techniques using heterologous antisera or on functional characteristics such as the presence of mature T cells of "receptors" for sheep erythrocytes. More recently, the development of monoclonal antibodies detecting a range of cell surface antigens has allowed a much more precise characterization of lymphocyte function and development (Fig. 57).

Much of our present knowledge has come from the study of relatively pure cell populations obtained from patients with leukemias and lymphomas. Indeed, cell marker analysis is important in helping the clinician select optimal therapy for patients. Although certain antigens detected on leukemic cells were initially thought to be "leukemia-specific," it is usually possible to detect small numbers of cells in normal persons that express the same antigens, and it is therefore more appropriate to consider them as normal markers of differentiation.

The most useful lymphocyte cell markers are surface membrane immunoglobulin (SmIg), terminal deoxynucleotidyl transferase, HLA DR and Ia antigens, sheep erythrocyte rosetting, the common ALL antigen (cALLa), and various antigens detected by monoclonal antibodies.

Surface Membrane Immunoglobulin (SmIg). B cells are most readily distinguished by their ability to synthesize immunoglobulin. At the very earliest stage of B cell differentiation, the immunoglobulin genes undergo rearrangement, and this can be detected by analysis of DNA after hybridization with suitable probes. The first overt evidence for immunoglobulin synthesis is the appearance of μ heavy chains in the cytoplasm at the pre-B cell stage. On the other hand, mature B cells are characterized by the presence of surface immunoglobulin, principally IgM and IgG. Individual cells synthesize Ig of only one specificity, this being the means by which they can recognize a wide range of foreign antigens. It follows that each cell produces only kappa or lambda light chains, and this itself is a useful marker for demonstrating clonality in neoplasms of B cell origin.

Terminal Deoxynucleotidyl Transferase. This cytoplasmic enzyme was first detected in thymic tissue, but raised levels were subsequently reported in lymphoblasts from patients with acute lymphoblastic leukemia (ALL). It has subsequently been detected in small numbers of normal bone marrow cells and is now thought to be expressed by cells at the earliest stages of lymphocyte development but to be lost early in the process of B cell differentiation. It is present in cortical thymocytes but cannot be detected in mature T cells. Its functional role is uncertain. Other intracellular enzymes that are useful in the study of lymphocyte development and leukemia include adenosine deaminase, hexosaminidase, acid phosphatase, and 5'-nucleotidase.

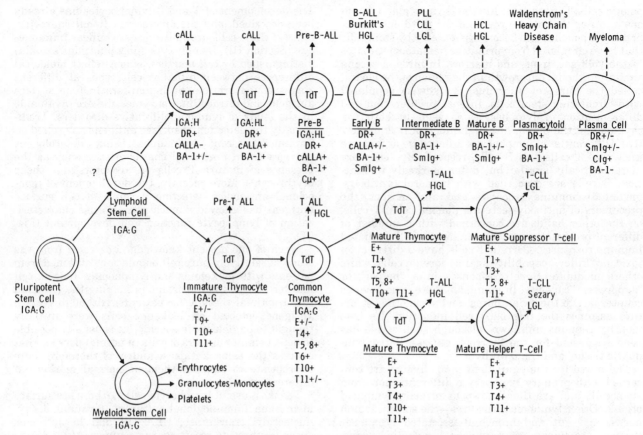

Figure 57. A scheme of lymphocyte differentiation based on surface markers, enzyme, and molecular studies. Each "cell" illustrated represents a phenotypically discrete stage in a continuum of differentiation. The pathways of differentiation are indicated by a solid arrow (→) and the relationship of various developmental stages with lymphomas and leukemias is indicated by a broken arrow (---→). The phenotypic characteristics are indicated beneath each cell. IGA indicates the arrangement of immunoglobulin genes as follows: G = germ line arrangement, H = heavy chain genes rearranged, L = light chain genes rearranged; T1, 3, 6, 8–11, and BA-1 represent reaction with monoclonal antibodies detecting various stages of T and B lymphocyte development, respectively; cALL = common acute lymphoblastic leukemia antigen; TdT = terminal transferase; DR = HLA DR expression; E = sheep erythrocyte, rosetting; Cμ = cytoplasmic μ heavy chain; SmIg = surface membrane Ig; CIg = cytoplasmic Ig (heavy and light chain); CLL = chronic lymphatic leukemia; PLL = prolymphocytic leukemia; HCL = hairy cell leukemia; HGL = non-Hodgkin's lymphoma (high grade); LCL = non-Hodgkin's lymphoma (low grade). (Modified from Foon, K. A., et al.: Blood 60:1, 1982.)

HLA DR and Ia Antigens. Products of the HLA-D locus and the closely related immune-associated (Ia) genes are expressed on the cell surface by early lymphocyte progenitors, B cells, and myeloid precursors. However, they are not specific for B lymphocyte differentiation, since the antigens are expressed by T cells responding to antigenic stimulation.

Sheep Erythrocyte Rosetting. Mature T cells of most species have surface receptors for an antigen present on sheep erythrocytes and can be identified in cell suspensions by their ability to form rosettes with these cells. B cells do not react with sheep erythrocytes in this way, although a percentage form rosettes with mouse erythrocytes.

The Common ALL Antigen (cALLa). Cells from patients with the common (non-T, non-B) variety of ALL (p. 273) have been used in rabbits to raise antisera that detect an antigen present on blast cells from 70 per cent of patients with ALL. Although this antigen is absent from normal peripheral blood lymphocytes, it can be detected in normal bone marrow cells that

are also TdT and Ia positive. Normal cALLa-positive cells are thought to be bone-marrow–derived lymphoid progenitors.

Antigens Detected by Monoclonal Antibodies. Monoclonal antibodies have been produced that react with a wide variety of lymphocyte and hemopoietic cell surface antigens. This is a rapidly expanding field, and the nomenclature can now confuse even the initiated. The most important antibodies differentiate between T and B cells and can identify functional subsets of T cells such as helper-inducer and suppressor-cytotoxic cells (Fig. 57).

THE PLASMA CELLS

Plasma cells are the immunoglobulin-secreting descendants of B lymphocytes that have been stimulated by antigen. They are normally confined to the lymphatic tissues, in particular to the germinal centers and medullary cords of the lymph nodes, and to the white pulp and periarteriolar sheaths of the spleen. They are also found throughout the lamina propria of the gut and bronchial mucosa. As lymphatic tissue is diffusely scattered throughout the marrow, plasma cells may constitute up to 4 per cent of the nucleated cells in a given marrow sample. They are rarely found in the peripheral blood or lymph and then only after antigenic stimulation or as part of a malignant process.

MORPHOLOGY AND PRODUCTION

Plasma cells are ovoid, larger than lymphocytes, and have an eccentric round nucleus with coarse chromatin distributed in a "cartwheel" pattern. The cytoplasm stains deeply basophilic because of its high RNA content, but there is a clear perinuclear halo. The electron microscope shows an extensive endoplasmic reticulum and a large distinct Golgi complex, in keeping with the cells' function in the synthesis of immunoglobulin.

Differentiation from a B lymphocyte to a plasma cell involves several mitotic divisions and takes seven to ten days, paralleling the time required to mount a primary immune response. Differentiation involves the development not only of a factory for packaging and secreting immunoglobulin but also of the ability to produce different immunoglobulin classes. B lymphocytes produce only IgD and IgM, which remain membrane-bound and are not secreted; plasma cells produce and secrete IgM, IgG, or IgA. It should be noted that a given plasma cell produces immunoglobulin of only one subtype and specificity.

PROLIFERATIVE DISORDERS OF THE LYMPHOCYTES

Lymphocytes proliferate as a result of antigenic stimulation or as a neoplastic process. In the former instance the result is appropriate, but in practice a widespread reactive proliferation can sometimes be difficult to distinguish from neoplasia, particularly when the responsible antigen cannot be identified. The clinical features of reactive proliferation depend on the nature and location of the antigen and the type of response invoked, but the hallmark is a tender enlargement of the lymphatic organs. For example, local skin infection may be followed by inflammation along the lymphatic vessels with tender enlargement of regional and possibly more central lymph nodes. With bacterial sepsis there is increased lymphocyte recirculation and proliferation within the node but not usually any detectable increase in lymphocytes in the blood, the leukocytosis being predominantly a neutrophilia.

Peripheral Blood Lymphocytosis. This condition is most commonly seen in the course of certain viral illnesses, particularly those in which the lymphocytes themselves are infected—for instance, infectious mononucleosis and cytomegalovirus infection. However, a moderate lymphocytosis may be seen in any of the viral exanthemata (rubella, measles, mumps, and so on) when large numbers of reactive lymphocytes undergoing proliferation may also be seen.

Infectious Mononucleosis. This is of particular interest because of an association between its causative agent, the Epstein-Barr (EB) virus, and Burkitt's lymphoma (p. 281). Infectious mononucleosis results from direct transmission of the virus to susceptible individuals during close physical contact such as kissing. The disease may be clinical or subclinical, but in either instance specific anti-EB virus antibodies are produced, and these can be taken as an indication of previous infection. The illness is characterized by sore throat, lymphadenopathy, and fever. Splenomegaly, hepatomegaly, rash, and jaundice occur with decreasing frequency. Symptoms persist for two to three weeks or occasionally longer, and recovery may be complicated by a prolonged period of lethargy and depression. Lymphocytosis is usual in the acute phase, and many of the lymphocytes are transformed, or "reactive." Neutropenia may occur in the early stages and thrombocytopenia is usually present to a mild degree, although it is rarely apparent clinically. In the early stages of infection the abnormal circulating lymphocytes are thought to be infected B cells; later, however, suppressor T cells appear in response to neoantigens on the surface of EB-virus–infected B cells. Associated with the condition is the appearance of a heterophilic antibody with affinity for horse or sheep erythrocytes. It can be detected in the serum in the vast majority of symptomatic cases. Specific EB virus antibodies can also be demonstrated, and the virus itself can be recovered from the throats of most patients. Virus excretion may persist for years. Infectious mononucleosis is considered by some to be a virally induced "neoplastic" lymphoproliferative process in which the transformed cells are successfully eliminated by the host's cell-mediated defenses.

Acute Infectious Lymphocytosis. This is a short self-limiting illness that occurs in outbreaks in young people. It is thought to be a result of a viral infection, although an infectious agent has not yet been isolated. It is characterized by a striking leukocytosis due mainly to an increase in the number of small lymphocytes. This lasts from three to five weeks and may be associated with eosinophilia.

NEOPLASTIC DISORDERS OF LEUKOCYTES

Neoplastic leukocyte disorders are traditionally classified as leukemias or lymphomas. The term "leukemia" implies that neoplastic leukocytes circulate in the blood, while the term "lymphoma" implies a disorder involving principally the lymphatic organs. This distinction is by no means mutually exclusive, and there can be considerable overlap between the two groups.

THE LEUKEMIAS

The leukemias are a group of neoplastic disorders characterized by abnormal clonal proliferation of hemopoietic cells arising from a malignantly transformed progenitor. They are broadly classified by this apparent differentiation as myeloid or lymphoid and by their kinetic behavior as acute or chronic.

Etiology and Pathogenesis. Although there are usually no etiologic clues to the individual case of leukemia, a number of predisposing factors are apparent from epidemiologic studies. The first to be recognized was exposure to ionizing radiation, when it was found that mortality from leukemia was particularly high among radiologists who worked with x-rays earlier in this century. Later, an increased incidence of chronic granulocytic and acute leukemias was noted in survivors of the atomic bomb explosions in Japan. These cases came to light some years after the event. A relationship with the dose of radiation received could be inferred from the distances of individual patients from the blast.

Damage to the marrow by drugs or chemicals has been implicated in the genesis of some human leukemias. The best documented example is that of leukemia developing after marrow damage by benzene or one of its derivatives, while less convincing reports have implicated the drugs chloramphenicol and phenylbutazone. A much closer association with cytotoxic drugs is emerging, as reflected by the increase in acute leukemia in patients who have received cytotoxic chemotherapy for other malignancies.

Genetic factors are also important. Studies of rodents clearly indicate the importance of genetic makeup in the expression of leukemia and suggest that its development is not the result of a single mechanism but involves the interaction of genes coding for susceptibility and resistance together with a variety of environmental factors. A similar picture is beginning to emerge for at least some, if not all, human leukemias and lymphomas. An increased familial incidence has been demonstrated for the acute leukemias and chronic lymphatic leukemia, although such observations do not necessarily indicate a genetic basis. A high degree of concordance for acute leukemia has been noted in identical twins; this is particularly striking in young children, who are liable to develop the disease within a year of their twin. The risk is not as great for nonidentical twins but is still significantly higher than for the general population.

Chromosomal abnormalities can be demonstrated in many but not all patients with leukemia (Table 51). About 50 per cent of patients with acute myelogenous leukemia (AML) have an increased modal number of chromosomes or karyotypic abnormalities. In earlier studies individual chromosomes appeared to be involved at random, but more recently certain nonrandom patterns have emerged. These include a translocation between the long arms of chromosomes 8 and 21 (t[8;21][q22;q22]) in a subset of patients with AML and a translocation between the long arms of chromosomes 15 and 17 (t[15;17][q25;q22]) in patients with acute promyelocytic leukemia. In the majority of patients with *chronic* myeloid leukemia a specific constant translocation is found (p. 276). Abnormalities are also common in acute lymphoblastic leukemia but have been less well characterized. However, a translocation identical to that in chronic myeloid leukemia is seen in some patients, and several cases of B cell ALL have been reported with a translocation identical to that associated with the phenotypically related Burkitt's lymphoma (p. 281).

A clear association is now recognized between infection with certain specific viruses and the development of leukemias and lymphomas in a variety of animal and avian species. The viruses implicated are C-type RNA retroviruses, so-called because they possess the enzyme *reverse transcriptase*. This is an RNA-dependent DNA polymerase that enables the host cell to generate a complementary DNA copy of the viral RNA template, which can then be integrated into the cellular genome. So far, only one type of human leukemia-lymphoma has been closely associated with a virus of this kind: some patients with a particularly aggressive form of T cell neoplasm with features of both leukemia and lymphoma have been found to have circulating antibodies to a retrovirus that is now known as the *human T-cell lympotropic virus (HTLV)*. Further evidence linking this virus with the pathogenesis of these neoplasms comes from observations of virus shedding from tumor cells in vitro.

A framework for understanding the pathogenesis of human leukemias and lymphomas is developing, although the precise alteration in the genetic machinery of the transformed progenitor cells that induces malignant properties remains unknown. It has been shown recently that fragments of DNA extracted from a variety of human tumors (including some leukemias and lymphomas) can induce transformation of certain cell lines in vitro. Analysis of the DNA capable of inducing such transformation has shown a remarkable degree of homology, if not identity, with genes present in the retroviruses associated with animal and avian neoplasms. The viral genes are called oncogenes (*v-onc*); their human homologs are called cellular oncogenes (*c-onc*). The latter are important in a variety of regulatory mechanisms including phosphorylation and the control of the cell cycle. It is believed that their abnormal function, caused either by mutation or translocation to other parts of the genome, may play a central role in neoplastic proliferation. As we shall see in later sections, specific translocations of cellular oncogenes have been found in several types of leukemia or lymphoma.

Two or more separate steps probably are involved in tumorigenesis. The first may involve an alteration in the kinetics of a cell population that simply enables the cells to go on growing indefinitely (immortalization), but subsequent transforming events seem to be required to enable the cells to grow in the completely unrestrained fashion that characterizes malignancy. In certain B cell lymphomas and leukemias immortalization of B cells may result from prior EB virus infection (infectious mononucleosis), and a further spontaneous mutation may be necessary to activate a cellular oncogene that then alters the kinetic behavior of the cell. This notion is discussed further on page 281.

TABLE 51. CHROMOSOMAL ABNORMALITIES IN ACUTE LEUKEMIAS

Acute myelogenous leukemia (AML)
Loss or gain of chromosomes, e.g., trisomy 8, monosomy 7
Structural rearrangements
    M2: 8 to 21 translocation (t[8;21] [q22;q22]) ± absent Y (males) or X (females)
    M3: 15 to 17 translocation (t[15;17] [q25;q22])
Acute lymphoblastic leukemia (ALL)
Ph¹ translocation: (t[9;22] [q34:q11]) may occur at presentation or in "lymphoid" blast crisis of chronic myeloid leukemia
B cell ALL: 8 to 14 translocation (t[8;14] [q24;q32])
Nonspecific abnormalities are common in all types.

M2, M3 = subgroups of FAB classification (see Table 52).

THE ACUTE LEUKEMIAS

The acute leukemias are characterized by an uncontrolled proliferation and accumulation of leukocyte precursors that are capable of only limited differentiation and are thus apparently "frozen" at a primitive stage of development. The clinical features can be attributed to the accumulation of abnormal cells and to a severe failure of normal bone marrow function. Acute leukemia is invariably fatal without treatment, but with modern management cure is possible in favorable cases, and a temporary but worthwhile remission of the disease can often be obtained in the remainder.

Acute leukemia is classified according to the nature of the blast cells present as *lymphoblastic* (ALL) or *myeloblastic* (AML). It may be further subdivided according to the presence or absence of certain differentiation markers and morphologic characteristics (Table 52). The majority of patients with ALL have a non-B non-T phenotype with blast cells that are positive for the cALL antigen (p. 270). The arrangement of the immunoglobulin genes in leukemic cells from some of these patients is compatible with the notion that they are derived from early B cell progenitors. ALL with a more mature B cell phenotype occurs but is rare and has an extremely poor prognosis. A T cell phenotype is found in about 20 per cent of patients: these are usually older children or young adults who often have massive lymphadenopathy with mediastinal involvement (Fig. 58), hepatosplenomegaly, and high circulating blast cell counts. In some instances this picture can be difficult to distinguish from malignant lymphoma, and occasionally a suppressor or helper T cell phenotype may be demonstrated. The prognosis is intermediate between cALL and B cell ALL. AML may be further classified by the morphologic characteristics of the blast cells (Table 52), but this has only limited prognostic value.

Cell Kinetics in Acute Leukemia. The functional defect in acute leukemia appears to be a failure of normal differentiation and maturation in a population of leukocyte precursors that proliferates uncontrollably at the expense of normal marrow function. Contrary to expectations, the leukemic cells turn over at a slower rate than do normal marrow precursors, and this fact is useful in planning treatment. Using in vitro culture

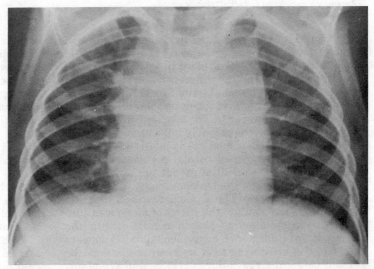

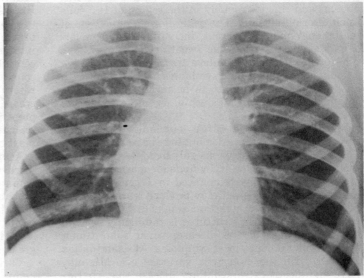

Figure 58. Massive mediastinal enlargement in a five-year-old boy with ALL at examination *(above)* and after treatment *(below)*. (From Callender, S. T. C.: The leukaemias. *Oxford Textbook of Medicine.* Weatherall, D. J., Ledingham, J. G. G., and Warrell, D. A. (eds.). Oxford, Oxford University Press.)

TABLE 52. CLASSIFICATION OF ACUTE LEUKEMIAS BY SURFACE MARKERS, HISTOCHEMISTRY, AND ENZYMES

	MORPHOLOGICALLY IDENTIFIABLE AS LYMPHOID OR MYELOID				SUDAN BLACK PEROXIDASE	FREQUENCY†
	Reaction with Anti-ALL Serum	Surface IgG	E − Rosettes	TdT*		
Lymphoblastic (ALL)						
Common ALL	+	−	−	+	−	75%
T Cell	−	−	+	+	−	10%
B Cell	−	+	−	−	−	<5%
Null Cell	−	−	−	±	−	10%
Myelogenous (AML)‡						
M1: Myeloblastic (undifferentiated)	−	−	−	−	±	62%
M2: Myeloblastic (differentiated)	−	−	−	−	±	
M3: Promyelocytic	−	−	−	−	+	5%
M4: Myelomonocytic	−	−	−	−	+	20%
M5: Monocytic	−	−	−	−	+	<5%
M6: Erythroleukemia	−	−	−	−	±	<5%

Morphologically unclassifiable
  <5% of all acute leukemias; some patients may show evidence of lymphoid origin with anti-ALL or positive TdT.
Acute transformation of chronic granulocytic leukemia
  Patients have positive Ph¹ chromosome but may be classified as either lymphoblastic or myeloblastic by the morphologic and functional criteria given above.

*Elevated levels of terminal deoxynucleotidyl transferase.
†Data from Chessels, J. M., et al.: Lancet 2:1307, 1977 (ALL) and Crowther, D., et al.: British Medical Journal 1:131, 1973 (AML).
‡M1 to M6 correspond to the FAB classification.

methods it can be demonstrated that some very limited capacity for differentiation persists, at least in AML, but this is generally less evident in vivo. The lack of commitment to terminal differentiation leads to a progressive accumulation of immature cells, with failure of marrow function resulting in anemia, thrombocytopenia, and neutropenia. The mechanism of marrow failure is not clear; it is probably not a simple physical "crowding-out" phenomenon but is more likely caused by a subtle disturbance of normal regulatory mechanisms, possibly as a result of production of inhibitors of cell proliferation by the leukemic cells.

Clinical Features. The clinical features of acute leukemia are the result of the effects of marrow failure and the accumulation of leukemic cells within the tissues. From studies with mouse leukemias it appears likely that a critical mass of leukemic cells must be present before marrow failure develops and symptoms appear, and this is probably in the region of 10^{12} cells in childhood leukemia. The general systemic effects of malignancy may be present, including fatigue, anorexia, weight loss, excessive sweating, and fever. The consequences of marrow failure are those of progressive anemia and its associated symptoms, neutropenia with an increased susceptibility to bacterial infection and thrombocytopenia with petechial or more extensive hemorrhage.

Tissue infiltration in acute leukemia is not often symptomatic at presentation but may be so later. There may be slight hepatosplenomegaly in AML and in ALL lymphadenopathy as well. Lymphadenopathy and hepatosplenomegaly may be marked in T cell ALL, and mediastinal enlargement may produce tracheal or superior vena caval obstruction (Fig. 58). Macroscopic involvement of other structures is commonly seen in the later stages of the disease, when solid tumor deposits may produce local symptoms. At examination patients with the monocytic varieties of AML may have significant extramedullary disease that charac-

teristically involved the gums (Fig. 59) and skin. Microscopic infiltration may be widespread at the onset of all types of the disease, and cells in certain sites may be relatively inaccessible to the action of cytotoxic therapy. The classic "sanctuary" site is the central nervous system, and meningeal leukemia develops at some time in the majority of patients with ALL and in a minority with AML, unless steps are taken to prevent its appearance. Thus most schedules for ALL now include a period of intensive prophylactic irradiation to the central nervous system; the usefulness of this in AML has not been demonstrated. Another sanctuary site in the male is the testis, and prophylactic irradiation of this site may also prove important in the prevention of late relapse.

Myeloblasts, and to a lesser extent lymphoblasts, are relatively rigid cells and when present in significant numbers can increase the viscosity of whole blood. Excessively high circulating blast cell counts (>100,000/μl) may result in a "hyperviscosity syndrome" with blockage of small blood vessels and tissue infarction. The brain and lungs are particularly susceptible, and the clinical features include clouding of consciousness, fits, focal neurologic signs, and respiratory distress. Death may occur suddenly. The increase in whole blood viscosity may be offset by the presence of anemia only to be precipitated by blood transfusion if this is undertaken before the circulating blast cell count has been reduced.

Acute hemostatic failure related to disseminated intravascular coagulation in addition to thrombocytopenia may occur in promyelocytic varieties of AML, probably owing to the release of lysosomal enzymes into the circulation from the abnormal cells (see also p. 312). This complication is most troublesome shortly after the start of treatment when cell breakdown is greatest.

Various metabolic problems may occur in acute leukemia. Hyperuricemia is common and reflects the

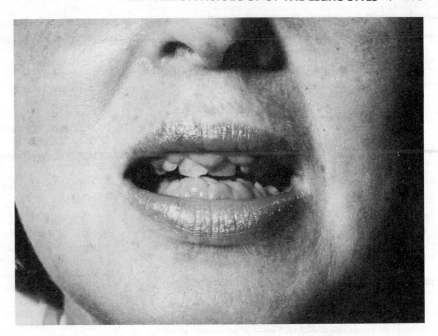

Figure 59. Gum hypertrophy in a patient with acute monocytic leukemia.

presence of a large proliferating cell mass. Gout may result, but a more serious consequence is acute renal failure following tubular obstruction with uric acid crystals. This is particularly a problem when large numbers of cells are destroyed at the start of treatment, but it can be prevented by adequate hydration, maintenance of a good urine output, and the administration of bicarbonate to render the urine alkaline, since uric acid crystallizes only in acid solution. Allopurinol also helps by preventing the conversion of xanthine to uric acid. Another unwanted effect of the rapid breakdown of a large tumor mass is hyperkalemia. This occurs most dramatically in T cell ALL when the leukemic mass may be extremely large and may be further aggravated by renal impairment. Sudden death from cardiac arrest may occur. Severe hypokalemia is sometimes seen in patients with monocytic forms of AML: in these patients large amounts of lysozyme are produced and excreted by the kidney, in which tubular damage may result. Significant lactic acidosis is seen occasionally in patients with extensive disease.

Blood Changes in Acute Leukemia. The blood picture at presentation is variable. There is usually a marked normochromic normocytic anemia with thrombocytopenia and neutropenia, although the total leukocyte count is influenced by the number of circulating blast cells and may be reduced, normal, or elevated, sometimes to very high levels. The hemoglobin and platelet counts can be normal at presentation. Occasionally patients have severe pancytopenia and a peripheral blood picture indistinguishable from aplastic anemia. The diagnosis of acute leukemia is confirmed by marrow aspiration or biopsy; the marrow is hypercellular and largely replaced by leukemic cells, which may represent over 90 per cent of the nucleated cells present. It is important for both prognosis and treatment that the type of acute leukemia be correctly characterized at presentation. This is often possible on cytologic grounds, but a variety of techniques are now available for cell marker analysis (Table 52).

Principles of Treatment. It is beyond the scope of this section to discuss the treatment of acute leukemia in detail, and only a brief outline of the underlying principles is given. The selection of optimal treatment depends first on accurate diagnosis and characterization of the type of leukemia and second on the establishment of realistic goals for therapy. For example, a cure may reasonably be expected in about 50 per cent of children with common ALL and perhaps 10 per cent of young patients with AML. However, to achieve this rate of cure requires intensive treatment, which itself involves a significant morbidity and mortality from infection and bleeding. In older patients the likelihood of cure is much less, and intensive treatment is often poorly tolerated. For many such patients it may be more realistic to aim for better quality in the patients' remaining life, rather than for a total cure.

There are two main aspects to the successful treatment of acute leukemia. First, the patient must be supported through periods of bone marrow failure, with blood and platelet transfusions together with prompt treatment of infection as appropriate. Second, cytotoxic drugs may be used in an attempt to eradicate or reduce the load of leukemic cells (Fig. 60). The cure of acute leukemia by chemotherapy depends on the successful exploitation of differences between normal and leukemic cells in their sensitivity to the drugs selected. The drugs most commonly employed are listed in Table 53 together with a brief description of their modes of action. Vincristine and prednisolone are particularly effective in the treatment of ALL, and this combination alone can produce remissions in over 90 per cent of cases. An advantage of these drugs is their lack of myelotoxicity. Unfortunately they are much less effective in AML, and myelotoxic drugs such as daunorubicin, cytosine arabinoside, and 6-thioguanine are commonly used.

Treatment of all forms of acute leukemia is more effective when drugs with different modes of action are used in combination rather than singly. Toxicity to

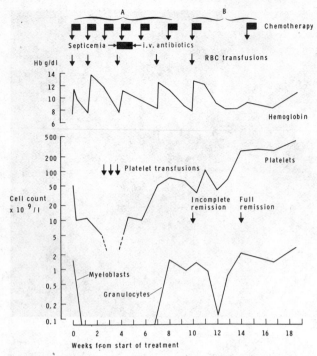

Figure 60. Hematologic course in a 44-year-old woman treated for acute myeloblastic leukemia. Chemotherapy A was with daunorubicin and cytosine arabinoside. Chemotherapy B was cyclophosphamide, vincristine, cytosine arabinoside, and prednisolone.

normal cells is minimized by cyclical drug administration; this exploits differences in cell cycle-time between normal and leukemic cells, since the faster generation time of the former allows them to regenerate more efficiently between courses of treatment. Development of resistance may be reduced by alternating schedules using different groups of drugs to which the leukemic cells show little cross-resistance.

Despite considerable refinements in cytotoxic therapy, the majority of patients with acute leukemia are not cured. In the majority of instances this is because the disease becomes resistant to the doses of cytotoxic drugs that can be safely given. The limiting toxicity of many drugs is to the hemopoietic system, and an alternative strategy is to use much higher doses of chemotherapy together with whole body irradiation, and to rescue the patient from the inevitable bone marrow failure by subsequent transplantation of hemopoietic cells from a normal donor. This approach is now possible but carries significant hazards in its own right. Nevertheless, in selected patients ablative therapy followed by bone marrow transplantation may offer a much improved chance of cure.

THE CHRONIC LEUKEMIAS

The chronic leukemias differ from the acute leukemias in that the neoplastic cell line retains a greater capacity for differentiation. The basic kinetic defect appears to be the input of inappropriate numbers of cells into the amplifying and differentiating compartments, which results in a huge expansion of the cell line involved. In chronic myeloid leukemia this is reflected in the appearance in the marrow and blood of large numbers of myeloid cells at all stages of development. Most of these are mature neutrophils, but less mature myeloid cells are seen as well. Similarly, in chronic lymphatic leukemia there is extensive infiltration of the marrow and lymph nodes together with peripheral blood lymphocytosis.

The discussion at this point is confined to chronic myeloid leukemia; chronic lymphatic leukemia has much in common with the lymphomas and is more conveniently discussed with them later in this section (pp. 278 to 283).

Chronic Myeloid (Granulocytic) Leukemia (CML)

Chronic myeloid leukemia accounts for about one fifth of all leukemias and is principally a disease of middle life, although it may occur at any age. The majority of patients have a characteristic chromosome abnormality known as Philadelphia (Ph[1]) chromosome (Fig. 61). This is a balanced translocation between the long arms of chromosomes 22 and 9 (t[9;22][q34;q11]) or occasionally of other chromosomes. Recent molecular studies indicate that the translocated fragment contains a cellular gene that is structurally related to the murine Abelson-leukemia-virus-transforming gene. The finding that the human homolog of this gene, *c-abl*, is translocated into the region of one of the immunoglobulin genes that is constantly rearranging as part of the normal mechanism for producing antibody diversity offers a possible mechanism for its abnormal activation as one of the events leading up to the genesis of this form of leukemia. The abnormal karyotype is also found in erythroid precursors and

TABLE 53. CYTOTOXIC DRUGS COMMONLY USED IN THE TREATMENT OF LEUKEMIA

Alkylating Agents	Alkylate guanine residues in DNA, preventing replication and impairing transcription; not cell-cycle specific.
Cylophosphamide	(AML, ALL, lymphomas)*
Busulfan	(CML)*
Chlorambucil	(CLL)*
Nitrogen mustard	(Hodgkin's lymphomas)
Anthracycline Antibiotics	Intercalate between DNA base pairs, impairing replication and transcription; not cell-cycle specific.
Daunorubicin	(AML)
Adriamycin	(ALL, lymphomas)
Antimetabolites	Various actions as metabolic inhibitors of DNA synthesis; cell-cycle specific.
Methotrexate	(ALL)
Cytosine arabinoside	(AML)
6-thioguanine	(AML)
6-mercaptopurine	(ALL)
Mitotic Inhibitors	Microtubular poisons. Interfere with mitotic spindle formation; cell-cycle specific.
Vincristine	(ALL, lymphomas)
Vinblastine	(lymphomas)
Vindesine	(lymphomas)

*AML = acute myelogenous leukemia; ALL = acute lymphoblastic leukemia; CML = chronic myeloid leukemia; CLL = chronic lymphatic leukemia.

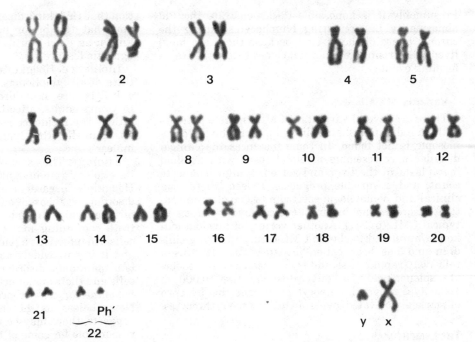

Figure 61. The chromosomes of a patient with chronic myeloid leukemia showing the typical Philadelphia (Ph¹) chromosome.

megakaryocytes, but the karyotype of somatic cells, fibroblasts, and the majority of lymphocytes is normal. This suggests that CML is a clonal disorder that has arisen from a single pluripotent hemopoietic stem cell. Further confirmation for this view has come from cytogenetic studies of mosaic individuals, from studies of patients heterozygous for glucose-6-phosphate dehydrogenase isoenzymes A and B (p. 232), and from patients undergoing blast transformation. The Ph¹ chromosome is not specific for CML and is seen occasionally in patients with ALL or AML.

The clinical features of CML include general systemic symptoms such as malaise, fever, weight loss, and sweating. At presentation there is usually anemia with a normal or elevated platelet count, but thrombocytopenia commonly develops later. Lymphadenopathy is exceptional, but the majority of patients have hepatosplenomegaly. This is often marked, and the spleen may fill the abdomen and enter the pelvis. Hypersplenism may aggravate the anemia and thrombocytopenia, and attacks of pain as a result of splenic infarction are common. Hyperuricemia is common and reflects increased cell turnover.

The hematologic findings in CML are characteristic. There is marked leukocytosis in the range 10,000 to 500,000/μl. The cells are predominantly mature neutrophils, but myelocytes, metamyelocytes, and smaller numbers of myeloblasts and promyelocytes are also present. An increase in the number of basophils is common. Anemia is variable in degree, and the platelet count is usually elevated at the onset but may be normal or occasionally reduced. An important finding is a marked reduction in the amount of neutrophil alkaline phosphatase, which is helpful in discrimination from leukemoid reactions (p. 262). In the later stages of the illness the blood may show changes typical of myelosclerosis (p. 247) or an acute leukemia.

The natural history of CML is one of progressive marrow failure with increasing hepatosplenomegaly and the general systemic features described above.

This picture may be modified by cytotoxic therapy with significant improvement in the quality if not the length of survival. Generally treatment with busulfan or similar agents reduces the total leukocyte mass and is associated with regression of symptoms and signs and an improvement in marrow function. Thus a clinical and hematologic "remission" of the disease may be obtained that may last for months or even years, although chemotherapy may be required from time to time to control the disease. Even in well-controlled patients the Ph¹ chromosomal abnormality persists; there have been occasional reports of its disappearance but usually only in patients who have been accidentally overtreated with busulfan. There is no evidence that the abnormal clone can be eradicated intentionally by aggressive treatment, although this can be achieved in selected cases with supralethal chemoradiotherapy followed by bone marrow transplantation. At any time the disease may be complicated by the development of an acute leukemia, the so-called "acute blast crisis," or by progressive myelosclerosis. Alternatively, it may progress to a more active accelerated phase, with little or no response to therapy, refractory anemia, and increasing transfusion requirements.

The transformation to an acute leukemia is of particular interest, since, contrary to expectations, the leukemic blast cells in about half the patients have lymphoid rather than myeloid characteristics. In most instances these lymphoid cells show evidence of B cell maturation, as shown by immunoglobulin gene rearrangements; rare cases of a T cell phenotype have been described. In contrast, cells from patients with a myeloblastic type of transformation retain a germ-line immunoglobulin gene pattern. The Ph¹ translocation is found in transformed blast cells of both lymphoid and myeloid type, which confirms that both types arise from the original malignant CML clone. The implications of these findings is that the transforming event responsible for CML occurs in a pluripotent stem cell capable of both myeloid and lymphoid differentiation.

Presumably it is impossible to demonstrate the Ph[1] abnormality in circulating lymphocytes during the chronic phase of the disease because these are long-lived cells arising from normal clones before the transforming event.

Variants of CML

There are several variants of CML. In some patients with an indistinguishable clinical picture the Ph[1] chromosome is not found. In some instances the clinical disorder may resemble myelosclerosis, with myeloid metaplasia in the liver and spleen, a high leukocyte count, and a variable prognosis. Indeed, there is a clinical and hematologic spectrum of "myeloproliferative" disorders ranging from typical myelosclerosis to typical CML (p. 247). Another variety of myeloid leukemia unrelated to classic CML occurs in young children and has been called *juvenile CML*. It runs a relatively rapid course and is characterized by moderate splenomegaly, a leukocytosis in the 10,000 to 100,000/μl range, thrombocytopenia, and the presence of markedly elevated levels of HbF in the erythrocytes.

THE LYMPHOMAS

The lymphomas are malignant disorders of lymphoid origin in which a major clinical feature is lymph node enlargement. The majority of lymphomas are thought to arise in the lymph nodes themselves and the remainder from lymphoid tissue in other sites such as the marrow, gut, skin, or lung. Lymphomas are broadly divided into two groups, which have many clinical similarities but different histologic appearances. The first group comprises those with the characteristic histological pattern known as Hodgkin's disease, and the second is a more heterogenous group of conditions that at the present are best classified simply as the non-Hodgkin's lymphomas. Major clinical differences between the two are shown in Table 54.

Hodgkin's Disease

In 1832 Thomas Hodgkin described a fatal condition characterized by generalized lymphadenopathy, splenomegaly, and absence of obvious inflammatory cause. The disease was not further studied until improved microscopic techniques became available and the presence of multinucleate giant cells led Sternberg in 1898 to believe that it was a form of tuberculosis. In 1902 Dorothy Reed dispelled this notion with the observation that Hodgkin's disease was a distant disease entity and that the bi- or multinucleate giant cells, now known as Reed-Sternberg cells, were an essential diagnostic feature.

Incidence. Hodgkin's disease accounts for about one third of all lymphomas. The age distribution is bimodal; it is rare in children and becomes more common in young adults, affecting about 25 per million population. The incidence rises in persons above the age of 50, as in the other lymphomas. It is more common in males.

Etiology. The exact nature of Hodgkin's disease and its etiology remain unknown. The earlier belief that Hodgkin's disease is an infectious or inflammatory disorder was based on the characteristic histologic picture, which includes a pleomorphic cellular infiltrate containing many normal or "reactive-looking" cells. No infectious agent has so far been demonstrated, and it is now widely accepted that Hodgkin's disease is a malignant disorder and that the Reed-Sternberg cells and their mononuclear counterparts (the *Hodgkin mononuclear cells*) represent the malignant cell line. Nevertheless, as the characteristic histologic picture suggests, there may be reactive features that could be responsible for some of the clinical features.

The malignant cells in Hodgkin's disease share some of the characteristics of both B lymphocytes and cells of monocyte-macrophage origin. There is much current interest in the possibility that the neoplastic proliferation may be a result of viral infection. There have been frequent reports of geographical and familial clustering, but most of these do not withstand critical statistical analysis and could be explained on the basis of random chance with a possible increase in hereditary susceptibility. One report does merit attention, however. In 1971 Vianna reported that a particular New York High School class had become the center of an "epidemic" of malignant lymphoma, with 34 people—either classmates themselves or their close friends and relatives from that period—developing lymphoma, including 31 cases of Hodgkin's disease. There have been reports of an association with previous Epstein-Barr virus (EBV) infection in some patients, but the numbers involved do not suggest that this is the causative agent, and attempts to demonstrate either EBV antigens or the EBV genome within Hodgkin's disease cells have been unsuccessful. The demonstration of an association between Hodgkin's disease and specific HLA-DR types has raised the possibility that the condition may be associated with an abnormal immune response, although whether to an infective agent or another form of antigen remains unclear. Chromosomal analysis of affected lymph nodes generally shows a mixture of normal and abnormal karyotypes. The latter appear to be confined to the Hodgkin's cells and lend further support to the belief that these are malignant.

Pathology. Hodgkin's disease is characterized by progressive enlargement of the lymph nodes followed by infiltration of other organs. As the disease progresses the general systemic effects of a neoplastic process become apparent. The first lymph nodes to be affected are most often the cervical group; the incidence of involvement of other groups is shown in Table 55. Extranodal involvement is usually confined to advanced disease and can affect any organ, although

TABLE 54. MAJOR CLINICAL DIFFERENCES BETWEEN HODGKIN'S AND NON-HODGIN'S LYMPHOMAS

HODGKIN'S	NON-HODGKIN'S
More often localized to one or more discreet groups of nodes	Commonly generalized
Waldeyer's ring and gut lymphatic tissue rarely affected	Waldeyer's ring and/or gut involvement common
Extranodal involvement (marrow, skin) uncommon	Extranodal involvement common

TABLE 55. PERCENTAGE INVOLVEMENT OF LYMPH NODE SITES AT PRESENTATION IN HODGKIN'S DISEASE*

Cervical	51%
Mediastinal	24%
Axillary	18%
Inguinal	16%
Abdominal	9%
Other nodes	2%
Multiple sites	26%

*Adapted from Smithers, D. W.: Brit Med J 2:263, 1967.

lung, liver, spleen, and marrow are the most commonly involved. The disease is thought to start at a single site and to spread via the lymphatics to contiguous nodal areas and hematogenously to noncontiguous and extranodal sites in advanced cases. In some patients with localized disease direct extranodal spread may be found.

Several different histologic patterns of Hodgkin's disease are recognized, but the presence of the Reed-Sternberg cell in a characteristic setting is necessary for definitive diagnosis. At present the most widely used classification is the Rye modification of that of Lukes and Butler, which recognizes four basic histologic patterns (Table 56). In the lymphocyte predominant pattern there is a variable alteration of lymph node architecture, scanty infiltration with Reed-Sternberg cells, and a diffuse or nodular, predominantly lymphocytic, reaction. In lymphocyte-depleted Hodgkin's disease the Reed-Sternberg cells are more abundant, and lymphocytes and normal histiocytes (macrophages) are scarce; there may also be extensive obliterative fibrosis. A halfway pattern is that of mixed cellularity, in which there is diffuse infiltration of lymphocytes as well as neutrophils, eosinophils, plasma cells, and histiocytes. Finally, in the nodular sclerosis pattern the lymphomatous tissue is divided into nodules by bands of fibrous tissue. This histologic pattern tends to occur in young women and commonly affects the mediastinum. The different histologic patterns are of prognostic significance: the lymphocyte predominant pattern is the most favorable and the lymphocyte-depleted the least.

Clinical Features. The cardinal clinical feature of Hodgkin's disease is lymphadenopathy, and in patients with widespread disease general systemic effects such as weight loss, fever, and sweating are common. Intense pruritus is also fairly common and may occur some time before lymphadenopathy develops. A peculiarly characteristic but uncommon symptom is pain localized to affected sites and precipitated by the ingestion of alcohol. This is not specific for Hodgkin's disease but can be diagnostically helpful at times. Fever may be marked and is often associated with drenching night sweats. Sometimes an undulating pattern of fever is seen; this is termed a *Pel-Ebstein fever,* although this fever pattern was originally described in a patient with brucellosis.

Lymphadenopathy may be massive but is rarely destructive. However, local pressure effects are common and may be dangerous in sites such as the mediastinum. Local discomfort may also be caused by splenomegaly. Extranodal spread can occur, particularly in the later stages of the disease, and the marrow, lungs, pleura, liver, meninges, renal tract, or gonads may be affected.

Most patients with Hodgkin's disease have impaired cell-mediated immunity that is manifested as absent or reduced delayed hypersensitivity and an increased susceptibility to viral infections such as herpes zoster. Humoral immunity is spared, and there may indeed be an increase in immunoglobulin levels. The mechanism of this immune incompetence is not clear, but since it is not marked in the early stages of the disease it is more likely to be a secondary phenomenon rather than a primary etiologic factor.

Hematologic abnormalities are seen frequently in Hodgkin's disease. Many patients with localized disease have a normal blood count, and the earliest change is the development of an anemia of chronic disorders (p. 228). Anemia may be aggravated by hypersplenism and the effects of treatment, but in contrast to the non-Hodgkin's lymphomas, autoimmune hemolysis is rare. Marrow infiltration occurs in advanced disease and may produce a leukoerythroblastic blood picture or one of progressive marrow failure. Lymphopenia is a characteristic finding in severe cases. It is caused by a parallel reduction in circulating B and T cell numbers but is insufficient to explain the degree of impairment in cell-mediated immunity. A blood eosinophilia is seen occasionally but is less impressive than the degree of tissue eosinophilia would suggest.

Prognosis. Until fairly recently, the prognosis in Hodgkin's disease was extremely poor. The key to successful management is accurate assessment of the extent of the disease, and the best treatment for localized disease is radiotherapy, which is usually curative. More extensive disease is difficult to manage successfully with radiotherapy alone, and systemic chemotherapy using a combination of cytotoxic drugs (such as nitrogen mustard, prednisolone, procarbazine, and vincristine) is more appropriate. Chemotherapy has unpleasant side effects, including intense nausea and vomiting induced particularly by nitrogen mustard, with the result that some patients have difficulty

TABLE 56. CLINICAL AND PATHOLOGIC STAGING OF HODGKIN'S DISEASE

CLINICAL (RYE CLASSIFICATION)

I. Disease confined to one anatomic site or to two contiguous anatomic sites on the same side of the diaphragm

II. Disease in more than two anatomic sites or in two noncontiguous sites and confined to one side of the diaphragm

III. Disease on both sides of the diaphragm but confined to lymph nodes, spleen, and Waldeyer's ring

IV. Involvement of extranodal sites other than by direct invasion from affected node

For each stage in the classification A = asymptomatic, B = with typical symptoms (fever, weight loss, night sweats, etc).

PATHOLOGIC CLASSIFICATION (LUKES AND BUTLER)

Lymphocyte predominant
Lymphocyte depleted
Mixed cellularity
Nodular sclerosing

completing an adequate period of treatment. Less toxic drugs such as chlorambucil may be substituted for nitrogen mustard but may be less effective.

It is now customary to grade involvement with Hodgkin's disease from stage I through stage IV (Table 56), with the suffix "B" for those with typical symptoms and signs (weight loss of more than 10 per cent body weight over the preceding six months, night sweats, and unexplained fevers above 38° C). Disease above the diaphragm is readily detected clinically and radiologically, but subdiaphragmatic involvement is less easily excluded. Lymphangiography has been employed extensively in the past, but computerized axial tomography is simpler and probably as informative. Neither of these investigations can completely exclude intra-abdominal disease, and a laparotomy with splenectomy, liver biopsy, and abdominal lymph node biopsy is necessary unless the known extent of the disease indicates that chemotherapy is the treatment of choice.

The prognosis in advanced Hodgkin's disease is less favorable than in localized disease, but a 50 per cent five-year survival is not unrealistic, and many patients may be cured. The histologic pattern also affects prognosis. In particular, lymphocyte depletion is more common in stages III and IV and has a worse prognosis than lymphocyte predominant disease, which is seen more often in stages I and II. Nodular sclerosis is commonly associated with mediastinal involvement and also appears to have a poor prognosis.

The Non-Hodgkin's Lymphomas

The non-Hodgkin's lymphomas are a heterogenous group of malignant lymphomas whose only common feature is the absence of the typical multinucleate and mononuclear cells of Hodgkin's disease. The classification of these disorders is fraught with difficulties. Traditionally, this has been descriptive, but more recently various immunologic and histochemical techniques have been applied to the analysis of the lymphomatous cells in the hope of producing a more logical basis for understanding these disorders. Problems in classification have arisen mainly from a failure in the past to identify correctly the origin of various cell types in normal lymph nodes, let alone in lymphomatous tissue. As a result there are now at least five different classifications in current use. Recently the United States National Cancer Institute sponsored a wide-ranging clinicopathologic study of non-Hodgkin's lymphoma that resulted in a "Working Formulation for Clinical Usage." This classification (which may well become standard over the next few years) can be seen in Table 57.

Apart from helping to broaden understanding of the cellular nature of non-Hodgkin's lymphoma, the various classification schemes appear to have some intrinsic prognostic value and thus help the clinician to determine optimal therapy and to communicate the results of treatment trials to others. All of the existing schemes can identify histologic patterns that have a particularly good or bad prognosis. In general, patients with a small-cell pattern have "low-grade" disease and follow a relatively benign clinical course, although cure is rarely obtained in patients with the more diffuse patterns of disease. On the other hand, large-cell or "high-grade" patterns tend to be more rapidly progressive, and the early mortality is high. However, an aggressive approach similar to that employed in Hodgkin's disease may produce long-term survival or

TABLE 57. A WORKING FORMULATION OF NON-HODGKIN'S LYMPHOMAS FOR CLINICAL USAGE*

LOW GRADE	HIGH GRADE
Malignant lymphoma	Malignant lymphoma
Small lymphocyte	Large cell, immunoblastic
Consistent with chronic lymphatic leukemia	Plasmacytoid
Plasmacytoid	Clear cell
Malignant lymphoma, follicular	Polymorphous
Predominantly small cleaved cell	Epithelioid cell component
Diffuse areas	Malignant lymphoma
Sclerosis	Lymphoblastic
Malignant lymphoma, follicular	Convoluted cell
Mixed, small cleaved and large cell	Nonconvoluted cell
Diffuse areas	Malignant lymphoma
Sclerosis	Small noncleaved cell
INTERMEDIATE GRADE	Burkitt's
Malignant lymphoma, follicular	Follicular areas
Predominantly large cell	Miscellaneous
Diffuse areas	Composite
Sclerosis	Mycosis fungoides
Malignant lymphoma, diffuse	Histiocytic
Small cleaved cell	Extramedullary plasmacytoma
Sclerosis	Unclassifiable
Malignant lymphoma, diffuse	Other
Mixed, small and large cell	
Sclerosis	
Epithelioid cell component	
Malignant lymphoma, diffuse	
Large cell	
Cleaved cell	
Noncleaved cell	
Sclerosis	

*From National Cancer Institute Sponsored Study of Classifications of Non-Hodgkin's Lymphomas. Summary and Description of a Working Formulation for Clinical Usage. Cancer 49:2112–2135, 1982.

even cure in a high percentage of cases, so that paradoxically the long-term prognosis may be more favorable than in the low-grade types of disease.

Functional Characteristics of Non-Hodgkin's Lymphoma. With a variety of immunologic techniques it is now possible to characterize the phenotype of the malignant cell in the vast majority of cases of non-Hodgkin's lymphoma, and in most instances the cells have a B cell phenotype, as judged by the presence of surface or cytoplasmic immunoglobulin. Furthermore, in a small number of patients a monoclonal paraprotein (pp. 283 to 284) may be found in the serum. A clonal origin for the neoplasm may also be inferred from the finding of only one light-chain type on the affected cells. In contrast, only about 5 to 10 per cent of cases of non-Hodgkin's lymphoma have a T cell phenotype. The recent development of a variety of monoclonal antibodies to different T cell subsets allows a more detailed characterization of this group of disorders, but unfortunately no definitive marker for T cell clonality is yet available.

True histiocytic lymphomas (that is, neoplasms of monocyte-macrophage origin) are even less common. These include *histiocytic medullary reticulosis,* which is an aggressive malignant disorder with widespread proliferation of malignant histiocytes. Phagocytosis of erythrocytes, granulocytes, and platelets is evident throughout the reticuloendothelial system and produces a severe pancytopenia. The term *"histiocytosis-X"* is used to describe a group of conditions characterized by abnormal histiocytic proliferation. Included are the relatively benign *eosinophilic granuloma* and the rapidly progressive malignant condition of diffuse histiocytosis or *Letterer-Siwe disease.*

Etiology of Non-Hodgkin's Lymphoma. The etiology of non-Hodgkin's lymphoma is unknown, although in common with the leukemias and Hodgkin's disease there is a strong suspicion that certain viruses may play a part in the pathogenesis of some if not all of these tumors. Of particular interest has been the relationship of Burkitt's lymphoma to infection with the Epstein-Barr virus (EBV). Burkitt's lymphoma is a high-grade lymphoblastic lymphoma of B cell origin that is unusually common in East African children, in whom it appears with tumors of the jaw and abdomen. The EB virus was first isolated from cultures of Burkitt's lymphoma cells and has since been shown to be the causative agent of infectious mononucleosis. This is primarily an infection of B cells, and resolution of the illness follows successful suppression of the infected cells by T cells. The virus is not completely eliminated, however, and remains latent. Furthermore, EBV-infected B cells undergo a change of kinetic behavior in vitro, which readily allows the establishment of "immortalized" cell lines. In areas of Africa where Burkitt's lymphoma is endemic, EB virus infections are extremely common in infancy or early childhood, when they are often subclinical. It seems most unlikely that EBV is directly responsible for malignant transformation, but latently infected cells may be more susceptible to subsequent transforming events. The geographical distribution of Burkitt's lymphoma in Africa is similar to that of malaria, and it has been suggested that persistent malarial infection during childhood chronically stimulates the immune system and further increases its susceptibility to a transforming event.

The majority of patients with Burkitt's lymphoma and phenotypically related acute leukemias and lymphomas have a consistent translocation between the long arms of chromosomes 8 and 14 (t[8;14][q24;q32]). It has recently been shown that the cellular oncogene *c-myc* is situated on chromosome 8, and this translocation carries the oncogene to a position in chromosome 14 close to the immunoglobulin heavy chain region. Activation of the *myc* oncogene following this translocation could thus represent the final step required for the development of this tumor.

However, Burkitt's lymphoma represents a small proportion of non-Hodgkin's lymphoma, and in the majority of cases no such obvious etiologic factors have been detected. There is an increased incidence in survivors of atomic bomb irradiation, in some families with inherited immune deficiency states, and also in patients who have had long-term immunosuppressive treatment for other disorders. Furthermore, nonrandom chromosomal abnormalities are being increasingly recognized, and it seems likely that a multistep process similar to that described for Burkitt's lymphoma is involved in the development of other kinds of lymphoma.

Clinical Features. The clinical picture of non-Hodgkin's lymphoma is broadly similar to that of Hodgkin's disease with the exception that the disease is often more widespread at initial examination (Table 54). Involvement of the gut lymphatic tissue, particularly in Waldeyer's ring (the tonsils and adenoids), and of the liver, spleen, and bone marrow are all common. Diffuse gut involvement may result in malabsorption with abdominal and digestive symptoms. Local pressure from nodal enlargement may produce mediastinal obstruction, bowel or urinary symptoms, or obstructive lymphedema in the extremities. Extranodal spread is common and may occur in any site, including the central nervous system.

Primary extranodal non-Hodgkin's lymphoma is seen occasionally. Primary intracranial disease is extremely rare, but an association with recent EB virus infection has recently been shown. Primary lymphoma involving the skin is more common and often shows a T cell phenotype; this may reflect the tendency for normal T lymphocytes to recirculate through the skin. One interesting but rare form of T cell lymphoma is the *Sézary syndrome.* This condition is related to the dermatologic curiosity *mycosis fungoides,* which is characterized by erythroderma and subsequent plaque formation in the skin, which may progress to actual tumors. Abnormal mononuclear cells (the Sézary cells) may be found in the blood. The Sézary syndrome itself consists of generalized erythroderma and lymphadenopathy with the appearance of similar abnormal cells in the skin and blood. These cells have the characteristics of T cells that in some instances may be of the helper variety.

Hematologic Findings. In patients with localized disease there may be no hematologic abnormality, but a normochromic anemia is common in more advanced disease. Autoimmune hemolysis, marrow infiltration, and hypersplenism all occur more frequently than in Hodgkin's disease. Lymphomatous cells may appear in the peripheral blood, particularly in the later stages of the disease when the picture may resemble a leukemia.

The majority of cases of non-Hodgkin's lymphoma are B cell neoplasms. Suppression of immunoglobulin production may be marked, and a monoclonal paraprotein may occasionally be detected. Cellular immunity is well preserved, in contrast to Hodgkin's disease, but this may be affected by treatment and may be impaired in patients with T cell disorders.

Course and Prognosis. The broad relationship between the histologic pattern of non-Hodgkin's lymphoma and ultimate prognosis has already been mentioned. Various clinical features also have some prognostic significance. The most important appears to be the presence or absence of constitutional symptoms such as fever, weight loss, and night sweats, since these considerably worsen the prognosis. The age of the patient is probably also important: non-Hodgkin's lymphoma becomes commoner with advancing age, and many patients with high-grade lymphomas that might ordinarily respond to aggressive chemotherapy may therefore be unsuitable for this form of treatment. Although many patients have apparently localized disease, it should be remembered that the non-Hodgkin's lymphoma is a disorder affecting cells that normally recirculate freely. It is therefore not surprising that successful treatment of localized disease by radiotherapy may be followed by later recurrence at a remote site.

CHRONIC LYMPHATIC LEUKEMIA

Chronic lymphatic leukemia is a neoplastic disorder characterized by clonal proliferation of lymphocytes at an intermediate stage of development. The affected cells are long-lived but unable to complete terminal differentiation to functionally competent cells. They thus accumulate in the bone marrow, peripheral blood, and lymphatic tissue and produce a clinical picture of variable severity ranging from asymptomatic lymphocytosis to a progressive fatal disorder with widespread lymphadenopathy, hepatosplenomegaly, and marrow failure. In 95 per cent of cases the malignant lymphocytes have a B cell phenotype, the majority of the remainder being of T cell origin. In the latter the disease tends to run a more aggressive course.

Chronic lymphatic leukemia is the commonest of the leukemias. It is principally a disease of later life and affects males twice as often as females. Unlike other forms of leukemia, no relationship with previous radiation exposure has been demonstrated. On the other hand, a strong genetic basis is recognized and familial cases are not uncommon. Recently a number of patients with T cell leukemia-lymphoma have been described in whom there was evidence for infection with a human retrovirus. This association is discussed on p. 272.

Clinical Features. Patients with chronic lymphatic leukemia may be entirely asymptomatic, the disease being discovered accidentally in the course of routine checks or investigation of unrelated symptoms. However, some degree of generalized lymphadenopathy is usual and in some instances this may be severe (Fig. 62). Lymph node biopsy shows histologic features of a diffuse lymphocytic or centrocytic lymphoma. Hepatosplenomegaly is common and in some patients splenomegaly may be a dominant feature. Mild to moderate normochromic anemia with a variable thrombocytopenia occurs in advanced cases, and autoimmune he-

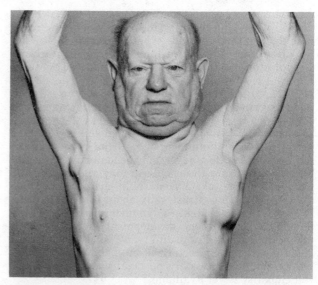

Figure 62. Generalized lymphadenopathy of exceptional degree in a patient with chronic lymphatic leukemia. The patient complained only of deafness and was unaware of the enlarged nodes.

molysis is not uncommon. The leukocyte count is elevated with an absolute lymphocytosis. The actual lymphocyte count correlates poorly with other features of the disease but may reach 100 to 200,000/μl or rarely higher. The lymphocytes have a mature appearance, although a proportion of cells are larger, and bare nuclei (smear cells) are frequent. Bone marrow examination shows a marked infiltration with lymphocytes, and in severe cases residual normal marrow cells may be infrequent. Hypogammaglobulinemia reflecting defective B cell function is almost always present, and recurrent infections, particularly with pneumococci and hemophilus, are common.

Course and Prognosis. Asymptomatic patients with minimal clinical disease or simply a peripheral blood lymphocytosis may progress slowly, if at all, and treatment is not required. The prognosis for such patients is excellent, and making allowances for the fact that such patients are often elderly, survival of 10 years is not exceptional. On the other hand, for symptomatic patients disease progression and response to treatment is similar to that in patients with low-grade diffuse non-Hodgkin's lymphoma. Cure is not possible, but relatively simple chemotherapy using an alkylating agent such as chlorambucil with or without corticosteroids can often control the disease effectively for many months or years. In some patients, however, the disease follows a more aggressive course and treatment may be unsuccessful.

Variants of Chronic Lymphatic Leukemia

Two rather uncommon lymphoproliferative disorders that appear to be variants of chronic lymphatic leukemia are *prolymphocytic leukemia* and *hairy-cell leukemia*. Prolymphocytic leukemia is characterized by massive splenomegaly and a markedly increased leukocyte count in which many of the cells are large nucleated cells with the characteristics of prolymphocytes. For some reason lymphadenopathy is minimal or absent. The disease does not respond well to chemotherapy, but splenectomy may afford considerable symptomatic relief.

Patients with hairy-cell leukemia also have marked splenomegaly and only trivial lymphadenopathy. In contrast to prolymphocytic leukemia, there is usually pancytopenia with an excess of mononuclear cells, which under light and electron microscopy have a number of villous projections that give them a "hairy" appearance. The exact origin of these cells is controversial. They have phagocytic properties but many of the characteristics of B cell origin. There is often increased reticulin fibrosis in the marrow, which may be difficult to aspirate. Again, treatment with chemotherapy is unrewarding, but splenectomy may be followed by remission of symptoms for several years. This condition may respond to α-interferon.

THE PARAPROTEINEMIAS

The paraproteinemias are monoclonal proliferations of B cells, plasma cells, or intermediates in which there is excessive production of immunoglobulin or immunoglobulin subunits. The abnormal immunoglobulin (paraprotein) migrates electrophorectically as a single narrow band, is of one class, and has only one type of light chain (Fig. 63). These features are taken as evidence for monoclonality; on the rare occasions that it can be demonstrated, the immunoglobulin has spec-

TABLE 58. CHARACTERISTICS OF MALIGNANT PARAPROTEINEMIAS

1. Progressive increase in amount of paraprotein
2. Immunosuppression: reduced levels of normal serum immunoglobulins, plasma cells in rectal biopsy, and normal circulating B cells
3. Morphologic plasma cell abnormalities
4. Urinary excretion of immunoglobulin light chains in addition to presence of serum paraprotein

ificity for only one or, at most, a very limited number of antigens.

Paraproteinemia is often an incidental finding and may not be associated with any clinical disturbance. Symptoms may arise from the physical properties of the paraprotein itself or as a result of the underlying cellular proliferation. While some of these disorders are clearly malignant, the neoplastic nature of some of the more benign paraproteinemias has not been proved. Useful criteria for the identification of malignant paraproteinemias are shown in Table 58.

MYELOMATOSIS

Myelomatosis is a malignant proliferation of plasma cells. It is principally a disease of late middle to old age, although it is occasionally seen in younger adults and rarely in children. The clinical picture ranges from a slowly progressive disorder that may be accidentally

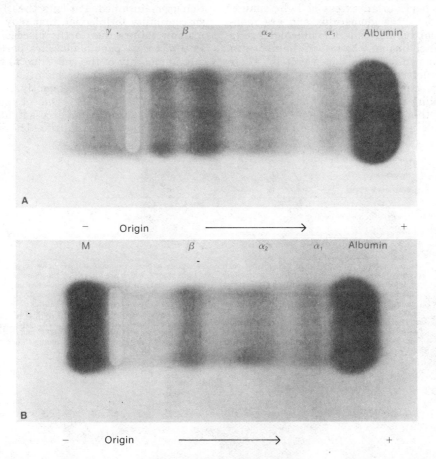

Figure 63. Multiple myelomatosis. *A,* A protein electrophoretic strip from an individual with infection and a diffuse increase in beta- and gammaglobulins. *B,* A protein electrophoretic strip from a patient with multiple myeloma showing a tight M component behind the origin.

discovered in the course of some other investigation to a rapidly progressive illness of grave prognosis.

Pathophysiology. The malignant proliferation is most evident in the marrow as a diffuse infiltration with abnormal plasma cells (Fig. 64), but multiple or solitary local osteolytic plasma cell tumors are equally characteristic. The malignant cells are not confined to the marrow, and although lymphadenopathy is unusual, abnormal plasma cells are found in lymph nodes at autopsy in many cases. Apparently normal lymph node lymphocytes may also show a monoclonal pattern of SmIg, suggesting that the neoplastic process may involve a population of B cells that circulates preferentially to, or originates from, the marrow and that retains the capacity to differentiate into recognizable secretory but functionally inept plasma cells.

Bone destruction (Fig. 65) may result in local pain, pathologic fractures, or vertebral collapse, often with neurologic damage. Hypercalcemia is common and produces the clinical picture of thirst, polyuria, constipation, and renal failure. It may be precipitated by a period of immobility, such as may follow a pathologic fracture or accompany an infective episode. Extramedullary plasmacytomas may develop, often as a direct extension of medullary disease—for example, in the chest wall or spine.

The abnormal clone of plasma cells usually secretes a monoclonal protein. This may consist of intact immunoglobulin molecules, but often an imbalance of chain production leads to an excess of light chains. These are filtered by the glomerulus and are reabsorbed by the renal tubular cells. Tubular damage is common and light-chains may be lost in the urine, in which they are known as Bence-Jones protein. Their presence may be detected simply by heating the urine—the protein precipitates at 40 to 50° C, redissolves on heating to boiling point, and reappears on cooling at about 70° C. Other urinary proteins precipitate at about 60° C and do not redissolve at the higher temperature. This test is insensitive to small quantities of light chains, which may be more readily detected by electrophoresis of concentrated urine. Immunoelectrophoresis shows the light chains of myeloma to be either kappa or lambda rather than both. In general, their presence suggests a functionally less well-differentiated tumor, and in some instances immunoglobulin production may be so deranged that only light chains are produced.

The presence of monoclonal immunoglobulin in the blood accounts for the characteristic elevation of the erythrocyte sedimentation rate. The paraprotein is most commonly IgG, but IgA and IgM myelomas are not infrequent. Very high levels of circulating paraprotein may increase blood viscosity and produce characteristic clinical symptoms. Because of its greater molecular size, IgM is the most likely to produce hyperviscosity, but the tendency for IgA to polymerize results in hyperviscosity in at least 15 per cent of patients with IgA myeloma. Very high levels of IgG are needed for similar problems to occur with this immunoglobulin (Fig. 66). The clinical effects of hyperviscosity include spontaneous bleeding or bruising, loss of vision due to retinal hemorrhage, and neurologic signs ranging from drowsiness to coma.

In common with other malignant B cell neoplasms, there is a reduction in normal immunoglobulin production, and this is a valuable point of distinction from the benign paraproteinemias, in which normal production is maintained. Patients thus have an increased susceptibility to infection that may be aggravated by marrow failure due to the disease or its treatment. Pneumococcal pneumonias are particularly common, and immobility of the chest due to painful rib lesions may contribute to the problem.

Renal failure occurs frequently in myeloma and is a common cause of death. One of the most important factors in hypercalcemia, excess light chain production may also cause renal failure. The mechanism is not

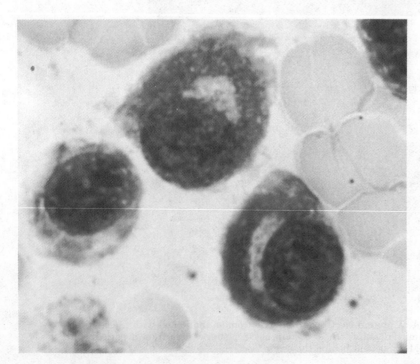

Figure 64. Abnormal plasma cells in the marrow of a patient with multiple myeloma.

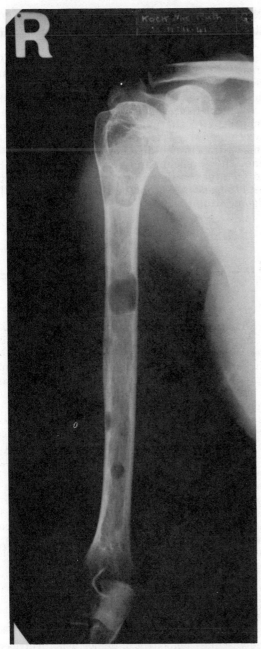

Figure 65. The humerus of a patient with multiple myelomatosis shows multiple punched out areas typical of the disorder.

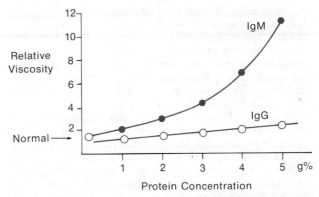

Figure 66. Effect of increasing levels of IgM and IgG on serum viscosity. Note the exponential increase in viscosity in IgM paraproteinemia as compared with the modest linear increase in IgG disorders. (From Fahey, J. L., et al.: J.A.M.A. 192:120, 1965.)

fragments of immunoglobulin light chains. Infiltration with this substance occurs in a variety of tissues, but when associated with the paraproteinemias it characteristically affects the kidneys, with development of a nephrotic syndrome, and also the tongue, heart, skeletal muscle, skin, gut, and nervous system.

Clinical Features. The clinical features of myelomatosis may be deduced from the above description. Certain features occur more frequently with a particular immunoglobulin class, as shown in Table 59. As mentioned above, the condition may be accidentally discovered and progression may be slow. A particularly bad prognosis is associated with the presence of renal impairment or anemia at diagnosis. Patients without these features may have a good prospect of survival for several years.

WALDENSTRÖM'S MACROGLOBULINEMIA

This condition is a slowly progressive B cell neoplasm in which the neoplastic cells do not differentiate fully to plasma cells, yet they secrete IgM. The disease

completely known; in the early stages hyaline bodies—presumably aggregated light chains—are seen in the tubular cells. Later, the tubular cells atrophy and there is dilatation of distal tubules and collecting ducts that appear to be obstructed by polychromatophilic casts surrounded by multinucleated giant cells. The glomeruli are usually spared unless there is associated amyloidosis, when a nephrotic syndrome is seen. Dehydration, from whatever cause, is often the precipitating factor in the development of renal failure.

Not uncommonly, patients with myeloma and other paraproteinemias develop amyloidosis. Amyloid substance consists of a network of fibrils that are, in fact,

TABLE 59. CLINICAL FEATURES OF MYELOMATOSIS RELATED TO IMMUNOGLOBULIN CLASS*†

	IgG	IgA	Bence Jones Only‡
Percentage of patients§	53	22	20
Mean doubling time myeloma protein/months	10.1	6.3	3.4
Mean serum M-protein concentration g/100 ml	4.3	2.8	—
Normal Ig < 20%	68	30	19
Infections requiring hospital admission	60	33	20
Osteolytic bone lesions	55	65	78
Hypercalcemia	33	59	62
Blood urea > 79 mg	16	17	33

*Data from Hobbs, J. R.: *In* Blood and Its Disorders. Oxford, Blackwell Scientific Publications, 1974; and Bergasel, D. E. *In* Cancer Therapy; Prognosis Factors and Criteria of Response. Staquel, M. J. (ed.): New York, Raven Press, 1975.
†Figures show percentage of patients affected unless otherwise stated.
‡Patients with light chain excretion without serum paraprotein.
§IgD, IgM, and IgE account for the remainder.

is one of later life and may be discovered accidentally. It often appears with symptoms of anemia or hyperviscosity, due to higher levels of circulating IgM. The disease may be considered as a B cell neoplasm intermediate between the non-Hodgkin's lymphomas and myeloma. There is widespread infiltration with lymphocytic cells showing variable plasmacytoid features, but only IgM and IgD are produced.

Renal insufficiency is much less common than in myeloma. Bone destruction and hypercalcemia do not occur, and although Bence-Jones protein may be detected in 25 per cent of cases, the amount is rarely sufficient to cause renal damage. However, a nephrotic syndrome can occur from glomerular deposition of IgM or as a feature of amyloidosis.

HEAVY CHAIN DISEASES

These are exceedingly rare but interesting monoclonal conditions in which there is proliferation of B cells that have lost the capacity to synthesize light chains. Thus they elaborate only fragments of immunoglobulin heavy chains of one type α, β, or γ. In some instances, there is a lymphoma-like illness. Perhaps as a reflection of the abundance of IgA-producing plasma cells in the gut, the Mediterranean type of heavy chain diseases are manifested as intestinal lymphomas with chronic diarrhea and a sprue-like syndrome. They predominantly affect patients who have lived in areas with a high incidence of intestinal infestation and may thus be related to chronic local antigenic stimulation.

Hemostasis and Thrombosis

The arrest of hemorrhage after damage to a blood vessel is a remarkably efficient protective mechanism. During human evolution the development of an efficient hemostatic mechanism must have been a vital adaptive function for early humans and their forebears in the wild. On the other hand, what appears to be a deviation of this process—pathologic thrombus formation—is a major cause of morbidity and mortality, particularly in the more affluent modern societies.

In this section the hemostatic mechanism and its relationship to pathologic bleeding and thrombosis are described. Many bleeding disorders can be readily explained in terms of definable lesions of blood vessels, platelets, or the coagulation pathway. On the other hand, thrombotic disease appears to be the end result of the interactions of a large number of ill-defined genetic and acquired abnormalities, some of which have no obvious connection with hemostasis. While this discrepancy undoubtedly reflects our current state of ignorance about the extraordinarily complex mechanisms that maintain the balance between hemostasis and thrombosis, the fact remains that it has not yet been possible to ascribe any of the common forms of arterial or venous thrombotic disease to primary abnormalities of the components of the hemostatic mechanism.

THE HEMOSTATIC MECHANISM

Hemostasis results from the interaction of a series of mechanisms that operate either immediately following injury to a blood vessel or over a longer period of time to consolidate the process. The immediate reaction to injury has two components: vasoconstriction caused by contraction of the muscle of the vessel wall and the formation of a hemostatic plug by masses of aggregated platelets. The consolidation process is the formation of a fibrin clot, or thrombus, which is the end result of a chain reaction involving the various factors that make up the coagulation system. It appears that platelet plug formation is particularly important in small ves-

sels, whereas vascular constriction and fibrin clot formation play a major role in achieving hemostasis in larger vessels.

The hemostatic system is balanced by an equally complex set of mechanisms that are designed to maintain blood in a fluid state. Both cellular and circulating components are involved. The cellular component consists of the reticuloendothelial system, the cells of which may be able to remove activated clotting factors without affecting their inactive precursors, and the vascular endothelium, which, while contributing to hemostasis, is also adapted to prevent inappropriate thrombus formation. These cellular mechanisms are supported by a series of enzymes designed to inactivate various components of the coagulation system. Presumably the hemostatic processes and those that counteract them are in a state of balanced equilibrium, the disturbance of which leads to bleeding or pathologic thrombosis.

THE VASCULAR COMPONENTS OF HEMOSTASIS

The vascular component of hemostasis involves contraction of the wall of blood vessels and a series of interactions with platelets and coagulation factors mediated by the constituents and products of the vessel wall and its endothelial lining.

COMPONENTS OF THE VESSEL WALL

Functionally, the important components of the vessel wall are the endothelial cells, the basement membrane, and the intercellular matrix, and smooth muscle cells.

The endothelial cells are elongated, with the long axis in the direction of blood flow. They are 25 to 50 μm long and 10 to 15 μm wide and overlap to some degree. Two types of junctions between these cells, tight and gap, have been described. The tight junctions are more common in arteries, but both types occur throughout the circulation, except in capillaries in which there are no gap junctions. It is thought that the form of junction is critical for limitation of trans-endothelial exchange of substances other than water and small molecules. The main function of the endothelial cell is to form a mechanical barrier with the facility for selective diffusion and transport. Its negative charge may be important in preventing the adherence of platelets, which are also negatively charged. These cells have a considerable capacity for protein synthesis. They are believed to produce angiotensin converting enzymes that are responsible for the cleavage of angiotensin I to produce angiotensin II, factor VIII–related antigen or the von Willebrand factor, plasminogen activator, antithrombin III, Hageman factor, and tissue thromboplastin. They are also involved in prostaglandin synthesis, and they metabolize exogenous nucleotides, ATP and ADP, with the production of AMP and adenosine. The functions of these various products and their metabolic activities are considered in the discussion of the different phases of hemostasis.

The basement membrane that underlies the endothelial layer contains three important components: collagen fibers, a filtering system of proteoglycans, and the cell-binding proteins laminen and fibronectin. These substances are probably synthesized by the endothelium; smooth muscle cells in the media of arteries produce similar components in the media and internal elastic lamina.

The main cellular components of the media of mammalian blood vessels are the smooth muscle cells. The adventitia also contains fibroblasts. The smooth muscle cells synthesize types I and III collagen and the glycosaminoglycans (GAG) chondroitin sulfate and dermatin sulfate. These cells have two main functions: synthesis of the vessel support matrix and contractility. Following damage to a vessel, there is a loss of differentiation of some of the smooth muscle cells with the appearance of mitoses and cell divisions. Proliferation, migration, and synthetic activities in smooth muscle cells are influenced by the number of plasma components, which include insulin, somatomedins, and lipoproteins as well as locally produced prostaglandins.

THE HEMOSTATIC FUNCTIONS OF THE VESSEL WALL

Injury to an artery is followed by vasoconstriction. This occurs in vessels of all sizes and may persist as a powerful spasm in larger arteries for up to 20 minutes or more and in smaller arteries for 5 to 10 minutes. The fact that this response occurs in denervated vessels suggests that it may result from the stimulation of local reflexes. The chemical messages that trigger it are poorly characterized; angiotensin II and prostanoids liberated from the arterial wall together with serotonin and thromboxane A_2 released by platelets are among the likely candidates.

Local mechanical factors may also play a role in hemostasis. Equalization of pressure between the interior of the vessel and the tissues may follow a rise in external pressure—by hematoma formation, for example—or a fall in the intraluminal pressure, which may occur locally or as part of the generalized fall in blood pressure that occurs in shock. These changes probably play a relatively minor part in the hemostatic process. However, the vessel wall probably plays a more fundamental role through its interactions with

platelets and by its participation in initiating both the intrinsic and extrinsic coagulation pathways.

Endothelial cells contain tissue thromboplastic activity in an inactive or sequestered form. After injury to a vessel, this material is activated and released by an unknown mechanism and hence is made available to help initiate the extrinsic pathway of coagulation. Subendothelial collagen fibers are involved in the intrinsic pathway of blood coagulation by participating in the activation of factor XII (see p. 302). The vessel wall is also closely involved with platelets in the hemostatic process, and interaction of platelets with subendothelial collagen triggers off the complex series of events that results in the formation of a hemostatic plug. The endothelial cells also synthesize the von Willebrand factor, a large glycoprotein with a molecular weight of greater than one million daltons, which is part of the factor VIII complex (see p. 303). This factor is essential for normal platelet function.

The vessel wall is also involved in the inhibition of platelet aggregation and blood coagulation. It may thus play an important role in limiting the local extension of thrombus and in preventing pathologic arterial and venous thrombosis. Endothelial cells synthesize and secrete plasminogen activator. This function may play a part in preventing thrombosis, particularly in the venous system. The vascular endothelium also produces several potent inhibitors of platelet aggregation, the most important of which is the prostaglandin PGI_2 or prostacyclin, which is derived from arachidonic acid via cyclic endoperoxides (Fig. 67). Prostacyclin synthesis is stimulated by thrombin, trypsin, or calcium ionophore. It has been suggested that basal prostacyclin production by intact vascular endothelium may be sufficient to prevent platelet aggregation in intact vessels and that increased production in response to mechanical injury or thrombin may provide a regulatory mechanism for the limitation of the extension of hemostatic plugs and thrombi after injury. This topic is discussed further with the relationship between prostaglandin metabolism and platelet function. The vessel wall also produces ADPase, which by reducing the local ADP concentration may play an important part in limiting platelet aggregation. Other products with potential antithrombotic effects include antithrombin III, heparin, and heparin sulfate and related sulfated substances.

Some of the hemostatic functions of vascular endothelium are summarized in Table 60. Clearly, the role of the vessel wall in hemostasis goes far beyond simple vasoconstriction. Rather, it is involved in activation of platelets and the coagulation pathway and in the neutralization of platelet action and thrombus formation.

DISORDERS OF THE VASCULAR PHASE OF HEMOSTASIS: NONTHROMBOCYTOPENIC PURPURA

The vascular purpuras are an extremely heterogenous group of conditions characterized by a tendency to bleed from small vessels in the absence of any demonstrable abnormality in platelet numbers or function or of the coagulation system. A partial list of these disorders is shown in Table 61. In the brief account that follows a few of the better defined vascular pur-

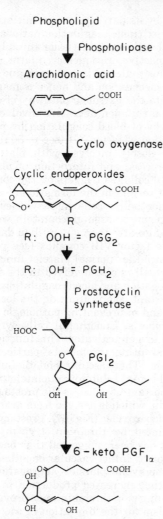

Figure 67. Synthesis of prostacyclin (PGI₂) by vascular tissues. (From Hardisty, R. M.: *Blood and Its Disorders*. 2nd ed. Hardisty, R. M., and Weatherall, D. J. (eds.). Oxford, Blackwell Scientific Publications, 1982.)

puras have been selected to illustrate some of the ways in which damage to the vessel wall is mediated.

Mechanical Purpura

Mechanical strain on small vessels may be increased in several ways, including raised intraluminal pressure and lack of adequate tissue support leading to increased shear stress.

Local purpura may occur as a result of increased intravascular pressure, particularly in small venules. There are several clinical examples of bleeding from this mechanism. It is responsible for the orthostatic purpura that occurs over the ankles of patients with varicose veins or other forms of venous insufficiency of the lower limbs and for the widespread purpura over the face and eyelids that occurs after bouts of coughing, vomiting, or after asphyxiation.

Senile purpura is the name given to the occurrence of ecchymotic lesions on the extensor surfaces of the arms and legs of elderly people. Because these occur in areas where the skin is normally freely mobile over deeper structures, they are thought to result from

TABLE 60. SOME HEMOSTATIC FUNCTIONS OF VASCULAR ENDOTHELIUM

Thrombogenic
  Synthesis
    Von Willebrand factor
    Tissue thromboplastin
    Collagen
    Fibronectin
    Mucopolysaccharides
Nonthrombogenic
  Synthesis
    Prostacyclin
    Antithrombin III
    Plasminogen activator
    Angiotensin converting enzyme
  Metabolism of released platelet aggregating substances
    ADPase
    Serotonin uptake
  Physical and binding properties
    Negative charge
    Heparin binding
    α2 macroglobulin binding

rupture of small vessels being subjected to increased shear strains because of a loss of subcutaneous tissue elasticity with age. It seems likely that the purpura that occurs in Cushing's syndrome or in patients receiving corticosteroids has a similar basis.

Scurvy

Vitamin C deficiency is characterized by perifollicular hemorrhages, ecchymoses, and in infancy by subperiosteal bleeding. Ascorbate deficiency leads to abnormal collagen formation as a result of defective hydroxyproline synthesis. This may be the basis for the abnormal vessel function in this disorder.

Allergic Purpura

The allergic purpuras are a group of nonthrombocytopenic purpuras characterized by a vasculitis involving the skin vessels, often in association with other

TABLE 61. MAIN GROUPS OF VASCULAR PURPURA

Mechanical
  Cough
  Orthostatic
  Asphyxiation
Allergic
  Henoch Schönlein
  Drug sensitivity
  Autoerythrocyte sensitization
  DNA sensitivity
Defective collagen synthesis
  Scurvy
Atrophic
  Senile
  Corticosteroids
  Cushing's syndrome
Paraproteinemia, Amyloidosis
Heredity
  Osler-Rendu-Weber
  Fabry's disease
  Inherited disorders of connective tissue
Disseminated intravascular coagulation
  Purpura gangrenosa

features of a hypersensitivity reaction such as urticaria, edema, and polyarthritis. These conditions occur in response to a variety of drugs or other allergens or may be part of an autoimmune disorder. In many forms of vascular purpura the putative sensitizing agent has not been identified.

The most well-defined form of allergic purpura is the *Henoch-Schönlein syndrome*. This condition is characterized by a slightly raised, symmetric, violaceous, macular eruption over the extensor surfaces of the limbs and buttocks, together with polyarthritis, abdominal pain, and in some cases nephritis. It occurs in several clinical forms, including an acute illness in childhood, which may be followed by complete recovery, a less common type with progressive renal disease, and a chronic relapsing type in adults. The pathogenesis is completely unknown. Microscopically, the characteristic lesion is a vasculitis that can be demonstrated by skin or renal biopsy. The renal lesion is a focal glomerular nephritis with fibrinoid deposition and mesangial proliferation. Deposits of IgA, C_{3c}, C_{3d}, and C_5, or, less commonly, IgM, C_4, and C_{3b} can be demonstrated by immunofluorescent analysis of skin lesions. C_{1q} and C_3 have not been found. These findings suggest alternate pathway activation of complement by IgA.

Vascular purpuras are also associated with drug therapy. Many drugs have been implicated, particularly the penicillins, sulfonamides, barbiturates, and thiazide diuretics. Although thought to have an allergic basis, very little is known about the pathophysiology of these conditions.

A curious type of sensitization purpura has been described in young women as *autoerythrocyte sensitization* or the *painful bruising syndrome*. This condition is characterized by the occurrence of spontaneous ecchymoses, often preceded by a tingling sensation and local edema at the site of the bruise. This condition may follow sensitization to components of the red cell membrane. A similar syndrome has been described in which lesions of this type can be produced by intradermal injection of autologous leukocytes or purified DNA but not by red cells.

Hereditary Vascular Purpuras

The best defined of the genetic purpuras is the autosomal dominant disorder *hereditary telangiectasia* or the *Osler-Rendu-Weber syndrome*. The vascular lesions are small angiomatous formations that occur on the skin of the face and lips, the mucous membrane of the mouth, and throughout the gastrointestinal tract. They often cause chronic gastrointestinal bleeding. They may not produce symptoms until adult life or even old age. In some cases they are associated with pulmonary arteriovenous fistulas.

Spontaneous bleeding into the skin is a feature of all the hereditary disorders of connective tissue.

Dysproteinemias and Amyloid Disease

The mechanism whereby the abnormal proteins that occur in macroglobulinemia, multiple myeloma, and cryoglobulinemia produce purpura is not understood. They may cause damage to vessel walls by producing capillary anoxia as a result of local hyperviscosity changes. They may also cause defective platelet function. In the syndrome of mixed cryoglobulinemia the vascular lesions result from immune complex damage to the vessels. The complexes consist of IgG and IgM, which has anti-IgG activity. The syndrome may be associated with a variety of underlying disorders, including infection and autoimmune conditions; in some cases no associated disease can be demonstrated.

Vascular purpura, particularly involving the eyelids, is occasionally seen in patients with amyloidosis.

Infection

Purpuric lesions occur commonly in patients with bacterial septicemia or viremia. The pathophysiology of the vascular damage is not fully understood. In some instances it probably follows small vascular infarcts, while in others it may result from immune complex damage to the vascular endothelium. More extensive damage to the skin may occur in septicemia or viremia following beta-hemolytic streptococcal, meningococcal, or varicella infections, for example. There is discoloration of the skin followed by extensive hemorrhage and, if the condition progresses, necrosis with full-thickness loss of skin. This condition, which is called *purpura gangrenosa,* is thought to result from local blockage of the skin vessels by fibrin deposition as part of the syndrome of intravascular coagulation (see p. 312). However, it is not clear why some patients develop localized gangrenous areas of the skin in association with intravascular coagulation, while others have generalized hemostatic failure without skin changes. This problem is discussed further with the consumption coagulopathies.

PLATELETS

Platelets play a major part in hemostasis by their ability to adhere to subendothelial collagen and aggregate to form a hemostatic plug. In addition, they are intimately involved in the process of blood coagulation. They may also play a role in other biologic processes, particularly in the response to infection.

STRUCTURE

On a well-stained peripheral blood film normal platelets appear as anucleate bodies about 2 to 4 μm in diameter with a volume of 7 to 8 fl. On Giemsa staining they are light blue and contain small purplish red granules. On electron microscopy they show three distinct structural zones, each of which appears to be related to a specific group of functions (Fig. 68). The peripheral zone is involved in adhesion and aggregation, the cytoplasmic or sol-gel zone in contraction, and the organelle zone in secretion.

The peripheral zone consists of a surface coat or glycocalyx made up of acid mucopolysaccharides and glycoproteins, a bilayer plasma membrane, and a submembranous area. The platelet surface also forms part of a surface-connected canalicular system that consists of invaginations of the surface membrane into the platelet cytoplasm. The glycocalyx is involved in platelet-platelet and platelet-surface interactions and provides the "trigger" mechanism whereby appropriate

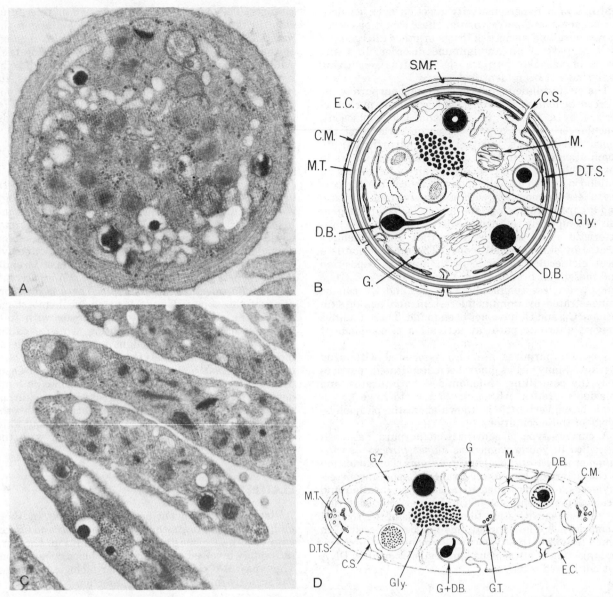

Figure 68. The fine structure of platelets. *A,* Electron micrograph of a platelet sectioned in the equatorial plane. *B,* Diagram of the platelet shown in *A.* EC = external coat; CM = cell membrane; SMF = submembranous microfilament; MT = microtubules; DTS = dense tubular system; CS = surface connected system; G = alpha granule; DB = dense body; M = mitochondrion; Gly = glycogen granules. *C,* Electronmicrograph of platelets sectioned transversely to the equatorial plane. *D,* Diagram of a platelet in transverse section. GT = tubules within an alpha granule; GZ = Golgi zone; other symbols are as in *B.* (From White, J. G.: *The Circulating Platelet.* Johnson, S. A., (ed.). New York, Academic Press. p. 45, 1971. Also from White, J. G.: *Platelet Aggregation.* Caen, J. (ed.) Paris, Maison et Sie, p. 15, 1971.)

stimuli are transmitted from the exterior to the interior of the platelet. There are specific binding sites for thrombin, ADP, epinephrine, plasminogen and the von Willebrand factor (factor VIIIR, p. 303). Analysis of the membrane glycoproteins by labeling and SDS-polyacrylamide gel electrophoresis shows that they consist of a series of components of different molecular weights. The nomenclature of these glycoproteins, together with their receptors and known functions, is summarized in Table 62. In a later section the rare genetic disorders that result from deficiencies of these different membrane components are considered, as well

as how their study is providing information about the functions of the membrane glycoproteins.

The phospholipid bilayer plays an important role in accelerating blood coagulation and contains enzymes involved in membrane transport and cyclic AMP metabolism.

In the submembranous region and cytoplasmic zone there are several fibrillary components. In the submembranous area bundles of microtubules composed of tubuli encircle the platelet and form a cytoskeleton, which serves to stabilize and maintain the shape of the cell. Microfilaments are distributed throughout the

TABLE 62. THE PLATELET MEMBRANE GLYCOPROTEINS WITH THEIR KNOWN FUNCTIONS

COMPONENTS	PROPERTIES	FINDINGS IN PLATELET FUNCTION DISORDERS
Ia (glycocalin) Ib	Sialic-acid–rich Thrombin receptor Drug-dependent antibody receptor	Deficient in Bernard-Soulier syndrome
IIa	—	—
IIb	—	—
IIIc	?Fibrin receptor PI^A antigenic site α-actin–related	Deficient in thrombasthenia
IIIb V	Thrombin receptor	—

platelet cytoplasm. They are composed of actin and myosin and are probably responsible for the coalescence of granules during platelet aggregation, contraction of pseudopods, and clot retraction. Platelet actin is similar in structure to muscle actin, but platelet myosin differs from muscle myosin in several respects.

The structural components of the organelle zone include glycogen-containing particles, mitochondria, and a variety of different types of membrane-enclosed granules. In a small proportion of platelets a distinctive Golgi apparatus can be seen. This region also contains a dense tubular system, which appears as an irregular series of channels lying under the band of microtubules and which may be analogous to the sarcoplasmic reticulum of muscle. There is evidence that this system is the site of synthesis of prostaglandin endoperoxides and thromboxane A_2. Finally, the surface-connecting canalicular system appears in this area as a series of spaces lined by a unit membrane with the glycocalyx on its inner surface.

The granules are the secretory bodies of the platelet. Three main types are recognized: alpha, dense, and lysosomal. These secretory organelles release their contents in response to stimuli such as thrombin, collagen, ADP, or adrenaline. Apparently the threshold for release of each type of granule is different; the sequence in order of increasing stimulation is alpha, dense, and lysosomal. The contents of these organelles are summarized in Table 63.

TABLE 63. PLATELET GRANULES AND THEIR CONTENTS

TYPE	CONTENTS
Dense bodies	ATP, ADP 5-HT Serotonin Epinephrine Ca^{++}
α granules	Platelet factor 4 β-Thromboglobulin Fibrinogen Fibronectin Growth factors Factor V von Willebrand factor
Lysozomes	Acid hydrolases
Peroxisomes	Catalase

In summary, the structure of the platelet is adapted to its hemostatic function. It has a complex membrane, which also forms part of a canalicular system involved in transport of various secretions to the surface, a cytoskeleton, a contractile system for its important motile functions, and series of secretory organelles, each separately adapted for specific functions.

THE FUNCTIONS OF PLATELETS IN HEMOSTASIS

Platelets play a central role in the sequence of events that follow injury to a vessel wall. In particular, they are able to adhere to structures in the wall, aggregate to form a hemostatic plug, and contribute to both local vasoconstriction and to blood coagulation. Since lack of platelets causes spontaneous purpura, they must also be essential for the maintenance of vascular integrity in the absence of injury. The mechanism of this important function is not understood; platelets may plug small gaps in the vascular endothelium that are caused by shedding of endothelial cells or minor trauma resulting from local changes in the caliber of the vessels.

The participation of platelets in the formation of a hemostatic plug occurs in several stages (Fig. 69) which, for descriptive purposes, can be divided into adhesion, release, aggregation, contribution to blood coagulation, and clot retraction. Platelet activation involves the interaction of an agonist with a membrane receptor and the transfer of the signal to the interior of the cell. The signal involves an increased local concentration of Ca^{++} and is modulated by cyclic AMP.

Adhesion. After injury to a vessel wall platelets adhere to subendothelial collagen and to a lesser extent to basement membranes. The regular-spaced free amino acid groups of collagen are of particular importance, and it has been suggested that fibronectin on the platelet surface may also interact with collagen. Thrombin, a product of the coagulation cascade, triggers platelet adhesion to tissues and increases the expression of the fibronectin antigen on platelet surfaces. From observations of patients with disorders characterized by defective platelet adhesion it appears

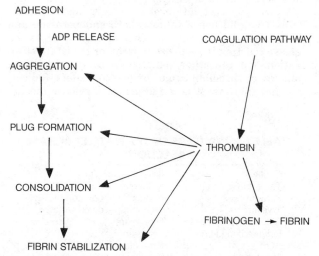

Figure 69. The main stages in the formation of a hemostatic plug. ADP = adenosine diphosphate.

that membrane glycoprotein 1 and factor VIIIR are essential for normal adhesion. Factor VIIIR, also known as the von Willebrand Factor (p. 303), has been shown to bind to both normal platelets in the presence of ristocetin (ristocetin cofactor activity, factor VIIIR:RC) and to arterial subendothelium. It may act as an agent for binding platelets to subendothelial structures. Platelet adhesion, unlike aggregation, is an irreversible process.

Release. After interacting with collagen, platelets release the contents of their granules in a process called "the release reaction." This reaction is also induced by thrombin and many other substances (Table 64); it is probable that both collagen and thrombin initiate release during hemostasis. The release reaction involves the contractile proteins within the cell and requires energy, which is derived from both the glycolytic pathway and the Krebs cycle. Both the release and aggregation mechanisms seem to be mediated by the concentration of cyclic AMP in the platelets, which is produced from ATP by adenylate cyclase and degraded by phosphodiesterase. Release is inhibited by agents such as prostacyclin that increase the concentration of cyclic AMP. On the other hand, other products of arachidonic acid metabolism (Figs. 67 and 70) play an important role in mediating the release reaction.

Both endothelial cells and platelets form PGG_2 and PGH_2 by a similar mechanism but the pathways then diverge; endothelial cells convert the endoperoxides to the aggregation inhibitor prostacyclin, while platelets form the aggregating agent thromboxane A_2 (Figs. 67 and 70). When platelets are stimulated by thrombin or ADP, free arachidonic acid is cleaved from platelet phospholipids by phospholipases C and A_2. Arachidonic acid is sequentially converted by cyclo-oxygenase to the cyclic endoperoxides PGG_2 and PGH_2. These are transformed to thromboxane A_2 by thromboxane synthetase. Thromboxane A_2 directly induces the release reaction, but being unstable it is rapidly transformed to thromboxane B_2, which is inactive. In the main alternative pathway for PGH_2 metabolism (Fig. 70) it is broken down to malonyl dialdehyde, but small amounts are converted to PGE_2, PGF_2, and PGD_2; the latter is an inhibitor of aggregation.

Aspirin, by acetylation of cyclo-oxygenase, renders it inactive and hence inhibits both endoperoxide and thromboxane A_2 formation. This in turn inhibits the release reaction in response to weak or moderate stimulation. On the other hand, high concentrations of collagen or thrombin can overcome this effect, indicating that there must be an alternative release mechanism.

TABLE 64. INDUCERS OF THE PLATELET RELEASE REACTION

Collagen	Bovine factor VIII
Thrombin	Ristocetin
Plasmin	Antigen-antibody complexes
Trypsin	γ-Globulin–coated surfaces
Calcium ionophores	Endotoxin
Polymerizing fibrin	Zymosan
ADP	Particulate fatty acids
Epinephrine	Viruses, bacteria
Arachidonic acid	Snake venoms

The precise consequences of the release reaction are not fully understood. ADP induces further aggregation, as mentioned below. Serotonin causes local vasoconstriction. Platelet factor 4 (see p. 293) neutralizes heparin, and the closely related protein β-thromboglobulin may inhibit prostacyclin generation in the vessel wall and thus contribute to the formation of the platelet plug and thrombus. Prostaglandin endoperoxides and thromboxane A_2 induce aggregation and stimulate further release, thus initiating a self-sustaining process. The physiologic function of platelet growth factor is not yet understood. This mitogenic protein, which has sequence homology with a recently defined oncogene, stimulates a variety of connective tissue cells, and its primary physiologic role may be in wound healing. This problem is treated later in the discussion of the role of platelets in the production of atheroma.

Aggregation. A major effect of the release reaction is to produce a high local concentration of ADP, which causes platelet aggregation leading to the formation of a hemostatic plug. The exact mechanism of the action of ADP on platelets is not clear. At low concentrations aggregation is reversible, whereas at higher concentrations it is irreversible. The initial step is thought to involve the binding of ADP to specific receptors on the platelet membrane. The first observable effect on platelets is a change in shape from smooth discs to spiny spheres with the formation of many pseudopodia. The process requires the presence of divalent cations and fibrinogen. Since the latter does not bind to thrombasthenic platelets, which are known to be deficient in membrane glycoproteins IIb and IIIa, it is possible that this glycoprotein complex carries a fibrinogen receptor that becomes exposed on the outer surface of the platelet in the course of its initial change in shape.

Apart from ADP there are a variety of other agents that cause platelet aggregation. These include thrombin, epinephrine, norepinephrine, 5-hydroxytryptamine (serotonin), cyclic endoperoxides and thromboxane A_2, vasopressin, and platelet activating factor (PAF). PAF is a lysolecithin analog, 1-0-alkyl-2-acetyl-sn-glyceryl-3-phosphorylcholine, derived from a variety of cells involved in the inflammatory response. PAF may be a mediator of an ADP- and arachidonic acid–independent pathway of platelet aggregation, but its role in platelet function remains to be further defined. Thrombin aggregates platelets at concentrations below those required to clot fibrinogen and, unlike ADP, does not require the presence of fibrinogen, possibly because it also stimulates the secretion of fibrinogen from platelets themselves. Low concentrations of epinephrine and thrombin also potentiate the aggregating activity of ADP.

Clearly, the interactions of the various mediators of release and aggregation are extremely complex and are not yet fully understood. The time course of aggregation and nucleotide release suggests that the former is not entirely dependent on the latter. Aggregation, thromboxane synthesis, and secretion from dense bodies act synergistically in the hemostatic process. All of these functions are energy-dependent and involve the breakdown of ATP, and they all can be inhibited by blocking glycolysis and oxidative phosphorylation. Progressively more energy is needed for the initial shape change of platelets, aggregation, thromboxane synthesis, secretion from alpha-granules and dense bodies,

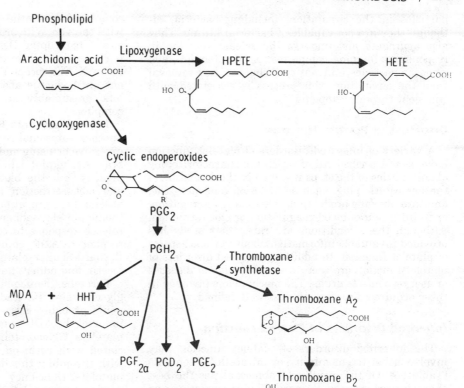

Figure 70. Pathways of arachidonic acid metabolism in human platelets. HPETE = 12-hydroperoxy-eicosatetranoic acid; HETE = 12-hydroxy-eicosatetranoic acid; MDA = malonyl dialdehyde; HHT = 12-hydroxy-hepatadecatrienoic acid. (From Hardisty, R. M.: *Blood and Its Disorders*. 2nd ed. Hardisty, R. M., and Weatherall, D. J. (eds.). Oxford, Blackwell Scientific Publications, 1982.)

and release of lysosomal enzymes. These functions are dependent on the intracellular mobilization of calcium, and it is likely that this is the main stimulus through which the binding of an aggregating agent to its receptor on the platelet membrane is coupled to these different responses.

Interactions with Blood Coagulation. Platelets interact with coagulation factors in several ways (see also later sections on coagulation). First, there is evidence that platelets can directly activate factor XI by bypassing the stage of contact activation (pp. 302 to 303). Second, activation of factor X by factors IXa and VIII is enhanced by their adsorption onto a phospholipid surface in the presence of calcium, and an appropriate surface is provided by the platelet membrane. Third, platelet factor (PF3) is the name given to a procoagulant activity that becomes available on the platelet membrane during aggregation and release. Stimulation by collagen and thrombin exposes active phospholipid sites on the platelet membrane, probably via a "flip-flop" mechanism by which phosphatidylserine and phosphatidylinositol are translocated from the inner to the outer leaflet of the membrane. Factor Va released from platelets binds to these sites and, in this state, forms a receptor for factor Xa in the presence of calcium; the binding of factor Xa is rapidly followed by thrombin formation on the platelet surface.

Various platelet factors (PFs) have been defined in terms of their interactions with the coagulation cascade. As platelet physiology has become better understood, it is clear that in some cases the "factors" reflect a particular platelet function or structural change rather than the production of a specific molecule. The platelet factors are distinguished from the coagulation factors by their designation with Arabic rather than Roman numerals. PF1 activity is attributable to adsorbed factor V, as mentioned above. PF2 accelerates the conversion of fibrinogen by thrombin and may neutralize antithrombin III. PF3 function has already been described. PF4, released from alpha-granules, is thought to neutralize heparin and also the inhibitory effects of fibrinogen degradation products on thrombin and on platelet aggregation. Platelets also have antithrombin activity and may play a role in the activation and inhibition of fibrinolysis (see below).

Clot Retraction. Platelets play a major role in clot retraction. This has been used as a test of platelet function for many years, although it is not clear to what extent it is a necessary component of hemostasis. Clot retraction depends on the contraction of actomyosin microfibrils in the platelet pseudopodia. This process is energy-dependent and is abolished by inhibition of glycolysis and oxidative phosphorylation. The actomyosin system is regulated by Ca++, which is stored in cytoplasmic vesicles. Extrusion of these vesicles is generated by prostaglandin endoperoxides and thromboxane A₂, which may act as physiologic calcium ionophores.

Other Functions. Platelets probably play a role in the inflammatory response, although its importance is not yet clear. They accumulate at sites of tissue damage and release several substances that increase vascular permeability and that are chemotactic or granulocytes. These include a cationic protein derived from the alpha-granules, which mediates its chemotactic effect through the fifth component of complement, and at least two products of arachidonic acid metabolism that increases vascular permeability. Platelets ingest particles in the circulation, including bacteria, although they are not capable of bacterial killing. They also aggregate and undergo the release reaction in response to immune complexes, aggregated IgG and zymosan particles, and may contribute to their removal from the circulation; this process is associated with transient thrombocytopenia.

DISORDERS OF PLATELET FUNCTION

A variety of inherited disorders of platelet function have been described, all of which are characterized by abnormalities of the steps involved in the formation of the hemostatic plug, such as adhesion, endoperoxide, and thromboxane production, release and aggregation, or in initiation of blood coagulation or clot retraction. Although these conditions are rare, their study has provided invaluable information about various aspects of platelet function. In addition, acquired disorders of platelet function are seen in a wide range of diseases or as a response to drugs. The mechanisms involved in these acquired disorders are less well defined.

Inherited Disorders of Platelet Function

The inherited disorders of platelet function may involve either the membrane or intracellular contents (Table 65). Of the membrane abnormalities the best characterized are the *Bernard-Soulier syndrome* and *thrombasthenia*. Of the intracellular defects, dense body and alpha-granule deficiencies and disorders of thromboxane synthesis are the most clearly defined.

Bernard-Soulier Syndrome. This is a rare autosomal recessive condition characterized by bleeding into the skin and mucous membranes, a prolonged bleeding time, a normal or reduced platelet count, defective prothrombin consumption, and unusually large platelets. The platelets adhere normally to collagen in vitro and aggregate and release normally in response to ADP or collagen. However, they do not aggregate in response to von Willebrand factor and ristocetin and do not adhere normally to the subendothelium of a rabbit aorta. The abnormality of adhesion and response to ristocetin-induced aggregation is caused by an inherited deficiency of the glycoprotein I complex of the platelet membrane. Presumably this

TABLE 65. INHERITED DISORDERS OF PLATELET FUNCTION

Membrane abnormalities
  Bernard-Soulier syndrome
  Thrombasthenia
  Platelet factor 3 deficiency
Intracellular abnormalities
  Storage-pool (dense body) deficiency
  Hermansky-Pudlak syndrome
  Wiskott-Aldrich syndrome
  Chediak-Higashi syndrome
  Thrombocytopenia with absent radii
  α-Granule deficiency
  Gray platelet syndrome
  Combined deficiency of dense bodies and α granules
Defects of thromboxane synthesis
  Cyclo-oxygenase deficiency
  Thromboxane synthetase deficiency
  Defective response to thromboxane

complex is essential for the interaction of platelets with the von Willebrand factor and hence may be the site of its receptor. Defective prothrombin consumption is caused by failure of the platelets to bind activated factor X. The receptor for quinine and quinine-dependent antibodies is absent from Bernard-Soulier platelets; presumably this is also on the glycoprotein I complex.

Thrombasthenia (Glanzmann's Disease). This is another autosomal recessive disorder characterized by excessive bruising and bleeding from the mucous membranes. The platelets are normal in number and morphology, but the bleeding time is greatly prolonged and clot retraction is defective. There is complete absence of aggregation in response to ADP. Thrombasthenic platelets adhere to collagen and show a normal release response to collagen or thrombin but do not respond to ADP, epinephrine, or 5-HT. In contrast to Bernard-Soulier platelets they are aggregated by ristocetin and adhere normally to the subendothelium.

Thrombasthenic platelets are deficient in membrane glycoproteins IIb and IIIa. These membrane components probably carry the fibrinogen receptor that is inducible by ADP on normal but not on thrombasthenic platelets. Glycoproteins IIb and IIIa also become associated with actin on stimulation of normal platelets with thrombin; this does not occur in thrombasthenic platelets. Deficiency of these glycoproteins may thus deprive the platelet of points of attachment of fibrinogen on the outer surface of the membrane and of actin on the inner surface. These changes presumably account, at least in part, for the abnormalities of aggregation and clot retraction. Glycoprotein IIIa also carries the Pl^A1 platelet antigen; this is partially or wholly absent on thrombasthenic platelets.

Platelet Factor 3 Deficiency. Only one patient has been reported in whom there appeared to be a primary defect of platelet procoagulant activity unassociated with any other abnormality of aggregation or secretion. The disorder was evidently caused by a deficiency of factor V binding sites on the platelet membrane, resulting in impaired binding of factor Xa.

Intracellular Defects. The disorders characterized by defective aggregation and failure of the release reaction fall into two groups: deficiency of storage organelles and abnormalities of induction of the release mechanism, which include disorders of thromboxane synthesis from arachidonic acid or of response to thromboxane. All these conditions are associated with a mild bleeding tendency. They are recognized by failure of the platelets to aggregate in response to collagen and the production of only a first phase aggregation pattern with ADP or epinephrine, that is, the absence of the second phase associated with the release reaction.

The storage organelle deficiencies may involve the dense bodies (storage pool deficiency) or the alpha-granules (the gray platelet syndrome). In the former, the 5HT content of the platelets is low, and they are unable to release labeled 5HT in response to thrombin. There is a paucity of dense bodies on electron microscopic examination. Storage pool disease may occur as an isolated abnormality, but it usually occurs as part of a more widespread genetic disorder, the Hermansky-Pudlak, Wiskott-Aldrich, and Chediak-Higashi syndromes, for example. In the rare gray platelet syndrome there is a specific deficiency of alpha-granules, the storage of beta-thromboglobulin, PF4, and other platelet proteins.

The other group of inherited defects involving the release reaction consists of disorders in which the adenine nucleotides and 5HT are present in normal amounts but the mechanism for their release is defective. These abnormalities mimic those caused by aspirin and hence are sometimes referred to as aspirin-like defects. In most cases the underlying mechanism has not yet been elucidated, although deficiency of platelet cyclo-oxygenase or thromboxane synthetase has been demonstrated in a few patients. The platelets show a defect of aggregation similar to the storage pool disorders but also fail to aggregate or to synthesize thromboxanes in response to sodium arachidonate.

Acquired Disorders of Platelet Function

Some acquired disorders of platelet function are summarized in Table 66. In many of them, in contrast to the genetic conditions described previously, the precise functional abnormalities of the platelets have not yet been worked out completely. The clinical relevance of the abnormal in vitro platelet function tests that have been described for these conditions is equally uncertain.

Renal Failure. The bleeding tendency that occurs in patients with renal failure may be due, at least in part, to defective platelet function. The bleeding time is often prolonged, and several abnormalities of platelet function have been demonstrated, including abnormal clot retraction and defects of ADP-induced aggregation and of the release mechanism. Some of these changes can be corrected by hemodialysis or peritoneal dialysis. Recently, uremic bleeding has been found to be associated with reduced prostaglandin endoperoxidase production and adenylate cyclase activity in platelets and with increased prostacyclin production by vessel walls. It has been suggested that the resulting imbalance between prostacyclin and thromboxane A_2 production may be responsible for the observed defects in platelet aggregation in uremia.

Myeloproliferative Disease. Several in vitro platelet function defects have been observed in patients with myeloproliferative disorders. In some studies the results of platelet function tests have correlated with clinical evidence of bleeding. The most consistent change is failure to respond to epinephrine or norepinephrine, which may be related to a deficiency of alpha-adrenergic receptors on the platelet membranes. Abnormal release reactions in response to collagen have also been described. The fact that platelet function usually returns to normal in response to myelosuppressive therapy suggests that these abnormalities

TABLE 66. ACQUIRED DISORDERS OF PLATELET FUNCTION

Uremia	Liver disease
Myeloproliferative syndromes	Valvular and congenital
Acute leukemias and	heart disease
preleukemic states	Severe burns
Dysproteinemias	Scurvy
Chronic hypoglycemia	Drugs

TABLE 67. DRUGS THAT MAY CAUSE BLEEDING BY INTERFERING WITH PLATELET FUNCTION

Acetylsalicylic acid
Other nonsteroidal anti-inflammatory agents
   Indomethacin
   Sulfinpyrazone
   Phenylbutazone
Dextrans
Heparin
Penicillins, cephalosporins

reflect the properties of an abnormal clone of platelets; the cellular mechanisms for these defects have not been established.

Drugs. There is a variety of drugs that interfere with platelet function (Table 67). The effects of aspirin were mentioned briefly in an earlier section. Aspirin has been shown to impair platelet aggregation by inhibiting the release reaction. This effect is mediated by its inhibition of cyclo-oxygenase, which leads to a failure of endoperoxide and thromboxane A_2 synthesis. Aspirin inhibits cyclo-oxygenase by acetylation, and because this reaction is irreversible the effect of a single pharmacologic dose can be detected for up to a week or more. Aspirin also inhibits prostacyclin production by vascular endothelial cells. However, unlike platelets, these cells can regenerate cyclo-oxygenase, and so the effect is shorter lived than in platelets. For this reason it is at least theoretically advisable that when designing antithrombotic regimens low doses of aspirin (2 to 3 mg/kg) should be given every 48 to 72 hours, rather than larger daily doses. So far, however, any benefit that has been demonstrated in clinical trials of the use of aspirin, in the prevention of myocardial infarction for example, has shown no evidence of a dose-dependent effect.

Other nonsteroidal anti-inflammatory drugs have an action similar but milder than aspirin's. Sulfinpyrazone acts like aspirin by inhibiting cyclo-oxygenase but also inhibits platelet endothelial interactions. Dipyridamole has complex actions on the vessel wall and platelets. It inhibits the activity of phosphodiesterase, thus raising the level of cyclic AMP, and appears to potentiate cyclic AMP elevation produced by prostacyclin and other adenylate cyclase stimulators.

A variety of abnormalities of platelet function has been observed in patients receiving high doses of penicillins or cephalosporins. These include defective adhesion to collagen and the subendothelium, abnormalities of aggregation and release, and defective clot retraction. These agents may act by coating the platelet surface. Dextrans cause a prolonged bleeding time and interfere with collagen-induced aggregation, perhaps by causing reversible platelet aggregation with subsequent refractoriness to further aggregating stimuli. A similar effect has been observed after low-dose heparin therapy. Other drugs that produce in vitro platelet function defects include antihistamines, phenothiazines, tricyclic antidepressants, and local anesthetics.

Other Conditions. In patients with liver disease there may be defective platelet aggregation in response to ADP and thrombin; the mechanism is uncertain, although in some cases high levels of circulating fibrinogen degradation products may play a role. A variety of defects, including reduced PF3 availability, aggregation, and release, have been described in patients with acute leukemia. Defective aggregation occurs in patients with type I glycogen storage disease.

TESTS OF PLATELET FUNCTION

The diagnosis of hereditary or acquired disorders of platelet function is suggested by bleeding associated with a platelet count that is either normal or only moderately reduced to a level at which bleeding would not be expected to occur (see later section).

The key investigation in establishing the diagnosis of a hemostatic disorder due to abnormal platelet function is the bleeding time. A prolonged bleeding time in the presence of a normal or only slightly reduced platelet count suggests that there is a disorder of vascular or platelet function.

A few simple platelet function tests that are within the capability of most clinical laboratories are sufficient to characterize the more common platelet disorders. Clot retraction is usually tested in whole blood or by adding thrombin to platelet-rich plasma and by observing the extent of retraction of the clot after one hour. Retraction is defective in thrombasthenia, but it is also abnormal if there is thrombocytopenia or hypofibrinogenemia. Assays for the various activities of the factor VIII complex are required for the diagnosis of von Willebrand's disease (see p. 310). Platelet aggregation in response to ADP, collagen, arachidonic acid, and ristocetin is assessed by adding various concentrations of these agents to continuously stirred platelet-rich plasma in a cuvette and recording the increase in light transmitted through the suspension after aggregation has occurred. Some typical aggregation patterns are shown in Figures 71 and 72.

The investigations outlined above serve to diagnose most disorders of platelet function. Confirmatory tests, which require the skills of a laboratory with a special interest in platelet disorders, include electron microscopy, estimation of the content and secretion of dense bodies and alpha-granules, platelet coagulant activities, and endoperoxide and thromboxane synthesis, and analysis of membrane glycoproteins by SDS-electrophoresis.

THE PRODUCTION AND FATE OF PLATELETS

Platelets are produced in the bone marrow from megakaryocytes. Very little is known about the early progenitors of megakaryocytes or about the regulation of thrombopoiesis.

Megakaryocytes and Thrombopoiesis

Megakaryocytes are polypoid cells that follow a pattern of maturation that is unique in mammalian biology. They are derived from a hierarchy of stem cells, which are as yet ill-defined. As mentioned earlier, clonal assay systems have been developed for the detection of pluripotent progenitor cells. The latter give rise to mixed colonies in methyl cellulose or plasma clot. It has been possible to grow megakaryocyte colonies from adult bone marrow or blood or from fetal liver: megakaryocytes can be identified in these colonies by their morphology and by specific staining

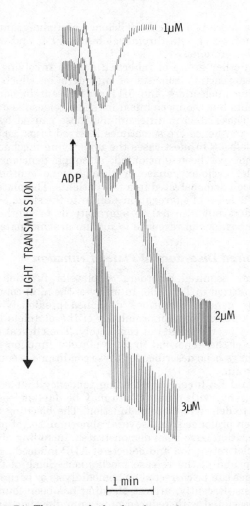

Figure 71. The normal platelet shape changes response and aggregation with the addition of ADP. 1 μM, first phase only; 2 μM, biphasic; 3 μM, maximal aggregation. The initial decrease in light transmission represents the shape change. (From Hardisty, R. M.: *Blood and Its Disorders*. 2nd ed. Hardisty, R. M., and Weatherall, D. J. (eds.). Oxford, Blackwell Scientific Publications, 1982.)

for platelet peroxidase. Megakaryocytic colony formation requires a large number of cells to be plated and the presence of erythropoietin, although rare spontaneous megakaryocytic colonies can be observed even in the absence of erythroid colonies. The megakaryocyte progenitor is called Mk-CFC. So far the Mk-CFC assay has not been applied widely to study defective platelet production.

The earliest promegakaryocytic cell that can be identified in the marrow is the size of a lymphocyte, stains positively for acetyl cholinesterase, and shares certain surface antigens in common with mature platelets. These cells are thought to undergo mitosis; thereafter the megakaryocyte enters what is called a "ploidy ladder," in which it goes through successive steps of chromosomal replication without cell division. During its further development the cell becomes intensely basophilic and granular. The development of megakaryocytes is divided into several stages defined by their level of ploidy and morphologic appearances. Stage 1 cells, or megakaryoblasts, are in the 4N, 8N,

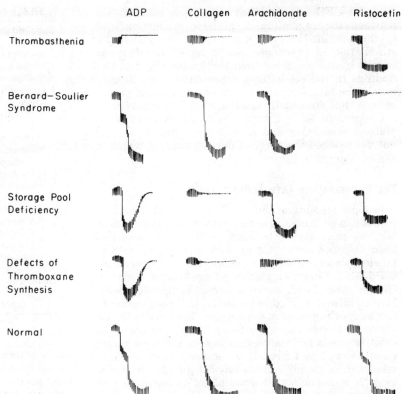

Figure 72. Some typical platelet aggregation curves in the various genetic disorders of platelet function. The normal aggregation pattern is shown in Figure 71. (From Hardisty, R. M.: *Blood and Its Disorders.* 2nd ed. Hardisty, R. M., and Weatherall, D. J. (eds.). Oxford, Blackwell Scientific Publications, 1982.)

and 16N ploidy classes. They synthesize DNA and have relatively high nuclear to cytoplasmic ratios. Stage 2 or basophilic megakaryocytes are characterized by the development of nucleolus and a well marked Golgi apparatus and the presence of numerous polyribosomes throughout their cytoplasm. The principal ploidy class at this stage is 16N. Stage 3 or granular megakaryocytes make up the majority of the identifiable megakaryocytes in normal human bone marrow. These cells are ameboid, with projections protruding into the marrow sinusoids. Cytoplasmic fragments and platelets are probably released into the sinusoids, although it has been postulated that a number of the platelets can be accounted for by shedding of the cytoplasm of megakaryocytes that have first traveled to the lungs.

Several theories have been proposed to explain the variability in the pattern of endomitosis during megakaryocytic maturation. Perhaps the most attractive is that the level of ploidy is related to the content of the internalized membrane system; cells of the 32N class have a much greater content of internalized membrane and a lower concentration of granules and mitochondria than do cells of the lower ploidy classes. It appears that cells with less membrane give rise to larger platelets and those with more membrane, smaller platelets. However, the biologic significance of these observations, which is a topic of heated debate, remains to be determined.

The circulating platelets vary greatly in size, density, biochemical characteristics, and morphology. This heterogeneity can be ascribed in part to the effects of platelet aging. However, the factors that govern the size distribution of platelets in the circulation are extremely complex. For example, in states of rapid platelet turnover such as idiopathic thrombocytopenic purpura platelet size shows a log-normal distribution, suggesting that both large and small platelets are being produced simultaneously. The megathrombocytes that are found in conditions of increased platelet turnover should probably be regarded as "stress platelets" with their own particular properties, in that like stress erythrocytes (see earlier section) they may not be the product of a normal maturation cycle.

Regulation of Platelet Production

Nothing is known about the regulation of the early megakaryocyte precursors. The platelet count is maintained at a fairly constant level in health, ranging from 150,000 to 400,000/µl. Depletion or infusion of platelets is followed by compensatory changes in platelet production. This is thought to be mediated by a humoral agent called *thrombopoietin*.

Thrombopoietin is a small glycoprotein which, like erythropoietin, is probably produced in the kidneys. However, bilateral nephrectomy does not result in sustained thrombocytopenia in humans. Experiments in rats have suggested that thrombopoietin may also be produced in the liver. Attempts to establish assay systems for thrombopoietin using cohort labeling of newly produced platelets have been difficult to standardize, and so far it has not been possible to arrive at a convincing model for the regulation of thrombopoiesis.

The observation that the platelet count is often raised in patients with hemolytic anemia and the fact that erythropoietin preparations are required to produce Mk-CFC suggests that there is a relationship between the regulation of platelet production and erythropoietin. However, it is equally likely that the stimulation of thrombopoiesis in hemolytic states is caused by factors other than erythropoietin, and the findings in the cell-culture experiments may simply reflect the lack of purity of the erythropoietin preparations that are usually used in studies of this type.

Clearly, little is known about the regulation of platelet production and a thrombopoietin assay has not yet reached the stage of development at which it can be applied in clinical practice.

THE SURVIVAL AND FATE OF PLATELETS

Isotopic labeling of platelets for survival measurements has been carried out by both cohort and random labeling techniques. The most useful information has been obtained from ^{51}Cr random labeling. The ^{51}Cr-labeled platelet disappearance pattern in normal individuals is linear, suggesting an age-related removal. On the other hand, survival curves of platelets with labeled diisopropylfluorophosphate (DFP) are curvilinear, suggesting random destruction. The results of ^{51}Cr survival studies suggest a finite lifespan of about 10 days, whereas DFP curves indicate a mean intravascular T½ to 3 to 4 days. It is not clear which of these results most closely reflects physiologic platelet turnover. It is possible that some platelets circulate and are removed after 7 to 14 days, whereas others, possibly a proportion of younger forms, are consumed in repairing minor vascular injuries that occur in response to trauma. In conditions of increased platelet turnover the pattern of ^{51}Cr labeling becomes exponential, suggesting random removal.

Labeling studies have also shown that there is a sizable splenic pool of platelets; in health approximately one third of labeled platelets disappear from the circulation in this pool, which is thought to exchange freely with the platelets in the circulation. The size of the splenic pool may increase considerably in patients with marked splenomegaly in whom as little as 10 per cent of an injected dose of labeled platelets may be recovered from the circulation.

QUANTITATIVE DISORDERS OF PLATELETS

A reduction of the platelet count below normal is called *thrombocytopenia,* and an increased platelet count, *thrombocytosis.* The term *"thrombocythemia"* is reserved for the myeloproliferative disorder in which there is an increased production of abnormal platelets, probably from a clone of precursors with properties similar to those of the other myeloproliferative disorders.

Thrombocytopenia

The thrombocytopenias can be classified into three main groups depending on their etiology: reduced platelet production; increased platelet destruction or utilization; and pooling or sequestration of platelets in an enlarged spleen (Table 68).

The clinical consequences of severe thrombocytopenia are spontaneous bleeding into the skin, mucous membranes, and elsewhere. Purpura, ranging from

TABLE 68. CAUSES OF THROMBOCYTOPENIA

Impaired production
  Marrow aplasia (acquired)
  Megaloblastic anemia
  Megakaryocytic abnormalities (congenital, acquired)
  Infiltration of marrow (leukemia, lymphoma)
Increased utilization or destruction
  Immune platelet destruction
    Primary (idiopathic)
    Secondary
    Drug-induced
  Intravascular coagulation
    Disseminated (malignancy, sepsis, obstetric accidents)
    Local (massive thromboembolism, giant hemangioma)
  Intravascular platelet utilization, deposition, or loss
    Thrombotic thrombocytopenic purpura
    Hemolytic-uremic syndrome
    Viremia
    Drugs (ristocetin, heparin)
    Extracorporeal circulation
    Hemorrhage
    Thrombocytopheresis
Distribution abnormalities
  Splenic pooling in splenomegaly
  Dilution by massive blood transfusion

small petechial lesions to large ecchymoses, is commonly found on the lower extremities and over pressure areas. Mucous membrane bleeding causes the formation of black hemorrhagic bullae in the mouth and epistaxis. With severe thrombocytopenia there may be serious gastrointestinal, uterine, or intracerebral bleeding. Retinal bleeding is less common unless the thrombocytopenia is associated with severe anemia.

There is a reasonably good relationship between the platelet count, the bleeding time, and the severity of bleeding. With platelet counts in excess of 50,000/μl, severe bleeding is unusual, while with platelet counts of less than 20,000/μl bleeding is common.

Defective Platelet Production

Some of the causes of thrombocytopenia due to defective production of platelets are shown in Table 68. This condition occurs in all forms of aplastic anemia, the causes of which are summarized earlier, and in any condition in which there is infiltration of the bone marrow, particularly the acute leukemias. A moderate degree of thrombocytopenia occurs in the megaloblastic anemias as a result of vitamin B_{12} and folate deficiency, reflecting defective nuclear maturation of the megakaryocytes. Thrombocytopenia also occurs commonly in the myelodysplasic syndrome. Some virus infections may cause thrombocytopenia just as they cause transient red cell aplasia; this phenomenon has been observed recently in parvovirus infections in patients with chronic hemolytic anemia.

Any of the drugs or toxins that cause marrow aplasia can cause thrombocytopenia. However, some drugs, the thiazide diuretics for example, may have a more specific effect on thrombopoiesis. Alcohol also causes mild thrombocytopenia, probably through the same mechanism.

There are some rare congenital and inherited disorders that are associated with thrombocytopenia. These are listed in Table 68.

Immune Thrombocytopenic Purpura

The immune thrombocytopenias make up a substantial number of all cases of thrombocytopenic purpura. The main varieties are summarized in Table 69. In addition to the primary acquired (autoimmune) thrombocytopenias, there are many conditions in which immune platelet destruction sometimes occurs, such as the lymphoproliferative disorders, systemic lupus erythematosus, virus infections, and drug reactions. Immune thrombocytopenia is characterized by purpura associated with a low platelet count, normal or increased numbers of megakaryocytes in the bone marrow, a shortened platelet survival, and the presence of antibodies directed against platelets.

Idiopathic thrombocytopenic purpura (ITP) is a condition in which thrombocytopenia occurs in the absence of any demonstrable underlying disorder and in which drug administration can be excluded. There are two main forms, acute and chronic. Since the classic experiments of Harrington, who produced severe thrombocytopenia by injecting himself with serum from a patient with idiopathic thrombocytopenic purpura, it has been believed that this disorder has an immune basis. Subsequent work has confirmed that Harrington's thrombocytopenic factor is an antiplatelet antibody that in adults appears to be exclusively of the IgG3 subclass. Recently, by use of a radio-labeled antigloblin test, it has been estimated that there are approximately 5×10^3 IgG–combining sites on normal platelets. In idiopathic thrombocytopenic purpura and other immune thrombocytopenias the quantity of platelet-bound IgG is increased up to ten times normal; the amount bound appears to correlate well with the severity of the disease and resistance to various forms of treatment. Platelet-bound immunoglobulin can also be demonstrated by immunofluorescence or by using immunoperoxidase techniques. One half to two thirds of patients with idiopathic thrombocytopenic purpura have demonstrable platelet-bound complement. Despite clinical differences between the acute form of this disease in childhood and in the adult form, the incidence of platelet-bound immunoglobulin and complement is similar in the two groups. Platelet survival as determined by isotope disappearance techniques is greatly decreased in all forms of idiopathic thrombocytopenic purpura. The spleen is a major site of platelet destruction and also appears to be involved in antibody production.

TABLE 69. IMMUNE THROMBOCYTOPENIAS

Primary (idiopathic)
  Acute
  Chronic
Secondary
  Systemic lupus erythematosus
  Chronic lymphocytic leukemia
  Lymphoma
  Hodgkin's disease
  Hashimoto's thyroiditis
  Hyperthyroidism
Drug-induced
Neonatal thrombocytopenia due to maternal antibody
  Passive—maternal autoantibody
  Active—maternal isoantibody
Posttransfusion purpura

Acute idiopathic thrombocytopenic purpura frequently follows a viral illness by a period ranging from a few days to three weeks. The disorder is characterized by the sudden onset of purpura with hemorrhagic bullae in the mucous membranes. In more severe cases there may be gastrointestinal hemorrhage, hematuria, severe epistaxis, and bleeding into the central nervous system. In chronic idiopathic thrombocytopenic purpura there is usually no antecedent history, and the first manifestation is unusual bruising or purpura, although menorrhagia or recurrent epistaxes are also common symptoms. Splenomegaly is most unusual in either form of the disease. The blood picture is characterized by severe thrombocytopenia associated with marked variation in size of the platelets. The rest of the blood count is usually normal unless there has been severe bleeding. The bone marrow shows normal or increased numbers of megakaryocytes with an increased number of immature forms.

Thrombocytopenic purpura is a common accompaniment of *systemic lupus erythematosus (SLE)*. Indeed, it may be the only manifestation of this disorder for many years before the typical clinical and serologic pattern of the disease emerges. The clinical and hematologic features are similar to those of idiopathic thrombocytopenic purpura. However, the antiplatelet antibody associated with systemic lupus erythematosus differs in some respects from that found in idiopathic thrombocytopenic purpura. It occurs in all the subgroups of IgG rather than just IgG3. Furthermore, it binds complement to the platelet membrane and requires the presence of complement for antibody-induced platelet damage.

A wide variety of drugs have been implicated in the production of immune thrombocytopenia. There are several mechanisms whereby a drug can produce immune destruction of platelets. It may bind to a plasma protein to form the primary antigen. Antibodies stimulated by this antigen bind the drug, and thrombocytopenia occurs when drug-antibody complexes with a high affinity for platelet membranes are formed. The best studied examples are quinidine and quinine. A more complex mechanism is involved in the thrombocytopenia caused by heparin. It is not certain whether the platelet damage is mediated by heparin itself or by contaminants. In some patients it is possible to demonstrate heparin-dependent antiplatelet antibodies, whereas in others it is thought that platelet consumption during heparin therapy may be the result of intravascular coagulation. Other drugs also seem to produce thrombocytopenia by more than one mechanism. For example, the thrombocytopenia associated with trimethoprim may be caused by interference with folate metabolism, but in some cases an immune mechanism appears to be involved.

There are several causes of increased platelet destruction in the neonatal period, some of which are summarized in Table 70. Passive immune thrombocytopenia may occur in infants born of mothers with idiopathic thrombocytopenic purpura or systemic lupus erythematosus. About 20 per cent of cases of purpura in the newborn result from active immunization. Neonatal alloimmune thrombocytopenia is most often caused by antibodies to the P1^A antigen on platelets. Since 97 per cent of the population are P1^A-positive, such immunization is rare. Histocompatibility alloim-

TABLE 70. NEONATAL THROMBOCYTOPENIA

Intrauterine infections
Rubella, cytomegalovirus, herpes
Toxoplasmosis
Syphilis
Platelet antibodies
Maternal idiopathic thrombocytopenic purpura and systemic
lupus erythematosus (autoantibody)
Fetomaternal incompatibility (isoantibody)
Drug-induced
Disseminated intravascular coagulation
Maternal pre-eclampsia
Hypothermia, asphyxia, shock, sepsis
Rhesus isoimmunization
Congenital megakaryocytic hypoplasia
Hereditary thrombocytopenias
Wiskott-Aldrich syndrome
Giant hemangioma
Congenital and neonatal leukemia and histiocytosis
Metabolic disorders: hyperglycinemia, methylmalonic acidemia,
etc.
Postexchange transfusion

munization probably occurs more commonly, although it seldom results in severe thrombocytopenia. Thrombocytopenia may also accompany intrauterine infections, particularly in the congenital rubella syndrome.

Occasionally, posttransfusion purpura may result from an antibody response to P1^A antigen in those who lack it.

Increased Platelet Utilization

Thrombocytopenia occurs commonly in all the intravascular coagulation syndromes, particularly disseminated intravascular coagulation (DIC), thrombotic thrombocytopenic purpura (TTP), and the hemolytic-uremic syndrome (HUS). Disseminated intravascular coagulation is discussed later.

Thrombotic Thrombocytopenic Purpura. This is a rare disorder characterized by thrombocytopenia, microangiopathic hemolytic anemia, fluctuating neurologic abnormalities, and renal impairment. The basic lesion is thrombotic vascular occlusion in arterioles and capillaries, particularly in the brain and kidneys. The vessels are also occluded by hyaline material associated with endothelial proliferation. The hyaline seems to be composed of fibrin and platelets, but complement and immunoglobulin have also been demonstrated in these lesions. The mechanism underlying these changes is unknown. The endothelial cell proliferation and subendothelial changes suggest that the primary event is vascular damage, with secondary platelet adhesion and aggregation. The thrombocytopenia and shortened platelet survival are not associated with evidence of intravascular coagulation. Some patients with thrombotic thrombocytopenic purpura have a platelet aggregating factor in the serum that can be reduced in amount by incubation with normal plasma, and clinical responses have been obtained with infusions of plasma. In addition, in severe cases a reduction in the level of prostacyclin activity has been observed. Thus this disease may result from a deficiency of a plasma component that inhibits a platelet aggregating factor or that stimulates prostacyclin production in vessel walls. This hypothesis remains to be confirmed.

Hemolytic Uremic Syndrome. This is an acute illness of childhood and is characterized by renal failure, thrombocytopenia, and hemolytic anemia. It often follows an infection; viruses, bacteria, and rickettsiae have been implicated in individual cases. There are microthrombi in the marrow, lungs, brain, kidneys, and elsewhere; the renal vessels show subendothelial hyaline deposits that stain for fibrin. Immune complexes cannot be demonstrated. Usually there is no evidence for disseminated intravascular coagulation, and the mechanism of the thrombocytopenia and hemolytic anemia is unclear. The frequent association with infection and the documented relationship with circulating endotoxin in some cases suggest that a viral or bacterial product may produce endothelial damage; there is some similarity between the endotoxin-mediated Shwartzman reaction and this condition. Intravascular deposition of platelets may result from a defect of prostacyclin production by the vessel wall; the plasma of several patients with hemolytic uremic syndrome has been shown to contain an inhibitor of PGI$_2$ synthesis.

Hemolytic uremic syndrome is a heterogeneous condition in which damage to vessel wall, probably mediated by different mechanisms, is followed by platelet consumption and microangiopathic red cell damage.

Thrombocytopenia Caused by an Enlarged Splenic Pool. Splenomegaly from any cause may be associated with thrombocytopenia. It occurs commonly in liver disease, myeloproliferative disorders, lymphomas, chronic leukemias, and the tropical splenomegaly syndrome associated with malaria, kala-azar, or schistosomiasis.

Other Causes of Loss of Platelets. The passage of blood through an extracorporeal circulation is associated with platelet adherence to foreign surfaces, activation of coagulation, and thrombocytopenia. This occurs within a few hours of initiation of cardiopulmonary bypass, for example, and is particularly marked when profound hypothermia has been induced. It seems likely that infectious agents such as bacteria, viruses, and rickettsiae can cause platelet destruction by nonimmune mechanisms.

Thrombocytosis

The main causes of a raised platelet count are summarized in Table 71. The differentiation between thrombocytosis and thrombocythemia is usually easy to make, since the latter is nearly always associated

TABLE 71. CAUSES OF A RAISED PLATELET COUNT

Myeloproliferative disorders
Essential thrombocythemia
Polycythemia vera
Myelosclerosis
Chronic myeloid leukemia
Secondary thrombocytosis
Bleeding
Inflammatory disorders
Malignant disease
Postsplenectomy or other surgery
Drugs—vincoids, epinephrine
Postthrombocytopenia
Hemolytic anemia
Iron deficiency

with features of a myeloproliferative disease affecting other cell lines. Occasionally, in patients with thrombocythemia the platelet line alone is affected, and if the spleen is not enlarged it may be difficult to distinguish the condition from reactive thrombocytosis. In these cases the magnitude of the platelet count, platelet morphology, and platelet function tests are useful guides to the diagnosis of thrombocythemia.

Thrombocytosis occurs most frequently after hemorrhage. It may also occur in association with inflammatory diseases, particularly rheumatoid arthritis, and in patients with carcinoma or lymphoma, including Hodgkin's disease. The mechanism of the thrombocytosis of inflammatory disease or neoplasia is not understood; it is not always associated with bleeding. Thrombocytosis occurs regularly after splenectomy, but the platelet count usually reverts to normal or near normal in 7 to 10 days. Persistent thrombocytosis may occur in patients who have undergone splenectomy for hemolytic anemia but who remain anemic after the operation. The thrombocytosis associated with vincristine therapy appears to result from a genuine increase in platelet production. The mechanism is

unknown. Similarly, the basis for the very high platelet counts that occur occasionally in patients with iron deficiency who are not bleeding is not known.

Thrombocythemia

This condition was considered in the discussion of myeloproliferative disease. It is characterized by a high platelet count, megakaryocyte hyperplasia, abnormal platelet morphology and function, and a thrombotic and bleeding tendency. Glucose-6-phosphate dehydrogenase isozyme studies have shown that the abnormal platelets are derived from a single clone of progenitors. Presumably the latter proliferate independently of the factors involved in the regulation of normal thrombopoiesis. The platelets show morphologic changes, including increased size dispersion, and hypertrophy of the dense tubular and open canalicular systems. There are also surface changes, including decreased glycoprotein I, alpha-adrenergic receptors, and prostaglandin A2 receptors. A variety of abnormalities of metabolism and granule formation have been reported. The associated abnormalities of platelet function were described earlier.

Blood Coagulation _____

The blood coagulation mechanism comprises a complex series of biochemical reactions involving a number of plasma proteins known collectively as *coagulation factors,* which normally circulate in an inactive state. In response to vascular injury, a "cascade" of reactions is set in motion in which factors activate one another in a sequential fashion (Fig. 73), leading to the generation of *thrombin,* a proteolytic enzyme that cleaves

plasma fibrinogen to form an insoluble fibrin clot. The individual coagulation factors (Table 72) are conventionally denoted by Roman numerals with activated forms indicated by the suffix a (IXa, Xa, and so forth). The cascade concept implies that the coagulation mechanism behaves as a biologic amplifier in which the activation of minute amounts of coagulation factors in the early stages of the cascade leads to the formation of substantial amounts of the end product, fibrin.

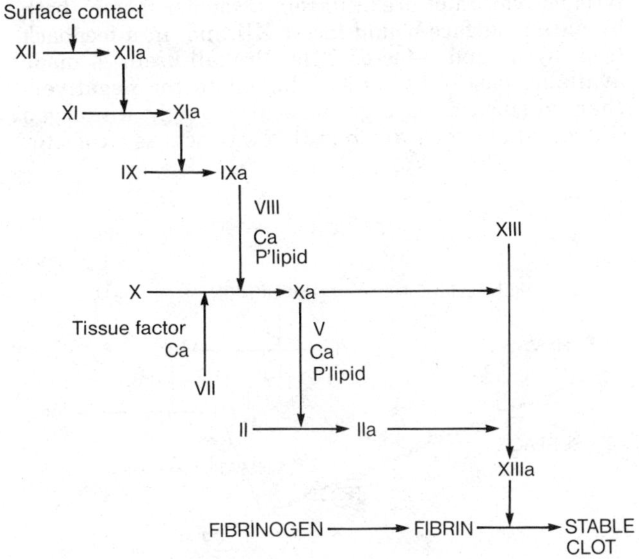

This amplification potential is illustrated by the fact that a sufficient amount of thrombin can be generated from the prothrombin in 2 ml of blood to clot the entire circulating volume. Protective mechanisms have thus evolved to ensure that this process does not get out of hand and that the circulating blood remains fluid. Several such mechanisms are indicated below in the discussion of interactions between individual coagulation factors, but one of the most important is the mechanism by which the coagulation process is localized to the site of vascular injury. Coagulation is normally activated after damage to the vascular endothelium. Platelet aggregation at the site of injury provides a suitable milieu of coagulation and thus helps to localize the production of fibrin. Indeed, activated coagulation factors (with the exception of VIIA) are rapidly cleared from the free circulation by the reticuloendothelial system, and certain plasma proteins, such as antithrombin III, protein C, α_2 macroglobulin and α_1 antitrypsin, specifically inactivate coagulation factors, as described below. Furthermore, a complementary process known as *fibrinolysis* is provided by a sequence of enzyme interactions that leads to the formation of *plasmin,* a proteolytic enzyme that dissolves fibrin clot. Like coagulation, fibrinolysis can

Figure 73. A simplified outline of the coagulation cascade. For further details see the text and Figures 74 to 78.

TABLE 72. THE BLOOD COAGULATION FACTORS

FACTOR	SYNONYMS	TYPE	VITAMIN K REQUIRED?	ACTIVE FORM	PLASMA HALF-LIFE*	MOLECULAR WEIGHT†	STORAGE-LABILE?
I	Fibrinogen	Polypeptide	No	Fibrin	3–4 d	340	No
II	Prothrombin	Zymogen	Yes	Thrombin (IIa)	2–3 d	69	No
III	Tissue factor	Lipoprotein	No	—	—	45	—
IV	Calcium	Co-factor	—	—	—	—	—
V	Proaccelerin‡	Co-factor	No	?	approx. 24 hr	330	Yes
VII	Proconvertin‡	Zymogen	Yes	?	< 6 hr	50	No
VIIIc	Antihemophilic	Co-factor	No	?	10 hr	360	Yes
IX	Christmas	Zymogen	Yes	IXa	18 hr	57	No
X	Stuart-Prower	Zymogen	Yes	Xa	3 d	67	No
XI	PTA	Zymogen	No	XIa	2–4 d	160	No
XII	Hageman	Zymogen	No	XIIa	2 d	80	No
XIII	Fibrin stabilizing	Transaminase	No	XIIIa	4–7 d	320	No

*d = day, hr = hours. These figures are approximate and are based on the biologic half-life of infused material in deficient subjects.
†Molecular weight × 1,000^{-1} daltons.
‡This name is no longer in common use.

be activated by surface contact, and the two systems proceed in parallel to provide an additional safeguard against unwanted thrombosis. Generalized activation of fibrinolysis is prevented by the potent plasma inhibitors α_1 antiplasmin and a_2 macroglobulin.

THE COAGULATION MECHANISM

Recent work has considerably clarified the role of individual coagulation factors, and certain generalizations may be made about their mode of action. First, three of the coagulation factors function as *cofactors* for other activation reactions, while the remainder circulate as inactive precursors that are activated during the process of coagulation. These precursors are known as *zymogens,* and their activation typically involves a limited proteolytic step that induces a change of shape within the molecule and exposes an active site containing a serine residue. The activated coagulation factors are known as *serine proteases* and are all homologous in structure and action with other proteolytic enzymes such as trypsin, chymotrypsin, and elastase.

Second, activation of coagulation factors does not normally occur within the free circulation, and an important feature of the coagulation mechanism is that the activation process only occurs where it is needed at a site of vascular injury. Activation of the early stages of the coagulation cascade is promoted by contact with any tissue other than the vascular endothelium—the activation of factor X and of prothrombin—both take place on the surface of activated platelets. Platelets only adhere to tissues exposed by endothelial damage, since endothelial cells themselves actively inhibit platelet adhesion. The assembly of these factors on the platelet surface is facilitated by calcium, which has long been recognized to be essential for blood coagulation. Four of the coagulation factors have calcium-binding sites, the synthesis of which is dependent on vitamin K.

It is convenient to discuss the biochemical reactions involved in the coagulation cascade in four stages: (1) the contact phase, (2) activation of factor X, (3) conversion of prothrombin to thrombin, and (4) formation and stabilization of the fibrin clot.

THE CONTACT PHASE (Fig. 74)

When blood comes into contact with a non-endothelial surface, the coagulation system is activated and the blood rapidly clots. Surfaces that are able to promote coagulation in this way have in common a negative surface charge, and include collagen, glass, and kaolin. The initial enzymatic reactions participating in this "contact phase" involve factors XII and XI together with prekallikrein, high molecular weight kininogen, and plasminogen.

Factor XII, also known as Hageman factor, is a single chain polypeptide of M_r 74,000 that binds readily to negatively charged surfaces, undergoing a conformational change that renders it considerably more susceptible to proteolytic activation. The initial step in its activation is the cleavage of the internal peptide bond, a step common to the activation of all of the coagulation zymogens. This gives rise to a dipeptide serine protease (α-factor XIIa), while further cleavage produces a smaller unbound peptide fragment (β-factor XIIa). The enzyme responsible for factor XII cleavage is kallikrein, which is generated as a result of proteolytic activation of prekallikrein (Fletcher factor), both by native surface-bound factor XII and, in a feedback loop, by α- and β-factor XIIa. Prekallikrein is made available locally by its attachment to the negatively charged surface via high molecular weight kininogen (Fitzgerald factor), which in this way acts as a cofactor

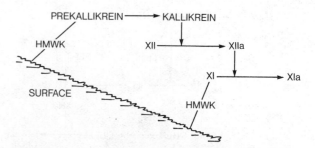

Figure 74. The contact phase of blood coagulation. HMWK = high molecular weight kininogen.

both in the activation of prekallikrein and in the subsequent activation of factor XI by factor XIIa.

Factor XI is a glycoprotein of M_r 160,000 comprising two very similar or identical peptide chains. Activation to the serine protease factor XIa follows cleavage of an internal peptide bond in each subunit by factor XIIa in the presence of high molecular weight kininogen and a negatively charged surface.

Much of our understanding of the contact phase has come from studies using artificial surfaces in vitro, the presumed physiologic counterpart of which is connective tissue collagen exposed after endothelial injury. Congenital absence of factors XI and XII is associated with a surprisingly mild defect in hemostasis, and other mechanisms of activation are thought to be important in vivo. One mechanism may involve activated platelets that are capable of activating factor XI directly. Furthermore, as described below, factor X may be activated either as a result of the contact mechanisms already described or independently by a mechanism involving factor VII.

ACTIVATION OF FACTOR X (Fig. 75)

Factor X is a two-chain glycoprotein M_r 67,000. Its activation involves a proteolytic cleavage within the heavy chain with the loss of a peptide fragment and may occur by one of two mechanisms, both of which are probably important clinically. *Intrinsic activation* occurs by a series of reactions involving factor XIa (generated following surface contact as already described), together with factors IX and VIII. This process is relatively slow, and a faster and more direct *extrinsic activation* results from the action of factor VII in the presence of a factor released from damaged tissue. As a result, small amounts of thrombin are rapidly generated that can subsequently amplify the intrinsic pathway by feedback activation of factor VIII.

Intrinsic Activation of Factor X involves first the activation of factor IX by factor XIa. Factor IX is a single-chain glycoprotein of M_r 57,000 that is dependent on vitamin K for its procoagulant properties. Cleavage of an internal peptide bond by factor XIa produces an inactive intermediate consisting of a heavy chain and a light chain that contains calcium-binding carboxyglutamic residues. A second cleavage within this heavy chain removes a polypeptide fragment to expose the active serine residue. Factor IX can also be activated by factors VIIa and Xa and (less physiologically) by an enzyme present in the venom of Russell's viper.

Factor X activation by factor IXa takes place in the presence of Ca^{2+}, phospholipid, and factor VIII. Calcium ions facilitate the binding of the carboxyglutamic residues of factor IXa to a phospholipid "surface" on the platelet membrane.

Factor VIII is a molecular complex consisting of two proteins that are under separate genetic control and that are most likely synthesized at different sites. The procoagulant protein is known as factor VIII:C and is deficient in patients with classic hemophilia. Because of difficulties in obtaining sufficient material, human factor VIII:C has only recently been purified to homogeneity. Its estimated M_r is 360,000. Its site of synthesis is uncertain; the liver has been implicated, but normal or increased levels in severe hepatic disease suggest that other sites may also be important.

The second component of the factor VIII complex is a large multimeric protein with a M_r typically over one million, known as factor VIII–related protein (VIIIR) or *von Willebrand factor*, since it is deficient in patients with von Willebrand's disease (p. 310). It is required for normal platelet adhesion. The physiologic significance of the complex between VIII:C and VIIIR is not clear, but probably the factor VIII–related protein protects the smaller procoagulant molecule from proteolytic degradation.

Factor VIII:C acts as a cofactor in the activation of factor X by factor IXa, probably by binding and orientating enzyme and substrate on the platelet surface. Prior proteolytic activation by VIII:C by thrombin is required, providing a further example of positive feedback.

Extrinsic Activation of Factor X depends on the interaction of factor VII with a tissue factor and Ca^{2+}. Blood drawn carefully into glass tubes generally takes 4 to 10 minutes to clot, but the addition of tissue extracts accelerates the process considerably, so that coagulation occurs in 10 to 15 seconds. This phenomenon was one of the earliest observations in biochemistry and has been extensively studied, yet only now is a detailed knowledge of the molecular events involved beginning to emerge. Not all tissues are able to promote coagulation in this manner; brain, lung, and placenta are notably active, but platelets have no such activity. Tissue factor has been partially characterized as a lipoprotein of M_r 50,000, the lipid portion of which is essential for its proper function. It appears to be devoid of intrinsic enzymatic activity and to act as a co-factor with factor VII.

Factor VII is a single-chain glycoprotein of M_r 50,000 whose synthesis is vitamin K–dependent. It is a serine protease with weak intrinsic proteolytic activity, but its ability to activate factor X is enhanced some 16,000-fold by the presence of tissue factor; the mechanism of this latter interaction is not clear. Unlike other serine procoagulant proteases, factor VII does not require prior proteolytic activation for its

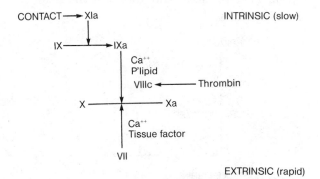

Figure 75. The activation of factor X.

function, and interaction with tissue factor is sufficient to trigger coagulation. This may resolve a dilemma with respect to how—in an enzyme system in which each component must apparently be proteolytically activated by other components—coagulation can start in the first place. Further enhancement of factor VII activity is obtained by proteolytic cleavage into a two-chain peptide. This can be mediated by factor Xa or thrombin, although further proteolytic cleavage by these enzymes results in the loss of coagulant activity.

THE CONVERSION OF PROTHROMBIN (Fig. 76)

Prothrombin (factor II) is converted to thrombin (factor IIa) by a complex activation step involving factor Xa, factor V, and calcium, bound together with phospholipid on the platelet membrane.

Factor V is a single-chain polypeptide of M_r 330,000. It is present both in plasma and on platelets. Like factor VIII, it is activated following limited proteolysis by thrombin but itself has no intrinsic enzymatic activity. It acts by binding factor Xa and prothrombin to a specific receptor on the platelet surface. The attachment of factor Xa and prothrombin is facilitated by their carboxyglutamic acid–calcium binding sites. The complex formed between platelet phospholipid, calcium, and factor Xa is known as the *prothrombin activator complex*.

Prothrombin (factor II) is a single-chain glycoprotein of M_r 70,000. Three different domains have been defined: Fragment 1, Fragment 2, and Prethrombin 2 (Fig. 77). Fragment 1 contains the calcium-binding carboxyglutamate region, and Fragment 2 contains a binding site for factor V. Cleavage by factor Xa first separates Prethrombin 2 from Fragment 2, but the two cleavage fragments remain associated until a second cleavage splits the bond between the two peptide chains of thrombin. Thrombin itself is able to split prothrombin between Fragments 1 and 2, slowing down its own generation.

THE FORMATION OF FIBRIN (Fig. 78)

Fibrin is formed from the enzymatic cleavage of fibrinogen by thrombin, followed by polymerization and stabilization. Fibrinogen is a rod-shaped dimeric glycoprotein of M_r 340,000 of which each dimer consists of three dissimilar chains, Aα (M_r 63,000), Bβ (M_r 56,000), and γ (M_r 47,000) joined at the N terminal region by disulfide linkages between pairs of α and γ

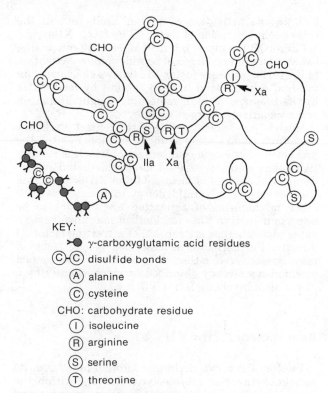

KEY:

- γ-carboxyglutamic acid residues
- Ⓒ–Ⓒ disulfide bonds
- Ⓐ alanine
- Ⓒ cysteine
- CHO: carbohydrate residue
- Ⓘ isoleucine
- Ⓡ arginine
- Ⓢ serine
- Ⓣ threonine

Figure 77. The secondary structure of prothrombin. The thrombin and Xa cleavage points are indicated by arrows. (Esnouf, M. P.: British Medical Bulletin 33:216, 1977.)

chains (Fig. 79). The action of thrombin on fibrinogen is to remove a peptide fragment from the N terminal end of each α chain (fibrinopeptide A) and each β chain (fibrinopeptide B) to yield *fibrin monomer*. This cleavage is associated with a change in the net molecular charge of the central domain of the fibrin molecule permitting spontaneous polymerization by side-to-side electrostatic bonding, with each molecule half overlapping the next. A strand of fibrin, initially two molecules thick, develops by elongation. At this stage the fibrin polymer is unstable and hemostatically ineffective, since it is particularly susceptible to proteolysis by plasmin; stabilization is achieved by the action of factor XIII.

Factor XIII is a dimer of M_r 320,000 that comprises two A and two B chains. Both thrombin and factor Xa

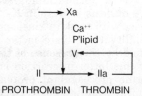

Figure 76. The conversion of prothrombin.

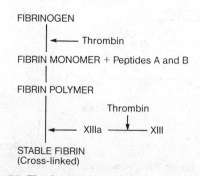

Figure 78. The formation and stabilization of fibrin.

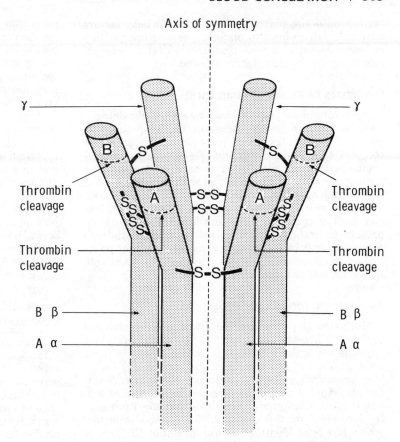

Figure 79. The N-terminal end of fibrinogen showing sites of cleavage by thrombin. (From Forbes, C. D., and Prentice, C. R. M.: Physiology and biochemistry of blood coagulation of fibrinolysis. In *Blood and Its Disorders*. 2nd ed. Hardisty, R. M., and Weatherall, D. J. (eds.). Oxford, Blackwell Scientific Publications, 1982.)

can activate factor XIII by a two-stage process involving calcium ions. Factor XIIIa promotes a stable clot by catalyzing the formation of isopeptide bonds or crosslinks between the γ chains of fibrin, forming a covalently linked macromolecule, which is considerably more resistant to proteolysis.

THE ROLE OF VITAMIN K IN COAGULATION

Vitamin K is the name given to a number of naphthoquinone derivatives that are widespread in plants. Most dietary vitamin K_1 comes from green vegetables, but this is supplemented to a variable and uncertain extent by de novo bacterial synthesis within the intestine. Vitamin K is essential for the production of factors II, VII, IX, and X, and the synthesis of at least three other plasma proteins depends on this vitamin. Two of these (protein C and protein S) have anticoagulant activity; protein C is activated by thrombin to a serine protease, which acts on factors V and VIII, effectively inhibiting the binding of Xa to platelets and the conversion of prothrombin to thrombin. Protein S may act as a co-factor in this reaction. Activated protein C also stimulates fibrinolysis.

The vitamin K–dependent proteins show considerable sequence homology in their N-terminal regions. A characteristic feature is that all contain 10 to 12 modified glutamic acid residues to which an extra carboxy group has been added post-translationally by a vitamin K–dependent process. This carboxylation step is dependent on vitamin K, reduced nicotinamide-adenine dinucleotide (NADH), molecular oxygen and

carbon dioxide, and an hepatic microsomal enzyme. In this process vitamin K is converted to its epoxide, and it may be the subsequent physiologic reduction of the epoxide back to vitamin K that is inhibited by oral anticoagulants of the coumarin group such as warfarin (Fig. 80). However, the precise site of action of these vitamin K antagonists has not yet been determined. In their presence carboxylation does not occur, and the descarboxy factors II, VII, IX, and X lack procoagulant activity and may indeed inhibit normal coagulation in a competitive manner. The carboxyglutamic residues formed in the presence of vitamin K have a high avidity for calcium, which serves to bind and localize

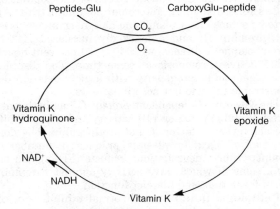

Figure 80. The vitamin K cycle.

factors onto the platelet surface. Descarboxy-factors therefore fail to bind to platelets, and although they possess otherwise normal structure they fail to interact efficiently in the coagulation cascade.

INHIBITORS OF BLOOD COAGULATION

Inhibitors of coagulation may be either physiologic, such as heparin or antithrombin III, or pathologic, such as the antibody to the prothrombin activator complex that is characteristic of systemic lupus erythematosus. Substances such as heparin or coumarin compounds may be administered with the intention of interfering specifically with the coagulation process. The existence of families in which an inherited deficiency of coagulation inhibitors (antithrombin III or protein C) coincides with a lifelong thrombotic tendency (thrombophilia) clearly demonstrates that physiologic coagulation inhibitors play an important role in the control of hemostasis.

Physiologic Inhibitors

Heparin. Heparin is a highly negatively charged sulfated glucosaminoglycan (mucopolysaccharide) of variable molecular weight. It is located chiefly in mast cells, particularly in the lungs, gut, and vessel walls. The precise physiologic significance of heparin is uncertain, since it cannot be detected in the circulation, but it has anticoagulant activities that are known to be dependent on the presence of a plasma co-factor, which has been identified as *antithrombin III*. This is one of a number of plasma proteins with antithrombin activity, which include α_1-antitrypsin and α_2-macroglobulin. Antithrombin III is a single-chain glycoprotein that is able to form a tight equimolar complex with thrombin and other serine esterases (XIIa, XIa, IXa, VIIa, and Xa), thus rendering them inactive. The formation of these complexes, which are between the active serine residues of the protease and an arginine residue on the antithrombin, is markedly accelerated by heparin. Heparin binds both to thrombin and to antithrombin, producing in each a conformational change that favors their interaction. Endothelial cells have heparin-like molecules protruding from their vascular surface, and it is postulated that this is where complexes between antithrombin III and active clotting factors are formed physiologically. Deficiency of antithrombin III occurs in about 1:2000 of the population and is inherited as an autosomal dominant trait. Affected persons have about one-half normal levels of antithrombin III and a markedly increased risk of thromboembolic disease, with 40 to 70 per cent developing active thrombosis at some time. The disorder shows genetic heterogeneity with a gene deletion demonstrable in some but not all patients.

The vitamin K–dependent *protein C* has both anti-factor V and anti-factor VIII activity and thus inhibits the activation of factor X and prothrombin. The degradation of fibrin by plasmin produces a number of products (fibrin degradation products [FDPs], see below), some of which have activity against thrombin, fibrin formation, and platelet function.

Pathologic Inhibitors. Abnormal inhibitors of coagulation may arise spontaneously in previously normal individuals or may develop in patients lacking a particular factor (such as factor VIII in hemophilia A), who are given infusions of normal plasma proteins and who react to the missing factor as to a foreign protein. Nonspecific inhibition of various aspects of coagulation, including platelet function, has also been noted in the presence of extreme plasma levels of monoclonal immunoglobulin. This is seen occasionally in patients with myeloma and macroglobulinemia. Spontaneously occurring antibodies are rare, but antibodies to factors V, IX, XI, XII, XIII, and more usually VIII have been reported in otherwise apparently normal individuals and in patients with collagen-vascular disorders such as lupus erythematosus and rheumatoid arthritis. In the former condition a more characteristic inhibitor with the properties of an antibody to the phospholipid portion of prothrombin activator complex is commonly seen. However, although the presence of this inhibitor produces prolongation of in vitro coagulation tests it is clinically associated with a thrombotic rather than a hemorrhagic tendency.

LABORATORY ASSESSMENT OF BLOOD COAGULATION

Laboratory tests of blood coagulation may be divided into simple screening tests for abnormalities in the intrinsic or extrinsic pathways of factor X activation or in the conversion of fibrinogen to fibrin, assays for individual coagulation factors, and tests for the presence of coagulation inhibitors. Blood for these tests is normally collected into a citrate solution in order to bind calcium, thus preventing activation of factors II, VII, X, and IX.

Screening Tests

The extrinsic blood coagulation pathway is tested by the one-stage *prothrombin time (PT)*. A quantity of standardized tissue thromboplastin (generally made from human or rabbit brain extract) is added to the test plasma, and the time taken to clot after recalcification is compared with that of normal plasma. The prothrombin time is prolonged in patients with deficiency of factors VII, X, V, prothrombin or fibrinogen, and is widely used in the control of therapeutic anticoagulation by the coumarin group of drugs.

The intrinsic pathway is tested by the *partial thromboplastin time (PTT)*, also known as the *kaolin-cephalin coagulation time (KCCT)*. First, kaolin is added to citrated platelet-poor plasma to activate the contact mechanism (factors XII and XI); subsequently calcium and phospholipid (cephalin) are added. The latter takes the place of platelets in the activation of factor X and prothrombin. The PTT is prolonged in patients with deficiencies or inhibitors of factors XII, XI, VIII, X, V, prothrombin or fibrinogen but is normal in patients with pure deficiency of factor VII.

The conversion of fibrinogen to fibrin is assessed by the thrombin time. This is the time taken for plasma to clot following the addition of thrombin. The thrombin time is prolonged in patients with reduced fibrinogen levels, abnormal fibrinogen, or inhibitors of fibrinogen conversion such as heparin or degradation products. A rough estimate of fibrinogen levels may be obtained by determining a thrombin time with double dilutions of test plasma and by observing the highest dilution at which a visible clot is formed. A more accurate method is to dry and weigh the clot formed from a standard volume of plasma.

Factor Assays

The activity of individual coagulation factors is assessed by comparing the ability of test and normal control plasma samples to shorten the prolonged PT or PTT of a plasma sample known to be specifically deficient in the factor to be assayed.

Tests for Inhibitors of Coagulation

In patients with coagulation factor deficiencies the abnormal coagulation time tests may be corrected by mixing 50 per cent test plasma with 50 per cent normal plasma. Failure to correct abnormal coagulation tests in this way indicates the presence of a pathologic coagulation inhibitor.

Platelets

Platelets play an important role in coagulation as well as in primary hemostasis. However, the coagulation tests described here are performed on platelet-free plasma so as to be independent of platelet numbers or activity. Full investigation of hemostasis must therefore include a platelet count, a bleeding time, and, if appropriate, tests of platelet function (p. 296).

FIBRINOLYSIS

By removing fibrin clot, the fibrinolytic system is possibly the major homeostatic mechanism for ensuring the continued patency of the vascular system (see Fig. 81). The initial event in fibrinolysis is the formation of the serine protease *plasmin* from its inactive zymogen *plasminogen,* a single chain β globulin of M_r 90,000, which is found in plasma and in other body fluids. Conversion of plasminogen to plasmin is promoted by a number of activators and involves a limited proteolytic step to produce a dipeptide molecule with marked proteolytic activity. After isolation from plasma, plasminogen can be found in two forms, *lys*-plasminogen and *glu*-plasminogen, differing in their composition at the N-terminal end (Fig. 82). *Glu-*

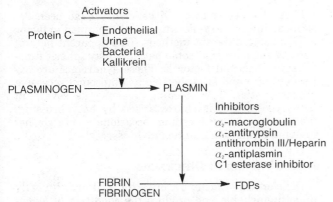

Figure 81. An outline of fibrinolysis. FDP = fibrin-fibrinogen degradation products.

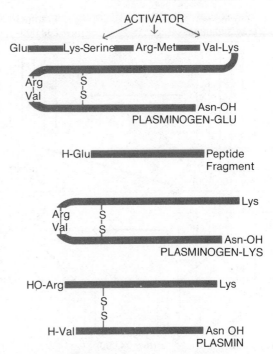

Figure 82. The activation of plasminogen.

plasminogen is a precursor of *lys*-plasminogen. Plasmin is particularly active in degrading fibrinogen and fibrin, although other coagulation factors are also susceptible to its action.

PLASMINOGEN ACTIVATION

Plasminogen activators are present in a wide variety of tissues and body fluids. Several different activators have been partially characterized. The most important appear to be associated with endothelial tissues, particularly in veins, and are released into the blood after tissue injury, stress, exercise, hyperpyrexia, or venous occlusion. A distinct activator *urokinase* is synthesized by renal cells and can be isolated from the urine, where it is important in maintaining the patency of the urinary tract. A variety of tumor cells produce plasminogen activators, and these may facilitate tumor spread. Activators are also produced by certain bacteria, notably streptococci, which produce *streptokinase*. This, like urokinase, has been isolated and is available for therapeutic use to aid the dissolution of pathologic thrombus. Plasminogen activators are inactivated by inhibitors in plasma and also by the liver, and enhanced fibrinolytic activity is thus sometimes seen in patients with chronic liver disease.

Plasminogen may also be activated following contact activation of the coagulation system. The mechanism involves kallikrein generated from prekallikrein by the action of factor XIIa (Fig. 74). In addition, thrombin itself releases plasminogen activator from perfused vascular beds and also activates protein C, another activator of the fibrinolytic system.

ACTIONS OF PLASMIN

Degradation of fibrinogen and fibrin by plasmin occurs in stages with the formation of a variety of fibrin-fibrinogen degradation products (FDPs) (Fig. 83),

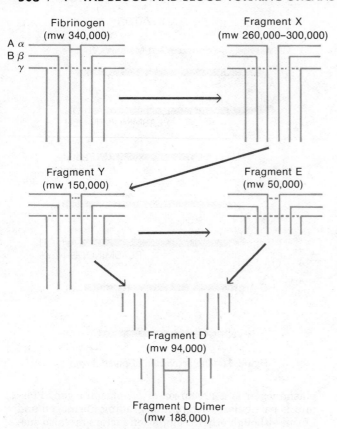

Figure 83. Fibrin(ogen) degradation products. (After Gaffney, P. J.: British Medical Bulletin 33:248, 1977.)

some of which have intrinsic biologic activity. Fibrinogen is more susceptible to the action of plasmin as the cross-linking within the fibrin polymer confers some resistance to degradation. FDPs are able to inhibit the action of thrombin, the polymerization of fibrin, and also platelet aggregation, adhesion, and release. They also have vasoactive properties and potentiate the vascular effects of bradykinin, serotonin, epinephrine, and angiotensin.

The proteolytic action of plasmin is not confined to fibrinogen and fibrin, and activity against other circulating coagulation factors can be demonstrated in vitro. However, plasma activity is suppressed in the circulation by the presence of high concentrations of inhibitors such as α_2-antiplasmin and α_2-macroglobulin. Indeed, under normal circumstances free plasmin cannot be detected in the circulation, and various explanations have been put forward for this apparent paradox of how intravascular thrombi can be lysed by the fibrinolytic system. Contact activation of both coagulation and fibrinolytic mechanisms simultaneously may ensure that activators are incorporated together with plasminogen into the developing clot, so that gradual dissolution could then proceed safe from circulating inhibitors. Both activators and plasminogen have marked affinity for lysine residues in fibrin and bind strongly to fibrin as it is formed. Plasminogen bound in this way is not only more susceptible to activation but is protected from the action of inhibitors as its lysine binding sites form complexes with fibrin. However, this effect is balanced by the covalent binding of α_2-antiplasmin to fibrin by factor XIIIa during

clot formation. Thus the subsequent rate of dissolution of the thrombus may well depend on the relative amounts of plasminogen and plasminogen activators, and antiplasmins laid down within the clot.

CONGENITAL DEFICIENCIES OF COAGULATION FACTORS

Congenital deficiencies have been described for each of the coagulation factors: these may take the form of a complete absence of the coagulant protein or the presence of a functionally defective form. The vast majority involve single factors, but a few patients have been described with deficiencies of two or more. The impact of these relatively uncommon disorders has been great. They have provided insight into the significance of individual steps in the coagulation cascade, and the management of affected patients has posed a considerable challenge to the resources of blood transfusion services.

Of these uncommon disorders factor VIII deficiency is most frequent, with factor IX deficiency occurring about one fifth as often. Deficiencies of other factors are quite rare.

CONTACT FACTOR DEFICIENCIES

Factor XII deficiency was first discovered in a patient named Hageman in the course of routine blood tests. Surprisingly, patients with this deficiency have little or no bleeding tendency, and indeed some, including Hageman himself, have died from thromboembolic disease. Deficiencies of prekallikrein (Fletcher factor) and high molecular weight kininogen (Fitzgerald factor) have been described but are not associated with any clinical bleeding tendency. Excessive bleeding after trauma occurs in *factor XI deficiency,* especially in homozygous cases that most frequently involve Ashkenazi Jews. In all of these disorders there is prolongation of the kaolin-cephalin clotting time (KCCT). The mild or nonexistent clinical defects of hemostasis associated with these deficiencies suggest that contact activation can be bypassed by other reactions in the physiologic processes of coagulation and platelet activation.

FACTOR X DEFICIENCY

Several types of factor X deficiency have been described, differences reflecting results obtained in factor assays using different methods. This apparent heterogeneity suggests that some patients may inherit functionally abnormal factor X. These syndromes are extremely rare and are inherited as autosomal recessive characteristics. The bleeding tendency is severe in homozygotes and is characterized by easy bruising, mucous membrane bleeding, occasionally muscle hematoma formation, and hemarthroses.

FACTOR VIII AND IX DEFICIENCIES

Deficiencies of factor IX or factor VIII are clinically indistinguishable and produce the condition of *hemophilia.* Both are inherited as x-linked recessive traits. About 30 per cent of cases may be caused by new mutations, since no relative with hemophilia can be traced. Their clinical severity attests to the importance of these factors in hemostasis. Both conditions produce a marked prolongation of KCCT, but they can be distinguished by assays of the respective factors. In Britain, factor VIII deficiency (classic hemophilia, hemophilia A) has an incidence of about 1:12,500 and is about five times more common than factor IX deficiency (Christmas disease, hemophilia B).

The molecular basis for factor VIII deficiency is not known. Recently, a gene probe has been developed that has made it possible to perform gene mapping studies on a number of patients with factor IX deficiency. In some cases a gene deletion has been demonstrated, but in the majority no lesion has been found. Further progress depends on successful cloning and sequencing of the factor IX gene.

The clinical severity of hemophilia reflects the level of residual factor VIII (or IX) activity. Thus patients with 15 per cent factor VIII activity may have little or no spontaneous bleeding, and the condition may only occur following accidental or surgical trauma. In contrast, patients with completely absent factor VIII activity have repeated and severe spontaneous hemorrhage that principally affects joints and soft tissue (Fig. 84). If untreated, these result in severe structural damage and functional disability; when vital organs are involved bleeding may be fatal.

The diagnosis of hemophilia is usually suspected from the family history. As an x-linked recessive disorder (Fig. 85), it affects males born of a female carrier. The disorder may thus be seen in the patients' brothers or maternal uncles. In a number of cases, however, there is no family history, and a spontaneous mutation may be assumed. The manifestations of severe hemophilia may appear shortly after birth with bleeding from the umbilical stump: excessive crying may result in severe hemorrhage from the lingula of the tongue, or the disorder may become evident after circumcision. Bruising is noted in the crib, but as soon as the infant becomes independently mobile, the characteristic pattern of repeated hemarthroses affecting particularly the knees, ankles, and elbows become evident. Re-

peated hemarthroses, especially when there has been some delay in instituting treatment, eventually lead to a destructive and crippling arthropathy. Soft tissue hemorrhage may occur anywhere, but the muscles of the leg, thigh, and the ileopsoas region are particularly affected. The diagnosis of hemophilia is confirmed in the laboratory by the finding of a markedly prolonged KCCT and demonstration of markedly reduced or absent activity of factor VIII or IX.

Replacement Therapy. Hemophilia is treated by replacing the missing coagulation factor by transfusion. However, factor VIII is labile, and its activity diminishes rapidly in stored blood. Furthermore, the use of whole blood is not appropriate for such a specific deficiency, and factor VIII concentrates are now available that permit correction of the coagulation defect for limited periods of time. Such concentrates may take the form of cryoprecipitate or freeze-dried concentrates. Cryoprecipitate is made from fresh plasma that has been frozen and then thawed at 4° C; under such conditions factor VIII precipitates together with fibrinogen and cold insoluble globulin and can be concentrated by centrifugation. A drawback is that this product must be stored frozen, whereas the newer freeze-dried preparations may be stored in a domestic refrigerator. The plasma half-life of factor VIII is short (10 hours), and twice-daily infusions are therefore necessary to maintain a normal level. Factor VIII concentrates are manufactured from plasma pooled from up to 5,000 donations, and the risk of transmitting hepatitis is virtually 100 per cent. The acquired immune deficiency syndrome (AIDS) may also be transmitted in this fashion. Similar concentrates are now available for the treatment of factor IX deficiency, although fresh-frozen plasma may suffice in mild cases. The plasma half-life of factor IX is 18 hours, and it is thus slightly easier to maintain adequate levels.

Immunologic Aspects of Factor VIII

Further information about the factor VIII molecule and the molecular basis of hemophilia A has come from the study of the reaction of patients to replace-

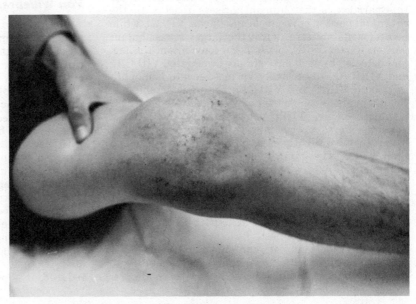

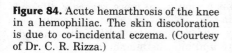

Figure 84. Acute hemarthrosis of the knee in a hemophiliac. The skin discoloration is due to co-incidental eczema. (Courtesy of Dr. C. R. Rizza.)

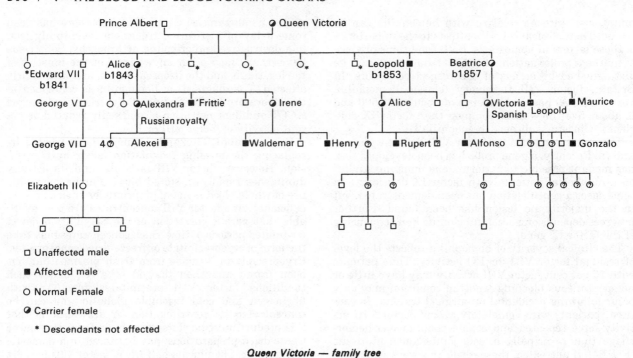

Queen Victoria — family tree

Figure 85. The inheritance of hemophilia in the family of Queen Victoria and Prince Albert. (From Jones, P. *Living with Haemophilia.* Lancaster, MTP Press, 1974.)

ment therapy. A small proportion of hemophiliacs treated with factor VIII infusions develop circulating inhibitors that complicate their treatment. In general, such patients are severe hemophiliacs with absent factor VIII activity. The inhibitors are antibodies to factor VIII, but they have different properties to the heterologous precipitating antisera raised in rabbits. When hemophiliac plasma is tested with human factor VIII antisera, antigenically cross-reacting material (CRM) can be detected in about 10 per cent of samples, and in a small number the amounts detected do not differ from normal. In contrast, CRM detected by heterologous antisera is present in similar amounts in hemophiliac and normal plasma. The explanation for this paradox is that human antisera react with the *coagulant* portion of the molecule (factor VIII:C), while heterologous antisera detect the larger noncoagulant portion (factor VIIIR, p. 303). By convention, the factors detected by such antisera are designated VIII:CAg and VIIIR:Ag, respectively. In most severe hemophiliacs, both VIII:C and VIII:CAg are undetectable, although in about one quarter of patients in whom VIII:C is undetectable, VIII:CAg is present in reduced amounts. Persons with mild to moderate hemophilia generally have slightly more immunoreactive material than VIII:C. The implication of these observations is that hemophiliacs with detectable VIII:CAg have an X-chromosome mutation that modifies the structure of VIII:C, while patients with absent VIII:C have either absent synthesis or produce a molecule that is so abnormal that its antigenic reactivity as well as its coagulant function are lost.

The development of immunologic assays for VIII:CAg and VIIIR:Ag has improved the ability to detect carriers of the disease and has also made pre-natal diagnosis feasible. Carrier women have normal VIIIR:AG levels but reduced VIII:C, since on the average only half of their chromosomes actively direct VIII:C synthesis. However, X-chromosome inactivation in females (lyonization) is a random process, and some carrier females have very low levels of VIII:C owing to inactivation of most of their *normal* X-chromosomes, whereas others have normal levels of VIII:C owing to inactivation of most of their *hemophiliac* X-chromosomes. The prenatal diagnosis of hemophilia can be obtained by analysis of fetal blood samples for VIII:CAg using VIIIR:Ag as a control protein.

Von Willebrand's Disease

Von Willebrand's disease represents a heterogeneous group of bleeding disorders characterized mainly by an autosomal pattern of inheritance, a prolonged bleeding time, abnormal platelet adhesion, and abnormalities of the factor VIII complex. Heterozygotes have a mild to moderate bleeding diathesis from early childhood that is characterized by easy bruising and mucous membrane bleeding. The homozygous state is much less common, but patients are more severely affected with hemophilia-like lesions such as hemarthroses, muscle bleeding, and retroperitoneal bleeding, in addition to purpura and mucous membrane bleeding.

The disorder is caused by an inherited defect of factor VIIIR (known as the von Willebrand factor) with secondary effects on factor VIII:C. Most commonly there is a reduction in levels of all components of the factor VIII complex with a prolongation of the bleeding time, and in homozygotes these findings are exaggerated. It is not clear why factor VIII:C levels should be reduced; it is possible that VIIIR protects VIII:C from inactivation in vivo (p. 303). Alternatively, it may affect synthesis of VIII:C or its release into the blood. The prolonged bleeding time is caused by defective platelet adhesion, which correlates with reduced levels of ristocetin co-factor activity (VIIIR:RC, pp. 291 to 292). In some patients there is a marked reduction in VIIIR:RC with normal or nearly normal levels of VIIIR:Ag. In these patients the VIIIR molecule may be nonfunctional, and recent evidence shows that this is related to a shift from large multimeric forms that are required for normal function to smaller less highly polymerized molecules.

FACTOR VII DEFICIENCY

A number of patients have been described with factor VII deficiency, but characterization of these disorders is far from complete. Inheritance is autosomal recessive with homozygotes being severely affected. The clinical disorder is similar to that associated with factor X deficiency.

FACTOR V DEFICIENCY

Factor V deficiency is rare and shows autosomal recessive inheritance. The disorder is often mild, and abnormal bleeding, if present, may appear as bruising or mucous membrane bleeding; fatal intracranial hemorrhage also has been recorded. The intimate association of factor V with platelets has made the disorder difficult to characterize, but platelet transfusions have been used to correct the bleeding diathesis, although they do not increase plasma levels of factor V.

FACTOR II DEFICIENCY

Congenital prothrombin deficiency is exceedingly rare and comprises a heterogeneous group of conditions showing an autosomal pattern of inheritance in which the prothrombin may be totally absent or functionally defective. The clinical picture resembles that seen with deficiencies of factors VII and X.

FIBRINOGEN DEFICIENCY

Fibrinogen may be deficient in quantity (hypofibrinogenemia or afibrinogenemia) or quality (dysfibrinogenemia). Congenital afibrinogenemia is rare and probably represents homozygous inheritance of an autosomal trait. Affected patients have a moderate to severe bleeding disorder that may be manifested shortly after birth with bleeding from the umbilical stump. In contrast to hemophilia, mucous membrane bleeding is common. However, hemarthroses do occur. The defect can be corrected by infusion of plasma or fibrinogen concentrates such as cryoprecipitate; fibrinogen has a long half-life, so infusions are not required as frequently as in hemophilia. Laboratory tests in affected patients show prolongation of all coagulation tests that depend ultimately on fibrin formation. In addition, biochemical and immunologic assays show absence of fibrinogen. Mild thrombocytopenia may occur, and platelet function is defective; this can be corrected by a low concentration of fibrinogen and presumably reflects a reduced intraplatelet fibrinogen pool. Parents of affected patients (who are thus heter-

ozygotes) show laboratory evidence of hypofibrinogenemia but little or no clinical defect. It is not known whether congenital afibrinogenemia represents a gene deletion or whether there is synthesis of a highly abnormal and unstable molecule.

A number of congenital dysfibrinogenemias have been described. These are thought to be caused by an inherited molecular defect that gives rise to a functionally abnormal molecule, although in most instances the exact defect has not been elucidated. These conditions are rare and are generally not associated with a serious bleeding disorder, but come to light principally through the discovery of abnormal coagulation during routine testing. The functional abnormalities observed in these patients have been classified as (1) affecting fibrinopeptide release, (2) affecting fibrin polymerization, and (3) affecting cross-linking of fibrin. Paradoxically some patients with dysfibrinogenemia have shown an abnormal tendency toward thrombosis. These structurally abnormal fibrinogens are named by their place of discovery—for example, fibrinogen Baltimore—using the same approach as that used to name hemoglobin variants.

FACTOR XIII DEFICIENCY

Deficiency of factor XIII is another rare but severe bleeding disorder with an autosomal recessive inheritance. Invariably it is first manifested as bleeding from the umbilical stump. Typically, hemostasis is normal immediately after trauma, and bleeding starts after some hours or days owing to failure to consolidate the initial thrombus through fibrin stabilization. Abnormal wound healing and spontaneous abortion are other characteristic clinical features. This condition can be treated by infusions of cryoprecipitate at biweekly intervals.

ACQUIRED DISORDERS OF BLOOD COAGULATION

VITAMIN K DEFICIENCY

Because dietary vitamin K is widely available from green vegetables and also from bacterial synthesis within the intestine, primary dietary deficiency is exceedingly uncommon. However, human milk is a poor source of the vitamin, and deficiency may occur in breast-fed infants. Naturally occurring vitamin K (phylloquinone, vitamin K_1) is fat soluble and its absorption from the intestine depends on the presence of bile salts. Secondary deficiency may thus be seen in patients with obstructive jaundice or external biliary fistulae as well as in general malabsorptive states. Reduced bacterial synthesis within the intestine may occur in patients given broad-spectrum antibiotics. This does not in itself produce clinically significant deficiency but may precipitate bleeding in patients with poor diet or malabsorption or in patients taking oral anticoagulant drugs (see later discussion).

Vitamin K deficiency results in impaired carboxylation of factors II, VII, IX, and X and protein C (p. 305). The noncarboxylated precursor molecules circulate normally but are ineffective or even antagonistic

TABLE 73. DRUG INTERACTION WITH WARFARIN AND SIMILAR COUMARIN ANTICOAGULANTS

ACTION	DRUGS
Increased Sensitivity to Warfarin	
(i) Displace warfarin from plasma binding sites	Aspirin and other nonsteroidal anti-inflammatory (NSA) drugs
(ii) Prolongs warfarin half-life	Metronidazole
(iii) Inhibit enteric bacterial synthesis of vitamin K	Broad spectrum antibiotics
(iv) Reduces absorption of vitamin K	Liquid paraffin
(v) Prolongs prothrombin time	Cimetidine
(vi) Platelet function inhibitors	Aspirin, NSA, dipyridamole, alcohol
(vii) Complex action	Clofibrate
Reduced Sensitivity to Warfarin	
(i) Drugs that induce hepatic microsomal enzyme activity and thus increase warfarin catabolism	Alcohol, phenytoin, barbiturates
(ii) Direct competition	Vitamin K

in the coagulation process. They are sometimes referred to as "proteins induced by vitamin K absence (PIVKA)." The presence of these nonfunctional proteins rather than functional coagulation factors leads to a severe bleeding disorder characterized by easy bruising, macroscopic hematuria, and extensive soft-tissue hemorrhage. Retroperitoneal and cerebral hemorrhage may occur. Coagulation tests show a markedly prolonged prothrombin time and a variably prolonged PTT. In the presence of adequate liver function, normal synthesis of deficient clotting factors may be restored by parenteral administration of vitamin K_1. Reversal of the coagulation defect, however, takes one to two days and may be achieved more rapidly by infusion of fresh frozen plasma.

Hemorrhagic Disease of the Newborn. This condition is characterized by persistent bleeding in the neonatal period, which can be corrected by vitamin K_1 administration. Affected infants may bleed from the umbilical stump, the intestine, or at sites of birth injury. The prothrombin and partial thromboplastin times are prolonged. The disorder is mainly caused by impaired synthesis of coagulation factors by the immature liver. It is thus most severe in premature infants but can be prevented by intramuscular administration of vitamin K_1, which should be given routinely to premature infants at birth.

Oral Anticoagulants. Oral anticoagulants of the coumarin group (warfarin and phenindione) interfere with the vitamin K cycle (p. 305) and produce effects identical to those seen with deficiency of the vitamin. They are used clinically in a variety of situations to prevent thrombosis, particularly within the venous system. By carefully controlling the dose of anticoagulant used—usually by means of the prothrombin time or a similar test—a safe and stable degree of anticoagulation may be achieved. However, numerous drugs and other factors can interfere with anticoagulant control (Table 73).

LIVER DISEASE

The liver plays a complex role in blood coagulation, being the site responsible for synthesis of fibrinogen, plasminogen, factors II, V, VII, and IX to XIII as well as antithrombin III and α_2-antiplasmin. Reticuloendothelial cells within the liver and elsewhere are responsible for clearance of circulating activated coagulation factors, and plasminogen activators are also cleared by the liver. Not surprisingly, therefore, a variety of coagulation abnormalities may be seen in patients with liver disease (Table 74), and abnormal bleeding is frequently encountered. Impaired synthesis of coagulation factors is mainly responsible, but thrombocytopenia (often associated with splenomegaly and portal hypertension), impaired platelet function, and enhanced fibrinolysis may contribute. Furthermore, portal hypertension is often associated with the development of marked venous distension at the lower end of the esophagus and around the stomach. These *esophageal varices* are particularly prone to sudden and dramatic bleeding.

DISSEMINATED INTRAVASCULAR COAGULATION

Under certain circumstances the coagulation system may be triggered into uncontrolled activity, producing the syndrome of *disseminated intravascular coagulation (DIC)*. A variety of consequences may result: deposition of fibrin within small blood vessels may lead to occlusion and loss of function of affected organs. Lesser degrees of fibrin deposition may result in hemolysis due to fragmentation of passing red cells, producing a *microangiopathic hemolytic anemia* (see

TABLE 74. HEMOSTATIC ALTERATIONS ASSOCIATED WITH LIVER DISEASE

Effects on Coagulation Factors
Reduced synthesis of vitamin K–dependent (II, VII, IX, X, protein C) and other factors (I, V, XI, XII, XIII)
Abnormal fibrin polymerization
Reduced clearance of activated factors
Effects on Platelets
Impaired aggregation to ADP, collagen, thrombin, and ristocetin
Thrombocytopenia (hypersplenism)
Effects on Fibrinolysis
Increased fibrinolysis
  Primary (reduced clearance of plasminogen activators)
  Secondary to DIC
Miscellaneous
DIC
Reduces synthesis of antithrombin III and α_2 antiplasmin
Effects of massive blood transfusion

p. 240). Often fibrinolytic activity is also increased so that intravascular thrombi may be rapidly lyzed. Thus critical organ damage may not occur, and the predominant clinical consequence may be acute hemostatic failure with bleeding as a result of increased consumption and exhaustion of coagulation factors and platelets. This state of affairs has been called the *defibrination syndrome* or, more appropriately, a *consumption coagulopathy*. The presence of increased fibrinolytic activity in such patients may be manifested clinically as reactivation of bleeding from recent venepuncture sites or similar sites of injury (Fig. 86).

DIC may occur in a wide variety of clinical settings (Table 75). The most common associations are with infections, particularly gram-negative septicemias, a number of rickettsial and viral diseases, malignant disease, and certain obstetric disorders.

Pathogenesis. A number of mechanisms are thought to be responsible for the development of DIC, and it is likely that different underlying conditions promote DIC in different ways. Activation of the contact pathways with associate kinin generation (leading to hypotension and shock), fibrinolysis, and complement activation are frequently seen in cases of DIC secondary to infection and in particular with gram-negative septicemia. It is not clear, however, whether any of these associated phenomena is responsible for activation of the coagulation pathways and thus the development of DIC. Considerable evidence points to bacterial endotoxin playing a key role, and in many respects DIC resembles the *Shwartzman reaction,* in which experimental animals develop a DIC-shock syn-

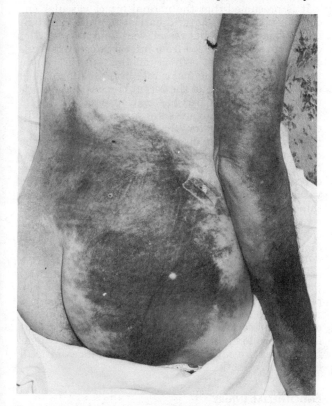

Figure 86. Extensive hemorrhage after venepuncture and bone marrow biopsy in a patient with disseminated intravascular coagulation caused by prostatic carcinoma.

TABLE 75. CLINICAL DISORDERS ASSOCIATED WITH DISSEMINATED INTRAVASCULAR COAGULATION

Infections
  Septicemia, especially gram-negative
  Viremia
  Malaria
Malignancy
  Carcinoma, especially prostate, pancreas, lung, mucus-secreting adenocarcinoma
  Acute promyelocytic leukemia
Immunologic
  Anaphylaxis
  Mismatched blood transfusion
Shock
  Hypovolemia
  Cardiac
  Septic
Snake venoms
Embolic disorders
  Fat embolism
  Amniotic fluid embolism
  Massive pulmonary embolism
Local tissue damage
  Intrauterine fetal death
  Premature placental separation
Disordered regulation
  Liver failure (see Table 74)

drome after two temporally spaced intravenous injections of bacterial endotoxin. The reaction can be induced after a single injection of endotoxin in the presence of reticuloendothelial blockade, following inhibition of fibrinolysis, or during treatment with cortisone. Moreover, it can be produced despite prior depletion of complement components but can be prevented, at least in rabbits, by prior removal of neutrophils with cytotoxic agents. In other infections, antigen-antibody complexes may be responsible for initiating DIC, possibly by inducing complement-mediated damage to vascular endothelium and/or platelets. Thrombocytopenia may occur in bacterial infections by such a mechanism in the absence of other features of DIC.

The most likely mechanism for the development of DIC in malignancy is the release into the bloodstream of substances with procoagulant or tissue factor-like activity, which activate the extrinsic pathway. In many patients this results in a chronic low-grade DIC, typically with recurrent thrombotic events but minimal laboratory disturbance. In most instances the malignancy is metastatic, and tumor microemboli within small vessels may contribute to the development of microangiopathic hemolysis. A more acute hemorrhagic form of DIC is typically seen with prostatic carcinoma and with acute promyelocytic leukemia, in which the abnormal lysosomal granules are probably the source of procoagulant material. Bleeding is a frequent cause of death in this latter condition, since not only is marrow replacement associated with thrombocytopenia, but treatment may profoundly aggravate the effects of DIC by destroying leukemic cells and releasing lysosomal contents.

DIC after snake bites is more obviously the result of the procoagulant material gaining access to the circulation. A similar mechanism may be responsible for DIC complicating amniotic fluid or fat embolism, and obstetric conditions such as intrauterine death, abruptio placentae, and retained placenta. Alterations in the function of the coagulation and fibrinolytic systems during pregnancy may contribute. The cause of DIC in pre-eclampsia and toxemia of pregnancy (like the cause of toxemia itself) is less clear.

Laboratory Diagnosis. The most sensitive laboratory indicator of the presence of DIC in a suitable clinical setting is the prothrombin time, which is prolonged in 90 per cent of patients. This test is by no means specific, but in 70 per cent of patients there is also a reduction in fibrinogen levels, and the presence of both abnormalities in the absence of liver disease is highly suggestive of DIC. The PTT is prolonged in a smaller number of patients and is thus less useful as a screening test. Confirmation of the DIC may be obtained by demonstrating raised circulating levels of FDPs, but assays for these are less widely available in an emergency. Surprisingly, tests for increased fibrinolytic activity such as the euglobulin lysis time are positive in only a few cases.

ACUTE HEMOSTATIC FAILURE FOLLOWING MASSIVE BLOOD TRANSFUSION

A severe hemostatic disorder may develop in patients with blood loss requiring a massive blood transfusion, irrespective of the cause of the hemorrhage. When blood is stored at 4° C there is a rapid loss of platelet viability and of factor V and VIII activity: transfusion of large amounts of stored bank blood may thus result in thrombocytopenia and coagulation abnormalities. This only becomes a significant problem after transfusion of more than five units of stored blood within a four-hour period and may be avoided if one or two units of platelet concentrate and fresh frozen plasma are transfused with every five units of stored blood. Toxicity related to a transfusion of large quantities of the citrate anticoagulant present in stored blood is rare, since normally the liver can metabolize citrate faster than it can be transfused. However, in the presence of severe liver disease citrate infusion may produce acute hypocalcemia. This is unlikely to affect blood coagulation in vivo but may have other undesirable consequences, which can be prevented by the administration of additional calcium intravenously at intervals during the course of any massive blood transfusion.

HEMOSTASIS AND PATHOLOGIC THROMBOSIS

A thrombus is a mass or deposit formed from the constituents of the blood on the surface of the lining of the heart or blood vessels. An occlusive thrombus occupies the entire lumen of a vessel and obstructs flow, whereas a mural thrombus is adherent to only one side of a vessel and flow continues past its free border. Occlusive thrombi tend to occur in medium-sized atheromatous arteries, smaller vessels in the microcirculation, and veins.

The anatomy of a thrombus reflects the state of blood flow in the affected vessel. Injury to a vein with slowed or arrested blood flow usually leads to the formation of a thrombus rich in fibrin and red cells. On the other hand, a thrombus that forms in the arterial circulation, particularly if the flow is relatively undisturbed, consists mainly of aggregated platelets and fibrin.

In 1856 Virchow suggested that three main factors determine the site and extent of thrombi: blood flow, the constituents of the blood, and the vessel wall. A great deal is now known about the role of the vessel wall and the constituents of the blood in hemostasis. There is also a mass of epidemiologic and experimental data about the various factors that might modify the normal hemostatic mechanism to increase the likelihood of pathologic thrombosis.

The evidence that suggests that pathologic thrombus formation is a perversion of the normal hemostatic mechanism is summarized briefly below.

THROMBOTIC MECHANISMS

VASCULAR COMPONENT

The vascular endothelium has both thrombogenic and antithrombotic activity. The thrombogenic factors produced by the vessel wall include tissue thromboplastin, Hageman factor activator, and the von Willebrand factor. The main antithrombotic components are the negative charge of the vascular endothelium, substances like adenosine diphosphatase that are involved in the metabolism of platelet aggregating agents, various proteinases such as plasminogen activator and antithrombin III, and, perhaps most important, prostacyclin, which inhibits local platelet aggregation and causes vasodilatation.

It is presumed that the normal intact vascular endothelium acts as a natural barrier to prevent thrombus formation on the vessel wall and to stop the constituents of the blood from interacting with subendothelial structures. Which of the antithrombotic mechanisms plays the major role in these functions is far from clear. Much of the recent clinical and experimental work in this area has concentrated on the role of prostacyclin. The results are inconsistent and difficult to evaluate. Prostacyclin levels are reduced in the vessel wall in certain disorders in which thrombosis is common. On the other hand, when prostacyclin synthesis in the vascular wall is artificially reduced in experimental animals, platelets do not adhere to the vascular endothelium; similar results have been obtained in in vitro experiments. Furthermore, the recently described genetic form of cyclo-oxygenase deficiency is associated with a very mild bleeding diathesis; there is no thrombotic tendency.

Thus, by virtue of its wide variety of antithrombotic activities, the vessel wall has considerable potential for providing a basis for inherent variability in the proneness to pathologic thrombosis. However, there is no evidence to date that abnormalities of these mechanisms per se are involved in thrombotic disease. It seems more likely that the events that actually trigger thrombosis are injury to the wall or changes in local blood flow, or both.

ENDOTHELIAL INJURY

Platelets adhere to damaged endothelium (Fig. 87), and adhesion to subendothelial collagen is an important trigger mechanism for the formation of a hemo-

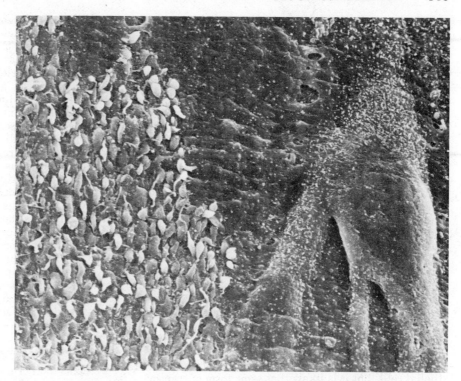

Figure 87. Scanning electron micrograph of rat carotid artery after endothelial cell injury. Large numbers of platelets are attached to the denuded surface on the left. Regenerating endothelium is spreading across the denuded surface from above. The bulge on the right contains an endothelial cell nucleus; the endothelial surface shows multiple small microvilli (× 2800). (By courtesy of Professors G. B. Ryan and D. G. Penington.)

static plug. The major problem is to define the factors that might cause endothelial cell injury as the prelude to pathologic thrombosis. There are many candidates. Under hypoxic conditions gaps form between endothelial cells, and platelet adhesion has been reported to follow local ischemia. Endothelial cells may be damaged by circulating agents such as thrombin, bacterial endotoxin, and neuraminidase. Homocystine, the amino acid produced in excess in hereditary homocystinuria, in which recurrent thrombosis is common, has been shown to promote atheromatous-like lesions and thrombosis in experimental animals. There is also some experimental evidence that hypercholesterolemia can cause endothelial damage. Many other substances have been implicated, including the products of tobacco smoke, viruses, bile salts, and immune complexes. However, it is in the pathogenesis of atheroma that the endothelial injury hypothesis is receiving most attention at the present time.

THOMBOSIS AND ATHEROMA

Thrombosis superimposed on a pre-existing atheromatous lesion, leading to arterial occlusion, is an important event in the natural history of atherosclerotic arterial disease. However, the thrombotic process may also be involved in the genesis of atherosclerosis. During the development of an atherosclerotic plaque, there is proliferation of modified smooth muscle cells in the arterial intima, the formation of a matrix of connective tissue elements, including collagen, elastin, and proteoglycans, and finally the deposition of both intra- and extracellular lipid. There is increasing interest in the possibility that many of these processes result from interactions between platelets and the arterial wall.

The idea that mural thrombi play an important role in atheromatous plaque production is not new. Re-

cently, a modification of this hypothesis has been developed that proposes that atherogenesis involves (1) endothelial cell injury, (2) the release into the subendothelium of factors that induce the migration of smooth muscle cells through the internal elastic lamina with subsequent proliferation in the intima, (3) the synthesis by muscle cells of collagen, elastin, and a variety of proteoglycans, (4) intracellular and extracellular lipid accumulation, and (5) associated thrombus formation. A growing body of experimental data is compatible with this mechanism of atherogenesis, although numerous doubts and discrepancies remain.

In animals the proliferative intimal lesions found in arteries after endothelial denudation are platelet dependent. For example, removal of the endothelial lining of an arterial wall is followed by platelet deposition in the subendothelium (Fig. 87) and intimal proliferation of smooth muscle cells. If animals are made thrombocytopenic, smooth muscle cell proliferation does not occur. In pigs that lack von Willebrand factor, there is impaired platelet adhesion to exposed subendothelium, and proliferative arteriosclerosis cannot be produced. A variety of possible mechanisms are possible for the observed smooth muscle cell proliferation. These include mitogenic stimuli derived from platelets, stimulation derived from the vessel wall itself owing to altered endothelial function, and loss of intrinsic growth regulation of smooth muscle cells owing to spontaneous cell mutation. Many potential sources of mitogenic growth factors are candidates for stimulators of smooth muscle cell proliferation. Among those that have been studied in detail are platelet-derived growth factor, an endothelial cell-derived growth factor, and several mitogens produced by macrophages, which are found in atherosclerotic lesions. Studies using glucose-6-phosphate dehydrogenase isozymes have shown that the proliferating muscle cells are derived from a single clone, which suggests that atheromatous plaques may be analogous to benign tumors, the cells of which continue to proliferate spontaneously and fail to respond to normal cellular regulatory mechanisms. However, the relative importance of the roles played by growth factors or autonomous cell proliferation in the process of muscle cell proliferation remains to be determined.

Morphologic and immunohistologic data, much of them conflicting, suggest that various platelet and fibrin components form part of atheromatous lesions. There is also evidence that thrombi occur on intimal surfaces in the absence of demonstrable atherosclerotic plaque. However, the nature of the primary endothelial injury that might allow platelets or their products, or other smooth muscle stimulants, through the endothelial wall is far from clear. The basal rate of replication of vascular endothelium is extremely low, although areas that are associated with vessel branching show focal increased replication. It has been reported that endothelial replication is increased in response to hypertension or hyperlipidemia; this work requires confirmation. In in vitro systems there is accelerated transport across replicating cells, and this might provide a mechanism for the movement of factors such as platelet growth factor or other mitogens across the vascular endothelium.

Very little is known about lipid flux across endothelial cells, but it is likely that some form of transcytosis occurs. These cells carry high affinity receptors for low density lipoprotein; lipid flux occurs at an increased rate in regenerating endothelial cells in culture. Whether this is true of the vessel wall in vivo is not known. Proteoglycans, which are found in atherosclerotic vessels and sites of endothelial regeneration, have a high affinity for low density lipoproteins. Whether this is a mechanism for the accumulation of lipid in atheromatous lesions remains to be determined.

While these observations provide a tentative working model for the generation of an atheromatous plaque, they leave open the question of the nature of the endothelial injury that initiates the process. Is it primary damage to the vessel wall, perhaps associated with diminished antithrombogenic activity of the wall, or does atheroma result from the interaction of abnormally activated platelets with lesions caused by the minor trauma that occurs to the endothelium of all normal vessels? Perhaps a combination of all of these mechanisms is responsible. Much of the recent work that has attempted to distinguish between these variables has concentrated on prostaglandin metabolism in vessel walls and platelet metabolism.

Prostacyclin (PGI_2) generation may be reduced in atherosclerotic vessels, both in experimental animals and humans. Synthesis of PGI_2 in biopsy specimens of forearm veins is reduced in diabetic patients as compared with nondiabetic subjects. Similar results were obtained from studies of the arteries of rats with experimentally induced diabetes. Much work has been carried out to determine whether there is "hyperactivity" of platelets in patients with atheroma. The platelets of patients with familial hypercholesterolemia are abnormally sensitive to aggregating agents, and the acquisition of cholesterol by platelets is also associated with increased sensitivity. In vitro, cholesterol-enriched platelets release more labeled arachidonic acid then do control platelets. Recent studies on Eskimo populations, in which there is a very low incidence of atheromatous disease, has provided some interesting insights into platelet metabolism. The Eskimo diet consists mainly of animal fat, but the phospholipid content is rich in linolenic rather than linoleic acid. Increased eicosapentaenoic acid is released by membrane phospholipases; in platelets the resulting prostaglandin intermediates that are formed, the trienoic series, are not aggregatory. On the other hand, endothelial trienoic-series prostaglandins retain antiplatelet-aggregation activity. Eskimos have a mildly prolonged bleeding time, and their platelets show reduced reactivity to aggregating agents.

In summary, although work over the last few years has revealed a series of tantalizing clues about potential mechanisms for atherosclerosis, there is no real understanding about its pathogenesis. The uncertainties are reflected in the disappointing results of the use of antiplatelet drugs and other agents for the primary or secondary prevention of coronary artery disease and other forms of atheromatous vascular disease.

HEMODYNAMIC FACTORS

It seems likely that hemodynamic factors play a role in thrombogenesis. One experimental model that has been used extensively is an extracorporeal shunt in which a branched plastic tube is inserted between the carotid arteries and jugular veins of pigs. Platelet microthrombi form downstream from flow dividers on the walls of the tube. The platelets are deposited at these sites of turbulent flow and not elsewhere on the tube surfaces. There is a striking similarity between the distribution of thrombi in this model and the siting of human thromboatherosclerotic deposits. Others have confirmed that there is a good relationship between hemodynamic changes and the distribution of platelet deposition. Two important factors in these models are shear rates and the presence of red cells. The latter provides a major force that contributes to the movement of platelets from the axial stream toward the vessel wall.

The rheologic characteristics of blood flow have also been studied in relationship to thrombotic disease. Patients with diabetic vascular disease and other forms of severe peripheral vascular disease have increased blood viscosity. Thrombotic episodes in patients with polycythemia occur more frequently in those with high hematocrits, an effect that may well be mediated by stasis, since small changes in the hematocrit lead to proportionately large changes in blood flow. There is strong circumstantial evidence that stasis and decreased blood flow encourage thrombosis on the venous side of the circulation. Pathologic studies have suggested that deep venous thrombi form preferentially at sites at which ligaments or tendons compress veins or valve cusps interrupt laminar flow.

THE PRETHROMBOTIC OR HYPERCOAGULABLE STATE

It has long been the goal of those who wish to prevent thromboembolic disease to define changes in the platelets or components of the coagulation system that

TABLE 76. POSSIBLE CAUSES OF HYPERCOAGULABLE STATES*

Increased concentrations of
  Clotting factors
  Platelets
  Inhibitors of activation or action of plasma
Decreased concentrations of
  Inhibitors of coagulation
  Plasminogen
  Activators of plasminogen
Circulating activated clotting factors
Synthesis of
  Clotting factors with increased susceptibility to activation
  Plasminogen with decreased susceptibility to activation
Impaired generation of activators of plasminogen
Impaired clearance of activated clotting factors from circulation

*After Ratnoff, Clin Haemat 10:265, 1981.

might increase the risk of arterial or venous thrombosis. There is a bewilderingly large number of clinical disorders and risk factors that seem to be associated with susceptibility to thrombosis (Tables 76 and 77). These observations have led to a rather vague concept of a hypercoagulable state common to all of these conditions or induced by various risk factors. In an attempt to define such a prethrombotic condition, platelet function and the levels of various clotting factors have been measured in patients who appear to be at increased risk for thrombotic disease or who have already had a thrombotic episode. One of the great difficulties in interpreting these studies is to make the distinction between those changes that precede thrombosis and those that occur only after a thrombotic episode has occurred.

Platelets

A variety of platelet function studies have been carried out in an attempt to demonstrate platelet

TABLE 77. SOME RISK ASSOCIATIONS FOR ARTERIAL DISEASE AND VENOUS THROMBOSIS*

ARTERIAL THROMBOSIS	ARTERIAL AND VENOUS THROMBOSIS	VENOUS THROMBOSIS
Atherosclerosis	Geography	Varicose veins
Male sex	Age	Malignancy
Smoking (positive)	Obesity	Infection
Blood pressure	Blood group A	Trauma
Diabetes	Oral contraceptives	Surgery (especially orthopedic)
	Homocystinemia	
Low-density lipoprotein cholesterol		
High-density lipoprotein cholesterol (negative)		General anesthesia Pregnancy
Triglyceride		Immobility
Family history		Heart failure
Hard water		Nephrotic syndrome
Alcohol (negative)		
Hematocrit		

*After Lowe, Clin Haemat 10:409, 1981.

reactivity in the thrombotic disease. The tests used have included aggregation, survival, release reactions, and analysis of platelet coagulant activity. Increased sensitivity to aggregating agents has been found in a variety of diseases, including myocardial infarction, diabetes mellitus, transient cerebral ischemia, and hyperbetalipoproteinemia. Platelet survival appears to correlate with the risk of subsequent thromboembolic complications following the insertion of cardiac valve prostheses, and a shortened survival has been found in a number of thrombotic states. The levels of two specific platelet proteins, β-thromboglobulin and platelet factor 4, may be significantly elevated in patients with established thrombosis. Apparent overactivity of the coagulant functions of platelets has been observed in a number of thrombotic states, although measurements of this kind do not appear to have been made in individuals before the development of thrombosis.

It appears therefore that the measurement of certain products of the platelet release reaction may be useful for confirming that there is an established thrombosis. On the other hand, the vast literature on abnormalities of platelet function in patients with thrombotic disease or who have disorders known to be associated with a high risk of thrombosis have provided little information about the pathogenesis of the thrombotic state.

Coagulation Factors

There has been considerable interest in the possibility that an increase in the concentration of one or more clotting factors might heighten the tendency to thrombosis. However, support for this view is scanty. Indeed, it seems to be based on rather dubious logic. Clotting factors are present in excess in normal plasma; there is no a priori reason that additional amounts should accelerate coagulation. There are, of course, many examples of protracted increases in the levels of clotting factors in conditions that appear to predispose to thrombosis. For example, elevated concentrations of fibrinogen, factor VIII, and the vitamin K–dependent clotting factors occur in normal pregnancy. Increased levels of factor VIII and fibrinogen occur in many pathologic states, including diabetes, renal disease, ischemic heart disease, and ulcerative colitis; these factors may be considered as acute phase reactants in these disorders. The same applies to the high levels of certain clotting factors in patients with malignancy or severe hepatic disease. Women who take oral contraceptives have higher levels of Hageman factor than do nonusers. Short-lived elevations of the concentration of factor VIII, fibrinogen, and possibly other factors occur after childbirth, surgical operations, other forms of trauma, myocardial infarction, and many acute illnesses. While these changes could form the basis for a prethrombotic state, there is no real evidence that an elevation in the level of one or more clotting factors is the primary cause of thrombotic disease.

Currently, efforts are being made to increase the sensitivity of techniques for demonstrating thrombin generation by employing sensitive assays for the demonstration of thrombin activity in the circulation. These methods may be valuable for diagnosing an established thrombosis. Whether they will be of any help for defining prethrombotic states is less clear.

Plasma Inhibitors of Clotting

The demonstration of an increased risk of thrombosis in individuals with inherited forms of antithrombin III deficiency and the apparent reduction in the incidence of thrombosis with the use of agents like stanozolol, which raise antithrombin III levels in such individuals, poses the question of how often a thrombotic tendency is caused by a relative deficiency of inhibitors of the coagulation system. Acquired antithrombin III deficiency has been described in the nephrotic syndrome (in which the protein is lost in the urine) or after asparaginase therapy for leukemia. There have been a few reports of deficiency of antithrombin III in the postoperative period or in association with malignancy. On the other hand, the measurement of antithrombin III levels preoperatively does not identify patients who subsequently develop postoperative thrombosis.

Recently, an association between venous thromboembolism and protein C deficiency has been reported. Protein C is the zymogen of a vitamin K—dependent serine protease. In its absence the inactivation of factors Va and VIII:C is impaired. So far, the deficiency has been reported in only a few isolated families.

Fibrinolytic activity has also been studied in a wide range of thrombotic and putative prethrombotic states. Reduced activity has been described in peripheral vascular disease, coronary artery disease, hypertriglyceridemia, diabetes, in contraceptive pill users, and in many other conditions. In a recent prospective study, men dying of coronary diseases had impaired fibrinolytic activity compared with the survivors, although the difference did not reach statistical significance. Inhibitors of plasminogen activation have been described occasionally in patients with gangrene, venous thrombosis, and Behçet's syndrome, although their significance is not yet clear.

SUMMARY OF THE CLINICAL ASSOCIATION OF THE PRETHROMBOTIC STATE

Some of the clinical disorders that are associated with a high incidence of arterial or venous thrombosis are summarized in Table 77. In no case is the mechanism for the thrombotic tendency absolutely clear.

Estrogen has already been considered. In summary, its administration has widespread metabolic effects, alters blood flow, and may damage vessel walls. It elevates plasma concentrations of fibrinogen and factors II, VIII, IX, and X and has measurable effects on platelet function. Plasma concentrations of antithrombin III are reduced, and vessel wall fibrinolytic activity is depleted. Similar changes have been noted in pregnancy.

There is a well-defined association between malignant disease and an increased tendency toward thromboembolism. There is evidence from animal experiments that material derived from tumor cells can activate platelets. Mucus, secreted by certain human adenocarcinomas, can activate factor X and cause intravascular coagulation when it is injected into experimental animals. The association between consumption coagulopathy and carcinoma has already been described.

A wide range of abnormalities of the vessel wall, platelets, and coagulation factors have been found in patients with diabetes. Which of these alterations increase the tendency toward thrombosis in this disorder and whether any of these alterations are of prime importance in the pathogenesis of the vascular lesions of diabetes remains uncertain.

Severe thrombotic episodes have been reported after administration of concentrates of the vitamin K–dependent clotting factors to patients with Christmas disease or liver disease or to premature infants. The responsible agents have not been defined. Low levels of antithrombin III seem to predispose to this complication.

The basis for the marked thrombotic tendency in disorders like paroxysmal nocturnal hemoglobinuria, Behçet's syndrome, and homocystinuria and the occurrence of thromboembolism in a number of patients with a circulating "lupus" anticoagulant is equally uncertain. It has been shown recently that the lupus anticoagulant inhibits the production of prostacyclin (PGI_2) by rat aorta. It has been suggested that these "antilipid" antibodies may interfere with the release of arachidonic acid from cell membranes. A similar type of antibody has been observed in patients with Behçet's syndrome.

SUMMARY

There is now a vast literature covering epidemiologic, clinical, and experimental studies on the pathogenesis of thrombotic and atherosclerotic disease. The picture is still very confusing. Undoubtedly, several genetic and environmental factors can interact to increase the likelihood of atheromatous change or pathologic thrombosis. Unfortunately, there is still no information about exactly how these processes are initiated or about the relative importance of the bewildering number of factors that appear to make them more likely to occur. The elucidation of these problems remains one of the most challenging problems for clinical practice in the affluent societies.

REFERENCES

General Textbooks Dealing with the Pathophysiology of the Blood

Beck, W. D. (ed.): Hematology. Harvard Pathophysiology Series. Vol. 2. Cambridge, MIT Press, 1977.

Hardisty, R. M., and Weatherall, D. J.: Blood and Its Disorders. 2nd ed. Oxford, Blackwell Scientific Publications, 1982.

Nathan, D. G., and Oski, F. A.: Hematology of Infancy and Childhood. 2nd ed. Philadelphia, W. B. Saunders Company, 1982.

Williams, W. J., Beutler, E., Erslev, A. J., and Lichtman, M. A.: Hematology. 3rd ed. New York, McGraw-Hill, 1983.

Wintrobe, M. M.: Clinical Hematology. 8th ed. Philadelphia, Lea and Febiger, 1981.

The Blood-Forming Organs and the Red Cell

Adamson, J. W., and Finch, C. A.: Hemoglobin function, oxygen affinity and erythropoietin. Ann Rev Physiol 37:351, 1975.

Bessis, M., Weed, R., and LeBlond, P. (eds.): Red Cell Shape, Physiology, Pathology, Ultrastructure. New York, Springer-Verlag, 1973.

Bird, G. W. G., and Tovey, G. H.: Blood groups and transfusion. In Hardisty, R. M., and Weatherall, D. J. (eds.): Blood and Its Disorders. 2nd ed. Oxford, Blackwell Scientific Publications, 1982, p. 1393.

Bowdler, A. J.: The spleen and its abnormalities. In Hardisty, R. M., and Weatherall, D. J. (eds.): Blood and Its Disorders.

2nd ed. Oxford, Blackwell Scientific Publications, 1982, p. 751.

Bunn, R. H., Forget, B. G., and Ranney, H. M.: Human Hemoglobins. Philadelphia, W. B. Saunders Company, 1977.

Chanarin, I.: The Megaloblastic Anaemias. 2nd ed. Oxford, Blackwell Scientific Publications, 1981.

Cooper, R. A., and Jandl, J. H.: Destruction of erythrocytes. In Williams, W. J., Beutler, E., Erslev, A. J., and Lichtman, M. A. (eds.): Hematology. 3rd ed. New York, McGraw-Hill, 1983, p. 377.

Crosby, W. H.: Structures and functions of the spleen. In Williams, W. J., Beutler, E., Erslev, A. J., and Lichtman, M. A. (eds.): Hematology. 3rd ed. New York, McGraw-Hill, 1983, p. 89.

Dacie, J. V.: The Haemolytic Anaemias. Vol. 1–4. London, Churchill Livingstone, 1960–1969.

Halliday, J. W., and Powell, L. W.: Serum ferritin and isoferritins in clinical medicine. In Brown, E. B. (ed.): Progress in Hematology, XI. New York, Grune and Stratton, 1979, p. 229.

Harris, J. W., and Kellermeyer, R. W.: The Red Cell. Cambridge, Harvard University Press, 1970.

Hoffbrand, A. V., and Wickremasinghe, R. G.: Megaloblastic anaemia. In Hoffbrand, A. V. (ed.): Recent Advances in Haematology. 3rd ed. Edinburgh, Churchill Livingstone, 1982, p. 25.

Hughes-Jones, N. C., and Bain, B.: Immune haemolytic anaemias. In Hardisty, R. M., and Weatherall, D. J. (eds.): Blood and Its Disorders. 2nd ed. Oxford, Blackwell Scientific Publications, 1982, p. 479.

Izac, G.: Erythroid cell differentiation and maturation. In Brown, E. B. (ed.): Progress in Hematology. Vol. 10. New York, Grune and Stratton, 1977, p. 1.

Jacobs, A.: Disorders of iron metabolism. In Hoffbrand, A. V. (ed.): Recent Advances in Haematology. 3rd ed. London, Churchill Livingstone, 1982, p. 1.

Keitt, A. S.: Diagnostic strategy in a suspected red cell enzymopathy. Clin Haematol 10:3, 1981.

Lajtha, L.: Cellular kinetics of haemopoiesis. In Hardisty, R. M., and Weatherall, D. J. (eds.): Blood and Its Disorders. 2nd ed. Oxford, Blackwell Scientific Publications, 1982, p. 57.

Marchesi, V. T.: The red cell membrane skeleton: Recent progress. Blood 61:1, 1983.

Miwa, S.: Pyruvate kinase deficiency and other enzymopathies of the Embden-Meyerhoff pathway. Clin Haematol 10:57, 1981.

Mlaeeovic, J., and Adamson, J. W.: Erythroid colony growth in culture: Analysis of erythroid differentiation and studies in human disease states. In Hoffbrand, A. V. (ed.): Recent Advances in Haematology. 3rd ed. Edinburgh, Churchill Livingstone, 1982, p. 95.

Mollison, P. L.: Blood Transfusion in Clinical Practice. 7th ed. Oxford, Blackwell Scientific Publications, 1982.

Moore, M. A. S.: Bone marrow culture: Leucopoiesis and stem cells. In Hoffbrand, A. V. (ed.): Recent Advances in Haematology. 3rd ed. Edinburgh, Churchill Livingstone, 1982, p. 109.

Schrier, S. L.: The red cell membrane and its abnormalities. In Hoffbrand, A. V. (ed.): Recent Advances in Haematology. 3rd ed. Edinburgh, Churchill Livingstone, 1982, p. 69.

Weatherall, D. J., and Clegg, J. B.: The Thalassemia Syndrome. 3rd ed. Oxford, Blackwell Scientific Publications, 1981.

White Cells and Lymphoma

Beeson, P. B., and Bass, D. A.: The Eosinophil. Philadelphia, W. B. Saunders Company, 1977.

Boggs, D. R., and Winkelstein, D. R.: White Cell Manual. 4th ed. Philadelphia, F. A. Davis, 1983.

Boxer, L. A., Coates, T. D., Haak, R. A., Wolach, J. B., Hoffstein, S., and Baehner, R. L.: Lactoferrin deficiency associated with altered granulocyte function. New Engl J Med 307:404, 1982.

Boxer, L. A., Greenberg, M. S., Boxer, G. J., and Stossel, T. P.: Autoimmune neutropenia. New Engl J Med 293:748, 1975.

Brouet, J.-L., Flandrin, G., Sasportes, M., Preud'Homme, J.-L., and Seligmann, M.: Chronic lymphocytic leukaemia of T-cell origin. Immunological and clinical evaluation in eleven patients. Lancet 2:890, 1975.

Butterworth, A. E., and David, J. R.: Eosinophil function. New Engl J Med 304:154, 1981.

Canellos, G. P., Whang-Peng, J., and DeVita, V. T.: Chronic granulocytic leukemia without the Philadelphia chromosome. Am J Clin Pathol 65:467, 1976.

Carter, R. L., and Penman, H. G.: Infectious Mononucleosis. Oxford, Blackwell Scientific Publications, 1969.

Catovsky, D., Pettit, J. E., Galton, D. A. G., Spiers, A. S. D., and Harrison, C. V.: Leukaemic reticuloendotheliosis ("hairy" cell leukaemia): A distinct clinico-pathological entity. Br J Haematol 26:9, 1974.

Cawley, J. C., and Hayhoe, F. G. H.: Ultrastructure of Haemic Cells. A Cytological Atlas of Normal and Leukaemic Blood and Bone Marrow. Philadelphia, W. B. Saunders Company, 1973.

Dale, D. C., Guerry, D., Wewerka, J. R., Bull, J. M., and Chusid, M. J.: Chronic neutropenia. Medicine 58:128, 1979.

Delamore, I. W.: Hypercalcaemia and myeloma. Br J Haematol 51:5–7, 1982.

Diamond, A., Cooper, G. M., Ritz, J., and Lane, M.-A.: Identification and molecular cloning of the human *Blym* transforming gene activated in Burkitt's lymphomas. Nature 305:112, 1983.

Epstein, M. A., and Achong, B. G.: Pathogenesis of infectious mononucleosis. Lancet 2:1270, 1977.

Fauci, A. S., Harley, J. B., Roberts, W. C., Ferrans, V. J., Gralnick, H. R., and Bjornson, B. H.: The idiopathic hypereosinophilic syndrome: Clinical pathophysiologic, and therapeutic considerations. Ann Intern Med 97:78, 1982.

Fialkow, P. J., Singer, J. W., Adamson, J. W., Vaidya, K., Dow, L. W., Ochs, J., and Moohr, J. W.: Acute nonlymphocytic leukemia: Heterogeneity of stem cell origin. Blood 57:1068, 1981.

Foon, K. A., Schroff, R. W., and Gale, R. P.: Surface markers on leukemia and lymphoma cells: Recent advances. Blood 60:1, 1982.

Galton, D. A. G., Goldman, J. M., Wiltshaw, E., Catovsky, D., Henry, K., and Goldenberg, G. J.: Prolymphocytic leukaemia. Br J Haematol 27:7, 1974.

Gunz, F. W., and Henderson, E. S.: Leukemia. 4th ed. New York, Grune and Stratton, 1983.

Jacob, H. S., Craddock, P. R., Hammerschmidt, D. E., and Moldow, C. F.: Complement-induced granulocyte aggregation. An unsuspected mechanism of disease. New Engl J Med 302:789, 1980.

Johnston, R. B.: Defects of neutrophil function. New Engl J Med 307:434, 1982.

Kaplan, H. S.: Hodgkin's disease: Biology, treatment, prognosis. Blood 57:813, 1981.

Kay, A. B.: Functions of the eosinophil leucocyte. Br J Haematol 33:313, 1976.

Klein, G.: The Epstein-Barr virus and neoplasia. New Engl J Med 293:1353, 1975.

Koeffler, H. P., and Golde, D. W.: Chronic myelogenous leukemia—new concepts (Part 1). New Engl J Med 304:1201, 1981.

Korsmeyer, S. J., Arnold, A., Bakhshi, A., Ravetch, J. V., Siebenlist, U., Hieter, P. A., Sharrow, S. O., LeBien, T. W., Kersey, J. H., Poplack, D. G., Leder, P., and Waldmann, T. A.: Immunoglobulin gene rearrangement and cell surface antigen expression in acute lymphocytic leukemias of T cell and B cell precursor origins. J Clin Investigat 71:301, 1983.

Krontiris, T. G.: The emerging genetics of human cancer. New Engl J Med 309:404, 1983.

Logue, G. L., and Shimm, D. S.: Autoimmune granulocytopenia. Ann Rev Med 31:191, 1980.

Murphy, P.: The Neutrophil. New York, Plenum Medical, 1976.

Nathan, C. F., Murray, H. W., and Cohen, Z. A.: The macrophage as an effector cell. New Engl J Med 303:622, 1980.

Purtilo, D. T.: Immunopathology of infectious mononucleosis and other complications of Epstein-Barr virus infections. Pathol Ann 15:253, 1980.

Rowley, J. D.: Do all leukemic cells have an abnormal karyotype? New Engl J Med 305:164, 1981.

Safai, B., and Good, R. A.: Lymphoproliferative disorders of the T-cell series. Medicine 59:335, 1980.

Salmon, S. E., and Seligmann, M.: B-cell neoplasia in man. Lancet 2:1230, 1974.

Segal, A. W., and Peters, T. J.: Characterisation of the enzyme defect in chronic granulomatous disease. Lancet 1:1363, 1976.

The Non-Hodgkin's Lymphoma Pathologic Classification Project: National Cancer Institute sponsored study of classifications of Non-Hodgkin's lymphomas. Summary and description of a working formulation for clinical usage. Cancer 49:2112, 1982.

Vincent, P. C.: The measurement of granulocyte kinetics. Br J Haematol 36:1, 1977.

Ziegler, J. L.: Burkitt's lymphoma. New Engl J Med 305:735, 1981.

Hypersplenism, Platelets, and Coagulation

Bloom, A. L., and Thomas, D. P.: Haemostasis and Thrombosis. Edinburgh, Churchill Livingstone, 1981.

Born, G. V. R.: Fluid-mechanical and biochemical interactions in haemostasis. Br Med Bull 33:193, 1977.

Bowdler, A. J.: Splenomegaly and hypersplenism. Clin Haematol 12:467, 1983.

Burstein, S. A., and Harker, L. A.: Control of platelet production. Clin Haematol 12:3, 1983.

Cederholm-Williams, S. A.: Control of fibrinolysis. Br J Hosp Med 30:107, 1983.

Chesterman, C. N., Gallus, A. S., and Penington, D. G.: Platelets, the vessel wall and antiplatelet drugs. Recent Advances in Haematology. 3rd ed. Edinburgh, Churchill Livingstone, 1982, pp. 253–284.

Collins, J. A.: Problems associated with the massive transfusion of stored blood. Surgery 75:274, 1974.

Colman, R. W., Robboy, S. J., and Minna, J. D.: Disseminated intravascular coagulation: A reappraisal. Ann Rev Med 30:359, 1979.

Davie, E. W., and Fujikawa, K.: Basic mechanisms in blood coagulation. Ann Rev Biochem 44:799, 1975.

Davies, J. A., and McNicol, G. P.: Blood coagulation and thrombosis. Br Med Bull 34:113, 1978.

de Gaetano, G.: Platelets, prostaglandins and thrombic disorders. Clin Haematol 10:297, 1981.

Esnouf, M. P.: Biochemistry of blood coagulation. Br Med Bull 33:213, 1977.

Esnouf, M. P.: Biochemistry of coagulation. Recent Advances in Haematology. 3rd ed. Edinburgh, Churchill Livingstone, 1982, pp. 285–299.

Ferrant, A.: The role of the spleen in haemolysis. Clin Haematol 12:489, 1981.

Gaffney, P. J.: Structure of fibrinogen and degradation products in fibrinogen and fibrin. Br Med Bull 33:245, 1977.

Gallop, P. M., Lian, J. B., and Hauschka, P. V.: Carboxylated calcium-binding protein and vitamin K. New Engl J Med 302:1460, 1980.

Gardner, F. H., and Bessman, J. D.: Thrombocytopenia due to defective platelet production. Clin Haematol 12:23, 1983.

Goldman, J. M., and Nolasco, I.: The spleen in myeloproliferative disorders. Clin Haematol 12:505, 1983.

Hardisty, R. M.: Hereditary disorders of platelet function. Clin Haematol 12:153, 1983.

Harker, L. A., Schwartz, S. M., and Ross, R.: Endothelium and arteriosclerosis. Clin Haematol 10:283, 1981.

Harlan, J. M.: Thrombocytopenia due to non-immune platelet destruction. Clin Haematol 12:39, 1983.

Hoyer, L. W.: The factor VIII complex: Structure and function. Blood 58:1981.

Kernoff, P. B. A.: Normal and abnormal fibrinolysis. Br Med Bull 33:239, 1977.

Kernoff, P. B. A., and Tuddenham, E. G. D.: Congenital and acquired coagulation disorders. Recent Advances in Haematology. 3rd ed. Edinburgh, Churchill Livingstone, 1982, pp. 301–322.

Koutts, J., Howard, M. A., and Firkin, B. G.: Factor VIII physiology and pathology in man. In Brown, E. B. (ed.): Progress in Hematology, XI. New York, Grune and Stratton, 1979, p. 115.

Lowe, G. D. O.: Laboratory evaluation of hypercoagulability. Clin Haematol 10:407, 1983.

Lowe, G. D. O., and Forbes, C. D.: Blood rheology and thrombosis. Clin Haematol 10:343, 1981.

Mannuccio, P. M., and Vigano, S.: Deficiencies of protein C, an inhibitor of blood coagulation. Lancet 2:463, 1982.

McKay, D. G., and Margaretten, W.: Disseminated intravascular coagulation in virus disease. Arch Intern Med 120:129, 1967.

McMillian, R.: Immune thrombocytopenia. Clin Haematol 12:69, 1983.

Meade, T. W.: Risk associations in the thrombotic disorders. Clin Haematol 10:391, 1981.

Moncada, S., and Vane, J. R.: Unstable metabolites of arachidonic acid. Br Med Bull 34:129, 1978.

Murphy, S.: Thrombocytosis and thrombocythaemia. Clin Haematol 12:89, 1983.

Nemerson, Y., and Pitlick, F. A.: Extrinsic clotting pathways. In Spet, T. H. (ed.): Progress in Hemostasis and Thrombosis. Vol. 1. New York, Grune and Stratton, 1974, p. 1.

Paglia, D. E., and Valentine, W. N.: Haemolytic anaemia associated with disorders of the purine and pyrimidine salvage pathways. Clin Haematol 10:81, 1981.

Rao, A. K., and Walsh, P. N.: Acquired qualitative platelet disorders. Clin Haematol 12:201, 1983.

Ratnoff, O. D.: Hemostatic mechanisms in liver disease. Med Clin North Am 47:721, 1963.

Schleider, M. A., Nachman, R. L., Jaffe, E. A., and Coleman, M.: A clinical study of the lupus anticoagulant. Blood 48:499, 1976.

Sharp, A. A.: Diagnosis and management of disseminated intravascular coagulation. Br Med Bull 33:265, 1977.

Slichter, S. J., and Harker, L. A.: Hemostasis in malignancy. Ann NY Acad Sci 230:252, 1974.

Vermylen, J., Badenhorst, P. N., Deckmyn, H., and Arnout, J.: Normal mechanisms of platelet function. Clin Haematol 12:107, 1983.

White, J. G.: Platelet morphology and function. In Williams, W. J., Beutler, E., Erslev, A. J., and Lichtman, M. A. (eds.): Hematology. 3rd ed. New York, McGraw-Hill, 1983, p. 1121.

Yoshikawa, T., Tanaka, K. R., and Guze, L. B.: Infection and disseminated intravascular coagulation. Medicine 50:237, 1971.

Zimmerman, T. S., and Ruggeri, Z. M.: Von Willebrand's disease. Clin Haematol 12:175, 1983.

Journals and Monograph Series Dealing with Pathophysiology of the Blood

Several journals and monograph series deal with various aspects of the pathophysiology of the blood. These include *British Journal of Haematology* (Oxford, Blackwell Scientific Publications); *Blood* (New York, Grune and Stratton); *Clinics in Hematology* (Philadelphia and London, W. B. Saunders Co.); *Seminars in Hematology* (New York, Grune and Stratton); *Recent Advances in Haematology* (London and New York, Churchill Livingstone); and *Progress in Hematology* (New York, Grune and Stratton).

METABOLISM

PHILIP FELIG, M.D.,
RICHARD J. HAVEL, M.D.,
and LLOYD H. SMITH, JR., M.D.

Introduction

FUEL HOMEOSTASIS

The human organism may be characterized not only in terms of its constituent organ systems but also with respect to the chemical and physical processes undertaken in these systems. In this sense, *metabolism* is central to all physiological processes carried out in every organ system of the body. However, as a discipline of medicine, *metabolism* generally deals with body fuel homeostasis, particularly the assimilation, interconversion, and degradation of carbohydrate, fat, and protein. Since the utilization of these various substrates is largely hormonally regulated, an understanding of various aspects of endocrine function, particularly the glucoregulatory, lipolytic, and protein anabolic and catabolic hormones, is essential to a discussion of metabolism.

In this section the metabolic pathways and endocrine control of carbohydrate, fat, and amino acid metabolism will be discussed. The synthesis, transport, metabolism, and pathophysiology of lipids are covered beginning on page 392. In the present section, lipids are discussed as metabolic fuels. Various vitamins and trace minerals that are involved in fuel homeostasis will also be covered.

METABOLIC PATHWAYS AND CYCLES

The breakdown or formation of organic compounds within cells occurs along a series of enzymatically catalyzed reactions that are generally referred to as metabolic pathways (for example, the glycolytic, or Embden-Meyerhof, pathway). In these sequences a given compound is converted by means of a variety of intermediate steps into an end product (for example, the conversion of glucose to lactate in the glycolytic pathway) (Fig. 1*A*). To ensure that the sequence of events progresses in a desired fashion, one or more reactions in a given pathway are essentially irreversible. This irreversibility is a consequence of a large loss of free energy. These irreversible steps constitute sites of metabolic control. In many (but not all) instances the first step in the pathway is the regulatory site and is termed the *committed step.*

A given precursor or series of intermediates may be common to a variety of metabolic pathways. Such pathways thus show branch points (Fig. 1*B*); for example, in addition to glycolysis, glucose may be converted to glycogen or (via the pentose pathway) to ribose. The initial step common to each of these pathways is the formation of glucose-6-phosphate. The committed step in glycolysis is consequently at a point distal to the formation of glucose-6-phosphate—namely, the formation of fructose-1,6-diphosphate (see Carbohydrate, p. 326).

In certain circumstances a reaction sequence involves the regeneration of the initial precursor. Such processes are termed metabolic cycles (Fig. 1*C*). These cyclic interconversions may take place within a given cell or subcellular compartment or may involve the interchange of precursors and intermediates between

A. Unbranched Pathway

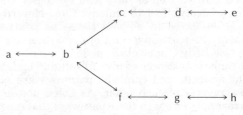

B. Branched Pathway

C. Cyclic Pathway

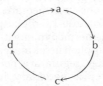

Figure 1. Various types of metabolic pathways: A, Unbranched; B, Branched; C, Cyclic Pathway. Each of the steps in all of the pathways is catalyzed by a specific enzyme requiring various cofactors.

different tissues. For example, in the oxidation of acetyl CoA to CO_2 via the tricarboxylic acid cycle (Krebs cycle), oxaloacetate condenses with acetyl CoA in the first step of the reaction sequence and is regenerated in the final step. The entire process occurs within the mitochondria. In contrast, in the Cori cycle, glucose is taken up by muscle tissue, where it is converted to lactate and pyruvate. The latter are released from muscle into the bloodstream and are extracted by the liver. Within the liver, lactate and pyruvate are reconverted to glucose. This recycling of glucose via pyruvate and lactate is quantitatively important in human subjects, accounting for 15 to 25 per cent of the total glucose turnover.

CATABOLISM AND ANABOLISM

Metabolic sequences may be characterized as catabolic or anabolic in nature. Catabolism refers to degradative processes in which larger, complex molecules such as proteins, carbohydrates, and lipids of endogenous origin (for example, liver glycogen) or exogenous origin (for example, a protein meal) are broken down to smaller molecules. The resultant smaller molecules may take the form of metabolic intermediates that remain within the body and undergo further transformations (for example, lactate or pyruvate). In addition, catabolic processes generate very small products that are irretrievably lost to the organism in expired air (CO_2 generated from carbohydrate, fat, or amino acid oxidation) or urine (urea formed from amino acids). Regardless of the end product formed, catabolic processes result in the liberation of energy, which is made available for other cellular processes by storage as ATP (adenosine triphosphate).

Anabolism refers to synthetic processes in which simple compounds are converted to more complex molecules such as proteins, lipids, and polysaccharides. Such synthetic reactions consume ATP. However, biosynthesis should not be viewed as a process resulting in a net loss of energy to the organism. The complex substances synthesized represent a reservoir of energy that is regenerated as ATP when the storage molecules are degraded; for example, ATP is consumed in the first, committed step of fatty acid synthesis, the conversion of acetyl CoA to malonyl CoA. Nevertheless, fatty acids stored in adipose tissue as triglycerides represent the most important storage reservoir of calories (see Body Composition, p. 364).

An important aspect of overall cellular metabolism is that anabolic and catabolic pathways are not the precise reverse of each other. As noted above, there are irreversible steps in these pathways that constitute points of metabolic control. Bypass of these irreversible reactions is achieved by means of separate enzymes and/or the formation of metabolic intermediates. For example, the synthesis of fructose-1,6-diphosphate from fructose-6-phosphate is a thermodynamically irreversible step catalyzed by phosphofructokinase. This transformation constitutes a key regulatory point in glycolysis. Reversal of this step is necessary in the gluconeogenic pathway and is achieved by means of a separate enzyme, fructose diphosphatase. In another glycolytic reaction, conversion of phosphoenolpyruvate to pyruvate by the enzyme pyruvic kinase is irreversible. This sequence is nevertheless reversed by initially converting pyruvate to oxaloacetate (by the enzyme pyruvate carboxylase), after which the oxaloacetate is converted to phosphoenolpyruvate (by the enzyme phosphoenolpyruvate carboxykinase). In this instance the biological reversal of a metabolic pathway requires two additional enzymes plus an intermediate (oxaloacetate) not present in the forward pathway.

INTEGRATION OF METABOLIC PATHWAYS

The individual chemical reactions that occur in intact cells can largely be duplicated in the laboratory test tube so long as the proper enzymes and cofactors are available. The in vivo situation differs, however, in that a variety of reactions progress simultaneously and may influence each other in a positive or negative manner. For example, the conversion of acetyl CoA to malonyl CoA (the first committed step in the pathway of fat synthesis) results in decreased ketone formation. This interaction is a consequence of inhibition of the acylcarnitine transferase reaction necessary for fatty acid oxidation (see Lipids, p. 337). In this manner changes in the metabolic pathway involved in fat synthesis have a negative feedback effect on fat oxidation and ketogenesis.

An example of a positive feedback in a reaction sequence is the interaction between fat oxidation and gluconeogenesis. Increased oxidation of fatty acids results in an elevation of mitochondrial acetyl CoA. The latter acts as an allosteric activator of the enzyme pyruvate carboxylase, which catalyzes the first step in the reversal of glycolysis, whereby glucose is formed from pyruvate. Stimulation of fat oxidation thus has the effect of enhancing gluconeogenesis.

Interactions between pathways may not only take the form of enzyme activation by intermediates but may also involve the production of substrates for the replenishment of intermediates in metabolic cycles. Such transformations are termed *anaplerotic reactions*. In the example cited above, carboxylation of pyruvate results in the formation of oxaloacetate, which is a necessary substrate for the operation of the tricarboxylic acid (Krebs) cycle.

It is thus apparent that the complexity of cellular metabolism derives not only from the multiplicity of pathways available but also from the diversity of interactions between these processes. Alterations in the metabolism of a given body fuel (for example, glucose) are thus likely to be accompanied by changes in the metabolism of other fuels as well.

HORMONAL REGULATION

Among the most important regulators of the various metabolic pathways are the hormones, chemical messengers secreted by specialized tissues that have effects at target cells distal to the site of their secretion. In terms of their chemical composition, the hormones may be divided into three subgroups: polypeptides, steroids, and amino acid derivatives. Examples of these three types are provided in Table 1.

A characteristic feature of hormone action is the initial interaction with *receptors*, specialized proteins that bind the hormone with high specificity and affinity (Fig. 2). In the case of polypeptide hormones (for

TABLE 1. CLASSIFICATION OF HORMONES BY CHEMICAL STRUCTURE

POLYPEPTIDES	STEROIDS	AMINO ACID DERIVATIVES
Insulin	Cortisol	Thyroxine
Glucagon	Aldosterone	Epinephrine
Growth Hormone	Testosterone	Norepinephrine
ACTH	Estrogen	Triiodothyronine
FSH	Progesterone	
LH	Vitamin D	
Prolactin		
Parathormone		
Calcitonin		
Somatostatin		
Oxytocin		
Vasopressin		
Gastrin		
Secretin		
Pancreozymin-Cholecystokinin		
TSH		
Somatomedins		

example, insulin and glucagon) and catecholamines, these receptors are located on the cell surface. In contrast, the lipid-soluble steroid hormones interact with cytoplasmic receptors, while thyroxine binds to the cell nucleus. The role of hormone receptors in regulating the cellular response to hormones is covered in detail in the discussion of insulin (see p. 356).

Following the interaction of the hormone with its receptor, changes in intracellular metabolism are mediated via a *second messenger* within the cell. In the case of glucagon and the beta-adrenergic effects of epinephrine, the second messenger has been clearly identified as 3'5' cyclic adenylic acid (cyclic AMP). The binding of the hormone to its receptor induces a conformational change in the cell membrane that activates a membrane-bound enzyme, adenylate cyclase, which in turn promotes the formation of cyclic AMP

from ATP. The increase in cyclic AMP results in the allosteric activation of a cytoplasmic protein kinase. The latter may activate a variety of intracellular enzymes. Cessation of these intracellular events when the hormone concentration is decreased is facilitated by the action of phosphodiesterase, an enzyme that catalyzes the hydrolysis of cyclic AMP to adenosine phosphate. This enzyme is inhibited by theophylline and caffeine, which can thereby amplify the action of cyclic AMP–dependent hormones.

An example of the cascade of enzymatic activations whereby glucagon or epinephrine stimulates glycogen breakdown within the liver is shown in Figure 3.

While cyclic AMP has been documented as the second messenger for a variety of hormones, in the case of insulin, a major regulator of intermediary metabolism, the nature of the second messenger remains to be established. In glucagon-stimulated or epinephrine-stimulated cells in which cyclic AMP levels are elevated, insulin will bring about a reduction in its concentration. However, in unstimulated cells, insulin induces a variety of effects without altering basal levels of cyclic AMP. The mechanism of insulin action is discussed in detail beginning on page 353.

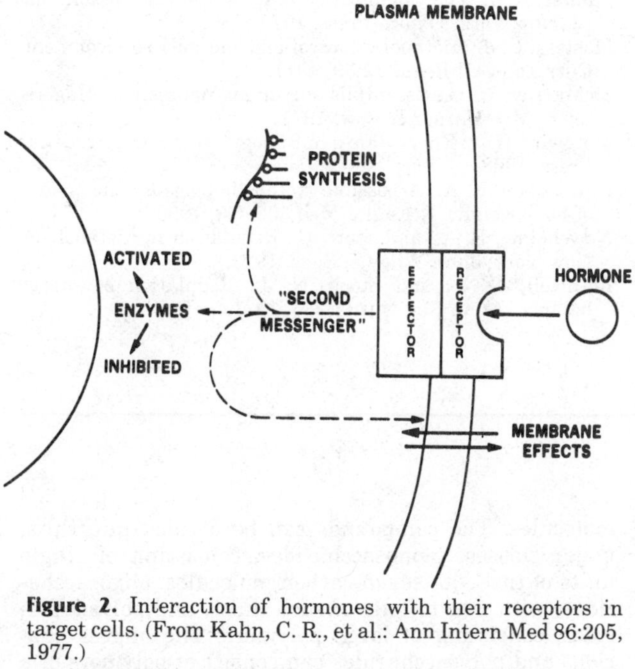

Figure 2. Interaction of hormones with their receptors in target cells. (From Kahn, C. R., et al.: Ann Intern Med 86:205, 1977.)

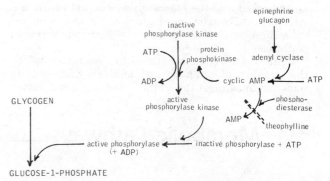

Figure 3. Metabolic sequence in the stimulation of glycogenolysis by epinephrine or glucagon. A hormonally mediated increase in cyclic AMP initiates a cascade of enzymatic reactions resulting in glycogen breakdown. (From Felig, P.: Disorders of carbohydrate metabolism. In Bondy, P. K., and Rosenberg, L. R. (eds.): Metabolic Control and Disease. 8th ed. Philadelphia, W. B. Saunders Co., 1980.)

Increases in hormone concentration alter metabolic activity by changing substrate concentrations or enzyme activity. Changes in substrate concentration may be brought about by alterations in transport processes. For example, the stimulation of glycogen synthesis in muscle and triglyceride formation in adipose tissue is the result of the stimulatory effect of insulin on the transport of glucose across the cell membrane of the muscle cell or adipocyte. In contrast, in the liver, which is freely permeable to glucose, glycogen synthesis is stimulated by insulin, which activates glycogen synthetase and induces the synthesis of glucokinase.

The nature of hormone action is such that a variety of processes are simultaneously affected so as to achieve a given end result. For example, the stimulatory effects of epinephrine on glycogenolysis are accompanied by simultaneous inhibition of glycogen synthetase and activation of gluconeogenesis. The overall result is an increase in blood sugar concentration. Similarly, insulin enhances triglyceride storage in adipose cells through a variety of mechanisms: stimulation of fatty acid synthesis, inhibition of lipolysis (triglyceride breakdown), and increased uptake of glucose and its conversion to α-glycerophosphate.

From the standpoint of body fuel homeostasis and intermediary metabolism, the most important hormones are insulin, glucagon, catecholamines, growth hormone, cortisol, and thyroid hormone. Each of these (other than thyroid hormone, which is covered in Section VIII, Endocrinology) is discussed in detail below.

DYNAMIC STATE OF METABOLISM

The intracellular and extracellular concentrations of substrates are generally maintained within relatively narrow limits. This constancy of the metabolic milieu is not due to a lack of activity along metabolic pathways but is a result of a dynamic equilibrium in which the rates of catabolic and anabolic processes are delicately balanced. Extracellular metabolites also show rapid turnover rates despite minimal changes in concentration. During exercise blood glucose is continuously extracted by the muscle, where it undergoes terminal oxidation. At the same time glucose is formed by gluconeogenesis and glycogenolysis within the liver and released into the bloodstream. The net result is a virtually unchanged blood glucose concentration despite three- to fivefold increases in total body turnover of glucose.

While steady-state conditions are characterized by the equality of catabolic and anabolic processes, in some circumstances the overall "metabolic set" favors either net catabolism or anabolism. Changes in substrate and/or hormone concentrations and in enzyme activity may favor either biosynthetic (anabolic) or catabolic processes, resulting in the accumulation or dissipation of complex molecules. For example, after the ingestion of a carbohydrate-containing meal the rise in blood glucose coupled with an elevation in plasma insulin stimulates glycogen and fat synthesis while reducing lipolysis. The result is an increase in glycogen and triglyceride synthesis. In contrast, during starvation, a fall in plasma insulin and glucose coupled with a rise in glucagon results in stimulation of glycogen and fat breakdown and cessation of fat synthesis.

The integrated nature of metabolic control is such that hormonal- and substrate-induced changes in synthetic and/or catabolic pathways are coordinated so as to avoid *futile cycles*. The latter may be described as increases in metabolic activity that fail to increase or decrease the concentration of complex or simple substrates yet may result in a net loss of ATP. For example, stimulation of glycogen synthetase by insulin and glucose would result in little accumulation of glycogen were there not a simultaneous inhibition of phosphorylase (conversion of the active to the inactive form). In some organisms, however, there may be futile cycling, as in the interconversion of fructose-6-phosphate and fructose-1,6-diphosphate. The purpose of such futile cycling may be the production of body heat. Whether such futile cycles, which have been observed in insects, occur in human cells and contribute to temperature regulation or dissipation of stored calories has not been established.

REFERENCES

Fuel Homeostasis

Bender, M. L., and Brubacker, L. J.: Catalysis and Enzyme Action. New York, McGraw-Hill Book Co., 1973.

Kim, E., and Grisohn, S. (eds.): Biochemical Regulatory Mechanisms in Eukaryotic Cells. New York, John Wiley & Sons, 1972.

Laidler, K. J.: The Chemical Kinetics of Enzyme Action. 2nd ed. New York, Oxford Press, 1973.

Masters, C. J.: Metabolic control and the microenvironment. Curr Top Cell Regul 12:39, 1977.

McMurray, W. C.: Essentials of Human Metabolism. Hagerstown, MD, Harper & Row, 1971.

Morowitz, H. J.: Energy Flow in Biology. New York, Academic Press, 1968.

Newsholme, E. A.: A possible metabolic basis for the control of body weight. N Engl J Med 302:400, 1980.

Newsholme, E. A., and Start, C.: Regulation in Metabolism. New York, John Wiley & Sons, 1973.

Rothwell, N. J., and Stock, N. J.: Regulation of energy balance. Annu Rev Nutr 1:235, 1981.

Metabolic Pathways

CARBOHYDRATE

DEFINITION

Carbohydrates are molecules of three or more carbons combined with hydrogen and oxygen in a proportion of CH_2O, or are simple derivatives of these basic molecules. The compounds can be divided into three major classes: monosaccharides, consisting of single units of three- to seven-carbon molecules; oligosaccharides, with two to four of such units; and polysaccharides, consisting of large polymers. The oligosaccharides and polysaccharides can consist of polymers of a single monosaccharide unit or of mixtures of several such units. Thus, maltose consists of two glucose molecules, whereas lactose consists of a glucose and a galactose molecule. The most important polysaccharides from a nutritional point of view—starch and glycogen—consist of only glucose polymers. Structural polysaccharides usually include units that are not pure carbohydrate but that have a carboxyl or esterified amino group. Hyaluronic acid, for example, is a polymer of glucuronic acid and *N*-acetyl-glucosamine. Mixed polymers with proteins also occur (mucoproteins).

Although carbohydrates are essential components of the nucleic acids and of structural compounds such as hyaluronic acid and although they are required as energy-producing substrates for certain organs such as the central nervous system and exercising muscle, all the necessary sugar units can be manufactured in the body from various precursors. These precursors may take the form of amino acids as well as glycolytic intermediates such as lactate, pyruvate, and glycerol. As a result, no carbohydrate is required in the diet, and it has been shown experimentally that human beings can survive in good health for months on a diet of meat and fats, which provides only very small amounts of sugar. In spite of this, the diets consumed in most parts of the world provide considerable amounts of carbohydrate, both as components of vegetable and grain foods, and as purified substances such as sucrose. Most Americans and Western Europeans obtain approximately 40 to 50 per cent of their calories from carbohydrate. In some parts of Asia, carbohydrate may account for over 80 per cent of dietary calories. Since it is more efficient and less expensive to use vegetables and grains for food than meats and dairy products, the proportion of carbohydrate in the diet tends to be higher when financial resources are restricted.

SITES AND FATE OF GLUCOSE METABOLISM

Since little, if any, glucose is present as such intracellularly, any glucose taken up by tissues undergoes metabolic transformation (Fig. 4). The major fates of glucose that enters the cell are (1) storage as glycogen; (2) oxidation via the glycolytic (anaerobic) pathway to pyruvate and lactate; (3) oxidation via the aerobic, tricarboxylic acid (Krebs) cycle to CO_2; (4) conversion to fatty acids and storage as triglyceride (fat synthesis); and (5) release from the cell as free glucose.

The major tissues in which glucose is metabolized are liver, muscle, fat, and brain. The extent of glucose uptake and the nature of its metabolic transformations depend on such factors as whether one is dealing with fasting, feeding, rest, or exercise. These various conditions are discussed in detail below.

In general, the brain is primarily a site of aerobic oxidation to CO_2 and adipose tissue is a locus of conversion of glucose to glycerol (an intermediate in the glycolytic pathway) and of fatty acid synthesis. Within muscle tissue there is active glycogen synthesis in the resting state after feeding as well as between meals. With exercise, anaerobic and aerobic oxidation are stimulated. Within the liver each of the potential fates of glucose is represented by active metabolic pathways.

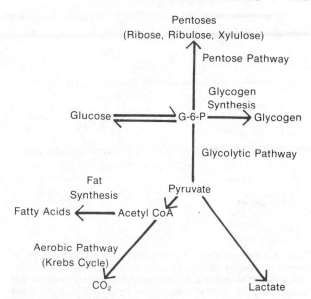

Figure 4. The metabolic fates of glucose. The metabolic transformation of glucose begins with the formation of glucose-6-phosphate (G-6-P). Thereafter, G-6-P may be utilized along the pentose pathway, for glycogen synthesis for glycolysis, for fat synthesis, or for oxidation to CO_2 via the aerobic pathway (Krebs cycle).

PHYSIOLOGY AND PATHOPHYSIOLOGY OF GLYCOGEN METABOLISM

The control of glycogen metabolism demonstrates several regulatory principles characteristic of a variety of metabolic pathways. First, the enzymatic steps involved in glycogen synthesis (Fig. 5) and breakdown (Fig. 6) are entirely different. In this manner biological reversal of thermodynamically irreversible steps is achieved. Second, hormonal signals stimulating glycogen breakdown (for example, epinephrine in muscle and liver or epinephrine and glucagon in liver) by activating phosphorylase cause a simultaneous inhibition of glycogen synthetase (Fig. 3). The reverse is true for signals that activate glycogen synthetase (for example, insulin and/or glucose). In this manner a futile cycle in which there is increased turnover of glycogen with neither net accumulation nor breakdown is avoided. Third, a deficiency in the enzymatic steps involved in these processes results in glycogen storage diseases characterized by the accumulation of abnor-

Glucose
   ATP ↓ Hexokinase, Glucokinase
Glucose-6-P
    ↓ phosphoglucomutase
Glucose-1-P
UTP ↓ uridine diphosphate glucose pyrophosphorylase
Uridine Diphospho Glucose (UDPG)
Primary Glycogen
  Residue   ↓ Glycogen Synthetase
   Glycogen Elongation
    ↓ Amylo (1, 4 → 1, 6) transglucosylase
   Glycogen Branching

Figure 5. Metabolic pathway for glycogen synthesis. Glucose must be converted to an "activated" form, uridine diphosphoglucose, in order for glycogen synthetase to catalyze its transfer to a primer residue of glycogen.

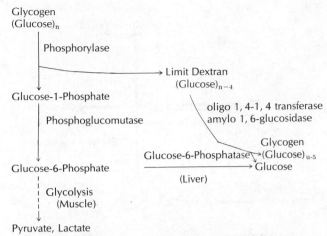

Figure 6. Glycogenolysis. The breakdown of glycogen by phosphorylase results in the formation of glucose-1-phosphate, which, after conversion to glucose-6-phosphate, may be released from the liver as free glucose by action of the enzyme glucose-6-phosphatase. In muscle tissue that lacks the enzyme glucose-6-phosphatase, the phosphorylated glucose enters the glycolytic pathway, resulting in the formation of lactate and pyruvate. A small amount of free glucose is formed directly from glycogen by action of the debrancher enzyme, amylo-1,6-glucosidase.

mal amounts or types of glycogen in liver and/or muscle tissue. At present, at least 10 varieties of glycogen storage disease have been identified. Three examples will be described briefly to illustrate clinical expression of enzyme deficiency states.

Type I glycogen storage disease, or von Gierke's disease, is the most common form of glycogenosis and is characterized by a deficiency of the hepatic enzyme glucose-6-phosphatase. Absence of this enzyme prevents the release of glucose from the liver, resulting in fasting hypoglycemia. Furthermore, the high concentration of glucose-6-phosphate within the liver stimulates the enzyme glycogen synthetase even when it is present in its active form, resulting in massive accumulation of liver glycogen. Since glucose-6-phosphatase is normally absent from muscle tissue, no abnormalities in muscle glycogen metabolism are observed.

In McArdle's syndrome there is selective deficiency of muscle phosphorylase. As a consequence, glucose is unavailable for glycolysis during the early phase of exercise, resulting in weakness and muscle cramps. The rise in blood lactate and pyruvate that normally accompanies exercise fails to occur in such patients. These findings contrast with Hers' disease (Type VI glycogenosis) in which there is a specific lack of liver phosphorylase. Such patients have no difficulty with exercise but may experience mild hypoglycemia in childhood.

An abnormality of the glycogen synthetic pathway is observed in Type IV glycogenosis (amylopectinosis). In this disorder the enzyme required for the formation of $\alpha 1,6$ glucosyl linkage (the brancher enzyme, amylo [1,4→1,6] transglucosylase) is deficient. The glycogen that accumulates in this disorder is abnormal, having a paucity of branch points. Hepatomegaly and decreased liver function are observed.

GLYCOLYSIS

The anaerobic catabolism of glucose to pyruvate and lactate is termed glycolysis. This catabolic process was the first enzymatic system to be elucidated and is often referred to as the Embden-Meyerhof pathway (Fig. 7). It provides the mechanism whereby the chemical energy stored as glucose is made available for cellular processes as high energy phosphate in the form of ATP via oxidative-reductive reactions that may occur in the absence of oxygen. Under anaerobic circumstances, the end product of glycolysis is lactate. In aerobic conditions the end product is pyruvate, which, following conversion to acetyl CoA, enters the tricarboxylic acid or Krebs cycle and is oxidized to CO_2 (Fig. 4). The enzymes involved in glycolysis are located within the cytoplasm and are widely distributed in virtually all cells throughout the body. However, glycolysis is quantitatively a major route of glucose utilization in only specific cell types: (a) red blood cells that lack the aerobic oxidative pathway; (b) skeletal muscle, particularly during vigorous exercise; and (c) heart muscle during circumstances of impaired perfusion (for example, coronary artery disease).

The overall catabolism of glucose to lactate involves three simultaneously coordinated processes: (1) breakdown of the 6-carbon skeleton of glucose, an aldehyde, via a series of enzymatic steps to a 3-carbon acid, lactic acid; (2) transfer of energy by the net synthesis of ATP; (3) transfer of electrons via a sequence of oxidoreductive reactions.

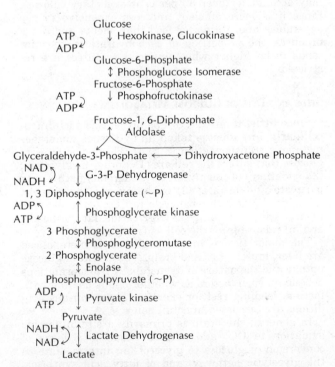

Figure 7. The glycolytic (Embden-Meyerhof) pathway. The major rate-limiting reactions are those catalyzed by hexokinase (or glucokinase), phosphofructokinase, and pyruvatekinase. Each glucose molecule gives rise to two triose phosphates, each of which is further metabolized to pyruvate and lactate.

The overall net balance of carbon skeletons in glycolysis may be summarized as follows:

$$Glucose \rightarrow 2 \; lactate + 2 \; H_2O$$

The lactic acid formed in glycolysis diffuses freely from the cell and enters the bloodstream. As a result, in circumstances of augmented glycolysis, such as severe exercise or decreased oxygenation of tissues, a rise in blood lactic acid is observed. It should also be noted that lactate formation is a metabolic cul-de-sac. Lactate can undergo no metabolic transformation unless it is first converted to pyruvate. Consequently, lactate will accumulate even in the absence of accelerated glycolysis in circumstances in which there is interference with the utilization of pyruvate (see below).

Energy Transfer. From a teleological standpoint the usefulness of glycolysis to the organism is the conversion of chemical energy stored in glucose to ATP, a form more readily utilizable for energy-requiring cellular processes (for example, muscle contraction).

Over the course of the glycolytic sequence, one ATP was consumed in the hexokinase reaction and one in the phosphofructokinase reaction. On the other hand, one ATP was formed in the phosphoglycerate kinase reaction and one in the pyruvate kinase reaction. Since each glucose molecule results in the formation of two trioses, a total of 4 moles of ATP is generated from each mole of glucose in the reactions between glyceraldehyde-3-phosphate and pyruvic acid. The overall balance of ATP in glycolysis is given by the following equation:

$$2 \; ATP + 2 \; Pi + 4 \; ADP \rightarrow 2 \; ADP + 4 \; ATP$$

By cancelling out common terms the net result is:

$$2 \; Pi + 2 \; ADP \rightarrow 2 \; ATP$$

Thus the result of glycolysis is the net formation of 2 ATP from each mole of glucose. Since the breakdown of ATP yields approximately 7.3 kcal mol^{-1} while the standard free energy exchange of and the conversion of glucose to lactate is -47 kcal mol^{-1}, the theoretical efficiency of glycolysis in conserving energy as ATP is 31 per cent.

It should be noted that the reactions in which ATP is formed in glycolysis involve the direct transfer of high energy phosphate ($\sim$P) from metabolic intermediates to ADP. This process has been termed *phosphorylation at the substrate level* and is to be differentiated from *oxidative phosphorylation*. In the latter process, which occurs in the mitochondria, ATP formation is coupled to the transfer of electrons to oxygen along the cytochrome pathway. No oxygen is required for the ATP formation that occurs at the substrate level in glycolysis; hence the term anaerobic glycolysis.

Electron Transfer. The conversion of glyceraldehyde-3-phosphate to 1,3-diphosphoglycerate is an oxidoreductive reaction in which NAD is converted to NADH. In order for additional glucose to undergo glycolysis, a steady supply of NAD is required. In the absence of oxygen, the regeneration of NAD is achieved by the conversion of pyruvate to lactate. In the latter reaction NADH is oxidized to NAD. Thus the importance of the final reaction in glycolysis (pyruvate→lactate) is that it permits the continued breakdown of glucose by providing NAD at the expense of lactate formation. The overall net result is the transfer of four electrons from glyceraldehyde-3-phosphate to pyruvate.

GLUCONEOGENESIS (Fig. 8)

Gluconeogenesis refers to the formation of glucose from noncarbohydrate sources. The principal precursor substrates from which glucose may be derived are pyruvate, lactate, glycerol, odd-chain fatty acids, and amino acids. With regard to the latter, all the constituent amino acids in protein tissue, except leucine, can ultimately be converted to glucose. However, the pattern of amino acid uptake by the liver is such that alanine is the principal glycogenic substrate released from peripheral protein reservoirs. It should be emphasized that conversion of even-chain fatty acids (accounting for over 95 per cent of total fatty acid content) to glucose is not possible in mammalian liver, because the enzymes necessary for the de novo synthesis of 4-carbon dicarboxylic acids from acetyl CoA are lacking.

With the exception of glycerol, each of the gluconeogenic precursors must be converted to pyruvate and/or oxaloacetate prior to formation of glucose.

The enzymatic steps involved in the formation of glucose from pyruvate differ from those involved in glycolysis at the three points in which thermodynamically irreversible reactions occur: (1) the dephosphorylation of phosphoenolpyruvate to form pyruvate; (2) the phosphorylation of fructose-6-phosphate to form fructose-1,6-diphosphate; and (3) the phosphorylation of glucose to glucose-6-phosphate. Biological reversal is achieved by means of enzymes unique to the gluconeogenic pathway. These enzymes constitute the key regulatory steps in gluconeogenesis (Fig. 8).

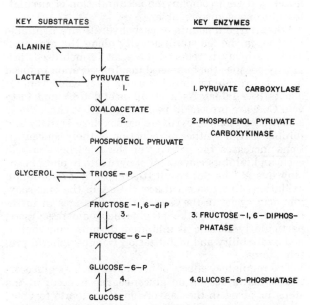

Figure 8. The gluconeogenic pathway. The major rate-limiting enzymes and the major substrates are shown in the figure.

The four regulatory enzymes unique to the gluconeogenic pathway are present in liver, kidney, and intestinal epithelium but not in muscle or heart. Quantitatively the liver is the most important site of gluconeogenesis in physiological circumstances such as an overnight or several day fast, and exercise, and in pathological conditions such as diabetes. The kidney, however, becomes an important gluconeogenic organ after prolonged starvation (see Starvation, p. 366).

The moment-to-moment regulation of gluconeogenesis depends on substrate availability, enzyme activity, and the hormonal milieu. In the postabsorptive state and during short-term starvation, protein is rapidly broken down and amino acids are mobilized, providing a large supply of glucose precursors. In this circumstance fatty acids serve as the major substrate for energy formation. As a consequence intrahepatic levels of acetyl CoA are elevated, resulting in increased activity of the key gluconeogenic enzyme, pyruvate carboxylase. As starvation continues for prolonged periods, availability of precursor substrate becomes the rate-limiting process, as peripheral release of alanine is markedly reduced.

The key role of the four rate-limiting gluconeogenic enzymes in glucose as well as in lactate metabolism is underscored by observations in patients with inborn deficiencies of these enzymes. The development of hypoglycemia and excessive accumulation of liver glycogen in infants with a deficiency of glucose-6-phosphatase (von Gierke's disease; Type I glycogen storage disease) has been discussed. In addition, hypoglycemia in association with lactic acidosis, hyperpyruvicemia, and hyperalaninemia has been reported in infants with a deficiency of fructose-1,6-diphosphatase, pyruvate carboxylase, or phosphoenolpyruvate carboxykinase. In each of these enzymatic disorders the utilization of alanine, pyruvate, and lactate by the liver for gluconeogenesis is defective, while the formation of these intermediates from glucose in muscle is normal. Consequently, as glycogen stores are depleted in fasting there is an inability to maintain normal blood glucose levels and an accompanying accumulation of circulating gluconeogenic precursors.

When large amounts of carbohydrate are available (that is, in the fed state) activity along the gluconeogenic pathway is reduced. Less fat is mobilized, primarily because the increased insulin secretion induced by carbohydrate inhibits release of fatty acids from fat depots (see later). As a result acetyl CoA and fatty acid CoA are present in reduced quantity. Since these substances promote pyruvate carboxylase activity and inhibit citrate synthesis, reduction of their concentrations increases the activity of the tricarboxylic acid cycle and inhibits movement of pyruvate to phosphoenolpyruvate. The net result, therefore, is to stimulate oxidation of pyruvate via acetyl CoA in the tricarboxylic acid cycle. In the face of these changes in intrahepatic events, uptake of gluconeogenic precursors, particularly alanine, is inhibited, despite their continued availability and mobilization from peripheral protein stores.

The regulatory effects of hormones such as glucocorticoids and glucagon on gluconeogenesis occur at the steps involved in the conversion of pyruvate to phosphoenolpyruvate. Glucocorticoids also influence gluconeogenesis by their catabolic effect on protein tissue, thereby increasing the availability of precursor amino acids.

INTEGRATION OF GLYCOLYSIS AND GLUCONEOGENESIS: THE CORI CYCLE

In the foregoing discussion of the glycolytic and gluconeogenic pathways the concentration of ATP, the oxidoreductive state of the cytoplasm (NAD:NADH ratio), and the hormonal milieu were emphasized as important in determining the direction of carbon flow (that is, toward lactate or toward glucose). While net movement of substrate is in one or the other direction within a given tissue such as the liver, in the organism as a whole both glycolysis and glyconeogenesis are generally proceeding simultaneously, albeit at different sites. The liver demonstrates gluconeogenic activity beginning approximately three hours after ingestion of a carbohydrate-containing meal and continuing throughout the postabsorptive state and during starvation. On the other hand, lactate is continuously produced by the formed elements of the blood, by resting muscle, and to a much larger extent by exercising muscle. The combined activity of gluconeogenesis and glycolysis results in a cycling of carbon skeletons as glucose and lactate between liver and muscle. This cycle was described first by Cori and is shown in Figure 9. Glucose is released by the liver into the bloodstream and is taken up by muscle tissue. Within muscle the glucose undergoes glycolysis and its carbon skeletons are released to the bloodstream as lactate and pyruvate. The liver extracts lactate and pyruvate from the blood and by the process of gluconeogenesis reconverts these substrates to glucose. The recycling of carbon skeletons between lactate and glucose has been estimated to account for 20 per cent of the total turnover of each of these substrates.

The Cori cycle fails to result in the net production of new glucose. It does, however, provide a means whereby the end products of glycolysis may enter an

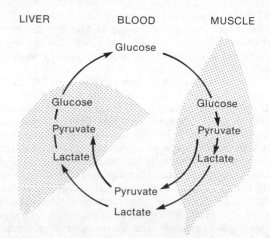

Figure 9. The Cori cycle. In this cycle pathway glucose is taken up by muscle and converted to lactate and pyruvate, which are released into the bloodstream. Pyruvate and lactate are taken up by the liver where they are reconverted to glucose, which is released into the bloodstream. The Cori cycle accounts for approximately 15 to 20 per cent of the total turnover of glucose.

anabolic process rather than accumulate within the bloodstream or undergo further oxidation. A similar cycle involving glucose and alanine (the glucose-alanine cycle) was described more recently and will be discussed in the section on amino acid metabolism.

Although lactate must be derived from pyruvate, the relative concentrations of these substrates in the bloodstream favor lactate in a ratio of 6:1 to 10:1. As noted above, lactate accumulation occurs in circumstances of increased anaerobic glycolysis whether they be physiological (for example, exercise) or pathological (cardiovascular collapse due to hypovolemia, sepsis, or cardiogenic shock). Lactate will also accumulate when substances that inhibit gluconeogenesis such as ethanol or fructose interfere with the Cori cycle. The *antigluconeogenic* effect of ethanol derives from a marked increase in the NADH:NAD ratio incident to the metabolism of alcohol by the enzyme alcohol dehydrogenase. As a result of the accumulation of excessive NADH, conversion of lactate to pyruvate is inhibited. In contrast, gluconeogenesis from glycerol, which enters the gluconeogenic pathway at the triosephosphate level (Fig. 8), is not inhibited by ethanol.

Gluconeogenesis is not the sole metabolic fate of lactate released into the bloodstream. Within the liver and to a much larger extent in heart muscle and kidney, lactate undergoes terminal oxidation to CO_2.

THE TRICARBOXYLIC ACID CYCLE

The degradation of glucose to lactate does not require the presence of oxygen nor does it result in the liberation of carbon dioxide. The enzymatic process whereby aerobic tissues utilize oxygen and produce carbon dioxide (that is, undergo cellular respiration) is termed the tricarboxylic acid (TCA) cycle. This pathway, first described by Sir Hans Krebs in 1937, is also known as the Krebs cycle or the citric acid cycle. This sequence of metabolic conversions represents the final common pathway of aerobic oxidation and CO_2 formation for all substrates, carbohydrates, fatty acids, and amino acids. The enzymes catalyzing the TCA cycle are located within the mitochondria. Within those organelles they are in close association with the respiratory chain, a sequence of proteins that permit the energy liberated in the various oxidative reactions of the TCA cycle to be coupled to the formation of ATP, the process of oxidative phosphorylation. The TCA cycle thus is quantitatively the most important pathway for the utilization of the energy available in various metabolic fuels.

The point of entry of all fuels into the TCA cycle is via the metabolic intermediate, acetyl CoA. The resultant products are two moles of CO_2, H_2O, and coenzyme A. In this manner there is terminal oxidation of the carbon skeleton of acetyl CoA. The cyclical nature of this pathway derives from the fact that the substrate combining with acetyl CoA in the first reaction of the cycle, oxaloacetate, is reconstituted in the final reaction (Fig. 10). The product of this initial reaction is citrate, a tricarboxylic acid; hence the terms tricarboxylic acid cycle or citric acid cycle. Because of the cyclical nature of this pathway the various tricarboxylic acids (citrate, cis-aconitate, isocitrate) and dicarboxylic acids (α-ketoglutarate, succinate, fumarate,

malate, and oxaloacetate) that compose the sequence serve a catalytic as well as substrate role. Thus the classic experiments of Krebs demonstrated that addition of these dicarboxylic or tricarboxylic acids to muscle suspensions stimulated oxygen utilization well beyond that attributable to the oxidation of the added acids alone. Thus it is apparent that the overall rate of aerobic oxidation will be influenced by (1) the availability of acetyl CoA; (2) the activity of the enzymes in the TCA cycle; and (3) the availability of the dicarboxylic and tricarboxylic acids that are formed during each turn of the TCA cycle.

Reactions of the TCA Cycle. The TCA cycle consists of eight individual, enzymatically catalyzed steps by means of which the following overall transformation occurs:

$$Acetyl\ CoA\ +\ Oxaloacetate\ +\ 2O_2 \rightarrow$$
$$2CO_2\ +\ H_2O\ +\ Oxaloacetate\ +\ CoA$$

The specific reactions involved in this sequence are shown in Figure 10 and are described here briefly.

1. The condensation of acetyl CoA and oxaloacetate to form citrate.
2. The conversion of citrate to isocitrate via the intermediate cis-aconitate. This process consists of an initial hydration and subsequent dehydration.
3. The oxidative decarboxylation of isocitrate to α-ketoglutarate. An unstable intermediate, oxalosuccinate, is formed as an intermediate. Reduction of NAD is linked with this oxidative process.
4. The oxidative decarboxylation of α-ketoglutarate to succinyl CoA. NAD is reduced to NADH.
5. The hydrolysis of succinyl CoA to succinate, which is coupled with the formation of GTP from GDP plus inorganic phosphate. The GTP then reacts with ADP to form ATP. This step represents phosphorylation at the substrate level analogous to that which occurs in the glycolytic pathway.
6. The oxidation (dehydrogenation) of succinate to fumarate. This is linked with the reduction of the flavoprotein, flavin adenine dinucleotide (FAD), to FADH.
7. Hydration of fumarate to form L-malate.
8. Oxidation of malate to oxaloacetate. In this reaction NAD is reduced to NADH.

The cycle consists of four oxidative steps, two of which are combined with decarboxylation. The major enzymatic control points with respect to the operation of the cycle and its relationship with other aspects of intermediary metabolism are those catalyzing steps 1 (citrate synthase), 3 (isocitrate dehydrogenase), 4 (α-ketoglutarate dehydrogenase), 6 (succinate dehydrogenase), and 8 (malate dehydrogenase).

The various allosteric modifications of the key rate-limiting enzymes in the TCA cycle indicate that increases in ATP inhibit activity of the cycle, while activation of the cycle accompanies a fall in ATP and an elevation in ADP levels.

Oxidative Phosphorylation. The operation of the TCA cycle provides not only a means of generating CO_2 and water from glucose, but also constitutes a mechanism whereby the energy in metabolic fuels is made available for cellular function. This process involves the conversion of energy released in oxidation-

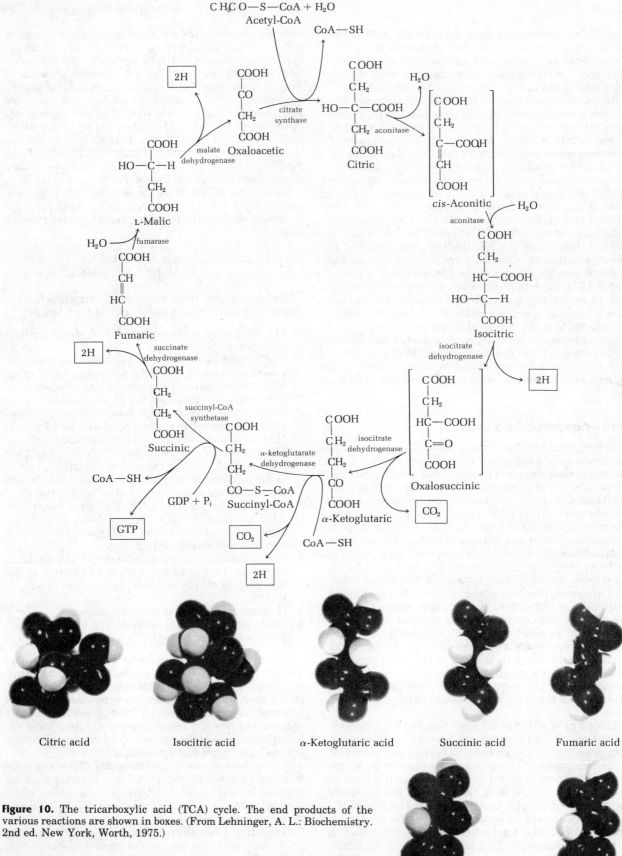

Figure 10. The tricarboxylic acid (TCA) cycle. The end products of the various reactions are shown in boxes. (From Lehninger, A. L.: Biochemistry. 2nd ed. New York, Worth, 1975.)

Citric acid   Isocitric acid   α-Ketoglutaric acid   Succinic acid   Fumaric acid

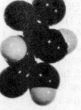

L-Malic acid   Oxaloacetic acid

reduction reactions to the high-energy phosphate bonds of ATP.

Oxidation-reduction reactions are involved in the formation of acetyl CoA from pyruvate, and in steps 3, 4, 6, and 8 of the TCA cycle. In each of these steps, save for step 6 of the cycle (succinate dehydrogenase) in which a flavoprotein is the cofactor, the electron acceptor for the oxidation reaction is the pyridine nucleotide NAD. Within the mitochondria, enzymes and cofactors are present that, through a sequence of steps, result in the transfer of electrons from reduced NAD to molecular oxygen. This series consists of flavoproteins, iron sulfur proteins, ubiquinone (coenzyme Q), and the cytochromes (Fig. 11).

The first reaction in the process is catalyzed by NADH dehydrogenase. The latter contains flavin mononucleotide (FMN) as the prosthetic group and catalyzes the transfer of electrons from NAD to an iron sulfur protein, which undergoes reversible $Fe^{++} \leftrightarrow Fe^{+++}$ reactions. The electrons are next transferred to ubiquinone, a lipid-soluble, electron-carrying coenzyme. Thereafter, the electrons are carried via the cytochromes to molecular oxygen. The cytochromes are proteins containing iron-porphyrin groups, which undergo reversible $Fe^{++} \leftrightarrow Fe^{+++}$ transformations. Several mitochondrial cytochromes have been identified that differ in their molecular weight and have distinctive spectral bands.

The formation of ATP occurs at three points of electron transfer in the respiratory chain: (1) from NAD to the flavoprotein via NADH dehydrogenase; (2) between cytochromic b and c; and (3) between cytochromic a and molecular oxygen. Thus a total of three ATP are generated in the oxidation of each NADH. In the case of enzymes such as succinate dehydrogenase, which use flavoprotein cofactors rather than NAD, their entry of electrons into the respiratory chain is at the level of coenzyme Q (Fig. 11). As a result, one ATP-generating step in the respiratory chain is bypassed and only two ATP are produced.

It should be noted that not all oxidations are accompanied by phosphorylation. The microsomes contain a cytochrome electron transfer system (cytochrome P450) that participates in a variety of hydroxylation reactions important in the metabolism of various drugs (for example, phenobarbital) and steroid hormones but that does not result in the generation of ATP.

Energy Balance. The overall production of ATP from pyruvate during aerobic oxidation is summarized in Table 2.

A total of 15 ATP are produced from each molecule of pyruvate. Of these, 14 are formed by oxidative phosphorylation and one is formed at the substrate level. It should be recalled that two moles of pyruvate are formed from each mole of glucose. In addition, in the glycolytic breakdown of glucose to pyruvate, two

TABLE 2. SYNTHESIS OF ATP DURING PYRUVATE OXIDATION

REACTION		ATP
Pyruvate ⟶	Acetyl CoA	3
Isocitrate ⟶	α-Ketoglutarate	3
α-Ketoglutarate ⟶	Succinyl CoA	3
Succinyl CoA ⟶	Succinate	1
Succinate ⟶	Fumarate	2
Malate ⟶	Oxaloacetate	3
	Total	15 ATP

moles of ATP are generated at the substrate level and two moles of NADH are formed. Oxidation of the cytosolic NADH produced in glycolysis contributes two or three ATP depending on the "shuttle" employed for the transfer of its electrons to the mitochondria. Thus an additional four or six ATP are generated as glucose is converted to pyruvate. The overall energy balance of glucose oxidation is indicated by the equation

$$Glucose + 6O_2 + Pi + 36\ ADP \rightarrow$$
$$6CO_2 + 36\ ATP + 6H_2O$$

The energy value of the ATP formed (263 kcal mol^{-1}) is approximately 40 per cent of the total energy available in glucose. While the efficiency of glucose oxidation with respect to energy conservation is thus considerably less than 100 per cent, the amount of ATP formed (36) is 18 times that produced by the glycolytic breakdown of glucose to lactate.

Anabolic Functions of the TCA Cycle. In addition to its catabolic functions and role in energy metabolism, the TCA cycle also provides precursors for a variety of biosynthetic reactions (Fig. 12). As discussed previously, oxaloacetate is a precursor substrate in the gluconeogenic pathway whereby it is initially converted to phosphoenolpyruvate. It should be emphasized that while the carbon atoms of acetyl CoA are incorporated into oxaloacetate with each turn of the TCA cycle, no net formation of glucose from acetyl CoA is possible. This is because two other carbon atoms are lost as CO_2 with each turn of the cycle. Oxaloacetate may also undergo transamination to form aspartate, which is a precursor in pyrimidine biosynthesis. Succinyl CoA condenses with glycine in the inital step of porphyrin formation. Transamination of α-ketoglutarate gives rise to glutamate and glutamine, which are important in ammonia production by the kidney. Finally, citrate is an important source of extramitochondrial acetyl CoA, which is necessary for fatty acid biosynthesis.

Since the mitochondrial membrane is impermeable to acetyl CoA and since pyruvate dehydrogenase (the

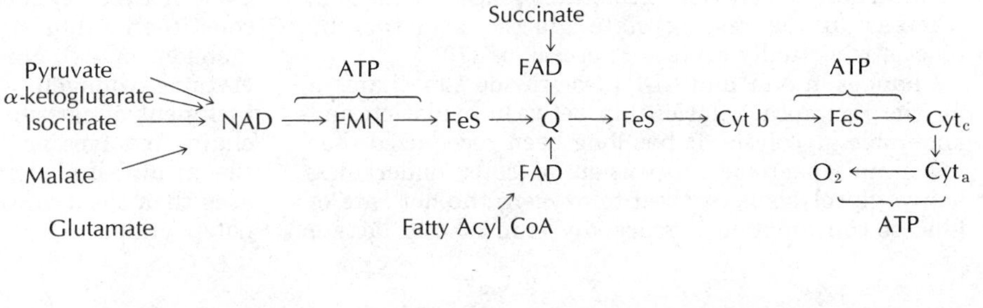

Figure 11. The electron transport chain. One ATP is generated at each of three sites in the transfer of electrons from NAD to molecular oxygen. FeS = Iron sulfur protein. Q = Coenzyme Q.

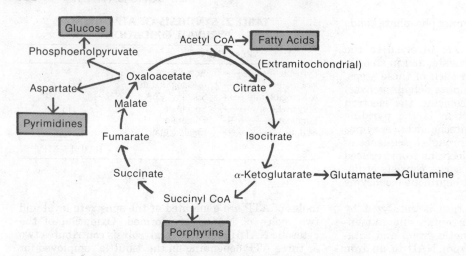

Figure 12. Anabolic reactions of the tricarboxylic acid (TCA) cycle. The major biosynthetic end products are shown in boxes.

enzyme necessary for acetyl CoA formation from glucose-derived pyruvate) is located within the mitochondria, while the enzymes required for the synthesis of fatty acids are in the cytosol, a mechanism is necessary for the transfer of glucose-derived acetyl CoA to the extramitochondrial space. This function is performed by citrate, which permeates the mitochondrial membrane and is acted upon by the enzyme ATP–citrate lyase to undergo the following reaction:

$$\text{Citrate} + \text{ATP} + \text{CoA} \rightarrow$$
$$\text{acetyl CoA} + \text{oxaloacetate} + \text{ADP} + \text{Pi}$$

The variety of anabolic processes in which TCA cycle intermediates may participate indicates that despite the regeneration of oxaloacetate within the cycle, there may be a net drain of these intermediates by biosynthetic reactions. Repletion of TCA cycle intermediates is achieved by means of *anaplerotic reactions*. The major pathway for the repletion of oxaloacetate is that catalyzed by the enzyme pyruvate carboxylase. This reaction has been discussed in the section on gluconeogenesis.

Regulation of the TCA Cycle. The overall activity of the TCA cycle is determined by the availability of ATP, substrate, the activity of enzymes, and the hormonal milieu. These controlling influences are largely interdependent. For example, when insulin levels are extremely low, gluconeogenic enzymes are markedly activated and oxaloacetate may be sufficiently drained so as to limit activity of the TCA cycle.

A major determinant of enzyme activity is the relative availability of ATP, ADP, and AMP. In circumstances of decreased ATP availability and increased levels of ADP, citrate synthase and isocitrate dehydrogenase activity is increased. In contrast, these enzymes are inhibited when ATP levels are increased and ADP is reduced. In this manner, the consumption of ATP by muscular contraction accelerates glucose oxidation, whereas in the resting state glucose oxidation by muscle is virtually nil (see Exercise, p. 370).

Changes in ATP and ADP also provide a mechanism for the reciprocal relationship between oxidation and anaerobic glycolysis. It has long been recognized that when an anaerobic suspension of cells undergoing active glycolysis is exposed to oxygen, the net rate of glucose consumption is markedly reduced and lactate

accumulation ceases. This phenomenon whereby oxygen decreases glucose utilization and lactate production is termed the *Pasteur effect*. The basis for this effect is the fact that in the presence of oxygen the formation of ATP from glucose (via aerobic oxidation) is accelerated. Furthermore, the amount of ATP generated per mole of glucose is 18 times greater than under anaerobic conditions (36 ATP vs 2 ATP). The increase in cellular ATP results in inhibition of phosphofructokinase, a key regulatory enzyme in the glycolytic pathway that is allosterically inhibited by ATP and activated by ADP. The increase in citrate accompanying activation of the TCA cycle also contributes to inhibition of phosphofructokinase.

THE PENTOSE PATHWAY AND OTHER METABOLIC FATES OF GLUCOSE

In addition to glycolysis and aerobic oxidation, glucose-6-phosphate may be oxidized by the enzyme glucose-6-phosphate dehydrogenase, resulting in formation of 6-phosphogluconate. The latter may then be converted via a sequence of intermediate reactions to the pentoses—ribulose, ribose, and xylulose. The major purpose of this pathway, which is located within the cytosol, is the formation of pentoses required for nucleic acid synthesis and the generation of reducing equivalents in the form of NADPH, which are necessary in the reductive synthesis of fatty acids and sterols. Consequently, the pentose pathway is of some importance in the glucose metabolism of liver (the major site of fatty acid biosynthesis in humans) and in adrenal tissue and testis (sites of sterol biosynthesis). In contrast, virtually no pentose pathway activity is demonstrable in muscle tissue.

The utilization of glucose and other carbohydrates in the biosynthesis of glycoproteins is another important metabolic fate of these substrates. Glycoproteins exist in a variety of forms, including circulating plasma constituents (fibrinogen, immunoglobulins), hormones (gonadotropins), enzymes (ribonuclease B), mucus secretions, collagen, and basement membrane. The attachment of carbohydrate moieties to the polypeptide chains involves an initial reaction with UTP to form the uridine-diphosphate derivative. Specific transferases then catalyze the transfer of carbohydrate to the polypeptide.

GLUCOSE BALANCE IN POSTABSORPTIVE MAN

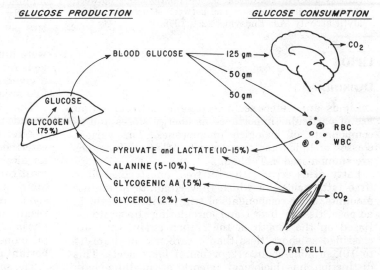

Figure 13. Glucose balance in normal humans in the postabsorptive (overnight fasted) state. The amounts shown for glucose consumption by brain, blood cells, and muscle represent 24-hour values in resting subjects.

Glucose or fructose may also be converted to the polyhydroxyl alcohol sorbitol by the following reactions:

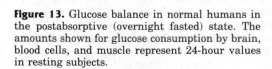

Glucose ⟷ Sorbitol ⟷ Fructose
Aldose Reductase   Ketose Reductase

The sorbitol pathway is widely distributed in mammalian cells, including such specialized structures as nerve tissue and vascular endothelium.

The significance of these alternate pathways of glucose metabolism derives from the fact that their activity is largely determined by the concentration of blood glucose and does not depend on the availability of insulin. Thus in the presence of hyperglycemia and insulin deficiency (as occurs in diabetes), an increase in glycosylation of basement membrane protein and of hemoglobin has been described. Increased accumulation of sorbitol has also been observed in the nerve tissue of diabetic animals. These changes in glucose metabolism have been implicated in the microvascular disease and neuropathy that occur with long-standing diabetes (see Diabetes Mellitus, p. 386).

Quantitative Aspects of Glucose Metabolism in Humans. From the foregoing it is clear that glucose can be actively metabolized in a variety of tissues. Under basal, postabsorptive conditions (overnight fast), the liver may be viewed as primarily an organ of glucose production. Glucose is released by the liver into the circulation at a rate of 2 to 3.5 mg/kg/min, or 200 to 350 grams/day. Under basal conditions, glycogen breakdown accounts for 75 to 80 per cent of hepatic glucose production; an additional 15 to 20 per cent is derived from lactate, and the remaining 5 to 10 per cent is produced from amino acids, particularly alanine. As fasting progresses and glycogen stores are depleted, the contribution from gluconeogenesis becomes increasingly important.

With regard to glucose uptake, terminal oxidation to CO_2 in nervous tissue accounts for utilization of 125 to 150 grams of glucose per day. An additional 50 grams is extracted by glycolytic tissues (formed elements of the blood and renal medulla), and a similar amount is consumed by resting muscle. These relation-ships are outlined in Figure 13. It is apparent that for the liver and fat cell to assume importance in glucose disposal they must do so primarily in circumstances of carbohydrate ingestion (the fed state).

REFERENCES

Carbohydrate

Boyer, P. D., Chance, B., Eruster, L., Mitchell, P., Racker, E., and Slater, E. C.: Oxidative phosphorylation and photophosphorylation. Annu Rev Biochem 46:955, 1977.

Buschiazzo, H., Exton, J. H., and Park, C. R.: Effects of glucose on glycogen synthetase, phosphorylase, and glycogen deposition in the perfused rat liver. Proc Natl Acad Sci 65:383, 1970.

Cahill, G. F., Jr., and Owen, O. E.: Some observations on carbohydrate metabolism in man. In Dickens, F., Randle, P. J., and Whelan, W. J. (eds.): Carbohydrate Metabolism and Its Disorders. Vol. 1. London, Academic Press, 1968.

El-Maghrabi, M. R., Claus, T. H., Pilkis, J., Fox, E., and Pilkis, S. J.: Regulation of rat liver fructose-2,6-bisphosphatase. J Biol Chem 257:7603, 1982.

Felig, P.: The glucose-alanine cycle. Metabolism 22:179, 1973.

Gabbay, K.: The sorbitol pathway and the complications of diabetes. N Engl J Med 288:831, 1973.

Hers, G. H.: The control of glycogen metabolism in the liver. Annu Rev Biochem 45:167, 1976.

Hers, H. G., and Hue, L.: Gluconeogenesis and related aspects of glycolyses. Annu Rev Biochem 52:617, 1983.

Kreisberg, R. A.: Glucose lactate inter-relations in man. N Engl J Med 287:132, 1972.

Mahler, R. F.: Disorders of glycogen metabolism. Clin Endocrinol Metab 5:579, 1976.

Mehlman, M. A., and Hanson, R. W. (ed.): Energy Metabolism and the Regulation of Metabolic Processes in Mitchondria. New York, Academic Press, 1972.

Newgard, C. B., Foster, D. W., and McGarry, J. D.: Evidence for suppression of hepatic glucose-6-phosphatase with carbohydrate feeding. Diabetes 33:192, 1984.

Pagliara, A. S., Karl, I. E., Keating, J. P., Brown, B. I., and Kipnis, D. M.: Hepatic fructose-1,6-diphosphatase deficiency. A cause of lactic acidosis and hypoglycemia in infancy. J Clin Invest 51:2115, 1972.

Ramiak, A.: Pasteur effect and phosphofructokinase. Curr Top Cell Regul 8:297, 1974.

Spiro, R. G.: Glycoproteins: Their biochemistry, biology and role in human disease. N Engl J Med 281:991, 1043, 1969.

Utter, M. F., Barden, R. E., and Taylor, B. L.: Pyruvate carboxylase: An evaluation of the relationships between structure and mechanisms and between structure and catalytic activity. Adv Endzymol 42:1, 1975.

LIPIDS

DEFINITION

Lipids are water-insoluble organic molecules that are of particular importance as energy stores and as components of biological membranes. The various classes of lipids and their major biological functions are summarized in Table 3.

Fatty acids occur either in free, unesterified form (free fatty acids), in which they circulate in minute amounts, or as components of triglycerides present in adipose tissue, liver, and circulating lipoproteins. Based on the length of the carbon chain, they are classified as short- (less than 4 carbons), medium- (4 to 10), or long-chain (12 or more) fatty acids. This distinction has biological import, as medium-chain fatty acids are absorbed via the portal route and can permeate the mitochondrial membrane. In contrast, long-chain fatty acids are absorbed via the lymphatics and require a carrier system (carnitine transferase) to gain entrance to mitochondria. Over 90 per cent of the fatty acids present in mammalian tissue have an even number of carbon atoms. Fatty acids also differ with respect to the number and location of double bonds. The most commonly occurring fatty acids are palmitic (16 carbons) and stearic acid (18 carbons), which are fully saturated. Oleic acid differs from stearic acid by the presence of a double bond between carbons 9 and 10. Linoleic acid contains two double bonds ($\delta 9$, $\delta 12$), linolenic acid contains three ($\delta 9$, $\delta 12$, $\delta 15$), and arachidonic acid, a C_{20} fatty acid important as a prostaglandin precursor, contains four double bonds.

Although most fatty acids are readily synthesized from glucose, this is not true for linoleic and linolenic acids, which are considered *essential* and are necessary components of the diet. In circumstances of dietary deficiency of these fatty acids (as may occur in patients treated for prolonged periods with fat-free intravenous hyperalimentation), a syndrome characterized by skin and hair changes may develop.

Fatty acids are stored in adipose tissue and other cells (liver) as esters of the trihydroxyalcohol glycerol, hence the name triglyceride, or, more properly, triacylglycerol (Fig. 14). The triglycerides constitute the most important storage form of energy available in mammals. This importance derives from their caloric density (9 calories per gram as compared with 4 calories per gram of carbohydrate or protein), as well as their not requiring water for storage in cells. Thus, were humans to store calories as carbohydrate (glycogen) rather than fat, the total mass required to store a given number of calories would be more than eightfold greater than that required as fat.

The phospholipids, or phosphoglycerides, are compounds in which one of the hydroxyl groups of glycerol is esterified to phosphoric acid and the other two are esterified to fatty acids. The phospholipids also contain an alcohol that is esterified to phosphoric acid. The most common types of phospholipids contain ethanolamine and choline (trimethylethanolamine) as the alcohol group that is esterified to phosphoric acid. The resultant compounds (phosphatidylethanolamine and phosphatidylcholine), which have been given the trivial names cephalin and lecithin respectively, are important components of cellular membranes.

The sphingolipids are compounds that contain sphingosine (a long-chain amino alcohol), one molecule of a long-chain fatty acid, and an additional, polar grouping that is esterified to phosphoric acid. The most abundant of these compounds are the *sphingomyelins,* which contain ethanolamine or choline as their polar groups. The *glycosphingolipids* contain one or more neutral sugars as their polar group. These compounds are important membrane components in neural tissue. In addition, they may accumulate in a variety of genetic disorders (for example, Tay-Sachs disease and Fabry's disease) in which the specific enzymes required for the breakdown of glycosphingolipids or sphingomyelins are lacking. These disorders are referred to as lipid storage diseases or as *lysosomal diseases,* since the degradative enzymes that are lacking are normally present in lysosomes, subcellular cytoplasmic organelles containing hydrolytic enzymes. Examples of the lipid storage diseases and the enzymes lacking are given in Table 4.

The biochemistry of other lipids and the lipoproteins, and of the sterols, is discussed in the chapter Lipids in Biological Systems, p. 392 and in Section VIII, Endocrinology, respectively.

BIOSYNTHESIS OF FATTY ACIDS

Although fat constitutes only 40 per cent of the calories in the diet, it accounts for over 80 per cent of

TABLE 3. CLASSIFICATION OF LIPIDS

TYPE	FUNCTION
Free fatty acids	Combustible, circulating fuel
Glycerides (acylglycerols)	Storage fuel
Lipoproteins	Transport to storage sites
Phospholipids (phosphoglycerides)	Cell membrane component
Sphingolipids	Cell membrane component
Sterols	Hormonal functions
Cholesterol	
Adrenal steroids	
Sex steroids	
Vitamin D	
Prostaglandins	Physiologic and metabolic regulators

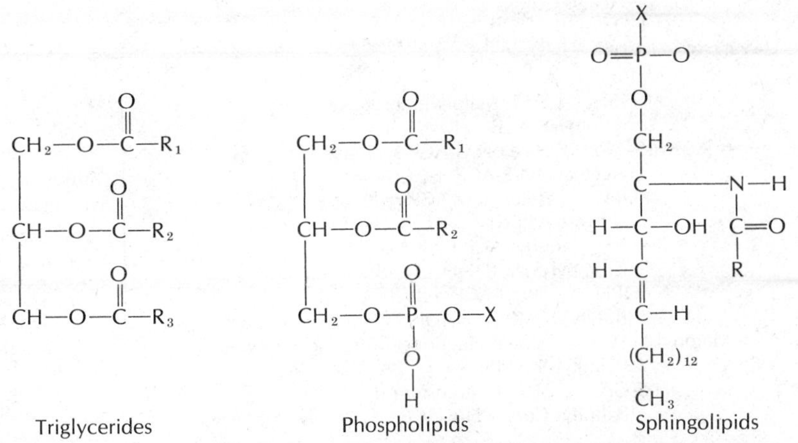

Figure 14. Chemical structures of triglycerides, phospholipids, and sphingolipids. The notation "R" denotes acyl groups of varying chain lengths. The designation "X" refers to the polar head groups in phospholipids and sphingolipids, which most commonly are phosphorylethanolamine and phosphorylcholine.

Triglycerides   Phospholipids   Sphingolipids

the calories stored in the human body. Furthermore, adipose tissue is in a state of dynamic equilibrium in which the half-life of depot lipid may be less than two days. It is thus clear that fatty acids are normally being synthesized by the organism. The metabolic pathway whereby fatty acids are synthesized involves a sequence of seven enzymatic steps (Fig. 15) that are cytosolic in location.

The initial precursor in the formation of fatty acids is acetyl CoA, which is derived from glucose via pyruvate by the pyruvate dehydrogenase reaction (see above) or by oxidation of amino acids or fatty acids (see below). The enzymes involved in all of the oxidative processes giving rise to acetyl CoA are located within the mitochondria, an organelle that cannot be traversed by acetyl CoA. The generation of cytosolic acetyl CoA is achieved by means of citrate (which readily escapes from the mitochondria) and the citrate cleavage enzyme, ATP–citrate lyase:

Citrate + ATP + CoA →
  acetyl CoA + ADP + Pi + oxaloacetate

The first step in the pathway for fatty acid synthesis in the cytosol is the carboxylation of acetyl CoA to form malonyl CoA. The enzyme catalyzing this reaction, acetyl CoA carboxylase, is the rate-limiting step in fat biosynthesis. The enzyme requires biotin as a cofactor and is allosterically activated by citrate. It is inhibited by free fatty acids and fatty acyl CoA derivatives. The levels of the enzyme are decreased in starvation and diabetes and are increased during refeeding.

For the storage of fatty acids as fat droplets in cells, esterification with α glycerolphosphate to form triglyceride is required (Fig. 16). Glycerol-3-phosphate may be generated by the glycolytic breakdown of glucose to dihydroxyacetone, which can then undergo reduction in the presence of NADH. Alternatively, glycerol-3-phosphate may be formed from free glycerol (liberated in the breakdown of triglyceride) in the presence of ATP and the enzyme glycerol kinase (Fig. 16). The latter is present in liver but is virtually absent in adipose tissue. Consequently the synthesis of triglyceride in adipose tissue requires not only the availability of fatty acyl CoA derivatives (either synthesized in situ or derived from circulating lipoproteins), but also the uptake of glucose and its utilization via the glycolytic pathway so as to generate glycerol-3-phosphate.

The enzymes required for fat synthesis are present

TABLE 4. THE SPHINGOLIPIDOSES

DISEASE	ONSET	ENZYME DEFICIENCY	PRODUCT STORED
Farber	Childhood	Ceramidase	Ceramide
Gaucher	Various	β-glucosidase	Ceramide glucoside (glucocerebroside)
Niemann-Pick	Infancy or childhood	Sphingomyelinase	Sphingomyelin
Krabbe	Infancy	β-galactosidase	Ceramide galactoside (galactocerebroside)
Metachromatic leukodystrophy	Various	Aryl sulfatases	Ceramide galactose-3-sulfate (sulfatide)
Lactosyl ceramidosis	Childhood	β-galactosidase	Ceramide lactoside
Fabry	Childhood	α-galactosidase	Ceramide trihexoside
Tay-Sachs	Infancy or childhood	Hexosaminidases	Ganglioside GM_2
Sandhoff-Jatzke	Infancy	Hexosaminidases	Globoside (plus ganglioside GM_2)
Generalized gangliosidosis	Infancy	β-galactosidase	Ganglioside GM_1

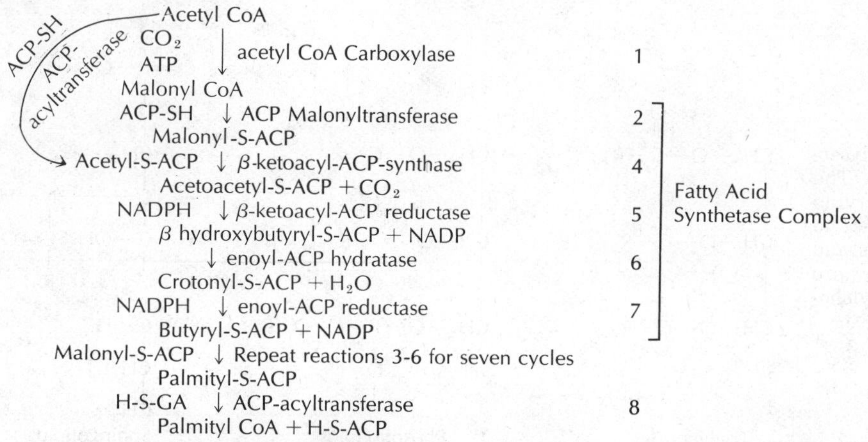

ACP-SH
ACP-acyltransferase
Acetyl CoA
CO_2
ATP
acetyl CoA Carboxylase
1
Malonyl CoA
ACP-SH ↓ ACP Malonyltransferase
2
Malonyl-S-ACP
Acetyl-S-ACP ↓ β-ketoacyl-ACP-synthase
4
Acetoacetyl-S-ACP + CO_2
NADPH ↓ β-ketoacyl-ACP reductase
5
β hydroxybutyryl-S-ACP + NADP
↓ enoyl-ACP hydratase
6
Crotonyl-S-ACP + H_2O
NADPH ↓ enoyl-ACP reductase
7
Butyryl-S-ACP + NADP
Fatty Acid Synthetase Complex
Malonyl-S-ACP ↓ Repeat reactions 3-6 for seven cycles
Palmityl-S-ACP
H-S-GA ↓ ACP-acyltransferase
8
Palmityl CoA + H-S-ACP

Figure 15. The metabolic pathway for fatty acid biosynthesis. Steps 2 to 7 are catalyzed by components of a multienzyme complex, collectively described as the fatty acid synthetase complex. ACP refers to the acyl carrier protein within the synthetase complex.

in a variety of tissues, notably liver, adipose tissue, and intestine. Studies with human adipose tissue have, however, revealed relatively slow rates of glucose incorporation into fatty acids. The available data suggest that fatty acids are synthesized in man largely in the liver, from which they are released to transport triglycerides to adipose tissue, where the enzyme lipoprotein lipase catalyzes their hydrolysis to free fatty acids (FFA) and glycerol, which enter the cell. The reesterification reaction within the adipose cell occurs between glucose-derived glycerol-3-phosphate and lipoprotein-derived fatty acids. The synthetic function of adipose tissue is thus primarily involved in the formation of glycerol-3-phosphate, while it is in the liver that acetyl CoA is converted to long-chain fatty acids.

Mobilization of Fatty Acids

Although fat is stored as triglyceride, its uptake and combustion by tissues (heart, muscle, liver) requires its release from depot stores as free fatty acids that are transported into the blood. The breakdown of triglyceride in adipose tissue is regulated by a tissue lipase that catalyzes the following reaction:

$$\text{Triglyceride} + 3H_2O \rightarrow 3\ \text{FFA} + \text{Glycerol}$$

The process, which is termed lipolysis, is under the regulation of a variety of hormones (epinephrine, growth hormone, insulin). The enzyme has consequently been termed a *hormone-sensitive lipase.* Activity of this enzyme is increased by epinephrine, glucagon, growth hormone, ACTH, and thyroid hormone. Its activity is reduced by insulin. In general, an increase in cyclic AMP accompanies (and may be the mechanism of modulation for) hormonal activation of the lipase, while a decrease in cyclic AMP is associated with inactivation. From a physiological viewpoint, epinephrine is the most important activator of the hormone-sensitive lipase, while insulin is the most important inhibitor. It is unlikely that ACTH or glucagon contributes to the physiological modulation of lipolysis, since extremely high concentrations of these hormones are required to increase lipase activity.

The net rate of lipolysis is also influenced by glucose utilization in adipose tissue. As indicated in Figure 16, triglycerides may be resynthesized as long as glycerol-3-phosphate is present for esterification with free fatty acids. Since adipose tissue lacks the enzyme glycerol kinase, the availability of glycerol-3-phosphate is determined by the rate of glycolysis. Consequently, in circumstances of increased glucose utilization, mobilization of fatty acids is reduced because of increased substrate availability for esterification of fatty acids, in addition to alterations in activity of the hormone-sensitive lipase.

Oxidation of Fatty Acids

Utilization of the chemical energy stored in fat tissue requires its aerobic oxidation, which is coupled to the formation of high energy phosphate in the form of ATP. The metabolic pathway for fat oxidation is not a reversal of the synthetic reactions, but involves a separate series of enzymes and intermediates. Furthermore, the oxidative process occurs within the mitochondria, while the synthetic reactions are located in the cytosol. The overall process whereby fatty acids are oxidized has been termed *beta-oxidation,* since it involves oxidation of the β-carbon to yield a β-keto acid that undergoes cleavage to produce acetyl CoA and a fatty acid that is shortened by two carbon atoms. The process is repeated until the entire fatty acid has been oxidized to acetyl CoA, which enters the TCA cycle for terminal oxidation to CO_2.

The initial step in the oxidation of fatty acids is their activation in the cytosol by formation of the acyl

Glycolysis
Glucose → Dihydroxyacetone -P
G-3-P-hydrogenase
→ Glycerol-3-phosphate
NADH
+
ATP
Triglyceride → Glycerol
glycerol kinase
3 Fatty Acyl CoA
acyl transferase
Triglyceride

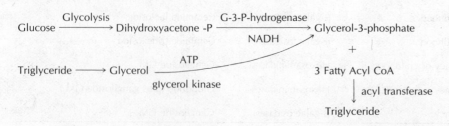

Figure 16. The synthesis of triglyceride from glycerol-3-phosphate and fatty acyl CoA. The glycerol moiety is derived from glucose (in fat tissue and liver) or by phosphorylation and glycerol released from triglyceride by the enzyme glycerol kinase (present in liver but not in fat tissue). G-3-P signifies glycerol-3-phosphate.

CoA derivative, a process that occurs at the expense of two ATP. However, the long-chain fatty acyl CoA derivatives (12 or more carbons), cannot penetrate the mitochondrial membrane. Consequently, a carrier molecule, carnitine, is required. The enzyme acylcarnitine transferase I catalyzes the formation of the fatty acylcarnitine derivative that crosses the inner mitochondrial membrane. The fatty acyl group is transferred to intramitochondrial CoA by the action of the enzyme acylcarnitine transferase II. Free carnitine is regenerated and is thus available for the shuttle of additional fatty acyl residues into the mitochondria. Recent data suggest that this is the rate-limiting enzymatic step in the beta-oxidative pathway. Furthermore, the acylcarnitine transferase I is inhibited by malonyl CoA, the first committed intermediate in the pathway of fatty acid biosynthesis. In this manner a reciprocal relationship is maintained between fat synthesis and fat oxidation.

The factors regulating the rate of fatty acid oxidation include (1) the availability of FFA, (2) the activity of the acylcarnitine transferase step, and (3) the availability of NAD. Each of these factors may be shown to have physiological or pathophysiological significance.

In prolonged exercise, contracting muscle uses less and less glucose and comes to rely almost exclusively on oxidation of fatty acids. The factor governing this progressive dependence on fatty acids is a progressive rise in the arterial level of free fatty acids. In contrast, muscle utilization of fatty acids either at rest or during exercise is reduced by glucose feeding. This is due to the reduction in fat mobilization that accompanies a rise in blood sugar.

The importance of the acylcarnitine transferase step is observed in a hereditary muscle disorder in which this enzyme is deficient. Such patients demonstrate impaired exercise capacity, marked increases in blood triglycerides and FFA, since FFA oxidation is impaired, and necrosis of muscle tissue with the appearance of myoglobin in the urine (myoglobinuria).

The requirement for NAD is indicated by the inhibition of fatty acid oxidation that accompanies a reduction in blood supply (ischemia) of heart muscle. In such circumstances a lack of oxygen interferes with the regeneration of NAD from NADH. As a result, the dehydrogenation reaction is inhibited. The net effect is an accumulation of fatty acyl CoA derivatives.

KETOGENESIS AND KETONE UTILIZATION

When there is an increase in fatty acid oxidation by the liver, the rate at which acetyl CoA is produced may exceed the rate at which it undergoes oxidation via the TCA cycle. In such circumstances, acetyl CoA is utilized for the production of acetoacetic acid, β-hydroxybutyric acid, and acetone. These substances are collectively termed *ketone bodies*. When present in marked excess as occurs in starvation or uncontrolled diabetes, the accumulation of acetoacetate and β-hydroxybutyrate leads to a metabolic acidosis, termed starvation ketosis or diabetic ketoacidosis. The large quantities of acetone present in various forms of ketosis do not contribute to the metabolic acidosis but impart a characteristic fruity odor to the patient's breath.

The formation of ketone bodies from acetyl CoA (Fig. 17) involves as its initial step the condensation of two molecules of acetyl CoA to form acetoacetyl CoA or (to a lesser extent) the oxidation of the final four carbon chains derived through the successive beta oxidation of long-chain fatty acyl CoA. The conversion of acetoacetyl CoA to acetoacetic acid requires its initial conversion to β-hydroxy-β-methylglutaryl CoA, which is cleaved to acetoacetic acid and acetyl CoA. Formation of β-hydroxybutyrate from acetoacetate involves a reversible oxidoreductive reaction employing NADH as the cofactor. Acetone is produced from acetoacetate by a nonenzymatic spontaneous decarboxylation.

The factors regulating the rate of ketogenesis have been the subject of intensive investigation. Clearly an increase in fatty acid delivery to the liver (augmented

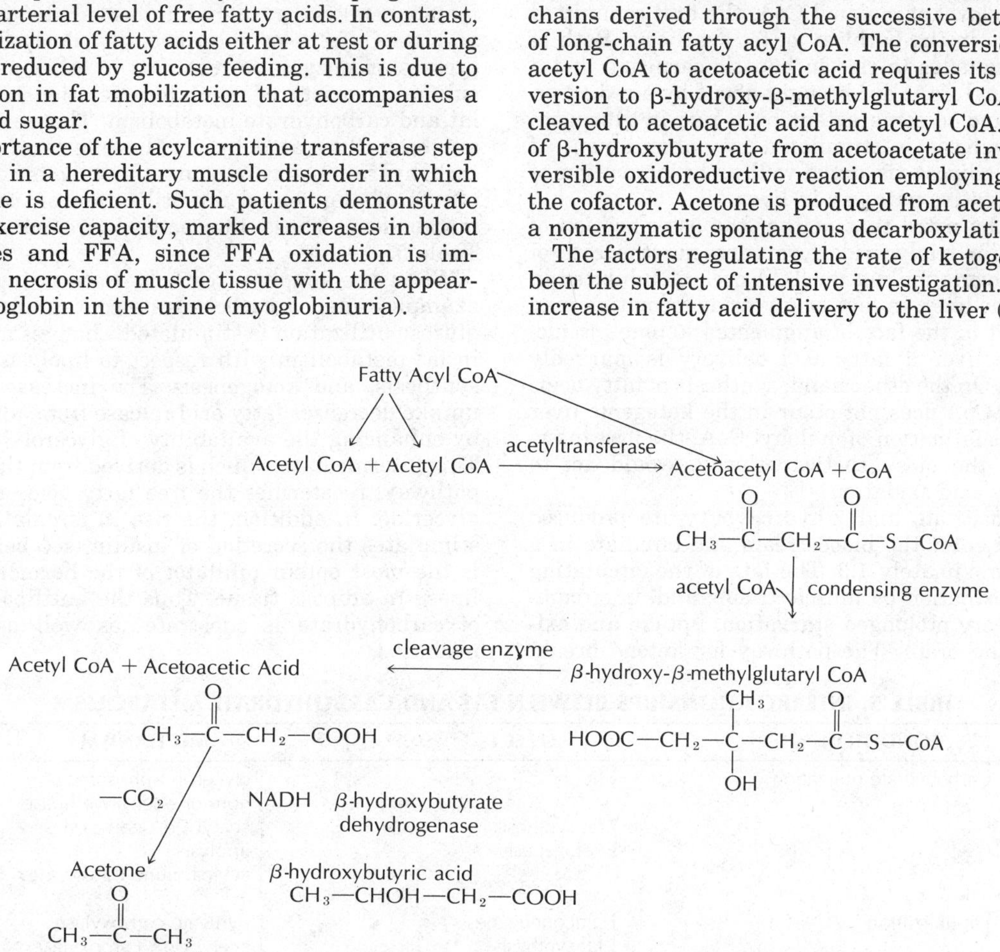

Figure 17. Ketogenesis. The end products of ketogenesis, which are released by the liver, are acetoacetate, β-hydroxybutyrate, and acetone.

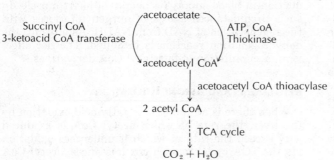

β-hydroxybutyrate

NAD $\downarrow$ β-hydroxybutyrate dehydrogenase

Succinyl CoA
3-ketoacid CoA transferase

acetoacetate

ATP, CoA
Thiokinase

acetoacetyl CoA

$\downarrow$ acetoacetyl CoA thioacylase

2 acetyl CoA

$\vdots$ TCA cycle

$CO_2 + H_2O$

Figure 18. Ketone oxidation. This process occurs in muscle tissue and after prolonged starvation in brain.

lipolysis) is a necessary factor. However, substrate delivery is not the sole determinant, since normal subjects in whom a rise in FFA is induced by administration of a fatty (triglyceride-containing) meal and an activator of lipoprotein lipase (heparin) fail to become ketotic. A second requirement is an increase in the rate of beta-oxidation within the hepatic mitochondria. In this manner fatty acids entering the liver are utilized for acetyl CoA formation rather than for triglyceride synthesis. As noted above, the rate-limiting step in beta-oxidation of fatty acids is the acylcarnitine transferase reaction. This reaction is activated by an increase in the availability of free carnitine and a fall in the level of malonyl CoA, the first committed intermediate in the pathway of fat synthesis. Both of these prerequisites (a rise in hepatic carnitine and a fall in malonyl CoA) are brought about by a reduction in insulin and to some extent by a rise in glucagon. Thus, ketogenesis is stimulated by enhancement of lipolysis in adipose tissue as well as by activation of the beta-oxidative pathway in liver.

It should be noted that neither the esterification of fatty acids for triglyceride formation nor the rate of acetyl CoA oxidation via the TCA cycle is inhibited in the ketogenic liver. In fact, triglyceride formation may be enhanced in the face of augmented ketone production by the liver if fatty acid delivery is markedly accelerated. On the other hand, synthesis of fatty acids from acetyl CoA does not occur in the ketogenic liver inasmuch as formation of malonyl CoA, the first intermediate in the biosynthetic pathway, would act to inhibit fatty acid oxidation.

The acetoacetate and β-hydroxybutyrate produced in the liver enter the bloodstream and circulate in a ratio of approximately 1:3. The fate of the circulating ketones is oxidation by muscle tissue, and, in circumstances of very prolonged starvation, uptake and oxidation by the brain. The pathway for ketone break-

down (Fig. 18) involves as its first step the oxidation of β-hydroxybutyrate to acetoacetate. Acetoacetyl CoA is then formed by a transferase reaction with succinyl CoA or by means of a thiokinase-requiring ATP. Acetoacetyl CoA is then cleaved to yield two moles of acetyl CoA. This reaction, catalyzed by a thioacylase, does not occur in liver but occurs in muscle.

INTERACTIONS OF FAT AND CARBOHYDRATE METABOLISM

The convergence of pathways in fat and carbohydrate metabolism via a shared intermediate (acetyl CoA) and the effects of intermediates derived from one process on enzymatic reactions in other pathways result in a variety of regulatory relationships between fat and carbohydrate metabolism. These relationships are best illustrated by (1) the effects of augmented carbohydrate utilization on fat metabolism, and (2) the effects of augmented fat utilization on carbohydrate metabolism. These interactions are summarized in Table 5.

When the supply of carbohydrate is increased (for example, after a carbohydrate-containing meal) and glucose utilization is stimulated, changes are observed in fat metabolism with respect to lipolysis, fatty acid synthesis, and ketogenesis. The increase in glucose uptake decreases fatty acid release from adipose tissue by enhancing the availability of glycerol-3-phosphate. This intermediate, which is derived from the glycolytic pathway, reesterifies the free fatty acids to form triglyceride. In addition, the rise in circulating glucose stimulates the secretion of insulin (see below), which is the most potent inhibitor of the hormone-sensitive lipase in adipose tissue. Thus the antilipolytic action of carbohydrate is substrate- as well as hormone-mediated.

TABLE 5. INTERRELATIONSHIPS BETWEEN FAT AND CARBOHYDRATE METABOLISM

CONDITION	EFFECT	MECHANISM
Carbohydrate utilization	$\downarrow$ lipolysis	$\uparrow$ glycerol-3-phosphate
		$\downarrow$ hormone-sensitive lipase
	$\uparrow$ fat synthesis	$\uparrow$ acetyl CoA carboxylase
	$\downarrow$ ketogenesis	$\downarrow$ lipolysis
		$\downarrow$ acylcarnitine transferase
Fat utilization	$\uparrow$ gluconeogenesis	$\uparrow$ pyruvate carboxylase
	$\downarrow$ fat synthesis	$\downarrow$ acetyl CoA carboxylase
	? $\downarrow$ glucose oxidation	$\downarrow$ phosphofructokinase
		$\downarrow$ pyruvate dehydrogenase

The utilization of carbohydrate also promotes the net synthesis of long-chain fatty acids. The rate-limiting enzyme in fat biosynthesis, acetyl CoA carboxylase, is increased in activity by carbohydrate feeding. This effect is mediated by hormonal changes (increased insulin) as well as the augmented availability of citrate, which is an activator of the enzyme, and the reduction in free fatty acids, which inhibit the enzyme. The utilization of glucose along the pentose pathway also provides the NADPH necessary for fat biosynthesis.

Ketogenesis is also markedly inhibited by carbohydrate utilization. This effect is mediated via the inhibition of lipolysis, which decreases the availability of fatty acids for oxidation by the liver. In addition, the enhancement of fat biosynthesis increases the availability of malonyl CoA, which inhibits acylcarnitine transferase I. Hormonal changes accompanying carbohydrate utilization (increased insulin, reduced glucagon) also reduce the availability of free carnitine necessary for the transport of fatty acyl derivatives across the mitochondrial membrane.

The effects of augmented carbohydrate availability and utilization on fat metabolism are thus a diminution in lipolysis, an increase in fat synthesis, and an inhibition of ketogenesis. The net effect is that an increase in carbohydrate uptake (as with a high carbohydrate diet) results in increased fat stores.

When fat utilization is increased, as occurs with restriction of dietary carbohydrate, in total starvation, and in disease states such as diabetes, a number of effects on carbohydrate metabolism are observed. An increase in gluconeogenesis generally accompanies augmented fat utilization and ketogenesis. The mechanism whereby fat oxidation stimulates gluconeogenesis probably derives from the allosteric activation by acetyl CoA of pyruvate carboxylase, the first step in the gluconeogenic pathway (Fig. 8). Thus, while fatty acids (other than the relatively rarely occurring odd-chain derivatives) cannot provide net carbon skeletons for glucose synthesis, their oxidation enhances gluconeogenesis by enzymatic activation.

Increases in fat oxidation are also accompanied by inhibition of fat synthesis from glucose-derived (or fat-derived) acetyl CoA. The activity of acetyl CoA carboxylase is inhibited by high levels of FFA and by the hormonal milieu (decreased insulin) that accompanies carbohydrate depletion.

In studies with the perfused rat heart an inhibitory effect of free fatty acids on glucose utilization via glycolytic and aerobic pathways has also been observed. The sites of inhibition of glucose utilization are the steps catalyzed by phosphofructokinase, the rate-limiting enzyme in glycolysis, and pyruvate dehydrogenase, the enzyme required for the formation of acetyl CoA from pyruvate. This relationship has been termed the glucose–fatty acid cycle and proposes that an elevation in circulating free fatty acids interferes with glucose oxidation. Whether this relationship applies to skeletal muscle in intact humans is controversial. For example, during exercise an increase in glucose utilization is accompanied by a rise in FFA and increased fat oxidation by the contracting muscles. Nevertheless, a reciprocal relationship between fat and glucose oxidation may apply to heart muscle or other conditions.

REFERENCES

Lipids

Bloch, K., and Vance, D.: Control mechanisms in the synthesis of saturated fatty acids. Annu Rev Biochem 46:263, 1977.

Brady, R. O.: Inborn errors of lipid metabolism. Adv Enzymol 38:293, 1973.

Cahill, G. F., Jr.: Starvation in man. N Engl J Med 282:668, 1970.

Foster, D. W.: From glycogen to ketones—and back. Diabetes 33:1188, 1984.

Fulco, A. J.: Metabolic alterations of fatty acids. Annu Rev Biochem 43:147, 1974.

Grey, N. J., Karl, I., and Kipnis, D.: Physiologic mechanisms in the development of starvation ketosis in man. Diabetes 24:10, 1975.

McGarry, J. D., and Foster, D. W.: Regulation of hepatic fatty acid oxidation and ketone body production. Annu Rev Biochem 49:395, 1980.

McGarry, J. D., Leatherman, G. F., and Foster, D. W.: Carnitine palmitoyltransferase I. The site of inhibition of hepatic fatty acid oxidation by malonyl CoA. J Biol Chem 253:4128, 1978.

Owen, O. E., Caprio, S., Reichard, G. A., Jr., Mazzoli, M. A., Boden, G., and Owen, R. S.: Ketosis and starvation: A revisit and new perspectives. Clin Endocrinol Metab 12:287, 1983.

Wakil, S. J., Stoop, J. K., and Joshi, V. C.: Fatty acid synthesis and its regulation. Annu Rev Biochem 52:537, 1983.

AMINO ACIDS AND PROTEIN

DEFINITION AND CLASSIFICATION OF AMINO ACIDS

Amino acids are the building blocks from which proteins are synthesized. A total of 20 different amino acids are commonly found in proteins, while additional nonprotein amino acids (ornithine, citrulline, homocysteine, homoserine) are important intermediates in amino acid metabolism. The two characteristic features common to amino acids are the presence of a free carboxyl group and a free amino group on the alpha carbon. In the case of proline an alpha imino group is present. The amino acids differ from each other with respect to their side chains.

The amino acids form subgroups based on the similarity of their carbon skeletons or substituent groups and the sharing of metabolic pathways. Valine, leucine, and isoleucine have in common a branched aliphatic side chain and are thus referred to collectively as the branched chain amino acids. In addition, these amino acids undergo similar metabolic transformations (see below). Methionine and cysteine are both sulfur-containing amino acids, while tyrosine and phenylalanine have an aromatic side chain.

Despite the constancy of the protein mass in the fully grown individual, there is a rapid turnover of body proteins and their constituent amino acids. In a healthy, well-fed adult a total of 12 to 15 grams of nitrogen appears in the urine each day, reflecting the breakdown of 70 to 90 grams of protein. This amount of protein must be resynthesized to maintain nitrogen balance. The amino acids from the diet provide the necessary substrate for protein synthesis.

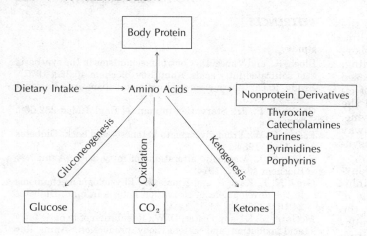

Figure 19. The metabolic fate of endogenous and dietary amino acids.

The amino acids released from body protein as well as those ingested in the diet may undergo a variety of metabolic fates, as shown in Figure 19. Synthesis of protein is obviously a most important fate of amino acids. The processes and regulation of protein synthesis are discussed in detail in Section II (Genetics). A small proportion of the total amino acid pool is used for nonprotein anabolic reactions such as the synthesis of purines, pyrimidines, and porphyrins, and for the formation of amino acid–derived hormones, thyroxine, and the catecholamines. The major catabolic fates of the amino acids are oxidation of CO_2, conversion to glucose (gluconeogenesis), and conversion to ketones. In addition to the degradative pathways, amino acids may be synthesized from carbohydrate precursors or from other amino acids.

BIOSYNTHESIS OF AMINO ACIDS

To support protein anabolism humans require an exogenous source of specific amino acids that cannot be synthesized from endogenous precursors. These amino acids have been termed *essential* and are listed in Table 6. In the absence of these eight amino acids growth or maintenance of body protein cannot be supported. In contrast, the remaining 12 amino acids contained in protein can be synthesized from glucose-derived or TCA cycle intermediates (pyruvate, oxaloacetate, α-ketoglutarate, or from other (essential or nonessential) amino acids. In the case of alanine, aspartate, and glutamate only a single step (transamination) is required in which an amino group is transferred to the alpha carbon (in place of the alpha keto group) on pyruvate, oxaloacetate, and α-ketoglutarate, respectively.

TABLE 6. THE ESSENTIAL AMINO ACIDS

AMINO ACID	APPROXIMATE DAILY REQUIREMENT (g)
Isoleucine	0.70
Leucine	1.10
Valine	0.80
Lysine	0.80
Methionine	1.10
Phenylalanine	1.10
Threonine	0.50
Tryptophan	0.50

CATABOLISM OF AMINO ACIDS

Transamination. The major degradative fates of amino acids are oxidation to CO_2, conversion to glucose (gluconeogenesis), and conversion to ketones (ketogenesis). In the catabolism of almost all amino acids (lysine and possibly threonine are exceptions), the initial catabolic step is transamination. This reaction involves the transfer of an amino group from the donor amino acid to the alpha carbon of an alpha keto acid. In this process the alpha keto derivative of the donor amino acid and the amino acid analogue of the recipient alpha keto acid are formed. The reaction is illustrated in Figure 20, in which the transamination of alanine and α-ketoglutarate is shown. The products of the reaction are pyruvate (the keto acid analogue of alanine) and glutamate, the amino acid analogue of α-ketoglutarate.

The enzymes catalyzing such reactions are known as transaminases or aminotransferases. They are present in the cytosol and mitochondria of liver as well as skeletal muscle and heart tissue. The reactions are freely reversible, requiring pyridoxal phosphate as a cofactor. The dietary requirement for trace amounts of pyridoxal phosphate (vitamin B_6) derives from its importance in transamination. Rarely, larger amounts of pyridoxal phosphate are required because of hereditary defects in the utilization of this cofactor. Such circumstances are described as *vitamin-dependency* syndromes.

For most amino acids, α-ketoglutarate acts as the amino group acceptor, so that the final disposition of the amino groups depends on the catabolism of glutamate. This amino acid is degraded by the enzyme glutamate dehydrogenase, which catalyzes the oxidative deamination of glutamate as shown by the following equation:

$$\text{Glutamate} + \text{NAD} + H_2O \longleftrightarrow \text{α-ketoglutarate} + NH_4^+ + \text{NADH}$$

This reaction is the most important pathway for the production of ammonia from the catabolism of amino acids, since no other amino acid has such an active dehydrogenase. Glutamate dehydrogenase is an allosteric enzyme that is activated by ADP and GDP and inhibited by ATP, GTP, and NADH. In this manner a fall in tissue ATP favors amino acid oxidation while the reverse is true when ATP levels are high.

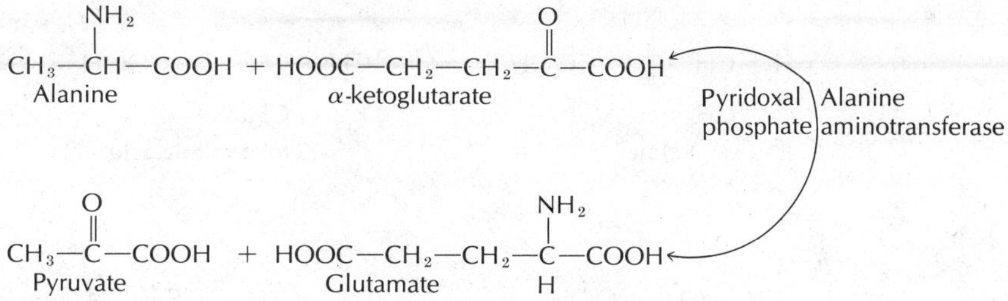

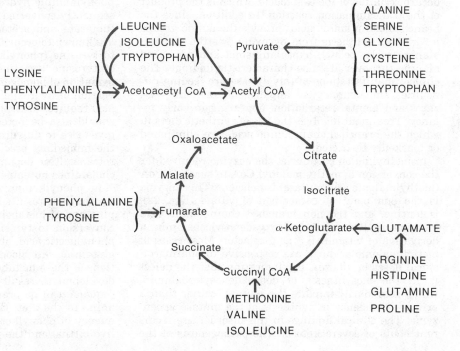

Figure 20. The alamine aminotransferase (transaminase) reaction. Pyridoxal phosphate (vitamin B_6) is required as a cofactor.

Oxidation.

Oxidation. Following removal of the amino group by means of transamination or oxidation, the carbon skeletons of each of the amino acids give rise either directly or via a series of reactions to pyruvate, various TCA cycle intermediates, or acetyl CoA, which can then undergo oxidation to CO_2 and water via the TCA cycle. The points of entry of each of the amino acids into the TCA cycle are shown in Figure 21.

Pyruvate is produced by the transamination of alanine and the degradation of serine, glycine, cysteine, and threonine. The catabolism of leucine, isoleucine, and tryptophan gives rise to acetyl CoA without the prior formation of pyruvate. Leucine, tryptophan, lysine, phenylalanine, and tyrosine give rise to acetoacetyl CoA, which is then cleaved to acetyl CoA. Transamination of glutamate produces α-ketoglutarate. The latter is also produced (by way of glutamate) in the catabolism of arginine, histidine, glutamine, and proline. Succinyl CoA is formed in the degradation of isoleucine, valine, and methionine. Fumarate is produced as an end product of phenylalanine and tyrosine metabolism. The transamination of aspartate yields oxaloacetate.

Although the individual steps in each of these catabolic pathways will not be covered here, their pathophysiological import derives from a host of inborn errors of metabolism that are ascribable to isolated enzymatic defects. These defects in catabolism result in the accumulation of intermediates prior to the metabolic block, which often have deleterious effects, particularly to the central nervous system. While the defects cannot be cured, early treatment with special diets that eliminate the amino acid whose catabolism is reduced (for example, a low phenylalanine diet in the treatment of phenylketonuria) or administration of large doses of vitamins in specific vitamin-dependency syndromes (for example, vitamin B_{12} in methylmalonic aciduria) may be helpful. As examples of these defects the catabolism of the branched chain amino acids and of phenylalanine and tyrosine will be described.

In Figure 22, the individual steps in the catabolism of the branched chain amino acid valine is shown. Although the end product is not the same for all three branched chain amino acids (succinyl CoA for valine and isoleucine, acetyl CoA for leucine, and acetoacetyl CoA for leucine and isoleucine), the initial steps of transamination and decarboxylation are identical. In fact, the same enzyme is involved in the oxidative decarboxylation of the α-ketoacids formed by transamination.

At least 14 specific enzymatic defects have been described involving the catabolism of one or more of the branched chain amino acids. Perhaps the best known of these defects is classic maple syrup urine disease, which involves the accumulation of all three

Figure 21. Points of entry of the carbon skeletons of amino acids into the tricarboxyl acid (TCA) cycle. Some of the amino acids enter at more than a single point (for example, isoleucine is catabolized to acetyl CoA and succinyl CoA).

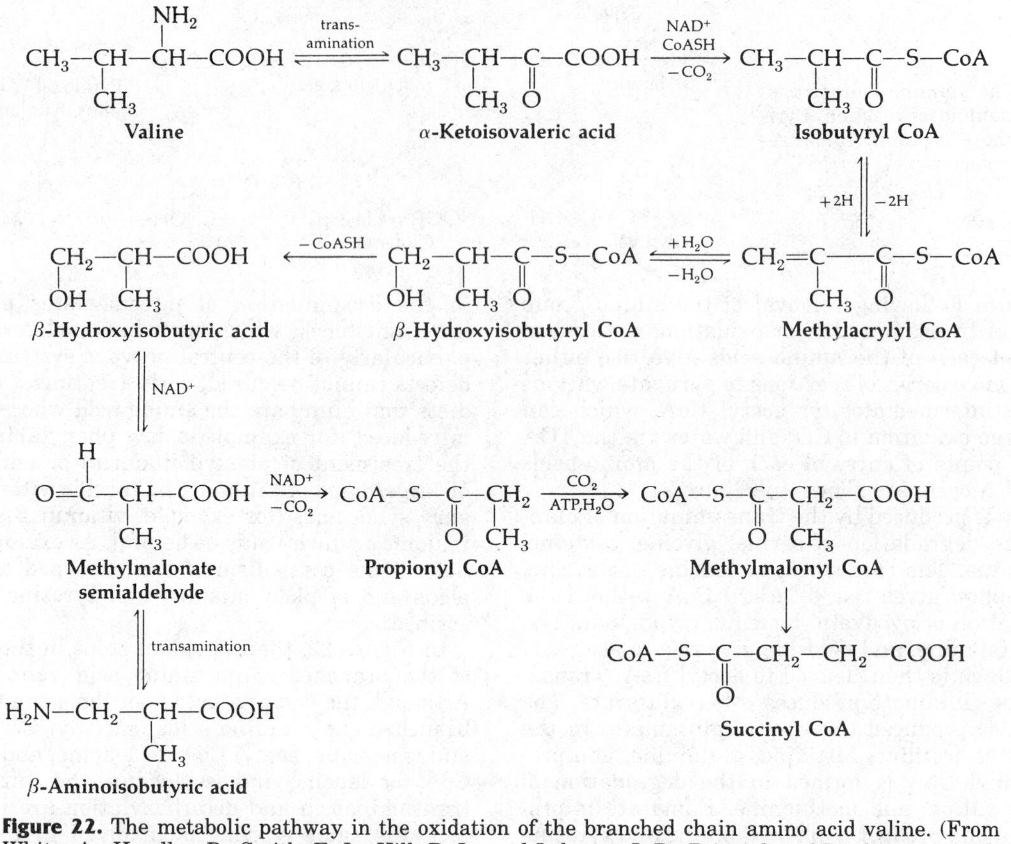

Figure 22. The metabolic pathway in the oxidation of the branched chain amino acid valine. (From White, A., Handler, P., Smith, E. L., Hill, R. L., and Lehman, I. R.: Principles of Biochemistry. 6th ed. New York, McGraw-Hill Book Co., 1978.)

branched chain keto acids (α-ketoisovaleric acid, α-ketoisocaproic acid, and α-keto-β-methylvaleric acid). These acids impart to the urine a characteristic odor, which resembles that of maple syrup. The disorder is due to a loss of the α-ketodehydrogenase, which, in the presence of NAD and CoA, catalyzes the oxidative decarboxylation of the α-ketoacid, which is the product of the transamination reaction. In addition, since the branched chain amino acids provide the amino groups for alanine synthesis from pyruvate (see the glucose-alanine cycle, below), hypoalaninemia and decreased alanine turnover are also characteristic findings. The clinical manifestations of this disease are feeding difficulties and neurological impairment, including seizures and mental retardation, appearing in early infancy. Treatment involves the use of synthetic diets in which the branched chain amino acids are eliminated or markedly restricted.

In methylmalonic aciduria, the enzyme required for the conversion of methylmalonyl CoA to succinyl CoA (methylmalonic acid mutase) is deficient. This enzyme is the end point of catabolism of valine (Fig. 22), isoleucine, and the non–branched chain amino acid methionine. It requires 5′ deoxyadenosylcobalamin, a derivative of vitamin B_{12}, as a cofactor. Most cases of methylmalonic aciduria are responsive to pharmacological doses of vitamin B_{12}, indicating that the defect is in the biosynthesis of deoxyadenosylcobalamin, which secondarily impairs the mutase, rather than a primary deficiency in synthesis of the mutase apoenzyme. The clinical findings in this disorder are recurrent bouts of severe ketosis. The pathogenesis of the

ketosis is uncertain but may relate to the inhibitory effect of methylmalonyl CoA on fat synthesis, thereby enhancing fatty acid availability for beta-oxidation.

In Figure 23 the pathway for the catabolism of phenylalanine and tyrosine metabolism is shown. Phenylalanine is initially converted (via the enzyme phenylalanine hydroxylase) to tyrosine, which is subsequently converted via several intermediate steps to fumarate and acetoacetate. Defects in this pathway are known to occur in the conversion of phenylalanine to tyrosine (phenylketonuria), in the transamination of tyrosine (tyrosinemia or tyrosinosis), and in the oxidation of homogentisic acid (alkaptonuria). The conversion of hydroxyphenylpyruvic acid to homogentisic acid requires ascorbic acid (vitamin C) as a cofactor. It should also be noted that oxidation of tyrosine also gives rise to dihydroxyphenylalanine (dopa), which is the immediate precursor in the synthesis of the neurotransmitter dopamine and a precursor of the catecholamines norepinephrine and epinephrine.

In phenylketonuria a deficiency of phenylalanine hydroxylase results in the accumulation of phenylalanine and of metabolites that do not require its initial conversion to tyrosine—namely, phenylpyruvic acid, phenylacetic acid, phenyllactic acid, and phenylacetylglutamine—in blood and urine. The high concentrations of these metabolites interfere with normal brain development, resulting in mental retardation. These sequelae can be prevented by restriction of phenylalanine in the diet. Because of the relatively high frequency of phenylketonuria (7 to 12 cases per 100,000 live births) and the prevention of its clinical sequelae

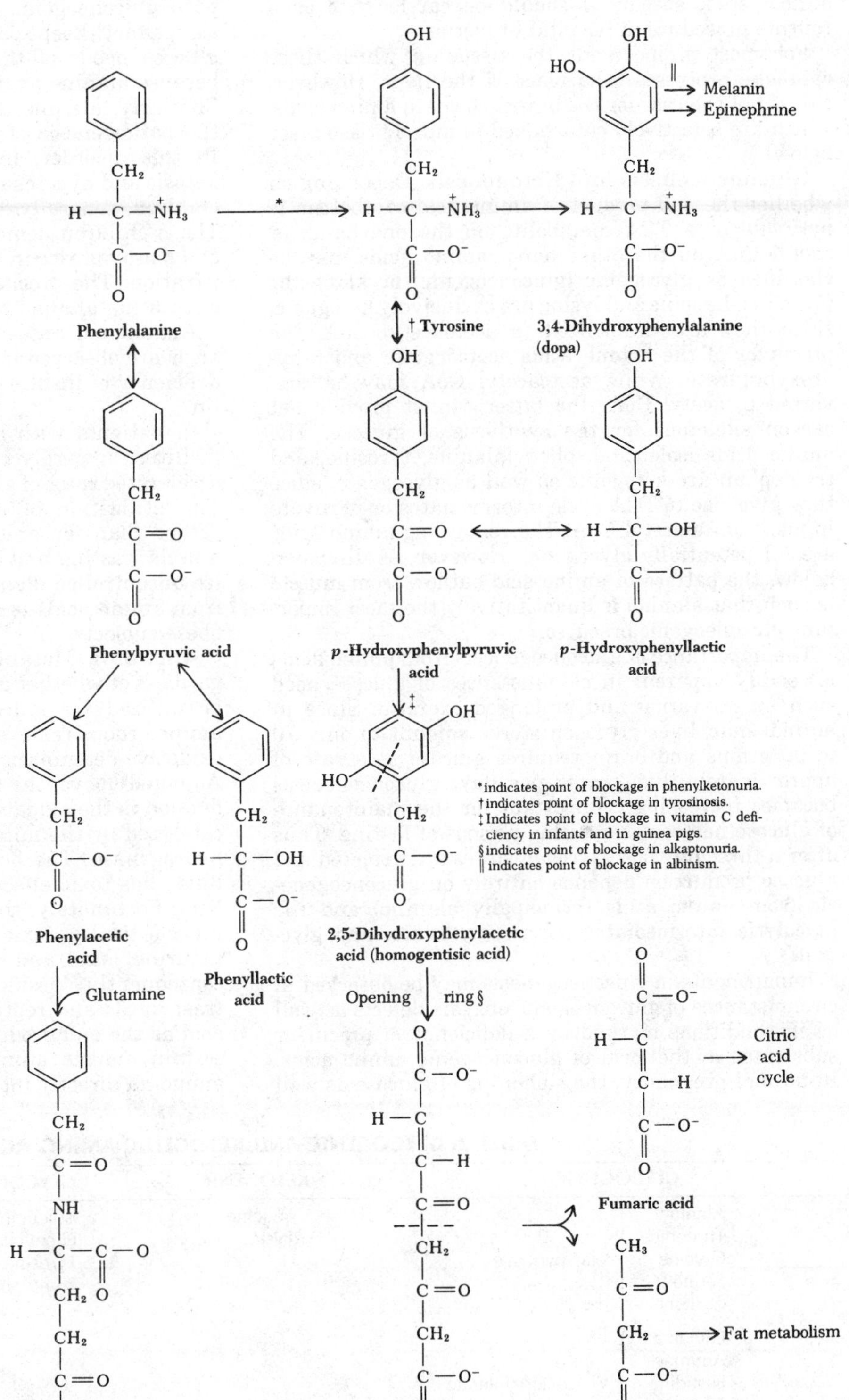

Figure 23. Metabolism of phenylalanine and tyrosine. In phenylketonuria there is a deficiency in the enzyme required for the conversion of phenylalanine to tyrosine (phenylalanine hydroxylase). As a consequence there is conversion of phenylalanine to phenylpyruvic acid, phenylacetic acid, phenyllactic acid, and phenylacetylglutamine, which appear in the urine. In tyrosinemia (or tyrosinosis) there is a deficiency in tyrosine transaminase. In alkaptonuria there is failure of oxidation of homogentisic acid. (From Orten, J. M., and Neuhaus, O. W.: Human Biochemistry. 9th ed. St. Louis, C. V. Mosby, 1975.)

*indicates point of blockage in phenylketonuria.
†indicates point of blockage in tyrosinosis.
‡indicates point of blockage in vitamin C deficiency in infants and in guinea pigs.
§indicates point of blockage in alkaptonuria.
∥indicates point of blockage in albinism.

by early dietary intervention, screening of newborns for high levels of phenylalanine in blood (by means of a heel stick specimen) should be carried out as a routine procedure in hospital nurseries.

For most amino acids the tissue in which these catabolic processes take place is the liver. However, this is not the case for the branched chain amino acids, which are selectively catabolized in muscle tissue (see below).

Gluconeogenesis and Ketogenesis. Depending on whether the end product of amino acid catabolism is pyruvate or a TCA metabolite on the one hand, or acetyl CoA on the other hand, amino acids may be classified as glycogenic (gluconeogenic) or ketogenic (Table 7). Leucine and lysine are exclusively ketogenic, since they are catabolized to acetoacetyl CoA, the precursor of the ketone acids acetoacetate and β-hydroxybutyrate. While acetoacetyl CoA may be converted to acetyl CoA, the latter cannot provide net carbon skeletons for the synthesis of glucose. The amino acids isoleucine, phenylalanine, tyrosine, and tryptophan are ketogenic as well as glycogenic, since they give rise to TCA cycle intermediates or pyruvate in addition to acetyl CoA. The remaining amino acids are all potentially glycogenic. However, as discussed below, the pattern of amino acid outflow from muscle is such that alanine is quantitatively the most important gluconeogenic precursor.

The importance of gluconeogenesis from amino acids is readily apparent in circumstances of glucose need such as starvation and prolonged exercise. Since in normal man liver glycogen stores amount to only 70 to 90 grams and brain requires glucose at a rate of approximately 125 grams per day, gluconeogenesis becomes increasingly important for the maintenance of glucose homeostasis during periods of fasting. Thus after a three-day fast glycogen stores are depleted and glucose production depends entirely on gluconeogenesis from amino acids (principally alanine) and the glycolytic intermediates lactate, pyruvate, and glycerol.

Impairments in gluconeogenesis may be observed in circumstances of gluconeogenic enzyme defects as well as in conditions marked by a deficiency of precursor substrates in the form of gluconeogenic amino acids. In normal pregnancy, the siphoning of glucose as well as alanine and other amino acids results in an acceleration of starvation hypoglycemia. Despite intact hepatic gluconeogenic enzymes, maternal gluconeogenesis cannot keep pace with the combined obligate glucose needs of the maternal brain and conceptus because alanine availability is reduced in the mother. Similarly, alanine deficiency has been implicated in the pathogenesis of ketotic hypoglycemia of infancy. In this disorder, hypoglycemia in association with ketosis and hypoinsulinemia is observed in infants and children, generally following a bout of gastroenteritis. These children demonstrate low alanine blood levels and a prompt rise in blood glucose after alanine administration. The precise mechanism of the reduction in circulating alanine has not been established.

Augmented rates of gluconeogenesis from amino acids are observed in disease states characterized by a deficiency of insulin or lack of responsiveness to insulin.

In patients with severely decompensated diabetes mellitus, hyperglycemia is due at least in part to accelerated rates of glucose synthesis from amino acids. The utilization of amino acids for gluconeogenesis rather than for protein synthesis contributes to the muscle wasting and negative nitrogen that characterize uncontrolled diabetes. Augmented gluconeogenesis from amino acids is also observed in insulin-resistant obese subjects.

Ammonia Metabolism and the Urea Cycle. Regardless of whether amino acids are catabolized to CO_2 or utilized for gluconeogenesis or ketogenesis, the amino groups removed by initial transamination or by oxidative deamination may be converted to ammonia. As noted above, the major pathway for ammonia production is the oxidative decarboxylation of glutamate, catalyzed by the mitochondrial enzyme glutamate dehydrogenase. The accumulation of ammonia in body fluids has toxic effects, particularly on brain metabolism. Fortunately, the end product of nitrogen in humans is the less toxic substance urea, which is excreted in urine. Man and other terrestrial vertebrates are consequently classified as ureotelic organisms. In contrast, birds and reptiles are uricotelic, excreting uric acid as the end product of nitrogen metabolism, while certain marine animals are ammonotelic, excreting ammonia directly into their aqueous environment.

TABLE 7. GLYCOGENIC AND KETOGENIC AMINO ACIDS

GLYCOGENIC		KETOGENIC	GLYCOGENIC AND KETOGENIC
Alanine Threonine Glycine Serine Cysteine	} Via* pyruvate	Leucine Lysine	Isoleucine via* succinyl CoA Phenylalanine } Via fumarate Tyrosine Tryptophan via pyruvate
Glutamate Arginine Histidine Glutamine Proline	} Via α-ketoglutarate		
Methionine Valine	} Via succinyl CoA		
Aspartate Asparagine	} Via oxaloacetate		

*Denotes intermediate through which carbon skeleton enters gluconeogenic pathway.

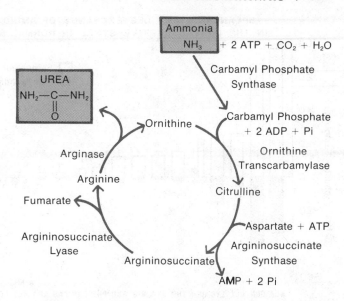

Figure 24. The urea (Krebs-Henseleit) cycle. The first two steps in the pathway (synthesis of carbamyl phosphate and condensation of the latter with ornithine to form citrulline) occur in the mitochondria and the remainder in the cytosol. With each turn of the cycle two amino groups (one entering as ammonia and the other as the amino group on aspartate) are converted to urea. Three ATP are converted in the process of ADP, AMP, and 4Pi (inorganic phosphate).

The formation of urea from ammonia involves a series of reactions known as the Krebs-Henseleit or urea cycle (Fig. 24). In this pathway carbamyl phosphate is the initial product formed by the condensation of ammonia and water at the expense of two ATP. Thereafter, carbamyl phosphate condenses with ornithine to form citrulline. The condensation of citrulline and aspartate at the expense of ATP gives rise to argininosuccinate. The latter undergoes an elimination reaction yielding arginine and fumarate. In the final step of the cycle two nitrogens are converted to urea, one having entered as carbamyl phosphate and the other as the amino group from aspartate.

The importance of the urea cycle in preventing the accumulation of toxic amounts of ammonia is indicated by the clinical sequelae accompanying genetic defects of urea cycle enzymes. Such patients demonstrate an intolerance to protein ingestion characterized by hyperammonemia and mental impairment. In acquired diseases of the liver, such as Laennec's cirrhosis, particularly when accompanied by portal hypertension and the shunting of blood from the portal to the systemic circulation, a similar accumulation of ammonia occurs. An intolerance of dietary protein and mental impairment (often accompanied by asterixis, a characteristic flapping tremor on extension of the wrists) are also observed. The precise mechanism whereby hyperammonemia interferes with brain metabolism has not been established. Reversal of the glutamate dehydrogenase reaction, resulting in depletion of α-ketoglutarate and interference with the TCA cycle, has been postulated.

An additional pathway for the transfer of amino groups out of muscle is provided by the synthesis of alanine. Alanine is formed in muscle tissue by transamination of glucose-derived pyruvate. The alanine released into the bloodstream is taken up by the liver, where it again undergoes transamination and its amino group is converted to urea. This sequence of reactions, which also involves the cyclic interconversion of the carbon skeleton of alanine to glucose (the glucose-alanine cycle), is discussed in greater detail below.

INTERORGAN AMINO ACID EXCHANGE

Maintenance of steady-state concentrations of circulating amino acids depends upon the net balance between release from endogenous protein stores and utilization by various tissues. Since muscle accounts for well over 50 per cent of the total body pool of free amino acids and since the liver is the repository of the urea cycle enzymes necessary for nitrogen disposal, these two organs would be expected to play a major role in determining the circulating levels and turnover of amino acids.

Muscle. Examination of amino acid exchange across the deep tissues of the human forearm demonstrates that in normal man in the postabsorptive state (that is, following a 12- to 14-hour overnight fast), there is a net release of amino acids from muscle tissue, as reflected in a consistent addition to the venous effluent. The pattern of this release is quite distinctive, the output of alanine and glutamine exceeding that of all other amino acids and accounting for over 50 per cent of total alpha amino nitrogen release. The same pattern is observed if one examines amino acid exchange across the leg by determining arteriofemoral venous differences (Fig. 25). In contrast to the net outputs from muscle tissue observed for most amino acids, small but consistent uptakes are demonstrable for serine, cystine, and glutamate.

Splanchnic Tissues. Complementing the negative balance of amino acids in muscle tissue is the consistent uptake of amino acids across the splanchnic bed. As in the case of peripheral output, alanine and glutamine predominate in the uptake of amino acids by splanchnic tissues. In fact, there is fairly close correspondence between the relative outputs of most amino acids from the periphery and their uptake by splanchnic tissues (Fig. 25). A notable exception is serine, which is extracted by peripheral tissues as well as the splanchnic bed. The source of the serine consumed by these tissues is the kidney (see below). In contrast to all other amino acids, a consistent release from the splanchnic bed is observed only for citrulline, a urea cycle intermediate. Within the splanchnic bed, the liver is the site of uptake of alanine and the gut is the

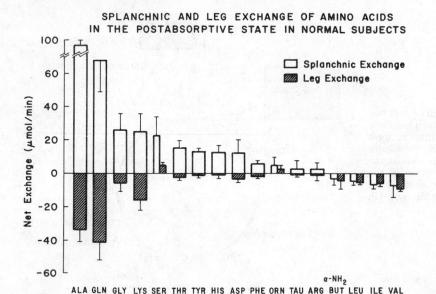

SPLANCHNIC AND LEG EXCHANGE OF AMINO ACIDS IN THE POSTABSORPTIVE STATE IN NORMAL SUBJECTS

☐ Splanchnic Exchange
▨ Leg Exchange

Net Exchange (μmol/min)

α-NH₂

ALA GLN GLY LYS SER THR TYR HIS ASP PHE ORN TAU ARG BUT LEU ILE VAL

Figure 25. Splanchnic and peripheral (arteriofemoral venous differences) exchange of amino acids in normal man after an overnight fast. (From Felig, P.: Amino acid metabolism in man. Annu Rev Biochem 44:933, 1975.)

site of utilization of glutamine. Most of the amino groups of the glutamine extracted by the gut are released as alanine or free ammonia.

Kidney. The net balance of amino acids across the kidney consists of an uptake of glutamine, proline, and glycine and an output of serine and alanine. As noted above, serine is extracted by liver as well as by peripheral tissues, indicating that the kidney is the major source of release of this amino acid into the systemic circulation. In contrast, the contribution by the kidney to total alanine release (10 to 20 μmol/min) is far smaller than that released from muscle (100 μmol/min). Precise data on the relative importance of the kidney and gut in the uptake and catabolism of glutamine are not available for man. However, studies with eviscerated, nephrectomized rats suggest that the gut may be quantitatively more important than the kidney in the clearance of glutamine from plasma.

Brain. An uptake of most amino acids by human brain tissue has been demonstrated by measuring arterial–jugular venous differences in normal subjects. The uptake of the branched chain amino acids, particularly valine, exceeds that of all other amino acids. Furthermore, the capacity of rat brain to oxidize the branched chain amino acids is fourfold greater than that of muscle and liver. Inasmuch as significant amounts of valine, leucine, and isoleucine are released

from muscle but not extracted by liver, it is likely that the brain constitutes an important site of utilization of these amino acids.

Summary. The observations on the net balances of amino acids across muscle, liver, gastrointestinal tissues, kidney, and brain in normal man in the postabsorptive state clearly demonstrate the key role of alanine and glutamine in the overall flux of amino acids among tissues (Fig. 26). Free amino acids are released from muscle and gut and are extracted by the liver. Alanine and glutamine account for more than 50 per cent of the total alpha amino nitrogen released by muscle. The gut also releases substantial amounts of alpha amino nitrogen, primarily as alanine. The major site of alanine uptake is the liver, where its extraction exceeds that of all other amino acids. The kidney and gut are the major sites of uptake of glutamine, which provides the nitrogen source for alanine synthesis in the gut and ammoniogenesis in the kidney. The branched chain amino acids, particularly valine, escape hepatic uptake and are utilized by the brain. The key role of alanine in this overall formulation is underscored by observations in the rat, dog, sheep, and reptiles, demonstrating the universality of this amino acid as a vehicle of nitrogen transport and as an end product of nitrogen catabolism in a variety of species.

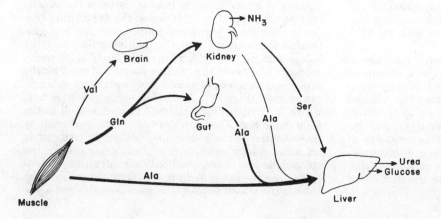

Figure 26. Interorgan amino acid exchange in normal, postabsorptive man. The key role of alanine and glutamine in amino nitrogen outflow from muscle is shown. (From Felig, P.: Amino acid metabolism in man. Annu Rev Biochem 44:933, 1975.)

THE GLUCOSE-ALANINE CYCLE

The primacy of alanine in the overall availability and uptake of amino acids by the liver immediately suggested the importance of this amino acid as the key protein-derived glucose precursor. Support for this hypothesis was obtained from studies in experimental animals as well as from observations in intact man. In the perfused liver, the rate of glucose synthesis from alanine and serine is far higher than that observed from all other amino acids. Gluconeogenesis from alanine has been demonstrated to increase in proportion to the availability of this amino acid. Furthermore, whereas glucose production from a mixture of amino acids is saturated at three times normal concentrations, gluconeogenesis from alanine does not reach saturation until an alanine concentration of 9 mM, which is 20 to 30 times the normal physiological level. In vivo incorporation of ^{14}C-labeled alanine into blood glucose in the rat occurs six times more rapidly than that of labeled serine and increases linearly as alanine levels are raised to tenfold above physiological concentrations.

The predominance of alanine in the outflow of amino acids from muscle to liver cannot be explained on the basis of its availability in constituent cellular proteins. Alanine composes no more than 7 to 10 per cent of muscle proteins yet accounts for 30 per cent or more of the net flow of alpha amino nitrogen from muscle to the splanchnic bed. This discrepancy led to the suggestion that alanine is synthesized de novo in muscle tissue by transamination of pyruvate. On the basis of the evidence implicating alanine as a glucose precursor, and the data indicating its synthesis in muscle tissue, a "glucose-alanine cycle" was proposed. This formulation holds that alanine is synthesized in muscle by transamination of glucose-derived pyruvate and is transported to the liver, where its carbon skeleton is reconverted to glucose (Fig. 27A). The branched chain amino acids were suggested as the origin of the amino

groups for muscle alanine synthesis inasmuch as extrahepatic tissues, particularly muscle, have been demonstrated as the site of their oxidation.

A variety of studies in man and experimental animals have subsequently appeared supporting the existence of the glucose-alanine cycle. In normal man, a direct linear relationship between plasma alanine and pyruvate levels has been observed; such a relationship does not exist between pyruvate and other amino acids. In association with the increased glucose utilization of muscular exercise, a specific increase in muscle production and circulating levels of alanine is observed. In addition, in acquired or congenital disorders of lactate and pyruvate metabolism characterized by hyperpyruvicemia, plasma alanine levels are elevated. In contrast, in patients with McArdle's syndrome, in whom glucose consumption by exercising muscle is limited and pyruvate levels fall during exercise, a simultaneous fall in alanine concentration has been noted. The addition of glucose or insulin to incubated rat diaphragm results in a two- to threefold increase in the release of alanine but fails to increase the release of other amino acids. Furthermore, studies using ^{14}C-glucose indicate that 60 per cent of the carbon skeletons of alanine released by muscle is derived from exogenous glucose, while virtually none of the carbon skeletons are derived from the in situ muscle catabolism of other amino acids. Quantitatively, recycling of carbon skeletons along the glucose-alanine cycle occurs at a rate approximately 50 per cent of that observed for the Cori (lactate) cycle.

Although the glucose-alanine cycle does not yield new carbon skeletons for de novo glucose synthesis, it is of importance in glucose homeostasis as well as nitrogen and energy metabolism. As discussed above, a deficiency of alanine has been implicated in the accelerated starvation observed in pregnancy, in ketotic hypoglycemia of infancy, and in hypoglycemia of maple syrup urine disease. Alanine also provides a

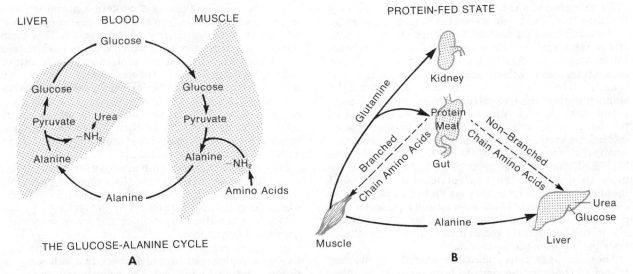

Figure 27. *A*, The glucose-alanine cycle. *B*, Influence of protein feeding on interorgan amino acid exchange. The branched chain amino acids in the ingested protein escape from the liver and are taken up by muscle tissue where they are utilized for protein synthesis or catabolized. In contrast, only a small proportion of the remaining amino acids in the ingested protein are transported as such to muscle. (From Felig, P., et al.: Arch Intern Med 137:507, 1977.)

nontoxic alternative to ammonia in the transfer of amino groups derived from the catabolism of branched chain amino acids in muscle to the liver. This carrier role of alanine in nitrogen metabolism may be of particular importance in circumstances characterized by augmented formation or inadequate disposal of ammonia. Contraction of muscle is known to increase ammonia production. During exercise, increased transfer of amino groups to pyruvate may serve to limit ammonia accumulation. Hyperalaninemia is also observed in a variety of disorders of urea cycle enzymes, where it may serve to mitigate the degree of hyperammonemia.

The glucose-alanine cycle may also be useful with respect to ATP production. Conversion of glucose to alanine provides 8 mol ATP compared with 2 mol provided by conversion to lactate. Furthermore, to the extent that alanine formation facilitates the oxidation of the branched chain amino acids, an additional 30 to 40 mol ATP will be generated per mol of amino acid oxidized.

PROTEIN REPLETION AND FEEDING

Since muscle tissue is in negative nitrogen balance in the fasting state, repletion of muscle nitrogen depends on a net uptake of amino acids in response to protein ingestion. Interestingly, it has long been recognized that following the ingestion of a protein meal, there are marked variations in the plasma increments of individual amino acids observed in peripheral blood. The largest elevations, amounting to increments of 200 per cent or more, are observed for the branched chain amino acid concentrations, which remain elevated for as long as eight hours. In contrast, other amino acids, such as alanine, show little change in plasma concentration after protein feeding. These effects of protein ingestion on circulating amino acids reflect their action on the interorgan exchange of amino acids.

In normal, healthy subjects ingestion of a protein meal (lean beef) is followed by a large output of amino acids from the splanchnic bed involving predominantly the branched chain amino acids. Valine, isoleucine, and leucine together account for more than 60 per cent of the total amino acids entering the systemic circulation despite the fact that they compose only 20 per cent of the total amino acids in the protein meal. Simultaneous with the release of amino acids from the splanchnic bed, peripheral muscle exchange of most amino acids reverts from the net output observed in the basal state to a net uptake. As in the case of splanchnic exchange, the uptake of amino acids across peripheral muscle tissue is most marked for the branched chain amino acids. The latter account for more than half of the total peripheral amino acid uptake in the first hour, and for 90 to 100 per cent at two to three hours. Most interestingly, alanine and glutamine are continuously released by muscle tissue, albeit at a transiently reduced rate, during the three-hour period after the protein meal.

These findings thus indicate a special role for the branched chain amino acids in body nitrogen metabolism, not only in the fasting state but after protein feeding as well. These amino acids demonstrate a unique tendency to escape hepatic uptake and/or metabolism after intestinal absorption. This observation is in keeping with the relative unimportance of the liver, as noted above, in branched chain amino acid catabolism. Furthermore, since the branched chain amino acids compose only 20 per cent of the amino acid residues in muscle proteins, it is likely that these amino acids are not utilized solely for protein synthesis but are largely catabolized within muscle. Thus, as in the fasting state, they provide a source of energy for muscle.

The effects of protein feeding on interorgan amino acid exchange and the key role of the branched chain amino acids are summarized in Figure 27B. A nitrogen "shuttle" is observed in which branched chain amino acids provide for nitrogen repletion in muscle tissue in the fed state. The nitrogen thus delivered is released as alanine and glutamine in the fed as well as the fasted condition. The high circulating and intracellular levels of branched chain amino acids induced by protein feeding may have importance beyond delivery of nitrogen. Recent data suggest that the branched chain amino acids, particularly leucine, may have a regulatory role in protein synthesis.

PROTEIN MALNUTRITION

As noted above, of the 20 amino acids commonly found in various proteins, 8 cannot be synthesized by man and are consequently referred to as essential amino acids (Table 6). The adequacy of dietary protein intake depends on the presence of these essential amino acids, their relative proportions, and the presence of additional nitrogen in the form of nonessential amino acids. Interestingly, the addition of large amounts of a single nonessential amino acid leads to an imbalance that may interfere with normal protein synthesis despite the presence of the essential amino acids. Clinically this circumstance may be observed in obese patients treated for prolonged periods with hypocaloric liquid protein diets made up of collagen hydrolysates containing large amounts of glycine.

The overall effectiveness of protein-containing foods in promoting growth (protein synthesis) may be expressed in terms of their *biological value*. This term refers to the efficiency with which a given food protein is retained and utilized for protein synthesis rather than catabolized and excreted as urinary nitrogen. The reference protein, whose biological value is by convention taken as 100, is whole egg protein. The biological value of other proteins compared with whole egg is determined on the basis of their effects on nitrogen balance or by comparing their chemical composition with that of whole egg protein.

In general, proteins of animal origin (egg, beef, milk) are of higher biological value than those of vegetable or plant origin, such as cereals (corn meal, oatmeal), wheat flour, nuts, or legumes. The inadequacy of plant proteins generally derives from their low content of lysine and tryptophan.

In underdeveloped areas of the world a spectrum of disorders is observed in which there is a deficiency of dietary protein and/or calories collectively described as *protein-calorie malnutrition*. A severe deficiency in the quantity and quality of protein despite an adequate intake of nonprotein calories results in *kwashiorkor*. In this syndrome, generally observed in children between the age of one and three years, there is marked growth retardation, muscle wasting and weakness, and dependent edema resulting from hypoalbuminemia. The circulating pattern of amino acids is characterized by a marked decline in essential amino acids and an elevation of nonessential amino acids. Depigmentation of the skin and hair (resulting in a characteristic red haired appearance) are also observed. The syndrome develops after weaning in children fed a diet composed almost exclusively of cereal grains.

In *marasmus* there is a very low intake of all nutrients, resulting in a marked caloric deficiency. The most prominent features are growth retardation and wasting of muscle and fat so as to give a "skin and bones" appearance. The edema and hypoalbuminemia of kwashiorkor are not observed. Most commonly, however, intermediate syndromes demonstrating features of both kwashiorkor and marasmus are observed.

REFERENCES

Amino Acids and Protein

Aikawa, T., Matsutaka, H., Takezawa, K., and Ishikawa, E.: Gluconeogenesis and amino acid metabolism. I. Comparison of various precursors for hepatic gluconeogenesis *in vivo*. Biochim Biophys Acta 279:234, 1972.

Buse, M. G., and Reid, S. S.: Leucine. A possible regulator of protein turnover in muscle. J Clin Invest 56:1250, 1975.

Cahill, G. F., Jr., and Owen, O. E.: The role of the kidney in the regulation of protein metabolism. In Munro, H. (ed.): Mammalian Protein Metabolism. New York, Academic Press, 1970, p. 559.

Chang, T. W., and Goldberg, A. L.: The origin of alanine produced in skeletal muscle. J Biol Chem 253:3677, 1978.

Felig, P.: Amino acid metabolism in man. Annu Rev Biochem 44:933, 1975.

Felig, P.: The glucose-alanine cycle. Metabolism 22:179, 1973.

Felig, P.: Starvation. In DeGroot, L. (ed.): Endocrinology. New York, Grune & Stratton, 1979.

Felig, P., Wahren, J., and Ahlborg, G.: Evidence for the uptake of amino acids by the human brain. Proc Soc Exp Biol Med 142:230, 1973.

Felig, P., Wahren, J., Sherwin, R. S., and Palaiologos, G.: Protein and amino acid metabolism in diabetes mellitus. Arch Intern Med 137:507, 1977.

Haymond, M. W., Ben-Galim, E., and Strobel, K. E.: Glucose and alanine metabolism in children with maple syrup urine disease. J Clin Invest 62:398, 1978.

Haymond, M. W., and Miles, J. M.: Branched chain amino acids as a major source of alanine nitrogen in man. Diabetes 31:86, 1982.

Mallette, L. E., Exton, J. H., and Park, C. R.: Effects of glucagon on amino acid transport and utilization in the perfused rat liver. J Biol Chem 244:5724, 1969.

Matsutaka, H., Aikawa, T., Yamamato, H., and Ishikawa, H.: Gluconeogenesis and amino acid metabolism. 3. Uptake of glutamine and output of alanine and ammonia by non-hepatic splanchnic organs of fasted rats and their metabolic significance. J Biochem (Tokyo) 74:1019, 1973.

Odessey, R., and Goldberg, A. L.: Oxidation of leucine by rat skeletal muscle. Am J Physiol 223:1376, 1972.

Pozefsky, T., Felig, P., Tobin, J., Soeldner, J. S., and Cahill, G. F., Jr.: Amino acid balance across the tissues of the forearm in postabsorptive man: Effects of insulin at two dose levels. J Clin Invest 48:2273, 1969.

Rosenberg, L. E., and Scriver, C. R.: Disorders of amino acid metabolism. In Bondy, P. K., and Rosenberg, L. E. (eds.): Disease of Metabolism. Philadelphia, W. B. Saunders Co., 1974, p. 465.

Snell, K.: Muscle alanine synthesis and hepatic gluconeogenesis. Biochem Soc Trans 8:205, 1980.

Tischler, M. E., DeSautel, M., and Goldberg, A. L.: Does leucine, leucyl-tRNA, or some metabolite of leucine regulate protein synthesis and degradation in skeletal and cardiac muscle? J Biol Chem 257:1613, 1982.

Wahren, J., Felig, P., and Hagenfeldt, J.: Effect of protein ingestion on splanchnic and leg metabolism in normal man and diabetes mellitus. J Clin Invest 57:987, 1976.

Hormonal Regulation _____

INSULIN

As discussed earlier, the rate of various metabolic reactions, as well as the availability of substrate for these reactions, is largely determined by the hormonal milieu. The major hormones influencing the moment-to-moment regulation of body fuel metabolism are insulin, glucagon, catecholamines, glucocorticoids, and growth hormone. The integrated action and coordinated secretion of these hormones facilitates either fuel storage or dissipation. For example, in the fed state, insulin augments the storage of triglyceride and glycogen by virtue of a multiplicity of effects: increased fatty acid synthesis, augmented formation of glycerol-3-phosphate, inhibition of lipolysis, augmented glycogen synthesis, and decreased glycogenolysis. In contrast, during exercise the coordinated secretion of epinephrine, glucagon, growth hormone, and cortisol combined with inhibition of insulin secretion allows for the mobilization of fat, breakdown of liver glycogen, and enhancement of gluconeogenesis necessary to meet the fuel requirements of contracting muscle.

In this section the biosynthesis, secretion, and action of insulin will be considered. A discussion of the other glucoregulatory hormones will follow.

BIOSYNTHESIS

The insulin molecule consists of two polypeptide chains, designated the A and B chains, connected by two disulfide bridges. There is, in addition, a disulfide bridge between the sixth and eleventh amino acid residues of the A chain (Fig. 28). The complete unit contains 51 amino acids and has a molecular weight of 5800.

Insulin is synthesized by the beta cells of the islets of Langerhans as a single-chain precursor, proinsulin, which has a molecular weight of about 9000. Recent studies using cell-free systems indicate that the immediate translation product of proinsulin messenger RNA is a larger peptide containing 23 additional amino acids residues at the NH_2-terminus designated as pre-proinsulin. Proinsulin consists of a spiral molecule in which the A and B chains are joined by a connecting

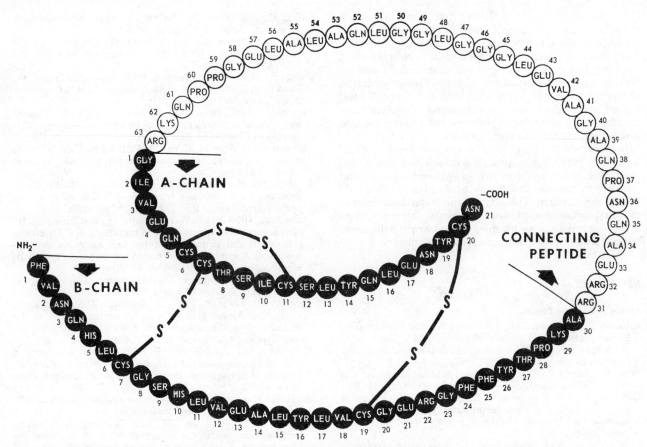

Figure 28. The chemical structure of proinsulin. (From Shaw, W. N., and Chance, R. E.: Diabetes 17:737, 1968.)

peptide (C-peptide) (Fig. 28). In contrast to the minor differences in the amino acid sequences of A and B chains in various species, considerably greater variability is observed in the structure of the corresponding C-peptides. Thus human and porcine insulins differ by a single amino acid, whereas human C-peptide, a 23 amino acid chain with a molecular weight of 3021, differs from porcine C-peptide by 10 residues and contains two fewer amino acids. This high mutation rate is in keeping with the lack of a specific hormonal function attributable to C-peptide. Proinsulin has only 3 to 5 per cent of the biological effectiveness of native insulin, its biological activity being more pronounced on the liver than on peripheral tissues.

The intracellular site of preproinsulin synthesis and its rapid cleavage to proinsulin is the rough endoplasmic reticulum (Fig. 29). Proinsulin is then transferred by an energy-dependent process to the Golgi apparatus (transfer step 1, Fig. 29). At the Golgi, packaging into smooth-surfaced microvesicles takes place so as to form storage or secretory granules (transfer step 2, Fig. 29). Beginning within the Golgi complex and continuing in the secretory granules, membrane-bound proteases cleave proinsulin into equimolar amounts of insulin and C-peptide.

Release of the contents of the mature secretory granules involves progressive migration of the granules to the plasma membrane of the cell followed by extrusion of insulin and C-peptide. Within the cytosol, microtubules, composed of dimeric 120,000 molecular weight subunits known as tubulin, act to guide granule movement to the plasma membrane. A series of microfilaments, which are thought to be composed of the contractile protein actin, form a network near the plasma membrane and surround the secretory granules. The "final common path" of beta cell secretion is believed to involve the intracellular entry of calcium, resulting in contraction of the microfilaments. As a result, the secretory granules are moved to the cell surface, where their membranes fuse with the plasma membrane and their contents are discharged into the extracellular space (transfer step 3, Fig. 29). This process of membrane fusion has been termed emiocytosis or exocytosis. Interestingly, the granule membranes added to the cell membrane during emiocytosis are recycled by a process of endocytosis in which membrane-bound vacuoles are transferred back to the cytoplasm.

CIRCULATING INSULIN

The pioneering studies of Berson and Yalow led to the development of radioimmunoassay techniques with which insulin and a variety of polypeptides are measured in blood. The concentration of insulin in peripheral venous or arterial plasma or serum in healthy subjects after an overnight fast is generally 10 to 20 μU per ml (0.5 to 0.8 ng/ml). As noted above, equimolar amounts of C-peptide are released with insulin during

BETA GRANULE FORMATION

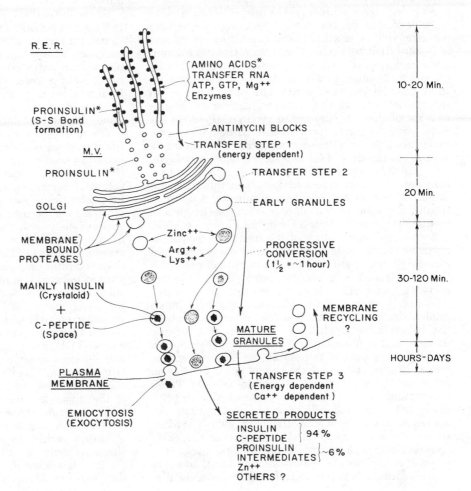

Figure 29. Insulin biosynthesis in the beta cells of the islets of Langerhans. (From Steiner, D. F., et al.: Fed Proc 33:2105, 1975.)

the secretory process and are present in concentrations of 0.9 to 3.5 ng/ml in the fasting state. The relatively greater amount of C-peptide as compared with insulin reflects the slower metabolic clearance and the negligible hepatic extraction of this substance. Since the drainage of the pancreatic islets is into the portal vein and since the liver removes 50 to 60 per cent of the insulin presented to it, the portal concentration of insulin is threefold higher than that in peripheral blood in the basal state. Following acute bursts of secretion (for example, in response to glucose or amino acids) the portal:peripheral gradient for insulin may increase to 10:1. This portal:peripheral gradient for insulin may account for the fact that small increments in insulin secretion alter hepatic glucose metabolism in the absence of changes in peripheral glucose utilization.

Although proinsulin may be found in peripheral plasma, it generally accounts for less than 15 per cent of total circulating insulin immunoreactivity. Familial hyperproinsulinemia is a recently described asymptomatic genetic defect with autosomal dominant inheritance in which 65 to 90 per cent of total plasma insulin immunoreactivity is accounted for by proinsulin. This defect may be caused by an abnormality in cleavage of proinsulin to insulin or a defect in proinsulin biosynthesis.

SECRETION

Carbohydrate. Among the factors capable of stimulating insulin secretion, the role of glucose is preeminent. Although the precise mechanism whereby glucose acts on the beta cells to cause insulin release has not been entirely clarified, metabolism of glucose within the islet cells probably initiates the response. The following observations favor the metabolic theory: (1) metabolizable sugars (hexoses or trioses) are more potent stimuli of insulin secretion than nonmetabolizable carbohydrates (for example, mannose); (2) glucose increases the concentration of glycolytic intermediates within islet cells; (3) compounds that inhibit glucose metabolism (mannoheptulose and 2-deoxyglucose) interfere with insulin secretion.

As in the case of a large number of intracellular processes, cyclic AMP participates in the insulin secretory process. Although early studies failed to demonstrate an increase in beta cell levels of cyclic AMP after glucose stimulation, more recent studies have clearly documented such increments. The increase in cyclic AMP is believed to act primarily as a positive modulator of a glucose-sensitive secretory step. However, an increase in cyclic AMP is not sufficient to stimulate insulin secretion, as indicated by the fact that theophylline (an inhibitor of phosphodiesterase) elevates cyclic AMP but has little stimulatory action on insulin secretion unless glucose is present.

As noted above, an increase in intracellular calcium is believed to be the final triggering mechanism whereby glucose or other stimuli result in the release of insulin from beta cells. These alterations in calcium are a consequence of an inhibition of calcium efflux by glucose and enhanced mobilization of stored intracellular calcium by cyclic AMP. The importance of an increase in intracellular calcium independent of glucose metabolism or changes in cyclic AMP levels derives strong support from studies using ionophores, molecules that act as membrane carriers for ion transport. In the presence of the heterocyclic monocarboxylic acid A23187, a specific divalent cation ionophore that transports calcium across biological membranes, addition of calcium to beta cells results in a burst of insulin secretion in the absence of a rise in glucose availability or an increase in intracellular cyclic AMP.

A characteristic feature of the insulin response induced by glucose is its biphasic nature. An initial rapid secretory burst begins within one minute of presentation of a glycemic stimulus, reaches a peak within two minutes, and declines over the ensuing three to five minutes. A second phase, characterized by a more gradual increase in insulin levels, commences about five to ten minutes after the initiation of a glucose infusion and continues over the next hour (Fig. 30). In the perfused pancreas, puromycin, an inhibitor of protein synthesis, attenuates the second phase but has no effect on the early phase of insulin release. These observations have led to the proposal that insulin exists with the beta cell as a two-pool system. An acutely releasable pool consisting of previously synthesized insulin is rapidly discharged during the early secretory phase. A second chronic-release pool, composed of newly synthesized insulin and small amounts of proinsulin, in addition to stored, preformed insulin, is gradually discharged during the second phase (Fig. 30).

Gastrointestinal Hormones. Glucose, in addition to its direct action on the beta cell, is a major stimulus to insulin secretion as a result of its interaction with receptors within the gastrointestinal tract. Thus, the plasma concentration of insulin is higher after administration of a given dose of glucose into the jejunum than when it is given intravenously, even though the arterial blood glucose remains lower after the intrajejunal glucose instillation.

The mechanism by which glucose administered into the intestinal tract stimulates insulin release is connected in some way with hormones released by cells of the stomach or upper small intestine. Among the potential hormones, current evidence supports a role for gastric inhibitory polypeptide (GIP). After an oral glucose load, serum GIP levels increase before or simultaneously with the rise in serum insulin. Intravenous infusion of purified GIP in amounts resulting in plasma concentrations (1 ng/ml) comparable to those observed after oral glucose causes an enhancement of glucose-induced insulin secretion. Furthermore, an insulinotropic effect of endogenous GIP is suggested by the observation that ingestion of corn oil, a potent stimulus of GIP secretion, increases the insulin response to intravenous glucose. The demonstration of elevated GIP levels in diabetics suggests that insulin may in turn exert a negative feedback influence on GIP secretion. The possibility remains, however, that other hormones (e.g., secretin, gastrin, pancreozymin) of the upper gastrointestinal tract may be insulinotropic and contribute to in vivo augmentation of glucose-induced insulin release.

Amino Acids. Ingestion of protein or infusion of single or multiple amino acids stimulates insulin secretion. When amino acids are infused individually they vary considerably in their ability to stimulate the

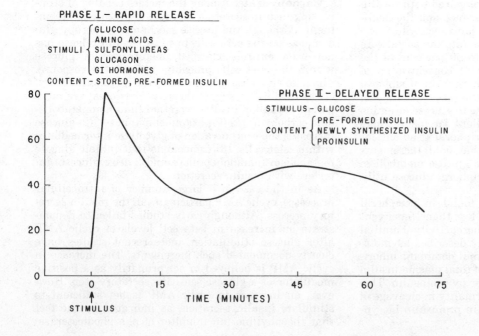

BIPHASIC INSULIN RESPONSE TO GLUCOSE

Figure 30. The biphasic secretory response of insulin to glucose stimulation. (From Felig, P.: Med Clin North Am 55:821, 1971.)

beta cells. As in the case of glucose, stimulation of insulin secretion by intraduodenal amino acids exceeds that of intravenous amino acids, suggesting enhancement by gastrointestinal hormones. Protein-stimulated secretion of cholecystokinin-pancreozymin and/or gastrin may mediate this effect. With respect to the mechanism whereby amino acids stimulate insulin secretion, more than one process may be operative, since pharmacological agents (for example, diazoxide) may inhibit insulin release after leucine but not after arginine. Nonmetabolizable analogues of leucine and arginine have been shown to stimulate insulin secretion, suggesting that membrane recognition (receptor interaction) rather than intracellular metabolism may trigger insulin secretion.

Autonomic Nervous System. The autonomic nervous system also participates in the control of insulin secretion. In experimental animals, simultaneous stimulation of both vagus nerves causes a release of insulin, which can be blocked by atropine, and vagotomy reduces the concentration of insulin in the pancreatic vein. However, the stimulating effect of glucose on insulin secretion is not altered by vagotomy. In man, a stimulatory effect of methacholine on insulin secretion is blocked by atropine.

In contrast to the effects of vagal stimulation, the sympathomimetic amines epinephrine and norepinephrine inhibit insulin release. The action of these catechols is mediated via alpha receptors in the islet cells. That beta adrenergic receptors are present as well is indicated by the stimulatory effect of isoproterenol, which in turn is inhibited by the beta-adrenergic blocking agent propranolol. Despite this dual receptor system in the beta cells, the alpha-adrenergic action of epinephrine predominates so that the net effect of this agent is inhibition of glucose-stimulated insulin secretion. As noted previously, the adrenergic receptors in the islet cells appear to influence insulin secretion via alterations in intracellular cyclic AMP.

It is likely that the diminution in insulin secretion noted with hypothermia and with exercise is a consequence of augmented epinephrine and norepinephrine release. In addition, endogenous overproduction of catecholamines appears to be responsible for the blunted insulin response observed in patients with pheochromocytoma.

Somatostatin. Somatostatin is a tetradecapeptide originally isolated from the hypothalamus as a growth hormone release–inhibitory factor and subsequently identified by immunofluorescent techniques in pancreatic islet cells and in stomach antral and jejunal cells in the gastrointestinal tract. In addition to interfering with release of growth hormone, somatostatin is a potent inhibitor of insulin as well as glucagon secretion. This effect of somatostatin on islet hormones represents a direct action that is demonstrable with in vitro techniques. Within the islets of Langerhans, somatostatin is localized to the D cells (A_1 cells) located at the periphery of the islets.

Although the precise role of endogenous somatostatin in the regulation of insulin secretion has not been established, recent evidence that pancreatic somatostatin release is affected by nutrients and other islet hormones supports the view that it serves as a physiological regulator. It is generally believed that somatostatin acts as a local rather than systemic hormone (paracrine). Indeed, there may be intercellular communications between B and D cells within islets.

ACTION OF INSULIN

Although the most dramatic effect of insulin is its ability to reduce the concentration of glucose in plasma, it is well established that insulin influences fat and protein metabolism in addition to its effects on carbohydrates. Besides lowering the blood sugar, it promotes the synthesis of glycogen in liver and muscle, and of fat in liver and adipose tissue. It also stimulates RNA, DNA, and protein synthesis and is essential for growth and maturation. Associated with these functions is a decrease in the circulating levels of free fatty acids and free amino acids. Despite the diversity of these effects, the actions of insulin on the major metabolic fuels are synergistic, so that the net result is conservation of body fuel supplies. Insulin thus functions as the primary storage hormone, serving as the body's signal for the fed or fasted state, depending on whether the concentration of this hormone is elevated or reduced. These effects of insulin are focused on three target tissues—liver, fat, and muscle (Fig. 31).

Effects on Carbohydrate Metabolism. Although a direct action of insulin on the liver was long the subject of debate, it is currently recognized that the liver occupies a central role in the action of insulin on carbohydrate homeostasis. The uniqueness of the liver derives from four properties: (1) in the basal state, glucose is continuously released at a rate of 2 to 3 mg/kg body weight/min; (2) the membrane of the liver cell

	LIVER	ADIPOSE TISSUE	MUSCLE
ANTICATABOLIC EFFECTS	Decreased glycogenolysis Decreased gluconeogenesis Decreased ketogenesis	Decreased lipolysis	Decreased protein catabolism Decreased amino acid output
ANABOLIC EFFECTS	Increased glycogen synthesis Increased fatty acid synthesis	Increased glycerol synthesis Increased fatty acid synthesis	Increased amino acid uptake Increased protein synthesis Increased glycogen synthesis

Figure 31. Target sites and metabolic actions of insulin. (From Sherwin, R., and Felig, P.: Med Clin North Am 62:695, 1978.)

is freely permeable to glucose; (3) the level of insulin in portal blood is three- to tenfold greater than in peripheral blood; (4) absorbed hexoses reach the liver via the portal vein prior to their delivery to peripheral tissues.

As a consequence of these characteristics, the actions of insulin on the liver differ from those on other target tissues: (a) insulin acts on the liver not only to promote glucose uptake but also to suppress intracellular processes involved in glucose production and release; (b) this action is mediated by altering enzyme activity rather than by directly influencing transport processes; (c) small increases in glucose concentration and insulin secretion result in an effect on the liver in the absence of stimulation of peripheral glucose utilization; (d) the liver is a major site of disposal of ingested glucose in humans.

In view of the permeability of the hepatocyte to glucose, uptake of glucose in the liver is not rate-limiting. The first potential control point occurs when metabolism is initiated by phosphorylation to glucose-6-phosphate. As mentioned previously, phosphorylation in the liver takes place under the influence of two enzymes, hexokinase and glucokinase. Hexokinase is essentially saturated at normal physiological glucose concentrations. On the other hand, glucokinase activity is only half-saturated when the blood glucose level reaches 180 mg/dl. Consequently, hepatic glucose uptake may be adjusted to changing blood glucose concentrations by alterations in glucokinase activity. The activity of this enzyme depends on the presence of insulin and a relatively high carbohydrate diet. Thus in the absence of insulin, or in subjects who are fasting or receiving a carbohydrate-free diet, glucokinase activity drops to low levels within less than 48 hours. The loss of this enzyme greatly reduces the ability of the liver to adjust its carbohydrate intake to variations of the plasma glucose concentration and thereby limits its ability to maintain the blood glucose within the normal range. Although observations on the effect of insulin and diet on glucokinase have mainly been made in animals, the livers of human beings with type 2 diabetes also have depressed glucokinase activity.

A second crucial step in the glycolytic pathway involves the phosphorylation of fructose-6-phosphate by phosphofructokinase (see Fig. 7). In the absence of insulin, the activity of this enzyme is diminished. This has significance not only with regard to glycolysis but also with respect to gluconeogenesis. A decrease in phosphofructokinase activity favors reversal of the glycolytic scheme, with formation of fructose-1-phosphate, and ultimate conversion to glucose.

The glycogen content of the livers of patients with diabetic acidosis is significantly reduced and is promptly restored following insulin administration. This effect of insulin is due to its ability to activate glycogen synthetase within a few minutes after it is administered. Glycogen accumulation is further facilitated by insulin's inhibition of phosphorylase, the enzyme catalyzing the rate-limiting step in glycogen breakdown.

Insulin diminishes the output of glucose from the liver not only by its action on glycogen synthesis and breakdown but also by virtue of its inhibitory effects on *gluconeogenesis*. Following the injection of insulin antiserum, glucose production from lactate is increased in the perfused liver. In contrast, insulin lowers hepatic glucose output while diminishing urea production, indicating a diminution in the conversion of amino acids to glucose. The key intermediary step in the gluconeogenic pathway lies between pyruvate and phosphoenolpyruvate, which depends on the enzymes pyruvate carboxylase and phosphoenolpyruvate carboxykinase (see Fig. 8). The latter is inhibited in the presence of glucose and insulin. Pyruvate carboxylase activity is also diminished by insulin, perhaps as a consequence of decreased release and breakdown of fatty acids (see below), resulting in lessened availability of acetyl CoA, a necessary cofactor for pyruvate carboxylase.

In addition to influencing gluconeogenesis by altering fatty acid availability, it has long been suspected that insulin diminishes gluconeogenesis by decreasing the supply of precursor amino acids. More recent studies, however, fail to show inhibition of alanine release, the key glycogenic amino acid, from peripheral muscle tissues. In contrast, glucose-stimulated insulin secretion results in a fall of hepatic alanine uptake despite unchanged arterial levels of this amino acid. The bulk of the evidence thus favors the notion that insulin regulates gluconeogenesis, primarily by altering intrahepatic processes rather than by influencing the rate of precursor supply.

The overall sensitivity of hepatic glucoregulatory mechanisms to insulin is indicated by the fact that a twofold increment in arterial levels (induced by infusing glucose at a rate of 150 mg/min) fails to augment peripheral glucose utilization, yet is accompanied by an 80 per cent reduction in hepatic glucose output. It is of interest in this regard that inhibition of gluconeogenesis requires greater amounts of insulin than are necessary for inhibition of glycogenolysis. Thus a 60 to 100 per cent increase in serum insulin results in virtually complete inhibition of glycogenolysis, yet hepatic uptake and conversion of alanine, lactate, and pyruvate to glucose persist in the face of such relatively minor increments of insulin.

A major question in the overall control of hepatic glucose metabolism concerns the relative importance of hyperinsulinemia and hyperglycemia as regulatory signals. Over 40 years ago Soskin and Levine proposed that the blood glucose concentration is the primary stimulus that determines glucose uptake or glucose output by the liver. More recent support of this hypothesis derives from studies demonstrating that (a) glycogen synthetase and phosphorylase are exquisitely sensitive to the ambient glucose concentration; (b) hyperglycemia in the absence of a change in insulin concentration can inhibit hepatic glucose output from the perfused liver; (c) in the absence of hyperglycemia, hyperinsulinemia fails to induce a net uptake of glucose by liver. In contrast, other data emphasize the importance of insulin in regulating hepatic glucose output: (a) in the diabetic, hyperglycemia induced by glucose infusion fails to inhibit hepatic glucose output; (b) in perfused liver insulin activates glycogen synthetase in the absence of added glucose; (c) much smaller increments in blood glucose (10 to 15 mg/dl) required to inhibit hepatic glucose output when insulin concentrations are kept at basal levels.

The overall data thus suggest that hyperinsulinemia as well as hyperglycemia contribute to hepatic glucose balance. A rise in insulin markedly increases the sensitivity of the liver to the inhibitory effects of glucose on hepatic glucose release. In a like manner, a rise in glucose concentration facilitates and is probably essential for insulin-induced hepatic uptake of glucose.

Unlike the situation in the hepatocyte, at physiological concentrations of plasma glucose, the rate of entry of the sugar into the *muscle* cell is the slowest (and therefore the rate-limiting) step. A major effect of insulin in this tissue is to control the transport of glucose across the cell membrane. In addition, insulin increases phosphofructokinase activity, probably as a consequence of its ability to promote the formation of ADP and AMP, which stimulate the enzyme, and to remove ATP, which inhibits it. A major end product of glucose uptake in nonexercising muscle is glycogen formation.

It should be emphasized that glucose uptake by exercising muscle does not depend on increased insulin secretion (see Exercise, p. 370). In resting muscle, glucose is a relatively unimportant fuel (as compared with fatty acids) in the fasting state. Nevertheless, elevations in plasma insulin (as occur with feeding) are an important determinant of glucose uptake by muscle.

In the *fat* cell, the situation is similar to muscle in that insulin acts primarily to stimulate transport of glucose across the cell membrane. An effect is also observed on glycogen synthetase and on phosphofructokinase. The major end products of glucose metabolism in the adipose cell are fatty acids (discussed below) and α-glycerophosphate. The latter is important in fat storage because it esterifies with fatty acids to form triglycerides, the major storage form of fat in the body.

Effect on Fat Metabolism. In the *liver* the synthesis of fatty acids is stimulated by an elevation in plasma insulin. This effect reflects several actions of the insulin. First, the increased flow of substrate down the glycolytic pathway into the tricarboxylic acid cycle increases the availability of citrate and isocitrate, which stimulate the liposynthetic pathways, particularly the activity of acetyl CoA carboxylase. Second, the reduction in free fatty acids removes the inhibitory influence that they exert on this enzyme. Third, the availability of reduced NADP, which is a necessary hydrogen donor for many of the steps of synthesis of fatty acids, is increased by insulin as glucose utilization along the pentose pathway is increased. The overall ability of insulin to stimulate fatty acid synthesis by liver is underscored by the fact that, in humans, lipogenesis occurs primarily in liver rather than in adipose tissue. The fatty acids synthesized in liver are then transported (as very low density lipoproteins) to adipose tissue, where they are stored as triglyceride.

An additional major effect of insulin on hepatic fat metabolism concerns its antiketogenic action. As discussed previously, ketosis occurs as a consequence of increased fatty acid mobilization from adipose tissue (lipolysis) as well as augmented beta oxidation of fatty acids in the liver. The rate-limiting step in fatty acid oxidation is the transfer of the fatty acyl derivatives across the mitochondrial membrane, a process catalyzed by the enzyme acyl carnitine transferase. Insulin inhibits this regulatory step by decreasing the availability of carnitine and by increasing the concentration of malonyl CoA, an inhibitor of acyl carnitine trans-

ferase. Since malonyl CoA is the first committed intermediate in the pathway of fat synthesis, the stimulatory action of insulin on fatty acid synthesis serves to augment its antiketogenic activity.

In adipose tissue, insulin acts to increase the storage of triglyceride by at least four mechanisms. First, the uptake of fatty acids from circulating lipoproteins is increased by stimulation of the enzyme lipoprotein lipase. Second, the activity of a hormone-sensitive lipase, which catalyzes the hydrolysis of triglyceride within the fat cell, is markedly inhibited by insulin. Third, augmented glycolysis increases the availability of glycerol-3-phosphate, which is necessary for esterification of fatty acids derived from circulating triglyceride. Since adipose tissue lacks the enzyme glycerol kinase, glycerol-3-phosphate cannot be formed from free glycerol released from triglycerides but must be derived by glycolysis. Finally, insulin stimulates fatty acid biosynthesis from glucose in a manner analogous to that occurring in liver. However, as noted above, relatively little in situ biosynthesis of fatty acids occurs in human adipose tissue. Most of the fatty acids stored as adipose tissue triglyceride have been synthesized in the liver.

Effects on Amino Acid and Protein Metabolism. Insulin increases the net uptake of most amino acids into muscle. This effect reflects combined actions in which transport into muscle and protein synthesis are stimulated while protein catabolism is inhibited. In intact man, intrabrachial arterial infusion of insulin in physiological amounts results in diminished output of amino acids from deep forearm tissues. This effect is particularly prominent with respect to the branched chain amino acids leucine and isoleucine, as well as tyrosine and phenylalanine. In the absence of adequate insulin—for example, in the diabetic in ketoacidosis—an elevation is observed in plasma levels of valine, leucine, and isoleucine. In addition, the uptake of these amino acids by muscle tissue after the ingestion of a protein meal is reduced in the absence of adequate amounts of insulin.

It has already been noted that insulin promotes the synthesis of certain specific proteins (for example, hepatic glucokinase). The effect of insulin on protein synthesis, however, is much more general than these limited examples might suggest. Diaphragms or heart muscle from animals deprived of insulin incorporate radioactive amino acids into protein to a much smaller extent than tissues from normal subjects. When insulin is added to the medium, protein synthesis is increased even when glucose is absent from the medium. If glycolysis is completely blocked, however, stimulation by insulin is abolished. It is not a result of increased amino acid transport, because the same effect can be seen with ribosomes isolated from diabetic myocardium under circumstances in which the availability of amino acids is not a limiting factor.

Adding insulin to ribosomes isolated from insulin-deficient animals does not restore activity, but administering insulin in vivo one hour before isolating the ribosomes completely restores their potency. The defect in protein synthesis is not a result of inadequate supplies of messenger RNA, but appears to be in the structure or function of the ribosome itself, since individual ribosomes from diabetic muscle either function normally or do not function at all. The difference between diabetic and normal muscle is therefore, that fewer ribosomes are functioning in the diabetic and not that all ribosomes function somewhat inadequately. The mediator by which insulin "turns on" ribosomes is probably a specific regulatory protein, synthesized by precharged ribosomes that require the presence of insulin to begin transcribing their message.

In addition to its action on protein synthesis, the overall anabolic action of insulin derives from its ability to inhibit protein catabolism. The oxidation of branched chain amino acids by muscle tissue is also inhibited by insulin and is accelerated in the diabetic state. Insulin thus increases body protein stores via at least four mechanisms: (1) increased tissue uptake of amino acids; (2) increased protein synthesis; (3) decreased protein catabolism; (4) decreased oxidation of amino acids.

Summary. The integrated and synergistic nature of these diverse metabolic effects of insulin at the various target tissues is striking. Inhibition of hepatic gluconeogenic enzymes decreases the liver's requirements for amino acids. Simultaneously, the anabolic action of insulin reduces the output of amino acids from muscle (diminishing their availability for hepatic gluconeogenesis) as amino acid incorporation into muscle protein is facilitated. Glucose uptake by muscle is also stimulated, providing an energy source to replace fatty acids whose release from adipose tissue is inhibited by the antilipolytic action. Fat accumulation is further enhanced by augmented hepatic lipogenesis and by increased formation of α-glycerophosphate in the adipose cell. Finally, the antilipolytic action at the adipose cell reinforces insulin's inhibition of hepatic gluconeogensis as well as insulin's stimulation of muscle glucose uptake by depriving tissues of an energy source (fatty acids) and cofactors (acetyl CoA).

INSULIN RECEPTORS AND THE MECHANISM OF INSULIN ACTION

Despite the diversity of insulin's actions, there is strong evidence that its effects are triggered by the binding of this hormone to a specific receptor on the cell membrane (see Fig. 2). As first shown by Cuatrecasas in the isolated fat cell, linkage of insulin to a synthetic polymer (sepharose) that prohibits its entry into the cell fails to prevent the hormone's action in stimulating glucose utilization and in inhibiting lipolysis. Insulin receptors have been identified not only in the classic target cells (liver, muscle, fat) but also in a variety of other cell types such as circulating monocytes, placenta, fibroblasts, and thymic lymphocytes. They comprise two alpha and beta subunits of 135,000 and 95,000 daltons, respectively. The properties of insulin receptors are as follows: (a) hormone binding is rapid and reversible; (b) hormone binding is specific (for example, receptors for insulin do not bind glucagon, and vice versa); (c) maximal biological action occurs when only a small fraction (10 per cent or less) of insulin receptors are occupied. The target cells thus have many more receptors than are necessary to elicit maximal responses, but all of the receptors are potentially functional ("spare receptor" theory); (d) the number of insulin receptors is regulated by the ambient insulin concentration such that hyperinsulinemia leads to a reduction in the number of insulin binding

sites. The mechanism of this "down-regulation" appears to involve an increase in the degradative rate of receptors.

The biological importance of the insulin receptor as a regulatory site of hormone action has gained support from the demonstration that conditions in which insulin resistance is present are often characterized by a decrease in the number of insulin receptors. Insulin resistance is generally recognized on the basis of diminished responsiveness to endogenous insulin (hyperinsulinemia in association with a normal or elevated glucose level) or exogenous insulin (diabetics requiring massive doses of insulin). The insulin-resistant state that has been most extensively studied is obesity. In obesity in humans as well as experimental animals a decrease in insulin binding has been observed in a variety of cells including monocytes, adipocytes, hepatocytes, and muscle cells. Altered receptor function has also been reported in hyperinsulinemic, nonobese type 2 diabetics, in lipoatrophic diabetics, and in patients with the syndrome of acanthosis nigricans and extreme insulin resistance. In the latter syndrome there is either a decrease in the number of receptors or the presence of a circulating antireceptor antibody that decreases receptor affinity.

It should be noted that a decrease in insulin binding may not be the sole or major mechanism of insulin resistance for a given target cell. For example, in obesity, a defect in intracellular glucose oxidation is demonstrable at maximal concentrations of insulin and cannot be accounted for by a diminution in insulin binding. Furthermore, during starvation, insulin binding to monocytes and adipocytes increases, yet intracellular utilization of glucose declines. These findings indicate that several mechanisms of insulin resistance may coexist in the same condition (for example, obesity) in which receptor as well as postreceptor intracellular abnormalities may be operative.

The major unsettled question with regard to the mechanism of insulin action concerns the identifying of events triggered in response to insulin-receptor association (see Fig. 2). The nature of this "second messenger" remains unclear, although a variety of theories have been propounded involving changes in cyclic nucleotides, cellular calcium flux, and tyrosine kinase activity. Recently, a mediator has been isolated from muscle that is generated by insulin and has insulin-like effects on glycogen synthase and pyruvate dehydrogenase. The chemical structure and actions of the mediator have not yet been identified. Furthermore, it remains unclear whether such a mediator can provide the molecular basis of the diverse intracellular biological actions attributable to insulin.

REFERENCES
Insulin

Abumrad, N. N., Jefferson, L. S., Rannels, J. R., Williams, P. E., Cherrington, A. D., and Lacy, W. W.: Role of insulin in the regulation of leucine kinetics in the conscious dog. J Clin Invest 70:1031, 1982.

Brown, J. C., and Otte, S. C.: Gastrointestinal hormones and the control of insulin secretion. Diabetes 27:782, 1978.

Chan, S. J., Keim, P., and Steiner, D. F.: Cell-free synthesis of rat preproinsulins: Characterization and partial amino acid sequence determination. Proc Natl Acad Sci USA 73:1964, 1976.

Chiasson, J. L., Liljenquist, J. E., Finger, F. E., and Lacy, W.

W.: Differential sensitivity of glycogenolysis and gluconeogenesis to insulin infusions in dogs. Diabetes 25:283, 1976.

Cuatrecasas, P.: Interaction of insulin with the cell membrane: The primary action of insulin. Proc Natl Acad Sci (Wash.) 63:450, 1969.

Czech, M. P., Richardson, D. K., and Smith, C. J.: The biochemical basis of fat cell insulin resistance in obese rodents and man. Metabolism 26:1057, 1977.

DeFronzo, R. A., Ferrannini, E., Hendler, R., Wahren, J., and Felig, P.: Influence of hyperinsulinemia, hyperglycemia, and the route of glucose administration on splanchnic glucose exchange. Proc Natl Acad Sci 75:5173, 1978.

Felig, P., and Wahren, J.: Influence of endogenous insulin on splanchnic glucose and amino acid metabolism. J Clin Invest 50:1702, 1971.

Felig, P., Wahren, J., Sherwin, R. S., and Palaiologos, G.: Protein and amino acid metabolism in diabetes mellitus. Arch Intern Med 137:507, 1977.

Fulks, R. M., Li, J. B., and Goldberg, A. L.: Effects of insulin, glucose and amino acids on protein turnover in rat diaphragm. J Biol Chem 250:290, 1975.

Gerich, J. E., Charles, M. A., and Grodsky, G. M.: Regulation of pancreatic insulin and glucagon secretion. Annu Rev Physiol 38:353, 1976.

Howell, S. L.: The mechanism of insulin secretion. Diabetologia 26:319, 1984.

Idahl, L. A., Rahemtulla, F., Shelin, J., and Taljedal, I. B.: Further studies on the metabolism of D-glucose anomers in pancreatic islets. Diabetes 25:450, 1976.

Kono, T.: Actions of insulin on glucose transport and cAMP phosphodiesterase in fat cells: Involvement of two distinct molecular mechanisms. Rec Progr Horm Res 39:519, 1983.

Larner, J.: Four questions times two: A dialogue on the mechanism of insulin action dedicated to Earl W. Sutherland. Metabolism 24:249, 1975.

Malaisse, W. J., Hutton, J. C., Kawazu, S., Herchvelz, A., Valverde, M., and Sener, A.: The stimulus-secretion coupling of glucose-induced insulin release. XXV. The links between metabolic and cationic events. Diabetelogia 16:331, 1979.

McGarry, J. D.: New perspectives in the regulation of ketogenesis. Diabetes 28:517, 1979.

Olefsky, J. M.: The insulin receptor: Its role in insulin resistance of obesity and diabetes. Diabetes 25:1154, 1976.

Orci, L.: The microanatomy of the isles of Langerhans. Metabolism 25:1303, 1976.

Permutt, M. A., Chirgwin, J., Rotwein, P., and Giddings, S.: Insulin gene structure and function: A review of studies using recombinant DNA methodology. Diabetes Care 7:386, 1984.

Pointer, R. H., Butcher, F. R., and Fain, J. N.: Studies on the role of cyclic guanosine 3'5'-monophosphate and extracellular Ca^{2+} in the regulation of glycogenolysis in rat liver cells. J Biol Chem 251:2987, 1976.

Polonsky, K. S., and Rubenstein, A. H.: C-peptide as a measure of the secretion and hepatic extraction of insulin: Pitfalls and limitations. Diabetes 33:486, 1984.

Raptis, S., Dollinger, H. C., Schroder, K. E., Schleyer, M., Rothenbuchner, G., and Pfeiffer, E. F.: Differences in insulin, growth hormone and pancreatic enzyme secretion after intravenous and introduodenal administration of mixed amino acids in man. N Engl J Med 288:1199, 1973.

Rubenstein, A. H., Kuzuya, H., and Horwitz, D. L.: Clinical significance of circulating C-peptide in diabetes mellitus and hypoglycemic disorders. Arch Intern Med 137:625, 1977.

Soskin, S., and Levine, R.: Carbohydrate Metabolism: Correlation of Physiological, Biochemical and Clincial Aspects. 2nd ed. Chicago, University of Chicago Press, 1952.

Wahren, J., Felig, P., Cerasi, E., and Luft, R.: Splanchnic and peripheral glucose and amino acid metabolism in diabetes mellitus. J Clin Invest 51:1870, 1972.

Wool, I. G., and Kurihara, K: Determination of the number of active muscle ribosomes: Effect of diabetes and insulin. Proc Natl Acad Sci (Wash.) 58:2401, 1967.

GLUCAGON

BIOSYNTHESIS

Glucagon is a polypeptide consisting of 28 residues, with a molecular weight of 3485 (Fig. 32). It has nothing in common with insulin, either in structure or in amino acid sequence. The terminal histidine group at the amino end of the molecule is necessary for biological activity. In contrast, the major binding site (with liver membranes) is at the carboxyl end of the molecule.

The alpha cells of the islets of Langerhans are the site of glucagon biosynthesis. Immunofluorescent studies indicate that these cells are situated in the outer rim of the islet. Within the islet cells, synthesis of glucagon involves the initial formation of a larger precursor (proglucagon) that has been estimated to have a molecular weight of 9000 and is devoid of glycogenolytic behavior. Following cleavage of this molecule to glucagon, the contents of the secretory granules within the alpha cell are discharged by the process of exocytosis (emiocytosis), which is analogous to that described for insulin.

CIRCULATING GLUCAGON

Studies of the physiology of glucagon have been clarified by the development in the laboratories of Unger and Hedding of antibodies for glucagon that demonstrate minimal cross-reactivity with gut peptides. With these antibodies, the concentration of plasma glucagon in the basal postabsorptive state is in the range of 75 to 150 pg/ml. The combined application of gel filtration and radioimmunoassay techniques reveals that the immunoreactive "glucagon" consists of four fractions: (1) true pancreatic glucagon (molecular weight 3485), which accounts for 40 to 50 per cent of total immunoreactivity; (2) big plasma glucagon (BPG), a substance with a molecular weight of 160,000 that is probably devoid of biological activity; (3) a 9000 molecular weight substance that is probably proglucagon; and (4) a 2000 molecular weight substance that may represent a glucagon fragment. Despite the heterogeneity of circulating glucagon in the basal state, it is primarily the biologically active true glucagon (molecular weight 3485) that varies in response to physiological stimulation or suppression of alpha cell secretion.

CONTROL OF SECRETION

The rate of pancreatic glucagon secretion in man is extremely small when compared with the doses of glucagon previously employed to study the metabolic effects of this hormone. Basal secretory rates of glucagon in normal man are not greater than 100 to 150 µg/day. These values are probably an overestimate when one takes into account that portion of glucagon immunoreactivity that is not biologically active.

Glucagon secretion demonstrates little fluctuation in normal subjects receiving mixed meals. The plasma glucagon level is thus fairly constant throughout the

His-Ser-Gln-Gly-Thr-Phe-Thr-Ser-Asp-Tyr-Ser-Lys-Tyr-Leu-Asp-Ser-Arg-Arg-Ala-Gln-Asp-Phe ⌐
                              Thr-Asn-Met-Leu-Tyr-Gln-Val ⌐

Figure 32. The chemical structure of glucagon. (From Felig, P.: Disorders of carbohydrate metabolism. In Bondy, P. K., and Rosenberg, L. R. (eds.): Metabolic Control and Disease. 8th ed. Philadelphia, W. B. Saunders Co., 1980.)

day (Fig. 33). This contrasts with insulin secretion, which shows an increase with ingestion of mixed meals. Increases in glucagon secretion in normal man generally result from the ingestion of large, purely protein meals or the infusion of amino acids. In contrast, glucagon secretion is reduced following the consumption of large amounts of carbohydrate.

While basal glucagon levels are rarely if ever suppressed in circumstances other than pure glucose ingestion, a number of physiological conditions are capable of increasing plasma glucagon concentration. Alpha cell hypersecretion is associated with acute hypoglycemia, prolonged heavy exercise, hypercorticism, and by stimulation of the ventromedial hypothalamus and the adrenergic nervous system. Neither spontaneous episodic release nor diurnal fluctuations in glucagon secretion have been reported in normal subjects. In starvation, a circumstance characterized by hyperglucagonemia, altered catabolism rather than hypersecretion is responsible for the elevated plasma levels. As noted above, somatostatin, a potent inhibitor of insulin as well as glucagon secretion, has been identified in the D cells of the islets. This peptide probably functions as a physiological modulator of pancreatic glucagon release.

ACTION OF GLUCAGON

Although a variety of biological effects have been attributed to glucagon, the *physiological* role of this hormone has been difficult to assess. The classic experimental approach of producing a hormone deficiency state by surgical extirpation has been precluded by the proximity of alpha and beta cells in mammalian pancreatic islets. A chemical agent with an alpha-cytotoxic effect comparable to that of alloxan on the beta cell has also been lacking. In addition, the problems in measuring endogenous glucagon have led to difficulties in estimating the secretory rate of the hormone. As a consequence, pharmacological doses of glucagon have often been employed in experiments designed to establish physiological effects.

A role for glucagon in maintaining hepatic glucose output in the basal state is suggested by the demonstration that hepatic glucose output falls in somatostatin-treated subjects in whom basal insulin levels are maintained by infusion of exogenous insulin. Studies involving the administration of physiological doses of glucagon (3 ng/kg/min) to human volunteers have demonstrated a 50 to 100 per cent rise in hepatic glucose output (Fig. 34). Furthermore, such doses of glucagon are capable of reversing insulin-mediated suppression of hepatic glucose output. It is noteworthy, however, that the stimulatory effects of glucagon on hepatic glycogenolysis are evanescent, lasting less than 30 minutes (Fig. 34). The basis of this transient responsiveness has not been established. It is not simply due to a compensatory increase in insulin secretion.

In addition to its action on glycogenolysis, a gluconeogenic effect of glucagon has been demonstrated with the perfused liver. An increase in fractional extraction of alanine has been demonstrated in the glucagon-infused state. In addition, using isotopic techniques alanine conversion to glucose was stimulated by glucagon even in the absence of changes in total net splanchnic uptake of alanine. Interestingly, glucagon's effect on gluconeogenesis persists even when total glucose production is no longer stimulated.

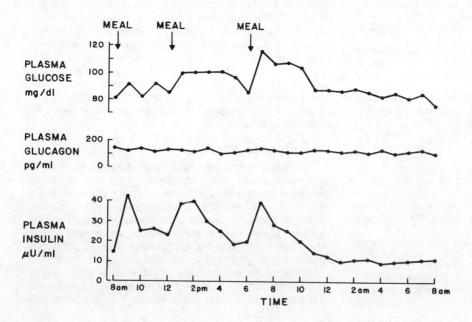

Figure 33. Plasma glucose, immunoreactive glucagon (IRG), and immunoreactive insulin (IRI) in normal subjects over a 24-hour period. (Modified from Tasaka, Y., et al.: Horm Metab Res 7:205, 1975.)

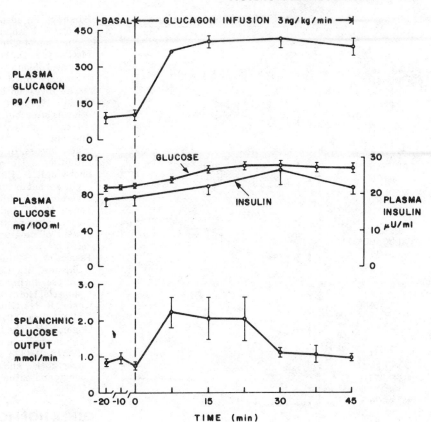

Figure 34. The evanescent effect of glucagon in stimulating hepatic (splanchnic) glucose release. (From Felig, P., et al.: Diabetes 25:1091, 1976.)

Glucagon is believed to enhance glycogenolysis and gluconeogenesis by interacting with a hormone-sensitive adenyl cyclase present in the plasma membrane of hepatic cells. The increase in intracellular cyclic AMP thus produced results ultimately in an elevation in phosphorylase activity (as described in Fig. 3), and in more rapid conversion of pyruvate to glucose. Although epinephrine has glycogenolytic and gluconeogenic effects that are also presumed to be mediated via cyclic AMP, discrete glucagon-responsive and epinephrine-responsive adenyl cyclase enzymes have been identified in mammalian liver. It should be emphasized that the acute hyperglycemic effects of glucagon do not involve alterations in peripheral glucose utilization. In keeping with this finding studies demonstrated that elevations in plasma glucagon to levels of 300 to 400 pg/ml (comparable to those observed in a variety of hyperglucagonemic states) fail to alter glucose tolerance in normal subjects. Glucagon-induced changes in glucose tolerance thus require either an absolute deficiency of insulin or pharmacological doses of this hormone or a glucagon-producing tumor (glucagonoma).

From the foregoing observations on the response to physiological doses of glucagon, the effects of somatostatin-induced glucagonopenia, and the factors regulating the secretion of glucagon, the following concept of this hormone emerges. In the postabsorptive state, ongoing secretion of glucagon is necessary for maintenance of hepatic glucose output in the face of basal levels of insulin. Following protein ingestion a rise in glucagon prevents the fall in hepatic glucose output and hypoglycemia that would otherwise result from

protein-stimulated secretion of insulin (Fig. 35). In response to acute hypoglycemia, prolonged exercise, or starvation, a rise in glucagon contributes to stimulation of hepatic glucose output. In contrast to the importance of increased glucagon secretion in maintaining glucose production, particularly after protein feeding, suppression of glucagon by glucose is not essential for normal glucose tolerance as long as insulin is available.

In addition to its action on carbohydrate metabolism, glucagon has been implicated in the regulation of ketogenesis. Livers obtained from rats given physiological doses of glucagon demonstrate augmented ketone production from precursors. In addition, in human diabetics administration of somatostatin markedly diminishes the ketogenic response to insulin withdrawal. These observations have led to the hypothesis that an increase in glucagon is essential for the alterations in intrahepatic metabolism that characterize ketogenesis (for example, augmented beta oxidation of fatty acids). Other in vivo studies, however, cast doubt on the primacy or essentiality of glucagon in hepatic ketogenesis. In normal subjects in whom free fatty acids are elevated by heparin administration, infusion of glucagon fails to induce hyperketonemia. Furthermore, in insulin-withdrawn, pancreatectomized humans, hyperketonemia develops in the absence of detectable circulating glucagon. These findings thus suggest that while glucagon may enhance the ketogenic capacity of the isolated perfused liver, in intact man physiological increments in glucagon are neither necessary nor sufficient to induce ketosis.

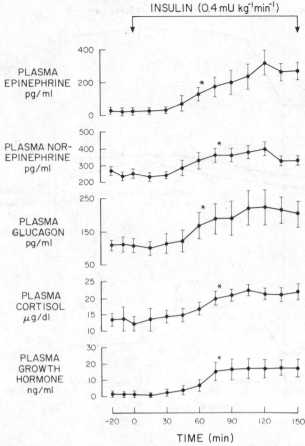

Figure 35. The counterregulatory hormonal response to insulin-induced hypoglycemia in normal man. The asterisks indicate the point at which the hormonal increments were statistically significant. (From Sacca, L., Sherwin, R., Hendler, R., and Felig, P.: J Clin Invest 63:849, 1979.)

REFERENCES

Glucagon

Barnes, A. J., Bloom, S. R., George, K., Alberti, G. M., Smythe, P., Alford, P. P., and Chisholm, D. J.: Ketoacidosis in pancreatectomized man. N Engl J Med 296:1250, 1977.

Cherrington, A. D., Chiasson, J. L., Liljenquist, J. E., Jennings, A. S., Keller, U., and Lacy, W. W.: The role of insulin and glucagon in the regulation of basal glucose production in the postabsorptive dog. J Clin Invest 58:1407, 1976.

Cherrington, A. D., Williams, P. E., Shulman, G. I., and Lacy, W. W.: Differential time course of glucagon's effect on glycogenolysis and gluconeogenesis in the conscious dog. Diabetes 30:1980, 1981.

Chiasson, J. L., Liljenquist, J. E., Sinclair-Smith, B. C., and Lacy W. W.: Gluconeogenesis from alanine in normal postabsorptive man. Intrahepatic stimulatory effect of glucagon. Diabetes 24:574, 1975.

Exton, J. H.: The effects of glucagon on hepatic glycogen metabolism and gluconeogenesis. In Unger, R. H., and Orci, L. (eds.): Glucagon, Physiology, Pathophysiology and Morphology of the Pancreatic A-Cells. New York, Elsevier, 1981, pp. 195–219.

Felig, P., Wahren, J., and Hendler, R.: Influence of physiologic hyperglucagonemia on basal and insulin-inhibited splanchnic glucose output in normal man. J Clin Invest 58:761, 1976.

Fisher, M., Sherwin, R. S., Hendler, R., and Felig, P.: Kinetics of glucagon in man: Effects of starvation. Proc. Natl Acad Sci USA 73:1735, 1976.

Kuku, S. F., Jaspan, J. B., Emmanouel, D. S., Zeidler, A., Katz, A. I., and Rubenstein, A. H.: Heterogeneity of plasma glucagon. J Clin Invest 58:742, 1976.

McGarry, J. D., Wright, P. H., and Foster, D. W.: Hormonal control of ketogenesis: Rapid activation of hepatic ketogenic capacity in fed rats by anti-insulin serum and glucagon. J Clin Invest 55:1202, 1975.

Raskin, P., Pietri, A., and Unger, R. H.: Changes in glucagon levels after four to five weeks of glucoregulation by portable insulin infusion pumps. Diabetes 28:1033, 1979.

Sherwin, R. S., and Felig, P.: Glucagon physiology in health and disease. In McCann, S. M. (ed.): Endocrine Physiology. Baltimore, University Park Press, 16:151, 1977.

Sherwin, R. S., Fisher, M., Hendler, R., and Felig, P.: Hyperglucagonemia and blood glucose regulation in normal, obese and diabetic subjects. N Engl J Med 294:455, 1976.

Tager, H. S., and Steiner, D. F.: Isolation of a glucagon-containing peptide: Primary structure of a possible fragment of proglucagon. Proc Natl Acad Sci USA 70:2321, 1973.

Tasaka, Y., Sekine, M., Wakatsuki, M., Chgawara, H., and Shizume, K.: Levels of pancreatic glucagon, insulin and glucose during twenty-four hours of the day in normal subjects. Horm Metab Res 7:205, 1975.

Unger, R. H.: Glucagon. In Freinkel, N. (ed.): The Year in Metabolism, 1976. New York, Plenum Press, 1976, p. 73.

Unger, R. H.: The Berson Memorial Lecture. Insulin-glucagon relationships in the defense against hypoglycemia. Diabetes 32:575, 1983.

Unger, R. H., and Orci, L.: Glucagon and the A-Cell. Physiology and pathophysiology. N Engl J Med 304:1518, 1575, 1981.

OTHER HORMONES

Although insulin and glucagon are the major glucoregulatory hormones, a variety of other hormones contribute to fuel homeostasis. These include the catecholamines epinephrine and norepinephrine, cortisol, and growth hormone. Somatostatin also has potent effects on body fuel metabolism. However, whether this action is physiological or pharmacological has not been established.

CATECHOLAMINES

The metabolism and action of these substances is considered in detail in Section VIII, Endocrinology. As noted previously, catecholamines influence carbohydrate metabolism by altering insulin secretion. In addition, epinephrine is an important factor in blood glucose homeostasis by virtue of its effects on glycogenolysis, gluconeogenesis, fat mobilization, and peripheral insulin effectiveness. When the blood glucose concentration falls below certain concentrations—about 55 mg/dl in man—a series of protective reactions occurs to prevent further fall and to restore the blood glucose concentration to normal. Epinephrine is one of the hormones secreted in response to hypoglycemia. The nature of its action, as well as the temporal pattern of its response, suggests that it has an important role in the response to hypoglycemia. The epinephrine released acts to raise the blood glucose via the following mechanisms: (a) decreased glucose uptake by muscle tissue; (b) stimulation of hepatic and muscle glycogenolysis; (c) stimulation of lipolysis; (d) inhibition of insulin secretion; and (e) stimulation of glucagon secretion.

In muscle tissue, the decrease in insulin-mediated glucose uptake appears to be mediated primarily via beta-adrenergic receptors. Since muscle lacks the enzyme glucose-6-phosphatase, stimulation of muscle glycogenolysis results in release of lactic acid rather than free glucose. This effect is also largely mediated via beta receptors. Since lactate released from muscle can be used by the liver for gluconeogenesis, epinephrine increases the supply of substrate for gluconeogenesis.

Epinephrine also activates glycogenolysis in the liver. Whether this effect is mediated via alpha or beta receptors is unsettled and may depend on the species examined. In the rat the glycogenolytic effect of epinephrine is primarily attributable to alpha-adrenergic stimulation, which occurs independent of elevations in cyclic AMP. In contrast, in the dog, a glycogenolytic effect is primarily mediated by beta-adrenergic receptors. In humans, a glycogenolytic effect of epinephrine is demonstrable in the face of both alpha- and beta-adrenergic blockade. However beta-adrenergic mechanisms again appear to predominate. The mechanism whereby epinephrine-mediated beta-adrenergic stimulation results in activation of hepatic phosphorylase has been discussed above (see Fig. 3).

While epinephrine and glucagon are similar with respect to the magnitude and transient duration of their hepatic glycogenolytic effects, the hyperglycemic action of physiological increments in epinephrine exceeds that of physiological increments in glucagon. This difference derives largely from the fact that epinephrine reduces peripheral glucose clearance whereas glucagon fails to exert a comparable effect.

Epinephrine also exerts a powerful beta-receptor mediated lipolytic effect via stimulation of a hormone-sensitive lipase in adipose tissue. Decreased glucose uptake also limits the availability of glycerol-3-phosphate for reesterification of free fatty acids in adipose tissue. Increased secretion of catecholamines is an important factor in the lipolytic response to exercise.

In contrast to its inhibitory effects on insulin secretion, epinephrine stimulates the secretion of glucagon. This occurs particularly when epinephrine is raised into the upper physiological range, such as during severe hypoglycemia. Under these conditions, the hyperglycemic effect of epinephrine is blunted when hyperglucagonemia is prevented by concomitant administration of somatostatin.

The importance of these adrenergic mechanisms in glucose homeostasis is underscored by the observations that the beta-blocking agent propranolol may precipitate hypoglycemia, augment peripheral insulin effectiveness, and dampen the rebound in plasma glucose during an insulin tolerance test in diabetic patients whose counterregulatory response is already impaired by a defective glucagon response to hypoglycemia.

GLUCOCORTICOIDS

It has been recognized since the classic experiments of Long and Lukens that the secretions of the adrenal cortex have a diabetogenic effect. Subsequent work by Long and colleagues established the gluconeogenic nature of adrenal corticosteroids; hence the term glucocorticoids. These hormones stimulate proteolysis while increasing gluconeogenesis and glycogen formation. In vitro, physiological increments in glucocorticoids are largely permissive in facilitating a gluconeogenic response to epinephrine or glucagon. More recent in vivo studies indicate that hypercortisolemia enhances the hyperglycemic response to epinephrine and glucagon by converting their transient glycogenolytic effects to a sustained stimulation of hepatic glucose production.

Glucocorticoids also tend to raise blood glucose levels by decreasing the responsiveness of muscle and adipose tissue to insulin-mediated glucose uptake. This effect appears to be mediated by an inhibition of postreceptor events. Thus, in Cushing's syndrome of spontaneous or iatrogenic origin, hyperinsulinemia and insulin resistance are characteristic findings. Whether such patients develop diabetes (either postprandial or fasting hyperglycemia) depends on their insulin secretory capacity, which, in turn, is probably genetically determined.

In contrast to the insulin antagonism induced by epinephrine, which is demonstrable within minutes, the effects of glucocorticoids require hours to days to become fully manifest. This time course of action suggests mediation via alterations in the synthesis of various proteins involved in the transport and metabolism of glucose.

Increased secretion of cortisol is characteristically observed in conditions of "stress" such as trauma (extensive body burns), severe infection, or diabetic ketoacidosis. The hyperglycemia that is known to occur in such circumstances is, at least in part, due to the excess of glucocorticoids.

The effects of the adrenal steroids are discussed further in Section VIII, Endocrinology.

GROWTH HORMONE

In the intact animal the effect of pituitary growth hormone is to decrease catabolism of protein—or to increase anabolism—by an action that requires the presence of insulin, to decrease the rate of deamination of amino acids, to increase lipolysis, and to reduce the effectiveness of insulin in increasing glucose transport. As a result of these actions it decreases utilization of both carbohydrate and protein as energy sources and forces the body to depend mainly on fat. In general the anti-insulin effects of growth hormone are countered by its beta-cytotropic action, resulting in an appropriate increase in insulin levels. However, if large enough quantities of growth hormone are involved, either from the pituitary or by injection, the blood glucose concentration may rise to abnormal concentrations. Furthermore, in diabetics who are unable to increase their endogenous insulin secretion, growth hormone produces profound hyperglycemia. In this situation the hyperglycemia involves a stimulation of hepatic glucose production, as well.

Striking changes in glucose and insulin concentrations are observed in the absence of growth hormone. During fasting, blood glucose levels fall to strikingly lower concentrations in growth hormone–deficient dwarfs than are observed in controls. Insulin levels in these subjects are also reduced. Thus it appears that growth hormone does have a primary role in setting the blood glucose concentration (a "glucostat" effect) and influences insulin secretion under basal and prolonged fasting conditions. It is noteworthy in this respect that acute hypoglycemia is a potent stimulus of growth hormone secretion.

The anabolic actions of growth hormone appear to derive from its induction of secondary substances in serum initially termed "sulfation factor" and more recently identified as a family of compounds termed somatomedins or insulin-like growth factors. The action of growth hormone in stimulating protein synthesis and growth is mediated via these peptides. There is now good evidence that the somatomedins are closely related to or identical with a component of the insulin-like activity in plasma that is nonsuppressible by insulin antibodies and is soluble in acid ethanol (NSILA$_s$). It has also been demonstrated that serum somatomedin activity is reduced in streptozotocin-diabetic rats and that this reduction is prevented or reversed by insulin therapy. Growth failure in diabetes may thus be related to decreased somatomedin activity.

NONSUPPRESSIBLE INSULIN-LIKE ACTIVITY

Using in vitro bioassay systems such as glucose uptake by the rat diaphragm or rat epididymal fat pad, insulin-like activity that is not inhibited by specific insulin antibodies is demonstrable in the blood of normal subjects and persists after pancreatectomy. Thus, of the total circulating insulin-like activity measurable in plasma by bioassay (200 µU/ml), only about 10 per cent corresponds to true, pancreatic insulin as determined by specific radioimmunoassay techniques. The remainder of the circulating insulin-like activity has been termed nonsuppressible insulin-like activity (NSILA). NSILA consists of two components: (1) NSILA-S, a single-chain polypeptide with a molecular weight of about 7500 that influences adipose tissue and diaphragm muscle in a manner analogous to pancreatic insulin. (2) NSILA-P, a large polypeptide with a molecular weight of approximately 100,000 that also mimics the action of insulin on adipose tissue and diaphragm. Increased levels of NSILA-S have been observed in 30 to 50 per cent of patients with extrapancreatic tumor hypoglycemia (for example, mesenchymal tumors, hepatomas, adrenal carcinomas) and thus may contribute to the pathogenesis of this syndrome.

As noted above, NSILA-S is now believed to be identical to somatomedin-C or insulin-like growth factor-I, the mediator of growth hormone action. Somatomedin-C levels are reduced in hypopituitarism and increase to normal after administration of human growth hormone, at which time blood glucose and FFA levels decline.

SOMATOSTATIN

This tetradecapeptide originally isolated from the hypothalamus was discussed earlier with respect to its inhibitory effects on insulin and glucagon secretion. Somatostatin-containing cells have been identified in the hypothalamus, gastrointestinal tract, and pancreatic islet cells.

Inhibition of growth hormone secretion was the first effect attributed to this substance and constitutes the basis for its name. Subsequent studies have shown an inhibitory effect on the secretion of a variety of gastrointestinal hormones (gastrin, secretin, motilin). In addition, somatostatin has been shown to interfere with carbohydrate absorption and may alter protein and fat absorption.

Studies measuring radioimmunoassayable somatostatin have demonstrated that glucose stimulates the release of somatostatin from perfused pancreas. These effects of feeding on circulating somatostatin coupled with its effects on gastrointestinal function have lead to the hypothesis that somatostatin is a physiological regulator of the rate of nutrient absorption. Whether *physiological* increments in somatostatin do in fact alter gastrointestinal function remains to be established.

Somatostatin has also been suggested as a potentially useful agent in the management of type I (insulin-dependent) diabetes in view of its glucagon-lowering effects. However, the studies on gastrointestinal function suggest that the seeming improvement in diabetes and reduction in insulin requirements may be in part attributable to interference with nutrient absorption rather than a consequence of hypoglucagonemia.

HORMONAL INTERACTIONS

The major hormones influencing body fuel metabolism may be classified as promoting either energy storage or energy dissipation (Table 8). In this regard, insulin is unique as the hormone that promotes the storage and anabolism of all the major body fuels, carbohydrate (as glycogen), fat (as triglyceride), and protein. In contrast, five hormones (epinephrine, glucagon, cortisol, growth hormone, and thyroid hormone) have major effects in promoting the dissipation of fat, glycogen, and/or protein stores. Four of these hormones (all but thyroid hormone) also cause an elevation of blood sugar by virtue of their glycogenolytic or gluconeogenic actions and/or their antagonism to insulin-mediated glucose uptake (Table 8). Thus with respect to glucose homeostasis, insulin is generally considered the major *regulatory* hormone and the hormones raising the blood sugar are described as *counterregulatory*.

The integrated nature of the hormonal milieu in maintaining fuel homeostasis is apparent from an examination of the secretory response to various physiological conditions of altered fuel supply or requirements (Table 9). In starvation, mobilization of body fat coupled with increased glycogenolysis, gluconeogenesis, and ketogenesis are the major changes in body fuel metabolism. These changes are brought about by a fall

TABLE 8. HORMONES AND ENERGY METABOLISM

ENERGY STORAGE	ENERGY DISSIPATION
Insulin	**Epinephrine**
Antilipolytic	Lipolytic
Glycogenic	Glycogenolytic
Antigluconeogenic	Gluconeogenic
Anabolic	Insulin antagonism
Protein synthesis	**Glucagon**
Fat synthesis	Glycogenolytic
	Gluconeogenic
	Cortisol
	Gluconeogenic
	Insulin antagonism
	Proteolytic
	Growth Hormone
	Lipolytic
	Insulin antagonism
	Thyroid Hormone
	Lipolytic

TABLE 9. HORMONAL RESPONSE TO ALTERED FUEL SUPPLY OR FUEL REQUIREMENTS

CONDITION	INSULIN	GLUCAGON	EPINEPHRINE	GROWTH HORMONE	CORTISOL
Starvation	↓	↑	↑ or ±	↑ or ±	↓
Acute hypoglycemia	↓	↑	↑	↑	↑
Exercise	↓	↑	↑	↑	↑
Glucose ingestion	↑	↓	±	±	±
Protein ingestion	↑	↑	±	↑	±
Mixed meal	↑	±	±	±	±

↑ Increased Secretion; ↓ Decreased Secretion; ± Unchanged

in insulin. Transient elevations in glucagon and growth hormone are also observed but are not necessary to mediate these changes in fuel mobilization. However, in response to acute hypoglycemia (induced by exogenous insulin), increases in counterregulatory hormones are the major factors responsible for the restoration of blood sugar concentration. While the secretion of all counterregulatory hormones is increased by hypoglycemia, the response of glucagon and epinephrine is the most rapid and most important in stimulating a rise in hepatic glucose output. During muscular exercise the fuel requirements of contracting muscle necessitate a supply of glucose as well as fat. Here too, a rise in each of the counterregulatory hormones as well as a fall in insulin is necessary for the mediation of this response.

The hormonal response to an increase in fuel supply is determined by the nature of the ingested nutrient. With glucose feeding a rise in insulin and a fall in glucagon is observed. As discussed above, the fall in glucagon is not essential for the normal uptake and storage of ingested glucose by liver, muscle, and adipose tissue. On the other hand, in the absence of a rise in insulin, as occurs in the diabetic, glucose uptake is reduced, resulting in hyperglycemia. With protein feeding, insulin, glucagon, and growth hormone levels are elevated. The basis for this multiple hormonal elevation is to facilitate anabolism from the ingested protein, which requires insulin and perhaps growth hormone secretion. The hypoglycemic effect of hyperinsulinemia is prevented by the concomitant elevation in glucagon, which facilitates ongoing release of glucose from the liver in the face of a rise in insulin (Fig. 36). When mixed meals are ingested (as is the case with the diets consumed in most areas of the world) the only hormonal change is a rise in insulin.

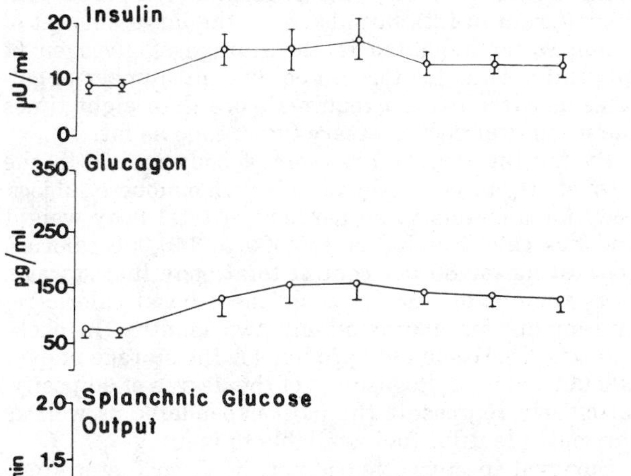

From the above considerations the following principles emerge regarding hormonal regulation of body fuel supply: (1) An increase in fuel storage accompanying nutrient supply is mediated by a rise in insulin. (2) A decrease in fuel storage accompanying fuel lack (for example, starvation) is mediated by a fall in insulin. (3) Accelerated mobilization of fuel stores as occurs in circumstances of acute fuel need (acute hypoglycemia, exercise, "stress") is mediated via a fall in insulin coupled with a rise in the counterregulatory hormones.

REFERENCES

Other Hormones

Effendic, S., and Luft, R.: Somatostatin, a classical hormone, a locally active polypeptide and a neurotransmitter. Ann Clin Res 12:87, 1980.

Eigler, N., Saccà, L., and Sherwin, R. S.: Synergistic interactions of physiologic increments of glucagon, epinephrine, and cortisol in the dog. A model for stress-induced hyperglycemia. J Clin Invest 63:114, 1979.

Felig, P., Marliss, E., and Cahill, G. F., Jr.: Metabolic response to human growth hormone during prolonged starvation. J Clin Invest 50:411, 1971.

Garber, A. J., Cryer, P. E., Santiago, J. V., Haymond, M. W., Pagliara, A. S., and Kipnis, D. M.: The role of adrenergic mechanisms in the substrate and hormonal response to insulin-induced hypoglycemia in man. J Clin Invest 58:7, 1976.

Gerich, J. E.: Somatostatin. Its possible role in carbohydrate homeostasis and the treatment of diabetes mellitus. Arch Intern Med 137:659, 1977.

Gerich, J. E., Lorenzi, M., Tsalikian, E., and Karam, J. H.: Studies on the mechanism of epinephrine-induced hyperglycemia in man. Evidence for participation of pancreatic glucagon secretion. Diabetes 25:65, 1976.

Hintz, R. L.: The somatomedins. In Barness, L. A. (ed.): Advances in Pediatrics. Chicago, Year Book Medical Publishers, Vol. 28:293, 1981.

Kinney, J. M., and Felig, P.: The metabolic response to injury and infection. In DeGroot, L. (ed.): Endocrinology. New York, Grune & Stratton, 1979.

Merimee, T. J., Felig, P., Marliss, E., Fineberg, S. E., and Cahill, G. F., Jr.: Glucose and lipid homeostasis in the absence of human growth hormone. J Clin Invest 50:574, 1971.

Figure 36. Influence of protein feeding on plasma insulin, plasma glucagon, and splanchnic glucose output in normal humans. The rise in glucagon prevents the rise in insulin from inhibiting splanchnic (hepatic) glucose output, thereby maintaining normoglycemia. (Based on the data of Wahren, J., Felig, P., and Hagenfeldt, L.: J Clin Invest 58:761, 1976.)

Oelz, O., Froesch, E. R., Bunzli, H. F., Humbel, R. E., and Ritschard, W. J.: Antibody-suppressible and nonsuppressible insulin-like activities. In Greep, R. O., and Astwood, E. B. (eds): Handbook of Physiology. Section 7, Endocrinology. Vol. 1. Endocrine Pancreas. Washington, D. C., American Physiological Society, 1972, p. 685.

Olefsky, J. M: Effect of dexamethasone on insulin binding, glucose transport, and glucose oxidation of isolated rat adipocytes. J Clin Invest 56:1499, 1975.

Phillips, L. S., and Young, H. S.: Nutrition and somatomedin. II. Serum somatomedin activity and cartilage growth activity in streptozotocin-diabetic rats. Diabetes 25:516, 1976.

Press, M., Tamborlane, W. V., and Sherwin, R. S.: Importance

of raised growth hormone levels in mediating the metabolic derangements of diabetes. N Engl J Med 310:810, 1984.

Sherwin, R. S., and Sacia, L.: Effects of epinephrine on glucose metabolism in humans: Contribution of the liver. Am J Physiol 247 (Endocrinol Metab 10):E157, 1984.

Unger, R. H.: Somatostatinoma (editorial). N Engl J Med 296:998, 1977.

VanWyk, J. J., Svoboda, M. E., and Underwood, L. E.: Evidence from radiology and assays that somatomedin C and insulin like growth factor I are similar to each other and different from other somatomedins. J Clin Endocrinol Metab 50:206, 1980.

Fuel-Hormone Interactions

STARVATION

Under normal circumstances a human feeds intermittently, the interval between meals generally extending no more than 12 to 14 hours. Occasionally, however, either because of voluntary cessation of intake, intercurrent disease interfering with feeding, or lack of food availability, man is faced with more prolonged periods of fasting. The metabolic response to starvation represents an integration of normal secretion and fuel utilization designed to (a) maximize utilization of the major storage fuel (triglyceride), (b) minimize dissipation of body protein, and (c) maintain glucose availability (glycogenolysis and gluconeogenesis) to meet the needs of obligate, glucose-consuming tissues. Although prolonged starvation is rarely encountered as a medical problem in Western civilization today, in various disease states characterized by debilitation (metastatic cancer, uremia, severe inflammatory bowel disease), starvation is often an important contributory cause of death. In such patients the following sequence of events is often encountered: decreased food intake → protein wasting → weakness of respiratory muscles → atelectasis → pneumonia → death. The inability to conserve body protein stores in such patients reflects a failure of the normal homeostatic mechanisms present in healthy subjects undergoing prolonged periods of food deprivation. In the discussion that follows, the normal response to starvation will be viewed as a continuum that can be divided into three phases: the postabsorptive state (9 to 15 hours after food intake); short-term starvation (lasting one to seven days); and prolonged starvation (two weeks or longer).

BODY COMPOSITION

The calories consumed in the typical American or Western European diet consist of about 45 per cent carbohydrate, 35 to 40 per cent fat, and 15 to 20 per cent protein. In some parts of Asia 80 per cent of the diet is carbohydrate. The composition of the fuels stored in the human body is, however, far different from that ingested in the diet (Table 10). Carbohydrate represents a calorically insignificant fuel store. The combined caloric value of liver glycogen (70 grams), muscle glycogen (200 grams), and circulating blood glucose (20 grams) amounts to approximately 1100 calories, well below the total caloric expenditure of a single day, even under basal conditions. Nevertheless, liver glycogen represents an important source of carbohydrate to meet the ongoing needs of the brain, particularly in the interval between the evening meal and breakfast and during bursts of augmented glucose utilization accompanying exercise. However, liver glycogen is rapidly depleted as starvation extends beyond 18 to 24 hours. The teleological basis of the limitation in stored carbohydrate derives not only from its decreased caloric density (4 kcal/gram as compared with 9 kcal/gram in fat), but also from the large amount of tissue water obligated in the storage of glycogen (4 ml/gram). Thus to store an equivalent number of calories as carbohydrate requires more than eight times the mass (weight) necessary for storage as fat.

By far the largest reservoir of body fuel is in the form of fat, stored as triglyceride. In a nonobese subject, body fat amounts to 20 per cent of total body weight and has caloric value of 130,000 to 140,000 calories, accounting for 80 per cent of total body fuel storage. This amount of calories could meet basal caloric requirements for approximately two months. In obese subjects, fat tissue may provide for the storage of over 500,000 calories. Regardless of the degree of adiposity, fat clearly represents the most expendable as well as the most plentiful fuel available to man.

Survival in starvation is not, however, determined by depletion of fat or carbohydrate, but rather by dissipation of protein. The major reservoir of body

TABLE 10. BODY COMPOSITION AND FUEL RESERVES IN A NORMAL 70-KG MAN

FUEL	TISSUE	Kg	PER CENT BODY WEIGHT	ENERGY VALUE (kcal)
Fat	Adipose tissue	11–17	15–25	100,000–150,000
Protein	Primarily muscle	8–12	12–17	32,000–48,000
Carbohydrate	Liver glycogen	0.070	<1	280
	Muscle glycogen	0.200	<1	800
	Blood glucose	0.020	<1	80

protein is in muscle tissue, amounting to 10 kg (exclusive of tissue water), or 40,000 calories. Because of protein's importance in body structure, in muscle function, and as a catalytic agent (enzymes), depletion of body protein by 30 to 50 per cent is incompatible with survival, despite residual, mobilizable fat tissue. Death in starvation results not from hypoglycemia, but, as noted above, from loss of respiratory muscle function leading to terminal pneumonia.

Of particular importance in the homeostatic response to starvation is the interchangeability of fuels. Body protein (by virtue of its constituent amino acids, other than leucine) is readily converted to glucose (gluconeogenesis). Carbohydrate availability for obligate, glucose-dependent tissues (for example, brain) does not cease with depletion of liver glycogen. On the other hand, fatty acids containing an even number of carbon atoms (comprising over 95 per cent of the total fatty acids stored as triglyceride) cannot be converted to glucose, since mammalian tissue lacks the enzymatic steps necessary for net gluconeogenesis from acetyl CoA. Thus to the extent that blood glucose is terminally oxidized in starvation and replenished by gluconeogenesis, there will be an obligate dissolution of body protein stores.

THE POSTABSORPTIVE STATE

The changeover from the fed to the fasted condition can best be examined in the context of the postabsorptive state—the condition that exists 9 to 15 hours after food ingestion. While this interval represents a nonsteady state, it is nevertheless a readily identifiable reference point. In the postabsorptive condition, adipose tissue releases free fatty acids to meet the fuel requirements of muscle and heart as well as parenchymal tissues (liver, kidney). Carbohydrate utilization in this circumstance occurs primarily in the brain, which terminally oxidizes glucose at a rate of about 125 grams per day. Smaller amounts of glucose are utilized by resting muscle, and by obligate anaerobic tissues such as the formed elements of the blood and the renal medulla (see Fig. 13). Maintenance of euglycemia depends on release of glucose from the liver at a rate equal to the combined utilization in brain and peripheral tissues (150 to 250 grams/day; 2 to 3 mg/kg body weight/min; 6 to 10 grams/hr). Approximately 75 per cent of the glucose released after an overnight fast is derived from glycogen, the remainder being formed by gluconeogenesis. Since as noted above, liver glycogen stores (70 grams) can sustain cerebral glucose requirements for less than 24 hours, as fasting extends beyond the postabsorptive state, greater reliance is placed on gluconeogenesis. In addition, the rates of lipolysis and ketogenesis are increased.

SHORT-TERM STARVATION

The integrated fuel-hormone response to relatively brief starvation (three to seven days) represents an acceleration of gluconeogenic, lipolytic, and ketogenic processes that are already functioning, albeit at a less rapid rate, in the postabsorptive condition. Stimulation of gluconeogenesis is necessitated by the rapid depletion of glycogen stores and the need to provide glucose for consumption by the brain. Lipolysis allows for the mobilization of the most abundant fuel supply available to the fasted individual, body fat. Ketogenesis may be viewed as a mechanism whose usefulness becomes apparent in prolonged starvation, at which point ketones function as fuel for the brain and as a possible signal for protein conservation in muscle.

The chief factors mediating the enhancement in gluconeogenesis and ketogenesis as fasting extends from 12 hours to three days or a week are a drop in plasma insulin and rise in glucagon (Fig. 37). The altered levels of insulin and glucagon accelerate gluconeogenic and ketogenic processes by virtue of their effects on hepatic and, in the case of insulin, peripheral tissues. The prime locus of the increase in gluconeogenesis is an augmentation in hepatic extraction of alanine despite a fall in plasma alanine levels. The augmented rate of alanine extraction in brief starvation is comparable to that observed in other insulinopenic states such as diabetes and prolonged exercise. The overall rate of gluconeogenesis increases two- to threefold above postabsorptive levels, and in view of the depletion in liver glycogen, accounts for virtually the entire output of glucose from the liver. An increase in proteolysis and amino acid mobilization from muscle (to supply glucose precursors) accompanies the rise in hepatic gluconeogenesis. This is reflected in negative nitrogen balance at the rate of 10 to 12 grams/day, indicating breakdown of 75 to 100 grams of protein per day. A progressive rise in the blood levels of the insulin-sensitive branched chain amino acids (valine, leucine, and isoleucine) is also observed, providing further similarity to the diabetic state.

Simultaneous with the increase in gluconeogenesis, ketone production by the liver is enhanced. The fall in insulin stimulates lipolysis, thereby increasing the delivery of FFA. In addition, changes in the beta-oxidative pathway within the liver induced by the change in insulin and glucagon favor ketone formation at the expense of alternate pathways of FFA disposal. The result is that the liver after a three day fast utilizes FFA at twice the rate observed in postabsorptive man and produces ketones at a rate of 75 to 100 grams/day. The lipolytic and ketogenic activity also serves to enhance gluconeogenesis by (a) providing FFA to meet hepatic energy requirements, (b) furnishing acetyl CoA, which stimulates pyruvate carboxylase (a rate-limiting enzyme in gluconeogenesis, see above), and (c) altering the hepatic redox state to favor glucose synthesis.

The overall sequence of events characterizing early starvation is shown in Figure 38 and may be summarized as follows. Ongoing glucose utilization by the brain results in depletion of liver glycogen and a small decline in blood glucose (5 to 10 mg/dl). As a result, beta cell secretion is reduced and insulin levels decline. An accompanying rise in glucagon is observed that may be mediated primarily by diminished hormonal catabolism rather than hypersecretion. The bihormonal changes influence intrahepatic events (augmented alanine uptake and conversion to glucose, increased acylcarnitine transferase activity) so as to accelerate gluconeogenesis as well as ketogenesis. Contributing to these effects are peripheral actions of hypoinsulinemia, enhancing the mobilization of FFA and amino acids from adipose tissue and muscle respectively.

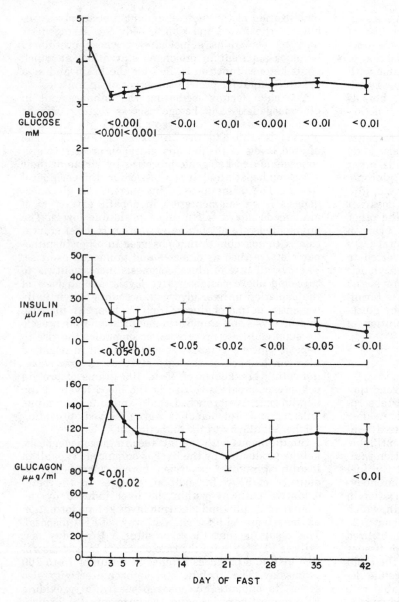

Figure 37. Influence of prolonged starvation on plasma glucose, insulin, and glucagon. (From Marliss, E., et al.: J Clin Invest 49:2256, 1970.)

PROLONGED STARVATION

Continuation of the events described in early starvation would facilitate the maintenance of euglycemia as well as dissipation of fat stores, but at the expense of body protein. As noted above, fatty acids cannot be converted to glucose; net gluconeogenesis occurs only from protein-derived precursors. Persistence of gluconeogenesis and proteolysis at rates observed early in starvation would result in dissipation of 30 to 50 per cent of body protein (a life-threatening situation) within four to six weeks, well before body fat stores have been fully mobilized. Studies in obese subjects (whose body protein mass is comparable to nonobese subjects) reveal that fasts lasting six weeks or more (in a hospital setting) can be tolerated without ill effect. The adaptive mechanism permitting such extended periods of starvation involves a progressive decrease in protein breakdown. As shown originally in the classic studies of Benedict in 1915 and repeatedly confirmed by others, the rate of urinary nitrogen loss in prolonged fasting falls progressively, reaching levels

as low as 3 grams/day, indicating dissolution of no more than 20 grams of body protein (Fig. 39). The nature of the nitrogenous end products also changes, from predominantly urea to primarily ammonia (Fig. 39).

Gluconeogenesis. A decline in protein breakdown necessitates a simultaneous reduction in gluconeogenesis. Direct measurements of glucose production in prolonged fasted subjects (three to six weeks) reveal that hepatic glucose production falls from postabsorptive rates of 150 to 250 grams/day to approximately 50 grams/day. An additional 40 grams of glucose is produced by the kidney, which in prolonged starvation contributes to gluconeogenesis in amounts equal to the liver. Theoretically, the marked decline in hepatic glucose production could be ascribed to inhibition of hepatic substrate conversion, diminished precursor (alanine) release from muscle, or a combination of these processes. In fact, the rate-limiting step is in the periphery, where a marked diminution in muscle release of alanine as well as other amino acids is observed

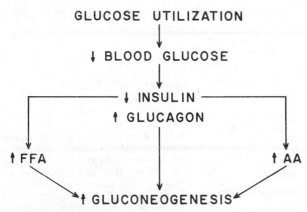

GLUCOSE UTILIZATION

↓ BLOOD GLUCOSE

↓ INSULIN
↑ GLUCAGON

↑ FFA   ↑ AA

↑ GLUCONEOGENESIS

Figure 38. Summary of the metabolic response to short-term starvation. The key hormonal change is a fall in plasma insulin, which leads to increased lipolysis, proteolysis, and gluconeogenesis.

(Fig. 40). Prolonged fasting thus clearly differs from early starvation (three-day fast), in which there is a rise in muscle alanine output. Accompanying this fall in alanine output is a progressive decline in circulating alanine levels (Fig. 40) that exceeds the fall observed in all amino acids. Underscoring the role of alanine availability in regulating gluconeogenesis are observations on hepatic alanine uptake. The fractional extraction of alanine by the liver in prolonged starvation is no less than that observed in the overnight fasted state. Furthermore, administration of exogenous alanine to prolonged fasted subjects results in a prompt rise in blood glucose, indicating unimpaired intrahepatic gluconeogenic pathways.

In contrast to the fall in glucose output from the liver, the kidney serves an important role as a site of glucose formation in prolonged fasting. This contrasts with the situation in postabsorptive man or in circumstances of augmented glucose production such as exercise or diabetes, in which conditions no net addition of glucose from the kidney to the bloodstream is observed. It has been suggested that the enhanced ammonia excretion dictated by the ketonuria of starvation (Fig. 39) serves as a stimulus of renal glucose production.

Ketone Metabolism. Despite the contribution of the kidney to gluconeogenesis, total glucose production in prolonged fasting (90 grams/day) is one half that observed in postabsorptive man. In the absence of adaptive changes in glucose consumption, severe hypoglycemia and attendant derangement in brain function would rapidly ensue. As shown in Figure 37, blood glucose levels reach a plateau of 50 to 60 mg/dl within three days of fasting and subsequently stabilize. Even more striking is the fact that prolonged fasted subjects have no problem in maintaining cerebral function in the face of a marked reduction in glucose production. This seeming paradox is resolved by the observation that ketone acids become a major fuel for the brain in prolonged fasting. The uptake of ketone acids by the brain is sufficient to account for 50 per cent or more of its fuel requirements. A corresponding decline in brain uptake of glucose permits euglycemia in the face of diminished glucose production.

The mechanism responsible for ketone utilization by the brain in prolonged starvation is primarily sub-

strate availability. Studies in experimental animals and man reveal that ketone-oxidizing enzymes are active in the brain after an overnight fast. The progressive increase in brain ketone utilization is thus a reflection of a rising arterial ketone concentration. It is of interest in this regard that blood ketone levels (particularly β-hydroxybutyrate) continue to rise for three to four weeks of starvation, while FFA levels as well as hepatic ketone production rates reach peak levels within three to ten days. The events of prolonged starvation thus appear to be directed at raising the arterial concentration of ketone acids so as to augment their availability to the brain without necessitating an increase in ketogenesis. This adaptation is achieved by a progressive decrease and/or saturation of extra-

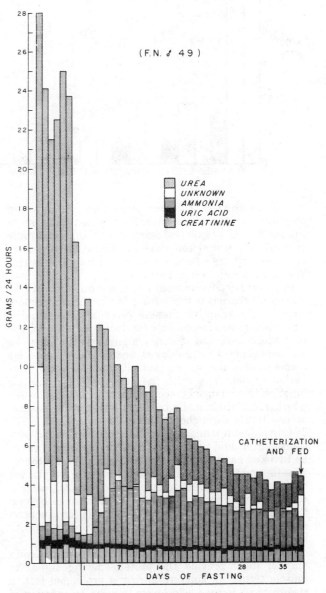

Figure 39. The effect of prolonged starvation on urinary nitrogen excretion. There is a progressive reduction in nitrogen loss, reflecting a reduction in the rate of protein catabolism. (From Owen, O. E., et al.: J Clin Invest 48:574, 1969.)

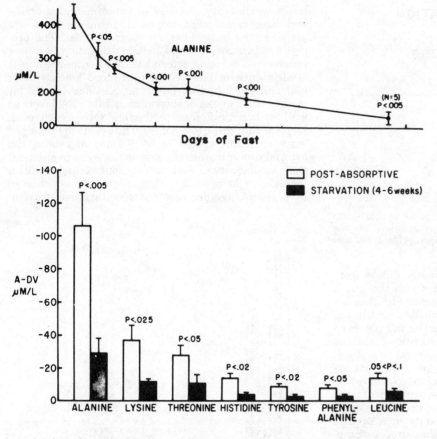

Figure 40. The effect of prolonged starvation on plasma alanine concentration (upper panel) and on muscle output (arterio–deep venous differences) of alanine and other amino acids. The plasma level of alanine progressively declines as its release (and that of other amino acids) from muscle tissue decreases. The decline in alanine availability is responsible for the reduction in hepatic gluconeogenesis observed after prolonged fasting. (Based on the data of Felig, P., et al.: J Clin Invest 48:584, 1969.)

cerebral pathways of ketone utilization as starvation continues beyond three days. Finally, a rapid rise in the net rate of ketone reabsorption by the renal tubule between three and ten days of starvation serves to diminish urinary ketone losses and thereby accentuate ketone accumulation in blood.

Regulatory Mechanisms. A major question in prolonged starvation is the nature of the signals responsible for the adaptive changes described. Specifically, what factors are responsible for decreased muscle protein catabolism and lessened alanine availability for gluconeogenesis in prolonged fasting? The key roles demonstrated for insulin and glucagon in early starvation immediately raise the possibility of a similar function in prolonged fasting. However, insulin levels, which reach their nadir in seven to ten days, remain at low levels throughout prolonged fasting (Fig. 37). The hypoinsulinemia responsible for accelerated gluconeogenesis and proteolysis in early starvation cannot be invoked as an explanation of diminished gluconeogenesis and protein conservation in prolonged starvation. In the case of glucagon, a return to basal, postabsorptive levels occurs as starvation continues beyond three days (Fig. 37). Furthermore, a role for glucagon in regulating muscle proteolysis or alanine availability has not been established.

Recently it has been suggested that hyperketonemia may of itself provide the protein-sparing signal to muscle tissue. In subjects during a prolonged fast, a rise in blood ketone acid levels induced by infusion of exogenous β-hydroxybutyrate has been accompanied by a reduction in urinary nitrogen losses. Furthermore, a selective effect of ketones in reducing alanine for-

mation and release from muscle and in inhibiting proteolysis and amino acid catabolism has been observed in in vitro studies. These observations suggest that ketones may act not only as substrate for the brain but as the "signal" to muscle tissue limiting proteolysis and secondarily reducing precursor (alanine) availability to the liver for gluconeogenesis. This view, however, remains controversial.

Other Hormonal Changes. The preceding discussion has emphasized the role of insulin and glucagon in the metabolic response to fasting, particularly in early starvation. A variety of other hormonal changes have, however, also been demonstrated. A transient increase in circulating growth hormone, diminished secretion of cortisol, a fall in serum triiodothyronine, and increased levels of catecholamines have all been noted in starvation.

In contrast to the changes in insulin and glucagon, hormones such as growth hormone and cortisol exert primarily a permissive rather than a regulatory role in starvation (that is, normal glucose homeostasis requires their presence but does not depend on changes in secretion). Growth hormone does not play an essential role in either the lipolytic effects of early starvation or the protein conservation of late starvation. On the other hand, growth hormone–deficient dwarfs have a greater decline in blood glucose than is observed in healthy subjects. Accompanying this hypoglycemic response is an exaggerated fall in serum insulin. Thus the normal glucose-insulin relationship of starvation does not depend on GH, but the setting of the blood glucose concentration at which this relation takes place is reduced in growth hormone–deficient subjects.

In starvation an increase in plasma and urinary norepinephrine and unchanged plasma epinephrine have been observed. However, neither the lipolytic nor the hyperglucagonemic response to fasting is altered by beta-adrenergic blockade. Thus while there is little doubt that sympathoadrenal mechanisms contribute importantly to the acute counterregulatory response engendered by an abrupt fall in blood glucose as manifested by glycogenolysis, this system is less important in the more gradual homeostatic response to fasting. Furthermore, in recent studies examining the turnover of myocardial catecholamines, a decrease in adrenergic activity has been observed in starvation.

Although serum thyroxin (T_4) is unchanged and free T_4 concentration remains within normal limits during starvation, studies have shown a profound decline (50 per cent) in free triiodothyronine (3,5,3'-triiodothyronine, free T_3) in fasted subjects. This reduction in free T_3 occurs in patients in whom endogenous thyroid hormone secretion has been suppressed by administration of replacement doses of exogenous hormone, suggesting an alteration in peripheral conversion of T_4 to T_3 rather than suppression of endogenous thyroid secretion of T_3. This conclusion is supported by studies in fasted rates showing decreased conversion of T_4 to T_3 in isolated liver as well as a reduction in the activity of the key enzyme regulating this step, 5'-deiodinase. Starvation results in a shift in the peripheral conversion of T_4 from the metabolically active T_3 to the calorigenically inactive form, reverse T_3, because the metabolism of reverse T_3 is also regulated by 5'-deiodinase. This effect of starvation on T_3 levels appears to be related to the carbohydrate content of the diet; it is demonstrable in anorexia nervosa as well. The physiological significance of the fall in serum free T_3 is that it provides an explanation of the well-recognized reduction in basal metabolic rate (oxygen consumption) that accompanies prolonged fasting.

ACCELERATED STARVATION

A number of physiological and pathological conditions exist in which the normal response to starvation is accelerated and exaggerated. Particularly striking changes in blood glucose and ketones are observed in normal pregnancy and in patients with alcoholic ketoacidosis.

Pregnancy. In pregnancy, the fuel requirements of the developing fetus are met primarily by the consumption of glucose, inasmuch as little, if any, transfer of free fatty acids occurs across the placenta. The rate of glucose utilization by the fetus at term is estimated at 6 mg/kg/min, well in excess of adult utilization rates of 2 mg/kg/min. In addition to glucose transfer, amino acids are actively transported across the placenta for fetal protein synthesis and possibly for oxidative processes as well. The ongoing siphoning of glucose and amino acids persists during periods of maternal fasting as well as feeding. As a consequence, the maternal response to starvation is characterized by an accelerated and exaggerated fall in blood glucose. Maternal hypoglycemia results in hypoinsulinemia and a concomitant exaggeration of starvation ketosis. In addition, the fall in plasma alanine is also accentuated in pregnancy as a result of ongoing transfer of alanine to the fetus. That maternal gluconeogenic mechanisms remain intact is indicated by the prompt rise in blood glucose after exogenous alanine is administered. Thus the maternal hypoglycemia of pregnancy is initiated by fetal siphoning of glucose and perpetuated by the transfer to the fetus of gluconeogenic precursors.

The starvation ketosis of pregnancy is of particular interest in view of the possible adverse consequences of hyperketonemia to the fetus. On the basis of indirect data in humans, it is likely that maternal ketones are transferred to the fetus, where the enzymes necessary for ketone oxidation have been identified in fetal brain tissue. In contrast to the seemingly innocuous effects of ketone uptake by the brain of the fasting adult (see above), it has been suggested that psychoneurological development of the fetal brain may be impaired by the transfer of ketones from the maternal to the fetal circulation. This underscores the importance of avoiding periods of fasting and fad diets involving severe carbohydrate restriction during pregnancy.

Alcoholic Ketoacidosis. In normal subjects, peak rates of ketone production and utilization observed in prolonged fasting are associated with blood ketone levels that remain below 8 mM, while serum bicarbonate generally remains above 14 mEq/liter. Briefer periods of fasting (one to three days) are accompanied by ketone levels of less than 3 to 4 mM. In contrast, in alcoholics a period of binge drinking accompanied by protracted vomiting and poor food intake may result in an exaggerated starvation ketosis in which ketone acids accumulate to levels of 8 to 12 mM and a metabolic acidosis is observed. Arterial pH is often reduced to less than 7.2 and the anion gap is increased. In about 25 per cent of cases the blood glucose level is less than 50 mg/dl. This is due to alcohol's inhibitory effect (via changes in the redox state) on key gluconeogenic enzymes in the liver. The nature of the metabolic acidosis is often not recognized or is mistakenly attributed to lactate, since the semiquantitative nitroprusside reaction for ketones (Acetest, Ketostix, Ames Co.) is often only faintly positive. This is due to the high ratio of β-hydroxybutyrate (which is not detected in the nitroprusside test) to acetoacetate. A variety of mechanisms may be responsible for the accelerated ketosis observed in alcoholics. Alcohol may exaggerate ketogenesis via (1) a direct lipolytic effect, (2) altered intramitochondrial redox potential resulting in conversion of oxaloacetate to malate and consequently decreased Krebs cycle activity, and (3) stimulation of intramitochondrial mechanisms involved in the transfer and oxidation of fatty acids. In most instances a prompt clinical response follows the administration of glucose-containing fluids. Treatment with insulin is generally not required and is contraindicated in patients with accompanying hypoglycemia.

REFERENCES

Starvation

Benedict, F. G.: A study of prolonged fasting. Washington, D.C., Carnegie Institute, 1915 (Publication No. 203).

Cahill, G. F., Jr., Herrera, M. G., Morgan, A. P., et al.: Hormone-fuel inter-relationships during fasting. J Clin Invest 45:1751, 1966.

Felig, P.: The metabolic events of starvation. Am J Med 60:119, 1976.

Felig, P.: Body fuel metabolism and diabetes mellitus in pregnancy. Med Clin North Am 61:43, 1977.

Felig, P.: Starvation. In DeGroot, L. (ed.): Endocrinology. New York, Grune & Stratton, 1979.

Felig, P., Kim, Y. J., Lynch, V., et al.: Amino acid metabolism during starvation in human pregnancy. J Clin Invest 51:1195, 1972.

Felig, P., Owen, O. E., Wahren, J., and Cahill, G. F., Jr.: Amino acid metabolism in prolonged starvation. J Clin Invest 48:584, 1969.

Garber, A. J., Menzel, P. H., Boden, G., and Owen, O. E.: Hepatic ketogenesis and gluconeogenesis in humans. J Clin Invest 54:981, 1974.

Gelfand, R. A., and Sherwin, R. S.: Glucagon and starvation. In Lefebvre, R. J. (ed.): Handbook of Experimental Pharmacology, Vol 66/II. Berlin, Springer-Verlag, 1983, p. 223.

Goodman, M. N., McElaney, M. A., and Ruderman, N. B.: Adaptation to prolonged starvation in the rat: Curtailment of skeletal muscle proteolysis. Am J Physiol 241 (Endocrinol Metab 4):E321, 1981.

Havel, R. J.: Caloric homeostasis and disorders of fuel transport. N Engl J Med 287:1186, 1972.

Hawkins, R. A., Williamson, D. H., and Krebs, H. A.: Ketone body utilization by adult and suckling rat brain in vivo. Biochem J 122:13, 1971.

Hultman, E., and Nilsson, L. H.: Liver glycogen in man. Effect of different diets and muscular exercise. Adv Exp Med Biol 11:143, 1971.

Levy, L. J., Duga, J., Girgis, M., et al.: Ketoacidosis associated with alcoholism in nondiabetic subjects. Ann Intern Med 78:213, 1973.

Marliss, E. B., Aoki, T. T., Unger, R. H., Soeldner, J. S., and Cahill, G. F., Jr.: Glucagon levels and metabolic effects in fasting. J Clin Invest 49:2256, 1970.

Owen, O. E., Caprio, S., Reichard, G. R., Jr., Mazzoli, M. A., Boden, G., and Owen, R. S.: Ketosis of starvation: A revisit and new perspectives. Clin Endocrinol Metab 12:359, 1983.

Owen, O. E., Morgan, A. P., Kemp, H. G., Sullivan, J. M., Herrera, M. G., and Cahill, G. F., Jr.: Brain metabolism during fasting. J Clin Invest 46:1589, 1967.

Page, E. W.: Human fetal nutrition and growth. Am J Obstet Gynecol 104:378, 1969.

Portnay, G. I., O'Brian, J. T., Bush, J., et al.: The effect of starvation on the concentration and binding of thyroxine and triiodothyronine in serum and on the response to TRH. J Clin Endocrinol Metab 39:199, 1974.

Pozefsky, T., Tancredi, R. G., Moxley, R. T., et al.: Effects of brief starvation on muscle amino acid metabolism in non-obese man. J Clin Invest 57:444, 1976.

Reichard, G. A., Jr., Owen, O. E., Haff, A. C., et al.: Ketone body production and oxidation in fasting humans. J Clin Invest 53:508, 1974.

Sherwin, R. S., Hendler, R. G., and Felig, P.: Effect of ketone infusion on amino acid and nitrogen metabolism in man. J Clin Invest 55:1382, 1975.

EXERCISE

Skeletal muscle constitutes 40 per cent of body weight in normal man and accounts for 35 to 40 per cent of total oxygen consumption in the resting state. During exercise the consumption of oxygen and metabolic fuels increases markedly so as to provide the ATP necessary for the contractile process. Changes in the circulating levels and/or turnover of all the major body fuels (carbohydrate, fat, amino acids) are observed in this circumstance. The outflow of fuel from the liver (glycogenolysis and gluconeogenesis) and from adipose tissue (lipolysis) is determined, at least in part, by hormonal signals. On the other hand, uptake of glucose by contracting muscle is largely related to the contractile process per se.

RESTING MUSCLE

In the resting state the respiratory quotient (RQ) of muscle is close to 0.7, indicating the virtually total dependence of muscle on the oxidation of fatty acids. Uptake of glucose accounts for less than 10 per cent of the total oxygen consumption by muscle. The overall rate of glucose utilization by muscle is about 20 to 25 mg/min, representing no more than 10 to 25 per cent of the total body glucose turnover. The major site of glucose consumption in the resting state is the brain.

EXERCISING MUSCLE

Carbohydrate and Fatty Acid Utilization. Uptake of blood glucose by exercising muscle has been recognized for almost 90 years. It is now clear that stored carbohydrate (muscle glycogen) and blood-borne glucose as well as free fatty acids contribute substantially to the energy needs engendered by exercise. The relative contribution of each of these fuels at any given time is largely determined by the duration and intensity of the exercise performed.*

During the earliest phase of exercise, muscle glycogen constitutes the major fuel consumed. The rate of glycogenolysis in muscle is most rapid in the first five to ten minutes of exercise. As exercise continues and blood flow to muscle increases, blood-borne substrates become increasingly important sources of energy. Dur-

---

*The intensity of exercise may be graded in absolute terms (watts or kilogram-meters/min; 1 watt=6.135 kg-m/min) or in terms of relative work capacity (per cent of maximal capacity). In the studies described in this review "mild" exercise refers to an intensity of 400 kg-m/min (65 W) or 50 per cent of maximal capacity, and "severe" or "heavy" exercise refers to a work intensity of 1200 kg-m/min (195 W) or 70 to 80 per cent of maximal capacity.

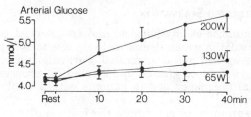

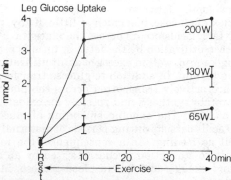

Figure 41. The effect of exercise of varying intensities on blood glucose and leg glucose uptake in normal subjects. Mild exercise = 65 watts (W). Moderate exercise = 130 W. Severe exercise = 200 W. (From Wahren, J., Felig, P., and Hagenfeldt, L.: Diabetologia 14: 213, 1978.)

ing exercise lasting 10 to 40 minutes, glucose uptake by muscle rises markedly above basal levels. The magnitude of this increment, varying from 7- to 20-fold, is determined by the intensity of the work performed (Fig. 41). The rise in glucose utilization is sufficient to account for 30 to 40 per cent of the total oxygen consumption by muscle. The dependence of muscle on blood glucose is thus comparable to free fatty acids, which provide an additional 40 per cent of the oxidizable fuels. Furthermore, by 40 minutes of exercise, blood-borne glucose is responsible for 75 to 90 per cent of the total carbohydrate consumed, reflecting the progressive decline in availability of muscle glycogen as exercise continues. Underscoring the overall importance of exercise as a stimulus to carbohydrate utilization is the observation that total body turnover of glucose is increased two-, three-, and five-fold during mild, moderate, and severe exercise, respectively.

As exercise is continued beyond 40 minutes, the rate of glucose utilization progressively increases, reaching a peak at 90 to 180 minutes and then declining slightly (Fig. 42). In contrast, fatty acid utilization progressively increases in prolonged exercise (Fig. 42). Between one and four hours of exercise there is a 70 per cent rise in the uptake of free fatty acids by muscle. As a consequence, after four hours of continuous mild exercise the relative contribution of fatty acids to total oxygen utilization is twice that of carbohydrate. This increase in uptake of free fatty acids (FFA) is in direct proportion to the inflow of FFA, expressed as the product of arterial concentration and plasma flow. These findings indicate that under normal circumstances FFA uptake by exercising muscle is not primarily regulated by the muscle itself but by external factors such as the rate of FFA mobilization from adipose tissue.

The overall pattern of fuel utilization during mild to moderate exercise extending for prolonged periods may thus be characterized as a triphasic sequence in which muscle glycogen, blood glucose, and free fatty acids successively predominate as the major energy-yielding substrate. With exercise at heavy work loads, there is a more persistent dependence on muscle glycogen. This is suggested by the observation that exhaustion coincides with depletion of muscle glycogen but is not accompanied by significant changes in other physiological parameters such as heart rate, blood pressure, blood levels of glucose and lactate, and muscle electrolyte concentrations. It is unclear, however, why glycogen depletion should coincide with fatigue when large amounts of circulating substrate in the form of fatty acids are still available.

Amino Acid Exchange. In the resting, postabsorptive state, muscle is in negative nitrogen balance. This is reflected by a net output of amino acids, in which alanine and glutamine predominate. The quantitative importance of alanine in muscle amino acid exchange has been ascribed to its synthesis in situ from glucose-derived pyruvate (the glucose-alanine cycle). During exercise, augmented glucose utilization is associated with a rise in alanine output from muscle that is proportional to the intensity of the exercise performed. That the production of alanine in exercise is related to glucose utilization and the availability of pyruvate is suggested by the direct linear correlation between arterial alanine and pyruvate levels. Further evidence of this relationship is provided by McArdle's syndrome, in which the deficiency in muscle phosphorylase and consequent inability to break down glycogen results in decreased levels of pyruvate in muscle tissue. This is accompanied by a net uptake rather than an output of alanine by the exercising leg. In addition, arterial levels of alanine as well as pyruvate and lactate fail to rise during exercise in this disorder.

With respect to the source of the amino groups for alanine synthesis, studies have demonstrated that the branched chain amino acids (leucine, isoleucine, and valine) are preferentially catabolized in muscle tissue rather than the liver. In prolonged exercise, selective uptake of these amino acids by the exercising limb and an accompanying equimolar output from the splanchnic bed have been demonstrated. Since oxidation of each mole of branched chain amino acids provides 32 to 42 moles of ATP, in prolonged exercise leucine, isoleucine, and valine may become important energy-yielding fuels. An additional source of nitrogen for augmented alanine formation in short-term as well as prolonged exercise is ammonia. It has long been recognized that exercise stimulates the formation and release of ammonia from muscle tissue. Recent studies indicate that ammoniagenesis in muscle occurs through a cyclic interconversion of the purine nucleotides adenosine monophosphate (AMP) and inosine monophosphate (IMP). The ammonia thus liberated may be used for the synthesis of glutamate (by the reductive amination of α-ketoglutarate), which subsequently undergoes transamination with pyruvate to form alanine. The functional significance of augmented alanine production may derive from the fact that it provides a nontoxic alternative to ammonia in the transfer of amino groups from the periphery to the liver.

Glucose Production and Blood Glucose Regulation. In mild to moderate exercise of short-term duration blood glucose concentration changes little

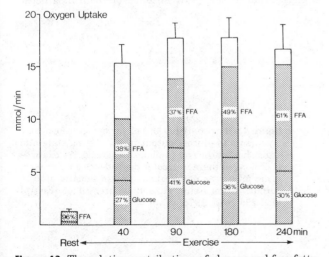

Figure 42. The relative contributions of glucose and free fatty acids (FFA) to total oxygen uptake by the leg during prolonged bicycle ergometer exercise. As exercise is prolonged there is greater dependence on fatty acid oxidation. (From Wahren, J., Felig, P., and Hagenfeldt, L.: Diabetologia 14:213, 1978.)

from the basal state (Fig. 41). With more severe exercise an increment in blood glucose of 20 to 30 mg/dl may be observed. In contrast, exercise extending 90 minutes or more results in a decline in blood glucose of 10 to 40 mg/dl below basal. Frank hypoglycemia (blood glucose <40 mg/dl) is, however, an uncommon occurrence, observed in rare instances in marathon runners, in subjects maintained on a low carbohydrate diet, and occasionally in exercising insulin-treated diabetics.

In view of the stimulation of glucose utilization that characterizes exercise, ongoing repletion of the blood glucose pool can be achieved only by an increase in glucose production by the liver. During short-term exercise, hepatic glucose output increases two- to fivefold depending on the intensity of the work performed and keeps pace with the increment in glucose utilization by muscle tissue. This increase in glucose production is almost entirely a consequence of augmented glycogenolysis inasmuch as splanchnic uptake of gluconeogenic precursors remains unchanged from the resting state, save for a transient rise in lactate consumption. As a consequence of the absolute increment in total glucose production, the relative contribution from gluconeogenesis falls from resting levels of 25 per cent to 16 per cent after 40 minutes of mild exercise (Fig. 43) and to less than 6 per cent with severe exercise. The total amount of glucose released from the liver during 40 minutes of heavy work is estimated to be 18 grams, representing no more than 20 to 25 per cent of the total hepatic glycogen stores in the postabsorptive state.

As exercise extends beyond 40 minutes, slight imbalances between hepatic production and peripheral utilization rates of glucose and increasing reliance on hepatic gluconeogenesis are observed which serve to spare liver glycogen. During prolonged mild exercise, glucose output doubles in the first 40 minutes and thereafter remains constant for the ensuing three to four hours. Since glucose utilization continues to rise for 90 minutes or more (Fig. 42), glucose production fails to keep pace with utilization and a modest decline

in blood glucose concentration is observed (Fig. 44). The relative contribution from gluconeogenesis to overall hepatic glucose output (as inferred from substrate balances across the splanchnic bed) increases from 25 per cent in the basal state to 45 per cent during prolonged exercise, representing a threefold rise in the absolute rate of gluconeogenesis (Fig. 43). Splanchnic uptake of alanine, lactate, and pyruvate is doubled, while glycerol utilization increases tenfold (Fig. 43). These increments are largely a result of augmented fractional extraction. In the case of alanine, fractional extraction by the splanchnic bed increases from resting levels of 35 to 50 per cent to almost 90 per cent in prolonged exercise, a rate that is well in excess of the 50 to 70 per cent extraction rates observed in other circumstances of augmented gluconeogenesis such as diabetes, obesity, and a three-day fast.

Glucoregulatory Hormones. The hormonal response to exercise is characterized by a fall in plasma insulin and an increase in plasma glucagon (Fig. 44). These findings are especially pronounced in prolonged or severe exercise. The decrease in insulin is particularly noteworthy in severe exercise, in which circumstance hypoinsulinemia occurs despite a modest rise in blood glucose. These findings suggest an inhibition in insulin secretion, probably mediated via the adrenergic nervous system. Other hormonal changes occurring in exercise include elevated levels of growth hormone, epinephrine, norepinephrine, and cortisol. Altered levels of catecholamines have been implicated in the hyperglucagonemia of exercise.

The stimulatory effect of exercise on glucose uptake in the face of hypoinsulinemia indicates that such enhancement of glucose consumption is not modulated by an increase in insulin secretion. Further support for this conclusion is provided by the observation of increased glucose utilization during exercise in insulin-withdrawn diabetics. On the other hand, there is evidence that insulin may exert a permissive effect on exercise-induced glucose uptake and that sensitivity to insulin is increased in exercise. In vitro studies suggest that in the total absence of insulin, glucose

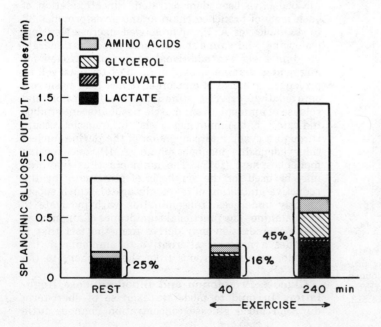

Figure 43. The contributions of various gluconeogenic precursors to glucose output in the resting state and after short-term and prolonged exercise. As exercise is prolonged there is greater dependence on gluconeogenic precursor uptake to maintain hepatic glucose output. (From Felig, P., and Wahren, J.: N Engl J Med 293:1078, 1975.)

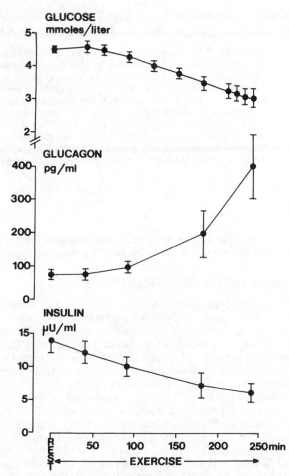

Figure 44. The effect of prolonged exercise on blood glucose, plasma glucagon, and plasma insulin. (From Felig, P., and Wahren, J.: N Engl J Med 293:1073, 1975.)

uptake is not enhanced by muscle contraction. The permissive action of insulin is demonstrable with concentrations of 0.2 to 1.2 μU/ml, which is below the circulating level observed in exercise (Fig. 44). More recent studies in intact man indicate that acute exercise increases the binding of insulin to receptors on monocytes. If similar changes can be shown to occur in muscle cells, augmented glucose uptake in exercise and after physical training may be mediated in part by enhanced sensitivity to insulin.

The physiological significance of the altered hormonal milieu in exercise relates more to the stimulation of hepatic glucose production than the enhancement of glucose utilization. Studies in intact man have demonstrated the exquisite sensitivity of hepatic glycogenolysis to the inhibitory action of small increments in insulin. The importance of the hypoinsulinemia of exercise thus derives from its enhancement of hepatic glycogenolysis. In prolonged or severe exercise, the rise in glucagon and the increments in growth hormone and catecholamines also contribute to the glycogenolytic and gluconeogenic response. However, neither hypoinsulinemia, hyperglucagonemia, nor altered adrenergic activity alone are solely responsible for the exercise-induced stimulation of hepatic glucose output. In short-term exercise, prevention of the usual fall in plasma insulin concentration by infusion of glucose

fails to abolish the rise in glucose output. In prolonged exercise, a doubling of splanchnic glucose output is demonstrable in mild exercise although elevations in epinephrine, norepinephrine and glucagon are not consistently noted with such workloads.

POSTEXERCISE RECOVERY

Glucose Metabolism. Upon cessation of exercise there is a redistribution of blood flow characterized by a fall in perfusion of the previously exercising limbs and increased flow to the splanchnic bed. The overall effect of the immediate recovery phase on glucose metabolism is to initiate repletion of glycogen stores in muscle as well as liver. Glucose uptake by muscle remains three- to fourfold above basal levels for at least 40 minutes after stopping exercise. In the absence of augmented lactate release or oxygen consumption, these findings suggest a resynthesis of muscle glycogen. Repletion of liver glycogen is facilitated by a fairly rapid decline in splanchnic glucose output, which reaches basal levels by 40 minutes. Simultaneously there is an augmented splanchnic uptake of gluconeogenic substrates. This is particularly prominent in the case of lactate and pyruvate. Splanchnic uptake of these glucose precursors during recovery exceeds the rates observed during exercise and is three- to fourfold greater than in the basal state. Smaller increments are observed for splanchnic alanine uptake. This augmentation in precursor utilization is a consequence of a rise in splanchnic blood flow and elevations in arterial levels as well as an increased fractional extraction rate. The net effect is a doubling of the proportion of glucose output attributable to gluconeogenesis as compared with the resting state. Repletion of liver glycogen thus appears to begin even in the absence of glucose ingestion by means of augmented recycling to glucose of glucose-derived carbon skeletons. In addition to glycogen synthesis, increased hepatic utilization of glycolytic intermediates has the effect of reducing arterial lactate levels, which may reach peak concentrations during exercise of 2 to 10 mmoles/liter depending upon the severity of the work performed and the training of the subjects.

The hormonal response in the early recovery period is characterized by a rapid increase in insulin levels within the first two to ten minutes of the recovery phase, perhaps mediated via a cessation of inhibitory adrenergic signals. In view of the marked sensitivity of hepatic glycogenolysis to insulin, the rise in insulin may be a major factor responsible for the decline in hepatic glucose output to basal levels. In contrast to the rapid changes in circulating insulin, glucagon concentrations remain elevated in the early recovery period and may thereby contribute to the augmented hepatic uptake of gluconeogenic precursors.

The effects of prior exercise on body fuel metabolism are observed not only during the immediate recovery period (10 to 40 minutes) but persists for at least 12 hours after exercise. These effects are particularly noticeable with regard to glycogen metabolism in liver and muscle tissue. During exercise there is depletion of muscle as well as liver glycogen. In the 12- to 14-hour period following exercise, muscle glycogen stores increase 50 per cent or more even in the absence of food intake. This repletion of muscle glycogen in the

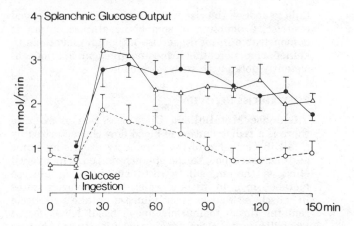

4 ┐ Splanchnic Glucose Output

m mol/min

Glucose
Ingestion

0   30   60   90   120   150 min

Figure 45. The stimulatory effect of prior exercise on the splanchnic glucose response to oral glucose ingestion. Nonexercised controls: ○----○; glucose ingestion immediately (●——●) or 14 to 15 hours after exercise (△——△). During the postexercise recovery period there was a doubling of the release of glucose from the splanchnic bed to peripheral tissues. The greater glucose release enhances repletion of muscle glycogen in the postexercise recovery period. (From Maehlum, S., Felig, P., and Wahren, J.: Am J Physiol 235:E255, 1978.)

face of starvation thus must occur at the expense of further depletion of liver glycogen or as a result of accelerated hepatic gluconeogenesis.

When carbohydrate is ingested in the postexercise recovery period, there also is selective uptake of glucose by muscle rather than hepatic tissues (Fig. 45). The extra glucose released to the periphery can be accounted for in its virtual entirety as being utilized for the repletion of muscle glycogen. The regulatory signals responsible for the siphoning of ingested glucose by muscle in the recovery period have not been established. Clearly, the insulin and glucagon response to ingested glucose in the recovery period is no different from that observed in unexercised subjects. Furthermore, since these effects of prior exercise persist for 12 to 14 hours they are unlikely to be due to acute exercise-induced elevations in catecholamines, which are only transient in nature.

Protein Catabolism and Anabolism. As noted above, prolonged exercise and the recovery period after brief exercise are associated with augmented utilization of alanine by the liver for gluconeogenesis. In addition, increased consumption of branched chain amino acids by muscle, presumably for oxidation as energy-yielding fuels, is observed in prolonged exercise. To the extent that there is a net flow of branched chain amino acids from liver to muscle, this catabolic effect occurs at the expense of liver rather than muscle protein. Regardless of the site of proteolysis, exercise would consequently be expected to result in negative nitrogen balance. Early studies, however, failed to demonstrate an increase in urinary nitrogen loss during exercise. More recent data, however, reveal a 60 per cent increase in urea production and in blood urea nitrogen concentration during prolonged, severe exercise in well-trained subjects (cross-country skiers). The failure to observe similar evidence of protein catabolism in earlier studies may relate to the sensitivity of the techniques employed. In addition, intermittent exercise of mild intensity may differ from more severe, sustained exercise with respect to its action on protein catabolism.

In contrast to the transient catabolic effects of continuous, prolonged exercise and the early postexercise recovery period, the long-term effect of repeated bouts of exercise is protein anabolism manifested by muscle hypertrophy. This hypertrophic action is demonstrable even in the face of starvation. The anabolic effects of repeated contraction have been shown to occur in resting muscle and to involve an inhibition in protein catabolism as well as stimulation of protein synthesis.

GLUCOSE FEEDING AND EXERCISE

The preceding discussion has indicated that during exercise changes in fuel metabolism and hormonal secretion are reminiscent of the response to starvation but occur in a much more rapid time frame. This concept of exercise as an accelerated form of starvation is underscored by the effects of glucose ingestion either prior to or during prolonged exercise.

When 100 grams of glucose are ingested prior to the initiation of prolonged exercise, the fuel as well as hormonal response to exercise is markedly altered. In glucose-fed subjects, arterial glucose levels are 30 to 40 per cent higher than in controls, while free fatty acid levels, which show a progressive threefold rise throughout exercise in controls, show little if any increment in the glucose-fed group. Glucose uptake by the exercising leg is 40 to 100 per cent higher in the glucose-fed subjects, accounting for 50 to 60 per cent of oxygen consumption as compared with 25 to 40 per cent in controls. Uptake of gluconeogenic substrates by the splanchnic bed is reduced by 60 to 100 per cent as compared with unfed controls. The hormonal response is characterized by plasma insulin levels that are two- to threefold higher than in controls, while plasma glucagon levels fail to demonstrate the fourfold increment observed in unfed, exercise controls. A similar effect on substrate and hormone levels is observed if glucose is fed after 90 minutes of exercise, which is then continued for an additional two hours.

Thus the effect of glucose feeding before or during exercise is further stimulation of glucose uptake by exercising muscle and inhibition of lipolysis and gluconeogenesis. These changes appear to be mediated by the hyperinsulinemia and relative hypoglucagonemia induced by glucose feeding. Provision of exogenous carbohydrate substrate thus overrides the stimulatory action of exercise on lipolysis and gluconeogenesis.

REFERENCES

Exercise

Ahlborg, G., and Felig, P.: Substrate utilization during prolonged exercise preceded by the ingestion of glucose. Am J Physiol 233:E188, 1977.

Ahlborg, G., Felig, P., Hagenfeldt, L., Hendler, R., and Wahren, J.: Substrate turnover during prolonged exercise in man. Splanchnic and leg metabolism of glucose, free fatty acids and amino acids. J Clin Invest 53:1080, 1974.

Berger, M., Hagg, S., and Ruderman, N. B.: Glucose metabolism in perfused skeletal muscle. Interaction of insulin and exercise on glucose uptake. Biochem J 146:231, 1975.

Felig, P., and Wahren, J.: Amino acid metabolism in exercising man. J Clin Invest 50:2703, 1971.

Felig, P., and Wahren, J.: Fuel homeostasis in exercise. (Seminars of the Beth Israel Hospital). N Engl J Med 293:1078, 1975.

Felig, P., Ali-Cherif, M. S., Minagawa, A, and Wahren, J.: Hypoglycemia during prolonged exercise in normal man. N Engl J Med 306:895, 1982.

Felig, P., and Wahren, J.: Role of insulin and glucagon in the regulation of hepatic glucose production during exercise. Diabetes 28(Suppl. 1):71, 1979.

Galbo, H., Holst, J. J., and Christensen, N. J.: Glucagon and plasma catecholamine responses to graded and prolonged exercise in man. J Appl Physiol 38:70, 1975.

Goldberg, A. L.: Relationship between hormones and muscular work in determining muscle size. In Alfred, N. (ed.): Cardiac Hypertrophy. New York, Academic Press, 1971, p. 39.

Hagenfeldt, L., and Wahren, J.: Metabolism of free fatty acids and ketone bodies in skeletal muscle. In Pernow, B., and Saltin, B.: Muscle Metabolism During Exercise. New York, Plenum Press, 1971, p. 153.

Hartley, L. H., Mason, J. W., Hogan, R. P., Jones, L. G., Kotchen, T. A., Mougey, E. H., Wherry, F. E., Pennington, L. I., and Rickets, P. T.: Multiple hormonal responses to graded exercise in relation to physical training. J Appl Physiol 33:602, 1972.

Hultman, E.: Studies on muscle metabolism of glycogen and active phosphates in man with special reference to exercise and diet. Scan J Clin Lab Invest 19: Supplement 94:1, 1967.

LeBlanc, J., Nadeau, A., Boulay, M., and Rousseau-Migneron, S.: Effects of physical training and adiposity on glucose metabolism and 125I-insulin binding. J Appl Physiol 46:235, 1979.

Lowenstein, J. M.: Ammonia production in muscle and other tissues: The purine nucleotide cycle. Physiol Rev 52:382, 1972.

Maehlum, S., Felig, P., and Wahren, J.: Splanchnic glucose and muscle glycogen after glucose feeding during post-exercise recovery. Am J Physiol 235:E255, 1978.

Refsum, H. E., and Stromme, S. B.: Urea and creatinine production and excretion in urine during and after prolonged heavy exercise. Scand J Clin Lab Invest 33:247, 1974.

Rennie, M. J., Jennet, S. M., and Johnson, R. H.: The metabolic effects of strenuous exercise: A comparison between untrained subjects and racing cyclists. Q J Exp Physiol 59:201, 1974.

Simonson, D. C., Koivisto, V., Sherwin, R. S., Ferrannini, E., Hendler, R., Juhlin-Dannfelt, A., and DeFronzo, R. A.: Adrenergic blockade alters glucose kinetics during exercise in insulin-dependent diabetics. J Clin Invest 73:1648, 1984.

Wahren, J., Felig, P., Ahlborg, G., and Jorfeldt, L.: Glucose metabolism during leg exercise in man. J Clin Invest 50:2715, 1971.

Wahren, J., Felig, P., Hendler, R., and Ahlborg, G.: Glucose and amino acid metabolism during recovery after exercise. J Appl Physiol 34:838, 1973.

Wahren, J., Hagenfeldt, L., and Felig, P.: Splanchnic and leg exchange of glucose, amino acids, and free fatty acids during exercise in diabetes mellitus. J Clin Invest 55:1303, 1975.

OBESITY

Obesity is one of the most common disorders of body fuel metabolism encountered in humans. While malnutrition and undernutrition remain important causes of mortality and morbidity in many parts of the world, obesity has become a progressively more important public health problem because of its association with diabetes, hypertension, hyperlipidemia, and coronary artery disease. It has been estimated that in the United States 30 per cent of men and 40 per cent of women are 20 pounds or more overweight.

DEFINITION

All forms of obesity are characterized by an increase in body fat. Under normal circumstances, body fat (triglyceride-containing adipose tissue) accounts for 15 to 20 per cent of body weight in men and 20 to 25 per cent in women. In obese subjects this value is abnormally increased. Inasmuch as large population studies fail to show a bimodal distribution in body fat mass with an abrupt cutoff between "normal" and "obese" subjects, the magnitude of the increase in adiposity that is necessary to constitute an "abnormal" increase is somewhat arbitrary.

Actuarial statistics reveal that the body weight (for a given height, frame, and sex) associated with the lowest mortality is the average body weight observed at age 25. This weight is generally referred to as the "ideal body weight" (beyond age 25 the average body weight increases progressively until the sixth or seventh decade and this cannot be equated with ideal weight). Since caloric storage as carbohydrate (glycogen) is virtually nil, and only a very moderate amount of calories are stored as protein, an increase in body weight (in the absence of fluid retention or marked muscular hypertrophy) is almost entirely due to an increase in body fat.

The quantitative considerations are such that for a 70 kg man, a 25 per cent increase in weight above ideal (17.5 kg) results in a doubling of body fat mass (14 kg → 28 kg) (Table 11). In more severe circumstances in which total body weight is twice ideal, there is a fivefold increase in body fat (Table 11). From a practical standpoint, an increase in body weight of 10 kg or more above ideal, which is generally associated with an increase in fat mass of 50 per cent or more, may be taken as evidence of obesity.

It should be noted that measurement of body fat is not easily accomplished in the clinical setting. Studies using isotopically labeled potassium (40_k) for measurements of lean body mass or body densitometric measurements using underwater weighing are time-consuming and require specialized techniques. Measurements of skin-fold thickness using calipers provide a more practical approach but are quite variable and difficult to standardize. Thus the most readily available means of diagnosing obesity is based on body weight and actuarial tables of ideal weight.

TABLE 11. BODY FAT MASS IN OBESITY

	NONOBESE	MILD OBESITY	MARKED OBESITY
Body weight, kg	70	90	140
Ideal weight, per cent	100	130	200
Body fat, kg	14	28	70
Body fat, kcal	132,000	264,000	658,000

Pathogenesis

An increase in body fat is a consequence of an imbalance in caloric homeostasis in which intake exceeds energy expenditure. Since, as noted above, the capacity for storage of calories as carbohydrate is extremely small (~1000 kcal), and since protein mass increases only moderately in response to dietary excess, virtually all of the calories stored when there is positive energy balance are in the form of triglyceride in adipocytes.

The factors influencing the storage of triglyceride are summarized in Figure 46. Intake of glucose or fat in the diet results in the delivery of fatty acids to adipose tissue. Most of the synthesis of fatty acids from dietary carbohydrate occurs in the liver. The fatty acids are released to the circulation as very low density lipoprotein (VLDL). Additional triglycerides derived from dietary fat absorbed in the intestine enter the circulation as chylomicrons. At the adipocyte the enzyme lipoprotein lipase catalyzes the release of fatty acids from circulating lipoproteins, permitting their uptake by the fat cell. Resynthesis of triglyceride within the adipocyte also requires the uptake of glucose, which is converted to α-glycerol-phosphate (glycerol-3-phosphate). The latter combines with free fatty acids to form triglyceride. Simultaneous with triglyceride synthesis there is ongoing breakdown of triglyceride to free fatty acids and glycerol, a reaction catalyzed by a hormone-sensitive tissue lipase. The free fatty acids released to the circulation are then taken up by skeletal muscle, heart, liver, and, to a lesser extent, kidney, where they are important oxidative fuels. The major factor determining fat synthesis is thus dietary intake. The major determinants of fat utilization are the basal metabolic rate and the extent of voluntary activity, notably muscular exercise.

Theoretically, an increase in body fat could result from an increase in caloric intake (overeating), a decrease in caloric expenditure (underactivity), or a combination of the two. While the role of these factors in the genesis of obesity is not fully established, the majority of evidence suggests that increased fat accumulation is in most cases due to an increase in caloric intake. Indeed the basal metabolic rate in obese subjects (by virtue of their increased body surface area) is greater than in lean individuals. On the other hand, the tendency for obese subjects to shun physical exertion may help *perpetuate* already existent obesity.

The possibility has long been considered that obese individuals have some metabolic abnormality that permits a more efficient utilization of food and consequently a greater storage of ingested calories. Indeed studies with lean individuals made obese by the ingestion of an extremely high caloric intake (5000 to 6000 kcal/day) reveal marked individual differences in the rate of weight gain despite identical food intake and similar physical activity. Differences in the thermic response to food ingestion (specific dynamic action) have been postulated as a possible mechanism for these variations in efficiency of storage of ingested calories but remain unproven. In a genetic form of obesity in the mouse (ob/ob mouse) lack of a thyroid-dependent sodium, potassium ATPase, has been observed, allowing for increased efficiency with which ATP is utilized. A similar defect in Na-K ATPase activity has been reported in red blood cells of obese patients. However, such an abnormality has not been consistently observed and does not appear to extend to metabolically active tissues (e.g., liver).

FAT HOMEOSTASIS IN MAN

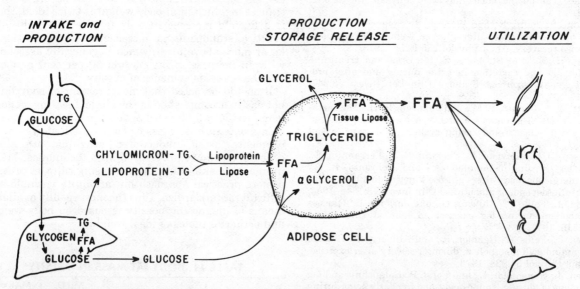

Figure 46. Fat homeostasis in normal man. TG = triglyceride. FFA = free fatty acids. The liver is a major site of the synthesis of fat, which is released as the triglyceride moiety of lipoproteins. The adipose cell is the major storage reservoir of fat. Release of fatty acids from the adipose cell depends on the activity of a hormone-sensitive tissue lipase. The free fatty acids released to the circulation are largely oxidized by skeletal and cardiac muscle and to a smaller extent by kidney and liver. (From Sherwin, R., and Felig, P.: Med Clin North Am 62:695, 1978.)

Regardless of whether the imbalance in caloric homeostasis is due primarily to changes in intake or expenditure, theoretically an increase in adiposity may result from an increase in size of fat cells, an increase in number, or a combination of the two. Studies of fat tissue obtained by biopsy technique have revealed that all forms of human obesity are characterized by an increase in fat cell size. On the other hand, an increase in cell number is generally observed in infantile or juvenile-onset obesity (hyperplastic, hypertrophic obesity). Except for massively obese patients, adult-onset obesity is characterized by a normal number of adipose cells (hypertrophic obesity). The corollary of these observations is that in youth-onset obesity the patient is destined to go through life with an increase in number of fat cells regardless of body weight. It has been suggested that this morphologic alteration through some undetermined mechanism may play a role in the perpetuation of obesity (the "adipose cell hypothesis").

INSULIN SECRETION

While a variety of hormones may affect the adipocyte, consideration of the various reactions in carbohydrate and fat metabolism that contribute to an increase in triglyceride storage (Fig. 46) indicates that insulin is the key hormone modulating an increment in body fat. An increase in insulin has the following effects: (a) stimulation of fatty acid synthesis from carbohydrate (a process that in humans occurs primarily in the liver); (b) stimulation of lipoprotein lipase allowing transfer of free fatty acids from circulating lipoproteins to the adipose cell; (c) stimulation of glucose uptake and utilization by the fat cell, thereby providing the α-glycerol-phosphate (glycerol-3-phosphate) necessary for esterification to form triglyceride; (d) inhibition of the hormone-sensitive tissue lipase within the adipocyte, thereby preventing the escape of fatty acids from adipose tissue.

A variety of studies have demonstrated that insulin secretion is increased in obesity (Fig. 47). The hyperinsulinemia is present in the fasting state as well as in the fed condition. An exaggerated insulin response is observed regardless of whether the stimulus is glucose, protein, or amino acids.

The precise mechanism whereby obesity results in hyperinsulinemia has not been established. Clearly adiposity rather than a change in lean body mass is the major factor, inasmuch as muscular weight lifters (who are above "ideal" weight) are not hyperinsulinemic. On the other hand, adiposity is not of itself a sufficient stimulus, since plasma insulin levels fall to normal in association with substantial weight loss and/or a restriction in carbohydrate intake well before body weight has reached normal levels. Thus it is both the patient's feeding behavior (hyperphagia, particularly involving carbohydrate) and increase in adipose tissue mass that are necessary for the development of hyperinsulinemia.

Since insulin promotes fat storage, it has been suggested that hyperinsulinemia may be the primary pathogenetic abnormality. Indeed in patients with insulin-producing tumors of the pancreas (insulinomas), weight gain is a characteristic finding. However, as noted above, a decrease in feeding results in a nor-

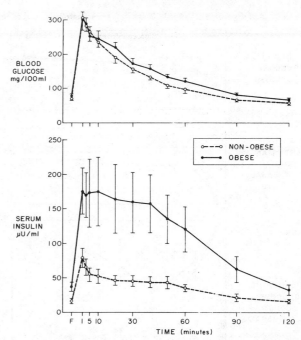

Figure 47. Blood glucose and serum insulin response to intravenous administration of glucose in nonobese and obese subjects. The obese subjects are hyperinsulinemic in the fasting state (F) as well as after glucose administration. (From Felig, P., et al.: N Engl J Med 281:811, 1969.)

malization of insulin secretion in obese subjects. Furthermore, in experimental obesity produced by a marked increase in caloric intake by lean subjects, the hyperinsulinemia of spontaneous obesity is reproduced. Thus, changes in insulin secretion in obesity are a metabolic consequence rather than a cause of overfeeding and fat accumulation.

INSULIN RESISTANCE

Despite the cardinal role of insulin in promoting the metabolic reactions necessary for fat storage, once obesity is manifest and is accompanied by hyperinsulinemia, there is a decrease in tissue sensitivity to the action of insulin. As shown in Figure 47, despite an increase in fasting plasma insulin concentration, obese subjects are not hypoglycemic.

The decrease in tissue sensitivity to insulin is manifest in all the target tissues of insulin action—namely, adipose tissue, muscle, and liver. In adipose tissue insulin resistance appears to be related to an increase in fat cell size. In muscle the decrease in insulin action not only interferes with glucose uptake but also enhances net amino acid release by muscle, thereby contributing to the hyperaminoacidemia of obesity. The resistance to insulin on the part of liver is indicated by the observation that comparable increments in insulin are less effective in inhibiting glucose output by the liver in obese subjects as compared with lean controls (Fig. 48).

With regard to the mechanism of insulin resistance in obesity, in experimental animals as well as human obesity a decrease in insulin binding to its receptor on adipocytes, liver, muscle, and circulating monocytes have been observed. Despite the fact that the monocyte

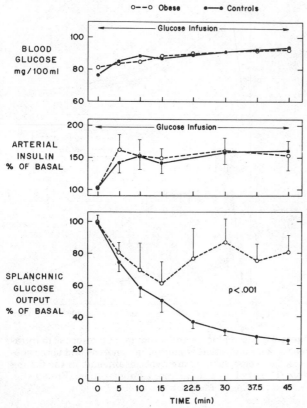

o--o Obese   •--• Controls

Figure 48. The splanchnic glucose response to equivalent increments in plasma glucose and insulin in obese and non-obese subjects. Whereas net splanchnic glucose output fell 75 to 80 per cent in controls, it declined no more than 40 per cent in the obese subjects. These findings provide evidence of resistance on the part of the liver to insulin action in obesity. (From Felig, P., et al.: J Clin Invest 53:582, 1974.)

is not a target cell of insulin action, decreased insulin binding to the monocyte correlates directly with in vivo insulin action in obese subjects in the postabsorptive state. However, studies in obese rats have provided evidence for postreceptor defects that are not correctable with maxillary effective doses of insulin. Thus it is likely that receptor as well as postreceptor events mediate the insulin resistance of obesity.

A major unresolved question in obesity is whether hyperinsulinemia is a cause or a consequence of insulin resistance. Studies demonstrating that an increase in the concentration of insulin may of itself reduce insulin binding suggest that hyperinsulinemia secondarily brings about insulin resistance. The studies demonstrating the requirement for hyperphagia in general and carbohydrate feeding in particular (potent stimuli of beta cell secretion), for hyperinsulinemia to be manifest in obesity, also suggest that hypersecretion is an antecedent of, rather than a response to, insulin resistance.

OBESITY AND DIABETES

It is well recognized that obesity is present in most non–insulin dependent diabetics and that the incidence of diabetes is significantly increased among obese patients. Since hyperinsulinemia and insulin resistance coexist in obesity, for most obese subjects the net result

is maintenance of normal glucose tolerance. However, in those subjects in whom hypersecretion of insulin cannot be maintained (presumably because of an inherited defect in beta cell function) diabetes ultimately develops. Obesity thus increases the likelihood of diabetes by increasing the demand for insulin secretion because of the accompanying insulin resistance. Although obese diabetics have been described as having an excess of insulin, hyperinsulinemia is more apparent than real. When comparison is made with weight-matched obese subjects with normal glucose tolerance, obese diabetics have a decreased insulin response. The relationship between insulin secretion, insulin resistance, and obesity is discussed further in Diabetes, pp. 379–381.

REFERENCES

Obesity

Bessard, T., Schutz, Y., and J'Equier, E.: Energy expenditure and thermogenesis in obese women before and after weight loss. Am J Clin Nutr 38:680, 1983.

Bray, G. A., Schwartz, M., and Rozin, R.: Relationships between oxygen consumption and body composition in obesity. Metabolism 19:418, 1970.

Bullen, B. A., Reed, R. B., and Mayer, J.: Physical activity of obese and nonobese adolescent girls appraised by motion picture sampling. Am J Clin Nutr 14:211, 1964.

Felig, P., Wahren, J., and Hendler, R.: Splanchnic glucose and amino acid metabolism in obesity. J Clin Invest 53:582, 1974.

Grey, N., and Kipnis, D. M.: Effect of diet composition on the hyperinsulinemia of obesity. N Engl J Med 285:837, 1975.

Hirsch, J.: The adipose cell hypothesis. N Engl J Med 295:389, 1976.

Hirsch, J., and Batchelor, B.: Adipose tissue cellularity in human obesity. Clin Endocrinol Metab 5:299, 1976.

Kolterman, O. G., Insel, J., Saekow, M., and Olefsky, J. M.: Mechanisms of insulin resistance in human obesity—evidence for receptor and postreceptor defects. J Clin Invest 65:1273, 1980.

Rabinowitz, D.: Some endocrine and metabolic aspects of obesity. Ann Res Med 21:241, 1970.

Rothwell, N. J., and Stock, M. J.: A role for brown fat adipose tissue in diet-induced thermogenesis. Nature (Lond.) 281:31, 1979.

Salans, L. B., Bray, G. A., Cushman, S. W., Danforth, E., Jr., Glennon, J. A., Horton, E. S., and Sims, E. A. H.: Glucose metabolism and the response to insulin by human adipose tissue in spontaneous and experimental obesity. J Clin Invest 53:848, 1974.

Salans, L. B., Cushman, S. W., and Weismann, R. E.: Studies of human adipose tissue: Adipose cell size and number in nonobese and obese patients. J Clin Invest 52:929, 1973.

Sims, E. A. H., Danforth, E., Jr., Horton, E. S., Bray, G. A., Glennon, J., and Salans, L. B.: Effects of experimental obesity in man. Recent Prog Horm Res 29:457, 1972.

Sims, E. A. H.: Experimental obesity, dietary-induced thermogenesis and their clinical implications. Clin Endocrinol Metab 5:377, 1976.

York, D. A., Bray, G. A., and Yukimura, Y.: An enzymatic defect in the obese (ob/ob) mouse: Loss of thyroid induced sodium and potassium dependent adenosine-triphosphatase. Proc Natl Acad Sci 75:497, 1978.

DIABETES MELLITUS

DEFINITION AND CLASSIFICATION

Diabetes mellitus is a generalized, chronic metabolic disorder manifesting itself in its fully developed form

TABLE 12. CLASSIFICATION OF DIABETES

	TYPE 1 DIABETES	TYPE 2 DIABETES
Synonyms	Juvenile Onset	Maturity Onset
Age of onset	Usually before 30	Usually after 40*
Type of onset	Frequently sudden	Usually gradual
Presentation	Polydipsia, polyuria	Often asymptomatic
Body weight	Thin	Usually (80%) obese
Ketoacidosis	Ketosis-prone	Ketosis-resistant
Control of diabetes	Difficult; brittle	Generally easy
Control by diet alone	Not possible	Frequent
Control by oral agents	Not possible	Frequent
Long-term complications	Frequent	Frequent

*When present in youngsters (before age 20), non-insulin dependent diabetes is often referred to as maturity onset diabetes of youth (MODY).

by hyperglycemia, glycosuria, increased protein breakdown, ketosis, and acidosis. If the disease is prolonged, it is usually complicated by degenerative changes of the blood vessels, the retina, the kidneys, and the nervous system.

It is common practice to divide diabetics into two major categories. *Type I diabetes* is characterized as an insulin-dependent, ketosis-prone state with onset generally before age 25 to 30 in individuals who are not obese. In *type 2 diabetes,* there is resistance to ketosis, treatment with insulin is generally not necessary, onset is usually after age 40, and 70 per cent or more of patients are obese (Table 12). Recently, a third type of spontaneous diabetes has been described under the term *maturity-onset diabetes of youth* (MODY). In this group a ketosis-resistant, non–insulin dependent, generally asymptomatic form of diabetes is present in individuals before age 25. These classifications admit many exceptions. For example, some older diabetics are ketosis-prone and insulin-dependent. While the different clinical types of diabetes have previously been thought to represent only quantitative differences in the disorder in insulin secretion or action, more recent findings suggest heterogeneity in spontaneous diabetes with respect to patterns of inheritance, and the relative importance of acquired factors such as viral infections, autoimmunity, and obesity in the etiology of these syndromes. Thus spontaneous diabetes is manifest not only in a variety of clinical patterns but probably is a consequence of a variety of etiological factors.

INSULIN SECRETION

The importance of insulin deficiency in the pathophysiology of diabetes mellitus has been firmly established since the studies of Minkowski in pancreatectomized animals and the epoch-making discovery of insulin by Banting and Best over 50 years ago. Later work by Houssay and by Long and Lukens indicated that pituitary and adrenal hormones interfere with the action of insulin and may contribute to hyperglycemia. The subsequent introduction of radioimmunoassay techniques for the measurement of polypeptide hormones led to the demonstration that insulin deficiency characterizes type 1 diabetes and most forms of type 2 diabetes. More recently, techniques have been developed for evaluating the in vivo action of insulin. Such studies have rekindled interest in the role of insulin resistance in type 2 diabetes. In addition, a host of new data have accumulated regarding the contribution of glucagon to the diabetic syndrome. Current evidence, however, favors the concept that a relative or absolute deficiency in the insulin secretory mechanism of the beta cell is the predominant or primary lesion in most forms of diabetes.

In type 1 diabetes, insulin secretion is either totally defective or severely impaired. Endogenous insulin production in these patients generally varies inversely with the duration of the disease. In fact, endogenous insulin secretion, as determined from circulating C-peptide levels, is generally not detectable in type 1 diabetics who have received exogenous insulin therapy for more than five years (Fig. 49). Correlating with this functional disability is the frequent anatomic evidence of hyalinization and fibrosis of the islets in type 1 diabetics of long standing. Despite its severity, the secretory deficiency in the type 1 diabetic is often temporarily reversible in its initial stages, as indicated by the tendency toward remission ("honeymoon phase" or Brush effect). This remission is characterized by a temporary partial restoration of insulin secretion as assessed by studies of C-peptide release. The extent to which residual insulin secretion is maintained in the insulin-requiring diabetic is perhaps the major factor that distinguishes the more readily manageable patient from the "brittle" diabetic.

In the type 2 diabetic the secretory failure is less severe. Basal insulin concentration is generally normal or increased, whereas glucose-stimulated insulin secretion is generally diminished. In its mildest forms the beta-cell defect involves only the initial secretory phase; the slower insulin response remains intact. In such individuals the loss of responsiveness to glucose is demonstrable despite normal responsiveness to secretagogues such as beta-adrenergic stimulation. These observations suggest a specific abnormality of glucose recognition in the beta cell in the earliest stages of diabetes. Of note is the fact that reduced insulin secretion in diabetes mellitus cannot be explained on the basis of diminished secretion of gastrointestinal hormones with insulinogenic activity. In fact, GIP release after glucose ingestion is augmented in diabetes.

It is of interest that the initial reports by Berson and Yalow regarding plasma insulin levels in type 2 diabetes emphasized the presence of hyperinsulinemia. The seeming hyperinsulinemia of the type 2 diabetic was subsequently shown to be more apparent than real when body weight and ambient blood glucose levels are considered. Approximately 80 per cent of type 2 diabetics are obese, and obesity per se is accompanied by hyperinsulinemia. In fact, when comparison is made between obese type 2 diabetics and an appropriate weight-matched nondiabetic control group, it

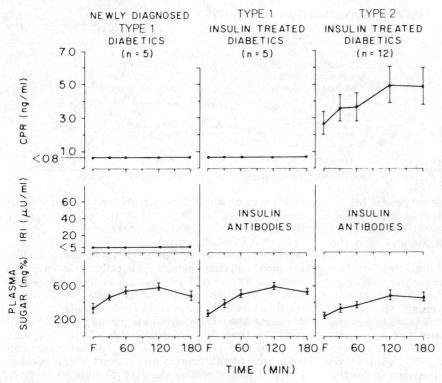

Figure 49. Influence of glucose administration on serum C-peptide reactivity (CPR) and insulin immunoreactivity (IRI) in type 1 and type 2 insulin-treated diabetic subjects. The presence of insulin antibodies precludes serum insulin measurement in the diabetics. However, measurement of serum C-peptide indicates that residual islet cell function is nil in the type 1 diabetics. (From Block, M. B., et al.: Diabetes 21:1013, 1972.)

becomes apparent that insulin levels in obese diabetics are clearly below those observed in obese subjects with normal glucose tolerance (Fig. 50). Obesity acts as a diabetogenic factor because the accompanying insulin resistance increases the demand for insulin.

In the nonobese type 2 diabetic, insulin secretion is somewhat variable. In most such patients, the seeming hyperinsulinism is a consequence of the accompanying hyperglycemia. In other words, when the glucose tolerance curve of the mild diabetic is simulated in the normal individual the insulin response is substantially greater than that of the diabetic. On the other hand,

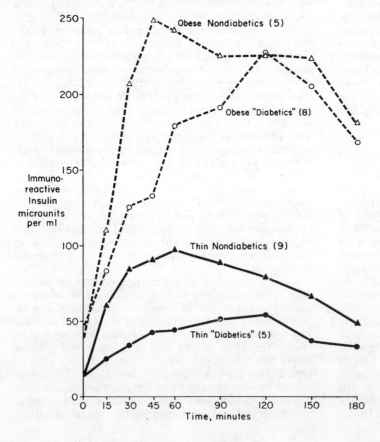

Figure 50. Serum immunoreactive insulin (IRI) responses to oral glucose administration in obese subjects with and without type 2 diabetes and in nonobese subjects with and without type 2 diabetes. When compared with weight matched controls, the type 2 diabetics are generally insulin deficient, particularly during the first hour after glucose administration. (From Bagdade, J. D., et al.: J Clin Invest 46:1549, 1967.)

in some mild type 2 diabetics hyperinsulinemia may not be accounted for by either obesity or hyperglycemia. In such patients altered sensitivity to insulin (insulin resistance) may be an important pathogenetic factor.

INSULIN RESISTANCE IN DIABETES MELLITUS

The biological action of insulin is not only related to the concentration of this hormone in the interstitial fluid of target tissues, but is also a function of the ability of insulin to activate cellular events. The first step in the cellular action of insulin is the binding of the hormone to a specific receptor on the cell surface. Resistance to endogenous and exogenous insulin in obese man is associated with a reduction in insulin receptors on adipocytes and circulating mononuclear cells. A decrease in the concentration of insulin receptors has also been reported in the plasma membranes of adipocytes, muscle cells, and hepatocytes from obese animals. On the basis of these studies it has been suggested that decreased insulin binding to target tissues contributes to the insulin resistance observed in obesity. Altered binding, however, is only one of many factors that may influence insulin action. For example, following starvation and refeeding the close relationship between insulin binding and insulin action is lost. The rate-limiting step in such circumstances involves postreceptor intracellular events.

With respect to insulin resistance in diabetes, reduced insulin binding to circulating mononuclear cells has been observed in type 2 diabetics, particularly when basal hyperinsulinemia is present. Furthermore, in vivo resistance to the action of insulin has been reported in such patients using a variety of insulin infusion techniques involving euglycemic hyperinsulinemia (Fig. 51). Because this resistance is not overcome by maximal doses of insulin, which should overcome a deficiency of insulin receptors, it is thought that an impairment of postreceptor events is a major component of insulin resistance in type 2 diabetes.

Overall, the available data suggest the presence of heterogeneity with respect to insulin sensitivity as well as insulin secretion in type 2 diabetes. In most circumstances, type 2 diabetes is brought about by a failure of insulin secretion to keep pace with the augmented demands for insulin engendered by obesity. However, in some patients insulin resistance may be present even in the absence of obesity and may bring about diabetes despite hypersecretion of insulin.

Severe resistance to the action of insulin may develop secondarily in diabetic patients who have been treated with insulin for months or years. This uncommon clinical event may be due to marked overproduction of antibodies to exogenous insulin. Even less commonly, severe insulin resistance may be due to a decrease in the number of insulin receptors on target tissues or the presence of a circulating antibody to the insulin receptor. For reasons that are unclear, such patients also have acanthosis nigricans, an increase in pigmentation and coarsening of skin folds in the neck and axilla. It is likely that future studies will uncover patients in whom severe insulin resistance is a consequence of postreceptor intracellular defects.

METABOLIC DYSFUNCTION

The metabolic alterations observed in diabetes primarily reflect the degree to which there is an absolute or relative deficiency of insulin. Viewed in the context of the role of insulin as the major storage hormone, a minimal deficiency results in a diminished ability to increase the storage reservoir of body fuels because of inadequate disposal of ingested foodstuffs (for example, glucose intolerance). With a major deficiency of insulin, not only is fuel accumulation hampered in the fed state, but excessive mobilization of endogenous metabolic fuels also occurs in the fasting condition (for example, fasting hyperglycemia, hyperaminoacidemia, and elevated fatty acids). In its most severe form (diabetic ketoacidosis) there is overproduction of glucose and a marked acceleration of catabolic processes (lipolysis, proteolysis).

Carbohydrate Metabolism. The blood glucose level is the most widely used means of assessing metabolic homeostasis in the diabetic. In its mildest forms diabetes is manifest as a decrease in glucose tolerance in association with normal fasting blood glucose concentrations. In this circumstance ingested glucose fails to elicit an early insulin response and this together with insulin resistance impairs glucose disposal in peripheral tissues and liver.

When absolute or relative insulin deficiency occurs in the basal state, an elevation in fasting blood glucose ensues. In this circumstance normal basal levels of insulin may be maintained, but only at the expense of fasting hyperglycemia. In such patients, glucose production (determined by radioactive tracer techniques)

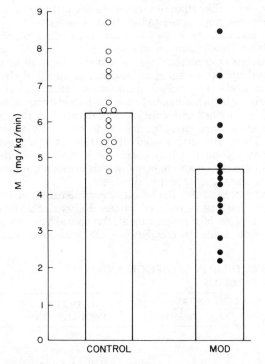

Figure 51. Insulin action in normal nonobese subjects and in nonobese type 2 diabetics. The decrease in insulin action in the type 2 diabetics is manifested as a reduction in insulin-mediated glucose metabolism (M). (Based on the data of DeFronzo R. A., et al.: J Clin Invest 63:939, May, 1979.)

is generally increased. Since only mild hyperglycemia in a normal individual is sufficient to inhibit hepatic glucose output, the diabetic with fasting hyperglycemia is always in a state of relative or absolute glucose overproduction. Furthermore, the relative contribution of gluconeogenesis to total hepatic glucose output is increased. This enhancement of gluconeogenesis with moderate deficiencies of insulin is in keeping with the relatively greater amounts of insulin necessary to inhibit gluconeogenesis as compared with glycogenolysis.

In the extreme situation of total beta cell failure, an ever-increasing fasting blood glucose level fails to elicit a secretory response. In the absence of the restraining influence exerted by insulin, glucose production by the liver increases threefold or more above normal, largely as a consequence of accelerated hepatic gluconeogenesis. The clinical correlate of this sequence of events is severe hyperglycemia as is observed in diabetic ketoacidosis or nonketotic hyperosmolar coma.

The various gradations of disordered carbohydrate metabolism in diabetes are summarized in Table 13.

Fat Metabolism. In the decompensated diabetic, the plasma free fatty acids, triglycerides, and, usually, the cholesterol are elevated. The increased free fatty acid concentration is a result of an increased flow of free fatty acids from the fat depots to the liver and other tissues.

This increase in lipolysis is a consequence of the loss of the normal inhibitory influence of insulin on a hormone-sensitive lipase in adipose tissue. In addition, decreased glucose utilization results in lessened availability of glycerol-3-phosphate for reesterification of fatty acids within the fat cell. The increase in plasma triglycerides in diabetes has been the subject of controversy. Decreased removal of these substances from the plasma has been described in poorly controlled diabetics presumably because of reduced activity of lipoprotein lipase, which is an insulin-dependent enzyme. However, some authors find an increased production of triglyceride. When insulin is given to the poorly controlled hyperglycemic diabetic, the plasma triglyceride concentration falls. This effect of insulin may derive from its stimulation of lipoprotein lipase as well as inhibition of lipolysis in adipose tissue. In contrast, in the mild, maturity-onset diabetic, hyperinsulinemia may contribute to hepatic overproduction of triglyceride.

With respect to cholesterol metabolism, a recent study in a small group of Pima Indians with diabetes revealed elevations in plasma cholesterol and in cholesterol synthesis in association with untreated hyperglycemia. Treatment with insulin reduced plasma cholesterol as cholesterol synthesis diminished.

Amino Acid and Protein Metabolism. Severe insulin deficiency is accompanied by negative nitrogen balance and marked protein wasting. Such changes are not surprising, since insulin is known to stimulate protein synthesis and muscle amino acid uptake, and to inhibit protein catabolism and the output of amino acids from muscle. The interface between diabetes and protein metabolism also involves gluconeogenesis, inasmuch as glucose overproduction in the diabetic depends in part on augmented utilization of protein-derived precursors. The alterations in amino acid metabolism that characterize the diabetic are observed in the fasted (postabsorptive) as well as the protein-fed state.

THE POSTABSORPTIVE STATE. In the insulin-dependent diabetic with mild to moderate hyperglycemia, changes in circulating levels, hepatic uptake, and muscle output of amino acids are demonstrable. A reduction in plasma concentrations of alanine and an elevation in branched chain amino acid concentrations have been repeatedly shown in spontaneous diabetes. Despite the reduction in plasma alanine, uptake of this glycogenic amino acid as well as other glucose precursors is increased twofold or more. As a consequence of this increase in substrate uptake, gluconeogenesis can account for over 30 to 40 per cent of hepatic glucose production as compared with 15 to 20 per cent in normal man. Since circulating alanine levels are reduced in the diabetic, augmented fractional extraction of this amino acid by the liver is responsible for the increase in alanine uptake. These findings in the diabetic thus indicate that changes in intrahepatic processes rather than in muscle are the primary factors responsible for augmented gluconeogenesis.

In addition to a decrease in circulating alanine levels, an elevation in plasma valine, leucine, and isoleucine is demonstrable in diabetes because of decreased uptake by muscle. Despite the elevated circulating levels of branched chain amino acids, studies in experimental animals indicate that oxidation of leucine, isoleucine, and valine is accelerated in the diabetic state once these amino acids enter the muscle cell. Thus, the augmented utilization of alanine by liver is accompanied by increases in situ catabolism by muscle of the amino acids, which provide the nitrogen necessary for alanine synthesis.

PROTEIN FEEDING. Repletion of muscle nitrogen after protein feeding is reduced in the diabetic. Following the ingestion of a protein meal, the splanchnic release of amino acids is comparable to that observed in

TABLE 13. CORRELATION BETWEEN CHANGES IN INSULIN SECRETION AND GLUCOSE REGULATION IN DIABETES

	INSULIN SECRETION		GLUCOSE UPTAKE		GLUCOSE PRODUCTION
	Early	Late	Hepatic	Peripheral	
Abnormal glucose tolerance	↓	N1	N1	↓	N1
Fasting hyperglycemia	↓	↓	↓	↓	↓
Ketoacidosis	↓↓	↓↓	↓↓	↓↓	↑↑

N1 = normal; ↑ = increased; ↓ = decreased

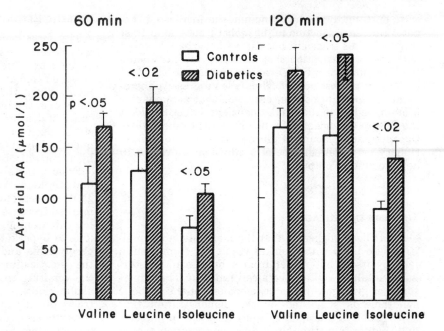

Figure 52. The effects of protein feeding on the arterial levels of the branched chain amino acids in normal and diabetic subjects. In the diabetics, insulin lack results in diminished muscle uptake of branched chain amino acids (valine, leucine, and isoleucine), resulting in their accumulation in plasma. (From Felig, P., et al.: Arch Intern Med 137:507, 1977.)

controls. However, the rise in arterial concentration of the branched chain amino acids is 30 to 50 per cent greater than in healthy control subjects (Fig. 52). Furthermore, in contrast to the persistently positive net uptake of these amino acids observed in normal controls, in the diabetics a net uptake is observed only transiently, at 60 minutes. These observations are in keeping with the known stimulatory effect of insulin on muscle amino acid uptake, which is most marked for the branched chain amino acids. The arterial accumulation and reduced uptake of these amino acids observed in the diabetic are thus likely to represent the effects of insulin deficiency. The metabolic defect in diabetes is thus characterized by protein as well as glucose intolerance.

The catabolic state of the diabetic during protein feeding is not only reflected by the failure of amino acid uptake but also by an accelerated rate of alanine release. In normal subjects, protein feeding results in a transient, but significant, 60 per cent reduction in peripheral alanine output. In contrast, in diabetic subjects alanine output is not reduced after a protein meal. The failure to reduce alanine output thus reflects ongoing protein catabolism and branched chain amino acid oxidation in the absence of an adequate insulin secretory response to a protein meal.

PROTEIN-CARBOHYDRATE INTERACTIONS. In addition to the abnormalities in amino acid metabolism, protein feeding exacerbates the changes in carbohydrate homeostasis characteristic of diabetes. In normal, healthy subjects after protein feeding, blood glucose levels and glucose output remain unchanged despite an elevation in plasma insulin concentration (Fig. 53). This constancy of hepatic glucose production and blood glucose concentration is a consequence of protein-stimulated glucagon secretion, which counteracts the effects of the concomitant rise in plasma insulin. In marked contrast, in diabetic patients protein feeding results in a 150 per cent increase in splanchnic glucose output (Fig. 53), as well as an exaggerated rise in plasma glucose. The stimulatory effect of protein feeding on

hepatic glucose production is a consequence of the rise in plasma glucagon concentration, which in the diabetic is exaggerated and, more importantly, occurs in a setting of absolute insulin deficiency. However, de-

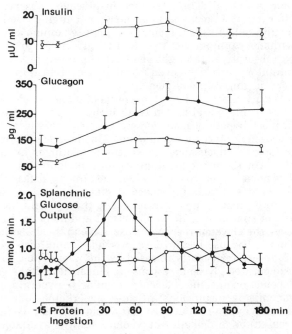

Figure 53. Arterial plasma insulin and glucagon levels and splanchnic glucose output in normal subjects (open circles) and insulin-dependent diabetics (closed circles). Insulin levels could not be measured in the diabetics. After protein feeding, splanchnic glucose output remains stable in normal subjects but rises by 150 per cent in the diabetics. The stimulatory effect of the protein meal on glucose production in the diabetics is due to the exaggerated rise in plasma glucagon in a setting of absolute insulin deficiency. (Based on the data of Wahren, J., Felig, P., and Hagenfeldt, L. J.: Clin Invest 57:987, 1976.)

spite ongoing hyperglucagonemia, the increase in hepatic glucose production in the diabetic does not persist (Fig. 53). This transient hepatic response is in keeping with the demonstration that physiological increments in glucagon have only an evanescent stimulatory effect on hepatic glucose output. Thus, the progressive increment in blood glucose concentration that accompanies protein feeding in the insulin-deficient diabetic reflects the failure (engendered by insulin lack) to metabolize the increased amount of glucose delivered to the periphery as a consequence of a transient elevation in hepatic glucose output.

THE ROLE OF GLUCAGON

It has been suggested that the metabolic abnormalities associated with diabetes result not from insulin lack by itself, but rather from a bihormonal disturbance of alpha cell and beta cell function. The importance of glucagon in the development of the diabetic syndrome is suggested by the demonstration that suppression of glucagon by glucose is lost in diabetes and that protein-stimulated glucagon secretion is augmented. However, recent studies indicate that glucagon contributes to the diabetic state primarily under circumstances of absolute insulin deficiency.

With respect to normal physiology, the major role of glucagon is to prevent hypoglycemia during non–glucose (for example, protein) stimulated insulin secretion. As noted above, the rise in glucagon observed after a protein meal permits the accompanying rise in insulin to facilitate the uptake of ingested amino acids without running the risk of hypoglycemia. In the postabsorptive state, glucagon acts to antagonize the inhibitory action of even basal levels of insulin on hepatic glucose production.

With respect to the pathogenesis of diabetes, elevations in plasma glucagon (within the range observed in most hyperglucagonemic states) have no effect on glucose tolerance in normal man or in diabetic patients so long as endogenous or exogenous insulin is available. On the other hand, glucagon contributes to endogenous hyperglycemia when insulin is deficient. While the stimulatory effect of glucagon on hepatic glucose production is transient (less than 45 minutes) and of similar magnitude in normal and diabetic subjects, the glycemic response is excessive in the diabetic. This is because insulin lack precludes rapid disposal of glucose transiently released by the liver. Thus, the exaggerated glycemic response to glucagon in diabetes depends on insulin deficiency. Similarly, hyperglucagonemia is insufficient to cause hyperketonemia in normal man (even if free fatty acid delivery is increased) or in diabetics in whom insulin is available. Glucagon, however, accelerates the development of ketosis in circumstances of absolute insulin lack. The contribution of glucagon to hyperketonemia derives from this hormone's capacity to augment the hepatic conversion of fatty acids to ketones. Thus, glucagon secretion may exaggerate the metabolic alterations accompanying insulin deficiency. However, relative or absolute insulin lack is the essential factor necessary for the changes in fuel mobilization and utilization that characterize the diabetic state.

DIABETIC KETOACIDOSIS (DKA)

The most severe clinical manifestation of insulin lack is the development of diabetic ketoacidosis. This is an acute, life-threatening, medical emergency requiring rapid diagnosis and institution of proper treatment. Since the advent of insulin therapy over 50 years ago, the importance of diabetic ketoacidosis as a cause of death in the diabetic population has progressively declined. Nevertheless, this condition is frequently encountered and continues to be characterized by a mortality rate of 5 to 10 per cent.

From a metabolic standpoint the major findings in diabetic ketoacidosis are the accumulation of the organic acids acetoacetate and β-hydroxybutyrate, and a marked increase in blood glucose. Clinically, the major life-threatening abnormalities are metabolic acidosis (due to hyperketonemia), hyperosmolarity (due to hyperglycemia and water loss), and dehydration (due to the osmotic diuresis accompanying hyperglycemia and the vomiting that generally accompanies severe metabolic acidosis). All of these abnormalities may be traced directly to an absolute or relative lack of insulin. Nevertheless, associated increases in all of the counterregulatory hormones undoubtedly contribute to the syndrome.

With respect to the pathogenesis of hyperglycemia, decreased tissue utilization of glucose and glucose overproduction by the liver characterize the insulin-deficient state. Whereas glucose is released by the liver at a rate of 150 to 200 mg/min (2 to 3 mg/kg/min) in normal, postabsorptive subjects, in DKA the rate of glucose production is increased to 400 to 600 mg/min. Hyperglycemia thus is mainly a result of overproduction of glucose from endogenous precursors. Consequently the diabetic may have had no intake of carbohydrate or other food for 12 to 24 hours yet manifest hyperglycemia in excess of 500 mg/dl. Since protein-derived amino acids are the only precursors available for de novo glucose synthesis, implicit in this increase in gluconeogenesis is a dissolution of body protein stores and the development of negative nitrogen balance. A more immediate threat to the patient, however, is the osmotic diuresis that accompanies severe hyperglycemia. This leads to dehydration as a result of urinary losses of water and sodium as well as to the development of hyperosmolarity.

Coincident with the increase in blood glucose, ketone acids (acetoacetic acid and β-hydroxybutyric acid) progressively accumulate in blood. The development of hyperketonemia is triggered and regulated by the rate of mobilization of fatty acids from adipose tissue as well as alterations in hepatic metabolism independent of fatty acid delivery.

As discussed above, hypoinsulinemia results in augmented lipolysis in adipose tissue. This is due to lack of the normal restraining effect of insulin on the hormone-sensitive lipase in adipose tissue. In addition, decreased glucose uptake by fat cells results in a deficiency of glycerol-3-phosphate, which is needed for in situ reesterification of fatty acids. However, the increase in fatty acid mobilization is not of itself sufficient to bring about hyperketonemia. When FFA levels are markedly increased in normal subjects (by administering a fat meal and heparin, an activator of lipoprotein lipase), hyperketonemia fails to develop.

In addition to increased fatty acid mobilization, the development of hyperketonemia requires an increase in the ketogenic capacity within the liver. The metabolic site within the liver that is responsible for this activation of ketogenesis has been suggested to reside at the carnitine acyl-transferase reaction. This enzyme catalyzes the transfer of long-chain fatty acids across the mitochondrial membrane. Since beta-oxidation of fatty acids occurs solely within the mitochondria, accelerated transfer of free fatty acids across the membrane results in augmented fatty acid oxidation and acetyl CoA production. The marked increase in acetyl CoA availability exceeds the capacity for its oxidation to CO_2 via the Krebs cycle, resulting in condensation of acetyl CoA molecules to form ketone acids. The mechanism whereby insulin deficiency leads to augmented activity of the carnitine acyltransferase reaction is believed to involve augmented transfer of carnitine from extrahepatic sites to the liver as well as a fall in intrahepatic levels of malonyl CoA, the first committed intermediate in the biosynthesis of fatty acids. Malonyl CoA has been demonstrated to be a potent inhibitor of the carnitine acyltransferase reaction. Since insulin lack interferes with fat synthesis, a deficiency in malonyl CoA is a characteristic finding in circumstances of insulin lack.

An elevation in glucagon concentration as well as insulin lack will markedly accelerate the ketogenic capacity of the liver. Hyperglucagonemia increases the level of carnitine, decreases the concentration of malonyl CoA, and increases the activity of carnitine acyltransferase in excess of that attributable to insulin deficiency alone. As a consequence, in pancreatectomized patients in whom glucagon as well as insulin is lacking, the magnitude of hyperketonemia is less than that observed with spontaneous diabetes. Furthermore, in insulin-withdrawn type 1 diabetics rendered hypoglucagonemic by administration of somatostatin, hyperketonemia is diminished, although not entirely prevented.

In addition to increased ketone production, hyperketonemia in diabetes is a consequence of decreased utilization of these organic acids by muscle tissue. Even in patients with mild insulin lack, a diminution in the ability to dispose of ketones is demonstrable.

The overall sequence of events leading to the development of hyperketonemia can thus be viewed as a three-pronged process involving adipose tissue, the liver, and muscle (Fig. 54). Insulin lack results in

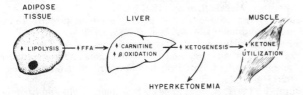

Figure 54. The pathogenesis of hyperketonemia in diabetes. Ketone accumulation is a consequence of three distinct metabolic events: 1, Accelerated lipolysis leading to increased delivery of free fatty acids (FFA) from adipose tissue. 2, Augmented beta-oxidation of free fatty acids to ketones as a result of activation of the acyl-carnitine transferase enzyme. The latter is stimulated by the increase in carnitine levels and decreased levels of malonyl CoA in the diabetic liver. 3, A reduction in ketone utilization by muscle. Each of these processes is reversed by the action of insulin.

augmented lipolysis in adipose tissue, leading to increased delivery of free fatty acids to the liver. Within the liver an increase in carnitine acyltransferase results in stimulation of the beta-oxidative pathway and augmented ketone production. The ketones released by the liver cannot be metabolized at normal rates by muscle tissue and thus accumulate within the blood. The end result is thus a metabolic acidosis in which β-hydroxybutyrate and acetoacetate are the predominant organic acids.

It should be noted that acetone, which does not contribute to acidosis, is also formed (by the spontaneous decarboxylation of acetoacetate) and circulates in a concentration that may reach 10 to 15 mM. Because of its low vapor pressure, excretion by the lungs, and characteristic fruity odor, the presence of acetone may be detected on the patient's breath and may serve as a useful diagnostic clue.

METABOLIC CHANGES AND DIABETIC COMPLICATIONS

Since the advent of insulin therapy, the major factors responsible for mortality in diabetes are not changes in body fuel metabolism (for example, hyperglycemia and/or hyperketonemia), but long-term complications characterized by small blood vessel disease (microangiopathy), accelerated atherosclerosis, and neuropathy. Diabetic microangiopathy affects the capillaries and precapillary arterioles throughout the body. However, the changes are most striking in the kidney and retina. In the kidney the earliest lesions consist of basement membrane and mesangial thickening that may progress generally so that the entire glomerulus is replaced by a sheet of amorphous material. Alternatively there may be coalescence of these thickened areas in the glomerulus into nodular masses as described by Kimmelstiel and Wilson. In the retina capillary changes eventually cause ischemia, which may lead to the growth of abnormal vessels (proliferative retinopathy). From a clinical standpoint, the major clinical expressions of these microvascular changes are impairment of renal function (proteinuria and ultimately renal failure) and decreased vision (due to proliferative retinopathy).

Neurological dysfunction is also frequently observed in the diabetic. Neuropathy may involve any portion of the neuraxis, extending from the spinal cord to the distal nerve endings. Clinically the most common manifestations are: (a) peripheral polyneuropathy—a symmetrical sensory loss generally involving the lower extremities; (b) mononeuritis multiplex—involvement of a simple, mixed, motor-sensory nerve causing pain and weakness; (c) autonomic neuropathy—afferent and efferent sympathetic and/or parasympathetic nerve involvement resulting in orthostatic hypotension, loss of sweating, diarrhea, impotence, and bladder dysfunction. Histologically, diabetic mononeuropathy is generally vascular in origin, resulting from occlusion of the vasa nervorum. However, in the case of peripheral polyneuropathy, degenerative changes are present in the absence of vascular occlusive disease. Segmental demyelination of nerve fibers has been observed in experimental as well as spontaneous diabetes. Furthermore, a decrease in nerve conduction time that is reversible by insulin is present in as many as 70 per cent of newly discovered diabetics in the absence of histological changes.

A major unresolved question concerns the mechanism whereby insulin deficiency and/or hyperglycemia contributes to or is responsible for the vascular and neuropathic complications of diabetes. Two schools of thought have emerged. One theory holds that microvascular disease occurs entirely independent of the changes in insulin and body fuel metabolism. By this hypothesis, diabetics inherit an abnormality in their blood vessels and nerves. The alternative concept proposes that insulin deficiency and/or its metabolic consequences result *secondarily* in functional and histological abnormalities in the microvasculature and nervous system. Although this controversy remains unsettled, a number of recent studies have provided intriguing observations regarding metabolic abnormalities in the target tissues affected by diabetic complications.

Chemical Composition of Diabetic Glomerular Basement Membrane. The renal glomerular basement membrane is an extracellular, collagen-like structure composed of glycoprotein. Chemical analysis of this material has shown that in diabetics there is an increase in the number of glucosyl-galactosyl moieties linked to the amino acid residues in the polypeptide chain. Interestingly, glycosylation of the basement membrane represents a postribosomal process that is influenced largely by the ambient glucose concentration. Since the number and position of the carbohydrate moieties affect the cross-linkage and shape of the glycoprotein molecule, it is speculated that an increase in glucose content may lead to increased porosity of the membrane that manifests clinically as proteinuria. In this manner hyperglycemia could conceivably contribute to diabetic glomerulosclerosis.

Glycosylation of Hemoglobin. Hemoglobin A_{1c} is one of three negatively charged minor hemoglobin components eluted on cation exchange resin chromatography before the main hemoglobin A peak (hence the term "fast hemoglobin"). The concentration of hemoglobin A_{1c} in poorly controlled diabetic patients is twice that observed in normal controls. More importantly, the level of hemoglobin A_{1c} is reduced with improvement of diabetic control. The glycosylation of hemoglobin A is a nonenzymatic process dependent, at least in part, on the level of blood glucose. The significance of the elevation in hemoglobin A_{1c} in diabetes thus lies not only in providing a potential marker of the efficacy of diabetic control but in suggesting the possibility that changes in structural proteins resulting from glycosylation reactions may provide a unifying metabolic basis for the long-term sequelae of diabetes.

Metabolism of Nerve Tissue. Metabolic changes in nerve tissue referable to insulin deficiency and/or hyperglycemia have been observed in experimentally induced diabetes in laboratory animals. Using incubated Schwann cells (the site of myelin synthesis) it has been demonstrated that incorporation of labeled precursors into lipid and protein components of myelin is influenced by the ambient insulin and glucagon concentration. Those studies raise the possibility that insulin deficiency and/or glucagon excess may alter the metabolism of Schwann cells so as to result in focal areas of demyelination.

Increased accumulation of sorbitol, a polyhydroxyalcohol formed from glucose, has been observed in nerve tissue obtained from animals with experimental diabetes. The enzyme induced in this reaction is aldose reductase. The sorbitol thus formed may be further metabolized to fructose. Aldose reductase has a relatively low affinity for glucose, having a K_m of 70 to 150 mM, and is localized to specific tissues: the Schwann cells, the lens, and vascular endothelium. Consequently a high intracellular glucose concentration in these non–insulin dependent tissues (as occurs with diabetic hyperglycemia) would be expected to result in sorbitol accumulation. An excess of sorbitol has in fact been implicated as the mechanism leading to "sugar" cataract formation in the diabetic eye. In addition, swelling of nerve endings and a reduction in nerve conduction velocity accompany the accumulation of sorbitol in experimental diabetes. More recently, studies have shown a decrease in myoinositol in diabetic nerve tissue. This appears to be due to interference with myoinositol uptake by hyperglycemia. Myoinositol supplements in the diet of diabetic animals prevent both the deficiency of this compound and the decrease in nerve conduction velocity. The implications of these studies to human diabetes are readily apparent.

While these studies suggest a variety of mechanisms whereby experimental diabetes leads to nerve disease, their relevance to human diabetes remains to be established. Nevertheless, these observations do raise the possibility that tissues whose metabolism is generally considered to be unaffected by insulin (that is, nerve tissue) may nevertheless undergo a variety of chemical changes as a consequence of the diabetic state.

REFERENCES

Diabetes Mellitus

Barnes, A. J., Bloom, S. R., Alberti, K. G. M. M., Smythe, P., Alford, F. P., and Chisholm, D. J.: Ketoacidosis in pancreatectomized man. N Engl J Med 296:1250, 1977.

Bennion, L. J., and Grundy, S. M.: Effects of diabetes mellitus on cholesterol metabolism in man. N Engl J Med 296:1365, 1977.

Block, M. B., Mako, M. E., Steiner, D. F., and Rubenstein, A. H.: Circulating C-peptide immunoreactivity. Studies in normals and diabetic patients. Diabetes 21:1013, 1972.

Brunzell, J. D., Porte, D., Jr., and Bierman, E. L.: Reversible abnormalities in postheparin lipolytic activity in diabetes mellitus. Metabolism 24:1123, 1975.

Bunn, H. F.: Nonenzymatic glycosylation of protein: Relevance to diabetes. Am J Med 70:325, 1981.

Buse, M. G., Herlong, H. F., and Weigand, D. A.: The effects of diabetes, insulin, and the redox potential on leucine metabolism by isolated rat hemidiaphragm. Endocrinology 98:1166, 1976.

Dunn, F., Petri, A., and Raskin, P.: Plasma lipid and lipoprotein levels with continuous subcutaneous insulin infusion in type I diabetes mellitus. Ann Intern Med 95:426, 1981.

Felig, P., Wahren, J., and Hendler, R.: Influence of maturity-onset diabetes on splanchnic glucose balance after oral glucose ingestion. Diabetes 27:121, 1978.

Felig, P., Wahren, J., Sherwin, R. S., and Hendler, R.: Insulin, glucagon, and somatostatin in normal physiology and diabetes mellitus. Diabetes 25:1091, 1976.

Gabbay, K. H.: The sorbitol pathway and the complications of diabetes. N Engl J Med 288:831, 1973.

Gabbay, K. H., Sosenko, J. M., Banuchi, G. A., Mininsohn, M. J., and Fluckiger, R.: Glycosylated hemoglobins: Increased glycosylation of hemoglobin A in diabetic patients. Diabetes 28:337, 1979.

Gerich, J. E., Lorenzi, M., Bier, D. M., Schneider, V., Tsalikian, E., Karam, J. H., and Forsham, P. H.: Prevention of human diabetic ketoacidosis by somatostatin. Evidence for an essential role of glucagon. N Engl J Med 292:985, 1975.

Greene, D. H., DeJesus, P. V., and Winegrad, A. J.: Effects of insulin and dietary myoinositol on impaired peripheral motor nerve conduction velocity in acute streptozotocin diabetes. J Clin Invest 55:1326, 1975.

Kipnis, D. M.: Insulin secretion in normal and diabetic individuals. Adv Intern Med 16:103, 1970.

Kolterman, O. G., Gray, R. S., Griffin, S., Burstein, P., Insel, J., Scarlett, J. M., and Olefsky, J. M.: Receptor and postreceptor defects contribute to the insulin resistance in non-insulin dependent diabetes mellitus. J Clin Invest 68:957, 1981.

The Kroc Collaborative Study Group: Blood glucose control and the evolution of diabetic retinopathy and albuminuria: A preliminary multicenter trial. N Engl J Med 311:365, 1984.

McGarry, J. D., and Foster, R. P.: Hormonal control of ketogenesis: Biochemical considerations. Arch Intern Med 137:495, 1977.

Nikkila, E. A., and Kekki, M.: Plasma triglyceride transport kinetics in diabetes mellitus. Metabolism 22:1, 1973.

Olefsky, J. M., Faouhar, J. W., and Reaven, G. M.: Reappraisal of the role of insulin in hypertriglyceridemia. Am J Med 57:5551, 1974.

Reaven, G. M., Bernstein, R., Davis, B., and Olefsky, J. M.: Nonketotic diabetes mellitus: Insulin deficiency or insulin resistance. Am J Med 60:80, 1976.

Robertson, R. P., and Porte, D., Jr.: The glucose receptor. A defective mechanism in diabetes mellitus distinct from the beta adrenergic receptor. J Clin Invest 52:870, 1973.

Schade, D. S., and Eaton, R. P.: Glucagon regulation of plasma ketone body concentration in human diabetes. J Clin Invest 56:1340, 1975.

Shamoon, H., Hendler, R., and Sherwin, R. S.: Altered responsiveness to cortisol, epinephrine, and glucagon in insulin-infused juvenile-onset diabetes: A mechanism for diabetic instability. Diabetes 29:284, 1980.

Sherwin, R. S., Fisher, M., Hendler, R., and Felig, P.: Hyperglucagonemia and blood glucose regulation in normal, obese and diabetic subjects. N Engl J Med 294:455, 1976.

Sherwin, R. S., Hendler, R., and Felig, P.: Effect of diabetes mellitus and insulin on the turnover and metabolic response to ketones in man. Diabetes 25:776, 1976.

Shima, K., Tanaka, R., Morishita, S., Tarui, S., Kumahara, Y., and Nishikawa, M.: Studies on the etiology of "brittle" diabetes: Relationship between diabetic instability and insulinogenic reserve. Diabetes 26:717, 1977.

Sidenius, P.: The axonopathy of diabetic neuropathy. Diabetes 31:356, 1982.

Spiro, R. G.: Search for a biochemical basis of diabetes macroangiography. Diabetologia 12:1, 1976.

Spritz, N.: Nerve disease in diabetes mellitus. Med Clin North Am 62:787, 1978.

Tatersall, R. B., and Fajans, S. S.: A difference between the inheritance of classical juvenile-onset and maturity-onset type diabetes of young people. Diabetes 24:44, 1975.

Unger, R. H.: Diabetes and the alpha cell. Diabetes 25:136, 1976.

Wahren, J., Felig, P., Cerasei, E., and Luft, R.: Splanchnic and peripheral glucose and amino acid metabolism in diabetes mellitus. J Clin Invest 51:1870, 1972.

Wahren, J., Felig, P., and Hagenfeldt, J.: Effect of protein ingestion on splanchnic and leg metabolism in normal man and in patients with diabetes mellitus. J Clin Invest 57:987, 1976.

Yalow, R. S., and Berson, S. A.: Immunoassay of endogenous plasma insulin in man. J Clin Invest 39:1157, 1960.

HYPOGLYCEMIA

Of the various substrates circulating in the blood, the concentration of glucose is one of the most tightly regulated. Under normal circumstances of mixed meal ingestion, the blood glucose level varies by less than 40 mg/dl over the course of a 24-hour period (Fig. 33). The basis for this minimization of glucose fluctuation is the feedback relationship between glucose concentration and insulin secretion (Fig. 33). A breakdown in this feedback loop due to a lack of insulin results in hyperglycemia as considered in the discussion on diabetes. In some circumstances, there is a failure of those mechanisms that prevent the blood sugar from falling to excessively low values. The result of such a breakdown is hypoglycemia.

DEFINITION

Hypoglycemia may be defined as that condition in which the plasma (or blood) glucose concentration falls to levels below normal. When such a reduction is accompanied by symptoms, clinical as well as chemical hypoglycemia is manifest. A major area of dispute concerns the precise definition of the lower limits of "normal." Recent studies indicate that normative values are affected by sex and age. In normal adult males the plasma glucose level remains above 65 mg/dl after a 24-hour fast and above 55 mg/dl after a 72-hour fast (Fig. 55). In normal females the values may be 10 mg/dl lower at 72 hours (Fig. 55). In healthy asymptomatic subjects monitored for five to six hours after oral glucose ingestion, the plasma glucose concentration generally falls to a nadir value at three to four hours, which is below the initial fasting value, but generally remains above 55 mg/dl. However, in some series as many as 35 per cent of normal subjects have

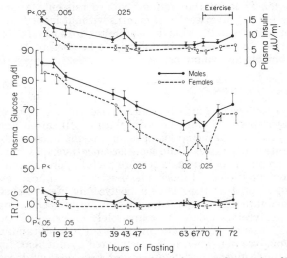

Figure 55. The effect of a 72-hour fast on plasma insulin, plasma glucose, and insulin glucose ratio (IRI:G) in healthy, nonobese male and female adult subjects. (From Fajans, S. S., and Floyd, J. C., Jr.: N Engl J Med 294:766, 1976.)

plasma glucose levels below 55 mg/dl and remain asymptomatic. Thus, while there is some dispute regarding definition, practical guidelines for the diagnosis of hypoglycemia are as follows: (a) in adult males and females after an overnight fast, a plasma glucose below 60 mg/dl (blood glucose <52); (b) in males fasted for 72 hours, a plasma glucose below 50 mg/dl; (c) in females fasted for 72 hours a plasma glucose less than 40 to 45 mg/dl; (d) in males and females given a 100-gram oral glucose load, a lowest plasma glucose less than 50 mg/dl.

CLINICAL FINDINGS

The symptoms of hypoglycemia may be divided into two categories, those related to neuroglycopenia and its attendant decrease in cerebral oxygen consumption and those due to increased activity of the adrenergic nervous system and secretion of catecholamines. The neuroglycopenic symptoms consist of headache, mental dullness, fatigue, confusion, hallucinations, bizarre behavior, and ultimately convulsions or coma. As a result hypoglycemic attacks may be confused with cerebral vascular disease in elderly patients, or with other types of organic psychoses. Chronic or repeated attacks of hypoglycemia cause loss of intellectual function. The adrenergic symptoms consist of palpitations, anxiety, sweating, tremulousness, and hunger, reflecting increased secretion of catecholamines. A characteristic feature of hypoglycemia regardless of its cause is its *episodic nature*. While symptoms may recur repeatedly, chronic disability in the form of ongoing fatigue or altered personality persisting (without remission) for days or weeks is not ascribable to hypoglycemia. The reason for this is that hypoglycemia will result within a finite period (of minutes to hours) to one of three outcomes: (1) the blood glucose will spontaneously revert to normal because of counterregulatory mechanisms (see below); (2) ingestion of food will result in normalization of plasma glucose; or (3) if both (1) and (2) fail to occur, the plasma glucose will continue to fall to levels that result in either syncope, seizures, or coma. Thus in the patient with persistent fatigue lasting for days, weeks, or months without identifiable episodic disability that is of minutes to hours in duration, hypoglycemia is unlikely to be present or responsible for symptoms.

CLASSIFICATION

Hypoglycemia may be characterized in a variety of ways based on alterations in glucose utilization and production, hormonal changes, or enzyme and/or substrate deficiencies. While such classifications may have some physiological basis, a more useful approach combines physiological mechanisms with the clinical setting of presentation. Thus hypoglycemia may be classified into three major categories (Table 14): (1) fasting hypoglycemia (when it occurs solely or primarily in the absence of nutrient ingestion); (2) postprandial hypoglycemia (when it is precipitated by nutrient, for example glucose or fructose, ingestion); and (3) induced hypoglycemia (when it is brought about by a drug or some other chemical, nonnutritive substance, for example, insulin or alcohol). Within each of these categories the mechanisms may differ widely, varying from

TABLE 14. CLASSIFICATION OF HYPOGLYCEMIA

A. Fasting Hypoglycemia
  1. Insulinoma
  2. Extrapancreatic tumors
  3. Counterregulatory hormone deficiency
    Hypoadrenalism
    Hypopituitarism
  4. Liver Disease
    Acute hepatic necrosis
    Glycogen storage disease
    Gluconeogenic enzyme defects
  5. Substrate Deficiency
    Kwashiorkor
    Ketotic hypoglycemia of infancy
  6. Autoimmune Hypoglycemia

B. Postprandial Hypoglycemia
  1. Alimentary
  2. Spontaneous, reactive
  3. Early diabetes
  4. Fructose intolerance

C. Induced Hypoglycemia
  1. Insulin
  2. Sulfonylurea
  3. Alcohol
  4. Akee nut poisoning (Hypoglycin)

hormone excess (insulinoma) to hormone deficiency (hypoadrenalism) or substrate lack (ketotic hypoglycemia).

FASTING HYPOGLYCEMIA

Since glucose uptake by the brain continues during starvation, maintenance of plasma glucose levels above 50 mg/dl during the course of a prolonged fast requires intact mechanisms of glucose production. As discussed previously, liver glycogen stores amounting to about 70 grams after an overnight fast are depleted within 24 to 48 hours of starvation, necessitating a progressive increase in gluconeogenesis. This process requires three factors: (1) a hormonal milieu characterized by a fall in insulin and elevated levels of glucagon; (2) intact hepatic gluconeogenic and glycogenolytic enzymes; (3) adequate mobilization of precursor gluconeogenic substrate (protein-derived alanine) and energy-yielding substrate (adipose tissue–derived free fatty acids). Fasting hypoglycemia thus may occur as a result of (1) an excess of insulin or insulin-like substances; (2) deficiencies of contrainsulin hormones; (3) congenital or acquired hepatic disease; or (4) substrate deficiency. Starvation per se does not of itself cause hypoglycemia in normal subjects. In the face of severe inanition (kwashiorkor, protein-calorie malnutrition) hypoglycemia may be observed in association with terminal infection, presumably due to a lack of mobilizable alanine from protein stores. Similarly, the combination of alcohol ingestion and starvation may produce hypoglycemia (see below). Prolonged carbohydrate restriction followed by severe, prolonged exercise may also bring about hypoglycemia. However, after a three-day fast, exercise of one to two hours' duration fails to cause hypoglycemia in normal subjects (Fig. 55).

Insulinoma. Excessive insulin secretion by beta-cell tumors of the pancreas may cause hypoglycemia. These tumors may be either benign or malignant, the latter representing about 10 per cent of the total. The tumors are very rare in patients less than ten years old, and about 90 per cent occur in patients over the age of 30. They may occur in any part of the gland. The histological appearance is of whorls of typical beta cells. Although the clinical picture produced by hypoglycemia in insulinoma is not different from that caused by administered insulin, it is characteristic in occurring particularly when the patient is fasting, or after exercise. In this respect it differs from the hypoglycemias induced by feeding various stimuli to insulin secretion, which are discussed later.

Diagnosis is usually made by finding a very low blood glucose concentration in the fasting state, in association with an elevated (>20 μU/ml) plasma insulin level. In about 50 per cent of patients with islet cell tumors, the overnight fasting plasma glucose will be less than 60 mg/dl and the plasma insulin level will exceed 20 μU/ml. In an additional 25 to 35 per cent of patients, hypoglycemia will be provoked by merely prolonging the fast for up to four hours (by withholding breakfast). In only 10 per cent of cases or less is a 72-hour fast followed by exercise necessary to provoke hypoglycemia. In rare instances hypoglycemia may be accompanied by a "normal" plasma insulin level. In such circumstances the insulin:glucose (I/G) ratio may be helpful. An I/G ratio in excess of 0.30 is indicative of inappropriate insulin levels (for the level of glucose) or relative hyperinsulinism. The episodic nature of insulin secretion by islet cell tumors may contribute to difficulties in making the diagnosis.

The basic pathogenetic defect in the patient with an islet cell tumor is excessive or inappropriate secretion of insulin relative to the circulating glucose level. This may take the form of episodic bursts of insulin secretion occurring spontaneously. Alternatively there may be failure to inhibit insulin secretion between meals or during exercise, thus necessitating provocative tests such as prolonged fasting and/or exercise. In those patients with absolute hyperinsulinemia there is combined excessive utilization and decreased production of glucose. However, in the patient in whom insulin levels fail to decline during a fast or exercise and in whom there is a relative hyperinsulinemia, the mechanism responsible for hypoglycemia is inhibition of glycogenolysis and gluconeogenesis. This inhibition derives from the exquisite sensitivity of the liver to small changes in circulating insulin.

The management of insulinomas involves surgical removal or, in the case of metastatic tumors, administration of beta cell cytotoxic agents such as streptozotocin.

In infants and children, hyperinsulinemic hypoglycemia not uncommonly occurs in the absence of an identifiable adenoma (or microadenoma). Careful histological evaluation of the pancreas in such cases often reveals *nesidioblastosis,* an increase in islet cell mass in which there is formation of islet cells from ductal epithelium. Rather than typical islets, clusters of endocrine cells of varying size and shape are observed in which there is a widespread infiltration of acinar tissue and continuity between endocrine cell groups and ductular structures. Treatment consists of subtotal pancreatectomy and, when necessary, diazoxide therapy or total pancreatectomy.

Extrapancreatic Tumors. Tumors arising outside the pancreas may cause hypoglycemia, in some instances by secreting an insulin-like material, in others by utilizing glucose at an accelerated rate, and in still others by inhibiting, in some way, the ability of the liver to release glucose. Most commonly these tumors arise from mesenchymal tissue (fibromas, fibrosarcomas, neuromas) and are retroperitoneal or occasionally mediastinal in location. In a recent study, 50 to 70 per cent of patients with extrapancreatic tumor hypoglycemia showed elevated levels of NSILA-S (nonsuppressible insulin-like activity) as determined by radioreceptor assay. Only in very rare instances have such tumors been shown to produce radioimmunoassayable insulin.

Counterregulatory Hormone Deficiency. In addition to the fall in insulin secretion, maintenance of glucose homeostasis requires intact secretion of growth hormone, cortisol, and glucagon. Clinical hypoglycemia may be observed in hypopituitarism, isolated deficiency of growth hormone or ACTH, and in Addison's disease. In each of these circumstances the plasma insulin level is appropriately reduced. Diagnosis depends on evaluation of pituitary and/or adrenal function. Although glucagon levels normally increase in starvation, clinical hypoglycemia due to deficiency of this hormone has not been documented.

Liver Disease. As mentioned previously, the major source of glucose in the fasting person is the liver. Hypoglycemia is not uncommon in patients with viral hepatitis, but the degree of hypoglycemia is rarely sufficient to cause symptoms. In patients with very severe liver disease, failure of gluconeogenesis may cause a rise in the concentration of plasma amino acids and a fall of blood glucose concentrations, but this is ordinarily seen only in the terminal phase of hepatic necrosis. In these patients the demand for glucose may be much larger than one would expect if simple replacement of the minimal glucose utilization of fasting were required, and it seems likely that an additional problem is the loss of the insulin-inactivating mechanisms that the normal liver possesses. The result is a combined increase of insulin activity and a decrease of gluconeogenesis.

Hypoglycemia may also occur as a result of inborn errors of metabolism characterized by a deficiency of hepatic *glycogenolytic* or *gluconeogenic enzymes.* As previously discussed, in type I glycogen storage disease (von Gierke's disease) there is excessive accumulation of liver glycogen and fasting hypoglycemia due to a deficiency of glucose-6-phosphatase. In patients with a deficiency of fructose-1,6-diphosphatase, a key enzyme in the gluconeogenic pathway, fasting hypoglycemia is the major clinical finding.

Substrate Deficiency Hypoglycemia. In addition to a reduction in insulin, availability of counterregulatory hormones and intact hepatic glycogenolytic and gluconeogenic mechanisms, glucose production in fasting requires the availability of precursor substrate, notably alanine. In normal subjects the rate of alanine release from muscle determines the rate of gluconeogenesis in starvation. A physiological reduction in alanine and accentuation of fasting hypoglycemia is observed in normal *pregnancy.* Alanine deficiency has also been implicated in the pathogenesis of *ketotic hypoglycemia* of infancy and childhood. In this disorder, hypoglycemia and hyperketonemia are generally provoked by a gastrointestinal upset. Plasma insulin levels are appropriately reduced. The children respond to glucose administration and the long-term prognosis is good, with disappearance of the attacks.

Insulin Autoimmune Hypoglycemia. A small number of patients have been reported from Japan and Scandinavia in whom hypoglycemia is associated with circulating antibodies to insulin despite the absence of a prior history of insulin treatment. Investigation of these antibodies has shown them to possess the properties of IgG and their light chains were exclusively of K-type. The postulated mechanism of hypoglycemia is the sudden release of free insulin from a large pool of antibody-bound insulin. The hypoglycemia may occur in the fasted state or after meals. This syndrome must be distinguished from factitious hypoglycemia due to surreptitious insulin injection, which is generally accompanied by insulin antibodies as well.

POSTPRANDIAL HYPOGLYCEMIA

In contrast to the preceding group of diseases, which are manifested clinically by hypoglycemia occurring in the fasted state, there is a large group of syndromes in which the blood glucose depression occurs only in response to some stimulus. The commonest agent that produces this pattern is food. In patients with the appropriate form of sensitivity, ingestion of carbohydrate, protein, or certain specific sugars may cause the blood glucose to fall to symptomatic levels.

Alimentary Hypoglycemia. After partial gastrectomy or gastrojejunostomy, ingested carbohydrate moves from the stomach remnant to the small intestine more rapidly than normal. This rapid transit may be associated with a variety of symptoms such as epigastric fullness, sweating, palpitations, and weakness, which can be produced whenever hyperosmolar material enters the jejunum rapidly. On the other hand, hypoglycemia is a common finding in patients after gastroenterostomy and gastric resection. The patients develop a very high absorptive peak, followed by hypoglycemia after an oral glucose tolerance test. The intravenous glucose tolerance test is normal, indicating that the mechanism of insulin secretion within the islet cells is not disturbed. Whether the hyperinsulinemia is due to rapid absorption of glucose or to excess release of some gastrointestinal secretagogue has not been established.

Spontaneous, Reactive Hypoglycemia. Patients with reactive hypoglycemia have normal fasting blood glucose concentrations but become mildly hypoglycemic within two to four hours after a carbohydrate-containing meal. It is unusual for the blood glucose concentration to fall below 40 mg/dl and coma or convulsions are virtually unknown in this syndrome. The chief complaints are weakness, palpitations, nervousness, and sweating. The symptoms are not caused by fasting or exercise and may be precipitated by an oral glucose tolerance test. In some but not all patients it has been possible to demonstrate that hypersecretion of insulin occurs after a carbohydrate-containing meal.

Although some of the patients with this syndrome have clear-cut hypoglycemia and physical disease, many patients who complain of tremulousness, weakness, and other nonspecific problems occurring toward the end of the morning or afternoon prove not to have low blood glucose concentrations. These patients often have psychosocial problems, and their symptoms are due to their emotional disturbance rather than to a reduced level of blood glucose. Unfortunately, they are often victimized by misguided physicians who make a diagnosis of hypoglycemia without adequate evidence and treat the patients with a variety of nostrums of little value. When reactive hypoglycemia is in fact present, treatment consists of a reduction in dietary carbohydrate and the use of frequent, small feedings.

Early Diabetes. In occasional patients with mild diabetes postprandial hypoglycemia may be the first clinical manifestation. The glucose tolerance test generally reveals abnormally high values at 60 to 90 minutes (160 to 220 mg/dl) followed by a decline to abnormally low levels at three or four hours. This pattern reflects loss of the initial phase of insulin secretion, resulting in early hyperglycemia. The latter then may result in a delayed "overshoot" of the secondary phase of insulin secretion that remains intact early in the course of type 2 diabetes.

Fructose Intolerance. Inborn errors of fructose metabolism may give rise to hypoglycemia when dietary fructose is ingested. In *hereditary fructosemia* a deficiency of fructose-1-phosphate aldolase results in accumulation of fructose-1-phosphate. The latter interferes with the enzyme fructose-1,6-diphosphate aldolase, a necessary step in the gluconeogenic (and glycolytic) pathway. In patients with *fructose-1,6-diphosphatase deficiency,* hypoglycemia occurs either in the fasting state or after the ingestion of fructose-containing foods.

INDUCED HYPOGLYCEMIA

Insulin and Sulfonylurea Agents. Hypoglycemia may be provoked by the administration of drugs, toxins, or alcohol. Overdosage with insulin during the course of treatment of diabetes is probably the most commonly encountered form of hypoglycemia. In insulin-treated patients hypoglycemia may occur because of a decrease in food intake, an inappropriate elevation in the dose, or moderate to severe exercise. Recent studies have shown that exercise-induced hypoglycemia is due, at least in part, to augmented mobilization of insulin from injection sites in the exercised extremity. This complication can consequently be prevented by ingesting extra carbohydrate prior to exercise and by using a nonexercised injection site (for example, the abdominal wall).

Hypoglycemia is occasionally observed in patients treated with sulfonylurea agents. This is more commonly observed with long-acting preparations.

In recent years a number of patients have been described in whom hypoglycemia was due to the surreptitious administration of insulin or sulfonylurea agents. The possibility of *factitious hypoglycemia* should receive particular consideration when dealing with medical personnel or individuals involved with diabetic patients (for example, family members of diabetics). Administration of insulin is suggested when antibodies to insulin are observed in a patient without prior history of insulin usage. Since antibodies to insulin may also occur in insulin autoimmune hypoglycemia (see above), the diagnosis rests on the demonstration of low to absent levels of C-peptide, a reflection of the suppression of endogenous insulin secretion. In circumstances of surreptitious ingestion of sulfonylureas, the drugs will be detectable in the plasma.

Alcohol. One of the most common forms of hypoglycemia observed in hospital emergency rooms is alcohol-induced hypoglycemia. It has been shown that pure ethyl alcohol can produce the same effect when it is given to undernourished subjects or to normal individuals after a prolonged fast. The immediate cause is a lack of release of glucose from the liver, because glycogen reserves are depleted and the rate of gluconeogenesis is inadequate to protect the blood glucose.

The mechanism of the alcohol effect is related to its metabolism. Ethanol is oxidized to acetaldehyde and acetate by enzymatic steps that require the presence of NAD as a hydrogen acceptor. When large amounts of ethanol are being oxidized, most of the cytoplasmic NAD is converted to NADH. Some of this can be reoxidized in the gluconeogenic pathway as diphosphoglycerate is reduced to glyceraldehyde phosphate; but if the amount involved is very large, NADH accumulates and is removed by the reversible reduction of pyruvate to lactate. Formation of glucose from either lactate or alanine (the quantitatively most important gluconeogenic precursors) requires their initial conversion to pyruvate, which is then converted via oxaloacetate to phosphoenolpyruvate. The accumulation of NADH during the metabolism of alcohol results in the removal of pyruvate (by rapidly reducing it to lactate) and thus interferes with substrate utilization along the gluconeogenic pathway. The oxidation of alcohol proceeds quite rapidly, so that, ordinarily, inhibition of gluconeogenesis does not persist long enough to cause trouble; but if the glycogen stores have previously been depleted by prolonged poor intake of carbohydrate, and if the intake of alcohol is large, hypoglycemia can occur. The syndrome is, therefore, seen almost exclusively in alcoholics after several days of drinking. When recognized, it can usually be treated adequately with intravenous glucose. Glucagon should not be used; these patients do not respond to the hormone because their livers are already glycogen depleted.

Akee Nut Poisoning (Hypoglycin). Ingestion of the ripe akee nut, fruit of the tree *Blighia sapida,* can cause a severe sickness associated with vomiting and hypoglycemia. The disease is particularly prevalent in Jamaica, although the tree is distributed throughout the tropics; it is therefore called "Jamaican vomiting sickness." The toxic element is a complex organic compound, hypoglycin (L-α-amino-β(methylenecyclopropyl)-propionic acid), which is converted in the body to methylenecyclopropylacetic acid by deamination and decarboxylation of the propionic acid residue. This latter product is the toxic material. It competes successfully with long-chain fatty acids for access to carnitine, which is necessary for transport of fatty acids into the mitochondria before they can be oxidized. Since fatty acid oxidation is necessary as an energy source to maintain gluconeogenesis, there is an inhibition of glucose synthesis. Furthermore, since fatty acids cannot be used efficiently for formation of ATP, increased demands are made on glucose utilization; but since gluconeogenesis is also blocked, glycogen stores are rapidly depleted and the blood glucose concentration cannot be maintained.

REFERENCES

Hypoglycemia

Boden, G., Soriano, M., Hoeldtke, R. D., and Owen, O. E.; Counterregulatory hormone release and glucose recovery after hypoglycemia in non-insulin dependent diabetics. Diabetes 32:1055, 1983.

Broder, L. E., and Carter, S. K.: Pancreatic islet cell carcinoma. 1. Clinical features of 52 patients. Ann Intern Med 79:101, 1973.

Cahill, G. F., Jr., and Soeldner, J. S.: A non-editorial on nonhypoglycemia. N Engl J Med 291:905, 1974.

Couropmitree, C., Freinkel, N., Nagel, T. C., Horwitz, D. L., Metzger, B., Rubinstein, A. H., and Hahnel, R.: Plasma C-peptide and diagnosis of factitious hyperinsulinism. Ann Intern Med 82:201, 1975.

Cryer, P.: Glucose counterregulation in man. Diabetes 30:261, 1981.

Fajans, S. S., and Floyd, J. C.: Fasting hypoglycemia in adults. N Engl J Med 294:766, 1976.

Heitz, P. U., Kloppel, G., Hacki, W. H., Polak, J. M., and Pearse, A. G. E.: Nesidioblastosis: The pathologic basis of persistent hyperinsulinemic hypoglycemia in infants. Diabetes 26:632, 1977.

Ichihara, K., Shima, K., Saito, Y., Nonaka, K., Tarui, S., and Nishikawa, M.: Mechanism of hyperglycemia observed in a patient with insulin autoimmune syndrome. Diabetes 26:500, 1977.

Koivisto, V. A., and Felig, P.: Effects of leg exercise on insulin absorption in diabetic patients. N Engl J Med 298:79, 1978.

Megyesi, K., Kahn, C. R., Roth, J., and Gorden, P.: Hypoglycemia in association with extrapancreatic tumors: Demonstration of elevated plasma NSILA-S by a new radioreceptor assay. J Clin Endocrinol Metab 38:931, 1974.

Melancon, S. B., Kachadurian, M. D., and Nadler, H. L.: Metabolic and biochemical studies on fructose-1,6-diphosphatase deficiency. J Pediatr 82:650, 1973.

Merimee, T. J., and Tyson, J. E.: Stabilization of plasma glucose during fasting. Normal variations in two separate studies. N Engl J Med 291:1275, 1974.

Pagliara, A. S., Karl, I. E., Haymond, M., and Kipnis, D. M.: Hypoglycemia in infancy and childhood. J Pediatr 82:365, 558, 1973.

Permutt, M. A.: Postprandial hypoglycemia. Diabetes 25:719, 1976.

Rizza, R. A., Haymond, M. W., Verdonk, C. A., Mandarino, L. J., Miles, J. M., Service, F. J., and Gerich, J. E.: Pathogenesis of hypoglycemia in insulinoma patients. Suppression of hepatic glucose production by insulin. Diabetes 30:377, 1981.

Sacca, L., Sherwin, R., Hendler, R., and Felig, P.: Influence of continuous physiologic hyperinsulinemia on glucose kinetics and counterregulatory hormones in normal and diabetic humans. J Clin Invest 63:849, 1979.

Tanaka, K., Kean, E. A., and Johnson, B.: Jamaican vomiting sickness: Biochemical investigation of two cases. N Engl J Med 295:461, 1976.

Lipids in Biological Systems

CHEMICAL AND PHYSICAL PROPERTIES

Lipids are organic compounds that can be dissolved in solvents of low polarity (that is, solvents that are immiscible in water). The major classes of lipids can be divided into two groups (Fig. 56). The first group, the *nonpolar* lipids, include the triacylglycerols (synonyms are "triglycerides" and "fat") and the cholesteryl esters. These lipids are virtually insoluble in water and do not enter directly into active metabolic pathways; rather they serve mainly to store fatty acids (in the case of triglycerides) and cholesterol (in the case of cholesteryl esters) as lipid droplets in tissues. As discussed in Lipids (p. 334), the fatty acids that are esterified to glycerol in triglycerides may be classified as short-chain (up to 4 carbon atoms), medium-chain (6 to 10 carbon atoms), and long-chain (12 or more carbon atoms). Milk triglycerides contain appreciable amounts of medium- and short-chain fatty acids, but most mammalian triglycerides are composed almost entirely of long-chain fatty acids. A common shorthand designation of fatty acids depicts carbon chain length and number of unsaturated bonds. Thus, the main fatty acids in human triglycerides are the saturated fatty acid palmitic acid (16:0), the monounsaturated fatty acid oleic acid (18:1), and the diunsaturated fatty acid linoleic acid (18:2).

The second group, the *amphipathic* or *polar* lipids, have limited solubility in water, owing to the presence of polar as well as bulky nonpolar hydrocarbon regions. At concentrations exceeding this limited solubility, they form aggregates (micelles) in which a number of molecules are organized so as to expose the polar regions to water and to shield the hydrocarbon regions. The major amphipathic lipids are (1) fatty acids, in which the polar region is a negatively charged carboxyl group; (2) cholesterol, in which the polar region is an uncharged hydroxyl (alcohol) group; (3) glycerophosphatides, in which the polar region is a phosphate-containing aminoalcohol or polyalcohol; (4) sphingolipids, in which a basic lipid, ceramide, is combined with phosphorylcholine (sphingomyelins) or various carbohydrates (glycosphingolipids). The glycerophosphatides and sphingomyelins are often grouped together under the rubric of "phospholipids." The polar "head group" of phospholipids may be negatively charged at physiological pH (as in phosphatidylserine), positively charged (as in phosphatidylethanolamine), or zwitterionic (as in phosphatidylcholine ["lecithin"] and sphingomyelin) (Table 15). Whereas fatty acids form spherical micelles when they aggregate in water, glycerophosphatides and sphingolipids, with their bulkier nonpolar regions, form "myelin figures," in which lamellar layers of liquid crystals of the lipid alternate with layers of water (Fig. 57). Unlike nonpolar lipids, amphipathic lipids enter directly into active metabolic pathways and, except for fatty acids and certain cholesterol derivatives (see below), they

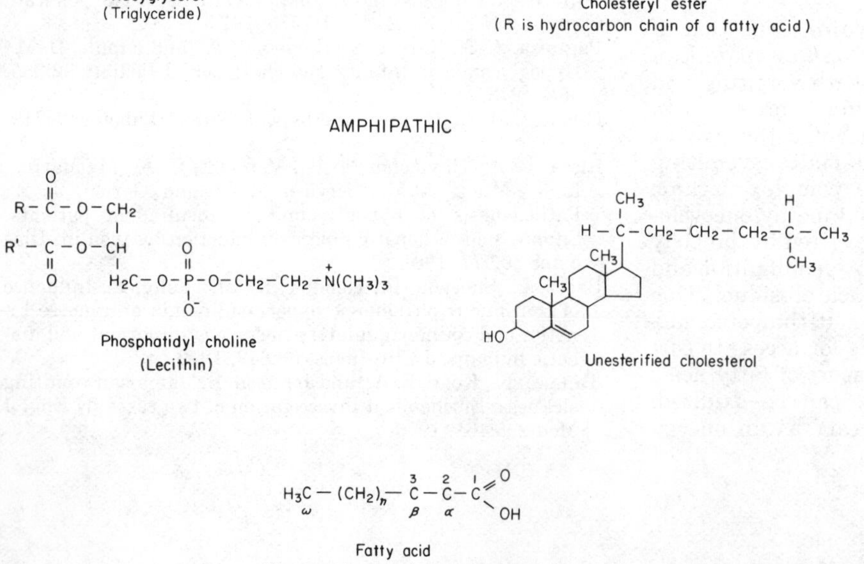

Figure 56. Major classes of lipids.

TABLE 15. SOME COMPLEX LIPIDS

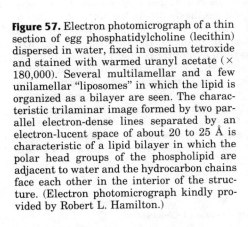

Glycerophosphatides
  Phosphatidylcholine (lecithin)
  Phosphatidylethanolamine (cephalins)
  Phosphatidylserine
  Phosphatidylinositol (lipositol)   "phospholipids"
  Cardiolipin (diphosphatidyl glycerol)
  Plasmalogens (ether-linked)
Sphingolipids
  Sphingomyelin (phosphorylcholine ceramide)
  Glycolipids
    Neutral: cerebrosides
    Acidic: gangliosides (sialocerebrosides)
             sulfatides (cerebroside sulfates)

REFERENCES

Chemical and Physical Properties of Lipids

Lehninger, A. L.: Lipids, lipoproteins and membranes. In Lehninger, A. L.: Biochemistry. 2nd ed. New York, Worth Publishers, 1975, p. 279.

Small, D. M.: Surface and bulk interactions of lipids and water with a classification of biologically active lipids based on these interactions. Fed Proc 29:1320, 1970.

van Golde, L. M. G., and van den Bergh, S. G.: Introduction: General pathways in the metabolism of lipids in mammalian tissues. In Synder, F. (ed.): Lipid Metabolism in Mammals. New York, Plenum Press, 1977, p. 1.

SOURCES OF FATTY ACIDS AND CHOLESTEROL

Although fatty acids can be synthesized in most tissues of the body by the pathway of "lipogenesis," this process contributes only a very small fraction of the fatty acid supply when the diet contains appreciable fat. Dietary fatty acids are derived mainly from dietary triglycerides and only to a small extent (except in eggs and organ meats) from complex lipids. The fatty acids in triglycerides are hydrolyzed in the small intestine by pancreatic lipase to yield two fatty acids

become major structural components of cell membranes, in which a lipid bilayer, resembling one lamella of a myelin figure, is associated with proteins.

Most of the fatty acids in the body are covalently bound to other compounds by ester, amide, or ether linkages. In lipids of blood plasma, most are bound as esters and it is this linkage that is attacked during the processes of lipid transport, described in Fatty Acid Transport (pages 401–404).

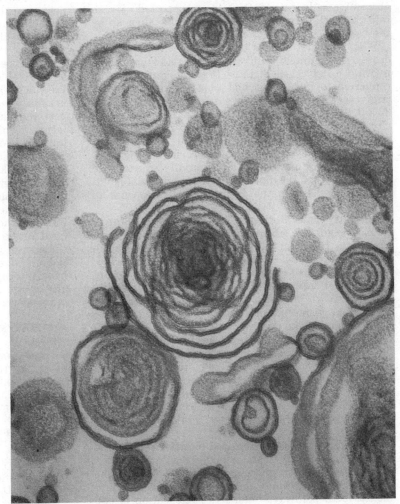

Figure 57. Electron photomicrograph of a thin section of egg phosphatidylcholine (lecithin) dispersed in water, fixed in osmium tetroxide and stained with warmed uranyl acetate (× 180,000). Several multilamellar and a few unilamellar "liposomes" in which the lipid is organized as a bilayer are seen. The characteristic trilaminar image formed by two parallel electron-dense lines separated by an electron-lucent space of about 20 to 25 Å is characteristic of a lipid bilayer in which the polar head groups of the phospholipid are adjacent to water and the hydrocarbon chains face each other in the interior of the structure. (Electron photomicrograph kindly provided by Robert L. Hamilton.)

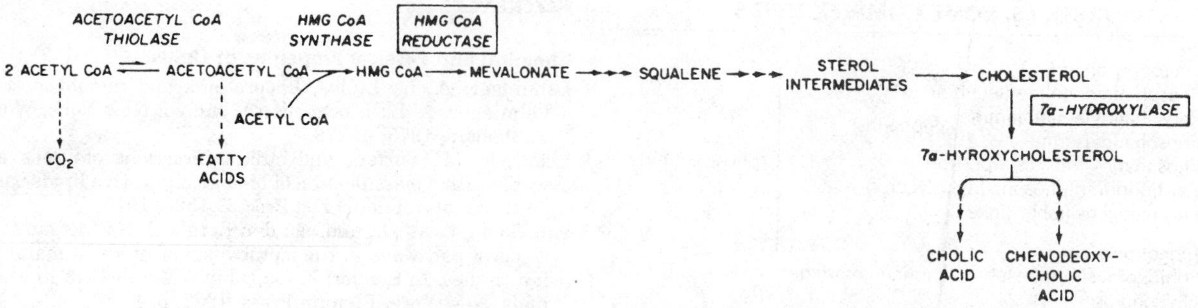

Figure 58. Pathway showing the major steps in the synthesis of cholesterol and bile acids and the steps at which metabolic regulation occurs. HMG CoA reductase is the major rate-controlling enzyme in the overall conversion of acetyl CoA to cholesterol. 7α-Hydroxylase is the major rate-controlling enzyme in the overall conversion of cholesterol to the two major bile acids, cholic acid and chenodeoxycholic acid.

and a monoglyceride. These lipolytic products associate with bile acids (which are polar products of hepatic cholesterol catabolism, as described below) to form mixed micelles, from which the fatty acids and monoglycerides diffuse readily into the microvillous membrane of intestinal absorptive cells. There, the fatty acids are reesterified to form triglycerides and then secreted as components of chylomicrons (see below) into the intestinal lymph. Short- and medium-chain fatty acids, produced by lipase action in the intestinal lumen, are not reesterified appreciably in intestinal absorptive cells; rather, they are transported as such into the portal venous blood and largely taken up by the liver.

When the diet is poor in fat (and rich in carbohydrates), the limited ability of the body to store carbohydrate as glycogen dictates that the remainder be converted to fatty acids and then esterified to form triglycerides by the pathways described in Lipids (pp. 334–339). In many mammals, adipose tissue is a major site of conversion of carbohydrates to fat, but in humans most lipogenesis occurs in the liver. Dietary carbohydrates are also converted to fat in the liver whenever caloric intake is substantially in excess of need, even when the diet also contains appreciable fat. Thus, lipogenesis is the final metabolic response to gluttony.

The fatty acids of dietary fats, whether of plant or animal origin, are efficiently absorbed, even with very high rates of intake (up to 300 or more grams daily). Dietary sterols, by contrast, are less well absorbed. Sterols in plants, such as sitosterol and campesterol (which differ only slightly from cholesterol chemically), are very poorly absorbed (less than 1 to 2 per cent). Absorption of cholesterol in humans is less limited. At low levels of intake (less than 300 mg daily), about 50 per cent is absorbed. At higher levels, absorption tends to fall, but net absorption increases with increasing intake up to very high levels (2000 mg daily). Cholesterol, like fatty acids, is also absorbed from mixed micelles in the intestinal lumen, esterified in the absorptive cells of the intestine and incorporated into chylomicrons that are secreted into the intestinal lymph.

Cholesterol can be synthesized by most cells of the body, and, like fatty acids, it is derived from a series of reductive steps beginning with acetyl CoA in the endoplasmic reticulum (Fig. 58). The first step is common to both pathways—namely, condensation of two

acetyl CoA units to form acetoacetyl CoA—but thereafter the pathways diverge, with that to cholesterol leading to the synthesis of β-hydroxy-β-methylglutaryl CoA (HMG-CoA) and thence, by the principal rate-limiting and regulated step, catalyzed by HMG-CoA reductase, to mevalonic acid. Steps beyond mevalonic acid in the biosynthetic sequence, including formation of squalene and then cyclization to form the complex cyclopentanoperhydrophenanthrene ring, are not ordinarily rate-limiting, but the activity of at least some of the enzymes that catalyze steps beyond mevalonic acid may also be subject to regulation.

Cholesterol is needed by cells as an essential component in the synthesis of membranes in tissues with rapid cell turnover. Thus, rapid cholesterol synthesis can be expected to occur in fetal life and in cells such as those of the hemopoietic system, which have a short life-span. The content of cholesterol in cell membranes is tightly regulated, as described in Cholesterol Transport and Catabolism (p. 404). One aspect of this regulation involves cholesterol synthesis, chiefly at the level of HMG-CoA reductase. Under most conditions, body cholesterol synthesis occurs mainly in the parenchymal cells of the liver and the absorptive cells of the small intestine. In humans, the limited absorption of dietary cholesterol evidently is insufficient to meet the needs of these tissues. Thus, although hepatic cholesterol synthesis varies inversely with dietary cholesterol intake, the liver continues to synthesize some cholesterol under most conditions. By contrast, although most tissues other than liver and intestine have the capacity to synthesize cholesterol, they usually obtain sufficient cholesterol from plasma lipoproteins, as described below.

REFERENCES

Sources of Fatty Acids and Cholesterol

Bloch, K.: The biological synthesis of cholesterol. Science 150:19, 1965.

Carey, M. C., Small, D. M., and Bliss, C. M.: Lipid digestion and absorption. Annu Rev Physiol 45:651, 1983.

Grundy, S. M.: Dietary fats and sterols. In Levy, R. I., Rifkind, B. M., Dennis, B. H., and Ernst, N.: Nutrition, Lipids and Coronary Heart Disease. New York, Raven Press, 1979, p. 89.

Turley, S. D., and Dietschy, J. D.: Cholesterol metabolism and excretion. In Arias, I., Popper, H., Schachter, D., and Shafritz, D. A.: The Liver: Biology and Pathobiology. New York, Raven Press, 1982, p. 467.

Lipid Transport and Catabolism

THE LIPOPROTEINS OF BLOOD PLASMA

Owing to the fundamental properties previously described, lipids do not exist to any extent in free solution in body fluids. Rather, they are carried almost entirely in complexes with proteins, known as lipoproteins. Some polar lipids, such as fatty acids and certain fat-soluble vitamins, are carried primarily by specific plasma proteins. For example, fatty acids (usually called "free fatty acids" to distinguish them from the esterified fatty acid residues found in other lipids) are carried in noncovalent association with plasma albumin, and vitamin A (retinol) is carried by a specific retinol-binding protein. However, nonpolar lipids, such as triglycerides, cholesteryl esters, retinyl esters, and carotenoids, are found in the "core" of large spherical lipoproteins, in which they are covered by a monolayer of polar lipids, chiefly phospholipids and cholesterol, together with variable amounts of proteins (Fig. 59). These lipoproteins possess the fundamental properties of a micelle composed of amphipathic lipids, but differ from such micelles in that they also contain a core region containing the nonpolar lipids and are therefore microemulsions. In these lipoproteins it is the core components that primarily are transported from one part of the body to another; the amphipathic lipids and

proteins compose the vehicle for transport, although they may also be taken up into cells, along with the nonpolar components, during lipoprotein catabolism. Small amounts of nonpolar lipids are dissolved in the surface monolayer, from which they can also move, via special transfer proteins, from one lipoprotein to another. At this site, they are also available for enzymatic attack.

The spherical lipoproteins are generally divided into two groups, according to the content of the major core components, triglycerides and cholesteryl esters. The two triglyceride-rich lipoprotein classes are the *chylomicrons* and the *very low density lipoproteins* (VLDL), and the two cholesteryl ester–rich lipoproteins are the *low density lipoproteins* (LDL) and the *high density lipoproteins* (HDL) (Fig. 60). Each of these lipoprotein classes, which have distinct functions in lipid transport, can be separated from plasma by various physical methods. The most generally useful of these methods is ultracentrifugation, which takes advantage of the differing hydrated densities of lipoproteins. In general, lipoproteins with the lowest density are the largest because they contain more nonpolar core lipids of low density relative to the surface components. The latter include the slightly more dense polar lipids and especially the much denser proteins. When blood plasma

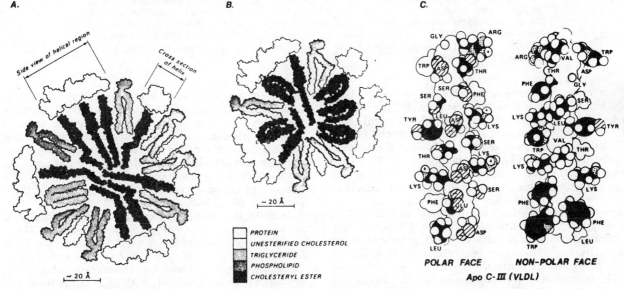

Figure 59. *A* and *B,* Cross sections of space-filling models of two fractions of human HDL. *A,* HDL₂ (density interval = 1.063–1.125 g/ml) and *B,* HDL₃ (density interval = 1.125–1.21 g/ml). The various components are drawn from projections of molecular models and the surface perimeters are divided into lipid and protein regions on the basis of compositional data. The surface contains helical portions of the proteins, the polar head groups of phospholipids, and the polar ring *A* of the sterol nucleus with its hydroxyl group. The nonhelical regions of the protein are not shown. Note that it is possible for the fatty acyl chains of cholesteryl esters to be in an extended configuration of HDL₂, whereas in HDL₃ they are folded upon the sterol nucleus. Most of these cholesteryl esters penetrate between the hydrocarbon chains of the phospholipids, 85 per cent of which are composed of lecithin (phosphatidyl choline). Panel *C,* orientation of amino acids at the polar and nonpolar faces of a single amphipathic helical region of C-III apoprotein shown in two projections. (HDL models are reproduced from Verdery and Nichols: Chem Phys Lipids 14:123, 1975; the model of an amphipathic helix is reproduced from Segrest, Jackson, Morrisett, and Gotto: FEBS Lett 38:247, 1974, with permission of the publishers.)

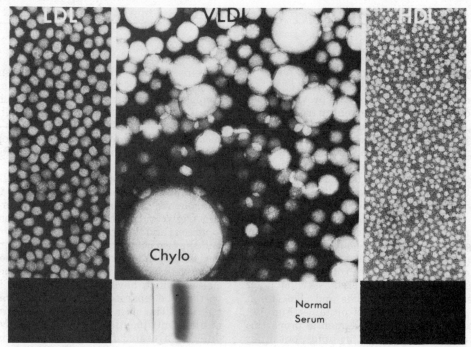

Figure 60. Major classes of human plasma lipoproteins. *Above:* electron photomicrographs of negatively stained preparations obtained by preparative ultracentrifugation. *Below:* agarose electropherogram of normal human plasma, stained for lipid with Sudan black. The upper left panel shows low density lipoproteins (LDL), about 200 Å in diameter, which correspond to β-lipoproteins (intensely staining band on electropherogram). The middle panel shows very low density lipoproteins (VLDL), 300 to 800 Å in diameter, which correspond to pre-β lipoproteins (middle band on electropherogram). A single chylomicron is also shown; upon electrophoresis in agarose gel, chylomicrons remain at the origin (line at left on electropherogram) because they are too large to enter the interstices of the gel particles. The right panel shows high density lipoproteins (HDL), about 100 Å in diameter, which correspond to α-lipoproteins (band at right on electropherogram). (Electron micrographs kindly provided by R. L. Hamilton.)

is subjected to ultracentrifugation (at forces of about 100,000 × gravity), the triglyceride-rich lipoproteins, which have densities less than 1.006 grams/ml, float to the top of the centrifuge tube, whereas the cholesteryl ester–rich lipoproteins sink toward the bottom. Chylomicrons and VLDL can be separated from each other by techniques that take advantage of the larger size of chylomicrons (rate centrifugation or gel filtration chromatography). The distinction by size of chylomicrons and VLDL is not absolute, but the usual cutting point is at a particle diameter of 800 Å. Ultracentrifugation at a density of 1.063 grams/ml floats the LDL, and subsequent centrifugation at a density of 1.21 grams/ml floats the HDL. Neither LDL nor HDL, so defined, are homogeneous, either structurally or physiologically. The least dense component of LDL (with density between 1.006 and 1.019 grams/ml) is usually called *intermediate density lipoprotein* (IDL) to distinguish it from the major, more homogeneous LDL with density between 1.019 and 1.063 grams/ml. HDL are often separated into two subclasses, HDL_2 (with density between 1.063 and 1.125 grams/ml) and HDL_3 (with density between 1.125 and 1.21 grams/ml). Some of the properties of the major lipoprotein classes are summarized in Table 16.

In certain disease states, lipoproteins of a quite different structure are found in blood plasma. These lipoproteins are composed mainly of amphipathic lipids

and proteins, with very few nonpolar lipids. These lipoproteins are composed of a lipid bilayer, as in a typical cell membrane, together with one or more of the same proteins found in spherical lipoproteins, and are consequently called *lamellar* lipoproteins. They occur in two principal forms. In the first the particles are coin- or disk-shaped and in the second they form a hollow vesicle or "liposome" (Fig. 61). Some of their properties are also shown in Table 16.

Each of the plasma lipoprotein classes contains a group of specific proteins, the *apolipoproteins*. These proteins have specific functions in lipoprotein synthesis, secretion, or catabolism. For purposes of convenience and presumed functional interrelationships, they are often grouped together, with each group receiving an alphabetical designation. In most cases, the apolipoproteins behave like the "peripheral" proteins of cell membranes. They are water-soluble when separated from the lipids and transfer readily between different lipoprotein classes, as well as among particles of the same class. The association of these proteins with lipids involves important hydrophobic forces. However, interactions between regions of these proteins and the polar "head" groups of phospholipids on the surface of lipoproteins seem to be critical to the lipid-binding property of these apolipoproteins. Molecular models of those apolipoproteins that have been sequenced indicate that they contain regions known as "amphipathic

TABLE 16. PROPERTIES OF NORMAL AND ABNORMAL HUMAN PLASMA LIPOPROTEINS

CLASS	DIAMETER (Å)	DENSITY (g/ml)	ELECTROPHORETIC MOBILITY	CHEMICAL COMPOSITION (% of Dry Mass)				
				"Core"		"Surface"		
				Triglyc-erides	Choles-teryl esters	Choles-terol	Phospho-lipids	Proteins
Spherical (normal)								
Chylomicrons	800–5000	0.93	α_2	86	3	2	7	2
VLDL	300–800	0.95 –1.006	pre-β	55	12	7	18	8
IDL	250–350	1.006–1.019	slow pre-β	23	29	9	19	19
LDL	216	1.019–1.063	β	6	42	8	22	22
HDL$_2$	100	1.063–1.125	α_1	5	17	5	33	40
HDL$_3$	75	1.125–1.210	α_1	3	13	4	25	55
Lp (a)*	300	1.055–1.085	slow pre-β	3	33	9	22	33
Lamellar (abnormal)								
Vesicles, LP-X	300–600	1.010–1.030	β	<2	<2	30	65	3
Discs, LCAT(−)	190–44	1.075–1.175	pre-β	4	1	29	45	21

*Lp(a) is a minor lipoprotein in most individuals, but in a few its concentration is substantial. It is also called "sinking pre-β lipoprotein." Its concentration is genetically determined.

helices," in which one face of the helix contains polar groups of amino acids and the other contains only nonpolar groups (Fig. 59). When these proteins are mixed with zwitterionic glycerophosphatides, heat is released and the helical content of the protein increases, suggesting that ionic interactions take place between the head group of the phospholipid and the polar face of the helix. Other portions of the protein are in intimate contact with nonpolar regions of the phospholipids and, in some lipoproteins, with the nonpolar core components as well.

One of the major apolipoproteins, known as apoli-

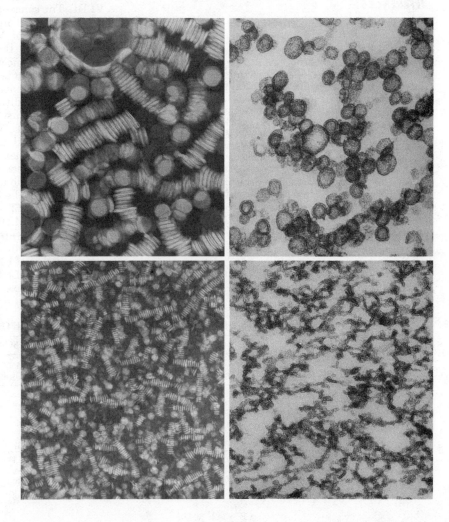

Figure 61. Lamellar lipoproteins. *Left:* electron photomicrographs of negatively stained preparations of vesicular (top) and discoidal (bottom) lamellar lipoproteins. *Right:* thin sections of osmium-fixed samples. In the thin sections it is evident that the vesicular lipoproteins (top) are spherical and that their wall is trilaminar (that is, like a lipid bilayer), whereas the discoidal lipoproteins (bottom), which stain similarly, are truly coin-shaped. The vesicular lipoproteins collapse when dried in the presence of potassium phosphotungstate for negative staining (top, left). The lamellar lipoproteins tend to associate in stacks (rouleaux) (top and bottom, left). (Electron micrographs from Hamilton, et al.: Science, 172:475, 1971; J Clin Invest 58: 667, 1976; reproduced with permission of the publishers.)

TABLE 17. THE HUMAN PLASMA APOLIPOPROTEINS

NAME	MOLECULAR WEIGHT	APPROXIMATE CONCENTRATION (mg/dl)
A-I	28,300	130
A-II	17,400	40
A-IV	46,000	15
B-100	~400,000	80
B-48	~210,000	0[a]
C-I	7,000	12
C-II	10,000	3
C-III[b]	9,300	12
D	32,500	10
E	34,100	5
Lp(a)	~645,000	3

[a]Present as component of chylomicrons during active fat absorption.
[b]Subspecies with 0, 1, 2, and 3 moles/ml of sialic acid are termed C-III-0, 1, 2, and 3, respectively.

poprotein B, does not behave as a peripheral protein, but rather more like an "intrinsic protein" of cell membranes. Little is yet known about the forces that bind this protein to lipid in the lipoproteins in which it occurs. Apolipoprotein B is found only in triglyceride-rich lipoproteins and LDL; it is not found in HDL or in lamellar lipoproteins. A list of the plasma apolipoproteins and some of their properties is given in Table 17.

REFERENCES

The Lipoproteins of Blood Plasma

Hamilton, R. L., and Kayden, H. J.: The liver and the formation of normal and abnormal plasma lipoproteins. In Becker, F. F. (ed.): The Liver: Normal and Abnormal Functions. New York, Marcel Dekker, 1974, p. 531.

Hatch, F. T., and Lees, R. S.: Practical methods for plasma lipoprotein analysis. Adv Lipid Res 6:1, 1968.

Havel, R. J.: Lipoproteins and lipid transport. In Kritchevsky, D., Paoletti, R., and Holmes, W. L. (eds.): Lipids, Lipoproteins, and Drugs. New York, Plenum Press, 1975, p. 37.

Jackson, R. L., Morrisett, J. D., and Gotto, A. M., Jr.: Lipoprotein structure and metabolism. Physiol Rev 56:259, 1976.

Kane, J. P.: Plasma lipoproteins: Structure and metabolism. In Snyder, F. (ed.): Lipid Metabolism in Mammals. Vol. I. New York, Plenum Press, 1977, p. 209.

QUANTIFICATION OF PLASMA LIPOPROTEINS

It is more convenient to measure the concentration of individual lipids in blood plasma than to measure them in individual lipoprotein classes (Table 18). Generally, the two lipids that are measured are "total cholesterol" and triglycerides. Total cholesterol is normally composed of about 75 per cent esterified cholesterol and about 25 per cent "free cholesterol" (so designated to indicate that the alcohol group of cholesterol is not in ester linkage with a long-chain fatty acid). Total phospholipids of plasma are not usually measured because their concentration follows closely that of total cholesterol. In general, the concentration of triglycerides in blood plasma provides a very good measure of the concentration of the triglyceride-rich lipoproteins. Normally, chylomicrons are absent from plasma in blood obtained in the postabsorptive state (that is, after individuals have not eaten for 9 to 15 hours). Thus, except for rare disorders associated with fasting chylomicronemia, measurement of the concentration of triglycerides is sufficient to estimate the concentration of VLDL. When chylomicrons are present, they can be detected after allowing the test-tube containing blood plasma or serum to remain in a refrigerator overnight. The larger chylomicrons, but not VLDL, will rise to the top of the tube as a creamy layer.

About two thirds of the plasma total cholesterol is normally carried in LDL so that the concentration of this lipid provides a reasonably good measure of the level of LDL in most people. However, with disease, a substantial fraction of cholesterol may be carried in VLDL. The concentration of LDL can still be estimated reasonably well in most cases from knowledge of the concentration of VLDL (estimated from plasma triglycerides) and that of total cholesterol. However, to estimate the concentration of LDL reliably and also to obtain an estimate of the concentration of HDL (which may also be important clinically), at least one measurement in addition to that of total cholesterol and triglycerides must be made: the concentration of cholesterol in HDL. This can be done rather simply by precipitating all lipoproteins other than HDL with a polyanion such as heparin and a divalent cation such as Mn^{++} and measuring the HDL-cholesterol that remains in solution. The concentration of LDL-cholesterol can then be estimated with accuracy in almost everyone (Fig. 62).

Estimates of LDL and HDL, based upon these three measurements, are useful because the composition of these lipoprotein classes varies less than does the concentration of LDL and HDL particles. However, the composition of LDL, and especially that of HDL, may vary with disease. In particular, when the concentra-

TABLE 18. DISTRIBUTION OF LIPIDS IN PLASMA LIPOPROTEINS

LIPOPROTEIN CLASS	CORE COMPONENTS (mg/dl)		SURFACE COMPONENTS (mg/dl)	
	Triglycerides	Esterified Cholesterol	Cholesterol	Phospholipids
VLDL	40	8	4	15
LDL (+ IDL)	22	97	37	95
HDL (HDL$_2$ + HDL$_3$)	8	40	9	85
VHDL*				25
Whole Plasma	70	145	50	220

Representative concentrations in unfractionated plasma for lean young men. Values for VLDL and LDL in particular vary widely in healthy individuals. Women of similar age have less VLDL and more HDL.
*Very high density lipoproteins (d > 1.21 g/ml). Most of the phospholipid in this class is lysolecithin, which is bound to albumin, but some lecithin associated with apolipoproteins is also present.

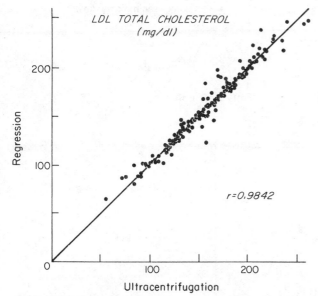

Figure 62. LDL-cholesterol concentration in 178 randomly selected healthy adults, determined directly by sequential preparative ultracentrifugation (abscissa) and estimated from three other lipid values: serum total cholesterol, serum triglycerides, and HDL-cholesterol (ordinate). There is no systematic difference between the two estimates of LDL-cholesterol (slope of regression line = 0.99) and the correlation coefficient is 0.984.

tion of triglycerides in chylomicrons or VLDL increases, LDL and HDL then contain fewer cholesteryl esters and more triglycerides in their cores owing to interchanges of nonpolar components among lipoproteins, as described below. Under these and some other circumstances, measurements of other lipoprotein components, such as one of the major apolipoproteins in a given class of lipoproteins, may provide more reliable and useful estimates of the concentration of lipoprotein particles.

REFERENCES

Quantification of Plasma Lipoproteins

Havel, R. J.: Classification of the hyperlipidemias. Annu Rev Med 28:195, 1977.

Myers, L. H., Phillips, N. R., and Havel, R. J.: Mathematical evaluation of methods for estimation of the concentration of the major lipid components of human serum lipoproteins. J Lab Clin Med 88:491, 1976.

Warnick, G. R., and Albers, J. J.: A comprehensive evaluation of the heparin-manganese precipitation procedure for estimating high density lipoprotein cholesterol. J Lipid Res 19:65, 1978.

LIPOPROTEIN BIOSYNTHESIS AND SECRETION

Triglyceride-rich lipoproteins are synthesized in two cells derived from the embryonic foregut: the absorptive mucosal cells of the small intestine and the parenchymal cells of the liver. As with most other proteins destined for export from cells, the protein components of these lipoproteins are synthesized on the ribosomes of the rough endoplasmic reticulum and transported into the cisternae of this organelle as a pro-protein. The lipid components are synthesized in the smooth endoplasmic reticulum and, by mechanisms not presently defined, are sequestered within the cisternae of this organelle as droplets that presumably consist of triglycerides and some cholesteryl esters, stabilized by a surface film of phospholipids. In the intestine, the triglycerides are synthesized mainly by the monoglyceride pathway (see Sources of Fatty Acids and Cholesterol, p. 393), in which the newly absorbed monoglycerides and fatty acids produced by the action of pancreatic lipase upon dietary fat are recombined following activation of the fatty acids with coenzyme A. In the liver, the triglycerides are synthesized by the phosphatidic acid pathway (Fig. 63). These two pathways have a high capacity and each is driven by the rate at which fatty acids enter (or are formed within) the cell. The major phospholipid of these droplets (lecithin) is formed in both cells by reactions that also lead from phosphatidic acid (Fig. 63). In the intestine, lecithin may also be formed from dietary lecithin by reacylation of lysolecithin produced by pancreatic phospholipase in the intestinal lumen. The cholesteryl esters that are found in these droplets are also synthesized by an enzyme (acyl CoA cholesterol acyltransferase; ACAT) that catalyzes the transfer of activated fatty acid to cholesterol.

The newly formed lipid droplet moves within the smooth endoplasmic reticulum and, presumably at or near the junction of the smooth and rough reticulum, joins with the newly formed protein to form the nascent lipoprotein. Apolipoprotein B is the key protein in this process. In the genetic disorder abetalipoproteinemia, the failure of this apolipoprotein to be synthesized normally or to bind to the lipid droplet results in complete failure of secretion of triglyceride-rich lipoproteins from both intestine and liver. Other apolipoproteins also become associated with the nascent lipoprotein particle. In the intestine, these "peripheral" proteins are those of the "A" group, including apolipoproteins A-I, A-II, and A-IV. In the liver, the major peripheral proteins associated with nascent VLDL are those of the "C" group (C-I, C-II, and C-III) and apolipoprotein E. After initial assembly the nascent lipoproteins move from the endoplasmic reticulum, enclosed within the membranous system, to the Golgi apparatus, where they accumulate in secretory vesicles. The secretory vesicle moves to the cell surface, with the participation of the microtubular system, and the membrane of the vesicle fuses with the plasma membrane, releasing the lipoprotein particles into the extracellular space. The basic processes involved are those described above for secretion of other proteins from the cell, differing from them mainly in the combined and evidently coordinate synthesis of lipids and specific proteins. The newly secreted chylomicrons enter the lacteals in the intestinal villi by moving between the lining endothelial cells and are thence transported to the blood via the thoracic duct. VLDL enter the blood through the fenestrae of the sinusoidal cells lining the hepatic microcirculation (Fig. 64).

The rates of triglyceride synthesis in gut and liver depend upon the fatty acid traffic. Secretion of chylomicrons is directly coupled to the rate of fat absorption. During active fat absorption, the rate of lymphatic triglyceride transport may be as high as 300 grams

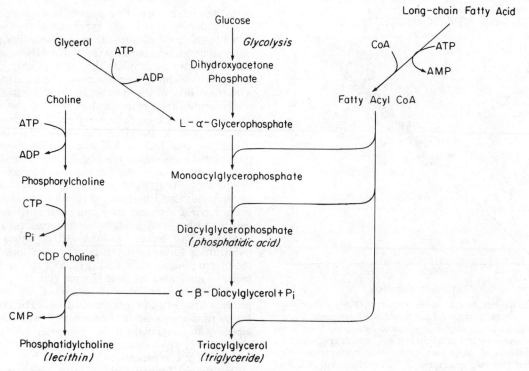

Figure 63. Pathways for the synthesis of triglycerides and lecithin in the endoplasmic reticulum of the liver. Diacylglycerol is the common lipid precursor of both products.

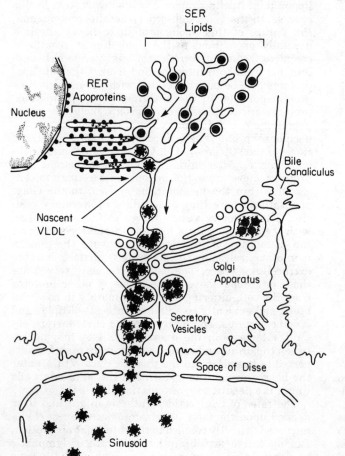

Figure 64. This diagram depicts the sites of synthesis and assembly and the pathway of secretion of VLDL in the liver (see text). RER = rough endoplasmic reticulum, with attached ribosomes. SER = smooth endoplasmic reticulum. The details of this diagram are discussed in the text.

daily. This large increase in transport rate is achieved in part by synthesis of a greater number of chylomicron particles, but it also depends upon the formation of larger particles. An increase in chylomicron diameter during active fat absorption, from an average of 500 Å to 2000 Å, is associated with a 64-fold increase in triglyceride mass per particle. In the postabsorptive state the rate of triglyceride secretion from the liver is about 15 grams per day. This rate can also be increased, according to the fatty acid traffic, to as much as 100 grams daily.

Normally, the absorptive mucosal cells of the small intestine have the capacity to secrete rapidly in chylomicrons virtually all of the triglycerides that they synthesize in response to a dietary fat load. This is not the case for the liver. This organ responds to an increased load of fatty acid not only by secreting more triglycerides in VLDL, but also by sequestering and storing triglycerides as large droplets in the cytoplasm, leading to the state known as "fatty liver."

In the formation of triglyceride-rich lipoproteins of varying size, the content of apolipoprotein B (the protein essential to the synthesis and secretion of these lipoproteins) in each particle remains constant. Thus, synthesis of this apolipoprotein is directly related to the rate at which particles are secreted and not necessarily to the rate of triglyceride secretion.

The surface of chylomicrons and VLDL is rapidly modified when these particles are exposed to other lipoproteins in lymph or blood plasma. Certain proteins, especially the C and E apolipoproteins, are rapidly transferred to chylomicrons from HDL, in exchange for phospholipids. As described below, these transfers are critical to the metabolism of these particles.

REFERENCES

Lipoprotein Biosynthesis and Secretion

Alexander, C. A., Hamilton, R. L., and Havel, R. J.: Subcellular localization of "B" apoprotein of plasma lipoproteins in rat liver. J Cell Biol 69:241, 1976.

Havel, R. J.: Caloric homeostasis and disorders of fuel transport. N Engl J Med 287:1186, 1972.

Havel, R. J.: Lipoprotein biosynthesis and metabolism. Ann NY Acad Sci 348:16, 1980.

Havel, R. J.: Origin of HDL. In Gotto, A. M., Miller, N. E., and Oliver, M. F. (eds.): High Density Lipoproteins and Atherosclerosis. Amsterdam, Elsevier/North-Holland Biomedical Press B. V., 1978, p. 21.

FATTY ACID TRANSPORT

Fatty acids are transported in plasma as triglycerides in lipoproteins that are synthesized in the small intestine and the liver. They are also transported in the unesterified ("free") form, bound to plasma albumin. The reasons that two distinct mechanisms for fatty acid transport have evolved may perhaps be deduced from their respective functions. Free fatty acids (FFA) are derived primarily from stored triglycerides in adipose tissue and are transported to other tissues, where they provide for energy needs. Triglycerides, by contrast, are transported to a large extent from the tissues of origin to adipose tissue to be stored.

Plasma FFA are derived from two sources: (1) from hydrolysis of stored triglycerides in adipose tissue by a hormone-sensitive lipase, as described in Lipids (p. 334); (2) from hydrolysis of plasma triglycerides by lipoprotein lipase at the endothelial surface of capillaries in many tissues, as described in detail below (Fig. 65). In the postabsorptive state, more than 90 per cent of the plasma FFA is derived from stored fat. Under these conditions, the rate of hydrolysis of triglyceride ("lipolysis") in fat cells of an adult male is about 9 grams per hour, an amount sufficient to supply all of the needs of oxidative metabolism at rest. By contrast, when insulin is secreted in response to carbohydrate ingestion, the rate of transport of FFA falls rapidly to about 2 to 3 grams per hour. Under these circumstances, a greater fraction of plasma FFA may be derived from hydrolysis of plasma triglycerides, owing in part to increased activity of lipoprotein lipase in adipose tissue, the synthesis of which is also promoted by insulin. In adipose tissue, the activities of lipoprotein lipase and the hormone-sensitive lipase are inversely related with changing nutritional state, in keeping with their respective functions of fat storage and mobilization.

Although FFA are tightly bound to albumin, they are rapidly taken up into most cells of the body, so that their life-span in plasma is only about three minutes. FFA taken up into at least some cells are initially bound to specific "fatty acid–binding proteins," the concentrations of which may influence the rate of uptake. However, minute-to-minute changes in the rate of uptake of FFA into tissues such as liver and muscle are determined mainly by the rate of local blood flow. In the postabsorptive state at rest, oxidation of FFA supplies almost all of the energy needs of muscle and most other tissues except the central nervous system and a few tissues with low or absent aerobic oxidative capacity, such as mature erythrocytes. Any FFA entering a cell in excess of the immediate need for energy is esterified to triglycerides that are stored in small droplets within the cell. These triglycerides, together with glycogen, form the main cellular energy stores. Because of the rapidly acting controls on lipolysis in adipose tissue, the FFA transport system is admirably suited to regulated delivery of the fatty acids stored in adipose tissue. For proper homeostasis, equally effective mechanisms for fat storage must exist.

The need for such storage is evident from the large rates at which triglyceride can be transported from the small intestine (up to 15 grams per hour) and the liver (up to 4 grams per hour). The role of these two tissues in triglyceride transport differs. In the intestine, transcellular transport of fatty acids constitutes the major pathway for fatty acid traffic, whereas, in the liver, it is an "overflow" pathway, used to the extent that entry of fatty acids (or their formation within the cell) exceeds the needs of oxidative metabolism. Thus, in the postabsorptive state, about 3 grams of FFA enters the liver hourly, but only about 0.6 gram leaves the liver as triglycerides in VLDL.

The catabolism of triglyceride-rich lipoproteins proceeds in two steps. The first of these occurs in extrahepatic tissues and constitutes the unique function of lipoprotein lipase, located at the surface of capillary endothelial cells in many tissues. The lipoprotein particles entering capillaries bind to these enzymes and,

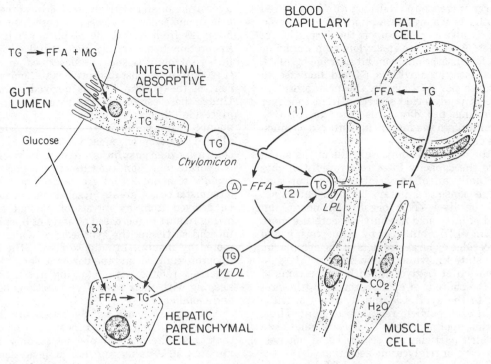

Figure 65. Sources and fate of plasma triglycerides. Triglycerides (TG) in chylomicrons are derived primarily from absorbed fatty acids (FFA) and monoglycerides (MG), whereas VLDL triglycerides are formed in liver from fatty acids that are derived from the following sources: (1) stored fat in adipose tissue; (2) hydrolysis of lipoprotein-triglycerides by lipoprotein lipase (LPL) on capillary endothelial cells; and (3) dietary carbohydrates converted to fatty acids in the liver. Fatty acids derived from the first two sources are transported in the blood bound to albumin (A). Fatty acids derived from triglycerides taken up by the liver in remnant lipoproteins also contribute to hepatic triglyceride synthesis (not shown). Whereas the rate of transport of triglycerides in chylomicrons is a direct function of dietary fat intake, transport of triglycerides in VLDL is an "overflow" pathway used to the extent that fatty acids are not needed by the liver for oxidative metabolism or synthesis of biliary lipids. Note that diversion of energy-rich substrates, such as FFA, to muscle can limit their availability for hepatic triglyceride snythesis.

in the presence of a specific apolipoprotein cofactor (C-II), the component triglycerides are efficiently hydrolyzed to form 2-monoglycerides and two molecules of FFA. Lipoprotein lipase is readily displaced from the capillary surface by negatively charged polyelectrolytes, including heparin, which suggests that these enzymes are bound to a similar molecule on the cell surface, possibly heparan sulfate. Removal of chylomicron triglycerides is so rapid that it seems likely that several enzyme molecules act simultaneously on each particle (Fig. 66). The average life-span of a chylomicron triglyceride is about 5 minutes. For VLDL triglycerides, the rate is slower, with an average life-span on the order of 30 minutes. Under most conditions, 80 to 90 per cent of the triglycerides contained in chylomicrons and VLDL is removed by the action of lipoprotein lipase. The monoglycerides produced are rapidly hydrolyzed by separate enzymes so that all three fatty acids are made available for uptake into the tissues or to "recycle" in the blood as albumin-bound FFA.

Lipoprotein lipase turns over rapidly and is subject to active regulation. The enzyme in adipose tissue is particularly responsive to nutritional state; its functional activity is increased by insulin secreted after ingestion of carbohydrate. This increase in activity promotes storage of fat in adipose tissue.

Most of the lipoprotein lipase in the body is normally found in adipose tissue and "red" muscle fibers (muscles that are rich in mitochondria and thus have high aerobic capacity). "White" muscle fibers that are poor in mitochondria and thus contract intermittently and mainly under anaerobic conditions contain little of the enzyme. Not all of the lipoprotein lipase in a tissue is located at the capillary surface. Some of it, presumably serving as a stored precursor of the endothelial species, must be transported to the endothelial surface to perform its normal function.

The fate of the fatty acids produced by the action of lipoprotein lipase is determined not only by the concentration of the active endothelial species but also by the activity of enzymes of fatty acid oxidation and esterification within tissues. In the postabsorptive state, a substantial fraction of the FFA produced from plasma triglycerides (about 50 per cent) is recycled in the blood bound to albumin; these FFA are handled as are those FFA derived from triglycerides in adipose tissue (Fig. 65). In the fed state, a larger fraction is esterified directly in the tissue containing the enzyme. The adaptation is most notable in adipose tissue and is required for effective storage of these FFA as fat.

The hydrolysis of the bulk of triglycerides in chylomicrons and VLDL by lipoprotein lipase is accompanied by concomitant modification of the surface of

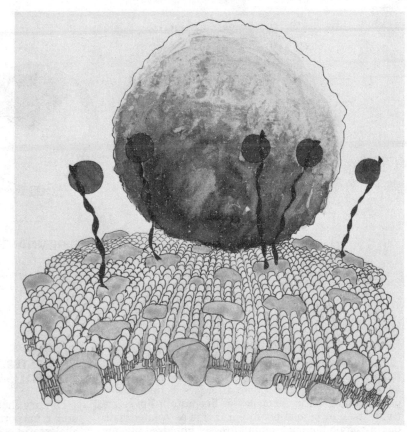

Figure 66. Model for the interaction of lipoprotein lipase with a substrate triglyceride-rich lipoprotein at the surface of the capillary endothelium. The enzyme (small dark spheres) is attached to a glycosaminoglycan (possibly heparan sulfate), which in turn is anchored to membrane proteins interspersed in the lipid bilayer that forms the plasma membrane of the endothelial cells. The length of the glycosaminoglycan molecules is 200 to 500 Å and the enzyme molecules are anchored at some distance from the membrane. Note that several enzyme molecules may act simultaneously on one lipoprotein particle and that the immediate environment is that of blood plasma rather than the cell membrane. (From Olivecrona, et al.: Fed Proc 36:60, 1977; reproduced with permission of the publisher.)

the particles. These modifications reduce the amount of surface so as to maintain the basic pseudomicellar structure of the particle. Thus, removal of 85 per cent of the core of a given particle reduces its diameter by a factor of two and requires a corresponding reduction of surface components of about 75 per cent to maintain a "tight" surface monolayer. This is accomplished in two ways. First, some of the lecithin on the surface is also attacked by lipoprotein lipase to yield lysolecithin, which, like FFA, leaves the surface and is bound to albumin. The remainder of the lecithin and most of the "A" and "C" apolipoproteins are transferred to HDL. The C apolipoproteins are utilized repeatedly in the metabolism of triglyceride-rich lipoproteins, cycling between newly secreted chylomicrons or VLDL and HDL. The fate of the phospholipids and A apolipoproteins (the latter derived only from chylomicrons) will be covered in the following discussion on Cholesterol Transport and Catabolism.

When the surface of chylomicrons and VLDL has been sufficiently modified, including the loss of the C-II apolipoprotein cofactor for lipoprotein lipase, this enzyme ceases to act effectively upon the partially degraded particle, which is now called a "remnant." Remnant catabolism constitutes the second step in the catabolism of these lipoproteins. Chylomicron remnants that leave the capillary surface are rapidly taken up by the liver. This efficient process involves binding of the remnant particle to a specific receptor on the surface of hepatic parenchymal cells. Recognition of remnants by hepatic receptors is facilitated by loss of the C apolipoproteins and seems to be mediated specifically by apolipoprotein E. The bound remnants are then taken up by endocytosis of coated pit regions. The endocytic vesicles fuse to form multivesicular bodies,

which in turn fuse with primary lysosomes. This leads to degradation of the component lipids and proteins of the particle by lipases and proteases that are active at the acid pH present within the endocytic compartment. In rats and certain other mammals, VLDL remnants are known to be metabolized by the liver in a similar manner, although a small fraction is further converted, by an ill-defined process, to form LDL. In this process, apolipoprotein B is conserved, but most of the remaining triglycerides and remaining "peripheral" proteins are removed (Fig. 67). In humans, this latter process normally accounts for a substantial fraction of total VLDL catabolism. The reason that VLDL can be converted to LDL whereas chylomicrons cannot may be that the B apoprotein of VLDL (B-100) differs from that of chylomicrons (B-48) (see Table 17). Remnant VLDL differ from their precursors not only by a reduced content of triglycerides but also by a substantially reduced number of C apolipoproteins. The latter change is associated with a less negative surface charge at the lipoprotein surface at physiological pH. By ordinary electrophoresis on supporting media, such as agarose gel, remnant VLDL can be distinguished from parent VLDL by their lower mobility. By this means, remnant VLDL can be found in the blood plasma of many humans. Some of these remnant particles remain in the same density range as their precursors (that is, less than 1.006 grams/ml), but some are more dense and are isolated as IDL. The process by which VLDL are converted to LDL accounts for all of the plasma LDL normally found in humans. Under most conditions, the number of LDL particles formed is a function of (1) the rate of secretion of VLDL particles from the liver, and (2) the extent to which VLDL remnants are taken up by the liver.

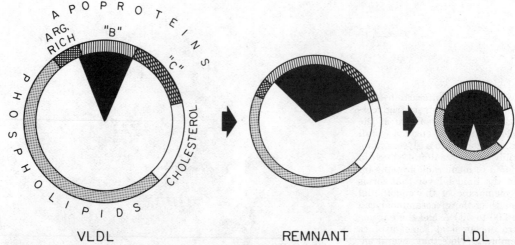

Figure 67. This diagram depicts the conversion of human VLDL, via VLDL remnants, to LDL. The relative size and the proportions of core and surface components are indicated. The mass of B apoprotein is the same in all three particles. Apoprotein E ("ARG, RICH") is conserved in remnants, but it and virtually all of the remaining C apoproteins are lost when LDL are formed. The mass of triglycerides (white region in the core) is reduced progressively at each step of the metabolism of VLDL.

The importance of lipoprotein lipase and apolipoproteins in catabolism of triglyceride-rich lipoproteins is evident in certain monogenic disorders of lipid transport. Thus, genetic deficiency of lipoprotein lipase activity itself or of apolipoprotein C-II is associated with fasting chylomicronemia and grossly impaired plasma triglyceride catabolism. Defective catabolism of remnant lipoproteins is observed in individuals with a mutant form of apolipoprotein E. This apolipoprotein is secreted from the liver in VLDL and is one of the proteins transferred to chylomicrons from HDL after they are secreted. It is retained in remnant lipoproteins, along with apolipoprotein B. Association of a mutant apolipoprotein E with defective remnant catabolism suggests that this protein is required for recognition of remnants by the liver.

REFERENCES

Fatty Acid Transport

Eisenberg, S., and Levy, R. I.: Lipoprotein metabolism. Adv Lipid Res 13:2, 1975.

Fielding, C. J.: Origin and properties of remnant lipoproteins. In Dietschy, J. M., Gotto, A. M., Jr., and Ontko, J. A. (eds.): Disturbances of Lipid and Lipoprotein Metabolism. Bethesda, Am Physiol Soc, 1978, p. 83.

Fielding, C. J., and Havel, R. J.: Lipoprotein lipase. Arch Pathol 101:225, 1977.

Havel, R. J.: Caloric homeostasis and disorders of fuel transport. N Engl J Med 287:1186, 1972.

Havel, R. J.: The fuels for muscular exercise. In Johnson, W. R., and Buskirk, E. R. (eds.): Science and Medicine of Exercise and Sport. New York, Harper and Row, 1974, p. 137.

Havel, R. J.: Lipoprotein biosynthesis and metabolism. Ann NY Acad Sci 348:16, 1980.

Olivecrona, T., Bengtsson, G., Marklund, S., Lindahl, U., and Höök, M.: Heparin-lipoprotein lipase interactions. Fed Proc 36:60, 1977.

Sigurdsson, G., Nicholl, A., and Lewis, B.: Conversion of very low density lipoprotein to low density lipoprotein. J Clin Invest 56:1481, 1975.

CHOLESTEROL TRANSPORT AND CATABOLISM

Dietary cholesterol is absorbed in the small intestine and transported, mainly after esterification to form cholesteryl esters, in chylomicrons. When chylomicron remnants are taken up into the liver, the cholesteryl esters are then hydrolyzed by acid lipases in lysosomes and the liberated cholesterol, together with the cholesterol present on the surface of the remnant particle, is transferred to various membranes of the liver cell. This cholesterol, by a process still poorly defined, leads to reduced activity of HMG-CoA reductase in the cell. Uptake of chylomicron cholesterol by the liver also leads to increased activity of cholesterol 17-α-hydroxylase, the first and rate-limiting enzyme in the pathway of conversion of cholesterol to bile acids (Fig. 58). These changes in enzymatic activity tend to maintain a constant content of cholesterol in the cell in the face of increased input of cholesterol from the blood. As discussed earlier, the parenchymal cells of the liver and absorptive mucosal cells of the small intestine normally account for most of the cholesterol synthesized in the body. Other tissues obtain most of their cholesterol from plasma lipoproteins. On a low cholesterol diet, a normal adult excretes about 550 mg of cholesterol (derived mainly from biliary cholesterol) and 250 mg of bile acids in the feces daily and loses about 100 mg of cholesterol during normal desquamation of skin. In the steady state, this means that 900 mg of cholesterol must be synthesized daily, mainly in the liver and small intestine. When cholesterol is present in the diet, hepatic cholesterol synthesis is repressed and more bile acids are synthesized. Individuals differ substantially in the extent to which they make each of these two responses to increased dietary cholesterol. Because chylomicron cholesterol is rapidly taken up by the liver, ingestion of cholesterol is not followed by a large increase in plasma cholesterol levels. However, increased intake of cholesterol in the diet generally leads gradually to increased levels of cholesterol in plasma lipoproteins, by mechanisms described below.

Almost all of the cholesteryl esters found in plasma lipoproteins in the postabsorptive state are produced within the blood itself by an enzyme secreted by the liver, lecithin-cholesterol acyltransferase (LCAT). This enzyme acts upon cholesterol and lecithin in a fraction of HDL to yield two products, cholesteryl ester (mainly cholesterol linoleate) and lysolecithin. As with lysolecithin produced by lipoprotein lipases during the catabolism of triglyceride-rich lipoproteins, the lysolecithin is transferred to albumin and transported to various cells, which take it up and acylate it to reform lecithin. The fate of the cholesteryl ester product will be discussed later.

The HDL upon which LCAT act are formed by complex mechanisms that are only partly understood. In rats, nascent HDL are secreted from the liver as lamellar discoidal lipoproteins. As with other lamellar lipoproteins, these disks contain very little nonpolar lipids, but rather are composed of a bilayer of phospholipids together with some cholesterol and certain apolipoproteins, including apolipoprotein A-I; this protein is a necessary cofactor for the efficient action of LCAT. These "nascent" HDL are converted by LCAT to spherical HDL, in which the product cholesteryl esters form the core of the particle, as shown in Figure 68. Apolipoprotein A-I is transferred from chylomicrons to HDL during the formation of chylomicron remnants, along with phospholipids and C apolipopro-

teins. Thus, surface components of triglyceride-rich lipoproteins contribute to the formation of plasma HDL. LCAT, by hydrolyzing the lecithin transferred from triglyceride-rich lipoproteins, contributes to the catabolism of these surface components.

By no means do all of the cholesteryl esters formed in HDL by LCAT remain in that lipoprotein class. Most of these esters are transferred by a transfer protein to VLDL, LDL, or other HDL particles. When VLDL are converted to LDL, a large fraction of the cholesteryl esters remain with the particle and this also contributes to the cholesteryl esters found in LDL which normally carry about two thirds of the cholesterol and cholesteryl esters in blood plasma.

LDL and HDL are catabolized in the liver and in a number of extrahepatic tissues. In contrast to triglyceride-rich lipoproteins, these cholesterol-rich lipoproteins remain in the blood for an average of several days, and some of these lipoproteins are gradually transported, presumably by pinocytosis, across the blood capillaries into many tissues. Considerable insight into the catabolism of LDL has come from studies of uptake by cells in tissue culture. When cells such as fibroblasts are grown for two days or more in the absence of lipoproteins in the growth medium, they develop the capacity to take up and degrade LDL (Fig. 69). This uptake depends upon a specific glycoprotein, which is a high affinity receptor for lipoproteins that contain apolipoproteins B or E. This "LDL receptor" is located in fibroblasts in restricted regions of the cell surface called "coated pits." The polymeric protein forming the coat on the cytoplasmic surface of the plasma membrane is called clathrin. Bound LDL or other lipoproteins are taken into the cell during endocytosis of the coated region and are then catabolized as described earlier for remnant lipoproteins. The cholesterol released by hydrolysis of cholesteryl esters in the core of LDL is free to transfer to other cell membranes and, in adrenal cortex and gonads, it can be used for synthesis of steroid hormones. The liberation of cholesterol within the cell also leads to reduction in

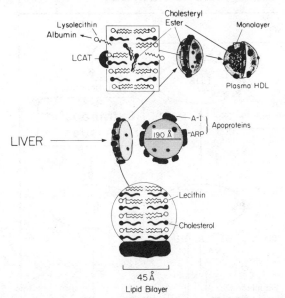

Figure 68. Formation of spherical HDL of blood serum from nascent discoidal HDL produced by the liver. In the presence of apolipoprotein A-1 cofactor, LCAT acts upon the lecithin and cholesterol in the bilayer of discoidal HDL to produce cholesteryl esters. These esters move into the nonpolar hydrocarbon region of the bilayer, causing it to swell, gradually producing a pseudomicellar HDL particle. The other product of the reaction, lysolecithin, leaves the surface of the particle and is bound to serum albumin. (From Hamilton: In Dietschy, J. M., Gotto, A. M., Jr., and Ontko, J. A. [eds.]: Disturbances of Lipid and Lipoprotein Metabolism. Bethesda, American Physiological Society, 1978, p. 164; reproduced with permission of the publisher.)

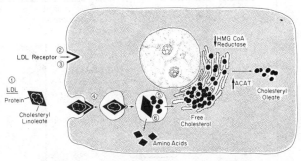

Figure 69. Sequential steps in the LDL pathway. The numbers indicate the sites at which mutations have been identified: (1) abetalipoproteinemia; (2) familial hypercholesterolemia, receptor-negative; (3) familial hypercholesterolemia, receptor-defective; (4) familial hypercholesterolemia, internalization defect; (5) Wolman disease; and (6) cholesteryl ester storage disease. HMG CoA reductase denotes 3-hydroxy-3 methylglutaryl coenzyme A reductase, and ACAT denotes acyl-CoA:cholesterol acyltransferase. (Modified from Brown and Goldstein: Science 191:150, 1976; reproduced with permission of the publisher.)

the activity of HMG-CoA reductase and activation of an ACAT, responses that tend to maintain the content of cholesterol in the cell. Not only are excessive amounts of cholesterol entering the cell stored as cholesteryl esters, but the liberation of cholesterol within the cell also leads to suppression of the synthesis of the high affinity receptor. By this means, the cell can regulate its uptake of LDL and consequently the accumulation of cholesteryl esters. In general, cells grown for sufficient time in the absence of lipoproteins in the culture medium make three responses designed to increase the availability of cholesterol: (1) they increase the activity of HMG-CoA reductase; (2) they increase the synthesis of the high affinity receptor for LDL; and (3) they decrease the synthesis of ACAT. Although the concentration of LDL in the extravascular space of tissues may be as low as 5 to 10 per cent of the concentration in blood plasma, studies with cultured cells indicate that such concentrations are more than sufficient to almost saturate the high affinity receptors. This presumably explains the very low rates of cholesterol synthesis generally found in cells when freshly isolated from the body. These facts provide the basis for a concept of "cholesterol homeostasis," in which the content of cholesterol in cell membranes is tightly regulated. It can be expected that conditions accompanied by rapid cell growth or division, as occurs normally in fetal and early postnatal life and in proliferative diseases such as hemolytic

states and rapidly growing cancers, will be accompanied by increased cellular synthesis of cholesterol and increased rates of uptake of LDL.

Although many cells of the body have the capacity to take up and degrade LDL via the LDL receptor, one half or more of LDL particles are normally catabolized in the liver, where they can readily pass through the fenestrae of the sinusoidal endothelium, thus gaining rapid access to the surface of the parenchymal cells. The cholesterol liberated during lysosomal catabolism of lipoproteins, such as LDL and chylomicron remnants, can be excreted in the bile as such or after oxidation to bile acids.

The best evidence that the "LDL receptor pathway" normally operates in vivo is the observation that mutations affecting the function of the receptor are associated with substantially increased concentrations of LDL in blood plasma (familial hypercholesterolemia). In individuals homozygous for deficiency of the receptor, the fractional catabolic rate of plasma LDL is 15 per cent daily, irrespective of the LDL level. By contrast, the fractional turnover rate in unaffected individuals is about 45 per cent per day. Catabolism of LDL in homozygotes is thought to occur by nonspecific pinocytosis, mainly in the liver. If this pathway is unaffected by the presence of mutant receptors for LDL, then it appears that about two thirds of LDL is normally catabolized via the LDL pathway.

Most of the cholesteryl esters produced by LCAT are

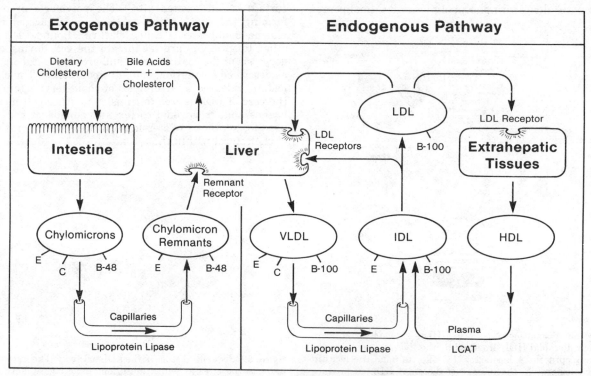

Figure 70. The two pathways of cholesterol transport in lipoproteins. Note that chylomicron remnants, which contain apoprotein B-48, enter the liver by receptor-mediated endocytosis. Some VLDL remnants (here indicated as "IDL"), which contain apoprotein B-100, also enter the liver, but a large fraction is converted instead to LDL. LDL are catabolized both in the liver and in extrahepatic tissues. Cholesterol in extrahepatic tissues can be returned to the liver ("reverse cholesterol transport") for excretion in the bile by a series of steps, which includes transfer to a fraction of HDL, esterification by LCAT, transfer of the esters to IDL (as shown here), VLDL or LDL, and uptake with these lipoproteins by the liver. This system can, however, also transfer cholesterol from one extrahepatic tissue to another. (From Goldstein et al.: N Engl J Med 309:288, 1983. Reprinted with permission of the publisher.)

catabolized with LDL. As LDL seem to be catabolized to a significant extent in extrahepatic tissues and the rate of transport of cholesterol in LDL is about 1.5 grams daily, it is clear that LDL can supply a substantial amount of cholesterol to various tissues.

The cholesterol used by LCAT comes from the surface of lipoproteins and from the plasma membrane of cells, and the LCAT system seems to prevent abnormal accumulation of cholesterol in plasma lipoproteins and tissues. In the rare monogenic disease familial LCAT deficiency, not only are plasma cholesteryl esters levels low, but discoidal HDL resembling nascent HDL and large abnormal lamellar lipoproteins accumulate in blood plasma. The cholesterol content of the plasma membrane of erythrocytes and certain other cells is also increased. Failure of cholesterol esterification in blood plasma therefore seriously interferes with the normal processes of cholesterol transport. Some HDL particles can accept cholesterol from cells; the cholesterol can then be converted to cholesteryl esters by LCAT. As mentioned above, most of these esters normally leave the blood with LDL. Thus it appears that cholesterol-rich lipoproteins provide the vehicles for transporting cholesterol to and from cells. LCAT, by forming cholesteryl esters, provides a concentration gradient that promotes movement of excess cholesterol onto HDL, whereas LDL and the LDL receptor system deliver the cholesterol as esters to cells that need cholesterol. For example, these combined mechanisms could transport cholesterol derived from dying cells, such as erythrocytes taken up in the spleen, to rapidly proliferating erythroblasts in the bone marrow, thus conserving the cholesterol molecule and maintaining cholesterol homeostasis.

Figure 70 summarizes the processes of cholesterol transport in plasma lipoproteins. There appear to be two major cycles of cholesterol transport. In one, dietary cholesterol is transported to the liver in chylomicron remnants and is then excreted in the bile as such or after conversion to bile acids. The biliary cholesterol is in part reabsorbed in the intestine and can therefore be reutilized. In the second, partially extrahepatic cycle, cholesterol taken up from cells or the surface of plasma lipoproteins onto HDL is transferred to LDL and then taken up into cells containing high affinity receptors for this lipoprotein. The cholesteryl esters of chylomicrons in the enterohepatic cycle are formed in the absorptive cells of the intestinal mucosa by ACAT, whereas the cholesteryl esters that participate in the extrahepatic cycle are produced by LCAT.

REFERENCES

Cholesterol Transport and Catabolism

Anderson, R. G. W., Brown, M. S., and Goldstein, J. L.: Role of the coated endocytic vesicle in the uptake of receptor-bound low density lipoprotein in human fibroblasts. Cell 10:351, 1977.
Brown, M. S., Anderson, R. G. W., and Goldstein, J. L.: Mutations affecting the binding, internalization, and lysosomal hydrolysis of low density lipoprotein in cultured human fibroblasts, lymphocytes, and aortic smooth muscle cells. J Supra Struc 6:85, 1977.
Brown, M. S., Kovanen, P. T., and Goldstein, J. L.: Receptor-mediated uptake of lipoprotein-cholesterol and its utilization for steroid synthesis in the adrenal cortex. Recent Prog Hormone Res 35:215, 1979.
Fielding, C. J., and Fielding, P. E.: Cholesterol transport between cells and body fluids. Med Clin North Am 66:363, 1982.
Glomset, J. A., Norum, K. A., Nichols, A. V., King, W. C., Mitchell, C. D., Applegate, K. R., Gong, E. L., and Gjone, E.: Plasma lipoproteins in familial lecithin: Cholesterol acyltransferase deficiency: Effects of dietary manipulation. Scand J Clin Lab Invest 35:3, 1975.
Goldstein, J. L., Kita, T., and Brown, M. S.: Defective lipoprotein receptors and atherosclerosis. N Engl J Med 309:288, 1983.
Hamilton, R. L.: Hepatic secretion and metabolism of high-density lipoproteins. In Dietschy, J. M., Gotto, A. M., Jr., and Ontko, J. A. (eds.): Disturbances in Lipid and Lipoprotein Metabolism. Bethesda, Am Physiol Soc, 1978, p. 155.
Havel, R. J.: Origin of HDL. In Gotto, A. M., Jr., Miller, N. E., and Oliver, M. F. (eds.): High Density Lipoproteins and Atherosclerosis. Amsterdam, Elsevier/North-Holland Biomedical Press, 1978, p. 21.
Nestel, P. J., and Poyser, A.: Changes in cholesterol synthesis and excretion when cholesterol intake is increased. Metabolism 25:1591, 1976.
Stein, Y., Stein, O., and Goren, P.: Metabolism and metabolic role of serum high density lipoproteins. In Gotto, A. M., Jr., and Oliver, M. F. (eds.): High Density Lipoproteins and Atherosclerosis. Amsterdam, Elsevier/North-Holland Biomedical Press, 1978, p. 37.

Nutritional Aspects of Lipid Transport and Metabolism

CALORIC INTAKE

As triglycerides contain little oxygen and are stored in cells in anhydrous droplets, fat provides an efficient means of storage of energy. Oxidation of one gram of triglyceride yields about 9 kilocalories. Fat storage in adipose tissue, which contains about 70 per cent triglycerides by weight, can therefore yield about 6 kilocalories per gram. Oxidation of one gram of carbohydrate, which contains much more oxygen than does fat, yields about 4 kilocalories per gram. As glycogen, the storage form of carbohydrate, is hydrated in tissues, only about 1.5 kilocalories is available for each gram of tissue glycogen.

Glycogen and triglycerides are stored to some extent in most cells and can be used directly for cellular energy metabolism. However, glycogen storage in the body is limited. Most glycogen is stored in liver and muscle. In each tissue, maximal glycogen stores are about 5 per cent of tissue mass, so that liver can store up to 75 grams and muscle as much as 1000 grams. Triglycerides are stored largely in adipose tissue. The extent of storage normally varies over a wide range. On the average, these triglycerides comprise about 15 per cent of body weight in adult men and about 20 per cent in adult women.

In humans, very little of the triglycerides in adipose tissue is synthesized there from carbohydrates or other precursors. Rather, they are derived from triglycerides delivered to adipose tissue via the blood, as described in the discussion on Lipid Transport and Catabolism. When the diet contains appreciable fat (that is, more than 10 to 20 per cent of caloric intake) almost all fat stores are derived directly from dietary fat (that is, chylomicron triglycerides). On low fat diets, lipogenesis from carbohydrates is activated in the liver. Hepatic lipogenesis increases especially when excessive amounts of carbohydrates are eaten and can yield 100 grams or more of triglycerides daily. This results in fat storage in the liver, which can occasionally amount to 10 to 30 per cent of hepatic mass. Transport of these triglycerides to adipose tissue is accomplished by secretion of VLDL, leading to increased VLDL levels in blood plasma. If ingestion of large amounts of carbohydrates persists, the activity of lipoprotein lipase in adipose tissue capillaries increases in most persons, resulting in efficient fat storage and reduction of hepatic and plasma triglyceride levels. When this does not occur, hyperlipemia and fatty liver may persist. It is thus evident that triglyceride stores in adipose tissue can increase as a result of increased intake of either fat or carbohydrate.

REFERENCES

Caloric Intake

Havel, R. J.: Caloric homeostasis and disorders of fuel transport. N Engl J Med 287:1186, 1972.

Wolfe, B. M., and Ahuja, S. P.: Effects of intravenously administered fructose and glucose on splanchnic secretion of plasma triglycerides in hypertriglyceridemic men. Metabolism 26:983, 1977.

SATURATED, MONOUNSATURATED, AND POLYUNSATURATED FATTY ACIDS

Triglycerides in foods contain a mixture of fatty acids, mainly of the long-chain variety. Plant fats derived from seeds usually contain mainly polyunsaturated fatty acids (examples are sunflower, sesame, cottonseed, and peanut oils), whereas plant fats derived from the coating of certain fruits are mainly monounsaturated, as in olive oil. Coconut and palm kernel fats, which contain mainly lauric acid (12:0)* and myristic acid (14:0), are exceptions. Fats derived from land mammals contain mainly saturated and monounsaturated fats and are generally more saturated than plant fats. Milk fats are similarly saturated, but also contain appreciable amounts of short-chain fatty acids. Fish fats contain mainly polyunsaturated fatty acids with chain lengths of 20 or more, which remain liquid at the low body temperature of these animals. The first unsaturated bond in fish fatty acids is three carbon atoms from the terminal methyl group, so that they

are designated as "omega-3" fatty acids. Polyunsaturated fatty acids from plants have the first unsaturated bond six carbon atoms from the methyl end ("omega-6" fatty acids). Solid cooking fats are often prepared from unsaturated vegetable oils by partial catalytic hydrogenation.

All of the fatty acids in food fats are readily oxidized and are roughly equivalent in terms of energy yield. However, they have differing effects upon lipid transport mechanisms. Saturated fats generally increase levels of VLDL and LDL, whereas polyunsaturated fats reduce them. The omega-3 fatty acids of fish are especially effective in lowering VLDL levels by decreasing VLDL synthesis in the liver. Monounsaturated fats, when substituted for carbohydrate in the diet, have no effect upon lipoprotein levels. The effect of adding 1 gram of a saturated fatty acid to the diet is approximately equivalent to removing 2 grams of polyunsaturated fatty acid. Diets rich in polyunsaturated fats also lead to higher rates of biliary excretion of sterols. In some individuals, increased excretion of cholesterol leads to a supersaturation of bile and predisposes to the formation of gallstones. It is uncertain whether the effects of polyunsaturated fat diets upon biliary sterol excretion are related to their effects on plasma lipoprotein levels.

The amount and type of dietary fat vary widely in different parts of the world. In many countries, such as China and India, fat intake (especially animal fat) is low. In Japan, fat intake is also low, and most animal fat is derived from fish (and hence is polyunsaturated). In most Western countries, intake of fat derived from land animals is relatively high. Whereas some populations have eaten large amounts of monounsaturated fat for centuries (mainly as olive oil), no population in the world has eaten comparably large amounts of polyunsaturated fats from plants. Comparisons of the effects of fat ingestion upon health and disease are confounded by the fact that total caloric intake is generally higher in countries in which the diet contains more saturated fats.

REFERENCES

Saturated, Monounsaturated, and Polyunsaturated Fatty Acids

Brignoli, C. A., Kinsella, J. E., and Wehrauch, J. L.: Comprehensive evaluation of fatty acids in foods. V. Unhydrogenated fats and oils. J Am Diet Assoc 68:224, 1976.

Grundy, S. M.: Dietary fats and sterols. In Levy, R. I., Rifkind, B. M., Dennis, B. H., and Ernst, N. (eds.): Nutrition, Lipids and Coronary Heart Disease. New York, Raven Press, 1979, p. 89.

Nestel, P. J., Connor, W. E., Reardon, M. F., Connor, S., Wong, S., and Boston, R.: Suppression by diets rich in fish oil of very low density lipoprotein production in man. J Clin Invest 74:82, 1984.

ESSENTIAL FATTY ACIDS

Cells of metazoa contain enzymes that catalyze the coordinate elongation and desaturation of long-chain fatty acids. Thus, palmitic acid (16:0) can readily be converted to oleic acid (18:1) and thence to certain polyunsaturated fatty acids, including eicosatrienoic

---

*The convention for describing fatty acids indicates number of carbon atoms:number of unsaturated bonds.

acid (20:3). However, linoleic acid (18:2) and linolenic acid (18:3) cannot be synthesized to any extent in higher organisms. Linoleic and linolenic acids as well as arachidonic acid (20:4), which is formed from linoleic acid, are called "essential" fatty acids because they are required in the diet for normal function of certain tissues. Essential fatty acid deficiency especially affects tissues with high rates of cell renewal. In rats, the deficiency is associated with retarded growth, scaly skin, and sterility. In human infants, dry skin is also observed but obvious abnormalities have been reported in adults only after prolonged parenteral alimentation with glucose and amino acids. This probably reflects the large stores of essential fatty acids in adipose tissue of adults and the low requirement for essential fatty acids, on the order of 1 gram daily. Such small amounts are present in most mixed diets, even those that are low in fat.

At a biochemical level, essential fatty acid deficiency is manifested by the accumulation of eicosatrienoic acid in lipids, owing to reduced availability of linoleic acid, which is normally converted to arachidonic acid by the same pathway that yields eicosatrienoic acid from oleic acid. Some of the symptoms of essential fatty acid deficiency result from deficient prostanoids, but others are thought to be caused by altered structure of cell membranes.

REFERENCE

Essential Fatty Acids

Alfin-Slater, R. B., and Aftergood, L.: Physiological functions of essential fatty acids. Progr Biochem Pharm 6:214, 1971.

CARBOHYDRATES

Excessive amounts of dietary carbohydrates are readily converted to triglycerides in the liver. Sucrose (a disaccharide containing glucose and fructose) is an important component of the diet in most Western countries, contributing as much as 10 to 20 per cent of caloric intake and as much as one half of carbohydrate calories. By contrast, in those countries in which carbohydrate-rich foods such as rice provide the greatest percentage of calories, the carbohydrates are usually composed almost entirely of starches and ingestion of sucrose is low. Diets rich in sucrose or fructose may lead to higher plasma triglyceride levels than diets rich in starch or glucose. This difference may be associated with a greater short-term tendency of fructose to promote hepatic lipogenesis and to a lesser stimulation of insulin secretion by fructose than glucose. The lower insulin secretion with fructose would be associated with less inhibition of hormone-sensitive lipase and less stimulation of lipoprotein lipase in adipose tissue, and thus with greater rates of fat mobilization and lower rates of fat storage. It is important to note that these effects of different carbohydrates are not observed in all individuals and may be influenced by other components of the diet.

REFERENCE

Carbohydrates

Little, J. A., McGuire, V., and Derksen, A.: Available carbohydrate. In Levy, R., Rifkind, B., Dennis, B., and Ernst, N. (eds.): Nutrition, Lipids and Coronary Heart Disease. New York, Raven Press, 1979, p. 119.

CHOLESTEROL

As cholesterol is readily synthesized in most mammalian tissues, it is not an essential dietary component, at least in adults. Intake of cholesterol varies widely, owing mainly to variation in ingestion of meats and dairy products. Most muscle meats and cheese contain about 0.05 to 0.10 per cent cholesterol by weight, whereas organ meats and egg yolks contain much more. One hen's egg contains about 250 mg cholesterol. Low fat diets usually contain less than 300 mg cholesterol daily, whereas diets rich in animal fats usually contain 500 to 1000 daily. Cholesterol intake influences the level of plasma cholesterol, especially that carried by LDL. This can come about in several ways. First, dietary cholesterol forms one of the sources of the cholesteryl esters produced by LCAT, most of which is carried by LDL. Second, when dietary cholesterol accumulates in the liver, this organ secretes VLDL that are enriched in cholesterol and cholesteryl esters. The extent to which this occurs in man is uncertain. Third, the accumulation of dietary cholesterol in cells leads to down-regulation of LDL receptors, thereby impairing LDL catabolism. Because dietary cholesterol is mainly in animal meats that contain adipose tissue, the effects of such diets upon LDL levels are attributable to the cholesterol as well as the saturated fatty acids present. The effect of the saturated fatty acids in meats is generally more important than that of cholesterol. However, the influence of dietary cholesterol on plasma cholesterol levels varies widely among individuals. The basis for this variability is not known.

During the first year of life, body stores of cholesterol increase rapidly, owing to continuing myelination of the brain. During this period of life, dietary cholesterol is usually derived mainly from milk. Whether cholesterol synthesis can adequately replace dietary cholesterol for myelin synthesis during this period is not known.

REFERENCES

Cholesterol

Connor, W. E., and Connor, S. L.: The dietary treatment of hyperlipidemia. Med Clin North Am 66:485, 1982.

Feeley, R. M., Criner, P. E., and Watt, B. K.: Cholesterol content of foods. J Am Diet Assoc 61:134, 1972.

Nestel, P. J., and Poyser, A.: Changes in cholesterol synthesis and excretion when cholesterol intake is increased. Metabolism 25:1591, 1976.

ALCOHOL

The major sources of dietary calories in most individuals are carbohydrate, fat, and protein. However, ethanol in alcoholic beverages provides about 6 kilocalories per gram and, in some population groups, ethanol regularly provides 10 to 20 per cent of caloric intake. Ethanol is initially metabolized almost exclusively in the liver, to yield acetic acid. Acetic acid is metabolized poorly in the liver, owing to the low activity of the thiokinase that converts acetic acid to acetyl CoA, so that the acetate produced is transported to extrahepatic tissues where it is readily and completely oxidized. Ethanol is oxidized in the liver in preference to most other substrates of energy metabolism, including fatty acids. Thus, when the liver burns ethanol, incoming fatty acids are oxidized to a lesser extent and esterified to form triglycerides to a greater extent. This in turn leads to accumulation of triglycerides in the liver and to increased secretion of triglycerides in VLDL. In most individuals, adaptive increases in plasma triglyceride catabolism prevent increases in plasma triglyceride levels, but in certain susceptible individuals large increases may ensue (alcoholic hyperlipemia).

Whether the fatty liver produced by ethanol contributes to the toxic effects of ethanol that lead to liver damage (alcoholic hepatitis and cirrhosis) is not known.

REFERENCES

Alcohol

Belfrage, P., Berg, B., Hägerstrand, I., Nilsson-Ehle, P., Tornqvist, H., and Wiebe, T.: Alterations of lipid metabolism in healthy volunteers during long-term ethanol intake. Eur J Clin Invest 7:127, 1977.

Hawkins, R. D., and Kalant, H.: The metabolism of ethanol and its metabolic effects. Pharmacol Rev 24:67, 1972.

Wolfe, B. M., Havel, R. J., Marliss, E. B., Kane, J. P., Seymour, J., and Ahuja, S. P.: Effects of a three-day fast and of ethanol on splanchnic metabolism of free fatty acids, amino acids and carbohydrates in healthy young men. J Clin Invest 57:329, 1976.

Hormonal Regulation of Lipid Transport and Metabolism

INSULIN

The effects of insulin upon lipid transport are consistent with its central role in fuel storage and anabolism. Thus, in adipose tissue, insulin reduces the activity of the hormone-sensitive lipase and increases the activity of lipoprotein lipase, thereby inhibiting fat mobilization and promoting storage of plasma triglycerides. In the liver, insulin promotes lipogenesis and synthesis of triglyceride and protein, all of which contribute to increased synthesis of VLDL. With short-term deficiency of insulin, increased mobilization of FFA from adipose tissue also leads to increased hepatic triglyceride synthesis and secretion of VLDL. However, uptake of VLDL-triglycerides in adipose tissue is impaired, owing to reduced activity of lipoprotein lipase and reduced capacity to esterify fatty acids. Consequently, VLDL levels in the blood rise. With longer term insulin lack, the capacity of the liver to synthesize VLDL falls, owing to impaired hepatic protein (and apolipoprotein) synthesis. As mobilization of FFA from adipose tissue continues, triglycerides formed from these fatty acids accumulate in the liver, leading at times to extraordinary degrees of fatty liver. Plasma triglyceride levels remain elevated, particularly if the diet contains appreciable fat, because of the impaired triglyceride catabolism. The hyperlipemia occurring in insulinoprivic diabetes mellitus therefore can result from increased VLDL secretion at the onset, but continuing hyperlipemia results mainly from impaired uptake of both VLDL and chylomicron triglycerides in adipose tissue.

REFERENCE

Insulin

Havel, R. J.: Caloric homeostasis and disorders of fuel transport. N Engl J Med 287:1186, 1972.

CATABOLIC HORMONES

The hormones of catabolism, including glucagon, growth hormone, cortisol, thyroid hormone, and norepinephrine, all increase the activity of the hormone-sensitive lipase in adipose tissue, and hence, tend to promote fat mobilization. Of these, norepinephrine is the most important under physiological conditions. Norepinephrine mediates the short-term regulation of lipolysis as, for example, in response to muscular activity. It is doubtful whether glucagon exerts an appreciable lipolytic effect in healthy individuals. The other catabolic hormones contribute to maintenance of the hormone-sensitive lipase, the adenyl cyclase–cyclic AMP system, or both, so that fat mobilization may be impaired in diseases in which synthesis or secretion of growth hormone, cortisol, or thyroid hormone is impaired. Among its hepatic effects, glucagon promotes fatty acid oxidation and thereby reduces the amount of fatty acids available for triglyceride synthesis and secretion in VLDL. The physiological importance of these actions of glucagon, which directly oppose those of insulin, is uncertain.

REFERENCES

Catabolic Hormones

Fain, J. N.: Biochemical aspects of drug and hormone action in adipose tissue. Pharm Rev 25:67, 1973.

Schade, D. S., and Eaton, R. P.: Modulation of fatty acid metabolism by glucagon in man. I. Effects in normal subjects. Diabetes 24:502, 1975.

INSULIN RESISTANCE

In obesity and in many disease states, tissues become resistant to the various actions of insulin. In some cases, this may result from down-regulation of the insulin receptor, but in others, effects distal to the insulin receptor seem to be impaired. These states of insulin resistance are often associated with endogenous hypertriglyceridemia (increased levels of plasma VLDL). In some of these conditions, such as uremia and certain lipodystrophies, the hypertriglyceridemia results from impaired catabolism of plasma triglycerides. In others, such as obesity, increased hepatic triglyceride synthesis and secretion of VLDL are accompanied by variably impaired plasma triglyceride catabolism. In genetically determined forms of hypertriglyceridemia (see discussion of Metabolic Disorders, p. 412), obesity greatly magnifies the severity of the hyperlipemia, presumably because the basic disorder impairs the capacity of one or more of the steps required for removal from the blood and storage in tissues to adapt to the increased triglyceride flux.

SEX HORMONES

Women generally have lower VLDL levels than men, owing to more efficient mechanisms for plasma triglyceride catabolism, including greater activity of lipoprotein lipase in adipose tissue. Rates of plasma VLDL-triglyceride transport tend to be higher in women, and exogenous estrogens increase VLDL levels and triglyceride transport rates. In susceptible individuals (for example those with genetically determined hyperlipemias) exogenous estrogens can lead to severe hyperlipemia.

Women also have higher HDL levels than men, beginning at puberty and continuing beyond the menopause. Administered estrogens increase HDL levels, whereas administered androgens reduce them. Whether these changes in HDL are related to the higher rates of triglyceride transport in women is not known. The sex differences in HDL may be related to differences in risk of atherosclerotic disease (see discussion of Metabolic Disorders, p. 412).

REFERENCE

Insulin Resistance

Havel, R. J., Goldstein, J. L., and Brown, M. S.: Lipoproteins and lipid transport. In Bondy, P. K., and Rosenberg, L. E. (eds.): Metabolic Control and Disease. 8th ed. Philadelphia, W. B. Saunders Co., 1980, p. 393.

REFERENCE

Sex Hormones

Havel, R. J., Goldstein, J. L., and Brown, M. S.: Lipoproteins and lipid transport. In Bondy, P. K., and Rosenberg, L. E. (eds.): Metabolic Control and Disease. 8th ed. Philadelphia, W. B. Saunders Co., 1980, p. 393.

Pharmacological Regulation of Lipid Transport and Metabolism

Increased levels of VLDL and LDL in blood plasma are associated with premature atherosclerotic vascular disease (see discussion of Metabolic Disorders, p. 412). Because LDL is a catabolic product of VLDL, measures that reduce hepatic secretion of VLDL should reduce not only VLDL levels, but those of LDL as well. When obesity is present, this can be accomplished best by reducing caloric intake. Alternatively, diets restricted in saturated fats may reduce VLDL and LDL levels. In individuals who do not respond to such dietary measures (or who will not adhere to them), treatment with drugs may be needed. The actions of the three classes of drugs in most common use and a fourth class that has great promise for reducing LDL levels will be described here.

ARYL-SUBSTITUTED ISOBUTYRIC ACIDS

The prototype of this class of drugs is p-chlorophenoxyisobutyrate. In large doses it has antilipolytic properties and it also increases the activity of lipoprotein lipase in adipose tissue. It regularly increases the rate of VLDL-triglyceride catabolism and it may also reduce the rate of VLDL synthesis. The latter effect may explain the modest reduction in LDL levels that often occurs. However, in individuals whose only lipoprotein abnormality is an elevated VLDL level, the level of LDL often increases when the level of VLDL is reduced.

This effect may result from an increase in the fraction of B apolipoprotein of VLDL-remnants that is converted to LDL (see discussion of Fatty Acid Transport, p. 401). This class of drugs also has a number of effects upon hepatic lipid metabolism that may contribute to its hypolipidemic effect. One of these is increased fatty acid oxidation. Another is augmented biliary excretion of cholesterol, which increases the risk of formation of gallstones. Long-term use of p-chlorophenoxyisobutyrate may also be associated with an increased incidence of gastrointestinal malignancies.

REFERENCES

Aryl-Substituted Isobutyric Acids

Havel, R. J., and Kane, J. P.: Drugs and lipid metabolism. In Elliott, H. W. (ed.): Annual Review of Pharmacology. Vol. 13. Palo Alto, Annual Reviews Inc., 1973, p. 287.

Oliver, M. F., Heady, J. A., Morris, J. N., and Cooper, J.: A cooperative trial in the primary prevention of ischaemic heart disease using clofibrate. Report from the committee of principal investigators. Br Heart J 40:1069, 1978.

NICOTINIC ACID

This B vitamin (and its congeners), when given in large doses, has an immediate antilipolytic effect, which leads to short-term reduction of VLDL levels. However, with sustained administration, nicotinic acid appears to reduce VLDL levels mainly by reducing the rate of VLDL-triglyceride formation. It thereby reduces LDL formation as well. Nicotinic acid, in pharmacological doses, produces cutaneous flushing, owing to release of prostaglandins in the skin. This unpleasant effect usually disappears with continued use.

REFERENCES

Nicotinic Acid

Grundy, S. M., Mok, H. Y. I., and Zech, L.: Effects of nicotinic acid on lipid metabolism in man. Circulation, Suppl. II:170, 1978.

Havel, R. J., and Kane, J. P.: Therapy of hyperlipidemic states. Annu Rev Med 33:417, 1982.

BILE ACID–BINDING RESINS

These nonabsorbable cationic acids, given in large oral doses, bind bile acids in the intestine, preventing their normal enterohepatic circulation. This results in activation of cholesterol-7-alpha-hydroxylase in the liver and increased catabolism of cholesterol. Although hepatic cholesterol synthesis also increases, administration of these resins regularly increases LDL catabolism by increasing the number of hepatic LDL receptors. LDL levels therefore fall, usually by 15 to 30 per cent

REFERENCES

Bile Acid–Binding Resins

Grundy, S. M., Ahrens, E. H., Jr., and Salen, G.: Interruption of the enterohepatic circulation of bile acids in man: Comparative effects of cholestyramine and ileal exclusion on cholesterol metabolism. J Lab Clin Med 78:94, 1971.

Havel, R. J., and Kane, J. P.: Therapy of hyperlipidemic states. Annu Rev Med 33:417, 1982.

HMG-CoA REDUCTASE INHIBITORS

Fungal metabolites, which contain an aliphatic group resembling mevalonic acid as well as a bulky naphthalene ring, are potent competitive inhibitors of HMG-CoA reductase. In small doses they inhibit hepatic cholesterol synthesis without impairing the synthesis of nonsterol products of mevalonate. Hepatic LDL receptors increase sufficiently to produce moderate reductions of LDL. In combination with bile acid–binding resins they can reduce LDL levels by 50 per cent or more.

REFERENCE

HMG-CoA Reductase Inhibitors

Tobert, J. A., Bell, G. D., Birtwell, J., James, I., Kukovetz, W. R., Pryor, J. S., Buntinx, A., Holmes, I. B., Chao, Y.-S., and Bolognese, J. A.: Cholesterol-lowering effect of mevinolin, an inhibitor of 3-hydroxy-3-methylglutaryl–coenzyme A reductase, in healthy volunteers. J Clin Invest 69:913, 1982.

Metabolic Disorders

GENETIC DISORDERS OF LIPOPROTEIN FORMATION

Three rare genetically determined diseases due to impaired formation of lipoproteins, each of which is inherited as an autosomal recessive, are important to our understanding of lipid transport in lipoproteins. The first of these, abetalipoproteinemia, primarily involves lipoproteins containing apolipoprotein B. In the other two, Tangier disease and LCAT deficiency, the primary defect involves HDL.

In abetalipoproteinemia, there is a profound defect in the synthesis or secretion of lipoproteins that contain apolipoprotein B, and virtually no triglycerides or LDL are found in blood plasma. As a result of this defect, severe malabsorption of fat and fat-soluble vitamins occurs, with fatty infiltration of the absorptive cells of the small intestine. Similarly, there is fatty infiltration of the parenchymal cells of the liver. Transport of cholesterol derived from LCAT is secondarily impaired and there is a high ratio of free cholesterol to phospholipids in HDL. Because the lipids of the plasma membrane of red blood cells are in equilibrium with those of plasma lipoproteins, this leads to a proportionately high ratio of cholesterol to phospholipids in red blood cells, which are abnormally shaped, with a spiculated surface (acanthocytes). More importantly, affected individuals develop degeneration of the cerebellum, spinal cord, and retina, as well as cardiac and skeletal muscles. The neurological symptoms are aggravated by vitamin E deficiency, and night blindness may result from deficiency of vitamin A. However, the abnormalities in nerve and muscle function may also reflect cellular membrane abnormalities similar to those observed in red blood cells.

Tangier disease, which is characterized by extremely low blood levels of apolipoprotein A-I and very low levels of HDL, leads to less severe clinical consequences than abetalipoproteinemia. This disorder results from an abnormality in the structure or metabolism of apolipoprotein A-I. This protein is secreted in normal amounts, at least from the intestine, but it consists mainly of the pro form of the protein and is not incorporated into normal HDL particles. Although the concentration of HDL is very low and HDL have abnormal composition, LCAT continues to be active. At a biochemical level, the defect leads to abnormalities of other lipoproteins, including increased levels and abnormal composition of VLDL and reduced levels of LDL. These abnormalities presumably result from severe impairment of the normal processes by which HDL participate in triglyceride and cholesterol transport. The lipoprotein changes are accompanied by deposition of large amounts of cholesteryl esters (mainly cholesteryl oleate) in tissues that are rich in reticuloendothelial cells (such as the tonsils and lymph nodes) and in Schwann cells of peripheral nerves. The major clinical consequence is peripheral neuropathy. The lipid deposition may result from phagocytic uptake of the abnormal lipoproteins or a defect in the normal mechanism by which HDL participate in the removal of cholesterol from cells.

Familial LCAT deficiency provides a contrasting picture of the result of a severe defect of the HDL-LCAT system for transport of cholesteryl esters. In this disorder, virtually complete lack of LCAT activity prevents the synthesis of cholesteryl esters in HDL. This in turn results in persistence of discoidal HDL and also in the accumulation of lamellar lipoproteins in VLDL and LDL, owing to failure to process cholesterol derived from these lipoproteins and from various cells of the body. The red blood cells contain excess cholesterol and anemia is common, owing to increased red blood cell destruction. Lipid-laden reticuloendothelial cells, containing lamellar deposits of cholesterol and phospholipids, accumulate. In the glomeruli of the kidneys, lipid deposition may be associated with nephrotic syndrome and renal failure.

Some similar, but usually less severe alterations of plasma lipoproteins occur in other diseases affecting formation of lipoproteins. Thus, severe malabsorption from any cause leads to decreased lipoprotein synthesis. This may be associated with various fat-soluble vitamin deficiencies, but the severe abnormalities of nerve and muscle function of familial abetalipoproteinemia are not seen. Any disease affecting the synthetic function of parenchymal cells of the liver also leads to hypolipidemia, owing to reduced lipoprotein synthesis. Often this is accompanied by fatty infiltration of the liver. In severe parenchymal liver disease, secretion of LCAT is impaired to the point that many of the lipoprotein changes of familial LCAT deficiency may be observed, as well as red blood cell abnormalities.

REFERENCE

Genetic Disorders of Lipoprotein Formation

Havel, R. J., Goldstein, J. L., and Brown, M. S.: Lipoproteins and lipid transport. In Bondy, P. K., and Rosenberg, L. E. (eds.): Metabolic Control and Disease. 8th ed. Philadelphia, W. B. Saunders Co., 1980, p. 393.

GENETIC DISORDERS OF LIPOPROTEIN CATABOLISM

The study of three genetically determined disorders of lipoprotein catabolism has played an important role in our present understanding of lipid transport in lipoproteins. Two of these, familial lipoprotein lipase deficiency and familial dysbetalipoproteinemia, are inherited as autosomal recessives and involve the major steps in the catabolism of triglyceride-rich lipoproteins. The third, familial hypercholesterolemia, is an important genetic disease of LDL catabolism, which is inherited as an autosomal dominant.

Familial lipoprotein lipase deficiency is a rare disorder in which the activity of lipoprotein lipases is severely impaired. The precise molecular defect that leads to the enzymatic deficiency is unknown. Triglyceride-rich lipoproteins, especially chylomicrons, accumulate in the blood owing to a block in the first step in plasma triglyceride transport. Levels of LDL and HDL are low, reflecting the failure of chylomicrons and VLDL to contribute to the normal formation of cholesterol-rich lipoproteins. Removal of triglyceride-rich lipoproteins from the blood of affected individuals may take place by reticuloendothelial phagocytosis or by the action of lipases on cell surfaces in the liver. In most cases, there are few clinical sequelae of lipoprotein lipase deficiency. The most important of these is acute pancreatitis, which can occur in any form of severe hypertriglyceridemia. Pancreatic inflammation may be the result of impaired blood flow in pancreatic capillaries, with consequent release of pancreatic lipase into a triglyceride-rich milieu. FFA produced by lipase action on these triglycerides can lead to increased capillary permeability and local thrombosis if insufficient albumin is available to bind the FFA, producing further lipase release and setting up a vicious circle. Patients with severe hypertriglyceridemia may also develop "eruptive xanthomas," which are papules in the skin containing lipid-laden phagocytic cells. These cells ingest chylomicrons that leak into the dermis at sites of increased capillary permeability. Individuals with lipoprotein lipase deficiency do well when dietary fat is restricted. Several kindreds have been found with a phenocopy of lipoprotein lipase deficiency, owing to lack of apolipoprotein C-II, the cofactor protein for the enzyme.

Familial dysbetalipoproteinemia results from a defect in the second step in the catabolism of triglyceride-rich lipoproteins, leading to the accumulation of remnant lipoproteins derived from chylomicrons and VLDL. Affected individuals are homozygous for point mutations of apolipoprotein E, usually substitution of cysteine for arginine at residue 158 of the protein. These mutations impair the interaction of apolipoprotein E with lipoprotein receptors that are required for hepatic uptake of remnants. Conversion of VLDL to LDL is also impaired. Heterozygotes, who comprise 10 to 15 per cent of the general population and have one half of the usual complement of normal apolipoprotein E, display only mild abnormalities of the plasma lipoproteins. The occurrence of hyperlipidemia is uncommon even among homozygotes and appears to require factors in addition to abnormal apolipoprotein E, such as a high rate of VLDL synthesis. Hyperlipidemic individuals with familial dysbetalipoproteinemia are prone to develop premature atherosclerotic vascular disease, with a special predilection for disease of the femoral artery. They also develop characteristic xanthomas, especially tuberoeruptive xanthomas over the elbows and knees and planar xanthomas in the palmar and digital creases. These xanthomas contain reticuloendothelial cells laden with cholesteryl esters, mainly cholesteryl oleate. The hyperlipidemia responds well to a low cholesterol, low fat diet, and also to aryl-substituted isobutyric acids.

Familial hypercholesterolemia is produced by various mutations that affect the high affinity LDL receptor on cell surfaces. The most common of these is a mutant receptor that is metabolically silent because it is not synthesized or is unable to reach the cell surface. The next most common is a receptor that has reduced affinity for LDL, and the rarest is associated with a receptor that has normal affinity but is not normally taken up into the cell. These defects can be detected in cultured cells, usually fibroblasts, in which LDL receptors have been derepressed by growing the cells in lipoprotein-deficient serum. In the first case, LDL and other lipoproteins containing apolipoprotein B or E are not bound at all to the mutant receptor. In the second case, less LDL are bound at the usual concentrations of LDL in the extracellular fluid. In the third case, the receptors bind LDL with normal affinity, but are randomly scattered on the cell surface, rather than concentrated in the coated pits, from which the bound lipoproteins are normally taken up into the cell (see Cholesterol Transport and Catabolism, p. 404). The heterozygous state affects about one in 500 individuals. In the much rarer homozygous state, lack of normal binding of LDL results in failure of clearance of LDL from the blood by the receptor-dependent pathway. LDL are catabolized only by the nonspecific pathways, including uptake of LDL into reticuloendothelial cells and into smooth muscle cells of the arterial intima (see discussion of Lipid Metabolism and Atherogenesis, p. 416). In homozygotes, removal of LDL is fixed at about 15 per cent of the LDL pool daily. Together with a substantial increase in LDL formation, probably from increased conversion of VLDL remnants to LDL, this results in plasma LDL levels about six times greater than normal. Consequently, there is severe atherosclerotic vascular disease in childhood and adolescence. In heterozygotes, reduction of effective receptor number to one half of normal leads to increased uptake of LDL by nonspecific pathways of lower efficiency. The LDL level is increased to the point that rates of LDL formation and removal are equal. This usually results in a concentration of LDL about twice the normal value. Premature atherosclerotic vascular disease, especially of the coronary arteries of the heart, is common in heterozygotes. In both heterozygotes and homozygotes, xanthomas containing cholesteryl esters in reticuloendothelial cells are common. In heterozygotes, these occur particularly in tendons such as the Achilles tendon.

REFERENCES

Genetic Disorders of Lipoprotein Catabolism

Cox, D. W., Breckenridge, W. C., and Little, J. A.: Inheritance of apolipoprotein C-II deficiency. N Engl J Med 299:1421, 1978.
Goldstein, J. L., and Brown, M. S.: LDL receptor defect in familial hypercholesterolemia. Med Clin North Am 66:335, 1982.
Havel, R. J.: Familial dysbetalipoproteinemia. Med Clin North Am 66:441, 1982.
Havel, R. J., Goldstein, J. L., and Brown, M. S.: Lipoproteins and lipid transport. In Bondy, P. K., and Rosenberg, L. E. (eds.): Metabolic Control and Disease. 8th ed. Philadelphia, W. B. Saunders Co., 1980, p. 393.

OTHER DISORDERS OF PLASMA LIPOPROTEINS

Most hyperlipidemic individuals in the general population do not have one of the well-defined monogenic disorders described above. Rather they have less well-defined, usually milder abnormalities that tend to occur in families (primary hyperlipidemias) or they have hyperlipidemia due to other disorders that affect lipid transport in lipoproteins (secondary hyperlipide-

mias). The lipoprotein disturbances produced by these disorders, as well as the other monogenic disorders described here, are summarized in Table 19.

In some of the poorly defined primary hyperlipidemias, a single mutant gene may dictate the occurrence of the disorder in families. The mutant gene may produce elevation of a single lipoprotein class (for example, VLDL in familial hypertriglyceridemia); in others, the abnormality may differ among affected individuals (for example, familial multiple lipoprotein-type hyperlipidemia, in which the level of VLDL, LDL, or both may be increased). As in familial dysbetalipoproteinemia, occurrence of hyperlipidemia often seems to be dictated by factors additional to the mutant gene. In such cases, hyperlipidemia may not be present before adult life and it may also be inconstant.

In many patients with hypertriglyceridemia, whether familial or not, obesity is common. Obesity may lead to hypertriglyceridemia in a predisposed host by increasing the rate of triglyceride transport. Increased triglyceride transport may result simply from increased caloric load, especially to the liver, with consequent increased secretion of VLDL-triglycerides (see Nutritional Aspects of Lipid Transport and Metabolism, p. 407).

Patients with primary but otherwise undefined hypercholesterolemia (due to elevated LDL) may be unusually sensitive to the effects of dietary fat or cholesterol upon LDL levels. In other cases, the basis for the unusual LDL levels is unknown.

Insulin deficiency or resistance contributes to many of the secondary forms of hypertriglyceridemia by the mechanisms described in Hormonal Regulation of Lipid Transport and Metabolism, p. 410. Insulin deficiency is of major importance in type I diabetes mellitus and in the glycogenoses associated with hypoglycemia. Insulin resistance is of major importance in the hypertriglyceridemia of the various lipodystrophies, in which adipose tissue is lost from part or all of the body, and it contributes to the hypertriglyceridemia produced by glucocorticoids, estrogens, and that observed in patients with uremia, as well as type II diabetes mellitus.

In the nephrotic syndrome, loss of albumin is accompanied by increased hepatic synthesis and secretion of VLDL and, consequently, by increased formation of LDL. This increased lipoprotein secretion seems to be part of an "unscheduled" increase in hepatic protein synthesis associated with hypoalbuminemia. Impaired lipoprotein catabolism may contribute to the hyperlipidemia of the nephrotic syndrome, but the mechanisms are poorly defined.

A peculiar form of lamellar hyperlipidemia occurs in patients with cholestasis. The major abnormal lamellar lipoprotein in such cases is a single-walled vesicle, the wall of which is composed of an equimolar mixture of cholesterol and glycerophosphatides. Certain of the normal plasma apolipoproteins are adsorbed to the vesicle surface. In cholestasis, similar vesicular structures can be observed in the obstructed bile ducts, and these may find their way into the blood by transport back through the liver cell (diacytosis).

In some patients with monoclonal gammopathies, lipoproteins are bound to the immunoglobulins, preventing normal access to catabolic mechanisms. The form of the hyperlipidemia depends upon the specific

TABLE 19. HYPERLIPIDEMIC DISORDERS

GENERIC DESIGNATION AND ELEVATED LIPO-PROTEIN CLASS	SYNONYM	PRIMARY DISORDERS	SECONDARY DISORDERS†
Exogenous hyperlipemia (chylomicrons)	Type I	Familial lipoprotein lipase deficiency Unclassified*	Dysglobulinemias Systemic lupus erythematosus
Endogenous hyperlipemia (VLDL)	Type IV	Familial hypertriglyceridemia (mild form) Familial multiple lipoprotein-type hyperlipidemia Sporadic hypertriglyceridemia Tangier disease	Diabetic hyperlipemia‡ Glycogenosis, type I Lipodystrophies Dysglobulinemias Uremia Hypopituitarism Nephrotic syndrome (Diabetes mellitus)§
Mixed hyperlipemia (VLDL + chylomicrons)	Type V	Familial hypertriglyceridemia (severe form) Familial lipoprotein lipase deficiency (during pregnancy)	(Alcoholism) (Estrogen use) (Glucocorticoid use) (Stress-induced)
Hypercholesterolemia (LDL)	Type II-a	Familial hypercholesterolemia (LDL receptor defects) Familial multiple lipoprotein-type hyperlipidemia Polygenic hypercholesterolemia (includes exogenous hypercholesterolemia)	Nephrotic syndrome Hypothyroidism Dysglobulinemias Cushing's syndrome Acute intermittent porphyria Hepatoma
Combined hyperlipidemia (LDL + VLDL)	Type II-b	Familial multiple lipoprotein-type hyperlipidemia Unclassified	Nephrotic syndrome Hypothyroidism Dysglobulinemias Cushing's syndrome (Glucocorticoid use) (Stress-induced)
Remnant hyperlipidemia (β-VLDL)	Type III	Familial dysbetalipoproteinemia Unclassified	Hypothyroidism Systemic lupus erythematosus
Lamellar hyperlipoproteinemia (Vesicular and discoidal lipoproteins)		Familial lecithin-cholesterol acyltransferase deficiency	Cholestasis (with LP-X) Hepatic failure (with lamellar HDL)

*Includes C-II apolipoprotein deficiency.

†Note: All conditions associated with elevated VLDL or β-VLDL are aggravated by hypertrophic obesity.

‡Denotes mixed hyperlipemia caused by severe, prolonged insulin deficiency.

§Parentheses indicate conditions that frequently aggravate a primary hyperlipemia, but seldom cause hyperlipemia, de novo. These conditions cause some cases of primary hypertriglyceridemia (mild form) to present as mixed hyperlipemia.

binding properties of the immunoglobulins and is highly variable.

REFERENCES

Other Disorders of Plasma Lipoproteins

Felker, T. E., Hamilton, R. L., and Havel, R. J.: Secretion of lipoprotein-X by perfused livers of rats with cholestasis. Proc Natl Acad Sci USA 75:3549, 1978.

Havel, R. J., Goldstein, J. L., and Brown, M. S.: Lipoproteins and lipid transport. In Bondy, P. K., and Rosenberg, L. E. (eds.): Metabolic Control and Disease. 8th ed. Philadelphia, W. B. Saunders Co., 1980, p. 393.

DISORDERS OF LIPID STORAGE

Certain disorders of lipid metabolism are not associated with abnormalities of plasma lipoproteins, but rather with abnormalities of lipid storage in tissues. These disorders can result from abnormalities in the transport of fatty acids from liver or adipose tissue (fatty liver and the lipodystrophies) or from abnormalities in the lysosomal catabolism of lipids ("lipidoses").

Storage of cholesteryl esters in arteries is covered in the following discussion on Lipid Metabolism and Atherogenesis.

Fatty liver is not a specific disease, but rather is the result of imbalance between the synthesis of triglycerides in the liver and triglyceride secretion in VLDL. As discussed earlier, increased triglyceride synthesis can lead to fatty liver in uncontrolled diabetes mellitus, obesity, and alcoholism, whereas fatty liver can result from defective secretion of triglycerides in a variety of disorders that impair protein synthesis or glycosylation of proteins in the liver, as well as in uncontrolled diabetes mellitus.

The lipodystrophies comprise several genetic and acquired disorders in which storage of fat in adipose tissue is impaired. The impaired storage can be regional (as in acquired partial lipodystrophy and familial lipodystrophy of limbs and trunk) or total, as in familial generalized lipodystrophy and acquired generalized lipodystrophy. Abnormalities of the hypothalamus are closely associated with the lipodystrophies and may cause dysfunction of central mechanisms that control lipolysis and fat storage in adipose tissue.

The lipidoses belong to the lysosomal storage diseases that result from defective cellular catabolism of polysaccharides as well as lipids. The site of deposition of the undegradable substrate determines the organ most affected. Most of the lipidoses are the result of defective catabolism of sphingolipids and lead to slow development and mental retardation in infancy. Some, which do not involve the central nervous system, are manifest later in life. All are inherited as autosomal recessives (except Fabry's disease, which is sex-linked) and many are genetically heterogeneous. Deficiencies of lysosomal acid lipases are associated with storage of cholesteryl esters and triglycerides in various tissues and also manifest genetic heterogeneity.

REFERENCES

Disorders of Lipid Storage

Brady, R. O., Johnson, W. G., and Uhlendorf, B. W.: Identification of heterozygous carriers of lipid storage diseases. Am J Med 51:423, 1971.

Havel, R. J., Goldstein, J. L., and Brown, M. S.: Lipoproteins and lipid transport. In Bondy, P. K., and Rosenberg, L. E. (eds.): Metabolic Control and Disease. 8th ed. Philadelphia, W. B. Saunders Co., 1980, p. 393.

Kolodny, E. H.: Lysosomal storage diseases. N Engl J Med 294:1217, 1976.

LIPID METABOLISM AND ATHEROGENESIS

Altered lipid transport in plasma lipoproteins plays an important and probably crucial role in the development of certain atherosclerotic lesions that underlie the major causes of death in Western countries. In populations that subsist on low fat, low cholesterol diets, lipoprotein levels, especially of LDL, are low and clinical sequelae of atherosclerosis are unusual. In Japan, development of an urbanized society has not led (at least until recently) to high levels of fat intake or to a high incidence of atherosclerotic coronary heart disease, although stroke is a common cause of death and disability (stroke in Japan evidently is the consequence of the high prevalence of hypertension, possibly due to the habitual high salt intake). However, hypertension, diabetes mellitus, and cigarette smoking, all of which are established risk factors for the development of coronary heart disease in populations in which LDL levels are high, do not lead to a high incidence of coronary heart disease in Japan.

In mammals fed fat- and cholesterol-rich diets and in affected humans, atherosclerotic lesions of the intima of arteries are composed of proliferating smooth muscle cells and connective tissue elements (collagen, elastin, and glycosaminoglycans). Cholesteryl esters are deposited in smooth muscle cells and macrophages and in association with the connective tissue elements.

In general, lipoproteins that contain apolipoprotein B are thought to be potentially atherogenic. Such lipoproteins are precipitated by negatively charged glycosaminoglycans in the presence of divalent cations. These lipoproteins include LDL and VLDL. However, all VLDL particles may not be equally atherogenic. In some families with genetically determined hypertriglyceridemia, the incidence of clinical sequelae of coronary atherosclerosis is not increased. Combined elevations of LDL and VLDL are commonly found in survivors of acute myocardial infarction. High levels of the remnant-like VLDL found in familial dysbetalipoproteinemia are also associated with premature atherosclerotic disease. The basis for differing atherogenicity of lipoproteins is not known, but remnant VLDL and LDL are richer in cholesteryl esters than the precursor form of VLDL. VLDL remnants also bind avidly to receptors on macrophages known as β-VLDL receptors. These receptors bind and take up the cholesterol-rich, beta-migrating VLDL that accumulate in certain animals fed cholesterol-rich diets, leading to the formation of foam cells.

The cholesteryl esters of atherosclerotic lesions are derived from plasma lipoproteins. As the arterial intima normally contains no blood capillaries, the endothelial cells of the artery normally constitute the barrier to the ingress of lipoproteins from the blood. It is thought that substantial uptake of lipoproteins into the subintimal space requires a breakdown of this barrier function of the endothelium, which may occur as a result of factors such as hypertension, tobacco smoking, and sustained hyperlipidemia. Such endothelial injury leads to adherence of platelets, followed by aggregation of platelets and release of platelet granules, some of which contain factors that promote proliferation of intimal smooth muscle cells. The stimulated smooth muscle cells also synthesize and secrete the connective tissue elements that accumulate in the lesion, and they take up LDL at a greater rate than unstimulated ones. Thromboxane A2, a major product of arachidonic acid metabolism in platelets, has a major role in the adherence of platelets to the injured intima. By contrast, prostacyclin, a major product of arachidonic acid metabolism in endothelial cells, prevents platelet adherence. Inhibitors of thromboxane synthesis have been found to reduce the formation of arterial thrombi in some patients with advanced atherosclerotic disease.

Although LDL may promote atherogenesis by their effects on endothelial integrity, it is not clear how they lead to the accumulation of cholesteryl esters in smooth muscle cells or macrophages to form foam cells. The LDL receptor is clearly not essential for lipid accumulation because patients with homozygous familial hypercholesterolemia develop fulminant atherosclerosis. One possibility is that complexes of LDL with glycosaminoglycans are taken into cells via receptors other than the LDL receptor. Receptors for acetylated LDL are present on endothelial cells, macrophages, and smooth muscle cells, and there is some evidence that chemically modified LDL may be present in atherosclerotic lesions. In some cases cholesteryl esters derived from chemically modified LDL can accumulate to form foam cells.

No matter how they are formed, once foam cells break down, the cholesteryl esters that they contain contribute to the formation of the debris that forms an atheromatous abscess within atherosclerotic plaques. The advanced "complicated" lesions of atherosclerosis are most liable to surface disruption and superimposed thrombosis.

When lipoprotein levels are reduced in animals with established diet-induced atherosclerosis, the cholesteryl esters of the lesions are gradually removed and the rate of cellular proliferation is substantially reduced. However, the connective tissue elements are removed very slowly and to a limited extent. Early lipid-rich lesions, which contain many foam cells and relatively little connective tissue, may resolve almost completely. The removal of cholesteryl esters from the lesions is thought to be mediated by LCAT. As described in the discussion on Cholesterol Transport and Catabolism, p. 404, cholesterol esterified by LCAT on the surface of HDL particles can be replaced by tissue cholesterol. In this way, the LCAT system may remove cholesterol from atherosclerotic lesions, provided that the stored cholesteryl esters are first hydrolyzed by the cholesterol esterases that have been identified in cells. If the level of LDL and other "antherogenic" lipoproteins is low, the action of the LCAT system may be sufficient to prevent cholesteryl esters from accumulating in the artery, even in the presence of endothelial injury. A high level of HDL is generally associated with a low risk of atherosclerotic disease. It is possible that such a high level is associated with an enhanced capacity for cholesterol removal. In accord with this concept, plasma HDL levels are inversely related to the risk of developing myocardial infarction, at any given LDL level.

Several studies have provided evidence that reduction of plasma cholesterol levels reduces the incidence of manifestations of coronary heart disease and of coronary atherosclerosis in hyperlipidemic persons. Acquisition of additional information on the effects of diets and drugs that affect plasma lipoprotein levels would be facilitated by the development of noninvasive methods to quantify atherosclerotic lesions.

REFERENCES

Lipid Metabolism and Atherogenesis

Armstrong, M. L.: Regression of atherosclerosis. In Paoletti, R., and Gotto, A. M. (eds.): Atherosclerosis Reviews. New York, Raven Press. Vol. 1, 1976, p. 137.

Brunzell, J. D., Schrott, H. G., Motulsky, A. G., and Bierman, E. L.: Myocardial infarction in the familial forms of hypertriglyceridemia. Metabolism 25:212, 1976.

Grundy, S. M., Bilheimer, D., Blackburn, H., Brown, W. V., Kwiterovich, P. O., Jr., Mattson, F., Schonfeld, G., and Weidman, W. H.: Rationale of the diet-heart statement of the American Heart Association. Circulation 65:839A, 1982.

The Lipid Research Clinics Program: The Lipid Research Clinics Coronary Primary Prevention Trial Results. I. Reduction in incidence of coronary heart disease. JAMA 251:351, 1984.

Purine and Pyrimidine Metabolism in Man

The purines and pyrimidines are complex cyclic bases that, as their respective nucleotides, constitute the chemical structure of genetic information and of the transcription and translation of that information into protein structure in living cells (Section II). As constituents of ATP, GTP, UTP, NAD, FAD, and other molecules, they also receive and selectively transfer energy for metabolic purposes. As cyclic AMP and cyclic GMP they serve as important regulatory systems, often as the final signal of hormone action. In a sense all genetic disorders are disorders of purine and pyrimidine "metabolism" as expressed in the linear sequencing of information expressed through the triplet code. In this section, however, the term will be used in a more restricted sense to apply to the abnormalities that have been demonstrated in the synthesis or degradation of purines or pyrimidines per se or of their respective nucleosides or nucleotides. As in other sections of this book, the description of the clinical syndromes associated with these metabolic abnormalities will be brief. More expanded treatment of these topics will be found in *Cecil Textbook of Medicine*, of which this is a companion volume.

PURINE METABOLISM

The purine bases of importance in human metabolism are shown in Figure 71, together with an indication of the ultimate sources of the constituent atoms. There is a limited utilization of preformed dietary purines and a considerable but not yet quantified reutilization of purine bases released during catabolism (see below) by a process known as "salvage synthesis" of purine nucleotides. Most purines are produced by de novo synthesis, however, at a rate of approximately 4 mmol per day for an average-size adult. At equilibrium a similar amount is metabolized to a nonutilizable form, largely uric acid (0.7 g), of which two thirds to three fourths is excreted in the urine. The remaining uric acid is secreted into the gastrointestinal tract to be destroyed there by bacterial metabolism.

BIOSYNTHESIS OF PURINES—DE NOVO SYNTHESIS

The de novo pathway for the synthesis of purine nucleotides is summarized schematically in Figure 72. The individual enzymatic steps, which can be found in any biochemistry textbook, will not be discussed in detail. Through this sequence the purine ring is progressively constructed on the skeleton of glycine and includes 2 amide-N's of glutamine, an amine group from aspartic acid, 2 formyl groups transferred from tetrahydrofolic acid, and a C from CO_2. The end product of this first stage of purine nucleotide synthesis is inosine 5'-phosphate (IMP).

The first steps in purine biosynthesis have attracted the most attention, since they represent sites of metabolic control that may be abnormal in certain disorders of purine metabolism in man. The high-energy compound 5-phosphoribosyl-1-pyrophosphate (PP-ribose-P) is a key reactant in both the de novo synthesis and in the "salvage synthesis" from their respective preformed bases of both purine and pyrimidine nucleotides. The supply of PP-ribose-P may therefore influence rates of synthesis. This phosphosugar is formed by the reaction

$$\text{Ribose 5-phosphate} + \text{ATP} \xrightarrow{\text{Mg}^{++}}$$

$$\text{PP-ribose-P} + \text{AMP}$$

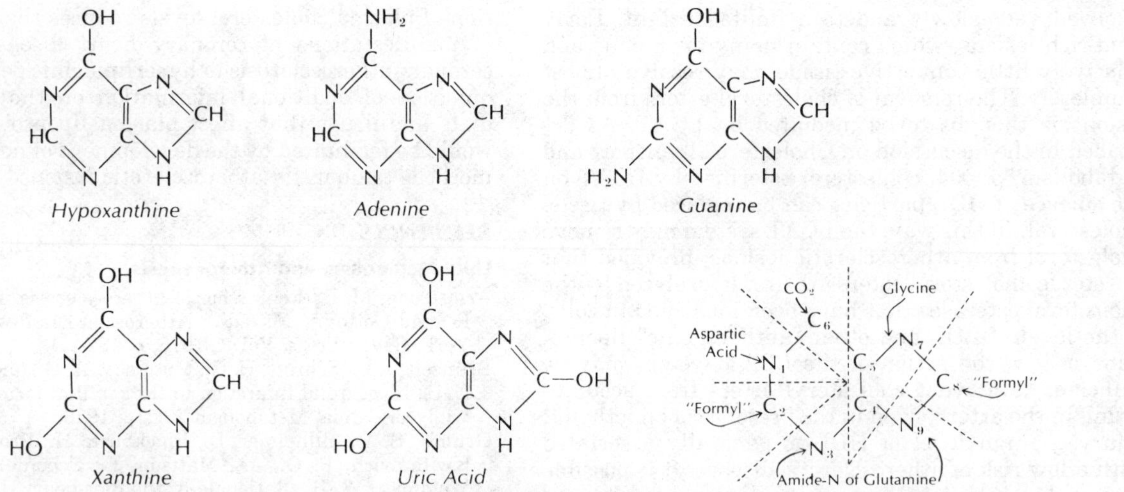

Figure 71. Structure of major purines and origin of the atoms of the purine ring.

catalyzed by PP-ribose-P synthetase. The enzyme is activated by inorganic phosphate and is subject to certain metabolic controls by nucleotides as noted below. In the first reaction unique to purine synthesis a labile amino sugar, 5β-phospho-D-ribosyl-1-amine, is formed by the displacement of the pyrophosphate of PP-ribose-P by the amide-N of glutamine:

$$\text{PP-ribose-P + glutamine + H}_2\text{O} \xrightarrow{\text{Mg}^{++}}$$
$$\text{phosphoribosylamine + glutamic acid + PP}_i$$

catalyzed by amidophosphoribosyl transferase. As the first unique compound in purine biosynthesis, the synthesis of phosphoribosylamine is normally under coordinated metabolic control (see below). From phosphoribosylamine the flow of synthesis then proceeds with the addition of glycine to form phosphoribosylglycineamide followed by the sequential but alternate additions of 1 C and 1 N groups (formyl, amide, CO_2, amine, formyl) until the structure is complete (Fig. 72).

All of the other purine nucleotides are derived from IMP as a precursor (Fig. 73). Adenosine 5′-phosphate (AMP) receives its amine group from a two-step exchange reaction with aspartic acid, the net result of which is the transfer of the amine group of aspartate to the 6-position of the purine ring at the cost of one high-energy phosphate group donated by GTP. IMP also serves as the precursor of guanosine 5′-phosphate (GMP) through a two-step reaction involving oxidation at the 2-position and transfer of an amide-N of glutamine to the 2-position.

AMP and GMP must be converted to their respective triphosphates prior to metabolic utilization. This conversion is carried out with the successive formation of the nucleoside diphosphate and triphosphate utilizing ATP as the source of the high-energy phosphate groups. These steps are catalyzed by the specific enzymes nucleoside monophosphate kinase and nucleoside diphosphate kinase.

The deoxyribonucleotides are necessary for the synthesis of DNA. They are derived from their corresponding purine or pyrimidine nucleoside diphosphates through a complex reduction at the 2′ carbon of the ribose moiety. The steps involved have not been fully elucidated, but include a protein cofactor (thioredoxin), a thioredoxin reductase enzyme, and two other components (B_1 and B_2) of the enzyme ribonucleoside diphosphate reductase:

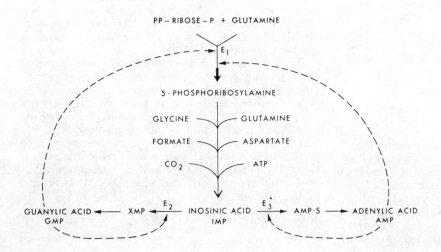

Figure 72. De novo pathway of purine nucleotide biosynthesis and the feedback control mechanisms (----------→). E_1, Amidophosphoribosyltransferase; E_2, inosine 5′-phosphate dehydrogenase; E_3, adenylsuccinic acid (AMP-S) synthetase; XMP, xanthosine 5′-phosphate. (Reprinted from Wyngaarden, J. B.: Gout. In Wyngaarden, J. B., and Smith, L. H., Jr.: Cecil Textbook of Medicine. 17th ed. Philadelphia, W. B. Saunders Co., 1985, p. 1134.)

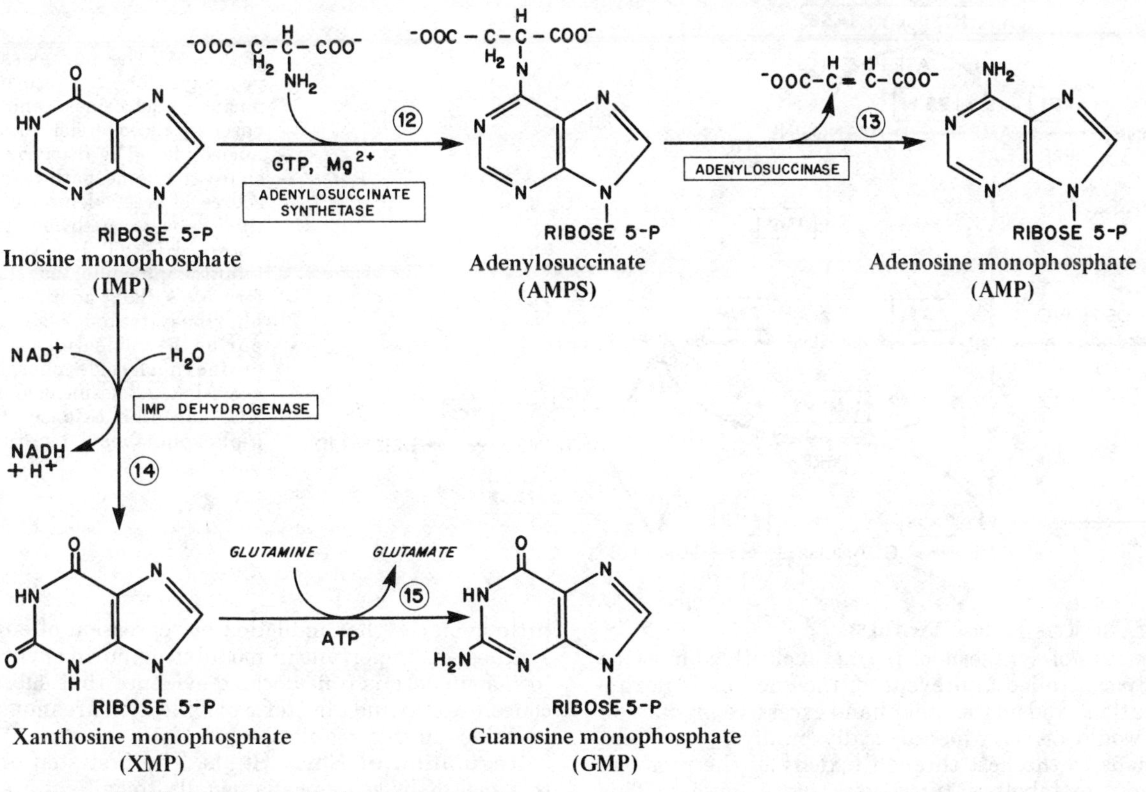

Figure 73. The synthesis of adenosine monophosphate and guanosine monophosphate from inosine monophosphate. (Reproduced, with permission, from Harper, H. H., et al. [eds.]: Review of Physiological Chemistry. 17th ed. Lange, 1979.)

Ribonucleoside diphosphate + reduced thioredoxin

$$\xrightarrow{B_1 \text{ and } B_2} \text{2'-deoxyribonucleoside diphosphate} + \text{oxidized thioredoxin}$$

Oxidized thioredoxin $\xrightarrow{\text{NADPH}}$ reduced thioredoxin

Through these steps of de novo synthesis all of the purine ribonucleotides and deoxyribonucleotides are synthesized from simple precursors, but at considerable energy cost.

SALVAGE SYNTHESIS

At equilibrium de novo synthesis of purines equals the irreversible oxidation of the purine ring to its end products, largely uric acid. Within this metabolic scheme, however, there is some reutilization of preformed purine bases by salvage pathways that are much more energetically efficient than total reliance on de novo synthesis. There are two general mechanisms for such salvage: (1) the reutilization of free purine bases by interaction with PP-ribose-P to form their corresponding nucleotides, and (2) rephosphorylation of purine nucleosides (Fig. 74). Of these the former is probably the most important quantitatively.

There are two enzymes that catalyze the salvage of free bases—adenine phosphoribosyltransferase (APRT) and hypoxanthine-guanine phosphoribosyltransferase (HGPRT), which carry out the salvage synthesis of

AMP and of IMP or GMP, respectively (Fig. 74). Of these two enzymes HGPRT appears to be the more active, or at least the more important in the body's economy as reflected in the syndromes produced by their respective deficiencies (see below).

The salvage of nucleosides may be more complex. There is an active and specific adenosine kinase that catalyzes the synthesis of AMP:

$$\text{Adenosine} + \text{ATP} \xrightarrow{\text{kinase}} \text{AMP} + \text{ADP}$$

Kinases for inosine and guanosine are more difficult to demonstrate and these purines may be recovered largely after release of their free bases by purine nucleoside phosphorylase (PNP) to be followed by salvage via PP-ribose-P (HGPRT pathway).

These cycles interact in complex ways, as shown in Figure 74. Adenosine may be converted to inosine directly, catalyzed by adenosine deaminase. This reaction is of obvious importance in some tissues in view of the immunological deficit that occurs when this activity is deficient, as noted below. The deoxynucleosides of adenine and guanine can be salvaged by direct phosphorylation catalyzed by adenosine kinase and deoxycytidine kinase, respectively.

There is now no method for selectively measuring the activities of the salvage pathways that spin around to recycle purines to their nucleotides at low energetic cost but indications are that (a) the pathways are overall quite active, and (b) their relative importance differs in various tissues.

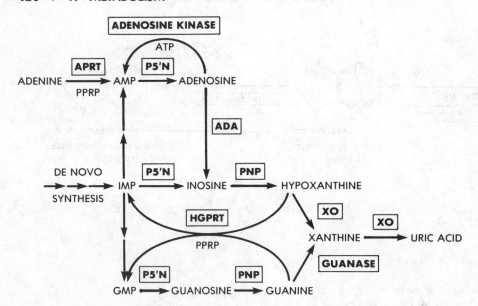

Figure 74. The purine salvage pathways for the recovery of purine nucleosides and free bases by reconversion to purine nucleotides. The deoxyribosides share the same pathways. The source of free adenine used in this salvage pathway is not known. HGPRT, hypoxanthine-guanine phosphoribosyltransferase; APRT, adenine phosphoribosyltransferase; P5'N, purine 5'-nucleotidase; PNP, purine nucleoside phosphorylase; ADA, adenosine deaminase; XO, xanthine oxidase; PPRP, 5-phosphoribosyl-1-pyrophosphate.

REGULATION OF PURINE SYNTHESIS

The rate of synthesis of purine nucleotides must be tightly controlled to prevent on the one hand "purine starvation" and on the other hand excessive production that would be both metabolically profligate and also injurious to the host through toxicity of the products of their metabolites (uric acid, for example). This control is exercised at various steps in the de novo pathway of purine synthesis and in the formation and interconversion of the specific nucleotides from a common origin in IMP. The most important of these regulatory steps are diagrammed in Figure 75.

Methods of Regulation. Enzymatic activity can be influenced by the concentration of substrates, by the amount of enzyme present (balance of synthesis and degradation), or by nonsubstrate compounds that influence the effectiveness of catalysis. The latter compounds, often distant products of the reactions, may compete with substrates for active sites or, more frequently, effect conformational changes in the three-dimensional structure of the enzyme protein in a way that modifies its action (allosteric control). There is

little evidence that induction or repression of enzyme synthesis is important in modulating purine synthesis in man. There is considerable evidence that substrate concentration and allosteric modification are important variables in this regulation.

Regulation of Early Steps. The first step unique to a metabolic sequence is usually the site of greatest feedback control. The first enzyme unique to purine synthesis is amidophosphoribosyl transferase (Figs. 72, 75), which catalyzes the formation of phosphoribosylamine from PP-ribose-P and the amide-N of glutamine. Control of purine synthesis, however, extends at least one step earlier at the formation of PP-ribose-P from ribose 5-phosphate and ATP. PP-ribose-P synthetase, which catalyzes this reaction, is stimulated by inorganic phosphate. ADP inhibits the synthetase competitively with respect to magnesium ATP. Many other nucleotides of both purines and pyrimidines, especially the di- and triphosphate derivatives, inhibit at a separate site through allosteric mechanisms. Both PP-ribose-P and 2,3-diphosphoglycerate inhibit the synthetase competitively with respect to ribose 5-phos-

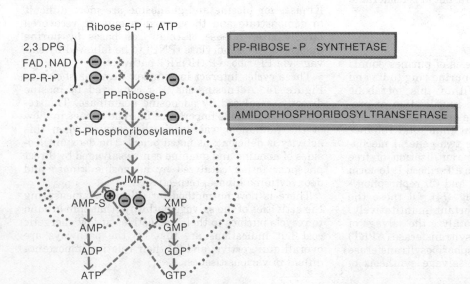

Figure 75. The regulatory mechanisms for the control of the de novo synthesis of purine nucleotides. The solid lines represent steps in biosynthesis. The dotted lines represent feedback regulation. (Modified from Harper, H. H., et al. [eds.]: Review of Physiological Chemistry. 17th ed. Lange, 1979.)

phate, but the significance of this has not been established. PP-ribose-P is a versatile reactant in de novo and salvage synthesis of purines and pyrimidines. Since it is not directly channeled for de novo purine biosynthesis, control at this step would seem lacking in specificity.

Amidophosphoribosyltransferase from human sources exists in two forms, an inactive aggregated form (molecular weight, 270,000) and a smaller, active, disaggregated form (molecular weight, 133,000). The interconversion of these two forms clearly influences catalytic activity, with PP-ribose-P promoting activation (Fig. 76). The adenine and guanine nucleotides act synergistically in this negative feedback allosteric control.

Regulation of Ribonucleotide Interconversions. The conversion of IMP to ATP and GTP also contains internal control mechanisms representing both restraint and activation (Fig. 75). AMP inhibits the condensation of IMP and aspartate to form adenylosuccinate, which requires the presence of GTP. GMP inhibits the formation of XMP from IMP, but the amination of XMP to GMP requires ATP. In studies using human tissues in vitro the intracellular level of GTP seems to be of particular importance in regulating the interconversions. Purine phosphoribosyltransferases are also inhibited by the ribonucleotide products of their reactions in the salvage pathway (Fig. 74). An additional point of control of ribonucleotide metabolism is that of cleavage by cytoplasmic 5'-nucleotidases to yield the corresponding ribonucleosides and orthophosphate. The control of cleavage has not been well elucidated.

Significance of Regulation. These regulatory steps presumably allow selective microadjustments within the overall scheme of purine synthesis. There are also specific controls for the reduction of the ribonucleoside diphosphates to their corresponding deoxyribonucleoside diphosphates as summarized in Figure 77. This will be discussed more extensively below concerning the purinogenic immunodeficiency syndromes.

Through these various regulatory mechanisms the supply of all of the functioning nucleotides is normally coordinated with reasonable precision for needs that

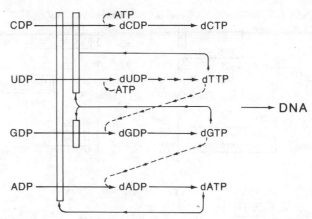

Figure 77. The physiological regulation of deoxyribonucleotide synthesis. In this scheme the broken arrows indicate positive effects and the open bars negative effects. (Reproduced, with permission, from Enzyme Defects and Immune Dysfunction, Ciba Foundation Symposium 68 (new series). Amsterdam, Excerpta Medica, 1979, pp. 1–289.)

are very disparate in differing cells—the hepatocyte versus the erythrocyte, for example. Do all human cells in fact make purines de novo? The mature erythrocyte is incapable of purine synthesis and depends on salvage mechanisms. There is some evidence, although not firmly established, that the liver may supply purines for other tissues, such as the brain. Data concerning the relative rates of synthesis of purines in different tissues and the relative importance of their respective regulatory devices are incomplete. Profound differences do exist, however, as noted below in the fact of the relative specificity of the effects of adenosine deaminase deficiency or purine nucleoside phosphorylase deficiency on the immunocyte.

CATABOLISM OF PURINES

The end product of purine catabolism in man is uric acid, all of which is synthesized by the sequential oxidations of hypoxanthine and xanthine catalyzed by xanthine oxidase (Fig. 78). Hypoxanthine is produced directly from inosine and deoxyinosine by the action of purine nucleoside phosphorylase and more remotely from adenosine and deoxyadenosine, which are converted to inosine and deoxyinosine catalyzed by adenosine deaminase. Guanine as a free base is derived from guanosine or deoxyguanosine, once again catalyzed by purine nucleoside phosphorylase, and then oxidatively deaminated to xanthine catalyzed by guanase. These pathways are pertinent for both exogenous (dietary) sources of purines and for endogenous sources. Xanthine oxidase is found in highest concentration in liver and intestine, but also exhibits trace activity in kidney, spleen, and muscle.

FATE OF URIC ACID

Uric acid is the end product of purine metabolism in man (and certain other higher primates, birds, and reptiles) in contrast to other mammals that hydrolyze relatively insoluble urate to highly soluble allantoin with the enzyme uricase. The pool size of extracellular urate varies with sex and size, being highest in the

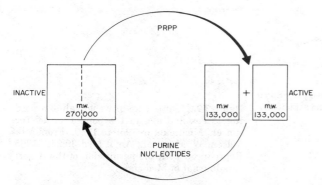

Figure 76. Model of the interconversion of small (active) and large (inactive) forms of amidophosphoribosyltransferase in the control of purine biosynthesis. (Reproduced, with permission, from Wyngaarden, J. B., and Kelley, W. N.: In Stanbury, J. B., Wyngaarden, J. B., Fredrickson, D. S., Goldstein, J. L., and Brown, M. S. (eds.): The Metabolic Basis of Inherited Disease. 5th ed. New York, McGraw-Hill Book Co., 1983, p. 1072.)

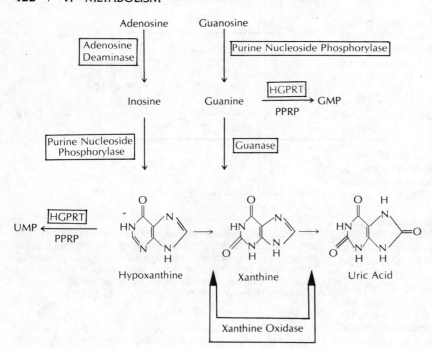

Figure 78. The catabolism of purine nucleosides and free bases to uric acid.

male, but generally is in the range of 600 to 1200 mg. Approximately two thirds of this pool turns over daily at steady-state equilibrium; that is, it is excreted and replaced by newly formed urate. Figure 79 illustrates normal serum urate levels in males and females according to age. It is probable that no more than 5 per cent of urate is bound to plasma proteins (albumin and an α_1-α_2-urate-binding globulin) in vivo. At pH 7.40 urate exists largely as its sodium salt.

Urate is excreted both by the kidney (two thirds to three fourths) and into the intestinal tract as a constituent of saliva, gastric juice, pancreatic juice, succus entericus, and bile. Urate that enters the intestine is destroyed by bacterial enzymes. If antibiotics are used to produce bacteriostasis, free urate may be recovered in the feces. Very little information is available about the variables in intestinal excretion of urate, including possible effects of pharmaceutical agents. Agents that would enhance the relative excretion of urate by the gut would be of obvious therapeutic importance in the reversal of hyperuricemia without the dangers of passing urate through the kidney. At present no such agents are known.

The excretion of urate by the human kidney is complex and cannot be considered here in detail. All, or virtually all (>95 per cent), of plasma urate is filtered by the glomerulus. Active tubular reabsorption of urate occurs in the proximal tubule closely linked with that of other components of filtrate, especially sodium. Simultaneously there is net tubular secretion of urate, followed still further by postsecretory reabsorption (Fig. 80). The net result of this intricate

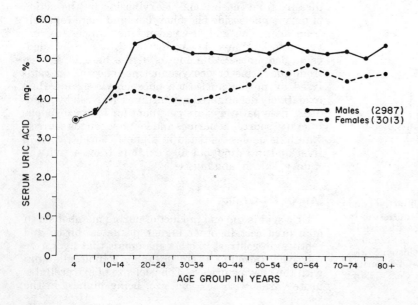

Figure 79. Mean serum uric acid values according to sex and age in the population of Tecumseh, Michigan, in 1959 to 1960. (From Mikkelsen, W. M., et al.: Am J Med 39:242, 1965. Reproduced with the permission of the American Journal of Medicine.)

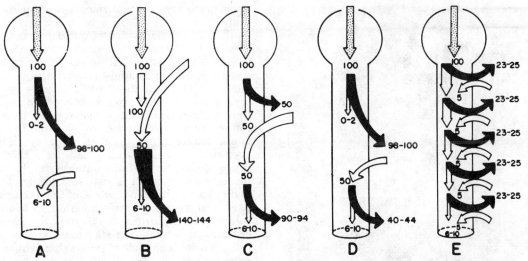

Figure 80. Five possible models for urate transport in man. The stippled arrows represent filtered urate, solid arrows represent urate reabsorption, and open arrows indicate either tubular secretion of urate or urate remaining in tubular fluid after reabsorption. Numerical values indicate hypothetical orders of magnitude of the transport processes. In *A,* the traditional view, wherein most filtered urate is reabsorbed and all secretion takes place subsequently, is depicted. Alternatively, no presecretory reabsorption takes place in *B;* all reabsorption occurs distally to secretion. In *C* and *D,* varying amounts of pre- and postsecretory reabsorption take place. Finally, secretion and reabsorption could occur simultaneously along a substantial length of the renal tubule *(E).* (From Rieselbach, R. E., and Steele, T. H.: Am J Med 56:665, 1974. Reproduced with the permission of the American Journal of Medicine.)

process of filtration and mingled reabsorption and secretion is a "clearance" that is approximately 6 to 8 per cent that of inulin.

DISORDERS OF PURINE METABOLISM

There are a number of disorders of purine metabolism that occur spontaneously in man either as genetic defects or as acquired abnormalities. Those that will be considered briefly in this section are listed in Table 20. Attention will be focused solely upon the pathogenesis of these disorders insofar as explanations are now available from current knowledge of normal purine metabolism.

Gout

Gout is by far the most important disorder of purine metabolism in man. Gout may be defined as a group

TABLE 20. DISORDERS OF PURINE METABOLISM

1. Gout
   a. metabolic (overproduction)
      primary and secondary
   b. renal (underexcretion)
      primary and secondary
2. Hypoxanthine-guanine phosphoribosyltransferase deficiency (Lesch-Nyhan syndrome and variants)
3. Adenine phosphoribosyltransferase deficiency
4. Purinogenic disorders of immune function
   a. adenosine deaminase deficiency
   b. purine nucleoside phosphorylase deficiency
5. Myoadenylate deaminase deficiency
6. Adenosine deaminase excess
7. Xanthinuria
8. Folate and vitamin B_{12} deficiencies
9. Uric acid stone diathesis

of disorders of purine metabolism productive of continuing hyperuricemia. When clinically manifest it is associated with one or more of the following: (1) acute, inflammatory arthritis; (2) deposition of sodium urate in a variety of tissues as tophi; (3) uric acid kidney stones; or (4) renal insufficiency. The pathophysiology of gout can be discussed as answers to two questions:

1. What causes the specific manifestations of this disease complex?
2. What causes the hyperuricemia that is the hallmark of gout?

The Manifestations of Gout. All of the manifestations of gout can be attributed to the excessive accumulation or concentration of urate in the body. There is no evidence that urate *in solution* is injurious to the host. Therefore all of the clinical features of gout result directly or indirectly from the crystallization of the sodium salt of urate in the body or of free uric acid in the urine. At pH 7.40 and 37° C saturation of human plasma by urate occurs at approximately 7.0 mg/dl. It is apparent that many patients with gout or asymptomatic hyperuricemia are chronically "supersaturated." Solubility of uric acid in urine is strongly pH-dependent. At pH 5 the saturation level is approximately 15 mg/dl; at pH 7 the solubility may be more than tenfold greater (160 to 200 mg/dl).

ACUTE GOUTY ARTHRITIS. Acute gouty arthritis is typically rapid in onset, is associated with marked signs of inflammation in and about the affected joint, and is severely painful. An attack often follows a stressful event, and the most frequent site of first involvement is the first metatarsophalangeal joint, a condition known since the time of Hippocrates as "podagra." Examination of synovial fluid from acute gouty arthritis routinely reveals fine negatively birefringent crystals of sodium urate, some of which have

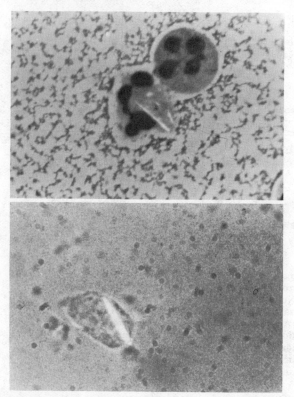

Figure 81. Sodium urate monohydrate crystals phagocytized by leukocytes in synovial fluid from acute gouty arthritis and examined by polarized light.

been phagocytized by polymorphonuclear leukocytes (Fig. 81). This finding is so constant as to be of diagnostic value.

An interaction of crystal and leukocyte appears to be necessary for the pathogenesis of acute gout, which is a special form of what has been termed microcrystalline synovitis (Fig. 82). Leukocytes phagocytize so-

dium urate crystals and release a chemotactic factor that attracts other leukocytes to the area of inflammation. The major action of colchicine, a drug widely used in the treatment of gout, may be to block the release of this factor. Within the leukocyte a phagolysosome is formed around the crystal in an attempt to digest it. Unfortunately, surface forces on the rigid crystal react by hydrogen bonding with the phospholipid membrane of the phagolysosome, disrupting its continuity to release lytic enzymes into the cytoplasm of the leukocyte. In brief, the leukocyte attacks the crystal in a manner appropriate for a bacterium but inappropriate for an inanimate crystal. In the process its digestive organelle is disrupted, leading to autolysis and release of its contents and of the unaltered crystal back into the area of inflammation. In addition to its role in the rupture of leukocytes, the sodium urate crystal can activate the Hageman factor and thereby set in motion a cascade of events that reinforce inflammation through the activation of kallikrein and the release of kinins. Vasodilatation, enhanced capillary permeability, and the margination and chemotaxis of leukocytes result. Urate crystals can also activate the complement system by activating C1 when incubated with the intact precursor macromolecule C1 qrs. Whether complement activation plays a role in spontaneous gouty arthritis has not been established.

Why does acute gouty arthritis so often appear as podagra? The answer is not known. The solubility of sodium urate is strongly temperature-dependent and the first metatarsophalangeal joint is distal and comparatively cool. This joint is also subject to considerable stress over years of weight-bearing and walking. In the reabsorption of joint effusions, water is more rapidly reabsorbed than urate. This tends to concentrate the urate, leading to saturation. It has been postulated that microeffusions occur secondary to degenerative joint disease and in the process of reabsorption urate is concentrated in a distal cool joint, leading to podagra. This postulate would be consistent with the fact that

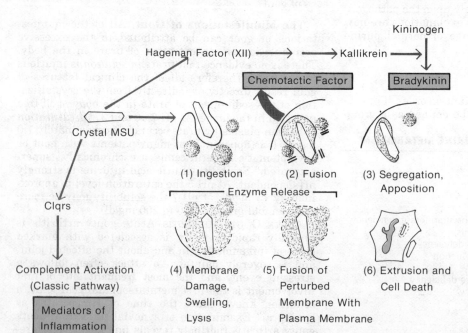

Figure 82. Scheme of postulated mechanisms by which sodium urate crystals may interact with leukocytes, Hageman factor, and the complement pathway to produce the acute inflammation characteristic of microcrystalline synovitis. It has not been proved that activation of the Hageman factor or of C1qrs is necessary for acute gouty arthritis. (Modified from Weissman, G.: Adv Intern Med 19:239, 1974.)

although hyperuricemia generally appears at puberty in the gouty patient, the first attack of arthritis most typically occurs about 25 to 30 years later, presumably when degenerative joint disease has made its appearance. Abnormalities of proteoglycan metabolism have also been postulated in the genesis of acute gout, since these complex protein polysaccharides of connective tissue have been shown to enhance urate solubility in in vitro studies.

Why is an attack of acute gouty arthritis self-limiting? Even without treatment the inflammation generally subsides over a few days. The mechanisms for spontaneous recovery are not clear. Inflammation itself may increase solubility by heat and by removing urate through increased blood flow. Leukocytes contain myeloperoxidase, which is capable of metabolizing some urate, although the importance of this has not been established. Stress-induced secretion of glucocorticoids may reduce inflammation. There are probably other processes of restraint and repair that are not yet evident.

In summary, acute gouty arthritis results from crystal-induced synovitis and requires the interaction of sodium urate microcrystals with polymorphonuclear leukocytes. Activation of the Hageman factor and of the complement cascade may play collateral roles. The factors that induce the seeding of a joint with crystals at a given time in the face of sustained hyperuricemia are unclear, as are the factors that induce spontaneous recovery. The crystal-leukocyte model of acute gout is an important advance in knowledge about the pathogenesis of this and other similar disorders.

TOPHACEOUS GOUT. The deposition of sodium urate monohydrate crystals, generally in connective tissue, results in tophi, one of the most striking manifestations of gout (Fig. 83). These masses of crystals induce a chronic mononuclear inflammatory reaction with foreign body granulomas and fibrosis. Tophi most frequently occur in cartilage, tendon sheaths, epiphyseal bone, subcutaneous layers of the skin, bursae, and the kidney. They may occur in virtually any tissue in the body except for the central nervous system, where the concentration of urate is reduced (<1.0 mg/dl in cerebrospinal fluid) by the blood-brain barrier. Tophi are also notably rare in liver, spleen, and skeletal muscle.

Little is known about the pathophysiology of tophi. Obviously they represent a storage disease, the crystallization of sodium urate from a supersaturated extracellular fluid. The reason why this crystallization is more likely to occur in cartilage than in skeletal muscle, for example, is unclear. Some patients may be crippled by massive tophi, while others with similar serum urate concentrations may be asymptomatic or have only a rare attack of acute gouty arthritis. Attempts to explain these differences in susceptibility to tophi on the basis of differences in protein binding of urate in plasma have not been convincing. Tophi can be remobilized by measures that reduce serum urate concentrations below the level of saturation over sustained periods of time.

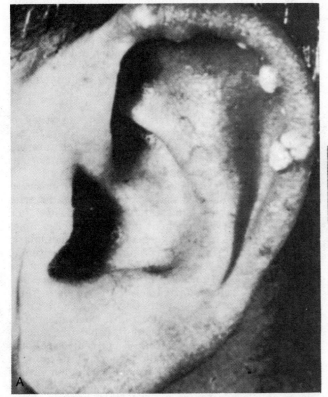

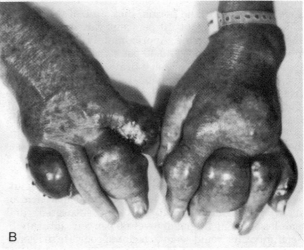

Figure 83. *A,* Multiple tophi of the helix of the ear. *B,* Chronic tophaceous gout of severe degree, with bulbous enlargements of several fingers. Note sparing of fourth finger of right hand. (Courtesy of Dr. R. Wayne Rundles, Duke University Medical Center.) (Reprinted with permission from Kelley, W. N.: Gout and related disorders of purine metabolism. In Kelley, W. N., Harris, E. D., Jr., Ruddy, S., and Sledge, C. B. (eds.): Textbook of Rheumatology. Vol. II. Philadelphia, W. B. Saunders Co., 1981, p. 1401.)

URIC ACID STONE FORMATION. Uric acid stones form more frequently in gouty than in nongouty individuals. On the other hand most uric acid stones occur in patients without gout. This manifestation of gout will be discussed briefly below under uric acid stone diathesis. The subject is covered more systematically in Section X in a general consideration of the pathogenesis of kidney stones.

RENAL INSUFFICIENCY. Renal failure sometimes occurs as a complication of gout. The pathogenesis of renal failure may be complex, but the most important factor is probably the interstitial deposition of sodium urate monohydrate crystals, especially in the medullary areas of the kidney. The result is chronic inflammation and fibrosis, which causes an interstitial nephritis often mistaken for chronic pyelonephritis in the past. Other features of the gouty kidney may include uric acid stone formation with obstruction and secondary pyelonephritis, nephrosclerosis, and possibly an early glomerular lesion. Acute renal failure may result from massive precipitation of uric acid in collecting tubules, usually in association with chemotherapy of malignancy and the sudden release of purines, which result in a pulse overload of urate.

The Cause of Hyperuricemia. All of the manifestations of gout result from the crystallization of sodium urate or uric acid from supersaturated solutions. The pathogenesis of the gouty syndromes is ultimately that of the pathogenesis of hyperuricemia and/or hyperuricosuria.

An increase in the concentration of a metabolite in the body can be caused by four variables that may act independently or in concert: (1) increased formation, (2) decreased metabolism, (3) decreased excretion, (4) increased absorption (from exogenous sources). Urate is not metabolized to a significant degree by human tissues because of the absence of uricase. It is metabolized by bacteria following its secretion into the gut, perhaps one fourth to one third being so metabolized. There is no evidence that this pathway of secretion-metabolism is impaired in gout. In fact it probably constitutes a safety valve for the disposition of urate when renal failure supervenes. There is very little preformed urate in the normal diet, and, of that added (C^{14}-urate), only about 10 per cent can be recovered unchanged in the urine. Approximately 25 per cent of ingested DNA purines and 50 per cent of RNA purines appear ultimately as urinary urate through degradative pathways outlined previously. Although the serum uric acid level can be raised somewhat by purine gluttony, there is no evidence that patients with gout absorb dietary purines more avidly as the pathogenesis of hyperuricemia. Sustained hyperuricemia in man, therefore, results only from excessive de novo synthesis of purines, reduced efficiency of renal excretion of urate, or both factors acting in concert.

In a sense, all human beings are in danger of gout. Normal adult males have a mean serum uric acid of about 5.0 mg/dl (over 70 per cent saturated) and females of about 4.3 mg/dl (over 60 per cent saturated). Certainly this would seem to be inappropriate uricemia with no known biological advantage. This condition of purine peril is secondary to two evolutionary events: (1) the loss of uricase, which would have converted urate to allantoin; and (2) the inappropriate reabsorption of urate from glomerular filtrate by the proximal renal tubule. There are rare individuals whose renal tubules fail to reabsorb urate as an isolated defect. They have urate clearances in excess of creatinine clearance, hypouricemia (often < 1.0 mg/dl), and excellent health.

METABOLIC (OVERPRODUCTION) GOUT. This form of gout results from continued excessive synthesis of purine nucleotides from simple precursors through the de novo pathway as described above and, at equilibrium, a corresponding irreversible oxidation of purine bases to uric acid. There are three general methods for estimating the rate of production of uric acid:

1. Measuring the 24-hour excretion of uric acid in the urine on a low purine diet. Since a significant but variable amount of uric acid is destroyed by uricolysis in the intestine, this simple method documents overproduction only when urinary urate is distinctly elevated on a low purine diet (> approximately 600 mg/day) or on a normal diet (> 800 mg/day). Some patients with normal or high normal excretions will actually be "overproducers" obscured by increased shunting of uric acid into the gut.
2. Measuring the pool size and turnover rate of urate in extracellular fluid. This is a research technique that requires the use of labeled uric acid (C^{14} or N^{15}) to determine the pool size by isotope dilution. From the progressive dilution of the isotopic urate with the newly formed unlabeled compound over time one can calculate the turnover rate of the miscible pool, and from these values the synthetic rate can be derived. This technique cannot be used to study patients with tophi, since the uneven exchange of the isotope with the solid phase urate introduces a major error in the measurement of pool size.
3. Measuring the rate of incorporation of labeled purine precursors into uric acid. The precursors most frequently used have been glycine or aminoimidazolecarboxamide.

These methods have been applied in the study of patients with gout, and approximately 10 to 15 per cent (the percentage varies in different laboratories) have been found to have overproduction of purines as the cause of hyperuricemia.

Overproduction can be *primary* (genetic) or *secondary* to some other disease process associated with enhanced synthesis and catabolism of tissues and therefore of their component nucleic acids. Examples of such diseases include agnogenic myeloid metaplasia and psoriasis. Primary overproduction hyperuricemia, however, is not associated with any evidence of increased tissue formation and destruction. It presumably results from inherited defects in purine metabolism that directly or indirectly enhance de novo synthesis. Some of these defects have been elucidated, but most have not. The disorders listed in Table 21 currently account for less than 5 per cent of patients with primary metabolic gout. Hypoxanthine-guanine phosphoribosyltransferase deficiency, though a form of metabolic gout, is distinctive enough to be discussed later as a separate entity. The other enzyme abnormalities associated with this form of gout will be presented briefly.

In theory excessive de novo synthesis of purines must result from one or more of four abnormalities at

TABLE 21. CLASSIFICATION OF THE PATHOGENESIS OF HYPERURICEMIA AND GOUT

1. Metabolic—continued excessive synthesis of purines
   a. primary—caused by a genetic defect (all such defects so far found account for <5 per cent of these patients)
      1. deficiency of hypoxanthine-guanine phosphoribosyltransferase
      2. PP-ribose-P synthetase variants
      3. glucose-6-phosphatase deficiency
   b. secondary—caused by increased tissue turnover-agnogenic myeloid metaplasia, psoriasis, leukemia, etc.
2. Renal—continued reduced efficiency of excretion by the kidney
   a. primary—genetic abnormalities have not been clarified at a chemical or biophysical level
   b. secondary—caused by renal disease or the effect of metabolites or drugs upon renal excretion of urate
      1. renal disease—most forms of renal failure, lead nephropathy
      2. metabolites—lactate, β-hydroxybutyrate
      3. drugs—pyrazinamide, thiazides, salicylates, etc.

the first step, that of the production of phosphoribosylamine catalyzed by amidophosphoribosyltransferase:

$$\text{PP-ribose-P + glutamine} \xrightarrow{Mg^{++}} \text{phosphoribosylamine + glutamic acid + PPi}$$

These abnormalities could include (1) increased concentration of a substrate, either PP-ribose-P or glutamine; (2) increased intrinsic activity or decreased sensitivity to feedback regulation; (3) a change in the concentration of a regulatory molecule, which affects enzyme activity either by competition with substrate for active sites or by allosteric changes in conformation; and (4) an increased amount of the transferase enzyme.

PP-ribose-P serves both as a substrate of the transferase and as an allosteric activator (Figs. 72, 75). PP-ribose-P synthetase, an enzyme coded for on the X chromosome, catalyzes its formation as noted:

$$\text{Ribose 5-P + ATP} \xrightarrow{Mg^{++}} \text{PP-ribose-P + AMP}$$

The activity of this synthetase under physiological conditions has been found to be increased in males with gout in several families, leading to overproduction of PP-ribose-P and, presumably, thereby enhancing purine synthesis. Interestingly, these individuals have exhibited distinct abnormalities in the enzyme: elevation of the Vmax, increased affinity for ribose 5-phosphate, and reduced affinities for purine nucleotide regulators, respectively. It has been speculated that the excessive purine production found in glycogen storage disease (Type I, von Gierke's disease) is due in part to the increased availability of ribose 5-phosphate because of shunting into this pathway secondary to deficiency of glucose-6-phosphatase. Increased tissue concentrations of PP-ribose-P in von Gierke's disease have not been demonstrated, however.

Glutamine is also a substrate in the synthesis of phosphoribosylamine. An increase in its intracellular concentration could also be a driving force for purine overproduction. Despite considerable speculation no genetic or acquired abnormality in glutamine metabolism has been firmly established as the biochemical basis of gout. Similarly, no intrinsic abnormalities of the enzyme amidophosphoribosyltransferase have so far been demonstrated in gouty subjects, although this would be a logical site for defects to occur comparable to those that have been described for PP-ribose-P synthetase.

RENAL (UNDEREXCRETION) GOUT. Most gout (85 to 90 per cent) results from a decreased efficiency in the ability of the kidney to excrete plasma urate. At equilibrium a normal amount of urate is excreted per unit time but at the cost of a higher plasma concentration. As in the case of metabolic gout, renal gout may be either primary (genetic) or secondary. As described above (Fig. 80), renal clearance of urate is a complex function of glomerular filtration and overlapping reabsorption and secretion by the renal tubule. By exclusion, gouty patients without overproduction of urate are assumed to have underexcretion (actually, decreased efficiency of excretion). A number of clearance studies have demonstrated reduced net clearance of urate in gouty patients, particularly in comparison with control subjects made hyperuricemic by dietary manipulations.

Secondary renal gout may result from any chronic renal disease resulting in generalized reduction in function. Since all or virtually all of the urate filtered by the glomerulus is normally reabsorbed, the hyperuricemia of uremia presumably represents reduced tubular secretory capacity rather than a reduced glomerular filtration rate. Several natural organic acids are known to inhibit renal tubular secretion of urate, especially lactate and β-hydroxybutyrate, and are capable thereby of inducing hyperuricemia. A number of pharmaceutical agents similarly inhibit tubular secretion, notably salicylates, pyrazinamide, and ethambutol. The metabolism of ethanol causes hyperuricemia in part by elevating plasma lactate as a coupled oxidation-reduction between alcohol dehydrogenase and lactic dehydrogenase. It also increases the synthesis of urate. The common occurrence of hyperuricemia during the use of potent diuretic agents, best studied for the thiazides, is most likely the result of enhanced tubular reabsorption coupled to that of proximal tubular reabsorption of sodium during the volume-contracted state. Lead nephropathy is the probable cause of the high incidence of gout associated with plumbism.

Primary renal gout occurs in some families with decreased efficiency of urate excretion in the absence of any other evidence of intrinsic renal disease or of any increased concentration of a metabolite or of the presence of a drug that might inhibit tubular function. It is presumed that such patients have an inherited impairment in tubular secretion of urate, but it is difficult to rule out enhanced postsecretory reabsorption. Elucidation of the biochemical basis for this abnormality awaits better definition of the mechanism for normal urate secretion and absorption. It is possible that such patients have some other genetic defect leading to the accumulation of a metabolite that secondarily inhibits tubular urate secretion (a lactate-like effect). No such metabolite has yet been found in these patients with heritable renal gout.

Summary. Four general causes of hyperuricemia are associated with the manifestations of clinical gout (Table 21). Because of excessive synthesis or reduced efficiency of excretion of urate (or rarely of both), supersaturation of sodium urate occurs in extracellular fluid. Sodium urate may then crystallize in and around joints, interacting with leukocytes to cause microcrystalline synovitis, or more generally in cartilage or connective tissues as tophi. Deposition of sodium urate in the kidneys leads to interstitial nephritis. Excessive urinary excretion of urate or increased urinary acidity may result in uric acid stone diathesis. Although much has been learned, many questions remain concerning the pathogenesis of hyperuricemia and clinical gout. Some of these are as follows:

1. What is the biochemical basis for urate overproduction in the vast majority (> 95 per cent) of patients with metabolic gout for whom no enzyme defects have so far been found?
2. What is the biochemical basis for reduced efficiency of renal tubular secretion (or enhanced postsecretory absorption) in patients with heritable renal gout?
3. What accounts for the marked differences in the clinical manifestations of gout in patients with similar levels of supersaturation? Some may have "essential hyperuricemia" throughout life, while others with the same serum level may be crippled by tophaceous gout and recurrent acute gouty arthritis.
4. Why are some tissues particularly susceptible to tophaceous deposits—cartilage, for example—while others are generally spared (liver, skeletal muscle)?
5. How can knowledge of the crystal-leukocyte model of acute gouty arthritis be used most effectively in the design of new therapeutic agents?

Other questions can be framed by the reader to which answers are missing or are incomplete.

HYPOXANTHINE-GUANINE PHOSPHORIBOSYLTRANSFERASE DEFICIENCY (LESCH-NYHAN SYNDROME)

A familial disorder was described by Lesch and Nyhan in 1964 characterized by marked overproduction of urate in association with a unique neurological syndrome in male children. The syndrome includes mental deficiency, spasticity, choreoathetosis, and compulsive self-mutilation. Some of the patients have had macrocytic anemia with megaloblastic marrow changes. The disorder is transmitted as a sex-linked recessive. Partial forms of the syndrome have been discovered in some adults with severe gout, some of whom exhibit minor neurological findings.

The Lesch-Nyhan syndrome results from a severe deficiency of hypoxanthine-guanine phosphoribosyltransferase (HGPRT) activity (Fig. 84), the defect having been found in erythrocytes, leukocytes, fibroblasts, brain, hair follicles, and cultured cells from amniotic fluid. Genetic heterogeneity has been found in the degree of residual activity of HGPRT (approximately 0.1 to 5 per cent of normal), the amount of cross-reactive immunological material (CRIM) to an antibody to normal HGPRT, relative activity of the enzyme with hypoxanthine and guanine and certain physical characteristics such as thermal stability of the enzyme. These differences represent different sites of mutation

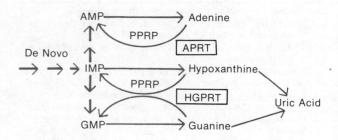

A. Normal

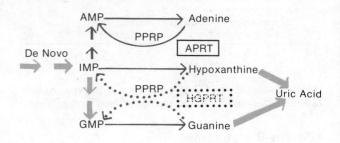

B. Lesch-Nyhan Syndrome

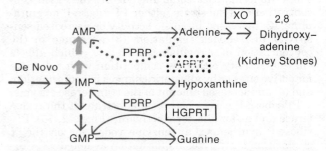

C. APRT Deficiency

Figure 84. Scheme that shows normal salvage pathways for purine bases *(A)* and the abnormalities that occur with deficiency of hypoxanthine-guanine phosphoribosyltransferase (HGPRT) in the Lesch-Nyhan syndrome *(B)* or of adenine phosphoribosyltransferase (APRT) *(C)*. Patients with APRT deficiency may be asymptomatic or may present with 2,8-dihydroxyadenine kidney stones. XO, xanthine oxidase.

within the same gene, affecting protein structure and therefore function. The human gene for HGPRT has been isolated and sequenced by the methods of recombinant DNA technology.

The result of the defect is a block in the salvage synthesis of IMP from hypoxanthine and of GMP from guanine. These free bases therefore cannot be reutilized and are converted to urate by the degradative pathways described earlier. In order to prevent "purine starvation," de novo synthesis must balance this pathological wastage. All methods for measuring the rates of purine synthesis, such as the excretion of uric acid or the incorporation of labeled precursors into urate, have documented massive overproduction of purines in such patients. The prevention of purine starvation is the teleological explanation for excessive synthesis. How is this effected at the regulatory level? The answer is not clear. A fall in tissue levels of IMP, GMP, and their derived nucleotides would be anticipated in the absence of salvage, which in turn would release PP-ribose-P synthetase and amidophosphoribosyltransferase from feedback inhibition (Fig. 85). An increased rate of de novo synthesis would result to restore the levels of the deficient nucleotides. Studies so far have not demonstrated low tissue levels of these nucleotides, but this may be the result of the effectiveness of the compensatory process. Levels of PP-ribose-P have been found to be elevated in erythrocytes and in cultured fibroblasts from patients with HGPRT deficiency, which would tend to drive purine synthesis both as a substrate in the synthesis of phosphoribosylamine and as a key activator of the amidotransferase (Fig. 85). Why does the PP-ribose-P accumulate? This is not clear. It has been speculated that this represents

underutilization in the salvage pathway, but assuming that the overall rate of purine nucleotide synthesis (salvage and de novo) is the same in the Lesch-Nyhan syndrome as in normals, the utilization of PP-ribose-P would be unchanged. Release of feedback inhibition by IMP and GMP might be expressed in an unbalanced manner leading to relatively greater activity of PP-ribose-P synthetase than of amidotransferase. Activity of adenine phosphoribosyltransferase (APRT) is elevated in erythrocytes from patients with HGPRT deficiency. This may be secondary to stabilization of APRT by PP-ribose-P.

The demonstration of defective purine salvage in the Lesch-Nyhan syndrome offers a rational explanation for the associated enhancement of de novo synthesis. The pathogenesis of the characteristic abnormalities of the function of the central nervous system has not

Figure 85. Purinogenic immunodeficiency syndromes. When adenosine deaminase (ADA) is reduced in activity, deoxyadenosine is shunted into deoxyATP, which inhibits the ribonucleotide reductase catalyzed conversion of pyrimidine and purine nucleotides to their corresponding deoxynucleotides (B, also see Fig. 77). Adenosine may also be shunted into S-adenosylhomocysteine and thereby inhibit a variety of methylation reactions. When purine nucleoside phosphorylase (PNP) is deficient, deoxyguanosine similarly accumulates as deoxyGTP and inhibits three of the ribonucleotide reductase catalyzed reactions (C).

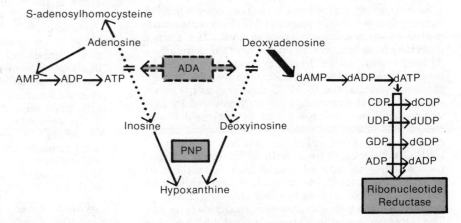

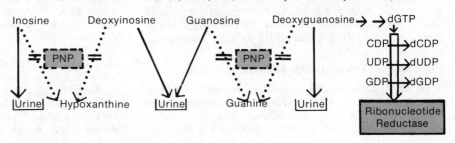

been established. De novo synthesis of purines is quite low in the brain, and, conversely, the activity of HGPRT is normally higher there than anywhere else in the body. The brain is, presumably, exceptionally dependent upon the recycling of preformed purine bases, either formed originally in situ by its limited de novo system or perhaps derived from circulating purines of hepatic origin. Loss of HGPRT activity may therefore create foci of cerebral purine starvation. No specific structural changes have been found in neuropathological studies. In the Lesch-Nyhan syndrome, the oxypurines hypoxanthine and xanthine are increased in cerebrospinal fluid, but not to levels higher than those found in patients with partial HGPRT deficiency who do not have dysfunction of the central nervous system. Self-mutilation has been experimentally produced in rats given massive amounts of caffeine, which is a methylated derivative of xanthine. The activity of dopamine-β-hydroxylase, which catalyzes the conversion of dopamine to norepinephrine, has been found to be high in the plasma of patients with HGPRT deficiency and self-mutilation. This observation is of interest in view of the fact that unilateral self-mutilation has been produced in rats with ipsilateral lesions in the nigrostriatal system produced by 6-hydroxydopamine. More recently, however, activities of both dopamine β-hydroxylase and monamine oxidase were found to be normal in brain tissue from patients with the Lesch-Nyhan syndrome obtained at autopsy. The pathogenesis of cerebral dysfunction in the Lesch-Nyhan syndrome is an important unresolved problem that has obvious therapeutic implications.

Adenine Phosphoribosyltransferase (APRT) Deficiency

Several families have been found that have exhibited varying degrees of deficiencies of APRT activity, transmitted as an autosomal recessive trait. The carrier state may be as frequent as 1 per cent of the population. Although gout and/or hyperuricemia were found in some of these patients and their families, the linkage of these abnormalities to APRT deficiency is not clear, since most of the cases have been discovered by surveying families with known gout for enzyme deficiencies, a bias of ascertainment. No neurological abnormalities have been noted, in contrast to those of HGPRT deficiency. Patients with APRT deficiency cannot normally salvage adenine, which is excreted in increased amounts in the urine. It is also oxidized by xanthine oxidase to 8-hydroxyadenine and 2,8-dihydroxyadenine, which also appear in the urine (Fig. 84). The latter compound is 50 times less soluble than uric acid and may result in crystalluria or even *2,8-dihydroxyadenine kidney stones*. These stones resemble uric acid stones, with which they are frequently confused. More needs to be learned about the seemingly analogous blocks of HGPRT and APRT salvage activities.

Purinogenic Disorders of Immune Function

In 1972 *deficiency of adenosine deaminase (ADA)* was discovered in erythrocytes of two patients with severe combined immunodeficiency disease—that is, collateral dysfunction of both T cells and B cells (see Section III). Subsequently, more than 50 patients have been found with this association, and this enzyme defect may account for as many as one third to one half of patients with autosomal recessive combined immunodeficiency. These patients have recurrent infections beginning in the first few months of life involving bacterial, viral, fungal, and protozoal agents representing failure of both cellular and humoral immunity. They also may have diarrhea, bony lesions, and failure to thrive, leading typically to early death. In 1975 a second disorder of purine metabolism, *deficiency of purine nucleoside phosphorylase (PNP)*, was discovered to be associated with another disorder of immune function, that of impaired T cell production and function, with retention of B cell function. This observation has been subsequently confirmed with a series of other patients. Both disorders are autosomal recessive in their inheritance pattern.

Figure 74 illustrates the metabolic pathway in which these sequential defects occur. Adenosine deaminase, for which the structural gene is found on the long arm of chromosome 20, catalyzes the irreversible deamination of adenosine and deoxyadenosine to inosine and deoxyinosine in the linked interconversion systems of the purines. Purine nucleoside phosphorylase (PNP), for which the structural gene is found on the long arm of chromosome 14, catalyzes the phosphorolysis of inosine to release the free base hypoxanthine, which can then be reconverted to IMP by the action of HGPRT. It is important to note that PNP is a versatile enzyme and also converts guanosine, deoxyinosine, and deoxyguanosine to their respective free bases, releasing ribose 1-phosphate or deoxyribose 1-phosphate in the process.

Three questions are of great interest concerning the purinogenic immunological disorders:

1. What is the biochemical linkage between the enzyme defects of ADA and PNP and immunocyte dysfunction?
2. What is the basis for the selectivity of expression as dysfunction of immunocytes in a disorder found in all cells? A subsidiary question would be whether the information obtained about selective immunocyte vulnerability could be used to suppress immunity when appropriate or to develop agents useful in the treatment of malignant disorders of B or T cell origin.
3. Are there additional defects of purine or pyrimidine metabolism that account for immunodeficiency in other patients who do not exhibit defects in ADA or PNP?

These questions can be answered in part, but are still under active investigation.

Adenosine Deaminase Deficiency. ADA deficiency causes a block in the further metabolism of adenosine. Some can be reconverted to AMP with adenosine kinase and ATP. More important, however, ADA deficiency leads to the intracellular accumulation of deoxyadenosine and even to its excessive excretion in the urine, reflecting the fact that the "adenosine cycle" is the *only* pathway available for the catabolism of deoxyadenine nucleotides. Deoxyadenosine can be phosphorylated by both adenosine kinase and deoxycytidine kinase. There is intracellular accumulation of deoxy AMP, deoxy ADP, and deoxy ATP. In nucleic acid metabolism the first step unique to DNA synthesis is the reduction of ribonucleotides to deoxyribonucleotides, catalyzed by the complex enzyme ribonucleotide reductase. This is an allosteric enzyme with an absolute requirement for specific effector molecules as well as being subject to inhibition by other products. These complex relationships are shown in Figure 77, which notes that dATP is a universal inhibitor of the reduction of all four purine nucleoside diphosphates by ribonucleotide reductase. In the absence of ADA, therefore, dATP accumulates and inhibits the first step unique to the synthesis of DNA (Fig. 85A, B). This is a gross distortion of the allosteric mechanisms that normally serve to regulate the production of the deoxynucleotides at a rate appropriate for DNA synthesis.

Other mechanisms of injury have been proposed and may play a role. The accumulation of adenosine will, in the presence of homocysteine, increase tissue levels of S-adenosylhomocysteine, a normal intermediary in methionine metabolism but one capable of inhibiting a variety of methylation reactions that utilize S-adenosylmethionine, its immediate precursor. It has also been found that 2'-deoxyadenosine irreversibly binds to and inactivates the enzyme S-adenosylhomocysteine hydrolase. This further enhances the intracellular concentration of S-adenosylhomocysteine with its adverse effect on methylation reactions. Adenosine may increase tissue concentrations of cyclic AMP through activation of cyclase with inhibition of immunocyte function. At this time, however, it seems most likely that inhibition of ribonucleotide reductase by accumulated dATP and S-adenosylhomocysteine toxicity are the major pathogenetic results of ADA deficiency.

Purine Nucleoside Phosphorylase Deficiency. PNP deficiency leads to a block in the further metabolism of inosine, guanosine, deoxyinosine, and deoxyguanosine to their corresponding free bases (Fig. 85C). All four metabolites are excreted in increased amounts in the urine. Of these compounds, deoxyguanosine is the only one for which a kinase has been identified for its phosphorylation, an enzyme identical to deoxycytidine kinase. In patients with PNP deficiency deoxyguanosine triphosphate (dGTP) is found in increased amounts in some cells (erythrocytes). The mechanism of toxicity of dGTP is probably analogous to that described for dATP above, inhibition of the ribonucleotide reductase catalysis of deoxyribonucleotide synthesis (Fig. 85C). As shown, this block occurs for the reduction of CDP, UDP, and GDP. There is evidence that inhibition of the conversion of CDP to dCDP is the limiting step in this overall inhibition of DNA synthesis. Patients with PNP deficiency also tend to have hypouricemia and hypouricosuria. This presumably results from the decreased availability of the free purine base uric acid precursors, hypoxanthine and guanine.

Selectivity of Tissue Expression. In patients with ADA or PNP deficiency the enzyme defects are found in all tissues. Why is the clinical expression largely confined to T and B cells or T cells, respectively, in these two disorders? Can this information be used for targeted suppression of T or B cell activity? There is evidence that the T cell has two characteristics to explain its relative sensitivity to the accumulation of deoxyadenine and its trapping as dATP, thought to be the ultimate toxic product. T cells have higher activities of deoxyadenosine phosphorylating activity combined with 10-fold lower levels of nucleotidase, leading to a combination of enhanced synthesis and decreased catabolism of dATP. Deoxyguanosine is phosphorylated to its toxic derivative dGTP by deoxycytidine kinase, which is particularly high in activity in T cells as well. Taken with low activities of T-cell nucleotidase noted above, this may account for the relatively selective accumulation of dGTP. In tissues with low activities for the phosphorylation of deoxyadenosine or deoxyguanosine, these metabolites are not sequestered to the same degree as their toxic triphosphates and presumably pass across cell membranes to be excreted in the urine. No new drugs have yet been developed on the basis of these recent insights into the biochemical patterns of T and B cells, but it is an area of active investigation.

No other specific genetic disorders of purine or pyrimidine metabolism have yet been found in patients with immunodeficiency syndromes. Several patients have been described with deficiency of transcobalamin II, a serum protein necessary for the delivery of vitamin B_{12} to tissues. Among other defects, agammaglobulinemia has been found. Whether this B cell dysfunction relates to diminished nucleic acid synthesis has not been established.

MYOADENYLATE DEAMINASE DEFICIENCY

Approximately 25 to 30 patients have been discovered to have deficiency of muscle AMP deaminase since this disorder was first described in 1978. Transmitted as an autosomal recessive trait, the disorder is associated with a comparatively benign myopathy characterized by easy fatigue, cramps, and myalgia occurring after vigorous exercise. The onset of symptoms is usually in early adult life but may occur in infancy or late in life. Some patients have also complained of weakness. The serum creatine kinase activity is frequently elevated, especially after exercise. Exercise fails to release ammonia and inosine monophosphate from muscle, as occurs normally, and muscle ATP falls excessively during exercise, with a slower recovery rate.

There is increasing evidence that the so-called purine nucleotide cycle plays an important role in muscle energetics (Fig. 86), but how it does so is not clear. AMP deaminase, perhaps the key participant in this 3-enzyme cycle, exists as several isoenzymes, one of which is specific for muscle. The function of the cycle, which is increased in exercise, may be (1) to prevent AMP accumulation, which would tend to displace the adenylate kinase reaction toward the synthesis of ATP; (2) to furnish NH_3 and/or IMP to activate phosphofructokinase and/or glycogen phosphorylase, respectively; (3) to furnish citric acid cycle intermediates; or (4) to preserve the purine nucleotide pool (as IMP) for use in the recovery phase. The abnormalities that occur in myoadenylate deaminase deficiency are shown schematically in Figure 87.

ADENOSINE DEAMINASE EXCESS

Two kindreds of patients have been described who exhibited hemolytic anemia, low levels of erythrocytic

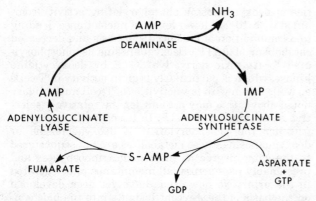

Figure 86. Purine nucleotide cycle. (Reprinted with permission from Swain, J. L., Sabina, R. L., and Holmes, E. W.: Myoadenylate deaminase deficiency. In Stanbury, J. B., Wyngaarden, J. B., Fredrickson, D. S., Goldstein, J. L., and Brown, M. S. (eds.): The Metabolic Basis of Inherited Disease. 5th ed. New York, McGraw-Hill Book Co., 1983, p. 1185.)

ATP, and marked elevations (45- to 70-fold) in the activity of adenosine deaminase (ADA). Those members of the family who do not exhibit hemolytic anemia have normal activities of adenosine deaminase. The purified enzyme from these patients has been found to have normal physical and kinetic characteristics, sug-

THE FATE OF CATABOLIZED AMP IN HUMAN SKELETAL MUSCLE

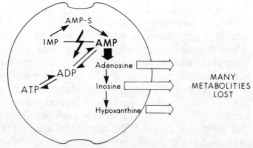

Figure 87. Comparison of purine metabolism in muscle from normal subject and patient with myoadenylate deaminase deficiency. (Reprinted with permission from Swain, J. L., Sabina, R. L., and Holmes, E. W.: Myoadenylate deaminase deficiency. In Stanbury, J. B., Wyngaarden, J. B., Fredrickson, D. S., Goldstein, J. L., and Brown, M. S. (eds.): The Metabolic Basis of Inherited Disease. 5th ed. New York, McGraw-Hill Book Co., 1983, p. 1190.)

gesting simple overproduction. ADA activities in leukocytes and cultured skin fibroblasts from these patients have been normal. The disorder has been detected in three generations transmitted as a mendelian dominant trait.

Hemolysis is presumed to result from the low levels of erythrocytic ATP and therefore to be analogous to that which occurs with a number of well-defined blocks in the glycolytic pathway within this specialized cell. The elevated level of ADA could potentially irreversibly deaminate adenosine to inosine, making adenosine unavailable for reconversion to AMP catalyzed by adenosine kinase (Fig. 74). The result is failure to replenish the crucial adenine nucleotide pool in a cell that cannot carry out de novo purine synthesis and therefore depends on salvage mechanisms. Although this formulation offers a rational explanation for the phenotypic expression as hemolysis secondary to deficiency of ATP, it does not explain why ADA activity is so markedly increased. Is this a primary genetic defect of too much enzyme production or is the production of ADA derepressed by an enzyme defect elsewhere? This remains to be demonstrated.

XANTHINURIA

The progressive oxidation of hypoxanthine to xanthine and of xanthine to uric acid is catalyzed by xanthine oxidase (Fig. 78), an enzyme found largely in human liver and intestinal mucosa. A number of patients have been described with deficiency of xanthine oxidase, transmitted as an autosomal recessive trait. As would be anticipated, they excrete increased amounts of hypoxanthine and xanthine in the urine and much less urate. Normal urinary xanthine is about 6 mg/24 hours, while patients with xanthinuria may excrete 50 times as much. Normal daily excretion of hypoxanthine is about 10 mg, but this does not increase as much as does xanthine with deficiency of xanthine oxidase. This probably reflects enhanced recycling of hypoxanthine to IMP catalyzed by HGPRT. A small amount of uric acid may be excreted, probably reflecting some residual activity of xanthine oxidase. The metabolic derangements of xanthinuria are simulated by use of the therapeutic agent allopurinol, which is both a substrate and a competitive inhibitor of xanthine oxidase.

Patients with xanthinuria are generally in good health. They are usually discovered through one of two mechanisms. On routine measurements their serum uric acids are found to be strikingly low (< 1.0 mg/dl), which may lead to further examinations. Alternatively, these patients may present with xanthine kidney stones. Xanthine is even less soluble in urine than is uric acid. Xanthine and hypoxanthine crystals have been described in muscle biopsies of patients with hereditary xanthinuria, and in three patients a myopathy was present. Two patients had recurrent polyarthritis, but neither xanthine nor hypoxanthine crystals have been described in synovial fluid as a possible cause of microcrystalline synovitis.

A second, very rare form of xanthinuria is associated with an abnormality of its molybdenum cofactor. This cofactor is also required for sulfite oxidase activity, the clinical features of which (neurological abnormalities, ocular lens dislocation) dominate the syndrome.

DEFICIENCY OF FOLATE AND/OR VITAMIN B₁₂

Folate is a cofactor in the synthesis of the purine ring, necessary for the insertion of the formyl C's at positions 2 and 8 (Fig. 71). Vitamin B_{12} is not known to play a direct role in the metabolism of purines, but in its absence tetrahydrofolate may be "trapped" as methyltetrahydrofolate because of a block in the methylation of homocysteine to methionine. Therefore purine biosynthesis may be deranged during deficiency of either of these two cofactors. Folate and B_{12} metabolism will not be discussed further here.

URIC ACID STONE DIATHESIS

In the United States, approximately 5 per cent of kidney stones contain uric acid as their main crystalloid constituent. There are two general causes of uric acid stones: increased uric acid excretion per 24 hours and increased urine acidity. Uric acid crystals may also constitute a nidus upon which a calcium oxalate stone is formed. Most uric acid stones do not represent the end result of disorders of purine metabolism per se. The topic of stone diathesis is considered in much more detail in Section X.

PYRIMIDINE METABOLISM

Pyrimidine metabolism has been less extensively studied than purine metabolism in man. This is the result of two factors: (1) the end products of pyrimidine metabolism are largely carbon dioxide and ammonia and are lost in the general pools of those metabolites; (2) there is no recognized disorder of pyrimidine metabolism that compares in importance with the gouty syndromes, so that less attention has been attracted to either its normal or abnormal metabolic pathways. Nevertheless, pyrimidines share equally with purines in the coding, transcription, and translation of genetic information. Pyrimidine nucleotides also have special functions in the intermediary metabolism of lipids and carbohydrates. Through indirect mechanisms (isotope incorporation into pseudouridine) it has been estimated

that the de novo synthesis of pyrimidines is 450 to 700 mg per day. On a molar basis this is approximately the same rate as that for purines. This section will summarize current knowledge about normal pyrimidine metabolism and then describe the abnormalities in metabolism so far detected.

DE NOVO SYNTHESIS OF PYRIMIDINES

As in the case of purines, pyrimidines are constructed from simple precursors—aspartate, bicarbonate, and ammonia (amide N of glutamine). In contrast to the purine pathway, the ring structure is formed first (orotic acid) before the interaction with PP-ribose-P to form a ribonucleotide.

The structural formulas for the four main pyrimidines are shown in Figure 88. The first sequence of steps in pyrimidine biosynthesis is summarized in Figure 89. The first step unique to pyrimidine synthesis is that of the formation of carbamyl phosphate (CAP):

$$2ATP + glutamine + HCO_3^- + H_2O \xrightarrow[Mg^{++}]{K^+}$$
$$CAP + 2\ ADP + P_i + glutamate$$

This reaction, catalyzed by carbamyl phosphate synthetase II, differs from that in mitochondria that forms CAP for citrulline synthesis in the urea cycle. CAP synthetase II, which forms pyrimidine-channeled CAP, exists in a cytoplasmic complex with the enzymes that catalyze the next two steps, aspartate transcarbamylase and dihydro-orotase. All three catalytic activities are synthesized from a common large mRNA template molecule.

Aspartate transcarbamylase catalyzes the irreversible transfer of the carbamyl group from CAP to the amine group of aspartate to form carbamylaspartic acid (Fig. 89), the first compound unique to pyrimidine synthesis. Both CAP synthetase II and aspartate transcarbamylase are sites for regulation of pyrimidine synthesis, as described further below. Carbamylaspartate undergoes a reversible dehydration to form the reduced pyrimidine ring dihydro-orotic acid (DHO),

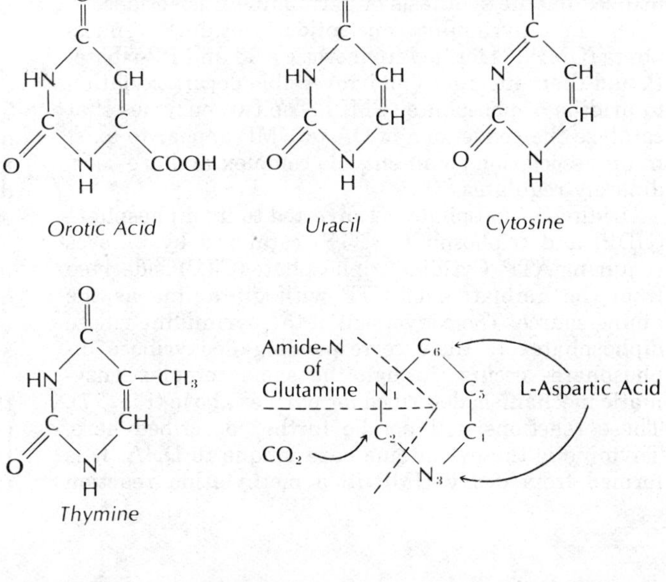

Figure 88. Structure of major pyrimidines and origin of the atoms of the pyrimidine ring.

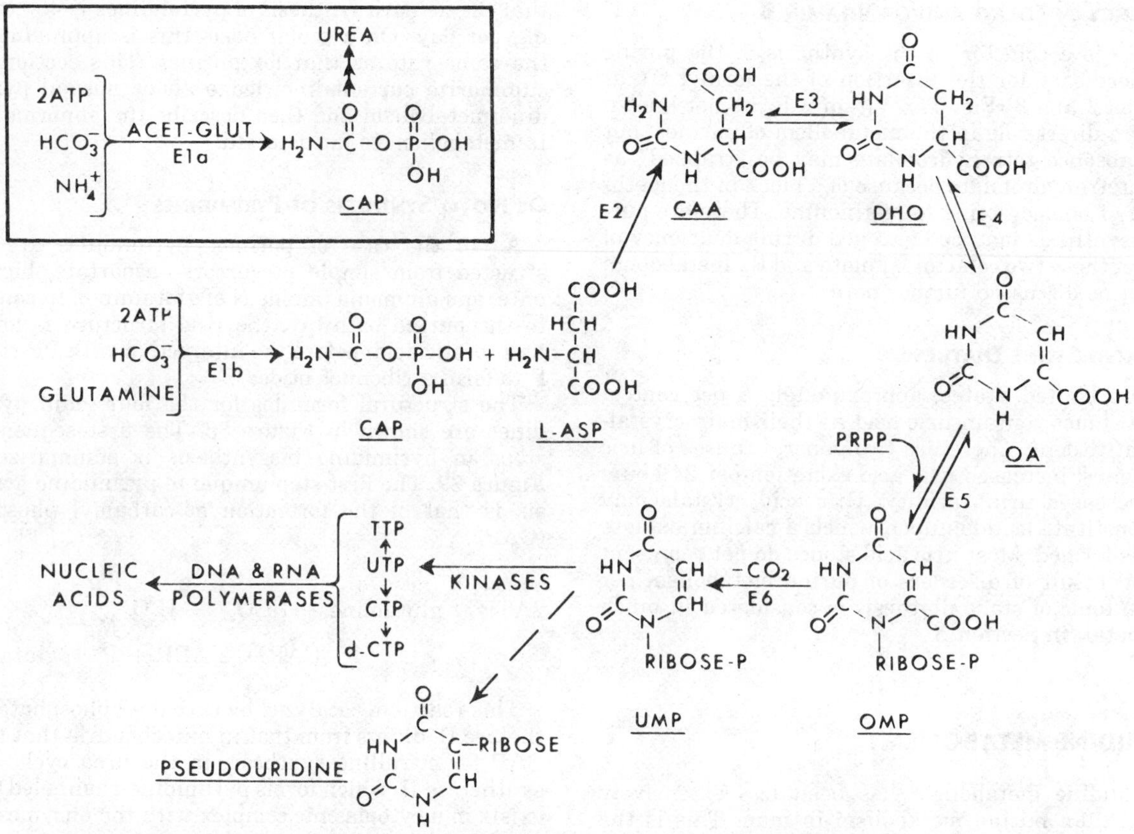

Figure 89. Pathway of pyrimidine biosynthesis. The synthesis of urea-channeled carbamyl phosphate is shown in the enclosed box. Acet-glut represents acetylglutamate, CAP carbamyl phosphate, L-ASP l-aspartate, CAA carbamylaspartate, DHO dihydro-orotic acid, OA orotic acid, OMP orotidine 5′-phosphate, UMP uridine 5′-phosphate, TTP thymidine triphosphate, UTP uridine triphosphate, CTP cytidine triphosphate, and dCTP deoxycytidine triphosphate. Of the enzymes: Ela indicates carbamyl phosphate synthetase (urea channel), Elb carbamyl phosphate synthetase (pyrimidine channel), E2 aspartate transcarbamylase, E3 dihydro-orotase, E4 dihydro-orotic dehydrogenase, E5 orotate phosphoribosyltransferase, and E6 orotidine 5′-phosphate decarboxylase. (From Smith, L. H., Jr.: N Engl J Med 288:764, 1973. Reproduced with the permission of the New England Journal of Medicine.)

which is then oxidized to orotic acid, the first pyrimidine, from which all others are derived. A small amount of orotic acid (approximately 1 to 2 mg per 24 hours) is excreted by the kidney, but most of it is utilized for the synthesis of pyrimidine nucleotides.

The first pyrimidine nucleotide, orotidine 5′-phosphate (OMP), is formed from orotic acid and PP-ribose-P, and then undergoes an irreversible decarboxylation to uridine 5′-phosphate (UMP). The two enzymes that catalyze the conversion of OA to UMP appear to exist in an association as an enzyme complex and are coordinately regulated.

Uridine 5′-phosphate is converted to its diphosphate (UDP) and triphosphate (UTP) catalyzed by kinases requiring ATP. Cytidine triphosphate (CTP) is derived from the amination of UTP with glutamine as the amine source. The conversion of the pyrimidine ribose diphosphates to their corresponding deoxyribose diphosphates occurs through the same complex enzymatic mechanism described for purines above (Fig. 77). These reactions will not be further described here. Thymine is the pyrimidine base unique to DNA. It is formed from deoxy UMP in a methylation reaction

catalyzed by thymidylate synthetase and requiring tetrahydrofolate and magnesium:

dUMP +

$$5,10\text{-methylene-}5,6,7,8\text{-tetrahydrofolate} \xrightarrow{Mg^{++}} TMP + 7,8\text{-dihydrofolate}$$

TMP is converted to TDP and TTP with kinases requiring ATP in a manner analogous to that described for UMP above. Folate interacts directly with pyrimidine synthesis only in the methylation reaction necessary for the synthesis of thymine, as a constituent of TMP. As far as is known, cobalamin (vitamin B_{12}) has no direct effect on pyrimidine synthesis. During B_{12} deficiency, however, there may be "folate trapping" and therefore a secondary impairment of thymidine synthesis.

In addition to the major pyrimidines so far described there are some trace pyrimidine bases. The most important of these is pseudouridine (Fig. 89), in which the ribose moiety is attached to C5 of the pyrimidine ring. This pyrimidine is found largely as a constituent of transfer RNA. It is not further metabolized in man and its excretion plus the rate of incorporation of labeled pyrimidine precursors into it has been used to assess the overall rate of pyrimidine biosynthesis.

SALVAGE SYNTHESIS

In analogy to purine metabolism, preformed pyrimidine bases, either released from endogenous sources or derived from the diet, are utilized in part for the synthesis of pyrimidine nucleotides. It is not known what fraction of pyrimidine nucleotide synthesis normally derives from such salvage mechanisms.

Uracil is a poor substrate for orotate phosphoribosyltransferase and in the presence of PP-ribose-P can be recovered directly as UMP. A more important reutilization pathway in mammalian systems, however, is the conversion of uracil first to uridine, catalyzed by uridine phosphorylase, and the subsequent phosphorylation of uridine to UMP by uridine kinase. Cytidine, or deoxycytidine, can be deaminated to the corresponding uridine derivatives, catalyzed by pyrimidine nucleoside deaminase, and then follow pathways described for uridine. Deoxycytidine can also be converted to its deoxynucleotide derivative directly by ATP and a specific kinase. Thymine can be salvaged with deoxyribose-1-P, catalyzed by the enzyme deoxythymidine phosphorylase, and then converted to thymidine 5'-phosphate by thymidine kinase. These recovery mechanisms for pyrimidines represent the biochemical basis for the use of various antineoplastic agents, such as 5-fluorouracil, 5-fluorocytidine, and 6-azauridine. As is the case with purines, there is some evidence, although not yet conclusive, that plasma uridine and cytidine perhaps derived from the liver may be an important source of preformed pyrimidines for other tissues.

CATABOLISM OF PYRIMIDINES

The catabolism of pyrimidine nucleotides largely flows through the release of uracil and thymine and the subsequent reduction, hydrolysis, and degradation of these free bases. Nucleotides are converted to nucleosides by 5'-nucleotidases, one of which at least is rather highly specific for pyrimidine nucleotides. Cytidine is then deaminated to uridine. The free bases, uracil or thymine, are released from the nucleosides, catalyzed by pyrimidine nucleoside phosphorylase. The ultimate end products are largely carbon dioxide and ammonia, although some β-aminoisobutyric acid of thymine origin is normally found in urine. As noted above, the lack of a specific end product comparable to uric acid has handicapped studies of pyrimidine metabolism in man.

REGULATION OF PYRIMIDINE SYNTHESIS

The rate of de novo synthesis of pyrimidine nucleotides must be appropriately controlled in view of their central role in nucleic acid structure and function and in intermediary metabolism and the varying requirements that must exist at different times and in different tissues. The control of the synthetic rate at a given point in the sequence could occur through changes in the concentration of a substrate (or substrates), the activity of an enzyme, or the total amount of enzyme available.

Almost invariably, rate control is exerted at the level of the first enzyme unique to a biosynthetic sequence. In mammalian systems the first unique enzyme in pyrimidine synthesis is carbamyl phosphate synthetase II, which catalyzes the formation of pyrimidine-channeled CAP (Figs. 89 and 90). The concentration of ATP, as a reactant, may strongly influence CAP synthesis, in contrast to HCO_3^- and glutamine, which appear to be at saturating concentrations. One of the end products of pyrimidine synthesis, UTP, is a feedback inhibitor of CAP synthetase, exhibiting competition with respect to ATP. In contrast PP-ribose-P activates CAP synthesis by decreasing the $S_{0.5}$ for ATP but without changing the overall Vmax of the synthetase. No regulation has been shown at the level of aspartate carbamyltransferase in mammalian systems—in contrast to bacteria, where this is the major site of control. Dihydro-orotase is inhibited by orotic acid, but the significance of this in vivo has not been established.

The rate-limiting step in pyrimidine nucleotide synthesis may be the conversion of orotic acid to orotidine 5'-phosphate, catalyzed by orotate phosphoribosyltransferase (Fig. 89). This reaction is highly sensitive to the concentration of PP-ribose-P as a reactant, further demonstrating the central role played by this compound in the regulation of the synthesis of both purine and pyrimidine nucleotides. Since the synthesis of OMP is reversible, the concentrations of OMP and of pyrophosphate also influence the net rate. The irreversible decarboxylation of OMP to UMP is also inhibited by a number of purine and pyrimidine nucleotides, including UMP itself.

There is some evidence for regulation of enzyme levels as well as of activity in pyrimidine nucleotide biosynthesis. In a patient with hereditary orotic aciduria (see below) levels of aspartate transcarbamylase and dihydro-orotase were elevated in erythrocytes, returning to normal following uridine therapy. In mammalian systems apparent coordinated induction

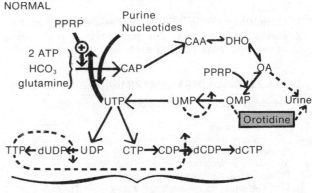

Figure 90. Normal regulatory mechanisms in pyrimidine biosynthesis. Arrows that cross those indicating the sequence of enzymatic reactions represent the major sites of feedback inhibition. The sequence is shown in more detail together with an explanation of the abbreviations in Figure 89.

of the first three enzymes has been noted—for example, after lectin-mediated transformation of human T lymphocytes. In other studies, apparent coordinated induction and repression of orotate phosphoribosyltransferase and orotidine 5'-phosphate decarboxylase have been described. In some experiments no distinction has been made between induction (new protein synthesis) and enzyme stabilization. Nevertheless there is considerable evidence now that the amount of enzyme protein available, as well as its activity per molecule or the substrate concentration, may be an additional method by which rates of pyrimidine nucleotide synthesis are appropriately modulated.

DISORDERS OF METABOLISM

A classification of disorders of pyrimidine metabolism in man is presented in Table 22. No one of these is a frequent cause of disease. A description of the associated pathophysiology, however, serves to elucidate human pyrimidine metabolism.

HEREDITARY OROTIC ACIDURIA

Hereditary orotic aciduria is a descriptive phrase for at least two disorders of pyrimidine biosynthesis associated with megaloblastic anemia, leukopenia, poor growth and development, and the continued excessive excretion of orotic acid in the urine. Only about 10 cases have been described in the past 25 years since its discovery. Orotic acid is relatively insoluble and may cause obstruction to urine flow through heavy crystalluria. The megaloblastic anemia fails to respond to folate, cobalamin, or a variety of other hematinic agents. In contrast, therapy with oral uridine leads to a prompt reticulocytosis, rise of the leukocyte count, and resumption of normal growth and development. There are several aspects that have added interest to the study of this rare group of disorders beyond that of another inborn error of metabolism per se:

1. In the most frequent form of the disease, hereditary orotic aciduria Type I, there is a double enzyme defect, which has raised a number of interesting questions about the molecular mechanisms involved.
2. Hereditary orotic aciduria represents "pyrimidine starvation" in man. The patient is a pyrimidine auxotroph, requiring an exogenous source of pyrimidines for the maintenance of health. It is the best example currently known of acquired auxotrophism in man.
3. The chemical abnormalities found in hereditary orotic aciduria illustrate the regulatory mechanisms normally at play in the control of pyrimidine synthesis.
4. The genetic abnormalities can be simulated by certain pharmacological agents.

In all patients with hereditary orotic aciduria so far studied, except one, the activities of both orotate phosphoribosyltransferase and orotidine 5'-phosphate decarboxylase have been markedly diminished (Fig. 91). This double enzyme defect, termed Type I, has been most frequently studied in erythrocytes, but similar defects have been demonstrated in leukocytes, liver homogenates, and cultured fibroblasts from skin. In a single patient the level of orotidine 5'-phosphate decarboxylase was markedly reduced in erythrocytes, but the level of orotate phosphoribosyltransferase was increased. There was an associated orotidinuria as well as orotic aciduria. This variant has been termed Type II (Fig. 92). Over the next two to three years, during therapy with uridine, the level of erythrocytic orotate phosphoribosyltransferase gradually fell to about 2 per cent of normal activity. Heterozygotes for hereditary orotic aciduria Type I can be conveniently detected by the measurement of the two specific enzymes in erythrocytes. They also exhibit modest increases in the excretion of orotic acid (about eight times normal—that is, about 10 to 12 mg per 24 hours), but no increase in urinary orotidine. The disease is transmitted as an autosomal recessive trait. One family was found (the "S" family) in which the propositus exhibited the double enzyme defect and had 15 to 20 times the normal amount of urinary orotic acid. Both parents had low normal activities of the two enzymes in their erythrocytes. It is postulated that the propositus is homozygous for a milder form of hereditary orotic aciduria, but it is possible that he represents a new mutation.

All patients with the Type I disorder and all obligate

TABLE 22. DISORDERS OF PYRIMIDINE METABOLISM

1. Hereditary orotic aciduria with double enzyme defect (Type I):
   a. symptomatic
   b. "S" family variant (not clearly established)
2. Hereditary orotic aciduria with selective orotidine 5'-phosphate decarboxylase deficiency (Type II)
3. Pyrimidine 5'-nucleotidase deficiency
4. Orotic aciduria secondary to other genetic defects:
   a. ornithine transcarbamylase deficiency
   b. purine nucleoside phosphorylase deficiency
   c. PP-ribose-P synthetase deficiency
5. Drug-induced orotic aciduria and orotidinuria
6. Beta-aminoisobutyric aciduria
7. Folic acid and vitamin B_{12} deficiency

Hereditary Orotic Aciduria, Type I

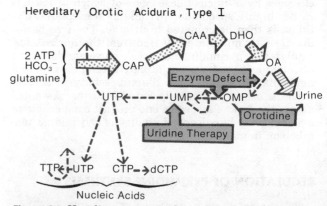

Figure 91. Hereditary orotic aciduria, Type I. The site of the double enzyme defect is indicated as orotate phosphoribosyltransferase and orotidine 5'-phosphate decarboxylase. The reduction in feedback inhibition and overproduction of orotic acid, with resulting orotic aciduria, are represented schematically by the increased size of the arrows before the site of the block. Abbreviations are as in Figure 89.

heterozygotes (with the exception of the parents in the "S" family) have exhibited deficiencies of both consecutive enzymes that catalyze the conversion of orotic acid to UMP (Fig. 89). There are many possibilities for such a double enzyme defect: a defect of a single protein with two catalytic functions, a defect in a common subunit, a defect in a regulatory gene, a single deletion involving two adjacent structural genes, or a failure of an enzyme to function normally to stabilize another enzyme in a complex. The latter explanation seems now to be the most plausible, although this has not been firmly established.

Patients with hereditary orotic aciduria require a source of preformed pyrimidines for the maintenance of health. When 2 to 4 grams of uridine is given orally to these patients there is a prompt improvement in all of their clinical and laboratory abnormalities and the resumption of normal growth and development. When uridine is withheld the complete syndrome returns. These patients are therefore "pyrimidine auxotrophs." This disorder is the best and virtually the only human example of auxotrophism for a biosynthetic intermediate. In phenylketonuria tyrosine becomes an essential amino acid because of a block in its synthesis from phenylalanine, but normal dietary sources suffice. Cysteine becomes an essential amino acid in homocystinuria and cystathioninuria. It is surprising that more examples of human auxotrophism have not been discovered. Possibly most auxotrophs fail to survive intrauterine life to live long enough to be recognized as such. Infants with hereditary orotic aciduria appear to be normal at birth. They may acquire sufficient maternal pyrimidines to maintain normal growth and development during gestation.

In the absence of uridine therapy the amounts of orotic acid excreted by patients with hereditary orotic aciduria may be increased 3000- to 5000-fold, exceeding by 10-fold the estimated total rate of pyrimidine synthesis by normal individuals. The orotic aciduria therefore results from two factors: (1) a block in its further metabolism, (2) massive overproduction. In part, the overproduction presumably results from pyrimidine starvation and therefore release of the feedback inhibition of carbamyl phosphate synthetase II described above (Fig. 90). The early enzymes in pyrimidine biosynthesis may be derepressed as well, leading to increased amounts of enzyme as well as increased activity for each enzyme molecule. Certain pharmaceutical agents have been developed, such as 6-azauridine and allopurinol, that inhibit orotidine 5′-phosphate decarboxylase and therefore simulate hereditary orotic aciduria Type II (Fig. 92). Patients who receive these agents have both orotic aciduria and orotidinuria, as would be anticipated from the site of the resulting metabolic block.

In summary, hereditary orotic aciduria is a rare syndrome representing at least two different enzyme defects in the synthesis of UMP from orotic acid. The study of its pathogenesis has clarified many aspects of pyrimidine metabolism in man.

Pyrimidine 5′-Nucleotidase Deficiency

Several patients have been described with hemolytic anemia and prominent basophilic stippling of erythrocytes on the stained blood smear (Fig. 93), abnor-

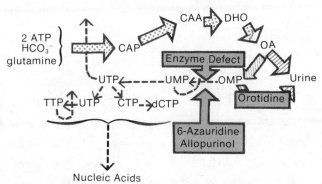

Hereditary Orotic Aciduria, Type II

Figure 92. Hereditary orotic aciduria, Type II. The enzyme defect is that of orotidine 5′-phosphate decarboxylase. The same enzyme is inhibited pharmacologically during 6-azauridine or allopurinol therapy. Orotidinuria occurs as well as orotic aciduria in patients receiving these agents and was found in the propositus of the Type II disorder.

malities transmitted as an autosomal recessive trait. These patients have marked increases in erythrocytic nucleotides, which on careful examination were found to be largely cytidine monophosphate (CMP) and uridine monophosphate (UMP). Their erythrocytes are deficient in the specific pyrimidine 5′-nucleotidase, which normally converts these compounds to their corresponding nucleosides (Fig. 94).

When RNA is degraded in the maturing reticulocyte, large amounts of purine and pyrimidine nucleotides are formed. They cannot escape the erythrocyte until they have been dephosphorylated. In the absence of normal pyrimidine nucleotidase activity these nucleotides accumulate and are thought to inhibit the degradation of ribosomes. Aggregations of these undegraded or partially degraded ribosomes are retained in the erythrocytes and constitute the stippling that is the hallmark of this form of inherited anemia. The mechanism of hemolysis has not been established. One possibility is that the pyrimidine nucleotides, present in abnormal concentrations, can compete with adenine nucleotides in a variety of reactions in intermediary metabolism. Anemia with basophilic stippling is also characteristic of lead poisoning. It is of great interest, therefore, that lead has been found to inhibit pyrimidine 5′-nucleotidase activity in erythrocytes. The anemia of lead poisoning may therefore represent an acquired disorder equivalent in its pathogenesis to the genetic disease, pyrimidine 5′-nucleotidase deficiency.

Drug-Induced Orotic Aciduria and Orotidinuria

As noted earlier, several drugs have been developed that inhibit the conversion of orotic acid to UMP and produce an associated orotic aciduria and orotidinuria. 6-Azauridine, following its conversion to 6-azauridine 5′-phosphate, is a specific competitive inhibitor of orotidine 5′-phosphate decarboxylase. Its use in patients as an antineoplastic agent is associated with massive orotic aciduria and orotidinuria, which disappear rapidly with discontinuation of therapy. Similarly, allopurinol and its product oxipurinol form ribonucleotides

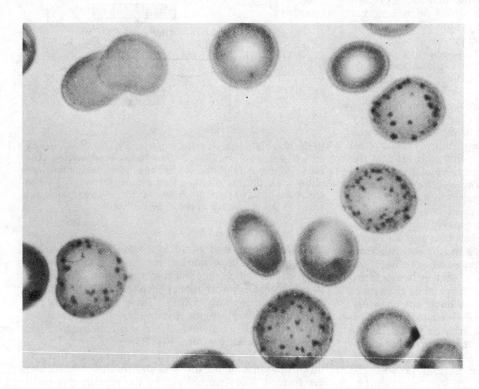

Figure 93. Prominent basophilic stippling on the stained blood smear of a patient with red cell pyrimidine 5'-nucleotidase deficiency. The stippling is thought to represent undegraded or partially degraded ribosomes. Similar stippling of red cells is seen in patients with lead poisoning. (From Valentine, W. N.: The Stratton lecture: Hemolytic anemia and inborn errors of metabolism. Blood 54:549, 1979. Reproduced with the permission of Blood.)

Figure 94. Pathogenesis of stippling and of hemolysis of erythrocytes in patients with deficiency of pyrimidine 5'-nucleotidase. The erythrocytes accumulate pyrimidine nucleotides, which are thought to inhibit the degradation of ribosomes, which are retained as material that gives stippling (see Figure 93). It is speculated that the abnormally elevated levels of pyrimidine nucleotides also inhibit the normal function of adenine nucleotides at a number of steps in energy metabolism, and in this way cause hemolysis.

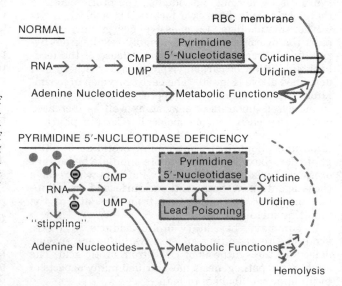

Thymine → →H_2N—C—C—COOH $\underset{\text{glutamate}}{\overset{\alpha\text{-ketoglutarate}}{\rightleftharpoons}}$ O=C C—COOH

(with H, CH_3 substituents)

β-AIB   methylmalonic acid semialdehyde

that inhibit OMP decarboxylase and cause orotic aciduria and orotidinuria, although the effect is less marked than that of 6-azauridine (Fig. 92).

BETA-AMINOISOBUTYRIC ACIDURIA

Beta-aminoisobutyric acid (β-AIB) is a metabolite formed in the catabolic pathway of thymine. It is normally converted to methylmalonic acid semialdehyde by transamination (see above). A number of individuals exhibit beta-aminoisobutyric aciduria, probably because of a defect in this transamination. This metabolic variation has no known biological disadvantage.

FOLIC ACID DEFICIENCY AND VITAMIN B₁₂ DEFICIENCY

Tetrahydrofolic acid is necessary for the methylation of deoxy UMP to form TMP. Vitamin B_{12} has no known direct effect on pyrimidine synthesis but is necessary to prevent "trapping" of folate due to a block in methionine synthesis. Either folate or B_{12} deficiency causes a block in the synthesis of TMP and therefore of DNA, as well as in the synthesis of the purine ring, as noted earlier. Abnormalities in the activities of enzymes in the synthesis of pyrimidines have been found in erythrocytes and leukocytes of patients with pernicious anemia, suggestive of derepression and returning to normal after therapy with vitamin B_{12}.

SUMMARY

There are a large number of disorders of purine and pyrimidine metabolism as outlined in Tables 20 and 22. They range from those that are very frequent and important, such as the various forms of gout, to those that are rare and obscure. Considering the variety of enzymes involved in the complex sequences for the synthesis of purine and pyrimidine nucleotides, and the many kinds of functioning nucleotides and nucleic acids in each cell, there are undoubtedly many more metabolic disorders in these pathways yet to be discovered.

REFERENCES

Purines

Edwards, N. L., Recker, D., and Fox, I. H.: Overproduction of uric acid in hypoxanthine-guanine phosphoribosyltransferase deficiency: Contribution by impaired purine salvage. J Clin Invest 63:922, 1979.

Fox, I. H., LaCroix, S., Planet, G., and Moore, M.: Partial deficiency of adenine phosphoribosyltransferase in man. Medicine 56:515, 1977.

Hirschhorn, R., and Martin, D. W., Jr.: Enzyme defects in immunodeficiency diseases. Springer Semin Immunopathol 1(3):65, 1978/79.

Kelley, W. N., and Wyngaarden, J. B.: Clinical syndromes associated with hypoxanthine-guanine phosphoribosyltransferase deficiency. In Stanbury, J. B., Wyngaarden, J. B., Fredrickson, D. S., Goldstein, J. L., and Brown, M. S. (eds.): The Metabolic Basis of Inherited Disease. 5th ed. New York, McGraw-Hill Book Co., 1983, p. 1115.

Valentine, W. N., Paglia, D. E., Tartaglia, A. P., and Gilsanz, F.: Hereditary hemolytic anemia with increased red cell adenosine deaminase (45- to 70-fold) and decreased adenosine triphosphate. Science 195:783, 1977.

Wyngaarden, J. B.: Gout. In Wyngaarden, J. B., and Smith, L. H. Jr. (eds.): Cecil Textbook of Medicine. 17th ed. Philadelphia, W. B. Saunders Co., 1985, p. 1132.

Wyngaarden, J. B., and Kelley, W. N.: Gout and Hyperuricemia. New York, Grune and Stratton, 1976.

Wyngaarden, J. B., and Kelley, W. N.: Gout. In Stanbury, J. B., Wyngaarden, J. B., Fredrickson, D. S., Goldstein, J. L., and Brown, M. S. (eds.): The Metabolic Basis of Inherited Disease. 5th ed. New York, McGraw-Hill Book Co., 1983, p. 1043.

Pyrimidines

Kelley, W. N.: Hereditary orotic aciduria. In Stanbury, J. B., Wyngaarden, J. B., Fredrickson, D. S., Goldstein, J. L., and Brown, M. S. (eds.): The Metabolic Basis of Inherited Disease. 5th ed. New York, McGraw-Hill Book Co, 1983, p. 1202.

Paglia, D. E., and Valentine, W. N.: Hereditary and acquired defects in the pyrimidine nucleotidase of human erythrocytes. Curr Top Hematol 3:75, 1980.

Smith, L. H., Jr.: Pyrimidine metabolism in man. N Engl J Med 288:764, 1973.

Valentine, W. N.: The Stratton lecture: Hemolytic anemia and inborn errors of metabolism. Blood 54:549, 1979.

PATHOPHYSIOLOGIC PRINCIPLES OF NUTRITION

DANIEL RUDMAN, M.D.,
and PATRICIA JO WILLIAMS, M.M.Sc., R.D.

The Scope of Nutritional Science

DEFINITION

All living creatures must continually take in from their environment the materials that provide the substrate and energy for growth, reproduction, and maintenance. These materials are oxygen, water, and food. The last two are the subject matter of nutritional science. Unless the intake of certain dietary constituents is within appropriate limits, the organism will deteriorate in structure and function.

THE QUESTIONS OF NUTRITION

In the attempt to understand the relationships between food, health, and disease, the nutritional scientist asks the following questions:

1. What are the chemical components of food?
2. Which components of food are digested and absorbed and by what mechanism? To what extent?
3. Of the absorbable food components, which are nutritionally essential and which are not?
4. For the essential nutrients, what is the minimal daily requirement? For both essential and nonessential nutrients what is the tolerance, that is, the largest amount that can be eaten without causing illness?
5. What are the manifestations of the various deficiency and toxic states corresponding to each food component?
6. How is each absorbable food component or nutrient processed in the body? What are its metabolic transformations, functions, and degradation products?
7. How does each species strive to achieve optimal intake of each nutrient, in order to maintain normal body composition as well as energy and elemental balances appropriate for the current stage of life cycle?
8. How does the body react in structure and function to variations in the intake of nutrients?
9. In the human, what quality and quantity of diet will minimize the incidence and prevalence of the common acute and chronic diseases and maximize longevity?

Nutritional science has had many important practical applications. In animal husbandry, nutrition has promoted cost-effective raising of livestock. In clinical medicine, the regulation of nutritional intake can cure or prevent some diseases, can symptomatically improve others, and can often minimize the tendency of chronically ill patients to become nutritionally depleted.

Chemistry of Foods

As members of the food chain, we eat the tissues of plants and animals that were recently alive. Our diet, therefore, has all the complexity of living tissue. In an attempt to achieve a logical and organized approach to the numerous components of food, two classifications are suggested:

1. Types of Food Components Consumed. Every food component can be placed in one of two broad classes: *nutrients* and *non-nutrients*. The nutrient class can be further divided into the categories protein, carbohydrate, fat, minerals, vitamins, energy source, and water. Each category of food can also be considered a macronutrient or micronutrient, nutritionally essential or nonessential, and organic or inorganic (Table 1). The non-nutrient class can be divided into the following categories: fiber, allergen, antibodies, toxins,

additives, and oxidants/antioxidants. Some non-nutrients probably have no effect on human health (some additives), others have a potentially favorable effect (fiber, antioxidants, and antibodies), and yet others may serve as risk factors over varying periods of time

TABLE 1. TYPES OF FOOD COMPONENTS

NUTRIENT	NON-NUTRIENT
Protein	Fiber
Carbohydrate	Allergen
Fat	Antibodies
Minerals	Toxins
Vitamins	Additives
Energy source	Oxidants/antioxidants
Water	

TABLE 2. THE NUTRIENT CONTENT OF THE FOUR FOOD GROUPS COMPARED WITH THE RECOMMENDED DIETARY ALLOWANCES (RDAs)*

FOOD	RECOMMENDED SERVINGS	ENERGY, kcal	PROTEIN (g)	FAT (g)	CARBOHYDRATE (g)	VITAMIN A (µg RE**)	VITAMIN E (mg)	ASCORBIC ACID (mg)	THIAMIN (mg)	RIBOFLAVIN (mg)	NIACIN (mg)	VITAMIN B_6 (mg)	VITAMIN B_{12} (µg)	FOLACIN (µg)	PANTOTHENIC ACID (mg)	CALCIUM (mg)	PHOSPHORUS (mg)	MAGNESIUM (mg)	IRON (mg)	ZINC (mg)	SODIUM (mg)	POTASSIUM (mg)	DIETARY FIBER (g)
MILK GROUP																							
2% low-fat	2 cups	288	20	10	29	117	0.19	5	0.2	1.0	0.5	0.19	1.9	5	1.6	698	547	62	0.5	1.9	298	854	0
MEAT GROUP																							
Egg	1	70	6	5	0	156	0.23	0	0.1	0.1	0.1	0.05	1.0	3	0.8	24	90	6	1.1	0.5	54	57	0
Meat, fish, poultry	4 oz	285	31	18	0	26	0.26	0	0.3	0.2	7.3	0.59	1.6	9	0.8	14	274	33	3.1	5.4	88	430	0
VEGETABLE-FRUIT GROUP																							
Leafy green and deep yellow	1/4 cup	12	1	0	2	254	0.47	20	0	0.1	0.3	0.08	0	22	0.1	34	22	13	0.6	0.3	12	127	2.0
Other vegetables	1/4 cup	19	1	0	4	35	0.16	7	0	0	0.4	0.05	0	14	0.1	19	22	13	0.5	0.2	30	105	1.4
Potato	1 med.	113	3	0	26	0	0.05	24	0.1	0	2.0	0.21	0	9	0.3	11	79	14	0.8	0.3	5	614	3.5
Citrus fruit	1 serving	44	1	0	10	12	0.04	44	0.1	0	0.3	0.03	0	3	0.2	19	17	11	0.3	0.1	1	174	0.4
Other fruit	1 serving	92	1	0	22	50	0.22	5	0	0	0.4	0.10	0	5	0.2	10	16	13	0.6	0.2	2	176	1.5
BREAD-CEREAL GROUP																							
Cereal, enriched or whole-grain	3/4 cup	135	4	1	29	0	0.22	0	0.1	0	1.3	0.04	0	15	0.2	13	75	21	1.1	0.5	303	73	3.8
Bread, enriched or whole-grain	3 slices	205	7	2	39	0	0.21	0	0.2	0.1	2.0	0.08	0	17	0.4	68	126	38	1.9	0.8	414	143	6.4
Fortified margarine	4 tsp	144	0	16	0	66	10	0	0	0	0	0	0	0	0	4	12	0	0	0	200	4	0
Totals		1300	75	62	161	716	12	105	1.9	1.5	14.6	1.42	4.5	102	4.7	914	1280	224	10.5	10.2	1407	2758	19
RECOMMENDED DIETARY ALLOWANCE†																							
Female (23–50 yr)		2000	44			800	12	60	1.0	1.2	13	2.0	3.0	400	4–7‡	800	800	300	18	15	1100–3300‡	1875–5625‡	
Male (23–50 yr)		2700	56			1000	15	60	1.4	1.6	18	2.2	3.0	400	4–7‡	800	800	350	10	15	1100–3300‡	1875–5625‡	

*Values represent the average nutrient content of a food group. In some cases, additional food selections may be necessary to fulfill requirements for energy and certain vitamins and minerals.

†Taken from Recommended Dietary Allowances.

‡Because there is less information on which to base an allowance, ranges of recommended intakes are given.

**RE, retinol equivalents.

for the production of disease (oxidants, toxins, and allergens).

NUTRIENTS. Nutrients are those constituents in food that promote growth and development and maintain health. The chemistry, metabolism, and functions of the five nutrient types (protein, carbohydrate, fat, minerals, and water) are discussed in detail in the rest of this section.

NON-NUTRIENTS. The non-nutrient class of food includes at least six types of material.

Dietary fiber contributes 15 to 25 g a day to the average diet in the United States and includes cellulose, hemicellulose, pectins, algae, polysaccharides, and lignin. The behavior of fiber in the intestine, its hydrophilic nature, gel-forming ability, and binding capacity for ions and salts have led to many claims for beneficial effects of fiber on diverticulosis, colonic cancer, gallstones, diabetes, and coronary artery disease. Much work is still needed in this area.

Food allergens constitute a well-known category of non-nutritive food components. Allergic reactions to food can be acute or chronic and can be mediated by cellular or humoral mechanisms. Common allergenic foods include milk, chocolate and cocoa, legumes, eggs, and citrus fruits.

Breast milk, especially the early colostrum, contains *antibodies* that may be significant to the infant. It is believed that infants do not absorb antibodies through the intestinal wall; thus the breast milk's antibodies may be important in inactivating bacteria or viruses in the intestinal tract.

There are numerous non-nutritive *food toxins*. Some are natural to the food item as harvested; others are added periodically by environmental pollution. Examples of natural toxins include oxalates and phytates, which interfere with mineral absorption by forming chelates with calcium, iron, zinc, and other minerals; antivitamins such as thiaminases and avidin, a biotin inhibitor; psychoactive substances, for instance, caffeine; toxins in some species of mushrooms. Microbial contaminants may be added during processing, such as the toxin of botulism.

Environmental toxicants may cause detrimental effects after ingestion. For example, our food now often contains insecticides, such as DDT and dieldrin, and the metals lead and mercury. The acute and chronic tolerance levels of such materials are unknown.

Food additives enhance flavor, appearance, and stability or preserve the quality of a food.

Some food substances can act as *oxidants* or *antioxidants*. Natural oxidants in food may function as mutagens through the generation of oxygen radicals.

2. Food Groups and Food Lists. The average individual eats about 200 food items on a regular basis. Many of these numerous food items are similar in nutrient content, such as broccoli and spinach or chicken and turkey. On the basis of these similarities, food groups can be developed. Four *food groups* are normally utilized: the meat-protein group, the fruit-vegetable group, the bread-cereal group, and the milk group. *Food lists* are utilized when an individual wishes to limit the intake of certain nutrients for a therapeutic purpose. For example, food lists are available for those foods high or low in sodium, high or low in fat, or low in oxalate.

The average individual can ensure adequate intake of all essential nutrients by consuming the proper number of servings every day from each of the four food groups (Table 2). For example, protein requirements can be met by eating the recommended number of servings of meat-protein foods and milk-dairy foods. Selection of calorically less dense foods within the same food group will allow for fewer calories but will not compromise nutrient intake. For example, lowfat milk has 90 fewer Kcal per serving than whole milk, yet the calcium content is similar.

Many disease states require the alteration of nutrient intake. Diabetics must limit their intake of simple sugars; people with hypertension should consume less sodium; and those with renal disease may need to limit protein, potassium, sodium, and phosphorus. In some cases, supplementation of a nutrient may be necessary when a disease state requires the virtual elimination of a food group. For example, calcium supplementation is necessary when the milk group is eliminated in those with lactose intolerance, because calcium ingestion is also markedly reduced by such a diet.

Essential and Nonessential Nutrients: Definition and Recognition

DEMONSTRATION OF ESSENTIAL DIETARY COMPONENTS

One of the goals of nutritional science has been to determine how many of the innumerable food components are actually nutritionally *essential* and how many (even though physiologically indispensable) are nutritionally *nonessential* because they can be synthesized endogenously. The problem is a practical one because in clinical situations it sometimes becomes necessary to feed a simplified, even synthetic diet either enterally or parenterally. Such "elemental" diets are constructed on the basis of our understanding of essential versus nonessential nutrients.

The essential nutrients have generally been described by placing an animal or person on a mixture consisting only of known, purified nutrients. The transition from mixed foods to the restricted diet often causes a failure of growth or other indication of illness, signifying that one or more essential nutrients have been withdrawn. Frequently utilized indicators have been (1) body weight gain and nitrogen retention by young, growing animals or by adult animals and (2) maintenance of zero nitrogen balance and constant body weight by healthy adult subjects. In addition, the purified restricted diet often led to specific lesions that indicated the withdrawal of an essential nutrient—for example, rachitic bone, scorbutic skin, beriberi opisthotonos, and canine black tongue. In the early twentieth century, crude lipid- and water-soluble extracts of liver were known to be required for the growth and integrity of rats on severely restricted purified diets. Subsequent work showed two or more essential factors in each of these extracts. Each factor corrected a different segment of the disorder induced by the restricted, deficient diet.

The longer the period on the restricted diet, the greater the tendency to develop signs of nutritional deficiency. Thus, long-term feeding of the restricted diets was required to demonstrate the essentiality of polyunsaturated fatty acids and the trace elements.

CLASSIFICATION OF ESSENTIAL NUTRIENTS

According to level of intake, the essential nutrients can be divided into macronutrients (for humans, more than 100 mg per day required) and micronutrients (less than 100 mg per day required). The essential nutrients can also be divided into organic factors (protein, calorie source, essential fatty acids, and vitamins) and inorganic factors (minerals and trace elements).

CONDITIONAL ESSENTIALITY

The distinction between essential and nonessential is not absolute. For example, the human body possesses

TABLE 3. CATALOGUE OF THE FORTY KNOWN ESSENTIAL NUTRIENTS

Energy	Vitamins	Elements
Water	Thiamin	Sodium
Amino Acids	Niacin	Potassium
L-Threonine	Riboflavin	Calcium
L-Valine	Pyridoxine	Magnesium
L-Isoleucine	Folic acid	Chloride
L-Leucine	B_{12}	Phosphorus
L-Lysine	Ascorbic acid	Iron
L-Tryptophan	Biotin	Copper
L-Methionine-cystine	Pantothenic acid	Zinc
L-Phenylalanine-	Vitamin A	Chromium
tyrosine	Vitamin D	Manganese
L-Histidine	Vitamin E	Selenium
Essential Fatty Acids	Vitamin K	Molybdenum
		Iodine
		Fluoride

some capacity to synthesize some clearly essential amino acids, such as the branched-chain amino acids, but at rates inadequate for growth and maintenance under normal circumstances. Similarly, arginine and histidine cannot be synthesized endogenously at a rate rapid enough to satisfy growth requirements. But in adulthood, the endogenous synthetic ability is probably sufficient, so that these two amino acids can be considered nonessential for the adult. The types of experiments described in the preceding paragraphs have led to the catalogue of 40 essential nutrients shown in Table 3.

Nutritional Thresholds: Minimum Daily Requirement (MDR), Recommended Daily Allowance (RDA), and Tolerance

DEFINITION OF MDR AND RDA

When other essential nutrients are not limiting, the smallest amount of an essential factor required to correct the corresponding deficiency is termed the MDR. Because of differences between individuals, a quantity equal to two to six times the MDR is designated as the RDA, the basis of dietary recommendations for the general population. The RDA values and estimated safe and adequate dietary intakes for the essential nutrients are given in Tables 4 and 5.

Many essential nutrients have a storage depot within the body. For example, the liver contains reserves of folic acid and vitamins A, D, and B_{12}. Reserves of iron are stored in the reticuloendothelial system, of iodine in the thyroid gland, of essential fatty acids in the adipose tissue, of thiamin and pyridoxine in muscle. These reserves undergo mobilization, turnover, and renewal at particular rates that may be under physiologic control. Each essential nutrient, moreover, is constantly exposed to degradation and/or excretion. The fractional rates of disposition of the body pool of each nutrient vary widely. For example, for folic acid the available pool is consumed at about 1 per cent per

day, whereas this percentage is much smaller for vitamin B_{12} because of its efficient conservation through the enterohepatic circulation. The MDR can be viewed as the amount of each nutrient that is required to replace the unavoidable daily loss that occurs by degradation and excretion.

After the intake or absorption of a specific nutrient has been interrupted, there is a period of time (t) during which the reserve of that nutrient (utilizable body stores, UBS) is utilized before deficiency signs and symptoms will appear:

$$t = \frac{UBS}{MDR}$$

FACTORS THAT INFLUENCE THE MDR AND RDA

Numerous factors influence the MDR and RDA and can either raise or lower these thresholds. The MDR and RDA of many nutrients are increased by growth, pregnancy, lactation, exercise, and exposure to cold.

TABLE 4. RECOMMENDED DAILY DIETARY ALLOWANCES[a]

AGE (yr)	WEIGHT (kg)	HEIGHT (cm)	ENERGY (kcal)	PROTEIN (g)	VITAMIN A (µg RE)[b]	VITAMIN D (µg)[c]	VITAMIN E (mg TE)[d]	ASCORBIC ACID (mg)	THIAMIN (mg)	RIBOFLAVIN (mg)	NIACIN (mg NE)[e]	VITAMIN B₆ (mg)	FOLACIN (µg)[f]	VITAMIN B₁₂ (µg)	CALCIUM (mg)	PHOSPHORUS (mg)	MAGNESIUM (mg)	IRON (mg)	ZINC (mg)	IODINE (µg)
Infants																				
0.0–0.5	6	60	kg × 115	kg × 2.2	420	10	3	35	0.3	0.4	6	0.3	30	0.5	360	240	50	10	3	40
0.5–1.0	9	71	kg × 105	kg × 2.0	400	10	4	35	0.5	0.6	8	0.6	45	1.5[g]	540	360	70	15	5	50
Children																				
1–3	13	90	1300	23	400	10	5	45	0.7	0.8	9	0.9	100	2.0	800	800	150	15	10	70
4–6	20	112	1700	30	500	10	6	45	0.9	1.0	11	1.3	200	2.5	800	800	200	10	10	90
7–10	28	132	2400	34	700	10	7	45	1.2	1.4	16	1.6	300	3.0	800	800	250	10	10	120
Males																				
11–14	45	157	2700	45	1000	10	8	50	1.4	1.6	18	1.8	400	3.0	1200	1200	350	18	15	150
15–18	66	176	2800	56	1000	10	10	60	1.4	1.7	18	2.0	400	3.0	1200	1200	400	18	15	150
19–22	70	177	2900	56	1000	7.5	10	60	1.5	1.7	19	2.2	400	3.0	800	800	350	10	15	150
23–50	70	178	2700	56	1000	5	10	60	1.4	1.6	18	2.2	400	3.0	800	800	350	10	15	150
51+	70	178	2400	56	1000	5	10	60	1.2	1.4	16	2.2	400	3.0	800	800	350	10	15	150
Females																				
11–14	46	157	2200	46	800	10	8	60	1.1	1.3	15	1.8	400	3.0	1200	1200	300	18	15	150
15–18	55	163	2100	46	800	10	8	60	1.1	1.3	14	2.0	400	3.0	1200	1200	300	18	15	150
19–22	55	163	2100	44	800	7.5	8	60	1.1	1.3	14	2.0	400	3.0	800	800	300	18	15	150
23–50	55	163	2000	44	800	5	8	60	1.0	1.2	13	2.0	400	3.0	800	800	300	18	15	150
51+	55	163	1800	44	800	5	8	60	1.0	1.2	13	2.0	400	3.8	800	800	300	10	15	150
Pregnancy			+300	+30	+200	+5	+2	+20	+0.4	+0.3	+2	+0.6	+400	+1.0	+400	+400	+150	[h]	+5	+25
Lactation			+500	+20	+400	+5	+3	+40	+0.5	+0.5	+5	+0.5	+100	+1.0	+400	+400	+150	[h]	+10	+50

[a]The allowances are intended to provide for individual variations among most normal persons living in the United States under usual environmental stresses. Diets should be based on a variety of common foods in order to provide other nutrients for which human requirements have been less well defined.

[b]Retinol equivalents; 1 retinol equivalent = 1 µg retinol or 6 µg beta-carotene.

[c]As cholecalciferol; 10 µg cholecalciferol = 400 IU vitamin D.

[d]Alpha-tocopherol equivalents; 1 mg d-tocopherol = 1 alpha-TE.

[e]Niacin equivalents; 1 NE = 1 mg niacin or 60 mg dietary tryptophan.

[f]The folacin allowances refer to dietary sources as determined by Lactobacillus casei assay after treatment with enzymes (conjugases) to make polyglutamyl forms of the vitamin available to the test organism.

[g]The RDA for vitamin B₁₂ in infants is based on average concentration of the vitamin in human milk. The allowances after weaning are based on energy intake (as recommended by the American Academy of Pediatrics) and consideration of other factors such as intestinal absorption.

[h]The increased requirement during pregnancy cannot be met by the iron content of habitual American diets or by the existing iron stores of many women; therefore, the use of 30 to 60 mg of supplemental iron is recommended. Iron needs during lactation are not substantially different from those of nonpregnant women, but continued supplementation of the mother for 2 to 3 months after parturition is advisable in order to replenish stores depleted by pregnancy.

TABLE 5. ESTIMATED SAFE AND ADEQUATE DAILY DIETARY INTAKES OF ADDITIONAL SELECTED VITAMINS AND MINERALS[a]

		VITAMINS		
	Age (years)	Vitamin K (μg)	Biotin (μg)	Pantothenic Acid (mg)
Infants	0–0.5	12	35	2
	0.5–1	10–20	50	3
Children and Adolescents	1–3	15–30	65	3
	4–6	20–40	85	3–4
	7–10	30–60	120	4–5
	11 +	50–100	100–200	4–7
Adults		70–140	100–200	4–7

		TRACE ELEMENTS[b]					
	Age (years)	Copper (mg)	Manganese (mg)	Fluoride (mg)	Chromium (mg)	Selenium (mg)	Molybdenum (mg)
Infants	0–0.5	0.5–0.7	0.5–0.7	0.1–0.5	0.01–0.04	0.01–0.04	0.03–0.06
	0.5–1	0.7–1.0	0.7–1.0	0.2–1.0	0.02–0.06	0.02–0.06	0.04–0.08
Children and Adolescents	1–3	1.0–1.5	1.0–1.5	0.5–1.5	0.02–0.08	0.02–0.08	0.05–0.1
	4–6	1.5–2.0	1.5–2.0	1.0–2.5	0.03–0.12	0.03–0.12	0.06–0.15
	7–10	2.0–2.5	2.0–3.0	1.5–2.5	0.05–0.2	0.05–0.2	0.10–0.3
	11 +	2.0–3.0	2.5–5.0	1.5–2.5	0.05–0.2	0.05–0.2	0.15–0.5
Adults		2.0–3.0	2.5–5.0	1.5–4.0	0.05–0.2	0.05–0.2	0.15–0.5

		ELECTROLYTES		
	Age (years)	Sodium (mg)	Potassium (mg)	Chloride (mg)
Infants	0–0.5	115–350	350–925	275–700
	0.5–1	250–750	425–1275	400–1200
Children and Adolescents	1–3	325–975	550–1650	500–1500
	4–6	450–1350	775–2325	700–2100
	7–10	600–1800	1000–3000	925–2775
	11 +	900–2700	1525–4575	1400–4200
Adults		1100–3300	1875–5625	1700–5100

[a]Because there is less information on which to base allowances, these figures are not given in the main table of RDA and are provided here in the form of ranges of recommended intakes.

[b]Since the toxic levels for many trace elements may be only several times usual intakes, the upper levels for the trace elements given in this table should not be habitually exceeded.

Sparing

The metabolism of some essential nutrients leads to a physiologically useful product. One of the functions of such an essential nutrient is to serve as a precursor for its metabolic product. The proportion of the nutritional precursor used for this purpose may vary from less than 2 per cent to as much as 50 per cent (examples are the tryptophan to niacin conversion and the methionine to cysteine conversion, respectively). If the synthetic diet is supplemented with a physiologically useful product, the MDR of the precursor will be reduced, or "spared." For example, the MDR of methionine can be reduced 50 per cent by an adequate cysteine supplement.

Nutrient-Nutrient Interactions

Sparing is one type of nutrient-nutrient interaction, a term signifying that the MDR of one nutrient is influenced by the dietary content of another nutrient. Many such interactions occur, and they operate at three different levels: gastrointestinal absorption, metabolic transformation, and renal excretion. Examples are as follows:

1. At the Absorption Level. Dietary phytates reduce the absorption of calcium and iron; the absorption of copper is inhibited by excess dietary zinc; and the absorption of non-heme iron is enhanced by dietary ascorbic acid.

2. At the Metabolic Level. The dietary requirement for protein is inversely related to caloric intake because, in times of calorie deficit, a portion of the amino acids is used for oxidative fuel. The dietary requirement for niacin is increased by deficiencies in vitamin B_6 or tryptophan because these nutrients are involved in niacin biosynthesis. The MDR values of thiamin and pyridoxine change with carbohydrate and protein intake, respectively, because these two vitamins function as coenzymes in pyruvate and amino acid metabolism. Moreover, the physiologic consequences of some deficiencies can be diminished by other nutrients. In animals fed diets lacking vitamin E, which helps protect membranes from free radicals, little damage to membranes is apparent when the animals consume other compounds such as sulfur amino acids and trace amounts of selenium, which help maintain membrane integrity.

3. At the Excretory Level. Excess intake of dietary protein causes hypercalciuria; the daily obligatory loss of water is related to the intake of dietary components producing urinary osmoles such as protein, which is converted into the main urinary osmole urea, and the minerals sodium, chloride, and potassium.

Drug-Nutrient Interactions

Drugs may cause nutrient malabsorption (e.g., aluminum hydroxide for phosphate), impaired nutrient utilization (e.g., isoniazid for pyridoxine), or excessive urinary excretion of a nutrient (e.g., cisplatin for magnesium).

Disease-Nutrient Interaction

Some diseases lower the MDR for certain nutrients because they reduce the rate of degradation or excretion. For example, the requirement for phosphorus is reduced in renal insufficiency. On the other hand, inborn metabolic errors may increase the requirement for vitamins because of impaired ability to absorb, activate, or utilize the vitamin. Furthermore, requirements are increased by acquired diseases if nutrient absorbability is reduced, as in the gastrointestinal malabsorption syndromes, or if nutrient loss is accelerated, as in burns, fistulas, or hypermetabolic states.

CONDITIONALLY ESSENTIAL NUTRIENTS

Many physiologically indispensable compounds are normally made from the limited number of essential nutrients. Metabolic pathways that carry out these conversions can be interrupted by genetic or by acquired enzymatic lesions or by immaturity in the formation of relevant enzymes. This will change the classification of the product from a nonessential to a "conditionally essential" nutrient. For example, cysteine is thought to be required in the neonate because of immaturity of the transsulfuration pathway, which synthesizes cysteine from methionine, or in the cirrhotic adult, in whom advanced liver disease may destroy most of the body's content of the transsulfuration enzymes, located in the liver.

NUTRIENT TOLERANCE

Nutrient tolerance is defined as the maximum amount of nutrient that can be consumed without causing ill effects. The maximum amount that can be tolerated acutely per day is greater than the amount that can be tolerated per day over longer periods of time; that is, evidence of toxicity may appear only after a prolonged exposure. Therefore, syndromes of excess can be acute or long term in nature. In some cases doses in the upper range of the tolerance level, if taken over prolonged periods of time, may possibly serve as risk factors for development of medical complications.

Just as the MDR can be raised or lowered by various disease states, the same is true of tolerance. Thus, any loss of ability to degrade or excrete the metabolite will reduce the tolerance.

FACTORS THAT INFLUENCE INDIVIDUAL TOLERANCE

Absorbability

If absorption is increased, as for iron in idiopathic hemochromatosis or as for calcium in hyperabsorptive hypercalciuria, tolerance will be reduced. On the other hand, if absorption is subnormal, then tolerance will be increased, as, for example, in the malabsorption of vitamin D.

Inborn Errors of Metabolism

If the metabolism of a nutrient is impaired, then tolerance may be lowered; for example, the congenital blocks of the urea cycle reduce tolerance for protein, and phenylketonuria decreases tolerance for phenylalanine. On the other hand, hereditary inability to hydroxylate vitamin D increases the tolerance for this nutrient.

Acquired Disease

If the ability to metabolize or excrete the nutrient or its products is reduced, tolerance will be lowered, as, for example, in the nitrogen accumulation diseases (cirrhosis and uremia), the sodium excretion diseases (edematous states), and the water excretion diseases (conditions such as advanced cirrhosis or heart failure associated with dilutional hyponatremia). If the ability to activate the nutrient has been impaired by acquired disease or if the rate of degradation of the nutrient is accelerated, then the tolerance may be increased; for example, vitamin B_6 is degraded abnormally fast in cirrhosis.

In some situations, the disease process reduces tolerance and at the same time increases the MDR, as, for instance, in the cirrhotic patient with hepatic encephalopathy and protein-calorie undernutrition. In this situation, the "window" between tolerance and requirement for protein is narrowed, and nutritional management of the patient becomes difficult or impossible.

Relation of Essential Nutrients to Intermediary Metabolism

In the body an organic nutrient joins one or more pathways of intermediary metabolism for (1) the biosynthesis of physiologically required products; (2) the incorporation of the nutrient or its metabolic products into structural macromolecules; (3) the hydrolysis or oxidation of the nutrient or its metabolic product with the release of utilizable chemical energy; (4) the storage of the nutrient or its metabolic product in polymeric form for subsequent hydrolysis, mobilization, and utilization; or (5) the degradation of the nutrient to a metabolic end-product in preparation for its excretion. For organic micronutrients, there may be conversion to a form that is active as a coenzyme for a particular apoenzyme in the body.

The flow of nutrients through the network of metabolic pathways is too vast a subject for comprehensive review here. Some pathways are described in the section on metabolism. Three aspects pertinent to nutritional requirements in health and disease will be discussed: (1) how biosynthetic pathways produce physiologically indispensable but nutritionally nonessential compounds; (2) how the organ distribution of enzymes influences the susceptibility of metabolic processes to acquired and congenital disease; and (3) how nutrients are removed from the body by metabolic degradation followed by excretion.

BIOSYNTHETIC PATHWAYS

The body contains at least 100,000 species of organic molecules. Probably the majority of these compounds are physiologically useful or indispensable, and their lack would create a handicap or disorder of some type. Yet only 30 organic molecules are nutritionally essential. This testifies to the amazing biosynthetic capacity of the healthy body: From the 30 required organic essential nutrients, the 100,000 nutritionally dispensable species are synthesized.

Consider the conversion of phenylalanine to tyrosine, in which both precursor and product are physiologically indispensable as building blocks of body proteins. Only phenylalanine, however, is nutritionally essential because the body's requirement for tyrosine can be readily satisfied by its biosynthesis from an adequate intake of phenylalanine. In the genetic disease phenylketonuria, however, the enzyme that converts phenylalanine to tyrosine is nonfunctional. Under these circumstances, tyrosine becomes nutritionally essential. We can therefore refer to tyrosine as a conditionally essential nutrient, that is, one that is ordinarily nonessential but one that, under certain circumstances, may become essential.

In the transsulfuration pathway (TSSP), an essential nutrient, methionine, is the precursor for several physiologically indispensable but nutritionally nonessential compounds. This pathway also illustrates the key role of cofactors for optimal operation of a metabolic process.

The first step in the TSSP pathway (Fig. 1), the formation of S-adenosylmethionine (SAM) from methionine and ATP, is mediated by S-adenosylmethionine synthetase. SAM is the main methylating agent in mammalian metabolism. Among the compounds that receive their methyl groups from SAM in reactions catalyzed by methyl transferases are histones, DNA, mRNA, melatonin, catecholamines, choline, carnitine, and creatine. Because their biosynthesis is so effective, these compounds are nutritionally dispensable. Deficiencies of choline, carnitine, or creatine do not occur in normal animals fed synthetic diets lacking these compounds, provided the diets furnish adequate amounts of the precursor (methionine) and the three vitamins (folic acid, B_{12}, and B_6) required by the TSSP. SAM is also pivotal in the biosynthesis of polyamines because it donates propylamino groups required for the synthesis of spermidine and spermine.

S-Adenosylhomocysteine is next cleaved by a specific hydrolase to form adenosine and homocysteine. Homocysteine lies at a critical junction in the transsulfuration pathway. It can undergo two conversions: It can be remethylated to methionine, or it can irreversibly proceed to form cystathionine. Remethylation is achieved by two reactions: one requiring N-methyltetrahydrofolate as a methyl donor and the other requiring betaine. The first reaction, mediated by methyltetrahydrofolate-homocysteine methyltransferase, requires cobalamin (vitamin B_{12}) as a cofactor and derives its methyl group from the one-carbon pool. This reaction is the site of interdigitation of folate, cobalamin, the one-carbon pool, and methionine and provides additional methyl groups besides those contributed by methionine for the endogenous synthesis of methylated compounds such as choline, carnitine, and creatine. This process of methyl neogenesis becomes especially significant during nutrition with synthetic diets lacking these compounds. It is as important for the regeneration of tetrahydrofolate as it is for the reformation of methionine. In the absence of this reaction, all the folate may be trapped as its N-methyl derivative. The second reaction, mediated by betaine-homocysteine methyltransferase, derives its methyl group from choline via betaine. The enzyme has a feedback regulatory mechanism and is inhibited by the reaction products methionine and dimethylglycine.

Homocysteine can also combine irreversibly with serine to form cystathionine. The reaction is mediated by cystathionine synthase and requires pyridoxal phosphate as a cofactor. Cystathionine, in turn, is cleaved by cystathionase to form the conditionally essential

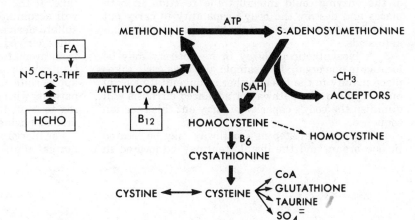

Figure 1. Transsulfuration pathway describing the conversion of methionine to cysteine.

amino acid cysteine; this reaction also requires pyridoxal phosphate.

In addition to its role as a building block in the synthesis of tissue proteins, cysteine is a precursor for another amino acid, taurine, and the tripeptide glutathione, both of which function in cellular metabolism throughout the body. Under normal conditions both of these derivatives are synthesized by hepatocytes in optimal quantities through the TSSP and are nutritionally nonessential. Taurine is required for normal retinal function and biliary secretion; glutathione influences redox potential in nearly all cells of the body.

This brief review shows how the single precursor methionine, as long as folate, vitamin B_{12}, and pyridoxine are present, can provide for the synthesis of a host of nutritionally "nonessential," although physiologically indispensable, compounds. Most of these are present in mixed foods but are lacking in the synthetic nutritional formulas often used in clinical therapeutics.

ENZYME DISTRIBUTION, SUSCEPTIBILITY TO ACQUIRED AND CONGENITAL DISEASES, AND THE INTER-ORGAN TRANSPORT OF NUTRIENTS AND THEIR METABOLIC PRODUCTS

The distribution of enzymes among organs in a pathway determines the susceptibility of this metabolic process to blocks by acquired and congenital disease and may establish an inter-organ journey in the flow of material through the pathway. Examples are as follows:

1. An enzyme may be located in one organ. For example, the hydroxylation of phenylalanine to tyrosine is virtually localized in the liver. The reaction will therefore be blocked either by acquired, severe hepatic disease (for example, hepatic insufficiency) or by a genetic abnormality in the structure of the enzyme.

2. An enzyme may be found in two or more organs. Branched-chain alpha-keto acid dehydrogenase activity is observed in the liver as well as in skeletal muscle. In this case, advanced disease of either organ would probably be insufficient to block the metabolic reaction in the body. However, an inborn error in the structure of the enzyme could interrupt the reaction in both places and destroy the body's capability to carry out oxidative decarboxylation of the branched-chain alpha-keto acids.

3. A biosynthetic pathway in its entirety may be located in one organ; for example, the urea cycle takes place mainly in the liver. Either a congenital block of one enzyme in the pathway or advanced cirrhosis will diminish the body's capacity to carry out this reaction sequence.

4. The proximal step in a pathway may be located in one organ, and the distal step may be located in another. Three examples are the biosynthesis of carnitine, the biosynthesis of creatine, and the dihydroxylation of the vitamin D molecule. In each case, both hepatic and renal steps are required. Acquired insufficiency of either liver or kidney will block the biosynthesis. Moreover, an inborn error in the activity of any enzyme involved in the process may block the biochemical reaction. Thus, in end-stage acquired renal disease, the conversion of 25-hydroxycholecalciferol to 1,25-dihydroxycholecalciferol is severely impaired. In addition, in pseudo–vitamin D–deficiency rickets, there is a genetic defect in the same hydroxylation reaction. In both cases, skeletal manifestations of vitamin D deficiency occur.

DEGRADATION AND EXCRETION OF NUTRIENTS

Every organic nutrient enters a metabolic pathway leading to its eventual degradation to end-products, which are then excreted by the ventilatory, urinary, or fecal route. To achieve zero balance for each nutrient, a prerequisite for health in the nongrowing adult, excretion of the end-products must equal intake of the nutrient. The most common end-products are carbon dioxide and water. For fatty acids and simple carbohydrates, these are the only end-products formed. (Incomplete oxidation of the fatty acids, of course, will lead in part to the urinary excretion of ketone bodies rather than to exhalation of carbon dioxide as the end-product.) The nitrogen component of amino acids is metabolized to urea. Amino acid sulfur is metabolized to sulfate and taurine. The breakdown of aromatic amino acids leads to the formation of several organic acids; for example, the tryptophan carbon skeleton is excreted in part as xanthurenic acid. Some micronutrients have unique end-products; for example, niacin $\rightarrow$ N-methylnicotinamide, and pyridoxine $\rightarrow$ pyridoxic acid. The end-product of the purines is urinary uric acid. In the metabolism of cholesterol, the end-products are the bile acids, which are excreted by the biliary and fecal routes.

The excretion of end-products is proportional to the amount of nutrient absorbed. Measurement of the end-product can provide a way of assessing a nutrient's intake within a population. Thus, daily urinary excretion of nitrogen or sulfate reflects protein intake, and daily pyridoxic acid excretion indicates pyridoxine intake. If the excretory route is impaired, the product will accumulate with potential toxicity. For example, sulfate derived from methionine and cysteine, guanidines derived from arginine, and organic acids derived from aromatic amino acids accumulate in uremic patients. With such patients, restricting the intake of the appropriate nutrient may be necessary. Likewise, in patients with primary overproduction of uric acid leading to gout, limited intake of the uric acid precursor, dietary purine, may be appropriate.

For inorganic nutrients, the rate of excretion (in the normal adult) must also equal intake.

Homeostasis of Nutrients

DEFINITION

At the RDA, in the healthy adult, the amount of nutrient absorbed equals the amount lost (degraded and excreted). As the intake of the nutrient increases or decreases, the body executes adaptive responses that minimize the change in body store of the nutrient. These responses represent homeostatic adaptations to the decreased or increased supply of the nutrient. The homeostatic responses are multiple and occur at the levels of intake, absorption, degradation, and excretion. If the adaptive responses are inadequate, syndromes of deficiency or excess will eventually result. The efficiency of the homeostatic responses is often impaired by disease.

MODULATION OF INTAKE IN RESPONSE TO AVAILABILITY OF NUTRIENT

Calories

Extirpation experiments showed hyperphagia when the ventromedial hypothalamus was removed and hypophagia when the ventrolateral hypothalamus was removed. These findings led to the concept of a ventromedial hypothalamic "satiety center" and a bilateral ventrolateral hypothalamic "feeding center" (Fig. 2). Food intake can be divided into two stages: the initiation and the termination of feeding. The former presumably represents increased activity of the feeding

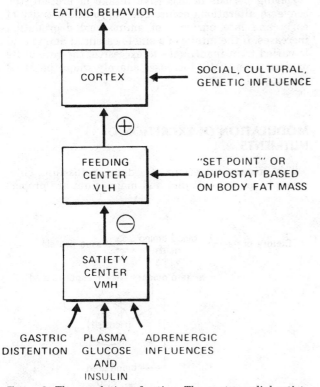

Figure 2. The regulation of eating. The ventromedial satiety center is considered to be inhibitory, and the ventrolateral feeding center stimulatory.

center and/or other stimulatory input into the cerebral cortex. Termination, on the other hand, represents increased activity of the satiety center.

What are the signals for activation of the feeding center?

1. The glucoprivation stimulus is potent but may be used only on an emergency basis and may not be a physiologic stimulus to eating.

2. It is possible that activation of the feeding center physiologically is determined primarily by declining activity of the satiety center.

3. Termination of eating and lack of appetite probably reflect activity of the satiety center. The signals to the satiety center arise from both preabsorptive and postabsorptive receptors. The preabsorptive receptors are located in the oropharyngeal, gastric, and intestinal regions. The mechanisms are both neural (afferent impulses) and endocrine (bombesin, cholecystokinin, and glucagon). Postabsorptive signals are thought to arise primarily in the liver and may involve alterations in glucose metabolism within that organ.

The satiety and feeding centers are also sensitive to amino acid intake. If the animal or human is provided with an imbalanced ratio of amino acids—for example, deficiency of an essential amino acid—then anorexia and hypophagia will result.

Feeding behavior occurs intermittently and tends to be initiated by caloric deficit and inhibited by caloric excess. If these mechanisms operate normally, the adult subject will achieve zero caloric balance, and the adipose mass will be maintained at about 15 to 30 per cent of total body weight.

Water

The intake of water is controlled by a hypothalamic thirst center, which is sensitive to osmolality of body fluids. Decrease in osmolality suppresses both the thirst center and the nearby center for the release of antidiuretic hormone; increase in osmolality has the opposite effect. The harmonious operation of these mechanisms results in a state of zero water balance, the maintenance of normal body fluid tonicity at about 280 mOsm/liter, and the maintenance of normal body water content at 70 to 75 per cent of lean body mass (see Section X for more detail).

MODULATION OF ABSORPTION IN RELATIONSHIP TO THE AVAILABILITY OF NUTRIENT

Calcium

When the RDA of calcium is being met in the healthy adult, its gastrointestinal absorption is 15 to 30 per cent of that ingested. As the calcium intake approaches the MDR or falls below it, the per cent of calcium absorption increases. These changes in calcium absorption are mediated by the parathyroid hormone–vitamin D system. Low calcium levels in the plasma cause an increase in parathyroid hormone, which in turn causes hydroxylation of 25-hydroxycholecalciferol (vitamin D) to the active form 1,25-dihydroxycholecalciferol in the kidney. The activated vitamin D acts in the intestine to increase calcium absorption by the formation of a calcium-binding protein.

Iron

Iron absorption is regulated by the ferrous ion concentration within the intestinal mucosal cell. As the ferrous ion concentration in the cell drops, the ferrous ions in the intestinal lumen are taken up by the mucosal cell and rapidly oxidized to ferric hydroxide, which combines with apoferritin (an iron-binding protein) to form ferritin. Within the mucosal cell, the breakdown of ferritin occurs and ferrous ions are released to the circulation.

MODULATION OF DEGRADATION

Calories

Under conditions of a negative caloric intake, the basal metabolic rate decreases. This adaptation reflects diminished availability of the two main calorigenic hormones of the body, norepinephrine and triiodothyronine (T_3). The turnover of catecholamines in the sympathetic fibers and the plasma norepinephrine level both decline. There is a diminished conversion of T_4 to T_3 and an increased conversion to reverse T_3 in the liver cells (see Section VIII). Conversely, states of temporary or chronic caloric excess, particularly of carbohydrate, are associated with increased activity of the sympathetic nervous system.

It is believed that these adaptive changes in metabolic rate in part reflect the decreased or increased actions of the adrenergic nervous system on brown fat cells. These adipocytes differ from white fat cells in possessing a substantial number of mitochondria and a multilocular distribution of triglycerides. Brown adipose sites are richly innervated by the sympathetic nervous system.

Lipolysis within brown fat cells is stimulated by the sympathetic nervous system during acclimation to cold. The free fatty acids released by the adrenergic stimulus are excellent metabolic fuel for oxidation, both within the adipocytes and elsewhere. In addition, the intracellular free fatty acids within the brown fat cells act on the mitochondrial membrane to activate a proton-conductive pathway, thereby uncoupling oxidative phosphorylation and greatly stimulating heat production. The resulting "nonshivering thermogenesis" serves to maintain body temperature during cold exposure. Calories are also dissipated as heat to a greater extent during periods of positive caloric balance than during zero or negative balance. This "thermic effect" of food represents a decreased metabolic efficiency that buffers the subject against excessive caloric balance. Several varieties of hereditary or acquired obesity in rodents appear to result from a deficiency either in cold-related thermogenesis or in calorie-related thermogenesis, or in both processes, with a resulting increase in metabolic efficiency and in adipose mass.

Amino Acids

The conservation of endogenous nitrogen during a low-protein diet is accomplished by regulating the activities of several key enzymes involved in nitrogen metabolism. The metabolic pool of endogenous nitrogen receives amino acids from two sources—the diet and the catabolism of endogenous protein (pathways 1 and 3 in Fig. 3); and it loses amino acids by two routes—the synthesis of tissue proteins (pathway 2) and the catabolism of amino acids (pathway 4) to urinary urea and other metabolites (pathway 6).

The urinary excretion of nitrogen falls significantly when protein intake is inadequate. This has been attributed at least in part to the reduced activities of argininosuccinase and arginase, two of the five enzymes of the urea cycle. In this manner the activities of the cycle are curtailed.

Low-protein diets also retard the metabolic flow through pathway 6 by altering several enzyme activities. For example, the conversion of methionine to cysteine via homocysteine (Fig. 1) is quite sensitive to the amount of protein ingested. When protein intake is inadequate, the activities of cystathionine synthetase and cystathionase (the enzymes converting homocysteine to cysteine) decline, and the activity of homocysteine methyltransferase (the enzyme converting homocysteine to methionine) increases. The result is conservation of methionine. Other effects of a low-protein diet include the reduced activities of phenylalanine hydroxylase, tyrosine transaminase, threonine dehydratase, and tryptophan oxygenase. The body thereby conserves these amino acids for protein synthesis.

During periods of excessive intake of protein, the converse alterations occur: The enzymatic activity of early and late enzymes of amino acid degradation increases. If the intake of a single essential amino acid is varied from inadequate to excessive, the rate of its oxidation generally increases sharply when the MDR is exceeded.

MODULATION OF EXCRETION OF NUTRIENTS

The urinary excretions of sodium, potassium, chloride, phosphate, calcium, and magnesium are propor-

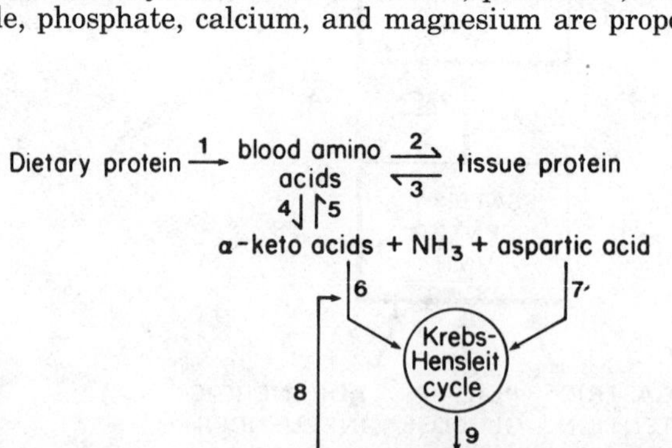

Figure 3. Overview of amino acid metabolism.

tional to intake. As the dietary intake and the quantity of each mineral that is absorbed increase, the result will be an increased filtered load of the nutrient, either because of an expansion of the extracellular fluid volume or because of an elevation in the plasma concentration of the mineral. The greater filtered load will tend to increase the daily urinary excretion. In addition, hormonal responses may adjust the net tubular reabsorption or secretion of the mineral. For example, during sodium deprivation, hypersecretion of aldosterone increases the tubular reabsorption of this cation. Antidiuretic hormone modulates the tubular reabsorption of water to adjust excretion to intake. Similarly, parathyroid hormone regulates urinary phosphate excretion according to the quantity absorbed by the small intestine. Thus an increase or decrease in the quantity of nutrient absorbed tends to be matched by a corresponding change in urinary excretion, thereby preventing any alteration in the total amount of nutrient found in the body.

Pathogenesis and Recognition of Nutrient Deficiency Syndromes

The broadest classification of the states of undernutrition is primary versus secondary. "Primary" undernutrition means that sufficient food is not available to the individual for socioeconomic reasons. In underdeveloped countries, this is the leading type. In "secondary" undernutrition, food is available, but because disease or medications have impaired the patient's ability to eat, absorb, utilize, or conserve his nutrients, or have raised the nutrient requirements, a deficiency syndrome develops. "Secondary," or "conditioned," deficiency syndromes are a major problem in the chronically ill and hospitalized groups in the developed countries.

The causes of nutrient deficiency can also be considered as exogenous and endogenous.

EXOGENOUS CAUSES OF DEFICIENCY SYNDROMES

Intake Level

Poverty, isolation, and old age are all risk factors for inadequate intake. The subject is too poor, weak, or discouraged to obtain and prepare an adequate diet. The "empty calories" phenomenon is a modern variation. An individual will ordinarily be satiated by 2000 to 3000 Kcal/day. If the calories are properly distributed among the four major food groups (Table 2), all RDAs will be met. But if the calories are taken in ultrarefined form (e.g., potato chips and soft drinks), some RDAs will not be met and deficiencies will develop. As a variation on this theme, in developing nations with poor diets, even the caloric content of the food (kilocalorie per kilogram) is inadequate. Most adults cannot eat more than 3000 Kcal of food a day. In the root-based diet, 3000 Kcal contains less than the MDR of calories, protein, or both, and protein-calorie undernutrition results even in persons who eat until satiated.

ENDOGENOUS CAUSES OF DEFICIENCY SYNDROMES

Intake

Disease often impairs the desire or ability to eat. Hypophagia is a major contributor to weight loss in the chronically ill.

Impaired Absorption (See Section XIV)

Malfunction or resection of the stomach, pancreas, bile duct, or small intestine impairs digestion, absorption, or both. The malabsorption usually affects fatty acids most severely; these substances then remove water and calcium, magnesium, sodium, and potassium as counterions to achieve the final fecal osmolality of about 300 mOsm/liter. Folate malabsorption and deficiency may aggravate the dysfunction of the gastrointestinal mucosa and may potentiate the malabsorption of other nutrients. Genetic transport errors may be present, as for tryptophan in Hartnup's disease.

Impaired Utilization

In acquired diseases—for instance, liver or kidney disease—vitamin D is not activated to the dihydroxy form. Another example is diabetes, a condition that impairs the utilization of glucose, which may therefore be excreted in the urine. In genetic diseases, vitamin cofactors may not be properly utilized.

Increased Destruction of Nutrients

Examples of nutrient destruction include increased metabolic rate resulting in accelerated protein breakdown, the accelerated breakdown of pyridoxal phosphate in cirrhosis, and the destruction of pyridoxal phosphate by such drugs as isoniazid or cycloserine.

Increased Excretory Losses of Nutrients

Examples of conditions causing excessive excretory nutrient loss include diarrhea, impaired renal conservation, and hemodialysis.

Inborn Errors of Metabolism

Some inborn errors of metabolism show the clinical and chemical characteristics of a specific nutrient deficiency, even though the intake of the nutrient is adequate. Several mechanisms are involved: impaired absorption of the nutrient; impaired transport; inability to convert the nutrient into its active form in the case of vitamins; and abnormality in the structure of the apoenzyme for which the nutrient acts as a cofactor, causing diminished affinity for the nutrient. In many disorders, we can view the condition as a genetic increase, sometimes as much as a 1000-fold, in the minimum daily requirement of the nutrient. Such conditions are often clinically benefited by megadoses of the nutrient ("vitamin-responsive inborn errors of metabolism").

STAGES OF NUTRIENT DEFICIENCY

Syndromes of nutritional deficiency evolve through three stages. Most essential nutrients have a storage reserve in the body; for example, calcium is stored in bone; thiamin and vitamin B_6 in muscle; iron and vitamins B_{12}, A, and D, and folate in liver; and essential fatty acids in adipose tissue. If the intake of an essential nutrient falls below the MDR, the utilization of these reserves will tend to maintain plasma levels and prevent a clinical deficiency syndrome. Thus consumption of the tissue reserves represents Stage I. In Stage II, as the reserves are extensively utilized, blood levels of the nutrient or nutrient-dependent factors decline, but the patient continues to be asymptomatic. In Stage III, the tissue reserves have been consumed, the blood levels have fallen, and clinical signs of the deficiency syndrome appear.

THE NATURE OF THE NUTRITIONAL DATA BASE

One purpose of the nutritional data base is to detect nutrient deficiencies in patients. There are two components: the physical findings and the laboratory findings. For each of the 40 essential nutrients, in theory, there is a specific nutrient deficiency state with its own set of physical and laboratory findings. Some of these will be discussed later.

Physical Findings

Physical findings include body weight as percentage of ideal (with attention to the fact that edema and ascites will tend to obscure the degree of weight loss), estimation of the mass of the adipose organ from measurements of skinfold thickness at several sites, estimation of the muscle mass from midarm circumference, and measurement of 24-hour urine creatinine excretion. In children as well as in adults, the quality of childhood nutrition is indicated by the height of the individual.

Laboratory Findings

Every nutrient deficiency and many nutrient excesses can be detected by one or several laboratory tests. Those assays designed to detect nutrient deficiency states can be placed in six categories.

1. **Plasma (Serum) Levels.** For example, a low level of serum B_{12} will indicate the presence of B_{12} deficiency.
2. **Low Levels of Nutrients in Circulating Cells.** For example, low levels of vitamin C in platelets and of folate in red blood cells may indicate deficiency.
3. **Urinary Excretion.** The urinary excretion of the unaltered nutrient or its metabolic product is a useful test for nutrient deficiency. For example, the excretion of urea and sulfate in the urine reflects the intake of protein; the excretion of pyridoxic acid is proportional to B_6 intake; and the excretion of methylnicotinamide is an indicator of niacin intake.
4. **Load Test with the Nutrient Under Consideration.** If the body reserve of a vitamin or mineral nutrient is reduced, then there is a strong tendency to retain a portion of the ingested nutrient in the body. On the other hand, if the body reserves are adequate, then a larger proportion of the factor will be excreted in the urine. This test is useful in demonstrating deficiencies of water-soluble vitamins.
5. **Nutrient-Dependent Enzymes.** The activity of those enzymes that utilize vitamins as cofactors, will tend to be reduced if the vitamin is deficient. However, if exogenous cofactor is added to the preparation, a substantial increase in enzyme activity will occur. An example is the effect of exogenous thiamin on the activity of erythrocyte transketolase, which uses thiamin as a cofactor.
6. **Load Test with a Nutrient-Dependent Metabolic Precursor.** Most pathways of amino acid metabolism utilize vitamins as cofactors at various steps. If the vitamin is deficient and a load of precursor is administered, then the metabolic intermediate that is a substrate for the vitamin-dependent step will tend to accumulate and be excreted in the urine. On the other hand, if the vitamin is present in adequate amount, the step under consideration will not be rate limiting and the intermediate will not accumulate. Examples are the excretion of formiminoglutamic acid after a load of histidine (folate deficiency) and the excretion of xanthurenic acid after a load of tryptophan (vitamin B_6 deficiency).

Pathogenesis of Syndromes of Nutrient Excess

NUTRIENT TOXICITY

Intake of a certain amount of excess nutrient over the RDA can be disposed of by the body's homeostatic mechanisms without a progressive or toxic increase in body content and therefore without illness. As noted, these homeostatic mechanisms include curtailing the fractional gastrointestinal absorption, increasing the rate of degradation, and raising the rate of excretion.

Above a certain level, however, tolerance is exceeded and illness will result. The ill effects can be immediate or delayed by weeks or years.

NUTRIENTS AS RISK FACTORS

Increased intake of a nutrient that is merely within the upper level of the habitual intake range of the general population and that does not cause obvious illness on an acute or subacute time scale may nevertheless act as a risk factor for late medical complications over a period of many years. Some examples are high sodium intake as a risk factor for hypertension, low calcium intake for osteoporosis and high calcium intake for kidney stones, high cholesterol intake for coronary artery disease, high saturated fat intake for coronary artery disease, and low fiber intake for gastrointestinal cancer.

DISEASES AS CONDITIONING FACTORS FOR NUTRIENT EXCESS

Just as deficiency syndromes are often conditioned by exogenous and endogenous factors that lower the MDR, so syndromes of nutrient excess are conditioned frequently by endogenous factors that lower the tolerance because they impair the body's ability to degrade or excrete the nutrient or because they enhance gastrointestinal absorption. Some examples of diseases as conditioning factors are as follows:

1. The nitrogen accumulation diseases—renal and hepatic insufficiency—reduce the tolerance to protein. Hepatic encephalopathy and uremia are specific conditions in which protein intolerance occurs.
2. Diseases of the heart, kidneys, and liver that predispose to edema lower the tolerance to sodium chloride. These diseases include congestive heart failure, nephrotic syndrome, and cirrhosis.
3. Renal insufficiency lowers the tolerance to potassium, magnesium, phosphate, and amino acids.
4. Inborn errors of metabolism may impair the tolerance for certain amino acids, such as phenylalanine in phenylketonuria or branched amino acids in maple syrup urine disease. In galactosemia the normally nontoxic sugar galactose cannot be metabolized and accumulates to cause disease.

OBESITY

Obesity is the most common nutritional disorder in the Western world. This condition of nutrient excess is a risk factor for hypertension, hyperlipidemia, type II diabetes, atherosclerosis, and osteoarthritis.

Homo sapiens, like other animals, evolved under conditions of restricted food intake, in which the intermittent unpredictable availability of calories and the threat of starvation were major challenges to survival. Consequently, mechanisms involving appetite, hunger, insulin, and the adipose organ were developed, including virtually complete gastrointestinal absorption of calories and renal conservation of glucose and amino acids. All of these factors provide the species with highly efficient mechanisms to absorb, conserve, and store energy in the form of adipose tissue triglyceride.

It is only within the last several generations in the Western world that unlimited availability of calories has been ensured for most members of the general population. The consequence of these changes without compensatory evolutionary adaptations has been a strong tendency toward the development of adiposity.

Obesity is defined as an excess of adipose mass in the body. Normally, 15 to 30 per cent of body weight should be adipose tissue. Adipose mass can be estimated by body density, by isotope dilution methods, or from skinfold measurements. About 25 per cent of men and 35 per cent of women in the United States are currently obese.

A positive caloric balance leads to the deposition of the excess calories as triglyceride in adipose tissue, regardless of whether the excess intake is in the form of carbohydrate, fat, or protein. The major factor in most cases of obesity is probably increased caloric intake. However, diminished caloric output due to the more sedentary way of life in developed nations probably contributes in many instances.

Obesity can result from hypothyroidism, hyperadrenalism, insulinoma, and hypothalamic disorders. These endocrine or neurologic causes, however, are involved in less than 1 per cent of obesity cases.

Basal metabolic rate, which accounts for about 75 per cent of caloric expenditure, is generally normal in obese individuals when referred to lean body mass. A subtle abnormality, however, may be present in the metabolic rate of some obese subjects. Obesity develops only during periods of positive caloric balance, so that it is in these periods that we must examine the difference between the obese and nonobese subject. In the nonobese individual, excess calories, particularly in the form of carbohydrate, induce a positive thermic effect. This calorie-induced thermogenesis can amount to 15 per cent of the metabolic rate, develops over a period of several weeks during sustained positive caloric balance, and represents an adaptive response tending to limit the caloric excess. This response is greater for protein and less for carbohydrate and fat. Besides satiety, it is the only adaptation available to *Homo sapiens* to prevent excess storage of calories. In some obese individuals, little or no rise in metabolic rate occurs during positive caloric balance.

Another hypothesis for a metabolic risk factor for obesity has to do with adipose tissue lipoprotein lipase. This enzyme is synthesized within fat cells and is then localized in the endothelium of the capillary walls of the adipose tissue. Its action promotes the deposition of circulating triglyceride fatty acid calories in adipose tissue. The lipoprotein lipase activity tends to be higher in the adipose tissue of some obese animal models. Increased activity of this enzyme could favor the deposition of fat calories into adipose tissue, thereby promoting obesity and actually stimulating appetite because of the siphoning off of ingested calories into the storage depot.

Nutrition in Clinical Therapeutics

Nutrition can be curative, preventive, palliative, or supportive.

THE CURATIVE USE OF NUTRITION

Dramatic examples of disorders that can be cured nutritionally are the classic monovalent deficiency diseases: scurvy, beriberi, pellagra, and rickets. For such patients, treatment with several times the RDA of the specific nutrient cures the disorder. Each of the essential nutrients, by definition, has such a monovalent deficiency syndrome. For some, such as selenium or biotin, a deficiency complex was heretofore seen only in the animal model receiving a restricted synthetic diet. The current extensive clinical use of "total parenteral nutrition," a synthetic diet that delivers only the known essential nutrients to individuals who often have increased nutritional requirements, is leading to a series of case reports of newly recognized trace element deficiencies.

THE PREVENTIVE USE OF NUTRITIONAL THERAPY

Some disorders of undernutrition—for example, goiter and rickets—were formerly quite prevalent. Addition of iodine to table salt in the first case and of vitamin D to milk in the second case has largely eradicated these diseases in many regions. These are dramatic examples of the worldwide application, in a highly feasible, cost-effective manner, of knowledge gained by nutritional research.

THE PALLIATIVE USE OF NUTRITIONAL THERAPY

Many diseases that are not primarily of nutritional origin impair the body's ability to process food at the gastrointestinal level or to metabolize and excrete certain nutrients and their metabolic products. Consequently, the unregulated intake of mixed foods in such individuals can worsen the patient's symptoms. Examples include the ingestion of unrestricted amounts of sodium worsening congestive heart failure and the ingestion of too much protein producing hepatic encephalopathy in cirrhotic patients.

THE SUPPORTIVE USE OF NUTRITIONAL THERAPY

Chronically and subacutely ill patients are characterized by debilitation, catabolic states, increased nutritional expenditures, and loss of the ability to eat because of anorexia or mechanical impediments to eating, digesting, and absorbing. Nutritional support systems have been developed to prevent progressive undernutrition in such individuals.

The Nasoenteral Approach

Two technical improvements—the modern, flexible, narrow-gauge Silastic tube and low-viscosity formulas—have made the nasoenteral approach generally applicable, provided that there is no intestinal obstruction and that some absorptive capability remains. Such patients can be nourished even despite total anorexia. If digestive capability has been lost, fat is omitted, protein is replaced by an appropriate mixture of essential and nonessential amino acids, and carbohydrate is furnished largely as glucose.

The Intravenous Approach

The intravenous approach can be either central or peripheral. The limitation of intravenous feeding is the osmotic tolerance of the veins. To provide all MDRs of the essential nutrients in a nearly fat-free mixture requires about 3600 mOsm/day; since the daily tolerance for water is about 3 liters, this would require solutions of about 1200 mOsm/liter. Unfortunately, solutions more concentrated than about 600 mOsm/liter will quickly cause chemical phlebitis in peripheral veins. This impasse has been circumvented in two ways: (1) The intravenous catheter may be placed in the central veins, which will tolerate up to 1800 mOsm/liter because of their high flow rate. (2) Alternatively, hypercaloric intravenous fluids can be infused in the peripheral veins, provided calories are shifted from osmotically active glucose and amino acids to osmotically inactive lipid emulsions.

A Synopsis of the Essential Nutrients

The 40 essential nutrients are listed in Table 3. What follows is a brief consideration of each. For each essential nutrient, there are at least eight questions that must be asked:

1. How was the essentiality of the nutrient identified or recognized? What was the human or animal model of the deficiency state? What served as the assay system for the original purification of the nutrient from mixed foods?

2. How is the essential nutrient distributed among the approximately 200 food items in the human diet?

3. What is the site, mechanism, and extent of the gastrointestinal absorption of the nutrient? In this connection, we must consider the bioavailability of the nutrient as it occurs in various foods; that is, merely because the nutrient is present in a particular food does not prove that it will survive premeal processing or that it will be fully absorbable or that its absorb-

ability may not be influenced by the presence of other food components.

4. How is the nutrient metabolized, transported, stored, and transformed in the body?

5. What are the physiologic functions of the nutrient and its metabolic products within the body?

6. By what mechanisms are the nutrient and its physiologically useful products degraded? By what means are the end-products excreted?

7. We come then to consideration of the deficiency syndrome which, by definition, applies to every essential nutrient. What are the MDR and RDA? What nutrient-nutrient, drug-nutrient, or disease-nutrient factors lower or raise these thresholds? What are the physical and chemical manifestations of the deficiency caused by absorption of less than the MDR?

8. What is the tolerance threshold for the nutrient? What exogenous and endogenous factors raise and lower the tolerance? What clinical disorder results when the tolerance is exceeded?

PROTEIN

Originally proteins were referred to as "albuminous matter." The word protein derives from the Greek root that means "to come first." Studies dating back to the 1800s have sought to delineate protein requirements. The recognition of the polymeric structure of proteins, based on peptide bonds connecting amino acids, and the subsequent determination of the structures of the 20 natural amino acids present in proteins led to improved understanding of protein requirements. Svedberg's studies with ultracentrifugation and the osmometer allowed measurements of the molecular weights of proteins. The first method to determine the unique amino acid sequence of a protein was developed by Sanger. Rose determined the minimum requirements of each essential amino acid in humans (Table 3) by feeding a balanced diet, including amino acids in pure form; eliminating specific amino acids, thereby producing negative nitrogen balance; and then replacing the amino acid until nitrogen balance was regained. Amino acid requirements, and what protein sources best meet these requirements, remain a major focus of interest today as the world population continues to be plagued by protein starvation.

Distribution of Protein in Food Groups

All foods contain proteins; animal products, however, contain more protein than plant products. Individual proteins differ in their efficiency for promoting growth or maintaining nitrogen balance. These differences in "biologic value" result from differences in the essential amino acid content (Table 3). Nearly optimal ratios of the nonessential and the essential amino acids are present in egg and milk protein, which consequently have the highest biologic value (approaching 100 per cent). Casein, lactalbumin, and ovalbumin are the usual reference standards. The world's major food products, in order of decreasing biologic value, are animal products, legumes, cereals (rice, wheat, and corn), and fruit. The adult RDA for protein of about 50 g is based on the assumption that the protein has a biologic value of 70, which would apply when the diet is based largely on animal products. The lower the biologic value, the higher the protein requirement. Plant proteins have a biologic value below 50; thus one or another essential amino acid is limiting. Corn is deficient in tryptophan, soybeans and green peas in lysine, rice in methionine, and wheat in lysine and threonine. Supplementing these proteins with the deficient amino acid enhances its biologic value.

Bioavailability of Protein

The coefficient of digestibility of an ordinary mixed food diet, with the protein source coming primarily from animal foods, is quite high, generally about 95 to 99. Apparent protein digestibility is calculated as nitrogen in the feces subtracted from the amount eaten, divided by the amount eaten, times 100. To determine true protein digestibility, the amount of fecal nitrogen excreted when no protein is fed must be considered. For example, with a 100-g protein diet (16 g N) and 1.7 g N in feces, apparent digestibility is $(16 - 1.7/16) \times 100$, or 89 per cent. The coefficient of digestibility, including the net percentage of protein digested and absorbed, of cereal, vegetables, and fruits is 85 to 90, whereas that of legumes may be as low as 75 to 80. Nitrogen loss is increased when diets contain a lot of indigestible matter, possibly because of bacterial growth resulting from the presence of these fibrous sources.

Cooking and food processing may alter the bioavailability of proteins. Legumes, for example, are more digestible after cooking, but protein denaturization may occur in most foodstuffs subjected to extreme temperatures. Acid or alkaline treatment may also denature an amino acid.

In addition, all the necessary amino acids must be present at the appropriate time for a protein source to be efficiently utilized. A sufficient quantity of calories must also be available to prevent the use of protein for energy.

Digestion and Absorption

The processes of digestion and absorption are discussed in Section XIV, including the participation of several specific amino acid and oligopeptide transport systems in the upper small intestine.

Metabolism of Protein

Biosynthesis of the Nonessential Amino Acids. Biosynthesis generally utilizes the nitrogen of ammonia, urea, or a nonessential amino acid. The carbon chain originates in glucose or in another nonessential amino acid. Cysteine and tyrosine are synthesized from the essential amino acids methionine and phenylalanine, respectively. For seven of the essential amino acids, the biosynthetic step lacking (which prevents *total* de novo production) involves the synthesis of the carbon skeleton. If the alpha-keto acids are provided in the diet, the essentials can be synthesized from them. This approach is now used in the treatment of uremia with nitrogen-poor diets.

By-products of Amino Acid Metabolism. Amino acids provide for the biosynthesis of a number of physiologically useful by-products. Among these are carnitine, choline, creatine, neurotransmitters, thyroxin, and pigmentary products.

Gluconeogenesis. During glucose starvation, amino acids donate their carbon skeletons for the synthesis of glucose. For this purpose, amino acids are mobilized from muscle during starvation, and the carbon skeletons of the gluconeogenic amino acids (Table 6) are transformed in the liver to glucose, which becomes available for nourishment of the brain (see Section VI).

Oxidative Fuel. During starvation, the carbon skeletons of amino acids are extensively utilized for oxidative metabolism. The gluconeogenic amino acids may pass through glucose en route to oxidation, or they may be oxidized directly.

Precursors for Lipogenesis. Under the condition of positive caloric balance, the carbon skeletons of the amino acids are degraded to acetate, incorporated into long-chain fatty acids, and stored as adipose tissue triglyceride. Thus an excess of calories ingested in the form of protein, just like excess calories eaten as carbohydrate or fat, will lead to an increase in adipose mass.

Incorporation into Protein. Amino acids serve primarily as building blocks of protein. Ribosomal protein synthesis involves initiation, elongation, and termination. Proteins are synthesized in the amino-to-carboxyl direction by the sequential addition of amino acids to the carboxyl end of the growing peptide chain (see Section I).

Degradation and Excretion. The carbon skeleton, the nitrogen moiety, and the sulfur moiety are handled separately. The carbon chains are oxidized to carbon dioxide and water, except that a portion of the aromatic amino acids are excreted as organic acids. The amino or amide groups are removed by transamination, deamination, or deamidation; enter the Krebs-Henseleit cycle; and emerge as the end-product urea, which is excreted into the urine. The sulfur moiety of the amino acids produces one of two end-products: If the sulfur remains attached to the carbon chain of cysteine, oxidation leads to the end-product taurine; if the sulfur is removed, the sulfur is oxidized to sulfate. Both products are excreted in the urine, generally in molar ratios of about 1 (taurine) to 4 (sulfate).

Minimum Daily Requirement of Protein. This varies with life cycle, biologic value of the protein, energy supply, and disease state.

In the natural proteins, a low biologic value is usually the result of a deficiency in an essential amino acid. Any alteration in the ratio of amino acids within a synthetic diet can alter the nutritional value of the mixture. For example, consider a particular mixture in which histidine is the deficient amino acid; if one adds additional amino acid mixtures that lack histi-

dine, rats become anorexic and cease growing. The amino acid imbalance can then be corrected by adding the most deficient amino acid, histidine. The addition of a structurally related amino acid to a diet in which a particular amino acid is deficient—for example, leucine for isoleucine—is certain to impair the biologic value. The addition of certain amino acids such as methionine and tyrosine to an otherwise balanced diet can cause toxic reactions.

Besides the quality of the protein, another factor that influences the protein requirement is the caloric intake. If calories are deficient, a larger portion of the protein must be used as fuel and as substrate for gluconeogenesis; the requirement is therefore greater.

Daily protein requirement is increased by growth, pregnancy, lactation, and repletion after weight loss. Fever, infection, and trauma, which cause greater breakdown of body protein and a negative nitrogen balance, likewise raise the amount of protein required to maintain zero balance. Gastrointestinal malabsorption causes increased loss of protein into the stools and thereby elevates the protein requirement. The need for protein is reduced by the several nitrogen accumulation diseases (uremia, cirrhosis, and inborn errors of the urea cycle).

Deficiency State

Epidemiology. Protein deficiency with or without calorie deficiency is the world's most common undernutrition syndrome. Indeed, the availability of protein of adequate amount and biologic quality is one of the factors that limit the size of the human population. In the developing nations, the main sources of protein are vegetables of low biologic quality, and the protein undernutrition is classified as primary or socioeconomic. In the United States, on the other hand, protein malnutrition is more often secondary to disease and is especially concentrated in the chronically ill population.

Because the protein requirement rises sharply if calories are restricted, protein and calorie undernutrition often occur together. This condition is termed *marasmus*. Protein undernutrition occurring with adequate caloric intake has been termed *kwashiorkor*.

Metabolic and Endocrine Aspects. When calories are restricted, the body adapts by reduced secretion of insulin, decreased peripheral conversion of T_4 to T_3, lowered activity of the adrenergic nervous system, and augmented secretion of glucagon and cortisol. The metabolic rate falls. The hypoinsulinemia mobilizes free fatty acids and amino acids to provide carbon for oxidative metabolism and for gluconeogenesis. In negative energy balance, oxidative metabolism becomes first priority for dietary protein. The use of amino acids in oxidation reduces the availability of amino acids for protein synthesis, which therefore declines; however, the rate of protein breakdown also diminishes. In protein-calorie undernutrition, or marasmus, free fatty acids are mobilized from adipose tissue; both lean body mass and adipose mass are consumed. The more successful the adaptation, which depends on curtailment of insulin secretion, the more successful the preservation of lean body mass at the expense of rapid consumption of adipose tissue.

Frequently protein intake is more restricted than that of calories—first, because dietary protein is more

TABLE 6. FATE OF AMINO ACIDS IN MAMMALS

Glucogenic	Glucogenic and Ketogenic
Alanine	Isoleucine
Arginine	Phenylalanine
Aspartic acid	Tyrosine
Asparagine	Histidine
Cysteine	Methionine
Glutamic acid	Proline
Glutamine	Serine
Glycine	Threonine
Ketogenic	Valine
Leucine	
Lysine	
Tryptophan	

expensive than carbohydrate or fat and, second, because animal protein, which has high biologic quality, is more expensive than vegetable protein, which has low biologic quality. Additional contributory factors are the tendency of persons to consume empty calories and the extensive hospital use of glucose infusions lacking amino acids. The latter type of treatment stimulates insulin secretion, and the hypoinsulinemia so vital to the adaptation to starvation is circumvented. Consequently, as in kwashiorkor, adipose mass is conserved. The extensive depot of metabolic fuel in adipose tissue cannot be readily utilized. The reduced availability of amino acids curtails the renewal of the tissue proteins and the synthesis of visceral proteins. Hypoalbuminemia, fatty liver, and muscle atrophy ensue.

Protein-calorie undernutrition affects every tissue in the body. The heart and kidneys, as well as muscle, lose mass; cardiac output declines; blood pressure, blood volume, and hematocrit are reduced; hypoalbuminemia occurs; and the gastrointestinal tract and pancreas atrophy. Involution of lymphatic tissues is associated with impaired cell-mediated immunity. Wound healing becomes defective. The lack of metabolic fuel adversely affects temperature regulation. Reproduction becomes difficult or impossible. Resistance to infection is lowered; urinary tract infection and bronchopneumonia are common. The mortality rate in the common infectious diseases increases. After lean body mass declines below 70 per cent of normal, the mortality rate is quite high.

Clinical Aspects. The clinical signs of protein-calorie undernutrition are underweight, stunted appearance (marasmus), edema (in kwashiorkor), "flaky paint dermatitis," pigmentary changes in skin and hair, pallor, and frequently physical signs of water-soluble or fat-soluble vitamin deficiencies in the eyes and mouth. In advanced stages, decubitus ulcers occur. Blood pressure, pulse, and temperature may be reduced. Anthropometric measurements show loss of adipose tissue and muscle mass.

Laboratory studies show reduced 24-hour urinary creatinine-to-height index and reduced nitrogen-to-creatinine and sulfur-to-creatinine ratios in the urine. Hypoalbuminemia, anemia, reduced serum levels of essential amino acids, and impaired T-lymphocyte cell function, as revealed by cutaneous anergy and peripheral lymphopenia, are often found. Plasma levels of cortisol may be raised, reverse T_3 is increased, and the metabolic rate is low.

Toxicity

The normal adult can degrade and excrete at least 200 g of protein a day without acute ill effects, but nausea and satiety will usually intervene to prevent this high an intake. Congenital or acquired nitrogen accumulation diseases, which impair degradation or excretion, can reduce this tolerance to as little as 20 g a day.

ENERGY

In order to maintain a constant body weight, energy balance in the adult must be zero and intake must equal output. The output can be divided into (1) *the*

basal metabolic rate (BMR), which is the rate of oxygen consumption or heat production in the fasting, resting stage; and (2) *increments of the metabolic rate above basal,* which are related to activity, food intake, or exposure to cold. After each meal, metabolic rate temporarily increases by 10 to 30 per cent ("specific dynamic action"). Positive caloric balance causes a prolonged increase in metabolic rate of similar magnitude. Metabolic rate during sleep falls by about 10 per cent. Mild, moderate, or severe exercise raises BMR by roughly 30, 50, or 100 per cent, respectively.

To estimate an individual's basal energy expenditure, we use the Harris-Benedict equation (Table 7) for sex, weight, height, and age. This measurement of basal energy expenditure takes into account BMR, specific dynamic action, and the reduction during sleep. To this basal expenditure we add 30, 50, or 100 per cent for sedentary, moderate, or strenuous activity, respectively.

Numerous clinical conditions alter the metabolic rate. Energy expenditure rises during fever, about 13 per cent for each degree Celsius over normal. Burns, trauma, and hyperthyroidism can increase the rate by 20 to 100 per cent. Gastrointestinal disease frequently impairs the absorption of calories. In such cases, the overall intake of calories must increase to compensate.

WATER (Also see Section X)

Water is clearly the most critical of all nutrients. Human beings will succumb to deprivation of water more quickly than to deprivation of any other nutrient. Water's unique chemical properties explain its essential role in human existence.

Because of its solvent properties, water is the milieu for most of the chemical processes in the body. Water's high specific heat and high latent heat of vaporization provide it with the ability to regulate body temperature. In addition, water is highly conductive and thus allows the even and rapid distribution of body heat and eventually the release of excess heat through vaporization.

Water is widely distributed in its natural form, ingested in liquids, present in solid foods, and formed in the cells as a result of the oxidation of foodstuffs. Water of oxidation accounts for approximately 15 per cent of the daily total available water, or 300 to 400 ml/day. For 100 g of foodstuff, the water of oxidation for protein, carbohydrate, and fat is approximately 41, 60, and 107 g, respectively.

Water is readily absorbed throughout the gastrointestinal tract. Approximately 70 per cent of the fat-free body is water. About 60 per cent of the total body water is found in the intracellular fluid, with the remaining 40 per cent in the extracellular fluid.

TABLE 7. CALCULATION OF BASAL ENERGY EXPENDITURE (BEE) BY HARRIS-BENEDICT EQUATIONS

WOMEN
BEE = $655.1 + (9.6 \times W) + (1.8 \times H) - (4.7 \times A)$

MEN
BEE = $66.5 + (13.8 \times W) + (5.0 \times H) - (6.8 \times A)$

W = actual body weight in kilograms; H = height in centimeters, A = age in years.

Requirement

An average of 2000 g (ml) of water a day is excreted by skin, colon, and kidney, the last being the major regulatory organ. Antidiuretic hormone adjusts the urinary excretion of water to the intake, which in turn is adjusted by the hypothalamic thirst center; thereby, zero water balance is maintained. A reasonable allowance for water is 1 ml/Kcal for adults and 1.5 ml/Kcal for infants. The minimum requirement, considerably less than the allowance, depends on solutes ingested, the normal concentrating ability of the kidney, and extrarenal losses. A helpful rule of thumb for daily water requirement is as follows:

100 ml/day/kg IBW*	First 10 kg
50 ml/day/kg IBW	Second 10 kg
20 ml/day/1 kg IBW	Remainder of weight

Thus a 15-kg infant would require

100 × 10	(First 10 kg)
+ 50 × 5	(Remainder)
1250 ml/day	

whereas a 70-kg man would need

100 × 10	
+ 50 × 10	
+ 20 × 50	
2500 ml/day	

This is a rough estimate and must be adjusted as the clinical situation dictates.

Pathophysiology of Water Excess or Deprivation. The metabolism of water in health and disease is discussed in detail in Section X.

MACROMINERALS

SODIUM (See Section X)

Since ancient times, sodium, which is the sixth most abundant element on earth, has been important as an item of commerce. It is used for flavoring, for food preservation, and in making glass. The name "sodium" comes from the medieval Latin word *sodanum,* which means headache remedy. In 1807 Davy first isolated the element by electrolysis of sodium hydroxide. In 1847 Liebig discovered that sodium was the main cation in blood and lymph, whereas potassium and magnesium were predominant in the soft tissues. In the Precambrian oceans in which unicellular organisms evolved, potassium was the major cation; by the time multicellular organisms with extracellular fluid were evolving in later geologic periods, sodium had become the predominant oceanic cation. This sequence may explain the differential distribution of sodium and potassium in animal tissues. Sodium was recognized to be a dietary essential in the late nineteenth century because experimental animals did not survive on salt-free diets.

Distribution and Bioavailability

Sodium is widely available in many foodstuffs; however, common table salt is responsible for most sodium intake in the United States. The amount of salt used in cooking, processing, and seasoning generally far outweighs the sodium content of natural foods. Fruits,

---

*Ideal Body Weight

vegetables, and grains are low in sodium; protein and dairy foods are better sources. Sodium is completely bioavailable in most foodstuffs. More than 95 per cent of sodium is absorbed from the intestinal tract.

Function

Sodium's main activities revolve around its role as the principal cation of the extracellular fluid. Maintenance of extracellular fluid volume and osmotic equilibrium are sodium's most important functions.

The human body contains about 1.8 g Na/kg fat-free body weight, the majority of which is present in extracellular fluid. The inorganic portion of the skeleton contains about one-third of the body's total sodium content. In bone, sodium is largely bound on the surface of the bone crystals. This sodium reservoir is apparently part of the active labile sodium pool in the body.

Requirement

In the healthy adult, sodium balance can be maintained with sodium intakes approximating 60 mEq/day (1380 mg). The usual intake of sodium, however, is far in excess of minimal needs and ranges between 100 and 300 mEq (2300 and 6900 mg). It is not uncommon to see sodium intakes as high as 30 to 40 g/day in Oriental countries. The possible link between sodium and hypertension has prompted further evaluation of sodium requirements. The current estimated safe and adequate daily dietary intake of sodium for adults is 1100 to 3300 mg. The sodium requirement is increased by heat exposure and excessive sweating.

Pathophysiology of Sodium Excess or Deficiency. Abnormalities of sodium metabolism are discussed in detail in Section X.

POTASSIUM

Potassium, the seventh most abundant metal in our planet, was discovered in 1807 by Davy, who obtained it by electrolysis from caustic potash (KOH). The Latin word *kalium* means "potash" and refers to the alkaline ash of vegetable substances. It was not until 1938 that McCollum demonstrated in rats that potassium is an essential nutrient.

Distribution

Potassium is highly bioavailable and is widely distributed in foods of both plant and animal origin. Meat and milk are good potassium sources. Most fruits, including tomatoes, and dark green, leafy vegetables are excellent potassium sources. Because of processing, cheese is a poor source of the element.

Absorption

Eighty to 90 per cent of potassium is readily absorbed from the intestinal tract. High concentrations of potassium in localized areas of the small bowel can cause ulceration and occasionally perforation.

Function

Because of its ionic nature, potassium, like sodium, is involved in the maintenance of normal water balance, osmotic equilibrium, and acid-base balance. Neuromuscular regulation is also an important activity in which potassium participates. The role of potassium in the normal operation of the conductive system of the heart is of vital importance, since malfunction of this system is a frequent cause of death.

Potassium is the chief cation of the intracellular fluid. The normal human body contains about 2.6 g/kg fat-free body weight, about 98 per cent of this being located in the intracellular space. Muscle and nerve cells are especially rich in potassium. The serum level of potassium is about 3.5 to 5 mEq/liter.

Requirement

No RDA for potassium intake has been established, but the estimated safe and adequate daily adult dietary intake of potassium is 1875 to 5625 mg. The healthy adult can maintain potassium balance with intakes of approximately 90 mg (2 to 3 mEq) per day. However, the usual adult intake of potassium is between 1950 and 5900 mg (50 to 150 mEq) per day.

The requirement for potassium is increased with diarrhea, with diabetic acidosis, or with the use of potassium-wasting diuretics. Renal failure greatly limits potassium excretion and so decreases potassium requirements.

Pathophysiology of Potassium Excess or Deficiency. This topic is discussed in detail in Section X.

CALCIUM (See also Section IX)

In the mid 1700s it was discovered that the principal part of the earthy matter of bones was actually calcium phosphate. Then in 1801 Berzelius determined the proportion of calcium to phosphorus in bones and suggested a chemical formula for the composition. In the earliest experiments on the effect of food on bone structure (1842), pigeons fed a restricted diet of wheat developed very porous bones. When the diet was supplemented with calcium carbonate, the osteoporosis resolved. By manipulations in diet, it was found that the amounts and the ratio of calcium and phosphorus in the diet influenced bone mass and density.

Distribution and Bioavailability

The most important sources of dietary calcium are milk and milk products. Two cups per day provide almost 75 per cent of the RDA (800 mg). With the exception of leafy vegetables, most foods are very poor sources of calcium.

Absorption

Most calcium is absorbed in the proximal small intestine, although the entire small bowel is involved in the process. Both an energy-dependent and a passive mechanism exist, and both are regulated by vitamin D. The efficiency of absorption varies between 10 and 40 per cent and is proportional to the availability of dietary calcium. The adjustment of absorption to body calcium stores is made by the parathyroid hormone–vitamin D system (see Section IX).

Function

Quantitatively, the most important function of calcium is to produce the material for the mineralized portion of bone. Calcium is initially deposited in bone as calcium phosphate and then undergoes a maturation process in which it is converted to hydroxyapatite with a higher calcium-phosphorus ratio. Ionic calcium is vital for muscle contraction, blood coagulation, platelet aggregation, gastric acid secretion, cellular adhesiveness, transmission of nerve impulses, activation of enzyme reactions, and hormone secretion.

Requirement

The oral RDA for calcium is 800 mg for adults and 1200 mg for children. RDA values for the intravenous route are only one third as great. Pregnancy and lactation increase the requirement by an additional 400 mg/day. Several groups of patients require an increased calcium intake—those with (1) end-stage renal disease (because deficiency of 1,25-dihydroxy vitamin D impairs absorption), (2) persistent diarrheal states with loss of calcium as the fatty acid soaps, and (3) senile osteoporosis resulting in part from reduced ability of the aging small intestine to absorb calcium. Low-calcium diets are used for those with idiopathic hypercalciuria and urinary stone formation.

Pathophysiology of Calcium Excess or Deficiency. This topic is discussed in detail in Section IX.

MAGNESIUM

Salts of magnesium, the eighth most abundant element in the earth, have been known for thousands of years for their healing properties. The Romans claimed that "magnesium alba," white magnesium salts from the district of Magnesia in Greece, cured many ailments. Magnesium's medicinal properties are still well known today in such products as "milk of magnesia" (magnesium hydroxide) and Epsom salts (magnesium sulfate), named after Epsom, a small village in London whose water supply was known to have wound-healing properties and a laxative effect.

It was not until 1926 that magnesium was shown to be an essential nutrient, with human magnesium deficiency documented a few years later. In 1964 Shils described magnesium deficiency in two adult male volunteers. The deficiency that developed after three months on the deficient diet was characterized by personality changes, muscle tremor, lack of coordination, and gastrointestinal disturbances. It is now obvious that human depletion occurs much more commonly than previously assumed.

Distribution and Bioavailability

Vegetables are particularly good sources of magnesium. About 30 per cent of the magnesium in a normal diet is found within the chlorophyll molecule in plant matter. Whole grains and raw, dried beans and peas are excellent sources. Cocoa, some nuts, soybeans, and some seafoods are also rich in magnesium. Magnesium absorption is reduced when the calcium and phosphorus content of foods is high, as in milk and milk products.

Absorption

Net gastrointestinal absorption normally is about 30 to 40 per cent of the magnesium ingested and is influenced by intestinal transit time; calcium, phosphorus, and lactose content in the diet; and total magnesium intake. Ingested magnesium appears to be absorbed mainly by the small intestine, particularly the ileum.

Function

Magnesium functions as a prosthetic group in many essential enzymatic reactions, specifically those that hydrolyze and transfer phosphate groups. Thus magnesium is intimately involved in adenosine triphosphate (ATP)-requiring reactions, including aerobic metabolism, oxidative phosphorylation, the citric acid cycle, the activation of amino acids, activities of alkaline phosphatases and pyrophosphatases, and the conversion of ATP to cyclic adenosine monophosphate (AMP). Magnesium also functions in protein synthesis, including ribosomal aggregation, binding of messenger RNA to 70S ribosomes, and the synthesis and degradation of DNA. Further, magnesium influences neuromuscular transmission and activity. It acts both synergistically and antagonistically with calcium in this role.

Transport and Storage

Magnesium exists in the plasma in free, complexed, and protein-bound forms. The approximate percentages are 55, 13, and 32, respectively. The average 70-kg adult contains approximately 24 g of magnesium. About 90 per cent of the body's magnesium is in bone (60 per cent) and muscle (30 per cent). The remainder of magnesium is distributed in nonmuscular soft tissues. Approximately 1 per cent of the total body magnesium content is extracellular.

In the bone, about 35 per cent of magnesium is associated with a surface-limited pool, whereas the larger fraction of magnesium is an integral part of bone crystal. The surface magnesium is probably sensitive to extracellular fluid levels, whereas the crystal component is dependent upon resorptive processes.

Excretion (See Section X)

Renal resorptive and excretory mechanisms appear to be the critical factors in maintaining magnesium homeostasis, as intestinal transport shows little adaptation to alterations of intake. About one third of the daily intake is excreted in the urine. Unbound plasma magnesium is filtered by the glomeruli and is reabsorbed by the renal tubules. Magnesium excretion, as well as that of calcium, potassium, and sodium, is enhanced by mercurial and thiazide diuretics. In high temperatures, sweat can account for 25 per cent of magnesium losses daily.

Requirement

The oral MDR ranges between 200 and 300 mg/day for adults. For the intravenous route, the MDR is only one third as great. The oral RDA is 300 to 400 mg/day for adult males and females. During pregnancy and lactation, 450 mg/day is recommended.

It is difficult to produce magnesium deficiency in healthy subjects because of the widespread distribution of the cation in most foods and the efficiency of renal conservation. Deficiency generally occurs coupled with other complicating diseases. Alcoholism, malabsorption, endocrine abnormalities, malnutrition, and some nephropathies (notably those caused by aminoglycoside antibiotics) can cause magnesium deficiency. In steatorrhea, there is extensive fecal loss of magnesium as soaps of the long-chain fatty acids. Magnesium is vitally important in parathyroid hormone (PTH) function, although the mechanisms are not clear, being necessary for osteoclast response to PTH, for renal sensitivity to the hormone, and probably for secretion of PTH by the parathyroid glands. As a result, magnesium deficiency can induce an intractable hypocalcemia. Other manifestations of magnesium deficiency are summarized in Table 8.

Magnesium should be replaced by the oral or intramuscular route unless the patient is actually symptomatic. Intravenous magnesium therapy must be carefully monitored to prevent respiratory arrest.

Toxicity

Hypermagnesemia and magnesium toxicity can occur when magnesium is used in patients with renal insufficiency and when magnesium is given to the eclamptic patient in large doses to control hypertension. The use of magnesium-containing antacids is a common cause of toxicity in individuals with renal insufficiency. In both renal insufficiency and eclampsia, serum levels over about 10 mEq/liter have been reported to cause central nervous system depression. Calcium infusion counteracts magnesium toxicity.

CHLORIDE (See Section X)

Distribution and Bioavailability

The distribution of chloride in foods is essentially the same as that of sodium. Table salt is probably the largest source of chloride in an average diet.

Absorption

Chloride is absorbed from the diet with greater than 95 per cent efficiency. There is a large enteroenteral circulation of chloride; that secreted by the stomach and pancreas is efficiently recovered by the lower intestine.

Transformation and Function

Chloride is the major extracellular anion. When measured in combination with serum bicarbonate, the sum of the two anion concentrations is roughly equal to that of sodium minus 12 mEq/liter. Any discrepancy reflects the presence of "unmeasured" anions—the so-

---

TABLE 8. CONSEQUENCES OF MAGNESIUM DEFICIENCY

Neuromuscular
  Lethargy, weakness, fatigue, decreased mentation
  Neuromuscular irritability, in part due to associated hypocalcemia
  Hyaline and vacuolar degeneration of myofibers with segmental necrosis
Gastrointestinal
  Anorexia, nausea, vomiting
  Paralytic ileus
Cardiovascular
  Increased sensitivity to digitalis glycosides
  Possible cause of tachyarrhythmias
Metabolic
  Hypocalcemia—probably due to the combined result of decreased PTH secretion and decreased end-organ responsiveness to PTH
  Hypokalemia—tendency toward renal potassium wasting

From Smith, L. H., Jr.: Disorders of magnesium metabolism. In Wyngaarden, J. B., and Smith, L. H., Jr. (eds.): Cecil Textbook of Medicine. 17th ed. Philadelphia, W. B. Saunders Co., 1985, p. 1165.

called anion gap. Chloride is also a significant component of gastric secretion, in which it is produced in the form of hydrochloric acid. Erythrocytes and gastric mucosa contain significant amounts of chloride. In both the intestine and the kidney, chloride-bicarbonate exchange "pumps" present in the cell membrane help control systemic pH by altering bicarbonate flux.

Excretion

Chloride is largely excreted by the kidney. It passively leaks into the renal interstitium through the proximal convoluted tubule, carrying large volumes of water with it. In the thick ascending limit of the loop of Henle, chloride is actively removed from the intraluminal filtrate. As a result, the fluid in the distal convoluted tubule is always hypo-osmotic, ready to be manipulated by antidiuretic hormone.

Requirement

Although no RDA for chloride has been established, an estimated safe and adequate daily dietary intake for adults is 1700 to 5100 mg. Most dietary chloride is provided by common table salt, sodium chloride. Generally, an average diet contains 2 to 5 g of chloride per day. When salt in the diet is restricted, chloride intake is thus reduced. Vomiting or use of diuretics may result in large chloride losses.

Deficiency

Because we ingest chloride mainly as the sodium salt, chloride deficiency is usually synonymous with sodium deficiency. Exceptions are continuous removal of gastric hydrochloric acid by prolonged nasogastric suction, with resulting hypochloremic alkalosis; and chloridorrhea, a hereditary disorder of chloride malabsorption characterized by life-long watery diarrhea and salt loss.

PHOSPHORUS (See Sections VI and X)

Phosphorus, from the Greek word *phosphoros,* meaning light-bearing, first interested chemists very much because in the free form it glows in the dark, is very toxic, and spontaneously bursts into flame. Phosphorus has been used for many varied purposes, such as matches, smoke bombs, detergents, fertilizers, glass, fine china, water softener, and baking powder.

Distribution

Phosphorus occurs in food and in the body almost exclusively as phosphate, mostly inorganic but also as organic esters. Phosphates can be joined in chains through the high-energy phosphate bond, which is vital for cellular energy distribution. Inorganic phosphate exists in the body as a pH-dependent mixture of HPO_4^{-2} and $H_2PO_4^-$.

An average diet contains 1500 to 1600 mg of phosphorus. Milk and milk products are a highly concentrated source of phosphorus, in the range of 1 mg/ml. Carbohydrates, fruits, vegetables, and fats are relatively poor sources, with meats and seafood in an intermediate position.

Absorption

Absorption of phosphate occurs in the small intestine; 70 per cent of ingested phosphate is absorbed in the absence of phosphate binders. Lipid phosphorus in ingested food must first be hydrolyzed to free phosphate before it can be absorbed. Vitamin D enhances phosphate and calcium absorption from the gut, and its deficiency causes hypophosphatemia, in part because of secondary hyperparathyroidism with enhanced renal clearance of phosphate.

Function

Phosphate is, in many ways, the currency of the energy economy of the cell. Through its ability to form diphosphate and triphosphate bonds with high potential energy, phosphate allows the cell to conserve energy in a readily usable form, perform chemical syntheses that would not otherwise be thermodynamically possible, and direct synthesis of chemicals by the differential distribution of phosphate bonds among precursors.

Although the uses of phosphate listed in the preceding paragraph are essential to life, the quantitatively most important use of phosphate in humans and other vertebrates is in the hydroxyapatite crystal in the mineralized portion of bone. Chronic phosphate deficiency causes rickets or osteomalacia, characterized by soft, poorly mineralized bone that is subject to fracture and distortion with minimal trauma.

Transport and Storage

About 1 kg of elemental phosphorus, almost exclusively in the phosphate form, is present in the normal adult. Over 85 per cent of this amount is in the skeleton, and the remaining 15 per cent is largely within cells of the soft tissues. Less than 1 per cent is present in the serum in various forms, making individual serum levels poor measures of total body phosphorus. Normal serum levels of phosphorus range from 2.8 to 4.0 mg/dl.

Relatively little phosphate is protein-bound, most being free in plasma. This pool of free phosphate is significant as a second-line pH buffer, next in importance to bicarbonate.

Excretion

The kidney is the major regulatory organ in phosphate metabolism. Normally vitamin D and parathyroid hormone influence the balance of secretion and reabsorption in the renal tubule. Thus the majority of excreted phosphorus is in urine; the presence of phosphorus in feces reflects unabsorbed dietary phosphorus.

Requirement

The recommended oral daily allowance of phosphorus in adults is 800 mg. In children, because of growth requirements, the RDA is somewhat higher (1000 to 1200 mg). The average diet more than adequately provides this level. During pregnancy and lactation, phosphorus demands may exceed supply, but the simple addition of milk or other high-phosphate food should suffice to meet increased needs. Hospitalized patients who have rapid tissue formation, healing burns, or rapidly growing tumors would be expected to require more phosphate.

Deficiency

Phosphate depletion resulting from inadequate absorption occurs in patients with diseases of the small

TABLE 9. CONSEQUENCES OF SEVERE HYPOPHOSPHATEMIA

Acute—"metabolic"
   Hematologic
      Red cell dysfunction and hemolysis
      Leukocyte dysfunction
      Platelet dysfunction
   Muscle
      Weakness
      Rhabdomyolysis
      Myocardial dysfunction
   Central nervous system dysfunction
   Hepatic dysfunction
Chronic—"structural"
   Osteomalacia or rickets

From Smith, L. H., Jr.: Phosphorus deficiency and hypophosphatemia. In Wyngaarden, J. B., and Smith, L. H., Jr. (eds.): Cecil Textbook of Medicine. 17th ed. Philadelphia, W. B. Saunders Co., 1985, p. 1163.

intestine, in patients with vitamin D deficiency, and in patients using excessive amounts of aluminum hydroxide antacids, which bind phosphate. In renal tubular disorders, phosphate depletion results from excessive urinary losses. Total parenteral nutrition with phosphate-free solutions causes acute phosphate deficiency. Phosphate deficiency, manifested by hypophosphatemia, has a variable clinical presentation, ranging from no symptoms to anorexia and muscle weakness to rhabdomyolysis, respiratory failure, hemolysis, and mental changes (Table 9).

Toxicity

Elemental phosphorus is present in three forms, of which the so-called white (or yellow) form is most toxic. It is fat soluble, and ingestion of as little as 50 mg can cause liver necrosis, which is frequently fatal.

A more common toxic condition from a nutritional viewpoint is hyperphosphatemia, most often seen in patients with chronic renal failure or hypoparathyroidism. Inadequate renal tubular function disrupts the major controlling mechanism for phosphorus balance. This can often be improved with phosphate binders and a low-phosphate diet.

ESSENTIAL FATTY ACIDS (EFA)

Fatty acids differ in their chain lengths and in the number and position of double bonds. The essentiality of certain fatty acids was first demonstrated by raising rats on a fat-free but otherwise complete diet; they developed severe dermatitis, swelling of the feet, and loss of hair, followed by nephropathy and renal insufficiency, all alleviated by the addition of unsaturated fats to the diet. In assays for EFA activity in the rat, arachidonic acid is found to be the most potent EFA; the essentiality of other fatty acids depends on the ease with which they can be converted to arachidonic acid in the body. As an exception, some odd-chain-length fatty acids of the omega 5 and omega 7 classes are as active as linoleic acid in alleviating the symptoms of fatty acid deficiency. In addition, although linolenic acid does not qualify as an EFA by structure or by the prevention of the EFA deficiency syndrome, it may be essential in other ways.

Chemistry

A polyunsaturated fatty acid is composed of a carbon chain with two or more double bonds, that terminates with a carboxyl group. The major essential fatty acids are polyunsaturated acids in straight-chain form of 16-, 18-, or 20-carbon length, with 2, 3, or 4 *cis* double bonds separated by a single methylene group. The structures of linoleic, linolenic, and arachidonic acids are shown in Figure 4. In the shorthand nomenclature used to designate a specific fatty acid, the number of carbon atoms is followed by the number of double bonds (e.g., 18:2). The positions of the double bonds are designated by prefixes denoting their distance from the carboxyl group (e.g., 9, 12–18:2) or by suffixes denoting the number of carbons from the distal double bond to the terminal (or omega) carbon (e.g., 18:2 omega 6).

Distribution and Bioavailability

Linoleic and linolenic acids are the major EFA in the diet. They are found to a greater extent in many vegetable oils, including safflower, sunflower, and peanut oils. There are also EFA in dairy products, in animal meats, and, to a lesser extent, in fruits and vegetables, although the avocado is an excellent source.

Absorption

EFA are absorbed from micelles in the small intestine, probably by simple diffusion. Once inside the cell, the fatty acids and 2-monoacyl glycerols of the micelles are esterified into triacylglycerols. These are then combined with protein and phospholipid coats to form chylomicrons, which enter the lymphatic system for transport to the thoracic duct and the circulation.

Transformation and Function

Unsaturated fatty acids are metabolized in higher animals to produce four distinct series of polyunsaturated fatty acids. These are derived from palmitoleate (omega 7), oleate (omega 9), linoleate (omega 6), and

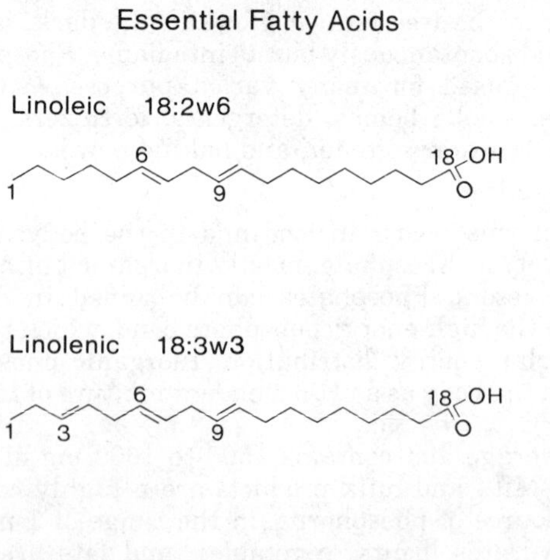

Essential Fatty Acids

Figure 4. Essential fatty acids.

linolenate (omega 3). Their major metabolic products are carbon-20 and carbon-22 trienes, tetraenes, pentaenes, and hexaenes formed by alterations occurring in the carboxy terminal region of the parent molecule.

The metabolic alterations consist of desaturation, in which additional double bonds are inserted between existing double bonds, and chain elongation, in which two carbon units are added to the carboxy terminus. The methyl end of the precursor fatty acid remains unchanged during these transformations. Thus linoleic acid (18:2 omega 6) is transformed to arachidonic acid (20:4 omega 6), retaining the distance between the methyl end and the nearest double bond.

The major polyunsaturated fatty acids formed in the body arise as the transformation products of dietary linoleic and linolenic acids (the omega 6 and omega 3 series). Normally the conversions of palmitoleate and oleate to polyunsaturated fatty acids represent relatively minor pathways in mammals. In severely fat-deficient animals, however, the transformation products of palmitoleate and oleate (primarily trienes) displace those of linoleate (tetraenes) and linolenate (pentaenes and hexaenes) as the major polyunsaturated fatty acids of animal tissues. Therefore the 20:3 omega 9 (triene)–to–20:4 omega 6 (tetraene) ratio is often used as an indicator of EFA deficiency.

Essential fatty acids maintain the liquid state of the interior portion of the hydrocarbon chains in cell membranes. They also function as precursors for the prostaglandins (PG). The common PGs are derived from three 20-carbon polyunsaturated acids having three, four, and five double bonds. These are transformation products of both linoleic and linolenic acids. Their synthesis depends on the release of the precursor fatty acid from cellular phospholipids by the enzyme action of phospholipase A_2. Their conversion involves the formation of a central cyclopentane ring through an endoperoxide intermediate and results in two fewer carbon atoms than the precursor molecule. The E series PGs contain ketone and hydroxyl groups on the cyclopentane ring, whereas the F series PGs contain two hydroxyl groups. The subscripts as in PGE_1, PGE_2, and PGE_3 refer to the number of double bonds.

Linoleic and linolenic acids are not interchangeable; their actions are nonequivalent and somewhat species specific. Although linoleic acid has little effect on the essential fatty acid syndrome seen in rats, it does prevent this syndrome in fish. Linolenic acid, on the other hand, has little or no effect on this syndrome in fish. These acids also give rise to discrete active metabolites whose actions are varied and often antagonistic. The prostaglandins (E and F series) and their products (thromboxanes), which are monoenes, dienes, or trienes, are derived from both linoleic and linolenic acids.

Linolenic acid may function in additional ways in rats and humans. One of its transformation products, eicosopentaenoic acid, has specific actions on platelet function, causing a decrease in platelet aggregation and an increase in bleeding. Its 22:6 w 3 product is concentrated in nervous tissue and in the retina, constituting the major fatty acid incorporated into phosphatidylethanolamine in the membranes of these tissues. A decrease in this fatty acid, brought about by dietary restriction of linolenic acid, has been correlated with a reduction in physical activity and learning ability in the rat. A syndrome of sensory and motor deficits was observed recently in a child on total parenteral nutrition containing linoleic acid but not linolenic acid. Gradual but complete resolution of this syndrome was achieved after administration of linolenic acid. It would appear, then, that both linoleic and linolenic acids are required for normal development and are essential, since neither can be synthesized by the body.

Transport and Storage (See Section VI)

Dietary EFA are transported through the circulation as chylomicron triglycerides. If not utilized for synthesis of phospholipids or cholesterol esters, they are stored in adipose tissue. When the chylomicrons reach the endothelial membranes of the capillaries perfusing adipose tissue, the EFA are liberated by lipoprotein lipase, enter the adipocytes, and are stored as triglycerides.

Polyunsaturated fatty acids are degraded in the body to carbon dioxide by beta oxidation. The presence of the *cis* double bonds, however, requires that structural modifications be made in the fatty acids in order for degradation to proceed to completion. These changes are accomplished by various isomerases. Without these additional enzymes, beta oxidation would proceed until a *cis* double bond, or D isomer, was encountered and then cease.

Requirement and Deficiency State

An adult man is thought to require at least 7.5 g of linoleic acid per day. Deficiency states are usually diagnosed by the triene-tetraene ratio in plasma and tissues. If this value exceeds 0.4, a deficiency is usually indicated. Some symptoms of deficiency are severe dermatitis, loss of hair, and impaired water balance reflecting membrane dysfunction. Deficiency states are most common in the developing stages of life when body stores have not yet appreciably accumulated. Once an animal reaches maturity, it becomes quite difficult to produce a deficiency. However, if EFA are not provided during the hyperalimentation of undernourished patients, EFA deficiency develops within weeks because the hyperinsulinemia stimulated by the infused glucose prevents mobilization of EFA stored in the fat cells. Conditioning factors contributing to a deficiency state include dietary cholesterol at 1 per cent or more and saturated fats at 2 per cent or more of the total caloric intake.

Toxicity

Although a toxic level for the EFA has not been determined, there are reports on the toxicity syndromes associated with high intakes. The antioxidant ability of the body is affected, as is indicated by cholesteryl linoleate hydroperoxide isolated from atheromas, apparently produced by auto-oxidation. High ratios of polyunsaturated to saturated fatty acids have been correlated with gallstone formation.

WATER-SOLUBLE VITAMINS

THIAMIN

Deficiency of thiamin causes beriberi, a syndrome with cardiac and neurologic manifestations. The disease was widespread in East Asia during the nineteenth century, coincident with the introduction of steam-powered rice mills. This milling process produced highly polished rice at the expense of the thiamin-rich outer hulk. In 1897 Eijkman, a Dutch physician, was able to create the neurologic form of the disease in birds raised on highly polished rice and cure it by the feeding of rice bran. A highly concentrated form of this curative factor was isolated in 1911 by Funk, who introduced the term "vitamin" to denote the newly recognized class of organic micronutrients. It was later named vitamin B_1 and later yet thiamin, when its structure was determined (1936).

Chemistry. Thiamin is an organic molecule consisting of a pyrimidine ring and a thiazole ring joined by a methylene bridge (Fig. 5). Microorganisms and plants, but not animals, can synthesize this vitamin.

Distribution and Bioavailability. Thiamin is concentrated in the outer layers of seeds. Fairly high concentrations are found in the outer layers of cereal grains, peas, beans, yeast, and animal tissues. Because of its instability at an alkaline pH and its water solubility, thiamin tends to be destroyed or removed when vegetables are cooked. The milling of cereal grains essentially strips away the vitamin through removal of the bran. As a result, wheat flour is a poor source of thiamin, whereas white bread made with enriched flour is an important dietary source. Raw fish and animal tissues contain thiaminases, both thermostabile and thermolabile, which can reduce the dietary content of thiamin.

Absorption. Thiamin is absorbed in the upper small intestine by a sodium- and ATP-dependent active transport system. Absorption is rapid as long as the intake is low (5 mg/day). At higher intake, a passive diffusion becomes increasingly important.

Transformation and Function. After absorption, thiamin is phosphorylated in the intestinal mucosa by an ATP-dependent phosphorylase; the body store of about 30 mg consists of a mixture of free thiamin and of the mono-, di-, and triphosphates. About 80 per cent is in the active diphosphate form, largely in muscle. This compound is formed from thiamin in the liver by direct transfer of diphosphate from ATP. Thiamin triphosphate may be involved in neurologic function.

Thiamin diphosphate serves as coenzyme for two general types of reactions involving cleavage of carbon-carbon bonds and the so-called "active aldehyde trans-fers." Examples are the decarboxylation of pyruvate, alpha-ketoglutarate, and the branched-chain alphaketo acids, and the transketolase reaction of the pentose phosphate pathway. In each of these reactions, the carbon-carbon bond adjacent to an alpha-keto group is cleaved, resulting in the formation of an "active" aldehyde group. This group is linked to the second carbon of the thiazole ring, and it is subsequently transferred to coenzyme A.

Transport and Storage. Thiamin is distributed widely throughout the body and is present in all tissues, with highest concentrations in the heart, liver, and kidneys. The body has a limited ability to store the vitamin, and when intake is inadequate, tissue stores are rapidly depleted.

Degradation and Excretion. Thiamin is either excreted in the urine intact or degraded to its pyrimidine and thiazole moieties.

Requirement. The MDR of thiamin is estimated at 0.27 to 0.33 mg/1000 Kcal, and the RDA is 0.5 mg/1000 Kcal of diet. The requirement, however, varies with physical activity and with the amount and composition of the diet. Intake of proteins and lipids decreases the requirement, whereas ingestion of carbohydrates increases it.

Deficiency Syndrome. The absence of thiamin in the diet leads to several deficiency syndromes with various combinations of cardiac, peripheral, and central neurologic components: beriberi (dry and wet), alcoholic polyneuritis, Wernicke's encephalopathy, and the Korsakoff syndrome. Beriberi is generally found in the Orient, where the diet is based on polished rice. In Asia, dietary thiaminases have also been incriminated as precipitating factors. In the Western world, thiamin deficiency is found most often in chronic alcoholics, who may not absorb the vitamin because of folate deficiency. Some evidence suggests genetic polymorphism of transketolase; a form with relatively lower affinity for thiamin diphosphate may predispose to clinical beriberi.

In "dry beriberi," peripheral neuritis develops, with resultant muscle wasting. When cardiac enlargement and congestive heart failure are involved, the generalized edema may obscure the muscle wasting ("wet beriberi"). There tends to be high-output cardiac failure with peripheral vasodilatation, causing the edematous extremities to be erythematous and warm. The central neurologic lesions of thiamin deficiency in both

Vitamin B_1

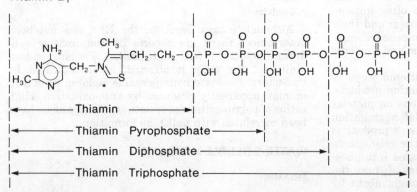

Figure 5. Structure of thiamin (vitamin B_1).

* functional site

humans and pigeons involve tissues close to the third and fourth ventricles of the brain.

Laboratory manifestations of thiamin deficiency are (1) reduced erythrocyte transketolase activity, which is abnormally stimulated by the addition of thiamin diphosphate and (2) subnormal urinary excretion of thiamin metabolites.

Several congenital metabolic errors respond to megadoses of thiamin and represent genetic increases in thiamin requirement: thiamin-responsive megaloblastic anemia (mechanism unknown); thiamin-responsive lactic acidosis (subnormal activity of hepatic pyruvic decarboxylase); thiamin-responsive branched-chain ketoaciduria (low activity of branched-chain keto-acid dehydrogenase); and intermittent cerebellar ataxia (abnormal pyruvic dehydrogenase).

Toxicity. Only isolated instances of toxicity have been reported for thiamin and apparently result from hypersensitivity.

NIACIN

In a classic study conducted by Dr. Joseph Goldberger and his colleagues on the widespread disease pellagra, a function for niacin was found. Prison inmates fed a corn diet developed pellagra; Goldberger cured the pellagra by enriching the diet with animal protein. Dr. Goldberger then fed deficient diets to dogs and produced "black tongue," the canine equivalent of pellagra. Addition of liver to the diet cured the disease. The substance that cured black tongue was later shown to be nicotinic acid, with nicotinamide being equally effective. The term niacin encompasses both forms of the vitamin.

Chemistry. Nicotinic acid (pyridine-3-carboxylic acid) is easily converted into nicotinamide (Fig. 6). Both compounds are soluble in water and stable in solution at temperatures less than 120° C. Nicotinic acid is the form found most often naturally.

Distribution and Bioavailability. The main food sources for niacin—liver, meat, whole-grain cereals, and fish—contain the vitamin mainly as nicotinamide adenine dinucleotide (NAD$^+$) and nicotinamide adenine dinucleotide phosphate (NADP$^+$). Niacin can be synthesized from tryptophan; thus tryptophan must be taken into account when calculating amounts of niacin available in a particular diet. A portion of dietary niacin is protein bound and ordinarily not available for absorption. Because the metabolic conversion of tryptophan to niacin is inhibited by leucine, the pellagragenic effect of a particular diet is enhanced by its leucine content; those species of corn with a higher leucine-tryptophan ratio are more pellagragenic.

Absorption. Both nicotinic acid and nicotinamide are readily absorbed by all portions of the small intestine.

Transformation and Function. In the liver, tryptophan is converted into nicotinic acid and then into nicotinamide. The latter compound reacts with 5-phosphoribosyl-1-pyrophosphate to form nicotinamide mononucleotide; successive reactions with ATP then yield NAD$^+$ and NADP$^+$ (Fig. 6). The nicotinamide moiety in NAD$^+$ or NADP$^+$ is utilized by numerous oxidoreductases throughout the body. The enzymes can catalyze alcohols to aldehydes or ketones, aldehydes to acids, and certain amino acids to their keto-analogues.

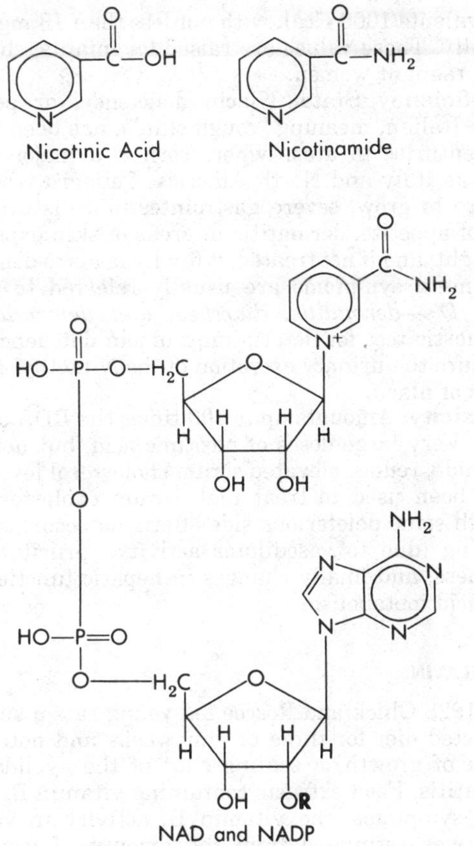

Figure 6. Structure of nicotinic acid, nicotinamide, NAD, and NADP.

There is a common mechanism for all these reactions: *First* a hydride ion is transferred from the substrate to the pyridine ring of the nucleotide coenzyme; and *second,* the hydronium ion from the oxidized substrate is removed simultaneously as a proton and exchanges as hydronium ion. Most oxidoreductases utilizing NAD$^+$ or NADP$^+$ function in a reversible fashion.

NAD$^+$ functions as the coenzyme for alcohol dehydrogenase, glycerol phosphate dehydrogenase, lactic dehydrogenase, and glyceraldehyde-3-phosphate dehydrogenase. Either NADP$^+$ or NAD$^+$ can act as a coenzyme for isocitric dehydrogenase and glutamic dehydrogenase. NADP$^+$ is coenzyme for malic enzyme and glucose-6-phosphate dehydrogenase.

Transport, Degradation, and Excretion. Nicotinamide and nicotinic acid can be transported in the circulation to the various tissues where the formation of NAD$^+$ occurs. The principal route of metabolism of nicotinic acid and nicotinamide is by the formation of *N*-methylnicotinamide, which is metabolized to pyridones. The main urinary metabolites of niacin are *N*-methylnicotinamide, the pyridones, and nicotinuric acid.

Requirement. The dietary requirements for niacin can be satisfied by nicotinic acid, nicotinamide, or tryptophan. Sixty mg of tryptophan can be converted into 1 mg of niacin. To provide for this conversion, "niacin-equivalent," a term that includes all three sources, is used. In general, the MDR is 4.4 mg niacin-equivalents/1000 Kcal and the RDA is 6.6 mg niacin-equivalents/1000 Kcal, with not less than 13 mg taken in daily. These values are raised for infants, children, and pregnant women.

Deficiency State. Niacin deficiency, or pellagra (from Italian, meaning "rough skin"), has been known for centuries in areas where corn is a major staple, such as Italy and North America. Pellagra results in failure to grow, severe gastrointestinal disturbances, loss of appetite, dermatitis in areas of skin exposed to sunlight; and if not treated, it finally leads to dementia. The main symptoms are usually referred to as the *three D's—dermatitis, diarrhea, and dementia.* The diagnostic test for determining niacin deficiency is to measure the urinary excretion of the *N*-methyl metabolites of niacin.

Toxicity. Amounts up to 100 times the RDA are not toxic. Very large doses of nicotinic acid, but not nicotinamide, reduce elevated serum cholesterol levels and have been used to treat high serum cholesterol, although some deleterious side effects do occur, such as flushing (due to vasodilator activity), pruritus, nervousness, and finally changes in hepatic function and uric acid metabolism.

RIBOFLAVIN

In 1928 Chick and Roscoe fed young rats a suitably restricted diet for three or four weeks and noted cessation of growth, a sealing shut of the eyelids, and dermatitis. Food extracts containing vitamin B_2 cured these symptoms; the vitamin B_2 activity in various foods was estimated from the amount of food that would produce a weight gain of 10 to 12 g/week. Concentration of the vitamin B_2 activity led to heat-stable preparations with yellow pigmentation. In 1932

Warburg and Christian described a yellow oxidation coenzyme in yeast. This factor was identified as a ribose derivative of riboflavin. The latter compound was then shown to be highly active in the Chick-Roscoe rat assay and proved to be vitamin B_2.

Chemistry. Riboflavin contains isoalloxazine and *D*-ribose. It is a yellowish, fluorescent compound that is widely present in naturally occurring flavins. Flavin mononucleotide (FMN) and flavin-adenine dinucleotide (FAD) are the major forms of the cofactor (Fig. 7).

Distribution and Bioavailability. Dairy products and organ meats are excellent sources of riboflavin. Other rich sources are eggs, green leafy vegetables, yeast, and wheat germ. Cereals are poor sources. The amount of riboflavin in milk is reduced by irradiation carried out to increase vitamin D content.

Absorption. The noncovalently bound coenzymes FAD and FMN are released by gastric acidification. Nonspecific pyrophosphatase and phosphatase act on the coenzymes in the upper gut. Covalently attached riboflavin is also released by these enzymes after proteolysis. Free riboflavin is primarily absorbed in the proximal small intestine by a transport system saturable by about 25 mg of riboflavin. Bile salts appear to facilitate riboflavin uptake.

Transformation and Function. Conversion of riboflavin to coenzymes occurs in the cellular cytoplasm of most tissues and primarily in the small intestine, liver, heart, and kidney. Flavoxinase catalyzes the phosphorylation of riboflavin to flavin mononucleotide (FMN) by ATP. FMN may function in several flavoproteins, or it may be further adenylated by ATP, under the influence of FAD synthetase, to flavin-adenine dinucleotide (FAD). The biosynthesis of FMN and FAD is stimulated by thyroxin and triiodothyron-

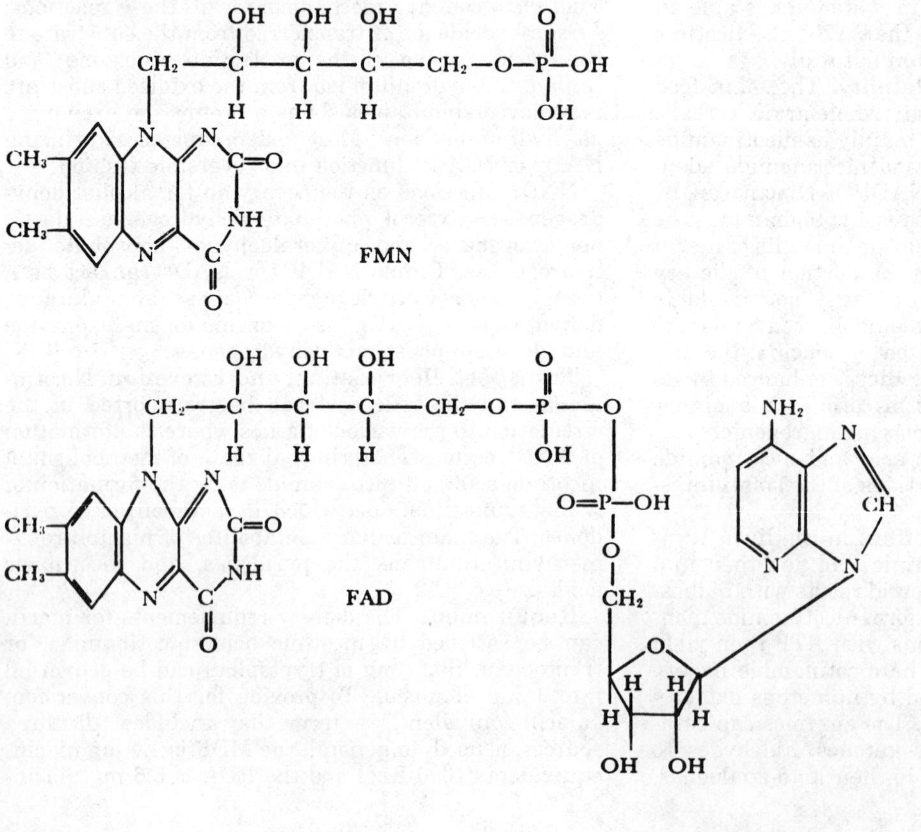

Figure 7. Structure of flavin mononucleotide (FMN) and flavin adenine dinucleotide (FAD).

ine and inhibited by chlorpromazine and tricyclic antidepressants.

FMN and FAD are utilized in energy production via the respiratory chain and in many metabolic pathways, including the Krebs cycle, beta-oxidation of fatty acids, oxidative phosphorylation, purine catabolism, oxidative deamination of amino acids, and reduction of O_2 to hydrogen peroxide. All of these pathways utilize the oxidation-reduction properties of the riboflavin coenzymes. The oxidation-reduction processes can take place via a one-electron transfer in which oxidized quinone of flavin is half reduced to a radical semiquinone and a two-electron transfer in which quinone is converted to hydroquinone.

Transport and Storage. Water-soluble riboflavin is transported freely in plasma. Tissue concentrations are low and little is stored.

Degradation and Excretion. Since there is little storage of riboflavin, urinary excretion reflects dietary intake. Smaller amounts of side-chain degradation products are also excreted and may largely result from intestinal microorganisms. Any riboflavin in the feces probably is synthesized by intestinal bacteria and is not absorbed.

Requirement. Riboflavin requirements are based on the relationship of dietary intake to overt signs of hyporiboflavinosis. The assessment of riboflavin nutriture has been primarily based on urinary excretion, the relationship of dietary intake to the production of signs of ariboflavinosis, red cell riboflavin, and, more recently, erythrocyte glutathione reductase activity. Riboflavin requirements are computed as 0.6 mg/1000 Kcal for people of all ages. However, a minimum intake of 1.2 mg/day is suggested for all people whose caloric intake is below 2000 Kcal. The RDA for women over age 22 is, therefore, 1.2 mg/day, and 1.6 mg/day is suggested for men over 22.

Deficiency State. CAUSES. Riboflavin deficiency is usually accompanied by other vitamin deficiencies; it is frequently present in randomly selected hospital patients, in the poor, and in alcoholics.

SIGNS AND SYMPTOMS. The usual first symptom of riboflavin deficiency is angular stomatitis, or fissures at the corners of the mouth. Other symptoms of riboflavin deficiency are sore throat; glossitis; cheilosis; dermatitis; normochromic, normocytic anemia; neuropathy; and visual problems ranging from corneal vascularization to opacities and corneal ulceration. Oral supplements of 5 to 10 mg riboflavin/day correct deficiency symptoms.

DIAGNOSTIC TESTS. Assessment of the adequacy of riboflavin stores is made by correlating dietary history with clinical and laboratory findings. Excretion of less than 50 µg riboflavin/day (normally greater than 120 µg) is indicative of a deficiency. Urinary riboflavin is measured both fluorometrically and microbiologically. The use of antibiotics and phenothiazines can increase urinary riboflavin. A decrease in red blood cell glutathione reductase activity also correlates with riboflavin deficiency. Other tests to evaluate riboflavin status include load tests and measurement of red blood cell riboflavin concentration.

Toxicity. Toxic effects of riboflavin have not been described.

PYRIDOXINE

Pyridoxine, or vitamin B_6, was originally delineated by Szent-Györgyi in 1934 as the unknown dietary factor that would, when added back into the restricted diet, prevent skin lesions in the rat. Pyridoxine was isolated and synthesized in 1938, and pyridoxal and pyridoxamine, the naturally occurring alternative forms of vitameric B_6, were identified in 1945.

Chemistry. The three forms of vitamin B_6—pyridoxine, pyridoxal, and pyridoxamine—differ only in their constituents on carbon 4 of the substituted pyridine nucleus (Fig. 8). Pyridoxine is a primary alcohol, pyridoxal is the aldehyde, and pyridoxamine contains an aminomethyl group. All three forms are readily utilized by humans. Pyridoxine is water soluble and stable to heat and acidic solutions but is unstable in alkaline solutions.

Distribution and Bioavailability. All three forms of vitamin B_6 are found in foods. Pyridoxine is found predominantly in plants, whereas pyridoxamine and pyridoxal are the principal forms found in animal tissues. The best sources for B_6 are whole grains, yeast, wheat germs, legumes, oatmeal, and potatoes. Pork and glandular meats, especially liver, are also good sources. Some B_6 is present in milk, eggs, vegetables, and fruits. (Cooking or processing may destroy up to 50 per cent of B_6 activity.) There is probably also some gut synthesis of B_6 by intestinal flora.

Absorption. Pyridoxine is rapidly absorbed by passive diffusion, in a relatively unlimited manner, in the upper small intestine.

Transformation and Function. The active form of vitamin B_6 is the coenzyme pyridoxal phosphate (PLP) (Fig. 8). By the actions of an oxidase and an ATP-dependent kinase, all three forms of B_6 are converted to PLP. PLP functions as a coenzyme in a large number of reactions involved in metabolism of proteins, carbohydrates, and lipids. Enzymes that require PLP as coenzyme include transaminases, decarboxylases, racemases, desulfhydrases, synthetases, amine oxidases, deaminases, dehydrases, and hydroxylases. The following types of reactions in amino acid metabolism are catalyzed by PLP-dependent enzymes: (1) replacement of substituents on alpha-carbon atoms (e.g., cleavage

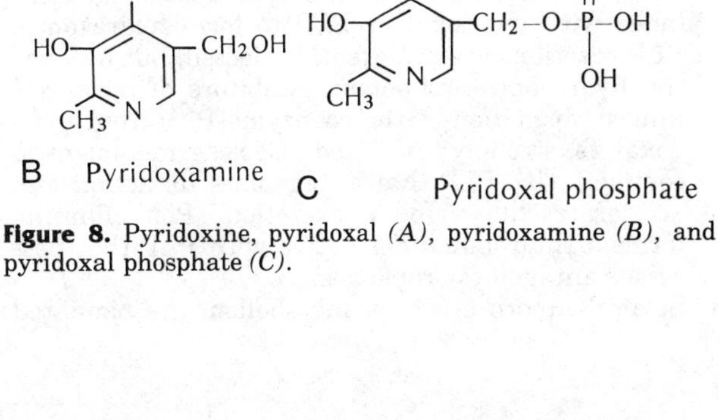

Figure 8. Pyridoxine, pyridoxal (A), pyridoxamine (B), and pyridoxal phosphate (C).

of C—N, C—H, and C—C bonds); (2) replacement of substituents, on beta-carbon atoms (e.g., cleavage of alpha-C—H and beta-C—Y bonds where Y is a polar substituent, and cleavage of beta—C and Y—C bonds); and (3) replacement of substituents on gamma-carbon atoms (e.g., cleavage of gamma C—X and beta-C—H bonds).

A common mechanism for all the reactions is the formation of a Schiff base between the aldehyde moiety of PLP and the amino group of an amino acid. This process weakens all bonds of the alpha carbon of the amino acid and facilitates its cleavage by the enzyme.

A general reaction involving PLP appears to occur in all enzymatic conversions requiring this coenzyme. PLP is tightly bound to the epsilon-amino group of lysine of the apoenzyme molecules, thus forming a Schiff base.

Transport and Storage. Most of the plasma PLP is bound to albumin. A substantial proportion of the body's vitamin B_6 is bound to glycogen phosphorylase in liver and muscle; the vitamin appears to stabilize the structure of the enzyme.

Degradation and Excretion. PLP is cleaved by a phosphatase to pyridoxal, which is then oxidized to 4-pyridoxic acid, the principal urinary excretory product. Also excreted in the urine are pyridoxal, pyridoxamine, PLP, pyridoxamine phosphate, and traces of pyridoxine.

Requirement. The MDR for vitamin B_6 increases as the amount of dietary protein increases. The MDR for an average adult is 1.5 mg/day based on an intake of 100 g protein/day. The RDA for B_6 is 2.0 mg/day for women, with greater requirements during pregnancy and lactation. For men, the RDA is 2.2 mg/day.

Deficiency Syndrome. A vitamin B_6 deficiency syndrome has been produced experimentally in humans and other mammalian species by a low-B_6 diet and sometimes with addition of the B_6 antagonist, 4-deoxypyridoxine. The deficiency syndrome includes growth failure or weight loss, skin lesions, stomatitis, anemia, peripheral neuropathy, and abnormal electroencephalogram (EEG), sometimes with convulsions. Demyelinating lesions are found in the peripheral and central nervous systems. There is also increased synthesis and urinary excretion of oxalate.

Because B_6 is so widely distributed in food groups, B_6 deficiency in the United States is usually secondary, or conditioned. An exception is infantile B_6 deficiency caused by lack of the vitamin in processed foods. Some conditioning factors that can raise the MDR are the folowing.

1. In alcoholics, excessively rapid metabolic clearance of PLP occurs.
2. Nutrient-drug interactions can raise the MDR. The antituberculous drug isoniazid, a hydrazine, combines with pyridoxal or PLP to form hydrazones. PLP reactions are not greatly affected, but because the hydrazones are potent inhibitors of pyridoxal kinase, formation of the coenzyme PLP from pyridoxal is strongly inhibited. Cycloserine forms a complex with PLP that antagonizes its action and accelerates its urinary excretion. Penicillamine forms a thiazolidine derivative with PLP that possesses antagonist properties.
3. Several inborn errors of metabolism are benefited

by pharmacologic doses of vitamin B_6 because of an abnormal structure of an apoenzyme that utilizes B_6 as a cofactor. The result is a 100 to 1000 times increase in the MDR:

a. Some infants with convulsions respond to megadoses of B_6. The apoenzyme for glutamic acid decarboxylase apparently is abnormal and has a decreased binding affinity for PLP. The consequence is a deficiency of gamma-aminobutyric acid, a physiologic inhibitor of neural activity in the brain.

b. Pyridoxine-responsive chronic anemia has been reported; the biochemical mechanism is not certain but may relate to the synthesis of delta-aminolevulinic acid in the biosynthetic pathway for heme.

c. Homocystinuria and cystathioninuria result from genetic abnormalities in the enzymes responsible for the synthesis and cleavage of cystathionine, respectively. Although homocystinuria shows little or no response to B_6, cystathioninuria is frequently improved remarkably in response to megadoses.

d. One variety of congenital xanthurenic aciduria reflects an altered enzyme, the activity of which can be enhanced by megadoses of B_6.

e. The synthesis and excretion of oxalate in primary hyperoxaluria may be reduced by large amounts of pyridoxine.

Laboratory Tests for the Diagnosis of the B_6-Deficient State. In vitamin B_6 deficiency, urinary excretion of the tryptophan metabolite xanthurenic acid is increased after tryptophan loading. In analogous fashion, urinary cystathionine excretion is abnormally large after administration of a methionine load test. Erythrocyte transaminase activity declines with inadequate intake of B_6 and is stimulated by added PLP. Finally, plasma levels of PLP and the urinary excretion of B_6 and 4-pyridoxic acid are reduced.

Toxicity. Sensory neuropathy has been reported to follow high levels of pyridoxine consumption—2 to 6 g/day, or 1000 to 2700 times the RDA, for 2 to 40 months.

FOLIC ACID

Folic acid was first recognized as a required nutrient in the work of Dr. Lucy Wills in 1931 in Bombay, India. A macrocytic anemia, present in a group of her pregnant patients, was found to be simulated in monkeys fed a diet similar to that of her patients. The disease could be cured with an autolysed yeast extract and crude liver extract, which had also proved effective in pernicious anemia. Purified liver extract was ineffective because the "Wills factor" was lost in purification of the anti–pernicious anemia factor. Folic acid, a factor isolated from foliage that is essential to the growth of *Lactobacillus casei*, was later shown to be identical to the Wills factor.

Chemistry. The folate molecule is composed of a substituted pteridine ring covalently linked to p-aminobenzoic acid and glutamic acid residues (Fig. 9). The basic structure may be varied at any of the three places labeled R_1, R_2, and R_3, and the number of glutamyl residues that can be substituted at position R_1 also

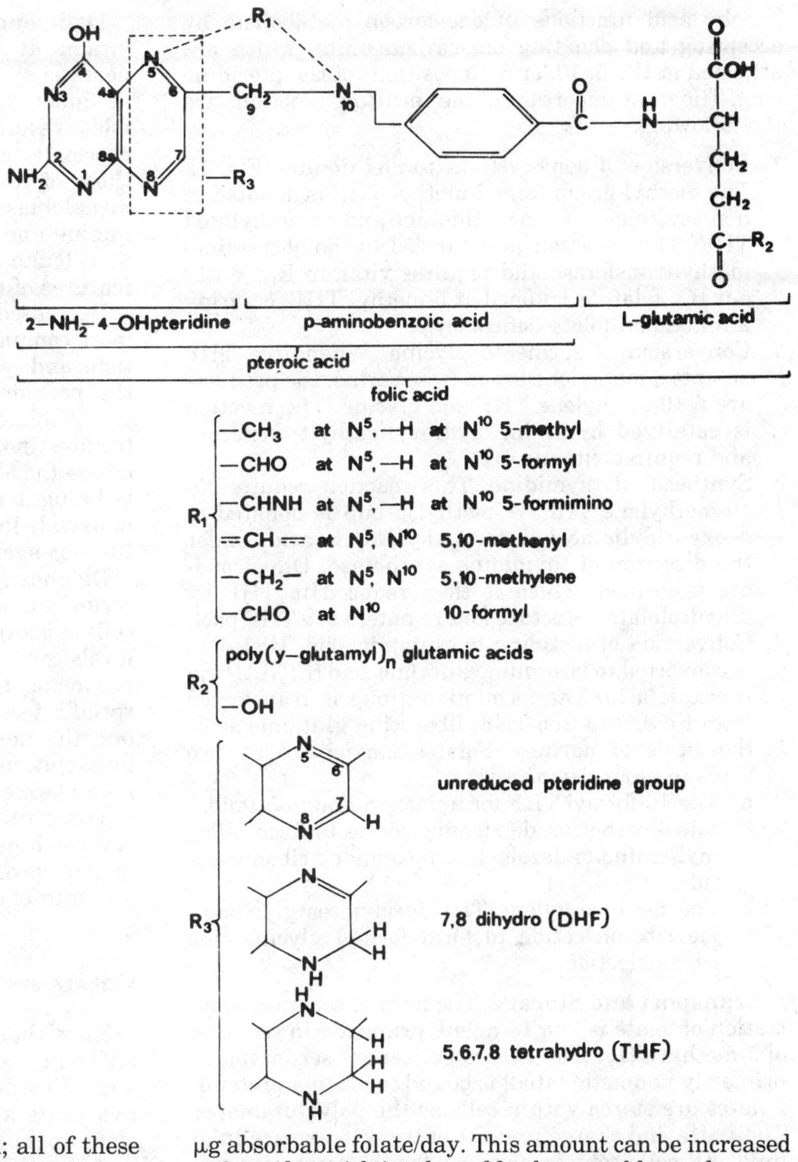

Figure 9. Schematic representation of the structure of folic acid and its derivatives.

varies. Up to seven residues can be found; all of these except one are cleaved during intestinal absorption. Three different states of reduction of the pyrazine ring of the pteridine moiety, shown as R_2, can be found. Two of these forms are found in the body: dihydrofolate (DHF), in which the 7—8 bond of the pteridine moiety is reduced; and tetrahydrofolate (THF), in which the 5—6 and 7—8 bonds are reduced. Six different one-carbon groups can substitute on the positions labeled R_1. These include 10-formyl; 5,10-methenyl; 5,10-methylene; and 5-methyl THF; all function physiologically as carriers of one-carbon units.

Folic acid is relatively stable above pH 5.0, and little destruction occurs at 100° C for an hour. The tri- and heptaglutamates, however, are much less stable in heat. Folic acid is stabilized by reducing agents such as ascorbate, and its destruction is catalyzed by copper.

Distribution and Bioavailability. Folates are essential to life and are found in all living systems, including viruses and bacteria. They occur naturally as the polyglutamates. Particularly good dietary sources include liver, yeast, fresh green vegetables, and some fruits. A standard diet can provide 50 to 500 µg absorbable folate/day. This amount can be increased to 2 mg/day with intakes of fresh vegetables and meats. Prolonged cooking of food, however, can destroy up to 90 per cent of the folate.

Absorption. Most of the folates present in food are in polyglutamate linkages. Before absorption can occur, the excess glutamates must be removed by conjugases present both on the brush border surface and within lysosomes of mucosal cells. The monoglutamate is absorbed primarily from the upper one third of the small intestine. When ingested alone, 90 per cent of the monoglutamate is absorbed; absorption of folate in foods is less efficient because some foods (yeast and beans) contain unidentified substances that limit absorption through inhibition of conjugases and folate transport.

Transformation and Function. Once the monoglutamate is absorbed, it is promptly reduced and methylated by enzymes present in the duodenum and jejunum. THF is the predominant form found in plasma, liver, and food sources. Plasma folate is largely monoglutamate, whereas intracellular folate is mostly polyglutamate.

Folic acid functions in one-carbon metabolism by accepting and donating one-carbon units, which are attached at the 5, 10, or 5-10 positions of the pteridine ring. The most important of the resulting reactions are the following:

1. Conversion of homocysteine to methionine (Fig. 1). The methyl group from 5-methyl THF is donated to homocysteine to form methionine and unmethylated THF. This reaction is catalyzed by homocysteine-methyltransferase and requires vitamin B_{12}. Without B_{12}, folate is trapped at 5-methyl THF, creating a functional folate deficiency.
2. Conversion of serine to glycine. When free THF accepts a methylene group from serine, the products are 5-10-methylene THF and glycine. The reaction is catalyzed by serine hydroxylmethyltransferase and requires vitamin B_6.
3. Synthesis of thymidine. This reaction requires 5-10-methylene THF. A methyl group is donated to deoxyuridylic acid to form thymidylic acid, under the direction of thymidine synthetase. Dihydrofolate is formed, which is then reduced to THF by dihydrofolate reductase and re-enters the THF pool.
4. Conversion of histidine to glutamic acid. Histidine is converted to formiminoglutamic acid (FIGLU) via urocanic acid. The formimino group is transferred from FIGLU to free THF, liberating glutamic acid.
5. Synthesis of purines. Folates participate at two steps in purine synthesis:
   a. The 10-formyl THF formylates 5-amino-5-imidazole-4-carboxamide ribonucleotide to form 5-formyl-aminoimidazole-4-carboxamide ribonucleotide.
   b. The 5-10-methylene THF formylates glycinamide ribonucleotide to form formyl glycinamide ribonucleotide.

Transport and Storage. The normal serum concentration of folate is 7 to 16 ng/ml, primarily in the form of 5-methyl THF. Less than 5 per cent of serum folate, primarily nonmethylated, is bound to plasma proteins. Folates are stored within cells as the polyglutamates. Their size and charge prevent entry into extracellular fluid. All cells contain enzymes for the formation (polyglutamate synthetase) and hydrolysis (gamma-glutamylcarboxypeptidase) of these polyglutamates. Total body store of folate is in the range of 5 to 10 mg, about half of which is in the liver. About 100 μg of folate is excreted into the bile daily. This enterohepatic circulation is impaired by alcohol. Folate stores are depleted three to six months after cessation of intake.

Degradation and Excretion. The major breakdown product of folate found in the urine is acetamidobenzoylglutamate, formed by acetylation of the p-aminobenzoyl moiety by the liver. Ten-formylfolate is found in the urine of scorbutic patients owing to irreversible oxidation of 10-formyl THF. Normally only 1 per cent of the folate dietary intake is excreted into the urine.

Requirement. The RDA ranges from 30 to 40 μg/day for infants to 100 to 300 μg/day for children to 400 μg/day for adults. Requirements are increased by hypermetabolism (as with infections and hyperthyroidism), increased cell turnover (as with hemolytic anemia, fetal growth, and malignant tumors), and alcohol consumption, which interferes with folate utilization.

Deficiency State. Folic acid deficiency resembles vitamin B_{12} deficiency in its manifestations outside the nervous system. This is due to the trapping of folate as 5-methylfolate when B_{12} is deficient. Deficiency of folate results in megaloblastosis in all cells of the body, especially cells undergoing rapid replication, such as those of the bone marrow and alimentary tract. The megaloblastosis reflects the block in synthesis of thymidine and therefore of DNA. Retarded growth, anemia, leukopenia, and thrombocytopenia are the main features of the deficiency.

Decreased intake in times of increased need is the most common cause of folate deficiency. Other conditions and syndromes, however, can create deficiency in the presence of normal intakes. For example, functional folate deficiency occurs in B_{12} deficiency. Gastrointestinal malabsorption and alcohol ingestion decrease the absorption of folate. Drug-induced deficiency is brought about by the use of anticonvulsant, antimalarial, immunosuppressant, antibacterial, and antitumor agents.

Diagnosis is made on the basis of folate levels in serum and red blood cells. The folate level in red blood cells is more reliable because rapid increase in serum levels can occur after ingestion of a few folate-containing meals, thereby obscuring the diagnosis. Other less specific tests include the use of folacin-loading tests and the measurement of urinary excretion of formiminoglutamic acid (FIGLU), urocanic acid, or aminoimidazolecarboxamide.

Toxicity. Folic acid is considered nontoxic up to several hundred times the RDA. Oral doses over 15 mg, however, may cause convulsions; therefore, the strength of oral tablets is 1 mg or less.

COBALAMINS (VITAMIN B_{12})

More than 150 years ago, Combe and Addison described an anemia associated with gastric and neurologic disorders, with death usually occurring two to five years after onset. Successful treatment of pernicious anemia was not achieved until 1926, when Minot and Murphy showed the effectiveness of feeding whole liver (Nobel Prize, 1934). Shortly thereafter, Castle demonstrated the need for both an extrinsic, dietary factor and an intrinsic, gastric factor. The structure of isolated, crystallized vitamin B_{12} was determined by Dorothy Hodgkins using x-ray diffraction (Nobel Prize, 1964).

Chemistry. The stable pharmaceutical form of vitamin B_{12}, and the form first isolated, is cyanocobalamin. It is not the natural form of the vitamin, however. The molecule consists of two major parts, a corrin nucleus similar to heme and a nucleotide, 5,6-dimethylbenzimidazole (Fig. 10). At the center of the corrin nucleus is an atom of cobalt. The major parts of the molecule are linked by a bridge consisting of D-1-amino-2-propanol and a bond between cobalt and one of the nitrogens of the nucleotide. Also attached to the cobalt atom is one of several anionic $(R-)$ groups that distinguish the various congeners. Cobalamin is the term used to describe the molecule in the absence of an $R-$ group. In its presence, the name of the particular $R-$ group is prefixed to cobalamin.

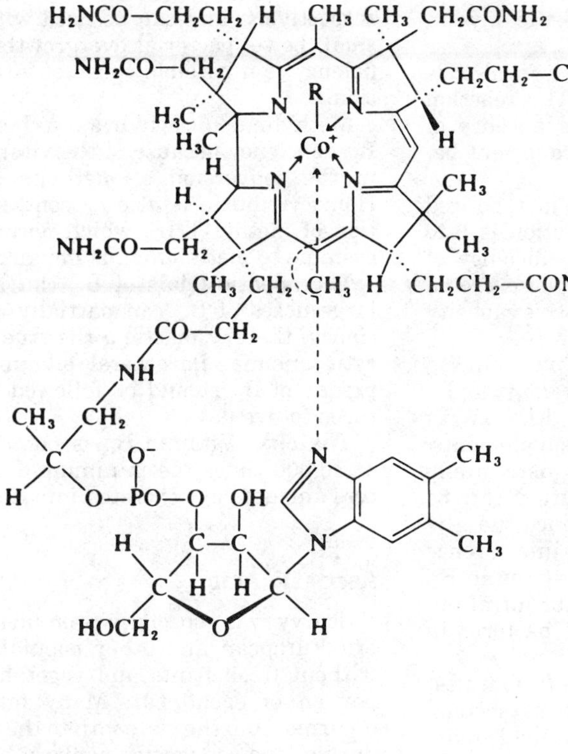

Figure 10. Vitamin B_{12}.

Substance	R
Vitamin B_{12}	—CN
Vitamin B_{12a}	—OH
Methylcobalamin	—CH_3
5'-Adenosylcobalamin (Coenzyme B_{12})	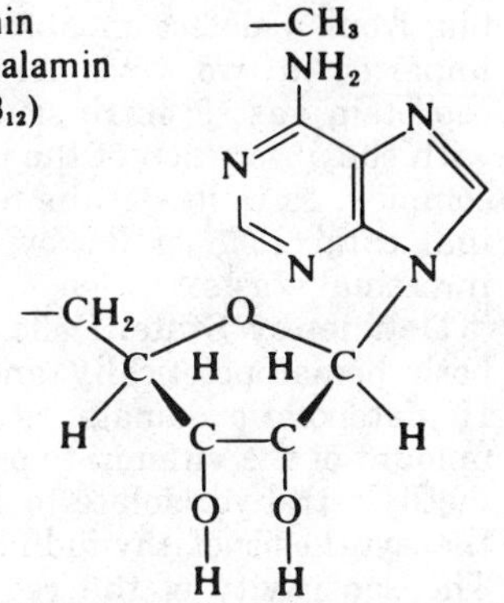 NH_2

Distribution and Bioavailability. The sole source of vitamin B_{12} in nature is synthesis by microorganisms. Plants are totally devoid of the vitamin unless contaminated by microorganisms. The usual dietary sources are the organs of domestic animals, which absorb the vitamin produced by microorganisms in the gastrointestinal tract. Vitamin B_{12} is also synthesized in the colon of humans, but it is not absorbed. Prime dietary sources include beef liver, kidney, whole milk, eggs, oysters, fresh shrimp, pork, and chicken. The average American diet supplies 7 to 30 μg of the vitamin per day.

Absorption. Vitamin B_{12} is absorbed by two mechanisms. Pharmacologically, 1 per cent of any dose of the free vitamin is absorbed by diffusion along the entire small intestine. Physiologically, a maximum of 1.5 to 3 μg of the vitamin is absorbed. The vitamin in food is released from its polypeptide linkage by gastric and intestinal enzymes and combines with the gastric intrinsic factor. Dimerization occurs, and a complex is formed consisting of two molecules of intrinsic factor and two molecules of vitamin B_{12}. The complex subsequently attaches to the brush border of the ileum. In the presence of calcium ions and a pH greater than 6.0, the complex enters the mucosa cell and B_{12} is released. It then enters the bloodstream, where it is bound by vitamin B_{12}–binding proteins.

Transport and Storage. The normal plasma concentration of vitamin B_{12} is 200 to 900 pg/ml. The vitamin is bound by three proteins in plasma, transcobalamin (TC) I, II, and III. Most of the B_{12} in plasma is bound to TC I, but it appears to be nonfunctional. Transcobalamins I and III are glycoproteins synthesized primarily by granulocytes and appear to serve a storage function. They are referred to collectively as cobalophilins. Unlike the cobalophilins, transcobalamin II is the vitamin B_{12} transport protein. It is a beta-globulin synthesized by the liver, and it delivers B_{12} to liver, bone marrow, lymphoblasts, fibroblasts, and tumor cells. It has a molecular weight of 38,000 compared with 60,000 for the cobalophilins, and it is not a glycoprotein.

The body stores of B_{12} range from 1 to 10 mg, 90 per cent of which is stored in the liver. Virtually the only loss is through excretion into bile. B_{12} is excreted into the bile and reabsorbed in the ileum with an enterohepatic circulation of 3 to 8 μg/day. The stored form of B_{12} is deoxyadenosylcobalamin, and the plasma form is methylcobalamin. Because of the efficiency of the enterohepatic circulation, B_{12} stores are not totally depleted until five to six years after cessation of intake or absorption.

Transformation and Function. In the body, vitamin B_{12} is reduced and converted to two active coenzyme forms, deoxyadenosylcobalamin and methylcobalamin. Only two metabolic pathways are known to require this cofactor.

1. 5-Deoxyadenosylcobalamin is required for hydrogen transfer and isomerization of methylmalonyl CoA to succinyl CoA. This reaction is involved in both fat and carbohydrate metabolism and may be related to

the abnormality of the lipid portion of the myelin sheath seen in B_{12} deficiency.

2. Methylcobalamin acts as coenzyme in synthesis of methionine from homocysteine (Fig. 1). This reaction also regenerates tetrahydrofolate. In the absence of B_{12}, the body becomes functionally folate deficient because folate is trapped as methyl THF.

Excretion. Vitamin B_{12} is not further metabolized in the body, and the major route of excretion is into bile. Losses at this step depend on the efficiency of reabsorption in the ileum. The vitamin is not excreted into urine until the renal tubular reabsorptive capacity has been exceeded.

Requirement. Only small amounts of vitamin B_{12} are required by the body. The MDR is 1 μg/day, and 1 to 1.5 μg is absorbed from the 3 μg/day RDA. With the exception of vegetarian diets without supplements, most deficiencies do not result from inadequate intake but from a defect in absorption. Absorption can be impaired in two ways: (1) failure to produce the glycoprotein gastric intrinsic factor and (2) interference with the absorption of the intrinsic factor–vitamin B_{12} complex, as in loss of the terminal ileum or intraluminal catabolism of B_{12} by overgrowth of bacteria in intestinal stasis.

Deficiency State. Deficiency is clinically manifest both hematopoietically and in the nervous system. Hematopoietic damage is caused by an inadequate amount of the vitamin to promote demethylation of N-methyltetrahydrofolate to THF, which is required for the synthesis of thymidine (and therefore of DNA). The sensitivity of the red blood cell to vitamin B_{12} deficiency is due to its rapid turnover rate. Vitamin B_{12} deficiency is suggested by large red blood cells (mean corpuscular volume > 95 fl) and is highly likely if the mean erythrocyte volume is > 110 fl and abnormally large numbers of segments (> 6) exist in nuclei of neutrophils. Deficiency in the nervous system can cause irreparable damage. Demyelination, cell death, and swelling of myelinated neurons are often seen.

Deficiency may be determined in several ways: (1) determination of plasma concentration of B_{12}; (2) gastric function tests; (3) excretion of methylmalonate; and (4) demonstration of reticulocytosis after a therapeutic dose of vitamin B_{12}. The simplest screening test is the serum B_{12} level, usually by a radioimmunoassay, which unfortunately has a decreasing accuracy at low levels of serum B_{12}.

The Schilling test is more sensitive for conditions that prevent proper cyanocobalamin absorption. It has four parts, of which only the first two are usually necessary: (1) The subject is given a known amount of radiolabeled vitamin B_{12} by mouth and a parenteral dose of 1 mg nonlabeled B_{12}. This saturates vitamin B_{12}–binding proteins and facilitates maximal urinary excretion of absorbed radioactive B_{12}. More than 7 per cent of the ingested radioactive cobalt should be recovered in the urine if normal absorption occurs. (2) The Schilling test is similarly repeated but with the ingested radiolabeled vitamin B_{12} attached to intrinsic factor. A normal result this time, after an abnormal result from the first part, confirms the presence of a gastric disorder causing insufficient production of intrinsic factor.

Parts three and four of the Schilling test involve treatment with antibiotics and pancreatic enzymes, respectively, and can be used with patients in whom small bowel bacterial overgrowth or pancreatic insufficiency is a possible cause of vitamin B_{12} malabsorption.

Methylmalonic aciduria is a chemical sign of vitamin B_{12} deficiency because of the vitamin's role as cofactor in the conversion of methylmalonate to succinate. Homocystinuria is also present, since the demethylation of methyl THF, which normally converts homocysteine to methionine, is impaired.

Therapeutic trials of B_{12} can be misleading, since large doses of B_{12} can partially correct a folate deficiency, thereby masking the true cause of the macrocytic anemia. Parenteral administration of 1 to 10 μg/day of B_{12} should be followed by reticulocytosis in three to five days.

Toxicity. Vitamin B_{12} is nontoxic in humans even at 10,000 times the minimum daily requirement. Excess amounts are excreted into the urine.

ASCORBIC ACID

Scurvy was especially prominent among the Northern European and other populations who had to do without fresh fruits and vegetables for a significant portion of each year. Many fatalities from scurvy occurred from the sixteenth to the eighteenth centuries during long sea-voyage explorations that deprived the crews of their nutritional requirements for the vitamin. In 1535 a dietary cure for scurvy was introduced by the Indians of Canada to Jacques Cartier with a concoction of spruce leaves. Yet it was 1747 before a systematic study by Lind, a physician of the British Royal Navy, tested the relationship of nutrition to scurvy.

Most animal species do not have a dietary need for vitamin C and cannot serve as test species. Humans, monkeys, and guinea pigs are exceptions in being unable to synthesize the vitamin. Their inability to convert gulonolactone to ascorbic acid blocks the biosynthesis of the vitamin.

Chemistry. L-Ascorbic acid, structurally related to glucose, exists in equilibrium with its oxidized form, dehydroascorbic acid, in a reversible reaction (Fig. 11). Both forms possess full nutritional activity as vitamin C. The reduction of dehydroascorbic acid to ascorbic acid is aided by glutathione in mammalian tissues.

Distribution and Bioavailability. Vitamin C exists in food primarily as ascorbic acid. Among the food groups, it is found mainly in fruits and vegetables.

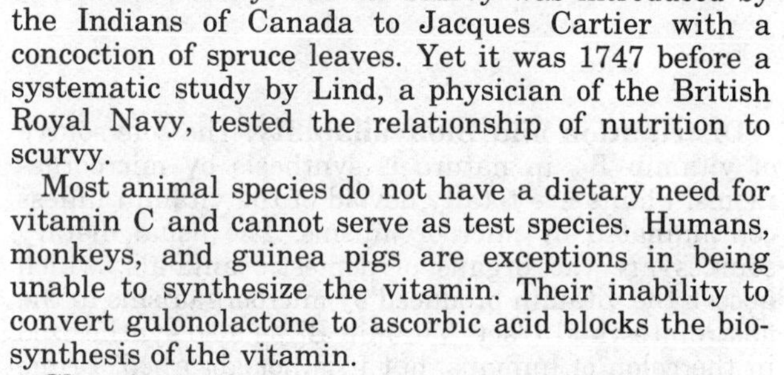

Figure 11. Ascorbic acid.

Citrus fruits, tomatoes, and green vegetables are the best sources; animal protein and grains are poor sources. Cooking and canning tend to destroy dietary vitamin C.

Absorption. The guinea pig possesses a Na^+-dependent carrier mechanism for absorbing ascorbic acid. Dehydroascorbic acid does not share this specific transport system. In humans, ascorbic acid is readily absorbed in the jejunum, in amounts exceeding 1000 times the RDA.

Function. In the tissues, ascorbic acid and dehydroascorbic acid are in equilibrium. They are essential to numerous biologic oxidation processes.

Ascorbic acid is a cofactor for hydroxylation of prolyl and lysyl residues of peptides of connective tissues (cartilage, collagen, dentin, and bone). Other major ascorbate-requiring reactions are as follows:

1. 3,4-Dihydroxyphenylethylamine → norepinephrine.
2. 4-Butyrobetaine → carnitine.
3. When large amounts of tryosine are being metabolized, ascorbic acid protects *p*-hydroxyphenylpyruvic acid oxidase from inhibition by its substrate, enabling tyrosine to continue through its pathway.
4. Tryptamine → 5 hydroxytryptamine.
5. Improved absorption of iron (as Fe^{+2}) in the gastrointestinal tract. In addition, ascorbic acid facilitates the removal of iron from ferritin, the form stored in the liver, spleen, and bone marrow.
6. Maintenance of folic acid in its reduced form.

Transport and Storage. Ascorbic acid is present in plasma and in all cells. The total body pool in normal adults is about 1.5 g to 3.0 g. The adrenal cortex and corpus luteum maintain high concentrations, apparently for steroid synthesis.

Degradation and Excretion. Two metabolites of ascorbic acid have been found in urine, oxalate and ascorbic acid-2-sulfate. Ascorbic acid is rapidly excreted when the concentration exceeds the 1.5 mg/dl plasma renal threshold.

Requirement. Thirty mg/day is the generally accepted MDR, and 60 mg/day is the RDA. Stress, infection, surgery, and pregnancy raise the RDA two- to three-fold.

Deficiency Syndrome. Infants are at risk because processed milk formulas have inadequate vitamin C content. Elderly adults living alone, rarely eating fresh vegetables and fruit, are also a vulnerable group. Deficiencies result in scurvy, a disease state characterized by a degeneration of collagenous tissues with clinical symptoms of stomatitis, glossitis, and petechiae. The abnormality in collagen synthesis is believed to cause weakening of the capillary walls, leading to bleeding, as well as poor wound healing and pathologic changes in the teeth, gums, bones, and joints. In scurvy, an abnormal collagen, deficient in hydroxyproline and hydroxylysine, is formed. Chemical tests revealing subnormal levels of ascorbic acid in plasma and in leukocytes and subnormal urinary excretion of the vitamin after an oral load confirm the presence of the deficiency state. The anemia of scurvy may reflect loss of the effects of ascorbic acid in releasing stored iron from ferritin and in folate metabolism.

Toxicity. There is very little, if any, toxicity with huge doses (a few grams or more per day) of this water-soluble, quickly metabolized, and rapidly excreted vitamin. Some patients exhibit increased urinary excretion of oxalate, however.

BIOTIN

The discovery of biotin, a water-soluble vitamin of the B complex, was the result of research in two unrelated areas: a toxic syndrome caused by raw eggs and the growth requirement of yeast. Rats fed a diet of raw egg whites as the only source of protein develop an "egg white injury" syndrome characterized by dermatitis, loss of hair, and neuromuscular disorders. The syndrome can be prevented either by cooking the egg or by administering yeast or liver extracts. In 1936 a crystalline factor essential to yeast growth was isolated from egg yolk and called biotin, from *bios* (Greek for "life"). Soon thereafter, biotin and the "anti–egg white injury factor" were demonstrated to be the same substance, and the structure of biotin as a ureido ring containing a sulfur atom and a valeric acid side chain was elucidated (Fig. 12).

Chemistry. Biotin, a compound relatively stable to heat in cooking, processing, and storage, has been isolated in at least five active forms. One of these forms, biocytin, is a covalent combination of biotin and lysine. The other forms are biotin sulfone (a potent antagonist), biotinal, and the D- and L-sulfoxides of biotin.

Distribution. Biotin is present in almost all foods, particularly those known to be good sources of the B complex vitamins, such as yeast, liver and other organ meats, grains, and some vegetables. Synthesis of biotin by microorganisms that normally inhabit the intestinal tract of animals and human beings contributes to the amount available for metabolic needs.

Absorption. Avidin, a glycoprotein found in eggs, can limit the availability of biotin by preventing its absorption from the small intestine. Denaturation of avidin, however, destroys its binding capacity.

Function. Biotin forms the prosthetic group for two types of carboxylation reactions:

1. Most mammalian biotin-requiring reactions are ATP dependent and involve cleavage of ATP to ADP and inorganic phosphate. Four enzymes have been identified: acetyl CoA carboxylase, which converts acetyl CoA to malonyl CoA and plays a role in the biosynthesis of fatty acids; beta-methylcrotonyl CoA carboxylase, which converts beta-methylcrotonyl CoA into beta-methylglutaconyl CoA in the degradation of leucine to acetoacetate; propionyl CoA carboxylase,

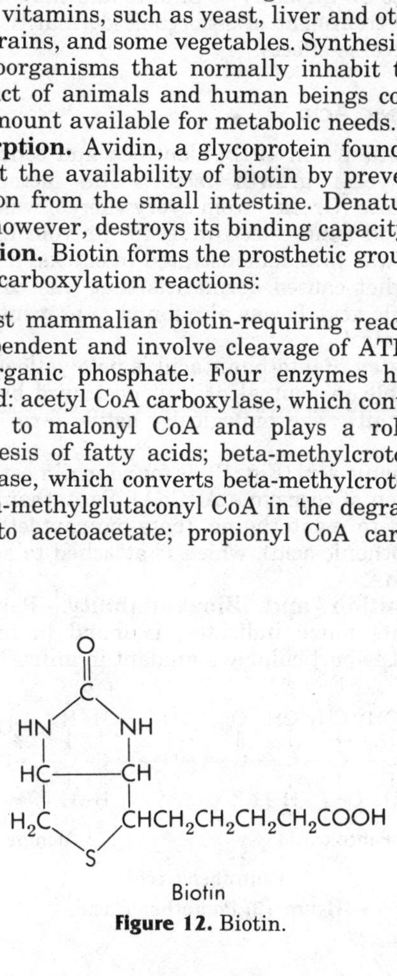

Biotin

Figure 12. Biotin.

which changes propionyl CoA to methylmalonyl CoA in the degradation of isoleucine and the oxidation of odd-numbered fatty acids; and pyruvate carboxylase, which converts pyruvate to oxaloacetate.

2. The second type of biotin-dependent reaction involves an exchange of carboxyl groups. The only known enzyme in this type is methylmalonyl CoA pyruvate carboxyltransferase.

Biotin action involves a two-step process: first, the binding of carbon dioxide to the ureido-1-nitrogen of biotin in combination with the apoenzyme and, second, the release of carbon dioxide to another substance.

Degradation and Excretion. In human urine, the principal excretory product is intact biotin, with lesser amounts of the metabolites bis-norbiotin and biotin sulfoxide.

Requirement. The body uses approximately 150 μg of biotin per day, an amount that appears to be adequately provided in most diets, even without the biotin supplied by intestinal microorganisms. Dietary intake is believed to be 100 to 300 μg daily.

Deficiency State. Biotin deficiency is rare in humans, although it can be induced. The symptoms are scaly dermatitis, graying of mucosal membranes, dry skin, depression, lassitude, muscle pains, nausea, and electrocardiogram abnormalities. Microbiologic assays with *Saccharomyces cerevisiae* and *Lactobacillus plantarum* can measure the amount of biotin present in whole blood and urine.

Toxicity. Biotin has little or no toxicity. The injection of 5 to 10 mg daily to infants less than 6 months of age for treatment of seborrheic dermatitis has not caused adverse effects.

PANTOTHENIC ACID

R.J. Williams, in 1919, identified and concentrated a novel yeast growth factor. The factor, called pantothenate (Greek, "from everywhere") was isolated in 1938 and synthesized in 1940. Its role in animal nutrition was first demonstrated in chicks, in whom a deficient diet caused dermatitis that was cured with pantothenic acid. It was also found to prevent graying in black rats.

Chemistry. Pantothenic acid, a pale yellow, viscous oil, is stable in neutral pH but destroyed by heat at any other pH. The biologically active form is the D isomer.

Pantothenic acid (Fig. 13) is found in almost all foods as a portion of coenzyme A (CoA). Pantothenic acid is converted to pantetheine (beta-mercaptoetholamine and pantothenic acid), which is attached to adenosine to form CoA.

Distribution and Bioavailability. Pantothenic acid, as its name indicates, is found in most food sources. It is particularly abundant in animal sources,

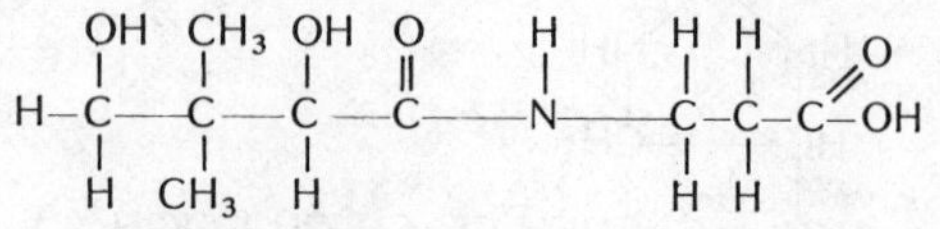

such as kidney and liver; egg yolks; legumes; whole-grain cereals; and yeast in amounts of 100 to 200 μg/g dry weight. Fair sources (35 to 100 μg/g dry weight) include broccoli, lean beef, skim milk, sweet potatoes, and molasses. Significant amounts are lost when foods are canned, cooked, frozen, or processed.

Absorption. Pantothenic acid is readily absorbed in the gastrointestinal tract. The main form found in foods, CoA, is hydrolyzed by intestinal phosphatases to pantetheine, which enters the circulation along with pantothenate.

Transformation and Function. Pantothenic acid is a major component of one of the most important catalysts of acyl transfers, coenzyme A. It is unusual in the vitamin family because it does not possess the reactive site of the coenzyme. The terminal thiol group of beta-mercaptoetholamine is the reactive site; pantothenate connects beta-mercaptoetholamine to adenosine. Through the terminal thiol group, coenzyme A forms a large number of acyl thiol esters, which are of great significance in the catabolism of lipids, carbohydrates, and ketogenic amino acids. The high energy of the thiol ester permits acylations, hydrolysis, and condensation reactions to proceed spontaneously. Pantothenic acid, as a phosphopantetheine moiety, is also a component of the acyl carrier protein, which functions during fatty acid biosynthesis to bind specific intermediates.

Transport and Storage. Eighty per cent of the vitamin, present in all tissues, is CoA; the rest is phosphopantetheine and phosphopantothenate. Circulating forms of the vitamin are pantothenate or pantetheine.

Excretion. Pantothenate is not metabolized by the body; over 70 per cent of the absorbed vitamin is excreted unchanged in the urine. CoA is degraded in the following steps: CoA → dephospho CoA → 4′ phosphopantetheine → pantothenate + cysteamine. Urinary excretion of less than 1 mg/day of pantothenate is abnormally low.

Requirement. No RDA for pantothenic acid has as yet been established. The National Research Council suggests 5 to 10 mg daily as adequate for adults, with 10 mg for pregnant and lactating women.

Deficiency State. No spontaneous, uncomplicated deficiencies of pantothenic acid occur in humans. Chronically malnourished people and poorly nourished alcoholics have low blood, urine, and serum levels, as measured by microbiologic assays. By administering a semisynthetic diet low in pantothenic acid—together with an antagonist, omega-methylpantothenic acid—a syndrome can be produced in humans characterized by fatigue, headaches, sleep disturbances, nausea, abdominal cramps, and vomiting.

Toxicity. Pantothenic acid is essentially nontoxic in humans. As much as 10 g/day has been administered with no symptoms.

FAT-SOLUBLE VITAMINS

VITAMIN A

The topical application of raw liver and the consumption of roasted liver were used as remedies for night blindness as early as 1500 BC. A cause-and-effect

Pantoic acid   β-Alanine

Pantothenic acid

Figure 13. Pantothenic acid.

relationship between the condition and the diet was suggested in the late 1800s by reports of the development of night blindness in Orthodox Russian Catholics as a result of fasting during Lent.

The discovery of vitamin A, however, was the result of observations made in an experimental setting. In 1913 it was noted that rats raised on a diet of purified protein, carbohydrate, and lard as the sole sources of fat were retarded in growth and developed xerophthalmia. The condition was correctable if butter, egg yolks, and cod liver oil were added to the diet. McCollum and Davis isolated the preventive factor from animal fats and fish oils and called it "fat-soluble A."

The isolation of the vitamin from plants resulted from the observation that vitamin A activity was associated with the pigmentation of plants. One of the pigments, carotene, was not only found to be structurally related to vitamin A but also was converted to the vitamin in vivo. Vitamin A was synthesized in 1947, and in 1967 Wald received the Nobel Prize for the elucidation of the biochemical function of the vitamin in vision.

Chemistry. Vitamin A, a primary alcohol, consists of a beta-carotene ring and a nine-membered hydrocarbon chain of alternating single and double bonds (Fig. 14). Of the number of existing isomers, the completely *trans* form predominates and is the most active. Vitamin A is insoluble in water but is soluble in fat and organic solvents. Activity is destroyed by oxidation by air or ultraviolet light, generally resulting in decarboxylation of the side chain.

The two natural forms of vitamin A are retinol (vitamin A_1), the mammalian form, and 3-dehydroretinol (vitamin A_2), the fish form. Vitamin A_2 has half the potency of vitamin A_1 in mammals. Retinol is oxidized to the aldehyde retinal and, to a lesser extent, to retinoic acid. Retinol and retinal undergo reversible interconversion, but retinoic acid is not appreciably converted to the other forms in the body. Vitamin A occurs as the provitamin in plants, in the form of the carotenoid pigments. Beta-carotene, the most common and active form, consists of two molecules of retinol attached by a double bond.

Distribution and Bioavailability. Vitamin A is found in various forms in all food groups except cereal and grains. Retinol occurs in esterified form in animal tissues, 3-dehydroretinol is present in fresh-water fish, and provitamin A is found in yellow and green fruits and vegetables. Major sources include liver, butter, cheese, whole milk, egg yolk, fish, and various yellow and green fruits and vegetables.

Absorption. Ninety per cent of the preformed vitamin A in the diet is in the form of retinol esters, usually as the palmitate. It is extensively absorbed by a carrier-mediated process in the intestinal tract. The retinol esters are hydrolyzed in the lumen of the intestine by retinyl ester hydrolase, a pancreatic enzyme. The vitamin is then absorbed into the mucosal cell in micellar form, where it is re-esterified with fatty acids and incorporated into chylomicrons.

Carotene is hydrolyzed at the central double bond in the wall of the small intestine by beta-carotene 15, 15'-dioxygenase. The reaction requires oxygen and yields two molecules of retinal. Some of the retinal is reduced to retinol and esterified. The rest is further oxidized to retinoic acid. Some of the carotene is absorbed intact, however, and excess intake can result in yellow discoloration of the skin. This condition is nontoxic and readily reversible by decreased intake.

Function. The best understood function of vitamin A is in vision. Circulating *trans*-retinol is isomerized and dehydrogenated by retinol dehydrogenase and NAD, in the cells of the retina, to 11-*cis*-retinol. This substance then reacts with the epsilon-amino group of lysine in opsin to form rhodopsin. Upon illumination, photoisomerization occurs, and all *trans*-retinol can isomerize back to 11-*cis*-retinol and once again combine with opsin, creating a vision cycle (Fig. 15).

Vitamin A participates in growth and reproduction as well. Its role in the synthesis of glycoproteins is thought to operate through donation of mannose via a retinol-phosphate-mannose glycolipid complex present in cell membranes. Vitamin A is also believed to work in association with vitamin E in the stabilization of membranes. Retinoic acid can replace retinol for growth purposes but is inactive in vision.

Transport and Storage. Retinyl esters in chylomicrons enter the bloodstream through the thoracic duct and are stored in the liver. The concentration of the vitamin in the liver is around 100 µg/g. The hepatic retinol esters are hydrolyzed, and the free retinol is associated with retinol-binding protein (RBP), an alpha$_1$-globulin. It is transported in plasma as a complex consisting of one molecule of RBP and one molecule of prealbumin. The normal body retinol pool, largely located in the liver, is 300 to 900 mg. The normal plasma concentration of vitamin A is 30 to 70 µg/dl. The plasma level of vitamin A is not proportional to liver stores and does not fall until the liver stores are depleted.

Some of the retinol released is conjugated to beta-glucuronide and excreted into bile. A small portion is reabsorbed, but most is hydrolyzed by enteric bacteria and excreted.

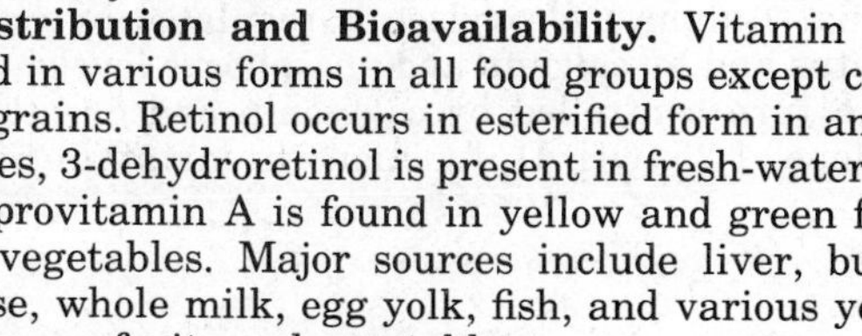

Figure 14. Vitamin A.

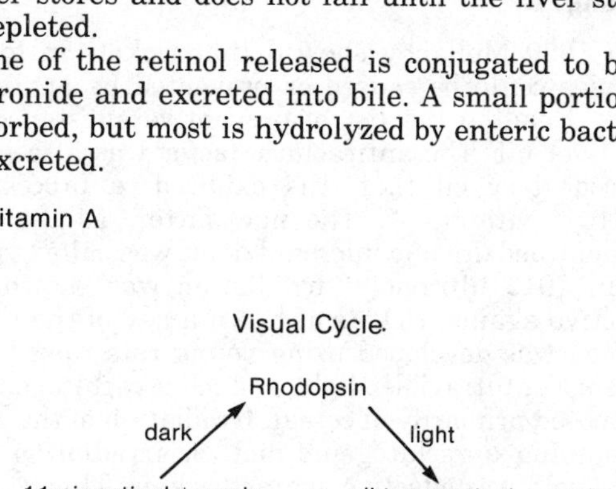

Figure 15. Visual cycle of vitamin A.

Degradation and Excretion. The main degradation pathway appears to be irreversible oxidation to retinoic acid, which is excreted in feces and urine as such or further metabolized in the liver to 5,6-epoxy-retinoic acid and retinyl beta-glucuronide and excreted. Approximately equal amounts of vitamin A catabolites are excreted in urine and in feces.

Requirement. The RDA of retinol is 4000 IU for women and 5000 IU for men. Exact requirements vary with age, growth, caloric intake, pregnancy, and lactation. Twice as much beta-carotene is needed owing to the inefficiency of its conversion to retinol.

Deficiency State. Deficiencies of vitamin A are characterized by degenerative changes in the eyes and skin. In developing nations, where green, leafy vegetables and other sources of the vitamin are lacking, vitamin A deficiency is still the major cause of blindness. In advanced liver disease or protein-calorie undernutrition, the liver may be unable to secrete retinol-binding protein and therefore is unable to mobilize the hepatic stores of vitamin A. In patients with gastrointestinal malabsorption, vitamin A deficiency is not uncommon.

The first sign of vitamin A deficiency is night blindness, followed by retinal degeneration and dryness of the conjunctivae (xerosis). These changes can be totally reversed with vitamin A treatment. However, in later stages, necrosis of the cornea occurs and may lead to blindness. Hyperkeratosis of the skin is also present.

The most definitive demonstration of vitamin A deficiency depends on accurate measurements of adaptation to darkness and of retinal function by electroretinography. Hepatic content of vitamin A is depleted, but serum concentration may still be normal.

Toxicity. Ingestion of 10 or more times the RDA will eventually lead to chronic toxicity in many individuals, characterized by discomfort in the extremities, skin dryness, loss of hair, anorexia and weight loss, intracranial hypertension, and hepatic enlargement. Serum vitamin A is then elevated, and the excess retinol esters are transported by lipoproteins rather than by the retinol-binding protein mechanism.

VITAMIN D

In 1920 Mellanby showed that rickets in growing puppies could be caused or prevented by appropriate diets. Heading the list of preventive substances was cod liver oil. The antirachitic factor was also present in cod liver oil that was oxidized, a process that destroys vitamin A. The new factor, as the fourth unidentified organic micronutrient, was called vitamin D. In 1919 ultraviolet irradiation was shown to be effective against rickets also. An assay of the vitamin in food was developed using young rats raised in the absence of ultraviolet light and fed a rachitogenic diet composed primarily of cereal. Irradiation of the animal consuming a rachitogenic diet, or irradiation of the diet itself, was effective against rickets. This led to the discovery that vitamin D was present in provitamin form in the sterol fraction of animal and plant fats and that the provitamin form could be converted to the vitamin by irradiation. Vitamin D (the sunshine vitamin) was the name given to the first product isolated after irradiation of the plant provitamin ergosterol. It was later shown to consist of many active congeners.

Chemistry. Provitamin D occurs in two sterol forms: 7-dehydrocholesterol is the provitamin found in animal tissue, and ergosterol is the provitamin found in plants, yeast, and fungi. They differ only in that ergosterol has a double bond between carbon 22 and 23 and a methyl group at carbon 24. 7-Dehydrocholesterol and ergosterol are photochemically converted to cholecalciferol (vitamin D_3) and calciferol (vitamin D_2), respectively (Fig. 16).

Distribution and Bioavailability. Vitamin D is found in the inactive provitamin form in skin and in plants. The availability of the active vitamin D_3, produced in skin, is seasonal owing to variations in sunlight. Preformed vitamin D_3, however, is found in the liver and oils of fish, eggs, fatty fish, and butter. Plants contain no preformed active vitamin; upon irradiation, however, they are good sources of vitamin D_2. Vitamins D_2 and D_3 are equally active in humans, rats, and most other mammals, but D_2 is less active in chicks and some species of monkeys. Vitamin D_2 is the form found in commercial vitamin preparations and in irradiated bread and milk.

Vitamin D is not affected by oxidation or by temperatures below $140°$ C. In acid media the vitamins are relatively unstable, the instability increasing with a rise in temperature.

Absorption. Vitamin D is efficiently absorbed in the small intestine and initially appears in lymph bound to the chylomicron fraction. Bile is essential for adequate absorption.

Transformation and Function. Vitamin D must be further metabolized in the body to calcitriol to exert its effects. This is accomplished by two successive hydroxylations, one occurring in the liver and the other in the kidney. In the liver, D_2 and D_3 are hydroxylated at the terminal side chain to form the 25-hydroxy derivative. The hepatic enzyme involved appears to be a mixed function oxidase requiring oxygen and NADPH. The second hydroxylation, occurring at the first carbon, takes place in the kidney and is catalyzed by an enzyme complex consisting of a mixed function oxidase, cytochrome P-450, and ferredoxin. This hydroxylation also requires oxygen and NADPH.

Renal 1-alpha-hydroxylase is regulated by vitamin D status and by calcium and phosphorus levels, which are in turn controlled by calcitonin and parathyroid hormone. $1,25-(OH)_2D_3$ functions to maintain normal

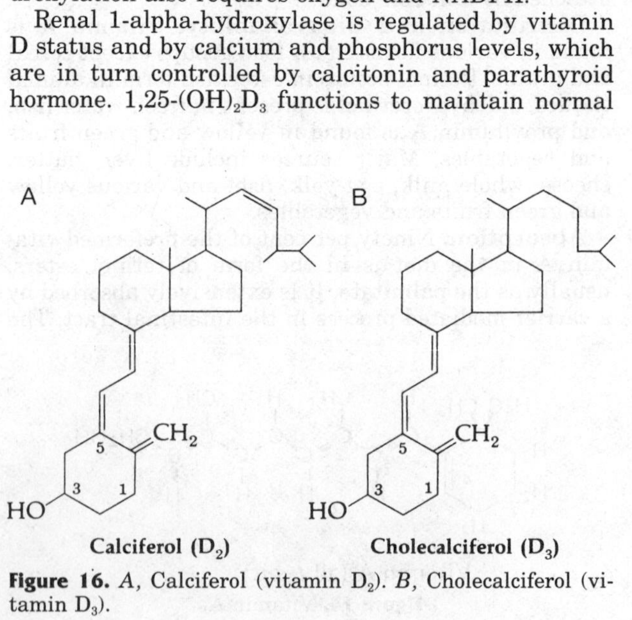

Figure 16. A, Calciferol (vitamin D_2). B, Cholecalciferol (vitamin D_3).

plasma concentrations of calcium and phosphorus by two mechanisms: facilitation of their absorption by the small intestine and enhancement of their mobilization from bone.

In the mucosal cell of the small intestine, the active vitamin binds to a cytosolic receptor protein and then enters the nucleus, where it binds to a chromatin receptor. There it acts on DNA-dependent RNA polymerase II to mediate synthesis of a calcium-binding protein and acid phosphatase.

Failure of bone mineralization in rickets is caused by inadequate absorption of calcium and phosphorus. Calcitriol promotes the mineralization of rachitic bone by enhancing the gastrointestinal absorption of both elements (see also Section IX).

Transport and Storage. Vitamin D circulates in plasma bound to a specific vitamin D–binding alpha-globulin. The globulin has the highest affinity for the 25-hydroxy derivatives. This complex constitutes the major vitamin D form in plasma and has a half-life of 19 days. The half-life of calcitriol is three to five days. Provitamin D has a plasma half-life of 19 to 25 hours but is stored for six months or longer in fat deposits throughout the body.

Degradation and Excretion. Three other metabolites of vitamin D have been identified: $1,24,25(OH)_3 D_3$; $24,25(OH)_2 D_3$; and $25, 26(OH)_2 D_3$. All are formed by a renal hydroxylase that is stimulated by calcitriol and inhibited by 1-alpha-hydroxylase stimulators. They are less active than calcitriol and are thought to represent metabolites destined for excretion. The principal route of excretion is in the bile; only a small amount appears in urine.

Requirement. An adequate daily supply of vitamin D is 400 IU. This level will promote maximum calcium absorption, is well below toxicity levels for children up to age six, and is adequate for periods of pregnancy and lactation. However, as the rate of skeletal growth and calcium need decrease, the daily requirement is reduced. One hundred IU is adequate from age seven on. In such diseases as uremic osteodystrophy and autosomal recessive vitamin D dependency, daily requirements are increased to the pharmacologic range of 1200 to 2000 IU.

Deficiency State. The deficiency state of vitamin D, resulting in rickets in children and osteomalacia in adults, is discussed in detail in Section IX.

Toxicity. Prolonged ingestion of large doses of vitamin D_2 or D_3, such as 50,000 to 100,000 IU/day, leads to a number of clinical syndromes. Some cases of toxic intake result from the administration of large doses of the vitamin to treat conditions that are wrongly purported to benefit from the vitamin. Other cases are a result of excessive doses used in the treatment of hypoparathyroidism, accidental ingestion by children, or excessive administration by their parents. Vitamin D toxicity has become more common since the highly active 1, 25-dihydroxy vitamin D preparation has become available.

Initial symptoms, which largely result from hypercalcemia, include weakness, fatigue, lassitude, headache, nausea, vomiting, and diarrhea. In infants, supravalvular aortic stenosis and mental retardation can result. Other clinical manifestations of toxicity are impaired renal function, nephrolithiasis, nephrocalcinosis, hypertension, and localized and generalized osteoporosis. The laboratory findings are hypercalcemia, hypercalciuria, and elevated serum 25-hydroxy vitamin D.

VITAMIN E

The "antisterility vitamin," vitamin E, was discovered by Evans and Bishop in 1922 as a fat-soluble factor necessary for normal pregnancy in female rats fed a high-fat diet. Rats deficient in this factor conceived normally, but fetal death and resorption occurred. It was called vitamin E but was not actually isolated from wheat germ oil until 1936.

Chemistry. Two classes of compounds make up the vitamin E group: (1) Tocopherols, from the Greek *tokos* (childbirth) and *phero* (to bring forth), derive from *tocol* containing a 16-carbon saturated isoprenoid side chain; and (2) tocotrienols, which contain a triply unsaturated side chain (Fig. 17). The active compound most often called vitamin E is alpha-tocopherol.

Distribution and Bioavailability. The most important sources of vitamin E are vegetable oils such as soybean, cottonseed, safflower, sunflower, and wheat germ oils. Olive, coconut, and peanut oils are low in vitamin E. The amount of alpha-tocopherol present is related to the percentage of linoleic acid found. Safflower oil is 80 per cent linoleate and is one of the best sources for vitamin E. An exception to this is corn oil, which contains 50 per cent linoleic acid but has about 90 per cent of the tocopherol in the gamma form, which cannot be utilized.

Function. A coenzyme function for vitamin E has not been shown. It is a strong antioxidant, and it is thought to function in protecting other nutrients such as vitamin A and polyunsaturated fatty acids from destructive oxidation. When the levels of alpha-tocopherol in the plasma are low, the erythrocyte has a decreased ability to withstand peroxidative degradation by hydrogen peroxide. This is the basis for the peroxide hemolysis test, which is most often positive if the plasma alpha-tocopherol level is below 0.5 mg/dl. There is little actual evidence, though, that vitamin E is of nutritional significance in humans. Alpha-tocopherol has a structure very similar to another potent antioxidant, coenzyme Q.

Degradation and Excretion. The urinary metabolites of vitamin E are glucuronides of tocopheronic acid and its gamma-lactone.

Requirement. A daily intake of 10 to 30 mg is sufficient to maintain plasma concentrations at a normal level. The level may vary depending on the amounts of polyunsaturated fats and other antioxidants in the diet.

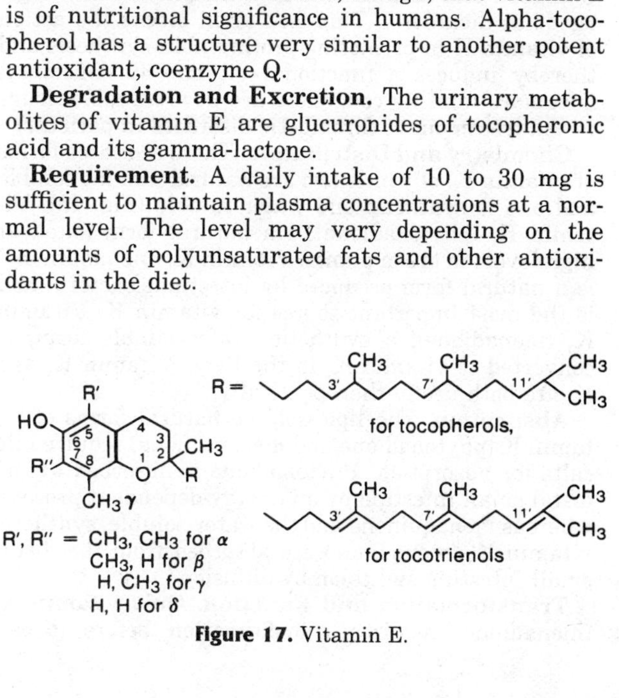

Figure 17. Vitamin E.

Deficiency State. The plasma concentration of vitamin E decreases significantly only after months on a deficient diet with no associated clinical symptoms. Deficiencies have been reported, however, in newborn infants, in association with protein-calorie malnutrition, and in some cases of fat malabsorption.

In male rats prolonged deficiency causes sterililty, and in pregnant females fetal death occurs. In many species—most notably herbivores such as rabbits, sheep, and cattle—a vitamin E deficiency can lead to muscular dystrophy, which can be prevented or reversed with one of several lipid-soluble antioxidants, including coenzyme Q.

Diagnosis is based on serum or plasma tocopherol levels and erythrocyte hemolysis tests.

Toxicity. Vitamin E has little or no toxicity in humans. Chicks given very high doses have demonstrated a number of deleterious effects, including depressed growth and interference with thyroid function, but no similar effects have been shown in humans.

Vitamin K

In 1929 Dam noticed that chickens maintained on an inadequate diet developed spontaneous bleeding, found later to be cured by an unidentified fat-soluble substance that he called vitamin K *(Koagulation)*. The substance isolated from alfalfa was called vitamin K_1 and that isolated from fish meal was called vitamin K_2.

Researchers were also studying the hemorrhagic tendency in patients with obstructive jaundice and diseases of the liver. Quick and coworkers noted in 1935 that this coagulation defect was due to a decreased amount of prothrombin. A combination of vitamin K and bile salts was found to be effective in treating hemorrhage associated with obstructive jaundice.

In 1924 Schofield noted a hemorrhagic disorder in cattle fed spoiled sweet clover, later shown to be associated with a decreased plasma prothrombin level. Campbell and Link in 1939 identified the hemorrhagic agent as dicumarol. This food toxin blocks the action of vitamin K in promoting prothrombin synthesis and thereby induces a functional vitamin K deficiency. Dicumarol and its congeners are now valuable drugs in the treatment of thrombotic disorders in patients.

Chemistry and Distribution. There are three forms of vitamin K, of which two are natural and fat soluble and one is synthetic and water soluble (Fig. 18). Vitamin K_1 (phytonadione) is a natural form found at high levels in green plants. Vitamin K_2 (menaquinone) is a natural form produced by intestinal bacteria and is the most important source for vitamin K. Vitamin K_3 (menadione), a synthetic, water-soluble form, is converted to vitamin K_2 in the liver. Vitamin K_1 and K_3 are both useful therapeutically.

Absorption. The lipid-soluble natural forms of vitamin K (phytonadione and menaquinone) require bile salts for absorption. Phytonadione is absorbed at the distal small intestine by an energy-dependent process, whereas menaquinone and the water-soluble, synthetic vitamin K_3 (menadione) are absorbed from the distal small intestine and colon by diffusion.

Transformation and Function. Only vitamin K_3 (menadione) requires transformation before it can

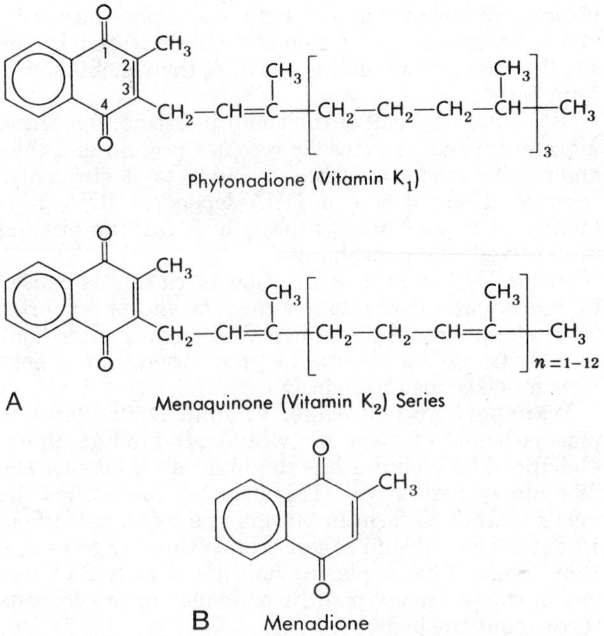

Figure 18. Structure of vitamin K, phytonadione (vitamin K_1), menaquinone (vitamin K_2) *(A)*, and menadione (vitamin K_3) *(B)*.

function. Vitamin K_3 is transported to the liver in the portal circulation and there converted to vitamin K_2.

Vitamin K carboxylates glutamic acid residues in a protein to produce gamma-carboxyglutamyl residues. The vitamin K cycle starts when the quinone is reduced by an NADH-dependent flavoprotein system to the hydroquinone. The hydroquinone can couple to oxygen and carbon dioxide and effect the gamma-carboxylation of glutamyl residues of proteins such as prothrombin. A 2,3-epoxide intermediate may be formed and subsequently reduced to the starting quinone. This final step is antagonized by the coumadin anticoagulants (dicumarol and warfarin).

Vitamin K is necessary for the hepatic biosynthesis of factors II (prothrombin), VII (proconvertin), IX (plasma thromboplastin component, or Christmas factor), and X (Stuart factor). The carboxylation enables these proteins to bind calcium ion and subsequently adhere to a phospholipid membrane. Other proteins with gamma-carboxyglutamyl residues that bind calcium are found in bone, kidney, urine, kidney stones, and blood. The synthesis of osteocalcin, found in bone, is regulated by 1,25-dihydroxy D_3 and acts through its specific binding to hydroxyapatite.

Transport and Storage. Vitamins K_1 and K_2 are transported from the intestine to the liver. Vitamin K_3 is carried to the liver in the portal circulation and there converted to vitamin K_2. Vitamin K circulates in association with beta-lipoproteins.

The small body store of vitamin K is found primarily in the liver. This supply is slowly degraded; vitamin K deficiency leads to hypoprothrombinemia in a matter of weeks.

Degradation and Excretion. Vitamin K_1 is rapidly converted to more polar metabolites, which are excreted in the bile and urine. Coumarin increases the phytonadione-2,3-epoxide form of vitamin K_1, and the degradation of this form increases total urinary excretion of vitamin K. Vitamin K_3 is excreted as glucuronide and sulfate conjugates.

Requirement. Healthy adults typically require no vitamin K in the diet, since intestinal bacteria produce adequate amounts. Neonates require vitamin K until the intestinal flora becomes established. However, in patients with gastrointestinal malabsorption or in those receiving long-term antibiotics, an intake of 70 to 1400 µg/day is suggested. This amount of vitamin K is provided by the average mixed diet, which contains 300 to 500 µg vitamin K/day. Patients experiencing hemorrhage associated with obstructive jaundice should receive 10 mg vitamin K/day.

Deficiency State. CAUSES. Deficiency of vitamin K is relatively common in the newborn because the intestinal flora is not established in the first week and mother's milk provides little vitamin K. The most serious nutritional complication of newborns is hemorrhagic disease. Approximately 1 of 400 infants born alive has some signs of hemorrhagic disease. A small prophylactic dose of 0.5 to 1 mg of vitamin K_1 is usually given parenterally to the infant at birth to prevent hemorrhagic disease.

Vitamin K supplementation for adults is required in predisposing conditions such as a starvation diet, long-term antibiotic therapy, and fat malabsorption. Coumadin anticoagulants interfere with the action of vitamin K by blocking the NADH-dependent reduction of the epoxide form to the hydroquinone form.

SIGNS AND SYMPTOMS. Vitamin K deficiency is manifested by prolonged prothrombin time, ecchymoses, epistaxis, hematuria, gastrointestinal bleeding, and operative wound bleeding. In cases of extreme deficiency, hemorrhage may affect vital structures like the brain and lead to death.

DIAGNOSTIC TESTS. Vitamin K levels can be measured both directly and indirectly. Direct methods include spectrophotometry of the extracted and chromatographed forms of vitamin K_1, colorimetry reactions involving the quinoid nucleus, and spectrophotometry of chemically reduced K. Prothrombin time is the indirect measure of vitamin K, which is the time required for plasma to clot once tissue thromboplastin, a platelet substitute, and calcium are added. For prothrombin time to increase by more than 30 seconds, the prothrombin concentration must decrease to less than 30 per cent of normal. If an oral vitamin K supplement corrects a prolonged prothrombin time, a vitamin K deficiency is confirmed. A failure to correct suggests either that the vitamin K was not absorbed or that the hypoprothrombinemia is caused by intrinsic liver disease.

Toxicity. Vitamins K_1 and K_2 are essentially nontoxic to animals. Vitamin K_3 can cause hemolysis in patients deficient in glucose 6-phosphate dehydrogenase.

TRACE ELEMENTS

IRON

Sydenham is credited with being the first to recognize that iron deficiency is the specific cause of chlorosis, an anemia that used to be prevalent in female adolescents. As early as 1713, the presence of iron in blood was demonstrated.

Distribution and Bioavailability. Iron, the fourth most abundant element, is generally found in the ferrous or ferric form because of the slow oxidation in the earth's atmosphere. Rocks and soil usually contain the ferric form in crystalline structure. This form must be made soluble by acid. Alkaline and high-phosphate environments reduce the bioavailability of iron.

In developed countries, dietary intake of iron is generally around 6 mg/1000 Kcal. Additional iron, however, may be contributed by iron cooking utensils, fermented beverages, and canned foods.

Absorption. Food contains two forms of iron, heme iron and non-heme iron. Heme iron is much more readily absorbed, and its absorption is independent of other factors present in foods. Non-heme iron is greatly affected by alkalinization, phosphates, phytates, ingested alkaline clays, or antacid preparations. Absorption is increased by ascorbic acid and by weak chelating agents such as succinic acid, sugars, and sulfur-containing amino acids. Orally administered medicinal iron is usually in the form of ferrous sulfate. The ferrous salts are absorbed about three times more efficiently than the ferric salts.

Iron is absorbed most efficiently in the upper small intestine. The relative amount is determined by internal stores. Only 5 to 10 per cent of the available iron is normally absorbed. This increases to 20 per cent in the deficient state.

Heme iron and non-heme iron are absorbed differently (Fig. 19). Heme iron must first be freed from its globin combination. Heme is absorbed intact, and the iron is removed from the heme by heme oxygenase, a heme-splitting enzyme in the mucosal cells. It is released into the plasma in a form that can be bound by transferrin. Non-heme iron is made soluble and ionized by gastric secretions and is then chelated and absorbed into mucosal cells. A portion is rapidly released into the bloodstream. The portion that exceeds transport capacity of circulating transferrin remains within the mucosal cell and combines with apoferritin. Some is later released, but most remains in the mucosal cells until the end of their two- to three-day life span.

Function. Iron serves as an electron carrier or as a ligand carrier in several non-heme and heme proteins.

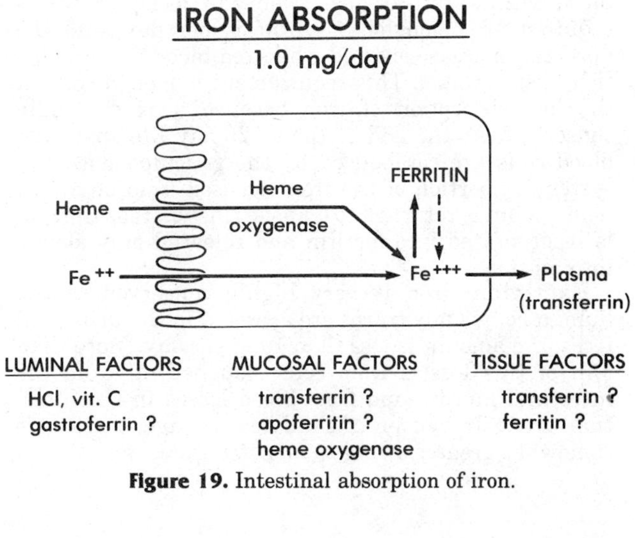

IRON ABSORPTION
1.0 mg/day

LUMINAL FACTORS	MUCOSAL FACTORS	TISSUE FACTORS
HCl, vit. C	transferrin ?	transferrin ?
gastroferrin ?	apoferritin ?	ferritin ?
	heme oxygenase	

Figure 19. Intestinal absorption of iron.

Non-heme proteins usually contain from two to eight iron atoms per molecule. Many participate in photosynthesis and nitrogen fixation reactions. In mammals, they are associated with, or are subunits of, flavin-linked dehydrogenase, such as NADH and succinate dehydrogenase, in which they act as electron acceptors. Their subsequent reduction is accompanied by bleaching of the red or pink oxidized form.

The iron in heme can function both as an electron and ligand carrier depending on the protein. Heme is a chelate linkage of iron with protoporphyrin, in which its four ligand groups form a square-planar complex with iron. In hemoglobin and myoglobin, the fifth iron position is bound to the imidazole group of histidine, and the sixth is either unoccupied or occupied by oxygen or other ligands such as carbon monoxide or cyanide. In the cytochromes, both the fifth and sixth positions are bound to specific amino acid residues of the protein. In these proteins, iron does not transport ligands but undergoes reversible changes between the ferric and ferrous forms, thereby functioning as an electron carrier.

Iron in hemoglobin and myoglobin does not undergo a valence change as oxygen is bound or lost. It is, however, oxidized to the ferric form by oxidizing agents. This oxidation is accompanied by a change in color from red to brown. In this form, iron can no longer function as a ligand carrier.

Transport and Storage. Body iron is compartmentalized into two pools, essential iron and stored iron. Essential iron amounts to 70 per cent of the total and is found in hemoglobin, myoglobin, metalloenzymes, and transferrin. The remainder is stored in ferritin and hemosiderin (an aggregated form of ferritin) in the liver and in the reticuloendothelial system. The plasma concentration of iron is 70 to 180 μg/dl. It is transported by transferrin, a beta$_1$-globulin containing two binding sites for ferric iron. Transferrin delivers iron to specific receptors on tissue membranes and accepts iron from the intestinal tract, from storage, or from hemoglobin catabolism. Stored iron is bound intracellularly to ferritin, a protein composed of 24 polypeptide subunits with a storage cavity for hydrous ferric oxide phosphate.

Eighty per cent of plasma iron is transported to bone marrow for hemoglobin synthesis. Hemoglobin contains four atoms of iron per molecule and circulates in blood within erythrocytes. Twenty to 25 mg of iron is required for hemoglobin synthesis per day, and the need can increase six-fold when red blood cell production is stimulated. This requirement is met in spite of the low absorption of iron because it is so avidly conserved. At the end of their 120-day life span, red blood cells are catabolized by the reticuloendothelial system. A portion of the iron released from degraded hemoglobin is returned to transferrin, whereas the rest is incorporated into ferritin and released only slowly into plasma.

Excretion. Iron is very highly conserved in the human body. Only traces are excreted in the urine and feces; the amount is less than 1 mg per day. More than half of this loss is from cells sloughed off from the intestinal mucosa and from blood losses in the intestinal tract. In women of child-bearing age, the loss is somewhat greater owing to menstruation.

Requirement. The amount of iron absorbed from a normal diet is approximately equal to the amount excreted per day (1 mg); thus a balance is maintained in the normal man and menopausal woman. The requirements for iron are dictated by physiologic losses and growth. Demands are greatest during infancy, pregnancy, and menstruation. Iron deficiency results from three conditions: inadequate intake, blood loss, and malabsorption. The RDA of 12 to 18 mg/day reflects the 10 per cent absorption capacity of the normal nondeficient adult.

Deficiency State. The result of severe iron deficiency is hypochromia and microcytosis of the red cells. Iron deficiency proceeds through several stages, from simple iron deficiency without anemia to the severe case of iron deficiency anemia. The natural history is as follows:

Stage I. Iron stores are depleted; iron absorption and the serum iron-binding capacity increase. At this stage, serum iron and hemoglobin levels are normal.

Stage II. The plasma iron level falls, erythropoiesis is impaired, and the amount of protoporphyrin in red blood cells increases.

Stage III. There is overt anemia characterized by hemoglobin-deficient red cells.

Diagnosis of iron deficiency is based on the evaluation of the biochemical changes that characterize each stage.

Toxicity. Large amounts of iron are toxic. Amounts from 2 to 10 g given acutely are fatal. Generally, such levels are reached by accidental ingestion of medicinal iron by children between the ages of 12 and 24 months or through suicidal attempts. Iron overload can occur, however, as a result of parenteral treatment and excessive dietary intake. An increase in tissue iron stores is known as hemosiderosis. Tissue damage caused by such increased iron storage is characteristic of the genetic disorder of excessive iron absorption, hemochromatosis. The classic abnormalities are cirrhosis, diabetes, and hyperpigmentation of the skin. Additional abnormalities are a particular form of arthritis, myocardiopathy, and anterior pituitary insufficiency.

COPPER

Distribution and Bioavailability. Dietary copper is most highly concentrated in beans, peas, and nuts, in which levels can be as high as 7 mg/kg. This source is a modest contributor to daily copper intake in Western diets, the majority coming from meat, poultry, and potatoes and other vegetables. A notably poor source of copper is milk and milk products. Copper in ingested food is probably hydrolyzed in the stomach in order to become available for absorption.

Absorption. Estimates of efficiency of absorption range from 25 to 60 per cent. Zinc is probably competitive for binding sites in intestinal mucosa. The exact mechanism of absorption is not known but may involve a receptor on intestinal mucosal cells or a component of pancreatic secretion that binds copper.

Transformation and Function. Copper is a cofactor in approximately 25 metalloenzymes, most of which are oxidases. These are vital in the synthesis of hemoglobin, elastin, collagen, tyrosine (and therefore melanin), and norepinephrine. Copper also acts in the reduction of superoxides, a major mechanism of drug toxicity, and influences iron absorption and mobilization from liver and other tissue stores.

Transport and Storage. Copper is initially bound to albumin, which acts as a buffer to prevent rapid increases in free copper. Ceruloplasmin then receives the ion, and it may be the carrier of copper to the cells. Ceruloplasmin must be chemically altered before it will release the ion.

Approximately 1.5 to 2.5 μg/g nonadipose weight is copper, mostly in liver, heart, and brain. A large fraction is present in erythrocytes. Of the copper in plasma, 90 to 95 per cent is bound to ceruloplasmin.

Excretion. The major routes of excretion are through the bile and sweat. The presence of copper in urine is quantitatively insignificant.

Requirement. The daily requirement for copper is difficult to define because it depends on the simultaneous intake of protein and zinc. It has been estimated that on a high-protein, low-zinc diet the daily requirement is as low as 0.83 mg/day. Humans on low-protein, high-zinc diets require more than twice that amount.

Deficiency State. Most Western diets provide 2 to 5 mg/day of copper, but some diets are marginal at best in copper intake, in the range of 1.0 mg/day. Even so, dietary copper deficiency is rare in the absence of predisposing factors. Copper deficiency has been recognized in infants receiving only milk and in rats, sheep, and pigs. The manifestations are as follows:

1. Copper deficiency causes diminished iron absorption, which leads to microcytic anemia with decreased iron content in tissues.
2. If the iron deficiency is corrected in the copper-deficient animal or human, one is then left with a macrocytic anemia that appears to reflect the intrinsic effect of copper deficiency on the bone marrow.
3. Prolonged copper deficiency leads to four additional manifestations in various animal species such as sheep, rats, humans, and pigs: dystrophic changes in bone, demyelinating neurologic disease, reproductive failure, and abnormal elastin in the artery walls due to inadequate cross-linking in elastin structure.

The rare Menkes' syndrome, or kinky hair disease, is associated with inadequate ability to absorb oral copper. Clinically, it is manifested by early neurologic degeneration, friable hair, and arterial fragility.

Toxicity. Wilson's disease is characterized by hepatic cirrhosis, neuropsychiatric symptoms, and characteristic brown or green copper deposits on the cornea known as a Kayser-Fleischer ring. The heritable disorder is due to an inability of intracellular enzymes to excrete copper once it is absorbed by hepatocytes. As a result, there is diffuse copper deposition, initially in the liver and later throughout the body.

Cirrhosis in East Indian children can probably be attributed to ingestion of excess copper resulting from the use of copper-containing cooking utensils.

A normal newborn has, at birth, what would be considered a toxic level of copper in the liver for an adult. This apparent copper reserve is slowly depleted over the first year of life as ion levels drop to normal.

ZINC

Distribution and Bioavailability. Zinc, present in most food groups, is extensively complexed with protein. The binding of zinc to protein is an important factor in its bioavailability.

Zinc in animal-derived foods is generally more available than zinc from plant sources. Phytic acid, a component of many Middle Eastern breads, inhibits zinc absorption and so may be an etiologic factor in the zinc deficiency syndrome seen in that area. The fiber content of foods also has a significant negative influence on zinc availability.

Other organic metals can compete with zinc for absorption, notably copper and iron. Conversely, edetate (EDTA) and soy protein appear to increase zinc absorption.

Absorption. Net absorption of dietary zinc is 10 to 40 per cent. Absorption is hindered by the absence of pancreatic secretion, so it has been postulated that there is a component of pancreatic secretion, "zinc-binding ligand," that aids in zinc absorption. Several intestinal disorders that decrease the ability of the body to absorb zinc include cystic fibrosis, Crohn's disease, other types of gastrointestinal malabsorption, and alcoholic cirrhosis.

Transport and Storage. Albumin is the major carrier protein, although some zinc may also be transported by transferrin. Zinc is present in most tissues of the body, with highest concentrations found in the choroid of the eye and in male reproductive organs. There is evidence for an enteropancreatic circulation of zinc; that is, large amounts of zinc are secreted in pancreatic juices and later absorbed by the intestine and returned to the pancreas.

Function. Zinc is present in a large number of metalloenzymes, among which are alcohol dehydrogenase, which oxidizes primary and secondary alcohols; carbonic anhydrase, which functions to maintain equilibrium between carbon dioxide and carbonic acid; and both carboxypeptidase A and B from pancreatic juice, which hydrolyze peptide bonds at the carboxy terminals of proteins. Zinc is also found bound to RNA to stabilize secondary and tertiary structures and thus has a role in protein and RNA metabolism.

Excretion. Zinc is excreted mainly through the feces. Small amounts can be found in the urine and in the perspiration.

Requirement. The average efficiency of absorption of zinc in food is 10 to 40 per cent. The estimated RDA for zinc is 15 mg/day, which increases during pregnancy and lactation.

Deficiency State. Because zinc is distributed in most food, the occurrence of zinc deficiency in humans usually requires a conditioning factor such as chronic diarrhea or a diet unduly rich in cereals and particularly in unleavened bread. The presence of phytic acid in unleavened bread reduces the absorption of zinc, calcium, and iron. A leavening process of yeast greatly reduces the phytic acid content. In the Middle East, where diets high in phytic acid are common, the result is a mixed picture of calcium, iron, and zinc deficiency. The manifestations of zinc deficiency in children are reduced growth and delayed puberty. Hypogeusia and anorexia have been attributed to zinc deficiency. A zinc deficiency has also been produced by nearly zinc-free diets in the rat and pig. The manifestations are a failure to thrive and skin lesions.

Acrodermatitis enteropathica, a human hereditary disorder of zinc malabsorption, is manifested by alopecia, eczematoid skin lesions, diarrhea, and growth retardation. Patients are prone to infection owing to defective phagocytosis. All of these features are also found in experimental zinc deficiency. A dose 10 times the normal daily zinc intake is required for maintenance of health in acrodermatitis enteropathica.

Toxicity. Zinc has relatively little inherent toxicity, but taken in large quantities it can compete with copper, iron, cadmium, and calcium for intestinal absorption.

CHROMIUM

Chromium was named from the Greek word *chroma*, meaning color. In 1957 Schwarz and Mertz postulated the existence of a dietary "glucose tolerance factor" (GTF), which contains chromium as an active component. Brewer's yeast is the richest known source of this compound. Chromium salts do not have any effect on glucose tolerance. In chromium deficiency in rats, the first sign is impaired glucose tolerance. The deficiency then develops into a syndrome consisting of impaired growth, fasting hyperglycemia, glycosuria, and elevated serum cholesterol levels.

Distribution and Bioavailability. Chromium exists in food as inorganic chromium and as the biologically active GTF form. Food analysis is extremely difficult, and the GTF form cannot be distinguished from the inorganic form at present. Few foods have appreciable amounts of chromium. Spices have the highest concentration. Lesser amounts are found in meats, vegetables, and fruits. Yeast is the best-known dietary source. Seafoods are poor sources. Water is not a reliable source, since its chromium content varies. Highly processed foods are essentially devoid of chromium. Some chromium may be supplied by stainless steel cookware, which contains chromium that can be leached out during the cooking of acidic foods.

Absorption. Inorganic trivalent chromium salts are poorly absorbed. Chromates are better absorbed; however, it is probable that any chromates present in the diet are reduced in the gastrointestinal tract from the 6^+ to 3^+ valence. Less than 1 per cent of orally administered labeled chromic chloride has been shown to be absorbed; however, absorption was increased two to four times in subjects with diabetes requiring insulin. Ten to 25 per cent of the chromium in yeast extracts has been shown to be absorbed.

Function. Chromium seems to play an important role in carbohydrate and lipid metabolism, at least in rats. Chromium by itself does not stimulate glucose metabolism, but as part of the organic complex GTF it has been found to enhance the stimulatory effects of insulin. It is thought to act in the binding of insulin to cell membranes by forming a bridge between the insulin molecule and the membrane.

Storage. At least two different forms of chromium circulate in the plasma: (1) Some chromium, probably trivalent, is bound to transferrin; and (2) the other is presumed to be GTF-bound chromium. The adult human body contains only about 6 mg of chromium. Highest concentrations are found in skin, fat, adrenal glands, brain, and muscle. Serum concentrations are less than 10 ng/ml.

Excretion. Chromium is almost entirely excreted in the urine. In fact, urinary excretion appears to be a better reflection of chromium status than does plasma concentration.

Requirement. The average chromium intake is estimated to be 52 µg/day. Data are not sufficient to establish an MDR or RDA.

Deficiency State. Chromium deficiency has been documented both accidentally and experimentally in animals. The hallmark of chromium deficiency in animals is impaired glucose tolerance. That chromium deficiency may occur in humans is suggested by the fact that glucose tolerance improves in malnourished individuals whose diets have been supplemented with chromium.

MANGANESE

Manganese—named from the Latin *magnes*, meaning magnet—is used to form many alloys and is responsible for the true color of amethyst. The essentiality of inorganic manganese for the rat has been known since 1931. Later it was shown to be essential for poultry, swine, guinea pigs, and other animals.

Distribution and Bioavailability. The foods that contain the highest amount of manganese are nuts, whole grains, and dried fruits, followed by leafy vegetables, whose manganese content may vary. Poultry, meats, and seafoods may also have a variable manganese content. Tea is an exceptionally rich source of manganese. High dietary concentrations of calcium, phosphorus, iron, or soy protein decrease manganese bioavailability.

Absorption. About 30 to 50 per cent of ingested manganese is absorbed from the intestinal tract. Apparently manganese is absorbed equally well throughout the length of the small intestine.

Function. Manganese is a cofactor or component in a large number of metal-enzyme complexes involving transferase, hydrolase, lyase, kinase, decarboxylase, isomerase, and ligase reactions. Manganese is not specific for these reactions, since other metals, especially magnesium, may substitute. The affinity of manganese for the apoenzyme varies from strong (metalloenzymes) to weak (metal-enzyme complexes). The number of manganese-containing metalloenzymes is limited, whereas the number of metal-enzyme complexes, or enzymes that can be activated by manganese, is extensive. The activating function of manganese is related to its electrophilic character, which facilitates proton departure.

Transport and Storage. Manganese is presumably transported in the plasma by binding to a $beta_1$-globulin termed transmanganin. Transmanganin has not been clearly shown to differ from transferrin, which has been shown to bind manganese, copper, and iron. The plasma concentration of manganese in the normal adult is about 2.5 µg/dl, with an approximately equal distribution between cells and plasma.

The highest concentrations of manganese (2 to 3 µg/g) in mammalian tissues are found in bone, pituitary, liver, pineal, and lactating mammary gland;

lowest concentrations occur in connective tissue and muscle. The manganese content of the adult human body is about 20 mg, and the concentrations in individual organs tend to remain constant throughout life. Both the nucleus and the cytoplasmic organelles contain manganese, with turnover rate and concentration being relatively high in mitochondria and low in the nucleus. Injected labeled manganese tends to localize in the cytoplasm of the liver and pancreas.

Excretion. Manganese excretion appears to play a major role in manganese homeostasis, with little regulation at the site of absorption. The liver is the primary tissue in this regulation, with the bile serving as the major route of excretion. Pancreatic juice also contains manganese, which contributes to excretion. Urinary excretion of manganese is very small.

Requirement. An estimated safe and adequate daily dietary intake of 2.5 to 5.0 mg/day has been established for manganese. This allowance is based on several balance studies in adult humans that have shown that equilibrium or accretion of the element occurs at intakes of 2.5 mg/day or greater, whereas an intake of 0.7 mg/day resulted in negative balance. The American adult's daily intake of manganese usually varies from 2 to 9 mg/day. Gastrointestinal malabsorption or diarrhea causes abnormal losses of manganese in the stools and thus raises the intake requirement.

Deficiency State. Deficiency has been demonstrated in a variety of animals but not yet in humans. Deficiency symptoms in animals include ataxia, alterations in coat color, and tendon and bone disorders. An inability to grow and reproduce and to produce normal offspring has also been documented. In both mice and mink, an inborn error of manganese metabolism producing symptoms similar to those found in nutritional manganese deficiency has been described.

Toxicity. Manganese toxicity has been demonstrated in miners who inhale large quantities of manganese dust over long periods. The disease is characterized by headaches, apathy, impotence, and leg cramps, progressing to a syndrome resembling Parkinson's disease.

SELENIUM

Selenium, which derives its name from the Greek word *selene,* or moon, is a member of the sulfur family and resembles sulfur in its various forms and compounds. Selenium's role in animal nutrition became apparent in 1957 as the unknown "compound factor 3," a compound that was capable of preventing and curing symptoms of vitamin E deficiency in rats and chicks.

Distribution and Bioavailability. Selenium occurs in several forms in food. Very little information is available about these forms or their bioavailability. In wheat that was grown in (^{75}Se) selenate-labeled soil, over 40 per cent of the ^{75}Se was present as protein-bound selenomethionine. The form of the remainder of the selenium in the wheat was unknown. The selenium content of food is related to protein content and geographic origin. Generally, selenium is found in the protein fraction of foods. Low-protein foods such as fruits have very little selenium. Animal and plant products vary as sources of selenium, since there is marked variability in the selenium content of soil. Fish products are known to be rich in selenium.

Absorption. When dissolved in water, 90 to 95 per cent of a 1 mg dose of selenium as selenite is absorbed. Only 20 to 40 per cent absorption of solid sodium selenite occurs. It has been suggested that the dietary ratio of selenium to sulfur may affect selenium absorption.

Function. Selenium's synergistic role with vitamin E suggests that selenium may serve as an antioxidant. Selenium is an integral part of the erythrocyte enzyme glutathione peroxidase. Glutathione peroxidase activity decreases in direct proportion to reductions in selenium intake. Selenium in glutathione peroxidase is present as a low molecular weight organic prosthetic group. The enzyme is composed of four identical subunits, each probably containing one selenium atom. It is proposed that the glutathione peroxidase pathway protects the red blood cell from oxidative damage caused by hydrogen peroxide and other peroxides. Glutathione peroxidase also may play an antioxidant role in phagocytic cells, platelets, and plasma and in lipid peroxidation.

Storage. The highest concentrations of selenium are found in the liver, kidney, heart, and spleen; the concentration is about 0.22 μg/ml, primarily occurring as selenocysteine or selenomethionine residues within proteins.

Excretion. When large quantities of selenium are ingested, some of the selenium is expired as dimethyl selenide; in other circumstances, this route of excretion is negligible. Urinary excretion of selenium accounts for about half the dietary intake. Fecal losses do not appear to be governed by intake, suggesting that gastrointestinal absorption is not adaptive.

Requirement. Although no MDR or RDA has been established for selenium, an estimated safe and adequate daily dietary intake of 50 to 200 μg/day has been established. The average American diet contains about 100 μg/day of selenium.

Deficiency State. Three deficiency diseases in animals due to selenium deficit have been clearly documented. Ten deficiency states that are responsive to both selenium and vitamin E have also been defined. Selenium deficiency in animals produces a wide range of symptoms, including liver necrosis, growth retardation, muscular dystrophy, sudden death, hemorrhages, infertility, nonmotile sperm, pancreatic lesions, cataracts, alopecia, and muscle calcification.

In humans, cardiomyopathy in children (Keshan disease) attributable to selenium deficiency has been described. Keshan is a province in China that has low selenium levels in its soil. Controlled supplementation of children with sodium selenite dramatically lowered the incidence of the disease in this area. Cases of selenium deficiency have now also been reported in the United States.

Toxicity. Both acute and chronic selenium toxicity occur in animals. Although reports of selenium toxicity have been proposed in humans, none are conclusive.

MOLYBDENUM

Molybdenum—named from the Greek word *molybdas,* meaning lead—is essential for the growth of higher plants. It was discovered in animal tissues in 1932.

Distribution. Inorganic molybdenum is widely distributed in foods in minute quantities. Legumes, cereals, organ meats, and yeast are the best known sources of molybdenum. Soil content of molybdenum varies widely, and thus food content is variable.

Absorption. Molybdenum is believed to be readily absorbed from the gastrointestinal tract. Interactions among copper, sulfate, and molybdenum may occur in the gut.

Function. Xanthine oxidase was the first enzyme to be characterized as a molybdenum-containing protein. In humans the enzyme activity is located in the liver and the gastrointestinal epithelium. The enzyme catalyzes the oxidative hydroxylation of a number of purines, pteridines, pyrimidines, and other heterocyclic nitrogenous aromatic molecules. The molybdenum atom is apparently reduced from the hexavalent state (Mo (VI)) to the (Mo (IV)) state. The electrons are transferred to FAD. In mammals, the level of xanthine oxidase in the liver has been shown to be related to the dietary intake of protein, riboflavin, molybdenum, and iron and inversely related to the vitamin E status of the animal. Xanthine oxidase catalyzes the last step in uric acid synthesis.

The second molybdenum-containing enzyme is sulfite oxidase, which catalyzes the oxidation of sulfite to sulfate. A genetic deficiency of sulfite oxidase has been described. The enzyme is necessary to prevent the accumulation of the toxic metabolite sulfite.

Transport and Storage. The molybdenum content of tissues in the body is very low. It ranges from 0.14 to 3.2 ppm, as measured in liver, kidney, muscle, brain, lung, and spleen. It is probably transported in the blood bound to molybdoenzymes or binding proteins.

Excretion. The main route of molybdenum excretion is via the urine.

Requirement. An MDR and RDA have not yet been established for molybdenum. However, an estimated safe and adequate daily dietary intake of 0.15 to 0.5 mg/day has been suggested.

Deficiency State. True molybdenum deficiency has yet to be achieved in experimental animals. Efforts to produce a molybdenum deficiency through administration of a low-molybdenum diet have resulted in reducing rat liver xanthine oxidase activity to 10 per cent of normal, but the health of the animals was not affected. It is possible to produce biochemical molybdenum deficiency, judged by low tissue levels of molybdenum and low xanthine oxidase and sulfite oxidase activities, by feeding a molybdenum antagonist such as tungstate or sulfate.

In humans, a deficiency disease exists that is marked by loss of both xanthine oxidase and sufite oxidase activities. Molybdenum supplementation does not, however, alter the disease.

Toxicity. Molybdenum toxicity has been observed in a number of animal species. Certain animals such as cows and sheep show extraordinary sensitivity to dietary molybdenum. Symptoms vary but generally include failure to thrive. The toxicity appears to be the result of reactions that occur in the gastrointestinal tract among copper, sulfur, and molybdenum. Molybdenum toxicity in humans, with blood molybdenum content five times higher than that of controls, has been reported in a province of Armenia.

IODINE

The ancient Chinese and Egyptians knew of the efficacy of several extracts in treating goiter. Only in the past 150 years has the significance of the high iodine concentration in such extracts been appreciated. The first intentional therapeutic use of iodide was in 1816 in England for the treatment of simple goiter. During the later nineteenth century, epidemiologic studies proved the association between endemic goiter and iodine deficiency. In this century, the discovery and synthesis of the thyroid hormones explained the physiologic role of iodine.

Distribution. Iodine is a halogen having several oxidation states, of which I^- (iodide) is most important in human metabolism. The most commonly ingested form is sodium iodide (NaI), a yellowish, salty crystalline substance added to table salt.

The concentration of iodine in foods is widely variable and depends in part on the soil content of the area where foodstuffs are grown. The highest iodine concentrations are found in seafoods. Iodized salt is an important source and, depending on salt intake, can provide roughly 400 µg I/day (5 g salt).

Absorption. In order to be absorbed, all ingested iodine must be converted to iodide. Intestinal absorption is highly efficient. No carrier protein or active transport mechanism for absorption is known.

Transformation and Function (See also Section VIII). The ion is actively taken up by the thyroid gland, oxidized, and then coupled to tyrosine residues present in thyroglobulin, the large protein that fills the thyroid acini. Two iodotyrosine molecules are then joined, producing thyroxine (T_4) and triiodothyronine (T_3). Under the influence of thyroid-stimulating hormone, the T_4 and T_3 hormones are then cleaved from the large globulin molecule and released into the circulation.

Transport and Storage. The vast majority of iodine is found in the thyroidal colloid. It is also present in salivary glands, lactating mammary glands, and gastric mucosa.

A significant portion (99.95 per cent) of total T_4 present in plasma is bound to a specific protein, thyroxine-binding globulin. Thus, most extrathyroidal T_4 is found in the plasma. T_3, in contrast, is mostly located in peripheral tissues, where it is derived from local deiodination of T_4.

Degradation and Excretion. Free iodine lost through the action of dehalogenases is avidly resorbed by the thyroid. However, a small portion is excreted by the kidneys. There is no conservation mechanism available to regulate the renal excretion of iodine.

Requirement. The RDA of iodine is 150 µg, which is easily obtained in an average diet if iodized salt is used. Pregnancy has essentially no effect on the iodine requirement, but lactation almost doubles it.

Deficiency. Iodine deficiency produces the well-known syndrome of endemic goiter. This entity is discussed in Section VIII.

Toxicity. Free iodine, as in tincture of iodine, is a corrosive agent, which, when swallowed, can cause esophageal damage. Iodides, on the other hand, are essentially nontoxic in an acute situation. On a chronic basis, however, high levels of iodide intake are, in a fraction of people, associated with inhibition of thyroid hormone synthesis and the development of a goiter (Wolff-Chaikoff effect). This effect is reversible by withdrawal of the iodide.

FLUORIDE

The benefit of the halogen anion fluoride in prevention of dental caries has been known since the 1930s. It was not until 1960 that its role in bone homeostasis was appreciated.

Distribution. Seafood and tea contain the highest concentration of fluoride (5 to 10 μg/g for seafood). Fluoridated drinking water is probably the most important source. The fluoride content of water and soil differs depending on the geographic region. However, the distribution of foods from one region to another in the United States tends to negate this difference.

Absorption. Fluoride is readily absorbed from the intestine.

Function. Fluoride helps prevent dental caries when given before eruption of the teeth and possibly even after their full development. Fluoride supplementation is used in treating osteoporosis as well. The ion is also known to enhance the intestinal absorption of iron. Adenyl cyclase is one of several enzymes activated by fluoride.

Storage. Fluoride is widely distributed in the body, with the highest concentration in the teeth and bones, where it occurs chiefly as fluorapatite. The concentration of fluoride in the bones and teeth may reach 0.5 per cent, on a dry basis. The average male has 2.6 g of fluoride in his skeleton.

Excretion. The urine is the main route of excretion, with about 98 per cent of ingested fluoride excreted in adults and about 80 per cent in children.

Allowance. The estimated safe and adequate daily dietary intake of fluoride is 1.5 to 4.0 mg for adults. For younger individuals it is recommended that fluoride intake not exceed 2.5 mg/day.

Deficiency State. Fluoride is so ubiquitous that it is difficult to produce a deficiency state. In rats, anemia and impaired fertility have been noted. Children on fluoride-deficient diets have a five-fold increase in the incidence of dental caries compared with those taking a fluoride supplement.

Toxicity. Only those people consuming over 20 mg/day develop the toxicity syndrome fluorosis. This is seen predominantly in arid desert regions and is manifested by exostoses, sometimes causing compression of neural structures. Acute fluoride toxicity causes transient nausea and abdominal pain without apparent long-term complications. In areas where the drinking water is high in fluoride content, the enamel of the teeth may be mottled, i.e., covered with black or gray spots. No other symptoms are found, and although the disfigurement is esthetically unattractive, tooth decay appears to occur less frequently than in other areas.

NICKEL

There is evidence that nickel is an essential nutrient for rats and chicks. Nickel is present in trace amounts in human tissues, but essentiality for humans has not yet been shown. A nickel metalloprotein named nickelplasmin has been isolated from both human and rabbit serum.

SILICON

Silicon has been shown to be essential for animals only as recently as 1972. Silicon may have an important role in connective tissue metabolism as a cross-linking agent contributing to the stability of mucopolysaccharides. Human umbilical cords have been shown to contain high levels of bound silicon as hyaluronic acid and chondroitin sulfate. Human cartilage also contains bound silicon as chondroitin sulfate and keratin sulfate. Silicon deficiency has not thus far been described in humans; no silicon allowance has been recommended as yet. Unrefined plant foods are good sources of silicon. Beer is the most concentrated source of this element.

VANADIUM

Vanadium has been shown to be essential for animals, although a requirement for humans has not yet been documented. Vanadium may have a role as a cofactor in controlling one or more enzymatic or catalytic reactions. Vanadium may act in oxidation-reduction reactions, in cholesterol metabolism, and in hard-tissue metabolism or formation. Human intake has been estimated to be 2 mg daily. Whole grains are reported to be good sources. Food processing depletes the vanadium content of foods.

TIN

Although reported to be necessary for the growth of rats, tin has not been definitely proved to be essential. No naturally occurring tin deficiency has been shown in either animals or humans. It has been proposed that tin may contribute to the tertiary structure of proteins or may be involved in oxidation-reduction reactions. So little is known about tin nutrition that requirements are not established.

ACKNOWLEDGMENTS

We gratefully acknowledge valuable advice and help of Ms. Carol Berry, Ms. Bettye Hollins, Ms. Martha Beard, Drs. Rajender Chawla and Brian Wallace, Mr. William Heath, Mr. Robert Roy, and Mr. Gary Shapira during the preparation of this section.

REFERENCES

General

Briggs, G. M., and Calloway, D. H.: Bogert's Nutrition and Physical Fitness, 10th ed. Philadelphia, W. B. Saunders Co., 1979.

Committee on Dietary Allowances, Food and Nutrition Board: Recommended Dietary Allowances, 9th ed. Washington, D. C., National Academy of Sciences, 1980.

Goodhart, R. S., and Shils, M. E. (eds.): Modern Nutrition in Health and Disease, 6th ed. Philadelphia, Lea and Febiger, 1980.

Hegsted, D. M., Chichester, C. O., Darby, W. J., et al. (eds.): Nutrition Reviews' Present Knowledge in Nutrition, 4th ed. Washington, D. C., The Nutrition Foundation, 1976.

Pike, R. L., and Brown, M. L.: Nutrition: Integrated Approach, 3rd ed. New York, John Wiley and Sons, 1984.

Schneider, H. A., Anderson, C. E., and Coursin, D. B. (eds.): Nutritional Support of Medical Practice, 2nd ed. Philadelphia, Harper and Row, 1983.

Essential Nutrients, Non-Essential Nutrients, and Nutritional Thresholds

Fernhoff, P. M., Danner, D. J., and Elsas, L. J., II: Vitamin-responsive disorders. In Garry, P. J. (ed.): Human Nutrition: Clinical and Biochemical Aspects. Washington, D. C., American Association for Clinical Chemistry, 1981, p. 219.

Horowitz, J. H., Rypins, E. B., Henderson, J. M., et al.: Evidence for impairment of transsulfuration pathway in cirrhosis. Gastroenterology 81:668, 1981.

Jelliffe, E. F. P., and Jelliffe, D. B. (eds.): Adverse Effects of Foods. New York, Plenum Press, 1982.

Rosenberg, L. E.: Vitamin-responsive inherited metabolic disorders. Adv Hum Genet 6:1, 1976.

Scriver, C. R.: Vitamin-responsive inborn errors of metabolism. Metabolism 22:1319, 1973.

Relation of Essential Nutrients to Intermediary Metabolism

Bondy, P. K., and Rosenberg, L. E. (eds.): Metabolic Control and Disease, 8th ed. Philadelphia, W. B. Saunders Co., 1980.

Chipponi, J. X., Bleier, J. C., Santi, M. T., et al.: Deficiencies of essential and conditionally essential nutrients. Am J Clin Nutr 35:1112, 1982.

Rudman, D., Kutner, M., Ansley, J., et al.: Hypotyrosinemia, hypocystinemia, and failure to retain nitrogen during total parenteral nutrition of cirrhotic patients. Gastroenterology 81:1025, 1981.

Nutrient Deficiency Syndromes

Herbert, V.: The five possible causes of all nutrient deficiency: Illustrated by deficiencies of vitamin B_{12} and folic acid. Am J Clin Nutr 26:77, 1973.

Sauberlich, H. E., Dowdy, R. P., and Skala, J. H.: Laboratory tests for the assessment of nutritional status. CRC Crit Rev Clin Lab Sci 4:215, 1973.

Syndromes of Nutrient Excess

Hodges, R. E.: Megavitamin therapy. Primary Care 9:605, 1982.

Woolliscroft, J. O.: Megavitamins: Fact and fancy. DM 29(5):1, 1983.

Nutrition in Clinical Therapeutics

Bethel, R. A., Jansen, R. D., Heymsfield, S. B., et al.: Nasogastric hyperalimentation through a polyethylene catheter: An alternative to central venous hyperalimentation. Am J Clin Nutr 32:1112, 1979.

Chipponi, J. X., Bleier, J. C., and Rudman, D.: Current status of peripheral alimentation. Ann Intern Med 95:114, 1981.

Heymsfield, S. B., Bethel, R. A., Ansley, J. D., et al.: Enteral hyperalimentation: An alternative to central venous hyperalimentation. Ann Intern Med 90:63, 1979.

Isaacs, J. W., Millikan, W. J., Stackhouse, J., et al.: Parenteral nutrition of adults with a 900 milliosmolar solution via peripheral veins. Am J Clin Nutr 30:552, 1977.

McCollum, E. V.: A History of Nutrition: The Sequence of Ideas in Nutrition Investigations. Boston, Houghton Mifflin Company, 1957.

Essential Nutrients

Alfin-Slater, R., and Kritchevsky, D. (eds.): Human Nutrition: A Comprehensive Treatise. Vol 3A, Nutrition and the Adult: Macronutrients. New York, Plenum Press, 1980.

McCormick, D. B.: Vitamins. In Tietz, N. W. (ed.): Textbook of Clinical Chemistry. Philadelphia, W. B. Saunders Co., 1985.

McCormick, D. B., and Wright, L. D. (eds.): Methods in Enzymology. Vols. 66 and 67, Vitamins and Coenzymes. New York, Academic Press, 1980.

Mead, J. F., and Fulco, A. J.: Unsaturated and Polyunsaturated Fatty Acid in Health and Disease. Springfield, Ill., Charles C Thomas, 1976.

Prasad, A. S., and Oberleas, D. (eds.): Trace Elements in Human Health and Disease. Volume 1, Zinc and Copper. New York, Academic Press, 1976.

Prasad, A. S., and Oberleas, D. (eds.): Trace Elements in Human Health and Disease. Volume II, Essential and Toxic Elements. New York, Academic Press, 1976.

Rose, J. (ed.): Trace Elements in Health: A Review of Current Issues. Boston, Butterworths, 1983.

Rudman, D., and Williams, P. J.: Megadose vitamins: Use and misuse. N Engl J Med 309:488, 1983.

Schaumburg, H., Kaplan, J., Windebank, A., et al.: Sensory neuropathy from pyridoxine abuse: A new megavitamin syndrome. N Engl J Med 309:445, 1983.

Stanbury, J. B., Wyngaarden, J. B., Fredrickson, D. S., et al.(eds.): The Metabolic Basis of Inherited Disease, 5th ed. New York, McGraw-Hill, 1983.

ENDOCRINOLOGY

General Introduction

MICHAEL ROSENBLATT, M.D.

DEFINITIONS

The hormones of the endocrine system have generalized metabolic and biochemical effects on all the tissues of the body. Hence, endocrine disease is often manifest by multiorgan disturbances with diffuse and systemic consequences. In this chapter we will review endocrine physiology and pathophysiology on an endocrine organ–based approach. The hypothalamus, pituitary, thyroid, adrenal, parathyroid, and reproductive glands and the hormones they secrete will be discussed. Antidiuretic hormone, the gastrointestinal hormones, and the carbohydrate regulatory hormones (insulin, glucagon, etc.) are discussed elsewhere in this volume.

A *hormone* is classically defined as a substance made in one organ that is secreted into the circulation in order to act on another organ or tissue. While this concept has proven too narrow to include all of the physiological roles of hormones and all the anatomical arrangements in which hormones are found, this definition does emphasize the integrative physiological role served by hormones. Although the organs of the body have fundamental and discrete physiological and structural roles, certain generalized functions, such as energy consumption, utilization and mobilization of body fuels, control of the ionic milieu bathing tissue, response to stress, and integration of behavior and physiology in reproductive function, require a system of biologically active substances moving through the circulation and regulating multiple target tissues.

The endocrine system that has evolved is based in several organs. Originally, substances currently considered to be hormones or "intercellular" mediators may have functioned as intracellular messengers in unicellular organisms. Hormones such as insulin and adrenocorticotropin (ACTH) are found in single-cell organisms and even plants and may serve important integrative functions. Possibly these substances were later co-opted and their physiological role extended when it became necessary for one cell to communicate with another and eventually for whole tissues and organs to be in communication in a complex organism.

FUNCTION OF THE ENDOCRINE SYSTEM

Regulation of most of the physiological functions under the control of hormones is based principally on a single hormone or a pair of hormones, each of which has opposite effects that together form a counter-regulatory system. The endocrine system itself is also interlocking and interdependent. Virtually each of the hormones requires the appropriate physiological environment established by the others for its own action. For instance, normal growth requires not only growth hormone and somatomedin C but also appropriate levels of insulin, thyroid, adrenal, and reproductive hormones. Similarly, maintenance of blood calcium levels within the normal physiological range requires parathyroid hormone and vitamin D principally, but also normal sodium and water metabolism and appropriate levels of steroid and thyroid hormones.

The homeostatic function of the endocrine system is served by rapid (seconds to hours) hormonal responses, the consequences of which are continuously monitored. For the most part, monitoring is based on straightforward feedback control. Levels of the final hormone in a cascade of hormones secreted by a series of endocrine glands is monitored by the cells of the gland secreting the initial hormone in the cascade.

If a hormone alters the level of an ion, such as sodium or calcium, then the absolute level or the change in level of that ion feeds back to modulate hormonal secretion by the regulating gland. When the level achieved is sensed as appropriate, hormonal secretion is arrested until the ion level drifts beyond the tolerance permitted by the regulatory hormone.

The rapid on-and-off effects of hormones are made possible not only by rapid onset of hormone action after interaction with target tissue, but also by relatively short duration of biological activity at the end organ or rapid degradation and inactivation of hormone. The phenomena taken together permit rapid, sensitive, and flexible regulation of physiological function. Along these lines, the circulating concentration of most hormones normally is very low (often in the picomolar range), facilitating rapid and large adjustments in circulating levels of biologically active hormone and reflecting the potency of the biological properties that evolution has concentrated in the hormones.

The pathophysiology of endocrine disorders is almost always related to abnormal regulation of endocrine gland function, i.e., the presence of too much or too little of a hormone. Too much hormone may be secreted as a result of the biosynthetic activity of an endocrine tissue or another tissue, which normally does not secrete hormone but under certain circumstances ectopically biosynthesizes and secretes abundant quantities of hormones. In some cases, a genetic defect or the trophic effects of other hormones on a tissue lead to oversecretion. Too little hormonal activity may result from inadequate biosynthesis or secretion of hormone, secretion of an abnormal or ineffective hormonal variant, or a hormone-resistant state at the level of the target tissue.

The hormones can be grouped into three classes: polypeptides, steroids, and thyroid hormones. The members of each class share common features in terms of the nature of receptor interaction and mechanism of hormone action.

POLYPEPTIDE HORMONES

Polypeptide hormones circulate free (unbound to larger carrier proteins) in the extracellular fluid, tend to have short half-lives and durations of action, and interact with cell-surface receptors present on target tissues. The binding of a peptide hormone to its specific receptor results in a change (presumably allosteric) in the receptor, which in turn activates an "effector" system. Activation of the plasma membrane–bound effector system causes an increase in intracellular levels of "second messenger," such as 3′,5′-cyclic adenosine monophosphate (cAMP) or calcium-calmodulin (Fig. 1). Until recently, it was thought that polypeptide hormones exert their effects entirely by interaction with receptors at the cell surface, leading to the generation of "second messengers," and that the hormones themselves are unable to enter into cells. It has now been demonstrated that a number of peptide hormones, when associated with their receptors, are able to enter cells. In some cases, the hormone-receptor complex is metabolically active and serves as a kinase, promoting phosphorylation of intracellular enzymes and other proteins. In other instances, cellular internalization of hormone with receptor is the first step toward degradation of the hormone; in such cases, the internalization event may play an important regulatory role in controlling levels of active hormone and available

receptor. Hormone-receptor internalization not only may regulate some acute metabolic events but may have long-term regulatory and trophic effects on target cells.

The classic peptide hormone–receptor interaction leads to the activation of membrane-bound adenylate cyclase and the production of cAMP. When one considers that hormone, receptor, nucleotide regulatory protein, and adenylate cyclase must interact to generate cAMP, and that each of these complex proteins may be composed of multiple components, nearly a dozen protein subunits or membrane components may be involved in the transduction and expression of peptide hormone biological activity (Figs. 1 and 2). The structures of several receptors have now been elucidated. In general, receptors are complex membrane-bound proteins, often composed of several subunits and often containing carbohydrate or lipid moieties. Interestingly, the receptor itself is often as highly conserved by evolution across species and target tissue as is the hormone. The interaction of hormone with receptor is presumed to cause an allosteric change in receptor, which in its resting stage binds the nucleotide regulatory subunit (N), which in turns binds guanyl nucleotide diphosphate (GDP). Association of hormone with receptor leads to dissociation of GDP from N. The N protein then binds guanyl nucleotide triphosphate (GTP). The GTP-N complex then associates with adenylate cyclase, activating its enzymatic activity, which converts adenosine nucleotide triphosphate (ATP) to cAMP. The cAMP binds to a cAMP-binding protein intracellularly, perhaps in functional compartments, to activate protein kinases and eventually regulate intracellular metabolic events (Fig. 2).

The process of transduction of hormonal activity is one of amplification. Consequently only a small number of receptors need to be occupied to effect full biological activity (Fig. 3), leading to the concept of spare receptors, each of which is indistinguishable from the receptors originally occupied and each of which is fully functional. Receptors are mobile on the cell surface and can move about to interact with different "effector system" components. In fact, in some systems, one of the early events following hormone-receptor interaction is a moving together of neighboring receptors on the membrane surface into a "coated pit," followed by receptor internalization (Fig. 4). In other systems, hormone-receptor complexes move to a position inside the membrane volume. This loss of available receptor is termed "down-regulation." In fact, the interaction of a single hormone molecule with a single receptor can lead to a subsequent decline in the accessibility of a number of neighboring receptors. In other instances, interaction of hormone with receptor results in a dissociation of other receptors from the effector system (such as adenylate cyclase). Such "desensitization" of target cells may be a response evolved to protect target cells from the effects of high levels of hormone in the circulation. Whatever the teleology of the phenomenon, it illustrates the importance of receptor number as well as hormonal concentration in modulating hormone activity. The simple chemical equation, $[H] + [R] \rightleftharpoons [HR] \rightarrow$ hormonal response, emphasizes the critical importance of both hormone and receptor concentrations in hormonal signaling and expression of biological activity.

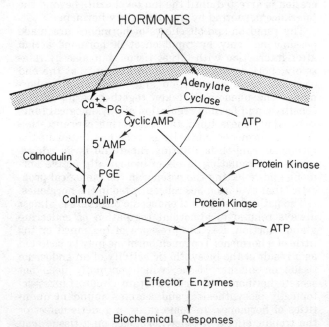

Figure 1. The interaction of a hormone agonist with cell surface receptors leads to generation of intracellular second messengers and a cascade of intracellular metabolic events, ultimately leading to expression of hormone bioactivity.

Figure 2. The stimulation of cyclic AMP production by hormone involves dissociation of the receptor from the guanyl nucleotide regulatory protein and association of the latter with adenylate cyclase, resulting in stimulation of the enzyme and production of cyclic AMP. Subsequent intracellular events leading to biological responses are depicted.

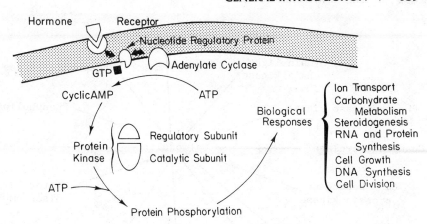

The nature of the hormone-receptor interaction itself varies widely from system to system. In most cases, hormone-receptor interaction is reversible, and hormone agonists and antagonists can often be distinguished on the basis of the rapidity with which they dissociate from the receptor (agonists tend to dissociate from receptor more rapidly than antagonists). In other systems, the hormone-receptor association is essentially irreversible.

The generation of cAMP is not the only mechanism by which peptide hormones communicate their messages intracellularly. In some instances, the receptor itself becomes an active kinase as a result of hormone interaction and may autophosphorylate as the first step in hormonal mode of action. In other systems, hormone-receptor interaction opens transmembrane calcium channels. The incoming calcium ions bind to an intracellular calcium-binding protein, calmodulin. The calcium-calmodulin complex then can activate adenylate cyclase or protein kinases, activate or inhibit phosphodiesterase (which degrades cAMP), or otherwise regulate important intracellular enzymes and proteins (Fig. 5). Other "second messenger" schemes are still being elucidated. Phospholipids and phosphoinositol may also serve "second messenger" roles in hormonal mode of action. In summary, the peptide hormone class, and indeed any single peptide hormone, may employ several effector systems at one or more target tissues to generate a biological response.

Steroid Hormones

A steroid hormone enters the cell and binds to intracellular receptor molecules. For many years it was thought that the steroid receptor was in the cytoplasm and that the steroid hormone-receptor complex moved from the cytoplasm to the nucleus, where it bound to nuclear acceptor sites. Recent studies suggest an alternative possibility: the steroid receptor is not cytoplasmic but rather intranuclear; therefore, relocation of receptor from the cytoplasm to the nucleus is not necessary—the hormone may diffuse through the cytoplasm to the nuclear binding sites. In any event, the steroid hormone-receptor complex influences the process of transcription, whereby RNA is synthesized (transcribed) from the DNA template. The consequences are alterations in the rates of synthesis of specific proteins. Thus, the steroid modifies the phenotypic expression of the genetic information. This mechanism of action appears to be applicable to all steroid hormones, including glucocorticoids, mineralocorticoids, sex hormones, and 1,25-dihydroxyvitamin D.

The mechanism of action of steroid hormones is distinct from that of peptide hormones, in which the peptide hormone binds to a receptor on the cell surface and thereby initiates a sequence of events, as described above. Our knowledge of the mechanism of action of steroid hormones, involving the intracellular formation of a hormone-receptor complex, appears to explain certain important physiological observations. For example, the duration of action of a steroid hormone is

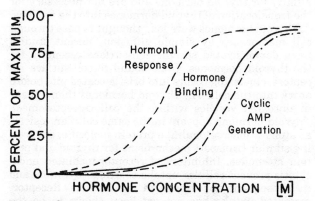

Figure 3. Comparison of log dose-response curves for hormone action, binding, and generation of cyclic AMP. A maximal hormone response can be elicited when only a fraction of the total number of available receptors is occupied (demonstrating "spare" receptors) and when submaximal quantities of cyclic AMP are generated.

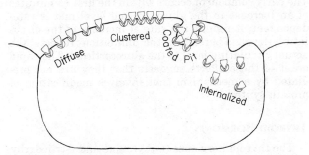

Figure 4. Events following hormone-receptor interaction leading to internalization of hormone-receptor complexes.

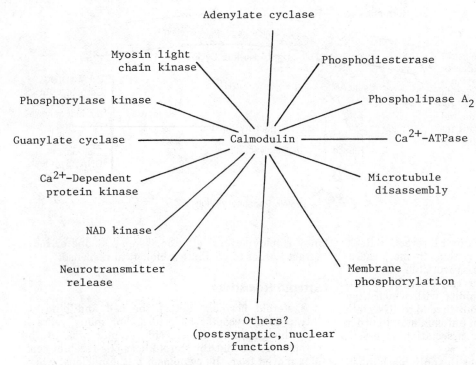

Figure 5. Intracellular enzymes and functions potentially regulated by calcium-calmodulin. (Adapted from Cheung, W. Y.: Calmodulin plays a pivotal role in cellular regulation. Science 207:19–27, 1980).

often much longer than one would predict from the circulating half life of that steroid in the circulation, assuming first order kinetics (in which one would expect the duration of action to be approximately equal to five times the circulating half-life). This discrepancy is attributable to the fact that the duration of action of the steroid reflects events that occur after the steroid has left the circulation. Thus, the durations of action of different glucocorticoids correlate better with their affinities for the intracellular receptor molecule than with the circulating half-life. The duration of action may also reflect the duration of the biological effects of the protein products synthesized in response to the steroid hormone.

The mechanism of action described above can also account for the fact that certain actions of a glucocorticoid do not begin until several hours after the administration of the steroid hormone. This is consistent with the time course and multistep process leading to effects of the steroid hormone on protein synthesis.

While this mechanism of action appears to account for numerous effects of steroid hormones, it probably does not account for all effects. For example, the glucocorticoid-induced feedback inhibition of ACTH secretion by the pituitary gland has two components. The early component occurs within the first 15 minutes of an increase in the glucocorticoid level and is rate-dependent; it reflects the rate of increase of the circulating level. Thereafter, the inhibition reflects the actual circulating level of the glucocorticoid. The rapid onset of these effects suggests that they are not mediated by a mechanism that involves modification of protein synthesis.

THYROID HORMONES

The thyroid hormones (L-thyroxine and L-triiodothyronine) are specialized (iodinated) amino acids that have diverse biological effects, influencing many but not all tissues. The mechanisms of action of the thyroid hormones are still being elucidated; certain features superficially resemble the actions of both steroid and peptide hormones.

The principal locus of action of thyroid hormone appears to be the cell nucleus. Sensitive target tissues possess high affinity nuclear binding sites (receptors) for thyroid hormones on the nonhistone chromatin proteins. Nuclear receptor occupancy leads to the synthesis of specific messenger RNA's, probably as a consequence of increased transcription of DNA.

Nuclear receptor occupancy by thyroid hormone has been closely correlated with its thyromimetic activity; less active thyroid hormone analogues in general bind less well to nuclear receptors.

Cytoplasmic receptors for thyroid hormone have been demonstrated as well, but these do not appear to be biologically important. These receptors have low affinity for thyroid hormone and are not necessary for the translocation of thyroid hormones into the nucleus.

Thyroid hormones were long thought to pass through cell membranes by simple diffusion. Recent studies have demonstrated specific cell-surface receptors for the thyroid hormones. Once bound to cell-surface receptors, clustering occurs into bristle-coated pits before entry into the cell. The thyroid hormones then appear in uncoated vesicles within the cell (receptosomes). Thyroid hormone appears in the same cellular vesicles as alpha-2-macroglobulin, a protein molecule, suggesting similar transport mechanisms for thyroid and protein hormones. Inhibitors of receptor-mediated endocytosis prevent cellular uptake of triiodothyronine and its subsequent appearance in the nucleus. Receptor-mediated uptake has not yet been shown to be the exclusive entry pathway for thyroid hormone. Furthermore, the number of thyroid hormone target tissues tested for this mechanism has been limited. Differences in cellular uptake by thyroid hormone analogues may explain differences in nuclear binding of these analogues by isolated nuclei, as opposed to intact cells.

Thyroid hormone has been shown to stimulate directly the transport of certain amino acids and sugars into the cell; this stimulation is independent of new protein synthesis. Although transport stimulation requires supraphysiologic concentrations of thyroid hormone in vitro, such actions of thyroid hormone may have physiological relevance in vivo. The relation between receptor-mediated thyroid hormone uptake and thyroid hormone–mediated amino acid and sugar uptake has not yet been investigated.

Lastly, high affinity mitochondrial receptors for thyroid hormones have been demonstrated. Thyroid hormone–induced increase in oxygen consumption or ATP synthesis appears to be independent of new protein synthesis in the system studied. This may represent yet a third, independent locus for the direct action of the thyroid hormones.

SOME FUTURE DIRECTIONS— NEUROPEPTIDES

During the last decade, considerable clinical and research interest in endocrinology has focused on the central nervous system. Many of the peptide hormones once thought to function exclusively as hormones (in that they are secreted into the circulation by an endocrine organ in order to alter the metabolism of other organs and tissues) have now been identified in the brain and demonstrated to serve in neurotransmitter or neuromodulatory roles.

The discovery of these hormones in the brain has broadened the definition of endocrinology to include the study of substances involved in cell-to-cell communication in general. Using this definition, multiple anatomical arrangements have been found which involve intercellular communication using hormones (Fig. 6). The specialized cells of the hypothalamus are neuronal at one end and endocrine-secretory at the other. They receive chemical and electrical signals from several regions of the brain which modulate their secretory activity. When stimulated, they release factors into the hypothalamic-pituitary portal circulation, or, in the case of cells producing antidiuretic hormone and oxytocin, the neurosecretory cells release these peptide hormones directly into the systemic circulation. At other central nervous system sites, neuropeptides may be synthesized and released across synapses to serve a highly localized neuroregulatory role on only one target cell. In the pancreas, "neuropeptides" (there is considerable overlap between the group of peptides found in the gastrointestinal tract and those present in the central nervous system) may modulate the activity of a group of cells, such as the cells of the islets of Langerhans, in a paracrine fashion. In this anatomical arrangement, high local concentrations of hormone may affect neighboring cells, but the levels of hormone attained in the general circulation are too low to produce systemic activity. Neuropeptides may also be secreted at one location directly into the cerebrospinal fluid to circulate and act at distant central nervous system sites, analogous to the transport of hormones in blood. Finally, locally produced neuropeptides such as angiotensin and bradykinin may turn on and off blood flow to regions of the brain in a precise fashion, thus directing metabolic and neuronal activity of certain regions of the central nervous system.

Much of the interest in the neuropeptides arises

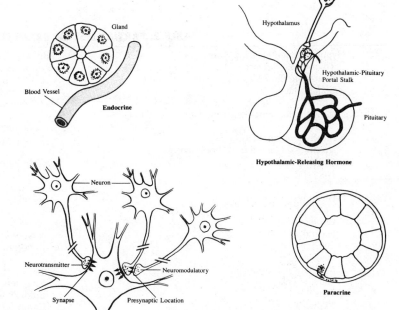

Figure 6. Various anatomical arrangements in which peptide "hormones" are involved in signaling.

TABLE 1. SOME BIOLOGICAL EFFECTS ATTRIBUTED TO NEUROPEPTIDES

Specific release of hypothalamic or pituitary hormones
Stress response
Memory and learning
Appetite/thirst
Sexual behavior
Psychiatric disorders—depression, schizophrenia
Seizures
Pain/analgesia
Sleep
Temperature regulation
Ventilation regulation
Blood pressure
Addiction/habituation

from their wide distribution in the body and their possible role in basic physiological functions and in disorders affecting large numbers of people. Many of the most common public health problems, such as obesity, smoking, alcoholism, and sleep disorders, have a prominent behavioral component to their etiology. The study of the physiological role of these peptide hormones in the central nervous system holds the promise of generating therapeutic agents and approaches for many common disorders. Therefore, the study of the neuropeptides lies at a growing interface between medicine, neurology, and psychiatry and represents an important new opportunity for biomedical research efforts to focus on basic functions such as appetite regulation, sleep, response to stress, and memory and learning. Further clinical interest in these compounds arises from the diverse biological properties and fundamental physiological roles attributed to them (Table 1).

The function of peptides as neurotransmitters and neuromodulators is a new one, discovered only within the last decade. Thirty to 40 neuropeptides have been found thus far in the brain—a number several-fold larger than the number of classic neurotransmitters (i.e., acetylcholine, dopamine, serotonin, etc.), and the expectation is that 200 to 400 neuropeptides ultimately will be identified. Although many of these substances function as hormones when present peripherally (Table 2), their biological activities in the central nervous system may be quite different from their properties as hormones in the systemic circulation. For instance, antidiuretic hormone (ADH) is involved systemically in control of water metabolism and serum osmolarity, but centrally ADH facilitates memory and learning; angiotensin II, which participates systemically in regulation of blood pressure, centrally may be responsible for thirst. Hence, the biological properties of these substances lie not only in their chemical structure but also in their anatomical site of action.

Often the hormonal and behavioral properties of the neuropeptides seem linked. Corticotropin-releasing factor (CRF) is a hypothalamic hormone that mediates release of adrenocorticotropin (ACTH) by the pituitary, which in turn leads to cortisol secretion by the adrenal glands. When given directly into the brain, CRF causes stresslike behavior; attentiveness and motor activity are increased in animals (Fig. 7). Cholecystokinin (CCK) stimulates gallbladder contraction and gut motility, but its central effect is to decrease feeding by producing early satiety, a property that may prove useful in the future in treating obesity. Gonadotropin-releasing hormone (GnRH or LHRH) stimulates release of the pituitary gonadotropins, luteinizing hormone (LH), and follicle-stimulating hormone (FSH). Given centrally, this peptide induces sexual posturing and sexual activity in rats.

Although it is not possible to catalogue all of the biological properties attributable to each of the neuropeptides in this chapter, a few important examples should be highlighted because of their potentially significant clinical implications.

TABLE 2. PARTIAL LIST OF BRAIN PEPTIDES

Hypothalamic-Releasing Hormones
Thyrotropin-Releasing Hormone (TRH)
Gonadotropin-Releasing Hormone (GnRH)
Somatostatin
Corticotropin-Releasing Hormone (CRF)
Growth Hormone–Releasing Hormone (GRF)

Neurohypophyseal Hormones
Vasopressin (antidiuretic hormone, ADH)
Oxytocin
Neurophysin(s)

Gastrointestinal Peptides
Vasoactive Intestinal Polypeptides (VIP)
Cholecystokinin (CCK-8)
Gastrin
Substance P
Neurotensin
Methionine Enkephalin
Leucine Enkephalin
? Insulin
? Glucagon
Bombesin
Secretin

Pituitary Peptides
Adrenocorticotropic Hormone (ACTH)
β-Endorphin
α-Melanocyte-Stimulating Hormone (α-MSH)
? Prolactin
? Growth Hormone
? Luteinizing Hormone
? Thyrotropin

Opioid Peptides
β-Endorphin
α-Endorphin
γ-Endorphin
Enkephalin
Dynorphin
α-Neo-endorphin
Rimorphin

Other
Angiotensin II
Bradykinin
Carnosine
Sleep Peptide(s)
α-Melanocyte-Stimulating Hormone (α-MSH)

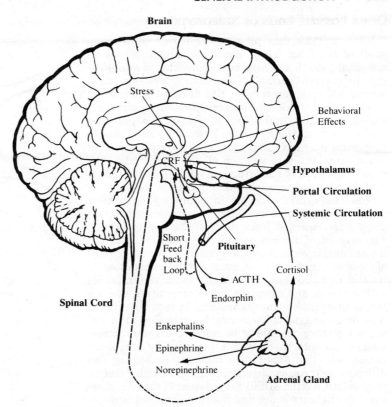

Figure 7. Hormonal response to stress based on corticotropin-releasing factor (CRF). (Reprinted with permission from Rosenblatt, M.: Neuropeptides: Future implications for medicine. Med Times 111:31–37, 1983.)

ENDOGENOUS OPIATES

Diverse clinical phenomena, such as the response to placebo, acupuncture-mediated analgesia, stress-induced amenorrhea, and the pathogenesis of shock, may all reflect actions of the enkephalins and endorphins. Beta-endorphin is synthesized by the pituitary gland and released together with adrenocorticotropin (ACTH) in response to physiological stimuli such as low cortisol levels, but also in response to stress, shock, exercise, etc. The endorphins (a contraction of "endogenous morphine") and enkephalins (meaning "in the head") were discovered only after opiate receptors were identified in the brain. Researchers reasoned that these receptors must interact with "endogenous opiates" rather than being intended to interact with exogenous substances such as the extract of the poppy plant.

The enkephalins and the endorphins, whose structures were elucidated shortly afterward, are twenty- to several hundred–fold more potent than morphine in producing analgesia. Acupuncture analgesia appears to be endorphin- or enkephalin-mediated; administration of the opiate antagonist naloxone reverses acupuncture analgesia. The analgesic response to placebo may simply represent successful recruitment of one's own endogenous opiate system. Depression and certain components of schizophrenia, such as auditory hallucinations, may be linked to altered levels of endorphins. The endorphins also suppress secretion of the pituitary gonadotropins (FSH and LH). Since endorphin levels increase with stress or strenuous physical activity, endorphins may be responsible for the commonly observed irregular or absent menses seen in women under stress or engaged in athletic training. Endorphin levels also increase in pregnancy and peak at the time of labor and delivery, perhaps providing some analgesic effects at that time.

Finally, endorphin is released together with ACTH by the pituitary in response to stresses such as hemorrhage, septic shock, and neurogenic shock. Under these circumstances, the endorphin secreted by the pituitary gland may have the adverse effect of exacerbating hypotension. Several studies of septic shock have now demonstrated restoration of normal blood pressure and increased survival in animals or patients treated with the opiate antagonist naloxone. Opiate antagonists may soon be added to the regimen of fluids, antibiotics, and corticosteroids used in treating septic shock.

ANTIDIURETIC HORMONE AND LEARNING

Antidiuretic hormone (ADH) may find important new clinical utility. Given centrally, ADH facilitates memory and learning. Rats genetically deficient in ADH learn new tasks more slowly and retain new knowledge for a shorter period than normal rats. Rats given antibodies to, or antagonists of, ADH directly into the cerebrospinal fluid (CSF) learn at a slower rate than normal rats. Interestingly, there is a circadian rhythm to ADH levels in the CSF that is completely dissociated from levels found in the blood. The ease of learning at different times of the day may correlate with CSF levels of ADH. Along the same lines, inappropriate levels of ADH in the CSF at certain times may contribute to the "jet-lag" syndrome or related clinical phenomena. Finally, long-acting, super-potent analogues of ADH are being evaluated for potential use in the treatment of human senility.

OTHER POSSIBLE ROLES OF NEUROPEPTIDES

Neuropeptides may play a crucial role in development of the CNS. They may have trophic effects on neuronal growth and may be responsible for establishing the correct "wiring" of neuronal tracts—i.e., neuropeptides may function in the developing brain as markers that guide one neuron to another, directing the location and establishment of some synapses and inhibiting formation of others. Eventually such trophic properties may have important clinical applications in stimulating the regeneration of damaged brain cells or perhaps even stimulating and guiding transplanted CNS tissue to appropriate anatomical positions.

Some important concepts in neurology have been overturned and some new principles in neuroendocrinology have emerged from study of the neuropeptides. The concept of distinct neuronal systems (such as the dopaminergic or cholinergic system) in which groups of neurons make only a single neurotransmitter is invalid in many instances. Many neurons synthesize both a classic and a peptide neurotransmitter, or even two neuropeptides simultaneously. In fact, classic and peptide neurotransmitters can be packaged into the same secretory granule to be released together across a single synaptic space, where they stimulate the same target cell. The duplication inherent in having two different neurotransmitters present in a single synapse may reflect a kind of fail-safe system (Table 3). However, the neuropeptides and the classic neurotransmitter often produce qualitatively different responses and possess different durations of activity (Fig. 8 and Table 4), suggesting differences in the signals each is intended to communicate. This multiplicity of agents and actions at many sites within the CNS is consistent with the complexity of functions that the brain is capable of conducting.

This complexity is further amplified by the finding that several different receptor types can be found within the central nervous system for any given class of neuropeptides. For instance, there are several types of opiate receptor present in the brain. The quantity of receptors also may be regulated. In addition, the neuropeptides themselves are biosynthesized in precursor forms that are much larger than the actual neuropeptides. This large protein template often contains the sequences of several other neuropeptides. The structures of the peptides were not known until the nucleotide sequence of the precursor of the original neuropeptide was elucidated. In many cases, these

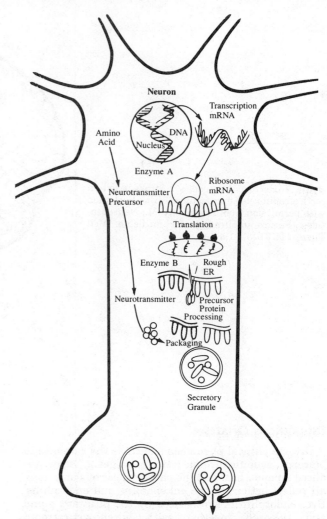

Figure 8. Different biosynthetic pathways for classic and neuropeptide neurotransmitters, both of which may be packaged into the same secretory vesicle by a single neuron to be released across the same synapse. (Reprinted with permission from Rosenblatt, M.: Neuropeptides: Future implications for medicine. Med Times 111:31–37, 1983.)

peptides (when synthesized and biologically evaluated) have been found to possess overlapping but nonidentical properties. In other cases, the structures are unrelated and the function of the so-called cryptic peptides is unknown. Furthermore, any or all of these peptides may be carved out of the precursor protein and secreted. Since there are often several cryptic peptides present in the precursor to the known neuropeptide, the total number of biologically active neuropeptides that exists may be considerably greater than originally estimated.

TABLE 3. NEUROPEPTIDES VS. CLASSIC NEUROTRANSMITTERS

Peptide
Biosynthesis: DNA→RNA→Peptide
Lower concentration: 10^{-15}–10^{-12} M
Slow frequency of response
Long duration of response
Termination by peptidase degradation

Classic
Biosynthesis: Series of enzymatic steps
Higher concentration: 10^{-9}–10^{-6} M
Rapid neuronal firing elicited
Short duration of response
Termination by reuptake

TABLE 4. EXAMPLES OF NEUROPEPTIDES AND CLASSIC NEUROTRANSMITTERS PRESENT IN THE SAME NEURON

Enkephalin	Catecholamines
Cholecystokinin (CCK)	Dopamine
Substance P	Serotonin
Vasoactive Intestinal Polypeptide (VIP)	Acetylcholine
Thyrotropin-Releasing Hormone (TRH)	Serotonin
Somatostatin	Norepinephrine

Many advances in future understanding and treatment of clinical disorders are likely to emerge from the study of neuropeptides. One of the most important principles to be established comes from the instances in which receptors have been discovered before the endogenous substance with which they interact has been characterized. Receptors exist for drugs such as tricyclic antidepressants or benzodiazepine tranquilizers. It is likely that endogenous "antidepressants" or "tranquilizers" are present in the central nervous system. These substances may be more potent and have fewer side effects than drugs we currently use. Some psychiatric disorders may originate from excesses or deficiencies of these endogenous substances or their receptors. And disorders of menstruation and reproduction may be attributable to inappropriate neuropeptide regulation.

The ability to design and synthesize analogues of neuropeptides should provide many new drug candidates of enhanced or selective activity. In addition, many human central nervous system pathways have not been fully identified. Until recently, information regarding these pathways has been obtained only through clinical correlations with central nervous system lesions. Detailed mapping of neuronal pathways by immunofluorescent or immunocytolocalization methods is now possible and should elucidate interrelations between the brain and the endocrine system, as well as guiding pharmacological or electrical therapy to very specific CNS locations, thus avoiding side effects produced by systemic administration of therapeutic agents. Finally, understanding of the role and mechanism of action of the neuropeptides should greatly extend our understanding of the interrelations of endocrinology, neurology, and psychiatry.

REFERENCES

Alberts, B., Bray, D., Lewis, J., Raff, M., Roberts, K., and Watson, J. D.: Molecular Biology of the Cell. New York, Garland Publishing, 1983.

Brown, M. S., and Goldstein, J. L.: Receptor-mediated endocytosis: Insights from the lipoprotein receptor system. Proc Natl Acad Sci USA 76:3330–3337, 1979.

Carr, D. B., Bergland, R., Hamilton, A., et al.: Endotoxin-stimulated opioid peptide secretion: Two secretory pools and feedback control in vivo. Science 217:845–848, 1982.

Carr, D. B., Bullen, B. A., Skrinar, G. S., et al.: Physical conditioning facilitates the exercise-induced secretion of beta-endorphin and beta-lipotropin in women. N Engl J Med 305:560–563, 1981.

Catt, K. J., and Dufau, M. L.: Peptide hormone receptors. Annu Rev Physiol 39:529–557, 1977.

Cheung, W. Y.: Calmodulin plays a pivotal role in cellular regulation. Science 207:19–27, 1980.

Felig, P., Baxter, J. D., Broadus, A. E., and Frohman, L. A.: Endocrinology and Metabolism. New York, McGraw-Hill Book Co., 1981.

Greengard, P.: Phosphorylated proteins as physiological effectors: Protein phosphorylation may be a final common pathway for many biological regulatory agents. Science 199:146–152, 1978.

Guillemin, R.: Hypothalamic hormones: Releasing and inhibiting factors. In Krieger, D. T., and Hughes, J. C. (eds.): Neuroendocrinology: The Interrelationships of the Body's Two Major Integrative Systems in Normal Physiology and in Clinical Disease. Sunderland, Mass., Sinauer Associates, 1980, pp. 23–32.

Hökfelt, T., Johansson, O., Ljungdahl, Å., et al.: Peptidergic neurones. Nature 284:515–521, 1980.

Krieger, D. T., and Martin, J. B.: Brain peptides. N Engl J Med 304:876–885, 944–951, 1981.

Potts, J. T., Jr., Kronenberg, H. M., and Rosenblatt, M.: Parathyroid hormone: Chemistry, biosynthesis, and mode of action. Adv Protein Chem 35:323–396, 1982.

Rigter, H., and Crabbe, J. C.: Modulation of memory by pituitary hormones and related peptides. Vitam Horm 37:153–241, 1979.

Rodbell, M.: The role of hormone receptors and GTP-regulatory proteins in membrane transduction. Nature 284:17–22, 1980.

Ross, E. M., and Gilman, A. G.: Biochemical properties of hormone-sensitive adenylate cyclase. Annu Rev Biochem 49:533–564, 1980.

Snyder, S. H.: Brain peptides as neurotransmitters. Science 209:976–983, 1980.

Vale, W., Spiess, J., Rivier, C., and Rivier, J.: Characterization of a 41-residue ovine hypothalamic peptide that stimulates secretion of corticotropin and β-endorphin. Science 213:1394–1397, 1981.

The Pituitary and Hypothalamus

E. CHESTER RIDGWAY III, M.D.

The pituitary gland, located at the base of the brain under the hypothalamus, is the "master gland" of the endocrine system. Its unique location is important to the integration of the endocrine system, because it serves to transduce information from the central nervous system to the peripheral endocrine glands. It has broad functions and widespread effects on many organ systems. The pituitary gland controls growth, metabolism, reproduction, and sexual function. It regulates these functions by the secretion from the pituitary of hormones that interact at specific sites in the periphery. All of the hormones from the pituitary are peptides or glycoproteins. Once secreted from the anterior pituitary, they all circulate freely in the serum and mediate their action by interacting with specific receptors on the surface of target organs.

The pituitary can be divided into two parts (Fig. 9). The larger portion is called the *anterior pituitary (adenohypophysis)* and consists of 80 per cent of the entire gland. The anterior pituitary secretes six major hormones: somatotropin (GH), prolactin (PRL), corticotropin (ACTH), thyrotropin (TSH), luteinizing hormone (LH), and follicle-stimulating hormone (FSH). The anterior pituitary is regulated by both positive and negative influences from the hypothalamus and peripheral target glands. The regulation from the hypothalamus is accomplished by the secretion of hypothalamic-releasing hormones that enter the hypophyseal-portal blood system, descend to the anterior pituitary cells, and interact with specific receptors on the anterior pituitary cells. The hypothalamic factors may be peptides or catecholamines (Table 5). In general, these

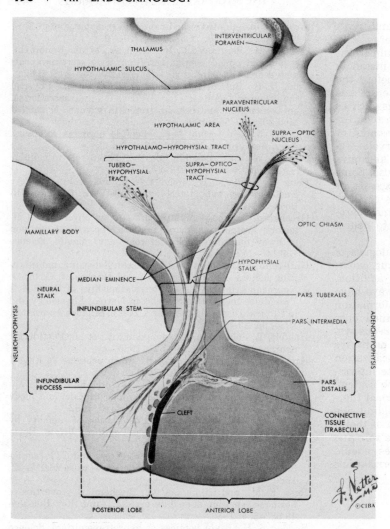

compounds have very short half-lives and are characterized by a highly specific interaction with a particular cell type of the anterior pituitary. For instance, the hypothalamic factor, which controls the gonadotropins LH and FSH, is called gonadotropin-releasing hormone (GnRH). This hypothalamic factor is secreted from the hypothalamus and interacts only with gonadotrope cells in the anterior pituitary. As a result of the interaction between GnRH and its target cells in the anterior pituitary, LH and FSH are secreted into the peripheral circulation. In the circulation LH and FSH stimulate the production of the sex steroid hormones

estrogen and testosterone. These peripheral sex steroid hormones mediate their effects on reproductive and sexual function and, in addition, feed back negatively or positively on both the anterior pituitary and the hypothalamus to modulate LH and FSH secretion. All of the pituitary hormones from the anterior pituitary are regulated by a variation of this same process (Fig. 10). In some instances, the hypothalamus not only will exert positive effects on anterior pituitary hormone secretion but also will regulate in a negative fashion. For instance, prolactin secretion is stimulated by thyrotropin-releasing hormone (TRH) but is inhibited by

TABLE 5. HYPOTHALAMIC HORMONES AFFECTING ANTERIOR PITUITARY FUNCTION

HYPOTHALAMIC HORMONE	STRUCTURE	PITUITARY HORMONE
Thyrotropin-releasing Hormone (TRH)	3 amino acids	Stimulates TSH and PRL release
Gonadotropin-releasing Hormone (GnRH, LHRH)	10 amino acids	Stimulates LH and FSH release
Growth Hormone–releasing Factor (GRF, Somatocrinin)	44 or 40 amino acids (isolated from pancreatic tumor)	Stimulates GH release
Corticotropin-releasing Hormone (CRF)	41 amino acids (isolated from ovine hypothalami)	Stimulates ACTH and β-LPH release
Growth Hormone–inhibiting Hormone (SRIF, Somatostatin)	14 amino acids	Inhibits GH (and TSH) release
Dopamine (PIF)	Catecholamine	Inhibits PRL (and TSH) release

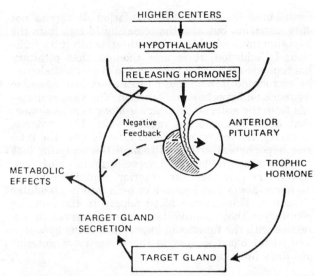

Figure 10. Relationship of anterior pituitary hormone secretion to regulation by hypothalamic factors that modulate their secretion. Target gland hormones exert metabolic effects and feedback, either negatively or positively, at the pituitary or hypothalamus. (From Hall, R., et al.: Fundamentals of Clinical Endocrinology. London, Pitman Medical, 1974.)

dopamine. The resulting secretion represents a balance between the oppositely directed forces. To understand the importance of the hypothalamus in controlling pituitary function, it is useful to consider the consequences of sectioning the pituitary stalk, thus depriving the pituitary of its regulation by the hypothalamus. Such an event leads to a decrease in the secretion of all anterior pituitary hormones except prolactin, which increases. Thus, the predominant net hypothalamic influence on GH, TSH, ACTH, LH, and FSH is *stimulatory*, while that on PRL is *inhibitory*. Complex diagrams can be drawn for each of the pituitary hormones, reflecting their integrated regulation by the hypothalamus and by peripheral hormones. These interesting regulatory features will be discussed briefly in this chapter and in more detail in subsequent chapters on the thyroid, adrenal, and reproductive glands.

The *posterior pituitary (neurohypophysis)* consists of less than 20 per cent of the entire pituitary and is distinct morphologically and functionally from the anterior pituitary. The posterior pituitary consists of the terminal axonal projections of cells that originate in the supraoptic and paraventricular nuclei of the hypothalamus and descend by long tracts within the pituitary stalk to the posterior pituitary. The posterior pituitary hormones are antidiuretic hormone (ADH) and oxytocin (Table 6). Both are peptides, and each is synthesized in cell bodies located in the hypothalamus. In association with unique binding proteins, the *neu-*

rophysins, ADH and oxytocin are transferred down the axonal projections to the posterior pituitary, where they are stored in secretory granules. Unlike the anterior pituitary, the posterior pituitary hormones are not regulated by hypothalamic factors secreted into the hypophyseal-portal blood system. In addition, they do not appear to be regulated in a negative feedback manner by circulating target gland hormones, such as thyroid, adrenal, or sex steroid hormones. These hormones will be discussed in subsequent chapters.

ANATOMY

The pituitary gland in a normal adult weighs approximately 500 mg. During certain physiological and pathological states, the pituitary can enlarge dramatically. For instance, during pregnancy, it may double its weight to 1 gm in size. Furthermore, in certain pathological states, such as primary hypothyroidism, unrestrained thyroid hormone deficiency may cause the pituitary to enlarge secondary to hyperplastic and hypertrophic growth of the thyrotropes. Hyperplastic pituitary growth is usually entirely reversible if the stimulus for growth is removed. Pathologically, pituitary tumors are the most important cause of pituitary enlargement. The exact prevalence of pituitary tumors is difficult to ascertain. In autopsy studies, the examination of pituitary glands has shown an incidence of microadenomas ranging from 2.7 to 22.5 per cent. This remarkably high figure is greater than the prevalence of pituitary tumors detected clinically in the population.

Cell Types. The anterior pituitary has at least five distinct cell types: somatotropes, lactotropes, corticotropes, thyrotropes, and gonadotropes. The different cell types are distinguished by morphology and by

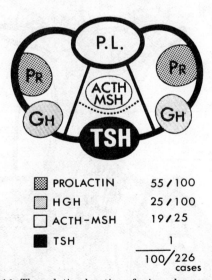

▨ PROLACTIN	55 / 100
▦ HGH	25 / 100
□ ACTH – MSH	19 / 25
■ TSH	1
	100 / 226 cases

Figure 11. The relative location of microadenomas of various cell types within the anterior pituitary. Note that prolactin microadenomas are the most frequent. Both prolactin and growth hormone–producing microadenomas are localized to the lateral aspect of the pituitary; ACTH microadenomas tend to be more centrally located. (From Hardy, J.: In Rand, R. W. (ed.): Microneurosurgery, 3rd ed. St. Louis, C. V. Mosby Co., 1978, p. 125.)

TABLE 6. POSTERIOR PITUITARY HORMONES

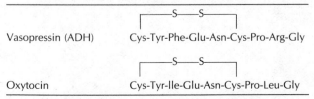

Vasopressin (ADH)   Cys-Tyr-Phe-Glu-Asn-Cys-Pro-Arg-Gly

Oxytocin   Cys-Tyr-Ile-Glu-Asn-Cys-Pro-Leu-Gly

immunohistocytochemistry. Although strict divisions within the anterior pituitary are not present, there does appear to be a regional localization of the different cell types. For instance, GH- and PRL-secreting microadenomas tend to concentrate on the lateral aspects of the pituitary, whereas those secreting ACTH localize in the midline (Fig. 11). The number of each cell type within the anterior pituitary has been estimated on morphological and immunohistocytochemical studies. In general, GH cells are the most frequent and account for 30 to 50 per cent of the cells. PRL cells are the next most frequent, accounting for 10 to 40 per cent of the cells. ACTH-secreting cells account for 5 to 15 per cent, and thyrotropes and gonadotropes each account for 5 to 10 per cent of the total cells.

Blood Supply. The blood supply to the anterior pituitary is quite substantial (Fig. 12). Arterial blood arrives from the superior hypophyseal artery, which originates from the internal carotid artery and ends in capillaries in the median eminence. These capillaries fuse into long portal vessels that descend as the hypophyseal-portal circulation to the anterior pituitary. The purpose of this portal circulation is to provide a critically important vascular connection between the hypothalamus and the pituitary. The majority of the blood supply to the anterior pituitary appears to be contributed by this portal circulation. It carries not only nutrients but also the releasing factors from the hypothalamus which regulate anterior pituitary function. In addition, it is now thought that pituitary hormones may be able to ascend to the hypothalamus by retrograde flow to exert ultra-short loop negative feedback on hypothalamic function. The venous drainage from the anterior pituitary is along venous sinuses that enter the internal jugular vein. The posterior pituitary derives arterial blood directly from the inferior hypophyseal artery. Although the posterior lobe consists of nerve fibers and nerve terminals with neurosecretory granules, the anterior pituitary contains no nerve fibers and appears to be a purely glandular structure. This unique blood supply to the anterior pituitary without concomitant neural innervation correlates with the functional importance of the hypophyseal-portal blood system to the integrity of anterior pituitary function.

FUNCTIONAL CONSIDERATIONS

In discussing the hormones of the anterior pituitary, their diverse functions, and the diseases that abnormalities in their secretion can produce, certain general principles are recurrent themes. First, the pituitary

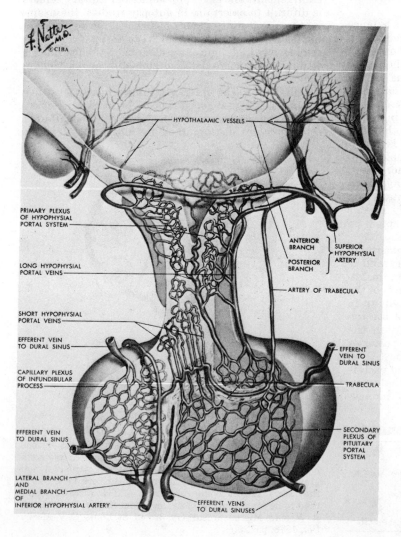

Figure 12. The blood supply to the pituitary gland, showing the dependence of the anterior pituitary (adenohypophysis) on the hypophyseal-portal system. In contrast, most of the posterior pituitary (neurohypophysis) derives its blood supply from the inferior hypophyseal artery. (© Copyright 1965, CIBA Pharmaceutical Company, Division of CIBA-GEIGY Corporation. Reprinted with permission from THE CIBA COLLECTION OF MEDICAL ILLUSTRATIONS, illustrated by Frank H. Netter, M.D. All rights reserved.)

hormones are all peptides or glycopeptides; they circulate free and all interact with specific receptors on target glands. The specificity of their action is determined not only by their chemical structure but also by the presence of receptors specific for them on target gland cells.

Second, the secretion of the anterior pituitary hormones is regulated by the hypothalamus. The hypothalamic regulation may involve stimulation, suppression, or both. In addition, the production of the pituitary hormones is also regulated by feedback from target glands. In most, the feedback is negative (i.e., thyroxine on TSH secretion), whereas in others it may be negative or positive (i.e., estrogen on LH secretion). Normal secretion of the pituitary hormones depends on a synchronous integration of the signals from the hypothalamus and from peripheral hormones.

Third, many of the pituitary hormones have secretion that is characterized by pulsatile or diurnal rhythms. These rhythms are entrained to the hypothalamus and central nervous system, which modulates their secretion by the hypothalamic-releasing hormones. In some instances, a disturbance of diurnal rhythm can produce disease (i.e., Cushing's disease with abnormal diurnal variation of ACTH and cortisol). In other cases, an abnormality in the amplitude or frequency of hypothalamic pulsations can produce significant clinical disorders (i.e., hypothalamic amenorrhea with abnormal GnRH and gonadotropin pulsations). In both of these examples *basal* secretion of the pituitary hormone may be normal, but *rhythm* abnormalities are producing functional disturbances. Thus, a correct diagnosis depends on a precise clinical presentation and blood tests that probe functional capacity rather than static basal concentrations.

Fourth, primary diseases of the pituitary gland generally produce clinical problems from mass effects or functional disturbances. The mass effects are usually related to pituitary tumors expanding within or growing out of the sella turcica. The functional disturbances relate to either hypersecretory or hyposecretory states. To make the diagnosis of an overproduction state, one must demonstrate evidence of excessive hormonal production as well as defects in the feedback suppression of the pituitary hormone in question. Conversely, underproduction states are diagnosed by the demonstration of decreased hormone production and defects in the stimulation of the anterior pituitary hormone. In all states of functional pituitary tumors, the hormone production by the tumor is relatively autonomous. Therefore, variable abnormalities in suppressibility always exist; in some instances, abnormalities of stimulation are also present. In underproduction states, decreases in the stimulation of pituitary hormones may be partial or complete. The utility of suppression and stimulation tests for each of the pituitary hormones will be discussed in relation to overproduction or underproduction states.

GROWTH HORMONE

CHEMISTRY AND PRODUCTION

Growth hormone (GH) is the major anterior pituitary hormone responsible for linear growth. Quantitatively,

GH is one of the most dominant of the anterior pituitary hormones; a normal anterior pituitary gland contains 5 to 10 mg of GH. Children secrete more GH than adults. Production rates of GH have been estimated to be between 500 and 1000 µg daily in children or adolescents and approximately 400 µg daily in adults. Like most peptides, GH circulates free in plasma and has a short half-life of between 30 and 60 minutes. The secretion of GH during a 24-hour period fluctuates significantly. In the fasting and basal states, most adults have plasma GH concentrations of less than 2 ng/ml, and in many instances the values are undetectable. Peaks of GH secretion occur after meals, and most predominantly during stages III and IV of sleep. Generally, the sleep-entrained GH secretion accounts for the majority of GH production during a 24-hour period (Fig. 13).

GH is composed of a large single polypeptide chain, with a molecular weight of 21,500, containing 191 amino acids. Chemically, GH contains two intramolecular disulfide bonds that, along with the amino-terminal end of the molecule, appear to be critical for achieving the biological effects of the hormone. Structurally, GH has considerable amino acid homology

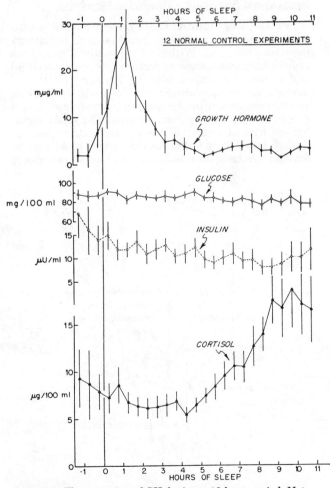

Figure 13. The secretion of GH during a 12-hour period. Note the increases in GH levels that occur during the early phases of Stage III or IV sleep. (From Takahashi, Y., et al.: J Clin Invest 47:2079, 1968. Reproduced by copyright permission of the American Society for Clinical Investigation.)

with human placental lactogen, also known as chorionic somatomammotropin, which also is a 191 amino acid peptide. Human placental lactogen has 161 amino acids that are identical to those of GH; however, despite this striking degree of homology, it contains less than 1 per cent of GH's biological effect. In addition, PRL, which has 198 amino acids, has considerable structural homology with GH. This high degree of homology between GH, PRL, and placental lactogen has suggested that all three hormones originated from a common gene. The GH and PRL genes have been shown to have similar intervening sequences. As is common with many proteins that are destined for secretion, GH is synthesized as part of a larger precursor with a molecular weight of 28,000 daltons. A very interesting smaller form of GH [20K], with a molecular weight of 20,000 daltons and a 15 amino acid deletion between amino acid residues 32 and 46, has also been isolated. Paradoxically, this form of GH, with its deletion that occurs at an intervening sequence, has some of the biological properties of GH (growth promotion) but lacks other features of GH action (glucose and free fatty-acid metabolism).

REGULATION OF GROWTH HORMONE SECRETION

Peptide Regulation. The secretion of GH is intimately associated with two hypothalamic regulatory peptides (Fig. 14). Within the hypothalamus, both growth hormone–releasing factor (GRF, somatocrinin) and growth hormone–inhibiting hormone (SRIF, somatostatin) are synthesized. They mediate their effects on GH secretion by interacting with specific membrane receptors on pituitary somatotropes. The exact structure of hypothalamic GRF is currently unknown, although two potent GH-releasing factors of 44 and 40 amino acids have been isolated from human pancreatic

tumors. Synthesis of the pancreatic GRF has provided a potent new tool for the evaluation of GH secretion. Somatostatin is a tetradecapeptide that is present not only in the hypothalamus but also in the D cells of the pancreas and throughout the gastrointestinal tract. The secretion of GH represents a balance between these two opposing forces. Many central nervous system and peripheral factors influence the minute-to-minute secretion of GRF and SRIF, thus altering the net effect on GH secretion. Since measurements of portal blood GRF and SRIF concentrations have not been quantitated relative to GH levels, the understanding of the modulation of GH secretion remains incomplete. Thus, the current discussion of GH regulation by neurotransmitters is limited to the *net* effect on GH secretion. Table 7 summarizes the important modulators of GH production.

Adrenergic Regulation. In general, α-adrenergic stimulation results in increased GH secretion. The administration of the α-adrenergic agonists (norepinephrine, clonidine, apomorphine, L-dopa) stimulates, whereas the α-adrenergic antagonist (phentolamine) inhibits GH secretion in man and laboratory animals. In contrast, the β-adrenergic antagonist (propranolol) increases and the β-adrenergic agonist (isoproterenol) inhibits GH secretion. Adrenergic neurotransmitters are thought to act primarily by increasing GRF secretion from the hypothalamus, since norepinephrine has no effect in vitro on GH secretion from pituitary cultures. Conversely, SRIF modulation of GH secretion is not currently thought to be influenced by the adrenergic neurotransmitters. Many of the physiological stimuli for GH secretion are mediated through these adrenergic influences, including stress, exercise, and the postprandial period by causing hyperaminoacidemia or relative hypoglycemia. Despite the importance of the adrenergic system in modulating *physiological*

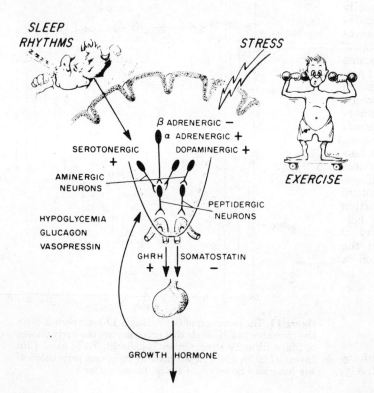

Figure 14. The regulation of GH secretion is related predominantly to hypothalamic GH-releasing factor (GRF) and somatostatin (SRIF). Adrenergic, dopaminergic, and serotonergic influences from the central nervous system modulate hypothalamic GRF and SRIF secretion, which determines the net secretion of GH from the anterior pituitary. (From Reichlin, S.: In Williams, R. H. (ed.): Textbook of Endocrinology. 6th ed. Philadelphia, W. B. Saunders Co., 1981, p. 618.)

TABLE 7. FACTORS AFFECTING GROWTH HORMONE SECRETION

STIMULATION	SUPPRESSION
Peptides	
1. GRF	1. SRIF
2. TRH, LHRH (acromegaly)	2. Growth hormone
3. Vasopressin	3. Somatomedins
4. Glucagon	
5. Enkephalins	
6. VIP	
7. α-MSH	
Biogenic Amines	
1. α-Adrenergic agonists (norepinephrine, clonidine, L-dopa, apomorphine)	1. α-Adrenergic antagonists (phentolamine)
2. Dopaminergic agonists (L-dopa, apomorphine, bromocriptine)	2. Dopaminergic antagonists (phenothiazines)
3. Serotonergic precursors (tryptophan, 5-hydroxytryptophan)	3. Serotonergic antagonists (cyproheptadine)
4. β-Adrenergic antagonists (propranolol)	4. β-Adrenergic agonists (isoproterenol)
	5. Dopaminergic agonists in acromegaly (L-dopa, dopamine, bromocriptine)
Substrates of Intermediate Metabolism	
1. Hypoglycemia (postprandial or after insulin)	1. Hyperglycemia
2. Hyperaminoacidemia (arginine)	2. Increased free fatty acids
Other	
1. Gamma amino hydroxybutyric acid	1. Hypothyroidism
2. Prostaglandins	2. Glucocorticoids
3. Histamine H_2 receptor antagonists	3. Progesterone
4. Cholinergic agonists	
5. Thyroid hormones (in vitro)	

GH release, blockade of α-adrenergic receptors does not inhibit elevated GH secretion in *pathological* states, particularly from pituitary tumors.

Serotoninergic Regulation. Serotoninergic stimulation, produced by the administration of the precursors (tryptophan and 5-hydroxytryptophan) of serotonin synthesis, generally has a positive effect on GH secretion. Antagonism of serotoninergic stimulation by cyproheptadine or methysergide inhibits the GH response to these precursors. Serotoninergic antagonism inhibits GH stimulation from a variety of pharmacological factors, including not only the serotonin precursors but also insulin-induced hypoglycemia and arginine infusion. In addition, serotonin appears to play an important role in modulating exercise and sleep-induced GH secretion, possibly involving both GRF stimulation and SRIF inhibition. A clinical finding, consistent with a serotonin-mediated decrease in SRIF secretion, is the occasional acromegalic patient who has decreased GH secretion following administration of the serotonin antagonist cyproheptadine.

Dopaminergic Regulation. Dopaminergic stimulation provides important modulation of GH secretion. Unlike serotoninergic and adrenergic influences, which mediate their effects at the level of the hypothalamus, dopaminergic stimulation has opposing effects at the hypothalamus and pituitary. At the hypothalamic level, dopaminergic agonists increase GH secretion, presumably by producing a positive effect on GRF secretion. Apomorphine, L-dopa, and bromocriptine all increase GH secretion by this mechanism. The effect is blocked by the dopaminergic receptor antagonists (phenothiazines) and glucose administration, the latter suggesting that stimulation of glucoreceptors in the hypothalamus can overcome dopaminergic stimulation of GH. In contrast, dopaminergic stimulation in vitro inhibits GH secretion directly at the pituitary, an effect that is mediated by specific dopamine receptors on anterior pituitary cells. Furthermore, dopaminergic stimulation causes an unexpected reduction in GH levels in approximately 75 per cent of acromegalic patients. These observations form the basis for the use of bromocriptine in the therapy of acromegaly.

Other Factors. Other factors that stimulate GH secretion are outlined in Table 7. Two important aspects of intermediate metabolism are particularly relevant. Hypoglycemia following insulin administration or decreases in the blood sugar in the late postprandial period are potent stimulators of GH release. This effect is thought to be mediated via hypothalamic glucoreceptors, thus enhancing GRF release. Likewise, hyperaminoacidemia causes a similar rise in GH. These physiological findings have been used to create the standardized "insulin tolerance test" and "arginine infusion test," which are routinely used in the diagnostic evaluation of GH secretory reserve. Of all the stimulation tests available for GH reserve, the insulin tolerance test has been considered to be the most reliable (Fig. 15). With the recent discovery and availability of pancreatic GRF, the future evaluations of pituitary GH reserve will most likely be improved by intravenous GRF stimulation tests (Fig. 16).

Factors that suppress GH secretion are also detailed in Table 7. SRIF is the most important hypothalamic substance that inhibits GH release. In addition, both GH and somatomedin C have been implicated in the negative feedback inhibition of GH release. These hormones may directly inhibit pituitary release of GH, or, alternatively, stimulate hypothalamic SRIF release, which mediates the inhibition at the pituitary level. Hyperglycemia also has potent suppressive effects on GH secretion. Elevated levels of blood sugar

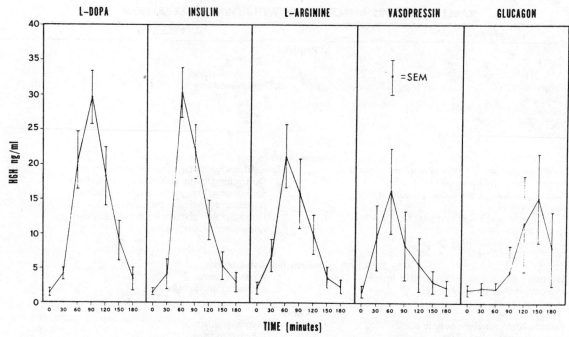

Figure 15. Comparison of GH secretory responses to a variety of physiological and pharmacological manipulations. The response to insulin-induced hypoglycemia is the standard against which other responses are compared. (From Eddy, R. L., Gilliland, P. F., and Ibarra, J. D., Jr.: Am J Med 56:179, 1974.)

interact with hypothalamic glucoreceptors and may mediate the inhibitory effects on GH by decreasing GRF release.

MECHANISMS OF ACTION

GH mediates its major effects on growth by stimulating the production of *somatomedins*; in addition, it

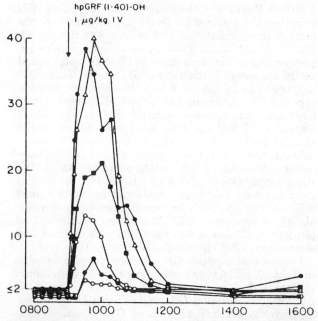

Figure 16. Serum GH responses (vertical axis) to intravenous administration of pancreatic GRF (hpGRF, 1-40) in six normal men. The increases in serum GH concentrations are specific, and GRF did not cause increases in the serum concentrations of other pituitary hormones. (From Thorner, M. O., Rivier, J., and Spiess, J.: Lancet 1:24, 1983.)

may have direct effects on adipose and hepatic cells, producing lipolysis and changes in intermediate metabolism. GH interacts with specific glycoprotein receptors on hepatic cells, stimulating somatomedin production and release. The somatomedins represent a class of proteins circulating in plasma which have been termed "growth factors." These proteins have wide biological effects that predominantly regulate linear skeletal growth as well as exert insulin-like actions on muscle and adipose tissue. Somatomedins include five separate peptides: somatomedin A, somatomedin C, insulin-like growth factor-1 (IGF_1), insulin-like growth factor-2 (IGF_2), and multiplication stimulating activity (MSA). Somatomedin C and IGF_1 appear to be identical and are the most sensitive growth factors stimulated by GH. These peptides usually consist of an amino acid chain of 60 to 70 residues with intrachain disulfide bridges, giving them a structural conformation similar to that of the A and B chains of insulin. Somatomedins do not exist free in plasma but rather are associated with carrier proteins.

Somatomedins have two basic functions: they are mitogenic for chondrocytes and are stimulators of cell growth. In general, somatomedin levels parallel GH levels. Values increase during childhood, reaching adult levels at adolescence. GH administered to hypopituitary patients causes a rise in somatomedin C within hours, with peak values being observed after approximately one week of therapy. In circumstances of excess GH secretion, such as acromegaly, somatomedin C levels are elevated and thus become an important additional test in the diagnostic evaluation of GH disorders. Somatomedin C levels generally correlate with growth velocity and are elevated in tall children and lower in patients of short stature. In addition to regulating growth velocity and certain aspects of intermediate metabolism, the somatomedins

TABLE 8. CLASSIFICATION OF GROWTH FAILURE

NAME	SITE OF DEFECT
I. Hypothalamic Disorder 　1. Congenital or idiopathic GH deficiency 　2. Hypothalamic tumors (craniopharyngioma)	I. Hypothalmus (GRF deficiency)
II. Pituitary Disorders 　1. Pituitary tumors 　2. Pituitary dysplasia 　3. Production of abnormal GH molecule	II. Pituitary (deficient or defective GH)
III. Tissue Resistance 　1. Laron's dwarf = high GH, low somatomedin C, 　　low IGF_2 (Kwashiorkor disease) 　2. Pygmy = Normal GH, low somatomedin C, 　　normal IGF_2	III. Liver (deficient or ineffective somatomedin C)

may regulate GH secretion by negative feedback. In vitro experiments have shown that somatomedin C will stimulate somatostatin release, resulting in inhibition of GH secretion.

GROWTH HORMONE DEFICIENCY

In children, GH deficiency results in retardation of linear growth, and, in some circumstances, insulin sensitivity; in adults, GH deficiency contributes to insulin sensitivity but does not further influence linear growth. In children, primary pituitary dwarfism is due to GH deficiency, which can be due to primary destructive or congenital lesions of the hypothalamus or pituitary (Table 8). This disorder is quite rare and occurs with a frequency of between 1:1,000 and 1:10,000 of the population. The most frequently encountered destructive lesions of the hypothalamus or pituitary include craniopharyngioma, trauma, granulomatous disorders, and pituitary tumors (Fig. 17). Patients with isolated congenital (or idiopathic) GH deficiency have a family history most compatible with an autosomal recessive pattern of inheritance. The disorder is thought to be due to defective GRF production by the hypothalamus. In this circumstance, dwarfism is as-

sociated with insulin sensitivity. In other families with dwarfism, the insulin sensitivity is absent and the pattern of inheritance is autosomal dominant. The diagnosis of congenital hypothalamic-pituitary dwarfism depends on the family history, an absence of other structural defects in the hypothalamus and pituitary, and low serum GH and somatomedin C levels.

It is important to distinguish hypothalamic-pituitary GH deficiency from the syndromes of end-organ resistance to GH. The Laron dwarf is characterized by insulin sensitivity, short stature, and a pattern of inheritance similar to that found in primary pituitary dwarfism (i.e., autosomal recessive). However, in these children, GH levels are elevated, but somatomedin C (IGF_1) levels are undetectable. Exogenous GH administration fails to increase somatomedin C levels or growth velocity (Fig. 18). Thus, the Laron dwarf represents an example of generalized tissue resistance to the actions of GH, possibly due to a defect in GH receptors or a postreceptor abnormality. Ironically, this disorder is similar to that seen in kwashiorkor disease, in which high GH levels, low somatomedin C levels, and delayed growth are found. In this latter circumstance, protein refeeding reverses the abnormality. These examples of generalized tissue unresponsiveness

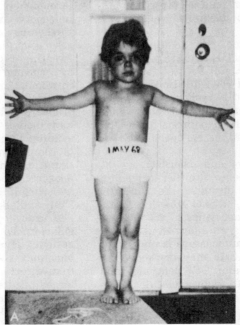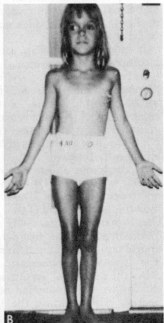

Figure 17. A six-year-old female with growth failure due to a craniopharyngioma before (A) and after (B) 15 months of GH therapy. (From Daughaday, W. H.: In Williams, R. H. (ed.): Textbook of Endocrinology. 6th ed. Philadelphia, W. B. Saunders Co., 1981, p. 98.)

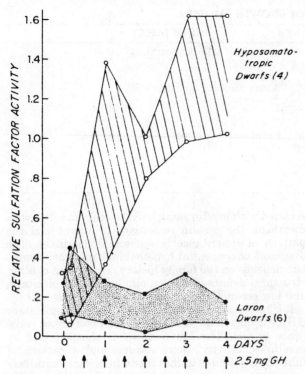

Figure 18. The response of somatomedin (sulfation factor) to GH administration in Laron dwarfs compared to children with growth retardation due to growth hormone deficiency. Note the tissue resistance in the Laron dwarfs compared to the tissue responsiveness in GH-deficient children. (From Daughaday, W. H., et al.: Trans Assoc Am Phys 82:129, 1969.)

to GH must be distinguished from the pygmies, in whom GH values are normal and somatomedin C levels are undetectable. This defect is felt to be due to an isolated failure in the generation of somatomedin C, which results in short stature. Other somatomedins, such as IGF_2, are normal. As with the Laron dwarf, additional GH administration fails to correct somatomedin C levels and does not restore normal growth velocity.

It is possible that in some patients the anterior pituitary can produce forms of GH that are biologically inactive to account for short stature associated with increased immunoactive GH concentrations and low somatomedin C levels. In this circumstance, when exogenous GH is given, somatomedin C levels rise and growth velocity increases. The hypothesis to account for these observations is that the endogenous GH is biologically inactive.

In summary, short stature and dwarfism can be caused by primary GH deficiency of either congenital or structural origin. These disorders are clinically indistinguishable from other forms of growth retardation in which pituitary GH deficiency is not present. To distinguish these disorders, an informed use of GH and somatomedin C radioimmunoassays is important. The discovery of pancreatic GRF may markedly improve the therapy of hypothalamic GRF deficiency, and the large-scale production of GH by molecular engineering will facilitate the therapy of pituitary GH deficiency.

GROWTH HORMONE EXCESS

Causes of GH Excess. Elevations in GH production due to GH-secreting pituitary tumors are the most common cause of acromegaly in adults or gigantism in children. GH-producing pituitary tumors are the second most common pituitary neoplasm encountered in clinical medicine. Rarely, acromegaly may be caused by hyperplasia of the somatotropes within the pituitary, which is secondary to the ectopic production of GRF by neoplasms. Acromegaly occurs in males and females equally and generally presents in middle age. The diagnosis is usually delayed a decade after symptoms have first appeared. This is due to the insidious development of symptoms that are usually not recognized by the patient. Untreated acromegaly results in considerable morbidity and reduces life expectancy. Death directly attributable to acromegaly generally results from cardiovascular complications.

The pituitary tumors causing acromegaly are generally larger than 1 cm. In over 80 per cent of cases, the tumors are considered to be macroadenomas. Approximately 20 per cent of GH-secreting tumors will also hypersecrete prolactin and contain lactotropes in the tumor. Pathologically, the adenomas contain densely granulated acidophilic granules that stain positively by immunocytochemistry for GH.

Clinical Manifestations. The clinical presentation of excessive GH secretion is largely attributable to high somatomedin C levels, which have diverse effects on the body. If the disorder occurs before puberty, acceleration of linear growth and gigantism result. If the disorder occurs after puberty, then acral enlargement of the bones is the predominant finding. This results in the classic physical features of acromegaly (Fig. 19), including prognathism, frontal bossing, enlargement of the mandible, widely spaced teeth, enlargement of the hands and feet, expansion of the ribs, crippling osteoarthritis, generalized enlargement of the skull, and increased size of the frontal sinuses (Table 9). In addition, soft tissue overgrowth results in swelling, puffy facial features, weight gain, and enlargement of the visceral organs, including hepatosplenomegaly and cardiomegaly. There is generalized thickening of the skin with increased activity of the sebaceous glands, resulting in oiliness and excessive sweating. Skin tags and papillomas are common, as are acne and sebaceous cysts. Hyperthecosis is common in women, and acanthosis nigricans may be observed. A variety of symptoms including sweating, heat intolerance, and fatigue are present. Neuropathic symptoms may include paresthesias secondary to carpal tunnel syndrome, as well as other neurosensory defects due to compression of nerves as they exit the cervical, thoracic, and lumbar spine. The lipolytic and gluconeogenic effects of GH lead to glucose intolerance and hyperinsulinism in over 50 per cent of the patients. Clinical diabetes mellitus is less common, and diabetic ketoacidosis is rarely seen. Hyperprolactinemia and galactorrhea may be seen in 20 per cent of female patients. Hypogonadism, infertility, and decreased libido may result either from hyperprolactinemia or from direct compression of gonadotropes by the enlarged pituitary tumor. Thyrotropin and corticotropin deficiencies are less commonly seen (less than 10 per cent of cases).

Radiologic Findings. Radiologic assessment of the pituitary to demonstrate a pituitary adenoma is now most efficiently performed by computerized tomography, with and without enhancement. Older methods, including routine films of the skull, polytomography of the sella turcica, and pneumoencephalography, have largely been supplanted by the technological advances provided by CT scanning. Only in special circumstances are additional studies, such as angiography, venography, metrizamide CT scanning, and polytomography, necessary.

THERAPY OF GROWTH HORMONE—PRODUCING TUMORS

A variety of options is available for the treatment of acromegaly. The immediate goal of therapy should be the complete removal of all abnormal tissue producing GH. Unfortunately, most of the tumors associated with acromegaly are large, and this goal is rarely achieved with a single modality of therapy. Therefore, combinations of the various therapeutic options are usually necessary. They will be summarized briefly, since this book is largely devoted to pathophysiology. The long-term objective of treatment is to arrest all progression of the acromegalic process, to normalize somatomedin C levels, and to reduce GH values to less than 2 ng/ml. Ideally, one would want to achieve GH values in the undetectable range.

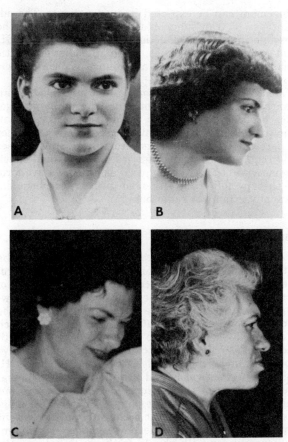

Figure 19. The development of changes in a patient with acromegaly. *A,* At age 16 the features are normal. *B,* At age 27 a profile shows normal fine nasal and jaw structure. *C,* At age 38, after birth of only child, early prognathism and coarsening of the features are present. *D,* At age 57 obvious acromegalic features are present in profile compared to *B.*

Laboratory Studies. The diagnosis of acromegaly depends on the demonstration of elevated levels of GH, which are usually greater than 5 ng/ml and may be as high as 500 ng/ml. The elevated levels of GH are associated with increased levels of somatomedin C (Fig. 20). Somatomedin C levels may, in fact, correlate better with clinical indices of disease activity than do GH values. Therefore, somatomedin C measurements have become an integral part of the diagnosis and follow-up of acromegalic patients. The regulation of GH secretion is also abnormal in acromegaly. GH values fail to suppress with an oral glucose load and fail to stimulate with insulin-induced hypoglycemia. Dopaminergic stimulation by bromocriptine administration reduces GH secretion in approximately 75 per cent of acromegalic patients, a feature different from that found in normal subjects, in whom dopaminergic stimulation increases GH secretion. Thyrotropin-releasing hormone and gonadotropin-releasing hormone paradoxically increase GH secretion in acromegaly in 25 per cent of cases but have no effect on GH secretion in normal subjects. Other less direct, nonspecific tests suggesting augmented GH activity include the demonstration of hypercalcemia, hypophosphaturia, hyperphosphatemia, hyperglycemia, and an abnormal glucose tolerance test.

TABLE 9. CLINICAL MANIFESTATIONS OF ACROMEGALY IN 100 PATIENTS*

MANIFESTATIONS OF GH EXCESS	PERCENTAGE
Acral enlargement	100
Soft tissue overgrowth	100
Hyperhidrosis	88
Lethargy or fatigue	87
Weight gain	73
Paresthesias	70
Joint pain	69
Photophobia	46
Papillomas	45
Hypertrichosis	33
Goiter	32
Acanthosis nigricans	29
Hypertension	24
Cardiomegaly	16
Renal calculi	11
DISTURBANCE OF OTHER ENDOCRINE FUNCTIONS	
Hyperinsulinemia	70
Glucose intolerance	50
Irregular or absent menses	60
Decreased libido or impotence	46
Hypothyroidism	13
Galactorrhea	13
Gynecomastia	8
Hypoadrenalism	4
LOCAL MANIFESTATIONS	
Enlarged sella	90
Headache	65
Visual deficit	20

*From Findling, J. W., and Tyrrell, J. B.: In Greenspan, F. S., and Forsham, P. H. (eds.): Basic and Clinical Endocrinology. Los Altos, CA, Lange Medical Publishers, 1983, p. 77.

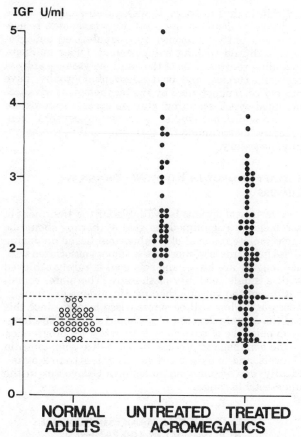

IGF U/ml

Figure 20. Serum IGF (somatomedin) levels in untreated and treated acromegalic patients compared to normal controls. There is excellent separation of untreated acromegaly from normal controls. (From Rieu, M., et al.: J Clin Endocrinol Metab 55:147, 1982.)

Surgical transsphenoidal hypophysectomy is generally the first line of approach. Microadenomas, which account for less than 20 per cent of all cases, can be cured by this approach in approximately 80 to 90 per cent of cases. However, tumors that are greater than 10 mm in diameter are completely resected with less success, although 50 to 60 per cent of these cases are cured. If the initial tumor is large with suprasellar extension or invasion into the cavernous sinus, then the cure rate drops to less than 10 per cent.

Radiotherapy offers a valid alternative or adjunctive modality for therapy of acromegaly. Conventional supervoltage radiation in doses of approximately 5,000 rads will reduce GH values in 75 per cent of patients. However, this reduction in GH values to less than 10 ng/ml takes approximately one decade to achieve. During this period of time, elevated GH and somatomedin C values persist. In addition, the incidence of hypopituitarism, secondary to radiation, is not minimal. Heavy particle or proton beam irradiation has the advantage of being able to deliver higher doses (7,000 to 12,000 rads) to the pituitary with corresponding greater effectiveness. Unfortunately, patients with suprasellar extension or optic nerve involvement cannot be treated initially with these forms of radiotherapy. Furthermore, the degree of hypopituitarism in these patients is significant, and there remains at least a two- to five-year delay before significant clinical im-

provement can be expected in most patients. The advantages of transsphenoidal resection, including the possible immediate reduction or normalization of GH and somatomedin C levels, make all radiotherapeutic modalities most useful as an adjunctive form of therapy.

Medical therapy of acromegaly consists predominantly of the administration of the dopaminergic agonist bromocriptine, which suppresses GH levels in approximately 75 per cent of these patients. Since suppression of GH levels is incomplete in most cases and requires extremely high doses for maximal effect, bromocriptine is generally used as an adjunctive form of therapy following either surgical transsphenoidal hypophysectomy or radiotherapy.

DIFFERENTIAL DIAGNOSIS

Acromegaly can also be caused by hyperplasia of the pituitary somatotropes. This is a rare cause of acromegaly, since over 90 per cent of the autopsy cases of acromegaly are, in fact, due to pituitary tumors. However, hyperplasia can cause acromegaly and should be recognized pathologically at the time of surgery. Such a diagnosis should lead to a search for ectopic GRF secretion. As noted earlier, two pancreatic tumors have now been independently described that produce GH-releasing peptides of 44 and 40 amino acids. The actual true incidence of this phenomenon is unknown, but careful attention should be paid to this possible diagnosis, since the therapeutic options for such a patient are entirely different. The development of radioimmunoassays for GRF should facilitate this diagnosis. Additionally, acromegaly occurring in patients with other malignant processes, such as pancreatic tumors, should be routinely screened for possible ectopic GRF production.

PROLACTIN

CHEMISTRY AND PRODUCTION

Prolactin (PRL) is the anterior pituitary hormone that regulates lactation in the postpartum period. The prolactin-secreting cells (lactotropes) are located in the lateral aspects of the anterior pituitary. In the past, they were considered to be chromophobic because of their failure to stain histologically with acidophilic or basophilic dyes; however, they are easily identifiable by their dense granules as seen on electron microscopy and with immunocytochemical stains. The number of PRL cells in the anterior pituitary is approximately one tenth the number of GH-secreting cells when assessed by electron microscopy. However, when studied by immunofluorescent techniques, PRL and GH cell numbers appear to be similar (i.e., each being 20 to 50 per cent of the total cell population). In the total pituitary, however, the PRL content is approximately 100 μg, which is 100-fold less than that of GH. In pregnancy, the size and number of lactotropes increase dramatically, as does the total PRL content of the pituitary, accounting for most of the increased size of the pituitary.

The normal pituitary PRL production rate is between 200 and 500 μg per day; thus, there is a rapid daily turnover of the pituitary PRL stores. PRL has a serum half-life of approximately 30 minutes and a metabolic clearance rate of 80 ml per minute. Both serum PRL concentration and pituitary PRL production rates are slightly, but significantly, higher in women than in men. Basal serum concentrations of PRL range from 0 to 20 ng/ml.

The human PRL molecule, like that of GH, is a single polypeptide chain of 198 amino acids (mol. wt. ~23,000). The amino acid sequence for PRL has a 16 per cent structural homology with GH and is somewhat less homologous with placental lactogen. PRL is synthesized in the lactotrope as a precursor of approximately 26,000 daltons (preproprolactin), which then undergoes post-translational cleavage. In the circulation, a variety of heterogeneous forms of PRL exists. The predominant species is the native 198 amino acid peptide, which comprises 80 per cent of the total immunoactive prolactin. Larger forms of prolactin, accounting for 10 to 20 per cent of the total immunoactive prolactin, are also present, but their biological significance is unknown. These forms may represent noncovalent binding of PRL to serum proteins, nonspecific aggregation of PRL molecules, or abnormal PRL polypeptide chains. The bigger PRL species are present more frequently in patients with pituitary prolactin-secreting tumors.

PROLACTIN REGULATION

The predominant hypothalamic influence on pituitary PRL secretion is tonic inhibition, which is unique among the anterior pituitary hormones (Fig. 21). For example, following pituitary stalk secretion, the secretion of all other anterior pituitary hormones decreases while PRL secretion increases. Furthermore, transplantation of the pituitary to a distant site in the body results in elevated PRL secretion from the transplanted pituitary, presumably due to the absence of hypothalamic inhibitory effects.

Dopaminergic Regulation. The major hypothalamic PRL inhibitory factor is dopamine, originating from dopaminergic neurons in the median eminence. Dopamine inhibits both PRL synthesis (by inhibiting DNA transcription) and PRL release. Dopamine acts via specific dopamine receptors on the surface of the lactotrope. Compounds that block dopamine receptors (metoclopramide, haloperidol, or the phenothiazines) or deplete hypothalamic dopamine content (α-methyldopa, reserpine) cause PRL secretion to increase. Whether other factors from the hypothalamus are important in inhibiting PRL secretion is a question that is currently under active investigation. Somatostatin does not appear to have major regulatory effects on PRL secretion.

Estrogen Effect. A variety of central and peripheral hormones increases pituitary PRL production. In these instances, the stimulation of PRL production either overcomes or interferes with the tonic inhibition by dopamine. Estrogen is one of the most potent stimulators of PRL production by the anterior pituitary, acting at multiple sites (Fig. 22). Estrogen directly stimulates PRL DNA transcription and stimulates PRL release into the circulation. Furthermore, chronic exposure to estrogens has a mitogenic effect on the lactotrope, thereby increasing the total number of these cells. Finally, estrogen may antagonize hypotha-

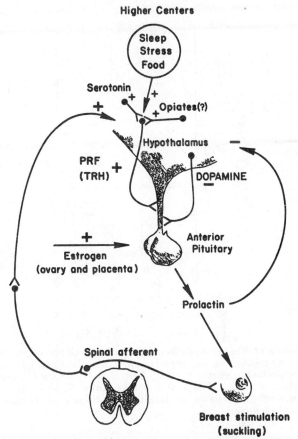

Figure 21. Regulation of prolactin (PRL) secretion from the anterior pituitary. The primary hypothalamic influence on PRL secretion is the inhibitory effect of dopamine. Stimulation of PRL secretion is mediated through estrogens and hypothalamic PRL releasing factors (PRF); TRH is one of the important releasing hormones. Breast suckling induces PRL release by stimulating complex afferent pathways, as illustrated.

lamic dopamine by inhibiting dopamine binding to its receptor. The positive effect of estrogen on PRL production causes PRL levels to be slightly higher in women than in men and increases the PRL responses to other stimuli such as TRH, serotonin, stress, and dopaminergic antagonism.

Thyrotropin-releasing Hormone (TRH) Effect. TRH is another major regulator of PRL secretion. Like estrogen, TRH has been shown to have a direct effect on both PRL DNA transcription and on PRL secretion. TRH increases PRL secretion in a dose-dependent fashion, similar to its effect on TSH release. The TRH effect on PRL release is ultimately related to an increase in the intracellular calcium, which is mediated by stimulation of specific TRH receptors. The extent to which TRH plays a functional role in PRL regulation is uncertain. For instance, the rise in PRL that occurs during suckling is not associated with a rise in TSH, suggesting that PRL release is not mediated by TRH. In hypothyroidism, the PRL response to TRH increases, whereas it decreases in hyperthyroidism, suggesting that thyroid hormones modulate the PRL response to TRH stimulation. In hypothyroidism, the augmented PRL response to TRH may be due either to an increased

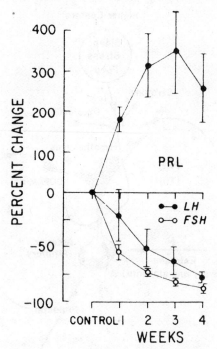

Figure 22. The positive effect of estrogen on prolactin secretion is in contrast to the negative effect that estrogen has on gonadotropin secretion. (From Yen, S. S. C., Ehara, Y., and Siler, T. M.: J Clin Invest 53:652, 1974. Reproduced by copyright permission of the American Society for Clinical Investigation.)

number of TRH receptors on the lactotropes or to a decreased dopaminergic tone from the hypothalamus.

Serotonin Effect. Serotonin also releases prolactin, and serotonin blockers (methysergide or cyproheptadine) can inhibit the rise in PRL due to serotonin. Administration of the serotonin precursors, L-trypto-

phan or 5-hydroxytryptophan, has been reported to increase PRL levels. The possible importance of serotonin in regulating PRL secretion is uncertain. PRL levels, like those of GH, rise during sleep, although at a later time (usually between 4:00 A.M. and 7:00 A.M.). In addition, PRL is secreted in a pulsatile fashion, with approximately four to nine pulses occurring during a 24-hour period. At least half of these pulses occur during sleep, with highly variable pulse amplitude. The nocturnal increase in PRL is not associated with a specific stage of sleep and can be blunted by serotonin antagonists (Fig. 23). Similarly, the PRL increase following stress (surgery, infection, hypoglycemia) can be reduced by serotonin antagonism.

Other Factors. Other central nervous system neurotransmitters may be important in modifying PRL secretion, including opiates and opiate peptides, gamma-aminobutyric acid and its analogues, histamine (H_1 receptor antagonists), the H_2 receptor blocker cimetidine, and vasoactive intestinal polypeptide.

FUNCTION OF PROLACTIN

The breast is the most important locus of PRL action. Specific PRL receptors are located on the surface of alveolar cells, and these receptors can be induced by prolactin. During normal pubertal development, PRL acts with glucocorticoids, mineralocorticoids, progesterone, and insulin to stimulate breast growth (Fig. 24). However, prolactin alone does not cause the breast to grow, and gynecomastia does not result from hyperprolactinemia. After the breasts have fully developed, PRL in association with estrogen, progesterone, glucocorticoids, and possibly chorionic somatomammotropin causes the breast to grow during pregnancy. In addition to effects on mammogenesis, PRL specifically stimulates milk production in the estrogen-primed breast, a process involving stimulation of the synthesis

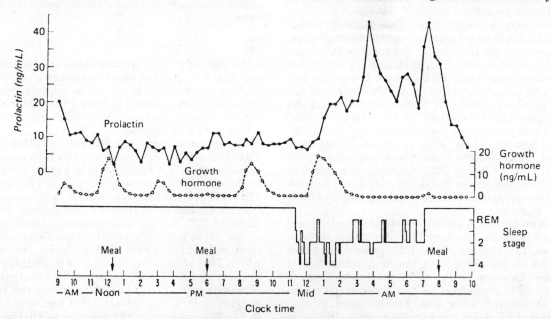

Figure 23. Changes in prolactin (PRL) and growth hormone (GH) during a 24-hour period. Note that PRL secretion is pulsatile and diurnal, with striking elevations in PRL secretion occurring during sleep. The increase in GH secretion during sleep is associated with Stages III and IV of sleep. (From Sassin, J. F., et al.: Science 177:1205, 1972. Copyright 1985 by the AAAS.)

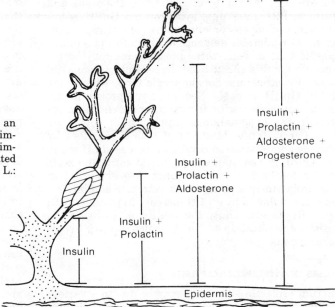

Figure 24. The development of the breast is dependent on an interaction of many hormonal factors. Ductal growth is stimulated by PRL and insulin, whereas mineralocorticoids stimulate branching of ducts, and secretory activity is stimulated by all hormones including progesterone. (From Ceriani, R. L.: Develop Biol 21:506, 1970.)

of the specific milk protein casein and alpha-lactalbumin.

During the course of normal pregnancy, PRL levels steadily increase and reach peak values of 100 to 300 ng/ml at the time of parturition (Fig. 25). The increase

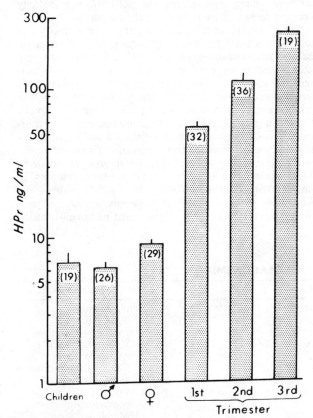

Figure 25. Prolactin concentrations during the various stages of pregnancy compared to normals. (From Jacobs, L., et al.: J Clin Endocrinol Metab 34:484, 1972.)

in prolactin during pregnancy is mediated by placental estrogens, which paradoxically block the effects of prolactin on the breast by reducing PRL receptor numbers, thereby preventing lactation during pregnancy. After parturition, there is a dramatic fall in estrogen levels, which restores normal sensitivity of the breast to prolactin. Immediately post partum, suckling induces an increase in prolactin levels. The basal and peak prolactin responses to suckling then diminish over time. By three to six months post partum, basal prolactin levels are nearly normal, and suckling is accompanied by only a small increase in prolactin or by no increase at all. During the early postpartum period, the suckling-induced increase in prolactin is a complex physiological event. Afferent nerves from the nipple to the brain are coupled to neurosecretory events at the level of the hypothalamic-pituitary axis. Interruption of this complex nervous innervation blocks prolactin release. Conversely, galactorrhea has been described in patients with herpes zoster infection, following chest surgery or trauma, and with spinal cord tumors. These diseases are thought to stimulate the afferent pathways, causing release of prolactin by mechanisms similar to those found in suckling.

Many other tissues (prostate, seminal vesicles, gonads, liver, adrenal, and kidney) have specific receptors for PRL, but the precise role for prolactin in these organs in humans is debated. PRL receptors appear to be important for progesterone production in female rodents, and in male rodents the growth of the seminal vesicles and prostate gland is modulated by PRL. In the kidney PRL acts synergistically with aldosterone and vasopressin to regulate salt and water retention. In the liver, it has a weak stimulatory effect on somatomedin C production. For example, hyperprolactinemic humans with low growth hormone levels have significantly higher somatomedin C levels than patients with low levels of both PRL and GH. In the brain, PRL stimulates maternal behavior in certain species; for instance, it will cause nonlaying hens to incubate eggs. At the level of the hypothalamus and pituitary, PRL interrupts synchronized GnRH secretion, which dampens or eliminates gonadotropin pulsations. Considerable evidence in animals and humans suggests that at least three mechanisms may be responsible for this effect. First, hyperprolactinemia increases hypothalamic dopaminergic tone, which may inhibit GnRH release. Second, hyperprolactinemia may be associated with increased endogenous opiate levels in the hypothalamus which inhibit GnRH release. For instance, blockade of opiate receptors by naloxone administration results in increased LH secretion. Third, the mechanisms by which estrogen exerts positive feedback on LH secretion are abnormal in hyperprolactinemia. Exogenous estrogen administration is not followed by an LH increase in patients with high PRL levels. Thus, the ability of estrogens to sensitize the pituitary to GnRH is defective in hyperprolactinemia.

CAUSES OF HYPERPROLACTINEMIA

Serum prolactin elevations may be due to a variety of physiological, pharmacological, and pathological conditions. These are outlined in Table 10.

Physiological Hyperprolactinemia. The most important physiological reason for hyperprolactinemia is pregnancy or breast feeding in the postpartum period. Other less important physiological causes of mild hyperprolactinemia include hypoglycemia, stress, and sleep.

Pharmacological Hyperprolactinemia. The important pharmacological compounds that produce hyperprolactinemia are high doses of estrogens, psychotropic drugs, particularly phenothiazine and butyrophenone derivatives, and thyrotropin-releasing hormone.

Pathological Hyperprolactinemia. The most important pathological cause of hyperprolactinemia is a prolactin-secreting pituitary tumor (*prolactinoma*). Prolactin-producing pituitary tumors are the most common type of pituitary tumor, accounting for more than 50 per cent of all pituitary neoplasms. These tumors may be small microadenomas, which are less than 10 mm in diameter, or they may be quite large (macroadenomas), extending above the sella turcica into the area of the optic chiasm or laterally into the cavernous sinuses. The circulating level of PRL correlates roughly with the size of the tumor; microadeno-

mas have less elevation of blood PRL concentrations than do large macroadenomas. From a practical viewpoint, PRL levels greater than 100 to 200 ng/ml are almost always associated with a pituitary tumor in the nonpregnant state. PRL elevations of 20 to 100 ng/ml are often found in patients with microadenomas but are also found in patients with hyperprolactinemia of other causes. *Primary hypothyroidism* is commonly associated with mild degrees of hyperprolactinemia, particularly in females. Both *renal failure* and *hepatic cirrhosis* can produce hyperprolactinemia, presumably as a result of either delayed clearance of PRL or delayed estrogen metabolism. The latter effect could stimulate an increase in PRL production. *Hypothalamic or pituitary diseases* other than prolactinoma can interrupt the tonic inhibitory signals from the hypothalamus and cause hyperprolactinemia. Hypothalamic diseases include metastatic tumors, craniopharyngiomas, or granulomatous diseases. Other pituitary tumors, particularly acromegaly, may be associated with hyperprolactinemia in 10 to 20 per cent of cases. In this circumstance, the cellular elements of the tumor are mixed, being composed of both prolactin-secreting and growth hormone–secreting cells.

CONSEQUENCES OF HYPERPROLACTINEMIA

Two extremely important physiological consequences result from hyperprolactinemia: galactorrhea and hypogonadism.

Galactorrhea. Galactorrhea (milk production in the absence of pregnancy) is present in approximately 80 per cent of hyperprolactinemia patients, particularly when it is searched for diligently on physical examination. Despite careful questioning, the patient frequently denies a history of galactorrhea, yet on physical examination, hyperprolactinemic patients are often found to have galactorrhea. Galactorrhea is particularly common in hyperprolactinemic females but is rarely seen in males. Surprisingly, the severity of the galactorrhea does not correlate with serum PRL levels. Although galactorrhea is extremely common in hyperprolactinemic patients, it is neither a sufficient nor a necessary condition for the diagnosis of hyperprolactinemia. For instance, hyperprolactinemia can occur in the absence of galactorrhea in prepubertal females, in females with delayed puberty, or in adult males. Furthermore, patients without hyperprolactinemia may have galactorrhea; up to 25 per cent of normal multi-

TABLE 10. CAUSES OF HYPERPROLACTINEMIA

PHYSIOLOGICAL	PHARMACOLOGICAL	PATHOLOGICAL
Pregnancy	Thyrotropin-releasing hormone (TRH)	Prolactinoma
Postpartum nursing	Estrogen administration	Acromegaly
Sleep	Psychotropic drugs (phenothiazines)	Hypothalamic diseases
Stress	Metoclopramide	Craniopharyngiomas
Sex (i.e., estrogens)	Alpha-methyldopa	Metastatic tumors
Hypoglycemia	Reserpine	Granulomatous diseases
Newborn	Sulpiride	Infiltrative diseases
Intercourse	Opiates	Pituitary stalk section
Nipple stimulation	Cimetidine	Hypothyroidism
	Vasoactive intestinal polypeptide	Liver failure
	L-Tryptophan, 5-hydroxytryptophan	Renal failure
	Gamma aminobutyric acid	Chest wall trauma

parous females may have slight degrees of galactorrhea. Thus, although galactorrhea is very common in hyperprolactinemia, it is neither a specific nor a sensitive indicator of abnormal blood PRL levels.

Hypogonadism. Hypogonadism, which is manifested by amenorrhea or anovulation in females and decreased libido or impotence in males, is another common sequela of hyperprolactinemia. In female patients presenting with amenorrhea, approximately 20 per cent will be found to have hyperprolactinemia due to a pituitary prolactin-secreting tumor. If the patient is found to have galactorrhea as well, her chances of having a prolactinoma rise above 75 per cent. There are few comparable statistics for males having impotence or decreased libido, but probably 1 to 5 per cent have a prolactinoma. There are a variety of postulated mechanisms by which hyperprolactinemia causes hypogonadism: (1) PRL may directly influence hypothalamic centers that govern pulsatile GnRH secretion. High PRL levels dampen or obliterate GnRH pulsations that interrupt the normal communication between the hypothalamus and the pituitary. This hypothesis is consistent with the observed data in humans, which show absent or abnormal LH pulsations in hyperprolactinemic females which normalize after therapy. Whether this effect is mediated directly by high PRL levels or by altered dopamine or opiate tone at the hypothalamus is uncertain. (2) The prolactinoma may directly compress or destroy normal gonadotropes or the pituitary stalk. This mechanism may be operative in patients with very large macroadenomas; however, it cannot account for the hypogonadism seen in association with microadenomas or in patients with hyperprolactinemia unassociated with tumors. (3) The high PRL levels may have a direct effect on gonadal function. This hypothesis is supported by findings in experimental animals that gonads have receptors for PRL and that ovarian progesterone production is inhibited in vitro by PRL. Furthermore, high levels of PRL in antral fluid have been associated with follicular atresia. However, a direct effect of PRL on the ovary would not explain the abnormal or absent LH pulsations seen in hyperprolactinemic females.

Whatever the mechanism, gonadal sex steroid production and gametogenesis are abnormal in hyperprolactinemia. In females, the low serum estrogen levels cause decreased libido, menstrual disorders (oligomenorrhea and amenorrhea), an atrophic vagina, and osteoporosis. In males, decreased libido and impotence are associated with diminished serum testosterone concentrations and decreased sperm counts. In addition to effects on ovarian function, a significant minority of female patients will also complain of hirsutism and mild obesity. The hypothesis to account for these clinical phenomena has been postulated to be a direct effect of PRL on the production of adrenal androgens, resulting in hirsutism and mild obesity. Dihydroepiandrosterone sulfate (DHEAS) is the adrenally secreted androgenic steroid that is found in excessive amounts in hyperprolactinemic patients. This syndrome, which is similar to polycystic ovary disease, is also associated with lowered concentrations of sex steroid–binding globulins and an elevation of free testosterone levels. The exact mechanisms for these findings are unknown, but one explanation would be a direct effect of PRL on the $\Delta 5$ pathway for steroid biosynthesis.

LABORATORY EVALUATION OF HYPERPROLACTINEMIA

The most important measurement for the evaluation of hyperprolactinemia is a random basal blood sample for PRL. The normal range for most laboratories is between 0 and 20 ng/ml. Females have slightly higher values than males. Serum PRL levels above 100 to 200 ng/ml in a nonpregnant individual are most commonly associated with prolactin-secreting tumors. Difficult diagnostic problems occur in patients with PRL elevations between 20 and 100 ng/ml. In these circumstances, the exclusion of other physiological, pharmacological, and pathological processes elevating serum PRL concentrations is mandatory. A reliable PRL suppression test has not been developed; therefore, alternative provocative tests to evaluate the autonomy of the PRL secretion have been investigated. In this regard, the TRH test has been used to investigate the functional status of the lactotrope in hyperprolactinemia (Fig. 16). In most physiological and pharmacological causes of hyperprolactinemia, serum concentrations of PRL increase by two-fold or more following stimulation with TRH. In contrast, patients with prolactin-secreting tumors, or those with hypothalamic disease causing hyperprolactinemia, almost always have a less than two-fold increment in PRL (Fig. 26). The TRH test can, therefore, be useful in the assessment of hyperprolactinemic patients with basal PRL levels between 20 and 100 ng/ml, in whom no other obvious cause for hyperprolactinemia is found. An absent PRL response to TRH stimulation generally suggests that a pituitary microadenoma or another hypothalamic pituitary disease process is present, while a greater than two-fold increase of PRL would make prolactinoma less likely.

If hyperprolactinemia due to a pituitary tumor is suspected, a variety of radiologic studies is available to assess the structural integrity of the pituitary. As mentioned earlier, the most useful procedure to assess the presence of a pituitary tumor is the high-resolution CT scan. This technique has replaced polytomography and encephalography in most situations in which a pituitary tumor is suspected. The role of more formal pituitary function testing in hyperprolactinemia is debated. If a large tumor is present, there are valid reasons for estimating other pituitary functions, such as ACTH, TSH, GH, FSH, and LH reserve prior to therapeutic intervention. In contrast, most patients with small microadenomas have normal anterior pituitary function, and specific testing is generally unnecessary.

TREATMENT OF HYPERPROLACTINEMIA

The proper therapy of hyperprolactinemia is dictated by its etiology. Pharmacological elevations of PRL may require the discontinuance of the offending drug. In primary hypothyroidism, thyroid hormone replacement completely normalizes PRL serum concentrations, whereas a hypothalamic-pituitary disease process requires an approach directed at the structural defect. For prolactinomas, three highly effective therapies are available: transsphenoidal surgery, modulation of dopaminergic tone, and radiotherapy.

Transsphenoidal surgery can cure 80 to 90 per cent

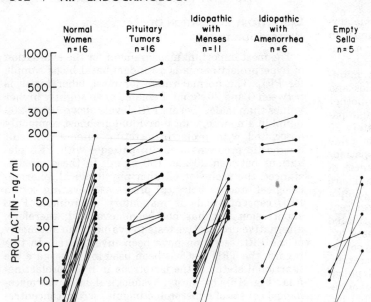

Figure 26. Prolactin (PRL) responses to TRH stimulation in patients with galactorrhea and pituitary tumors (second column) compared to responses seen in controls or patients with galactorrhea but without hyperprolactinemia. Note the relatively absent PRL response to TRH in patients with hyperprolactinemia and pituitary tumors. (From Kleinberg, D. L., et al.: N Engl J Med 296:589, 1977. Reprinted with permission.)

of patients with hyperprolactinemia due to pituitary microadenomas, but less than 30 per cent of macroadenomas are cured. In addition, there appears to be a significant recurrence rate (10 to 40 per cent) in patients originally thought to be cured by transsphenoidal surgery. Despite the reduced cure rate, most patients with macroadenomas and suprasellar extension with visual field defects require transsphenoidal surgery in order to preserve visual integrity.

Medical therapy of hyperprolactinemia centers on the use of dopamine agonists, especially bromocriptine (2-bromo-α-ergocryptine), an ergot derivative (Fig. 27). The realization that ergot derivatives could suppress lactation dates back to medieval accounts of infant death due to lack of milk in mothers with gangrenous ergotism (Saint Anthony's fire). Presumably, the mothers were ingesting rye flour contaminated with the fungus *Claviceps purpurea*, which produced the ergot compounds. Bromocriptine was developed specifically to have maximal antiprolactin effects combined with minimal vasospastic properties, a characteristic of most ergot compounds. Bromocriptine in relatively small doses normalizes PRL secretion in almost all patients with hyperprolactinemia, including those with pituitary tumors. Somewhat surprisingly, bromocriptine administration is also often associated with dramatic shrinkage of the tumor. Thus, treatment of patients with large tumors causing visual field defects with bromocriptine may result not only in normalization of PRL levels but also in a decrease in tumor size in approximately 75 per cent of patients. This observation suggests that large tumors could be reduced by bromocriptine to a size that would make surgical therapy more successful.

The mechanism by which bromocriptine causes a decrease in tumor size is debated. PRL synthesis and lactotrope size are both reduced by bromocriptine, but the actual number of cells remains constant. When bromocriptine is discontinued, these effects are rapidly reversed, with immediate increases in both serum PRL concentrations and tumor volume. Long-term therapy of patients with microadenomas has shown that PRL levels can be normalized, with resultant normalization of gonadal function and fertility in females. Some investigators prefer bromocriptine therapy in patients with presumed microadenomas that cannot be readily identified by CT scanning, since transsphenoidal surgery is "blind" in these circumstances. Bromocriptine may also be preferred even when the CT scan suggests a microadenoma, because the risks of surgery are avoided. The disadvantages of long-term bromocriptine therapy include its expense and the fact that a permanent cure has not been effected.

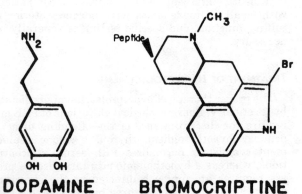

Figure 27. Structures of dopamine and bromocriptine showing relative chemical similarity. (From Barbieri, R. L., and Ryan, K. J.: Fertil Steril 39:727, 1983. Reprinted with permission of the American Fertility Society.)

With successful reduction of the serum PRL levels, gonadal function is restored within weeks, and ovulatory menstrual periods may be re-established within the first one to two months of therapy. In addition, galactorrhea ceases within this time frame. If pregnancy is desired, this can be achieved at any time after normal cycles are restored.

Radiotherapy for prolactin-secreting tumors is also an effective therapeutic modality for reducing serum PRL concentrations. This therapy is usually given adjunctively with surgery in patients with large macroadenomas with or without suprasellar extension or invasion into the cavernous sinus. Both conventional radiotherapy (4,000 to 5,000 rads) and proton heavy particle irradiation (5,000 to 10,000 rads) have been utilized. Radiotherapy is usually not given as the primary therapy. In circumstances in which a large prolactin-secreting tumor is being treated with radiotherapy, bromocriptine therapy can also be used until the effects of radiation are maximal, generally within two to five years.

CAUSES OF HYPOPROLACTINEMIA

The most important cause of hypoprolactinemia is pituitary infarction (Sheehan's syndrome or postpartum necrosis of the pituitary). In this circumstance, lactational insufficiency is present, which is often the first clinical clue that a pituitary defect exists. Other causes of hypopituitarism, such as pituitary tumors, hemochromatosis, or granulomatous diseases, are rare. In addition, previous radiotherapy to the pituitary for other pituitary disorders may result in hypoprolactinemia. All of these causes have only one significant clinical consequence, namely, lactational insufficiency. The diagnosis of this disorder is based upon the finding of low PRL levels that are unresponsive to TRH stimulation. At present no therapy is available for this rare condition.

CORTICOTROPIN

CHEMISTRY AND PRODUCTION

Corticotropin (ACTH) is the pituitary hormone responsible for the stimulation of growth and function of the adrenal gland. In the adult human pituitary, most cells that produce ACTH are located in the medial region at the posterior boundary of the anterior lobe. Corticotropes in the anterior pituitary comprise between 5 and 15 per cent of all pituitary cells. These cells are typically basophilic because of the carbohydrate content in the ACTH precursors. ACTH consists of 39 amino acids with a molecular weight of approximately 4,500 daltons. This molecule is derived from a large precursor, originally called "big-ACTH" or "pre-pro-ACTH," which has now been named pro-opiomelanocortin (POMC). This polypeptide is a single-chain peptide of approximately 31,000 daltons that is derived from a single mRNA. The large precursor undergoes specific proteolytic cleavage within corticotropes, giving rise to ACTH and other peptides. As depicted in Figure 28, ACTH itself can be further cleaved into two peptides: α-MSH, which is a 13 amino acid peptide, and another peptide consisting of amino acids 18 to 39, designated as "CLIP" (corticotropin-like intermediate lobe peptide). The "CLIP" peptide is found only in the intermediate lobe of the pituitary in species in which the intermediate lobe is developed, such as the rat or sheep. It has corticotropin-like activity in rats but is not found in humans. Another large derivative peptide is β-lipotropin (β-LPH), which contains 91 amino acids and has a molecular weight of 11,000. This peptide is cleaved to λ-LPH (1-58) and β-endorphin (61-91). The function of β-LPH and β-endorphin is a topic of considerable current interest. Both ACTH and β-LPH are secreted in equimolar amounts and appear to be regulated by the same modulators of secretion. For instance, both ACTH and β-LPH are stimulated by stress, insulin-induced hypoglycemia, and fever. Furthermore, they are cosecreted in many pathological states, such as Cushing's disease, Nelson's syndrome, and Addison's disease. The intriguing aspect about β-LPH and β-endorphin is their possible function as endogenous opiates with a specific role in pain perception. Additional broad biological functions, such as learning, appetite control, and stress responses, may be modified by endogenous endorphins. Furthermore, they may function to regulate other anterior pituitary hormones.

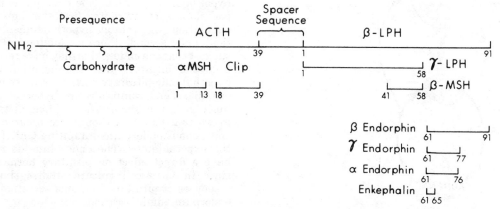

Figure 28. ACTH is derived from proteolytic cleavage of the large 31,000 dalton pro-opiomelanocortin. Other important peptides derived from the same precursor molecule include β-lipotropin (β-LPH, 1-91) and β-endorphin (61-91). α-MSH and "CLIP" are derived from the processing of ACTH in the intermediate lobe of the pituitary. (Modified from Roberts, J. L., et al.: Proc Natl Acad Sci USA 74:5300, 1977. In Williams, R. H. (ed.): Textbook of Endocrinology. 6th ed. Philadelphia, W. B. Saunders Co., 1981, p. 78.)

The normal anterior pituitary gland contains approximately 250 μg of ACTH and has a daily ACTH secretory rate of 25 μg. ACTH circulates free in plasma in concentrations that vary between 10 and 100 pg/ml. Its secretion is both diurnal and pulsatile, with peak levels being observed in the early morning hours and lower values being seen in the late afternoon and evening. In plasma, ACTH has a short half-life of less than 15 minutes.

REGULATION OF CORTICOTROPIN SECRETION

The secretion of ACTH from the pituitary is regulated by the hypothalamic peptide, corticotropin-releasing factor (CRF), which is produced by cells in the medial basal hypothalamus (Fig. 29). This releasing factor has been isolated and synthesized for the ovine species and consists of 41 amino acids (see Table 5). In humans, ovine CRF has a dose-dependent effect on pituitary ACTH secretion. It is hypothesized that the secretion of both CRF and ACTH is entrained to diurnal and pulsatile rhythms. The pulsatile release of CRF results in pulsatile pituitary secretion of ACTH and eventual cortisol secretion from the adrenal gland. There are approximately five to eight ACTH pulses per 24-hour period. The peak ACTH levels are found in early morning hours and decrease by afternoon and evening. The peripheral cortisol levels in turn feed back and inhibit not only ACTH release from the pituitary but also CRF release from the hypothalamus.

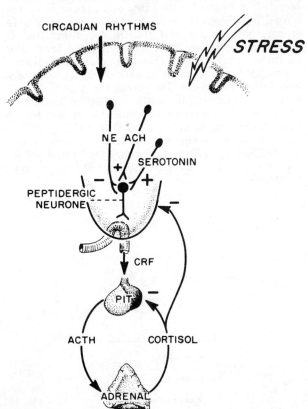

Figure 29. Diagrammatic representation of the regulation of ACTH secretion. ACTH secretion is stimulated by hypothalamic CRF and suppressed by negative cortisol feedback inhibition. (From Martin, J. B., et al.: Clinical Neuroendocrinology. Philadelphia, F. A. Davis, 1977.)

In addition to the daily diurnal and pulsatile release of ACTH, many other factors stimulate ACTH release. Any emotional or physical stress, such as insulin-induced hypoglycemia, surgery, injury, or emotional trauma, will stimulate ACTH release from the anterior pituitary, with concomitant increases in the plasma cortisol levels. These stimuli generally overcome the negative feedback effects of cortisol, although long-term, high-dose glucocorticoid therapy can suppress these responses. These generalized stress responses are thought to be mediated by stimulation of CRF release. Other factors that may mediate ACTH secretion include antidiuretic hormone, which has been shown both in vivo and in vitro to stimulate ACTH and β-LPH release from the anterior pituitary. Stimulation of ACTH release by antidiuretic hormone may be synergistic with that of CRF. α-Adrenergic stimulation increases ACTH and β-LPH release in vitro but inhibits CRF release. Both serotoninergic and cholinergic stimulation is thought to increase CRF release. Somatostatin may also be important to ACTH production, since it appears to inhibit the secretion of ACTH in vitro, whereas dopaminergic stimulation has no effect when given as L-dopa in man. In summary, the observed ACTH secretion found in man is a result of combined influences from CRF, negative feedback from cortisol, and other important central nervous system influences.

MECHANISM OF ACTION OF CORTICOTROPIN AND RELATED PEPTIDES

ACTH mediates its effect on adrenal function by interacting with specific receptors on the adrenal gland to stimulate not only growth of the adrenal gland but also the cascade of enzymes responsible for adrenal steroid biosynthesis. The interaction of ACTH with its receptor on adrenal tissue most likely involves the production of cyclic AMP and the ultimate phosphorylation and activation of specific enzymes responsible for steroid biosynthesis.

β-LPH and β-endorphin appear to function by interacting with specific endogenous opiate receptors. In addition to modulating pain perception and, possibly, other cortical functions, they influence pituitary hormone secretion by a short-loop feedback inhibition of hypothalamic function. The endorphins reach the hypothalamus by two routes: first, they enter the general circulation and inhibit hypothalamic-pituitary function, and, second, there is anatomical evidence to suggest that the endorphins may have retrograde entry from the pituitary into the hypothalamus via the hypothalamic-pituitary-portal circulation. A possible example of endorphins altering hypothalamic-pituitary function is the amenorrhea of long-distance running in women, which is thought to occur as a result of endogenous endorphins inhibiting GnRH release from the hypothalamus. The endorphins do not appear to have a direct effect on pituitary hormone secretion, since in vitro cell culture studies show negligible responses of pituitary hormone secretion following β-endorphin administration.

EXCESS ACTH PRODUCTION

Causes of Overproduction. The overproduction of ACTH may occur because of corticotrope hyperplasia (as in primary adrenal insufficiency or Addison's disease) or because of neoplasms, pituitary and nonpituitary, that produce ACTH. Pituitary tumors producing ACTH are associated with excesses of glucocorticoids, mineralocorticoids, and adrenal androgen production, resulting in the clinical syndrome known as "Cushing's disease." The pathophysiological description of this entity and its differential diagnosis are detailed in the chapter dealing with the Adrenal Cortex. Harvey Cushing was the first to document that pituitary tumors could produce hypercortisolism. Over 90 per cent of the cases of Cushing's disease are due to small pituitary tumors that secrete ACTH and its related peptides. These tumors are small and usually located in the midline of the pituitary. They range from 1 to 10 mm in diameter and have characteristic basophilic staining. In a rare minority of cases, hyperplasia of the pituitary may be seen rather than a discrete pituitary adenoma. Whether the diffuse hyperplasia or a discrete pituitary adenoma is due to primary pituitary pathology or chronic stimulation from hypothalamic centers secreting CRF is unknown.

Cushing's Disease. The laboratory diagnosis of Cushing's disease depends on the demonstration of elevated ACTH and cortisol production as well as abnormal and characteristic responses to suppression and stimulation tests. Plasma ACTH levels are inappropriately normal or elevated relative to the level of cortisol overproduction. Patients with Cushing's disease generally have ACTH values ranging from 70 to 250 pg/ml, compared with a normal range of 10 to 100 pg/ml. Because of this overlap with the normal range, basal plasma ACTH levels have not proved useful in establishing the diagnosis of Cushing's disease. In contrast, ACTH levels can be quite useful in the differential diagnosis of Cushing's syndrome; adrenal adenomas have undetectable values, pituitary tumors have normal or slightly elevated values, and ectopic tumors have extremely high levels of ACTH (Fig. 30). β-Endorphin levels have not been widely studied in the diagnosis of Cushing's disease despite their potential usefulness as an indicator of corticotrope activity. However, as shown in Figure 31, β-endorphin levels in Cushing's disease have a lesser degree of concordance with the normal range than do basal plasma ACTH levels. Therefore, the determination of β-endorphin levels may provide information that is helpful in establishing the diagnosis of Cushing's disease due to an ACTH-producing pituitary tumor.

The ACTH secretion in Cushing's disease is characteristically not totally autonomous. High doses of glucocorticoids can suppress ACTH secretion, thereby lowering endogenous plasma cortisol levels. Furthermore, the administration of CRF causes ACTH levels to rise in Cushing's disease (Fig. 32). The potential usefulness of CRF stimulation tests in differentiating patients with Cushing's disease from those with other disorders of the hypothalamic-pituitary-adrenal axis is under investigation. Patients with ectopic ACTH secretion do not generally respond to CRF administration, although exceptions have been reported. Patients with autonomous adrenal adenomas do not respond to CRF, suggesting that the negative feedback of excessive cortisol upon pituitary ACTH production prevents the response to exogenous CRF. Further experience with CRF will be necessary to determine its ultimate use-

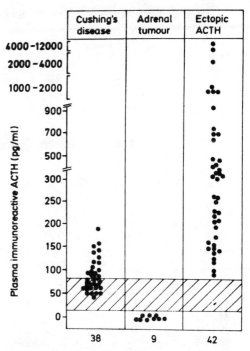

Figure 30. Plasma ACTH values in patients with various causes of hypercortisolism. ACTH levels in Cushing's disease significantly overlap with the normal range (hatched area), whereas patients with ectopic ACTH secretion or adrenal tumors have plasma ACTH values outside the normal range. (From Rees, L. H., et al.: In Some Aspects of Hypothalamic Regulation of Endocrine Functions. Symposium, Vienna, June 3–6, 1973. Stuttgart, F. K. Schattauer Verlag, 1974. Reprinted with permission.)

fulness in the evaluation of patients with suspected Cushing's disease. It is conceivable that ACTH and cortisol responses to CRF could improve the current laboratory methods for evaluating patients with disorders of the pituitary and adrenal gland.

Nelson's Syndrome. Nelson's syndrome refers to the clinical entity of large ACTH-producing pituitary tumors occurring in patients who have had bilateral adrenalectomy for Cushing's disease. These pituitary tumors occur following adrenalectomy, presumably because of unrestrained corticotrope growth and activity following the removal of the negative feedback imposed by the high levels of cortisol in Cushing's disease. Between 20 and 50 per cent of adrenalectomized patients will eventually progress to develop an ACTH-producing macroadenoma of the pituitary consistent with Nelson's syndrome. The patients characteristically have extremely high ACTH levels associated with hyperpigmentation and variable deficits of other anterior pituitary functions. Visual field defects due to suprasellar extension may be present, as well as extension of the tumor into the cavernous or sphenoid sinus. Prophylactic conventional radiation to the pituitary following adrenalectomy does not prevent the occurrence of this syndrome. The clinical diagnosis of this disorder is usually obvious from the history and physical examination, which reveals a generalized increase in pigmentation, particularly on scars, palmar creases, elbows, buccal mucosa, and areola. Serum ACTH levels are usually greater than 750 to 1000

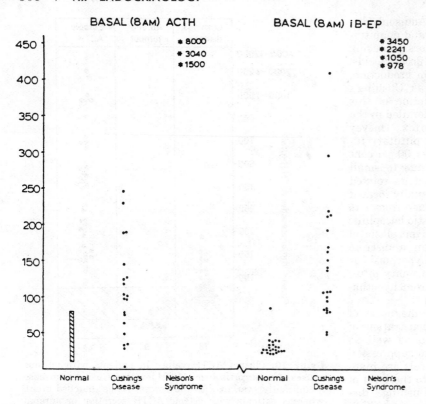

Figure 31. Basal plasma β-endorphin and ACTH levels (pg/ml) in patients with Cushing's disease and Nelson's syndrome compared to normal controls. Note the lesser degree of overlap of plasma β-endorphin levels in Cushing's disease with normal controls compared to plasma ACTH levels. (From Carr, D. B., et al.: Secretory Tumors of the Pituitary. New York, Raven Press, 1984.)

pg/ml. Dramatic elevations in serum β-LPH and β-endorphin levels are also present.

TREATMENT OF ACTH-SECRETING PITUITARY TUMORS

As with most pituitary hypersecretory syndromes, *transsphenoidal hypophysectomy* is the therapy of choice for pituitary tumors causing Cushing's disease or Nelson's syndrome. If a microadenoma is removed, a 90 to 95 per cent cure rate is observed. The exact incidence of relapse following cure is uncertain; however, recurrences have been reported in up to 10 to 20 per cent of patients. Patients who have had successful removal of microadenomas for Cushing's disease may have temporary but long-term ACTH deficiency due to

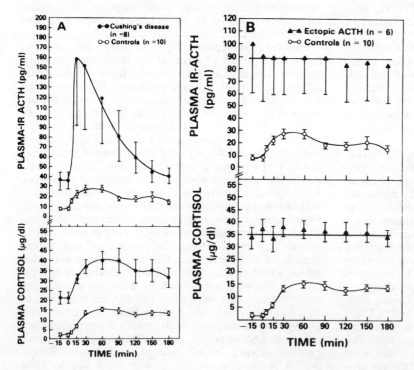

Figure 32. Plasma ACTH and cortisol levels after CRF administration (1 μg/kg body weight intravenously at 8 P.M.) in patients with *(A)* Cushing's disease or *(B)* ectopic ACTH syndrome compared to normal controls. The low plasma cortisol and ACTH levels in the normal controls are due to the timing of the CRF administration (i.e., 8 P.M.). (From Chrousos, G. P., et al.: N Engl J Med 310:622, 1984. Reprinted with permission.)

the prolonged effects of hypercortisolism on the hypothalamus and/or normal pituitary corticotropes. Partial or complete ACTH deficiency may persist for 6 to 24 months following removal of pituitary tumors, necessitating replacement glucocorticoid therapy during this time.

Pituitary irradiation by conventional or heavy particle modalities is a valuable adjunctive form of therapy in the treatment of ACTH-secreting pituitary tumors. Remission rates of 60 to 85 per cent are observed with radiotherapy, although the time lag to achieve these results varies from 2 to 10 years. *Medical treatment* of Cushing's disease includes the use of the serotonin antagonist cyproheptadine, which variably inhibits ACTH secretion and lowers serum cortisol levels. In the best series, 60 to 65 per cent of patients will gain a remission with cyproheptadine therapy, but the condition relapses after discontinuance of the medicine. Bromocriptine has also been used in the treatment of Cushing's disease with variable results. Other medical forms of therapy for Cushing's disease are discussed under the Adrenal Cortex.

ECTOPIC ACTH SECRETION

ACTH secretion may also occur from nonpituitary malignancies. Classically, these include oat cell carcinoma of the lung, a bronchial or thymic carcinoid, pancreatic carcinoma, and medullary carcinoma of the thyroid. Depending on the aggressiveness of the primary neoplasm, these patients may or may not have the classic clinical features of Cushing's disease. The patients with pancreatic or primary lung carcinoma usually do not have a "moon" facies, centripetal obesity, buffalo hump, plethora, or purple striae. Instead, their disease may be characterized by profound weakness, hypokalemia, weight loss, increased pigmentation, and anemia. In fact, any patient with a primary pulmonary or pancreatic carcinoma who presents with weakness, cachexia, and electrolyte disturbances should be considered a possible candidate for the ectopic ACTH syndrome. The muscle wasting, fatigue, and weakness may be due to a primary steroid myopathy or to hypokalemia and metabolic alkalosis. The hypokalemia is generally not a result of aldosterone secretion but rather the mineralocorticoid effect of corticosterone and deoxycorticosterone. Other features include hyperpigmentation, glucose intolerance, edema, and hirsutism.

The laboratory diagnostic characteristics of the ectopic ACTH syndrome include elevated levels of glucocorticoids, mineralocorticoids, and adrenal androgens. The glucocorticoids fail to suppress with either low or high doses of dexamethasone. However, exceptions have been reported, particularly with the more indolent bronchial or thymic carcinoids, which may behave like pituitary adenomas producing ACTH, i.e., suppression with high-dose dexamethasone. Therefore, the most important diagnostic test is the strikingly elevated plasma ACTH level (see Fig. 30). In most cases, the ACTH elevation is much higher than that seen with Cushing's disease. Finally, the ACTH secretion is generally autonomous and does not respond to CRF stimulation, although rare exceptions have been reported.

THYROTROPIN

CHEMISTRY AND PRODUCTION

Thyrotropin (TSH) is the pituitary hormone responsible for the growth and function of the thyroid gland. It is a glycoprotein hormone weighing 28,000 daltons. Unlike the other pituitary hormones, the glycoprotein hormones are composed of two dissimilar subunits, termed alpha and beta, which are noncovalently associated. The alpha subunit of TSH is identical to that in the other glycoprotein hormones (luteinizing hormone, follicle-stimulating hormone, and placental chorionic gonadotropin). It consists of 92 amino acids with two complex asparagine-linked carbohydrate side chains and weighs 14,000 daltons. The TSH-β subunit is different from the other beta subunits of the glycoprotein hormones, having only 30 to 40 per cent homology with them. It consists of 112 amino acids and has a single complex carbohydrate side chain, resulting in a molecular weight of 14,000 daltons.

The biosynthesis of TSH begins with the transcription of two distinct genes on different chromosomes, resulting in the production of separate mRNAs for the subunits (Fig. 33). These mRNAs are translated in the rough endoplasmic reticulum to the pre-alpha and pre-TSH-β subunits, which consist of the apoprotein plus

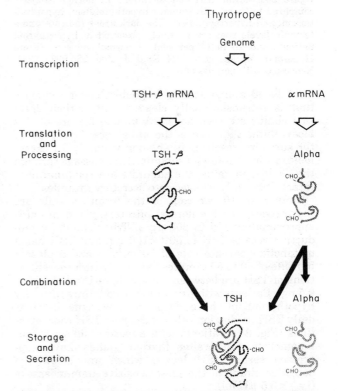

figure 33. Biosynthesis of TSH in pituitary thyrotropes begins with the transcription of two distinct genes that encode the alpha and TSH-β subunits. The mRNAs are translated in the endoplasmic reticulum into pre-subunits. Following cleavage of the leader sequences, glycosylation (-CHO) occurs. Further modifications and folding of the subunits result in protein configurations that associate noncovalently into the intact TSH molecule. Normally, both TSH and free alpha subunit are secreted by the thyrotrope, whereas the TSH-β subunit is rate-limiting for TSH synthesis.

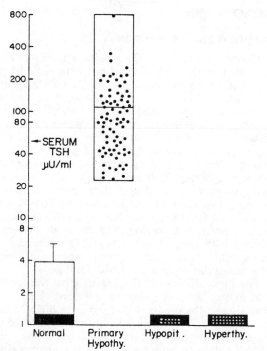

Figure 34. Serum TSH concentrations in normal subjects compared to those with primary hypothyroidism, hypopituitarism, and hyperthyroidism. The dark areas indicate undetectable levels that are routinely observed in hyperthyroid patients and 10 to 15 per cent of normal subjects. (From Hershman, J. M., et al.: N Engl J Med 285:997, 1971. Reprinted with permission.)

a 20 to 30 amino acid hydrophobic leader sequence that is cotranslationally cleaved. The carbohydrate side chains are then added. A unique feature of this biosynthetic sequence is the unbalanced synthesis of the subunits, resulting in an approximately 3:1 excess molar ratio of the alpha subunit. After passage through the Golgi apparatus, the subunits are combined into intact TSH and packaged in secretory granules.

Only 5 to 10 per cent of the pituitary cells are thyrotropes, and the normal pituitary gland contains approximately 100 to 200 µg of TSH. The daily production rate of TSH is 50 to 100 µg, and TSH has a metabolic clearance rate of 50 ml/min and a plasma half-life of 50 to 60 minutes. Normal serum concentrations of TSH are between 0.5 and 3.5 µU/ml (1 µU ≅ 0.5 ng). Patients with primary thyroid failure (primary hypothyroidism) have dramatic elevations in their daily TSH production rates and serum TSH concentrations (Fig. 34). Patients with hyperthyroidism or autonomously functioning thyroid glands have suppressed serum TSH levels, which are below the detection limits of the most sensitive immunoassays (i.e., <0.5 µU/ml).

The normal pituitary contains 100 to 500 µg of unassociated free alpha subunit, which is synthesized in both thyrotropes and gonadotropes. The daily production rate of the free alpha subunit is 100 to 200 µg, resulting in serum free alpha subunit levels of 0.5 to 2.5 ng/ml. The metabolic clearance rate of free alpha subunit is 120 ml/min. Human subjects with primary hypothyroidism or primary gonadal failure have a three-fold elevation in their production rates and serum concentrations of the free alpha subunit.

The amount of free TSH-β in the normal pituitary is low or undetectable, since most TSH-β subunit is processed directly into intact TSH. Thus, it is likely that TSH-β subunit synthesis is rate-limiting for TSH production. The daily production rate and serum concentration of *free* TSH-β in normal subjects is therefore undetectable. In primary hypothyroidism, free TSH-β is found in both the pituitary and serum.

REGULATION OF TSH SECRETION

The secretion of TSH is thought to be nonpulsatile and has only a minor diurnal variation involving a two-fold increase during the night. The primary regulation of TSH is from two oppositely directed forces: the positive stimulation of hypothalamic thyrotropin-releasing hormone (TRH) and the negative inhibition exerted by the thyroid hormones, thyroxine (T_4) and triiodothyronine (T_3) (Fig. 35).

Thyrotropin-releasing Hormones. TRH is a tripeptide (pyroglu-His-ProNH$_2$) with a molecular weight of 365. It is synthesized in the paraventricular and preoptic nuclei of the hypothalamus, secreted into the hypophyseal portal vessels, and transported to the

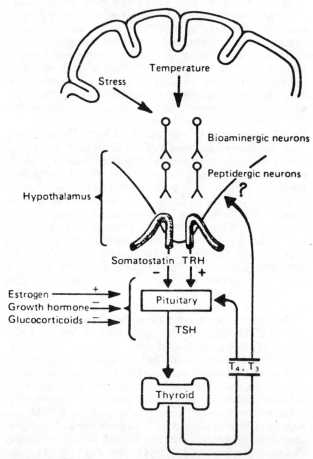

Figure 35. Regulation of the hypothalamic-pituitary-thyroid axis, illustrating the positive effect of TRH and the negative effect of thyroid hormones on TSH production. Other modulators from the central nervous system and peripheral circulation also contribute to the regulation of TSH. (From Martin, J. B., et al.: Clinical Neuroendocrinology. Philadelphia, F. A. Davis, 1977.)

anterior pituitary. The regulation of TRH secretion from the hypothalamus is complex and poorly understood. Thyroid hormones have a possible role in regulating both TRH synthesis and release. Cold exposure in animals or human neonates causes an increase in serum TSH concentration, which is thought to be mediated by TRH. The putative cold-induced increase in TRH is mediated by α_1-adrenergic stimulation, since α_1-adrenergic blockade will inhibit the response. The synthesis of TRH by hypothalamic fragments in vitro is augmented by both norepinephrine and dopamine, the latter being somewhat paradoxical, since dopamine inhibits TSH release from the pituitary. Serotonin and somatostatin both inhibit the production and/or release of TRH from the hypothalamus. At the pituitary, TRH interacts with specific membrane receptors that have a high affinity for TRH. Interaction of TRH with its membrane receptors initiates a cascade of events that result in the release of TSH into the circulation. One important result of the interaction between TRH and its receptor appears to be an acute change in cytosolic Ca^{++} concentrations that precedes TSH release by the thyrotrope. This event occurs within 15 seconds after TRH binds to its receptor. Although TRH may also be internalized into the cell and may eventually be located in the nucleus, the time frame of these events precludes their role in the acute release of TSH. TRH causes a dose- and time-dependent rise in TSH from the thyrotropes and PRL from the lactotropes. In humans, intravenous administration of TRH in doses above 100 μg will produce maximal TSH and PRL responses within 10 to 30 minutes. In addition, TRH may be given orally in high doses to produce TSH release. The triple ring chemical structure of TRH renders it partially resistant to digestion and destruction by gastrointestinal proteolytic enzymes.

Effect of Thyroid Hormones. The thyroid hormones, T_4 and T_3, exert the major negative influence on TSH secretion at the level of the pituitary, where they inhibit both biosynthesis and release of TSH. The major effect of thyroid hormones on TSH biosynthesis appears to be a direct effect on alpha subunit and TSH-β subunit gene expression. Administration of thyroid hormones to hypothyroid animals rapidly inhibits transcriptional events, leading to decreases in the intracellular mRNA concentrations encoding the alpha and TSH-β subunits. The production of TSH is exquisitely sensitive to small changes in ambient thyroid hormone concentrations. Decreases in circulating thyroxine levels of as little as 1 $\mu g/dl$ may be associated with a ten-fold increase in pituitary TSH secretion. Likewise, increments in serum thyroxine concentrations as small as 1 to 2 $\mu g/dl$ may completely inhibit TSH secretion. Complete suppression of pituitary TSH production by exogenously administered L-thyroxine occurs at doses of 100 to 200 $\mu g/day$.

T_4 is converted to T_3, which then interacts with thyroid hormone receptors within the nucleus of the thyrotrope cells. The anterior pituitary has been shown to have a very active 5' monodeiodinase, which converts T_4 to T_3. Inhibition of this conversion results in decreased intrapituitary T_3 formation, decreased TSH inhibition, and increased pituitary TSH release. The intrapituitary conversion of T_4 to T_3 within the thyrotrope contributes substantially to the intrapituitary T_3 pool. This contrasts with other peripheral sites of thyroid hormone action, where intracellular T_4-to-T_3 conversion contributes less to the intracellular T_3 pool. In these other peripheral tissues, circulating serum T_3 is the major source of T_3 that interacts with thyroid hormone receptors. These findings suggest that locally produced intrapituitary T_3 is the primary iodothyronine responsible for the rate of TSH biosynthesis and secretion.

Effect of Other Hormones. TSH secretion from the anterior pituitary is also regulated by a wide variety of other hormones. Dopamine and somatostatin have strong inhibitory effects on TSH secretion, decreasing TSH secretion in vitro and in vivo in a dose- and time-dependent manner. In contrast, α_1-adrenergic stimulation directly causes the release of TSH from normal pituitary cells in culture. Thus, α_1-adrenergic stimulation in vivo could theoretically stimulate TSH release by two mechanisms: release of TRH from hypothalamic centers and direct pituitary TSH release. Of these two, release of TRH from the hypothalamus into the portal circulation appears to be the more important mechanism. Glucocorticoids inhibit both basal and TRH-stimulated TSH release, while estrogens potentiate the TSH release by TRH. As a result, women generally have higher TSH responses to TRH than males. In summary, TSH secretion from the anterior pituitary is regulated predominantly by thyroid hormones and TRH. Other important central and peripheral hormones interact in this system to produce an integrated and highly regulated response.

TSH HYPERSECRETION

Primary thyroid failure is the most common cause of an elevated serum TSH level. The prevalence of this condition is much greater than previously thought. In America and Europe, 0.5 per cent of the population has primary hypothyroidism; in the elderly, 10 to 20 per cent of subjects will have elevated serum TSH levels, indicating varying degrees of primary thyroid failure. The causes of primary hypothyroidism are discussed under Thyroid Pathophysiology, but in most studies the two most common causes are Hashimoto's (autoimmune) thyroiditis and ablative treatment (radioactive iodide or thyroidectomy) of Graves' disease.

In hypothyroidism, the serum TSH levels are inversely correlated with the levels of serum T_4, but not with serum T_3 levels. This paradoxical finding is due to the fact that normal serum T_3 concentrations are maintained during the early phases of hypothyroidism, while serum T_4 levels fall. However, as serum T_4 levels continue to fall, less T_4 is available to the pituitary thyrotropes for intrapituitary conversion to T_3. Consequently, the intracellular T_3 concentration in the thyrotropes decreases, with a concomitant fall in thyroid hormone receptor occupancy. The inhibition of TSH production then decreases and TSH biosynthesis and secretion increase. This secretion of TSH is so sensitive to minor changes in thyroid hormone levels that serum TSH levels will increase before serum concentrations of T_4 and T_3 are discernibly low (Fig. 36). Furthermore, in many circumstances, the rise in TSH secretion occurs before symptoms of hypothyroidism appear. The finding of an elevated serum TSH level, but normal serum T_4 and T_3 levels, in patients with few or no symptoms of hypothyroidism has been called "subclin-

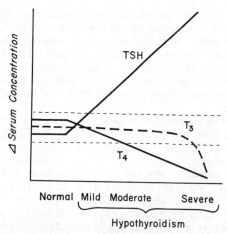

Figure 36. Changes in basal serum TSH, T_3, and T_4 concentrations in progressively worsening primary thyroid failure. Serum T_3 levels are well maintained during the early phases of thyroid failure, whereas serum T_4 levels are inversely correlated with the rising serum TSH levels.

ical hypothyroidism." Although very common, it remains controversial whether these modest increases in TSH merely reflect the sensitivity of the thyrotrope to thyroid hormone, or whether true, but mild, degrees of tissue hypothyroidism are also present in peripheral tissues.

TSH-Secreting Pituitary Tumors

Pituitary tumors that autonomously produce TSH are a rare cause of hyperthyroidism (Table 11). Probably less than 1 per cent of pituitary tumors produce TSH; only 40 to 50 cases have been reported in the medical literature. Most cases present with symptoms of hyperthyroidism that are difficult to distinguish from Graves' disease (see Thyroid Pathophysiology). Unlike Graves' disease, however, cases of hyperthyroidism due to TSH-secreting pituitary tumors are distributed equally between males and females. Patients with TSH-secreting tumors do not have the ophthalmopathy and dermopathy associated with Graves' disease and do not have thyroid-stimulating immunoglobins in their serum. In about 50 per cent of TSH-secreting pituitary tumors, either GH or PRL is coproduced by separate cells in the tumor.

The serum TSH levels are always elevated relative

TABLE 11. TSH-SECRETING PITUITARY TUMORS*

Total number of cases	46
Male:female ratio	21:25
Age range	17–64
Number hyperthyroid	43
Number with acromegaly	11
Number with hyperprolactinemia	7
Visual field defects (n = 29)	20
Suprasellar extension (n = 23)	19
Serum TSH (by RIA, n = 38)	1.6 to 480 μU/ml
Serum alpha subunit (n = 16)	1.1 to 105 ng/ml
Serum alpha:TSH molar ratio >1	14 of 16

*Clinical and biochemical characteristics of 46 cases reported in the literature between 1958 and 1983. Modified from Ridgway, E. C.: Glycoprotein Hormone Producing Tumors in Secretory Tumors of the Pituitary. New York, Raven Press, 1984.

to the serum T_4 and T_3 concentrations. In most, dramatic elevations are found; in some, the serum TSH level may be within the normal range but is "inappropriate" for the elevated thyroid hormone levels. Absolute values for serum TSH levels reported in the literature range from 1.6 to 480 μU/ml. Approximately one third of the cases had TSH values below 10 μU/ml. Therefore, it is important to employ RIA technology that can accurately measure TSH levels in the range of 0 to 10 μU/ml, thereby discriminating normal (but "inappropriate") values from the undetectable serum TSH levels (i.e., <0.5 μU/ml) that are routinely found in Graves' disease. One of the useful and characteristic features of TSH-secreting pituitary tumors is the cosecretion of excessive free alpha subunit. In over 85 per cent of cases, serum free alpha subunit levels have been elevated; in most of these, the elevation in free alpha subunit concentration has been extremely high, so much so, in fact, that more free alpha is being secreted on a molar basis than is intact TSH. The excessive molar ratio of free alpha to TSH secretion (i.e., free alpha:TSH >1) distinguishes patients with pituitary tumors from all other causes of elevated TSH levels. For instance, the molar free alpha:TSH ratio in primary thyroid failure is always less than unity.

The secretion of TSH and free alpha subunit from pituitary tumors is relatively autonomous. TRH administration has failed to increase by two-fold either TSH or free alpha subunit release in over 85 per cent of patients tested. Similarly, thyroid hormone administration fails to decrease serum TSH or free alpha subunit levels, a finding that distinguishes autonomous from nonautonomous TSH secretion.

The treatment of TSH-secreting tumors generally involves pituitary surgery and radiotherapy. The tumors are usually large and in many cases have suprasellar extension with visual field defects.

Pituitary Resistance to Thyroid Hormone

Two further important but unusual syndromes that have been reported are characterized by "inappropriate" but nonautonomous elevations of TSH secretion. These are contrasted with inappropriate TSH secretion from a pituitary tumor in Table 12. The first is "selective pituitary resistance" to thyroid hormones, which has been described in a small number of patients. In these cases, only the pituitary has a defect in the feedback suppression of TSH secretion by thyroid hormones. As a result, TSH secretion increases, causing the thyroid to grow and produce excessive quantities of T_4 and T_3; the high levels of thyroid hormone produce clinical hyperthyroidism. These cases may be familial or sporadic; the familial cases are inherited as an autosomal dominant disorder. As with pituitary tumors, there is an equal male-to-female distribution and an absence of Graves' ophthalmopathy and dermopathy. Unlike the situation with pituitary TSH-secreting tumors, the TSH production is not autonomous, and serum free alpha subunit levels are normal or minimally increased. Following TRH administration, both TSH and free alpha subunit levels increase despite the high thyroid hormone levels. Furthermore, exogenous thyroid hormone administration in high doses partially suppresses serum TSH levels. Finally, there is no radiographic evidence for a pituitary tumor.

TABLE 12. LABORATORY STUDIES IN SYNDROMES OF INAPPROPRIATE TSH HYPERSECRETION

	CLINICAL STATE	T4, FT4 T3, FT3	BASAL TSH	TSH p̄ TRH	α-SUBUNIT	α-SUBUNIT p̄ TRH	PITUITARY TUMOR
Hyperthyroidism secondary to TSH-secreting pituitary tumors	hyper	↑	nl/↑	→	↑	→	yes
Hyperthyroidism secondary to selective pituitary resistance to thyroid hormone	hyper	↑	nl/↑	↑	nl	↑	no
Euthyroidism with total peripheral and pituitary resistance to thyroid hormone	eu/hypo	↑	nl/↑	↑	nl	↑	no

Taken together, the responses of TSH and free alpha subunit to TRH and thyroid hormone administration suggest a defect in the ability of thyroid hormones to inhibit TSH secretion. The data are consistent with an altered set point, with higher than normal thyroid hormone levels necessary for complete suppression of TSH secretion.

The second is "generalized pituitary and peripheral resistance" to thyroid hormone that, although rare, is more common than selective pituitary resistance. The first kindred reported with this syndrome also displayed somatic defects, including deaf-mutism, stippled epiphyses, and skeletal abnormalities that were inherited in an autosomal recessive fashion. Since the original description, many other cases have been reported that appear to have an autosomal dominant inheritance pattern in 50 per cent of cases, and most of these do not have the somatic abnormalities. The clinical features of this syndrome include an equal male-to-female occurrence, modest thyroid enlargement, and, most importantly, clinical euthyroidism in the presence of elevated thyroid hormone levels. In many of these cases, inappropriate treatment for presumed hyperthyroidism will have been performed. The diagnosis depends on documenting peripheral euthyroidism in association with elevated thyroid hormone and TSH levels. The dynamics of TSH secretion are similar to those seen with selective pituitary resistance. The elevated basal TSH levels and normal free alpha subunit levels respond to both TRH stimulation and thyroid hormone suppression.

One of the early hypotheses offered to explain the pathophysiology of thyroid hormone resistance was the possibility of defective thyroid hormone receptors. Most recent studies have concluded, however, that both receptor affinity and maximal binding capacity are normal. Other theories, including possible abnormalities in the uptake of thyroid hormones into cells or defects in T_4-to-T_3 conversion within cells, have not been adequately explored. Thus, the molecular mechanism for thyroid hormone resistance at either the pituitary or peripheral level is unknown.

The therapy of the thyroid hormone resistance syndromes is controversial. In cases of "selective pituitary resistance," the patients have hyperthyroidism and benefit from normalization of the thyroid hormone levels. Whether lowering of thyroid hormone levels will produce unrestrained and autonomous (i.e., tumorous) TSH secretion is currently unknown. This raises the therapeutic possibility that dopaminergic modulation may have a potential role in controlling TSH secretion in thyrotrope-resistant states, thereby preventing tumor formation. In cases of "generalized pituitary and peripheral resistance," it is extremely important to make the correct diagnosis. These patients require high levels of thyroid hormones to remain clinically euthyroid, and attempts to lower thyroid hormone levels will produce hypothyroidism. Although these patients have minimal to moderate thyroid enlargement, there are no indications for treatment.

GONADOTROPINS

CHEMISTRY AND PRODUCTION

The gonadotropins, luteinizing hormone (LH) and follicle-stimulating hormone (FSH), are the glycoprotein hormones that are responsible for sexual and reproductive function. Both hormones have subunit structures similar to those described for TSH. The alpha subunits of LH and FSH are identical and, in turn, are identical to that found in TSH. The LH-β subunit contains 112 amino acids and has a single carbohydrate linked to the asparagine amino acid at position 30. Its molecular weight is approximately 14,000. The FSH-β subunit contains 118 amino acids and has two carbohydrate side chains: one homologous to that in TSH-β and LH-β, the other close to the N-terminus at position 7. There is only 40 per cent amino acid homology between the beta subunit of FSH and that of LH. The molecular weight of intact LH is 29,000 and that of intact FSH is 32,000. In a manner similar to TSH, the beta subunits of the gonadotropins confer biological specificity upon the intact hormones, whereas the individual subunits, alpha or beta, do not have any intrinsic biological activity. The concept that beta subunits confer biological specificity arises from elegant recombination experiments (Fig. 37). In this type of experiment, the subunits of one glycoprotein hormone are dissociated, separated, and then recombined with those of another glycoprotein hormone. For example, the beta subunit of TSH is first separated and then recombined with the alpha subunit derived from LH or FSH. The resulting "hybrid" recombinant molecule has the biological specificity of TSH and not that of the gonadotropins. Similar experiments have been done with the beta subunits of LH and FSH,

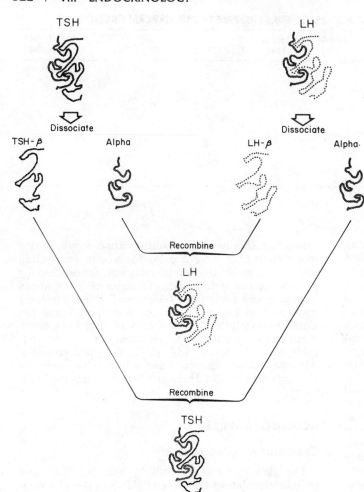

Figure 37. Schematic presentation of a classic recombination experiment, showing that the beta subunit determines the biological activity of the intact molecule. The recombinant molecule of TSH-β from TSH and alpha subunit from LH has the biological activity of TSH.

resulting in an identical finding, namely, that the beta subunit confers the biological specificity.

The biosynthesis of LH and FSH appears to be similar to that of TSH (Fig. 38). The genes for the alpha subunit and the FSH-β or LH-β subunits are on different chromosomes. Transcription results in the production of separate mRNAs. In rodents the beta subunits for LH, FSH, chorionic gonadotropin, and perhaps TSH may be located in a cluster on a single chromosome. Following transcription, the mRNAs are translated in the rough endoplasmic reticulum. Glycosylation and combination of the subunits occur in the endoplasmic reticulum and Golgi apparatus, followed by packaging of the hormones into secretory granules.

Five to 10 per cent of normal pituitary cells are gonadotropes. It appears that both FSH and LH are secreted predominantly from the same cell. In certain circumstances, one cell may secrete either LH or FSH, but generally both hormones are found in the same cell. The normal pituitary gland contains between 10 and 20 mg of LH and between 5 and 10 mg of FSH. The pituitary content is similar in males and females but is approximately two-fold greater for both hormones following castration or menopause. The daily production rate of LH and FSH is approximately equivalent to the pituitary content, thus indicating that the pituitary gonadotrope pool turns over at least once

daily. Estimates of pituitary secretory rates for LH in premenopausal women are approximately 20 mg per day (1000 IU/d) and for FSH are 10 mg per day (200 IU/d). The half-life of LH is one half that of FSH (30 versus 60 min), and the metabolic clearance rate of LH is 25 ml/min and that of FSH is 15 ml/min. The delayed clearance of FSH has been attributed to the higher sialic acid content of the carbohydrate sidechains on FSH.

The secretion of LH and FSH has different characteristics from that observed for TSH. Serum concentrations of the gonadotropins change dramatically with age. Immediately following birth, both LH and FSH are detected in plasma: in males LH predominates, and in females FSH predominates. Shortly thereafter, both LH and FSH plasma concentrations drop to undetectable levels and remain there until the prepubertal period. At the onset of puberty, nocturnal non-REM–associated pulsatile secretion of LH starts and is followed shortly by pulsatile FSH. As puberty progresses, the pulses increase in frequency and amplitude. Following puberty, adult women have well-defined LH pulses at approximately 60- to 90-minute intervals throughout the day. FSH pulses are more difficult to detect but follow a similar pattern. LH and FSH pulsations reflect the secretory bursts of gonadotropin-releasing hormone (GnRH) release from the hypothalamus. In females, the largest LH and FSH

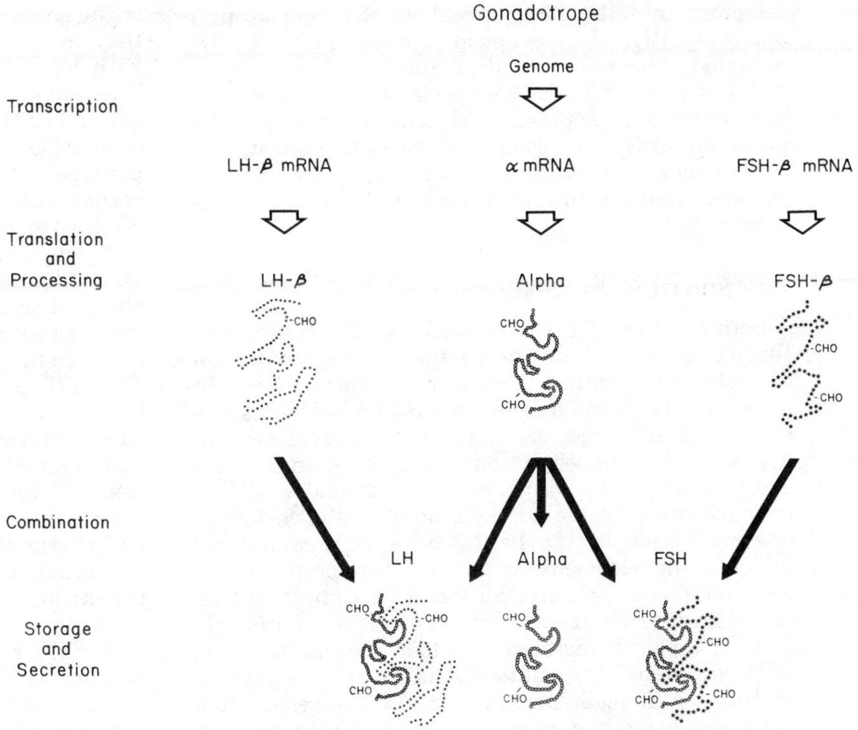

Figure 38. Biosynthesis of the gonadotropins. The separate genes for the beta subunits may reside on the same chromosome, whereas the gene for the alpha subunit is on a different chromosome. The genes are transcribed, resulting in separate mRNA, which are translated in the rough endoplasmic reticulum. The pre-subunit peptides are processed and carbohydrate side chains (-CHO) are added. Combination of the subunits occurs in the Golgi apparatus, and the intact hormones are stored in secretory granules.

peak occurs at the time of ovulation at midcycle. Following menopause or castration, serum LH and FSH concentrations both increase dramatically.

REGULATION OF GONADOTROPINS

Regulation of LH and FSH secretion from the anterior pituitary represents an intricate balance primarily between gonadotropin-releasing hormone (GnRH) and the sex steroids. An absence of GnRH due to hypothalamic disease or stalk secretion will reduce pituitary LH and FSH secretion to undetectable values. In contrast, castration or menopause causes an increase in both LH and FSH secretion. Within the framework of this basic positive and negative feedback system, highly complex interactions occur.

GnRH Effect. The cell bodies in the hypothalamus responsible for GnRH synthesis are located in the anterior, posterior, and medial portions of the hypothalamus. Axonal projections from these hypothalamic cells innervate the median eminence, where they terminate on portal hypophyseal blood vessels. From this system, GnRH is secreted in a pulsatile fashion at 60- to 90-minute intervals in women and approximately 120-minute intervals in males. GnRH reaches the pituitary in the portal blood supply and interacts with specific receptors on gonadotropes. Following each pulse of GnRH, LH and sometimes FSH can be detected in the peripheral circulation.

The secretion of LH and FSH is also determined by the characteristics of the GnRH stimulation. Orderly LH and FSH pulses follow specific GnRH pulses. If the GnRH arrives at the pituitary in a nonpulsatile manner (i.e., by constant infusion), LH and FSH secretion decreases, and the gonadotrope becomes refractory to GnRH pulses. This effect is consistent with either

down-regulation of GnRH receptors or desensitization of the gonadotrope. Knowledge of this physiology has resulted in valuable therapeutic options for patients with a variety of reproductive problems. For instance, fertility in some patients with hypogonadotropic hypogonadism can be restored with pulsatile GnRH administration. Furthermore, children with precocious puberty have augmented and abnormal LH and FSH secretion. Suppression of gonadotropin secretion in these children by the constant infusion of GnRH has resulted in a beneficial delay in pubertal progression.

Sex Hormone Effect. The effect of GnRH on the secretion of LH and FSH is highly dependent on the sex steroid milieu bathing the anterior pituitary cells and the frequency and amplitude of the GnRH pulsations. For instance, chronic exposure to high levels of estrogen or testosterone will inhibit LH and FSH release by GnRH. In contrast, estrogens can also exert a positive effect on gonadotropin secretion. As estrogen concentrations slowly rise within the physiological range during the follicular phase of the menstrual cycle, pituitary gonadotrope cells become primed to the effect of GnRH. The midcycle ovulatory LH surge results from an interaction between slowly increasing estrogen concentrations priming pituitary gonadotropes and GnRH pulses descending from the hypothalamus. In fact, the timing of ovulation is probably determined more by the pace and extent of the estrogen priming than by an intrinsic hypothalamic signal.

Other Factors. Other factors originating in the central nervous system and peripheral circulation can also modify gonadotropin secretion. In a manner similar to TSH, α_1-adrenergic stimulation augments LH secretion by stimulating both GnRH release from the hypothalamus and LH secretion directly from the anterior pituitary. Specific inhibition of the α_1-adrenergic receptors inhibits these effects. Cholinergic stimuli release GnRH, whereas opioid peptides inhibit GnRH secretion. The effects of dopamine are controversial and poorly understood. Hyperprolactinemia stimulates hypothalamic dopamine, which may contribute to the inhibition of GnRH release. As a result, gonadotropin pulsations are diminished in both frequency and amplitude, resulting in amenorrhea in females and impotence in males.

Function of Gonadotropins

Both LH and FSH interact with specific receptors on the gonad and mediate their action by the stimulation of cyclic AMP within testicular or ovarian cells. In females, LH stimulates ovulation and promotes the production of progesterone in the corpora lutea. In addition, LH is important for the stimulation of estrogen production by follicular cells. In males, LH is primarily responsible for the stimulation of testosterone production by the Leydig cells. FSH stimulates follicular development in females and prepares the follicle for ovulation. In addition, FSH stimulates thecal cells to synthesize and secrete estrogens. Both FSH and LH appear to increase prior to ovulation. In males, FSH stimulates spermatogenesis as well as sperm maturation. In addition, FSH appears to be responsible for stimulating the production of androgen-binding protein by the Sertoli cells. This protein binds to testosterone, allowing high concentrations of testosterone to be present at the site of spermatogenesis, possibly providing a permissive role for this important function.

Excess Gonadotropin Secretion

Primary Hypogonadism. Primary ovarian or testicular failure is the most common cause for elevated LH and FSH blood concentrations in humans. In all women undergoing menopause or oophorectomy, LH and FSH levels will rise dramatically concomitant with a two- to three-fold increase in LH and FSH production rates. In men, there are lesser but discernible decreases in testicular testosterone production after the age of 60, with small but detectable increases in serum LH and FSH concentrations. Other diseases with altered LH and/or FSH secretion, such as those found in precocious puberty or the polycystic ovary syndrome, will be discussed under Reproductive Endocrinology.

Pituitary Tumors Secreting the Gonadotropins. Pituitary tumors producing the gonadotropins are rare, accounting for only 2 to 5 per cent of all cases. Their detection has been difficult because they do not present with a classic clinical syndrome, such as acromegaly or the amenorrhea-galactorrhea syndrome. In addition, they do not produce clinical illness, such as that found with hyperthyroidism due to TSH-secreting tumors. The gonadotropic tumors may secrete only LH, both LH and FSH, or only FSH (Table 13). Pituitary tumors with isolated LH secretion are extremely rare, and perhaps only one well-documented case has been reported. This case occurred in a middle-aged male with a large tumor and visual field defects. The patient had few, if any, symptoms related to the LH hypersecretion. Testicular Leydig cell hyperplasia was associated with elevated serum testosterone levels and normal libido, whereas spermatogenesis was reduced. Serum LH levels were increased by GnRH administration, a feature that differs from the autonomous TSH secretion in thyrotrope pituitary adenomas. Furthermore, LH-β subunit levels were elevated and responded to GnRH administration. In a manner similar to TSH-secreting tumors, the serum alpha subunit concentration was extremely high and responded only minimally to GnRH stimulation. Whether LH-secreting tumors will be more frequently identified as patients with pituitary tumors are screened with gonadotropin radioimmunoassays is uncertain. Tumors that produce both LH and FSH are also quite rare. In these cases, the patients have normal or elevated serum testosterone levels in association with high levels of both serum LH and FSH. In vitro cultures of the tumor cells validated that the tumors produced both LH and FSH, and immunofluorescent studies on the tumor cells showed the presence of both LH and FSH.

Tumors producing only FSH are much more common than the LH-only or LH- and FSH-producing tumors. In fact, pure FSH-producing tumors may account for more cases than all other glycoprotein hormone–producing tumors combined. Most of these cases occur in males, and the patients classically present with hypogonadism, headaches, and visual field defects. The serum testosterone is low, and x-rays of the pituitary generally reveal large tumors with suprasellar extension. The diagnosis depends on demonstrating not only high serum FSH levels but also production of FSH by the pituitary tumor, usually by immunofluorescent localization in the resected tumor tissue. The production of FSH by the tumors has different characteristics than those previously discussed for TSH-secreting tumors. First, both FSH and its subunits are increased by GnRH stimulation, suggesting that FSH-producing tumors are not totally autonomous. Second, there is augmented secretion of the FSH-β subunit and normal secretion of the alpha subunit. Third, approximately 50 per cent of cases will respond aberrantly to TRH stimulation, a finding that is similar to the GH response to TRH in acromegaly. The responsiveness of

TABLE 13. CHARACTERISTICS OF GONADOTROPIN-PRODUCING PITUITARY ADENOMAS

	LH ONLY	LH AND FSH	FSH PREDOMINANT
Sex	M	M	M>>F
Tumor size	macroadenoma	macroadenoma	macroadenoma
Visual field defect	yes	yes	common
Serum LH	↑	nl- ↑	nl- ↓
Serum FSH		↑	↑
Serum α-subunit	↑	nl	nl- ↑
Serum testosterone	↑	nl- ↑	↓
LH or FSH p̄ GnRH	↑	↑	↑ (→)

the gonadotrope tumors suggests that some of these cases may respond to physiological manipulations. Unfortunately, only a limited experience is available, and the response of these tumors to other regulatory modulators, such as dopamine, somatostatin, or glucocorticoids, has not been well defined.

Alpha Subunit–Secreting Pituitary Tumors. In recent years, a subset of patients with pituitary tumors has been found to secrete the alpha subunit of the glycoprotein hormones without concomitant production of intact TSH, LH, or FSH. In some circumstances, excessive alpha subunit secretion has been found in association with growth hormone or prolactin-secreting tumors. When examined by immunofluorescence, the alpha subunit localizes in different cells than either growth hormone or prolactin. In other patients, only the alpha subunit is produced, making it the sole tumor marker being secreted. Patients with alpha subunit–secreting pituitary tumors usually present clinically with large tumors, visual field defects, and varying degrees of hypogonadism. The responses of the alpha subunit to dynamic testing suggest that its secretion is autonomous. In most cases studied, there is no response to TRH or GnRH stimulation nor to thyroid or sex steroid hormone suppression. Minimal decreases in serum alpha subunit concentrations have been reported following acute somatostatin and dopamine infusions, suggesting partial responsiveness to some regulators of glycoprotein hormone secretion.

Treatment of Tumors Producing the Glycoprotein Hormones. Surgical transsphenoidal hypophysectomy has been the treatment of choice in most tumors producing the glycoproteins. The tumors are usually large, producing visual defects in the patients. Although surgery has been successful in reducing tumor size and the serum concentrations of the glycoproteins, normalization of LH, FSH, or alpha subunit levels has generally not been achieved. Radiotherapy is a valuable therapeutic option, particularly as an adjunct to surgery or in cases in which surgery cannot be performed.

HYPOPITUITARISM

Hypopituitarism is a condition in which there is decreased pituitary hormone production due to deficient function of the pituitary. There is a wide spectrum in the clinical presentation of hypopituitarism, and the disease may be partial or complete. The pituitary gland has a large reserve capacity, and greater than 75 per cent destruction must occur before clinical signs of hypopituitarism develop and greater than 90 per cent destruction before panhypopituitarism occurs. In addition, defects may involve only one or all of the pituitary hormones. Separate monotropic pituitary deficiencies that occur in a familial or sporadic pattern have also been reported. Because the spectrum of pituitary deficiencies is wide, the clinical presentations are not uniform. Some patients may be virtually asymptomatic and become sick only at times of severe stress, whereas others may rapidly become seriously ill. Hypopituitarism either may be caused by primary disease in the pituitary or may be secondary to disorders in the hypothalamus. Many times, both the hypothalamus and the pituitary are involved by a path-

ological process, giving rise to hypopituitarism. Pinpointing the exact location of the defect by appropriate diagnostic studies has importance for understanding the etiology of the hypopituitarism and, more importantly, for its therapy. For instance, primary disease in the pituitary is treated by replacing either the pituitary hormone (i.e., gonadotropins for infertility and GH for growth failure) or the target gland hormones (thyroid, cortisol, or sex steroid hormones). In contrast, disease originating in the hypothalamus can in some instances be treated by replacing the hypothalamic factors (GnRH for the hypogonadotropic hypogonadism of Kallman's syndrome or possibly, in the future, GRF in certain types of hypothalamic growth failure).

Hypopituitarism may develop abruptly, as in Sheehan's postpartum necrosis, or gradually, as in the natural history of nonfunctioning pituitary tumors. If the hypopituitarism develops gradually, then defects in pituitary hormone secretion occur in a relatively predictable manner. The secretion of GH and gonadotropins appears to be the most sensitive to hypothalamic-pituitary disease. Thus, defects in growth and reproductive or sexual function occur early in the course of diseases involving the hypothalamus and pituitary. TSH and ACTH are generally well-preserved during the early stages of hypothalamic-pituitary disease and decrease later in the course of the disease. PRL generally is the last pituitary hormone to decrease in hypopituitarism. Although the anatomical or physiological reasons for the sequence of developing pituitary deficiencies are unknown, a knowledge of them is useful in the evaluation of patients. Men with normal sexual function and women in the premenopausal age range with normal menses generally have normal pituitary function. In contrast, complete PRL deficiency reflects total primary hypopituitarism in most cases.

ETIOLOGY OF HYPOPITUITARISM

Hypopituitarism can be caused by processes in the pituitary or hypothalamus or both (Table 14). In many instances, defects at both levels are present. A useful rule of thumb is that hypothalamic processes generally interrupt dopaminergic tone; thus, serum PRL concentrations rise, whereas the secretion of all other pituitary hormones decreases. Conversely, in hypopituitarism due to primary pituitary disease, all pituitary hormones, including PRL secretion, decrease.

1. Neoplasms. Tumors of either the pituitary or the hypothalamus can cause hypopituitarism. Pituitary tumors are the most common cause of hypopituitarism in adults. They disrupt pituitary function by displacing or destroying normal pituitary tissue or by interrupting the hypothalamic-pituitary communication of the hypophyseal-portal blood system. Microadenomas are rarely a cause of complete hypopituitarism, although PRL-secreting tumors commonly produce hypogonadotropic hypogonadism owing to the negative feedback of PRL on GnRH pulsations. Thus, pituitary tumors may directly cause hypopituitarism by altering hypothalamic function. The most common hypothalamic tumor is the craniopharyngioma. These are epithelial tumors originating in Rathke's pouch of the hypothalamus. They are most commonly observed in children

TABLE 14. ETIOLOGICAL CLASSIFICATION OF HYPOPITUITARISM

A. Neoplasms
  1. Pituitary tumors
  2. Hypothalamic tumors (craniopharyngioma, meningioma, epidermoid tumor, optic gliomas, chordomas)
  3. Metastatic tumors
B. Vascular
  1. Postpartum pituitary necrosis (Sheehan's syndrome)
  2. Hemorrhagic necrosis of a pituitary tumor
  3. Carotid aneurysm
C. Infiltrative
  1. Sarcoidosis
  2. Hemochromatosis
  3. Histiocytosis X
D. Ablative
  1. Pituitary surgery
  2. Pituitary irradiation
E. Injury
F. Infection
  1. Tuberculosis
  2. Syphilis
  3. Brucellosis
  4. Granulomata or inflammation
G. Monotropic pituitary deficiencies

but may also occur in adults. They usually produce hypopituitarism by interrupting hypothalamic function. Occasionally, they can grow into the sella and directly compress sellar contents. Craniopharyngiomas are nonsecretory tumors and, therefore, produce symptoms by compressing adjacent structures. Most present with headaches, visual field defects, and diabetes insipidus. Varying degrees of hypopituitarism are present. The tumors may become calcified, and speckled calcifications can be seen in the suprasellar region on routine skull x-rays. The tumors grow slowly and are generally quite large at the time of discovery. For that reason, complete resection is usually impossible. Following decompressive surgery, adjuvant therapy is usually accomplished by radiotherapy. Other tumors, which may involve the hypothalamus, include meningioma, epidermoid tumors, optic gliomas, and chordomas. Metastatic tumors, particularly those originating in the breast, may spread to the hypothalamus, producing varying degrees of hypothalamic hypopituitarism.

2. Vascular. There are three important vascular reasons for hypopituitarism. Pituitary necrosis was originally documented by Sheehan in a woman following postpartum hemorrhage and hypotension. Many additional cases have since been reported. The mechanism for the pituitary necrosis is unclear. During pregnancy, the pituitary usually enlarges and has an increased blood flow, thereby predisposing it to ischemic necrosis if hypotension occurs during the course of delivery or during the postpartum period. Generally, this event is catastrophic and severe hypopituitarism occurs. Occasionally, failure of postpartum lactation will be the only clinical sign of the disease.

The second important vascular cause of hypopituitarism involves the hemorrhagic degeneration of pituitary tumors. Like many benign endocrine tumors, the natural history of their evolution may involve hemorrhagic necrosis and degeneration. Like vascular postpartum necrosis, this event may be catastrophic, associated with severe hypopituitarism, vascular collapse, hypotension, headache, nausea, vomiting, and obtundation. In some circumstances, pituitary adenoma infarction is the first clinical sign of a silent pituitary adenoma, particularly a nonsecretory adenoma. Generally, treatment of this catastrophic illness involves evacuation of the sellar contents in addition to the acute administration of glucocorticoids and appropriate treatment of the hypotension. Following resolution of the acute episode, complete or partial hypopituitarism may be present.

The third vascular cause for hypopituitarism is a carotid aneurysm producing compression of the anterior pituitary contents as well as distortion of the hypophyseal-portal blood system. Differentiating this process from a pituitary adenoma is critical, since treatment of the two disorders is different.

3. Infiltrative. Three important infiltrative processes cause hypopituitarism. Sarcoidosis can produce hypopituitarism by infiltrative lesions in either the hypothalamus or the pituitary. In most cases, the lesions are located in the hypothalamus and can be demonstrated by CT scanning. Hemochromatosis may produce hypopituitarism due to iron infiltration in the pituitary or hypothalamus, with subsequent hypothalamic-pituitary dysfunction. Finally, histiocytosis X is associated with involvement of multiple organs, including the hypothalamus, by infiltration with well-differentiated histiocytes. These patients may also have diabetes insipidus.

4. Ablative Therapy. Following the treatment of pituitary tumors with surgery or ionizing radiation, hypopituitarism can develop. Following irradiation with conventional doses of 4,000 to 5,000 rads, hypopituitarism can develop. The hypopituitarism in this circumstance may be due either to the death of pituitary cells or to the destruction of hypothalamic cells, producing hypothalamic hypopituitarism. The hypothalamic damage is usually more important than the death of pituitary cells, since it takes between 8,000 and 12,000 rads to destroy normal adult pituitary cells, whereas hypothalamic cells are much more radiosensitive. For this reason, hypothalamic hypopituitarism is more likely to occur after conventional irradiation, since the hypothalamus receives considerable radiation with this mode of therapy. In contrast, focused heavy particle or proton beam irradiation delivers higher doses to the pituitary, but much less radiation is given to the hypothalamus. Therefore, hypopituitarism following proton beam therapy is usually due to the death of pituitary cells. Hypopituitarism following transsphenoidal surgery is distinctly unusual, particularly transsphenoidal surgery for microadenomas.

5. Other Causes. Head injury caused by trauma may create a tear in the hypophyseal-portal stalk, resulting in hypothalamic hypopituitarism. Infectious diseases, such as tuberculosis and other granulomatous processes, may also produce hypopituitarism, although these are distinctly unusual causes.

6. Monotropic or Isolated Pituitary Deficiencies. Isolated deficiencies of GH, PRL, ACTH, TSH, and LH or FSH have all been reported. Some of these occur in familial distribution, such as GH and LH or FSH deficiency, and appear to be due to deficient hypothalamic-releasing hormones. For instance, monotropic gonadotropin deficiency (Kallman's syndrome) is most commonly due to deficient GnRH production, which is an X-linked, dominantly inherited disorder. Others, such as ACTH, TSH, and PRL deficiencies, are usually isolated nonfamilial deficiencies. In monotropic TSH deficiency, the etiology is generally hypothalamic TRH insufficiency, whereas in isolated ACTH or PRL absence, the etiology is ambiguous.

CLINICAL AND LABORATORY DIAGNOSIS OF HYPOPITUITARISM

The clinical presentation observed in patients with hypopituitarism ranges from mild monotropic deficiencies to severe panhypopituitarism. In children, pituitary tumors are unusual and hypopituitarism is usually due to hypothalamic disorders that present as monotropic deficiencies, such as growth failure or delayed or absent puberty. In adults, pituitary tumors are more common, and the clinical presentation usually involves symptoms of a mass lesion in the sellar region. Endocrinologically, most of these patients will initially present with a defect in sexual or reproductive function. Total panhypopituitarism occurs later with further growth of the mass lesion or, in some instances, as a result of treatment (i.e., surgery or radiotherapy). These patients are usually older and demonstrate a generalized failure to thrive, with symptoms including decreased appetite, anorexia, weight loss, dry skin, constipation, cold intolerance, weakness, postural hypotension, and obtundation.

Diagnostically, a few simple rules are helpful in evaluating patients suspected of having hypopituitarism. Normal sexual and reproductive function in a premenopausal woman or man makes hypopituitarism unlikely. Likewise, elevated gonadotropins in postmenopausal women suggest that the hypothalamic-pituitary axis is functioning normally. In contrast, normal or low-normal *basal* thyroid and adrenal function should never be construed as evidence for normal pituitary function. Thyroid and adrenal function are well preserved during the early phases of hypothalamic-pituitary failure. For precise delineation of pituitary functional reserve, the laboratory procedures outlined in Table 15 are those of potential utility. The important general principle in evaluating possible hypopituitarism is that decreased secretion of the pituitary hormones is properly evaluated by *stimulation tests*. Basal hormonal secretion is thereby correlated with the functional reserve capacity of the pituitary. If the response to stimulation is negligible or absent, then hypopituitarism is due to primary pituitary disease. If, however, the responses are present but basal secretion is low, then the pituitary is normal and hypopituitarism must be due to a hypothalamic defect. For example, a hypothyroid patient with decreased thyroid hormone levels and an absent TSH response to TRH has hypopituitarism due to primary pituitary disease (Fig. 39). In contrast, the same patient who has a positive TSH response to TRH may have hypothalamic hypopituitarism due to conditions such as a craniopharyngioma, radiation to the hypothalamus, or a metastatic tumor of the hypothalamus. However, in some circumstances, the distinctions are less clear, and defects at both pituitary and hypothalamic loci contribute to the clinical presentation. For instance, an impotent male with a low plasma testosterone level may have both a positive LH response to GnRH (suggesting hypothalamic disease) and an elevated PRL level that is unresponsive to TRH (indicating the

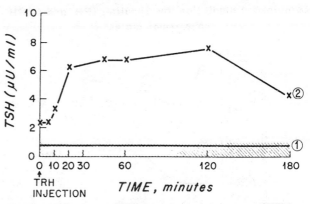

Figure 39. The serum TSH response to intravenous TRH in a patient (1) with hypopituitarism due to a pituitary tumor contrasted with a patient (2) with hypopituitarism due to a hypothalamic tumor. Note the delayed peak TSH response to TRH (120 minutes) in the patient with the hypothalamic tumor.

TABLE 15. LABORATORY DIAGNOSIS OF HYPOPITUITARISM

GONADOTROPINS	GROWTH HORMONE	CORTICOTROPIN
1. Plasma testosterone (males), LH, FSH	1. Serum somatomedin C and GH	1. Plasma cortisol and ACTH
2. GnRH stimulation (100 µg IV)	2. Insulin tolerance test (0.10–0.15 units CZI IV). Blood sugar and GH at 0, 30, and 60 min	2. Insulin tolerance test with ACTH and cortisol at 0, 30, and 60 min
	3. GRF stimulation (100 µg IV); GH at 0, 10, 20, 30, 60 and 120 min	3. Cortrosyn test, ACTH (1-24) (0.25 mg IV). Cortisol at 0, 30, and 60 min
		4. Metyrapone: 2–3 gm P.O. at midnight; plasma cortisol and deoxycortisol at 8 A.M.

THYROTROPIN	PROLACTIN	
		5. CRF stimulation (100 µg IV); ACTH at 0, 10, 20, 30, 60 and 120 min
1. T₄, T₃ resin uptake, TSH	1. Prolactin	
2. TRH (200 µg IV); TSH at 0, 10, 20, 30, 60, and 120 min	2. TRH (200 µg IV); Prolactin at 0, 10, 20, 30, 60 and 120 min	

Combined Stimulation by Insulin, TRH, and GnRH in Normal Males*

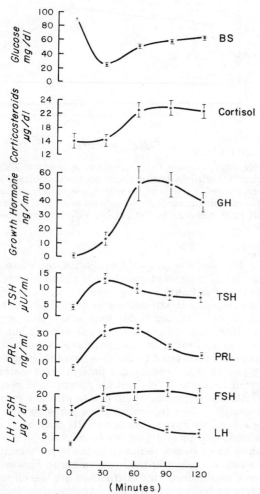

Figure 40. Hormonal responses to a combined TRH-GnRH-insulin–induced hypoglycemic stimulation test in normal males. (The data were derived from Table 2 in Lufkin, E. G., et al.: Am J Med 75:471, 1983.)

presence of a PRL-secreting pituitary tumor). In this case, the pituitary tumor produces excessive PRL; the elevated PRL produces the hypogonadism by altering hypothalamic GnRH secretion. Similar examples can be given for each of the pituitary hormones.

Traditionally, the workup for hypopituitarism was time-consuming and costly. The availability of the hypothalamic-releasing factors has simplified this evaluation enormously. The evaluation can now be carried out as an outpatient procedure in a short period of time. The individual provocative tests may be given on individual days, the same day, or, in fact, simultaneously by a combined insulin-TRH-GnRH stimulation test. The response of normal males to such combined stimulation testing is shown in Figure 40. The discovery and availability of CRF and GRF may make these evaluations even more specific and simple by eliminating the necessity for utilizing insulin-induced hypoglycemia.

Insulin-induced hypoglycemia has been considered the "gold standard" for testing GH and ACTH reserve. In fact, PRL is also released by hypoglycemia, but TSH and the gonadotropins are not. Insulin-induced hypoglycemia should be performed only by experienced clinicians who have performed many such tests. It is safely done in children and young adults. It carries hazard and risk to elderly patients or those with seizure disorders, hypertension, or cardiac disease. In contrast, the administration of TRH and GnRH is generally a benign procedure. However, complications and side effects of the administration of these agents, including severe headaches, seizure, and transient unconsciousness, have been reported in rare patients. These side effects are usually of very short duration and without permanent sequelae. Interestingly, most of these have occurred during the evaluation of patients with large intrasellar tumors, and most complications have occurred when combination testing has been performed.

THE EMPTY SELLA SYNDROME

The empty sella syndrome is an extremely common finding, and variations of it may be present in up to

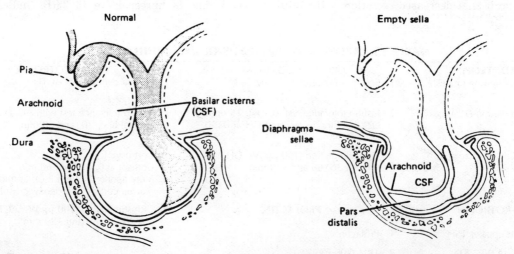

Figure 41. The primary empty sella syndrome (right) compared to normal pituitary anatomy (left). Compression of the anterior pituitary gland by an invagination of the diaphragma sella containing cerebrospinal fluid (CSF). (From Jordan, R. M., et al.: Am J Med 62:569, 1977.)

25 per cent of otherwise normal patients. In the vast majority of cases, the patient is asymptomatic. In others, the empty sella syndrome will be discovered during the course of evaluating an enlarged sella or in middle-aged, slightly obese women with mild hypertension. The defect appears to be in an invagination of the sellar diaphragm, perhaps due to congenital weakness, into the sella, such that sellar contents become exposed to cerebrospinal fluid pressures (Fig. 41). Investigators have theorized that the exposure to central nervous system pressure over long periods of time slowly expands the sella in a symmetrical fashion; focal defects in the sella are not found. Pituitary function in these cases is normal. Thus, the demonstration of an empty or partially empty sella by appropriate computerized tomography should eliminate the concern over hypopituitarism. The empty sella syndrome can also occur secondary to involution or cystic necrosis of a pituitary tumor. In this circumstance, a primary secretory adenoma may be present in association with a partially empty sella. The total pituitary function will then depend on the size and extent of the pituitary tumor, not the presence of the empty sella. Since the empty sella syndrome itself does not cause pituitary deficiency, this condition does not require specific treatment.

REFERENCES
General
Black, P. M., Zervas, N. T., Ridgway, E. C., and Martin, J. B. (eds.): Secretory Tumors of the Pituitary Gland. New York, Raven Press, 1984.
Daughaday, W. H.: The adenohypophysis. In Williams, R. H. (ed.): Textbook of Endocrinology, 6th ed. Philadelphia, W. B. Saunders Co., 1981, p. 73.
DeGroot, L. J., et al. (eds.): Endocrinology. Vol. 3. New York, Grune & Stratton, 1979.
Findling, J. W., and Tyrrell, J. B.: Anterior pituitary somatomedins: I. Anterior pituitary. In Greenspan, F. S., and Forsham, P. H. (eds.): Basic and Clinical Endocrinology. Los Altos, CA, Lange Medical Publications, 1983, p. 38.
Frohman, L. A.: Diseases of the anterior pituitary. In Felig, P., Baxter, J. D., Broadus, A. E., et al. (eds.): Endocrinology and Metabolism. New York, McGraw-Hill Book Co., 1981, p. 151.

Growth Hormone
Clemmons, D. R., Van Wyk, J. J., Ridgway, E. C., et al.: Evaluation of acromegaly by radioimmunoassay of somatomedin-C. N Engl J Med 301:1138, 1979.
Eddy, R. L., Gilliland, P. F., Ibarra, J. D., Jr., et al.: Human growth hormone release: Comparison of provocative test procedures. Am J Med 56:179, 1974.
Thorner, M. O., Rivier, J., Spiess, J., et al.: Human pancreatic growth-hormone-releasing factor selectively stimulates growth-hormone secretion in man. Lancet 18:24, 1983.
Van Wyk, J. J., and Underwood, L. E.: Relation between growth hormone and somatomedin. Annu Rev Med 26:427, 1975.

Thyrotropin
Bigos, S. T., Ridgway, E. C., Kourides, I. A., et al.: Spectrum of pituitary alterations with mild and severe thyroid impairment. J Clin Endocrinol Metab 46:317, 1978.

Chin, W. W., Habener, J. F., Kieffer, J. D., et al.: Cell-free translation of the messenger RNA coding for the α subunit of thyroid-stimulating hormone. J Biol Chem 253:7985, 1978.
Larsen, P. R.: Thyroid-pituitary interaction: Feedback regulation of thyrotropin secretion by thyroid hormones. N Engl J Med 306:23, 1982.
Shupnik, M. A., Chin, W. W., Ross, D. S., et al.: Regulation by thyroxine of the mRNA encoding the α subunit of mouse thyrotropin. J Biol Chem 258:15120, 1983.
Weintraub, B. D., Gershengorn, M. C., Kourides, I. A., et al.: Inappropriate secretion of thyroid-stimulating hormone. Ann Intern Med 95:339, 1981.

Gonadotropins
McCann, S. M.: Luteinizing-hormone–releasing hormone. N Engl J Med 296:797, 1977.
Peterson, R. E., Kourides, I. A., Horwith, M., et al.: Luteinizing hormone– and α-subunit–secreting pituitary tumor: Positive feedback of estrogen. J Clin Endocrinol Metab 52:692, 1981.
Ridgway, E. C., Klibanski, A., Ladenson, P. W., et al.: Pure alpha-secreting pituitary adenomas. N Engl J Med 304:1254, 1981.
Snyder, P. J., and Sterling, F. H.: Hypersecretion of LH and FSH by a pituitary adenoma. J Clin Endocrinol Metab 42:544, 1976.
Yen, S. S. C., and Jaffe, R. B. (eds.): Reproductive Endocrinology: Physiology, Pathophysiology and Clinical Management. Philadelphia, W. B. Saunders Co., 1978.

Prolactin
Chiodini, P., Liuzzi, A., Cozzi, R., et al.: Size reduction of macroprolactinomas by bromocriptine or lisuride treatment. J Clin Endocrinol Metab 53:737, 1981.
Frantz, A. G.: Prolactin. N Engl J Med 298:201, 1978.
Friesen, H., and Hwang, P.: Human prolactin. Annu Rev Med 24:251, 1973.
Kleinberg, D. L., Noel, G. L., and Frantz, A. G.: Galactorrhea: A study of 235 cases, including 48 with pituitary tumors. N Engl J Med 296:589, 1977.
Klibanski, A., Neer, R. M., Beitins, I. Z., et al.: Decreased bone density in hyperprolactinemic women. N Engl J Med 303:1511, 1980.

Corticotropin
Aron, D. C., Findling, J. W., Fitzgerald, P. A., et al.: Cushing's syndrome: Problems in management. Endocr Rev 3:229, 1982.
Crapo, L.: Cushing's syndrome: A review of diagnostic tests. Metabolism 28:955, 1979.
Krieger, D. T., Liotta, A. S., Suda, T., et al.: Human plasma immunoreactive lipotropin and adrenocorticotropin in normal subjects and in patients with pituitary-adrenal disease. J Clin Endocrinol Metab 48:566, 1979.
Roberts, J. L., and Herbert, E.: Characterization of a common precursor to corticotropin and β-lipotropin: Cell-free synthesis of the precursor and identification of corticotropin peptides in the molecule (peptide analysis/messenger RNA/immunoprecipitation). Proc Natl Acad Sci USA 74:4826, 1977.
Vale, W., Spiess, J., Rivier, C., et al.: Characterization of a 41-residue ovine hypothalamic peptide that stimulates secretion of corticotropin and β-endorphin. Science 213:1394, 1981.

Reproductive Endocrinology

ANNE KLIBANSKI, M.D.

NEUROENDOCRINE CONTROL OF REPRODUCTION

LHRH

Luteinizing hormone–releasing hormone (LHRH) or gonadotropin hormone–releasing hormone (GnRH) is the hypothalamic decapeptide responsible for the initiation and maintenance of normal reproductive function. LHRH is synthesized in hypothalamic-neuronal cells, from which it is transported along neuronal axons, stored in secretory granules, and released at the nerve terminals into the hypothalamic-hypophyseal portal circulation. The LHRH molecule has a "kink" or beta-turn in its center that allows it to fold back upon itself. This configuration is thought to be necessary for LHRH receptor binding activity. High concentrations of LHRH are found in the median eminence, the preoptic area, and the suprachiasmatic nucleus of the hypothalamus. LHRH is also found in other areas of the brain and hypothalamus and in the gonads; however, the biological significance of extrahypothalamic LHRH is unclear.

LHRH interacts with specific receptors on the pituitary gonadotrope plasma membrane to cause synthesis and release of LH and FSH. Peptides such as TRH, vasopressin, and the pituitary glycoproteins do not interact with these LHRH receptors. Although LHRH stimulates both LH and FSH, it is a more potent stimulus for LH release. Alterations in hypothalamic LHRH secretion are critical in determining the synthesis and secretion of gonadotropins. Calcium appears to play an important role in the mechanism by which LHRH increases gonadotropin secretion. In in vitro experiments calcium is required for LHRH-induced LH release from the gonadotrope. Cyclic nucleotides may act as second messengers in modulating LHRH action.

In the adult, LHRH is secreted in an episodic or pulsatile manner quite uniformly throughout the day and night and is responsible for the pulsatile release of LH and FSH into the circulation. These pulses occur at critical intervals and concentrations, and abnormalities in their release can disrupt normal reproductive function. During pulses, concentrations of LHRH in the hypophyseal-portal blood of experimental animals have been found to fluctuate between 20 and 800 pg/ml. Peripheral concentrations of LHRH in the human can be measured; however, they vary widely owing to pulsatile secretion and do not accurately reflect portal concentrations. The serum half-life of LHRH is several minutes. It is degraded throughout the body, its degradation in the brain being enhanced by sex steroids.

High concentrations of gonadal steroids exert a negative feedback effect that serves to inhibit LHRH secretion and subsequent gonadotropin release from the pituitary. Similarly, low concentrations of gonadal steroids have a positive feedback effect and stimulate LHRH. In experimental animals, castration causes an increase in LHRH portal blood concentrations. Gonadal steroids have also been shown to regulate LHRH receptor number without affecting binding affinity.

In addition to the modulating effect of gonadal steroids, several classic neurotransmitters, norepinephrine, dopamine, and serotonin, influence the synthesis and release of LHRH. It is unknown whether catecholamines modulate LHRH secretion by direct effects on LHRH synthesis or by affecting either the frequency or the amplitude of LHRH release. Norepinephrine is thought to play a stimulatory role in LHRH secretion, while dopaminergic compounds may have a dual effect on LHRH release. Depending on the experimental model, dopamine may either stimulate or inhibit LHRH release. The concentration of dopamine in the portal system is affected by the concentration of gonadal steroids, and hypothalamic catecholamine turnover rates change during the menstrual cycle. The interaction between gonadal steroids and LHRH in modulating LHRH secretion, mediated indirectly by dopamine, remains to be more clearly defined (Fig. 42). The opiates have also been shown to affect reproductive function. For example, endorphins can inhibit LHRH secretion and suppress gonadotropin pulsations. It is likely that some reproductive disorders may be caused

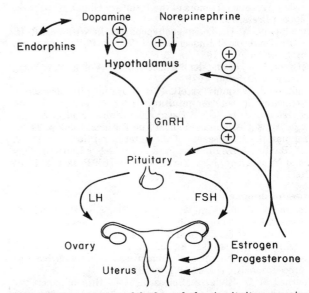

Figure 42. An overview of the hypothalamic-pituitary-ovarian axis. LHRH release is affected by neurotransmitters; norepinephrine can stimulate its release, whereas dopamine may either stimulate or inhibit its secretion depending on the experimental model. The opiates can inhibit LHRH secretion, and the effects of both the endorphins and dopamine are modulated by gonadal steroids. The pulsatile release of LHRH by the hypothalamus stimulates the release of LH and FSH by the pituitary gonadotrope at critical intervals and concentrations. Ovarian folliculogenesis and steroidogenesis occur as a result of gonadotropin stimulation. The gonadal steroids estradiol and progesterone have both positive and negative dose-dependent feedback effects on gonadotropin synthesis and release.

by abnormalities in endogenous catecholamines; however, at the present time, this has not been clearly defined.

GONADOTROPINS

Biosynthesis. The pituitary gonadotropins, LH and FSH, are synthesized and released by the pituitary gonadotropes and are responsible for ovarian sex steroid hormone production. LH and FSH are glycoprotein hormones composed of two noncovalently linked subunits, α and β. The α subunit of LH and FSH is identical with the α subunit of the other glycoprotein hormones, thyroid-stimulating hormone and human chorionic gonadotropin. The β subunit is unique to each of the glycoprotein pituitary hormones and confers both biological and immunological specificity. For example, when combined with the α subunit of either FSH, TSH, or hCG, the β subunit of LH provides the resulting hormone with LH bioactivity. The synthesis of LH-β and FSH-β is regulated by separate DNA molecules, coding for separate mRNAs. It is likely that the production of the β subunit of the glycoprotein is the rate-limiting step in the biosynthetic process. Gonadal steroids that influence LH and FSH secretion most likely do so by first altering gonadotropin biosynthesis, i.e., the rate of production of LH-β and FSH-β.

When studied in cell-free translation systems, the glycoprotein subunits are first synthesized as nonglycosylated large molecular weight presubunits (pre-α and pre-β), which are then processed to mature forms via signal peptide cleavage and glycosylation. The signal peptide is an amino terminal extension that may be important in transport of the subunit from the ribosome to the endoplasmic reticulum. Processing of the presubunits occurs co-translationally upon the ribosome as well as post-translationally once the subunits are transported to other intracellular organelles. Following linkage of the subunits to form the complete hormone, terminal sugars are added to the molecule prior to secretion. Glycosyl transferases are specific intracellular enzymes that transfer these sugars from a lipid donor to the nascent polypeptide. The function of the carbohydrate moiety is unknown, but it may relate to secretion, receptor binding, and peripheral degradation in the circulation. In summary, the α and β chains of LH and FSH are synthesized independently by separate mRNAs. The biosynthesis of the β subunit of LH and FSH appears to be the rate-limiting step in gonadotropin production and is regulated by sex steroid hormones, LHRH, and other factors. See The Pituitary and Hypothalamus for a further discussion of the chemistry of the gonadotropins.

Gonadotropin Regulation. Secretory bursts of LHRH are followed within minutes by release of LH and FSH into the peripheral circulation. Pulsatile gonadotropin secretion appears to be critical for normal gonadal function. In males, LH pulses are relatively frequent, occurring every 90 to 120 minutes. Pulsatile LH secretion in females is influenced by the varying estradiol and progesterone concentrations throughout the menstrual cycle. The LH and FSH response to physiological LHRH administration (0.025 ng/kg) every two hours, demonstrating large LH pulses, is shown in Figure 43. Circulating LH has a half-life of approximately 30 minutes, while the half-life of FSH is considerably longer at approximately 300 minutes. The shorter half-life of LH explains why LH pulses are easier to identify than those of FSH. The longer half-life of FSH is thought to be due to the higher sialic acid content of the FSH molecule. Continuous stimulation of the gonadotrope with LHRH depletes the gland of releasable LH and FSH; however, significant quantities of gonadotropins are still present within the pituitary gland. There is, therefore, a readily releasable gonadotropin pool as well as a storage pool within the pituitary. Gonadal factors act directly upon the pituitary gland or indirectly through LHRH to determine the relative quantities of the releasable and storage gonadotropin pools.

Two important concepts that have increased our understanding of gonadotropin release by LHRH are (1) LHRH priming, and (2) gonadotropin desensitization by LHRH. The ability of the pituitary gland to secrete LH and FSH after LHRH administration increases after previous LHRH exposure. This is called LHRH priming and requires estrogen exposure. The combination of LHRH and estrogen increases the availability of LHRH receptors on the anterior pituitary and increases their responsiveness to subsequent LHRH administration. The second concept is termed gonadotropin desensitization and refers to the decrease in gonadotropin secretion that occurs during continuous LHRH administration. In this situation, there is a decreased responsivity of the gonadotrope without a change in receptor number. In contrast, pharmacological doses of LHRH can lead to pituitary LHRH receptor down-regulation. In this case, LH and FSH secretion is decreased because of a reduction in LHRH receptor number.

In women, the gonadal steroids, estradiol and progesterone, have both positive and negative feedback effects on gonadotropin synthesis and release. Estradiol and progesterone can both alter gonadotropin secretion, by direct effects on either the gonadotrope or LHRH or both. The two critical factors that determine the feedback effects of gonadal steroids are the dose and the duration of exposure. Low concentrations of estradiol can inhibit LH and FSH secretion, although higher concentrations induce a surge in LH secretion. A serum estradiol concentration in women of over 200 pg/ml must be maintained for approximately 50 hours to stimulate LH secretion. Estradiol concentrations of this magnitude, sustained for several days, will also enhance the LH response to LHRH stimulation, as shown in Figure 44. Sustained supraphysiological amounts of gonadal steroids will inhibit gonadotropin secretion, as seen in menopausal women. Small amounts of progesterone enhance the LH response to LHRH; however, high concentrations of progesterone inhibit LHRH secretion and may interfere with the gonadotropin response to LHRH.

In the male, low concentrations of circulating testosterone stimulate LHRH and LH secretion. Higher concentrations of testosterone exert a negative feedback effect by decreasing hypothalamic LHRH secretion and by inhibiting the gonadotropin response to LHRH.

Developmental Aspects. Gonadotropin secretion occurs throughout fetal life, childhood, and adulthood. LHRH is detectable in the hypothalamus by 10 weeks of gestation, and LH and FSH are produced by the

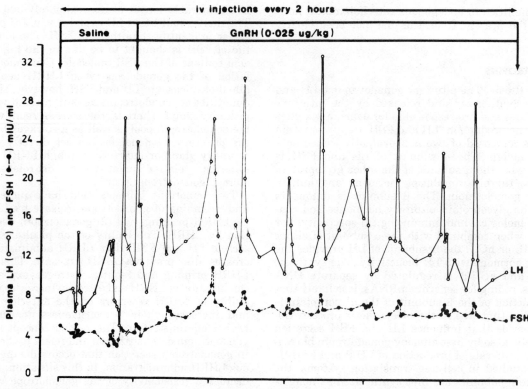

Figure 43. Plasma LH and FSH in a normal male with samples obtained every 20 minutes for two 3-hour periods as the baseline, followed by GnRH (0.025 μg/kg) every 2 hours I.V. Note the well-defined LH pulses in response to administration of physiological doses of GnRH. (From Valk, T. W., Corley, K. P., Kelch, R. P., and Marshall, J. C.: J Clin Endocrinol Metab 53:188, 1981.)

gonadotropes by 10 to 13 weeks. The concentrations of LH and FSH continue to rise until approximately midgestation, when there is a decrease in gonadotropin secretion because of increasing inhibition by gonadal steroids. An increase in gonadotropins is seen in the newborn because of withdrawal of placental steroids and hCG, which are cleared from the neonatal circulation within a few days. In female infants, gonadotropin secretion continues to rise until approximately three months of age, by which time serum FSH concentrations may be as high as those seen in castrates or postmenopausal women. Gonadotropin secretion during this period causes an increase in the number of antral follicles and a small rise in serum estradiol and 17-α-hydroxyprogesterone. LH and FSH levels subsequently decrease and reach a nadir at two to three years of age. Although gonadal steroids may play a role in the observed decrease in gonadotropin levels, there is probably a second mechanism whereby LHRH secretion is inhibited, since infants born without gonadal tissue will also show a decrease in gonadotropin levels during this time. Although the precise mecha-

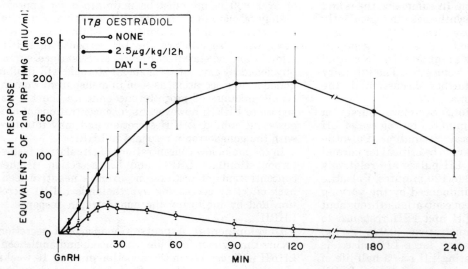

Figure 44. The increase in serum LH (mean ± SEM) following GnRH (100 μg) at time 0 on day 7 of the menstrual cycle after 7 days of treatment with estradiol benzoate 5 μg/kg/day (●——●). A control group LH response is also shown (○——○) of women who did not receive estradiol. The estradiol-treated group had a markedly enhanced LH response to GnRH stimulation. (From Jaffe, R. B., and Keye, W. R., Jr.: J Clin Endocrinol Metab 39:850, 1974.)

nism whereby LHRH and gonadotropin secretion is suppressed during the subsequent prepubertal years is unknown, the key timing of release of this suppression allows for normal pubertal and reproductive development.

Gonadotropin function differs in males and females. In the male fetus, LH and FSH concentrations are lower than those seen in the female. In newborn male infants, serum LH and FSH concentrations rise and reach a peak at approximately one to two months of age and then show a decrease into the prepubertal range by approximately four months. The sex difference in gonadotropin secretion probably reflects the influence of testicular androgens.

OVARIAN STRUCTURE AND FUNCTION

EMBRYOLOGY AND ANATOMY

During early embryonic development, primordial germ cells migrate from the yolk sac to the genital ridge. Initially, ovarian and testicular development proceeds in an "indifferent" gonad, which does not show signs of sexual differentiation until the fetus is approximately 15 mm in size. In the genetically determined female, the primordial germ cells are in a superficial cortex, and the inner medulla atrophies. At six to eight weeks of fetal life, there is rapid mitotic multiplication of oogonia, reaching a peak of six to seven million germ cells by midgestation. At midgestation, the gonadal cellular cortex of oogonia and oocytes is gradually subdivided into smaller segments by the appearance of vascular channels. The oocytes, which are in a state of arrested prophase, are covered by a layer of pregranulosa cells and an outer matrix of mesenchymal cells. The residual mesenchymal cells are present between the follicles and form a primitive ovarian stroma. Identifiable follicles appear in the fourth month of gestation, and they undergo different degrees of development. Most follicles become atretic, and at the time of birth, the 1-cm ovary has already depleted its cell mass by some four to five million germ cells.

The prepubertal ovary contains primary follicles. Further development will occur only in the approximately 400 oogonia selected for further monthly maturation throughout reproductive life. By puberty, the number of germ cells has been further reduced to approximately 100,000 to 300,000. The factors that determine which one of the many thousand germ cells is selected for further development are unknown.

The adult ovaries are located near the end of the fallopian tubes in the mesovarium of the pelvic broad ligaments. Each ovary measures approximately 2.5 to 5 cm in length, 1.5 to 3 cm in width, and 0.5 to 1.5 cm in depth. The ovarian cortex is composed of oocytes contained in follicles that are surrounded by connective tissue. The ovarian medulla consists of connective tissue and blood vessels.

FOLLICULAR DEVELOPMENT

The *immature follicle* or *primordial follicle* contains a primary oocyte in a state of arrested prophase surrounded by a single layer of granulosa cells and is separated from the surrounding ovarian stroma by a basement membrane. Follicular development of the dominant follicle is outlined in Figure 45. The rare follicle selected for further development develops a progressively larger oocyte and is called a primary follicle. The transition from a primordial to a primary follicle is thought to be gonadotropin-independent. The surrounding granulosa cells proliferate, and the adjacent ovarian stromal cells outside the basement membrane become arranged in concentric perifollicular layers called the theca. The part of the theca adjacent to the follicle is called the theca interna, and the part that is subsequently incorporated into the remainder of the ovarian stroma is called the theca externa. The growth of the primary follicle is dependent upon FSH, estrogen, and testosterone. In studies in experimental animals, specific estradiol receptors have been found

Figure 45. Stages of follicular development from a primordial follicle to a preovulatory follicle.

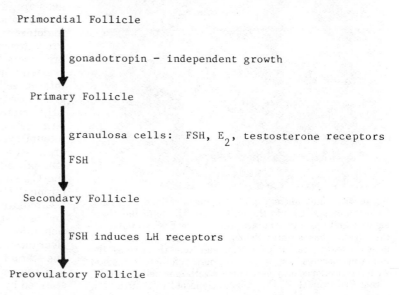

Follicular Development

Primordial Follicle

↓ gonadotropin - independent growth

Primary Follicle

↓ granulosa cells: FSH, E_2, testosterone receptors

FSH

Secondary Follicle

↓ FSH induces LH receptors

Preovulatory Follicle

in cytosol and nuclear fractions of rat granulosa cells of primary follicles. Estrogen increases the concentration of its own receptor and increases the sensitivity of the granulosa cell adenylcyclase system to FSH.

The secondary follicle, formed from the primary follicle under the influence of FSH and to a lesser degree LH, is approximately 0.2 mm in diameter and has fluid-filled spaces among the granulosa cells (Fig. 46). Estrogen is also important for this stage of follicular development by mediating granulosa proliferation, by enhancing the ability of FSH to stimulate synthesis of its own receptor, and by acting with FSH to stimulate ovarian LH receptor number. The fluid-filled spaces among the granulosa cells merge to form the antrum, and the follicle can grow up to 10 mm in size and is called a *graafian follicle.* The antral fluid of the graafian follicles contains a steroid hormone–rich plasma transudate from the granulosa cells. Follicular estradiol concentrations are critical in determining which follicle will become the dominant, or ovulatory, follicle. The dominant follicle has the high-

est intrafollicular estradiol concentration as well as the highest estrogen/androgen ratio. Although low concentrations of androgens serve as estrogen precursors (through aromatization), high intrafollicular androgen levels are associated with follicular atresia. The dominant follicle is also most responsive to available FSH and contains more aromatase enzyme necessary for androgen-to-estrogen conversion. By gonadotropin-independent mechanisms, the ovulatory follicle suppresses other available follicles in both ovaries. The underlying mechanisms are unclear, but it has been shown that the effluent from the human ovary containing the dominant follicle can suppress gonadotropin-stimulated steroidogenesis in animals. Once the dominant follicle is selected, other follicles no longer respond to stimulation by LH and FSH.

Following the preovulatory LH surge, the dominant follicle releases an oocyte from the surface of the ovary near the fallopian tube. Following ovulation, the remainder of the follicle forms the corpus luteum, which synthesizes progesterone and estrogen and persists for 14 days in the absence of conception. The formation of the corpus luteum is marked by the breakdown of the basement lamina, vascular invasion of the granulosa cells aided by an angiogenesis factor, and luteinization of the granulosa. The corpus luteum secretes progesterone in response to LH, and its LH receptors decrease as it ages. By eight to nine days after ovulation, the corpus luteum decreases in size and the granulosa cells become vacuolated. The degenerating corpus luteum is ultimately replaced by connective tissue and is termed a corpus albicans.

OVARIAN STEROID HORMONES

In a normal premenopausal woman, the rate of ovarian steroidogenesis varies with the menstrual cycle. The ovary produces estrogens, progestogens, and androgens (see Fig. 47). Estrogens are responsible for the development of female secondary reproductive characteristics; they stimulate the breast and exert a widespread systemic influence with effects on bone, skin, liver proteins, carbohydrate and lipid metabolism, and central nervous system function. Progestogens are important in preparing the endometrium for maintenance of pregnancy. Androgens are important in determining facial or body hair in the adult female. Progestogens and ovarian androgens also serve as precursors for ovarian biosynthesis. For example, the ovarian follicle contains granulosa cells and theca interna cells. Estrogens are formed primarily in the granulosa cells. The theca interna cells, stimulated by LH, secrete androgens, which are then aromatized to form estrogens in the granulosa cells. The corpus luteum synthesizes progesterone and, to a lesser degree, estrogen. The ovarian interstitium contains stromal cells and hilar cells, which mainly synthesize the C_{19} steroids, androstenedione, dehydroepiandrosterone (DHEA), and testosterone.

Circulating concentrations of estrogens, androgens, and progestogens are a reflection of (1) gonadal secretion rates, (2) adrenal secretion rates, (3) metabolic clearance rates, and (4) peripheral conversion rates of one steroid hormone to another. The secretion rate of a hormone is defined as the amount of a hormone secreted by a gland per unit time (milligram/day). The

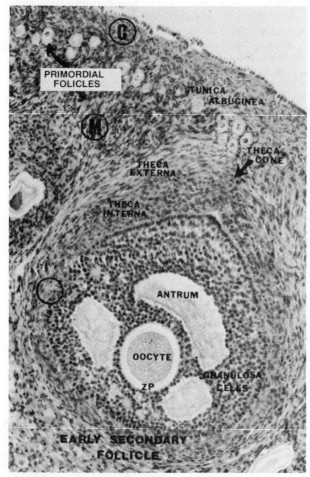

Figure 46. Light micrography showing a follicle migrating from the cortex (C) into the media (M). The follicular theca externa and theca interna are seen. Under FSH stimulation, the antrum has formed. Primordial follicles are seen in a band beneath the tunica albuginea. Note the size of the immature oocytes seen in these primordial follicles compared with the developed oocyte—complete with zona pellucida (ZP). (From Erickson, G. F.: Clin Obstet Gynecol 21:37, 1978.)

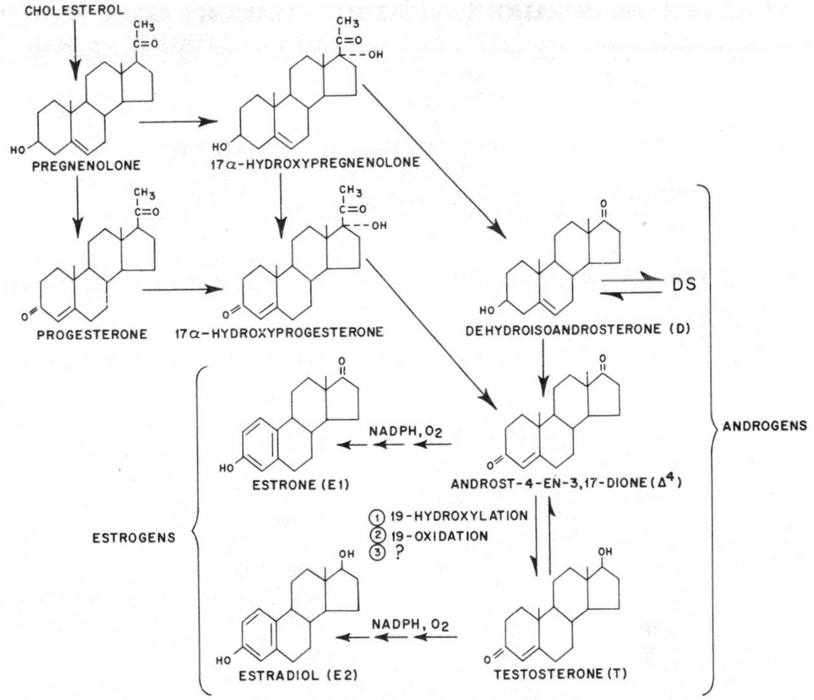

Figure 47. Ovarian biosynthesis of estrogens, androgens, and progestogens. (From Sitteri, P. K., and Febres, F.: In DeGroot, L. J., et al. (eds.): Endocrinology. Vol. 3. New York, Grune and Stratton, 1979, p. 1402. Reprinted with permission.)

Pathways of ovarian steroid hormone biosynthesis.

production rate of a hormone is the total amount of a hormone present in the circulation (amount derived from direct organ secretion plus the amount derived from peripheral conversion of other hormones). For example, in normal women circulating estradiol is almost entirely derived from direct secretion by the ovarian follicle, with a very small amount derived from the conversion of testosterone. Therefore, the production rate of estradiol is fairly comparable to its secretory rate. However, for testosterone, which is derived almost entirely from peripheral conversion of other hormones, such as androstenedione, the secretory rates are low, whereas the production rates are high. Peripheral conversion of a steroid hormone to another occurs in multiple locations in the body, including fat, muscle, liver, and brain. The final factor influencing the concentration of these hormones in the blood is the metabolic clearance rate (MCR) of the hormone, which is defined as the volume of blood that is cleared of a specific hormone per unit time. The concentration (C) of a hormone is therefore equal to its production rate (PR) divided by its metabolic clearance rate (C = PR/MCR).

Circulating gonadal steroids are bound to plasma proteins. The biological potency of a hormone in vivo is dependent upon how much of a hormone is bound to protein and how much is unbound or free and, therefore, "bioavailable." Sex hormone–binding globulin (SHBG) is a circulating low-capacity, high-affinity protein made in the liver, which binds many sex steroids. The greater the affinity of a hormone for SHBG, the lower its MCR. Physiological and pathological states that alter SHBG can influence the amount of free hormone present. For example, the concentration of SHBG in women is twice the amount found in men and is increased by estrogen administration, pregnancy, hyperthyroidism, and liver disease. SHBG can

be thought of as a physiological regulator of sex hormone action, by providing peripheral tissues with a relatively constant amount of available hormone. Since most hormone determinations measure the bound circulating hormone, SHBG must be considered in their interpretation. The concentrations, production rates, and metabolic clearance rates of the ovarian steroid hormones are shown in Table 16.

ESTROGENS

All natural estrogens contain phenolic-A rings and are derived from cholesterol, as shown in Figure 47. The most important ovarian estrogen, estradiol, is produced by the ovaries in variable amounts during the menstrual cycle. Serum estradiol concentrations are at their lowest amount during the early part of the menstrual cycle and increase slowly, reaching a peak just prior to ovulation. A second estrogenic compound, which is of lesser importance, is estrone. A small amount of estrone is secreted by the ovaries; however, most circulating estrone is derived from the peripheral conversion of androstenedione. A small amount of estrone may also be derived by conversion from estradiol. The liver is the major site of estrogen degradation, where it is conjugated with sulfate and glucuronate prior to entering the enterohepatic circulation. Estriol is a metabolic breakdown product of estradiol and estrone, and it is also formed from peripheral conversion of androstenedione and other androgens in the peripheral tissue. In addition to its known effects on maintenance of vaginal, uterine, and breast tissue, estrogens have other widespread systemic effects. Estrogens stimulate the production of plasma proteins by the liver, elevate concentrations of thyroid-binding globulin and cortisol-binding globulin, play a role in blood pressure regulation, and stimulate

TABLE 16. CONCENTRATIONS, METABOLIC CLEARANCE RATES, PRODUCTION RATES, AND OVARIAN SECRETION RATES OF STEROIDS IN BLOOD

COMPOUND	"MCR"* OF COMPOUND IN PERIPHERAL PLASMA (liters/day)	PHASE OF MENSTRUAL CYCLE	CONCENTRATION IN PLASMA (μg/dl)	PR** OF CIRCULATING COMPOUND (mg/day)	SR+ BY BOTH OVARIES (mg/day)
Estradiol	1350	Early follicular	0.006	0.081	0.07
		Late follicular	0.033–0.070	0.445–0.945	0.4–0.8
		Midluteal	0.020	0.270	0.25
Estrone	2210	Early follicular	0.005	0.110	0.08
		Late follicular	0.015–0.030	0.331–0.662	0.25–0.50
		Midluteal	0.011	0.243	0.16
Progesterone	2200	Follicular	0.095	2.1	1.5
		Luteal	1.13	25.0	24.0
20α-hydroxyprogesterone	2300	Follicular	0.05	1.1	0.8
		Luteal	0.25	5.8	3.3
17-hydroxyprogesterone	2000	Early follicular	0.03	0.6	0–0.3
		Late follicular	0.20	4.0	3–4
		Midluteal	0.20	4.0	3–4
Androstenedione	2010		0.159	3.2	0.8–1.6
Testosterone	690		0.038	0.26	
Dehydroisoandrosterone	1640		0.490	8.0	0.3–3

*Metabolic clearance rate.
**Production rate.
+Secretion rate.
From Williams, R. H. (ed.): Textbook of Endocrinology. 6th ed. Philadelphia, W. B. Saunders Co., 1981, p. 365.

angiotensinogen. Estrogenic compounds also have significant effects on plasma lipoproteins. Estrogen deficiency in menopause is associated with an increase in LDL cholesterol and a decrease in the ratio of HDL/LDL cholesterol. Estrogen administration causes a significant rise in HDL, primarily within the HDL-2 subclasses, and a decrease in LDL cholesterol. The mechanisms whereby estrogen affects lipoproteins and specifically HDL levels are unclear; however, it is known that hepatic lipase activity is significantly lower in women than in men and is decreased by the administration of estrogen.

PROGESTERONE

Progestogens, which include progesterone, 20α-hydroxyprogesterone and 17-hydroxyprogesterone, circulate throughout the menstrual cycle (Table 16). In the second half or luteal phase of the menstrual cycle, progesterone is secreted directly from the corpus luteum. During the early phase of follicular development, most progesterone is derived from extraglandular conversion of adrenal pregnenolone sulfate to progesterone. During the later stages of follicular development, the dominant follicle will secrete increased amounts of 17α-hydroxyprogesterone into the circulation. Aside from their effects on the endometrium, progestogens also have other systemic effects. The natural progestogens increase urinary nitrogen excretion and renal tubular absorption of sodium and may compete with aldosterone for receptor sites at the distal renal tubule. Progesterone can cause alterations in serum lipids and

carbohydrate metabolism. Respiratory drive is increased by progesterone, and this may be of therapeutic benefit in some patients with hypoventilation syndromes.

ANDROGENS

Serum concentrations of androgens in normal women reflect direct ovarian secretion, direct adrenal secretion, and peripheral conversion of one androgen to another. The sources and relative androgenicity of serum androgens in normal women are shown in Table 17. The ovary secretes androstenedione and smaller amounts of testosterone and DHEA. The majority of circulating testosterone is derived from peripheral conversion of Δ4-androstenedione, as well as from conversion of DHEA to testosterone. Androstenedione is secreted in relatively equal amounts by the ovaries and the adrenals. Androstenedione is only 10 to 20 per cent as potent an androgen as testosterone, as determined by bioassay. DHEA, which arises 80 per cent from the adrenal and 20 per cent from the ovary, is only 5 per cent as androgenic as testosterone. The blood production rate of testosterone in women is approximately 0.2 mg per 24 hr, whereas those of androstenedione and DHEA are 2 to 3 mg per 24 hr and 5 to 7 mg per 24 hr, respectively. The most potent androgen, dihydrotestosterone, is one and a half to three times more potent than testosterone and is derived almost entirely from peripheral conversion of androstenedione and testosterone. In the female, the major prehormone for the formation of dihydrotestosterone is androstenedi-

TABLE 17. ANDROGEN METABOLISM IN NORMAL WOMEN

| | PERCENT ARISING FROM | | | |
COMPOUND	Adrenal	Ovary	Peripheral Conversion	RELATIVE ANDROGENICITY(%) (based upon testosterone = 100%)
Dihydrotestosterone	—	—	100	125–300
Testosterone	0–30	5–20	50–70	100
Androstenedione	50	50	—	10–20
DHEA	80	20	—	5
DHEA sulfate	>90	<10	—	—

one. Because androgens may be converted through peripheral conversion to other androgens, it is important to remember that the secretion of any given androgen may result in increases in other circulating androgens with potency greater than or less than that of the parent compound. Androgens in women are important for stimulation of hair growth, maintenance of a positive nitrogen balance, muscular strength, and libido. At abnormally elevated concentrations, they can have masculinizing or virilizing effects and lead to an increase in muscle development, temporal balding, deepening of the voice, and enlargement of the clitoris.

PUBERTY

Puberty is a period lasting several years during which secondary sexual characteristics develop, somatic growth accelerates, and reproductive capacity begins. In the United States, puberty in girls usually begins between 8 and 13 years of age, and in boys between 9 and 14 years of age. The terms used to describe pubertal development include thelarche or breast development, adrenarche or the development of axillary and pubic hair, and, finally, gonadarche. Gonadarche in males is the development of testicular function, and in females it is the onset of menstrual periods (also called menarche). The pubertal process now begins earlier than it did a century ago; in 1900, European females began menarche more than two years later than girls do today. Although the timing of puberty is determined largely by genetic factors, it is also affected by general physical health, weight, and the degree of athletic activity. For example, delayed puberty is seen with malnutrition, chronic diseases, and vigorous endurance sports training. In contrast, moderate obesity is associated with an earlier menarche.

SECONDARY SEXUAL CHARACTERISTICS
Female

It is important to use objective criteria in the description of secondary sexual characteristics. This permits the establishment of normative data, which are important in diagnosing pubertal disorders. In females, the onset of breast development and the development of sexual hair occur several years prior to the onset of menarche. Breast changes typically constitute the first signs of puberty in a girl and usually become apparent somewhat prior to the appearance of pubic hair. The time required for completion of maturation is usually approximately four years for breast development and

three years for complete development of pubic hair. The following criteria for classification of breast and pubic hair development are adapted from Marshall and Tanner:

Stage 1: No palpable glandular breast tissue, and the areolae are unpigmented.
Stage 2: Glandular tissue is palpable in the diameter of the areola, and the nipple and glandular tissue project together from the chest.
Stage 3: Increased glandular tissue and visible breast enlargement; the areolae become larger and more darkly pigmented.
Stage 4: Further enlargement of breast tissue occurs, and there is increased areolar pigmentation. The areola and nipple now form a secondary projection above the level of the breast.
Stage 5: Adult breast development, in which the nipple and areola have a smooth contour on profile view.

The developmental criteria of pubic hair are as follows:

Stage 1: None
Stage 2: The presence of occasional hairs along the labia.
Stage 3: Darker, coarser hair extending upward over the pubis.
Stage 4: Darker, coarser hair covering the mons pubis in an adult pattern but not extending to the inner thighs.
Stage 5: Mature hair pattern. Hair extends to the thighs but remains in a female distribution.

The rate of progression from one stage of either breast or pubic hair development to another averages about five to nine months from the beginning through stage 4; however, completion of the final stages is more variable. The appearance of breast changes marks the onset of the pubertal growth spurt, which is the maximal rate of linear growth. Maximal linear growth has been achieved by about 75 per cent of normal girls by the time breast development has reached stage 3. The final stage of puberty is the onset of menarche or the onset of menstrual periods. The age range during which menarche occurs in North America is approximately 9.1 to 16.2 years. Although exceptions do occur, the first few menstrual periods in normal girls are typically anovulatory, because the positive feedback effect of estrogen on LH secretion is not yet established.

Male

Growth of the testes is usually the first sign of pubertal development in the male, and it occurs about six months later than the beginning of puberty in girls. The five stages of genital development in boys, adapted from Marshall and Tanner, are as follows:

Stage 1: Prepubertal.

Stage 2: Enlargement of the testes and scrotum begins, and some reddening of the scrotal skin is seen. Testicular length is greater than 2 cm and less than 3.2 cm.

Stage 3: Growth of the penis occurs, and there is continued testicular and scrotal enlargement. Testicular length is greater than 3.3 cm and less than 4.0 cm.

Stage 4: Further enlargement of the penis and the development of the glans as well as testicular and scrotal enlargement. Testicular length is greater than 4.1 cm and less than 4.9 cm.

Stage 5: Adult genitalia. Testicular length is greater than 5 cm. The mean age of onset of stage 2 genital development is 11.6 years, with a range of 9.5 to 13.8 years. The age of completion of genital development in boys occurs at a mean of 14.9 years, with a range of 12.7 to 17.1 years.

Physiology of Normal Puberty

The years between late infancy and the onset of puberty are characterized by inhibition of pulsatile LHRH secretion, decreased pituitary sensitivity to LHRH, and a highly sensitive negative feedback of gonadal steroids on gonadotropin release. Estrogen suppression of gonadotropin secretion in children is approximately five-fold greater than in adults. Prior to any physical evidence of secondary sexual development, there is an increased LH response to LHRH in the peripubertal period. The initiation of pulsatile LHRH secretion causes an enhanced response by LH and FSH to subsequent LHRH stimulation, i.e., an LHRH priming effect. There is also evidence to suggest that early in puberty the gonads may become more sensitive to stimulation by gonadotropins. Prior to puberty, LH and FSH serum concentrations are apulsatile and uniform throughout the day and night. An important maturational change seen in early puberty is enhanced LH secretion during sleep. Children born

without gonadal tissue will also have a sleep-associated increase in LH secretion. This indicates that the alterations in LHRH and LH secretion, which occur prior to puberty, are not dependent upon gonadal function, but are due to unknown central nervous system mechanisms responsible for the hypothalamic control of gonadotropin secretion.

When sexual maturation is completed, LH and FSH are secreted in pulses throughout the day and the night. The final stage in the maturation of gonadotropin secretion is the development of a positive feedback effect of gonadal steroids on gonadotropin release. Prepubertal or early pubertal girls will exhibit no increase in LH secretion despite estradiol levels comparable to those seen in the follicular phase of the menstrual cycle in adult women. Therefore, in early puberty, LHRH and LH pulses are maintained independent of steroid feedback. Positive estrogen feedback is established only in midpuberty, just prior to menarche. The pulsatile secretion of gonadotropins in boys and girls will lead to increases in testosterone and estradiol secretion, respectively. In girls, the maturation of the positive feedback relationship between estradiol and LH occurs in late puberty and leads to the establishment of ovulatory cycles. A delay in this maturational process will lead to continued anovulatory cycles and dysfunctional uterine bleeding. The changes in negative gonadal steroid feedback on gonadotropin secretion and the development of positive feedback effects during late puberty are shown in Figure 48.

Adrenarche

At the time of puberty, the growth of pubic and axillary hair is due to a progressive increase in adrenal androgen secretion that occurs in late childhood and early adolescence. The adrenal androgens, dehydroepiandrosterone (DHEA) and androstenedione, are not under gonadotropic control. In normal boys, adrenal androgens have a relatively weak masculinizing role relative to testicular androgens. Adrenarche and gonadarche appear to be independent maturational events regulated by different mechanisms, since adrenarche occurs without gonadarche in patients with absent gonadal tissue or in patients with gonadotropin defi-

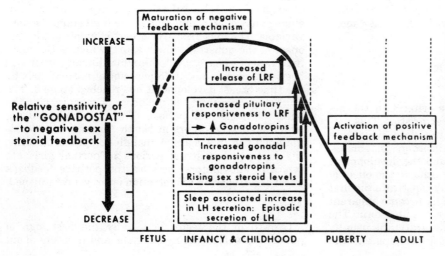

Figure 48. Representation of hypothalamic-pituitary gonadal maturation from fetal life to adulthood. The hypothalamic-pituitary axis is very sensitive to the negative feedback effects of gonadal steroids during infancy and early childhood, and sensitivity decreases as puberty progresses. During puberty LH secretion increases and the positive feedback effects of gonadal steroids on LH secretion gradually become established. (From Grumbach, M. M., Roth, J. C., Kaplan, S. C., and Kelch, R. P.: In Grumbach, M. M., Grave, G. D., and Mayer, E. F. (eds.): Control of the Onset of Puberty. New York, John Wiley and Sons, 1974, p. 115.)

ciency. Similarly, children with adrenal insufficiency secondary to Addison's disease will have normal onset of puberty and a normal growth spurt.

PHYSIOLOGY OF THE MENSTRUAL CYCLE

The menstrual cycle occurs in three general stages: the follicular phase, ovulation, and the luteal phase. The follicular phase lasts approximately 14 days, from the first day of the onset of the menstrual period until the LH surge of ovulation. It is characterized by the growth and development of the dominant follicle and increasing estradiol production predominantly under the influence of FSH. Ovulation, or rupture of the dominant follicle, occurs after the midcycle LH surge. This LH surge is the most important event in the menstrual cycle, since without it ovulation does not occur. The last part of the cycle or the luteal phase is characterized by the formation of the corpus luteum from the ruptured follicle and secretion of progesterone for approximately 14 days until the cycle ends with the onset of a new menstrual period.

Follicular Phase. During the follicular phase of the cycle, FSH increases very slowly (Fig. 49) and is essential for folliculogenesis. Although both FSH and LH are important throughout the menstrual cycle, the follicular phase can be thought of as FSH-dominant. Estrogen levels are at their lowest concentrations early in the follicular phase; however, they steadily increase as follicular development occurs under gonadotropin stimulation. As estradiol production by the granulosa cells increases, there is a small drop in serum FSH, just prior to ovulation, due to the negative feedback of estrogen and other factors on FSH. Under the influence of estrogen, LH pulses in the follicular phase occur every 60 to 90 minutes. Estradiol levels peak at approximately day 14 of the cycle. These rising estradiol levels have a positive feedback effect on LH secretion and are responsible for the initiation of the LH surge. The LH surge triggers ovulation within 28 to 32 hours. Gonadal steroids have a direct positive feedback on LH release by the pituitary gonadotrope in initiating this LH surge, with LHRH having a permissive role. Progesterone levels are very low in the early and mid-follicular phase. There is a preovulatory increase in progesterone that facilitates the positive effect of estradiol on FSH secretion and allows the midcycle FSH peak to occur. The normal midcycle gonadotropin surge is also accompanied by increases in other ovarian steroids. 17α-Hydroxyprogesterone exhibits a midcycle peak, and increased concentrations of androstenedione and testosterone are also seen.

In response to rising estradiol concentrations, the endometrium increases three- to five-fold in thickness. An increase in cellular mitosis and stromal cell numbers characterizes the histological picture of the endometrium in the "proliferative phase." If follicular development is abnormal, or if there is no increase in LH following increasing amounts of estradiol, ovulation will not occur. In this case, the reproductive system can be thought of as being in a chronic "follicular state," with varying degrees of follicular development accompanied by changing estradiol concentrations. Uterine bleeding can also occur without ovulation because the proliferative endometrium will sometimes partially shed in response to these changing

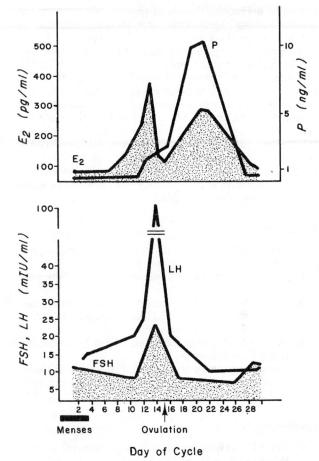

Figure 49. Changes in serum concentrations of LH and FSH (lower panel) and estradiol and progesterone (upper panel) throughout the normal menstrual cycle.

estrogen levels. This "anovulatory state" is important because it causes dysfunctional uterine bleeding and infertility.

Luteal Phase. The formation of the corpus luteum signals the luteal phase of the cycle. This part of the cycle can be thought of as progesterone- and LH-dominant. Progesterone concentrations surge following ovulation and reach a peak five to seven days later. Progesterone causes specific endometrial differentiation. Glandular vacuolization occurs, and four to five days following ovulation secretion occurs into the glandular cell lumen. This is termed a "secretory" or "ovulatory endometrium." Progesterone levels slowly decrease with declining corpus luteum function if conception does not take place. Progesterone is also important in suppressing new follicular growth during the luteal phase. There is evidence that prostaglandins may play a role in ovulation, particularly in maintaining corpus luteum function by an effect on steroidogenesis and ovarian vascular tone. Sustained low-level LH secretion in the luteal phase is important for continued progesterone production by the corpus luteum. Under the influence of progesterone, LH pulses show a marked decrease in frequency, slowing to one LH pulse every 3 to 4 hours in the mid- to late luteal phase. FSH levels slowly decline following ovulation but begin to increase toward the very end of the cycle owing to decreasing levels of gonadal steroids as the corpus luteum ages. This new increase in FSH is important for the initiation of folliculogenesis in the next menstrual cycle. Following ovulation, estradiol levels decline rapidly, only to increase again in the midluteal phase. Toward the end of the luteal phase, both estradiol and progesterone rapidly fall. Under the influence of falling progesterone and estradiol concentrations at the end of the luteal phase, the endometrium becomes invaded by lymphocytes, the endometrial spiral arteries constrict, interstitial hemorrhage occurs throughout the upper two thirds of the endometrium, and another menstrual period begins.

The important events during the menstrual cycle can be summarized as follows:

Follicular

1. Follicular growth occurs under gonadotropin, primarily FSH, stimulation.
2. Progessive estradiol production by the dominant follicle.
3. Increasing estradiol concentrations exert a positive feedback effect on LH secretion and an inhibitory effect on FSH secretion.
4. Peak estradiol concentrations, prior to ovulation, trigger an LH surge.
5. The preovulatory increase in progesterone facilitates the estrogen feedback effect, and the midcycle FSH surge begins.

Ovulation

1. The LH surge triggers follicular rupture, or ovulation, within 28 to 32 hours.
2. The midcycle FSH surge occurs and is progesterone-dependent.

Luteal

1. Granulosa cells form the corpus luteum, and progesterone production increases under continued LH stimulation.
2. Progesterone levels increase rapidly and peak at approximately day 21 of the menstrual cycle.
3. Progesterone suppresses new follicular growth.
4. Corpus luteum function declines, and both progesterone and estradiol concentrations fall rapidly at the end of the luteal phase.
5. Declining steroid hormone concentrations permit a new increase in serum FSH and the onset of a new menstrual cycle.

The documentation of abnormalities in ovulatory function is important in the evaluation of many reproductive disorders. Clinically, some women experience cramps around the time of ovulation. Changes that occur prior to menstruation are called moliminal symptoms and include breast swelling, cramping, and fluid retention. In addition, cervical mucus changes can be noted throughout the menstrual cycle. The methods used to document the occurrence of ovulation are (1) basal body temperature charts, (2) serum progesterone levels, and (3) an endometrial biopsy.

Progesterone has a thermogenic effect and can cause a small increase in body temperature, which is utilized in the basal body temperature chart. In normally ovulating women, there is a small decrease in temperature just prior to ovulation, followed by an increase that persists throughout the luteal phase for approximately 14 days. Although this is a simple way to document ovulation, women may differ in their sensitivities to the effect of progesterone so that these charts are sometimes inaccurate. In addition, charting requires a high degree of patient compliance. A second method of determining ovulatory function is a serum progesterone determination. Since the luteal phase is characterized by the secretion of progesterone from the corpus luteum, sustained elevations of serum progesterone are indicative of ovulation. A serum progesterone of approximately 5 to 25 ng/ml, drawn on day 21 of the cycle, is consistent with prior ovulation. In some women, the progesterone level is indicative of ovulation; however, the luteal phase of the cycle is "inadequate" in that adequate corpus luteum function is not sustained for two weeks and can result in infertility. In this case, one may not be able to diagnose this abnormality using a single progesterone level, and multiple determinations may be needed. For most women, the combination of basal body temperatures and a day 21 progesterone concentration represents a good initial way to determine whether ovulation has occurred. A final way of documenting ovulation is through an endometrial biopsy to determine whether characteristic histological changes consistent with ovulation are present in the current menstrual cycle. It also enables one to determine whether the histological changes of the endometrium are "in phase" with the chronological day of the cycle. This may be appropriate in some patients in whom further validation of ovulatory function is needed.

DISORDERS OF THE HYPOTHALAMIC-PITUITARY-OVARIAN AXIS

LHRH Deficiency States

LHRH deficiency may be either congenital or acquired, and its clinical presentation is critically dependent upon the time of its development in relation to puberty. LHRH deficiency before puberty will present with failure to develop normal secondary sexual characteristics. Adrenarche, however, usually occurs normally in these patients. Women with acquired postpubertal LHRH deficiency typically present with secondary amenorrhea. Specific disorders resulting in LHRH deficiency are listed in Table 18.

Although any congenital disorder affecting the hypothalamus can result in LHRH deficiency, *Kallman's syndrome* is a well-defined disorder. It may be transmitted as an autosomal dominant disorder with incomplete expressibility, or it may occur sporadically. It affects both women and men, with women typically presenting with primary amenorrhea associated with anosmia. Partial forms also exist in which LHRH is deficient rather than completely absent and hyposmia rather than anosmia is found. These patients typically have low serum gonadotropins, absent gonadal steroids, and a normal response to LHRH administration. Chronic administration of LHRH in a physiologically pulsatile manner stimulates normal pubertal development and ovulatory function in these women. At the present time, most girls with this disorder are given

TABLE 18. LHRH DEFICIENCY

A. Congenital
    1. Kallman's syndrome
    2. Hypothalamic lesions
B. Acquired
    1. Hypothalamic destruction
       a. tumors
       b. infiltrative lesions
       c. surgery
       d. radiotherapy
    2. Functional disorders
       a. weight-related
          i. anorexia nervosa
          ii. simple weight loss
       b. stress
       c. drugs
       d. chronic diseases

replacement doses of gonadal steroids, i.e., cyclic estrogens and progestogens. In the future, pulsatile administration of LHRH will most likely become the therapy of choice for women and men with LHRH deficiency interested in fertility.

Acquired LHRH deficiency can result from hypothalamic destruction or from functional deficiency of LHRH secretion without a demonstrable anatomical abnormality. Hypothalamic destruction causing LHRH deficiency may be secondary to tumors or infiltrative lesions affecting the hypothalamus, such as sarcoid. LHRH deficiency may also follow surgery in the hypothalamic area, or it may follow radiotherapy for pituitary or extrasellar tumors. In these cases, it may be difficult to distinguish gonadotropin insufficiency secondary to gonadotropin destruction from LHRH deficiency occurring at the hypothalamic level.

The most common LHRH deficiency states in adults appear to be functional disorders; i.e., there is evidence of LHRH deficiency without anatomical evidence of a hypothalamic lesion or injury. They are also "functional" in the sense that they are often reversible once the underlying cause has resolved. A common cause of this state is weight loss or, in its extreme form, anorexia nervosa. Anorexia nervosa is a relatively common psychiatric disorder in young women characterized by weight loss of 25 per cent of body weight, or weight 15 per cent below normal, amenorrhea, body image distortion, and bizarre eating habits. It can be associated with relative hypotension, bradycardia, edema, vomiting, lanugo hair, constipation, and the inappropriate use of diuretics or laxatives. Serum electrolyte and hematological abnormalities may occur. Hormonal disturbances include low serum gonadotropins, elevated cortisol levels, low serum T_3, and high reverse T_3. The amenorrhea in these patients is thought to be due to LHRH deficiency, since (1) ovulatory periods are restored with pulsatile LHRH administration, (2) serum LH pulses are lost during the illness but are reestablished with weight gain (see Fig. 50), and (3) blunted LH response to LHRH administration that normalizes with weight gain is seen in severely affected patients. The diagnosis is based upon its typical clinical presentation and the exclusion of other disorders such as hyperprolactinemia or a pituitary tumor. Amenorrhea can also result from simple weight loss due to dieting in individuals who are obese or of normal weight. In these cases, body image distortion and/or underlying psychopathology is absent. Crash dieting, food faddism, and bulimia (self-induced vomiting) are all relatively common eating abnormalities in young women. Since these disorders may be subtle, may occur without abnormalities on physical examination, and can be

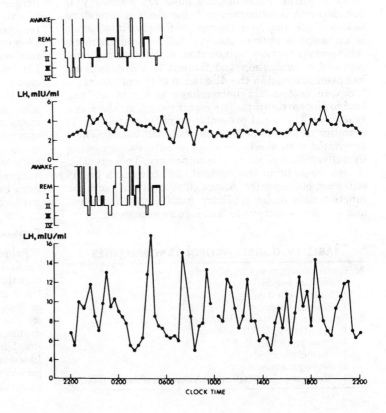

Figure 50. Plasma LH concentrations every 20 minutes for 24 hours during an acute exacerbation of anorexia nervosa (upper panel) and after clinical remission with return of normal body weight and restoration of normal pulsatile LH secretion (lower panel). (From Boyar, R. M., Katz, J., Finkelstein, J. W., et al.: N Engl J Med 291:863, 1974. Reprinted with permission.)

concealed by the patient, they should be specifically looked for.

The recent widespread popularity of exercise and endurance sports training in young women has resulted in a marked increase in exercise-induced amenorrhea. Many runners and athletes note menstrual irregularity or amenorrhea with progressive training which resolves during periods of inactivity. Mechanisms that appear to be involved in amenorrhea in this setting include (1) exercise-induced increase in endorphins, which suppress LHRH, (2) abnormalities in prolactin secretion, and (3) changes in body fat. A decrease in the amount or the frequency of exercise may normalize menstrual function.

Finally, severe emotional stress may cause amenorrhea in some women, and a history of a precipitating event should be searched for.

GONADOTROPIN ABNORMALITIES

Gonadotropin abnormalities can be secondary to gonadotropin insufficiency caused by LHRH insufficiency, to loss or damage of gonadotropes, or, more commonly, to hormone excess states or abnormalities in the feedback effects of gonadal steroids on gonadotropin secretion. Common causes of gonadotropin abnormalities are listed in Table 19. Gonadotropin loss is usually caused by large pituitary tumors, infiltrative lesions such as sarcoid, or postpartum pituitary infarction. Gonadotropin insufficiency secondary to pituitary adenomas can be seen with pituitary tumors hypersecreting any of the pituitary hormones, particularly prolactin or growth hormone. Nonfunctioning pituitary or extrasellar tumors, such as craniopharyngiomas, can also cause gonadotrope loss. In cases of a suspected pituitary adenoma or in the presence of hyperprolactinemia, further radiological studies are necessary. If gonadotropin insufficiency in these cases is secondary to loss of gonadotropes, therapy of the pituitary tumor is unlikely to reverse gonadal failure and hormone replacement therapy is indicated. A detailed explanation of the evaluation and therapy of these patients has been outlined in the discussion of the pituitary.

Severe postpartum hemorrhage and/or shock can lead to postpartum pituitary insufficiency, or *Sheehan's syndrome*. The usual presentation of this syndrome is inability to lactate because of prolactin insufficiency, associated with slowly developing features suggesting hypothyroidism or adrenal insufficiency. This disorder is less frequent in the modern obstetrical era but is still seen occasionally. Although recovery of hormone function may occur, pituitary insufficiency is typical and requires appropriate hormone replacement.

TABLE 19. GONADOTROPIN ABNORMALITIES

A. Primary gonadotropin insufficiency
   1. Pituitary tumors
   2. Infiltrative lesions
   3. Pituitary infarction
B. Functional gonadotropin insufficiency
   1. Secondary to LHRH deficiency
   2. Hyperprolactinemia
   3. Thyroid disorders
   4. Androgen excess
   5. Abnormalities in feedback—dysfunctional uterine bleeding

More commonly, normal gonadotropin secretion is impaired because of abnormalities in LHRH secretion and/or in the feedback effects of gonadal steroids on gonadotropin release. These disorders are usually functional; i.e., they do not represent actual gonadotropin loss and are reversible with treatment of the underlying disorder. The classic example of such a deficiency is that seen in hyperprolactinemia, which is discussed elsewhere.

Thyroid disorders can also disrupt normal gonadal function by interfering with normal gonadotropin release. Both hyperthyroidism and hypothyroidism are associated with anovulatory states and frank amenorrhea. In hypothyroidism, accompanying hyperprolactinemia may partly explain some of the reproductive abnormalities found. In hyperthyroidism, although the exact mechanism of amenorrhea is unclear, loss of positive feedback of estradiol on LH secretion has been observed. These reproductive abnormalities are functional and resolve when thyroid function is normalized.

A subset of women with anovulatory periods or amenorrhea is seen in whom an etiology is not apparent after a detailed history and in whom other hormone abnormalities such as hyperprolactinemia, thyroid disease, and androgen excess have been excluded. Many of these patients will prove to have abnormalities in the positive feedback of estrogen on the LH surge. In normal women, rising concentrations of estradiol in the late follicular phase of the cycle trigger a midcycle LH surge leading to subsequent ovulation. This capacity for positive feedback effect of estrogen on LH secretion often does not develop in early adolescence, but it is seen once the hypothalamic-pituitary-ovarian axis matures. In women with anovulatory bleeding or dysfunctional uterine bleeding, the midcycle gonadotropin surge does not occur, often despite normal follicular phase estradiol concentrations. In the absence of ovulation, uterine bleeding becomes irregular in response to the fluctuating estradiol concentrations. This defect in estrogen positive feedback on LH secretion has been documented by studies in which serum LH levels did not increase in patients with dysfunctional uterine bleeding despite rising estrogen production (Fig. 51). A normal increase in LH does not occur after an estrogen challenge in these women. Severe anemia may sometimes occur as a result of excessive uterine bleeding. Such patients can often best be treated by attempting to mimic the luteal phase of the cycle with cyclic progestogen therapy. The patient is advised to take Provera 10 mg daily for five to seven days every month. This will usually lead to regular withdrawal bleeding despite the absence of ovulation.

PRIMARY OVARIAN FAILURE

Primary ovarian failure is defined as a deficiency of normal ovarian function accompanied by markedly elevated serum gonadotropins. Ovarian failure may be the result of a common chromosomal abnormality such as gonadal dysgenesis or an enzymatic deficiency such as the 17α-hydroxylase deficiency of Biglieri's syndrome, or it may be acquired during adult reproductive life. Disorders resulting in primary ovarian failure are listed in Table 20. When ovarian failure occurs before puberty, the patient will usually present with delayed pubertal development and primary amenorrhea. Gon-

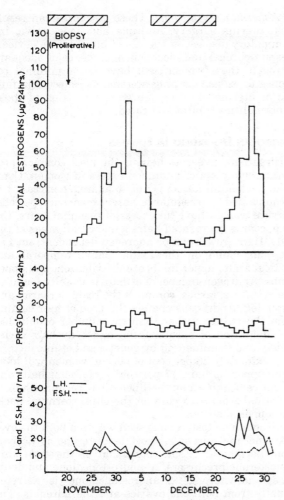

Figure 51. Daily urinary excretion of estrogens (upper panel), pregnanediol (middle panel), and concentrations of plasma LH and FSH (bottom panel) in a 19-year-old woman with dysfunctional uterine bleeding. Despite increasing estrogens, there is no midcycle LH ovulatory peak, and uterine bleeding (hatched area) occurs as a result of estrogen withdrawal. (From Fraser, I. S., Michie, E. A., Wide, L., and Baird, D. T.: J Clin Endocrinol Metab 37:411, 1973.)

adal failure occurring after puberty causes secondary amenorrhea.

Turner's syndrome is the most common cause of prepubertal ovarian failure. It is usually due to an XO chromosomal abnormality and occurs in approximately

TABLE 20. PRIMARY OVARIAN FAILURE

A. Congenital
  1. Gonadal dysgenesis
    a. Turner's syndrome
    b. XY gonadal dysgenesis
  2. Gonadal agenesis
  3. Enzymatic defects
    Biglieri's syndrome (17α-hydroxylase deficiency)
B. Acquired
  1. Autoimmune
  2. Chemical or radiation destruction
  3. Oophoritis
  4. Surgical removal
C. Resistant ovary syndrome

1 in 2700 live births. Classically, these patients exhibit a variety of phenotypical findings including short stature, webbed neck, shield chest, and associated cardiac and renal malformations (Fig. 52); however, some women have few phenotypical abnormalities. Occasionally, patients can have chromosomal mosaicism that refers to several cell lines with different cell chromosomes. XX/XO karyotypic individuals can have some functioning ovarian tissue and may have spontaneous menstrual periods for some time. These women will eventually develop secondary amenorrhea and elevated gonadotropins. Patients with mosaicism including a Y chromosome can virilize at the time of puberty and are at risk for the development of gonadal malignancies. Gonadectomy should, therefore, be done at the time of diagnosis. To guard against this possibility, it is essential to obtain a karyotype on all patients with primary ovarian failure. In a sense, gonadal dysgenesis can be viewed as "accelerated follicular atresia," since such patients will have a normal complement of oocytes at 20 weeks of gestation; how-

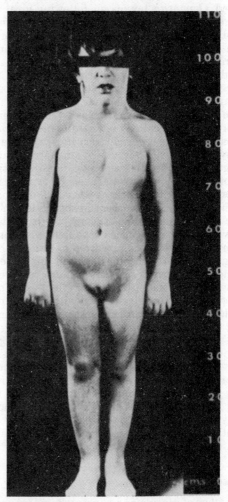

Figure 52. Nine-year-old girl with OX Turner's syndrome. Characteristic facies, low-set ears, shield chest, and low, widely spaced nipples are seen. This child was also found to have a horseshoe kidney and coarctation of the aorta. (From Ducharme, J. R., and Collu, R.: Clin Endocrinol Metab 11:76, 1982.)

ever, none is present at the time of birth. Such accelerated follicular atresia can also be seen in women who develop premature ovarian failure. A rare cause of ovarian failure is 17α-hydroxylase deficiency or Biglieri's syndrome. These phenotypic females present with hypertension as well as sexual infantilism.

Autoimmune ovarian disease is an important cause of primary failure in the adult. It is associated with other autoimmune disorders, including hypoparathyroidism, hypoadrenalism, and hypothyroidism; there is also an association of this syndrome with mucocutaneous candidiasis, pernicious anemia, diabetes mellitus, and myasthenia gravis. Patients with a normal karyotype and primary ovarian failure should be clinically evaluated for other autoimmune states. Premature ovarian failure in the adult may also result from a number of physical or chemical factors. *Radiotherapy* for Hodgkin's disease or *chemotherapy* with cyclophosphamide and other alkylating agents may cause ovarian failure. In these cases, the hypogonadism may be transient and is related to the dose and duration of therapy. Therefore, patients should be reassessed after a period of time to see whether ovarian function has returned. *Oophoritis* may occur following viral or bacterial illnesses. *Surgical removal* of a significant amount of ovarian mass for ovarian cysts or other benign abnormalities can likewise lead to premature ovarian failure.

A subset of patients with primary ovarian failure has been identified in whom ovarian biopsies show immature follicles with normal morphology, in contrast to the small inactive ovaries typically seen. This condition has been called the *resistant ovary syndrome*. Such patients have a normal karyotype and characteristically present with secondary amenorrhea and elevated gonadotropins. In women who desire fertility, it is important to make this diagnosis by ovarian biopsy, since pregnancies have been reported in some patients after therapy with high doses of exogenous gonadotropins or with estrogen. The etiology of this condition is unknown; however, because of the follicular unresponsiveness to endogenous gonadotropins, an abnormality of the gonadotropin receptor has been implicated.

Women with primary ovarian failure require gonadal steroid replacement therapy. Patients who present prepubertally are usually treated with several months of cyclic estrogen therapy alone, usually beginning at 0.3 mg of a conjugated estrogen per day, with gradual increases in order to maximize breast development. Following this, cyclic administration of estrogens and progestogens is chronically given, an oral contraceptive being a useful method of hormone replacement therapy. In women who develop premature ovarian failure during midreproductive life, hormone replacement therapy is also indicated to treat hot flashes and to prevent the long-term consequences of estrogen deficiency, especially osteoporosis.

Müllerian Abnormalities

A number of uterine and vaginal disorders may also cause amenorrhea. In these cases, ovarian function remains normal although the patient is amenorrheic. Agenesis of the müllerian structures may result in vaginal hypoplasia or agenesis and may cause primary amenorrhea. Acquired intrauterine strictures are seen in *Asherman's syndrome*. These strictures can result from uterine surgery, multiple abortions, pelvic inflammatory disease, or the use of intrauterine devices. Despite clinical and biochemical evidence of adequate estrogen, these women will have no or minimal response to exogenous progesterone, as reflected in failure of uterine bleeding. Surgical correction of these abnormalities is often indicated.

Androgen Disorders in Females

Hirsutism, or excess hair, is the most common presenting symptom of androgen excess in women. Commonly, when hirsutism is due to androgen excess, it is accompanied by irregular or absent menstrual periods. Hirsute women have an excess of terminal hairs, the long, coarse, pigmented hairs found on all areas of the body. Hair growth can be androgen-dependent, such as the hair found on the axilla, pubis, temporal and vertical scalp, upper lip, beard distribution, and upper limbs. Androgen-independent hair is usually found in the eyebrows, lashes, corona of the scalp, forearm, and lower leg. Androgens change the type of hair coming from the follicle rather than the number of follicles. The definition of normal facial and body hair varies widely and is influenced by genetic and ethnic factors. Approximately 26 per cent of normal women will have some upper lip hair, 17 per cent periareolar hair, and 35 per cent hair along the linea alba. Terminal hair is abnormal when it occurs on the chin, sternum, back, and upper abdomen.

Although testosterone is secreted from both the ovaries and the adrenals, most testosterone is derived from peripheral tissue conversion of the two main testosterone precursors, Δ^4-androstenedione and dehydroepiandrosterone. Δ^4-androstenedione is secreted equally from both the ovaries and the adrenals. The majority (approximately 80 per cent) of dehydroepiandrosterone is derived from the adrenals. Androgen excess in women is usually due to an increase in the secretion of testosterone or its precursors from the ovaries and/or adrenals. Since most testosterone is bound tightly to sex hormone–binding globulin, the free testosterone is the most sensitive reflection of the testosterone production rate. Increased glandular androgen secretion will cause a decrease in sex hormone–binding globulin and an increase in the concentration of free testosterone. A total serum testosterone determination, which measures both bound and unbound testosterone, may therefore not adequately represent testosterone production. Small changes in free hormone concentrations may have very significant biological effects on target tissues. As testosterone production rates and free testosterone concentrations rise, women will demonstrate progressive signs of androgen excess, from mild hirsutism to frank virilization, as shown in Table 21. Small increases in tes-

TABLE 21. SIGNS OF ANDROGEN EXCESS

| Increasing testosterone production ↓ | Increased body hair Increased facial hair Anovulation Amenorrhea Clitoromegaly Temporal balding Increased muscle mass | Virilization |

tosterone production will lead to increases in body hair and facial hair and may be associated with anovulation or amenorrhea. Severe androgen elevations, in which the testosterone level approaches that of normal men, results in virilization. Signs of virilization are clitoromegaly, temporal balding, and increased muscle mass. It is important to determine if virilization is present, since it is a biological marker of strikingly elevated androgen production. Exclusion of an ovarian or adrenal tumor is essential in the evaluation of such patients.

In most patients, androgen excess reflects increased androgen biosynthesis from the ovary and/or adrenal gland. The common etiologies of androgen hypersecretion in women are listed in Table 22. Ovarian androgen production can increase owing to the ovarian hyperplasias, polycystic ovaries, and hyperthecosis, or, less commonly, owing to androgen-secreting ovarian tumors.

Polycystic ovary disease is a syndrome of hirsutism, abnormalities of menstrual function, and infertility. Obesity is often seen as well. Clinical symptoms usually develop after puberty, and virilization is rare but has been reported. Typically, the ovaries are enlarged, with multiple follicular cysts and a thickened collagenized external capsule. Disorders of ovulation range from anovulatory periods to amenorrhea. Testosterone, free testosterone, and androstenedione levels are typically elevated. Serum LH concentrations are tonically elevated, LH pulsations have an increased amplitude, and FSH concentrations are normal or decreased. The pathogenesis of this common syndrome is unknown, and it has not as yet been determined whether the primary defect is in ovarian androgen biosynthesis or gonadotropin secretion and regulation. A subset of patients with ovarian androgen excess have hyperthecosis. In this disorder the ovaries may be normal in size, and the higher androgen levels can result in frank virilization. Hyperthecosis and polycystic ovary disease are often seen in several family members. Hyperthecosis may be associated with acanthosis nigricans and insulin resistance. Because of their high serum androgen concentrations, it may be difficult to distinguish these patients from women with androgen-secreting tumors, and the diagnosis is made by ovarian exploration and biopsy. The diagnosis of an androgen-secreting ovarian tumor should be suspected when hirsutism and/or virilization develops progressively and serum testosterone levels exceed 200 ng/dl.

TABLE 22. ANDROGEN-DEPENDENT HIRSUTISM

Ovary:	Ovarian Hyperplasias
	Polycystic ovaries
	Hyperthecosis
	Androgen-Secreting Tumors
	Arrhenoblastomas
	Hilus cell
	Lipoid cell
	Metastatic
Adrenal:	Congenital Adrenal Hyperplasias
	21-OH deficiency
	11-OH deficiency
	Adrenal Adenoma or Carcinoma
	Cushing's Syndrome
Iatrogenic:	Anabolic Steroids
	19-Nor Progestins
	Danazol

Cushing's disease, adrenal adenomas, and carcinomas can all cause adrenal androgen hypersecretion. Clinical stigmata of Cushing's syndrome, hypertension, and the presence of an adrenal mass may be seen in these patients. Diagnostic testing should be done to exclude these entities in clinically suspected cases. Enzymatic abnormalities in adrenal biosynthesis can also result in excess androgen secretion. Patients with 21-hydroxylase deficiency are unable to convert 17-hydroxyprogesterone to 11-deoxycortisol. They typically present early in life with masculization and may have associated salt wasting as well. Serum 17-hydroxyprogesterone concentrations are elevated, and 17-ketosteroid metabolites and pregnanetriol levels are elevated in the urine. These patients show an excellent response to treatment with glucocorticoids, such as dexamethasone, and the resulting suppression of ACTH secretion should normalize adrenal androgen overproduction. Recently, patients with attenuated or partial forms of 21-hydroxylase deficiency have been identified. Hirsutism and/or menstrual abnormalities appear after puberty, and urinary 17-ketosteroids and pregnanetriol are typically normal. This autosomal recessive trait is diagnosed by a marked hyperresponse of 17-hydroxyprogesterone following stimulation with ACTH.

Many women presenting with hirsutism and/or abnormalities in menstrual function will be found to have slight elevations in serum androgen levels without identifiable ovarian or adrenal pathology. This syndrome, called "idiopathic hirsutism," is characterized by pubertal onset, nonprogressive course, absence of virilization, and slight elevations in free serum testosterone concentrations. Identifiable abnormalities in androgen physiology in these women include increased testosterone production rates, increased testosterone metabolic clearance rates, and increased androstenedione production rates. The ovary is the main source of androgen excess in these women by either direct testosterone secretion or secretion of androstenedione, which is subsequently metabolized to testosterone in peripheral tissues. Increased utilization of testosterone or other androgen precursors at peripheral androgen target sites, such as the hair follicle, may also play a role in the development of hirsutism in some patients. A subset of hyperprolactinemic patients may also show signs of androgen excess. Increased prolactin may stimulate adrenal androgen biosynthesis, particularly DHEA. In such patients, normalization of the serum prolactin level will usually restore serum androgen concentrations to normal.

THERAPY OF HYPERANDROGENISM

The therapy of androgen disorders in women is a complex issue and is dependent upon factors that include the etiology of the androgen excess, associated menstrual function abnormalities, the degree of hirsutism, and fertility concerns. Patients found to have Cushing's syndrome or adrenal or ovarian tumors as a cause of excess androgens will respond to surgical and other therapy of their primary disease. For most patients, however, treatment is directed toward suppression of androgen production and/or antagonism of androgen action on peripheral tissues.

Oral contraceptives and glucocorticoids will decrease androgen production. An estrogen and progestogen combination pill will (1) decrease testosterone, androstenedione, LH, and FSH, (2) increase sex hormone–binding globulin, and (3) compete with the cytosol receptor for dihydrotestosterone in peripheral target cells, such as the hair follicle. Oral contraceptives are a good therapy for young women with polycystic ovary disease or idiopathic hirsutism, particularly if contraception is also an issue. Glucocorticoids in small doses, i.e., prednisone 5 mg/day or dexamethasone 0.5 mg/day, can suppress adrenal androgens and are therefore an appropriate therapy for adrenal hyperandrogenism. Patients with congenital adrenal hyperplasia or adult-onset 21-hydroxylase deficiency or women who have predominant hypersecretion of DHEA sulfate can be expected to respond well to glucocorticoids.

Another class of drugs, the antiandrogens, can act to decrease androgen biosynthesis and/or impair androgen target tissue effects. Spironolactone, an antihypertensive drug, impedes both testosterone biosynthesis and peripheral actions. This is a good therapeutic choice for women with polycystic ovary disease or idiopathic hirsutism, particularly if these patients have contraindications or a poor clinical response to oral contraceptives. Cimetidine, a histamine H_2 receptor antagonist, acts by competing with androgens for binding to target tissue androgen receptors. It causes a decrease in hair growth without altering serum androgen concentrations and has been used successfully in some patients.

The response to therapy of these disorders is slow. Hirsutism, in particular, rarely resolves. Improvement or stabilized hair growth may be seen after several months; however, signs of chronic androgen exposure usually persist. Because of this, it is important to start therapy as soon as these disorders are diagnosed, preferably in the teenage years, even if the clinical signs are mild.

DIAGNOSIS OF AMENORRHEA AND ANOVULATORY STATES

Disorders of the hypothalamic-pituitary-ovarian axis often present as amenorrhea or anovulation. Amenorrhea is arbitrarily defined as the absence of menstrual periods for four to six months in a nonpregnant woman. Dysfunctional uterine bleeding refers to irregular or excessive uterine bleeding without an underlying uterine abnormality. The aim of the patient's evaluation is (1) to exclude a structural or functional abnormality in the central nervous system and/or pituitary, (2) to exclude primary ovarian failure, androgen excess, or other endocrinopathies, (3) to offer prognosis on fertility, and (4) to determine the need for replacement or other drug therapy.

Patients may present with primary amenorrhea, which indicates that they have never had a menstrual period, or secondary amenorrhea, which refers to amenorrhea in a woman who has had previous menstrual periods. Although there is a great deal of etiologic overlap in these two conditions, a higher incidence of genetic defects and congenital abnormalities is present in the former group. The majority of patients presenting with secondary amenorrhea will be found to have gonadotropin regulatory defects, i.e., functional abnormalities in the hypothalamic-pituitary axis with impaired LHRH secretion and/or abnormalities in the positive and negative feedback systems of gonadal steroids, without evidence of an anatomic lesion in the hypothalamus, pituitary, or ovaries. Approximately one third of amenorrheic patients will be found to be hyperprolactinemic. The two other major causes of amenorrhea and/or anovulation are primary ovarian failure and androgen excess. The latter has been previously considered in a separate section.

The *history* is of primary importance in the diagnostic evaluation of amenorrhea. Knowledge of the patient's previous menstrual history is crucial, particularly the occurrence of regular menstrual periods and past pregnancies. Since some amenorrheic patients have estrogen deficiency, questions regarding hot flashes and pain on intercourse (dyspareunia) should be asked. A medication history is important, particularly the past use of birth control pills, tranquilizers, or antihypertensive drugs that could induce hyperprolactinemia. An evaluation of psychiatric status is also important, since stress of emotional factors can lead to functional amenorrhea and anovulation. Since low body weight or changes in body weight are an important cause of amenorrhea, it is important to ascertain the weight at which a woman had a normal period in the past. It is also important to establish if the patient has a history of vigorous exercise. To determine the possibility of a pituitary tumor, the patient should be questioned as to the presence of headaches, visual disturbances, or galactorrhea. Hyperthyroid or hypothyroid symptoms should be looked for. Symptoms of androgen excess to be considered include excess body hair and acne. A history of prior pregnancy is important, particularly a postpartum history, to assess the possibility of postpartum pituitary insufficiency. Past gynecological surgery and a history of repeated uterine curettage or abortions are important to determine possible structural damage to the reproductive tract.

On *physical examination,* one should pay particular attention to blood pressure, weight, emotional status, thyroid examination, the presence of galactorrhea, signs of androgen excess such as hirsutism, acne, or clitoromegaly, and signs of estrogen deficiency, such as vaginal mucosal or breast atrophy.

LABORATORY EVALUATION

The laboratory evaluation of amenorrheic and anovulatory women consists of assessing (1) serum gonadotropins, (2) serum prolactin levels, (3) estradiol levels, (4) androgen levels, and (5) thyroid function tests. Serum gonadotropins are most useful in the diagnosis of primary ovarian failure. Since it is most sensitive to the feedback effects of estrogen, a serum FSH measurement is the best method of diagnosing ovarian failure. Although both LH and FSH will be elevated in this case, overlap is occasionally seen between serum LH concentrations in premature menopause and other causes of amenorrhea, such as polycystic ovary disease. Markedly elevated FSH concentrations occur in a number of disorders, leading to primary ovarian failure. This elevation is accompanied by low serum estradiol concentrations in the postmenopausal range. Patients with the resistant ovary syndrome may present similarly, with the diagnosis being made only by assessment of follicular status on ovarian biopsy if fertility is a question. Undetectable levels of both LH and FSH are most compatible with pituitary tumors and/or pituitary insufficiency. A common pattern is a low LH with a normal FSH, which is often seen in hypothalamic amenorrhea due to stress or undernutrition, and in some patients with hyperprolactinemic amenorrhea. A slightly elevated LH, accompanied by a normal or somewhat decreased FSH, is commonly seen in patients with androgen excess disorders, such as polycystic ovary disease. Owing to the pulsatile release of gonadotropins by the pituitary, a single set of serum gonadotropins may not accurately reflect secretion; therefore, more information should be sought by obtaining a series of samples and pooling them. Gonadotropin determinations are much more useful in amenorrheic patients than in women who are cycling normally or who have irregular menstrual periods. Given the wide fluctuations of gonadotropins throughout the menstrual cycle, gonadotropin determinations in women with menstrual periods have to be evaluated in relation to the day of the cycle in which they were drawn. Although it was initially thought that LHRH testing might prove to be a useful way of distinguishing hypothalamic from pituitary causes of amenorrhea, this has not proved to be the case, since patients with both disorders can respond identically.

A serum prolactin level should be determined in all women with amenorrhea, anovulation, galactorrhea, or infertility. Many women with hyperprolactinemia will not have galactorrhea. If there is any clinical suspicion of thyroid disease, thyroid function tests should be done. An assessment of estrogen status is important in the diagnosis of amenorrhea and in determining which patients will need hormone therapy. Estrogen status in the amenorrheic woman can be determined by (1) vaginal smear for maturation index, with a greater than 10 per cent level of superficial cells demonstrating a good estrogen effect, (2) serum estradiol concentrations, and (3) response to a progestogen challenge. Uterine bleeding following five days of a progestogen, such as Provera 10 mg, indicates uterine estrogen exposure and demonstrates that the endometrium is capable of functioning. A negative response indicates very low estrogen concentrations or a uterine abnormality.

MENOPAUSE

In normal women, menopause is a physiological consequence of the aging process that marks the end of female reproductive capacity. It is a gradual process, lasting up to two years, marked by a progressive decline in ovarian function. As women approach menopause, there is a gradual decrease in the length of the menstrual cycle, so that by 40 to 50 years of age the cycle length often shortens to 21 days. This decrease in cycle length is often attributable to a decrease in the follicular phase of the cycle and may reflect inadequate folliculogenesis. The perimenopausal period is also typically characterized by irregular menstrual cycles, finally leading to the amenorrhea of the menopause. The average age of menopause remains at approximately 50 years of age. Smoking, malnutrition, and chronic disease states may be associated with an earlier age of menopause. The age of menarche and previous childbearing do not appear to influence the time of menopause.

Clinical Syndrome

Most of the clinical symptoms and consequences of the menopausal period are a direct reflection of the profound estrogen deficiency that characterizes this period. The two most common menopausal symptoms are hot flashes and symptoms due to atrophy of the female reproductive tract. Menopausal hot flashes are episodes of vasomotor instability, usually lasting several minutes, associated with peripheral vasodilation, increased skin temperature, and a relative tachycardia. They may occur as infrequently as several times a week; however, they can occur up to several times an hour. Hot flashes occur in approximately 80 per cent of women who undergo menopause and can last as long as five years. Although the exact mechanism of hot flashes is controversial, they can be relieved by estrogen administration. The onset of the hot flash is associated with dramatic increases in serum gonadotropin concentrations, which presumably reflect enhanced LHRH secretion. Neurotransmitters, particularly the adrenergic nervous system, and the endogenous opiate peptides have also been implicated in the pathogenesis of hot flashes. It is likely that the increased levels of gonadotropins, cortisol, and other hormones during the hot flashes are epiphenomena rather than etiologic events. It is of interest that estrogen priming is needed for the development of hot flashes. For example, girls born with gonadal dysgenesis, such as Turner's syndrome, do not experience hot flashes unless thay have received prior estrogen replacement therapy.

The second most common symptom of menopause is related to estrogen deficiency in the female reproductive tract. Estrogen receptors are found throughout the reproductive tract, and estrogen deficiency will affect the vagina, cervix, uterus, and breast. The vaginal epithelium is highly estrogen-sensitive, and the menopause is associated with atrophic vaginitis, which causes pain during sexual intercourse. The bladder and urethra can also show atrophic changes, and frequent urinary tract infections may occur as a consequence. In addition, urinary incontinence may result from atrophy of the pelvic supporting structures.

Hormonal Changes in the Menopause

The hormonal changes associated with menopause reflect (1) the depletion of ovarian follicles, (2) a decreased ovarian sensitivity to gonadotropins, and (3) a decreased sensitivity to negative steroid feedback. In midreproductive life, estrogen is derived from ovarian follicular secretion of 17-beta estradiol as well as from the peripheral conversion of androstenedione to estrone, arising from both the ovaries and the adrenals. Progressive loss of follicles leads to the changes that characterize menopausal estrogen deficiency. Almost all estrogen produced after the menopause (approximately 400 µg of estrone per day) is derived from peripheral conversion of adrenal androstenedione. The earliest sign of menopause is an increase in serum FSH concentrations. An increase in FSH first occurs during the follicular phase of the menstrual cycle several years prior to actual menopause and is not associated with changes in serum LH. In time, both FSH and LH rise significantly into the menopausal range, and low serum concentrations of progesterone reflect an insufficiency of the corpus luteum. Finally, the ability of estrogen to induce a midcycle LH surge via positive feedback is lost, and ovulation ceases. Following the menopause, serum FSH levels are up to 20-fold higher than they are during midreproductive life, and LH increases three- to five-fold. The diagnosis of menopause can, therefore, be made if a patient has amenorrhea associated with menopausal symptoms and biochemically confirmed by the findings of estrogen deficiency and appropriately elevated gonadotropins (particularly FSH).

Menopausal Consequences

Two important medical problems associated with the menopause are the development of osteoporosis and atherosclerotic heart disease. Osteoporosis appears to be a consequence of estrogen deficiency, aging, and other factors associated with bone formation and reabsorption. The loss of ovarian function has been shown to be a key factor in osteoporosis, and radiological studies have established that menopause is followed, within a variable period of time, by excessive loss of bone mineral. Postmenopausal women have an increased risk of clinical fractures, and the morbidity and mortality rates associated with fractures in these women are well established. It has been found that loss of ovarian function before the age of 45 is associated with an increased risk of osteoporosis within three to six years; therefore, premature menopause is an indication for hormone replacement therapy. Not all normal postmenopausal women develop osteopenia. Oriental and northern European women are most susceptible to its development. Factors increasing the risk of postmenopausal osteoporosis include malnutrition, alcoholism, cigarette smoking, decreased physical activity, poor dietary calcium, and disorders that interfere with normal calcium and vitamin D metabolism. The development of osteoporosis is an important factor in determining which postmenopausal women are candidates for hormone replacement therapy, since it is well established that hormone replacement therapy started within three years of menopause prevents bone mineral loss.

The issue of postmenopausal coronary artery disease is more complex. Although the incidence of atherosclerotic heart disease increases after menopause, the etiological role of estrogen deficiency is not firmly established. The link between estrogen deficiency and cardiovascular disease is most clearly established for women who undergo premature or surgical menopause prior to the age of 35. Loss of ovarian function in this age group has been associated with a seven-fold increase in the risk of myocardial infarction compared with control women. Large population studies have also found that women with coronary artery disease are most likely to have an early menopause. One potential etiological factor in the development of coronary artery disease is the alteration in plasma lipid levels that occurs following the menopause. Menopause is associated with a decrease in the high density lipoprotein to low density lipoprotein cholesterol ratio, a known risk factor for coronary artery disease. Estrogen administration causes a significant increase in high density lipoprotein, primarily within the high density lipoprotein-2 subclasses, and a decrease in low density lipoprotein cholesterol. Hormone replacement therapy in this age group may have a beneficial effect, reducing the development of coronary artery disease.

Hormone Therapy

Postmenopausal hormone replacement therapy is a controversial issue, and it is important to select those women who will benefit from its administration. Women who have entered the menopause because of premature ovarian failure or surgical removal of the ovaries are prime candidates for hormone replacement therapy to prevent the immediate and long-term consequences of estrogen deficiency. In menopausal women, the specific benefits of hormone replacement therapy include the relief of vasomotor symptoms, the treatment of urogenital atrophy and its associated problems, and the prevention and treatment of osteoporosis. The main risk of estrogen replacement therapy is a three- to four-fold risk for the development of endometrial cancer; however, the development of endometrial cancer during estrogen replacement is dependent on the dose and duration of therapy. Previous hormone replacement regimens for postmenopausal women made almost exclusive use of estrogen without progesterone. Given the important effects of progesterone in inducing cyclic differentiation of the endometrium, women treated with estrogen alone develop a chronic proliferative endometrium with a risk of hyperplasia. The risk of endometrial cancer does not appear to increase in women who are treated with both cyclic estrogen and cyclic progesterone for a duration sufficient to mimic normal luteal phase length. Other risks of hormone replacement therapy include the possible development of hypertension and gallstones. There is no evidence that postmenopausal hormone replacement therapy increases the risk of breast cancer. Estrogen replacement therapy is contraindicated in women with estrogen-dependent tumors such as breast cancer and in patients with liver disease, cerebrovascular or coronary artery disease, chronic thrombophlebitis, or a history of pulmonary emboli. Relative contraindications to estrogen administration include hypertension, fibrocystic breast disease, severe obesity, hyperlipidemia, gallbladder disease, and cigarette smoking.

It is critical to evaluate the risks versus the benefits of hormone replacement therapy in all women. Estrogen replacement therapy affords an excellent relief of hot flashes, although oral progesterone alone may be useful in women who are not candidates for estrogen therapy. The protective effect of estrogen on bone loss is dose-dependent, and the minimal effective dose appears to be 0.625 mg of a conjugated estrogen, such as Premarin. A typical replacement regimen involves the administration of a conjugated estrogen in a dose of 0.625 mg daily for three weeks every month. During the last 10 to 14 days of the estrogen course, an oral progestogen, such as Provera 5 or 10 mg a day, should also be given. The duration of the progestogen course is more important than the dose given to protect the endometrium from the deleterious effects of unopposed estrogen.

HYPOTHALAMIC-PITUITARY-TESTICULAR AXIS

REGULATION OF TESTICULAR FUNCTION

The pulsatile release of LHRH in the male is critical for the pulsatile release by the gonadotrope of LH and FSH, which, in turn, stimulate testosterone production and spermatogenesis. An overview of this axis is shown in Figure 53. The precise way in which LHRH is regulated by testosterone is poorly understood, but testosterone concentrations appear to be critical. Low concentrations of testosterone have a positive feedback effect to stimulate LHRH release. Supraphysiological concentrations of testosterone act in a negative feedback manner by inhibiting LHRH and LH secretion. In addition, testosterone can also inhibit the effect of LHRH on the gonadotrope.

LH is the most important hormone regulating tes-

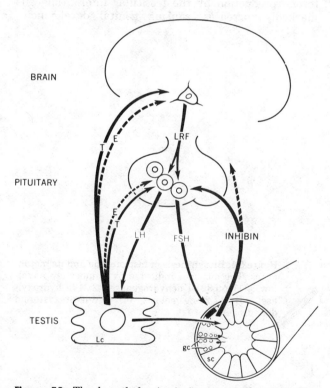

Figure 53. The hypothalamic-pituitary-testicular axis. The testis is functionally divided into the Leydig cells (Lc), which produce testicular steroids, and the seminiferous tubules composed of Sertoli cells (sc) and their germ cells (gc) necessary for spermatogenesis. Leydig cell steroidogenesis and Sertoli cell function are predominantly under the control of LH and FSH, respectively. Testosterone (T) and estradiol (E) have both positive and negative feedback effects on the hypothalamic-pituitary axis. The testicular peptide inhibin selectively inhibits FSH secretion. (From Bardin, C. W.: In Yen, S. S. C., and Jaffe, R. B. (eds.): Reproductive Endocrinology. Philadelphia, W. B. Saunders Co., 1978, p. 111.)

tosterone secretion by the testicular Leydig cell. Leydig cells also have membrane receptors for prolactin and LHRH. The role of these hormones in directly regulating testicular function is, however, as yet unknown. LH binds to specific hormone receptors on the Leydig cell membrane and stimulates steroidogenesis by mechanisms involving cyclic AMP. A pulse of LH is followed within minutes by an increase in testosterone secretion. A decrease in LH secretion, due to hypothalamic or pituitary disease, will result in a decrease in testosterone secretion. Similarly, a decrease in testosterone due to testicular damage will cause an increase in serum LH concentrations. LH is also important for spermatogenesis, since adequate testosterone production is required for normal sperm development. The seminiferous tubules are surrounded by interstitial fluid containing concentrations of testosterone 20- to 50-fold higher than those seen in serum, and spermatogenesis is dependent upon maintenance of these concentrations.

FSH is the hormone primarily responsible for maintaining Sertoli cell and seminiferous tubular function, and it is the key regulator of spermatogenesis. FSH stimulates the conversion of primary spermatocytes into more mature sperm forms. FSH is less sensitive than LH to the negative feedback effect of testosterone. A testicular polypeptide called inhibin is made by the Sertoli cells and is thought to be important in FSH regulation. In castrate males, both LH and FSH rise. If only the seminiferous tubules are damaged and testosterone concentrations remain normal, FSH increases, although LH remains unchanged. The selective increase in FSH after seminiferous tubule damage is thought to be due to a loss of inhibin.

Estrogen also appears to have a role in the regulation of LH secretion in men. In prepubertal and pubertal boys, estradiol administration will have a negative feedback effect on LH release. However, in adult men, estrogen administration will initially suppress LH release, followed by a positive feedback effect in most patients. Estrogen administration in adult men will also decrease gonadotrope responsiveness to LHRH stimulation.

TESTICULAR EMBRYOLOGY AND ANATOMY

The testes, like the ovary, develop from an undifferentiated gonad. In the male fetus, the XY karyotype will lead to medullary prominence within gonadal tissue and the subsequent development of sex cords and interstitial cells. This differs from an XX or female karyotype, where the gonadal cortex develops. The HY antigen, a protein synthesized if a Y chromosome is present, is a marker of fetal testicular development. The indifferent or undifferentiated gonad can be stimulated to develop either wolffian or müllerian structures. Wolffian structures are those that lead to the development of male accessory organs such as the vas deferens, epididymis, and seminal vesicles. Müllerian duct derivatives develop into female organs such as the uterus, the fallopian tubes, and the upper one third of the vagina. In normal male development, the müllerian duct structures are inhibited and wolffian duct structures will progressively develop.

By the twelfth week of gestation, Leydig cells can make testosterone, which stimulates development of wolffian duct structures. Testosterone becomes converted to its more potent metabolite, dihydrotestosterone or DHT, by an enzyme called 5-α-reductase. It is DHT that induces male external genital development, such as the fusion of the genital folds to form a scrotum, lengthening of the genital tubercle, and fusion of the folds to form a penis. The fetal testes also produce a peptide called müllerian inhibitory factor, or MIF. MIF is necessary to prevent müllerian duct structures from developing, and it enables normal male development to occur. Any abnormality interfering with the synthesis or action of male hormones on this system will lead to a phenotypical female.

The testes normally are found within the scrotum and measure 4 by 3 by 2.5 cm. The majority of testicular mass is composed of tightly coiled seminiferous tubules. The testes are suspended in a serous sac, the tunica vaginalis, and are covered by extensions of peritoneum and the abdominal wall. The testes have descended into the scrotal sac in approximately 90 per cent of male infants at the time of birth and in 98 per cent of infants by the end of the first year.

Androgen biosynthesis occurs in the Leydig cells, and spermatogenesis occurs in the seminiferous tubules. The Leydig cells are located in the connective tissue stroma between the seminiferous tubules, and the Sertoli cells are present on the basal lamina of the seminiferous tubules. The Sertoli cells are important

TABLE 23. TESTOSTERONE EFFECTS

A. Genital development
   Increase in penis, scrotum, testis, prostate, seminal vesicles
B. Hair growth
   Increased facial and body hair
C. Muscle development
D. Deepening of voice
E. Increased growth during puberty
F. Increased libido and potency

in maintenance of spermatogenesis. Undifferentiated spermatogonia line the seminiferous tubules and undergo six stages of maturation lasting approximately 74 days, during which time a mature sperm cell develops. The Sertoli cells also synthesize a protein called androgen-binding protein, the function of which has not yet been clearly characterized.

TESTICULAR ANDROGENS

Testosterone is the main androgen produced by the testes, and its production and effective peripheral action are necessary for normal male sexual development. A summary of testosterone effects is shown in Table 23. In males, adrenal androgens contribute little to overall androgen production. After puberty, testosterone production by the testicular interstitial cells markedly increases, causing genital development,

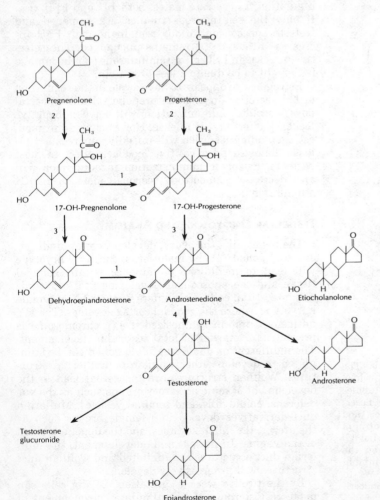

Figure 54. Biosynthesis of testosterone and its metabolites. The enzymes indicated by number are as follows: (1) Δ5,3β-ol dehydrogenase; (2) 17α-hydroxylase; (3) 17,20-desmolase; (4) 17β-hydroxysteroid dehydrogenase.

muscular growth, weight gain, deepening of the voice, pubic, axillary, and facial hair, positive nitrogen retention, development of libido, and fertility.

Testosterone is the major testicular androgen produced, and its production rate is approximately 5 to 7 mg per day. Normal circulating testosterone levels in males are 5 to 10 ng/ml, as compared with 0.3 to 1 ng/ml in females. The biosynthesis of testosterone and its metabolites is shown in Figure 54. The rate-limiting step in testosterone biosynthesis is the conversion of cholesterol to pregnenolone, a reaction regulated by LH secretion. Androstenedione, an important estrogen precursor in males, is produced at a rate of approximately 2 mg per day. The testes secrete other steroid hormones, including progesterone and 17α-hydroxyprogesterone. Dihydrotestosterone (DHT), an androgen with more than twice the potency of testosterone, is also secreted at a rate of approximately 0.3 mg per day.

The major pathway of testosterone metabolism is oxidation at position 17 in the liver, with ultimate conversion to form the 17-ketosteroids. Testosterone accounts for approximately 20 per cent of the total urinary ketosteroid production; most is derived from metabolism of dehydroepiandrosterone (DHEAS) and androstenedione. 17-Ketosteroids in the urine are a poor reflection of overall androgen metabolism. A small amount of testosterone is metabolized to DHT and androstenediol, which are important for local tissue effects. A small amount of testosterone is also excreted in the urine as a glucuronide. Testicular androgens are also the major source of serum estrogens, such as estrone and estradiol. Peripheral aromatization of androgens, specifically testosterone and androstenedione, accounts for approximately 45 μg per day of estradiol, and 10 to 15 μg per day of estradiol is directly secreted by the testes. The extratesticular metabolism of androgens and estrogens is shown in Figure 55.

In many developing tissues, such as the brain and pituitary, as well as in wolffian duct structures, such as the fetal epididymis, seminal vesicle, and vas deferens, testosterone is the dominant androgen. In other tissues, including the penis, scrotum, and prostate, testosterone is readily converted to dihydrotestosterone by the enzyme 5α-reductase. This enzyme can also convert androstenedione and DHEAS to DHT.

MALE HYPOGONADISM

Male hypogonadism refers to Leydig cell failure and testosterone deficiency. Hypogonadism can be a consequence of either primary or secondary testicular failure. Primary testicular failure is due to a testicular disorder, whereas secondary failure usually results from pituitary or hypothalamic dysfunction. The clinical manifestations of hypogonadism depend upon the time of its development in relation to puberty. If hypogonadism occurs prior to puberty, normal sexual maturation and development will not occur. The typical features of prepubertal hypogonadism are called

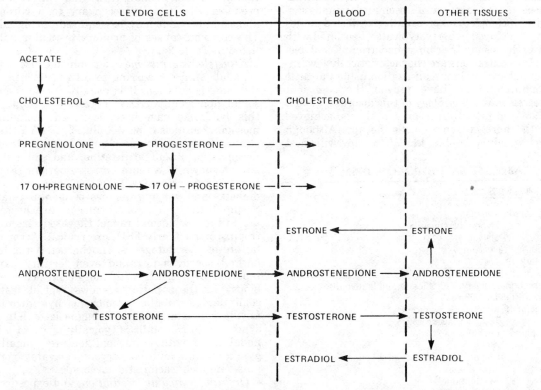

Figure 55. Testicular androgen secretion and extraglandular conversion. Testosterone is the major secretory product of the testis, and in man the major biosynthetic pathway is via the Δ⁵ pathway including pregnenolone, 17-hydroxypregnenolone, and androstenediol. Testosterone and androstenedione are secreted into the blood and converted to estrone and estradiol, respectively, at extraglandular sites in peripheral tissues. (From Bardin, C. W.: In Yen, S. S. C., and Jaffe, R. B. (eds.): Reproductive Endocrinology. Philadelphia, W. B. Saunders Co., 1978, p. 113.)

eunuchoidism, and their recognition is useful in determining the time of onset and duration of hypogonadism. These factors include prepubertal genitalia, decreased muscle development, and absence of facial and body hair. If adrenarche is normal, patients will have some pubic and axillary hair. Since testosterone-induced thickening of the larynx and vocal cords does not occur, these males typically have a high-pitched voice. The delay in epiphyseal closure results in a hallmark feature of the eunuchoidal male: an arm span at least two inches greater than height, and the distance from the soles to the symphysis pubis more than two inches greater than the distance from the symphysis to the head. In contrast, the development of testosterone deficiency in the adult may occur gradually and can be more difficult to detect. Patients usually present with impotence, decreased libido, or infertility. Testosterone deficiency will usually lead to a decrease in body hair and frequency in shaving. The testes become small and atrophic. In addition, gynecomastia or glandular breast enlargement may occur, and, very rarely, galactorrhea may be present. An overview of the differential diagnosis of male hypogonadism is shown in Table 24.

HYPOGONADOTROPIC HYPOGONADISM

Hypogonadotropic hypogonadism can result from LHRH and/or gonadotropin insufficiency, and it may be congenital or acquired. Common examples of these disorders are listed in Table 24. Kallman's syndrome is a congenital deficiency of LHRH. It is often familial and can be inherited as an autosomal dominant disorder with incomplete expressibility. Affected males present with delayed puberty, typically associated with anosmia or hyposmia. Serum gonadotropins and testosterone concentrations are characteristically low. Induction of puberty and masculinization using pulsatile LHRH administration have proven that deficient LHRH secretion is the etiology of this disorder. Sexual maturation and masculinization can also be achieved solely with androgen replacement therapy. Although not as yet widely available, LHRH therapy will most likely become the preferred treatment for achieving fertility in these patients. LHRH deficiency due to hypothalamic damage may also be acquired postpubertally from tumors, surgery, or radiotherapy effects on the hypothalamic area. Although extremely rare, hypogonadism in males with anorexia nervosa has been reported, and this is most likely due to functional LHRH deficiency.

Acquired gonadotropin insufficiency in adult males is most commonly due to pituitary tumors. Hypogonadism may result from actual destruction of pituitary gonadotropes by large tumors. It may also result from functional gonadotropin impairment as seen in hyperprolactinemia. Hyperprolactinemia can cause relative gonadotropin insufficiency without gonadotrope destruction by impairing the pulsatile release of LH from the pituitary gland. This may be corrected by normalization of serum prolactin concentrations by either surgery, bromocriptine, or radiation therapy. Hyperprolactinemia has been increasingly recognized as a cause of acquired male hypogonadism. Many patients present with advanced tumors and are brought to the attention of a physician because of mass effects causing headaches or visual field defects. An early sign of hyperprolactinemia in the male is decreased libido and/or impotence.

PRIMARY TESTICULAR FAILURE

Primary hypogonadism is defined as Leydig cell failure accompanied by elevated serum gonadotropin concentrations. Primary testicular failure can occur prepubertally, usually secondary to a chromosomal abnormality, or it may be acquired during adult life. The common causes of primary testicular failure are listed in Table 24.

Klinefelter's syndrome is a common cause of primary gonadal failure, occurring in 0.15 to 0.24 per cent of the male population. It is usually due to the chromosomal abnormality XXY; however, variant forms of this syndrome have been described, including chromosomal mosaicism, poly-X plus Y, or XYY. Its typical clinical features include a eunuchoid appearance, gynecomastia, absent virilization, and small testicular size as shown in a representative patient (Fig. 56). It has been associated with other disorders, including diabetes and varying degrees of mental retardation. Serum testosterone concentrations are decreased or are in the low normal range. Elevated serum gonadotropins, particularly FSH, are typical. Azospermia or failure of spermatogenesis is characteristic; however, normal sperm counts and even fertility have been reported in patients with mosaicism. The testicular biopsy in these patients shows typical features of seminiferous tubular membrane hyalinization and Leydig cell clumping. The diagnosis of Klinefelter's syndrome in the adult is typically made in a hypogonadal male with eunuchoid features, small testes, gynecomastia, low testosterone, elevated gonadotropins, and a characteristic karyotype.

Orchitis, testicular irradiation, and exposure to *chemotherapy* can all lead to varying degrees of testicular failure. Typically, seminiferous tubule function and spermatogenesis are more likely to be impaired by these agents than is Leydig cell function. Orchitis due to mumps in the pubertal or adult male can lead to

---

TABLE 24. MALE HYPOGONADISM

A. LHRH Deficiency
    Congenital: Kallman's syndrome
     Acquired: Tumors
               Hyperprolactinemia
               Starvation
B. Gonadotropin Deficiency
    Pituitary tumors
    Hypopituitarism
    Destruction—surgery, radiotherapy, infiltrative diseases
C. Primary Testicular Failure
    Congenital: Klinefelter's syndrome
                Testicular agenesis
     Acquired: Orchitis
              Alcohol
              Chemical or radiation destruction
              Liver disease
              Autoimmune
              Hemochromatosis
D. Disorders of Testosterone Biosynthesis
E. Androgen Receptor Disorders
    Testicular feminization
    Reifenstein's syndrome

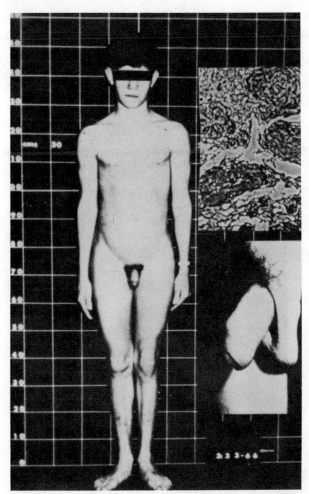

Figure 56. A 15-year, 7-month-old boy with XXY Klinefelter's syndrome. Note the small testes. The right upper panel shows the typical seminiferous tubule hyalinization and clumps of Leydig cells seen on testicular biopsy. (From Ducharme, J. R., and Collu, R.: Clin Endocrinol Metab 11:75, 1982.)

permanent seminiferous tubular destruction, and because of this, the testes are usually small. Leydig cell function may be unaffected, or testosterone may be deficient in severe cases. Irradiation for cancer and several chemotherapeutic drugs can lead to decreased testicular function. Spermatogenesis is extremely sensitive to the effects of radiation. Testicular failure resulting from radiation or chemotherapy may be transient; therefore, when testosterone replacement therapy is indicated, it is important to retest these patients after a period of time. Men with multiple *autoimmune endocrinopathies* may develop autoimmune testicular failure. Associated disorders may include hypothyroidism, hypoadrenalism, hypoparathyroidism, diabetes, and pernicious anemia.

Hypogonadism may also result from drug abuse or alcoholism. In addition to the direct toxic effect of alcohol upon testicular testosterone biosynthesis, it can impair the normal hypothalamic-pituitary axis. In patients with alcoholic liver disease, testicular androgen metabolism is impaired as well. Hypogonadal men with documented testosterone deficiency due to primary testicular failure are candidates for testosterone

replacement therapy. The usual form of testosterone replacement therapy is a testosterone ester (such as an enanthate), which is given intramuscularly, and these preparations are typically given every three weeks with an average dose of 200 to 300 mg per injection.

DISORDERS OF TESTOSTERONE METABOLISM AND ANDROGEN ACTION

Normal virilization requires adequate testicular androgen secretion, conversion of testosterone to dihydrotestosterone by the enzyme 5α-reductase, and end-organ responsiveness to available androgens, as shown in Figure 57. Abnormalities in testosterone biosynthesis, metabolism, and end-organ receptors can all result in abnormal male sexual development. Genetic males who have absent or incomplete masculinization in utero are called male pseudohermaphrodites. Testosterone enzymatic biosynthetic defects are very rare and are due to deficiencies of cholesterol desmolase, 3β-hydroxysteroid dehydrogenase, 17α-hydroxylase, and 17,20-desmolase. Inadequate masculinization also occurs if the conversion of testosterone to dihydrotestosterone is impaired. Testosterone- and dihydrotestosterone-dependent structures are listed in Table 25. In the fetus, dihydrotestosterone is necessary for male external genital development, such as the formation of the penis, scrotum, and prostate. A rare inherited disorder of 5α-reductase deficiency was first identified

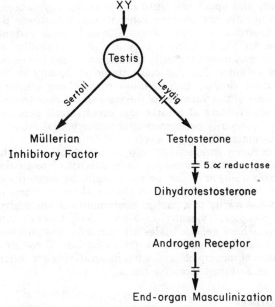

Figure 57. In a genetic male, the testis is composed of Sertoli and Leydig cells. The Sertoli cells secrete müllerian inhibitory factor, which causes regression of the müllerian (female) duct structures. The Leydig cells produce testosterone, which is converted to dihydrotestosterone and binds to tissue androgen receptors. Normal androgen action at the peripheral tissue level leads to masculinization and a phenotypic male. An absence of testosterone secretion leads to a phenotypic female. Impaired conversion of testosterone to dihydrotestosterone due to 5α reductase deficiency results in male pseudohermaphroditism. A defect in the androgen receptor may be complete (testicular feminization), resulting in a female phenotype, or partial, causing inadequate masculinization.

TABLE 25. TESTOSTERONE- AND DIHYDROTESTOSTERONE-DEPENDENT STRUCTURES

$$Testosterone \xrightarrow{5\alpha\text{-Reductase}} Dihydrotestosterone$$

Seminal vesicles	Penis
Vas deferens	Scrotum
Epididymis	Prostate

in a community in the Dominican Republic. These genetic males have normal testosterone levels; however, they cannot form dihydrotestosterone. They are born with ambiguous genitalia, since they cannot develop dihydrotestosterone-dependent structures normally.

A spectrum of disorders also exists in which testosterone secretion and metabolism by 5α-reductase are normal; however, an abnormality of the androgen receptor is present so that there is little or no end-organ response to available testosterone and its metabolites. The most striking example of this disorder is called *testicular feminization*. These patients are genetic males with functioning testes who lack androgen receptors, and therefore they exhibit a congenital insensitivity to androgens. Clinically, these phenotypical females usually present with primary amenorrhea; a representative patient is shown in Figure 58. Affected individuals have female external genitalia but lack normal axillary and pubic hair. Since the fetal testes are able to produce müllerian inhibitory factor, müllerian duct structures, such as the uterus, fallopian tubes, and upper one third of the vagina, are absent. The plasma testosterone concentrations in these patients are in the male range. Although these patients have an XY karyotype, they are phenotypically, socially, and psychologically females and must be considered as such. The testicular tissue is usually in the inguinal canals, and inguinal masses are common. Because of the tendency of the testicular tissue to form gonadal tumors at a later age, prophylactic gonadectomy is usually performed after puberty, and estrogen replacement therapy is given.

Androgen insensitivity can be complete, as in the case of the total androgen insensitivity of testicular feminization, or it can be incomplete. In these disorders, there is a more subtle abnormality in androgen response owing to a partial abnormality of the androgen receptor. Typically, as seen in Reifenstein's syndrome, these genetic males are partially masculinized but have hypospadia and gynecomastia. These syndromes of incomplete androgen insensitivity are inherited as X-linked recessive traits.

IMPOTENCE

Impotence is one of the most common problems in male reproduction and may be the presenting symptom of endocrine, neurological, systemic, or psychiatric disorders. Complete impotence or a significant decrease in the ability to maintain an erection should be investigated when it persists for more than three months. Common causes of impotence are listed in Table 26. Normal erectile capacity requires (1) intact central and peripheral nervous system function, (2) normal testosterone concentration, and (3) adequate arterial blood supply to the erectile tissues of the penis, the corpora

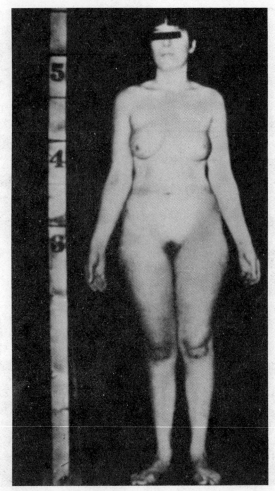

Figure 58. A patient with testicular feminization, a genetic male and phenotypic female. The breasts are well developed and she has scant pubic hair. (From Ducharme, J. R., and Collu, R.: Clin Endocrinol Metab 11:78,1982.)

cavernosa and corpus spongiosum. The parasympathetic arc originates in the genital area, passes through spinal cord synapses (S2 to S4), and returns to the penis by parasympathetic tracts. Other less well-defined pathways, influenced by psychological factors, originate in the cerebral cortex and descend down the thoracolumbar sympathetic tracts to the penis. Dysfunction of the central or peripheral nervous system can cause impotence, and diabetic neuropathy is a common example of this type of disorder. Testosterone

TABLE 26. CAUSES OF IMPOTENCE

A. Testosterone deficiency
B. Hyperprolactinemia
C. Disorders of the autonomic nervous system
    Neurologic disease
    Diabetes
D. Cardiovascular disease
E. Drugs
    Psychoactive agents
    Antihypertensives
    Alcohol
    Antiandrogens
F. Psychogenic

deficiency is a major cause of impotence, occurring in approximately 30 per cent of impotent men, and a serum testosterone determination is the most important laboratory test to obtain. If decreased, further evaluation must be done to distinguish primary from secondary testicular failure. Hyperprolactinemia, usually secondary to a pituitary tumor, must also be excluded, since it commonly presents with impotence as a symptom. Hyperprolactinemia impairs libido and erectile function by causing testosterone deficiency and through unknown central effects. Hyperprolactinemic men can have persistent impotence despite testosterone administration unless prolactin levels are normalized. Impotence can be seen in hyperthyroid men; however, it is unlikely to be the sole manifestation. Cardiovascular disease, specifically atherosclerosis, can lead to vascular insufficiency with resulting impotence.

Drugs are a common cause of impotence, and their use should be carefully looked for in the evaluation of the impotent patient. Many classes of psychotropic drugs can impair sexual function by effects on the central and peripheral nervous system and by induction of hyperprolactinemia. Antihypertensive drugs cause impotence by a number of mechanisms, including effects on the central nervous system and androgen action. Aldactone and cimetidine, for example, compete with androgens for binding to target tissue androgen receptors. In addition, aldactone interferes with testosterone biosynthesis. A number of chronic diseases, including renal failure, malignancy, and liver disease, may all lead to impotence by a variety of different mechanisms. Finally, depression can result in impotence and sexual dysfunction and may be an important presenting complaint of this disorder. Psychological factors have a critical influence on normal sexual function. The goal of the clinical evaluation should be to exclude and treat possible organic etiologies of this common problem.

REFERENCES

Female Reproductive Physiology

Flamigni, C., and Givens, J. R. (eds.): The Gonadotropins: Basic Science and Clinical Aspects in Females. New York, Academic Press, Inc., 1982.

Givens, J. R. (ed.): Clinical Use of Sex Steroids. Chicago, Year Book Medical Publishers, 1980.

Knobil, E.: The neuroendocrine control of the menstrual cycle. Rec Prog Horm Res 36:53, 1980.

Vande Wiele, R. L., Bogumil, J., Dyrenforth, I., et al.: Mechanisms regulating the menstrual cycle in women. Recent Prog Horm Res 26:63, 1970.

Yen, S. S. C., and Jaffe, R. B. (eds.): Reproductive Endocrinology: Physiology, Pathophysiology and Clinical Management. Philadelphia, W. B. Saunders Co., 1978.

Puberty

Cacciari, E., and Prader, A. (eds.): Pathophysiology of Puberty. London, Academic Press, Inc., 1980.

Faiman, C., and Winter, J. S. D.: Gonadotropins and sex hormone patterns in puberty: Clinical data. In Grumbach, M. M., Grave, G. D., and Mayer, F. E. (eds.): Control of the Onset of Puberty. New York, John Wiley and Sons, Inc., 1974.

Odell, W. D.: The physiology of puberty: Disorders of the pubertal process. In DeGroot, L. J., et al. (eds.): Endocrinology. Vol. 3. New York, Grune and Stratton, 1979.

Female Reproductive Disorders

Crosignani, P. G., and Robyn, C.: Prolactin and Human Reproduction. New York, Academic Press, Inc., 1977.

Givens, J. R.: Hirsutism and hyperandrogenism. Adv Intern Med 21:221, 1976.

Hull, M. G. R., Murray, M. A. F., Franks, S., et al.: Female hypogonadism—therapy oriented diagnosis of secondary amenorrhoea. In James, V. H. T., Serio, M., and Giusti, G. (eds.): The Endocrine Function of the Human Ovary. London, Academic Press, Inc., 1976.

Sherman, B. M., and Korenman, S. G.: Hormonal characteristics of the human menstrual cycle throughout reproductive life. J Clin Invest 55:699, 1975.

Male Reproductive Physiology

Burger, H., and de Kretser, D. (eds.): The Testis. New York, Raven Press, 1981.

Lipsett, M. B.: Physiology and pathology of the Leydig cell. N Engl J Med 303:682, 1980.

Steinberger, E.: Hormonal control of mammalian spermatogenesis. Physiol Rev 51:1, 1971.

Wilson, J. D., George, F. W., and Griffin, J. E.: The hormonal control of sexual development. Science 211:1278, 1981.

Male Reproductive Disorders

Bardin, C. W., and Paulsen, C. A.: The testes. In Williams, R. H. (ed.): Textbook of Endocrinology. 6th ed. Philadelphia, W. B. Saunders Co., 1981.

Carter, J. N., Tyson, J. E., Tolis, G., Van Vliet, S., Faiman, C., and Friesen, H. G.: Prolactin-secreting tumors and hypogonadism in 22 men. N Engl J Med 299:847, 1978.

Griffin, J. E., and Wilson, J. D.: The syndromes of androgen resistance. N Engl J Med 302:198, 1980.

Thyroid Pathophysiology

GILBERT H. DANIELS, M.D.

OVERVIEW

The thyroid gland utilizes iodine to synthesize the two iodothyronine hormones, thyroxine (T_4) and triiodothyronine (T_3). Quantitatively, the predominant hormone released from the thyroid gland is T_4; most circulating T_3 is derived from peripheral monodeiodination of T_4 after the T_4 has been secreted by the thyroid gland.

The thyroid gland is under the control of the pituitary gland, via the secretion of TSH (thyroid-stimulating hormone, thyrotropin), which controls most steps in the biosynthesis, storage, and release of thyroid hormone. Thyroid size and vascularity seem to be under the control of TSH as well.

When the thyroid gland fails, is destroyed, or is removed, the circulating level of TSH rises in an attempt to compensate for the loss of thyroid hormones

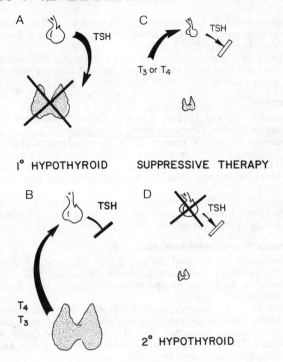

Figure 59. Pituitary-thyroid axis. *A*, Primary hypothyroidism. *B*, Hyperthyroidism. *C*, Suppressive therapy with thyroid hormone. *D*, Secondary hypothyroidism.

(primary hypothyroidism) (Fig. 59*A*). Conversely, when an excess of thyroid hormone is secreted by the thyroid gland (hyperthyroidism), TSH release is suppressed (Fig. 59*B*). When exogenous thyroid hormone is administered, TSH release is similarly suppressed and the thyroid gland decreases in size (Fig. 59*C*). Such suppressive therapy is used in the treatment of enlarged thyroids (goiters) and thyroid nodules.

The hypothalamus secretes a TSH-releasing hormone (TRH, thyrotropin-releasing hormone), which is necessary for TSH release. Destruction or removal of either the hypothalamus or the pituitary gland leads to thyroid gland atrophy and failure (secondary hypothyroidism) (Fig. 59*D*).

Hyperthyroidism is a clinical state characterized by excess thyroid hormone and its clinical consequences. Hyperthyroidism may result from excessive administration of exogenous thyroid hormone, excess thyroid gland stimulation, intrinsic thyroid abnormalities leading to excess thyroid hormone release, excess release of thyroid hormone from inflammatory conditions, or excess production of thyroid hormone by abnormal thyroid tissue at distant sites.

Hypothyroidism refers to inadequate circulating levels of thyroid hormone and its clinical consequences. It may result from primary thyroid gland failure (natural or induced biosynthetic defects, inflammatory disease, ablation) or be secondary to hypothalamic or pituitary failure.

The thyroid gland has a tendency to form nodules for reasons that remain obscure. Hundreds of millions of individuals throughout the world have enlarged, nodular thyroids, although most maintain normal thyroid gland function (euthyroid state). Thyroid cancers are uncommon but increase in incidence after the thyroid has been exposed to ionizing external radiation. Thyroid cancer may be treated with ¹³¹I, a radioactive isotope of iodine.

EMBRYOLOGY, ANATOMY, AND PHYSIOLOGY

The thyroid gland begins as an outpouching of the pharyngeal floor, which subsequently migrates in a caudal direction and fuses with the ventral aspect of the fourth pharyngeal pouch. The thyroid develops into a bilobed organ; hence, its name thyroid, or shieldlike. The connection between the base of the tongue and the thyroid gland (thyroglossal duct) usually disappears. However, remnants may remain, leading to cystic structures that can swell and may become inflamed (thyroglossal duct cysts). The upward movement of these cysts with protrusion of the tongue helps in their diagnosis and reminds us of their embryological origins. The lower portion of the duct gives rise to thyroid tissue, which forms the pyramidal lobe of the thyroid gland.

Maternal TSH, T_4, and T_3 do not cross the placental-fetal barrier. The fetal thyroid gland begins to concentrate iodine at about 10 weeks. Inadvertent administration of radioactive iodine to pregnant women beyond this stage may result in fetal thyroid destruction. At about this time, TSH appears in the fetal pituitary, and TSH, T_4, and thyroid hormone–binding protein appear in the fetal circulation.

The thyroid gland is organized into discrete follicles, the lumina of which contains colloid, the storage form of thyroid hormone. The adult thyroid in North Americans weighs about 20 grams, with the right lobe exceeding the left in size.

Blood flows through the thyroid gland at about 100 ml per minute. In patients with severe hyperthyroidism, the thyroidal blood flow may reach 2 to 10 liters per minute, the increased flow being recognized clinically with the stethoscope as a bruit ("whooshing" noise) or palpably as a "thrill" or vibration over the thyroid gland.

THYROID HORMONE BIOSYNTHESIS

The thyroid gland produces two active iodothyronine hormones (Fig. 60), T_4 and T_3. The biosynthesis of these two hormones requires iodide. Iodide's major role in human physiology is as a substrate for thyroid hormone biosynthesis. The structural unit of hormone synthesis is the thyroid follicle cell.

Iodide is derived predominantly from dietary sources; however, many pharmaceuticals and diagnostic agents also have high iodine contents. Iodide deficiency no longer exists in the United States. In the past, iodide deficiency goiter was common in the midwestern United States and currently remains an important international public health problem in underdeveloped nations. The average daily iodide intake in the United States is about 500 μg, with wide regional variations (200 to 900 μg/day). The minimum daily requirement for iodide is approximately 100 μg. In Japan, foods with high iodide content are commonplace, and intake may be as high as several milligrams per day.

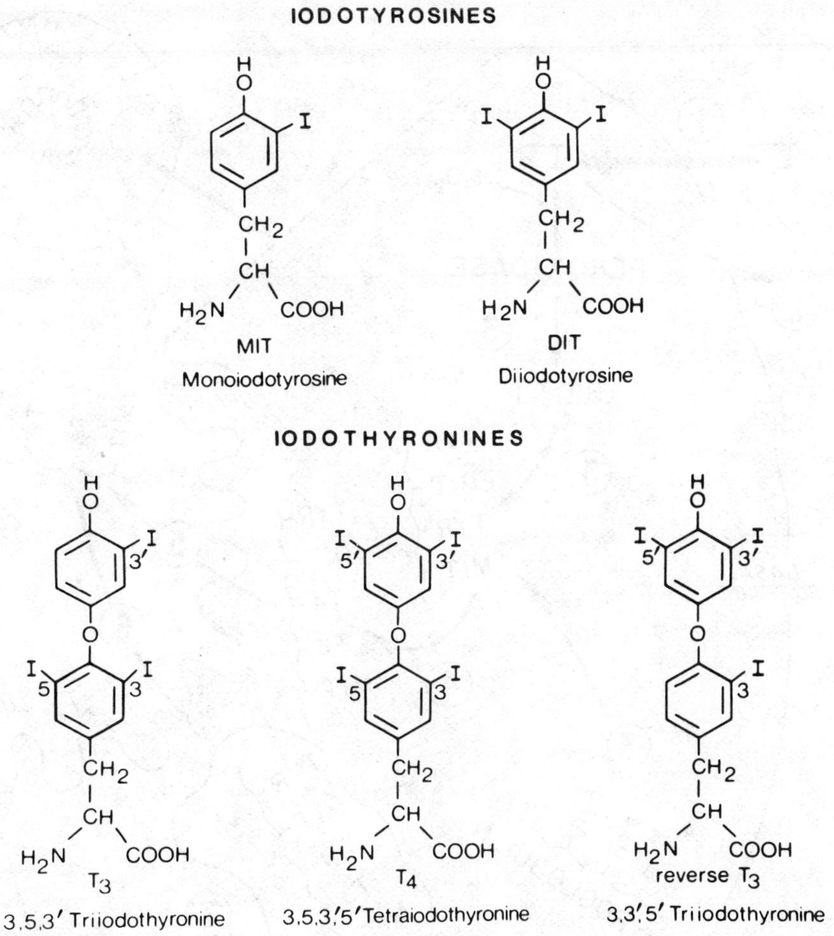

IODOTYROSINES

MIT
Monoiodotyrosine

DIT
Diiodotyrosine

IODOTHYRONINES

T₃
3,5,3′ Triiodothyronine

T₄
3,5,3′,5′ Tetraiodothyronine

reverse T₃
3,3′,5′ Triiodothyronine

Figure 60. Structure of iodotyrosines and iodothyronines.

Iodide is concentrated in gastric secretions and saliva and is rapidly absorbed by the gastrointestinal tract into the blood stream and cleared and excreted by the kidneys. In the steady state, the renal excretion of iodide equals the dietary intake.

Iodide Transport

The thyroid gland concentrates iodide against an electrochemical gradient (Fig. 61); this property is shared by the salivary glands and the gastric mucosa. Other anions, such as perchlorate and thiocyanate, inhibit this iodide trap. Pertechnetate competes for this trapping function and is itself concentrated by the thyroid gland. This property is utilized clinically by administering radioactive isotopes of pertechnetate (⁹⁹Tc) for functional imaging (radioisotope scanning) of the thyroid gland. The iodide trapping function is stimulated by TSH and inhibited by excess intraglandular organic iodine.

Organification

Free intrathyroidal iodide is able to diffuse rapidly out of the thyroid gland. However, intrathyroidal iodide does not remain free but is rapidly bound into an organic form. Such organification is unique to the thyroid gland; it does not occur in the stomach or salivary glands. Under ordinary circumstances, the intrathyroidal iodine pool contains about 8,000 μg of iodine, 90 per cent of which is organic iodine.

The organic fixation of iodide allows us to scan the thyroid gland with radioactive isotopes of iodine (¹²³I and ¹³¹I) 24 hours after their administration. In general, the 24-hour uptake of iodine correlates with thyroid gland function. The organification reaction is clinically important for a second reason. This reaction is inhibited by the drugs propylthiouracil and methimazole (thioamide drugs), which are used to treat hyperthyroidism by inhibiting thyroid hormone production.

Tyrosine is the organic substrate for iodination yielding mono- and diiodotyrosine (Fig. 60). Free tyrosine is not well iodinated, the tyrosine moieties being iodinated within the backbone of a large precursor protein molecule thyroglobulin (mol. wt. 660,000). Iodination yields mono-iodotyrosine (MIT) and diiodotyrosine (DIT), both within peptide linkage. This reaction is catalyzed by a peroxidase and requires a source of hydrogen peroxide. Iodide is oxidized to a higher valence state (possibly the iodinium ion, I⁺), which in turn iodinates the thyroxine moieties. This reaction probably occurs at the interface between the luminal surface of the thyroid cell and the colloid or storage space within the thyroid follicle.

Coupling Reaction

The coupling of two iodotyrosine molecules gives rise to iodothyronines: two DIT molecules give rise to T₄; an MIT plus DIT yields T₃. The reaction requires at

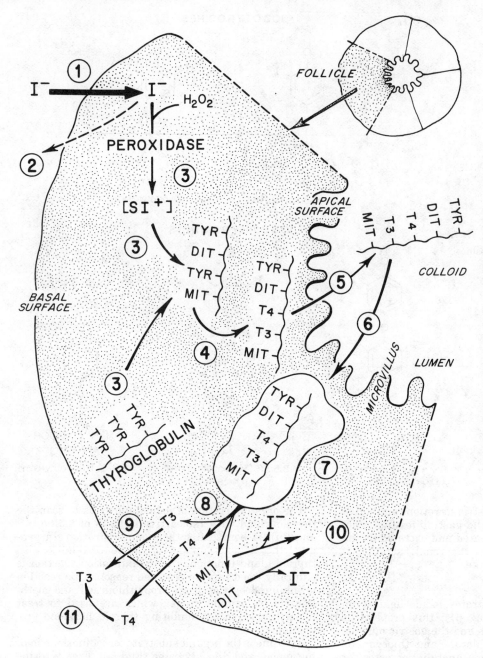

Figure 61. Thyroid hormone biosynthesis. (1) Iodide concentration (active transport). (2) Passive back diffusion of inorganic iodide. (3) Organification of iodide (MIT + DIT production). (4) Iodotyrosine coupling (T_3 and T_4 production). (5) Release of thyroglobulin to follicular lumen. (6) Pinocytosis (thyroglobulin reuptake). (7) Phagolysosome. (8) Digestive release of iodotyrosines and iodothyronines (proteolysis of thyroglobulin). (9) Release of thyroid hormone. (10) Deiodination of iodotyrosines. (11) Peripheral deiodination of T_4 to T_3. (From Daniels, G. H., and Maloof, F. M.: In Frohlich, E. D. (ed.): Pathophysiology. Altered Regulatory Mechanisms in Disease. Philadelphia, J. B. Lippincott, 1984, p. 365.)

least one of the DIT molecules to be within the thyroglobulin peptide linkage. There is controversy over the nature of the second coupling iodotyrosine; whether it is free or part of the same thyroglobulin molecule is still uncertain. The reaction appears to be catalyzed by a thyroid peroxidase, probably the same enzyme responsible for the organification reaction. The coupling reaction too is quite sensitive to inhibition by the antithyroid drugs propylthiouracil (PTU) and methimazole (Tapazole).

Colloid Storage

The thyroid gland is unique among endocrine glands because it has a large hormonal reservoir stored in the form of thyroid colloid. The iodinated thyroglobulin or colloid is the storage form of thyroid hormone and provides up to three months supply of hormone. When hyperthyroid patients are treated with antithyroid drugs (PTU and methimazole), this storage function becomes important. Although inhibition of hormone synthesis may be immediate, clinical improvement may take weeks to months until the thyroid hormone stores are depleted.

Although the thyroglobulin molecule contains about 120 tyrosine residues, relatively few iodotyrosines and iodothyronines are formed. (The actual numbers vary with the iodine content of the thyroid gland; however, there are approximately 20 DIT, 10 MIT, 3 T_4, and 0.3 T_3 moieties per molecule of thyroglobulin.)

For years, thyroglobulin was thought to be a sequestered antigen; however, small concentrations of thyroglobulin are found in the circulation in normal individuals. Thyroglobulin release is increased with thyroidal stimulation and decreased with thyroidal suppression. Well-differentiated thyroid malignancies (papillary and follicular carcinoma) are often found to have increased circulating concentrations of thyroglobulin; the measurement of serum thyroglobulin may be a useful tumor marker in following the progress or regression of the disease. The thyroglobulin released seems to be less well iodinated than the mature thyroglobulin within the gland.

RELEASE OF THYROID HORMONES

Thyroglobulin is taken up into the thyroid follicular cells by pinocytosis and combines with lysosomes to yield phagolysosomes. These digest the thyroglobulin molecule to yield free iodotyrosines and iodothyronines. A potent thyroidal deiodinase strips the mono- and diiodotyrosines of their iodine, which is reclaimed for future use in thyroid hormone biosynthesis. The T_4 and T_3 released from the thyroglobulin are then secreted into the circulation. In hyperthyroidism, T_3 secretion seems to be preferential (i.e., the secretion rate for T_3 is proportionately higher than its content in thyroglobulin).

Proteolysis and release of thyroid hormones are stimulated by TSH and inhibited by lithium and excess iodine. Increased iodination of thyroglobulin stabilizes its tertiary structure, making it more resistant to proteolysis. Clinically, iodide administration may lead to rapid improvement of severe hyperthyroidism by inhibition of hormone release. Lithium has been used with similar results as an experimental mode of therapy.

THYROID HORMONES IN THE CIRCULATION

The major hormone released from the thyroid gland is L-thyroxine (tetraiodothyronine), whose structure is shown in Figure 60. Under normal circumstances, approximately 60 to 80 µg per day are released from the thyroid gland. The majority of circulating T_4 (99.97 per cent) is tightly protein bound, but it is only the free hormone (free T_4 = 0.03 per cent of total) that is metabolically active. Thyroxine has an extremely long half-life of about seven days, in large part due to its tight protein binding.

Thyroxine-binding globulin (TBG) has an extremely high affinity for T_4 ($2.2 \times 10^{10} M^{-1}$) and accounts for approximately 75 per cent of the protein-bound thyroxine. There is one binding site for T_4 or T_3 per TBG molecule, with a total capacity for T_4 binding of 15 to 25 µg/dl. Thyroxine-binding prealbumin (TBPA) has a lower affinity for thyroxine ($1.3 \times 10^8 M^{-1}$), but it has higher total capacity, binding approximately 15 per cent of the total bound thyroxine. Albumin binds thyroxine in a relatively nonspecific fashion and accounts for 10 per cent of the total bound thyroxine.

Triiodothyronine (T_3) is largely protein bound as well (99.7 per cent), but less so than T_4. The majority of T_3 is bound to TBG (binding affinity, $10^9 M^{-1}$), with smaller quantities being bound to albumin and little or none to TBPA. T_4 and T_3 compete for the same binding site on TBG. As with T_4, the free hormone (free T_3 = 0.3 per cent) is the metabolically active form: the serum half-life of T_3 is relatively long (one day) but is much shorter than that of T_4 (seven days).

The T_4 and T_3 half-lives are quite long when compared to the half-lives of most protein hormones (minutes) or steroid hormones (hours).

All of the circulating T_4 is derived from the thyroid gland. In contrast, only 15 to 20 per cent of the 30 µg of T_3 produced each day is secreted by the thyroid gland. The majority of circulating T_3 (80 to 85 per cent) comes from T_4 after an iodine atom (5' iodine) has been removed by peripheral tissues. Many tissues are capable of deiodinating T_4 to T_3, including the liver, kidney, brain, and pituitary gland.

T_3 is at least three to four times as potent as T_4, and most evidence points to receptor-bound nuclear T_3 as the active thyroid hormone species. In this regard, T_4 serves as a precursor or prohormone for T_3. Approximately 35 per cent of T_4 is metabolized to T_3 under normal circumstances. Given the ratio of T_3 to T_4 potency of three or four to one and the fact that three T_4 molecules are necessary to produce one T_3 molecule, T_4 does not seem to have much intrinsic potency.

The conversion of T_4 to T_3 is not an automatic, passive process. The reaction is catalyzed by a series of 5' deiodinases that have different characteristics in different tissues. A number of conditions have been shown to alter T_4-to-T_3 conversion. Starvation, for example, is associated with a dramatic decrease in T_4-to-T_3 conversion. This appears to be homeostatic in the sense that less active hormone (T_3) is produced, with concomitant decrease in the basal metabolic rate and sparing of body tissues from unnecessary breakdown. Many other situations are associated with marked lowering of serum T_3 concentration (Table 27). Although decreases in metabolic rate may be helpful under such circumstances (e.g., severe trauma), clinicians continue to argue about whether such patients are euthyroid or hypothyroid.

Some studies suggest that T_3 concentrations rise slightly during prolonged cold exposure. This potential homeostatic mechanism would provide increased warmth and thermogenesis to protect against the cold. It is not clear if these increases in T_3 serum concentrations are due to increased thyroidal secretion or increased peripheral conversion of T_4 to T_3.

Figure 62A suggests that an iodine atom can be removed from the inner ring of T_4 to yield an isomer of T_3 called reverse T_3 ($3,3'5'$ T_3), an inactive molecule. Virtually all conditions associated with impaired T_4-to-T_3 conversion are associated with a rise in serum reverse T_3 concentrations. This appears to be due to a decrease in reverse T_3 clearance (Fig. 62B). In severe illnesses, the serum thyroxine concentration may decline, and the elevated reverse T_3 concentrations may be an important clue that we are dealing with nonthyroidal illness rather than hypothyroidism.

TABLE 27. IMPAIRED T_4-TO-T_3 CONVERSION

1. Neonates
2. Starvation
3. Severe illness, surgery, trauma
4. Medications
   Propylthiouracil
   Glucocorticoids
   Iodinated compounds including
      ipodate and amiodarone
   Propranolol

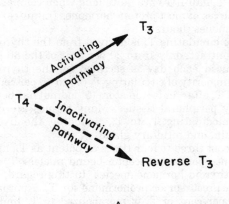

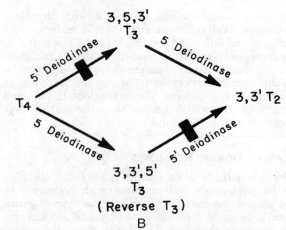

Figure 62. *A,* Although we can draw simple alternative paths from T_4 to T_3 or to reverse T_3, the actual situation is more complicated. *B,* Inhibition of the 5′ deiodinase will result in inhibition of T_3 production (with a fall in serum T_3) and a decrease in reverse T_3 *clearance* (with a rise in serum reverse T_3 concentration). T_2 is diiodothyronine.

Figure 63 summarizes the thyroidal and peripheral contributions to T_4, T_3, and reverse T_3 production.

THYROIDAL AUTOREGULATION

TSH is the dominant influence on the thyroid gland. However, iodide, the major substrate for thyroxine and triiodothyronine synthesis, is an important modulator of thyroid function as well.

In the 1920s and 1930s many individuals living in the midwestern United States had iodide-deficient diets; as a consequence, goiters were very common in these areas. Iodide deficiency has now been eliminated in the United States by the presence of iodide in salt, in many breads, in food coloring, in radiographic contrast material, and in other substances. However, many areas of the world are still plagued with iodine deficiency and its resulting goiters.

The thyroid gland adapts to iodine deficiency in two important ways (Table 28): (1) increased iodide trapping and (2) a change from a predominantly T_4-secreting gland to one that secretes a higher proportion of T_3. Increased T_3 secretion is quite important because it allows the thyroid gland to use only three-quarters as much iodide, yet produce a three- to four-fold more potent hormone. Thus, the thyroid hormone effect remains close to normal despite marked decreases in iodine intake. Eventually, as T_4 secretion declines, TSH rises, leading to a goiter; when severe, iodine deficiency will lead to hypothyroidism.

Iodide excess is a more frequent finding in the United States. Under normal circumstances, the thyroid gland adjusts to increased iodide intake without increasing output of thyroid hormone. A number of mechanisms have evolved to damp down thyroid hormone production and secretion in the face of excess iodide. Increases in serum iodide concentration ultimately lead to decreased iodide trapping by the thyroid; therefore, a lower percentage of iodide gets into the gland. The ability of excess iodide to inhibit iodide trapping has led to the suggestion that individuals who reside near nuclear power plants keep iodide tablets or solutions in their homes in case of inadvertent release of radioactivity. Under these circumstances, the radioactive iodide (^{131}I) released from the nuclear plants would not enter the iodide-blocked thyroid gland and thyroidal damage could be prevented. A net increase in organic iodide within the thyroid causes an inhibition of the coupling reaction, the so-called Wolff-Chaikoff effect. Furthermore, excess iodide stabilizes the thyroglobulin molecule, inhibiting proteolysis, and hence decreases

Figure 63. Summary of thyroidal and peripheral contributions to thyroid hormone economy. (From Schimmel, M., and Utiger, R. D.: Ann Intern Med 87:760, 1977.)

TABLE 28. THYROID GLAND ADAPTATIONS TO PATHOLOGICAL CONDITIONS

IODIDE DEFICIENCY	IODIDE EXCESS
1. Increased iodide trapping	1. Decreased iodide trapping
2. Increased secretion of T_3 relative to T_4	2. Decreased iodide organification (Wolff-Chaikoff effect)
	3. Inhibition of thyroid hormone release
	4. Increased secretion of T_4 relative to T_3

release of thyroid hormones from the gland. Lastly, the iodide-loaded thyroid gland secretes predominantly T_4, the less active hormone, rather than T_3, the more active hormone. The relative iodide excess in our diets may explain the current predominant secretion of T_4 by the thyroid. Normal thyroid physiology in the early twentieth century may have been quite different from the current situation, with a different proportion of T_3 to T_4 secreted (Table 28).

In normal individuals, the net result of excess iodide is a transient decrease in the output of thyroid hormone and a minimal fall in serum thyroxine concentration, followed by very rapid return to normal output despite continued iodide exposure. Although normal thyroid glands adapt well to iodide excess, abnormal thyroid glands have lost that flexibility. Damaged thyroid glands (e.g., radiation damage or autoimmune damage) are turned off by excess iodide, leading to hypothyroidism. In contrast, nodular thyroid glands may lose their ability to be regulated by iodides and may quantitatively turn iodide into thyroid hormone, leading to hyperthyroidism.

HYPOTHALAMIC-PITUITARY AXIS

Thyroid-stimulating Hormone (TSH, Thyrotropin). TSH controls virtually every step in the biosynthesis, storage, and release of thyroid hormone. In addition, thyroid size and thyroid vascularity are dependent upon TSH. Many, but not all, of the effects of TSH on the thyroid gland are mediated by cyclic AMP. The feedback relationship between the pituitary and the thyroid gland has been recognized for over a century: (a) falling thyroid hormone secretion leads to an increase in TSH secretion (primary hypothyroidism); (b) falling TSH secretion leads to thyroid gland failure (secondary hypothyroidism); and (c) administration of excess thyroid hormone leads to inhibition of TSH release and decrease in the size of the thyroid gland (Fig. 59). This simple system is complicated by the important controlling influence of the hypothalamus on the pituitary.

Thyrotropin-releasing Hormone (TRH). TRH is a simple tripeptide (L-pyroglutamyl-L-histidinyl-L-proline amide) that stimulates the release of TSH from the pituitary gland. TRH is necessary for the release of TSH. In the absence of TRH (e.g., hypothalamic destruction or pituitary stalk section in humans or anti-TRH antibodies in rats), TSH release does not occur and hypothyroidism ensues (so-called tertiary or hypothalamic hypothyroidism). TRH is now commercially available and is commonly employed for physiological or clinical testing. Figure 64 demonstrates the rise in serum TSH concentration after the intravenous administration of TRH in normal humans.

The pituitary is exquisitely sensitive to TRH, with nanogram quantities of TRH stimulating TSH synthesis and release of TSH in vitro. Specific, high-affinity TRH receptors are found on the pituitary gland; their numbers seem to decrease with continued TRH binding. The mechanism of TRH stimulation of TSH is still uncertain; however, effects on calcium ion flux may be of importance. TSH release after TRH administration does not require protein or nucleic acid synthesis. In humans, synthetic TRH will increase serum TSH concentrations after parenteral (microgram) or oral (milligram) dosages.

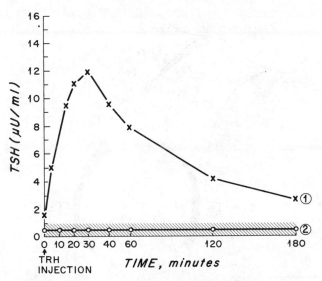

Figure 64. Rise in serum TSH concentration after intravenous injection of TRH. (1) Euthyroid patients. (2) Hyperthyroid patients or normals after administration of exogenous thyroid hormone.

The effect of TRH on prolactin has been reviewed in The Pituitary and Hypothalamus. The minimum quantity of TRH that is capable of TSH release also releases prolactin. The response of prolactin to TRH is decreased in hyperthyroidism and exaggerated in hypothyroidism. In the clinical setting, the release of prolactin and TSH are easily dissociable: pregnancy and suckling increase prolactin but not TSH; primary hypothyroidism elevates TSH but generally not prolactin. TRH does not usually cause the release of growth hormone, follicle-stimulating hormone (FSH), luteinizing hormone (LH), or adrenocorticotropic hormone (ACTH). Pathological growth hormone release may occur after TRH administration in patients with acromegaly, anorexia nervosa, or renal failure.

Thyroid Hormone Feedback. Is the major site of feedback control by thyroid hormones at the hypothalamic level? Using TRH, the major site of thyroid hormone feedback can be localized. If supraphysiological doses of thyroid hormone are administered prior to TRH injection, the release of TSH is completely inhibited, as shown in Figure 64. Prolonged infusion of high concentrations of TRH cannot overcome this inhibition of TSH release. This strongly suggests that the major site of feedback of thyroid hormone is at the pituitary level (Fig. 65). If hypothalamic feedback were of prime importance (leading to inhibition of TRH release), then continued TRH administration should result in TSH release. In general, patients with hyperthyroidism have no rise in TSH concentration after TRH injection. Thyroid hormone inhibits pituitary TSH secretion through an active process involving protein synthesis. The nature of the inhibitor produced has not yet been determined.

While the dominant influence of thyroid hormone at the pituitary level is quite clear, the presence of hypothalamic feedback is uncertain in humans. The solution to the problem of hypothalamic feedback is complicated by the rather short half-life of TRH in the systemic circulation, the presence of proteases that

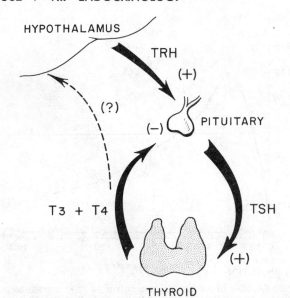

Figure 65. The normal hypothalamic-pituitary-thyroid axis. (From Daniels, G. H., and Maloof, F.: In Frohlich, E. D. (ed.): Pathophysiology. Altered Regulatory Mechanisms in Disease. Philadelphia, J. B. Lippincott, 1984, p. 36.)

destroy TRH, and the widespread distribution of TRH in the gastrointestinal tract and areas of the brain apart from the hypothalamus. Although hypothalamic TRH is the releasing hormone for TSH, extrahypothalamic TRH seems to serve an independent neurotransmitter function. In rats, cold exposure leads to increased TSH release, an effect apparently mediated by TRH and blocked by anti-TRH antibody. Anti-TRH antibody does not prevent the cold-induced release of prolactin. In humans, cold-induced TSH release is most convincingly demonstrated in the neonate.

Figure 66 schematically pictures the requirement of TRH for the tonic release of TSH, with the actual amount of TSH released from the pituitary gland being modulated by the serum concentration of thyroid hormones.

The oral ingestion of either T_4 or T_3 inhibits pituitary TSH release. Although thyroid hormone action correlates best with nuclear receptor occupancy of T_3, oral T_4 is relatively more effective than T_3 at producing TSH inhibition. Furthermore, in hypothyroid states, the serum TSH concentration correlates inversely with serum T_4 concentrations, but not with serum T_3 concentrations. Patients with iodine deficiency, with low-normal T_4 and high-normal or elevated T_3 concentrations, will have elevated TSH concentrations. Although T_3 can enter the pituitary, it enters less well than T_4. Under normal circumstances, approximately 50 per cent of intrapituitary T_3 is derived from T_4 by conversion to T_3 *within the pituitary gland itself*. For the pituitary gland, T_4 seems to be a better way to deliver T_3 than circulating T_3 itself. In contrast, the liver

derives most, if not all, of its nuclear T_3 from circulating T_3 rather than from circulating T_4. The pituitary enzymes that are responsible for T_4-to-T_3 conversion do not respond to the same inhibitory influences as peripheral (e.g., liver) 5′ diodinases. In starvation, for example, when serum T_3 concentrations markedly decline, serum TSH concentration does not rise, suggesting continued intrapituitary T_4-to-T_3 conversion. In a teleological way, this makes sense: if TSH concentrations were to rise during starvation, increased thyroidal secretion would occur and would overcome the (presumably beneficial) decline in basal metabolic rate.

Other Factors. Somatostatin (growth hormone–releasing inhibitory factor) and dopamine inhibit the secretion of TSH; the role of this inhibition in normal physiology is currently under investigation. During growth hormone therapy of patients with isolated hormone deficiency, secondary hypothyroidism may develop. Growth hormone leads to somatomedin production; both somatomedin and GH stimulate somatostatin production. The secondary (pituitary) hypothyroidism leads to growth failure and requires thyroid hormone therapy. Somatostatin inhibition of TSH release appears to cause the hypothyroidism.

Chronic therapy with L-dopa or dopamine agonists, such as bromocriptine, decreases the elevated TSH concentrations in patients with primary hypothyroidism. Dopamine receptor blockers increase TSH concentrations in normals as well as hypothyroid patients.

Glucocorticoids in pharmacological doses inhibit the release of TSH in response to TRH injections. Conversely, patients with primary adrenal (glucocorticoid) insufficiency tend to have elevated TSH concentrations, which return to normal with cortisol therapy.

TSH

TSH is a glycoprotein hormone with a molecular weight of 28,000 to 30,000. It contains two noncovalently bound subunits, alpha and beta. The amino acid sequence of the alpha subunit is virtually identical to that of luteinizing hormone (LH), follicle-stimulating hormone (FSH), and human chorionic gonadotropin (HCG). The beta subunit confers biological and immunological specificity on these molecules.

TSH is synthesized in specific thyrotropes (β_1 basophils) that comprise about 5 per cent of anterior pituitary cells. The normal pituitary contains about 165 mU, with a normal TSH production rate of 100 mU per day. Circulating TSH has a half-life of 58 minutes. A minor diurnal variation has been noted in TSH concentrations, with concentrations being highest prior to the onset of sleep.

ACTIONS OF THYROID HORMONE

The role of the thyroid hormones in normal physiology is best appreciated when the physiology is de-

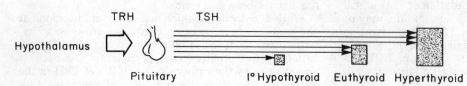

Figure 66. TRH is necessary for the tonic release of TSH. Rectangles represent circulating thyroid hormone concentrations.

ranged, as in patients with overactive and underactive thyroids. It is clear that the thyroid gland and its hormones are designed "for the long haul" rather than for sudden acute changes. Several months' supply of thyroid hormones is stored in the thyroid gland; circulating thyroxine has a plasma half-life of one week.

What functions are subserved by this long-lived, relatively stable system? Thyroid hormone is necessary for the development of the central nervous system. Children born without thyroid glands develop irreversible mental retardation if not treated within a short time after birth. Thyroid hormone is necessary for the development of the skeleton as well. Hypothyroidism results in marked delay in linear growth; hyperthyroidism accelerates bone growth.

Thyroid hormones stimulate calorigenesis, with a marked increase in oxygen consumption by many tissues. Although thyroid hormone has been shown to stimulate sodium-potassium ATPase (adenosine triphosphatase: the membrane-bound sodium pump) in the liver and kidney, it is not clear whether this stimulation is sufficient to account for the increased oxygen consumption that occurs in hyperthyroidism.

Thyroid hormones have important effects influencing the metabolism of fats, carbohydrates, and proteins. It is still not certain which effects are primary and which are secondary to general changes in energy metabolism. The complicated role of thyroid hormone in intermediary metabolism is illustrated by the diverse effects on lipid metabolism. Thyroid hormone directly stimulates lipolysis and facilitates lipolysis induced by other hormones. It stimulates hepatic synthesis of triglycerides and increases triglyceride removal from the circulation, probably through stimulation of lipoprotein lipase. Cholesterol synthesis may be accelerated; however, LDL (low density lipoprotein) receptors are increased in hyperthyroidism, which accelerates cholesterol degradation and removal and leads to a net lowering of serum cholesterol.

Thyroid hormones directly stimulate myocardial contractility and may render the heart muscle more sensitive to catecholamines as well. This increased sensitivity to the catecholamines is due to an increased number of beta-adrenergic receptors in some, but not all, tissues. Changes in catechol sensitivity induced by thyroid hormone appear to vary from tissue to tissue, and the mechanism of the change in sensitivity is far from uniform.

Mechanism of Thyroid Hormone Action

Despite intensive studies over many years, investigators have failed to uncover a single mechanism of action of thyroid hormone. Indeed, many cellular actions have been called "the mechanism of action." Thyroid hormones pass through cell membranes and induce gene transcription. High-affinity nuclear receptors for T_3 are generally conceded to be of major importance in thyroid hormone action. T_3 nuclear receptor occupancy correlates well with many, but not all, of the metabolic actions of thyroid hormone. Recent studies have disclosed high-affinity specific mitochondrial receptors for T_3 and suggest a direct stimulation of oxygen consumption by T_3 at the mitochondrial level. The situation is further complicated by the data that

support a direct effect for T_3 and specific binding sites for T_3 at the cell membrane. Transport of sugars and amino acids can be rapidly stimulated by T_3 in various animal tissues in the absence of new protein synthesis. On the basis of these studies, it seems likely that multiple sites of action of thyroid hormone exist and account for the variety of effects attributed to thyroid hormone.

TESTING THYROID FUNCTION

Thyroxine (T_4) has a stable plasma concentration (4 to 12 μg/dl), which is easily measured; all the circulating T_4 is produced by the thyroid gland. Hence, serum thyroxine concentration has evolved as the "standard" test of thyroid function. However, the vast majority of circulating T_4 (99.97 per cent) is protein bound; it is the very low concentration of free hormone (0.8 to 2.4 ng/dl) that is metabolically active.

Serum Thyroxine

A simple equilibrium expression for the binding of thyroxine to thyroxine-binding globulin (TBG) molecules would be:

$$T_4 + TBG \rightleftharpoons TBG\ T_4 \qquad (1)$$
$$\text{or}$$
$$TBG\ T_4 = K\ (T_4)\ (TBG) \qquad (2)$$

Virtually all of the circulating T_4 is bound to TBG; hence, the measured serum thyroxine can be substituted for TBG T_4. (T_4) represents the concentration of free thyroxine and (TBG) represents the available binding sites on TBG (Fig. 67). (For these simplified equations, binding to other binding proteins is not included.)

$$T_4\ (\text{serum thyroxine}) = K\ (\text{free } T_4)\ (TBG) \qquad (3)$$

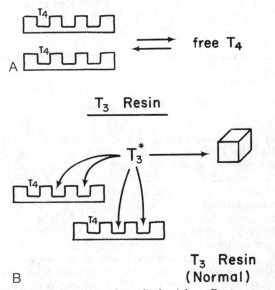

Figure 67. *A*, Normal (euthyroid) physiology. Boats represent thyroxine-binding proteins. *B*, T_3 resin test. T_3^* represents radiolabeled T_3. Cube represents resin or sponge. See text for details.

If the TBG concentration remains constant, then T_4 is indeed proportional to the free thyroxine concentration. However, under certain circumstances, serum TBG concentration can vary considerably. Equation 3 suggests that the serum T_4 concentration can rise as a consequence of an overactivity of the thyroid gland with an increase in free T_4 concentration; alternatively, an increase in the TBG concentration will result in an increase in the total serum thyroxine concentration if free T_4 remains normal. With an intact hypothalamic-pituitary-thyroid axis, free T_4 is maintained at a constant level, and any increase in TBG concentration results in an increase in serum T_4 concentration.

Serum thyroxine is measured simply and specifically with radioimmunoassays or with competitive binding protein assays: the former use specific anti-T_4 antibodies to bind radioactive T_4; the latter utilizes the high affinity binding of TBG as a ligand.

Free Thyroxine and Free Thyroxine Index

Based on the above considerations, it should be clear that some measure of the free thyroxine concentration is required. Although the technical approaches to measuring the low concentrations of the free hormone are rapidly changing, it is important to understand the currently available methods.

Measurement of serum free thyroxine by equilibrium dialysis remains the "gold standard." The percentage of dialyzable T_4 is determined; the product of the T_4 concentration times dialyzable percentage equals the free T_4 concentration. The method is tedious and expensive and is not universally available. Recently a series of direct radioimmunoassays for free T_4 has been developed. These have variable reliability and have not yet gained universal acceptance. Even the best of the methods (dialyzable free T_4) may give spuriously high or low values in certain clinical situations. The basis for these discrepancies is not always clear. It is, therefore, important to remember that laboratory measurements must always be interpreted in the light of the clinical findings. Furthermore, measurements in vitro will not always correspond to the situation in vivo.

Transposing equation 3 yields the following expression for free T_4:

$$\text{free } T_4 = K'(T_4) \times \frac{1}{\text{TBG}} \qquad (4)$$

The most commonly used test to assess (1/TBG) is called the T_3 resin or T_3 uptake test. In this test (Fig. 67B), a small amount of radioactive T_3 is added to a test tube with the patient's serum. This radioactive T_3 competes for the T_4 binding sites on TBG (and other binding proteins as well). Radiolabeled T_3 is chosen for convenience rather than radiolabeled T_4. The radioactive T_3 that does not bind to the binding proteins is taken up by a resin (or a sponge or tanned red cell). The T_3 resin test, therefore, gives an inverse measure of the available thyroid hormone binding sites. Since T_3 resin is proportional to 1/TBG, we can derive equation 5:

$$\text{free } T_4 = K''(T_4) \, (T_3 \text{ resin}) \qquad (5)$$

The product of the T_4 times the T_3 resin is known as the free thyroxine index and is proportional to the free T_4. It is a generally useful and inexpensive index of the free thyroxine concentration and, as such, is widely used. Although direct radioimmunoassays for TBG are available, these are more tedious and more expensive than the indirect T_3 resin test.

Abnormal Binding Proteins

Normal thyroid physiology is depicted in Figure 67A. (Although there is only one T_4 binding site per molecule, and TBG is normally one third saturated, for convenience these figures are drawn with three binding sites per molecule.) An elevated serum (total) thyroxine can be due to overproduction of thyroid hormone by the thyroid gland (Fig. 68A) (hyperthyroidism). Under these circumstances, the free hormone concentration will be elevated and the TBG will be relatively saturated. Alternatively, patients may have an excess of TBG. Under these circumstances, the hypothalamic-pituitary-thyroid axis maintains a normal concentration of free thyroxine, but the total T_4 is elevated (Fig. 69A). TBG excess is not a disease; these patients are euthyroid. Elevated T_4 due to TBG excess is merely a source of confusion for the clinician. TBG may be elevated as a hereditary X-linked condition, as a consequence of estrogen excess (either exogenous or from pregnancy), in hepatitis, and as an effect of 5-fluorouracil, a chemotherapeutic agent. When faced with an elevated serum thyroxine, some measure of free thyroxine is necessary to separate hyperthyroidism from an abnormality of the binding proteins. In hyperthyroidism, the T_3 resin will be elevated, since the binding proteins are relatively saturated (Fig. 68B). In TBG excess, the T_3 resin will be decreased due to the increased number of available TBG binding sites (Fig. 69B).

An analogous situation exists when the clinician is faced with a decreased serum T_4 concentration. This

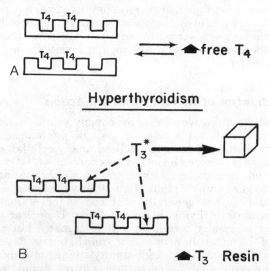

Figure 68. *A,* Elevated serum thyroxine due to hyperthyroidism. *B,* T_3 resin test in hyperthyroidism.

TBG Excess

TBG Deficiency

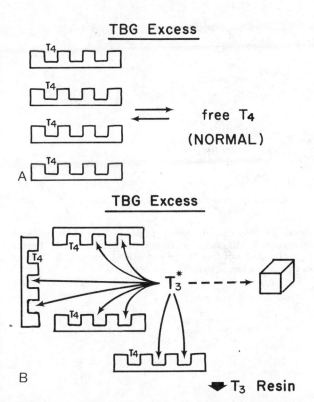

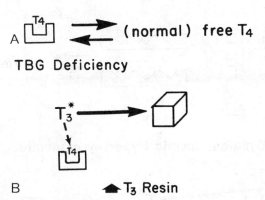

Figure 69. *A,* Elevated serum thyroxine due to TBG excess. *B,* T₃ resin test in TBG excess.

Figure 71. *A,* Low serum thyroxine due to TBG deficiency. *B,* T₃ resin test in TBG deficiency.

could be due to hypothyroidism with a diminished free T_4 concentration (Fig. 70*A*) or, alternatively, due to a decreased concentration of TBG, a situation in which the patient is healthy with a normally maintained free thyroxine concentration (Fig. 71*A*). TBG deficiency is most commonly an hereditary condition inherited as a X-linked trait. It occasionally accompanies states of severe protein loss, such as nephrotic syndrome. In

Hypothyroidism

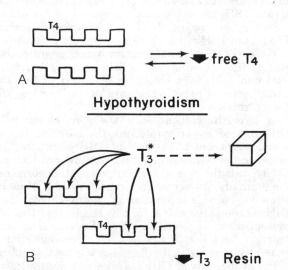

Figure 70. *A,* Low serum thyroxine due to hypothyroidism. *B,* T₃ resin test in hypothyroidism.

hypothyroidism, the T_3 resin tends to be diminished (Fig. 70*B*), whereas in TBG deficiency, the T_3 resin is markedly elevated (Fig. 71*B*).

A simple general rule emerges in the use of this test. In *thyroid* disease, the T_4 and the T_3 resin tests "move in the same direction"; i.e., both are elevated in hyperthyroidism and both tend to be low in hypothyroidism. In binding protein abnormalities, the T_4 and the T_3 resin tests "move in opposite directions" (Table 29). Although the free thyroxine index ($T_4 \times T_3$ resin) may occasionally give misleading answers, "looking at the directions" in which the T_4 and T_3 resin move will often yield an important clue to help define the clinical situation.

Recently, an abnormal protein has been described that binds T_4 but not T_3 (Fig. 72*A*). This protein is an abnormal albumin, and its appearance in patients is inherited as a dominant trait. Patients with this abnormal albumin are euthyroid with normal free thyroxine concentrations; however, the conventional laboratory studies yield confusing results. The total thyroxine is markedly elevated owing to the protein binding (so-called dysalbuminemic familial hyperthyroxinemia). However, T_3 does not bind well to the abnormal albumin. The T_3 resin will, therefore, be normal (Fig. 72*B*) (or occasionally elevated, as some of these patients seem to have a slight compensatory reduction in TBG). The free thyroxine index (elevated $T_4 \times$ normal or elevated T_3 resin) is elevated, leading to confusion about the diagnosis. If a T_4 resin test (analogous to T_3 resin, but using radiolabeled T_4) were employed, its value would be low, but this test is not generally available. When faced with an elevated T_4 and free T_4 index in a clinically euthyroid individual,

TABLE 29. DIAGNOSTIC INDICATIONS OF T₄ AND T₃ TESTING

	T₄	T₃ RESIN
Hyperthyroidism	↑	↑
Hypothyroidism	↓	↓
TBG Excess	↑	↓
TBG Deficiency	↓	↑

Dysalbuminemic Hyperthyroxinemia

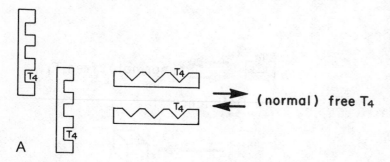

A

Dysalbuminemic Hyperthyroxinemia

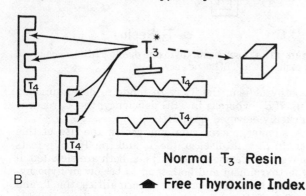

Normal T_3 Resin

Free Thyroxine Index

B

Figure 72. Dysalbuminemic hyperthyroxinemia. Boats with triangular binding sites represent abnormal albumin. Serum T_4 is elevated, but free T_4 concentration is normal. B, T_3 resin in dysalbuminemic hyperthyroxinemia.

the solution is to use the equilibrium dialysis method, which yields a normal free thyroxine concentration. Research laboratories would be able to directly identify the abnormal protein.

Serum Triiodothyronine (T_3)

T_3 is a "peripheral hormone," largely derived from conversion of circulating T_4. The measurement of the serum T_3 concentration is generally less useful in assessing thyroid gland function or secretion. T_3 is measured directly by a radioimmunoassay (75 to 195 ng/dl). The serum T_3 concentration is much lower than that of T_4 (4 to 12 µg/dl); hence, it is more difficult to measure. The serum free T_3 concentration (around 0.4 ng/dl) is about 20 per cent that of free T_4. Increases in serum TBG will also increase the serum T_3 concentration, but to a lesser extent than with T_4.

Measurements of serum T_3 are usually unnecessary. Certain hyperthyroid patients, however, will have normal concentrations of T_4 and free T_4 with increased thyroidal production and serum concentrations of T_3. Such patients have been called "T_3-toxic." Early hyperthyroidism may be "T_3-toxicosis."

T_3 measurements are of little use in the early diagnosis of hypothyroidism. As the thyroid gland fails and TSH secretion increases, T_3 production is preserved at the expense of T_4 production; hence, the excellent inverse correlation between T_4 and TSH concentrations, but the poor correlation between T_3 and TSH concentrations. Furthermore, a very low T_3 concentration is more often a reflection of a nonthyroidal illness than of hypothyroidism.

Serum TSH and the TSH Response to TRH

Although the normal level of serum T_4 concentration is wide ranging among individuals (4 to 12 µg/dl), each individual's level of T_4 concentration remains fairly constant. Early thyroid gland failure, therefore, is characterized by falling serum T_4 and free T_4 concentrations, with values remaining "within normal limits" for long periods of time. Eventually these concentrations may enter the "hypothyroid" or low range. However, the serum TSH concentration begins to rise with small decreases in serum T_4 (and free T_4), with elevated serum TSH concentrations (normal = <3.5 µU/ml) occurring long before the T_4 is definitely "abnormal." The serum TSH concentration is, therefore, important in the early diagnosis of primary hypothyroidism. It is also useful in distinguishing primary hypothyroidism (elevated TSH) from secondary (pituitary or hypothalamic) forms of hypothyroidism ("normal" or low TSH concentration).

In hyperthyroidism (with the rare exception of TSH-induced hyperthyroidism), the elevated thyroid hormone concentrations inhibit TSH secretion; TSH concentrations should be unmeasurably low. Unfortunately, as is the case with many polypeptide hormones, the normally low serum concentrations of TSH do not allow for reliable separation of "normal" from "low" TSH concentrations. It is for this reason that the TSH concentration in secondary hypothyroidism is often "normal" and that a baseline TSH determination is generally of no use in the diagnosis of hyperthyroidism.

The availability of TRH has allowed a multiplication factor to be applied to the "normal range" of TSH concentrations. Whereas basal TSH concentrations are

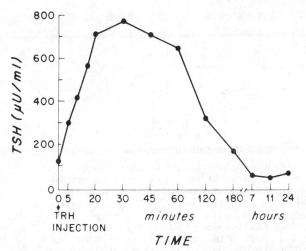

Figure 73. TRH test in primary hypothyroidism. Note elevated basal TSH concentration.

firms the diagnosis of primary hypothyroidism. If TSH concentration is normal, the TRH test will rarely be of help but may occasionally demonstrate an exaggerated TSH response. There does not seem to be a reliable way to diagnose early secondary hypothyroidism.

Radioactive Iodine Uptake

In recent years, the measurements of circulating thyroid hormone concentrations have largely replaced the use of isotopic studies in the assessment of thyroid function. However, once the diagnosis of hyperthyroidism has been made, the radioactive iodine uptake is important in the differential diagnosis (see Table 32). Radioactive iodine uptakes are of little use in the assessment of hypothyroid patients.

The thyroidal uptake of radioactive isotopes of iodine (^{123}I or ^{131}I) is measured 24 hours after the administration of the test dosage. Very little carrier (nonradioactive iodine, ^{127}I) is administered with the tracer. In general, the 24-hour RaI uptake is proportional to the avidity of the thyroid for iodine and inversely proportional to the iodide pool. In iodide deficiency states, the TSH rises and iodide avidity is increased; furthermore, the iodide pool is decreased, and, hence, the 24-hour RaI uptake is elevated. Conversely, with excess iodide administration, the trapping by the thyroid gland is diminished and the tracer is diluted in a pool of inorganic iodide. Inorganic iodide 100 mg by mouth is sufficient to reduce the radioactive iodine uptake to nil. The increasing iodine content in our diets explains the gradual decline in the normal values of 24-hour RaI uptake, with our current normals being 10 to 30 per cent uptake at 24 hours (Fig. 75).

Thyroid images (scans) with radioactive iodine or with technetium-99 are still quite important. These allow a picture of the thyroid configuration and the identification of nodules and their separation into "cold" (less functional than normal tissue) or "hot" (more active than normal tissue) nodules.

often around 1 μU/ml, after intravenous injection of TRH, TSH rises to a mean peak value of around 13 μU/ml, an easily measured value (TRH test). In contrast, with hyperthyroidism (see Fig. 64), the low basal TSH does not rise after TRH injection. Twenty minutes after a TRH injection, one can now easily distinguish "normal" from hyperthyroid values. In primary hypothyroidism, the elevated TSH concentrations rise further after TRH injection as well (Fig. 73). However, in the face of an already elevated TSH concentration, TRH stimulation becomes superfluous. In very early primary hypothyroidism, as the TSH concentration rises but still remains "within normal limits," one would expect an exaggerated response to TRH injection as well.

Figure 74 provides a simple approach to the assessment of thyroid function. Serum T_4 and T_3 resin are simple screening tests. If both are elevated and the patient is clinically hyperthyroid, the diagnosis is confirmed. If the patient is clinically hyperthyroid and the serum T_4 and T_3 resin tests are normal, a T_3 by radioimmunoassay should be measured. If all tests are equivocal, a normal TSH response to TRH excludes the diagnosis of hyperthyroidism. If the patient is clinically hypothyroid and the serum T_4 and T_3 resin are normal, then an elevated TSH concentration con-

Tests of Thyroid Hormone Effect

Serum measurements of the thyroid hormone concentration accurately assess the quantity of hormone in the blood. Accurate assessment of thyroid hormone effect would be preferable under certain circumstances. Thyroid hormone resistance syndromes, for example,

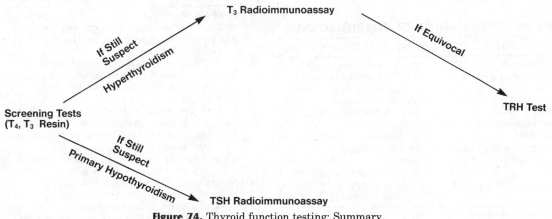

Figure 74. Thyroid function testing: Summary.

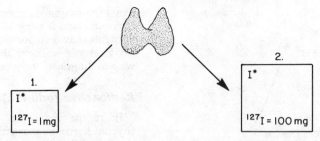

Figure 75. Radioactive iodine uptake. Assume the same thyroid gland in two patients, (1) and (2). Arbitrarily assume that the thyroid has the capacity to take up 1 mg of iodine in 24 hours. In the first patient, the total iodine pool (^{127}I) is 1 mg. Radioactive ^{123}I (I*) is added but does not increase total iodide. At 24 hours, all of the iodide (and hence all of the radioactive iodine) will be in the thyroid gland. The 24-hour radioactive iodine uptake will be 100 per cent. In patient (2) the radioactive iodine is now diluted in a pool of 100 mg of ^{127}I (non-radioactive iodine). In this patient, when the thyroid gland takes up 1 mg of iodide it will be only 1/100 or 1 per cent of the iodide pool and hence 1 per cent of the radioactive iodine added. The radioactive iodine uptake in this case will be 1 per cent. Note that the absolute amount of iodide taken up by the thyroid has not changed. The 24-hour radioactive iodine uptake measures only the *proportion* of the radioactive tracer taken up by the thyroid gland. Under ordinary circumstances, the excess iodide will also decrease the iodide trapping by the thyroid gland, further lowering the 24-hour RaI uptake.

may be confusing, with elevated thyroid hormone concentrations but without increased hormone effect.

A number of biological and biochemical assays are generally proportional to thyroid hormone effect but are relatively insensitive. These tests include basal metabolic rate (oxygen consumption at rest), speed of Achilles tendon relaxation, tests of myocardial contractility, and measurement of sex hormone–binding globulin. All increase in hyperthyroid states and decrease in hypothyroid states but are too crude for diagnostic purposes in most patients.

HYPERTHYROIDISM

Hyperthyroidism is a clinical syndrome, or group of diseases, characterized by an increased concentration of circulating thyroid hormones and their clinical effects. The excess hormone may be T_4 and/or T_3. Thyrotoxicosis is another term for hyperthyroidism.

Thyroid hormone enters all cells, and many cells have specific receptors for T_3 and T_4. It is, therefore, not surprising that thyroid hormone excess causes an array of clinical symptoms (Table 30). Increased sensitivity to catecholamines may account for part of this clinical picture as well. Increased oxygen consumption and increased calorigenesis make patients feel warm; weight loss develops despite an increased appetite and increased food intake. Increased myocardial rate and force of contraction lead to palpitations and may, ultimately, cause heart failure. Shortness of breath is in part a consequence of weakness of the respiratory muscles; arm and leg muscle weakness occurs as well. Bowel movements increase in frequency, and the menstrual flow diminishes. Emotional lability, nervousness, sleeplessness, and irritability are commonplace. The physical findings of hyperthyroidism are summarized in Table 30.

Although younger patients may demonstrate many of these findings, older patients may present with disease limited to a single organ system. A common presentation in older patients would be heart failure or arrhythmias in the presence of a goiter. Hyperthyroidism can cause heart disease or can exacerbate underlying coronary, valvular, or other heart disease.

Differential Diagnosis of Hyperthyroidism

There are many causes of hyperthyroidism, and these can be separated into several general classes, summarized in Table 31. The most common causes are

TABLE 30. MANIFESTATIONS OF HYPERTHYROIDISM

HISTORY	PHYSICAL EXAMINATION
Heat intolerance	Warm, moist skin
Weight loss with preserved appetite	Rapid pulse rate. Increased systolic, decreased diastolic blood pressure
Palpitations	Exophthalmos (proptosis)*
Shortness of breath	Goiter†
Increased frequency of bowel movements	Forceful precordium
Diminished menstrual flow	Muscle weakness
Emotional lability	Tremor
Anxiety	Brisk deep tendon reflexes
	"Constant motion"
	Pretibial myxedema*

*Found only in Graves' disease.
†Depending on etiology of hyperthyroidism.

TABLE 31. PATHOGENESIS OF HYPERTHYROIDISM

A. Excessive thyroid stimulation
  1. Graves' disease (IgG thyroidal stimulator)
  2. TSH-induced hyperthyroidism (TSH)
    a. Pituitary tumor
    b. Pituitary resistance to thyroid hormone
  3. Molar pregnancy thyroid stimulator (? HCG)
B. Autonomous thyroid gland function
  1. Toxic adenoma
  2. Toxic multinodular goiter
C. Excessive release of thyroid hormone from the thyroid gland
  1. Subacute thyroiditis (granulomatous thyroiditis; De Quervain's)
  2. Lymphocytic hyperthyroidism (spontaneously resolving hyperthyroidism, silent thyroiditis)
D. Nonthyroidal source of thyroid hormone
  1. Factitious hyperthyroidism (exogenous)
  2. Struma ovarii (ovarian teratoma)
  3. Metastatic follicular carcinoma of the thyroid

Graves' disease, toxic adenoma, toxic multinodular goiter, and lymphocytic hyperthyroidism.

Factitious Hyperthyroidism

The simplest form of hyperthyroidism is that due to ingestion of excess thyroid hormone. This often occurs in medical or paramedical personnel who surreptitiously consume large amounts of T_4 and/or T_3 in the hope of losing weight. These increased concentrations of T_4 or T_3 inhibit TSH release and cause the thyroid gland to decrease in size (Fig. 76). On physical examination, the thyroid gland is usually not palpable in such cases. The 24-hour radioactive iodine uptake is low or zero, an important clue to the diagnosis and a consequence of TSH inhibition. The finding of a decreased serum thyroglobulin concentration may be quite helpful for two reasons: (1) thyroglobulin is generally elevated in all other forms of hyperthyroidism, and (2) a low or zero radioactive iodine uptake is not specific for factitious hyperthyroidism (Table 32).

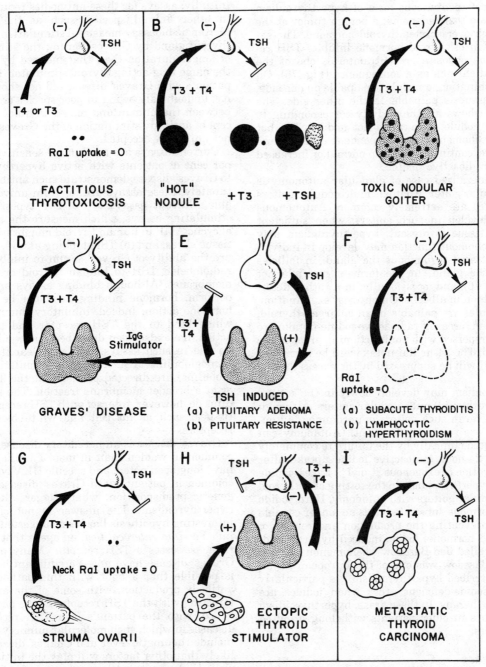

Figure 76. Pathogenesis of hyperthyroidism. (From Daniels, G. H., and Maloof, F.: In Frohlich, E. D. (ed.): Pathophysiology. Altered Regulatory Mechanisms in Disease. Philadelphia, J. B. Lippincott, 1984, p. 373.)

TABLE 32. HYPERTHYROIDISM WITH LOW OR ABSENT RADIOACTIVE IODINE UPTAKE*

1. Factitious (exogenous)
2. Subacute thyroiditis
3. Lymphocytic hyperthyroidism
4. Iodide-induced hyperthyroidism
5. Struma ovarii
6. Metastatic follicular carcinoma of the thyroid

*Any hyperthyroid patient recently exposed to large amounts of exogenous iodide may have a low or absent RaI uptake.

Toxic Adenoma and Toxic Multinodular Goiter

The simplest spontaneous form of hyperthyroidism is that due to a toxic adenoma, a benign tumor of the thyroid, which oversecretes thyroid hormone. The excess production of thyroid hormone inhibits TSH release, and the opposite or contralateral lobe of the thyroid gland shrinks as a consequence (Fig. 76). On physical examination, a nodule is palpable on one side; no thyroid tissue is palpable on the other side. The thyroid scan shows all the activity corresponding to the palpable nodule, a so-called hot nodule. The hot nodule is autonomous (i.e., independent of TSH) and will, therefore, continue to take up normal or increased amounts of (radioactive) iodine.

A more generalized case of glandular autonomy is the toxic nodular goiter. Nontoxic multinodular goiters (see page 578) are extremely common. Autonomous areas may develop in such goiters; when sufficient autonomous tissue is present, hyperthyroidism may develop. Autonomous function may develop in individual cells scattered throughout the gland, in follicles throughout the gland, in the form of multiple hot nodules (Fig. 76), and, occasionally, in a rather heterogeneous fashion in all cells. On physical examination, multiple nodules are palpable in an enlarged thyroid; on thyroid scan, areas of radioactive iodine uptake are variably interspersed with nonfunctioning areas of the thyroid gland. The 24-hr RaI uptake will be normal or elevated; TSH will be suppressed by the excess thyroid hormone.

Hyperthyroidism may develop slowly in the setting of nontoxic (euthyroid) multinodular goiters. Although hyperthyroidism in such goiters is uncommon, autonomous areas are relatively frequent. (Autonomy can be demonstrated clinically by the failure to completely suppress the 24-hour radioactive iodine uptake after the administration of exogenous T_4 or T_3.) Excess iodide may induce hyperthyroidism in the setting of euthyroid (nontoxic) nodular goiters with autonomy. Here, iodide serves as a hormone substrate but is no longer capable of normally preventing the production and release of excess thyroid hormone. Iodide-induced hyperthyroidism [the so-called Jod-Basedow phenomenon (Jod = iodide; Von Basedow was one of the European physicians who described hyperthyroidism)] is particularly common in iodide-deficient areas when iodides are introduced as therapy. In these areas, hyperthyroidism typically occurs in older patients with long-standing nodular goiters.

Graves' Disease

Graves' disease is an autoimmune disease and is the most common type of hyperthyroidism. This hyperthyroidism appears to be due to a class of immunoglobulins (polyclonal IgG) that interact with the TSH receptor and stimulate the thyroid gland to produce thyroid hormone and to enlarge. The growth-stimulating activity and the thyroid hormone–stimulating activity may not reside on the same immunoglobulin molecule.

The presence of these thyroid-stimulating antibodies was first suspected when mothers with active Graves' disease gave birth to newborns who were also hyperthyroid (neonatal Graves' disease). The neonatal hyperthyroidism spontaneously disappears over about three months, a time course consistent with the disappearance of maternal antibodies in the newborn. Initially, assays for these antibodies required bioassay in other animal species, such as the mouse. The McKenzie bioassay measured stimulation of the mouse thyroid gland by Graves' serum; the stimulation was of longer duration than that induced by TSH; hence, the name long-acting thyroid stimulator (LATS). Many patients with Graves' disease did not show such activity, undoubtedly owing to poor species cross-reactivity between the human and mouse thyroid, and the concept of antibody stimulation of the Graves' thyroid was not uniformly accepted.

Current assays are much more sensitive; at least 90 per cent of patients with active hyperthyroidism due to Graves' disease demonstrate such antibodies. Unfortunately, these assays are far from universally available. Current assays are of two types: (a) thyroid-stimulating assays, which measure the accumulation of cyclic AMP in human thyroid membranes or thyroid tissue slices, and (b) TSH-binding assays, which measure the ability of Graves' serum to inhibit binding of radiolabeled TSH to human thyroid or other tissue membranes. Although binding assays are simpler to perform, hormone binding need not be identical to hormone action. Indeed, inhibitory immunoglobulins, which bind to the TSH receptor and prevent TSH action, have also been described and would be demonstrated in such assays. It is not clear if Graves' immunoglobulins (TSI or thyroid-stimulating immunoglobulins) are directed precisely at the TSH receptor or at a broader membrane fraction. The immunoglobulins do, however, interact with TSH receptors in other tissues, such as fat cell and white blood cell TSH receptors.

Graves' disease is an hereditary disease that is more common in women than in men. Familial clusterings have long been noted, and specific HLA types are more common in patients with Graves' disease. Given this genetic predisposition, what triggers the episode of hyperthyroidism? The answer is not clear, but an interesting hypothesis has been suggested. The bacterium *Yersinia enterocolitica*, an agent that causes diarrhea, possesses a TSH receptor. Many patients with Graves' disease have anti-Yersinia antibody titers. It is possible that a bout with this pathogen leads to antibody production, with some of the antibodies interacting with the TSH receptor of the bacterium, and hence, with the patient's own TSH receptor. Other diseases in which such molecular mimicry is important include rheumatic fever and Chagas' disease. It seems likely that other factors will play the initiating role as well. Under certain circumstances, the TSI may disappear, leaving normal thyroid function.

Graves' disease is more than just hyperthyroidism.

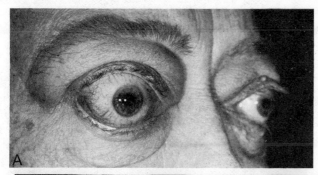

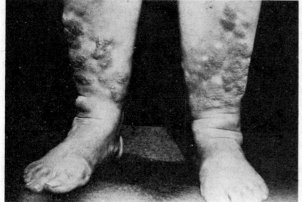

Figure 77. *A,* Exophthalmos (proptosis) in a patient with Graves' disease. *B,* Pretibial myxedema in a patient with Graves' disease.

Patients may develop inflammatory disease of the eye muscles and retro-orbital space, leading to "pop-eyes" (exophthalmos or proptosis) (Fig. 77*A*). This may be a cosmetic problem or it may lead to severe eye irritation, double vision, corneal exposure, and/or loss of vision due to optic neuropathy. Rarely, Graves' patients may develop a deposition of mucopolysaccharide over their anterior legs and dorsum of their feet, so-called pretibial myxedema (Fig. 77*B*). We are still ignorant of the pathogenesis of these eye and skin findings; they do not seem to be mediated by Graves' immunoglobulins. The eye findings appear to be autoimmune in nature, requiring cell-mediated immunity. Graves' disease is the only form of hyperthyroidism in which these changes occur.

Patients with active Graves' disease demonstrate a decrease in the suppressor-to-helper T-lymphocyte ratio. Other autoimmune diseases, such as pernicious anemia, myasthenia gravis, and Addison's disease, are more common in patients with Graves' disease as well.

The TSI stimulate the thyroid gland to overproduce thyroid hormone, which, in turn, inhibits the release of TSH from the pituitary gland. The thyroid gland is diffusely enlarged, often with a bruit due to the increased blood flow. The radioactive iodine uptake is elevated owing to TSI stimulation.

TSH-Induced Hyperthyroidism

TSH-induced hyperthyroidism is relatively rare, but increasing recognition is dependent upon the availability of sensitive TSH radioimmunoassays.

TSH-producing pituitary tumors account for about half of the reported cases. Some of these tumors make other hormones, and acromegaly or prolactin excess may occur simultaneously. These pituitary tumors appear to produce TSH autonomously and often overproduce the alpha subunit of the glycoprotein hormones (TSH-alpha). TSH output is fixed and generally does not increase with TRH stimulation or decrease with thyroid hormone administration.

Pituitary resistance to thyroid hormone is a somewhat more complicated entity. In this syndrome, the pituitary is uniquely resistant to thyroid hormone (Fig. 78), leading to a failure of the usual thyroid-pituitary feedback and continued TSH secretion. Thyroid hormone concentrations rise and eventually are able to partially restrain TSH production. The price paid, however, is a marked increase in serum concentrations of T_4, T_3, and their free hormones. Peripheral tissues are not resistant to the thyroid hormones, and clinical hyperthyroidism develops. The situation, although not necessarily the pathology, is analogous to pituitary Cushing's disease. The pituitary resistance is not absolute: further TSH suppression can result from the administration of exogenous T_3 or T_4; further TSH stimulation often occurs after TRH injection. The thyroid gland is often diffusely enlarged, but exophthalmos does not occur. The radioactive iodine uptake may be elevated or normal (Fig. 76). (See The Pituitary and Hypothalamus for a discussion of this rare entity.)

Subacute Thyroiditis (Granulomatous Thyroiditis; De Quervain's Thyroiditis (Fig. 76)

Subacute thyroiditis presents with a relatively acute thyroid inflammation; however, because the disease unfolds over several months, it is called *subacute* thyroiditis. In the wake of a viral illness or upper respiratory infection, the thyroid gland becomes painful, tender, and swollen, with pain often radiating to one or both ears. The involvement may be symmetrical or asymmetrical. In keeping with the inflammatory

ISOLATED PITUITARY RESISTANCE
TO THYROID HORMONE

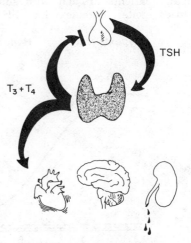

TSH

$T_3 + T_4$

Figure 78. Pituitary resistance to thyroid hormone leading to hyperthyroidism.

nature, the erythrocyte sedimentation rate is markedly elevated. Pathologically, the thyroid gland demonstrates follicular destruction with giant cells present.

Hormone leakage from the thyroid gland results in hyperthyroidism, its duration being limited by the thyroid hormone stores. T_4, T_3, and inactive iodinated compounds leak out of the thyroid gland. The increased T_4 and T_3 lead to hyperthyroidism and suppressed TSH release. The radioactive iodine uptake is low or zero, and new hormone synthesis does not occur. The thyroid gland shows intense inflammatory reaction with granuloma formation and giant cells.

As the thyroid gland damage progresses, the thyroid hormone stores are dissipated, and hypothyroidism ensues; if untreated, the hypothyroidism may last for several months (Fig. 79). Eventually, despite the severe inflammatory reaction, the thyroid regains normal function. The entire course (hyperthyroid, hypothyroid, euthyroid) may take up to a year but rarely recurs subsequently. The clinical clues to the diagnosis include the painful, exquisitely tender, often stony hard thyroid gland, the markedly elevated ESR, and the low or zero radioactive iodine uptake.

Lymphocytic Hyperthyroidism (Spontaneously Resolving Hyperthyroidism, Silent Thyroiditis)

The laboratory findings in patients with lymphocytic hyperthyroidism superficially resemble those of subacute thyroiditis. Here, too, the thyroid gland leaks thyroid hormone, leading to hyperthyroidism with a low or zero radioactive iodine uptake. Hypothyroidism then ensues, and then thyroid function returns toward normal (Fig. 79). Many important differences separate this entity from subacute thyroiditis, however.

Lymphocytic hyperthyroidism is not a postviral illness; it appears to be an autoimmune disease. The thyroid gland is infiltrated with lymphocytes and resembles that of Hashimoto's thyroiditis (chronic lymphocytic thyroiditis). Lymphocytic hyperthyroidism has a predilection for the postpartum period and may afflict as many as 5 per cent of all pregnant women in Japan. The postpartum prevalence has not been determined in the United States. As the disease runs its course, many patients are left with subtle thyroid abnormalities (goiter, chronic mild TSH elevation).

Furthermore, the entire sequence of hyperthyroid-hypothyroid-euthyroid may repeat itself again and again over many years. This disease is newly recognized and appeared to have increased in incidence during the late 1970s.

Clinical clues include a nontender, modestly enlarged thyroid, no exophthalmos, and a low or zero radioactive iodine uptake in the face of clinical hyperthyroidism. The sedimentation rate is normal or only moderately elevated.

Struma Ovarii

Struma ovarii is an extraordinarily rare entity with an interesting pathophysiology (Fig. 76). An ovarian tumor, usually a teratoma, develops thyroid elements that autonomously overproduce thyroid hormone. Pituitary TSH secretion is inhibited, and the thyroid shrinks. The radioactive iodine uptake over the thyroid gland is low or zero but will be normal or elevated if the pelvis is scanned.

The clue of a nonpalpable thyroid gland with hyperthyroidism and a low radioactive iodine uptake would ordinarily suggest factitious hyperthyroidism. An elevated thyroglobulin level would exclude that diagnosis and should lead to scanning over the pelvis for struma ovarii.

Molar Pregnancy

Trophoblastic moles secrete a substance that stimulates the thyroid gland and may cause hyperthyroidism. HCG shares a common alpha subunit with TSH, and many investigators believe that HCG is the thyroid stimulator in this condition. Recent evidence has shed some doubt on this concept; the true nature of the thyroid stimulator in this condition remains uncertain.

The thyroid gland is enlarged, and the radioactive iodine uptake is normal or elevated (Fig. 76). In a hyperthyroid pregnant patient, the presence of an abnormally enlarged uterus with an ultrasonogram suggesting molar pregnancy suggests this diagnosis.

Metastatic Follicular Carcinoma

Thyroid carcinoma tends to be an inefficient producer or a nonproducer of thyroid hormone. Occasionally,

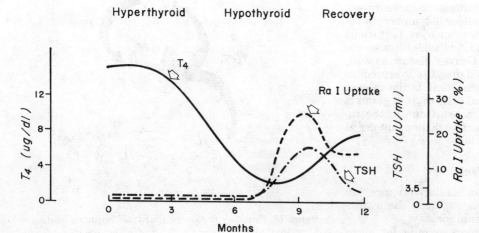

Figure 79. Time course of subacute thyroiditis or lymphocytic hyperthyroidism.

however, well-differentiated follicular carcinomas may be present in sufficient bulk to lead to hyperthyroidism. The excess thyroid hormone inhibits TSH and thyroidal secretion, leading to a low radioactive iodine uptake (Fig. 76).

Ectopic Thyroid Hormone Production

Although struma ovarii and metastatic thyroid carcinoma are "ectopic sources" of thyroid hormone, they represent ectopic thyroid tissue rather than "ectopic hormone production." Although polypeptide hormones are often overproduced by malignancies, thyroid (and steroid) hormones are not. The complicated series of enzymes and cofactors necessary for thyroid hormone production are unlikely ever to be reproduced in a nonthyroidal neoplasm.

LABORATORY EVALUATION OF HYPERTHYROIDISM

Hyperthyroidism is generally associated with an elevated serum thyroxine and free thyroxine or free thyroxine index. Patients with Graves' disease, toxic adenoma, or toxic multinodular goiter demonstrate disproportionately increased thyroid secretion of T_3; hence, the ratio of T_3 to T_4 in the circulation increases. Thus, hyperthyroidism is characterized by increased concentrations of both T_4 and T_3. Occasionally, the serum T_4 and free T_4 or free T_4 index are normal in hyperthyroidism, with T_3 alone being elevated, so-called T_3-toxicosis. Patients with hyperthyroidism who develop concurrent medical illnesses may have impaired peripheral conversion of T_4 to T_3, lowering the serum T_3 concentration to the normal range. Such hyperthyroid patients with elevated T_4 and free T_4, but normal T_3 concentrations, are called "T_4-toxic."

Although TSH is suppressed in almost all patients with hyperthyroidism, basal measurements are of little use apart from the diagnosis of TSH-induced hyperthyroidism. A TRH test is a useful means of excluding conventional hyperthyroidism, with a normal TSH response to TRH excluding all but the rare TSH-induced hyperthyroidism.

The radioactive iodine uptake and scan is of great value in the differential diagnosis of hyperthyroidism. The hyperthyroid syndromes with low or absent 24-hour RaI uptake are summarized in Table 32. In addition, any hyperthyroid patient recently exposed to large amounts of iodide (e.g., angiography or intravenous pyelography) will have a spuriously low or absent RaI uptake.

THERAPY OF HYPERTHYROIDISM

The therapy of hyperthyroidism depends upon the etiology. It will be discussed only briefly in this book, which is largely devoted to pathophysiology. Stopping thyroid hormone is sufficient in factitious hyperthyroidism; delivery of the trophoblastic mole will eliminate the hyperthyroidism due to a molar pregnancy. The hyperthyroidism of subacute thyroiditis and lymphocytic hyperthyroidism will spontaneously abate, although glucocorticoids may accelerate the return to normal in the latter instance. TSH-secreting pituitary tumors will require pituitary surgery or radiation; struma ovarii will require ovarian surgery.

Graves' disease, toxic adenoma, and toxic nodular goiter require specific therapy with medication, radioactive iodine, or surgery. The antithyroid drugs propylthiouracil and methimazole block thyroidal synthesis of thyroid hormones. They effectively treat the hyperthyroid state, with a delay of weeks to months due to the release of preformed stored thyroid hormone. When Graves' hyperthyroidism is treated with these drugs, the TSI may disappear; when the drugs are stopped, patients may remain euthyroid (up to 50 per cent of patients). Although current data *suggest* that these agents are directly immunosuppressive, the change from the hyperthyroid to the euthyroid state may itself change T lymphocyte cell function. The benefits of the antithyroid drugs are temporary when used to treat toxic adenoma or toxic nodular goiter; hyperthyroidism will recur when these agents are stopped. Iodide-induced hyperthyroidism is an exception to this rule; after therapy of the hyperthyroidism with antithyroid drugs, patients may remain euthyroid once the excess iodide has left the thyroid gland and the circulation.

Ablative therapy with ^{131}I is safe and effective and has been used for more than 40 years. The principal particle release by ^{131}I is a beta emission (90 per cent of the energy), which has an extremely short path length. This allows large amounts of radiation (5,000 to 10,000 rads) to enter and stay in the thyroid gland with relatively small amounts of radiation passing through surrounding tissues. ^{131}I therapy in Graves' disease radiates the entire thyroid gland. Most patients become euthyroid by three months. After one year, approximately 50 per cent of the patients will be hypothyroid; after 20 years, 75 per cent or more will be hypothyroid.

With radioactive iodine therapy of the toxic adenoma, all of the radioactive iodide enters the active side. In such cases, the contralateral (suppressed) side eventually resumes normal function and permanent hypothyroidism is rare. With toxic nodular goiters, autonomous and suppressed areas coexist. Hypothyroidism is uncommon after radioactive iodine therapy for toxic nodular goiter.

Surgery for Graves' disease requires great skill; if sufficient tissue is removed to treat the hyperthyroidism, hypothyroidism usually develops. Care must be taken to protect the parathyroid glands as well as the recurrent laryngeal nerves. The removal of a toxic adenoma is a simpler operation, requiring surgery on only one side of the thyroid gland. The suppressed side would be expected to return to normal function. Patients with toxic nodular goiters can be treated with subtotal thyroidectomy. Surgery is dangerous in patients with untreated hyperthyroidism. Patients should be pretreated with antithyroid drugs or with beta-adrenergic blocking agents for safe surgery.

Other forms of therapy are adjunctive or experimental: (1) Beta-adrenergic blocker agents provide immediate relief of some symptoms; they ameliorate the tachycardia, palpitations, tremor, nervousness, and occasionally the muscle weakness. Although the thyroid hormone concentrations do not dramatically change, the patients feel somewhat better. (2) The damaged thyroid gland is particularly sensitive to the inhibitory effects of iodides. After radioactive iodine therapy for Graves' disease, the addition of inorganic iodides (supersaturated solution of potassium iodide, SSKI) can accelerate the return to the euthyroid state. (3) Lithium has been used experimentally to inhibit thyroid hormone release as a primary modality of hyperthyroidism therapy or after the administration of radioactive iodide.

At this time, there is no absolutely specific therapy for Graves' disease; i.e., none of the therapies can reliably inhibit the production of TSI. Although the therapy for Graves' hyperthyroidism is effective if imperfect, the eye and skin changes of Graves' disease are not influenced by our therapy.

HYPOTHYROIDISM

PRIMARY HYPOTHYROIDISM

Primary hypothyroidism is a clinical syndrome characterized by thyroid failure leading to a decreased concentration of circulating thyroid hormone with a concomitant rise in TSH concentration. Whether patients with the low T_3 syndrome (i.e., inhibition of T_4-to-T_3 conversion) should be called "hypothyroid" is an interesting but unanswered question.

The symptoms of hypothyroidism are often vague or nonspecific. Most patients with weight gain, fatigue, constipation, depression, and/or apathy will not have thyroid gland failure. Cold intolerance, hair loss, dry skin, muscle cramps, failing memory, paresthesias (pins and needles), and poor balance are only slightly more specific. Menstrual irregularities, particularly heavy menses, are quite common. On physical examination, the presence of a goiter, puffy eyelids, and delay in the deep tendon reflexes may be the only clues (Table 33).

When profound hypothyroidism is present, the patient is said to have "myxedema" or to be "myxedematous" (myxedema = mucinous edema). Mucopolysaccharides deposit in the subcutaneous tissues of profoundly hypothyroid patients, their clearance being dependent upon thyroid hormone. This is a generalized phenomenon, not to be confused with the localized pretibial myxedema of Graves' disease. Such patients may develop deep husky voices and hearing loss. Profoundly hypothyroid patients may go into coma and die, particularly when given sedating agents or when coexisting diseases are present.

Although decreased cardiac output is common in primary hypothyroidism, cardiac failure is not. Profound hypothyroidism can lead to pericardial effusions, but pericardial tamponade is rare. The diastolic hypertension is probably due to increased total peripheral resistance, possibly related to decreased beta-adrenergic or increased alpha-adrenergic receptors. Low density lipoprotein cholesterol levels are elevated in hypothyroidism, presumably due to decreased clearance as a consequence of decreased LDL receptors. Hypothyroid patients with hypertension and elevated cholesterol are prone to accelerated atherogenesis. The clearance of digoxin is decreased in hypothyroid patients, making them much more sensitive to cardiac glycosides.

If hypothyroidism is present at birth and not diagnosed, irreversible mental retardation may develop. Children who develop hypothyroidism usually begin to lag in their school work. Growth fails in such children, and the epiphyses may become stippled if the hypothyroidism is severe and untreated.

Etiology of Primary Hypothyroidism

Primary hypothyroidism can be simply divided into cases with enlarged thyroid glands (goitrous) and those without. The most common forms of primary hypothyroidism are Hashimoto's thyroiditis (goitrous) and various forms of thyroid ablation, such as radioactive iodine and surgery (nongoitrous) (Table 34).

Hashimoto's Thyroiditis (Chronic Lymphocytic Thyroiditis, Autoimmune Thyroiditis)

Hashimoto's thyroiditis is the most common form of spontaneous hypothyroidism. This autoimmune disease occurs primarily in women and is often found in families in conjunction with Graves' disease. Antithyroid antibodies are present and are directed against various thyroidal components (e.g., thyroid microsomes, thyroid colloid, thyroglobulin) and are useful in the diagnosis of Hashimoto's thyroiditis when present in high titer. They do not appear to cause the hypothyroidism, however. The hypothyroidism appears to be due to cell-mediated immunity, although occasionally TSH receptor–blocking antibodies seem to play an important role.

The thyroid gland is usually diffusely enlarged with a prominent pyramidal lobe and a rubbery or firm consistency. The goiter is due to lymphocytic infiltra-

TABLE 33. MANIFESTATIONS OF HYPOTHYROIDISM

HISTORY	PHYSICAL EXAM
Fatigue	Slow pulse
Cold intolerance	Diastolic hypertension
Weight gain	Dry skin or puffy "myxedematous skin"
Menstrual irregularities, often with increased flow	Puffy eyes with loss of lateral third of eyebrows
Muscle cramps	Exophthalmos*
Paresthesias	Goiter or surgical scar or non-palpable thyroid†
Impaired hearing	
Ataxia	Delay in relaxation phase of deep tendon reflexes
Apathy, poor memory, depression	

*Previously treated Graves' disease; occasionally in Hashimoto's thyroiditis.

†See etiology of primary hypothyroidism.

TABLE 34. ETIOLOGY OF PRIMARY HYPOTHYROIDISM

GOITROUS	NON-GOITROUS
Hashimoto's thyroiditis (chronic lymphocytic thyroiditis)	Radioactive iodide for Graves' disease
Congenital biosynthetic defects	Surgical thyroidectomy
Goitrogens	Congenital athyreosis
Transient	External radiation for neoplasms
a. Subacute thyroiditis	Atrophic thyroiditis (? variant of Hashimoto's thyroiditis)
b. Lymphocytic hyperthyroidism	
Iodide deficiency*	

*Not in the United States.

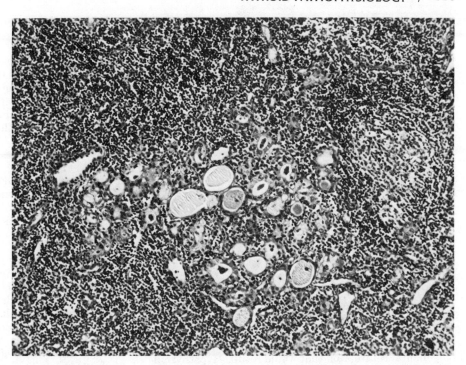

Figure 80. Pathology of Hashimoto's thyroiditis. There is a marked atrophy of the parenchyma, with shrunken residual follicles irregularly disposed in a stroma heavily infiltrated with lymphoid cells. Note the germinal center at the right (× 160).

tion (Fig. 80) as well as TSH stimulation of the remaining responsive thyroid cells. The thyroid gland is not tender or painful. Early in the disease, the TSH will be elevated, with normal T_4 concentrations. Later, more profound hypothyroidism may develop. Patients with Hashimoto's thyroiditis are particularly sensitive to the inhibitory effects of iodides; excess iodides can precipitate profound hypothyroidism.

Some patients with severe hypothyroidism are found to have thyroid atrophy, occasionally in association with circulating antithyroid antibodies. This situation may represent a variant of Hashimoto's thyroiditis.

Hashimoto's thyroiditis is more common in patients with other autoimmune diseases, such as pernicious anemia, vitiligo (autoimmune loss of pigment from the skin), Addison's disease, and others.

Hereditary Biosynthetic Defects

Hereditary defects in the biosynthesis of thyroid hormone are quite rare, but are important because of the insights they provide into the biochemistry of thyroid hormone biosynthesis. All are recessively inherited and lead to underproduction of thyroid hormone with increased TSH release and subsequent goiter development. The goiter is not present at birth but develops during the first few years of life. The following defects have been well described (see Fig. 61): (1) iodide transport defect with a failure of iodide trapping; (2) iodide organification defect; when associated with eighth nerve deafness it is known as Pendred's syndrome; (3) defect in the coupling of mono- and diiodotyrosine; (4) iodotyrosine dehalogenase defect, leading to a failure to reclaim iodide from MIT and DIT and an iodine deficiency type picture; (5) abnormal serum iodopeptides in which nonthyroglobulin iodinated proteins are released from the thyroid gland. This may be a defect in the synthesis or structure of thyroglobulin. Theoretically, the iodide transport defect and the iodotyrosine dehalogenase defect

might be treated with supplemental iodide; for simplicity, all these defects are treated with thyroid hormone.

Goitrogens

A goitrogen is any substance that interferes with thyroid hormone synthesis or release and leads to a goiter. Goitrogens rarely cause hypothyroidism. Certain foodstuffs, such as cabbage, contain a natural goitrogen, although the concentration is too low to cause goiters in humans. The antithyroid drugs (thionamides) propylthiouracil and methimazole can cause hypothyroidism. When hyperthyroid patients are overtreated with these agents, the TSH concentration may eventually rise with further goiter enlargement. Lithium inhibits thyroid hormone release and causes transient TSH elevations in as many as 30 per cent of patients chronically treated with this agent. The patients who develop more profound hypothyroidism on lithium often have positive antithyroid antibodies and may be a group with subclinical Hashimoto's thyroiditis. The sulfonylureas (used as oral hypoglycemic agents) and para-aminosalicylic acid (used in the therapy of tuberculosis) are weak goitrogens, inhibiting the synthesis of thyroid hormone. Iodide in excess can result in hypothyroidism in susceptible individuals, including those with Hashimoto's thyroiditis, Graves' disease treated with radioactive iodine, and those previously treated with external radiation for head and neck cancers. Rarely, individuals develop goiters and mild hypothyroidism upon exposure to iodide without demonstrable underlying thyroid disease. Whether these patients have subtle underlying organification defects is not clear.

Iodide Deficiency

Iodide deficiency is not a problem in the United States; however, endemic iodine deficiency goiter remains an important public health problem throughout the world. When iodide intake drops below 100 µg/day, iodide deficiency is said to be present. Mild deficiency occurs with 50 to 100 µg/day, moderately severe with 20 to 50 µg/day. Compensatory mechanisms prevent clinically important hypothyroidism until iodine intake falls below 20 µg/day, although goiters occur with mild iodide deficiency. The thyroidal compensations for low iodide uptake are reviewed in Table 28. As T_4 concentration begins to fall, TSH rises, a goiter develops, and the thyroid gland synthesizes relatively more T_3. With more profound iodine deficiency, serum T_4 and T_3 will decline and hypothyroidism may develop.

Transient Hypothyroidism

The transient hypothyroidism that occurs as part of subacute thyroiditis and lymphocytic hyperthyroidism has already been discussed. Some patients with lymphocytic hyperthyroidism will develop long-term mild hypothyroidism with goiter.

Nongoitrous Hypothyroidism

Approximately one in 5000 children will be born without a thyroid gland. Early detection of neonatal hypothyroidism through screening programs leads to prompt therapy and prevents the otherwise irreversible mental retardation that would result. Hypothyroidism is common after radioactive iodine therapy for Graves' disease, with thyroid failure continuing to appear for decades after such therapy. It is less well known that patients successfully treated with antithyroid drugs for Graves' disease may develop hypothyroidism decades after the drugs have been stopped (approximately 15 per cent). This is probably a consequence of autoimmune thyroid destruction, suggesting that Graves' disease and Hashimoto's thyroiditis may be different ends of a changing autoimmune spectrum. Many patients develop mild hypothyroidism after external radiation to the neck for malignancies such as Hodgkin's disease. This is particularly common if the patients have also undergone lymphangiography; the continued presence of the dye in lymph nodes leads to the release of iodide into the circulation, which serves to inhibit thyroid hormone biosynthesis and release.

Laboratory Diagnosis

The earliest and most sensitive indicator of thyroid gland failure is a rising TSH. The elevated serum TSH concentration rises even higher after TRH administration (Fig. 73). With a failing thyroid gland, serum thyroxine declines through the broad range of "normal" values and may eventually become "subnormal"; low T_4 concentrations are a relatively late finding. The thyroid gland often responds to a rising TSH with increased T_3 output; therefore, T_3 levels may remain normal until severe thyroid failure results. With T_3 concentrations being preserved, the patient may exhibit few clinical symptoms, a state that has been called "compensated hypothyroidism." The high TSH concentration is diagnostic of thyroid failure, however, and therapy is generally initiated when the elevated TSH concentration is discovered.

The presence of a goiter with positive antithyroid antibodies and an elevated TSH concentration is virtually diagnostic of Hashimoto's thyroiditis.

Occasionally, patients with profound primary hypothyroidism will develop myxedema of the pituitary gland. Although the basal TSH concentration is elevated, it may rise even higher after thyroid hormone replacement is initiated and then decline into the normal range. The concept of pituitary myxedema can be extended to other pituitary hormones, as some patients with profound primary hypothyroidism have impaired maximal release of growth hormone, gonadotropins, and ACTH. These abnormalities are usually reversed with thyroid hormone therapy.

With longstanding primary hypothyroidism, thyrotrope hypertrophy or hyperplasia may lead to pituitary and sella turcica enlargement. This may be confusing, leading to suspicion of a pituitary tumor. The elevated serum TSH, in the face of low or low-normal thyroid function, places the defect at the thyroid and not at the pituitary level. To confuse the matter further, serum prolactin may be modestly elevated in patients with profound hypothyroidism. Whether this is related to a TRH effect or has another mechanism is not clear at this time. In children, longstanding primary hypothyroidism may result in precocious puberty, galactorrhea, and striking enlargement of the sella turcica. All these abnormalities reverse with thyroid hormone therapy. The cause of the precocious puberty is still unclear; the galactorrhea is undoubtedly caused by prolactin excess.

Therapy of Primary Hypothyroidism

The therapy of hypothyroidism is a true replacement therapy. The long half-life of T_4, without significant day-to-day variation in serum T_4 concentrations, makes replacement therapy nearly perfect. Synthetic L-thyroxine is the therapy of choice. Approximately half the orally administered dosage is absorbed, making replacement dosage about twice the normal T_4 secretory rate (replacement therapy = 100 to 200 µg/day). Once absorbed into the circulation, T_4-to-T_3 conversion proceeds as it would with the naturally secreted hormone. Since thyroidal T_3 secretion is no longer contributing to serum hormone concentrations, adequately treated hypothyroid patients often have higher serum T_4 and free T_4 concentrations than do normal individuals, but have approximately normal T_3 concentrations (i.e., higher T_4 concentration is necessary with exogenous therapy to reach the same T_3 concentration). The dosage of L-thyroxine need not be adjusted for illnesses or for pregnancy.

Many other thyroid hormone preparations have been used over the years. Beef and pig thyroid extracts contain variable concentrations of T_4 and T_3 as well as other nonactive ingredients. Triiodothyronine-containing preparations result in peaks and troughs of T_3 concentrations, which are not at all physiological. There seems to be little place for these preparations in chronic therapy for most patients.

SECONDARY HYPOTHYROIDISM (PITUITARY HYPOTHYROIDISM) AND TERTIARY HYPOTHYROIDISM (HYPOTHALAMIC HYPOTHYROIDISM)

The secondary forms of hypothyroidism (pituitary and hypothalamic) cause thyroid failure as a conse-

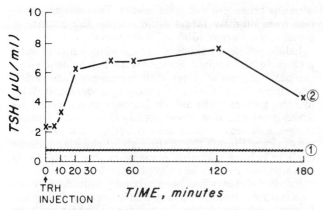

Figure 81. TRH test in secondary forms of hypothyroidism. (1) Pituitary (secondary) hypothyroidism. (2) Hypothalamic (tertiary) hypothyroidism. These are theoretical responses that may not be observed clinically.

quence of TSH insufficiency. With pituitary insufficiency, administration of TRH should not cause a rise in TSH concentration; in contrast, hypothalamic hypothyroidism reflects TRH deficiency and a delayed increase should be expected (Fig. 81). In the illustrations, the theoretical curves are depicted; however, in practice it is often impossible to separate hypothalamic from pituitary hypothyroidism on biochemical grounds.

Secondary hypothyroidism may be an isolated pituitary or hypothalamic defect. More commonly, however, multiple trophic hormone deficiencies are present. The hypothyroidism is usually less severe than that found with primary hypothyroidism. No goiter is present. Signs of decreased ACTH and cortisol, decreased gonadotropins in adults, and decreased growth hormone in children often coexist with signs of hypothyroidism.

Laboratory Diagnosis

Any patient with pituitary or hypothalamic disease should be screened for secondary forms of hypothyroidism. A low serum T_4 and free T_4 or free T_4 index in the presence of a "normal" or "low" TSH concentration is diagnostic of secondary forms of hypothyroidism. It is very important to exclude patients with TBG deficiency, since such patients will have a low T_4 and a normal TSH concentration. The diagnosis of TBG deficiency is based on the finding of an elevated T_3 resin test; with hypothyroidism, the T_3 resin test should be low.

When the diagnosis of secondary hypothyroidism is made, a TRH test adds little further diagnostic information. Attention should then be directed to the assessment of the other pituitary hormones. Cranial CT scanning will help delineate structural abnormalities if they are present.

Therapy of Secondary Hypothyroidism

The diagnosis of secondary forms of hypothyroidism was quite difficult before the TSH radioimmunoassay was developed. Initially, all patients with hypothyroidism were treated with thyroid hormone; most improved, but some died. The patients who died had secondary hypothyroidism. In patients with secondary hypothyroidism, the administration of thyroid hor-

mone may precipitate adrenal insufficiency. Thyroid hormone accelerates the metabolism (degradation) of cortisol; with an intact pituitary-adrenal axis, an increase in ACTH secretion and cortisol production should ensue. In patients with pituitary ACTH insufficiency, no such compensation can occur and adrenal crisis may develop. In the patient with known thyroid and adrenal insufficiency, cortisol replacement therapy should be given first. If a hypothyroid patient requires emergency treatment and it is not clear whether the hypothyroidism is primary or secondary, then glucocorticoid (cortisol) should be given along with thyroid hormone until the diagnosis has been clarified.

THYROID HORMONE RESISTANCE (END ORGAN REFRACTORINESS TO THYROID HORMONE)

A rare familial syndrome has been described with certain manifestations of hypothyroidism despite elevated circulating levels of T_4, free T_4, and T_3. TSH concentrations are normal or elevated in the face of high peripheral hormone concentrations; TSH concentrations rise further after TRH administration. Despite elevated circulating hormone concentrations, these patients are not clinically hyperthyroid, and, in fact, demonstrate several features suggesting hypothyroidism, including deaf-mutism and stippled epiphyses. These patients appear to have resistance to thyroid hormone involving the pituitary gland as well as peripheral tissues (Fig. 82). Although abnormalities of the nuclear T_4 and T_3 receptors have been postulated, when directly assayed, they appear to be normal. A post-receptor defect may explain the hormone resistance.

When peripheral tissues are normally responsive to thyroid hormone, but the pituitary gland is resistant to feedback, hyperthyroidism develops (see page 571 and Fig. 78). The combination of elevated T_4, free T_4, elevated T_3, and elevated TSH can suggest TSH-in-

PERIPHERAL TISSUE RESISTANCE TO THYROID HORMONE

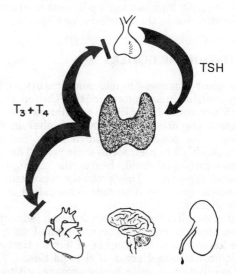

Figure 82. Resistance to thyroid hormone at the peripheral and pituitary levels.

duced hyperthyroidism or resistance to thyroid hormone (with hypothyroidism). The clinical assessment of the patient is extremely important if the laboratory studies are to be properly interpreted.

Low T$_3$ Syndromes and Sick Euthyroid Syndromes

Are patients with impaired T$_4$-to-T$_3$ conversion and low serum T$_3$ concentrations hypothyroid? During starvation, impaired T$_4$-to-T$_3$ conversion is associated with a decreased basal metabolic rate. When T$_3$ is physiologically replaced, the basal metabolic rate returns to normal. Despite falling concentrations of T$_3$, the serum T$_4$ remains normal and TSH does not rise. The pituitary at least does not sense hypothyroidism.

Critically ill patients with multisystem diseases, often associated with sepsis and hypotension, would be expected to have low serum T$_3$ concentrations. A surprising finding in some of these patients is a low serum T$_4$ concentration, the so-called sick euthyroid syndrome. The free thyroxine index and free T$_4$ by radioimmunoassay are often low as well; the serum free T$_4$ by equilibrium dialysis is usually normal. The low serum T$_4$ concentrations are in part related to decreases in binding proteins, in part to circulating inhibitors of T$_4$ binding, and in part are unexplained. There is no adequate explanation for the low free T$_4$ concentrations. The serum TSH is not elevated in these circumstances, and the TSH response to TRH is either normal or slightly blunted. The normal serum TSH concentration argues against, but does not exclude, a hypothyroid state. Serum reverse T$_3$ concentrations are markedly elevated in these patients, in contrast to subnormal values found in patients with primary or secondary hypothyroidism. Clinicians and scientists are still undecided about the proper approach to this syndrome. Many believe that any changes in serum hormone concentrations, and hence metabolic rate, under these circumstances are homeostatic. Others believe that thyroid hormone replacement should be instituted. All agree that the sick euthyroid patients with low T$_4$ concentrations are critically ill and have an exceedingly high (up to 90 per cent) mortality rate, presumably due to their underlying diseases.

MULTINODULAR GOITERS

The most common thyroid abnormality is the so-called multinodular goiter. In the United States at least 5 per cent of the living population carries this diagnosis; the prevalence is much higher in autopsy studies. This condition is much more common in women, with a 7 to 1 female-to-male ratio. The patients are generally euthyroid; hence, the name nontoxic multinodular goiter. This probably represents a heterogeneous group of disorders (also called colloid or simple goiters).

Pathologically these goiters contain adenomas or adenomatous changes, cystic areas filled with colloid or old hemorrhage, thick areas of fibrous tissue, areas of calcifications, and areas of thyroid tissue. The cellular population is quite heterogeneous, with areas of slowly dividing or rapidly dividing cells; some are capable of trapping and organifying iodide (hot areas),

whereas other are not (cold areas). Thyroids range in size from slightly larger than normal (20 grams) to massively enlarged (500 to 1000 grams).

Iodide deficiency was once the leading cause of such goiters in the United States. With iodide deficiency, the pathogenesis of goiter with decreasing T$_4$ secretion and rising TSH is relatively easy to understand. Why are the goiters nodular? The answer is not clear. As areas grow and new blood vessels form, small hemorrhages and scarification may develop, with extensive networks of fibrous tissue throughout the gland. Some authors believe that this network of scar tissue leads to a nodular pattern as cells proliferate.

Iodide deficiency has been virtually eliminated from this country through dietary and other iodine sources. Pockets of iodine deficiency goiter account for millions of patients with nodular goiter throughout the world.

The etiology of nontoxic multinodular goiters in iodide-*sufficient* areas is still uncertain. Many authors believe that decreased thyroidal secretion with concomitant TSH elevation lies at the heart of this process. Dietary goitrogens or biosynthetic defects, leading to impaired iodination of thyroglobulin, have been suggested as causes for this putative impaired thyroid function. According to this hypothesis, the thyroid gland grows and becomes nodular under the influence of TSH, as it does in the iodide deficiency setting. This sequence of events seems to account for the nodular goiters in patients with hereditary defects of thyroid hormone biosynthesis (see page 575). However, the concentration of TSH is not elevated in patients with nontoxic multinodular goiters. It is common to find elevations of serum thyroglobulin and increased serum ratios of T$_3$ to T$_4$ in patients with such goiters, suggesting defective thyroglobulin iodination. Before eliminating TSH as a factor in the development of these goiters, it should be noted that iodide deficiency and perhaps defective iodination of thyroglobulin renders the thyroid gland hypersensitive to TSH. It is possible that TSH hypersensitivity might exist in patients with multinodular goiters. During the early stages of these goiters, prior to extensive scarring, cystification, and hemorrhage, thyroid hormone suppression of TSH secretion will frequently lead to a decrease in goiter size.

TRH testing has been quite useful in the study of patients with multinodular goiters. If the "normal" TSH concentrations in these patients represent subtle TSH elevations within the normal range, then an exaggerated TSH response to TRH administration would be expected. In fact, the TSH response to TRH is either normal or blunted, strongly arguing against subtle basal TSH increases. Why should the TRH response be blunted or absent in as many as 25 per cent of these patients? This suggests TSH suppression by slightly supraphysiological concentrations of thyroid hormone. Thyroid hormone production in the absence of TSH stimulation implies autonomy of function at the cellular, follicular, nodular, or glandular level. These patients with autonomous function appear to be the ones who develop hyperthyroidism when exposed to excess iodide. Thyroid hormone suppression therapy for nodular goiters will not work in patients with autonomy and already suppressed TSH concentrations; such therapy will result in hyperthyroidism from the addition of exogenous to endogenous hormone. Glandular autonomy can be predicted by performing a TRH test (blunted TSH response) or measuring the failure of suppression of radioactive iodine uptake after administration of T_4 or T_3 for short periods of time.

The goiter in patients with Hashimoto's thyroiditis will often mimic multinodular goiter, with the bumpy texture of the Hashimoto's gland suggesting nodularity. An elevated serum TSH points strongly toward the diagnosis of Hashimoto's thyroiditis, being quite rare in patients with multinodular goiters.

THERAPY OF MULTINODULAR GOITERS

Suppressive therapy of multinodular goiters may prevent growth or allow shrinkage of the gland. If glandular autonomy is present, then thyroid hormone therapy should be avoided or discontinued if already begun. The vast majority of patients have no disability from nontoxic multinodular goiter. If the thyroid is large enough, tracheal compression with shortness of breath, esophageal compression with difficulty swallowing, or cosmetic embarrassment may necessitate surgical removal. Thyroid cancer rarely develops in multinodular goiters in the absence of a prior history of head and neck irradiation.

Hyperthyroidism is relatively uncommon in the large population of patients with multinodular goiters. As the goiters continue to grow and the patients get older, a higher percentage may develop hyperthyroidism. Autonomous thyroid cells continue to accumulate iodine even in the absence of TSH; normal thyroid cells may accumulate small amounts of iodide in the absence of TSH as well. If enough cells are present, as in a huge goiter, there may be sufficient thyroid hormone production to result in hyperthyroidism, either as a consequence of increased normal cells or more likely increased numbers of autonomous cells.

THYROID NODULES AND THYROID CANCER

Thyroid carcinoma is a clinically uncommon disease, with approximately 20 new cases per million people per year in the United States. In contrast, microscopic papillary carcinoma of the thyroid gland, like microscopic prostatic carcinoma, is quite common and of little clinical significance. When surgical or autopsied thyroid glands are subject to ultrathin sectioning, 10 per cent or more will have microscopic foci of papillary carcinoma.

When a clinically isolated thyroid nodule is discovered, the patient and the physician are concerned about the possibility of thyroid carcinoma. When multiple thyroid nodules are palpable, a multinodular goiter is diagnosed, with little additional concern about carcinoma.

The thyroid scan provides a straightforward triaging approach to the isolated thyroid nodule. A scan with either pertechnetate-99 or ^{123}I allows a thyroid image to be obtained. Occasionally, additional nodules are discovered on scanning, and the diagnosis is changed to multinodular goiter and treated accordingly. Isolated nodules may be "hot" or "cold."

A hot nodule is one that takes up more radioactivity than the normal surrounding thyroid tissue (Fig. 83A). As hot nodules grow, they tend to produce more thyroid

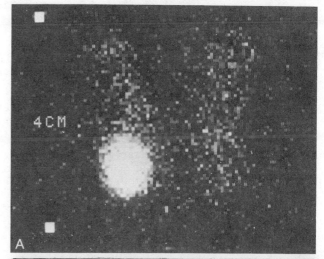

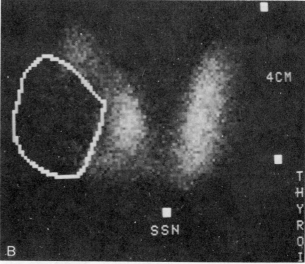

Figure 83. *A,* ^{123}I scan of a hot thyroid nodule (white circular area). The remainder of the thyroidal uptake is suppressed by the hyperfunctioning nodule. The distance between the white squares is 4 cm. *B,* ^{123}I scan of a cold thyroid nodule. The nodule is highlighted by the white circular marking. The nodule takes up less radioactive iodine than the remainder of the thyroid gland. SSN refers to suprasternal notch.

hormone and lead to progressive TSH suppression and shrinkage of the contralateral lobe. Hot nodules are "never" malignant. They may progress and cause hyperthyroidism; however, the vast majority are associated with the euthyroid state. When all of the radioactivity on a scan is localized to one side and the patient is euthyroid, additional studies are necessary to be sure that this is a hot nodule rather than agenesis of one lobe. Demonstration of a suppressed TSH response to TRH or a failure to suppress the radioactive iodine uptake after T_3 or T_4 administration confirms the diagnosis of a hot nodule. Fewer than 10 per cent of individuals with hot nodules go on to develop hyperthyroidism.

Cold thyroid nodules are those that take up less radioactive tracer than normal tissue (Fig. 83B). "All thyroid cancers are cold" on radioactive iodine scanning; however, most (90 to 95 per cent) cold nodules are benign. The benign cold nodules are usually follicular or cellular adenomas, which often develop central degeneration and cystification or hemorrhage. These nodules may be "cold" because they have lost their ability to trap iodine (the majority) or because they have lost their ability to organify the iodine already trapped (the minority). Despite the loss of synthetic function, these nodules often contain TSH receptors and may grow under the influence of TSH and shrink with the administration of thyroid hormone. Pertechnetate-99 (technetium thyroid scan) is trapped but not organified; hence, some thyroid nodules that are capable only of iodine trapping (rarely including thyroid cancers) are hot on technetium scanning but cold on radioiodine scanning.

Once an isolated thyroid nodule has been shown to be cold, the direct approach of needle aspiration for cytological examination or needle biopsy for histological examination should be carried out. This allows maximum selectivity in deciding which patients require surgery.

Radiation Therapy

Thyroid nodules, including benign and malignant thyroid neoplasms, are much more common in patients who have been exposed to low dose external radiation therapy. In years past, such therapy was commonly used for enlarged tonsils and adenoids, enlarged thymus glands, severe acne, and other benign diseases. Doses of several hundred to one thousand or more rads were commonly employed; however, even lower doses are associated with increased incidence of neoplasms, without a threshold dosage of radiation being demonstrated. Five to 40 years after such therapy, thyroid nodules appear with increased frequency. The annual incidence increases with the radiation dosage and with time, but seems to decrease again after 30 years. Up to 20 per cent of patients will develop such nodules, with a third of these being malignant; many of the malignancies are occult papillary thyroid carcinomas. It seems likely that these tumors develop slowly as a result of nuclear genetic damage. Primary hyperparathyroidism seems to be more common after such radiation; other benign and malignant head and neck tumors have been identified as well.

Higher doses of radiation (over 4000 rads) used to treat head and neck malignancies more commonly lead to hypothyroidism, but neoplasms are occasionally noted in this situation as well. In rats, external radiation therapy to the thyroid leads to elevated TSH levels and thyroid cancer. When thyroid hormone is given to suppress TSH after such radiation, cancer development is prevented. Whether TSH suppression will prevent neoplasms in previously irradiated patients is uncertain; it is not completely effective if many years have lapsed after the radiation therapy.

Fortunately, malignant thyroid neoplasms have not been reported to be increased in incidence after low (scanning) or high (therapeutic) doses of radioactive iodine.

THYROID CANCERS

Papillary carcinoma of the thyroid is the most common type of thyroid cancer and is one of the most benign. The tumor forms frondlike papillae and often has typical small areas of calcification known as psammoma bodies (Fig. 84). Papillary carcinoma typically spreads to regional lymph nodes; unlike other malignancies, the presence of nodal involvement does not adversely influence the patient's prognosis. If the primary tumor is contained within the capsule of the thyroid gland, it is hard to demonstrate a shortened life expectancy, even in the presence of nodal metastases. Microscopic papillary carcinoma is very common at surgery and at autopsy but is of no clinical conse-

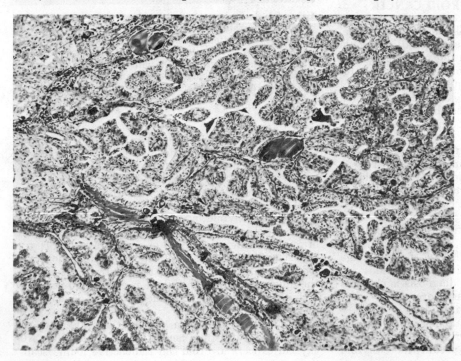

Figure 84. Papillary carcinoma of the thyroid: microscopic pathology (× 100). An almost pure papillary architecture is typically intermixed with an occasional follicle containing darkly staining colloid (center). Small calcifications (psammoma bodies) are scattered about, most evident in the lower right area.

quence. It is unusual for patients to die of papillary carcinoma of the thyroid; when death occurs, it is generally due to extensive local invasion in older patients.

Follicular carcinoma is the second most common type of thyroid carcinoma. Although papillary carcinoma may contain small or large amounts of follicular elements, such tumors behave biologically like papillary carcinoma if papillary elements are present. Although such tumors are called mixed papillary-follicular carcinoma by some authors, it is reasonable to refer to them all as papillary carcinomas.

Pure follicular carcinoma may be extremely well differentiated, mimicking normal thyroid follicles, the malignant nature being demonstrated only by showing capsular or vascular invasion or spread to distant locations. Occasionally, biopsies of lung nodules will be read as "normal thyroid tissue," only the location confirming the malignant nature of the lesion. Other follicular carcinomas are more cellular with less follicular differentiation. Follicular carcinoma tends to spread via the blood stream, with pulmonary and lytic bony metastases being most common. Although small follicular carcinomas with minimal vascular invasion have an excellent prognosis, the larger and more aggressive carcinomas are lethal.

The well-differentiated thyroid carcinomas can take up radioactive iodine and may be treated with therapeutic doses of ^{131}I. If these carcinomas present as "cold nodules," how can they take up radioactive iodine? First, "cold" is a relative term, referring only to uptake relative to the normal surrounding thyroid tissue. Second, some of these carcinomas are capable of trapping and organifying significant amounts of iodine only after they are stimulated by TSH. As a clinical problem, this means that one must remove all the normal thyroid tissue at surgery or destroy residual normal thyroid tissue with radioactive iodine. The patient is then allowed to become hypothyroid and is scanned with radioactive iodine (^{131}I) when the TSH is markedly elevated. Under these circumstances, distant metastases can often be induced to take up radioactive iodine. Occasionally, particularly in children, diffuse pulmonary metastases can be completely eradicated with repeated treatments with ^{131}I and cure can be achieved.

Both papillary and follicular carcinomas seem to grow in response to TSH. An integral part of the therapy for these tumors is TSH suppression to minimize growth. To be sure that adequate suppression is achieved, a TRH test might be performed. Measurement of the serum thyroglobulin may be of benefit in following such patients, high concentrations suggesting persistent or recurrent thyroid carcinoma.

Anaplastic thyroid carcinomas are among the most virulent tumors, with most patients dying in less than six months. *Medullary carcinoma* of the thyroid has an intermediate prognosis (better than anaplastic, but not as good as well-differentiated thyroid carcinomas). It is a malignancy of the parafollicular rather than follicular cells and is discussed in the Introduction. *Lymphomas* of the thyroid gland seem to be increasing in frequency and often develop in the setting of underlying Hashimoto's thyroiditis.

REFERENCES

Bernal, J., and Refetoff, S.: The action of thyroid hormone. Clin Endocrinol 6:227, 1977.

Chopra, I. J.: Euthyroid sick syndrome: Abnormalities in circulating thyroid hormones and thyroid hormone physiology in nonthyroid illness (NTI). Medical Grand Rounds 1:201, 1982.

Degroot, L. J., and Niepomniszcze, H.: Biosynthesis of thyroid hormone: Basic and clinical aspects. Metabolism 26:665, 1977.

Evered, D., and Hall, R. (eds.): Hypothyroidism and goitre. Clin Endocrinol Metab 8(1):1, 1979.

Ingbar, S. H.: Effects of iodine: Autoregulation of the thyroid. In Werner, S. C., and Ingbar, S. H. (eds.): The Thyroid. 4th ed. Hagerstown, Md., Harper and Row, 1978, p. 206.

Ingbar, S. H., and Woeber, K. A.: The thyroid gland. In Williams, R. H. (ed.): Textbook of Endocrinology. 6th ed. Philadelphia, W. B. Saunders Co., 1981, p. 117.

Jackson, I. M. D.: Thyrotropin-releasing hormone. N Engl J Med 306:145, 1982.

Kidd, A., Okita, N., Row, V. V., and Volpé, R.: Immunologic aspects of Graves' and Hashimoto's diseases. Metabolism 29:80, 1980.

Larsen, P. R.: Triiodothyronine: Review of recent studies of its physiology and pathophysiology in man. Metabolism 21:1073, 1972.

Larsen, P. R., Silva, J. E., and Kaplan, M. M.: Relationships between circulating and intracellular thyroid hormones: Physiological and clinical implications. Endocr Rev 2:87, 1981.

Moreley, J. E.: Neuroendocrine control of thyrotropin secretion. Endocr Rev 2:396, 1981.

Oppenheimer, J. H.: Thyroid hormone action at the cellular level. Science 203:971, 1979.

Studer, H., and Ramelli, F.: Simple goiter and its variants: Euthyroid and hyperthyroid. Endocr Rev 3:40, 1982.

Taurog, A.: Biosynthesis of iodoamino acids. In Greep, R. O., and Astwood, E. B. (eds.): Handbook of Physiology. Sec. 7, Endocrinology. Vol. III, Thyroid. Washington, D.C., American Physiological Society, 1974, p. 101.

Volpé, R. (ed.): Thyrotoxicosis. Clin Endocrinol Metab 7(1):1, 1978.

Wartofsky, L., and Burman, K. D.: Alterations in thyroid function in patients with systemic illness: The "euthyroid sick syndrome." Endocr Rev 3:164, 1982.

Williams, E. D. (ed.): Pathology and management of thyroid disease. Clin Endocrinol Metab 10(2):233, 1981.

Adrenal Cortex

LLOYD AXELROD

ANATOMY

The adrenal glands are paired triangular structures measuring approximately 5 by 2 by 1 cm and weighing 4 to 5 grams each in the normal adult. The adrenal glands are located in the retroperitoneal area, embedded in fat, sitting astride the upper pole of each kidney. The adrenal gland contains two distinct endocrine organs: the adrenal cortex and the adrenal medulla. The pathophysiology of the adrenal cortex is the subject of this chapter.

Embryologically, the adrenal cortex develops from the coelomic epithelium on the medial surface of the urogenital ridge. During the early stages of gestation, the adrenal cortex consists predominantly of the fetal adrenal cortex; the cells of the outer (permanent) cortex are immature at this time. The fetal adrenal cortex lacks the enzymatic ability to convert pregnenolone to progesterone, but in fetal life progesterone from the placenta is available to the fetal adrenal gland. Consequently, the enzymatic conversion of pregnenolone to progesterone is unnecessary and cortisol is synthesized using progesterone as the substrate. The outer adrenal cortex matures during the second half of gestation, but the fetal adrenal cortex persists until neonatal life. The fetal cortex involutes within a few weeks of birth, and rapid proliferation of the outer cortex occurs.

The mature adrenal cortex consists of three distinct zones: the outermost *zona glomerulosa,* the middle *zona fasciculata,* and the innermost *zona reticularis* (Fig. 85). The zona glomerulosa is composed of closely packed polygonal acidophilic groups of cells, which are the source of aldosterone. The zona fasciculata is a thick layer made up of large polygonal cells arranged in cords, one cell thick and surrounded by blood sinusoids. These basophilic cells are the source of cortisol and adrenal androgens. The zona reticularis contains groups of lightly and darkly staining cells in a reticular pattern.

FUNCTIONS OF THE ADRENAL CORTEX

The adrenal cortex synthesizes and secretes four classes of steroid hormone: *glucocorticoids, mineralocorticoids, androgens,* and *estrogens.* Cortisol is the principal glucocorticoid in man. Aldosterone is the principal mineralocorticoid. Dehydroepiandrosterone sulfate and androstenedione are the principal adrenal androgens. The adrenal cortex also synthesizes very small quantities of estrogens, specifically estradiol and estrone.

Cortisol is essential for life. Glucocorticoids have a host of biological and physiological effects, including the characteristic effect on plasma glucose, for which this class of compounds is named; effects on carbohydrate, protein, lipid and water metabolism; effects on blood pressure; a variety of effects on virtually every tissue and cell in the body; and characteristic ability to inhibit ACTH secretion. The mechanism of action of glucocorticoid hormones is described in the introductory chapter on endocrinology.

GLUCOCORTICOIDS

STRUCTURE AND BIOSYNTHESIS

Glucocorticoids are 21-carbon steroid molecules (Fig. 86). Glucocorticoids characteristically have hydroxyl groups at the 11, 17, and 21 positions, a keto group at the 3 position, and a double bond at the 4-5 position. The steroid hormones are derived from cholesterol; the term *steroid* reflects this origin. Although cholesterol used for steroid synthesis in the adrenal cortex is synthesized in part by the adrenal gland, it is derived predominantly from circulating low density lipoprotein (LDL) and high density lipoprotein (HDL) particles. The LDL particles bind to specific receptor sites on the cell surface and are internalized along with the receptors into vesicles that fuse with liposomes. The liposomes contain degradative enzymes that release cholesterol for use by the adrenocortical cell. The

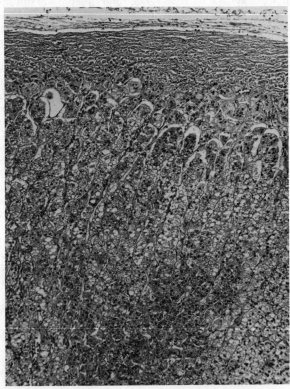

Figure 85. Photomicrograph of the normal human adrenal cortex, demonstrating the zona glomerulosa (beneath the capsule at top of figure), the zona fasciculata, and the zona reticularis. (Hematoxylin and eosin stain, × 340.) (Figure generously provided by Dr. Theodore H. Kwan, Beth Israel Hospital, Boston, Mass.)

mechanism of HDL uptake is not known. The pathways of steroid hormone synthesis in the adrenal cortex are presented in Figure 86. The shaded area in this figure depicts a common core of intermediates derived from cholesterol that are further converted to the characteristic products of the adrenal cortex: glucocorticoids, mineralocorticoids, androgens, and estrogens. The interconversions shown are enzymatically regulated. The rate-limiting step for cortisol synthesis is the conversion of cholesterol to pregnenolone. Adrenocorticotropic hormone (ACTH) acts at this step by stimulating the enzymatic cleavage of the side chain at carbon 20 (20α-hydroxylase or desmolase step).

PHYSIOLOGY OF CORTISOL SECRETION

In normal adult subjects in the basal state (i.e., not subjected to stress), the cortisol production rate is

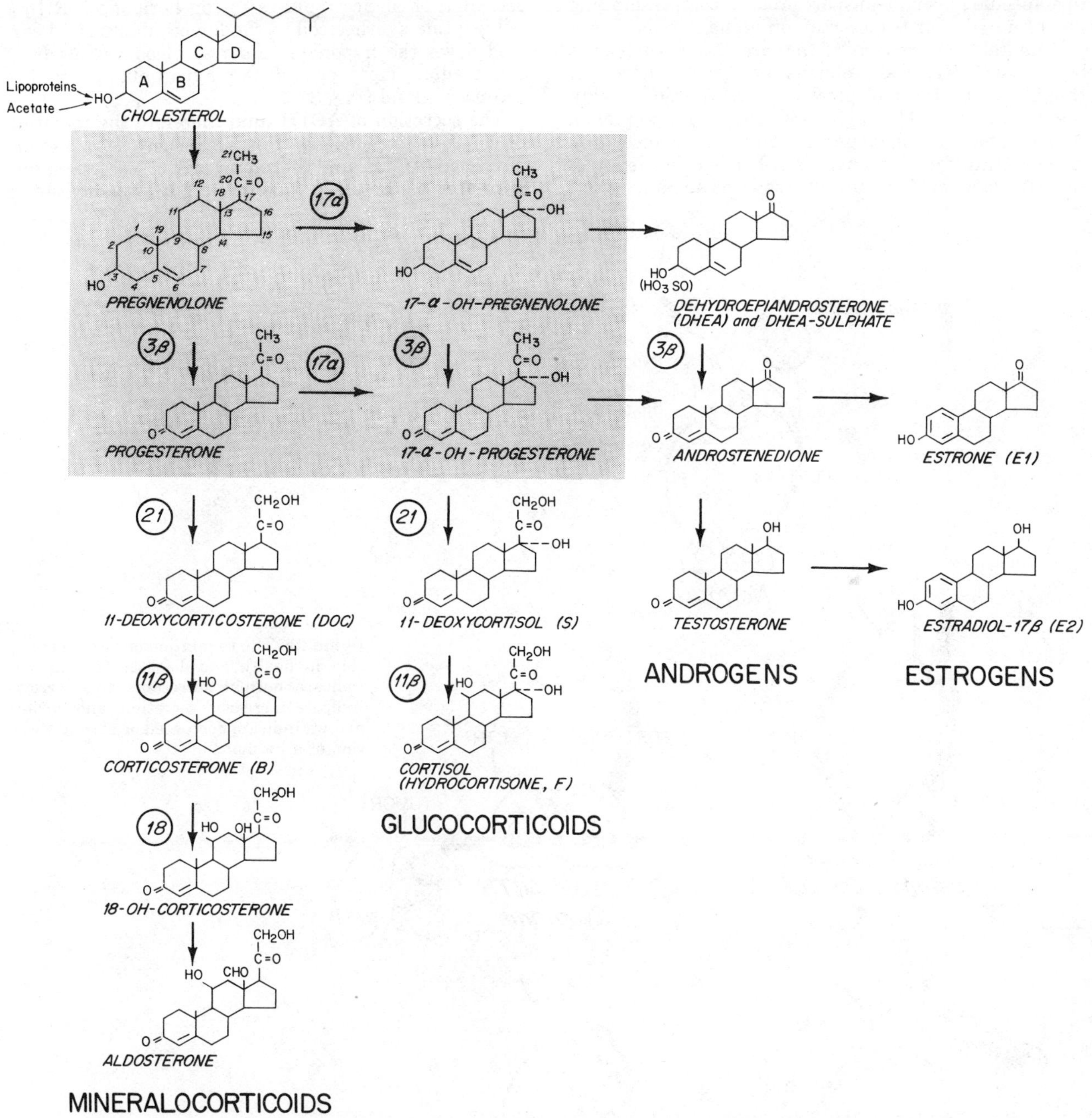

Figure 86. The structure and biosynthesis of steroid hormones in the human adrenal cortex. The letters designating the four rings of a steroid molecule are indicated for cholesterol; the numbers of the carbon atoms are shown for pregnenolone. Certain important enzymes are denoted as follows: 3β: 3β-hydroxysteroid dehydrogenase; 17α: 17α-hydroxylase; 21: 21-hydroxylase; 11β: 11β-hydroxylase; 18: 18-hydroxylase. The shaded area depicts a common core of intermediates that are further metabolized to produce the biologically active products of the adrenal cortex. The figure depicts in columns from left to right the synthesis of mineralocorticoids, glucocorticoids, androgens, and estrogens.

approximately 10 to 30 mg per day. The circulating half-life of cortisol is approximately 60 to 90 minutes. The biological duration of action of cortisol exceeds the duration of the steroid's presence in the circulation. This is consistent with the evidence that glucocorticoids bind to an intracellular receptor protein and exert their actions intracellularly by modifying the rate of transcription of RNA from the DNA template (see the introductory chapter in this section).

Within the circulation, cortisol is reversibly bound to a specific plasma transport protein, cortisol-binding globulin (CBG) or transcortin, an alpha$_2$ globulin. Approximately 90 per cent of the circulating cortisol is bound to CBG. The unbound or "free" cortisol is thought to be the biologically active fraction within the circulation. Although CBG may function as a reservoir for cortisol, its physiological role is uncertain, since certain families have an inherited deficiency of this transport protein with no apparent adverse effect.

REGULATION OF CORTISOL SECRETION
(see also Chapter on the Pituitary)

Since ACTH stimulates cortisol synthesis, cortisol secretion reflects ACTH secretion. ACTH is a 39-amino acid peptide secreted by the cells of the anterior pituitary gland. It is one of several biologically active peptides derived from pro-opiomelanocortin, a large precursor (see Fig. 36).

Secretion of ACTH is in turn regulated by the secretion of corticotropin-releasing hormone (CRH), a polypeptide synthesized in the hypothalamus and carried down the hypophyseal-portal blood vessels from the median eminence of the hypothalamus to the pituitary gland (Fig. 87).

The secretion of ACTH (and therefore the secretion of cortisol) is pulsatile (Fig. 88). There is a diurnal rhythm of ACTH (and therefore cortisol) secretion; this is related to the sleep-wake cycle but probably not to

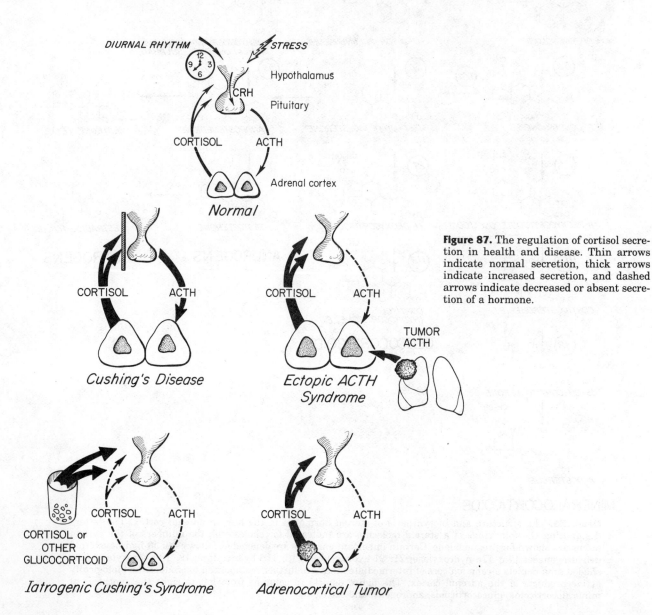

Figure 87. The regulation of cortisol secretion in health and disease. Thin arrows indicate normal secretion, thick arrows indicate increased secretion, and dashed arrows indicate decreased or absent secretion of a hormone.

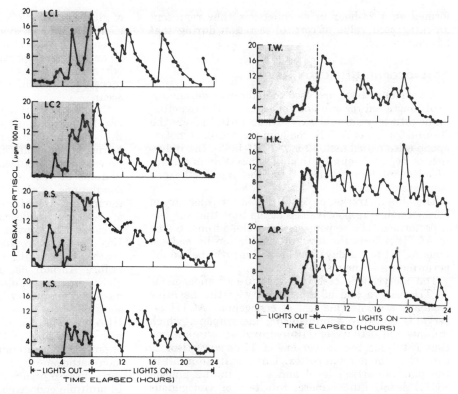

Figure 88. Episodic secretion of cortisol in man. The figure depicts the plasma cortisol values of normal subjects obtained every 20 minutes for 24 hours. The time period designated "lights out" is the sleep period available. (Reprinted from Weitzman, E. D., Fukushima, D., Nogeire, C., Roffwarg, H., Gallagher, T. F., and Hellman, M.: J Clin Endocrinol Metab 33:14–22, 1971.)

light. Thus, the pulsations of ACTH (and therefore cortisol) secretion occur more frequently and with greater amplitude early in the day than they do at the end of the day or in the early hours of sleep.

ACTH secretion is subject to negative feedback regulation by cortisol (or synthetic glucocorticoids). It is not known whether this occurs predominantly at the level of the pituitary or at the level of the hypothalamus, or both. Glucocorticoids inhibit ACTH secretion from isolated pituitary cells, but it is not known whether this is a major or minor component of the negative feedback regulatory system in vivo.

One cannot overemphasize the importance of the diurnal rhythm in adrenocortical physiology. The diurnal rhythm is disrupted only by stress or by Cushing's syndrome. The diurnal rhythm supersedes the negative feedback system. For example, during the first two to four hours after the onset of sleep, plasma cortisol levels fall to low or even undetectable levels, but this is not accompanied by a rise in ACTH secretion. A comparable fall of the plasma cortisol level just before the normal time of awakening or just after awakening is associated with a surge of ACTH secretion. An understanding of the diurnal rhythm is important in the evaluation of patients with adrenocortical disease and in the proper use of glucocorticoid therapy (see below).

Stress can override both the diurnal rhythm and the negative feedback system. Stress may take the form of emotional or physical stimuli, intercurrent illness, or hypoglycemia.

Glucocorticoids have the characteristic ability to inhibit ACTH secretion. The glucocorticoid-induced inhibition of ACTH secretion has two components. The early component of this feedback inhibition occurs within the first 15 minutes of an increase in the glucocorticoid level and is rate-dependent; it reflects the rate of increase of the circulating glucocorticoid level. Thereafter, the inhibition of ACTH secretion is dose-dependent; it reflects the circulating level of the glucocorticoid.

MEASUREMENT OF CORTISOL LEVELS AND OF CORTISOL SECRETION

Plasma cortisol levels are measured by radioimmunoassay. Under certain circumstances (i.e., when cross-reaction with other substances is a concern), a double isotope derivative assay may be used. Fluorescence methods and colorimetric methods have also been employed. The unbound or "free" cortisol in the circulation is excreted into the urine; measurements of urinary free cortisol are sometimes used in the evaluation of adrenocortical function.

A common method of estimating the cortisol production rate involves the measurement of urinary 17-hydroxycorticosteroids (17-OHCS). The major metabolites of cortisol are tetrahydrocortisol and tetrahydrocortisone, in which the double bonds in the A ring of cortisol or cortisone have been reduced. These metabolites are excreted in the urine as water-soluble conjugates of glucuronic acid. Prior to assay, the steroids are liberated from glucuronic acid by incubation with beta-glucuronidase. The metabolites are then measured by the phenylhydrazine reaction, which detects the presence of the 17, 20, 21-dihydroxyacetone side chain. Under most circumstances the urinary excretion of 17-OHCS is a reliable estimate of the cortisol secretory rate. Approximately one third of the cortisol that is secreted by the adrenal glands is excreted in the form of the metabolites measured by this reaction. Because these measurements are customarily performed on a 24-hour urine collection, they represent an integrated value of cortisol secretion during that 24-hour period.

ADRENOCORTICAL FUNCTION TESTS

A variety of tests are used to determine adrenocortical functional reserve and the status of the hypothalamic-pituitary-adrenal axis. These tests include the administration of ACTH, the administration of metyrapone (also called metopirone or SU-4885), the induction of hypoglycemia by the administration of insulin (insulin intolerance test), and the dexamethasone suppression test.

The administration of ACTH is a direct measure of adrenocortical responsiveness at the time that the test is performed. The responsiveness of the adrenal cortex to ACTH reflects the level of stimulation by endogenous ACTH in the days, weeks, and months before the performance of the test.

The metyrapone test is a measure of endogenous ACTH reserve and of the integrity of the negative feedback system. This test of endogenous ACTH reserve is done by administering metyrapone, which inhibits the activity of 11β-hydroxylase, the enzyme that catalyzes the conversion of 11-deoxycortisol to cortisol in the adrenal cortex. This results in a fall in the plasma cortisol level and a rise in the plasma ACTH level. Furthermore, this test of endogenous ACTH reserve is performed by measurement of adrenocortical secretions or their derivatives. That is, one uses the patient's own adrenal cortex as a bioassay organ for the measurement of endogenous ACTH. This test is sometimes performed by measuring the plasma level of 11-deoxycortisol, which accumulates behind the block induced by metyrapone if the ACTH level rises appropriately during the course of the test. In other circumstances, one measures the urinary 17-OHCS. This test measures not only the metabolites of cortisol but also those of 11-deoxycortisol. In short, this test of endogenous ACTH reserve is performed by inhibiting the last step in cortisol synthesis and by using the patient's own adrenal glands as bioassay organs for the determination of endogenous ACTH activity.

The dexamethasone suppression test employs this synthetic glucocorticoid to determine the suppressibility of ACTH secretion. The effects of dexamethasone are assessed by measurement of the adrenocortical response to endogenous ACTH using urinary 17-OHCS, urinary free cortisol, or plasma cortisol levels. Dexamethasone is not measured in these assays.

DISEASES OF THE ADRENAL CORTEX

HYPOFUNCTION OF THE ADRENAL CORTEX

Adrenocortical insufficiency may result from Addison's disease (primary adrenal insufficiency), secondary adrenal insufficiency, and congenital adrenal hyperplasia. In addition, one may encounter selective aldosterone deficiency (see below).

Primary Adrenal Insufficiency (Addison's Disease). Addison's disease denotes the clinical disorder caused by destruction or ablation of adrenocortical tissue from any cause. Typically, one has the features of glucocorticoid deficiency and mineralocorticoid deficiency. In women, evidence of adrenal androgen insufficiency (i.e., loss of axillary and pubic hair) may also be detectable. Approximately 90 to 95 per cent of total adrenocortical tissue must be destroyed by the disease process for the clinical features of Addison's disease to occur.

CAUSES OF PRIMARY ADRENAL INSUFFICIENCY (Table 35). Idiopathic (autoimmune) adrenal insufficiency is the commonest cause in the United States and Western Europe. In populations in which tuberculosis is highly prevalent, tuberculosis may be the leading cause. Populations at risk include recently arrived immigrant populations in the United States. Patients with autoimmune adrenal insufficiency have a high incidence of associated endocrine disorders, including thyroid disease (thyrotoxicosis, primary hypothyroidism, Hashimoto's thyroiditis), diabetes mellitus type I, idiopathic hypoparathyroidism, and premature ovarian failure. Antiadrenal antibodies occur with high prevalence in this population, and abnormalities in cell-mediated immunity are detectable. Idiopathic Addison's disease occurs in high association with certain HLA antigens, notably HLA-DR3 and DR4. The common association of these HLA antigens with other organ-specific autoimmune diseases suggests a common pathogenesis. In some patients, idiopathic Addison's disease occurs as part of two distinct disorders. In multiple endocrine insufficiency type I, the onset is typically in the first or second decade of life, and Addison's disease is associated with idiopathic hypoparathyroidism and mucocutaneous candidiasis. There is no association with specific HLA antigens. In multiple endocrine insufficiency type II the onset is typically in the middle years of life, and Addison's disease is associated with autoimmune thyroid disease and diabetes mellitus type I. There is in addition an association with the HLA-DR3 and DR4 antigens.

CLINICAL MANIFESTATIONS. Untreated Addison's disease is a fatal disorder. It may present insidiously with gradual progression of signs and symptoms, or it may present as an acute adrenal crisis, a medical emergency. Weakness (often profound), weight loss, anorexia, hyperpigmentation, hypotension, and hyponatremia are nearly always present. The hyperpigmentation is characteristically a bronze coloration most marked

TABLE 35. CAUSES OF ADRENAL INSUFFICIENCY

Primary (Addison's Disease)
  Idiopathic (autoimmune)
  Tuberculosis
  Bilateral total adrenalectomy
  Metastatic carcinoma
  Anticoagulant therapy
  Granulomatous disease (sarcoid, histoplasmosis)
  Sepsis
  Miscellaneous (amyloidosis, hemochromatosis)

Secondary
  Pituitary and hypothalamic disorders
  Glucocorticoid therapy
  Removal of adrenocortical tumor producing
    Cushing's syndrome with suppression of residual normal
    adrenal tissue

Congenital Adrenal Hyperplasia

over pressure points and in scars acquired after the onset of adrenal insufficiency. Salt craving, gastrointestinal symptoms, vitiligo, hypoglycemia, hyperkalemia, and azotemia are helpful when present but are frequently absent. In an acute adrenal crisis, the patient will have many of the above features, often in severe form, and in addition will have severe hypotension. An intercurrent illness or other stress may precipitate an adrenal crisis in a patient with Addison's disease.

DIAGNOSIS. The diagnosis of Addison's disease must be established with care, since this is generally a lifelong disorder with specific therapeutic implications. Addison's disease is uncommon, but the clinical features of Addison's disease occur in the differential diagnosis of many common clinical abnormalities. For this reason, an inexpensive and rapid screening test of high sensitivity is required. Fortunately, such a test exists: the rapid cosyntropin (Cortrosyn) test. In this test, synthetic alpha 1-24 ACTH is administered in a dose of 250 μg intravenously or intramuscularly. Plasma cortisol levels are obtained just before injection and 30 or 60 minutes later. A normal response is a plasma cortisol level of more than 18 μg/dl at 30 or 60 minutes. In addition, one may see an increment above the basal level in the plasma cortisol level of ≥ 7 μg/dl at 30 minutes and of ≥ 11 μg/dl at 60 minutes. These incremental values are applicable to normal, healthy, unstressed subjects. However, the cosyntropin screening test is often indicated in a patient with intercurrent illness. If the patient does not in fact have Addison's disease, he or she may have an increase in the basal plasma cortisol level due to the effects of stress on endogenous ACTH secretion. Thus, the absolute value at 30 and 60 minutes is a more reliable guide than the increment above the basal level. A normal response to this test rules out primary adrenal insufficiency; an abnormal result is an indication for further evaluation. These values are applicable to patients who may be ill but are not in shock or under comparable stress. In such patients, a plasma cortisol level of more than 30 μg/dl is expected.

If the screening test is abnormal, a definitive test for adrenal insufficiency is indicated. The screening test is not sufficient for this purpose. First, it would involve making the diagnosis of a lifelong disorder on the basis of a single laboratory determination. Second, when the patient with Addison's disease is properly treated, many of the clinical features are no longer apparent; a physician who sees the patient long after therapy has been instituted may be skeptical about the validity of the diagnosis. Thus, every patient with Addison's disease should have a definitive test performed and recorded once in his or her lifetime. In this test synthetic ACTH 25 units (250 μg) is infused in 500 ml of normal saline from 8:00 A.M. to 4:00 P.M. each day for three consecutive days; the 24-hour urine 17-OHCS or the plasma cortisol level at 4:00 P.M. is determined daily. Normal subjects achieve at least a three-fold increase over basal urinary steroid values and a plasma cortisol level above 45 μg/dl at 4:00 P.M. on the third day of the infusion. The ACTH must be administered in saline (to prevent water intoxication from a free water load in a patient with Addison's disease), and the patient must be treated with dexamethasone (e.g., 0.5 mg P.O. at 8:00 A.M. and 4:00 P.M.)

during each day of the test. This highly potent synthetic glucocorticoid prevents clinical deterioration while the test is performed and does not interfere with the determination of the plasma or urine steroid levels.

The differentiation between primary and secondary adrenocortical insufficiency is usually apparent from the clinical findings (such as hyperpigmentation and salt craving), from radiographic features (such as an enlarged sella turcica in secondary adrenal insufficiency), or from the plasma ACTH level if available. If not, the ACTH test may be extended for five days. Patients with primary adrenal insufficiency will fail to respond. Patients with secondary adrenal insufficiency will experience a gradual increase in response during the course of the test. Several modifications of this approach are in use.

In each instance, careful attention should be paid to the etiology of Addison's disease. This should include an evaluation for tuberculosis and for evidence of associated autoimmune disease.

TREATMENT. Addison's disease is a lifelong disorder with a normal life expectancy if properly treated. However, an adrenal crisis can be fatal and can deprive a patient of many years of otherwise healthy existence. Treatment includes the administration of a glucocorticoid such as cortisone acetate 15 to 50 mg per day, with half to two thirds given on arising and the balance in the early afternoon. Close attention must be paid to the total dose and to the timing of each dose to achieve optimal clinical results. Patients usually require fludrocortisone (9-α-fluorohydrocortisone, Florinef) 0.05 to 0.2 mg daily. In addition, patients must have an adequate intake of salt to provide substrate for the mineralocorticoid. Patients must have adequate identification such as a warning bracelet or necklace indicating the presence of Addison's disease and the necessity of steroid therapy. In addition, the patient and family must be educated about an appropriate response to intercurrent illness and other emergencies, including instruction in the method of injecting cortisol or another glucocorticoid in an emergency.

Secondary Adrenal Insufficiency. Secondary adrenal insufficiency refers to adrenal insufficiency resulting from lack of normal stimulation by ACTH. The causes of secondary adrenal insufficiency are listed in Table 35. Since aldosterone secretion is regulated primarily by the renin-angiotensin system, aldosterone secretion is usually normal in secondary adrenal insufficiency. Thus, the patient will have the signs and symptoms of glucocorticoid deficiency with no evidence of mineralocorticoid deficiency. Typical manifestations are weakness, fatigue, emotional lability, and hypoglycemia. Since these are relatively nonspecific, the diagnosis is often overlooked.

In patients with pituitary tumors, other abnormalities generally precede or accompany ACTH deficiency (growth hormone deficiency, gonadotropin deficiency, and prolactin excess). ACTH and TSH deficiencies occur relatively late. In Sheehan's syndrome (pituitary infarction due to hemorrhage during or after parturition), the patient generally has panhypopituitarism (see chapter on the pituitary). Isolated ACTH deficiency occurs but is quite uncommon (except with glucocorticoid-induced suppression).

The diagnosis of secondary adrenal insufficiency requires assessment of ACTH reserve, evaluation for deficiency or excess of other pituitary hormones, and evaluation of the cause of the ACTH deficiency. The assessment of ACTH reserve generally involves the use of insulin-induced hypoglycemia (insulin tolerance test) or the metyrapone test. The insulin tolerance test has the advantage that growth hormone reserve can be tested concurrently. The disadvantages of this procedure include the need to induce symptoms of hypoglycemia and the fact that this test is contraindicated by a seizure disorder or cardiac disease. The metyrapone test does not test growth hormone reserve and frequently causes gastrointestinal upset.

The management of secondary adrenal insufficiency is the same as that of primary adrenal insufficiency except that mineralocorticoid replacement and a generous salt intake are not necessary. Of course, one must also treat the cause of the ACTH deficiency when possible.

Congenital Adrenal Hyperplasia. The term congenital adrenal hyperplasia refers to a group of disorders, each of which is characterized by the deficiency of a single enzyme in the cortisol synthetic pathway. In each instance, cortisol production is diminished. Consequently ACTH secretion increases, since the negative feedback regulation of ACTH secretion is intact. The increase in ACTH secretion causes adrenocortical hyperplasia and results in increased synthesis of steroids produced proximal to the locus of the enzyme deficiency. The manifestations of each syndrome depend upon the level of the defect. In general, the manifestations of these syndromes are attributable to a deficiency of substances beyond the enzymatic defect (e.g., cortisol) and to excessive accumulation of biologically active products proximal to the level of the defect. Examples of the effects of congenital adrenal hyperplasia on steroid synthesis are depicted in Figure 89.

In *21α-hydroxylase deficiency,* there is a diminution in the production of glucocorticoids and mineralocorticoids (Fig. 89*B*). Patients may exhibit the features of glucocorticoid insufficiency and of salt wasting (there is a non–salt losing form as well). Because of accumulation of precursors proximal to the defect, the production of adrenal androgens is increased. This results in ambiguous secondary sex characteristics in females and pseudo-precocious puberty (accelerated linear growth, early appearance of secondary sex characteristics, premature closure of epiphyses, but minimal testicular development) in males. Previously thought to be uncommon, this disorder is described with increasing frequency as a cause of hirsutism, infertility, menstrual irregularities, and occasionally mild virilization in pubertal and adult women.

In *11β-hydroxylase deficiency,* cortisol production is again diminished (Fig. 89*C*). In this condition, in contrast to the previously described disorder, patients develop mineralocorticoid excess due to the accumulation of 11-deoxycorticosterone (DOC) proximal to the level of the enzymatic defect. Consequently these patients, as adults, have hypertension and hypokalemic alkalosis. Hypertension seldom occurs in the first decade; infants often present with vomiting suggestive of pyloric stenosis and hyperkalemia. Here, too, adrenal androgens accumulate, causing ambiguous genitalia or virilization in females and pseudoprecocious puberty in males.

In patients with *17α-hydroxylase deficiency,* the production of glucocorticoids, androgens, and estrogens is deficient; mineralocorticoids accumulate because pregnenolone and progesterone are produced in excess and are diverted to the mineralocorticoid pathway (Fig. 89*A*). These patients have evidence of mineralocorticoid excess. Females have primary amenorrhea and fail to develop secondary sexual characteristics. Males are born with ambiguous genitalia due to androgen production insufficient to fully virilize the target tissues in utero.

All of these disorders respond to glucocorticoid replacement therapy, which decreases ACTH secretion and thus diminishes the excessive production of byproducts such as mineralocorticoids and androgens. Lifelong replacement of mineralocorticoid deficiency may also be required depending on the defect in question, since glucocorticoid replacement therapy may suppress endogenous mineralocorticoid production. In the 17α-hydroxylase deficiency, sex steroid replacement is needed at adolescence.

HYPERFUNCTION OF THE ADRENAL CORTEX— CUSHING'S SYNDROME

Causes of Cushing's Syndrome. Cushing's syndrome is the clinical disorder that results from prolonged exposure to excessive quantities of cortisol or another glucocorticoid. Cushing's syndrome has several causes: bilateral adrenal hyperplasia due to excessive ACTH secretion by the pituitary, ectopic production of ACTH by a tumor, an adrenocortical adenoma, an adrenocortical carcinoma, or glucocorticoid therapy in pharmacological doses for a prolonged period (Fig. 87).

By convention, when Cushing's syndrome is due to bilateral adrenal hyperplasia as a consequence of excessive pituitary secretion of ACTH, it is called *Cushing's disease.* This is the commonest endogenous cause in adults. The etiology of Cushing's disease is unknown. It is not certain whether this is due to excessive hypothalamic stimulation of pituitary cells with consequent tumor formation, or whether this is primarily a disease of the pituitary. The finding that most patients with Cushing's disease respond to microsurgical removal of a pituitary adenoma suggests the latter. However, it is still possible that the tumor had its origin as a consequence of excessive hypothalamic activity. Possibly Cushing's disease is heterogeneous; perhaps some cases are due to hypothalamic dysfunction and others are due primarily to adenoma formation in the pituitary. Patients with Cushing's disease exhibit pulsatile release of ACTH; the pulses are larger than in normal persons. Characteristically, there is a loss of the diurnal rhythm of ACTH secretion. Cushing's disease is characterized by a set point elevation. That is, hypothalamic-pituitary suppression does not occur at low doses of dexamethasone (e.g., 0.5 mg by mouth every six hours for two days) but does occur at higher doses (e.g., 2.0 mg by mouth every six hours for two days; occasionally even higher doses are required). Patients with Cushing's disease are responsive to metyrapone, since central (hypothalamic-pituitary) function is enhanced.

The *ectopic ACTH syndrome* results from excessive

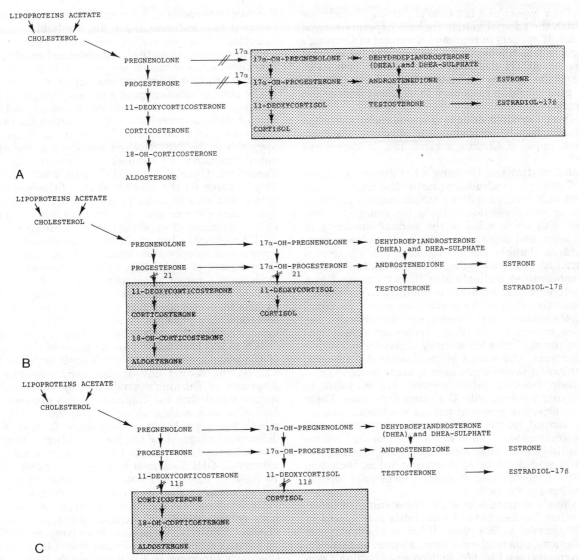

Figure 89. Syndromes of congenital adrenal hyperplasia: *(A)* 17α-hydroxylase deficiency, *(B)* 21-hydroxylase deficiency, and *(C)* 11β-hydroxylase deficiency. The layout of each panel corresponds to that of Figure 86, in which the structure of each steroid is displayed. In each panel the shaded area indicates those steroids located distal to the site of the enzymatic defect, the production of which is diminished. Steroids located proximal to the site of the enzymatic defect accumulate in excess (see text).

ACTH secretion by an ectopic (nonpituitary) tumor source (Fig. 87). The cushingoid habitus does occur in this syndrome but may be subtle or absent; this may reflect the often rapid onset and short duration of the syndrome. Hypokalemic alkalosis and proximal myopathy may occur out of proportion to other features of Cushing's syndrome. Some patients have hyperpigmentation. The baseline urinary and plasma steroid values are often among the highest seen in any form of Cushing's syndrome. Patients with the ectopic ACTH syndrome are usually unresponsive to dexamethasone (since ACTH production by the tumor is not suppressible) and unresponsive to metyrapone (owing to hypothalamic-pituitary suppression and to unresponsiveness of the tumor source of ACTH to reduced cortisol levels), but exceptions occur. For example, the ectopic ACTH syndrome due to a bronchial adenoma may behave like Cushing's disease, with suppression

in response to a high dose of dexamethasone and stimulation in response to metyrapone. The commonest causes of the ectopic ACTH syndrome are tumors of the lung, thymus (thymic carcinoid), and pancreatic islets; other tumors also cause this syndrome.

Adrenocortical tumors do not respond to dexamethasone or to metyrapone, since ACTH is already suppressed by excessive cortisol production by the tumor (Fig. 87). *An adrenocortical adenoma* is often characterized by basal secretion of 17-OHCS out of proportion to excretion of 17-ketosteroids. *An adrenocortical carcinoma* is the commonest cause of Cushing's syndrome in children and also occurs in adults. Virilization or feminization may occur owing to secretion of androgens or estrogens, respectively, by the tumor. Nearly half of all adrenocortical carcinomas are palpable at the time of diagnosis. Typically 17-ketosteroids are excreted out of proportion to 17-OHCS.

Nodular hyperplasia is a form of Cushing's syndrome in which the adrenal glands are both hyperplastic and nodular. It appears to represent a variant of Cushing's disease in which prolonged stimulation of the adrenal cortex by ACTH has resulted in nodule formation. Some of the nodules are autonomous. These patients may give variable responses to dexamethasone and metyrapone.

Cushing's syndrome due to *exogenous administration of glucocorticoids* for therapeutic purposes, the commonest cause of Cushing's syndrome, is considered below.

Manifestations of Cushing's Syndrome. Patients with Cushing's syndrome typically display a characteristic body habitus, with a rounded facial appearance (moon facies), deposition of fat in the supraclavicular spaces with obliteration of the normal concavity in these sites, and deposition of fat in the posterior cervical area (buffalo hump). Patients exhibit central obesity with relative wasting of the extremities (beetle-like appearance). Patients also display impaired glucose tolerance or frank diabetes mellitus, hypertension, osteoporosis (often with vertebral fractures), proximal muscle weakness, acne, menstrual disturbances, impotence, hirsutism or virilism, violaceous striae, thinning of the skin, easy bruisability, decreased resistance to infections, and a host of psychiatric disturbances varying from severe depression to acute psychosis.

Certain features, when present, are of value in identifying patients with Cushing's syndrome. These include objective proximal muscle weakness, osteoporosis, central obesity, spontaneous ecchymoses, and striae greater than 1 cm in width. Many of the features of Cushing's syndrome, although typical, are not sufficiently specific to be of diagnostic value, including obesity, hypertension, diabetes, menstrual disturbances, and plethora.

Cushing's syndrome is a life-threatening disorder. Untreated, the disorder has a mortality rate approaching 50 per cent in five years. Death is frequently due to infections, atherosclerotic heart disease, and suicide.

Diagnosis (see Fig. 90). Endogenous Cushing's syndrome is uncommon, but its clinical manifestations are similar to those of many common disorders. In addition, Cushing's syndrome has specific therapeutic implications. Thus, one needs a sensitive, cost-effective screening test to properly identify patients with this uncommon but treatable disorder. The test of choice is the *overnight dexamethasone suppression test*. One mg of dexamethasone is given by mouth at 11:00 or 12:00 P.M., and a plasma cortisol is obtained at 8:00 A.M. the following morning. A value of less than 5 µg/dl excludes the diagnosis of Cushing's syndrome. There are few false positives and virtually no false negative (normal) results. False positives may be due to failure to take dexamethasone, laboratory error, stress, and the effects of certain drugs. For example, phenytoin and other microsomal enzyme inducers accelerate the removal of dexamethasone, estrogens increase the CBG, and spironolactone may interfere when the fluorescence technique is used to measure the cortisol level. An alternative approach is to use the urinary free cortisol excretion (normal value less than 100 µg/24 hrs). The use of the 24-hour urine 17-OHCS as a screening test is unacceptable, since it will miss 10 to 15 per cent of patients with Cushing's syndrome.

Random or timed (e.g., 8 A.M. or 4 P.M.) plasma samples (without dexamethasone) are not a reliable means of detecting a loss of diurnal variation, owing to the pulsatile release of cortisol. An abnormal result of the overnight dexamethasone suppression test is an indication for further diagnostic evaluation.

The clinical assessment of a patient thought to have Cushing's syndrome does not depend on clinical findings or laboratory evaluation alone, but on the careful integration of clinical and laboratory findings. The approach to the definitive diagnosis and to the differential diagnosis of Cushing's syndrome is shown in Figure 90. Clinical evaluation must emphasize not only a search for the manifestations of Cushing's syndrome, but also for clues to the etiology of Cushing's syndrome. For example, special attention should be paid to evidence of hyperpigmentation (suggesting an ACTH-mediated form of Cushing's syndrome), to the presence or absence of an abdominal mass (suggesting the presence of an adrenocortical carcinoma), and to evidence of a tumor as an ectopic source of ACTH.

A *low-dose dexamethasone suppression test* (0.5 mg by mouth every six hours for two days) is used to determine the presence or absence of Cushing's syndrome. A normal response (suppression of urinary 17-OHCS to less than 3.5 mg per 24 hours or suppression of the plasma cortisol level to 5 µg/dl or below at 4 P.M. on the second day of the study) excludes the diagnosis of Cushing's syndrome; an abnormal response establishes the diagnosis of this disorder. The *high-dose dexamethasone suppression test* (2.0 mg by mouth every six hours for two days) is used in the differential diagnosis of Cushing's syndrome. Suppression with the high dose (to less than half of the basal urinary 17-OHCS value or to a plasma cortisol level of 10 µg/dl or below at 4 P.M. on the second day of the study) supports the diagnosis of Cushing's disease. Failure to suppress with this dose suggests that Cushing's syndrome is due to a cause other than Cushing's disease. Similarly, a *response to metyrapone* (750 mg by mouth every four hours for six doses) suggests that Cushing's syndrome is due to Cushing's disease. Failure to respond to metyrapone with an increase in urinary 17-OHCS secretion suggests that Cushing's syndrome is due to a cause other than Cushing's disease. Exceptions to these general guidelines occur, as noted above. For this reason, it is helpful to perform both the high-dose dexamethasone suppression test and the metyrapone test to obtain as much information as possible.

When the clinical and laboratory evaluation suggests a likely cause of Cushing's syndrome, further radiological studies are usually needed. For example, computerized body tomography of the adrenal glands may be helpful in localizing the cause of the disease. It should be emphasized that one does *not* make the diagnosis of Cushing's syndrome on the basis of radiological studies, since a patient may have a nonfunctioning adrenal nodule. Radiological studies are used for localization, not for diagnosis. If Cushing's disease appears to be present, computerized tomography of the sella and surrounding area is appropriate. However, most patients with Cushing's syndrome have a microadenoma, which may not be detected radiographically.

The treatment of Cushing's syndrome depends upon

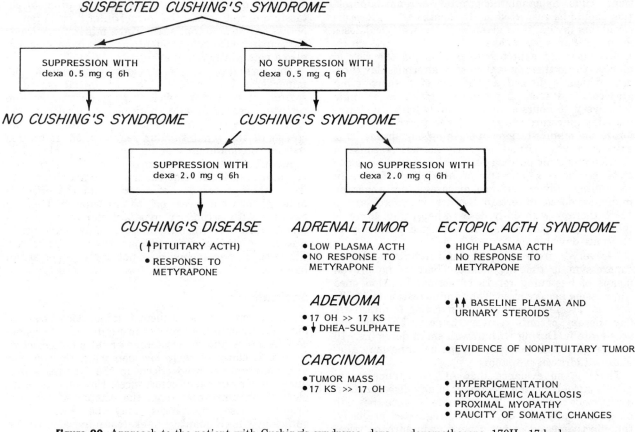

Figure 90. Approach to the patient with Cushing's syndrome. dexa = dexamethasone. 17OH = 17-hydroxy-corticosteroids. 17KS = 17-ketosteroids. Note that the responses to the diagnostic tests (e.g., to dexamethasone 2.0 mg P.O. every 6 hours or to metyrapone) depicted in the figure are typical but that exceptions do occur (see text).

the etiology determined by the above studies. At the present time, transnasal transsphenoidal adenomectomy is the treatment of choice for most patients with Cushing's disease. This is successful in the vast majority of patients without causing permanent pituitary insufficiency; transient secondary adrenal insufficiency often occurs. Since this procedure has only been in use for several years, long-term follow-up will be required before the recurrence rate following this procedure can be determined. Pituitary irradiation (proton beam or conventional radiation) and bilateral total adrenalectomy, which were used more extensively in the past, may have a role in selected patients. Cushing's syndrome due to an adrenal adenoma is treated with surgical removal of the tumor and the adrenal gland from which it arose and with glucocorticoid therapy until the contralateral adrenal cortex recovers function. An adrenal carcinoma is treated with surgical removal if possible. Drug treatment includes ortho, para-DDD, and aminoglutethimide. The treatment of the ectopic ACTH syndrome is directed at the underlying tumor. Occasional cases require control of cortisol secretion with metyrapone, aminoglutethimide, or bilateral total adrenalectomy.

GLUCOCORTICOID THERAPY

Glucocorticoids are frequently administered in pharmacological doses for anti-inflammatory and immuno-

suppressive effects in a host of disorders involving virtually every system in the body. However, glucocorticoid therapy can cause Cushing's syndrome and hypothalamic-pituitary suppression (with secondary adrenal insufficiency if the glucocorticoids are stopped before hypothalamic-pituitary-adrenal function has returned to normal). Cessation of glucocorticoid therapy can also cause the steroid withdrawal syndrome. This is a disorder in which patients have signs and symptoms of adrenal insufficiency, including hypotension, fever, arthralgias, myalgias, and abdominal pain, despite the fact that the hypothalamic-pituitary-adrenal axis is intact. Any therapeutic decision to use glucocorticoid therapy must weigh the potential benefits against the potential risks. In addition, every effort must be made to keep the risks to a minimum. Patients can develop evidence of hypothalamic-pituitary-adrenal axis suppression on commonly used doses (e.g., prednisone 25 mg P.O. twice a day) as early as five days after the onset of therapy. The rate of recovery from suppression depends on the total steroid dose to which the patient has been exposed and on the total duration of exposure. Recovery from a brief exposure to a high dose (e.g., 25 mg twice a day) may occur as early as five days after cessation of therapy. However, recovery from a prolonged exposure (e.g., for more than one year) to large doses may take as long as a year. The rate of recovery from an intermediate exposure is variable and difficult to predict in an individual patient. Thus, hypothalamic-pituitary-adrenal suppression should be suspected for 12 months after glucocorticoid therapy has been given in pharmacological doses for more than a few weeks.

An important approach to minimizing the risk of glucocorticoid therapy is the use of alternate-day therapy, which is defined as the use of a short-acting glucocorticoid such as prednisone given as a single dose every 48 hours at approximately 8:00 A.M. Alternate-day glucocorticoid therapy will prevent or ameliorate the manifestations of Cushing's syndrome. It is associated with normal or nearly normal response of the hypothalamic-pituitary-adrenal axis to provocative tests, and it is as effective or nearly as effective in controlling a diverse group of diseases as daily therapy in divided doses. In certain disorders it is necessary to begin therapy with daily doses; when the disorder is controlled the patient can be converted gradually to alternate-day therapy.

Recovery from hypothalamic-pituitary-adrenal suppression is time-dependent. There is no proven means of hastening return of normal function once suppression has occurred. The administration of ACTH does not accelerate recovery. Conversion to alternate-day therapy permits recovery to occur but does not accelerate it. During withdrawal, small doses (i.e., 10 to 20 mg) of hydrocortisone in the morning may alleviate withdrawal symptoms.

There is no evidence that ACTH is superior to glucocorticoids for the treatment of any disorder. Glucocorticoids are generally preferable because they can be given orally, the dose can be regulated precisely, the effectiveness does not depend upon adrenocortical responsiveness, and they produce a lower incidence of hypertension, acne, and hyperpigmentation than ACTH therapy.

MINERALOCORTICOIDS

Actions

Mineralocorticoids are 21-carbon steroid molecules that play an important role in the regulation of sodium, chloride, potassium, and hydrogen balance. Mineralocorticoids promote the transport of sodium from the lumen to the blood in the cortical collecting tubule of the kidney. Potassium and hydrogen ions move passively across the tubule from the circulation into the tubular lumen. Mineralocorticoids also exert similar actions on other epithelial cells, including salivary, sweat, and gastrointestinal glands. The consequences include decreased concentrations of sodium and chloride in saliva and in sweat and increased potassium secretion into the lumen of the gastrointestinal tract. The mechanism of action of mineralocorticoids is similar to that of other steroid hormones and appears to involve binding of the mineralocorticoids to an intracellular receptor protein and regulation of the rate of transcription of the genetic information. The consequence appears to be increased synthesis of proteins that influence ion transport by the target cells.

Mineralocorticoids function to conserve sodium and extracellular fluid volume under conditions of salt loss and volume depletion, circumstances that would otherwise result rapidly in volume depletion, hypoten-

sion, and death. Mineralocorticoids also promote potassium excretion and the intracellular distribution of potassium at nonrenal sites. Thus, mineralocorticoids participate in the body's defense against hyperkalemia, also a potentially lethal event.

The normal person has a defense against prolonged mineralocorticoid excess. After an initial period of sodium retention and weight gain, further sodium retention ceases despite continued mineralocorticoid excess *(the escape phenomenon)*. This is due to a decrease in the renal tubular reabsorption of filtered sodium (predominantly at the proximal tubule). Consequently, patients with primary hyperaldosteronism do not ordinarily develop edema. Patients with edema from other causes do not escape from the effect of mineralocorticoid excess on sodium balance. Thus, in patients with secondary hyperaldosteronism in edematous disorders, the mineralocorticoid excess contributes to the genesis of the edematous state (see below). The escape phenomenon does not apply to potassium balance.

Structure

Aldosterone is the principal mineralocorticoid in man. Its structure is depicted in Figure 86. 11-Deoxycorticosterone and corticosterone are also mineralocorticoids. Because of their low potencies, they do not exert mineralocorticoid effects in the quantities produced under normal circumstances. However, in pathological circumstances (e.g., the ectopic ACTH syndrome), these substances may be secreted in sufficiently high quantity to exert a mineralocorticoid effect. Certain steroids, although predominantly glucocorticoid in effect, have mineralocorticoid activity as well. Cortisol and cortisone exert such an effect, but generally only when secreted or administered in quantities exceeding 100 mg per day. Fludrocortisone (9α-fluorohydrocortisone) is a synthetic mineralocorticoid commonly used for therapeutic purposes.

Biosynthesis

The pathway of aldosterone biosynthesis is depicted in Figure 86. The mineralocorticoid synthetic pathway is derived from progesterone; thus, the molecules in this pathway are not hydroxylated in the 17α position. They undergo a sequence of enzymatically mediated steps including 21-hydroxylation, 11β-hydroxylation, 18-hydroxylation, and formation of the aldehyde at the C-18 position. Aldosterone is not synthesized in the zona fasciculata or the zona reticularis; only the zona glomerulosa contains 18-hydroxysteroid dehydrogenase, an enzyme required for aldosterone biosynthesis.

Degradation

The liver is the major site at which aldosterone is transformed to biologically inactive derivatives. About 30 to 40 per cent of aldosterone is converted by the liver to tetrahydroaldosterone glucuronide, in which the A ring is reduced at the site of the double bond. In addition, 4 to 10 per cent is converted by the liver to an 18-glucuronide derivative, which is acid hydrolyzable. Another 5 to 10 per cent is converted by the kidneys to this acid-hydrolyzable 18-glucuronide derivative. The remaining 40 to 50 per cent is rapidly converted by the liver to inactive metabolites that are for the most part excreted in the urine. All of the principal derivatives are water-soluble and rapidly excreted into the urine.

Aldosterone is inactivated by the liver so efficiently that it is virtually devoid of biological activity when administered orally. Thus, aldosterone is not used therapeutically. Instead, fludrocortisone, a mineralocorticoid that retains activity when given orally, is employed therapeutically.

Physiology

Normal adults who consume 100 to 150 mEq of sodium per day secrete approximately 40 to 160 μg of aldosterone per day. The production rate may rise tenfold or more in response to sodium depletion or in certain disease states. The aldosterone production rate falls toward zero in individuals who consume extraordinarily large quantities of sodium or in those who are exposed to excessive mineralocorticoid activity from exogenous administration or from a pathological process. Plasma aldosterone levels tend to be higher in the morning than in the afternoon and are higher with upright posture than with recumbency. Aldosterone is bound only loosely to plasma proteins (principally albumin). Approximately 70 per cent of this mineralocorticoid circulates in the free (unbound) form. In normal adults aldosterone has a circulating half-time of approximately 30 minutes.

REGULATION OF ALDOSTERONE SECRETION

Aldosterone secretion is regulated by angiotensin II, the potassium ion, and ACTH. Angiotensin II is the principal regulator of aldosterone secretion in man.

The feedback loop governing aldosterone secretion is depicted in Figure 91. When the blood pressure falls or the intravascular volume diminishes, renal perfusion decreases. In response to decreased renal perfusion pressure in the afferent arterioles, the juxtaglomerular cells release renin. Renin, a proteolytic enzyme, converts renin substrate produced in the liver to angiotensin I, a decapeptide. Angiotensin I is converted to angiotensin II, an octapeptide, by converting enzyme located in the lungs and in the vasculature. Angiotensin II stimulates aldosterone release from the zona glomerulosa of the adrenal cortex; it is also a potent vasoconstrictor. Enhanced aldosterone release results in increased sodium reabsorption in the cortical collecting tubule of the kidney. This response and the effect of angiotensin II on blood pressure lead to a physiological adjustment toward normal of the decreased intravascular volume and blood pressure, the stimuli that set this sequence of events in motion. The potassium ion and ACTH also stimulate aldosterone secretion. The effect of ACTH is relatively brief, lasting just a few days.

The rate-limiting step for aldosterone biosynthesis appears to be at the site of cleavage of the cholesterol side chain, where this precursor is converted to pregnenolone. This step is stimulated by angiotensin II,

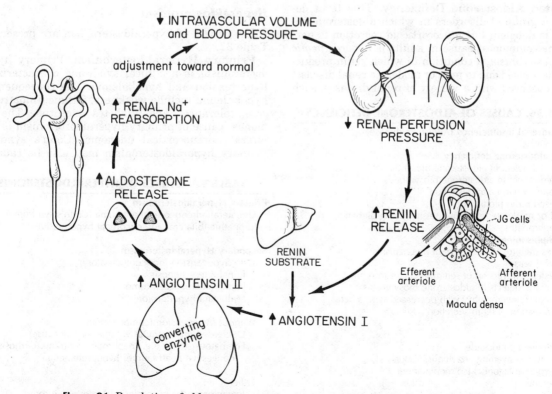

Figure 91. Regulation of aldosterone secretion in normal man. JG = juxtaglomerular.

potassium, and ACTH. Angiotensin II also stimulates later steps in the aldosterone synthetic pathway, such as conversion of corticosterone to 18-hydroxycorticosterone and aldosterone. Potassium also appears to stimulate both the early and the late steps in mineralocorticoid synthesis.

Angiotensin II is also converted to angiotensin III, a heptapeptide. Angiotensin III is as potent as angiotensin II with respect to the stimulation of aldosterone biosynthesis but circulates in lower concentration and probably has only a minor physiological role.

Measurement

Plasma aldosterone levels can be determined by radioimmunoassay, a competitive binding assay, or double isotope derivative methods. The urinary excretion of aldosterone actually reflects the excretion of the acid-hydrolyzable 18-glucuronide, which is cleaved by acid hydrolysis to remove glucuronic acid before measurement of the aldosterone. The aldosterone secretory rate can be determined by injection of a radioactively labeled steroid.

Renin levels are generally determined as plasma renin activity. This is usually measured by radioimmunoassay of the quantity of angiotensin I released during incubation of plasma under defined conditions for a specified period of time.

DISORDERS OF ALDOSTERONE PRODUCTION

Aldosterone Deficiency

The causes of aldosterone deficiency are depicted in Table 36.

Isolated Aldosterone Deficiency. This term describes a group of disorders in which aldosterone secretion is deficient but glucocorticoid secretion is normal. The commonest cause in adults is *hyporeninemic hypoaldosteronism*, a condition in which renin production is decreased due to mild or moderate renal disease. This is observed with a variety of renal diseases, such

TABLE 36. CAUSES OF ALDOSTERONE DEFICIENCY

Primary adrenal insufficiency (Addison's disease)

Selective aldosterone deficiency
  Congenital defect in aldosterone biosynthesis
  Acquired defect in aldosterone biosynthesis
    Chronic heparin administration
  Decreased renin production
    Mild or moderate renal disease, including diabetic
      nephropathy
    Lead poisoning
  Diabetes mellitus, due to several mechanisms:
    Renal disease
    Defective conversion of renin precursor to renin
    Enzymatic defects in aldosterone biosynthesis
    Autonomic neuropathy, with decreased sympathetic
      stimulation of renin secretion

Drugs
  Beta-adrenergic blockade
  Angiotensin-converting enzyme inhibitors
  Aldosterone antagonists (spironolactone)
  Triamterene
  Amiloride

as diabetic nephropathy and pyelonephritis. In infants, one encounters an enzymatic defect in the adrenocortical synthesis of aldosterone.

Diabetic patients may have this condition due to a variety of defects: (1) renal disease; (2) defective conversion of big renin (a relatively inactive precursor) to renin, manifesting itself as decreased renin *activity*; (3) enzymatic defects in aldosterone biosynthesis; and (4) autonomic neuropathy with decreased catecholamine secretion and decreased catecholamine-induced secretion of renin. Prolonged heparin administration may cause decreased aldosterone synthesis. Lead poisoning may cause decreased renin synthesis.

The manifestations of this disorder are hyperkalemia and its consequences: muscle weakness, cardiac arrhythmias, and central nervous system dysfunction. Salt wasting and hyperchloremic acidosis occur occasionally. Diagnosis of this entity requires the exclusion of other causes of hyperkalemia: volume depletion; diuretics that cause potassium retention such as spironolactone, triamterene, or amiloride; unrecognized potassium administration (in the form of potassium penicillin, for example), or thrombocytosis. Marked thrombocytosis causes hyperkalemia in serum due to release of potassium in vitro during platelet aggregation; hyperkalemia is not observed in plasma. Primary adrenocortical insufficiency must be excluded by a cosyntropin test (see above). The presence of the adult hyporeninemic form may be confirmed by demonstrating a blunted increase in plasma renin activity and the plasma aldosterone level in response to volume depletion (induced by a diuretic) and upright posture.

The disorder is treated with fludrocortisone and adequate salt intake.

Hyperaldosteronism

The causes of hyperaldosteronism are presented in Table 37.

Primary Hyperaldosteronism. Primary hyperaldosteronism is a clinical syndrome characterized by hypertension and hypokalemia. The consequences of hypokalemia include weakness, fatigue, impaired glucose tolerance, and diabetes mellitus. The commonest cause of primary hyperaldosteronism is a unilateral adrenocortical adenoma (Conn's syndrome). Primary hyperaldosteronism may also be caused by

TABLE 37. CAUSES OF HYPERALDOSTERONISM

Primary Hyperaldosteronism
  Unilateral adrenocortical adenoma (Conn's syndrome)
  Idiopathic (bilateral adrenocortical hyperplasia)

Secondary Hyperaldosteronism
  With hypertension (not compensatory)
    Renal artery stenosis
    Juxtaglomerular cell tumor
    Malignant hypertension

  Without hypertension (compensatory)
    Decreased intravascular volume (of any cause)
    Edematous states, e.g., nephrotic syndrome, cirrhosis,
      congestive heart failure, hypoproteinemia

  Other
    Juxtaglomerular hyperplasia (Bartter's syndrome)

bilateral adrenocortical hyperplasia (idiopathic hyperaldosteronism); this may account for 10 to 40 per cent of patients with primary hyperaldosteronism. Idiopathic hyperaldosteronism may be caused by increased circulating levels of a glycoprotein of anterior pituitary origin. The distinction between these forms of primary hyperaldosteronism is of therapeutic importance. When the syndrome is due to a unilateral adrenocortical adenoma, the hypertension usually responds to surgical removal of the adenoma. When primary hyperaldosteronism is due to bilateral adrenocortical hyperplasia, the hypertension usually does not respond to unilateral or bilateral adrenalectomy but may respond to mineralocorticoid antagonists such as spironolactone.

Primary hyperaldosteronism should be suspected when a patient with hypertension is found to have hypokalemia prior to the use of any diuretic agent or when the development of hypokalemia appears to be out of proportion to that expected from the use of the diuretic. The serum potassium level should always be measured prior to the initiation of a diuretic.

The evaluation of a patient for primary hyperaldosteronism requires, first of all, the exclusion of Cushing's syndrome (by an appropriate overnight dexamethasone suppression test, for example), since mineralocorticoid excess is a feature of certain forms of Cushing's syndrome. In addition, any further evaluation of a patient for primary hyperaldosteronism should be performed when the patient has been off all antihypertensive medication (and other medication) for at least two weeks, since the renin-angiotensin-aldosterone system is affected by diuretics, beta-adrenergic antagonists, converting enzyme inhibitors, and vasodilators.

The pathophysiology of primary hyperaldosteronism is depicted in Figure 92. Excessive secretion of aldosterone results in enhanced reabsorption of sodium at the cortical collecting tubule and enhanced potassium secretion into the urine. The increased sodium reabsorption results in expansion of the extracellular fluid volume and an increase in blood pressure. Consequently, renal perfusion pressure increases, renin release decreases, production of angiotensin I decreases, and production of angiotensin II falls. Thus, primary hyperaldosteronism occurs in the setting of diminished angiotensin II levels. This is in contrast to the normal situation, in which angiotensin II is the principal regulator of aldosterone secretion. The extent of the expansion of the extracellular fluid volume and of the increase in weight is limited by the mineralocorticoid escape phenomenon (see above).

The diagnosis of hyperaldosteronism depends upon exploitation of the pathophysiological features just described. Since renin activity is diminished, a useful approach is to determine whether renin activity is suppressed in response to physiological stimuli such as upright posture and the administration of a diuretic such as furosemide. If renin activity increases normally in response to these stimuli, the diagnosis of primary hyperaldosteronism can be excluded. Suppression of the response to upright posture and volume depletion is consistent with the diagnosis but not diagnostic, since approximately 20 to 25 per cent of patients with essential hypertension will also have suppressed renin levels.

Consequently, the diagnosis depends upon demonstrating that aldosterone secretion cannot be suppressed by physiological stimuli, such as the administration of a salt load. One can measure the plasma

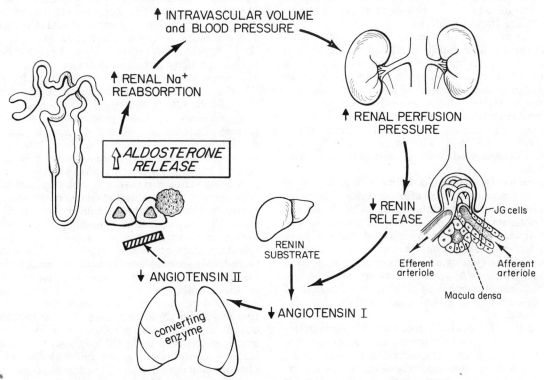

Figure 92. Pathophysiology of primary hyperaldosteronism. JG = juxtaglomerular.

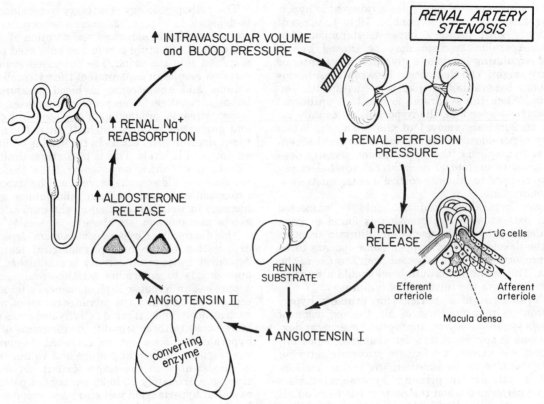

Figure 93. Pathophysiology of renal artery stenosis. JG = juxtaglomerular.

aldosterone level or the urine aldosterone excretion rate after the administration of a salt load to determine whether the aldosterone level fails to suppress appropriately under these conditions.

When the diagnosis of primary hyperaldosteronism has been confirmed by biochemical methods, it is then necessary to determine whether the patient has a unilateral adrenocortical adenoma or bilateral adrenocortical hyperplasia, because of the therapeutic implications described above. Selective adrenal vein catheterization with determination of aldosterone and cortisol levels in the effluent of each adrenal gland appears to be the most reliable procedure for this purpose. Computerized body tomography may also have a role.

Relation to Hypertension. Primary hyperaldosteronism is an uncommon cause of hypertension. Because plasma renin activity is diminished in 20 to 25 per cent of patients with essential hypertension, it was thought at one time that many of these patients have primary hyperaldosteronism. This does not appear to be the case. The genesis of low-renin hypertension is not known. Primary hyperaldosteronism must be distinguished from low-renin hypertension by studies of the suppressibility of aldosterone secretion, as described above.

Secondary Hyperaldosteronism. Hyperaldosteronism may also occur in response to nonadrenal disorders. These conditions are described collectively by the term secondary hyperaldosteronism. Secondary hyperaldosteronism may occur with hypertension, in which the hyperaldosteronism is not compensatory. Secondary hyperaldosteronism may also occur without hypertension, when the increased aldosterone secretion occurs in response to decreased effective intravascular volume. Renal artery stenosis is an example of secondary hyperaldosteronism with hypertension. The pathophysiology of this disorder is depicted in Figure 93. When the stenosis of the renal artery is hemodynamically significant, perfusion of the kidney on the affected side is decreased. This leads to enhanced renin release, increased production of angiotensin I, increased production of angiotensin II, increased aldosterone secretion, increased renal tubular sodium reabsorption, expanded intravascular volume, and increased blood pressure. A juxtaglomerular cell tumor producing renin will result in a similar picture.

Secondary hyperaldosteronism may occur in response to decreased intravascular volume in edematous states. Thus, in certain hypoalbuminemic states the decreased oncotic pressure results in decreased effective intravascular volume, with activation of the renin-angiotensin-aldosterone system. In congestive heart failure, volume may be sequestered on the right side of the circulation, with decreased renal perfusion. Again, the renin-angiotensin-aldosterone system is activated. Under these circumstances, the hyperaldosteronism results in sodium retention and volume expansion and contributes to the genesis of the edematous state. As noted earlier, the mineralocorticoid escape phenomenon does not occur in edematous patients with secondary hyperaldosteronism.

REFERENCES

Adrenal Gland

Baxter, J. D., and Tyrrell, J. B.: The adrenal cortex. In Felig, P., Baxter, J. D., Broadus, A. E., and Frohman, L. A. (eds.): Endocrinology and Metabolism. New York, McGraw-Hill Book Co., 1981, p. 385.

Glucocorticoids

Ashcraft, M. W., Van Herle, A. J., Vener, S. L., and Geffner, D. L.: Serum cortisol levels in Cushing's syndrome after low- and high-dose dexamethasone suppression. Ann Intern Med 97:21–26, 1982.

Axelrod, L.: Glucocorticoid therapy. Medicine 55:39–65, 1976.

Axelrod, L.: Glucocorticoids. In Kelley, W. N., Harris, E. D., Jr., Ruddy, S., and Sledge, C. B. (eds.): Textbook of Rheumatology. 2nd ed. Philadelphia, W. B. Saunders Co., 1985.

Crapo, L.: Cushing's syndrome: A review of diagnostic tests. Metabolism 28:955–977, 1979.

Frawley, T. F.: Adrenal cortical insufficiency. In Eisenstein, A. B. (ed.): The Adrenal Cortex. Boston, Little, Brown, and Co., 1967, p. 439.

Gold, E. M.: The Cushing syndromes: Changing views of diagnosis and treatment. Ann Intern Med 90:829–844, 1979.

Irvine, W. J., Toft, A. D., and Feek, C. M.: Addison's disease.

In James, V. H. T. (ed.): The Adrenal Gland. New York, Raven Press, 1979, pp. 131–164.

Liddle, G. W.: Tests of pituitary-adrenal suppressibility in the diagnosis of Cushing's syndrome. J Clin Endocrinol Metab 20:1539–1560, 1960.

Nerup, J.: Addison's disease—clinical studies. A report of 108 cases. Acta Endocrinol 76:127–141, 1974.

Urbanic, R. C., and George, J. M.: Cushing's disease—18 years' experience. Medicine 60:14–24, 1981.

Mineralocorticoids

Bravo, E. L., Tarazi, R. C., Dustan, H. P., Fouad, F. M., Textor, S. C., Gifford, R. W., and Vidt, D. G.: The changing clinical spectrum of primary aldosteronism. Am J Med 74:641–651, 1983.

DeFronzo, R. A.: Hyperkalemia and hyporeninemic hypoaldosteronism. Kidney Int 17:118–134, 1980.

Ferriss, J. B., Brown, J. J., Fraser, R., Lever, A. F., and Robertson, J. I. S.: Primary hyperaldosteronism. Clin Endocrinol Metab 10:419–452, 1981.

Perloff, D., and Schambelan, M.: Renovascular hypertension. Clin Endocrinol Metab 10:513–535, 1981.

Weinberger, M. H., Grim, C. E., Hollifield, J. W., Kem, D. C., Ganguly, A., Kramer, N. J., Yune, H. Y., Wellman, H., and Donohue, J. P.: Primary aldosteronism. Diagnosis, localization, and treatment. Ann Intern Med 90:386–395, 1979.

Hormonal Regulation of Calcium Metabolism

MICHAEL ROSENBLATT, M.D.

OVERVIEW OF CALCIUM METABOLISM

The maintenance of blood calcium levels within the narrow physiological range requires the action of at least two hormones acting on three organs. Parathyroid hormone, a polypeptide hormone, and vitamin D, a steroid hormone, act on bone, kidney, and gut in the regulation of calcium homeostasis. Calcium ion levels in blood and extracellular fluid are tightly controlled to ensure the normal functioning of cardiac muscle, nervous tissue, skeletal muscle, blood clotting factors, and various enzymes and hormones.

It is the ionized and unbound form of calcium that is closely regulated and circulates at a level approaching its saturation point, namely the solubility product constant for calcium phosphate. It also accounts for some of the major problems encountered in hypercalcemia, such as kidney stones and soft tissue calcification, which will be discussed later in this chapter. The amount of calcium that is closely regulated actually represents only a small fraction of the total calcium present in the body. The calcium present in blood and extracellular fluid is only 1 per cent of the total calcium; the remaining 99 per cent is found principally in bone. Furthermore, half of the calcium in the extracellular space is bound to albumin or other proteins. Hence, only approximately 0.5 per cent of the total calcium is ionized and serves a critical role in the physiological functions described above.

Although the quantity of calcium that is regulated is small, the fluxes of calcium at various organ interfaces is by comparison enormous (Fig. 94). The kidney filters large quantities of calcium, 5 to 7 grams per day. Normally, 96 to 98 per cent of the filtered calcium is reabsorbed. When maximally stimulated by para-

thyroid hormone, the kidney can come close to reabsorbing 100 per cent of the calcium that it filters; however, complete reabsorption is not possible. Therefore, there is always an obligatory leak of calcium at the level of the kidney. A substantial amount of calcium can be rapidly mobilized from bone; over a period of several hours, quantities of calcium comparable to the total amount of calcium present in the extracellular fluid can be released. While the calcium reservoir

CALCIUM HOMEOSTASIS

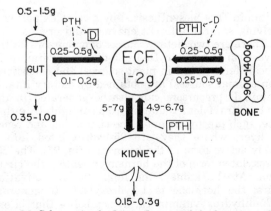

Figure 94. Schematic of calcium fluxes and the hormones that influence shifts in ionized calcium. Arrows indicate movement of calcium between the gut, bone, kidneys, and extracellular fluid (ECF). Principal modulation of this movement by vitamin D (D) or parathyroid hormone (PTH) is also shown. The numerical values indicate quantities of elemental calcium stored in bone and ECF, as well as the amount of elemental calcium typically transferred in a 24-hour period.

stored in bone can be used to prevent the development of hypocalcemia, over the long term, utilization of this mechanism for maintenance of normocalcemia can only incur negative calcium balance. Therefore, over time, the struggle for calcium homeostasis is won or lost at the level of the gut, which is the third principal site of calcium flux. The average American diet contains 0.5 to 1.5 grams of calcium (one quart of milk contains approximately 1 gram of calcium). However, the dietary intake of some individuals, particularly the elderly, falls well below this amount. The efficiency of calcium absorption is determined by the previous intake of calcium and circulating levels of parathyroid hormone and vitamin D, as will be discussed below. However, no matter how efficient the calcium absorption, there is an obligatory loss of calcium from the gut through the digestive juices and the shedding of luminar cells. Only dietary calcium intake can offset the obligatory negative calcium balance resulting from losses at the kidney and the gut.

The greatest challenge to calcium homeostasis in humans is defending against negative calcium balance and hypocalcemia. The two hormones that play the most important physiological role in this regard are parathyroid hormone and vitamin D, and the actions of each are to some extent dependent on the other. In addition, each hormone acts over a different time course and so has a different physiological role. Vitamin D has a prolonged action, measured in hours to days, and influences long-term maintenance of calcium balance. It stimulates the synthesis of the calcium-binding protein in the gut mucosal cell that is responsible for the transport of calcium from the intestinal lumen into the extracellular fluid. In contrast, parathyroid hormone has a half-life measured in minutes and causes rapid shifts in extracellular calcium through its action at the level of kidney and bone. Parathyroid hormone is responsible for the minute-to-minute regulation and "fine-turning" of calcium levels within the narrow physiological range.

BIOSYNTHESIS OF VITAMIN D

Vitamin D is biosynthesized by a complex pathway involving several different enzymes and organs (Fig. 95). There are two dietary sources of precursors for the active form of vitamin D, $1\alpha,25$-dihydroxyvitamin D. Ergocalciferol (found in plant sources) and cholesterol (from animal sources) are obtained by dietary intake. Vitamin D precursors can also be generated in the skin by ultraviolet irradiation from sunlight. By either route, such precursors enter the circulation and reach the liver, where they are 25-hydroxylated into a weakly active form of the hormone (Fig. 95). The 25-hydroxylated form of the hormone re-enters the circulation. At the kidney, the final step in activation occurs; the hormone is 1-hydroxylated to generate $1\alpha,25$-dihydroxyvitamin D_3, a metabolite that is one thousand times more potent than the 25-hydroxylated form. This form of the hormone stimulates the luminal cells of the gut to synthesize the calcium-binding protein responsible for the transport of calcium across the gut wall. The activity of the critical renal enzyme responsible for the 1-hydroxylation of 25-hydroxyvitamin D_3 to form $1\alpha,25$-dihydroxyvitamin D_3 is under

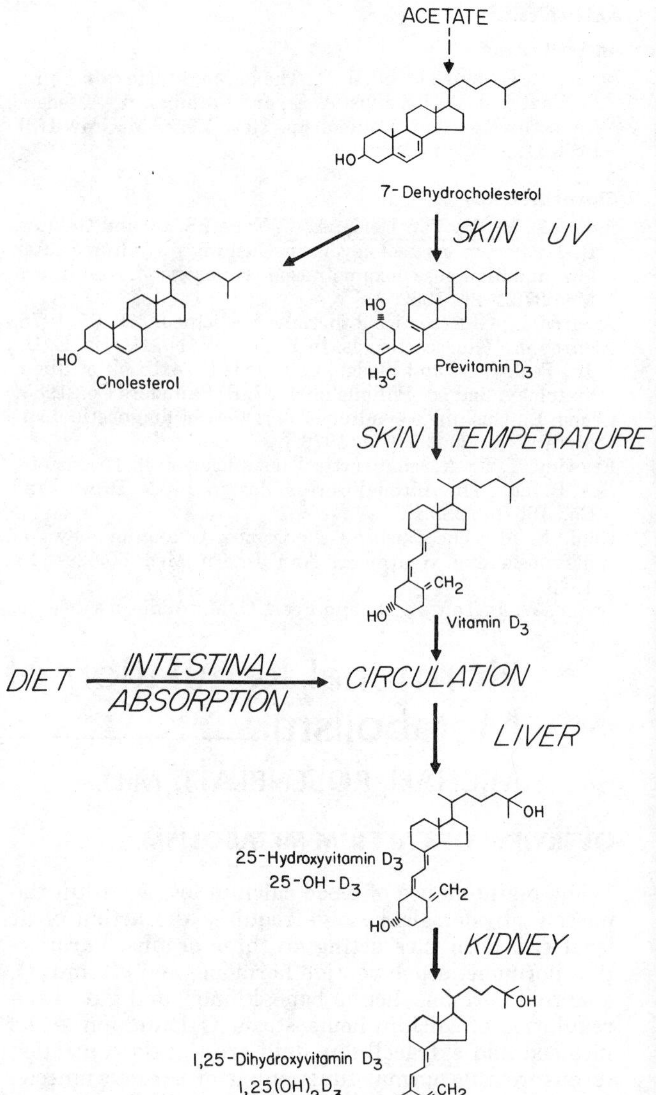

Figure 95. Biosynthesis of vitamin D. The precursor form of the hormone, 7-dehydrocholesterol, is converted to previtamin D_3 in skin by the action of ultraviolet light. With time and heat, the previtamin is converted in skin to vitamin D_3, which is transported through the circulation to liver. Alternatively, vitamin D_3 is available from animal sources in the diet. In the liver, 25-hydroxylation occurs. The 25-hydroxyvitamin D_3 formed is transported through the circulation to the kidney, where the final step in hormone activation (1α-hydroxylation) occurs, to generate $1\alpha,25$-dihydroxyvitamin D_3.

the regulation of parathyroid hormone (either directly or through parathyroid hormone's effects on phosphate fluxes). In addition, vitamin D in turn is necessary for parathyroid hormone's action; it is permissive for parathyroid hormone action on bone. Other metabolites of vitamin D are also generated, such as 24,25-dihydroxyvitamin D and several trihydroxylated derivatives. However, the physiological role of these other compounds is uncertain at this time.

Vitamin D is a hormone and not a vitamin, because it must be chemically modified from its precursor form in order to be active. Like all hormones, it is produced in one anatomical site and released into the circulation in order to act at another. Similar to steroid hormones, it has a long duration of action, circulates in the bloodstream bound to a specific binding protein, and then enters intracellularly into target tissue for expression of its bioactivity.

PARATHYROID HORMONE

The secreted form of parathyroid hormone is an 84-amino acid single chain polypeptide. However only a small portion of the structure, namely the amino-terminal one third, is necessary for full bioactivity as determined in multiple assay systems. The native hormone or the amino-terminal fragment of the hormone generated by cleavage of the hormone in the circulation in vivo interacts with receptors in kidney and bone. Through cyclic AMP and perhaps other postreceptor intracellular messengers, parathyroid hormone stimulates the release of calcium salts from bone and the reabsorption of calcium in the glomerular filtrate by the kidney, both actions causing an increase in blood calcium (Fig. 96).

Biosynthesis. The biosynthesis of parathyroid hormone begins with the transcription of the DNA of the gene encoding for preproparathyroid hormone. Precursor mRNA is processed into mature mRNA, which is translated into the nascent hormone. Although each of these steps (Fig. 97) is potentially regulated by the level of intracellular calcium (and hence hypocalcemia could theoretically stimulate these events, resulting in increased production of hormone), no evidence has yet been found for regulation by calcium at these steps.

Parathyroid hormone is first biosynthesized within the cells of the parathyroid gland in a larger precursor form termed preproparathyroid hormone (Fig. 98). Like other secreted proteins and peptide hormones, the precursor form contains an amino-terminal signal peptide or leader sequence thought to serve a critical role in identifying the protein by the cell as one destined for secretion, and then in facilitating its entry into the cisternae of the rough endoplasmic reticulum en route to ultimate secretion by the cell (Fig. 99).

After the leader sequence has served this role, and perhaps before the biosynthesis of the nascent hormone is complete, the leader sequence is cleaved from the remainder of the hormone. In the case of parathyroid

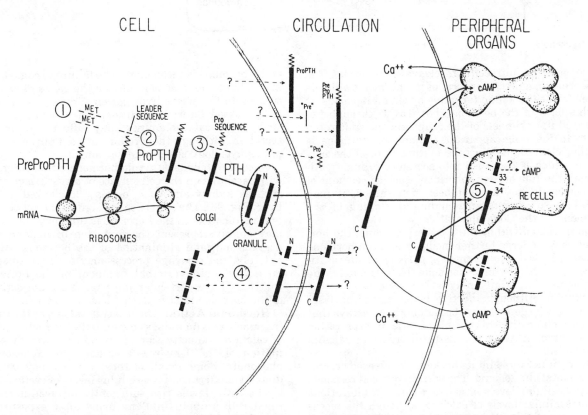

Figure 96. "Life cycle" of the parathyroid hormone molecule. The hormone is first biosynthesized in a precursor form, preproparathyroid hormone, by translation of mRNA on rough endoplasmic reticulum (RER). During biosynthesis of the nascent hormone, the two amino-terminal methionine residues are rapidly removed, followed by cleavage of the leader or signal sequence from the remaining hormone to generate the prohormone. Proparathyroid hormone moves intracellularly through the RER cisternae to the Golgi apparatus, where the prohormone-specific sequence is cleaved away and the native secreted form of the hormone is packaged into secretory granules. Few if any of the precursor forms of the hormone are secreted in normal physiology, although this possibility is indicated in the figure. In addition, some fragmentation of the hormone may occur within the secretory granules prior to secretion by the parathyroid cell. Once released into the circulation, the hormone may interact directly with its principal target tissues, kidney and bone, or may first be metabolized (by liver or kidney) into fragments, some of which are released back into circulation. An amino-terminal fragment generated by the liver would be an active form of the hormone.

PARATHYROID CELL

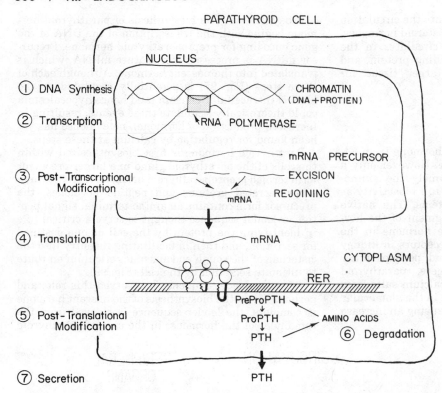

Figure 97. Schematic representation of potential control points in the regulation of biosynthesis and secretion of parathyroid hormone by the parathyroid cell. RER = rough endoplasmic reticulum. (Reprinted with permission from Rosenblatt, M.: Contrib Nephrol 33:163–177, 1982.)

hormone, this intracellular cleavage generates the prohormone, a precursor form of the hormone which is extended at the amino terminus by six amino acids. It is this form of the hormone that travels through the intracellular channels of the rough endoplasmic reticulum to the Golgi apparatus, where the hormone is further cleaved, yielding the mature form of the hormone, which is packaged into secretory granules. Although the role of the prohormone-specific segment of the molecule has not yet been determined, it may facilitate the events surrounding packaging of the hormone by the Golgi apparatus.

Once located within the secretory granule, the hormone may undergo further modification; the hormone may be cleaved into fragments, perhaps as an inactivation process for stored hormone. Unfortunately, the fragments so generated may later be released into the circulation. Although inactive biologically, the fragments may be detected by the radioimmunoassays that are used clinically. This complicates the interpretation of radioimmunoassay results in disorders of calcium metabolism.

Secretion. Stored intact hormone is released according to metabolic demand. The parathyroid cell responds to extracellular levels of calcium through alterations of intracellular levels of calcium, although the mechanism by which calcium regulates the secretion of parathyroid hormone is not known. The rate of parathyroid hormone secretion is inversely related to the concentration of ionized calcium in the extracellular fluid (Fig. 100). However, this relation is not linear. At calcium levels only slightly below the normal range (below 8 mg/dl), parathyroid hormone secretion increases dramatically. It is only over the narrow physiological range that relation of calcium to parathyroid hormone secretion is linear. At high calcium levels (11 to 18 mg/dl), suppression of parathyroid cell secretion

of the hormone is incomplete. The failure to completely arrest hormone secretion may be the cause of or may contribute to certain hypercalcemic disorders, as will be discussed later. In addition, other secretagogues, such as the catecholamines, may influence hormonal secretion, although their role in normal physiology or pathophysiology is still undetermined.

Once secreted, parathyroid hormone either interacts with receptors on the cell surface of target tissue cells, such as kidney and bone, or may be cleaved by the liver (Fig. 96). The physiological significance of peripheral metabolism of the hormone is unknown; cleavage may simply represent the first step in inactivation, degradation, and elimination of the hormone. Alternatively, the cleavage process may actually liberate an active amino-terminal fragment of the hormone that may have particular importance for the activity of the hormone in stimulating bone resorption.

Hormonal Action. The intact hormone, or its active fragment, acts on kidney to stimulate the reabsorption of calcium, the activation of vitamin D through stimulation of the 1-hydroxylase, and the excretion of phosphate. Some or all of these actions may be mediated via effects on intracellular levels of cyclic AMP. Cyclic AMP levels rise sufficiently intracellularly in renal cells to spill into the urine after exposure to parathyroid hormone, and detection of cyclic AMP in the urine can be used clinically as an indicator of parathyroid hormone activity. In response to parathyroid hormone, elevations in urinary cyclic AMP content and phosphate excretion occur rapidly in sequence and appear closely linked. The response of bone to parathyroid hormone typically occurs much more slowly, possibly reflecting a more complex pathway for expression of hormonal activity (Fig. 101). Ultimately, chronic stimulation of bone by parathyroid hormone leads to differentiation of cell types within bone and the stim-

Human
Pre – Proparathyroid Hormone

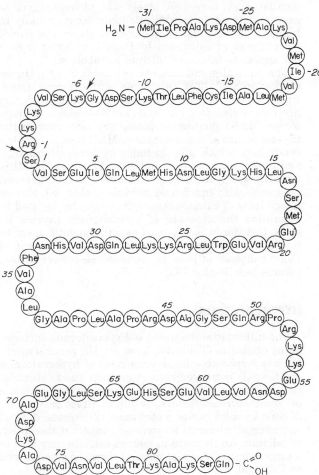

Figure 98. Structure of the 115-amino acid human preproparathyroid hormone molecule. Arrows indicate the sites where the leader or signal sequence is cleaved from the remaining molecule (between positions −7 and −6) and the prohormone is cleaved (between positions −1 and 1) to generate the native secreted form of the hormone, PTH-(1—84).

Figure 99. Events in biosynthesis, intracellular transport, processing, and secretion of parathyroid hormone. The leader or signal sequence of preproparathyroid hormone interacts with an intracellular signal receptor or signal recognition particle. This interaction is the step that ultimately commits the biosynthetic product of mRNA encoding for preproparathyroid hormone to secretion by the cell. The nascent molecule must traverse the membrane of the rough endoplasmic reticulum (RER) to gain access to the intracellular RER channels. On the interior side of the RER membrane is an enzyme, signal peptidase, that cleaves the signal sequence from the remainder of the hormone, generating proparathyroid hormone. After migration through the cisternae of the RER, proparathyroid hormone reaches the Golgi apparatus, where further cleavage and packaging of the hormone into secretory vesicles occur. The approximate time required for these events is indicated along the bottom of the figure. (Reprinted with permission from Rosenblatt, M.: Clin Orthop 170:260–276, 1982.)

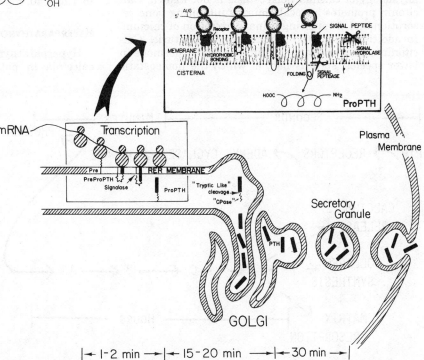

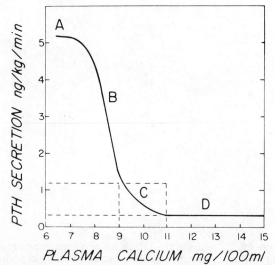

Figure 100. Plot of secretion of parathyroid hormone (PTH) by the parathyroid gland as a function of plasma levels of calcium. PTH secretion is inversely and approximately linearly related to calcium levels within the normal range of calcium (segment C). When calcium levels fall below normal, PTH secretion increases dramatically (segment B), until maximal glandular secretory rates (segment A) are achieved. At calcium levels above normal (segment D), PTH secretion is markedly, but incompletely, suppressed. (After G. P. Mayer, personal communication, 1973.)

ulation of reabsorption of the calcified matrix of bone by osteoclasts (see Section IX).

CALCITONIN

Although calcitonin, like parathyroid hormone, has potent effects on kidney and bone, its role in the human physiology of calcium homeostasis is not known. Calcitonin promotes hypocalcemia by inhibiting bone resorption and stimulating urinary excretion of calcium. In addition, calcitonin stimulates phosphaturia. Calcitonin is an important calcium regulatory hormone in lower species, such as fish, in which the homeostatic

challenge is maintenance of blood calcium levels in the presence of a calcium-rich environment such as sea water. In humans, it is unlikely that calcitonin serves an important physiological role: (1) calcitonin circulates at very low levels; (2) tachyphylaxis to exogenously administered calcitonin occurs rapidly in humans; (3) removal of the thyroid gland (the site of biosynthesis of calcitonin by C-cells) in humans does not appear to influence calcium metabolism.

The clinical significance of calcitonin is as a tumor marker in medullary carcinoma of the thyroid gland, which is one of the neoplasms associated with the hereditary disorders known as multiple endocrine neoplasia (MEN) syndromes. Medullary carcinoma of the thyroid occurs as a component of MEN type II (Sipple's syndrome), which also includes hyperparathyroidism and pheochromocytoma, and as a component of MEN type III, which includes pheochromocytomas, mucosal neuromas, and marfanoid habitus (Table 38). Stimulatory tests of calcitonin secretion can also be used to determine the presence of premalignant thyroid lesions. Calcitonin is also used as a therapeutic agent in treatment of hypercalcemia; its use in treatment of Paget's disease of bone is discussed elsewhere in this volume (see Section IX).

HYPERCALCEMIA

The differential diagnosis of hypercalcemia includes many etiologies (Table 39); however, the general mechanisms responsible for development of hypercalcemia are few: (1) increased bone resorption due to stimulation by humoral factors such as parathyroid hormone or tumor-secreted factors, or due to direct destruction of bone by solid tumor metastases; (2) decreased renal excretion of calcium; (3) increased intestinal absorption of calcium. An increase in ionized calcium may lead to a large number of symptoms and signs, as summarized in Table 40.

HYPERPARATHYROIDISM

Hyperparathyroidism is the leading cause of hypercalcemia in patients, with an incidence of 42 per

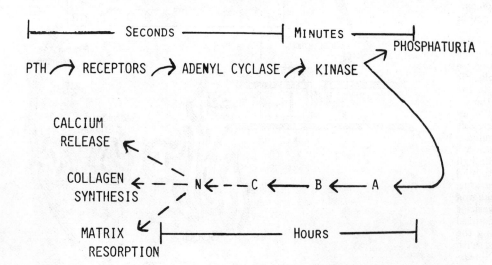

Figure 101. Postulated events in the expression of parathyroid hormone (PTH) biological activity. After interaction of PTH with hormone-specific receptors, a cascade of events occurs, including stimulation of adenylate cyclase activity and phosphorylation of proteins. The phosphaturic response to PTH occurs rapidly (within minutes) in kidney. Events in bone occur over a longer time period and are presumed to lead to several metabolic consequences of hormone action.

TABLE 38. MULTIPLE ENDOCRINE NEOPLASIA SYNDROMES

TYPE I	TYPE II	TYPE III
Hyperparathyroidism	Hyperparathyroidism	Medullary carcinoma of the thyroid
Pituitary tumors	Medullary carcinoma of the thyroid	Pheochromocytoma
prolactin-secreting	Pheochromocytoma	Mucosal neuromata
growth hormone–secreting		Marfanoid habitus
chromophobes		
Pancreatic tumors		
gastrin-secreting (Zollinger-Ellison)		
insulinoma		
glucagon-secreting		
vasoactive intestinal polypeptide–secreting		

100,000 per year in the United States. Although the majority of cases of hyperparathyroidism occur spontaneously, primary hyperparathyroidism is also one of the components of the multiple endocrine neoplasia (MEN) syndromes: MEN type I, when it is associated with pituitary adenomas and pancreatic neoplasms such as gastrinomas and insulinomas, and MEN type II (or IIa), when it is associated with medullary carcinoma of the thyroid and pheochromocytoma (Table 38).

Excess or inappropriate secretion of parathyroid hormone causes hypercalcemia directly by increasing bone resorption and stimulating reabsorption of calcium in the renal tubules, and indirectly by increasing absorption of dietary calcium through stimulating formation of the active metabolite of vitamin D by the kidney. The consequences of hyperparathyroidism, therefore, include bone demineralization (Fig. 102) and fractures, bone pain, development of kidney stones (hypercalciuria occurs as a result of the increased filtered load of calcium, despite the promotion of calcium reabsorption by the kidney due to parathyroid hormone), nephrocalcinosis, and a number of constitutional symptoms related to hypercalcemia and hypophosphatemia (Table 40).

As discussed earlier, each of the steps in biosynthesis and processing of parathyroid hormone, including transcription, translation, post-translational modification, and packaging (Fig. 97), represents a potential control point in the regulation of circulating levels of parathyroid hormone. As such, they also represent potential areas of dysfunction. Modulation of the levels of mRNA, the efficiency of transcription and translation, the conversion of precursor mRNA to mature mRNA, the stepwise conversion of preproparathyroid hormone

to proparathyroid hormone and of proparathyroid hormone to parathyroid hormone, and the intracellular degradation of stored hormone have each been examined in this regard, but seem not to be regulation points for the fine control of parathyroid hormone secretion displayed in vivo (Fig. 100). Rather, the release of the hormone into the circulation by the parathyroid cell appears inappropriately controlled in primary hyperparathyroidism.

Primary hyperparathyroidism results most frequently from an adenoma of a single parathyroid gland. Hyperplasia of four glands is seen in approximately 10 to 15 per cent of hyperparathyroidism and is often associated with the MEN syndromes (Table 38). A few cases of hyperparathyroidism (1 to 3 per cent) are caused by parathyroid carcinomas, to be discussed later.

Despite the anatomical differences in parathyroid adenomas and parathyroid hyperplasia (Fig. 103), the pathophysiological mechanism responsible for hypercalcemia in these disorders appears similar. Both hyperplastic and adenomatous tissues respond to some extent to changes in extracellular calcium concentra-

TABLE 39. HYPERCALCEMIA: DIFFERENTIAL DIAGNOSIS

Primary hyperparathyroidism (multiple endocrine neoplasia, types I and II)
Malignancy
Sarcoidosis or other granulomatous disease
Thyrotoxicosis
Adrenal insufficiency
Vitamin D intoxication
Hypervitaminosis A
Thiazide diuretics
Milk-alkali syndrome
Immobilization
Familial hypocalciuric hypercalcemia
Lithium-induced

TABLE 40. SYMPTOMS AND SIGNS OF HYPERCALCEMIA

Central nervous system
Drowsiness	Stupor or coma
Lethargy	Ataxia
Depression	Abnormal EEG
Organic psychosis	

Neuromuscular
Weakness	Hypotonia
Proximal myopathy	Diminished deep tendon reflexes

Cardiovascular
Hypertension	Short Q-T interval
Bradycardia	Potentiation of digitalis toxicity
Cardiac arrhythmia	

Renal
Polyuria
Hypercalciuria (stone diathesis)
Calcium nephropathy—nephrocalcinosis, sodium and potassium wasting, azotemia
Gastrointestinal
Nausea, vomiting, anorexia, constipation, increased gastric acidity and dyspepsia, pancreatitis
Metastatic calcification (when phosphorus is also elevated)
Band keratopathy, pruritus, ectopic conjunctival calcification

From Avioli, L. V.: Hypercalcemia. In Wyngaarden, J. B., and Smith, L. H., Jr. (eds.): Cecil Textbook of Medicine, 16th ed. Philadelphia, W. B. Saunders Co., 1982, p. 1329.

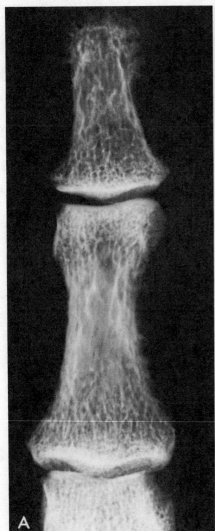

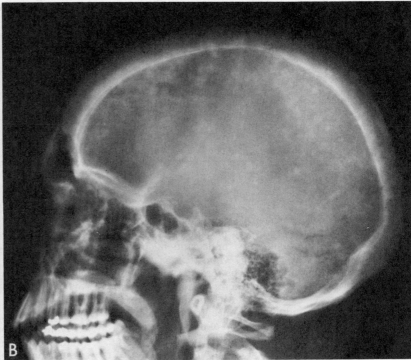

Figure 102. *A,* Magnified x-ray of index finger on fine grain industrial film, showing classic subperiosteal resorption in a patient with severe primary hyperparathyroidism. *B,* Skull x-ray from a patient with severe secondary hyperparathyroidism resulting from prolonged end-stage renal disease. Extensive areas of demineralization alternate with areas of increased bone density, resulting in an exaggerated picture of the "salt-and-pepper" skull x-ray, which used to be a classic finding in primary hyperparathyroidism. This is rarely seen now and cannot be visualized easily in x-ray reproductions. Although it is difficult to appreciate at this magnification, the dental lamina dura is absent, another classic x-ray finding in severe hyperparathyroidism. (Courtesy of Professor H. Genant, University of California, San Francisco, Department of Radiology.) (From Arnaud, C. D.: In Wyngaarden, J. B., and Smith, L. H., Jr. (eds.): Cecil Textbook of Medicine. 17th ed. Philadelphia, W. B. Saunders Co., 1985, p. 1437.)

tions—their secretion of parathyroid hormone is suppressed more than 50 per cent when exposed to high concentrations of calcium. In many instances, it appears as if a "set point" or "thermostat-like" error is present (Fig. 104). But the set point varies considerably in these tissues. Some of the similarities in response between hyperplastic and adenomatous tissue and the overall heterogeneous nature of the abnormal parathyroid cell response may relate to the etiology of parathyroid adenomas, which appear to arise from a multicellular origin. Hence, parathyroid adenomas may represent a kind of single-gland hyperplasia.

An abnormally high set point for calcium suppression of parathyroid hormone release may explain the pathophysiology of some hyperparathyroid disorders and may explain the finding of "normal" parathyroid hormone levels (by radioimmunoassay) in patients with hypercalcemia and hyperparathyroidism (Fig. 104). Other factors may also contribute to or entirely account for the clinical disorder, however. Because the secretion of parathyroid hormone by parathyroid cells cannot be completely suppressed, a simple increase in parathyroid tissue mass above a critical threshold

could theoretically produce hypercalcemia (Fig. 104). Increased parathyroid tissue in both hyperplasia and parathyroid adenomas could cause the nonsuppressible component of parathyroid hormone secretion to exceed this threshold. In fact, transplantation of several normal parathyroid glands into a single rat produces hypercalcemia. Hence, abnormally high calcium set points, or an increased component of nonsuppressible parathyroid hormone, may be responsible for the pathophysiology of hyperparathyroidism. Only cells from parathyroid carcinoma display autonomous parathyroid hormone secretion (failure to modulate parathyroid hormone release at even the highest calcium concentrations).

The pathophysiology of many of the symptoms and complications of hyperparathyroidism remains to be elucidated. Proximal muscle weakness occurs and is accompanied by specific neuromyopathic changes corresponding to loss of motor units under voluntary control evident by electromyography. These changes appear to be parathyroid hormone—mediated and reversible with correction of the disorder. Kidney stones may occur more frequently in a subset of patients with

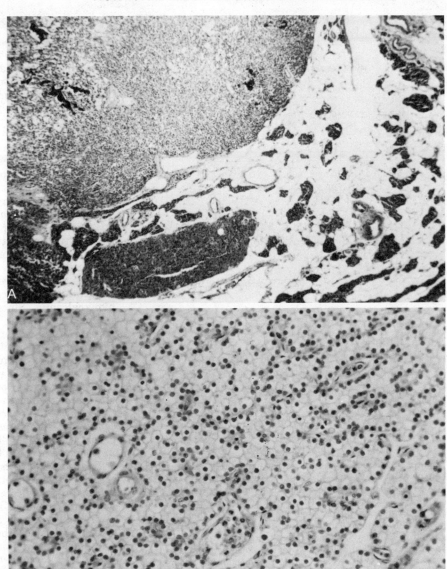

Figure 103. Photomicrograph of *(A)* parathyroid adenoma and *(B)* parathyroid hyperplasia. The adenoma has increased cellularity and decreased fat; a rim of normal tissue is seen at the border of the adenoma. In hyperplasia, all four parathyroid glands display a diffuse increase in cellularity.

hyperparathyroidism, namely those who have increased levels of $1\alpha,25$-dihydroxyvitamin D_3 in the circulation and hypercalciuria.

HYPERCALCEMIA OF MALIGNANCY

Several mechanisms may be operative in the production of hypercalcemia by malignancies. Osteolysis, or the direct destruction of bone by solid tumor metastases, such as those arising from breast or thyroid cancers, may cause hypercalcemia. Hematological malignancies may secrete locally active factors that stimulate bone resorption. For instance, in multiple myeloma the secretion of osteoclast-activating factor (O.A.F.) may produce hypercalcemia.

In the majority of cases of hypercalcemia of malignancy, hypercalcemia does not appear to be caused by local destruction of bone. Rather, the secretion by tumors of factors that stimulate bone resorption appears to be the more common mechanism. Some tumors

may secrete prostaglandins (especially those of the PGE_2 family) that stimulate bone resorption. The ectopic secretion of parathyroid hormone by renal cell carcinoma or squamous cell carcinoma of the lung has also been postulated. Although theoretically possible, this phenomenon appears to be exceedingly rare.

It now appears likely that approximately 80 per cent of the hypercalcemia of malignancy is mediated by secretion into the circulation of bone-resorbing factors by tumors. Although these factors are not parathyroid hormone, as demonstrated by their failure to react with anti–parathyroid hormone antisera and their larger molecular weight, these factors do appear to have many of the biological properties of parathyroid hormone. In addition to producing hypercalcemia, they stimulate excretion of cyclic AMP in the urine and decrease the renal threshold for phosphate clearance. However, $1\alpha,25$-dihydroxyvitamin D_3 levels are low or undetectable in the hypercalcemia of malignancy, which differs from the normal or high values observed

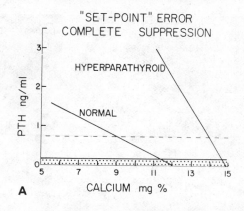

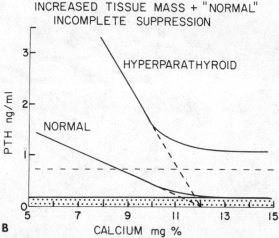

Figure 104. Possible mechanisms responsible for pathophysiology of primary hyperparathyroidism. *A*, A "set-point" or thermostat-type error accounts for abnormally increased secretion of parathyroid hormone (PTH) in hyperparathyroidism. In this case, higher levels of extracellular calcium must be achieved before hormonal secretion is suppressed, but the gland is responsive to modulation by plasma calcium. Hyperparathyroid individuals show steeper slopes of response owing to large mass of tissue. *B*, An alternate mechanism is depicted. The gland is "normally" responsive to plasma calcium levels in the hyperparathyroid state, but the increased mass of parathyroid tissue accounts for the increased amounts of PTH secreted. In addition, the normal incomplete suppression of PTH secretion that occurs at high levels of calcium is amplified because of the increased total mass of parathyroid tissue. Small amounts of hormone secretion persist despite elevated calcium; in the normal parathyroid, this secretion is small and insignificant, but in hyperparathyroidism the greatly increased tissue mass leads to persistent secretion of hormone above the normal range. The slopes of both the normal and hyperparathyroid glands extrapolate to the same calcium value. The dashed line indicates the upper limit of normal PTH secretion. Lower speckled space indicates undetectable range for PTH by radioimmunoassay.

in hyperparathyroidism. In preliminary studies, the bioactivity of tumor factors can be inhibited with synthetic antagonists of parathyroid hormone known to act by competitively occupying parathyroid hormone receptors. Taken together, this information suggests that some tumors secrete nonparathyroid hormone substances, perhaps growth factors, that may nevertheless produce hypercalcemia by interacting with and stimulating parathyroid hormone receptors on target tissue.

PATHOPHYSIOLOGY OF OTHER CAUSES OF HYPERCALCEMIA

Sarcoidosis or other granulomatous disease can cause hypercalcemia (Table 39). In the past, this was thought to be due to hypersensitivity to or decreased degradation of vitamin D. It now appears that granulomatous tissue itself performs the specialized reaction of converting 25-hydroxyvitamin D_3 to $1\alpha,25$-dihydroxyvitamin D_3.

Thyrotoxicosis can cause mild degrees of hypercalcemia but rarely causes severe hypercalcemia, and usually the thyrotoxic state is apparent clinically. Thyroid hormone–stimulated bone resorption appears to be the mechanism responsible for the hypercalcemia.

Acute adrenal insufficiency can cause hypercalcemia, but this is in large part a laboratory artifact resulting from dehydration causing hemoconcentration. The increased concentration of albumin binds calcium, so the total calcium is elevated, but the free or ionized form of calcium usually remains in the normal range.

Vitamin D intoxication produces a hyperabsorptive hypercalcemia. Since vitamin D metabolites are fat soluble, a reservoir of the hormone is established in adipose tissue, often leading to prolonged hypercalcemia. In addition, the availability for clinical use of $1\alpha,25$-dihydroxyvitamin D_3, the final active form of the hormone, which is positioned beyond the regulatory steps in activation of vitamin D, has made iatrogenic vitamin D intoxication more common.

Vitamin A intoxication can also produce hypercalcemia and symptoms similar to those of primary hyperparathyroidism. The mechanism of hypercalcemia in this case appears to be increased bone resorption.

Thiazide diuretics produce hypercalcemia by decreasing renal excretion of calcium. However, thiazide-induced hypercalcemia is transient and rarely persists for more than one month. If hypercalcemia persists after this period, it is likely that mild hyperparathyroidism or some other underlying cause of hypercalcemia has been unmasked.

The *milk-alkali syndrome* is decreasing in frequency as a cause of hypercalcemia. The syndrome was more commonly seen when the treatment regimen for peptic ulcer disease included consumption of absorbable calcium-containing antacids and large quantities of milk. This combination had the unfortunate effects of increasing calcium absorption from the gut while the basic pH decreased calcium salt solubility in the kidney and other soft tissues, leading to kidney stones or nephrocalcinosis.

Lithium, used for the treatment of certain psychiatric disorders, can produce hypercalcemia. The mechanism remains obscure, but it has been suggested that lithium alters the sensitivity of tissues, including the parathyroid glands, to calcium. The consequences of such an effect would be to raise the set point for suppression of parathyroid hormone secretion by the parathyroid gland, producing a mild but true hyperparathyroid state, which is reversible with discontinuation of lithium administration.

Immobilization can cause severe hypercalcemia. Without the stimulus of weight bearing and activity, bone formation is decreased relative to bone resorption. The increased bone turnover leads to hypercalcemia. This problem can be particularly manifest in growing children or adults with Paget's disease of bone.

Familial hypocalciuric hypercalcemia is a recently described hereditary disorder that can be very difficult to distinguish from hyperparathyroidism. As in primary hyperparathyroidism, blood calcium levels are elevated and the parathyroid hormone levels are either frankly elevated or detectable. There is no single biochemical marker for this disorder. In general, the parathyroid levels tend to be less than those seen in primary hyperparathyroidism for a comparable degree of calcium elevation. Other features of the syndrome include magnesium levels that are elevated or in the upper portion of the normal range and low urinary calcium excretion (<100 mg per 24 hours), especially for the level of hypercalcemia. The disorder tends to appear earlier in life than primary hyperparathyroidism, often in the first decade, although it may not be discovered until many decades later. It is inherited as an autosomal dominant disorder with nearly 100 per cent penetrance. In addition, it is associated with severe neonatal hypercalcemia, and newborns that are born into a kindred with this disorder need to be monitored closely during the first hours of life. Hypocalcemia also occurs in infants born to hypercalcemic mothers. Except for these latter rare features related to newborns, the disorder appears completely benign. There is no evidence of end-organ damage. Hence, the principal reason for clinical awareness of this disorder is to avoid sending a patient to needless parathyroid surgery. Surgical removal of one or more parathyroid glands does not restore calcium levels to normal, and since there are no known adverse sequelae of the disorder, surgery offers no benefit to the patient.

The pathophysiology of the syndrome has not yet been established. One suggested mechanism is a generalized insensitivity to calcium by tissues, comparable to the effects of lithium discussed above. In such a case, parathyroid hormone secretion would be increased because the level of calcium sensed by the parathyroid glands would be anomalously low. In addition, the long-term effects of hypercalcemia would be diminished in tissue that is relatively insensitive to calcium. The parathyroid glands are usually histologically normal.

TREATMENT OF HYPERCALCEMIA

The initial steps in the treatment of hypercalcemia are identical regardless of the etiology of the hypercalcemia. There are only a limited number of mechanistic approaches to the treatment of hypercalcemia (Table 41). Urinary excretion of calcium can be promoted by sodium loading or treating with furosemide. Gut absorption of calcium can be decreased by systemic administration of steroids or by binding calcium in the gastrointestinal tract by use of oral phosphates. The release of calcium into the bloodstream that results

TABLE 41. MECHANISTIC APPROACHES TO TREATMENT OF HYPERCALCEMIA

1. Block absorption from gut—diet, steroids, oral phosphate
2. Promote urinary calcium excretion—Na^+, furosemide
3. Block bone resorption—mithramycin, calcitonin, diphosphonates
4. Cause complexing of ionized Ca^{++}—intravenous phosphate, EDTA

from ongoing bone resorption can be blocked by mithramycin, calcitonin, or diphosphonates. Although rarely necessary, ionized calcium can be complexed intravenously by administering phosphate or EDTA. Finally, peritoneal dialysis or hemodialysis can be employed as a direct means of removing calcium from the extracellular fluid.

Severe hypercalcemia (calcium >14 mg/dl) can be life-threatening and should be treated urgently (Table 42). These patients are almost always dehydrated, which contributes to the hypercalcemia and impairs renal compensatory mechanisms to correct the abnormality. Intravenous rehydration with large quantities of saline-containing fluids is essential and must be accompanied by close monitoring of serum electrolytes, especially potassium and magnesium.

After infusion of 2 to 4 liters of fluid, intravenous furosemide can be added while a saline-containing infusion is maintained. The effect of saline and furosemide is rapid and substantial, but obviously unsatisfactory for long-term treatment. Since the remaining therapies often take several days to be effective, a decision has to be made at this early stage as to the appropriate additional intervention. Mithramycin inhibits bone resorption and is effective in treating hypercalcemia of all etiologies, including primary hyperparathyroidism. Its use is limited by a cumulative toxicity after multiple doses. Calcitonin inhibits bone resorption, but patients often develop tachyphylaxis to calcitonin, which appears to be delayed by the addition of steroids. Glucocorticoids alone are most effective in treating hypercalcemia associated with lymphomas and other malignancies, sarcoidosis, and vitamin D intoxication; steroids are ineffective in treating the hypercalcemia of primary hyperparathyroidism. Indomethacin is effective in diminishing hypercalcemia only in the rare instance in which a tumor is secreting prostaglandins responsible for the hypercalcemia. Intravenous phosphates are rapidly effective, but when the level of hypercalcemia is high, use of intravenous phosphates runs a high risk of exceeding the solubility product constant of calcium phosphate and causing ectopic (soft tissue) precipitation of calcium salts in the kidney and elsewhere. Dialysis is also rapidly effective but is fraught with complications and rarely needed. Finally, the long-term management of severe hypercalcemia requires that the underlying disorder be addressed; for instance, the best long-term treatment of hypercalcemia of malignancy is appropriate management of the tumor.

Moderate hypercalcemia, in the range of 12 to 14 mg/dl, is treated using the same modalities, but less aggressively. Salt, fluids, and furosemide can be given orally instead of intravenously. Oral phosphates may be useful, although caution must again be exercised to avoid long-term ectopic calcification. Oral phosphates are best used when the serum phosphate level is low initially, thus decreasing the risk of exceeding the solubility product constant for calcium and phosphate. Experience with the diphosphonates, which inhibit bone resorption, is still accumulating, and newer diphosphonate agents are being evaluated. Beta-blocking agents such as propranolol inhibit parathyroid hormone secretion to some extent and may have an ancillary role in managing primary hyperparathyroidism or maintaining a patient until surgery can be per-

TABLE 42. TREATMENT OF SEVERE HYPERCALCEMIA (>14 mg/dl)

THERAPY	ONSET	INDICATIONS	COMPLICATIONS
1. Rehydrate with saline (1–2 liters)	immed.	universal	congestive heart failure
2. Saline (4–12 L/day) + furosemide (20–80 mg I.V./day)	immed.	universal	↓K+, ↓Mg++
3. Mithramycin	48 hrs.	universal	cumulative toxicity: liver, bone marrow, kidney—monitor CBC, platelets, BUN, liver function
4. Calcitonin (100–200 units/day) + prednisone	6–48 hrs.	universal (best in immobilization)	rapid tachyphylaxis
5. Steroids (20–60 mg prednisone)	48 hrs.	breast carcinoma, lymphomas, leukemias, multiple myeloma, vitamin D poisoning, sarcoidosis	Cushing's syndrome
6. Indomethacin (25 mg q6h)	days–1 wk	suspected prostaglandin-mediated hypercalcemia	GI bleed, Na+ retention
7. Phosphate I.V.	immed.	almost never	high risk for ectopic calcification and renal failure
8. Dialysis	hours	universal, but rarely needed	many
9. Novel: diphosphonates (I.V.)	6–48 hrs.	universal	—

THEN ADDRESS UNDERLYING DISORDER

formed. Cimetidine decreases parathyroid hormone secretion, but the accompanying decline in calcium levels is usually small or insignificant.

Mild hypercalcemia (levels <12 mg/dl) usually requires no specific treatment. Again, the underlying disorder causing the hypercalcemia needs to be addressed. In the case of primary hyperparathyroidism, the decision to undertake surgical excision of the abnormal parathyroid gland or glands is a complicated one. Perhaps only 15 to 50 per cent of patients with primary hyperparathyroidism ultimately require surgical treatment because of the level of hypercalcemia attained or because of end-organ (bone, kindey) damage. However, this subset of patients is not readily identified, and the optimum means for monitoring integrity of bone and renal function has not been clearly established. In addition, the cost of monitoring patients with yearly follow-up for periods ranging up to decades can far exceed the cost of a surgical cure. Hence, the decision to undertake surgery versus medical management in primary hyperparathyroidism must be individualized to the patient and based on factors such as age, severity of hypercalcemia, surgical risk, and indicators of end-organ damage.

HYPOCALCEMIA

Hypocalcemia causes hyperpolarization of nervous and muscle tissue, resulting in the following signs and symptoms: seizures, circumoral and distal paresthesias, tetany, and prolonged Q-T interval on the EKG. On physical examination, Chvostek's and Trousseau's signs may be present.

The mechanisms responsible for hypocalcemia are principally inadequate parathyroid hormone levels and inadequate calcium absorption from the gut. Only rarely is an isolated renal calcium leak the cause of hypocalcemia.

The most common cause of hypocalcemia is surgically induced hypoparathyroidism, usually arising as a complication of total thyroidectomy (Table 43). Hypoparathyroidism also occurs on a hereditary basis associated with a multiple endocrine deficiency syndrome that includes hypothyroidism and adrenal insufficiency and accompanied by mucocutaneous candidiasis. Hypoparathyroidism is also a component of the DiGeorge syndrome, which includes lymphocytopenia and aplasia of the third branchial area. Hypoparathyroidism also occurs on an idiopathic basis.

Pseudohypoparathyroidism, although rare, is of considerable interest because of the insights its pathophysiology may provide into the mechanism of action of parathyroid hormone. The syndrome is named pseudohypoparathyroidism because, although the patient clinically is hypoparathyroid, parathyroid hormone ap-

TABLE 43. DIFFERENTIAL DIAGNOSIS OF HYPOCALCEMIA

Surgically induced hypoparathyroidism
Hypoparathyroidism (other causes)
  Familial
  Multiple endocrine deficiencies: hypothyroidism and hypoadrenalism; mucocutaneous candidiasis
  DiGeorge syndrome (lymphocytopenia + aplasia of third branchial area)
  Idiopathic
Pseudohypoparathyroidism
Malabsorption
Vitamin D deficiency
Hypomagnesemia
"Hungry bones" after parathyroidectomy
Medullary carcinoma of thyroid (exceptionally rare)
Hypoalbuminemia (ionized calcium normal)

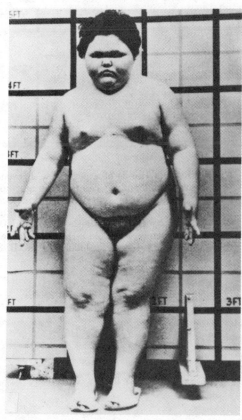

Figure 105. A patient with pseudohypoparathyroidism, showing typical round facies, obesity, and short stature. (From Potts, J. T., and Deftos, L. J.: In Bondy, P. K. (ed.): Duncan's Diseases of Metabolism. 6th ed. Philadelphia, W. B. Saunders Co., 1969, pp. 904–1082.)

pears present in adequate levels in the circulation. Accompanying features typically include short stature, obesity, round facies, and short fourth metacarpals and metatarsals (Figs. 105 and 106). The precise defect in this disorder has not yet been identified. There appears to be an end-organ resistance to parathyroid hormone in some kindreds with this disorder: parathyroid hormone levels are normal or elevated, and target tissue appears deficient in guanyl nucleotide regulatory protein, one of the essential components in the receptor-effector apparatus for parathyroid hormone. Other data suggest that an inactive form of the hormone may be secreted in some patients or that a circulating inhibitor of parathyroid hormone may be present. Such a variant form of the hormone could arise from incorrect excision of an intron during processing of the mRNA precursor encoding for preproparathyroid hormone.

Both vitamin D and calcium can be poorly absorbed in a variety of gastrointestinal disorders, causing hypocalcemia. Hypocalcemia itself causes diarrhea, which exacerbates the tendency toward malabsorption. Vitamin D deficiency can also occur on a dietary basis. Vitamin D deficiency can be very subtle; calcium levels are protected from becoming abnormally low by increased secretion of parathyroid hormone (secondary hyperparathyroidism). Vitamin D deficiency often accompanies the use of anticonvulsants such as pheny-

toin, since the drug induces increased degradation of vitamin D.

Hypomagnesemia, most typically seen in alcoholics, can cause hypocalcemia. Low magnesium levels impair parathyroid hormone secretion by parathyroid cells and also inhibit the action of the hormone at the target tissue, thus causing a "functional" hypoparathyroidism.

The syndrome of "hungry bones" can produce a prolonged period of hypocalcemia. The syndrome describes calcium metabolism in the period following surgery for longstanding and severe hyperparathyroidism. In this state, the bones undergo excessive resorption and compensatory coupled formation. The bones are also calcium-deprived. Sudden arrest of hyperparathyroidism leaves the bones able to accept large quantities of calcium without a rectifying bone resorption. The resulting shift produces acute hypocalcemia that is ineffectively opposed by the remaining "normal parathyroid tissue," since it has been chronically suppressed. The capacity of bones to absorb calcium excessively in the "hungry bone syndrome" is dramatic and may persist for months.

Although calcitonin is secreted in pathological excess in medullary carcinoma of the thyroid, this disease is rarely accompanied by hypocalcemia. Perhaps this results from opposing secretion of parathyroid hormone or from the tachyphylaxis that develops to calcitonin.

TREATMENT OF HYPOCALCEMIA

The treatment of hypocalcemia depends on the severity of the problem and its expected chronicity. Severe acute hypocalcemia can be treated with intravenous administration of a calcium salt. Less severe and chronic hypocalcemia can be treated with oral calcium supplements. If hypomagnesemia is the etiology of the hypocalcemia, normal physiology will not be restored until the (usually large) magnesium deficiency is corrected with either oral or intravenous magnesium replacement.

Unfortunately, parathyroid hormone is not available for treatment of hypoparathyroidism. Hence, a less satisfactory therapeutic approach using vitamin D preparations is taken. Vitamin D is given to increase gastrointestinal absorption of dietary calcium. To maximize the effectiveness of the therapy and minimize the dose of vitamin D, oral calcium supplements are also given. Often it is necessary to use $1\alpha,25$-dihydroxyvitamin D_3 or an analogue such as dihydrotachysterol, since the 1-hydroxylation of vitamin D precursors in the kidney is parathyroid hormone–regulated and is reduced in the absence of parathyroid hormone. In addition, phosphate levels are often high in hypoparathyroidism. To avoid ectopic calcification, phosphate levels may need to be diminished by administration of gastrointestinal phosphate binders, such as oral aluminum hydroxide, before calcium can be given. Furthermore, calcium levels should be brought only to the low normal range, since hypercalciuria is pronounced in the absence of parathyroid hormone, which normally enhances its renal tubular reabsorption. An increased filtered load of calcium under these circumstances can lead to formation of kidney stones.

Vitamin D deficiency in the absence of malabsorption can be treated by a variety of vitamin D preparations.

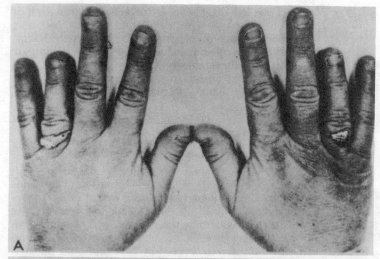

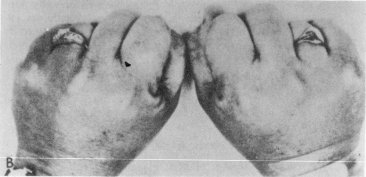

Figure 106. Hands of a patient with pseudohypoparathyroidism. *A,* The fourth finger appears short, owing to the shortened fourth metacarpal. When a fist is made *(B),* the fourth knuckle appears absent. (From Potts, J. T., and Deftos, L. J.: In Bondy, P. K. (ed.): Duncan's Diseases of Metabolism. 6th ed. Philadelphia, W. B. Saunders Co., 1969, pp. 904–1082.)

Patients who receive anticonvulsants should be given vitamin D and oral calcium prophylactically to prevent osteomalacia (see Section IX).

REFERENCES

Broadus, A. E.: Mineral metabolism. In Felig, P., Baxter, J. D., Broadus, A. E., and Frohman, L. A. (eds.): Endocrinology and Metabolism. New York, McGraw Hill Book Co., 1981, pp. 963–1080.

DeLuca, H. F.: Vitamin D endocrinology. Ann Intern Med 85:367, 1976.

Habener, J. F., and Potts, J. T., Jr.: Diagnosis and differential diagnosis of primary hyperparathyroidism. In DeGroot, L. J., et al. (eds.): Endocrinology. Vol. 2. New York, Grune & Stratton, 1979, pp. 703–712.

Heath, H., III, Hodgson, S. F., and Kennedy, M. A.: Primary hyperparathyroidism: Incidence, morbidity, and potential economic impact in a community. N Engl J Med 302:189, 1980.

Marx, S. J., Spiegel, A. M.,. Brown, E. M., et al.: Divalent cation metabolism: Familial hypocalciuric hypercalcemia versus typical primary hyperparathyroidism. Am J Med 65:235–241, 1978.

Neer, R. M., and Potts, J. T., Jr.: Medical management of hypercalcemia and hyperparathyroidism. In DeGroot, L. J., et al. (eds.): Endocrinology. Vol. 2. New York, Grune & Stratton, 1979, pp. 725–734.

Raisz, L. G., Yajnik, C. H., Bockman, R. S., et al.: Comparison of commercially available parathyroid hormone immunoassays in the differential diagnosis of hypercalcemia due to primary hyperparathyroidism or malignancy. Ann Intern Med 91:739–740, 1979.

Stewart, A. F., Horst, R., Deftos, L. J., Cadman, E. C., Land, R., and Broadus, A. E.: Biochemical evaluation of patients with cancer-associated hypercalcemia. N Engl J Med 303:1377–1383, 1980.

CONNECTIVE TISSUE

STEPHEN M. KRANE, M.D.,
and ROBERT M. NEER, M.D.

Connective tissues usually refer to those structures that are responsible for the form and shape of the animal body. The term is most often applied to tissues such as bone, cartilage, tendons, fascia, and the capsules of joints. Connective tissues also contribute to the major structures of large blood vessel walls. All organs, however, have some connective tissue component that is responsible not only for form but also for mechanical function. Connective tissues are composed not only of the specialized cells responsible for their formation but also of an extracellular matrix whose composition determines the properties of that tissue. The extracellular matrix, in turn, usually contains a fibrillar protein or proteins; globular proteins, some of which are glycoproteins; variable proportions of proteoglycans; and, in the case of a specialized connective tissue such as bone, a mineral phase as well. Some connective tissues, such as cartilage, are relatively avascular and turn over very slowly, whereas bone, even in adults, has a high metabolic rate and is continually being remodeled. Considerable information is now available concerning the composition, biosynthesis, and degradation of connective tissues and how disease states may alter their composition by affecting biosynthesis and degradation.

Composition

Connective tissues as organs are composed of vascular elements, specialized cells, and extracellular material (Fig. 1). Some connective tissues are exceedingly vascular, of which a good example is bone (Fig. 2). Bones possess a unique arrangement of blood vessels: The arterial supply is through a principal nutrient artery and periosteal arteries into the cortical venous channels and the central venous sinuses of the medulla of bone. The veins of bones drain the hematopoietic elements of the marrow, whereas cortical venous channels serve the nonmarrow-containing portions of compact bone. Bone cells (osteocytes) (Fig. 3) are connected to each other through microcanaliculi and depend upon continuous vascular supply for their nutrition. In contrast, cartilage is avascular, and cartilage cells must derive their nutrition from neighboring tissues. For example, the cells in articular cartilage obtain their nutrition by repeated compression and release of compression. By this means metabolic substrates can be delivered and metabolic products removed from the environment of the cells. Thus, chondrocytes have a low oxygen consumption and a high rate of glycolysis compared with bone cells, which depend upon an abundant arterial blood supply. With the possible exception of cartilage, the vasculature is usually intimately related to the function of most connective tissues. Indeed, blood vessel walls are themselves a form of connective tissue, and component cells are capable of synthesizing matrix components. Furthermore, the circulation may actually be the source of connective tissue cells. For example, circulating monocytes can, under some circumstances, differentiate into tissue osteoclasts. In bone, the specialized vascular areas that make up the sinuses in the marrow also contribute to skeletal function. Hematopoietic elements are thought to be responsible for precursor cells destined to become osteoclasts, whereas stromal elements of the marrow may be the source of precursor cells that differentiate into osteoblasts.

The cells of each connective tissue are responsible for the synthesis and organization of the extracellular matrix that characterizes that tissue. Thus, osteoblasts (Fig. 2) and chondrocytes (Fig. 4) synthesize and secrete the characteristic matrix of bone and cartilage, respectively. In other connective tissues the predominant cells that are responsible for the formation of connective tissue matrix are usually called fibroblasts (Fig. 5). However, all fibroblasts do not necessarily produce the same kind of matrix. Fibroblasts in tendons, for example, may produce the large, densely packed collagen fibers that are highly organized along their long axis with respect to each other, whereas fibroblasts may also synthesize the loosely woven stroma of parenchymal organs or other types of fibrous networks in tissues such as dermis. With respect to collagen, different cells—for example, osteoblasts and dermal fibroblasts—may produce the same protein with the same primary structure, yet other functions of each of these cells determine posttranslational modification of the primary structure of these proteins. The specialized cells of each connective tissue also produce other components of the extracellular matrix that determine the function of that tissue. In cartilage, for example, the chondrocyte secretes not only the specific type II collagen but also the proteoglycan. In bone, the osteoblast is also involved in the formation

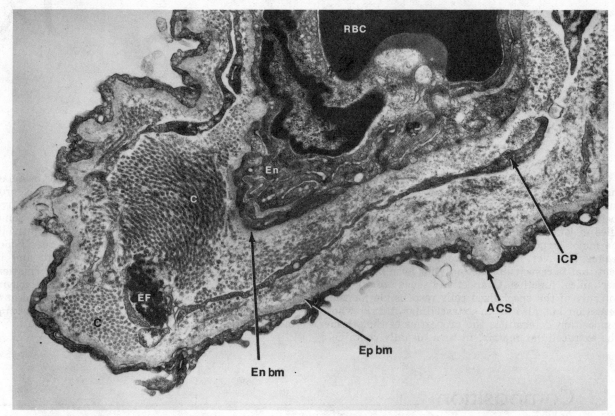

Figure 1. Electron micrograph of a portion of the alveolar diffusion organ of the lung illustrating relationships of cells to extracellular connective tissue matrices. The capillary is at the upper portion and the air space at the lower portion of the figure. An erythrocyte (RBC) is within the lumen of the capillary. A portion of an endothelial cell (En) and its surrounding basement membrane (En bm) is seen. An alveolar cell process lines the air space at the alveolar cell surface (ACS). A basement membrane (Ep bm) produced by these epithelial cells lies beneath the alveolar cell process. The process of an interstitial cell (ICP) is also shown. Collagen fibers (C) and elastic fibers (EF) are present in the extracellular matrix. (Courtesy of R. Trelstad.)

of the mineral phase, which must be deposited in an ordered fashion with respect to the matrix. A single fibroblast can stain with antibodies to both type I and type III collagen, implying that the same cell can synthesize and secrete two different macromolecules. Primitive mesenchymal cells may differentiate into cells that assume phenotypic characteristics of mature connective tissue cells. Such differentiation is under many different controls, including factors derived from immunocompetent cells, hormones, and neuronal influences. Connective tissues also underlie epithelial structures. These epithelial cells may synthesize specialized matrices such as basement membranes, which also contain specific collagens.

The extracellular matrices of connective tissues (Tables 1 and 2) contain not only substances formed by the cells of that connective tissue but also electrolytes and low molecular weight materials derived from the vascular system. The unique properties of each matrix in turn may determine the distribution of such substances. For example, the proteoglycans of articular cartilage with their large "domain" and high negative charge are responsible for the presence of large amounts of bound water. This water is responsible for the ability of cartilage to deform under stress and regain the original shape. On the other hand, when bone, cartilage, and dentin are calcified, water is lost as it is replaced by the inorganic mineral phase. Thus,

some extracellular tissues such as mineralized bone have an extracellular fluid volume considerably lower than that of other tissues. Some connective tissues also contain high molecular weight materials derived from plasma. The function of most of these components is unknown with respect to the character of the particular connective tissue. In the case of bone, there is evidence that specific glycoproteins derived from plasma are incorporated into the matrix.

FIBROUS PROTEINS

COLLAGENS

Collagen Structure

In most connective tissues, the major component of the organic portion is a fibrous protein such as collagen or elastin. Collagen is the major fibrillar protein of most connective tissues and indeed may be the predominant protein of such connective tissues as bone, where it represents approximately 95 per cent of the total organic material. The term collagen refers to a class of protein that is characterized by its amino acid composition and structural organization of the polypeptide chains. Most collagens have regions containing the specific collagen triple helix determined by the primary structure (that is, a glycine residue in every

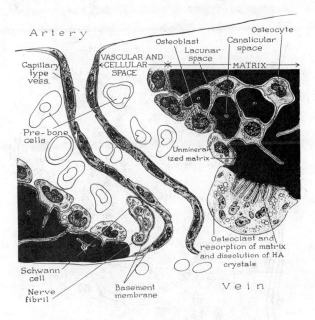

Figure 2. A schematic representation of a physiologic unit of bone tissue, with bone-forming and resorbing cells and their precursors intimately related to the vascular supply. (From Doty, S. B., Robinson, R. A., and Schofield, B.: Morphology of bone and histochemical staining characteristics of bone cells. In Aurbach, G. D., (ed.): Handbook of Physiology. Section 7. Endocrinology. Vol. VII. Parathyroid Gland. Washington, D.C., American Physiological Society, 1976, p. 3.)

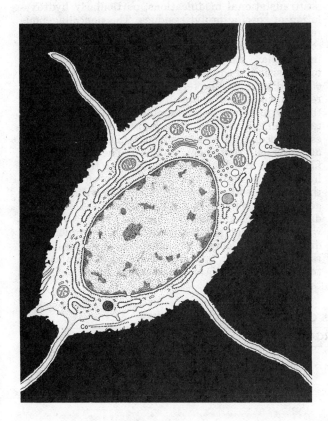

Figure 3. Drawing of a typical osteocyte shown encased in bone. Some unmineralized collagen fibers (Co) are shown in the extracellular space between the cell membane and mineralized bone. Extensions of the cytoplasm of the cell are seen within canaliculi (Ca). These cells are moderately active from the point of view of protein synthesis, as seen from the presence of the endoplasmic reticulum and Golgi apparatus. The Golgi apparatus and endoplasmic reticulum are more extensive in the osteoblast actively involved in formation and mineralization of the matrix. (From Lentz, T. L.: Cell Fine Structure: An Atlas of Drawings of Whole-Cell Structure. Philadelphia, W. B. Saunders Co., 1971.)

Figure 4. Drawing of a typical chondrocyte. These cartilage cells similar to bone cells lie within the lacunae, but, in contrast to the bone cells, the lacunae are not connected to a vascular supply and the cell processes do not connect through canaliculi. The chondrocytes synthesize both collagen and the proteoglycan of the surrounding extracellular matrix. (From Lentz, T. L.: Cell Fine Structure: An Atlas of Drawings of Whole-Cell Structure. Philadelphia, W. B. Saunders Co., 1971.)

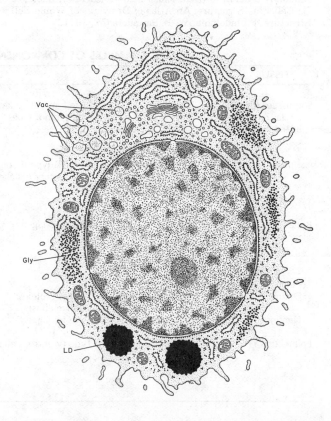

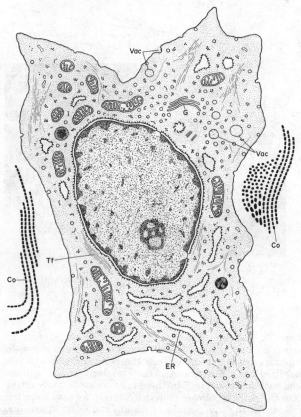

Figure 5. Line drawing of a typical fibroblast, the most common fixed cell of the soft connective tissue. These cells are responsible for synthesis of collagen and complex carbohydrates of the ground substance. They are highly ordered with respect to each other in tissues such as tendon but more randomly ordered in tissues such as dermis. (From Lentz, T. L.: Cell Fine Structure: An Atlas of Drawings of Whole-Cell Structure. Philadelphia, W. B. Saunders Co., 1971.)

TABLE 1. COMPONENTS OF CONNECTIVE TISSUES

Specialized cells
Vascular elements
Water and electrolytes
Other molecules derived from plasma (for example, glycoproteins)
Fibrillar extracellular matrix (for example, collagen, reticulin, elastin)
Ground substance (for example, hyaluronic acid, proteoglycans)
Other molecules formed locally (for example, GLA proteins, phosphoproteins)
Inorganic phases (for example, calcium-phosphorus mineral phase of bone)

third position) (Fig. 6). This structure is stabilized by posttranslational modifications, particularly hydroxylation of specific prolyl residues. The noncollagenous regions of the molecule may be integral parts of the collagen structure or may be present only during intermediate stages of biosynthesis and removed prior to deposition of the finished product. For the purposes of this discussion, the term procollagen will be used to refer to the completed precursor molecule stripped from the polyribosomes and assembled intracellularly. The term collagen molecule refers to the completely processed procollagen molecule from which the extensions at either end have been removed. The term collagen fiber refers to a higher order structure that is formed by a specific alignment of the collagen molecules and that must also have some relationship with noncollagenous components in tissues. Most tissues contain different kinds of collagens, each of which is a protein with a different primary structure determined by a different gene. Moreover, some of these collagens with the same primary structure may have unique posttranslational modifications that are characteristic of that organ or tissue.

TABLE 2. EXAMPLES OF COMPONENTS OF SOME CONNECTIVE TISSUES

TISSUE	CELLS	ORGANIC MATRIX		INORGANIC PHASE
		Fibrillar	*Nonfibrillar*	
Soft tissues (dermis, fascia, tendons, ligaments, joint capsule)	Fibroblasts Tendon cells	Type I and III collagen Other minor types	Hyaluronic acid Dermatan sulfate	
Cartilage	Chondroblasts Chondrocytes Chondroclasts	~>90% type II collagen <10% other collagens	Proteoglycans (chondroitin-4- and 6-sulfate) Chondronectin Other glycoproteins	Ca-P mineral in epiphyseal plate
Bone	Osteoblasts Osteocytes Osteoclasts	Type I collagen	Osteonectin Bone GLA-protein Bone proteoglycan α-2HS-glycoprotein	Ca-P mineral phase
Teeth Enamel	Enamel organ cells	Enamel proteins (enamelins)		Ca-P mineral phase
Dentine	Odontoblasts	Type I collagen		Ca-P mineral phase
Epithelium	Epithelial cells	Type IV and V collagen		Laminin Fibronectin Heparan sulfate proteoglycan Nidinogen

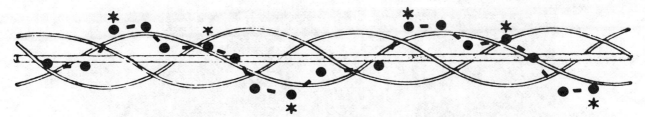

Figure 6. A schematic representation of the collagen triple helix. This pattern could be seen in the type I, II, or III collagens. The chains are shown around a central straight axis. The position of the amino acid residues in the backbone of one of the three chains is indicated by the closed circles. The presence of a glycyl residue regularly at every third position is indicated by the asterisk. The residue repeat distance would be about 0.28 nm.

The collagen molecule of the most common types of tissue collagens (interstitial collagens) can be considered as a long, rigid rod with dimensions of approximately 300×1.5 nm. Each collagen molecule, in turn, is composed of three individual polypeptide chains that have a unique helical structure. Each of the polypeptide chains contains a glycine residue at every third position; other abundant amino acids include alanine and proline. The interstitial collagens contain little tyrosine and phenylalanine and no tryptophan and, with the exception of type III collagen, usually lack cysteine in the body of the helical portion. Collagen chains also undergo posttranslational modification of amino acids (Fig. 7), unique for this class of proteins. The most important of these modifications involves an introduction of a hydroxyl group in the 4-*trans* position of critical prolyl residues. The 4-hydroxyproline formed appears to be responsible for the stabilization of the helical structure. In addition, there are small amounts of 3-hydroxyproline in most collagens; 3-hydroxyproline is more abundant in basement membrane collagens. In addition to modifications of prolyl residues, some lysyl residues are hydroxylated in the 5 position to form hydroxylysine.

Some of the ε-amino groups of lysines as well as hydroxylysines are also oxidized to their respective aldehydes to form derivatives known as allysine and hydroxyallysine, respectively. Hydroxylysines, lysines, and the aldehydes of these amino acids are involved in crosslinks from one collagen chain to another through side chain functions.

In the tissues the interstitial collagen molecules are aggregated with respect to their long axis and are usually staggered at a distance approximately one-quarter of the length of the molecules. This arrangement results in highly specific side chain interactions and predictable charge densities that in turn result in unique banding patterns observed by electron microscopy in some collagens (Fig. 8). The particular aggregation of collagen molecules also gives rise to regions in which molecules overlap and others in which there is no overlap. The latter results in voids or holes; it is probable that the mineral phase of bone is deposited initially in these hole zones.

Different connective tissues may contain a unique type of collagen or mixtures of collagens, most of which have the basic triple helical structure (Table 3). The commonest types of collagens are the interstitial collagens, types I to III. The most abundant collagen, such as is found in skin and bone, is composed of type I molecules, which are composed of two α1 chains (type I) and one α2 chain. The collagen of cartilage (type II) consists of three chains that are identical and are called α1(II). In addition, there are other collagens found in fetal skin, adult blood vessels, and parenchymatous organs that contain the trimer of another distinct polypeptide chain, α1(III). Small amounts of a type I trimer $(\alpha 1(I)_3)$ have also been identified. In addition to the interstitial collagens, basement membranes contain collagens with another primary structure called type IV. Type V collagen has a predominantly pericellular distribution. Other less abundant

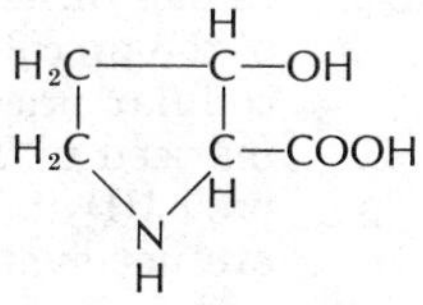

Figure 7. Structural formulas of unique amino acids in collagen, formed by posttranslational modifications of specific residues after incorporation into polypeptide chains.

3-Hydroxy-L-Proline

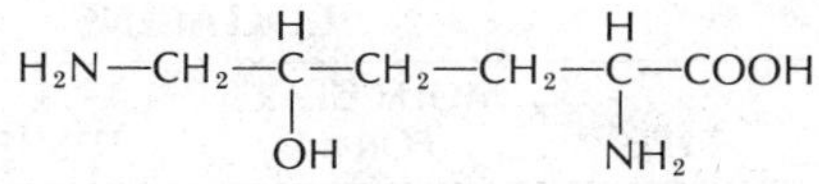

5-Hydroxy-L-Lysine

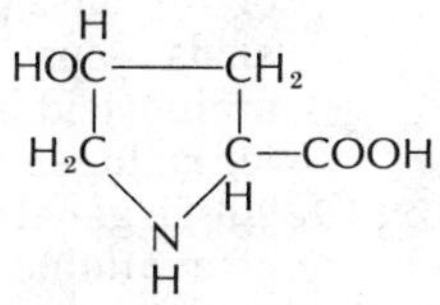

4-Hydroxy-L-Proline

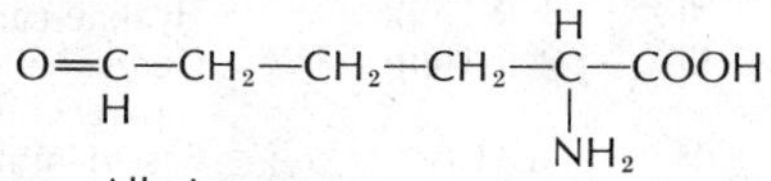

Allysine

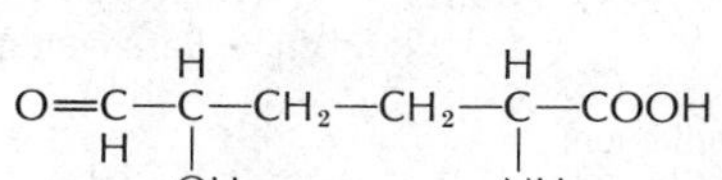

Hydroxyallysine

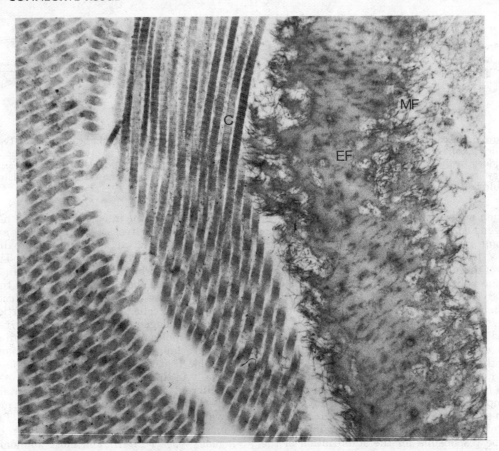

Figure 8. Electron micrograph of lung showing collagen fibers (C) with typical 66- to 68-nm banding lying in close proximity to elastic fibers (EF). These amorphous elastic fibers are surrounded by the microfibrillar component (MF). (Courtesy of R. Trelstad.)

types are found in several tissues, including cartilage, muscle, and placenta. Some of these are as follows: type VI, intimal collagen; type VII, long-chain collagen; type VIII, endothelial cell collagen; type IX, high molecular weight collagen; type X, short-chain collagen. Each of these collagens has a unique structure. There is sufficient information about some of these collagens, particularly type IV collagen, to construct models of higher order structure. A model for type IV collagen based on electron microscopic and chemical data is shown in Figure 9. The macromolecular structure consists of a network of individual molecules, each 390 nm long, which are aggregated and crosslinked via identical ends. This structure is very different from that of type I collagen illustrated in Figure 8. Collagen-like regions are also present in other proteins, such as the C1q components of hemolytic complement and the enzyme acetylcholinesterase.

Collagen Biosynthesis

Current information concerning the detailed steps in biosynthesis of procollagen molecules, the secretion of the procollagen molecules from the cell, their extracellular processing and formation into fibrils is summarized in Table 4 and Figure 10. The genes for the pro $\alpha 1$(I) and pro $\alpha 2$(I) chains of human type I collagen are not syntenic but are localized on chromosome 17 and 7, respectively. These genes are very large (approximately 40 kilobases) and complex, containing over 50 exons. The majority of these exons contain 54 or 108 base pairs, which would code for 18 or 36 amino acids. Most of the exons begin with codons for the amino acid glycine, suggesting that the ancestral gene for collagen was assembled by multiple duplications of single genetic units, each of 54 base pairs. On the basis of available information, it is unlikely that there is more than one copy of the pro $\alpha 2$(I) chain gene in the human haploid genome. The collagen mRNAs processed out of the primary gene transcript contain approximately 3000 bases.

TABLE 3. GENETICALLY DISTINCT MAJOR TYPES OF COLLAGENS

TYPE	MOLECULAR FORM	TISSUE DISTRIBUTION
I	$(\alpha 1[I])_2\alpha 2$	Bone, dermis, tendon, ligaments, fascia, arterial walls, parenchymal organs
II	$(\alpha 1[II])_3$	Hyaline cartilage
III	$(\alpha 1[III])_3$	Dermis, arterial walls, uterus, parenchymal organs
IV	$\alpha 1$(IV) $\alpha 2$(IV) $\alpha 3$(IV)	Basement membranes
V	$(\alpha 1[V]_2\alpha 2[V])$	Basement membranes, placenta, muscle
Complement Clq	A, B, C chains	Complement Clq

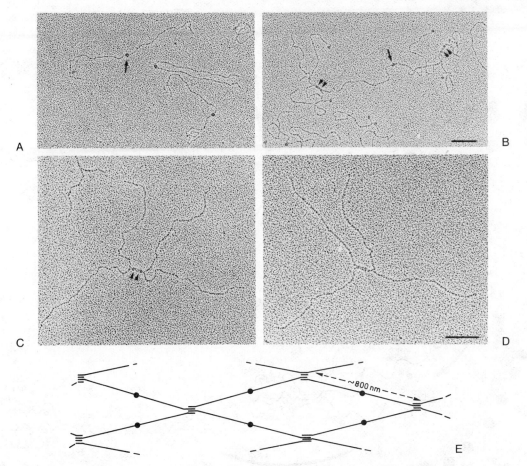

Figure 9. Electron micrographs (rotary shadowing technique) of different type IV collagen preparations from a mouse (EHS) tumor. *A, B,* Acid-extracted type IV collagen. In *A,* two molecular fragments 320 nm long are connected by the C-terminal globular domains *(arrow).* In *B,* polymeric molecules 400 nm in length are connected at the C-termini via their globular domains *(arrow)* and at the N-termini via their triple helical 30-nm long 7 S domains *(double arrow).* Bar = 100 nm. *C, D,* Pepsin-extracted type IV collagen. Four 390-nm long molecular fragments are connected at their N-termini via the triple helical 30-nm long 7 S domains *(double arrow).* The C-terminal globular domains have been digested by pepsin. Bar = 100 nm. *E,* Two-dimensional model of the supermolecular structure of type IV collagen in the extracellular matrix of basement membranes deduced from electron micrographs shown in *A* to *D.* (Courtesy of Professor K. Kühn.)

TABLE 4. SEQUENCE OF CELLULAR COLLAGEN BIOSYNTHESIS

1. Transcription of the gene for each collagen chain
2. Processing of the primary transcript to form the mRNA
3. Utilization of particular species of tRNA
4. Initiation of polypeptide α chains by formation of hydrophobic amino terminal leader sequence followed by assembly of proregion and helix
5. Hydroxylation of prolyl residues begins on nascent chains
6. Hydroxylation of lysyl residues
7. Glycosylation of hydroxylysyl residues
8. Formation of —S—S— bonds at carboxyterminal extension
9. Formation of triple helix
10. Packaging for secretion
11. Amino terminal extension cleavage
12. Carboxyterminal extension cleavage
13. Formation of microfibril
14. Lysyl and hydroxylysyl oxidation
15. Formation of reducible crosslinks
16. Maturation and growth
17. Further crosslinking and interaction with other components

Important control of the synthesis of any protein must be the entry of amino acid into the intracellular pool. In collagen-making cells it is possible that the size of the free proline pool or that of other amino acids may somehow be rate limiting for collagen biosynthesis. Following entry into the intracellular pool, amino acids must then be assembled into polypeptide chains attached to the polyribosome, where the sequence is coded for by the messenger RNA. The complement of the tRNA in a given tissue may be adapted for the synthesis of specific protein in that tissue. In the case of tissues making collagen, it appears that there is a preference for particular glycyl, alanyl, and lysyl tRNAs. Thus, the amount of a specific tRNA may well regulate the rate at which collagen is synthesized. Procollagen molecules synthesized by translating the collagen mRNA have an extra amino terminal extension (leader sequence) that is rapidly lost from the procollagen molecule. Thus, collagens, similar to certain other **proteins,** are synthesized as "prepro" pro-

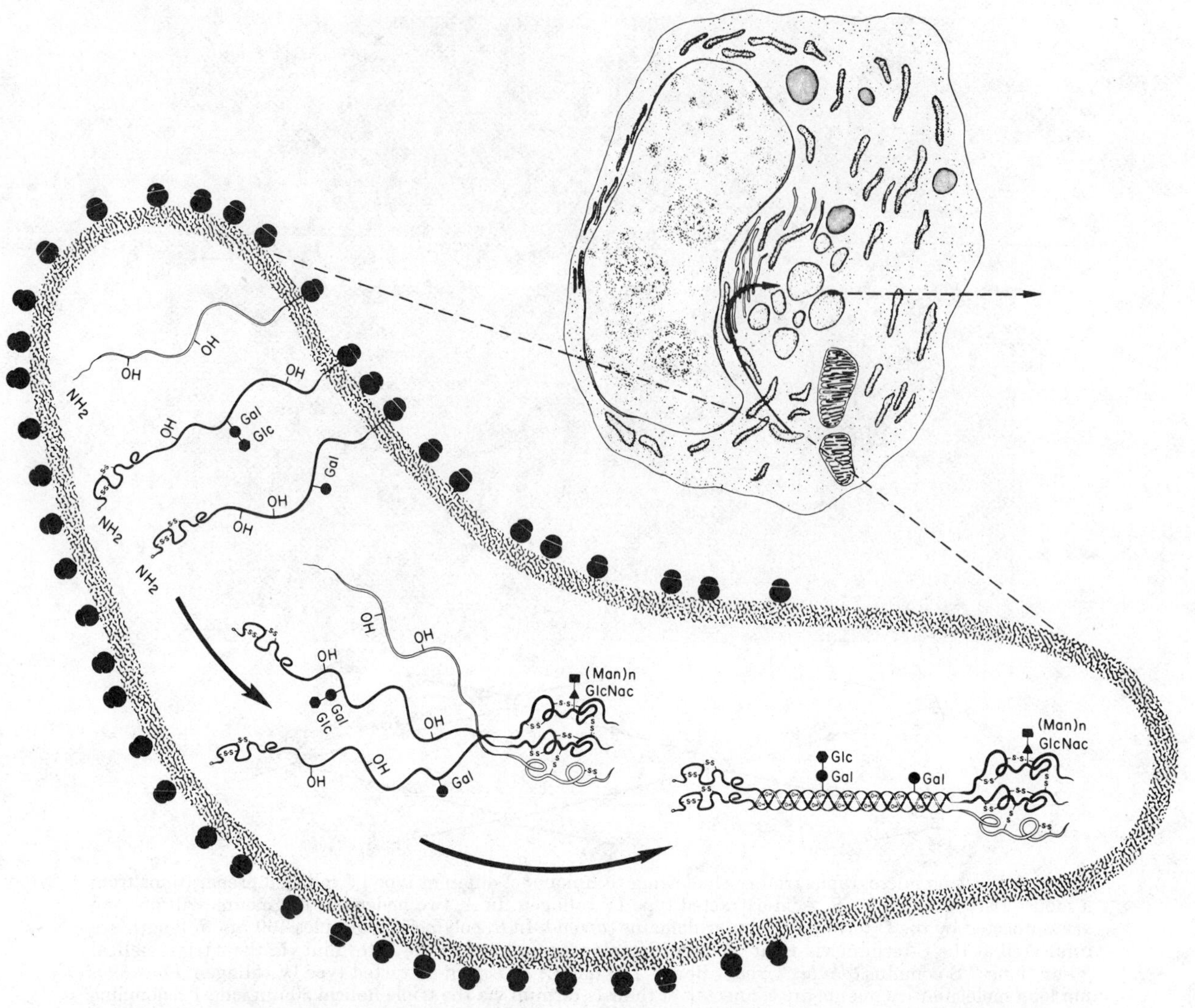

Figure 10. Schematic representation of some of the steps in collagen biosynthesis. One of the cisternae of the rough endoplasmic reticulum is enlarged in the lower portion of the figure. The ribosomes are pictured on the outer surface of the membrane with the growing chains inserted into the cisternae. The hydroxylation of prolyl and lysyl residues on the nascent chain is shown (OH) as well as subsequent additions of galactose (Gal) to some hydroxylysine residues and glucose (Glc) to some of the Gal residues. After release of fully formed chains, interchain disulfide (—S—S—) bonds are formed, some heteropolysaccharide is added at the extensions, and the molecules then fold into the triple helix prior to extrusion from the cell. (From Prockop, D. J., Kivirikko, K. I., Tuderman, L., Guzman, N. A.: The biosynthesis of collagen and its disorders. N Engl J Med 301:13, 77, 1979.)

teins. Once the amino terminal ends of the newly synthesized pro α chains enter the cisternae of the rough endoplasmic reticulum, hydroxylation of specific prolyl and lysyl residues begins. The enzymes —collagen prolyl 4-hydroxylase, collagen prolyl 3-hydroxylase, and collagen lysyl 5-hydroxylase—convert the amino acid residues in the polypeptide chains to the respective hydroxylated derivatives. These reactions require similar cofactors: an activated form of O_2, possibly superoxide ($\cdot O_2^-$); α-ketoglutarate (2-oxoglutarate); ferrous iron; and ascorbic acid. For each mole of proline or lysine hydroxylated, one mole each of succinate and CO_2 are released. The amino acid to be hydroxylated must be in the correct position in the

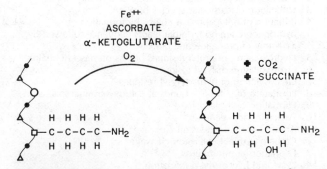

Figure 11. Formation of 5-hydroxylysine in collagen polypeptide chains. Glycine residues in the chain are indicated by the closed circles.

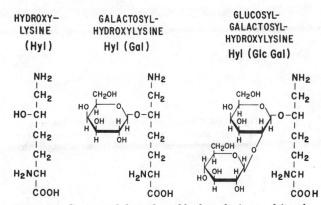

| HYDROXY-
LYSINE
(Hyl) | GALACTOSYL-
HYDROXYLYSINE
Hyl (Gal) | GLUCOSYL-
GALACTOSYL-
HYDROXYLYSINE
Hyl (Glc Gal) |

Figure 12. Structural formulas of hydroxylysine and its glycosylated derivatives. The hydroxylation and glycosylation reactions occur on lysyl residues incorporated into the polypeptide chains. These free modified amino acids are not reutilized for collagen biosynthesis.

polypeptide chain. In the case of the 4-prolyl hydroxylase, this is the Y position in the gly-X-Y triplet. Similarly, the lysyl hydroxylase usually hydroxylates lysines in the same position (Fig. 11).

As the polypeptide chain elongates, certain of the hydroxylated lysyl residues are then glycosylated, catalyzed by two different enzymes—a galactosyl transferase and a glucosyl transferase. Not every hydroxylysyl residue is glycosylated, and not every galactosylated residue is glucosylated (Fig. 12). The relative amount and type of carbohydrate in a partic-

ular collagen is characteristic of a tissue and not necessarily of the primary structure of the collagen chain. Thus, the compositions of the carbohydrates in type I collagens from human skin and bone are characteristic and different.

The disulfide bonds that join the carboxyterminal ends of the procollagen extensions are probably formed soon after translation is completed (Fig. 13). Shortly thereafter, the collagen molecules then assume the triple helical configuration. The newly synthesized procollagen molecules must then be packaged for secretion from the cell. It is probable that the collagen molecules within the cell assemble in linear arrays, laterally aligned, and that these arrays, or a similar form of bundle, leave the cell, where extracellular processing then begins. The amino terminal procollagen extension is probably removed first and the carboxyterminal procollagen extension later by separate endopeptidases. The collagens then begin to form microfibrils, where they are aligned in approximately quarter stagger, similar to the arrangement in the final native structure. At some point following this event, ϵ-amino groups of lysines or hydroxylysines can then be oxidized by a specific lysyl (hydroxylysyl) oxidase to their respective aldehydes (Fig. 7). As the collagen matures, these aldehydes can then interact either within a molecule or between molecules to form the Schiff base–type crosslink (Figs. 14 and 15). Most of these crosslinks require reduction for their stability, but stable Schiff base–type crosslinks have been demonstrated.

PROCOLLAGEN MOLECULE

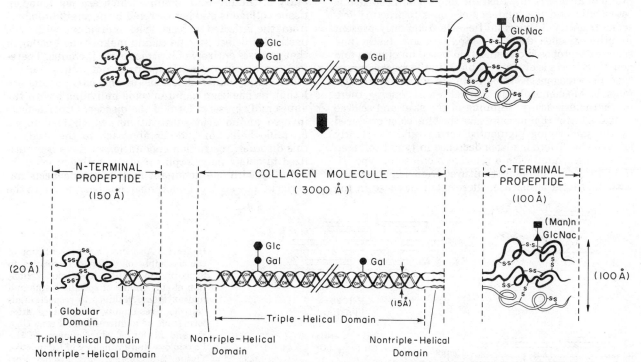

Figure 13. Schematic representation of the structure and processing of the procollagen molecule. Abbreviations are those used in Figure 12 in addition to Man = mannose; glcNac = N-acetylglucosamine. In this diagram measurements are given as Å, where 1Å = 0.1 nm. (From Prockop, D. J., Kivirikko, K. I., Tuderman, L., and Guzman, N. A.: The biosynthesis of collagen and its disorders. N Engl J Med 301:13, 77, 1979.)

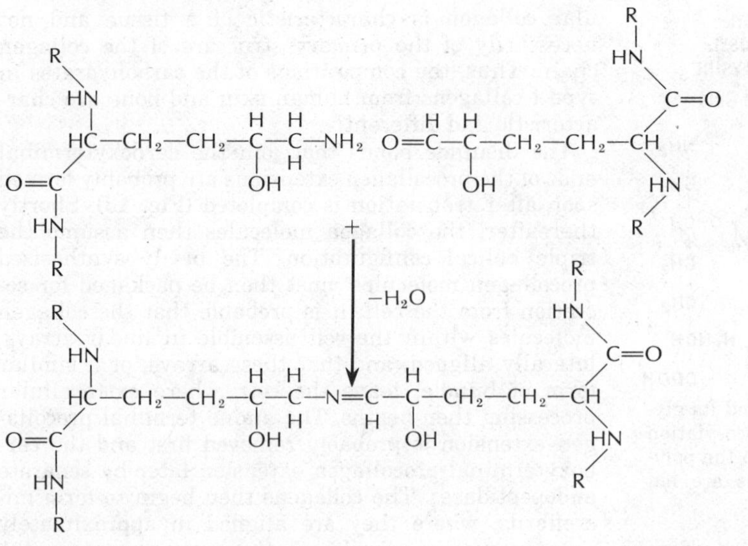

Figure 14. Formation of a Schiff base crosslink, in this case shown via the side chain of one hydroxylysine residue and a hydroxylysine aldehyde (hydroxyallysine).

DISEASES OF COLLAGEN STRUCTURE AND BIOSYNTHESIS

A large number of different human genetic diseases are characterized by defects in connective tissue. Most of these are relatively rare disorders. In a few disorders a molecular mechanism to explain the clinical problem has been established. Examples of these are as follows.

Osteogenesis Imperfecta

Osteogenesis imperfecta includes a heterogeneous group of disorders in which the major manifestation is osteopenia and the tendency of bones to fracture (osseous fragility). Abnormalities are frequently present in other tissues such as skin, tendons, teeth, and sclerae. A proposed classification based on clinical and genetic criteria is given in Table 5. In the most common type of osteogenesis imperfecta, in which there also must be biochemical and clinical heterogeneity, there is, characteristically, thinning of the skin and sclerae (it is the latter that accounts for the blue color produced by the underlying pigmented retina) and frequently joint laxity. There is also a decrease in type I collagen in skin associated with a relative increase in type III. In addition, in fibroblasts cultured from some patients with this form of disease, there is an increase in the amount of type III collagen synthesized relative to that of type I. The collagen fibers of bone are thinner than normal, and the collagen bundles have different dimensions.

In patients with different forms of the disorder, a variety of other defects are being uncovered. These involve deletions in portions of the gene coding for the helical regions or for the procollagen extensions. These deletions may prevent normal formation of collagen fibrils. In one instance a deletion in the carboxy terminal $\alpha2(I)$ propeptide has led to failure to align properly in the trimer and subsequently to an instability of the pro $\alpha2(I)$ chains, which are not found in tissue collagens and not secreted by dermal fibroblasts from the affected subject. The individual with this particular defect in gene coding makes type I collagen that consists entirely of a trimer of $\alpha1(I)$ chains. Therefore, an absence of $\alpha2(I)$ chains is not lethal. On the other hand, major deletions in the $\alpha1(I)$ chain are lethal, as has been found in some individuals with the autosomal recessive form of the disease. Other defects involve amino acid substitutions, which lead to an unstable helix. In another approach to the study of this disorder, restriction endonucleases have been utilized to detect polymorphism in the collagen gene. In a family with the dominant form of osteogenesis imperfecta, one such polymorphism has been found in the

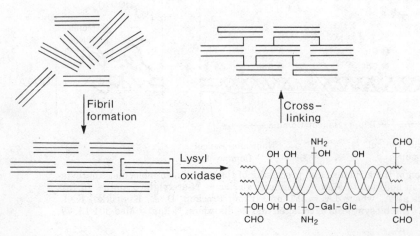

Figure 15. A schematic representation of the assembly of collagen molecules to form intermolecular crosslinks. Oxidation of side chains of specific lysine and hydroxylysine residues to respective aldehydes presumably takes place after formation of a microfibril. (From Gay, S., and Miller, E. J.: Collagen in the Physiology and Pathology of Connective Tissue. Stuttgart, Gustav Fischer Verlag, 1978.)

TABLE 5. CLASSIFICATION OF OSTEOGENESIS IMPERFECTA

TYPE	DESCRIPTION	PROBABLE INHERITANCE
I	Classic; moderately severe with blue sclerae and later deafness	Autosomal dominant
II	Lethal perinatal	Autosomal recessive
III	Progressive, deforming, with normal sclerae, frequently dentinogenesis imperfecta	Autosomal recessive
IV	Progressive, deforming	Autosomal dominant

5' half of the pro α2(I) gene. Now that such testing procedures are available, several new defects will be uncovered to account for the different forms of osteogenesis imperfecta.

Ehlers-Danlos Syndrome

A defect in collagen synthesis could be responsible for the clinical manifestations in some of the various forms of Ehlers-Danlos syndrome (Table 6). In most patients with Ehlers-Danlos syndrome, clinical problems involve varying degrees of hyperextensible skin, poorly formed scars, hyperextensible joints with multiple dislocations, formation of subcutaneous spherules, molluscoid pseudotumors, and, in some patients, vascular problems with rupture of major vessels or even rupture of viscera such as the large intestine.

In the best known classic form of Ehlers-Danlos syndrome (type I), no chemical abnormality of collagen has been demonstrated, although electron microscopy reveals that the collagen fibrils have an increased mean diameter and higher degree of variability in width and shape compared with controls. Such abnormalities could result from primary structural defects in collagen or from alterations in noncollagenous extracellular components that influence collagen fiber formation.

Most, but not all, forms of Ehlers-Danlos syndrome are inherited as an autosomal dominant. Patients with so-called type IV Ehlers-Danlos syndrome (Sack variety) have problems predominantly related to changes in blood vessels, including ecchymoses and, occasionally, vascular catastrophes. The cause of death in all types of Ehlers-Danlos syndrome often involves the rupture of a major blood vessel. In patients with type IV Ehlers-Danlos syndrome, problems with poor wound healing and joint dislocation are not as marked as in other variants. Several patients from a number of kindreds have had tissues analyzed either at autopsy or by biopsy. These patients have been found to lack type III collagen in their parenchymal organs and blood vessels. Furthermore, it has been found that fibroblasts cultured from collagenous tissues from some of these subjects fail to make type III collagen. It is therefore assumed that this problem is analogous to that of the most common form of osteogenesis imperfecta. Since type III collagen is a major component of medium-sized and large blood vessels, it is presumed that the walls of these blood vessels that are exposed to mechanical forces over a period of years can no longer stand stresses and are therefore subject to rupture. In addition, the subintimal connective tissue consists primarily of type III collagen, and it is possible that type III collagen present under certain circumstances (although not all) is a better substrate for platelet aggregation than type I collagen. It is still possible, then, that the absence of type III collagen in the subintimal

TABLE 6. CLASSIFICATION OF EHLERS-DANLOS SYNDROME

TYPE	DESCRIPTION	DEFECT
I Gravis	Classic severe form; skin hyperextensibility; friable skin and poor wound healing; severe hypermobility; subcutaneous spheroids; molluscoid pseudotumors	Unknown; large, variable-sized collagen fibers
II Mitis	All manifestations minor; musculoskeletal deformity may be absent	Unknown
III Benign hypermobile	Hypermobility generalized and gross; skin abnormalities minor	Unknown
IV Ecchymotic (Arterial; Sack)	Joint hypermobility limited to digits; skin thin, venous network prominent; ecchymoses prominent; cardiovascular and gastrointestinal catastrophes	Decreased type III collagen synthesis or secretion
V X-linked	Skin hypermobility prominent; joint hypermobility mild	?Decreased lysyl oxidase
VI Ocular	Thin, velvety skin; prominent skin hyperextensibility and joint hypermobility; joint dislocations; muscle tone poor, especially infants; scoliosis; ocular abnormalities, especially fragility	Decreased collagen hydroxylysine; defective lysyl hydroxylase
VII Arthrochalasis multiplex congenita	Marked joint hypermobility and subluxations; thin skin; torn ligaments; scooped out midfacies, epicanthal folds and hypertelorism	Incompletely processed procollagen, deficient procollagen endopeptidase, or structural defects in procollagen, preventing the action of the endopeptidase

region could be responsible, in part, for some of the hemorrhagic manifestations of this disease. Genetic and biochemical heterogeneity is also characteristic of this syndrome, since affected individuals from some of the reported kindreds make detectable type III collagen at levels varying from 10 to 30 per cent of normal. In some cells type III collagen is synthesized but not secreted from the cell. Thus, in several forms of osteogenesis imperfecta and the type IV Ehlers-Danlos syndrome, there are defects in the type I or III collagen genes, resulting in structural alterations or abnormalities in the regulation of gene expression.

Other individuals with Ehlers-Danlos syndrome have a clinical presentation consisting of skin hyperextensibility, hyperextensible joints, and, in some, severe structural scoliosis. In the kindreds described, the inheritance seems to be autosomal recessive rather than autosomal dominant. In some of these patients, ocular manifestations have been prominent. The skin from several of these patients has been found to be deficient in hydroxylysine content of the collagen. This deficiency of hydroxylysine has also been associated with a decrease in the number and distribution of covalent crosslinks that involve hydroxylysine. Skin fibroblasts cultured from these patients contain a lower activity of lysyl hydroxylase, accounted for by the presence of an abnormal enzyme protein. The defective enzyme is in turn responsible for decreased hydroxylation of specific lysyl residues. Hydroxylysine is critically involved in intermolecular crosslinking; if a lysyl residue has to be used instead of a hydroxylysyl residue, the resultant crosslink is less stable. The defect is heterogeneous and is not seen to the same extent in the collagens from different tissues despite the fact that the collagens have the same primary structure. This observation raises the possibility that in vivo lysyl hydroxylation is controlled by multiple forms of enzyme, each of which is specific for a tissue, or that the rate of polypeptide chain growth is critical for the rate at which specific lysyl residues can be hydroxylated. In one kindred it has been possible to effect clinical improvement by the administration of large doses of ascorbic acid, possibly accounted for by an apparent dissociation constant for ascorbic acid of the mutant lysyl hydroxylase higher than that of the normal enzyme.

In type V Ehlers-Danlos syndrome, the predominant manifestation is skin stretchability apparently associated with an X-linked form of inheritance. Decreased lysyl oxidase activity has been suggested. In one kindred of the inherited form of cutis laxa, in contrast to the acquired form, it has also been possible to demonstrate decreased activity of lysyl oxidase in cultured skin fibroblasts.

Patients have been described with a syndrome termed arthrochalasis multiplex congenita (Ehlers-Danlos syndrome type VII), which is characterized by hypermobile joints, recurrent joint dislocations, and scoliosis, in addition to a peculiar scooped-out facies, hypertelorism, and prominent epicanthal folds. Analyses of tissues from some of these individuals have revealed defective collagen fibers in which procollagen appears to persist outside the cell. In some individuals fibroblast sonicates contain decreased activity of procollagen aminoterminal (N) protease, the enzyme involved in cleavage of the aminoterminal extension peptides of type I procollagen. In another instance of this syndrome, however, the defect is in the amino acid sequence at the N protease cleavage site of the pro α2(I) chain. Since the pro α1(I) peptides do not dissociate from the pro α2(I) chains, the pro N molecules are still deposited extracellularly.

Homocystinuria

Homocystinuria, due to deficiency in cystathionine synthase, has several features similar to those of the Marfan syndrome. These patients may have ectopia lentis; long, thin extremities; and osteoporosis. However, joints are characteristically stiff, rather than hypermobile. Since there is a deficiency in cystathionine synthase, there is an accumulation of homocysteine behind the enzymatic block (Fig. 1, Section VII). This leads to increased concentrations of homocystine, which is excreted in excess in the urine. A number of studies have suggested possible explanations for the connective tissue defect based on aberrancies in collagen biosynthesis. Homocysteine itself can react with aldehydes of collagen and thus prevent formation of Schiff bases and subsequent crosslinking. However, the concentrations of homocysteine necessary to produce this defect are probably higher than those attained in the disease in vivo. It is also suggested that formation of the crosslinks themselves is abnormal or that homocysteine interferes with the activity of lysyl oxidase.

Menkes' Kinky-Hair Syndrome

In this disorder, which has an X-linked inheritance, there is a decrease in the intestinal absorption of copper and resulting low levels of serum copper. Affected individuals may have bone disease, often described as osteoporosis and having some resemblance to the bone disease of scurvy. Some of the manifestations of this disorder could be accounted for by decreased activity of lysyl oxidase, an enzyme that has an absolute requirement for tightly bound copper. Lysyl oxidase activity is decreased in experimental models of copper deficiency. However, studies to date have failed to demonstrate an abnormality in the formation of aldehydes in this disease, and thus no simple explanation currently available accounts for the bone disease.

ACQUIRED DISORDERS OF COLLAGEN STRUCTURE AND BIOSYNTHESIS

In addition to defects in collagen synthesis accompanying certain heritable disorders of connective tissue, there are acquired disorders in which collagen metabolism may be altered either at the level of transcription or translation or in the course of posttranslational modification (Table 7). Some of these abnormalities can be understood in terms of gene switching analogous to what may occur in some forms of osteogenesis imperfecta and Ehlers-Danlos syndrome type IV. Disorders such as idiopathic osteoporosis, in which thinning of the dermis accompanies decreased bone mass, might be candidates for such abnormalities. Circumstances that affect the rate of prolyl hydroxylation could also theoretically affect the rate of collagen synthesis. Modulations could occur at the level of the enzyme itself or in the concentration of cofactors such as α-ketoglutarate, O_2, or ascorbate that are necessary for the hydroxylation reaction or in

TABLE 7. ACQUIRED DISORDERS OR CONDITIONS ASSOCIATED WITH ALTERED COLLAGEN SYNTHESIS

CONDITION	DEFECT
Idiopathic osteoporosis	Decreased synthesis
Glucocorticoid excess	Decreased synthesis
Scurvy	Decreased synthesis (decreased prolyl hydroxylation)
Lathyrism (β-aminopropionitrile)	Decreased lysyl oxidase and crosslinking
Copper deficiency and ?Menkes' syndrome	Decreased lysyl oxidase and crosslinking
Ingestion of desferrioxamine	Decreased synthesis
Ingestion of proline analogues (for example, cis-4-hydroxyproline)	Decreased synthesis
Ingestion of penicillamine	Decreased crosslinking

the relative rate of chain elongation with respect to activity of the hydroxylases. Since 4-hydroxyproline stabilizes the collagen helix, under circumstances in which prolyl hydroxylation is insufficient, collagen is degraded within the cell and is not secreted. There has so far been no direct demonstration of alterations in collagen synthesis associated, for example, with hypoxia or iron-deficient states. Desferrioxamine, however, does decrease collagen synthesis in fibroblast cultures and may decrease hepatic fibrosis in patients with iron storage diseases.

Scurvy is accompanied by defective prolyl hydroxylation, which probably accounts for several of its abnormalities. Although it is possible that substances other than ascorbic acid could substitute in the hydroxylation reaction, deficiency of ascorbic acid does limit hydroxylation of prolyl residues, and in the presence of such deficiency, pro α chains do not form stable helices and are not secreted. Ascorbic acid also has a primary stimulatory effect on collagen synthesis that is apparently unrelated to hydroxylation. These effects could well account for the poor wound healing and thin connective tissues with poor support of blood vessels that characterize the scorbutic state. Although ascorbic acid is also a substrate for lysyl hydroxylase, hydroxylysine synthesis is less affected in ascorbic acid deficiency than is hydroxyproline synthesis. This may be accounted for in part by the higher K_m for ascorbic acid of the prolyl hydroxylase compared with that of the lysyl hydroxylase. Although there has been no demonstration that the activity per se of the hydroxylation enzymes is rate limiting for collagen synthesis, the rates of the hydroxylases measured in tissues and circulating blood cells reflect the overall rate of collagen synthesis; for example, in conditions of active hepatic fibrosis, blood prolyl hydroxylase activity is usually increased.

Glucocorticoids, in pharmacologic doses, are potent catabolic agents that decrease synthesis of DNA and proteins in general. The effects of high doses of glucocorticoids are particularly evident in skin and bone. In tissue in which collagen synthesis represents a large proportion of total protein synthesis, high doses of glucocorticoids decrease collagen synthesis (both types I and III) to a greater extent than that of other proteins. Although glucocorticoids inhibit amino acid uptake by cells, they also decrease the activity of the collagen hydroxylases and glycosyl transferases, and it is likely that the inhibition of collagen synthesis takes place at some step distal to amino acid uptake. Indeed, glucocorticoid-treated cells have decreased levels of type I procollagen mRNAs, suggesting that control could be at the level of transcription of the collagen gene or at some posttranscriptional step such as processing of the primary transcript or transport of the mRNAs from nucleus to cytoplasm.

In *hyperthyroidism,* there may be an associated decrease in bone mass and alterations in collagen synthesis in other tissues as well. The excretion of urinary collagen degradation products is increased in hyperthyroidism, although most of this increase probably represents increased collagen degradation. Indeed, there are suggestions that collagen synthesis may actually be increased in hyperthyroid states but to an extent insufficient to overcome the effects of increased degradation.

Compounds are derived from the common sweet pea, *Lathyrus odoratus,* the active principle of which is β-aminopropionitrile. Administration of this compound to experimental animals results in distorted bone structure, with resulting deformities in long bones and scoliosis, and dissecting aneurysm of the aorta. This state is termed lathyrism. The action of β-aminopropionitrile results from its interaction with lysyl oxidase to decrease its activity. The closest clinical analogy to the lathyrism produced by β-aminopropionitrile is that form of cutis laxa associated with a heritable defect in the activity of lysyl oxidase. In certain experimental animals, copper-deficient states can result in decreases in the formation of collagen and elastin aldehydes and defective crosslinking; copper is required for lysyl oxidase activity. Whether such abnormalities accompany copper-deficient states in humans has never been conclusively demonstrated.

Interference with crosslinking has also been shown to be associated with ingestion of D-penicillamine. This compound, used with a different rationale in the therapy of Wilson's disease, cystinuria, and rheumatoid arthritis, binds to aldehydes of lysine and hydroxylysine to form stable thiadiazolium rings. The reaction of the penicillamine in this complex with collagen side chains thus interferes with interactions of aldehydes and neighboring ε-amino groups and prevents the formation of Schiff bases and subsequent crosslinking. The mechanisms of the effects of D-penicillamine on collagen synthesis may be similar to those proposed for homocysteine. Abnormalities in solubility of collagen have been demonstrated in patients receiving penicillamine for Wilson's disease and can be explained by changes in collagen crosslinking.

Excessive Extracellular Deposition of Collagen

Several clinical conditions are characterized by *excessive extracellular deposition of collagen* (Table 8). Such *fibrosis* may interfere with mechanical function—for example, in the lung—or replace parenchymal cells—for example, in the liver.

General Mechanisms. It is not always possible to distinguish loss of cells from a tissue with subsequent fibrosis from primary fibrosis and secondary cellular loss. Excessive collagen deposition at any site would result from increased numbers of the cells (fibroblasts) that synthesize and secrete this protein and/or by increased function of cells already present. Fibroblasts,

TABLE 8. DISORDERS OR CONDITIONS ASSOCIATED WITH EXCESSIVE COLLAGEN DEPOSITION (FIBROSIS)

Silicosis
Idiopathic pulmonary fibrosis
Hepatic cirrhosis of various types
Atherosclerosis
Progressive systemic sclerosis
Fasciitis with eosinophilia
Fibrosis associated with
  paraquat
  bleomycin therapy

or cells capable of differentiating into fibroblasts, may be attracted to the site of potential fibrosis by products of other cells (lymphocytes or monocytes) or by components of the extracellular matrix itself, such as collagen or degradation products of collagen or fibronectin. Substances produced by mononuclear cells may also affect collagen synthesis by fibroblasts. Macrophages, following ingestion of silica particles, produce a factor that is capable of stimulating collagen synthesis by fibroblasts; these observations might be pertinent, for example, to the pathogenesis of the pulmonary fibrosis accompanying inhalation of silica particles. Extracts and culture supernatants of isolated egg granulomas obtained from the livers of mice infected with *Schistosoma mansoni* stimulate fibroblasts to proliferate. Similar substances present in hepatic granulomas might therefore explain the hepatic fibrosis that characteristically accompanies schistosomal infections in humans. Mononuclear cells also produce substances capable of increasing collagen synthesis by rheumatoid synovial cells, which might account for the fibrous ankylosis present in certain forms of rheumatoid arthritis. Prostaglandins of the E series inhibit collagen synthesis and thus could play a modulating role under normal and pathologic circumstances. Interference with prostaglandin formation might be accompanied by increased collagen synthesis.

Other substances may also be important in production of fibrosis. For example, β-adrenergic agonists inhibit and β-adrenergic antagonists stimulate collagen synthesis by cultured fibroblasts. Bleomycin, which may produce pulmonary fibrosis, increases prolyl hydroxylase activity and stimulates collagen synthesis in vitro. The herbicide paraquat, which also produces pulmonary fibrosis, stimulates collagen synthesis in vitro; this action is possibly related to formation of activated oxygen species (superoxide) required for collagen hydroxylations. Several of these substances not only might alter the rate and amount but also might influence which type of collagen is deposited.

Pulmonary Fibrosis. Several forms of pulmonary disease are characterized by *diffuse fibrosis at interstitial sites in the lung*. These disorders are associated with a variety of etiologic factors, most of which are unknown. In patients with idiopathic pulmonary fibrosis, there is an increase in both collagen types I and III. The initial event in interstitial lung disease is presumably an alveolitis characterized by infiltration of cells not present in the normal lung. The following sequence of events has been proposed to account for the fibrosis. Alveolar macrophages are activated, perhaps by immune complexes through Fc receptors, to lead to production of a chemotactic factor for neutrophils. The neutrophils contain a collagenase capable of degrading type I collagen. The macrophages also release fibronectin, which is a potent chemotaxin for fibroblasts, in addition to other factors that promote fibroblast proliferation. In forms of pulmonary fibrosis such as sarcoidosis and chronic hypersensitivity pneumonitis, an important role is assigned to T-lymphocytes, which, among other functions, release a lymphokine chemotactic for monocytes. The monocytes then localize in the lesion to contribute monokines capable of altering fibroblast proliferation and possibly collagen synthesis.

Cirrhosis. Scarring is also a feature of several forms of *liver disease, including alcoholic and postnecrotic cirrhosis*. It is presumed that the collagenous tissue replaces normal hepatic parenchyma and is responsible for decrease in hepatic function. It has still not been proved, however, whether the scarring is a secondary phenomenon or parenchymal cell loss is the primary or the most significant feature. At any rate, the presence of increased collagen content in several forms of liver disease may be important in the functional impairment immediately responsible for the clinical problem. In the initial phase of liver disease, loss of parenchymal cells leads to collapse of the reticular architecture and the formation of thin septa composed of pre-existing fibers presumably of type III collagen. Later in the course of cirrhosis, however, new collagen is synthesized that initially may be mostly type III collagen but is soon accompanied by the presence of type I collagen fibers as well. Thus, the increased collagen content of established cirrhosis includes both types I and III collagens and, in addition, some collagens of the basement membrane type deposited predominantly around bile ducts. In experimental forms of liver disease, the serum levels of several enzymes involved in posttranslational modifications of collagen, such as prolyl hydroxylase, glycosyl transferases, and lysyl oxidase, increase prior to the development of increased collagen deposition; similar increases have been observed in sera from patients with various forms of liver disease. It is likely that these enzymes serve as markers for increased activity of collagen-synthesizing cells.

The pathogenetic mechanisms could be similar to those in lung fibrosis. It is possible, however, that the hepatic parenchymal cells (epithelial cells), in addition to fibroblasts, may be able to synthesize the interstitial collagens (type I > III) deposited in cirrhosis. So-called Ito cells (lipocytes) may be another collagen-synthesizing cell, particularly for the type III collagen found early in the lesion.

Atherosclerosis. Certain aspects of the *atherosclerotic lesion* may also be considered with respect to abnormalities of control of collagen synthesis. Atherosclerotic lesions, especially early ones, contain not only increased numbers of smooth muscle cells but also an increased amount of connective tissue, composed of type I and III collagen molecules as well as type IV molecules. The presence of this heterogeneous connective tissue matrix precedes other features of the lesion, such as calcification and deposition of lipid. It has been proposed that increased synthesis of this collagen is initiated by endothelial injury and interaction of platelets with the collagen exposed in the denuded area. Aggregation of platelets by collagen (possibly associated with fibronectin) then results in release of a factor such as platelet derived growth factor capable of increasing the proliferation of smooth muscle cells that can synthesize both types I and III collagen. These smooth muscle cells can also synthesize elastin. The pathogenesis of atherosclerosis is discussed extensively in Section VI.

Progressive Systemic Sclerosis (Scleroderma). The increased collagen content of scleroderma is especially apparent in the skin but is also seen in the lung. The cause of the increased collagen deposition is not known, although it is presumably related to the vascular abnormalities that occur early in the disease. Fibroblasts cultured from the skin of patients with scleroderma, even after several passages, produce more collagen than do fibroblasts from normal subjects. This may be explained by selection in vivo of a population of cells that are relatively high collagen producers. It appears that type III collagen may be particularly prominent in early lesions, but more established lesions contain larger fibers of type I collagen as well. Some of the increased collagen deposition may be related to altered cellular immunity in scleroderma. For example, there is increased responsiveness to collagens of lymphocytes from patients with scleroderma compared with those from unaffected individuals. Products of lymphocytes and monocytes, cells found in the lesion, also alter collagen synthesis. Serum from some, but not all, patients with scleroderma contains a factor capable of stimulating proliferation of cultured endothelial cells. Such a factor might have a role in the pathogenesis of the proliferative vascular lesion.

Another disorder in which mononuclear cells might be important in modulation of collagen synthesis is the syndrome of *fasciitis with eosinophilia.* Extensive collagen deposition occurs in the deep subcutaneous tissue associated with a mononuclear cell infiltrate and peripheral blood eosinophilia; the dermal changes characteristic of scleroderma are not usually found.

Prevention of Collagen Deposition. Attempts have been made to *alter the extent of collagen deposition by pharmacologic means* in several of the clinical disorders associated with pathologic fibrosis. D-*Penicillamine* was initially used to treat patients with scleroderma on the basis of its properties of inhibiting formation of collagen crosslinks. However, convincing alteration of collagen deposition or amelioration of mechanical disabilities in scleroderma has not been demonstrated in therapeutic studies with this drug. β-*Aminopropionitrile* has also been introduced in the therapy of fibrotic contractures of the hands and in experimental animals to prevent the esophageal strictures that follow alkali burns. *Proline analogs,* such as *cis*-hydroxyproline, are recognized by prolyl tRNA and can replace proline in the polypeptide chain but do not stabilize the collagen helix. The collagen, thus synthesized, is degraded in the cell and not secreted. It is uncertain, however, whether serious toxicity from the use of such compounds might result from inhibition of synthesis of noncollagenous proteins. *Colchicine* inhibits secretion of collagen in several systems in vitro, presumably by interference with microtubule function. In addition, in cultures of rheumatoid synovium col-chicine increases collagenase synthesis and release. The use of colchicine to decrease collagen deposition has therefore been advocated in conditions such as scleroderma and hepatic fibrosis.

Collagen Resorption

It is probable that old collagen fibers are resorbed and new collagen deposited at very low rates in tissues such as dermis and fascia. However, collagen as the major component of the organic matrix is constantly resorbed in the physiologic process of bone remodeling. *Collagen resorption* is in part responsible for the decrease in size and weight of the uterus in postpartum involution. In several pathologic states, the rate of collagen resorption in specific tissues may be increased (for example, bone collagen in hyperparathyroidism), or resorption may take place when normally there is none (for example, corneal ulceration following alkali burns, resorption of alveolar bone in periodontal disease, and resorption of articular cartilage and bone in chronic rheumatoid synovitis). Collagenolysis is carried out by specific enzymes, collagenases, that have a number of properties in common. These collagenases are metalloenzymes that act at neutral pH and cleave collagens at specific sites in the polypeptide chain. In general, undenatured collagen molecules, collagen fibrils, and fibers are refractory to cleavage by proteolytic enzymes other than collagenases. These collagenases are usually not stored intracellularly in specific granules but are released into the extracellular milieu. The collagenase in polymorphonuclear leukocytes, however, is located in a granule fraction. Collagenases are usually released from cells in a latent form that requires activation before catalytic function can be detected. These enzymes preferentially attack native, rather than denatured, collagen molecules and cleave the polypeptides across the three chains at a locus three-quarters the distance from the amino terminal end of the helical portion of the collagen molecule (Fig. 16). The fragments produced are more soluble, peel off the collagen fibril, and undergo transformation to the denatured coil or gelatin structure. Once denatured, the cleaved fragments can be attacked by a variety of proteases that are incapable of cleaving the native molecules.

Collagen degradation is predominantly extracellular. Collagenases must thus be synthesized and secreted from the cell. Substances that increase collagenase production by cultured cells and tissues include soluble factors derived from other cells, such as mononuclear cells, as well as endotoxin and compounds such as colchicine, cytochalasin B, and phorbol myristate. Extracellular collagen may itself stimulate production of collagenases. Factors that inhibit collagenase production include the glucocorticoids and inhibitors of protein synthesis. Under some circumstances, optimal concentrations of prostaglandin E_2 are necessary for collagenase production.

Collagenase is secreted from many cells in an inactive, or latent, form. The production of active enzyme can be accomplished in vitro by exposure to other proteolytic enzymes. Latent collagenase is in the form of a proenzyme and is activated by another protease, a procollagenase activator. The latter is also secreted as an inactive zymogen that is activated by proteases. Among the proteolytic enzymes that are capable of

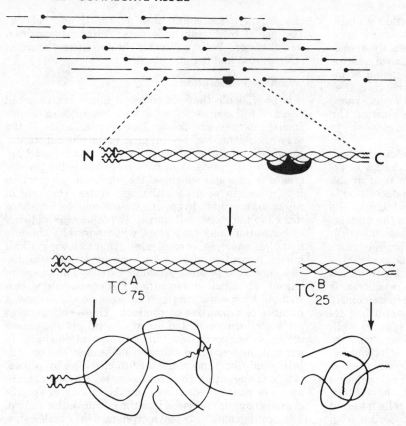

Figure 16. Schematic representation of mechanisms of animal collagenases. The collagen fibril is shown at the upper portion of the figure, where the bars represent collagen molecules with the amino-terminal end indicated by the closed circle. The collagenase enzyme is indicated by the dark figure attached to one molecule, an enlargement of which is connected by the dotted lines. After cleavage at a point three fourths of the distance from the amino (N)-terminal end, the fragments TC_{75}^A and TC_{25}^B are solubilized and then denatured (gelation), as shown in the bottom portion of the figure. (Modified from Harris, E. D., Jr., and Krane, S. M.: Collagenases. N Engl J Med 291:557, 605, 652, 1974.)

activation of the procollagenase-proactivator complex, plasmin produced by the action of plasminogen activator is a likely candidate. Inhibitors of collagenase are found in the plasma and extracellular fluid. These inhibitors in plasma include α2-macroglobulin and a protein of lower molecular weight with β-globulin mobility. The latter is related to a protein secreted by cells in several tissues that blocks the action of metalloproteases such as collagenase.

Collagens of different primary structure are attacked at different rates by collagenases; for example, whereas type I and type III collagen are cleaved at a similar rate, type II collagen is cleaved at a rate considerably slower than either of these two forms. Highly crosslinked collagens are also cleaved at rates lower than minimally crosslinked collagens, and other enzymatic mechanisms may be required to cleave such crosslinks. Bone collagen cannot be cleaved by collagenases as long as the mineral phase is present. If the mineral phase is removed, demineralized bone collagen is then readily cleaved by collagenases. The mineral phase stabilizes higher order collagen structure and protects the protein not only from enzymatic degradation but also from thermal denaturation. In bone resorption in vivo, therefore, a mechanism must exist for removal of the mineral phase prior to proteolytic attack on the organic portion.

Abnormal collagenolysis takes place in a number of pathologic conditions (Table 9). Possible examples include certain forms of corneal ulceration, the bone resorption that accompanies hyperparathyroidism and neoplastic processes, and the connective tissue resorption that is a characteristic feature of chronic periodontal disease. In the recessive dystrophic form of

epidermolysis bullosa, not only is there increased synthesis of collagenase but also the enzyme is biochemically distinguishable from normal. Several features of the regulation of collagenase production and action in these different conditions are common to all of them.

Rheumatoid Arthritis. Collagen degradation in rheumatoid arthritis is predominantly extracellular, and collagenase appears to be important in this degradation. Enzymatic activity has been demonstrated in synovial fluids from patients with rheumatoid arthritis, and the characteristic cleavage products of this collagenase have been identified. Synovial tissue obtained from patients with active joint disease cultured in vitro produces high levels of collagenase and, under certain conditions, large amounts of prostaglandin E_2 (PGE_2). Although cells with macrophage markers are also present during the early stages of culture, later the predominant cell is a large stellate cell that lacks macrophage markers, yet the cultures still produce collagenase and PGE_2. These fibroblast-like synovial cells can be stimulated to synthesize and release collagenase by a factor secreted by monocyte-macro-

TABLE 9. EXAMPLES OF INVOLVEMENT OF COLLAGENASES IN HUMAN DISEASES

Epidermolysis bullosa
Periodontal disease
Corneal ulceration
Neoplastic invasion
Cholesteatoma
Bone resorptive diseases
Inflammatory joint diseases (for example, rheumatoid arthritis)
Other destructive joint disease (for example, hemophilia, pigmented vilonodular synovitis)

phages, called mononuclear cell factor, which is homologous with interleukin 1. Thus, lymphocytes and monocytes present in the inflammatory cell mass from rheumatoid synovitis can modulate the production of factors by other cells, which in turn are capable of resorbing connective tissue. The lymphocytes and monocytes present in chronic periodontal lesions may also influence collagenase production in these tissues.

Hormones. Parathyroid hormone increases and calcitonin decreases bone matrix resorption, which is reflected in parallel changes in the urinary excretion of markers of collagen degradation products (hydroxyproline- and hydroxylysine-containing peptides and hydroxylysine glycosides) (Fig. 12). Estrogen and progesterone modulate collagenase in the involuting uterus. In pharmacologic doses, glucocorticoids inhibit collagenase release in several tissues. Nonsteroidal anti-inflammatory drugs that inhibit prostaglandin synthesis also inhibit collagenase production in some systems, but in other systems (for example, rheumatoid synovial cells), the synthesis and release of PGE_2 and collagenase can be dissociated.

ELASTIC FIBERS

Structure of Elastic Fibers

The other major fibrillar component of connective tissue is the elastic fiber, which consists of two distinct entities: (1) the amorphous elastin component and (2) a glycoprotein microfibrillar component (Fig. 8). Amorphous elastin component makes up the bulk of the elastic fiber, especially in mature tissue. The unit structure of elastin proper, known as tropoelastin, is a single polypeptide chain of about 800 amino acid residues (68,000 to 70,000 daltons), which has a characteristic amino acid composition that is similar in some respects to the collagens; approximately one third of the amino acid residues are glycine, and the proline concentration is approximately 12 per cent. In contrast to collagens, however, elastin contains relatively few residues of 4-hydroxyproline (approximately 1 per cent), no hydroxylysine, few charged residues such as aspartic and glutamic acids, lysine, and arginine, but a high content of the nonpolar amino acids, including alanine, valine, leucine, and isoleucine. Most of the

$$
\begin{array}{c}
\text{COOH} \\
| \\
\text{HC}-\text{NH}_2 \\
| \\
(\text{CH}_2)_3 \\
| \\
\text{CH}_2 \\
| \\
\text{NH} \\
| \\
\text{CH}_2 \\
| \\
(\text{CH}_2)_3 \\
| \\
\text{HC}-\text{NH}_2 \\
| \\
\text{COOH}
\end{array}
$$

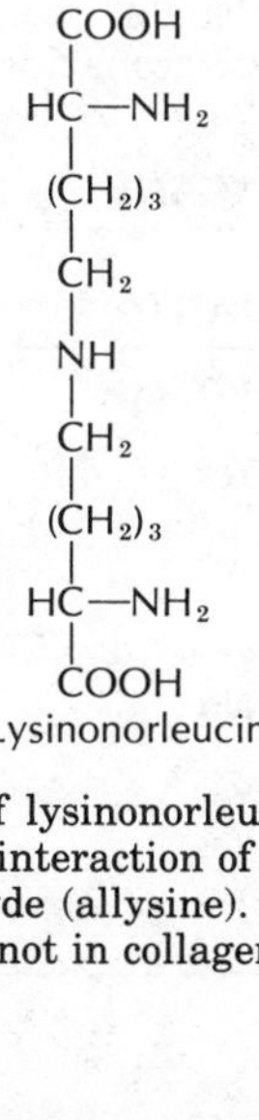

Lysinonorleucine

Figure 17. Structure of lysinonorleucine, the reduced Schiff base that results from interaction of a lysine side chain with that of a lysine aldehyde (allysine). This potential crosslink is found in elastin but not in collagen.

glycines are distributed randomly in elastin, although there are regions in tropoelastin that contain a collagen-like structure (-Gly-X-Y- repeat). Other regions are present where clusters of abundant residues may occur, such as triplets containing alanine or the repetition of a pentapeptide sequence Pro-Gly-Val-Gly-Val. By electron microscopy, elastic fibers from a variety of sources reveal no ordered structure and none of the periodicity found in collagens (Fig. 8). The elastic fibers behave physically as rubber-like elastomers. The polypeptide chains are highly crosslinked through lysyl and lysyl aldehyde residues. The simplest crosslink is formed from the reduced Schiff base of a lysine and lysyl aldehyde and is known as lysinonorleucine (Fig. 17). Other more complex crosslinks contain a pyridine nucleus also derived from lysine precursors. The latter crosslinked compounds, unique to elastin, occur as two isomers, designated as desmosine and isodesmosine.

Biosynthesis of Elastic Fibers

The predominant cell type involved in the biosynthesis of elastin is probably the smooth muscle cell, although it is possible that other cells can also synthesize this protein. The initial steps in biosynthesis involve the formation of a soluble proelastin (tropoelastin) with a molecular weight of approximately 72,000 and a characteristic amino acid composition. The tropoelastin mRNA, which codes for a protein of the expected size, contains approximately 3500 nucleotides, but the DNA sequences that hybridize to the elastin mRNA are composed of almost 30,000 nucleotides, suggesting either a large number of intervening sequences or multiple copies of the gene. In contrast to collagen, hydroxylation of specific protein residues in elastin is not essential to secretion of the protein, despite the presence of 4-hydroxyproline in mature elastin. Proelastin can be distinguished from the mature elastic fiber in its relatively high content of lysine and absence of the lysine-derived crosslinks. The formation of the crosslinks requires the oxidation of ε-amino groups of specific lysyl residues through the action of lysyl oxidase, probably the same enzyme involved in the oxidation of the lysyl and hydroxylysyl residues of collagens. Since the enzyme has an absolute requirement for copper and is inhibited by β-aminopropionitrile, experimental copper deficiency or administration of β-aminopropionitrile interferes with synthesis of mature elastin. Lysine is first incorporated into the polypeptide chain and then converted to allysine (the aldehyde of lysine) and subsequently to the reduced Schiff base compound termed lysinonorleucine (Fig. 17). The final crosslink compounds, desmosine and isodesmosine, are derived from four lysyl molecules.

The elastic fiber microfibrillar component probably is composed of more than one glycoprotein, with an amino acid composition distinct from that of the amorphous elastin. For example, the glycine, alanine, and valine contents are lower, there is no hydroxyproline, and cysteine is relatively abundant.

Disorders of Elastin Synthesis and Structure

There are several human disorders in which abnormalities in elastin structure or biosynthesis would be expected. Some of these conditions are characterized histopathologically by so-called fragmentation of elastic fibers, a prominent finding, for example, in pseudoxanthoma elasticum and in cystic medial necrosis of the aorta. The relationship of this histopathologic finding to proven chemical defects in elastin structure, however, has not been established. Interference with the formation of lysine-derived crosslinks results in biologic abnormalities. For example, copper deficiency in growing animals grossly impairs the integrity and functioning of the collagen and elastin network in the aorta. Repletion of copper in such animals restores lysyl oxidase activity, permitting the synthesis of lysyl derived crosslinks. It remains to be seen whether the low circulating copper levels in Menkes' kinky-hair syndrome are also associated with inadequate formation of elastin crosslinks. It has also not yet been demonstrated whether the use of compounds that chelate copper, such as D-penicillamine, results in significant decreases in lysyl oxidase activity.

Pseudoxanthoma elasticum, a genetic disorder usually inherited as autosomal recessive, is characterized by skin lesions, consisting of thickened redundant folds, yellowish plaques and papules, and changes in the ocular fundus known as angioid streaks. Vascular abnormalities, which are also characteristic features, consist of arterial calcification and occlusion and hypertension. In the skin lesions, elastic fibers appear swollen, clumped, and fragmented. Calcification of these elastic structures is also seen, and there is an abnormal accumulation of proteoglycans, yet there is no proof of chemical abnormalities either in the elastin itself or in associated extracellular material. A focal increase in elastic fibers is also seen in the skin lesions of *elastosis perforans serpiginosa,* but their significance is unknown. In the *Marfan syndrome,* characterized by arachnodactyly, tall stature, and ectopia lentis, the most serious manifestations are cardiovascular, such as aneurysms of the sinus of Valsalva, dissecting aneurysms, and dilatation of the aortic root with valvular insufficiency. The arterial lesions are characterized by fragmentation of elastic structures. Despite the analogies of Marfan syndrome to experimental lathyrism, no abnormal crosslinking of the elastin has been demonstrated. In one instance of the Marfan syndrome, aortic elastin was found to be low in desmosine content. In other cases, however, abnormalities in α2(I) chains of type I collagen have been demonstrated, as well as low content of the hydroxypyridinium crosslink. This is evidence that the Marfan syndrome must be genetically and biochemically heterogeneous, as are the other heritable disorders of connective tissue.

Proteolytic enzymes capable of degrading elastin, termed elastases, are serine proteinases that act at neutral pH. They are present in pancreas, where they are presumably involved in the digestion of dietary proteins. Elastases have also been demonstrated in human polymorphonuclear leukocytes and macrophages. The leukocyte elastase can degrade human lung elastin, arterial walls, and basement membranes. Whether or not such enzymes have a critical role in the degradation of elastic fibers in pathologic conditions such as pulmonary emphysema is uncertain, but enzymes of this sort may be critical for the tissue invasion and subsequent metastases of malignant tumor cells.

NONFIBRILLAR COMPONENTS

COMPLEX CARBOHYDRATES

Structure of the Complex Carbohydrates

Complex carbohydrates that make up the so-called ground substance of the interfibrillar matrix are major components of connective tissues. These substances may also be constituents of cellular materials. These complex polysaccharides of connective tissues, formerly known as mucopolysaccharides, are now termed glycosaminoglycans (the complex carbohydrate portion) and proteoglycans (those molecules in which the carbohydrate portion is covalently linked to polypeptides). In some tissues, such as articular cartilage, the proteoglycans may compose approximately half the dry weight of the tissue. Hyaluronic acid is the other major complex carbohydrate. The content of the complex carbohydrates varies, depending upon the site and function of the connective tissue. There is also considerable heterogeneity of chemical structure in different locations even within the same tissue. Glycoproteins, which by definition also contain variable proportions of carbohydrates, are usually of considerably lower molecular weight than the proteoglycans and hyaluronic acid and have carbohydrate side chains that differ chemically from those of glycosaminoglycan-containing macromolecules. Hyaluronic acid and the proteoglycans are high molecular weight linear polymers, usually consisting of disaccharide repeating units (Ta-

TABLE 10. COMPOSITION OF SOME GLYCOSAMINOGLYCANS

GLYCOSAMINOGLYCAN	DISACCHARIDE	SULFATED	APPROXIMATE MOLECULAR WEIGHT
Chondroitin-4-sulfate (chondroitin sulfate A)	Glucuronic; N-acetylgalactosamine	Yes	20,000–50,000
Chondroitin-6-sulfate (chondroitin sulfate C)	Glucuronic; N-acetylgalactosamine	Yes	20,000–50,000
Chondroitin-4,6-disulfate (chondroitin sulfate E)	Glucuronic; N-acetylgalactosamine	Yes	200,000
Dermatan sulfate	Iduronic; N-acetylgalactosamine (glucuronic)	Yes	20,000–50,000
Hyaluronic acid	Glucuronic; N-acetylglucosamine	No	50,000–5,000,000
Keratan sulfate			
Cartilage	Galactose; N-acetylglucosamine	Yes	8000–12,000
Cornea	Galactose; N-acetylglucosamine	Yes	4000–19,000
Heparin	Iduronic; N-acetylglucosamine (glucuronic)	Yes	5000–40,000
Heparan sulfate	Iduronic; N-acetylglucosamine (glucuronic)	Yes	10,000–50,000

ble 10), whereas the carbohydrate portion of the glycoproteins usually contains three or more sugar residues in a branched structure.

Hyaluronic acid, a constituent of most connective tissues, is a linear, nonsulfated polysaccharide, the repeating unit of which is 2-acetamido-2-deoxy-3-O-β-D-glucopyranosyl glucuronic acid. The disaccharides are linked β1–4. Most hyaluronic acids have very high molecular weights, are not covalently linked to proteins, and exist in solution as solvated spheres with a somewhat stiff but random coil configuration. Most hyaluronic acids have a molecular weight of approximately 1,000,000 and contain approximately 2500 repeating units. Hyaluronic acid is the major complex polysaccharide in synovial fluid and accounts for its high viscosity.

The proteoglycans contain repeating disaccharide units that are different from those in hyaluronic acid. The proteoglycans of cartilage are large molecules composed of a core protein to which chondroitin sulfate and keratan sulfate chains are linked covalently through xylose to seryl residues in the polypeptide chain (Fig. 18). The core proteins in turn are bound along with "link" glycoproteins through electrostatic forces to a linear molecule of hyaluronic acid, resulting in the so-called proteoglycan aggregates. Chondroitin sulfate and keratan sulfate are two glycosaminoglycans that have their own unique structure, consisting of repeating disaccharide units of an amino sugar and a uronic acid or galactose. The amino sugar in chondroitin sulfate is N-acetylgalactosamine, compared with N-acetylglucosamine in hyaluronic acid. These glycosaminoglycans are sulfated either in the 4 or the 6 position, resulting in so-called chondroitin-4-sulfate (chondroitin sulfate A) and 6-sulfate (chondroitin sulfate C), respectively. Keratan sulfate, on the other hand, contains N-acetylglucosamine rather than galactosamine; galactose replaces glucuronic acid in the repeating unit.

In a connective tissue such as cartilage, the glycosaminoglycans are covalently linked to the polypeptide core protein. The proteoglycans are polydispersed with a molecular weight of several million. They probably exist in the matrix of tissues such as cartilage as proteoglycan complexes, joined in association with glycoproteins to hyaluronic acid in a noncovalent fashion. The presence of these substances in large quantities in a tissue such as cartilage accounts for many of the mechanical properties of that tissue.

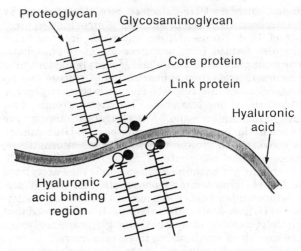

Figure 18. A diagram of possible structure of the proteoglycan aggregate.

Biosynthesis of the Complex Carbohydrates

The complex carbohydrates of the extracellular matrix are probably synthesized by the same cells (fibroblasts, chondrocytes, and smooth muscle cells) that synthesize the fibrillar components of connective tissue. In the biosynthesis of the proteoglycans, the formation of the protein core of the proteoglycan subunit precedes the formation of the glycosaminoglycan polysaccharide chains. Since the amino acid sequence of the core protein is not known, the precise mechanism of biosynthesis of this important component of proteoglycans remains unclarified. The polypeptide chain is synthesized on polyribosomes in a fashion similar to that of other proteins. The core protein synthesized in cell free translation systems is of very high molecular weight.

Sugar nucleotides are key intermediates in the synthesis of the polysaccharide chains as well as the oligosaccharide linkage region (Fig. 19). Critical reactions involve the formation of glucose-6-phosphate, the conversion to glucose-1-phosphate by the mutase reaction, and the formation of uridine-diphosphate-glucose by the interaction of uridine triphosphate (UTP) and glucose-1-phosphate. Several important interme-

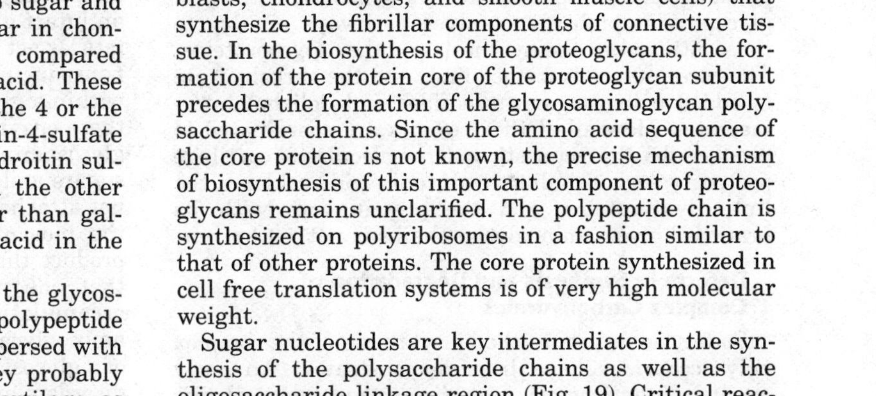

Figure 19. Formation of precursors of the glycosaminoglycans. Glc = glucose; GlcN = glucosamine; GlcNAc = N-acetylglucosamine; Gal = galactose; GlcUA = glucuronic acid; Xyl = xylose; GalNAc = N-acetylgalactosamine; IUA = iduronic acid. (From Silbert, J. E.: Biochemistry and Metabolism of the Mucopolysaccharides. Bull Rheum Dis 22:680, 1972.)

diates, such as UDP-galactose, are then formed by epimerases; UDP-glucuronic acid is an oxidation product of UDP-glucose. Other nucleotide intermediates are also formed from precursor glucose-6-phosphate. For example, the galactose and N-acetylgalactosamine precursors arise from epimerization of glucose and N-acetylglucosamine, respectively, while these sugars are linked to uridine phosphate. The acetyl groups of N-acetylglucosamine and N-acetylgalactosamine are added to the precursor sugar phosphates. Glucosamine is converted to glucose-6-phosphate or, alternatively, glucosamine-6-phosphate is formed from fructose-6-phosphate; glucosamine-6-phosphate is then acetylated to N-acetylglucosamine-6-phosphate. The UDP-N-acetylglucosamine is then converted through an epimerase to UDP-N-acetylgalactosamine. It is presumed that all cells capable of synthesizing glycosaminoglycans are capable of synthesizing these precursors.

Following the synthesis of the linkage oligosaccharide, the glycosaminoglycan side chains elongate by the alternate addition of sugars derived from nucleotide intermediates. For example, UDP-glucuronic acid and UDP-N-acetylgalactosamine are the precursors of chondroitin sulfate and dermatan sulfate. Sulfation of the glycosaminoglycans, which contributes to the high negative charge of these macromolecules, takes place after the sugars have been added to the growing polysaccharide side chains. The sulfate donor is phosphoadenosine phosphosulfate. The synthesis of the link glycoprotein probably involves pathways similar to those utilized in the synthesis of other glycoproteins. The core protein is formed first, and the carbohydrate is added using sugar nucleotides and dolichol intermediates. How all of these events are coordinated to produce the characteristic macromolecules of cartilage proteoglycans, including hyaluronic acid backbone, the link glycoproteins, and the protein core with its branched glycosaminoglycan chains is not yet known.

Defects in Synthesis and Degradation of Complex Carbohydrates

So far, no defects in the biosynthesis of the complex polysaccharides have been demonstrated. An early event in *inflammatory joint disease* and osteoarthritis is loss of proteoglycans from the articular cartilage. Following insult to the joint, such as removal of the synovial membrane or immobilization, cartilage proteoglycan is depleted. Although the loss results from degradation of the macromolecular component, the synthesis of new proteoglycan usually replaces that lost. There is thus considerable turnover of the glycosaminoglycan and protein portion of the proteoglycans. Enzymes described as hyaluronidases actually have much broader substrate specificity and might best be termed glycosaminoglycanylases. There is no convincing evidence that such enzymes, which can degrade the glycosaminoglycan portion under certain in vitro conditions, are operative in vivo. Hyaluronidases isolated from tissues such as testes have an acid pH optimum, and it is unlikely that such enzymatic reactions occur outside the cell at neutral pH. Even in inflammatory joint disease it is unlikely that so-called hyaluronidases are involved in the loss of the cartilage proteoglycan. However, limited proteolysis in vitro of the protein core of the proteoglycan can result in drastic reduction of the size and shape of the proteoglycan molecule. Proteases acting on cartilage fragments in this fashion can result in depletion of proteoglycan. Although lysosomal proteases such as cathepsin D can degrade the protein core of proteoglycans, it is unlikely that cathepsin D has significant proteolytic activity against the proteoglycan core protein or other proteins when the pH is greater than 6. There are several other proteases characterized from chondrocytes, polymorphonuclear leukocytes, and macrophages that can act at neutral pH to degrade the proteoglycan core protein of cartilage and result in solubilization of the remainder of the macromolecule. The enzymes from human granulocytes have been best characterized and have been identified as an enzyme with elastase properties as well as a chymotrypsin-like enzyme. It is probable that enzymes of this type are involved in the loss of cartilage proteoglycans in inflammatory arthritis as well as osteoarthritis.

Mucopolysaccharidoses. These disorders are the only pathologic conditions in which specific defects in the degradation of the proteoglycans have been demonstrated. Most of these disorders involve genetic defects in the formation of specific lysosomal glycosidases and sulfatases involved in the degradation of the glycosaminoglycans and result in the accumulation of an abnormal glycosaminoglycan within the cell. The glycosidases are exoglycosidases, which have the capacity only to cleave terminal, nonreducing sugar residues. These enzymes cannot cleave glycosidic bonds within an intact glycosaminoglycan chain. Similarly, the sulfatases act primarily on sulfate residues located at the nonreducing end of oligosaccharides and not on sulfates within a glycosaminoglycan chain. It is presumed that these enzymes acting in concert can degrade an entire glycosaminoglycan molecule by sequentially removing sugars and sulfate from the nonreducing end, which is not attached to the protein core. If there is a defect in the biosynthesis of any one of these enzymes, the product that would accumulate in the cell would be that one just before the block. Thus, intracellular accumulation of specific structurally abnormal glycosaminoglycans can be attributed to a defect in the action of a glycosidase or sulfatase. Examples of some of these disorders are given in Table 11.

An additional disorder associated with excessive storage of glycosaminoglycans is *I cell disease*. This disorder results not from the deficiency of a specific glycosidase or sulfatase but from the failure of biosynthesis of a particular membrane-bound mannose phosphate involved in recognition and uptake by the cell of the degradative enzymes. The very existence of this disease implies that there may be continuous release and uptake of degradative enzymes in order to account for the accumulation of the glycosaminoglycans. It is presumed that the presence of large amounts of these abnormal glycosaminoglycans within lysosomes somehow results in defects in cellular metabolism and secondarily produces the specific clinical picture associated with each enzymatic defect.

OTHER CONNECTIVE TISSUE COMPONENTS

Other Organic Components

Connective tissues also contain characteristic matrix components other than the proteoglycans and the fibrillar proteins. For example, dental enamel contains a

TABLE 11. A CLASSIFICATION OF MUCOPOLYSACCHARIDE STORAGE DISEASES*

DESIGNATION MUCOPOLYSACCHARIDOSES		CLINICAL FEATURES	PRESUMED STORAGE POLYSACCHARIDE	ENZYME DEFICIENT
MPS I H	Hurler syndrome	Early clouding of cornea, grave manifestations (dysostosis multiplex, mental retardation, heart disease); death usually before age 10	Dermatan sulfate Heparan sulfate	α-L-iduronidase
MPS I S	Scheie syndrome (formerly MPS V)	Stiff joints, cloudy cornea, aortic valve disease, normal intelligence, normal life-span (?)	Dermatan sulfate Heparan sulfate	α-L-iduronidase
MPS I H S	Hurler-Scheie compound	Phenotype intermediate between Hurler and Scheie	Dermatan sulfate Heparan sulfate	α-L-iduronidase
MPS II, severe	Hunter syndrome, severe	No clouding of cornea, milder course than in MPS I H but death usually before 15 years	Dermatan sulfate Heparan sulfate	Iduronate sulfatase
MPS II, mild	Hunter syndrome, mild	Survival to 30s to 60s, fair intelligence	Dermatan sulfate Heparan sulfate	Iduronate sulfatase
MPS III A	Sanfilippo syndrome A	Indistinguishable phenotype; mild somatic, severe central nervous system effects	Heparan sulfate	Heparan N-sulfatase
MPS III B	Sanfilippo syndrome B		Heparan sulfate	N-acetyl-α-D-glucosaminidase
MPS III C	Sanfilippo syndrome C		Heparan sulfate	Acetyl CoA:α-glucosamide N-acetyltransferase
MPS IV	Morquio syndrome (probably several forms with different enzyme deficiencies and possibly allelic forms of each)	Severe bone changes of distinctive type, cloudy cornea, aortic regurgitation	Keratan sulfate	Galactosamine 6-sulfatase
MPS V	Vacant			
MPS VI, severe	Maroteaux-Lamy syndrome, classic severe form	Severe osseous, soft tissue, and corneal change; valvular heart disease; striking white cell inclusions; normal intelligence; survival to 20s	Dermatan sulfate	Arylsulfatase B (N-acetylgalactosamine 4-sulfatase)
MPS VI, intermediate	Maroteaux-Lamy syndrome, intermediate form	Moderately severe changes	Dermatan sulfate	Arylsulfatase B (N-acetylgalactosamine 4-sulfatase)
MPS VI, mild	Maroteaux-Lamy syndrome, mild form	Severe osseous and corneal change, normal intellect	Dermatan sulfate	Arylsulfatase B (N-acetylgalactosamine 4-sulfatase)
MPS VII	β-Glucuronidase deficiency	Hepatosplenomegaly, dysostosis multiplex, mental retardation variable, white cell inclusions	Dermatan sulfate Heparan sulfate	β-Glucuronidase
MPS VIII	Glucosamine-6-sulfate sulfatase deficiency	Short stature, mental retardation, hepatomegaly	Keratan sulfate Heparan sulfate	N-acetylglucosamine-6-sulfate sulfatase

*Adapted from McKusick, V. A., Neufeld E. F., and Kelley, T. E.: The Mucopolysaccharide Storage Diseases. In Stanbury, J. B., Wyngaarden, J. B., and Fredrickson, D. S. (eds.): The Metabolic Basis of Inherited Disease. New York, McGraw-Hill, 1978, p. 1282.

unique set of noncollagenous proteins, some of which are phosphoproteins. Although some of these proteins are present in only small amounts in the adult tooth, their content is high early in the course of dental development.

Fibronectin is a cell surface glycoprotein that also circulates in plasma; the cellular and plasma forms are similar in structure but not identical. These types of fibronectin are both composed of two similar polypeptide subunits of 220,000 to 250,000 daltons, linked by disulfide bonds. There is no evidence yet for more than one fibronectin gene; therefore, differences in various tissue forms of fibronectin would probably result from differential processing of the primary transcript or some other posttranscriptional event. The relationship of different structural domains in fibronectin to functions such as binding to cell membranes, collagens, and heparin has been established (Fig. 20). Fibronectin probably has a role in the adherence of cells to collagen and proteoglycans in the extracellular matrix. In tissues studied with immunofluorescence, there is costaining of type III collagen and fibronectin in small fibers that also take silver stains and would be considered reticulin. Fibronectin can also act as a chemotactic agent and alter cell proliferation. Differences in amounts of fibronectin on cells, such as de-

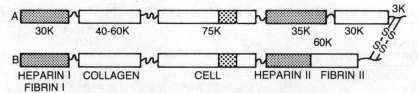

Figure 20. A model of the functional domains in the structure of fibronectin. K = kilodaltons. Note that there is a difference in the size of the A and B chains located at the carboxyterminal end. Differences among the forms of tissue fibronectin are accounted for by changes in this portion of the molecule, yet only a single gene for fibronectin has been identified. (From Yamada, K. M.: Cell surface interactions with extracellular materials. Annu Rev Biochem 52:761, 1983.)

creases on cancer cells and increases in synovial fluid in forms of arthritis have been documented. Whether these and other abnormalities are specific markers for disease has yet to be proved.

Laminin, a glycoprotein located in the basement membranes of epithelia and blood vessel walls, binds to heparin and type IV collagen; it may serve as an attachment factor for epithelial and endothelial cells and may be important in controlling the growth of cells such as neuronal cells. Laminin is composed of three A polypeptide chains, each about 200,000 daltons and a single B polypeptide chain of about 400,000 daltons. These are arranged in the form of a cross (Fig. 21). Laminin, type IV collagen, and a unique heparan sulfate proteoglycan interact to form a complex in basement membranes. This complex is presumably responsible for the specific properties of the basement membrane, e.g., acting as a permeability barrier for charged molecules (Fig. 22). Alterations in the relative amounts of these and other components may be found in disease. For example, the heparan sulfate proteoglycan content is reduced in glomerular basement membranes in experimentally produced diabetes mellitus. Autoantibodies may be directed against some of these components, such as the Goodpasture antigen, which may be within a globular domain of type IV collagen.

Bone also contains unique noncollagenous proteins. One of these is a low molecular weight (5700 daltons) peptide that contains three residues of γ-carboxyglutamic acid (GLA). This peptide has been called *osteocalcin* or bone *GLA-protein*. GLA is a modified amino acid whose synthesis depends upon the presence of vitamin K. This GLA-protein has been shown to be synthesized in bone and has a structure that is different from that of the better known vitamin K–dependent, GLA-containing proteins such as prothrombin. The formation of the GLA results from the posttranslational modification of critical glutamic acid residues. Enzymes involved in this reaction that require vitamin K for their full activity are present in

bone and utilize bicarbonate as the donor. Under circumstances in which vitamin K is unavailable or in the presence of a vitamin K antagonist such as coumadin, this γ-carboxylation does not occur. Whether or not these transcarboxylation reactions are important in human skeletal metabolism remains to be demonstrated. Proteins containing GLA are present in ectopic calcifications and in the matrices of certain renal calculi. Bone GLA protein circulates in human plasma, and levels have been determined by radioimmunoassay. These levels are elevated in states of high bone turnover, although it has not been established whether the antigens are by-products of synthesis or are released when bone is resorbed.

Other proteins are also found among the noncollagenous bone proteins. The most abundant is *osteonectin* (32,000 daltons), which is synthesized by bone cells and binds to apatite mineral and type I collagen. A unique bone proteoglycan has also been demonstrated. Other noncollagenous proteins in bone matrix are derived from plasma, such as albumin and α_2-HS glycoprotein. Glycoproteins are also found in cartilage. One of these is called *chondronectin,* a disulfide-linked multimer of 180,000 daltons. Chondronectin appears specifically to bind chondrocytes to type II collagen. Although this protein was first identified in serum, a related protein is synthesized by chondrocytes. Proteins such as chondronectin, laminin, osteonectin, and fibronectin may serve much broader functions than attachment and may prove to have significant roles in determining spreading of cells, replication, and synthetic functions characteristic of cell phenotypes. Disease-specific alterations in these proteins and their function will probably be found on further study.

Inorganic Mineral Phase

Another major component of the extracellular portion of some connective tissues is an inorganic mineral phase. Such a phase is characteristic of bone and indeed

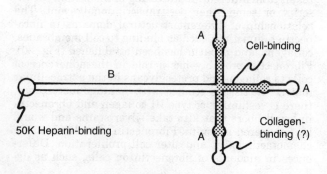

Figure 21. A model of the functional domains in the structure of laminin. K = kilodaltons. The A chains are of the same size ($\sim$ 200,000 daltons), whereas the B chains have a molecular weight of $\sim$ 400,000. Laminin can be attacked by several different proteases, but the shaded areas indicate protease-resistant fragments. (From Yamada, K. M.: Cell surface interactions with extracellular materials. Annu Rev Biochem 52:761, 1983.)

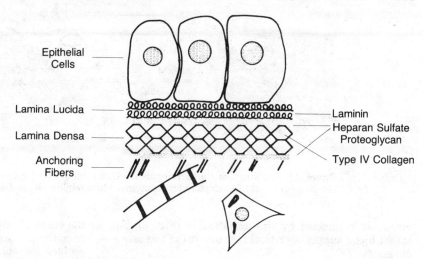

Figure 22. Schematic representation of the structure of an epithelial basement membrane, showing a possible arrangement of the component molecules. All of these components may interact with and bind to one another. (From Martin, G. R., Rohrbach, D. H., Terranova, V. P., and Liotta, L. A.: Structure, function, and pathology of basement membranes. In Wagner, B. M., Fleischmajer, R., and Kaufman, N. (eds.): Connective Tissue Disease. Baltimore, Williams and Wilkins, 1983, p. 16.)

accounts for approximately two thirds of its dry weight and is responsible for many of its physical properties. A calcium-phosphate phase is also deposited in the growth plate of cartilage during endochondral ossification, but in a manner different from that in bone.

The calcification of cartilage is a temporary phase that is usually replaced as the core of calcified cartilage is covered by new bone matrix. An inorganic mineral phase occurs also in teeth that is composed of calcium and phosphate in the crystal lattice.

Function, Composition, and Remodeling of Specific Connective Tissues and Mineral Ion Homeostasis

BONE

STRUCTURE AND COMPOSITION

The structure and composition of bone appear to be ideally suited for its function. Bone provides the rigid framework for body form and serves as the point of attachment for ligaments, muscles, and tendons, which surround and stabilize the joints. Bone is also important as a protective covering for neural structures and for certain viscera. The mechanical demands on the skeleton require a structure that will not deform under stress yet will not crack when exposed to forces that would shatter more brittle materials. Bone is also characterized by a high tensile strength despite its lightness. Since mechanical forces applied to the skeleton vary, mechanisms exist for bone to respond and adapt to those new demands. The properties of bone are determined by its chemical structure and organization of an organic portion intimately associated with an inorganic mineral phase. The mineral phase, which makes up two thirds of the dry weight of bone, is composed of calcium and phosphorus in the form of a mixture of poorly crystalline hydroxyapatite, brushite, and another solid, which has a lower calcium-phosphate ratio than pure hydroxyapatite and has been termed amorphous calcium phosphate. Mature bone contains a higher proportion of the poorly crystalline hydroxyapatite, whereas embryonic bone contains predominantly amorphous calcium phosphate and brush-

ite. The organic phase of mature bone contains 95 per cent collagen, all of which is type I collagen. The primary structure of this collagen is identical to the type I collagen of skin, but bone collagen in humans differs in certain posttranslational modifications, particularly the ratios of the di- and monoglycosylated hydroxylysines. Other components of the organic phase include the noncollagenous proteins synthesized locally (bone GLA-protein, heparan sulfate proteoglycan, osteonectin, and phosphoproteins) and derived from plasma (α_2-HS glycoprotein).

The mineral phase of bone is intimately associated with the collagen. The majority of the mineral is located in the so-called hole zones, which are produced by the particular packing arrangement of the collagen molecules that make up the collagen fiber. Indeed, some of the calcium of the mineral phase may be tightly linked to phosphate and carboxy groups in bone phosphoserine peptides or in collagen itself. In addition, the more highly structured mineral phase is partially oriented with the long axis of the crystals parallel to the long axis of the collagen molecules within the fiber. This basic structure is similar for all types of adult bone. For example, the cortex of bone contains more tightly packed collagen with its associated mineral phase (compact bone), whereas areas of bone toward the metaphyseal ends have a looser structure (cancellous bone). The extracellular matrix of bone encases the bone cells proper (osteocytes). These osteo-

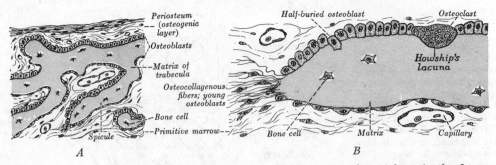

Figure 23. Drawings of the development of intramembranous (membrane) bone in the fetus. (From Arey, L. B.: Developmental Anatomy. Philadelphia, W. B. Saunders Co., 1965.)

cytes are connected by fine canaliculae (Fig. 3). An intact blood supply is critical for survival of the osteocytes.

Bone Development and Remodeling

In the embryo, bone is either formed as membrane bone (Fig. 23) or formed on cartilaginous models (Fig. 24). In early embryos, prior to the histologic appearance of cartilage, the most primitive mesenchymal cells can produce type I collagen as the extracellular matrix. At the stage when cartilage as such is recognizable, there is a switch to another gene that codes for type II collagen, the type characteristic of cartilage throughout life. With further maturation, the cartilaginous rudiment takes on the gross appearance of a bone. During fetal life, the cartilaginous precursor then increases in size by interstitial growth of the chondrocytes as well as appositional growth from new cartilage cells in the perichondrium. With continued growth, a change appears in the organization of the cartilage cells at the center of what will be the anlage of the bone shaft. In this region the cells become larger and are surrounded by a less dense matrix; soon thereafter an area of calcified cartilage appears as a collar around what is destined to become the bone shaft. The initial calcification is in cartilage, however, not in bone. The earliest calcification in cartilage appears to be contained within membrane-bound vesicles, most of which are unassociated with the cartilage collagen. Following

the stage of calcified cartilage, other cells differentiate from the periosteal region and surround and eventually replace the calcified cartilage to form a different matrix, which also becomes calcified. This is now bone as distinct from cartilage matrix and, as in the adult, is composed of type I collagen. The calcification process is also associated with loss of cartilage-specific proteoglycans in the matrix. The formation of bone matrix is carried out by cells that are brought in from the vascular supply and are of stromal origin and include primitive osteoblasts. This first cuff of bone is called the primary ossification center (Fig. 24). Shortly thereafter, a similar sequence of events is observed in the cartilage covering the ends of bones as well as the epiphyseal growth plates. The maturation of the epiphyseal plate is characterized by cell hypertrophy, calcification of the cartilaginous matrix, death of some cells, invasion of blood vessels that bring in osteoblasts, followed by deposition of bone matrix, which then becomes mineralized. The areas at the ends of the bone are termed the secondary centers of ossification. Proliferation of the cells at the epiphyseal plate and the subsequent endochondral ossification are responsible for growth in length of the long bones (Figs. 24 and 25). The change in the shape of the ends of the bone is due to a similar sequence of events occurring beneath the articular cartilage surfaces of the bone. In the process of growth, first calcified cartilage and then bone itself is resorbed through the action of chondroclasts and osteoclasts (Fig. 26), following which new

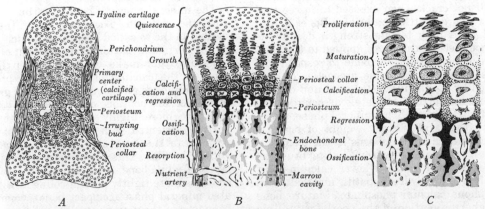

Figure 24. Schematic representation of endochondral bone formation. *A*, Formation of primary center of ossification in an early cartilaginous rudiment. *B*, Later stage of development of the sequence at the epiphyseal plate. *C*, An enlargement of the epiphyseal plate region shown in *B*. (From Arey, L. B.: Developmental Anatomy. Philadelphia, W. B. Saunders Co., 1965.)

Figure 25. Schematic representation of ossification and growth in a long bone. *A* represents the early cartilaginous rudiment before the development of the primary center of ossification. The latter is first seen as the dark area at the center of the shaft in *B*. Secondary centers of ossification are shown to appear first in *D*. In *F*, the epiphyseal growth plates are closed (fused), which occurs when adulthood is reached. In *G* is superimposed a drawing of the human femur at birth in the marrow cavity of an adult femur to show relative sizes resulting from bone deposition and remodeling during growth. *H* shows two periods in the elongation of a femur, illustrating the shape (stippled area) that would have resulted had resorption and deposition of bone (modeling and remodeling) not taken place. (From Arey, L.B.: Developmental Anatomy. Philadelphia, W. B. Saunders Co., 1965.)

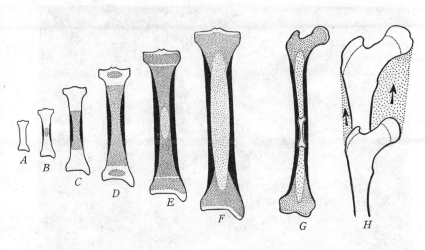

bone is deposited in its place. The bone grows in thickness by the action of osteoblasts in the cuff at the center of the shaft, whereas bone is resorbed centrally, resulting in formation of the medullary canal. Bone increases in thickness owing to the fact that the deposition of bone from the periosteal surface occurs at a rate faster than that at which it is removed at the endosteal surface. In many compact bones, new bone is formed in relationship to blood vessels that run longitudinally throughout the shaft in a somewhat spiraling fashion. The formation of new bone by osteoblasts surrounding these blood vessels gives origin to these haversian systems. Each blood vessel with its surrounding bone is termed an osteon, the basic unit of compact bone in the shafts. The final form of bone depends upon the ordered sequence of events described.

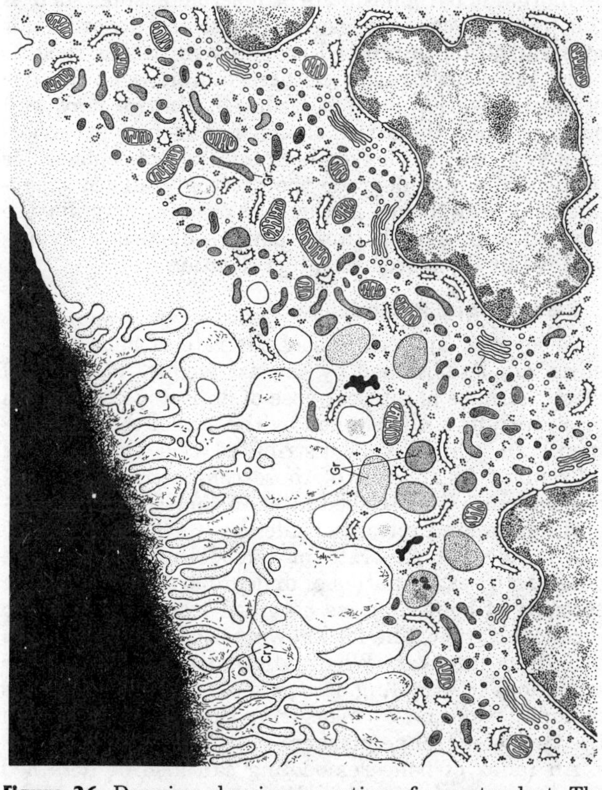

Organizational Types of Bone

Microscopically, bone can be classified on the basis of its organization as woven or lamellar bone. *Woven bone* is characteristic of that which is first deposited in the embryo (Fig. 23); it is seen in adults only in response to inflammation or injury, or in the primitive bone formed by neoplasms, such as osteosarcoma. Woven bone is formed rapidly and can be recognized by the relatively high proportion of cells to matrix and random organization of the collagen fibers. Almost all of the bone in adults, whether in compact or cancellous regions, is *lamellar bone* and is characterized by the parallel array of the collagen fiber bundles, arranged in sheets with alternation in the fiber direction of successive sheets. This gives rise to a layered pattern (Fig. 27).

Remodeling of Adult Bone

In adult bone, even after longitudinal growth has ceased, remodeling continues. The initial event in remodeling of adult bone appears to be a focal resorption carried out by osteoclasts, which are usually multinucleated. The resorptive process involves relatively few cells and is usually intense. On the other hand, soon after the resorption of bone, osteoblasts appear that lay down new bone matrix that subsequently calcifies. The deposition of bone involves relatively more cells than are necessary for resorption and lasts longer than resorption. Bone remodeling may be considered to occur in units or packets in which the initial resorptive phase is tightly coupled in time and space to the formative phase. The mechanism of this formation-resorption coupling that characterizes physiologic, as well as pathologic, remodeling is not known, although it is presumed that some soluble ligand

Figure 26. Drawing showing a portion of an osteoclast. The bone surface is to the left in the figure in contact with the ruffled border of the cell. Crystals (Cry) are shown liberated from bone matrix in this diagram, although it is uncertain whether this is a preparative artifact. Granules (Gr) may contain substances such as proteases, which are secreted by the osteoclasts. Golgi complexes (G) are numerous in active osteoclasts. (From Lentz, T. L.: Cell Fine Structure: An Atlas of Drawings of Whole-Cell Structure. Philadelphia, W. B. Saunders Co., 1971.)

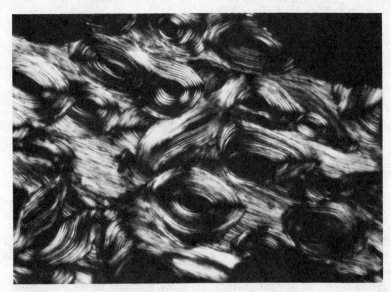

Figure 27. A photomicrograph of secondary haversian bone taken under polarized light. This illustrates the typical appearance of lamellar bone produced by the higher ordered packing arrangement of the collagen fibers. (From Jowsey, J.: Metabolic Diseases of Bone. Philadelphia, W. B. Saunders, Co., 1977.)

produced locally is responsible. Several factors have been isolated from bone and cartilage that can stimulate replication of skeletal tissue cells or collagen synthesis and could possibly serve this complexing function.

The sequence of events in remodeling of cancellous bone is as follows. A portion of the bone surface is involved in either formation or resorption or appears to be inactive. Active formation surfaces can be recognized by the presence of a narrow region of hypocalcified matrix (osteoid) covered with plump osteoblasts. The thickness of the osteoid seam is usually less than 12 to 13 μm. Some formation surfaces appear to be inactive, with the narrow osteoid seam covered by flattened cells. Resorption areas, on the other hand, are recognized by their scalloped appearance and the presence of cells with the characteristic appearance of osteoclasts. At the junction of the osteoid seam with mineralized bone is a narrow band that contains lipid and stains with metachromatic dyes (mineralization front); it is at this site that tetracyclines bind by interacting with the mineral phase and the matrix. Under ultraviolet light the deposition of tetracyclines in undemineralized histologic sections produces the appearance of a narrow band of intense fluorescence that persists for the lifetime of that particular region of bone.

Mineralization

The deposition of the mineral phase in bone requires the synthesis by osteoblasts of a calcifiable bone matrix that contains type I collagen with bone-specific post-translational modifications in addition to the other organic components of the matrix. Some of the matrix components may require modifications prior to mineralization, which include, for example, phosphorylation of specific seryl residues of bone phosphoproteins, or γ-carboxylation of other protein(s). Precipitation of the mineral phase can occur only in the presence of optimal concentrations of calcium and phosphate ions at the mineralization site. It is possible that concentrations of these ions are regulated by the activity of the osteoblasts. An optimal pH is necessary for the formation of the mineral phase. The pH at mineralization sites in cartilage is ~7.6, but no information is available regarding bone. Since the extracellular fluid is probably supersaturated with respect to the bone mineral phase, it is probable that mineralization does not occur normally in other collagenous matrices because of the presence of either circulating or local inhibitors of calcification. These inhibitors may involve ions such as inorganic pyrophosphate or macromolecules such as the proteoglycan aggregates. Therefore, in order for mineralization to proceed normally in tissues such as bone, the concentration of these inhibitors at the site of mineralization must be reduced. Control may well occur through the action of enzymes such as pyrophosphatases, which cleave inorganic pyrophosphate, or proteases, which degrade the proteoglycans by cleavage of peptide bonds in the core protein. Any disease that interferes with this orderly sequence of events will result in disordered mineralization.

Rate of Bone Remodeling

An overall appreciation of the rate of bone remodeling can be obtained by several means. The rate of disappearance of a tracer dose of an isotope of calcium or strontium is determined by the size of the compartments in which it is distributed and the rates of movement in and out of those compartments. These phenomena are described later in the section on skeletal uptake and release of calcium.

An index of the rate of remodeling can also be obtained by examination of undemineralized histologic sections of bone biopsies obtained from patients who received tetracycline for known periods of time with a drug-free interval. When allowances are made for variations in sampling, it is possible to determine rates of bone formation by measuring the distance between the two tetracycline markers.

An index of bone remodeling can also be obtained from an analysis of matrix degradation products. When collagen is resorbed, the 4-hydroxyproline and hydroxylysine released are not reutilized for collagen biosynthesis. Small peptides containing 4-hydroxyproline are rapidly cleared by the kidneys and excreted in the urine. Free 4-hydroxyproline, liberated by iminopeptidases, is metabolized in the liver by hydroxyproline oxidases. Under normal circumstances, therefore, little free 4-hydroxyproline circulates in plasma or is excreted in the urine. Thus, urinary excretion of 4-hydroxyproline represents only a small proportion of the total released from collagen breakdown (~10 to 20 per cent). These estimates have been derived in part from studies of individuals with hydroxyprolinemia, a disorder associated with deficient hydroxyproline oxidase. Affected individuals have high blood and urinary levels of free hydroxyproline. In normal individuals, bone is the major collagen-containing tissue that turns over, and it is likely that most of the 4-hydroxyproline excreted in the urine is derived from the breakdown of bone, rather than other tissue collagen. Normal adults excrete up to 40 mg/day of 4-hydroxyproline in the form of small peptides. Higher levels are observed during periods of rapid growth, in acromegaly, and in hyperthyroidism. Levels decrease when growth is slowed—for example, in hypopituitarism or hypothyroidism. Increased excretion is found in patients with excessive bone turnover, such as Paget's disease of bone, hyperphosphatasia, extensive fibrous dysplasia, and hyperparathyroidism associated with osteitis fibrosa. Patients with extensive burns also excrete increased amounts of 4-hydroxyproline peptides.

From a compositional point of view, there are a number of potential markers besides 4-hydroxyproline that can be utilized to estimate collagen metabolism. Potentially, these would include repetitive sequences of amino acids in the collagen peptide chain (Gly-X-Y-Gly) and the presence of a number of other modified amino acids essentially unique to collagen. In addition to 4-hydroxyproline, these include 3-hydroxyproline, hydroxylysine, and the aldehydes of lysine and hydroxylysine. The pattern of hydroxylysine glycosides is also tissue-collagen specific. Since the biosynthesis of these modified amino acids and hydroxylysine glycosides also takes place after amino acid assembly into the polypeptide chains, none of these compounds is reutilized after collagen degradation, and all could serve as markers for collagen metabolism.

DISTURBANCES IN GROWTH AND DEVELOPMENT

Clinically, there are many disturbances of growth and development that may be considered in terms of aberrations in the orderly sequence of bone growth and remodeling. These disorders usually produce decreased stature or abnormal shape of bones of the entire skeleton or a portion of the skeleton. A complete description or classification is not possible here, but a few examples serve to illustrate features of the pathophysiology. It is possible to discuss the skeletal dysplasias in two major groups.

The *osteochondrodysplasias* result from abnormal growth and development of cartilage and/or bone, whereas the *dysostoses* may be considered as malformations of individual bones, singly or in combination. The osteochondrodysplasias may be further divided into (1) the chondrodystrophies, which represent defects of growth of tubular bones and occasionally the spine—for example, achondroplasia; (2) disordered development of cartilaginous and fibrous components of the skeleton—for example, multiple cartilaginous exostoses; and (3) abnormalities of density and/or cortical diaphyseal structure and metaphyseal remodeling—for example, osteogenesis imperfecta. In most of these disorders the ultimate cause is unknown. In some, an accumulation of an abnormal proteoglycan within the cells may so alter function that a form of skeletal dystrophy results. In others, an abnormality of matrix biosynthesis may be the ultimate cause—for example, certain types of osteogenesis imperfecta in which synthesis of type I bone collagen is decreased. Last, there may be an identifiable hormonal abnormality as the basis of the underlying dysplasia. In cretinism, a lack of thyroxine and triiodothyronine leads to delayed appearance of secondary centers of ossification as well as abnormal structures of those centers that do appear. Thus, not only is growth in length retarded, but also failure of the normal endochondral sequence results in abnormally retarded growth at the ends relative to the shafts of bone. Since appositional growth at the diaphyses is retarded less than that of the endochondral sequence, the resulting bones become shorter and thicker.

In the *Morquio syndrome* there is a disordered and asymmetric pattern of growth in the cartilaginous ends of the bone, including the articular cartilage. The appearance of secondary centers of ossification is also delayed. The asymmetric pattern of growth leads to distortion of the ends of the bone and the development of secondary osteoarthritis. Vertebral growth is also affected, leading to a short trunk and angular deformities of the spine. These clinical problems in the Morquio syndrome are probably all due to defective degradation of keratan sulfate, which accumulates within cartilage cells and somehow interferes with their function. The intracellular content of this glycosaminoglycan is increased as a result of deficiency in a sulfatase required for its biodegradation. In *achondroplasia,* there is a marked decrease in the rate of proliferation of cells in the growth plate, which results in shortening of the bones and relative thickening, since appositional growth at the shafts is not affected.

In *osteopetrosis* of the autosomal recessive type, there is increased density of bones because of abnormal remodeling, in this case probably ascribable to decreased functional activity of bone-resorbing cells or failure to form osteoclasts. Osteoclasts are derived from hematopoietic cells, possibly related to those that are the precursors of mononuclear phagocytes. This decreased activity may be due to malfunctioning of some immunocompetent cell required for complete maturation of the osteoclasts. In a few instances, the disorder has been cured by bone marrow transplantation. In one instance of congenital osteopetrosis, there has been clinical improvement induced by treatment with 1,25 dihydroxyvitamin D (1,25-$(OH)_2D_3$). This hormone can stimulate bone resorption as well as induce maturation of monocyte precursor cells, presumably to functioning osteoclasts. Osteopetrosis has also been associated with renal tubular acidosis in several kindreds in which an almost complete absence of carbonic anhydrase II was found in the erythrocytes from affected individuals. Carbonic anhydrase has been demonstrated histochemically in osteoclasts, and there is evidence that carbonic anhydrase inhibitors can block the effects of hormones such as parathyroid hormone (PTH) on bone resorption.

Diseases of abnormal remodeling also occur in the adult skeleton after the cartilaginous growth plate has closed and longitudinal growth has ceased. In some of these disorders, the skeletal effects are generalized such as in osteoporosis and osteomalacia, but in others, of which *Paget's disease* is the best example, the abnormal remodeling is focal, always sparing some normal bone. Remodeling defects in the adult skeleton can result either in decrease or increase in bone mass or in the abnormal shape of a bone. In addition, both increases and decreases in bone mass are usually accompanied by abnormalities in the form and distribution of the remodeled bone. Although in most states of abnormal remodeling, there is still some direction to the remodeling according to mechanical forces (Wolff's law), the structure of the remodeled bone may be sufficiently poor that the bone is unable to withstand usual stresses and thus becomes prone to fracture. The mechanisms of pain that frequently are associated with abnormally remodeled bone are unknown.

Hormonal Effects

Maximum adult bone mass is usually attained at the end of the second decade at the time of sexual maturation, with resultant closure of the cartilaginous growth plates. After this time the only regions where reactivation of the endochondral sequence can occur are at the ends of bones at the articular cartilage. If sexual maturation is delayed or gonadal function ceases prior to epiphyseal closure, proliferation of the growth plate continues, resulting in continued longitudinal growth, although at a reduced rate. Precocious puberty, in contrast, is associated with increased maturation and a period of accelerated skeletal growth. Suppression of the pituitary-gonadal axis with an inhibitor of luteinizing hormone release is accompanied by slowing of excessively rapid growth and skeletal maturation. It would follow that castration in either sex would lead to a delay in skeletal maturation, which can be assessed by radiographic analysis of secondary centers of ossification. Retarded skeletal growth in children who do not experience normal sexual maturation can be corrected by administering sex hormones.

Thyroid hormones are also involved in maturation as well as growth. In hypophysectomized animals, thyroxin alone produces only slight changes in activation of chondrogenesis at the growth plate but markedly accelerates growth in the presence of added growth hormone.

Growth hormone in turn does not have direct effects on stimulation of epiphyseal cartilage but acts through the production of somatomedins. It may well be that a transient secretion of growth hormone produces a sustained secretion of somatomedins and has prolonged effects on growth. The so-called sexual ateliotic dwarf has an isolated deficiency of growth hormone. This results in individuals who are normal in all other respects and have a skeleton normal in its proportion. However, individuals resembling the sexual ateliotic dwarfs may actually be synthesizing and releasing growth hormone as demonstrated by provocative tests but may fail to respond to growth hormone. The problem in the so-called Laron-type dwarf results from a failure to produce somatomedins despite sufficient levels of growth hormone. On the other hand, the African pygmy retains child-like proportions because he is unresponsive to the effects of somatomedin, even though this factor is produced in response to normal secretion of growth hormone.

Children with craniopharyngioma frequently have delayed skeletal growth and short stature. Levels of somatomedins (insulin-like growth factors I and II) and insulin are low in these children. However, other children with craniopharyngiomas grow normally; levels of insulin-like growth factors are sufficient to permit normal growth. In children with craniopharyngioma and hyperphagia, hyperinsulinemia results, which may be accompanied by excessive growth. Presumably, insulin in high concentrations produces effects similar to those of insulin-like growth factors, possibly by interacting with their cellular receptors. In situations in which growth hormone secretion is excessive, resulting in increased production of somatomedin, cartilaginous growth and endochondral ossification may be stimulated. In the child, in whom epiphyseal growth plates are still present, this acceleration of cartilaginous growth results in gigantism. In adults, reactivation of the endochondral sequence can occur only in the thin rim of cartilage cells lying just beneath the articular cartilage. Thus, in acromegaly (excessive production of growth hormone in adults), increased size is observed only in short bones, where the activation of endochondral ossification at the articular cartilage occupies a proportionately larger fraction of total skeletal volume than it does in the large bones. Increase in thickness also occurs by stimulation of periosteal growth in the diaphysis. This, then, accounts for the appearance of the somewhat enlarged, thick bones in the acromegalic. If growth hormone secretion is normal and puberty is premature, then decreased stature results, since the effects of the sex hormones on maturation of the epiphyses predominate. On the other hand, if sexual function is delayed, then the unopposed action of growth hormone on endochondral ossification results in longer bones. Since these effects are more dramatic in the long bones than in the spine, individuals develop abnormal proportions, with arm span increased to a greater extent than height. Growth hormone and the somatomedins are discussed more extensively in Section VIII, Endocrinology.

MINERAL ION HOMEOSTASIS

Skeletal Uptake and Release of Calcium

The skeleton is the major reservoir of the mineral ions calcium and phosphorus. Therefore, in any consideration of skeletal remodeling, it is important to understand the factors that regulate the metabolism of these ions. In a normal adult, 99 per cent of the calcium is contained in the skeleton, and radioactive calcium injected intravenously localizes in the skeleton within minutes. This skeletal uptake of calcium occurs predominantly in areas adjacent to osteocytes or bone surfaces. By measuring the amount of radioactive calcium taken up by the skeleton in 24 hours, and simultaneously measuring the ratio of radioactive calcium to calcium in blood, one can determine that 30 to 40 g of calcium moves from blood to bone each day in a normal adult. Since the plasma calcium concentration varies only within a 5 per cent range in normal adults, an approximately equivalent amount of calcium must move in the reverse direction from bone to blood daily. A variety of indirect evidence suggests that this large efflux of calcium occurs from the same areas of the skeleton, those adjacent to bone surfaces and osteocytes. Calcium transfers into and out of the skeleton occur more rapidly in trabecular bone than in cortical bone, in part because of its greater surface-to-volume ratio.

These exchange processes occur so rapidly that the blood calcium is functionally one unit with at least part of the skeletal calcium, and consideration of the "total extracellular fluid calcium" is not operationally useful in discussing the kinetics of calcium distribution within the body. For example, the dilution of an intravenously injected tracer dose of ^{47}Ca produces an apparent calcium "pool" size of 1.2 g within one minute and 2.5 g within one hour in healthy young adults, amounts of calcium exceeding the total calcium in plasma and all interstitial fluids. It is conceptually important to distinguish the small blood-bone calcium fluxes associated with bone remodeling (200 to 300 mg Ca/day) from the much larger fluxes described previously. For clarity we will use the term *mineralization* to refer to ion movements into incompletely mineralized bone matrix, *bone removal* to refer to the destruction and dissolution of bone mineral and matrix, and *skeletal influx* and *skeletal efflux* to refer to the much larger movements of ions between bone crystals and blood. Exchange of calcium (or phosphorus) between blood and preformed skeletal mineral involves only a substitution process, with no net skeletal uptake or release of calcium or phosphorus. Mineralization and removal of bone require precipitation or dissolution of bone mineral and necessarily involve net uptake or release of both calcium and phosphorus. Some potential cellular processes involved in bone removal and new bone mineralization (remodeling) are considered elsewhere in this section; the cellular processes responsible for skeletal calcium efflux and influx, however, are as yet very poorly understood. The cell covering on mature bone surfaces appears discontinuous on electron microscopy, and large molecules rapidly gain access to the bone surfaces after intravenous administration. Such observations suggest that uptake of calcium by mature mineralized bone may be governed primarily by physicochemical processes rather than by cellular transport of calcium. The fact that skeletal calcium influx is linearly proportional to the serum calcium concentration at total serum calcium levels above 2.75 mM (11.0 mg/dl) is consistent with this possibility. On the other hand, bone mineralization requires cellular activity, as do calcium efflux from bone and bone removal, and extensive studies of ion movements into and out of bone show as too simplistic the view that calcium movements to and from the skeleton reflect simple chemical equilibria.

The fluxes of calcium into and out of the skeleton are normally equal or almost equal in a variety of normal and pathologic situations. Even when bone remodeling and skeletal calcium efflux and influx are augmented as much as 20 to 30 times above normal (as occurs in severe Paget's disease of bone), these fluxes remain in approximate balance. This remarkable "coupling" of calcium movements into and out of the skeleton is, in part, a reflection of the fact that skeletal calcium uptake is directly proportional to the serum calcium concentration: Increases in skeletal calcium efflux raise the serum calcium level slightly, leading to a greater bone uptake of calcium. In addi-

tion, it is likely that bone-resorbing and bone-forming cells influence each other reciprocally by locally secreted paracrine factors.

These skeletal processes are influenced by circulating levels of PTH and 1,25-(OH)$_2$ vitamin D, both of which increase bone removal and calcium efflux from the skeleton. Their effects are synergistic, and both are needed to maintain normal rates of calcium efflux from bone. In vitamin D–deficient subjects, PTH is not able to maintain normal rates of skeletal calcium efflux, and hypocalcemia may develop. Likewise skeletal calcium efflux is low in hypoparathyroid subjects even during treatment with 1,25-(OH)$_2$ vitamin D. The mechanisms by which these hormones act are discussed in Section VIII. Parathyroid hormone and 1,25-(OH)$_2$ vitamin D also stimulate skeletal calcium influx, at least in part by increasing serum calcium levels. These hormones also stimulate new bone formation (and hence bone mineralization) indirectly, presumably by stimulating cells in the skeleton to secrete growth factors. PTH and 1,25-(OH)$_2$D can thus augment directly or indirectly both phases of bone remodeling (bone removal and bone mineralization) and skeletal calcium efflux and skeletal calcium influx. The balance between these effects is dose dependent. High levels of PTH or 1,25-(OH)$_2$D stimulate bone resorption more than bone formation and mineralization and thus result in hypercalcemia and catabolic effects on bone. Smaller amounts of these hormones are probably not catabolic and are, in fact, needed for normal bone remodeling and growth and for maintenance of a normal serum calcium concentration.

The movements of calcium into and out of bone are also significantly affected by calcium deficiency, circulating levels of inorganic phosphate and calcitonin, and other factors. Severe dietary calcium deficiency or intestinal malabsorption of calcium produces defective skeletal mineralization (osteomalacia). If mineralization is profoundly impaired, there is inhibition of the effects of PTH on bone, resulting in hypocalcemia, analogous to that of vitamin D deficiency. Since calcium repletion of vitamin D–deficient animals, and vitamin D repletion of calcium-deficient animals, only partially restores the effects of PTH on skeletal calcium mobilization, it is apparent that calcium deficiency and vitamin D deficiency separately affect skeletal responsiveness to PTH and separately interfere with the skeleton's contribution to serum calcium homeostasis.

Hyperphosphatemia increases calcium deposition in the skeleton, owing in part to the formation of the calcium-phosphate mineral phase in bone. Phosphate depletion, on the other hand, decreases skeletal calcium influx and interferes with bone mineralization. Severe phosphate depletion also enhances bone removal and calcium efflux from bone, via direct skeletal effects that are not well characterized and by augmenting the blood levels of 1,25-(OH)$_2$D (see Section VIII). In consequence, phosphorus depletion tends to elevate the serum calcium concentration and hyperphosphatemia tends to lower it. Compensatory changes in PTH secretion will counteract these effects and maintain a normal serum calcium concentration unless renal function is impaired.

Skeletal removal and skeletal calcium efflux are inhibited by calcitonin, and administration of this hormone leads to a transient hypocalcemia in patients whose rates of bone remodeling and calcium efflux from bone are elevated (e. g., growing children, immobilized adults, and individuals with Paget's disease of bone, hyperparathyroidism, or certain malignancies). In normal adults, however, calcitonin has little effect on the serum calcium concentration, although more potent inhibitors of bone calcium efflux (e.g., the drug mithramycin) can cause profound hypocalcemia within hours. The heparin antagonist protamine also inhibits the efflux of calcium from bone and, if given in large doses, rapidly lowers the serum calcium concentration of humans or experimental animals. This lowering may result from interference with the effects of locally secreted heparin on bone cells.

These internal exchanges of calcium between blood and bone lead to a complete turnover of the plasma calcium approximately every hour. Simultaneously, relatively small amounts of calcium are absorbed from the intestine and excreted in the feces and urine. These exchanges with the external environment involve only 300 to 600 mg calcium/day, whereas the internal exchanges total 30 to 40 g/day and involve equilibration with large masses of skeletal calcium. Calcium absorption and excretion are so slow relative to internal calcium redistribution that changes in renal calcium clearance or intestinal calcium absorption can alter the serum calcium concentration only slowly, over days to weeks. In contrast, changes in skeletal calcium influx or efflux can alter the serum calcium concentration within hours. Figure 28 illustrates the fluxes of calcium that determine the serum calcium concentration.

Intestinal Absorption of Calcium

The amount of calcium absorbed from the intestines depends upon the amount in the diet and the efficiency

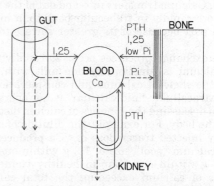

CALCIUM TURNOVER

Figure 28. Calcium turnover. Schematic outline of serum calcium input *(solid arrows)* and output *(dashed arrows)*. Arrows on the left represent input from and output to the intestine. Arrows on the right represent input from and output to the skeleton. The arrow inferiorly placed represents output to the glomerular filtrate, whereas the hooked arrow represents input to the blood from the proximal and distal renal tubules. The effects of $1,25\text{-}(OH)_2$ vitamin D, PTH, and lowered or raised serum Pi are indicated above the appropriate arrows. Vertical shading to the left of the rectangle representing bone indicates that only small portions of bone calcium are available for rapid exchange with blood. (From Parsons, J. A. (ed.): Endocrinology of Calcium Metabolism. New York, Raven Press, 1982.)

of intestinal calcium absorption. Normal adults in the United States consume a variable amount of dietary calcium, ranging from 200 to 1800 mg/day. Such intakes lead to calcium concentrations of 0.3 to 8.5 mM within the intestinal lumen. At high luminal calcium concentrations total calcium transfer across the intestinal mucosa is almost linearly proportional to the

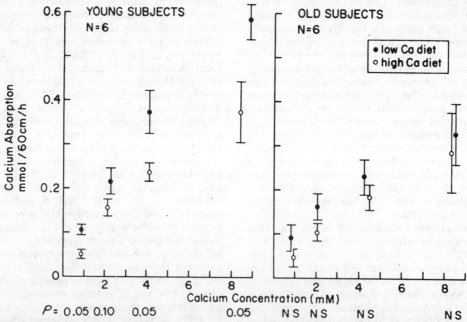

Figure 29. Intestinal calcium absorption as a function of luminal calcium concentration in healthy young and old adults, studied after their adaptation to low or high dietary calcium intakes. The illustrated measurements were made in the jejunum using a triple-lumen intestinal intubation technique. The postprandial luminal calcium concentrations in persons on low-calcium diets normally range from 0.3 to 2.0 mM, and from 3.0 to 8.5 mM in those with very high dietary calcium intakes. (From Ireland, P., and Fordtran, J. S.: Reproduced from *The Journal of Clinical Investigation,* 1973, vol. 52, p. 2672, by copyright permission of The American Society for Clinical Investigation.)

calcium concentration in the lumen (Fig. 29). Thus, total calcium absorption might vary widely as a function of dietary intake, were it not for the fact that the efficiency of intestinal calcium absorption changes inversely with the calcium intake. These changes in intestinal absorptive efficiency are important homeostatic adaptations and are mediated by alterations in the synthesis and secretion of 1,25-$(OH)_2$ vitamin D by the kidneys. When adults consume low-calcium diets, blood levels of 1,25-$(OH)_2D$ rise and the efficiency of intestinal calcium absorption increases (Fig. 29). As a result, the amount of dietary calcium absorbed into the blood decreases only slightly. At the same time, PTH secretion increases and blood levels of PTH rise, stimulating renal conservation of calcium and skeletal release of calcium into the blood. The extent to which the increase in 1,25-$(OH)_2D$ secretion depends upon the increase in PTH secretion has not yet been established. As a result of these homeostatic responses, the serum calcium concentration declines only transiently when an individual switches from a normal diet to one lower in calcium. However, serum calcium levels are sustained only by the mobilization of calcium from bone, and bone mass will decline if blood levels of parathyroid hormone remain very high, as occurs in normal adults when dietary calcium is less than 400 to 500 mg/day.

In individuals with renal insufficiency and in otherwise normal elderly people, renal secretion of 1,25-$(OH)_2D$ is limited, and intestinal absorption of calcium cannot be augmented (Fig. 29). Such individuals adapt to customary calcium intakes (400 to 800 mg/day) only by excessive increases in parathyroid hormone secretion and excessive bone resorption. This leads to osteopenia. The frequency with which this sequence of events contributes to age-related bone loss is not yet known. Treatment with oral 1,25-$(OH)_2D$ supplements is thus beneficial in certain patients with renal insufficiency, but its effectiveness in preventing age-related bone loss remains uncertain.

When normal adults consume diets high in calcium, 1,25-$(OH)_2D$ secretion and intestinal calcium absorptive efficiency decline. In a subset of the population, however, this adaptive mechanism is defective, and 1,25-$(OH)_2D$ secretion and intestinal calcium absorption efficiency fail to decrease sufficiently to compensate for the high dietary calcium. In such individuals, the kidneys play an important role in the adaptation to high-calcium diets; consequently, urinary calcium excretion increases substantially when these people consume high-calcium diets (1500 to 2000 mg/day). Such individuals are predisposed to develop calcium-containing renal calculi, wholly or in part because of their excessive urinary calcium excretion, as are persons with a more extreme form of this disorder who absorb from their diet and excrete in their urine excessive amounts of calcium even while consuming normal diets (700 to 1000 mg calcium/day). The mechanisms responsible for excessive 1,25-$(OH)_2D$ secretion in both these groups are unclear.

Renal Excretion of Calcium

The amounts of calcium filtered by the renal glomeruli and reabsorbed by the renal tubules each day are approximately one sixth of the daily calcium fluxes into and out of the skeleton. With a glomerular filtration rate of 100 ml/min (144 liters/day), approximately 8.8 g of calcium are filtered and 8.6 g are reabsorbed. Under normal circumstances, that fraction of calcium bound to plasma proteins is not filtered by the renal glomerulus. The remainder of plasma calcium (roughly half the total) is almost totally filtered. Sixty per cent of the filtered calcium is reabsorbed in the proximal tubule, mostly by passive transport but to some extent also by active transport. This reabsorption changes in parallel with tubular reabsorption of sodium under conditions of extracellular volume expansion or contraction. Thus urinary excretion of calcium tends to increase with high-salt diets and decrease with low-salt diets or during extracellular fluid depletion. Calcium reabsorption in the cortical thick ascending limb of Henle's loop and in the distal tubule is stimulated by PTH via a cyclic AMP-dependent pathway. The characteristics of the transport process (active transport versus voltage-driven diffusion) have not been established. In the distal tubule, an estimated 10 per cent of the filtered calcium is reabsorbed by active transport (which is also stimulated by PTH via a cyclic AMP-dependent mechanism). Calcitonin also increases renal tubular reabsorption of calcium, probably in the ascending limb of Henle's loop and in the distal tubule, but in pharmacologic doses, calcitonin has the opposite effect and increases urinary calcium excretion. Hydrochlorothiazide increases distal tubular reabsorption of calcium as well and is therefore effective clinically in reducing renal calcium clearance in patients with hypoparathyroidism or with hypercalciuria of renal origin. It is not certain if vitamin D metabolites in physiologic doses have important effects on renal tubular reabsorption of calcium. Bicarbonate administration also increases renal tubular reabsorption of calcium, and the ingestion of large amounts of alkali, if combined with the simultaneous intake of large amounts of calcium, can lead to hypercalcemia (the milk-alkali syndrome), particularly if the glomerular filtration rate is mildly reduced.

Acidosis, on the other hand, reduces renal tubular reabsorption of calcium and so tends to increase renal calcium clearance. Renal tubular reabsorption of calcium is also decreased by the administration of glucose, amino acids, or protein, probably because of the hyperinsulinemia that these agents provoke. Thus urinary calcium excretion increases after meals, particularly those with a high content of carbohydrate or protein. The mechanism by which insulin reduces renal tubular reabsorption of calcium is unclear. Renal tubular reabsorption of calcium is also lowered after the administration of furosemide or sulfate salts, effects that have found clinical application in the treatment of hypercalcemia. Furosemide functions by blocking calcium reabsorption in the thick ascending limb of Henle's loop, whereas sulfate probably acts by complexing calcium in the renal tubule, thus making the ion unavailable for reabsorption.

The effects of PTH on renal calcium clearance are such that in the steady state subjects with either hypoparathyroidism or hyperparathyroidism can excrete similar amounts of calcium in the urine each day, despite differences of 0.4 to 0.8 mM in their respective levels of ionized calcium in blood (differences of 3 to 6 mg/dl total calcium) (Fig. 30). This wide range of blood calcium levels for a given urinary calcium

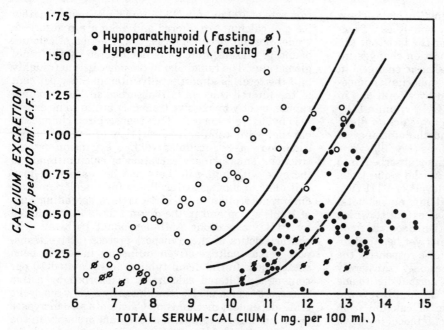

Figure 30. Urinary calcium excretion per 100 ml of glomerular filtrate as a function of the simultaneous total serum calcium concentration in hypoparathyroid and hyperparathyroid humans. The solid lines represent the mean, 5, and 95 per cent confidence limits for healthy males and females. The serum calcium level in the patients and normal volunteers was varied by oral and/or intravenous calcium loading. (From Peacock, M., Robertson, W. G., and Nordin, B. E. C.: Lancet 1: 384, 1969.)

level indicates the major degree to which the steady state serum calcium concentration of humans can be affected by the actions of PTH on the renal tubules. These actions are apparent within minutes if urinary calcium is measured and disappear equally rapidly when the hormone is withdrawn. Even these fast changes in renal tubular function, however, affect the serum calcium concentration relatively slowly because the increments and decrements in renal tubular calcium reabsorption are small relative to the skeletal calcium fluxes and the size of the miscible calcium pool.

If PTH stimulated only renal tubular reabsorption of calcium, the serum calcium concentration would increase until the extra calcium filtered across the glomeruli (serum calcium concentration × glomerular filtration rate [GFR]) exactly equalled the extra calcium reabsorbed by the renal tubules. At this point there would be no further increase in the serum calcium concentration. PTH would thus have no effect on the steady state urinary excretion of calcium. In reality, however, parathyroid hormone administration usually increases the steady state urinary calcium excretion by stimulating calcium absorption from the intestine and calcium removal and efflux from bone, changes independent of those affecting renal tubular calcium reabsorption. Similarly, diuretics could not lower the steady state excretion of calcium merely by reducing the renal clearance of calcium, since such an effect would only increase the serum calcium concentration and would leave urinary calcium excretion unaffected (except for a transient decrease until the new steady state was achieved). Although serum calcium concentration does rise transiently after administration of thiazide diuretics, PTH secretion is thereby suppressed until the serum calcium level returns to baseline. This combination of thiazide-induced decreases in renal calcium clearance and suppression of PTH secretion causes urinary calcium excretion to remain low during chronic administration of the drug. If PTH secretion is not suppressible, or if the serum calcium concentration is being maintained independ-

ently of PTH, chronic thiazide treatment can cause persistent hypercalcemia and may not reduce urinary calcium excretion.

When the serum calcium concentration is elevated (to levels that suppress normal PTH secretion to zero or to constant basal levels), nearly 15 per cent of the calcium filtered at the glomerulus appears in the urine, and the kidneys are critical to serum calcium homeostasis. In such a situation, any decrease in GFR or in calcium clearance will provoke marked worsening of the hypercalcemia in a few days. This situation can develop as a consequence of dehydration in hypercalcemic subjects with hyperparathyroidism, osteolytic bone disease, or intestinal hyperabsorption of calcium. The inability of such patients to suppress calcium efflux and removal from the skeleton, and/or calcium absorption from the intestines, makes them particularly vulnerable to reductions in renal calcium clearance.

Homeostatic Efficiency of the Parathyroid Glands

Blood levels of PTH increase from minimum to maximum values as the blood level of ionized calcium declines from 1.35 to 1.00 mM (about 10.8 to 8.0 mg/dl total calcium) in normal adults. Above and below these blood calcium levels, PTH secretion changes very little in normal adults, although in most patients with hyperparathyroidism blood levels of PTH and ionized calcium remain inversely related at higher levels of blood calcium. Consequently, it is within this narrow range that blood PTH levels can vary homeostatically. In contrast, skeletal uptake and renal excretion of calcium continue to increase as the blood calcium level is elevated above 1.35 mM. The relative importance of the parathyroid glands in calcium homeostasis therefore diminishes in normal adults as the blood calcium level rises above normal. This fact can be shown experimentally by giving a standardized intravenous infusion of calcium to normal and hypoparathyroid adults and by comparing the resultant increments in the blood calcium concentration. The difference is less than two-fold, indicating that the "homeostatic efficiency" of the parathyroid glands is relatively low in normal adults with hypercalcemia.

Analogous experiments have been done with intravenous edetate (EDTA) infusions to assess the homeostatic efficiency of the parathyroid glands during hypocalcemia. In thyroparathyroidectomized dogs, the resultant decrement in blood calcium is twice as great as in normal dogs; similar, but less well-controlled, results have been obtained in humans. All these results indicate that buffering of calcium and EDTA loads by the skeleton and the very large size of the miscible calcium pool in the skeleton are as important as the parathyroid glands for serum calcium homeostasis over short time intervals. However, the homeostatic efficiency of the parathyroid glands is presumably greater between the limits of 1.05 and 1.35 mM of ionized calcium in blood, since it is within this range that parathyroid hormone secretion is normally so variable.

Renal Excretion of Phosphorus

A variety of factors affect renal phosphate clearance (Table 12). PTH inhibits phosphorus reabsorption by a cyclic AMP-dependent mechanism in the proximal tubule (where 60 to 70 per cent of filtered phosphorus is normally reabsorbed), in the pars recta, in the distal convoluted tubule (where 10 per cent of filtered phosphorus is probably reabsorbed), and perhaps in the collecting duct. Increased renal phosphate clearance is thus characteristic of hyperparathyroidism, and the serum inorganic phosphate concentration is often low or low-normal in patients with that disorder. At puberty the serum level of inorganic phosphate declines from the high levels of childhood to the lower ones characteristic of adults. At menopause or after castration in either sex, mean levels of serum inorganic phosphorus rise again but rapidly decline after replacement doses of gonadal steroids. These changes in serum inorganic phosphate levels result from the effects of gonadal steroids on renal phosphate clearance, emphasizing the major role of the kidney as the regulator of the serum inorganic phosphate concentration. Glucocorticoids increase renal phosphate clearance significantly and are largely responsible for the diurnal rhythm in renal phosphate clearance and serum inorganic phosphate concentration. Starvation also increases renal phosphate clearance, perhaps secondary to the associated mild ketoacidosis and suppression of insulin secretion (see Table 12).

Hypocalcemia decreases renal phosphate clearance. This effect is most clearly demonstrated when intravenous calcium infusions are given to correct hypocal-

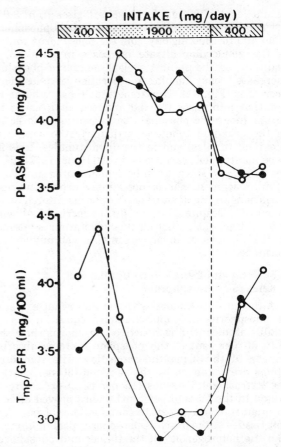

Figure 31. Response of the plasma inorganic phosphate concentration and the maximum inorganic phosphate input from the renal tubules to variations in the dietary phosphorus in two normal adults. (From Bijvoet, O. L. M., and Morgan, D. B.: In Hioco, D. J. (ed.): Phosphate et Métabolisme Phosphocalcique. Paris, L'Expansion Scientifique Française, 1971, p. 153.)

cemia in hypoparathyroidism. Such treatment rapidly increases renal phosphate clearance and lowers the elevated level of serum inorganic phosphate. It is difficult to appreciate this effect in subjects with intact parathyroid glands because hypocalcemia stimulates parathyroid hormone secretion, and the combined influence of hypocalcemia and hyperparathyroidism on renal phosphate clearance greatly complicates the interpretation of the changes in renal phosphate handling that occur after treatment of the hypocalcemia. The effects of 1,25-$(OH)_2$D on renal phosphate clearance are probably mediated by its influence on the serum calcium level.

Humans normally absorb from their intestines approximately two thirds of the phosphorus they ingest, over the entire range of normal phosphorus intakes (500 to 2200 mg/day). The absorptive mechanism is essentially unregulated, although it is to a slight extent stimulated by 1,25-$(OH)_2$D. The diet-induced variations in phosphorus absorption are normally compensated for by variations in the renal excretion of phosphorus, so that total body phosphorus remains nearly constant. These changes in renal phosphorus excretion are due in part to alterations in the phosphorus content of the glomerular filtrate (e.g., the

TABLE 12. FACTORS INFLUENCING RENAL TUBULAR CLEARANCE OF PHOSPHORUS

INCREASE CLEARANCE (inhibit tubular reabsorption)	DECREASE CLEARANCE (enhance tubular reabsorption)
High-phosphorus diet	Low-phosphorus diet
Parathyroid hormone, c-AMP	Growth hormone, insulin
Gonadal steroids	Low serum calcium
Glucocorticoids	EHDP (etidronate)
Volume expansion	
Chronic metabolic acidosis	
Increased pCO_2	

serum level of inorganic phosphate rises from 3.6 to 4.4 mg/dl after an increase in the dietary phosphorus from 400 to 1900 mg/day, and the phosphorus content of the glomerular filtrate increases in parallel). In addition, as the serum level of inorganic phosphate increases, renal tubular reabsorption of phosphorus decreases (Fig. 31). This important renal tubular adaptation minimizes the diet-induced changes in the serum inorganic phosphate concentration and occurs in the proximal tubules (particularly the superficial proximal tubules) and in the distal tubules. It is not dependent upon variations in PTH or 1,25-$(OH)_2D$ secretion, and since it can be demonstrated in isolated tubular segments, it is not simply dependent upon variations in the amount of phosphorus filtered at the glomeruli. Despite a large body of experimental work, it is still not clear whether this adaptation is intrinsic to the kidneys or involves some as yet unidentified hormone.

Skeletal and Extraskeletal Uptake and Release of Phosphorus

Although intestinal absorption and renal excretion of phosphorus are approximately equal in normal adults, studies with radioactive phosphorus show that only 50 per cent of the phosphorus atoms absorbed appear in the urine the same day. The remaining atoms are taken up by the skeleton (30 per cent) or the extraskeletal tissues (15 per cent) or are re-excreted in the feces (5 per cent). It has proved difficult to quantitate the separate contributions of bone and soft tissues to the miscible phosphorus pool in humans, and the heterogeneity of the tissues and phosphorus-containing molecules involved has made extensive study of phosphorus kinetics seem unrewarding. As a result, it is difficult to define quantitatively the role of the skeleton in human phosphorus homeostasis, except insofar as this can be inferred from animal experiments or from measurements of the parallel calcium movements when the two ions are deposited together in bone or removed together when bone dissolves.

As mentioned previously elevations in the serum inorganic phosphate concentration are associated with increased deposition of calcium (and phosphorus) in bone, leading to a decline in the blood calcium concentration. This sequence of events can result in severe hypocalcemia if the serum level of inorganic phosphate rises well above normal, as occurs, for example, when there is rapid and massive cell necrosis during acute hemolysis or rhabdomyolysis, or after extensive muscular injuries, or after cytolytic chemotherapy for leukemia or other malignancies. A chronic form of this syndrome has been produced in animals (and a few patients) by the chronic administration of large daily oral phosphate supplements. Such treatment leads to calcium and phosphate deposition not only in bones but also in the heart and kidneys, marked secondary hyperparathyroidism, increased skeletal remodeling, net bone loss, and osteopenia. In the disease familial hyperphosphatemia, renal phosphate clearance is impaired for unknown reasons despite normal glomerular filtration rate, resulting in ectopic calcifications (here termed tumoral calcinosis). In chronic uremia, renal phosphate clearance is also impaired, owing to decreases in glomerular filtration rate, with the occasional occurrence of a similar sequence of events.

The decrease in blood calcium levels caused by hyperphosphatemia stimulates PTH secretion, which in turn augments renal phosphorus clearance and so lowers the serum inorganic phosphate level toward normal. At the same time, PTH stimulates the removal of bone mineral and the efflux of calcium (and phosphorus) from bone. The mobilization of phosphorus from bone would aggravate or perpetuate the hyperphosphatemia, were it not for the fact that, in normal humans, the effects of PTH on renal phosphorus clearance are quantitatively more important than those on mobilization of bone phosphorus. In patients with severe uremia, however, the effects of PTH on renal tubular phosphate clearance are quantitatively less important because of the reduction in functioning renal mass. If the effects of the hormone on bone persist, with continued mobilization of bone phosphate and calcium, and if the mobilized phosphate cannot be excreted efficiently because of renal insufficiency, progressive hyperphosphatemia results. In this situation, continued PTH secretion aggravates the hyperphosphatemia, rather than limiting it. In such patients, parathyroidectomy decreases the serum inorganic phosphate concentration, whereas in normal people or patients with mild renal insufficiency, parathyroidectomy increases the serum inorganic phosphate concentration.

Chronic phosphate depletion has complex effects on the skeleton and on the secretion of PTH and 1,25-$(OH)_2D$. Phosphorus depletion may develop in individuals with intestinal malabsorption syndromes, in alcoholics with chronic diarrhea and a low-protein, low-phosphorus diet, and in individuals consuming excessive amounts of antacids containing aluminum hydroxide or aluminum carbonate (which bind phosphorus and prevent its intestinal absorption or reabsorption). Renal phosphate clearance falls to zero, and phosphorus disappears from the urine, owing to marked renal tubular conservation of the ion. Skeletal calcium influx and new bone formation and mineralization all decrease, and bone resorption increases because of direct skeletal effects produced by the phosphorus depletion. These changes help sustain phosphorus levels in extraskeletal tissue, at the expense of bone phosphorus. They also tend to shift calcium to the extraskeletal tissues and lead to a suppression of PTH secretion. Bone resorption continues, however, and 1,25-$(OH)_2D$ secretion is stimulated, despite the absence of PTH, because of the direct skeletal and renal effects of the low phosphorus levels. The greater 1,25-$(OH)_2D$ secretion further increases the mobilization of phosphorus and calcium from bone and augments the intestinal absorption of calcium (and to some extent phosphorus) from the diet. The release of calcium from bone and its increased intestinal absorption lead, in the absence of PTH, to a normal serum calcium concentration and a greater urinary calcium excretion. The full-blown phosphorus depletion syndrome is therefore characterized by an absence of urinary phosphorus excretion, low blood levels of phosphorus but normal blood levels of calcium, increased urinary calcium excretion, greater blood levels of 1,25-$(OH)_2D$ and low or absent blood levels of PTH.

In certain individuals, chronic phosphate depletion arises because of a defect in renal tubular reabsorption of phosphorus, rather than intestinal malabsorption of phosphorus. The pathophysiologic sequence and the laboratory findings are identical to those just described, except for the persistence of significant amounts of phosphorus in the urine despite severe hypophosphatemia. This syndrome of renal phosphate wasting is commonly familial, with the onset in childhood. In many affected persons, renal tubular synthesis and secretion of 1,25-(OH)$_2$D are also defective, and serum 1,25-(OH)$_2$D levels and urinary calcium excretion remain normal instead of rising, as would be expected in severe hypophosphatemia. The defect in 1,25-(OH)$_2$D secretion can be confirmed in such individuals by showing that their blood 1,25-(OH)$_2$D levels fail to increase during an intravenous infusion of PTH. A similar acquired syndrome develops spontaneously in adults and in some children. The acquired syndrome sometimes results from a hemangioma or benign mesenchymal tumor of bone or soft tissue, the removal of which eliminates the syndrome within days. The nature of the humoral factor or factors elaborated by such tumors and responsible for the renal tubular dysfunction is one of the intriguing unanswered questions of modern physiology.

DISORDERS OF REMODELING OF ADULT BONE

Osteoporosis

Disorders of remodeling in adults usually result in decrease in bone mass. The best example of this is the group of disorders termed osteoporosis (Fig. 32), in which the composition of the bone (matrix components and ratio of mineral to matrix) is indistinguishable from normal bone. There are multiple causes of osteoporosis, such as those listed in Table 13. In general, there are no changes in the plasma concentrations of calcium and inorganic phosphorus in patients with osteoporosis except when associated with hyperpara-thyroidism. Urinary calcium excretion may or may not be excessive. This is in contrast to osteomalacic states, which are usually associated with hypophosphatemia and hypocalcemia. Some features that distinguish osteoporosis from osteomalacia are listed in Table 14.

No one explanation accounts for the abnormality in all instances of osteoporosis. The pathogenesis in the largest group of patients with osteoporosis may be as follows. After longitudinal growth has ceased and the epiphyses have closed, the total skeletal mass remains constant. Although there is continued remodeling, the rates of bone formation and resorption are nearly equal. Approximately at the fifth decade, however, total skeletal mass begins to fall in both sexes and in all populations, as measured by such techniques as quantitation of metacarpal thickness or, more accurately, by photon absorption densitometry or quantitative computerized tomography. It is presumed that at some point the total mass falls to such an extent that individual bones, particularly those of the distal forearm, the proximal femurs, and the vertebral bodies can no longer withstand ordinary mechanical force and become subject to fracture with trauma that would be insufficient to fracture bones in younger individuals (Fig. 33). Since the total bone mass is decreasing, the rate at which bone is resorbed exceeds that at which it is formed, although there is not complete agreement on how the absolute rates of these functions are affected. The results of radiocalcium kinetics do not indicate a decrease in bone formation; the results of quantitative microradiography, which includes cortical as well as trabecular bone, also suggest that age-related bone loss is characterized by increased resorption surfaces and normal formation surfaces, presumably reflecting increased bone resorption rates and normal bone formation rates, respectively. On the other hand, the results of quantitative morphometric

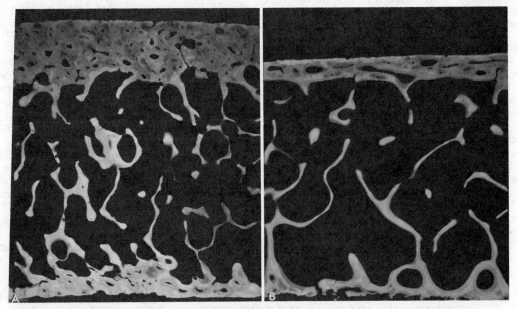

Figure 32. Microradiograph of iliac crest bone from a normal 43-year-old woman *(A)* and a 51-year-old woman with osteoporosis *(B)*. The periosteal surface is at the upper portion of the figure. In the osteoporotic sample the cortex is thinner and there is less cancellous (trabecular) bone as well. Most of the resorption is from the endosteal surface, although in these photographs the periosteal surfaces of the two samples are not aligned. (From Jowsey, J.: Metabolic Diseases of Bone. Philadelphia, W. B. Saunders Co., 1977.)

TABLE 13. CLASSIFICATION OF OSTEOPOROSIS*

Disorders of unknown cause in which osteoporosis is the major clinical abnormality
   Idiopathic osteoporosis
     Juvenile
     Adult
   Involutional osteoporosis

Disorders that contribute to osteoporosis in which the mechanism is partially understood
   Hypogonadism
   Hyperadrenocorticism
   Hyperthyroidism
   Intestinal malabsorption syndromes
   Scurvy
   Calcium deficiency
   Immobilization
   Systemic mastocytosis
   Chronic heparin administration
   Chronic ingestion of anticonvulsant drugs
   Adult hypophosphatasia
   Associated with other metabolic bone diseases such as osteomalacia (of various causes) or hyperparathyroidism

Heritable connective tissue disorders associated with osteoporosis
   Various forms of osteogenesis imperfecta
   Homocystinuria due to cystathionine synthase deficiency
   Menkes' syndrome

Other systemic disorders associated with osteoporosis, possibly more frequently than accounted for by chance alone
   Rheumatoid arthritis
   Diabetes mellitus
   Chronic hepatic disease
   Alcoholism
   Down's syndrome
   Chronic pulmonary disease
   Waldenström's macroglobulinemia
   Methotrexate therapy

*Modified from Krane, S. M.: Osteoporosis. In Rubenstein, E., and Federman, D. D. (eds.): Scientific American Medicine. Scientific American, New York, 1978, p. 15-XI-8.

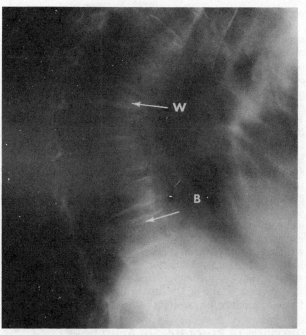

Figure 33. Lateral radiograph of the thoracic spine of a 67-year-old woman with osteoporosis, which was first evident after the menopause. Exaggerated biconcavity due to fracture of the superior plate (B) is seen as well as anterior wedging (W) of another vertebral body.

measurements that include only cancellous bone have suggested that rates of bone formation are lowered to account for the decrease predominantly in the trabecular bone mass. The mechanisms for the increased bone resorption are not known, although it is assumed that in postmenopausal women, in whom the process is clinically most apparent, the effects are due to decrease in secretion of female sex hormones. Age-related bone loss is also seen in men in whom no alteration in gonadal function can be demonstrated. Even if the rate of bone formation is normal compared with individuals in other age groups, the rate at which new bone is being formed is still insufficient to keep pace with the excessive resorption.

The osteoporosis that has its apparent onset after the age of 50 is heterogeneous. There may be at least two different subsets: Type I includes a small group of women, age 51 to 65, with primarily vertebral or wrist fractures (these bones are predominantly cancellous); type II comprises that group of women and men, usually over the age of 75, who fracture bones such as the femoral neck, humerus, and tibia (these bones are both cancellous and compact [cortical] in type). Some groups have reported that levels of immunoreactive PTH tend to be low in type I osteoporosis, possibly accounted for by accelerated bone loss with increased egress of calcium from the bone and suppression of parathyroid gland function. In type II osteoporosis, higher circulating levels of PTH may be a cause of the bone loss. The reasons for the secondary hyperparathyroidism may be related to abnormal vitamin D metabolism, as discussed earlier. However, even in type II other factors could contribute to the excessive bone resorption.

Patients with osteoporosis are frequently of small body habitus with poor musculature. The effects of muscular activity are important in the maintenance of normal skeletal mass. Lack of exercise contributes to development of osteoporosis, and prolonged immobilization can induce osteoporosis in normal subjects. How mechanical forces acting on the skeleton are translated into biologic responses has not been elucidated.

TABLE 14. DIFFERENTIAL FEATURES OF OSTEOPOROSIS AND OSTEOMALACIA

	TOTAL BONE MASS	BONE MINERAL/ MATRIX	PLASMA, CALCIUM AND PHOSPHORUS	PLASMA, ALKALINE PHOSPHATASE	RADIOGRAPHIC PSEUDOFRACTURES (Looser's zones)
Osteoporosis	Reduced	Normal	Usually normal	Usually normal	Absent
Osteomalacia	Reduced, normal, or increased	Reduced	Frequently abnormal	Usually elevated	Frequently present and diagnostic

There are increased numbers of mast cells in the bone marrow from patients with osteoporosis compared with age-matched controls. It is possible that secretion of heparin or similar complex polysaccharides by these cells could sensitize the resorbing cells to the effects of parathyroid hormone. Resorptive bone disease is observed in patients receiving chronic heparin therapy as well as in individuals with systemic mastocytosis. In postmenopausal women, the administration of estrogens can decrease the rate of bone resorption and retard loss of bone mass. Estrogen therapy in postmenopausal women is linked with decreased bone resorption and retardation in the rate of bone loss. PTH levels increase in patients with type I osteoporosis who are treated with estrogens, in association with elevated circulating levels of 1,25-$(OH)_2D_3$. The decrease in bone resorption resulting from estrogen therapy, however, is accompanied by a decrease in rates of bone formation, reflecting the normal process of resorption-formation coupling. Other maneuvers that decrease bone resorption, such as high calcium intake or administration of calcitonin, are associated with coupled decreases in bone formation as well.

Increased circulating levels of glucocorticoids are also associated with osteoporosis, in which there is a marked decrease in bone formation accompanying the increased bone resorption; collagen synthesis in extraskeletal sites such as dermis is also decreased. Abnormal metabolism of vitamin D is associated with glucocorticoid excess as well as alterations in the metabolism of parathyroid hormone. Increased levels of carboxyterminal immunoreactive parathyroid hormone have been found in patients with chronic glucocorticoid excess; increased levels of circulating immunoreactive parathyroid hormone can also result from acute infusions of glucocorticoids to normal subjects. Despite decreased intestinal calcium absorption and abnormal vitamin D metabolism, mineralization defects are not seen in bones of patients with uncomplicated glucocorticoid excess, probably because of the accompanying low rates of bone formation.

Hyperthyroidism may also be accompanied by a skeletal disorder with characteristics of osteoporosis. Thyroxin and triiodothyronine have direct effects on increasing skeletal resorption. This excessive resorption may be sufficient to result in hypercalcemia; more commonly, there is increased release of calcium from the skeleton into the extracellular fluid to produce a decrease in parathyroid hormone secretion and increased renal calcium clearance. The skeleton is usually able to respond with increased bone formation, and significant loss of bone mass is avoided. However, the superimposition of excess thyroid hormone levels on the postmenopausal state usually accelerates the loss of bone mass and the appearance of clinical manifestations of osteoporosis.

Focal Bone Resorption

In addition to the generalized bone loss that characterizes conditions such as osteoporosis and the focal type of bone loss of Paget's disease, *focal bone resorption* is characteristic of a number of different states. These include tumors, cysts, and traumatic and inflammatory lesions. In the so-called "expanding" lesions of bone, resorption of bone takes place at the periphery

TABLE 15. SOME FACTORS STIMULATING BONE RESORPTION

High PO_2	Heparin
Low pH	Vitamin A
Prostaglandins (PGE_2 particularly)	Cyclic AMP
Parathyroid hormone	Interleukin 1
25-hydroxy vitamin D	Platelet-derived growth factor
1,25-dihydroxy vitamin D	
Thyroxin, triiodothyronine	Epidermal growth factor
Osteoclast activating factor(s)	Fibroblast growth factor
Endotoxin	Transforming growth factor
Tumor cell products	

of the lesions. It should be appreciated, however, that "expansion" should not be construed in the mechanical sense, since bone is a rigid structure; biologic "expansion" results from cell-mediated resorption at the points of greatest pressure. These cellular responses to mechanical forces have to be translated in some way, although the mechanism is unknown. It has been postulated that mechanical stresses produce piezoelectric effects that can be recognized by cells. Even cells in culture respond directly to pressure by alteration in rates of proliferation. Tumors may stimulate focal resorption by the production of soluble factors that increase the rate of recruitment of osteoclasts from precursor cells or increase the resorptive function of osteoclasts already present. Such resorption-stimulating factors (Table 15) include parathyroid hormone or parathyroid hormone–like peptides, substances related to epidermal growth factor and transforming growth factor, prostaglandins of the E series, and osteoclast activating factor. Osteoclast activating factor, a polypeptide formed by activated lymphocytes, is also secreted in excess in hematopoietic malignancies such as multiple myeloma. Prostaglandins of the E series, capable of stimulation of bone resorption, are often produced in excess by solid tumors. In inflammatory lesions such as chronic periodontal disease or rheumatoid arthritis, production by mononuclear cells of bone-resorbing factors such as prostaglandins may be involved in formation of focal bone erosions as well as more diffuse bone loss in regions surrounding the lesions. Interleukin 1, produced by monocytes and possibly other cells, can induce bone resorption in vitro. Malignant tumors—for example, breast carcinoma—may also have direct lytic effects on bone not mediated by osteoclasts or related mononuclear cells such as macrophages.

Rickets and Osteomalacia

Abnormally remodeled bone may be characterized not only by alterations in mass and form but also by *alterations in the relationship of the mineral phase to the matrix*. The most significant abnormality characterized by defective mineralization results in bone in which the ratio of mineral to matrix is abnormally low. Mineralization defects occur in the growing skeleton (rickets) as well as in the adult skeleton. When there is functioning epiphyseal growth cartilage, mineralization defects also result in decrease in cartilage calcification accompanied by disorganization in the arrangement of the cells in the growth plate, increase in thickness and diameter of the growth plate, as well

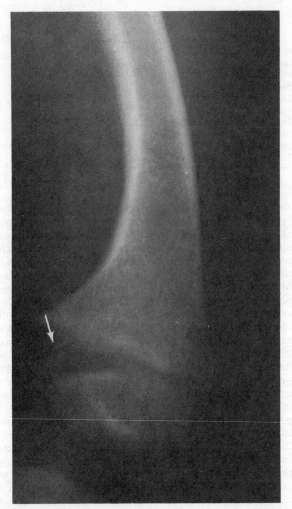

Figure 34. Radiograph of the distal femur of a 6-year-old girl with vitamin D–resistant rickets. The end of the femur is splayed, and a portion of the epiphyseal plate has a typical fuzzy appearance *(arrow)*.

the mineralization fronts. These mineralization fronts are reduced or absent in osteomalacia. Different disorders will produce defects at different stages in the process of mineralization. Normal osteoblast function is essential for mineralization, since formation, posttranslational modification, and secretion of matrix proteins and possibly of phospholipids are presumably initial events. Mineralization is critically dependent upon the supply of mineral ions from the extracellular fluid. Whether a local increase in concentration of one or other of these ions (particularly phosphate) is required at sites of mineralization has never been clarified. It has been postulated that alkaline phosphatase could function in this regard by controlling the local hydrolysis of organic phosphate esters, although there is no convincing evidence that the supply of organic phosphate esters is sufficient to provide additional inorganic phosphate. It is also conceivable that local "pump" mechanisms may exist for concentrating ions at mineralization sites. It is also necessary for the pH to be sufficiently high (approximately 7.6). Possibilities whereby disease states may interrupt these mineralization sequences are shown in Table 16. Since there are multiple causes for osteomalacia, the pattern of

as a splaying of the ends of the bones (Fig. 34). In adults, when endochondral ossification has ceased, mineralization disorders are manifested exclusively by defects in mineralization of newly forming bone (osteomalacia) (Fig. 35). (In neither osteoporosis nor osteomalacia is the bone "demineralized" in the sense that mineral is removed, leaving behind bare matrix.) Histologically, the bone reflects the abnormal mineralization, the major consequence of which is a decrease in deposition of mineralized bone. Since matrix is secreted but not fully mineralized, there is a widening of the osteoid seam usually present at sites of bone formation. Whereas normally the osteoid seams do not exceed 12 μm, the seams in osteomalacia are characteristically increased, occasionally exceeding several hundred μm. Not only is there increased thickness but also there is increased volume of osteoid and an increase in the bone surface covered by osteoid. In normal bone-forming surfaces, a calcification or mineralization front is evident at the junction of the mineralized bone and the osteoid. This can be demonstrated by stains such as toluidine blue and by the sharp fluorescence of administered tetracyclines that are concentrated at

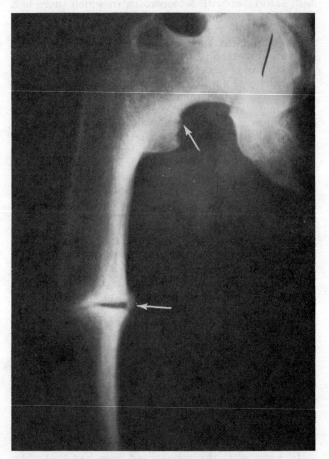

Figure 35. Radiograph of the proximal femur of a 36-year-old man with vitamin D–resistant osteomalacia and rickets since childhood. Pseudofractures or Looser's zones are seen at two typical locations in the inner aspect of the femur *(arrows).* The upper lesion is barely visible in this radiograph. These pseudofractures often occur at points where major arteries cross the bone.

TABLE 16. POSSIBLE MECHANISMS RESPONSIBLE FOR PRODUCTION OF OSTEOMALACIA

MECHANISM	EXAMPLE
Matrix synthesis faster than rate of mineralization	Postoperative hyperparathyroidism (preoperative osteitis fibrosa)
Abnormal matrix synthesis	Fibrogenesis imperfecta ossium
Insufficient phosphate at sites of mineralization as a consequence of low extracellular fluid phosphate levels	Renal tubular phosphate leaks
Insufficient calcium *and* phosphate at mineralization sites	Vitamin D deficiency, malabsorption syndromes
(?) Inadequate levels of vitamin D metabolites at mineralization sites	Vitamin D deficiency, vitamin D-refractory states
pH too low at mineralization sites	Systemic acidosis
Excessive concentration of mineralization inhibitors	Hypophosphatasia, aluminum intoxication

biochemical abnormalities measurable in plasma and urine depends upon the specific condition underlying the skeletal disorder. Most, but not all, of these conditions are accompanied by hypophosphatemia and several by hypocalcemia. The major exception is in chronic renal failure, in which severe osteomalacia may be found on bone biopsy in the presence of hyperphosphatemia and normo- or hypocalcemia. Examples of the patterns found in the more common forms of osteomalacia are listed in Table 17.

Ectopic Deposition of Calcium

Deposition of a mineral phase in regions that are normally not mineralized can be differentiated in several respects, such as whether the mineral phase is identical in composition to that normally found in bone or is a distinct phase—for example, the crystals deposited in cartilage and synovium in calcium pyrophosphate deposition diseases. In some disorders of aberrant mineralization, the inorganic phase is not deposited in the pattern identical to that of bone or cartilage with respect to its structure or its relationship to the organic matrix. The abnormality in these conditions is termed *ectopic calcification*. On the other hand, bone as a tissue may appear in areas where bone is not normally present (*ectopic ossification*). It is probable that each of these problems arises de novo, and that it is not necessary for ectopic ossification to pass through a preliminary phase of ectopic calcification.

Ectopic calcification, in which the mineral phase consists of both amorphous calcium phosphate and poorly crystalline hydroxyapatite, occurs under two general circumstances. In the first, the deposits are associated with increased levels of calcium and/or inorganic phosphate ions in the extracellular fluid. In all of these instances, hyperphosphatemia is critical for formation of the deposits. Prolonged hypercalcemia alone associated, for example, with primary hyperparathyroidism, in which serum phosphate levels are depressed, is not accompanied by ectopic calcification. On the other hand, if hypercalcemia is associated with renal failure—for example, with hypervitaminosis D or the milk-alkali syndrome—hyperphosphatemia coexists and ectopic calcification can then occur. In the milk-alkali syndrome, the associated alkalosis also favors deposition of the ectopic calcium-phosphate deposits. Such deposits are usually located in areas surrounding large joints and, when extensive, are also located in gastric mucosa, conjunctiva, renal parenchyma, and the walls of blood vessels. The calcium in these deposits is exchangeable with calcium ions in the extracellular fluid, and when serum inorganic phosphate levels are reduced, the deposits are usually mobilizable. In the condition termed tumoral calcinosis, hyperphosphatemia is associated with a normal serum calcium level and normal renal function. The calcium deposits, which can be massive in tumoral calcinosis, may also be reduced in size by inducing phosphate depletion with nonabsorbable antacids. In other disease states, ectopic calcification is associated with normal levels of calcium and inorganic phosphate in the extracellular fluid. Such calcifications also tend to occur in subcutaneous tissues around joints. The formation of these deposits does not depend upon the driving force of high circulating concentrations of calcium and inorganic phosphate ions and presumably involves some alteration of the matrix. The resultant calcification could occur either by (1) alteration in the concentration of local inhibitors that normally prevent calcification at normal circulating levels of mineral ions or (2) the presence of specific matrix components that have a role in induction of the mineralization. These deposits are usually not associated with a collagenous matrix but rather with noncollagenous proteins, some of which are GLA-containing proteins. Whether the latter have a primary role in inducing the mineralization or are adsorbed to the mineral phase after deposition has not yet been determined.

In *ectopic ossification,* the aberrant mineralized tissues grossly and microscopically have the appearance of bone, with osteoblasts and osteocytes embedded in a typical, often lamellar collagenous matrix. Marrow elements may also be identified. The mechanism of the

TABLE 17. BIOCHEMICAL CHANGES IN MORE COMMON FORMS OF OSTEOMALACIA

DISORDER	PLASMA				URINARY CALCIUM EXCRETION
	Calcium	Inorganic Phosphorus	Bicarbonate	Alkaline Phosphatase	
Classic vitamin D deficiency malabsorption syndrome	N*	L*	N or L	N or H*	L
Renal phosphate leak X-linked forms sporadic forms associated with tumors	N	L	N or L	N or H	N
Acidotic disorders	N or L	L	L	H	N or H
Renal glomerular osteodystrophy	L or N	H	L	H	L

*N = normal; L = low; H = high

formation of ectopic bone is unknown. It is presumed that local mesenchymal cell precursors must be induced to differentiate into bone cells or that the bone cells are derived from circulating osteogenic precursors. There are several animal models for producing this ectopic ossification. One involves the implantation of demineralized bone particles that contain an osteogenic factor (bone morphogenetic protein). Such particles are useful in inducing bone to fill in osseous defects, particularly in children. Ectopic ossification may be found associated with cutaneous neoplasms, pseudohypoparathyroidism, and myositis ossificans. Such deposits may also be formed around joints in various neurologic conditions, including paraplegic states, in which the ectopic ossifications are always seen below the level of paralysis.

CARTILAGE

Cartilages are avascular tissues that have in common the presence of a collagenous matrix intimately associated with proteoglycan in high concentration. The extracellular matrix is particularly abundant with respect to the number of component cells. In most hyaline cartilages, the fibrillar component is more than 90 per cent type II collagen, whereas in some fibrocartilages type I collagen may also be present. In the cartilage-like structures of the intervertebral disk, the outer portion of the disk contains mostly type I collagen as it merges imperceptibly with the annulus fibrosus, whereas the central portion of the nucleus pulposus contains almost exclusively type II collagen. The function of all cartilages is not the same. For example, the cartilages of the epiphyseal growth plates are involved predominantly in the lengthwise growth of bones in the embryo and throughout childhood and adolescence. Nasal cartilages maintain form yet permit deformability. The hyaline cartilages covering the articular ends of the bone of diarthrodial joints are particularly suited to the requirement as a shock absorber and a bearing surface for the movable joint.

Articular Cartilage

Articular cartilage has no nerve supply, lymphatics, or direct contact with the vascular system. Nutrients must diffuse from the vascular plexus in the synovium and pass through the synovial fluid and then through the cartilaginous matrix to reach the chondrocytes. Although the extracellular matrix is freely permeable to low molecular weight substances, the presence of the proteoglycan affects the character of the extracellular fluid of the cartilage. Components of the synovial fluid also influence the characteristics of extracellular fluid solutes reaching the chondrocyte. The concentration of high molecular weight hyaluronic acid in the synovial fluid confers properties of a gel filtration system that prevents high molecular weight materials from reaching the surface of the cell. In addition, the presence of the negative charge on the proteoglycan and the hyaluronic acid also affects movement of macromolecules in this milieu. Articular cartilage contains abundant extracellular water. When the articular cartilage is deformed under load, water is forced out from the extracellular matrix and then drawn back in when the load is removed. Normal articular cartilage has the ability to regain its shape when load is removed. This alternate compression and decompression permits movement of extracellular fluid and provides nutrition for the chondrocytes.

Articular cartilage is bathed on its surface by *synovial fluid*. This fluid is formed by filtration of various components from the vascular plexus of the synovium, accounting for the presence of water, electrolytes, and low molecular weight proteins such as albumin. Other components of the synovial fluid are synthesized by the synovial lining cells, including hyaluronic acid, which is responsible for its high viscosity and so-called lubricating glycoproteins. Serum proteins of high molecular weight are excluded from normal synovial fluid possibly because of the gel filtration effect of the hyaluronic acid. Thus, molecules such as α2-macroglobulin and fibrinogen are not found in normal synovial fluid. Other circulating proteins are present in synovial fluid in concentrations inversely proportional to their molecular weight.

The intrinsic properties of articular cartilage with its surface bathed in synovial fluid are responsible for the low coefficient of friction upon movement of the joint. Although the viscous hyaluronic acid is a good lubricant for the synovial membrane, this constituent is not essential for the lubrication of the articular cartilage itself. The major components responsible for articular cartilage lubrication are the lubricating glycoproteins and not hyaluronic acid. These glycoproteins interact with the surface of the articular cartilage, providing a type of boundary lubrication.

Injury to Cartilage

When articular cartilage sustains mechanical or chemical injury, changes occur in its composition. Early in the course of such injury, there is a decrease in the content of proteoglycan of the extracellular matrix and an alteration in the mechanical properties of the articular cartilage, manifested predominantly by increased strain—that is, the tendency to deform under load, as well as loss in the ability to regain form after the load is removed. On the other hand, the collagenous fibrillar component of articular cartilage is lost only late in the course of injury. The collagen of articular cartilage is primarily responsible for form and thickness. In response to injury, the articular chondrocytes can resynthesize the proteoglycan portion of the matrix. If the insult is only temporary (for example, following arthrotomy or bleeding into a joint), the synthetic capacity of the chondrocytes is sufficient to restore normal proteoglycan content, and the function of the articular cartilage returns to normal. The matrix synthesized in response to injury, however, is not always the same as that present initially, especially with respect to the composition of the glycosaminoglycan side chains. Cartilage cells can also proliferate in response to injury. The capacity to resynthesize normal collagenous components of the matrix, however, is very limited. If mechanical injury to articular cartilage is of great depth and reaches to blood vessels deep to the tide mark, mesenchymal cells accompanying vascular elements can enter the lesion. This results in a more fibrous matrix that contains type I, rather than type II, collagen. Whether or not chondrocytes, in reacting to injury, actually switch collagen synthesis from type II to type I is uncertain, although this has been demonstrated in vitro, in response to changing ambient calcium levels or having chondrocytes grow in adherent monolayers instead of in suspension.

In *human osteoarthritis* there is also an early decrease in the content of proteoglycan, especially in the superficial portions of the articular cartilage. This is associated with an increase in the number of chondrocytes, often occurring in clusters, suggesting clonal proliferation. As the disease progresses, there is a tendency for vertical clefts to form beginning at the surface of the articular cartilage and later extending deeper into the cartilage to the calcified zone, producing fibrillations. With further progression of osteoarthritis, the proteoglycans disappear completely, leaving the cartilage entirely eroded and the joint surface made up of subchondral bone (eburnation). The subchondral bone may increase in thickness, presumably because of reactivation of the endochondral sequence in regions deep to the articular cartilage. Osteophytes are thus formed at the margin of the joints. It is probable that proteoglycan depletion occurs through the action of proteases that cleave the protein portion of the proteoglycan. Convincing demonstration of hyaluronidases that can act at the pH of the extracellular fluid has not been obtained. The late loss of cartilage collagen is presumably due to the action of collagenases that can be produced by a number of different cells present in joint structures. Although articular chondrocytes can replicate and synthesize new proteoglycan matrix, they have a limited capacity to resynthesize normal type II collagen, which is the limiting factor in the repair process. What is called osteoarthritis, or degenerative joint disease, is not one disorder but a group of different problems with a similar end result and pattern of degradation of articular cartilage. The mechanisms whereby this degeneration is brought about are probably different in each of the conditions responsible.

In *inflammatory joint disease* there is also degradation of articular cartilage. This is particularly evident in a disorder such as rheumatoid arthritis, in which the degradation of cartilage is associated predominantly with the mass of inflammatory cells known as the pannus. These cells appear initially in the recesses of the joint at the reflection of the synovium at the bone–articular cartilage junction. The inflammatory cell mass then appears to proliferate over the surface of the articular cartilage; in areas adjacent to the pannus, cartilage and subchondral bone may be resorbed. Early in disease, proteoglycan is depleted in cartilage in areas remote from the edge of the proliferating cell mass, but the thickness of the cartilages, with the possible exception of some of the superficial layer, remains intact. In the articular cartilage remote from the pannus, these effects are probably produced by enzymes or other substances released from polymorphonuclear leukocytes, the predominant cell in the synovial fluid in inflammatory arthritis. Several neutral proteases from polymorphonuclear leukocytes have the capacity to degrade proteoglycans by cleaving peptide bonds in the protein core. Collagenases are also found in granular fractions from polymorphonu-

clear leukocytes. In addition, these cells release superoxide free radical and hydroxide free radical, which are capable of direct degradative effects on the glycosaminoglycans. The heterogeneous cell mass of the proliferating pannus includes synovial cells, which produce large amounts of collagenase as well as other proteolytic enzymes. Some of these proteases, such as plasmin produced by the action of plasminogen activator, can activate the proactivator-procollagenase complex. Others, such as neutral elastase, can cleave the globular regions of the interstitial collagen fibers, which contain the crosslinks, and attack the types IV and V collagens located in basement membranes and around cells. The synovial fibroblast-like cells synthesize and release collagenase and other proteases when stimulated by interleukin 1–type molecules. Articular chondrocytes are also target cells for interleukin 1 and produce collagenase as well as proteases capable of degrading proteoglycans by acting on the protein core. In order for bone erosion to occur, however, some mechanisms must exist for removal of the mineral phase, since none of the collagenases are capable of attacking completely mineralized collagen in tissues such as bone. The proliferating cell mass and the synovium itself produce large amounts of prostaglandin, particularly PGE_2, interleukin 1, and factors derived from lymphocytes that are capable of stimulating osteoclasts to resorb bone as well as stimulate differentiation of osteoclasts from precursor cells. Indeed, most of the bone-resorbing activity of rheumatoid synovial fluids and cultured synovium can be accounted for by the PGE_2. However, it remains uncertain whether bone is resorbed by osteoclasts stimulated by components of the proliferating cell mass or by inflammatory cells themselves, which have the capability of resorbing bone. Interactions among the mononuclear cells of the lesion are important in the production of substances that can stimulate the synovial cells to produce collagenase and prostaglandins and may also be important in other aspects of the chronic proliferative lesion.

REFERENCES

General

Arey, L. B.: Developmental Anatomy: A Textbook and Laboratory Manual of Embryology. 7th ed. Philadelphia, W. B. Saunders Company, 1965.

Caplan, A. I., Fiszman, M. Y., and Eppenberger, H. M.: Molecular and cell isoforms during development. Science 221:921, 1983.

Dingle, J. T., and Gordon, J. L. (eds.): Cellular Interactions. Amsterdam, Elsevier/North-Holland Biomedical Press, 1981.

Doty, S. B., Robinson, R. A., and Schofield, B.: Morphology of bone and histochemical staining characteristics of bone cells. In Greep, R. O., and Astwood, E. B. (eds.): Handbook of Physiology. Section 7. Endocrinology. Vol. VII. Parathyroid Gland. Washington, D.C., American Physiological Society, 1976, p. 3.

Glimcher, M. J.: Composition, structure, and organization of bone and other mineralized tissues and the mechanism of calcification. In Greep, R. O., and Astwood, E. B. (eds.): Handbook of Physiology. Section 7. Endocrinology. Vol. VII. Parathyroid Gland. Washington, D.C., American Physiological Society, 1976, p. 25.

Peck, W. A. (ed.): Bone and Mineral Research: Annual, Vol. 1. A Yearly Survey of Developments in the Field of Bone and Mineral Metabolism. Princeton, N.J., Excerpta Medica, 1983.

Raisz, L. G., and Kream, B. E.: Regulation of bone formation. N Engl J Med 309:29, 83, 1983.

Urist, M. R., DeLange, R. J., and Finerman, G. A. M.: Bone cell differentiation and growth factors. Science 220:680, 1983.

Wuepper, K. D., Holbrook, K. A., Pinnell, S. R., et al.: Supplemental issue: Structural elements of the dermis. J Invest Derm 79(Suppl. 1): 1S, 1982.

Mineral Ion Homeostasis

DeGroot, L. J., et al. (eds.): Endocrinology. Vol. 2. New York, Grune and Stratton, 1979.

Henry, H. L., and Norman, A. W.: Vitamin D: Metabolism and biological actions. Am Rev Nutr 4:493, 1984.

Klahr, S., and Hrushka, K.: Effects of parathyroid hormone on the renal reabsorption of phosphorus and divalent cations. In Peck, W. (ed.): Bone and Mineral Research Annual, Vol. 2. Princeton, N.J., Excerpta Medica, 1984, p. 65.

Kunin, A. S., and Simmons, D. J. (eds.): Skeletal Research: An Experimental Approach. Vol. 2. New York, Academic Press, 1983.

Lawson, D. E. M.: Vitamin D. London, Academic Press, 1978.

Simmons, D. J., and Kunin, A. S. (eds.): Skeletal Research: An Experimental Approach. New York, Academic Press, 1979.

Talmage, R. V., Cooper, C. W., and Toverud, S. U.: The physiological significance of calcitonin. In Peck, W. A. (ed.): Bone and Mineral Research. Annual, Vol. 1. Princeton, N.J., Excerpta Medica, 1983, p. 74.

Collagen Structure, Biology, Biosynthesis, and Degradation

Bornstein, P., and Sage, H.: Structurally distinct collagen types. Annu Rev Biochem 49:957, 1980.

Eyre, D. R.: Collagen: Molecular diversity in the body's protein scaffold. Science 207:1315, 1980.

Gay, S., and Miller, E. J.: Collagen in the Physiology and Pathology of Connective Tissue. Stuttgart, Gustav Fischer Verlag, 1978.

Kühn, K.: Chemical properties of collagen. In Furthmayr, H. (ed.): Immunochemistry of the Extracellular Matrix. Vol. I. Methods. Boca Raton, Fla., CRC Press, 1982, p. 1.

Merlino, G. T., McKeon, C., de Crombruggheo, B., et al.: Regulation of the expression of genes encoding types I, II, and III collagen during chick embryonic development. J Biol Chem 258:10041, 1983.

Nimni, M. E.: Collagen: Structure, function, and metabolism in normal and fibrotic tissues. Semin Arthritis Rheum 13:1, 1983.

Piez, K. L., and Reddi, A. H. (eds.): Extracellular Matrix Biochemistry. New York, Elsevier, 1984.

Prockop, D. J., Kivirikko, K. I., Tuderman, L., and Guzman, N. A.: The biosynthesis of collagen and its disorders. N Engl J Med 301:13, 77, 1979.

Woolley, D. E., and Evanson, J. M. (eds.): Collagenase in Normal and Pathological Connective Tissues. Chichester, John Wiley and Sons, 1980.

Elastin

Ross, R.: The elastic fiber. A review. J Histochem Cytochem 21:199, 1973.

Sandberg, L. B., Soskel, N. T., and Leslie, J. G.: Elastin structure, biosynthesis, and relation to disease states. N Engl J Med 304:566, 1981.

Uitto, J.: Biochemistry of the elastic fibers in normal connective tissues and its alterations in disease. J Invest Derm 72:1, 1979.

Proteoglycans and Cartilage

Brandt, K. D.: Glycosaminoglycans. In Kelley, W. N., Harris, E. D., Jr., Ruddy, S., et al. (eds.): Textbook of Rheumatology. Philadelphia, W. B. Saunders Co., 1981, p. 239.

Hascall, V. C. Proteoglycons: structure and function. In Ginsburg, V., and Robbins, P. (eds.): Biology of Carbohydrates. New York, John Wiley and Sons, 1981, p. 1.

Höök, M., Kjellén, L., and Johansson, S.: Cell-surface glycosaminoglycans. Annu Rev Biochem 53:847, 1984.

Howell, D. S., and Talbott, J. H. (eds.): Osteoarthritis symposium, Palm Aire, Florida, October 20–22, 1980. Semin Arthritis Rheum 11(Suppl. 1):1, 1981.

Mankin, H. J.: The reaction of articular cartilage to injury and osteoarthritis. N Engl J Med 29:1285, 1335, 1974.

Radin, E. L., and Paul, I. L.: A consolidated concept of joint lubrication. J Bone Joint Surg 54A:607, 1972.

Sledge, C. B.: Structure, development, and function of joints. Orthop Clin North Am 6:619, 1975.

Sokoloff, L.: Pathology and pathogenesis of osteoarthritis. In McCarty, D. J. (ed.): Arthritis and Allied Conditions. A Textbook of Rheumatology. 9th ed. Philadelphia, Lea and Febiger, 1979, p. 1135.

Swann, D. A., Hendren, R. B., Radin, E. L., Sotman, S. L., and Duda, E. A.: The lubricating activity of synovial fluid glycoproteins. Arthritis Rheum 24:22, 1981.

Connective Tissue Disease

Akeson, W. H., Bornstein, P., and Glimcher, M. J. (eds.): American Academy of Orthopaedic Surgeons. Symposium on Heritable Disorders of Connective Tissue. St. Louis, C. V. Mosby Co., 1982.

Hollister, D. W., Byers, P. H., and Holbrook, K. A.: Genetic disorders of collagen metabolism. Adv Human Genet 12:1, 1982.

McKusick, V. A.: Heritable Disorders of Connective Tissue. 4th ed. St. Louis, C. V. Mosby Co., 1972.

Prockop, D. J., and Kivirikko, K. I.: Heritable diseases of collagen. N Engl J Med 311:376, 1984.

Wagner, B. M., Fleischmajer, R., and Kaufman, N. (eds.): Connective Tissue Diseases. Baltimore, Williams and Wilkins, 1983.

Wuepper, K. D., Holbrook, K. A., Pinnell, S. R., and Uitto, J. (eds.): Supplemental issue: Structural elements of the dermis. Proceedings of the 31st Annual Symposium on the Biology of Skin. J Invest Derm 79(Suppl. 1):1S, 1982.

Noncollagenous Connective Tissue Proteins

Delmas, P. D., Stenner, D., Wahner, H. W., Mann, K. G., and Riggs, B. L.: Increase in serum bone γ-carboxyglutamic acid protein with aging in women. Implications for the mechanism of age-related bone loss. J Clin Invest 71:1316, 1983.

Kleinman, H. K., Klebe, R. J., and Mann, G. R.: Role of collagenous matrices in the adhesion and growth of cells. J Cell Biol 88:473, 1981.

Lindahl, U., and Höök, M.: Glycosaminoglycans and their binding to biological macromolecules. Annu Rev Biochem 47:385, 1978.

Price, P. A., Parthemore, J. G., and Deftos, L. J.: New biochemical marker for bone metabolism: Measurement by radioimmunoassay of bone GLA protein in the plasma of normal subjects and patients with bone disease. J Clin Invest 66:878, 1980.

Ruoslahti, E., Engvall, E., and Hayman, E. G.: Fibronectin: Current concepts of its structure and functions. Coll Relat Res 1:95, 1981.

Termine, J. D., Belcourt, A. B., Conn, K. M., and Kleinman,

H. K.: Mineral and collagen-binding proteins of fetal calf bone. J Biol Chem 256:10403, 1981.

Termine, J. D., Kleinman, H. K., Whitson, S. W., Conn, K. M., McGarvey, M. L., and Martin, G. R.: Osteonectin, a bone-specific protein linking mineral to collagen. Cell 26:99, 1981.

Veis, A. (ed.): The Chemistry and Biology of Mineralized Connective Tissues. New York, Elsevier/North-Holland, 1981.

Yamada, K. M.: Cell surface interactions with extracellular materials. Annu Rev Biochem 52:761, 1983.

Metabolic Bone Disease

Avioli, L. V., and Krane, S. M. (eds.): Metabolic Bone Disease. Vols. I and II. New York, Academic Press, 1977, 1978.

Cohn, S. H. (ed.): Non-invasive Measurements of Bone Mass and Their Clinical Application. Boca Raton, Fla., CRC Press, 1981.

DeGroot, L. J., Cahill, G. F., Jr., Martini, L., Nelson, D. H., Odell, W. D., Potts, J. R., Jr., Steinberger, E., and Winegrad, A. I.: (eds.). Endocrinology. Vol. 2. New York, Grune and Stratton, 1979.

DeLuca, H. F., Frost, H. M., Jee, W. S. S., et al. (eds.): Osteoporosis: Recent Advances in Pathogenesis and Treatment. Baltimore, University Park Press, 1981.

Dixon, A. St. J., Russell, R. G. G., and Stamp, T. C. B. (eds.): Osteoporosis: A Multidisciplinary Problem. London, Academic Press, 1983.

Frame, B., and Potts, J. T., Jr. (eds.): Clinical Disorders of Bone and Mineral Metabolism. Amsterdam, N.J., Excerpta Medica, 1983.

Jowsey, J.: Metabolic Diseases of Bone. Philadelphia, W. B. Saunders Co., 1977.

Smith, R.: Biochemical Disorders of the Skeleton. London, Butterworths, 1979.

Connective Tissue Degradation

Dingle, J. T., and Gordon, J. L. (eds.): Cellular Interactions. Amsterdam, Elsevier/North-Holland Biomedical Press, 1981.

Gordon, J. L., and Hazleman, B. L. (eds.): Rheumatoid Arthritis. Cellular Pathology and Pharmacology. Amsterdam, North-Holland Publishing Company, 1977.

Hamilton, J. A.: Hypothesis: *In vitro* evidence for the invasive and tumor-like properties of the rheumatoid pannus. J Rheumatol 10:845, 1983.

Krane, S. M., Goldring, S. R., and Dayer, J. -M.: Interactions among lymphocytes, monocytes, and other synovial cells in the rheumatoid synovium. In Pick, E. (ed.): Lymphokines: A Forum for Immunoregulatory Cell Products. Vol. 7, 1982, p. 75.

Weissmann, G.: Activation of neutrophils and the lesions of rheumatoid arthritis. J Lab Clin Med 100:322, 1982.

Fibrosis

Berk, P. D., Castro-Malaspina, H., and Wasserman, L. R. (eds.): Myelofibrosis and the Biology of Connective Tissue. New York, A. R. Liss, 1984.

Crystal, R. G., Bitterman, P. B., Rennard, S. I., Hance, A. J., and Keogh, B. A.: Interstitial lung diseases of unknown cause: Disorders characterized by chronic inflammation of the lower respiratory tract. N Engl J Med 310:154, 235, 1984.

Gay, S., and Miller, E. J.: Collagen in the Physiology and Pathology of Connective Tissue. Stuttgart, Gustav Fischer Verlag, 1978.

Müller, P. K., Kirsch, E., Gauss-Müller, V., et al.: Some aspects of the modulation and regulation of collagen synthesis in vitro. Mol Cell Biochem 34:73, 1981.

Rojkind, M., and Dunn, M. A.: Hepatic fibrosis. Gastroenterology 76:849, 1979.

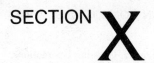
THE KIDNEY

PETER S. ARONSON, M.D., *and* SAMUEL O. THIER, M.D.

The kidneys are vital organs traditionally associated with the excretion of waste products. These complex organs, however, have numerous other critical functions. They are primarily concerned with maintaining the volume and composition of the body fluids within narrow acceptable physiologic limits. They also function in the regulation of blood pressure and the maintenance of red blood cell volume. They are key determinants of the pharmacokinetics of many drugs and the primary target of pharmacologic agents such as diuretics. Loss of any or all renal function produces pathophysiologic consequences that range from asymptomatic biochemical changes to death.

GROSS ANATOMY

The kidneys are paired retroperitoneal organs, approximately 12 cm in length, lying alongside the first through the third lumbar vertebrae; the right is lower than the left. These organs weigh about 150 g each.

A cross section of the kidney reveals the pale, approximately 1-cm cortex with the darker medullary area divided into pyramids by columns of cortex (the columns of Bertin) (Fig. 1). The bases of the pyramids abut the cortex and contain the medullary rays, which are actually composed of straight segments of the proximal and distal tubules as well as the collecting ducts. The apices of the pyramids form the papillae (8 to 18 per kidney), which are perforated by the openings of the collecting ducts of Bellini. The papillae drain into calyces, which coalesce to form the renal pelvis, which in turn drains into the ureter. The ureters course down the retroperitoneal area over the pelvic brim and into the bladder, which excretes urine via the urethra.

MICROSCOPIC ANATOMY

The kidney is divided into functional units termed nephrons. There are over one million nephrons per kidney. A nephron is composed of a glomerulus and the tubule that drains it. The tubule is divided into a proximal convoluted tubule, proximal straight tubule, descending limb of Henle's loop, ascending thin limb of Henle's loop, ascending thick limb of Henle's loop, distal convoluted tubule, connecting segment, cortical collecting ducts, and medullary collecting ducts. There is not, in fact, a single population of nephrons that is uniform, but rather at least two distinct populations. One group of nephrons (85 per cent of the total) is located in the outer cortex and has loops of Henle that either fail to descend into the medulla or at least do not descend into the inner medulla. The division of the loop of Henle into thin and thick segments is not well defined. The second group of nephrons has glomeruli in the juxtamedullary area, and has well-developed thin descending and ascending limbs of Henle's loop that reach to the innermost portions of the medulla (Fig. 2).

The microscopic structure of the glomerulus, which is predominantly vascular, will be described after a discussion of the blood supply to the kidney. At this point we will describe the tubule. Attempts to correlate structure and function have been facilitated by subdividing the proximal tubule into segments termed S_1, S_2, and S_3. These segments are more readily distinguishable in rats and mice than in humans. In man it is difficult to divide the proximal tubule into more than the convoluted and straight segments. The S_1 segment, corresponding to the earliest portion of the proximal convoluted tubule, has taller cells than seen

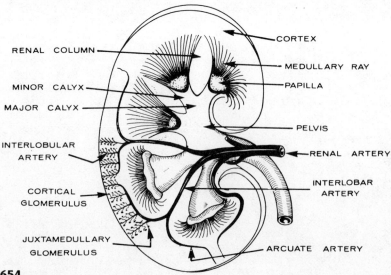

RENAL COLUMN

MINOR CALYX

MAJOR CALYX

INTERLOBULAR ARTERY

CORTICAL GLOMERULUS

JUXTAMEDULLARY GLOMERULUS

CORTEX

MEDULLARY RAY

PAPILLA

PELVIS

RENAL ARTERY

INTERLOBAR ARTERY

ARCUATE ARTERY

Figure 1. Sagittal section of the kidney. The upper half depicts the overall gross anatomic arrangement. The lower half demonstrates the arterial supply. (From Papper, S.: Clinical Nephrology. Boston, Little, Brown and Co., 1971, p. 36.)

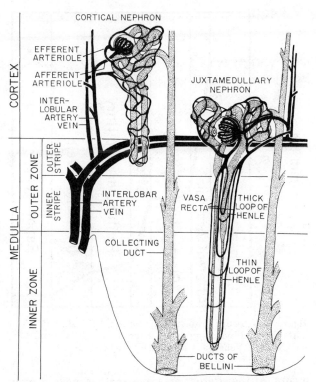

CORTICAL NEPHRON

JUXTAMEDULLARY NEPHRON

CORTEX

EFFERENT ARTERIOLE

AFFERENT ARTERIOLE

INTER-LOBULAR ARTERY VEIN

MEDULLA

OUTER ZONE — OUTER STRIPE

INNER STRIPE

INTERLOBAR ARTERY VEIN

VASA RECTA

THICK LOOP OF HENLE

COLLECTING DUCT

THIN LOOP OF HENLE

INNER ZONE

DUCTS OF BELLINI

Figure 2. Comparison of the blood supplies of cortical and juxtamedullary nephrons. (From Pitts, R. F.: Physiology of the Kidney and Body Fluids. 3rd ed. Chicago, Year Book Medical Publishers, 1974.)

in S_2 and S_3, with extensive lateral interdigitations and basal invaginations. These mitochondria-rich cells have a villous structure at their luminal surface known as the brush border. At the brush border surface the cells are joined by tight junctions. The S_2 segment begins at the distal portion of the convoluted segment and extends into the straight segment. The brush border is less developed, and there are fewer lateral interdigitations, basal invaginations, and mitochondria. The S_3 segment corresponds to the distal straight segment. Cells are now clearly cuboidal, have a richer brush border than the S_2 cells, and are virtually devoid of lateral interdigitations and basal invaginations. There are few mitochondria.

In the thin descending limb of Henle's loop the cuboidal cellular shape has disappeared and given way to flat squamous cells poor in mitochondria. There is now little in terms of brush border or basal invagination. The cells of the descending limb include intramembranous particles in greater numbers than the cells of the ascending thin limb of Henle's loop. There is little else to distinguish microscopically between the two thin limbs of Henle's loop. The cells of the thick ascending limb of Henle's loop regain cuboidal shape but differ from the cells of the proximal convoluted tubule by having far less brush border and fewer basal invaginations. The cells of the thick ascending limb do have much more extensive—that is, longer areas of—tight junctions between them. The more extensive tight junctions correlate with the markedly lower permeability to water in the thick ascending limb of Henle's loop as compared with the proximal tubule. As the thick ascending limb approaches the glomerulus,

there is a segment of tubular epithelium characterized by closely packed nuclei, giving it a dense appearance; the name macula densa is applied to this region.

The cells of the macula densa have a characteristic relationship with the base of the glomerulus. They lie in approximation to the efferent and, to a lesser extent, afferent glomerular arterioles. They are in close contact with specialized granular (lacis) cells and agranular (myoepithelioid) cells of the region of the mesangium that extends beyond the glomerular stalk (see below). The arterioles, the cells of the extraglomerular mesangium, and the macula densa form the juxtaglomerular apparatus. The macula densa marks the beginning of the distal convoluted tubule. The cells of the distal convoluted tubule differ from those of the proximal convoluted tubule by being lower, though still cuboidal, and by lacking brush borders. These cells do, however, have significant basal invaginations and are relatively rich in mitochondria. The transition from the distal convoluted tubule to the collecting duct through a connecting segment is gradual, and it is difficult to define striking changes in cell type. What does emerge at the collecting duct is a series of cells with little in terms of brush border or basal infolding. There are at least two types of cells, with one group of cells being intercalated dark cells that reach their highest density in the collecting duct. The intercalated cells first appear in the connecting tubule and are present in the collecting duct. They are rich in mitochondria and have microvilli in the cortex. These cells may have extensive basal invaginations. The principal or light cells of the collecting duct are relatively devoid of mitochondria and have rather simple contours; the number of microvilli increases according to their depth in the medulla.

BLOOD SUPPLY AND REGULATION OF BLOOD FLOW

The kidneys receive 25 per cent of the resting cardiac output via the renal arteries, which are the fifth branches of the abdominal aorta. The renal arteries lie anterior to the renal veins and divide in the hilum of the kidney into anterior and posterior branches. These major branches divide into the lobar arteries, supplying the upper, middle, and lower thirds of the kidney. The arteries further subdivide into interlobar arteries that course peripherally between the pyramids. At the cortical medullary junction, the arterial supply arches across the base of the pyramids as the arcuate arteries, and then gives rise to the more perpendicular interlobular arteries that again course toward the periphery. The interlobular arteries give rise to the afferent glomerular arterioles. The afferent glomerular arteriole divides into four to eight capillary loops, which then rejoin to form the efferent vessel. The vascular pattern of the postefferent arteriolar branches differs with the location of the glomeruli. In the outermost portion of the cortex, which contains the vast majority of glomeruli, the efferent vessel forms a capillary network associated primarily with the tubule serving the same glomerulus. In the midcortical area the postglomerular capillary network may serve several nephrons. In the juxtamedullary area the postglomerular arteriole may divide into a capillary network at the corticomedullary junction or may form the straight vessels (vasa recta) that follow the course of Henle's loop into the medulla. Capillaries serving the medulla branch from these vessels. Ascending vasa recta return to the cortex to reenter the venous system. The venous system throughout the kidney follows the arterial pattern in reverse direction, ultimately forming renal veins that enter the inferior vena cava (Fig. 2).

The vascular supply of the kidney permits delivery of a large volume of blood and is organized to permit effective ultrafiltration of plasma through the glomeruli, maximal secretion of solutes through the tubular epithelium into the lumen, and maximal reabsorption of solutes and water from tubular lumen to blood. The vascular organization in conjunction with the tubular structure also permits maintenance of a hypertonic medulla for dilution and concentration of the urine.

The kidneys receive blood under systemic hydrostatic pressure. The blood flow to the kidney is maintained nearly constant over a wide range of systemic pressures (80 to 180 mm of mercury) by autoregulatory adjustments. For autoregulation to be maintained the resistance to flow of blood through the kidney must be varied in direct proportion to the arterial pressure. Thus, as pressure falls, intrarenal vascular resistance will fall so as to maintain a constant flow rate of blood. Autoregulation of renal blood flow and intrarenal distribution of flow is a complex process dependent upon (1) myogenic arteriolar responses, (2) angiotensin II, (3) catechol stimulation, and (4) prostaglandins.

(1) There is growing evidence that the afferent arteriole of the glomerulus responds to increased pressure by maintaining or constricting its lumen to produce constant flow. The pressures at which this myogenic response occurs are those at which autoregulation is most effective. The response occurs in isolated vessels (excluding a requirement for a tubular feedback mechanism), occurs in the absence of angiotensin, and is blocked by smooth muscle relaxants.

(2) Angiotensin II appears to have its primary effect on the efferent glomerular arteriole. It would therefore play a role in renal hemodynamics and would alter glomerular ultrafiltration, but would not contribute directly to the autoregulatory response of the afferent arterioles.

(3) Beta catechols, as well as baroreceptors and chemoreceptors in the kidney, appear to act via cyclic 3',5'-adenosine monophosphate (AMP)–mediated renin release, and therefore via an angiotensin II mechanism (primarily efferent arteriolar response). Alpha catechols have a direct vasoconstrictor effect on afferent and efferent arterioles, but no clear role in autoregulation.

(4) Prostaglandins have the potential to produce vasodilation or vasoconstriction. Though these substances play a major role in protecting renal circulation during states of hypovolemia and high renin production, they have little importance under physiologic conditions.

The important areas of resistance to flow through the kidney reside at two serial control points: the afferent and efferent glomerular arterioles (Fig. 3). There is little change in hydrostatic pressure until the afferent arteriole is reached. The pressure falls across the afferent arteriole and then plateaus across the glomerulus, where little change in hydrostatic pressure

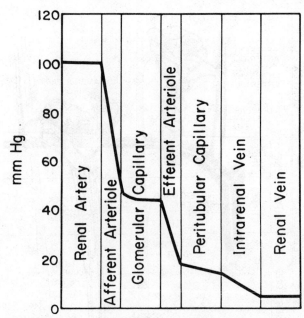

Figure 3. Pressure gradients in the renal circulation. (From Pitts, R. F.: Physiology of the Kidney and Body Fluids. 3rd ed. Chicago, Year Book Medical Publishers, 1974.)

occurs. At the efferent arteriole another major drop in pressure occurs, with little more than a modest slow decline of hydrostatic pressure beyond that point.

Virtually all renal blood flow passes through the glomeruli, and the majority perfuses the cortex. Less than 10 per cent of renal blood flow is directed to the medulla, and only about 1 per cent to the papillae. The distribution of renal blood flow has been most accurately determined using techniques of radioisotope washout and radioactive microsphere distribution.

The composite picture that emerges from the use of all of these techniques is of the delivery of approximately 25 per cent of resting cardiac output to the kidney. Of the plasma delivered to the kidney, approximately 20 per cent is ultrafiltered in the glomeruli. The renal blood flow is predominantly to the outer cortex with less to the inner cortex, still less to the medulla, and the least to the papillae. Under conditions of decreased arterial pressure or increased sympathetic nervous stimulation when total renal blood flow is reduced, relatively more flow is directed to the inner cortex and medulla and relatively less to the outer cortex. Thus, medullary blood flow is maintained more effectively than cortical flow. As blood flow to the kidney diminishes, the amount of plasma ultrafiltered per minute decreases less than does the total renal plasma flow. Thus, the fraction of plasma ultrafiltered tends to increase as the total plasma flow decreases.

PROSTAGLANDINS

Under physiologic conditions it is difficult to demonstrate a role for prostaglandins in regulating renal blood flow. However, in states of reduced renal perfusion, prostaglandins have an important regulatory and compensatory action. As renal blood flow falls, the vasodilatory prostaglandins PGE_2 and prostacyclin (PGI_2) are produced in increased quantities and protect renal perfusion. The importance of this compensatory phenomenon is demonstrated when prostaglandin synthesis inhibitors are given to patients with impaired renal perfusion. Compensatory vasodilation is prevented, and deterioration of renal function occurs. The important role of prostaglandins therefore requires a brief review. Renal prostaglandins are formed from arachidonic acid that is released by the action of phospholipase A_2 on membranes. The arachidonic acid is metabolized by cyclo-oxygenases to endoperoxides, which are subsequently converted to PGE_2, $PGF_{2\alpha}$, PGD_2, PGI_2, and thromboxane. Prostaglandin synthesis varies throughout the kidney with respect to the specific metabolites produced and the capacity for their production. The glomerulus synthesizes primarily PGI_2, which is a vasodilator and inhibitor of platelet aggregation. Prostacyclin is also synthesized in cortical and medullary arterioles. The cortical collecting tubule produces PGE_2, which is a vasodilator but in addition inhibits sodium chloride reabsorption. Both PGI_2 and PGE_2 stimulate renin release via cyclic AMP. There is therefore a potential feedback interaction of vasodilation and vasoconstriction. When vasodilatory prostaglandins are produced, they stimulate the production of vasoconstrictors via the renin-angiotensin system; in completing the loop, states of high renin-angiotensin production stimulate the production of vasodilatory prostaglandins.

The capacity for prostaglandin synthesis in the medulla is greater than in the cortex. Cells of the medullary interstitium, thick ascending limb, and medullary collecting duct all produce PGE_2, which acts as described above and in addition inhibits the effect of antidiuretic hormone, thus enhancing water excretion. Thromboxane A_2, a potent constrictor and stimulator of platelet aggregation, is produced in both the cortex and the medulla.

The circulatory effects of prostaglandins predominantly increase renal blood flow when it is compromised. Thus, when angiotensin II is increased, and in states of urinary tract obstruction, there is stimulation of prostaglandin synthesis. Prostaglandin synthesis will also predictably alter sodium reabsorption and antidiuretic hormone action. Therefore one can predict that inhibition of prostaglandin synthesis will have the following important effects on the kidney: (1) impair the vasodilatory response to reduced renal perfusion, thus producing renal damage; (2) inhibit the effectiveness of diuretics such as furosemide and ethacrynic acid; and (3) reduce the ability to excrete free water. Further, inhibition of prostaglandin synthesis may reduce the release of renin and the production of angiotensin sufficiently to produce an increase in serum potassium. With reduced renal perfusion, serum potassium may rise to dangerous levels.

On the positive side, inhibition of prostaglandin synthesis has been used with reasonable effectiveness to reduce the salt wasting seen in Bartter's syndrome, and has been used to reduce free water production in nephrogenic diabetes insipidus.

MICROSCOPIC ANATOMY OF THE GLOMERULUS

The glomerulus is formed as the afferent glomerular arteriole breaks up into a network of four to eight capillary loops in the shape of a tuft approximately 200 μ in diameter. The glomerular capillary tuft in-

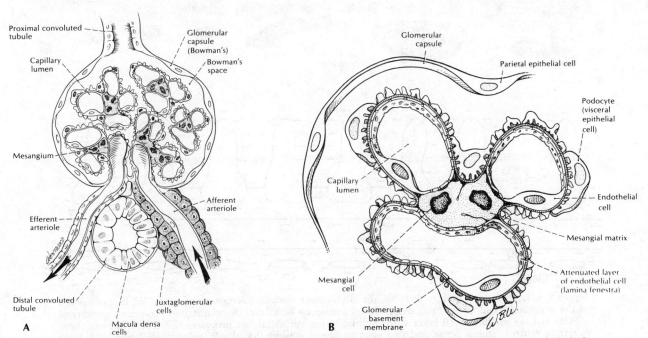

Figure 4. *A,* Microscopic anatomy of glomerulus illustrating the three major cell types (endothelial, mesangial, epithelial) and relationships of distal convoluted tubule to afferent and efferent arterioles. *B,* Schematic representation of a portion of a glomerular lobule. Note mesangium and its relationship to capillary loops. Note also that basement membrane is reflected away from mesangium. Mesangial cells are separated from capillary lumen by extensions of endothelial cell along capillary wall. (From Holley, K. E.: Anatomy of the kidney. In Knox, F. G. (ed.): Textbook of Renal Pathophysiology. Hagerstown, Md., Harper and Row, Publishers. Copyright 1978 by Mayo Clinic/Foundation.)

vaginates the epithelium of Bowman's capsule, so that the capillary tuft has a single layer of epithelial cells around it. The glomerular apparatus now consists of the capillaries, a basement membrane, and the lining epithelial cells separated by a space from the remainder of Bowman's capsule. The space, known as Bowman's space, is lined by epithelial cells and is continuous with the lumen of the tubule (Fig. 4).

The glomerulus now assumes the characteristics of a multilayered apparatus through which plasma ultrafiltrate may pass (Fig. 5). It is easiest to picture the structure of the glomerulus by tracing the pathway of ultrafiltrate. The plasma that enters the glomerular capillary loops must first pass through the endothelial cell layer with its large intercellular apertures. The endothelial cell layer retains cells but allows even large macromolecules to penetrate. The filtrate next reaches the glomerular basement membrane, which is the major barrier to the passage of macromolecules. The glomerular basement membrane is further subdivided into zones of differing density. The lamina densa is a central dense area sandwiched between two, more

electron-lucent, areas, the lamina rara interna and the lamina rara externa. For the remainder of our discussion we will consider the glomerular basement membrane as a single entity. Beyond the glomerular basement membrane are the epithelial cells that abut upon the basement membrane through a series of foot processes. The foot processes are separated from each other by a space called a filtration slit: the final barrier to the entry of macromolecules into Bowman's space. The glomerular structure is enmeshed in an extracellular matrix that has a high content of polyanionic material. It has been suggested that the negative charge around the foot processes of the epithelial cells prevents them from fusing. Fusion of foot processes does occur in a number of disease states, such as nephrotic syndrome, and may also occur under experimental conditions that diminish the negative charge on the foot processes.

The mesangium is the axial portion of the glomerulus. It is composed of a matrix traversed by intercellular canals and of at least three cell types. At the interface of the mesangium with the glomerular capillary there is no basement membrane. Thus the fe-

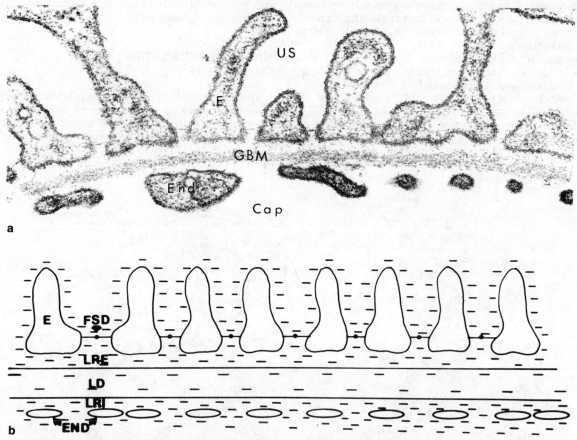

Figure 5. *a,* Glomerular capillary wall (GCW). High-power electron micrograph of rat GCW. It is composed of the endothelial cell layer *(End)* traversed by numerous fenestrae, the glomerular basement membrane *(GBM)* and the epithelial cell layer with interdigitating epithelial foot processes *(E).* The GBM has three layers, a central lamina densa and two electron-lucent subendothelial and subepithelial layers. A faint glycocalyx or cell coat material covers endothelial cell membranes. *Cap* = capillary lumen; *US* = urinary space. ×72,000. *b,* Schematic representation of the GCW indicating the distribution of polyanionic substances (−) in the glomerular extracellular matrix. The concentration is greatest over the epithelial and endothelial cell coats, and in the outer and inner layers of the GBM. *END* = endothelium; *LRI* = lamina rara interna or subendothelial layer of the GBM; *LD* = lamina densa; *LRE* = lamina rara externa or subepithelial layer of the GBM; *FSD* = filtration slit diaphragm; *E* = epithelial foot process. (Reprinted from Structural determinants of glomerular permselectivity. Fed Proc 36:2619, 1977.)

nestrations of the capillary allow access of filtrate directly to the mesangial matrix. This matrix, which is similar to but distinct from the glomerular basement membrane, extends to the base of the glomerular stalk and comes into direct apposition to the macula densa and the lacis and myoepithelioid cells of the juxtaglomerular apparatus. Glomerular filtrate entering the mesangium may exit via the stalk or distal tubule, or it may be disposed of by mesangial cells.

The intrinsic mesangial cell is most similar to a capillary pericyte and is of mesenchymal origin. It has numerous capabilities including (1) regulation of blood flow and filtration, a role facilitated by receptors for angiotensin II, presence of contractile proteins, and the ability to synthesize vasoactive prostaglandins; (2) production and metabolism of the mesangial matrix; (3) the ability to internalize and metabolize macromolecules; and (4) an ability to interact with inflammatory cells. A second resident cell demonstrated in rats is the bone marrow–derived Ia antigen-bearing cell. The role of these cells in the mesangium is not clear. Finally, there are transient monocyte-macrophages, which may be called to the mesangium in large numbers by appropriate stimuli.

There is much speculation that the mesangium plays a role in response to toxins, to immune-mediated stimuli, and to altered circulatory states. The accumulation of macromolecules in the mesangium appears to be a function of (1) plasma concentration—saturation of the reticuloendothelial system with a rise in plasma concentration leads to greater accumulation in the mesangium; (2) molecular size—complexes of larger molecular size are more likely to be localized in the mesangium than are smaller complexes; (3) molecular structure; and (4) electrical charge. The role of these macromolecules in producing mesangial disease is less clear. There does not appear to be any significant damage produced when macromolecules are localized to the mesangium, as opposed to the inflammatory response they evoke when lodged in the more peripheral aspects of the glomerular capillary loops. In the latter circumstance, however, the ensuing inflammatory response frequently involves the mesangium. The proposed role of the mesangium as a focus for the development of glomerular sclerosis in states of heavy proteinuria requires further definition.

The organization of the glomeruli and their more than 1.5 m² of filtering surface area allows the kidney to receive large volumes of blood each minute and to produce large volumes of plasma ultrafiltrate free of cells and protein. The ultrafiltrate passes directly into the lumen of the tubule, where it is exposed to the processes of reabsorption and secretion. A description of these processes is the topic of the next chapter.

NEPHRON FUNCTION

The function of the nephron is to ultrafilter plasma and then to modify the ultrafiltrate by reabsorbing substances from it or by secreting material into it so that the volume and composition of the body fluids are maintained within narrow physiologic limits. Specifically the kidneys regulate the volume and tonicity of body fluids, contribute to acid-base regulation, regulate potassium balance, regulate phosphate balance, con-

tribute to the regulation of calcium and magnesium homeostasis, excrete waste products such as urea and uric acid, and conserve important nutrients such as glucose and amino acids.

To accomplish these myriad regulatory functions requires the nephron to balance the processes of filtration, reabsorption, and secretion for several substances simultaneously and to accomplish several separate functions in the same nephron segment. Obviously several of the nephron functions are interrelated. However, for clarity, these functions are best dissected and discussed separately.

One of the key problems in dissecting the various nephron functions is assigning relative importance to the processes of filtration, reabsorption, and secretion in the excretion of any substance.

Unfortunately, measuring the urinary content of a substance tells little about the renal mechanism involved in its excretion. To assess the contribution of the kidney to altered excretion requires an understanding of the concepts of clearance. Clearance will provide the basis for measuring glomerular filtration, reabsorption, and secretion.

CLEARANCE

The original concept of renal clearance referred to urea, but it is applicable to any substance: "the volume of blood that one minute's excretion suffices to clear of urea when the urine volume is large enough to permit maximum urea output." From this concept it follows that the clearance of a substance that is freely filtered at the glomerulus and is neither reabsorbed nor secreted will be a measure of glomerular filtration rate (volume filtered/time). The polysaccharide inulin meets these criteria and is routinely used as the best measure of glomerular filtration rate (GFR). Creatinine, produced in relatively constant amounts by the muscles of the body, provides an endogenous substance that is freely filtered, is not reabsorbed, and is not secreted except at very high plasma concentrations. Clinically, measurement of creatinine clearance is used as an adequate measure of GFR. The clearance of any substance (S) can be calculated according to the equation:

$$\text{Clearance S} = \frac{\text{Urinary Conc. of S} \times \text{Vol. of Urine/time}}{\text{Plasma Conc. of S}}$$

When S is creatinine, the clearance of S is approximately equal to GFR. The Urinary Conc. of creatinine × Vol. of Urine/time is equal to the amount of creatinine excreted per unit time. Under steady-state conditions, in which the plasma concentration of creatinine is constant, the amount of creatinine excreted per unit time must equal the amount of creatinine metabolically produced per unit time. Thus,

$$\text{GFR} = \frac{\text{Production Rate of Creatinine}}{\text{Plasma Conc. of Creatinine}}$$

The production rate of creatinine is primarily a function of total muscle mass and is relatively constant in any individual whose muscle mass is stable. In such an individual, fractional changes in GFR will therefore be reflected by equivalent but oppositely directed fractional changes in plasma concentration of creatinine. That is, whenever GFR declines by 50 per cent the steady-state plasma concentration of creatinine will double.

Once GFR is known, the filtered load of a substance can be calculated. The filtered load is the quantity filtered/unit time. If a substance is freely filtered, the filtered load will be equal to the plasma concentration × GFR. If the substance is 80 per cent protein bound, then only 20 per cent will be freely filterable, and the filtered load will be equal to 0.2 × plasma concentration × GFR. The ability to measure the filtered load permits determination of net reabsorption or secretion. If the amount excreted in the urine is less than the filtered load, net reabsorption has occurred; if the amount excreted exceeds the filtered load, net secretion has occurred.

Net Reabsorption =
   Plasma Conc. × GFR − Urinary Excretion

Net Secretion =
   Urinary Excretion − Plasma Conc. × GFR

The terms *net reabsorption* and *net secretion* are used to indicate that the processes of filtration, reabsorption, and secretion may all proceed simultaneously. Net reabsorption does not indicate the absence of secretion but rather indicates the sum of all processes.

The clearance of a substance that is virtually completely removed from arterial plasma by filtration and secretion and that is not reabsorbed will be a measure of the minimal effective total plasma flow to the kidney. Para-aminohippurate (PAH) is such a substance. Any substance with a clearance in excess of PAH clearance must be assumed to be produced within the kidney. The ratio of the clearance of inulin (C_{IN}) to that of PAH (C_{PAH}) indicates the fraction of total renal plasma flow that is filtered (filtration fraction).

Clearance measurements depend upon accurate collections of adequate volumes of urine and permit only gross determinations of renal functions. Localization of tubular functions and independent quantitation of simultaneous secretion and reabsorption require more elaborate techniques, such as micropuncture of localized tubular segments, microperfusion of nephrons and peritubular capillaries, and perfusion of isolated tubular segments. Slices of renal tissue, isolated cell preparations, and even preparations of renal brush borders and basal lateral cell membranes have been used to study the biochemistry and kinetics of transport. Unfortunately the more elaborate techniques sample very few of the nephrons and do not provide an adequate view of the integrated function of the total kidney. Therefore our concepts of renal function are the product of a composite of clearance and more specific techniques.

GLOMERULAR FILTRATION

The glomerular capillary tuft ultrafilters plasma into Bowman's space. Fluid collected from Bowman's space is relatively protein free but contains electrolytes such as sodium, potassium, and chloride; and organic molecules such as urea, creatinine, and glucose in concentrations equal to those in plasma. Thus the glomerulus is selectively permeable to solutes. Ultrafiltration requires a driving force (glomerular capillary hydrostatic pressure) adequate to overcome the oncotic pressure in the glomerular capillaries and the hydrostatic pressure in Bowman's space. Let us dissect what is known of glomerular permeability and of the net driving force for filtration.

GLOMERULAR PERMEABILITY

The permeability of the glomerulus to a series of molecules is a function of the size, shape, and charge of the molecules as well as of the structure of the glomerulus.

Molecules of molecular weight less than 10,000 pass easily across the glomerulus; molecules of molecular weight greater than 50,000 are almost completely restricted from passing through the glomerulus. For solutes between 10,000 and 50,000 molecular weight, there is progressive exclusion from the ultrafiltrate. The shape of molecules, referred to as their effective molecular radius, allows correction for the differences in configuration that affect the rate of glomerular passage of two equal-weight molecules. Finally, charge is important in permeability. If a series of molecules are of comparable size, those that are negatively charged will cross the glomerulus less readily than those that are neutral, which in turn will be less permeant than the positively charged forms.

The structure of the glomerulus is such that plasma molecules first come in contact with the endothelium, which contains large pores of approximately 1000 Å diameter. Next in series is the glomerular basement membrane, which is the major barrier to the passage of macromolecules, and, finally, the foot processes with their filtration slits act as a final barrier to the molecules that have crossed the basement membrane. The glomerular extracellular matrix contains polyanionic material that selectively excludes negatively charged molecules while facilitating the passage of positively charged molecules (Fig. 5).

HYDROSTATIC PRESSURE

Blood flow to the kidney is relatively constant despite wide variations in systemic pressure. This autoregulation permits the kidney to maintain constant blood flow over the range of systolic pressure of 80 to 180 mm Hg and to maintain constant GFR over an even wider range of perfusion pressures (Fig. 6). There is no complete explanation of autoregulation, but myogenic responses of interlobular and afferent glomerular arterioles probably play an important role. The roles of angiotensin II, prostaglandins, alpha catechols, and distal tubule feedback control remain to be defined.

The kidney receives blood at systemic arterial pressure. The glomerular afferent and efferent arterioles are the two points of resistance that account for virtually all of the total fall in pressure between renal artery and vein. The pressure drop between the end of the afferent arteriole and the beginning of the efferent arteriole (that is, across the glomerulus) is negligible. Though the change in hydrostatic pressure across the

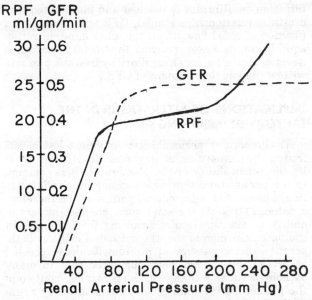

Figure 6. Autoregulation of glomerular filtration rate *(GFR)* and renal plasma flow *(RPF)* in the dog. (From Pitts, R. F.: Physiology of the Kidney and Body Fluids. 3rd ed. Chicago, Year Book Medical Publishers, 1974. [Adapted from Ochwadt, B.: Prog Cardiovasc Dis 3:501, 1961.])

glomerulus is negligible, the absolute hydrostatic pressure within the glomerulus will vary, depending upon the relative changes in resistance in the afferent and efferent glomerular arterioles. Reduced afferent arteriolar or increased efferent arteriolar resistance will increase glomerular hydrostatic pressure. Increased afferent or decreased efferent arteriolar resistance will decrease glomerular hydrostatic pressure. The changes in glomerular hydrostatic pressure will affect filtration fraction.

INTERACTION OF FACTORS DETERMINING GLOMERULAR FILTRATION

The ultrafiltration of plasma across the glomerular capillary wall is a function of capillary permeability and net hydrostatic pressure (Fig. 7). Capillary wall permeability is expressed as K_f, the coefficient of ultrafiltration that takes into account hydraulic permeability and surface area. K_f relates net filtration pressure to filtration rate and has the dimensions of milliliters per minute per millimeters of mercury. The higher the K_f, the more permeable the glomerular capillary wall. Net hydrostatic pressure is equal to the capillary hydrostatic pressure (p_c~50 mm Hg) favoring ultrafiltration minus the sum of the hydrostatic pressure of Bowman's space (P_{BS}~15 mm Hg) and capillary oncotic pressure (P_{CO}~30 mm Hg) opposing it. These relations can be expressed by the equation

$$GFR = K_f (P_C - [P_{BS} + P_{CO}])$$

The process of glomerular filtration can be viewed as similar to the process by which fluid traverses systemic capillaries (see Section XII) with a few important differences. Glomerular capillaries have a higher hydrostatic pressure than systemic capillaries, the pressure drop across the glomerulus is minimal, and the permeability of glomerular capillaries is greater than that of systemic capillaries. These properties of the glomerular apparatus favor greater ultrafiltration.

Let us examine the events of glomerular filtration (Fig. 8). Plasma enters the glomerulus at a relatively high hydrostatic pressure. That pressure will remain relatively constant along the length of the glomerulus. The hydrostatic pressure in Bowman's space will also remain relatively constant. Even accounting for oncotic pressure, net hydrostatic pressure will favor ultrafiltration at the earliest portions of the glomerulus. As ultrafiltration proceeds, the proteins are concentrated along the length of the glomerulus. For any initial protein concentration, oncotic pressure will rise along the length of the glomerulus as a function of K_f or plasma flow or both (see below). When the concentration of protein rises sufficiently to raise plasma oncotic pressure to a level that counterbalances the difference between capillary and Bowman's space hydrostatic pressure, glomerular filtration will cease (Fig. 8, curves A and B); filtration equilibrium has been reached.

Figure 7. Starling forces regulating glomerular filtration. Net filtration pressure *(ΔP)* is the result of opposing hydrostatic pressure *(HP)* in the glomerular capillary and of the sum of hydrostatic pressure in Bowman's space and plasma oncotic pressure *(OP)*. Net filtration pressure is maximal at the afferent arteriolar site of the capillary and approaches zero toward the efferent arteriolar site, because of increasing plasma oncotic pressure as a direct consequence of ultrafiltration. (From Frohnert, P. P.: Glomerular filtration. In Knox, F. G. (ed.): Textbook of Renal Pathophysiology. Hagerstown, Md., Harper and Row, Publishers. Copyright 1978 by Mayo Clinic/Foundation.)

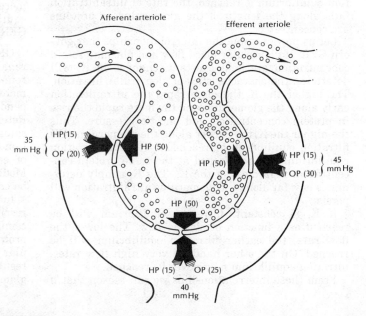

Glomerular Intracapillary Dynamics

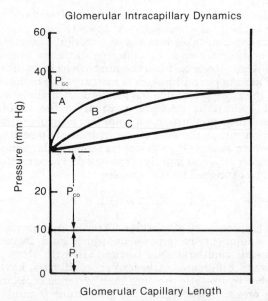

Figure 8. The hydrostatic pressures and colloid osmotic pressure along an idealized glomerular capillary in the strain of Wistar rats with glomeruli on the surface of the kidney. P_{GC} is the hydrostatic pressure in glomerular capillaries, P_T the hydrostatic pressure in the early proximal tubule assumed to be the same as that in Bowman's capsule, P_{CO} the colloid osmotic pressure in arterial blood entering the glomerular capillaries. Curves A, B, and C represent the colloid osmotic pressure at various points along the glomerular capillary as the protein concentration increases as a consequence of the loss of glomerular filtrate from the plasma. The difference between P_{GC} and the curves A, B, and C represents the net filtration pressure at each point, and the area between P_{GC} and curves A, B, and C represents the net filtration pressure. (From Brenner, B. M., Deen, W. M., and Robertson, C. R.: MTP International Review of Science, Physiology Series 1, vol. 6. Kidney and Urinary Tract Physiology. University Park Press, Butterworths, and MTP Medical and Technical Publishing Co., Ltd., 1974, p. 335.)

Filtration equilibrium is not always reached, and ultrafiltration may proceed along the entire length of the glomerulus (Fig. 8 curve C). Whether or not filtration equilibrium is reached, the rate of ultrafiltration falls along the length of the glomerulus as proteins are concentrated.

Let us now examine the interrelationships that govern GFR. If glomerular blood flow and plasma protein concentration are kept constant, changes in K_f will determine the characteristics of glomerular filtration. The higher the K_f the more rapid the ultrafiltration early along the glomerulus and the more rapid the rise in protein concentration and oncotic pressure. Thus the higher the K_f the earlier along the glomerulus will filtration equilibrium be reached. Note that filtration equilibrium will be reached at the same protein concentration regardless of the K_f. The K_f simply determines how far along the glomerulus ultrafiltration will persist.

If K_f is constant, filtration equilibrium will be reached as a function of plasma flow. The lower the flow rate, the earlier filtration equilibrium will be reached. On the other hand, at very high flow rates, filtration equilibrium may never be reached.

From these interrelationships we can reason that if

filtration equilibrium is reached and maintained (hydrostatic relationships stable), GFR will change as a function of blood flow. If, on the other hand, filtration equilibrium is never reached (hydrostatic pressures never reaching balance), capillary hydrostatic pressure will be the key determinant of GFR.

IMPLICATIONS OF ALTERATIONS IN THE FACTORS DETERMINING GFR

(1) Glomerular permeability: Anatomic lesions affecting the glomerulus, as in glomerulonephritis, modify the permeability of the glomerulus. It is common to see circumstances in which glomerular inflammation is associated with reduced perfusion and therefore a reduced GFR. At the same time, changes in permeability to macromolecules resulting from changes in the basement membrane, the epithelial cells, or both, permit greater passage of macromolecules expressed as proteinuria. It has been suggested that in many pathologic states a change in the polyanionic milieu of the glomerulus permits greater permeation by negatively charged proteins.

(2) K_f: The K_f will also be altered by pathologic processes affecting the glomerulus. A rise in K_f reflects increased permeability, and a fall in K_f reflects decreased permeability.

(3) Capillary hydrostatic pressure: The capillary hydrostatic pressure will be altered by changes in afferent and efferent glomerular arteriolar resistance. A rise in afferent arteriolar resistance or a fall in efferent arteriolar resistance will result in a decrease in GFR, particularly in states in which filtration equilibrium has not been reached.

(4) Bowman's space hydrostatic pressure: The hydrostatic pressure in Bowman's space becomes clinically important under conditions of anatomic or functional obstruction to urine flow. The former may occur, for example, as the result of a stone in the ureter, while the latter might occur as the result of diuresis resulting in a urine flow rate high enough to increase resistance in the nephron. In either case GFR may be reduced.

(5) Oncotic pressure: The capillary oncotic pressure will vary with the serum protein. Oncotic pressure is more likely to change the point at which filtration equilibrium will be reached than it is likely to affect GFR in any important way.

GFR is used as one of the prime means of assessing renal function. In addition to defining the extent of renal impairment, a reduced GFR warrants reassessment of the patient's entire status. Many solutes depend upon adequate glomerular filtration for excretion. Retention of these solutes triggers a series of compensatory responses, which will be considered in the section on uremia. Glomerular filtration is also the route of excretion of many drugs and their metabolites. Modification of drug therapy as a function of GFR may be critical in patient care.

Increases in GFR and renal blood flow occur in response to increased protein intake and to hyperglycemia. Brenner et al. have recently proposed that high protein intake or hyperglycemia may result in glomerular hyperfiltration with changes in permselectivity, resulting in proteinuria, mesangial cell injury, and glomerular sclerosis. The sequence of events might accelerate renal aging or the deterioration of function in renal insufficiency.

TUBULAR TRANSPORT PROCESSES

Tubular transport of various substances arises from passive diffusion, active reabsorption, active secretion, or a combination of these processes, as illustrated by the following examples.

UREA

Passive diffusion of a substance is said to occur when the movement of that solute across the tubule does not require energy, is a function of the concentration gradient of the substance across the tubule, and is nonsaturable. Passive transport of solute may occur in any segment of the nephron. All that is required is that a concentration gradient for the diffusion of the solute exist and that the tubular segment be permeable to that solute. An example of the passive transport of a substance is the reabsorption of urea from the proximal tubule. In the glomerulus, urea is filtered at a concentration equal to that in plasma. As salt and water are reabsorbed in the proximal tubule, the concentration of urea within the lumen rises, creating a concentration gradient from lumen to blood. Urea then diffuses down its concentration gradient and is reabsorbed by passive diffusion. The greater the extent of proximal tubular salt and water reabsorption, the greater the extent of concentration of urea and the more the urea will be reabsorbed by passive transport. Thus, in any state (e.g., extracellular fluid volume depletion) in which there is an increase in the fraction of salt and water that is reabsorbed in the proximal tubule, there will be a corresponding increase in urea reabsorption and decrease in urea clearance. This in turn will lead to an increase in the plasma urea concentration that is greater than expected on the basis of any observed decline in GFR. As already discussed, creatinine does not undergo appreciable reabsorption in the proximal tubule, and its plasma concentration, although inversely proportional to GFR, is independent of proximal tubular salt and water reabsorption. Thus an increase in the plasma concentration ratio of urea/creatinine may be observed in states characterized by increased fractional salt and water reabsorption in the proximal tubule. Reabsorption of urea by passive diffusion also occurs in the collecting duct, as will be discussed later.

NONIONIC DIFFUSION OF WEAK ACIDS AND BASES

Several weak acids and bases can undergo passive diffusion when they are uncharged, but not when they are ionized. This process of nonionic diffusion is illustrated for the case of a weak acid, HA, in Figure 9. Only the undissociated form of the acid, HA, being uncharged and lipid soluble, can diffuse across the cell membranes of the tubule. The tubule is far less permeable to A^-. Thus, net transport of the weak acid across the tubule proceeds according to the HA concentration gradient. If the H^+ concentration is higher in the tubular fluid than in the peritubular space, HA con-

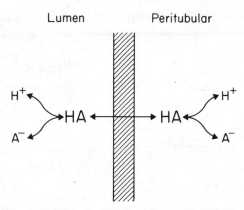

Figure 9. Nonionic diffusion of a weak acid, HA.

centration will also be higher and transport will be driven in the direction of net reabsorption. Conversely, alkalinization of the tubular fluid with respect to the peritubular space will promote net secretion of the acid. In the latter circumstance, augmentation of the tubular fluid flow rate will further increase secretion by preventing a rise in the concentrations of A^- and HA in the tubular fluid. In cases of poisoning with such weak acids as salicylate and phenobarbital, induction of alkaline diuresis is often used to increase drug excretion.

GLUCOSE

Glucose is freely filtered through the glomerulus and at physiologic filtered loads is reabsorbed in the proximal tubule so that the luminal concentration of glucose is far below that in the peritubular plasma. By definition, then, glucose is being transported against a chemical gradient, and the process should require energy. A number of studies utilizing systems ranging from brush border preparations to intact cells and intact kidneys have yielded results most consistent with the cotransport of sodium and glucose occurring in the tubule.

It is believed that there is a carrier in the luminal membrane of the renal tubule that moves most effectively when it contains both glucose and sodium (Fig. 10). The concentration of sodium in the proximal tubular lumen is far higher than that in the intracellular water. In addition, the intracellular space is electrically negative to the lumen. Thus, sodium will move down an electrochemical gradient from lumen into cell. If sodium and glucose occupy the same carrier, it is possible for glucose to ride the sodium electrochemical gradient into the cell. This electrochemical gradient will provide the driving force to move glucose against its own concentration gradient into the cell. Once in the cell, the sodium would be actively extruded into the lateral intercellular space, moving water into that space as well (see p. 670). While the extrusion of sodium from the cell requires energy, the sugar now exists at higher concentrations within the cell than within plasma. The final step of reabsorption of sugar, then, may be simply the passive diffusion of sugar across the basal lateral cell membrane and ultimately into the capillaries.

Because glucose reabsorption is carried out by a finite number of membrane carriers, one may observe

LUMEN   CELL   PERITUBULAR

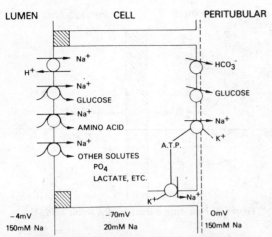

Figure 10. Sodium cotransport systems in the proximal tubule. (From Burg, M. B.: Renal handling of sodium, chloride, water, amino acids and glucose. In Brenner, B. M., and Rector, F. C., Jr. (eds.): The Kidney. 2nd ed. Philadelphia, W. B. Saunders Co., 1981, p. 335.)

saturability of the reabsorptive process as the load of glucose presented for reabsorption increases. This is shown in Figure 11. The amount of glucose filtered, reabsorbed, or excreted per unit time is plotted as a function of the plasma glucose concentration. As plasma glucose is increased from 100 to 200 mg/dl, glucose excretion remains unmeasurable. As plasma glucose rises above 200 mg/dl, glucose begins to appear in the urine, and glucose excretion thereafter increases linearly as plasma glucose is further increased. Since glucose is freely filtered, we can compute the filtered glucose as GFR times plasma glucose concentration.

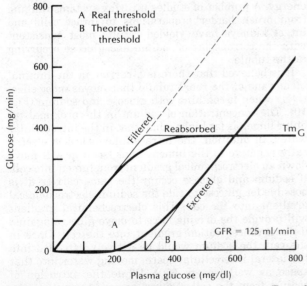

Figure 11. Titration curve for glucose to determine T_m and threshold. *A*, Actual threshold for glucose; *B*, calculated (predicted) threshold for glucose. (From Dousa, T. P.: In Knox, F. G. (ed.): Textbook of Renal Pathophysiology. Hagerstown, Md., Harper and Row, Publishers. Copyright 1978 by Mayo Clinic/Foundation. Originally from Pitts, R. F.: Physiology of the Kidney and Body Fluids, 3rd ed. Chicago, Year Book Medical Publishers, 1974.)

Filtered glucose increases linearly with increasing plasma glucose. The glucose reabsorbed is computed as the difference between the glucose filtered and the glucose excreted. At plasma glucose concentrations below 200 mg/dl the glucose excreted is negligible and the glucose reabsorbed equals the glucose filtered. However, when plasma glucose exceeds 200 mg/dl, reabsorbed glucose plateaus at a constant rate called the tubular maximum (T_m). Presumably the carriers for glucose reabsorption are fully saturated and cannot respond to further increases in filtered glucose once the T_m has been reached. The actual data for excreted and reabsorbed glucose follow curved lines as the T_m is approached, and do not have perfectly sharp breaks. This is referred to as splay in the curves. The phenomenon may reflect heterogeneity among proximal tubules in their capacity to reabsorb glucose. Because of the splay, glucose appears in the urine even before the T_m has been reached. The plasma glucose concentration at which glucose begins to "spill" into the urine is called the glucose threshold. In normal humans the glucose threshold is 180 to 200 mg/dl. Thus, diabetics will not usually have sugar in the urine unless the plasma glucose concentration exceeds this value. The glucose reabsorptive mechanism may be impaired as an isolated genetic defect (renal glycosuria) or as part of a generalized transport dysfunction affecting the proximal tubule (Fanconi syndrome).

AMINO ACIDS

Amino acids are freely filtered at the glomerulus and undergo net reabsorption in the proximal tubule such that 95 per cent or more of the filtered load is reabsorbed. The amino acids are reabsorbed by saturable, Na-cotransport systems in the brush border, similar to that described above for glucose. Thus the various amino acids achieve maximal reabsorptive rates. There exist at least five distinct, stereospecific transport systems for amino acids that recognize (a) neutral amino acids, (b) diamino amino acids, (c) the imino acids and glycine, (d) the dicarboxylic amino acids, and (e) the beta amino acids. In addition to active reabsorption there appears to be back leak or secretion of amino acids that is not evident under physiologic conditions. However, under conditions in which the reabsorptive mechanism for an amino acid is impaired, evidence of back leak or secretion may appear as net secretion. Impairment of amino acid transport may result in failure to reabsorb a group of structurally related amino acids, failure to reabsorb a specific amino acid, or impairment of the reabsorption of all amino acids as in Fanconi syndrome. In addition, with severe impairment of renal tubular reabsorption of amino acids, net secretion of involved amino acids may appear.

ORGANIC ANIONS

The brush border membrane of the proximal tubular cell contains at least two distinct Na-cotransport systems for reabsorbing organic anions that are metabolic intermediates in the oxidation of carbohydrates and lipids. One system is shared by such monovalent organic anions as lactate, acetoacetate, and beta-hydroxybutyrate. A second system is shared by such

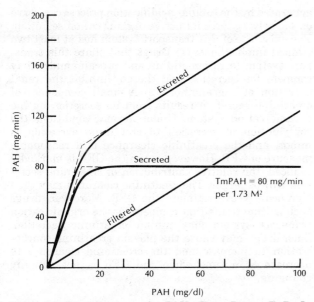

Figure 12. Titration curve for PAH. (From Dousa, T. P.: In Knox, F. G. (ed.): Textbook of Renal Pathophysiology. Hagerstown, Md., Harper and Row, Publishers. Copyright 1978 by Mayo Clinic/Foundation. Originally from Pitts R. F.: Physiology of the Kidney and Body Fluids. 3rd ed. Chicago, Year Book Medical Publishers, 1974.)

dicarboxylic and tricarboxylic intermediates of the Krebs cycle as alpha-ketoglutarate, succinate, malate, and citrate. Normally, reabsorption of all of these substances is virtually complete. However, because these transport mechanisms are saturable, the reabsorptive rates for organic anions achieve tubular maxima. Thus in diabetic ketoacidosis the filtered loads of acetoacetate and beta-hydroxybutyrate (ketone bodies) exceed their tubular transport maxima, and these anions appear in the urine in appreciable quantities.

A variety of other organic anions undergo net, active secretion in the proximal tubule. The best studied representative of this group is PAH. This compound is primarily secreted in the late proximal convoluted tubule and early pars recta (S_2). The uphill step in PAH secretion occurs across the basolateral membrane, probably by Na-cotransport. Downhill transport of PAH into the tubular lumen then occurs across the brush border membrane. Because PAH is transported by a saturable process, there exists a T_m for secretion of this substance, as shown in Figure 12. As the plasma concentration of PAH is raised from 0 to 10 mg/dl, excreted PAH increases much faster than does filtered PAH. Under these conditions the majority of excreted PAH is contributed by secretion. However, as the plasma concentration of PAH increases above 20 mg/dl, the rate of PAH secretion reaches a plateau (T_m), and further increments in excretion are due only to the rise in filtered PAH. The binding of PAH for secretion is so avid that at low concentrations virtually all of the PAH in the peritubular plasma is removed and secreted into the urine.

URIC ACID

Urate is freely filtered at the glomerulus and undergoes net reabsorption in the proximal tubule; over 90 per cent of the filtered load is reabsorbed. Although net reabsorption is the rule, mediated secretion of urate also occurs in the proximal tubule by a mechanism similar or identical to that responsible for active PAH secretion. Uric acid reabsorption occurs both by simple passive diffusion and by active transport. In states of enhanced proximal tubular reabsorption of salt and water (e.g., extracellular fluid volume depletion), urate excretion is depressed, probably because the resulting increase in the intratubular concentration of urate serves to enhance the passive and active components of urate reabsorption. Recent evidence suggests that the active reabsorption of urate across the luminal membrane of the proximal tubular cell occurs not by a mechanism of Na-cotransport, as is the case for many other reabsorbed organic anions, but by a mechanism of anion exchange, as shown in Figure 13. Any anion that shares this transport system and for which a cell-to-lumen gradient is present can serve to drive urate reabsorption. One anion sharing the exchanger is OH^-: A cell-to-lumen gradient is generated by the tubular acidification process. Other anions that can exchange with urate include lactate, beta-hydroxybutyrate, and acetoacetate, which are accumulated within the cell by Na-cotransport across the luminal membrane. Urate can also exchange with certain anions such as PAH that are accumulated within the cell by Na-cotransport across the basolateral membrane.

The existence of such a roundabout mechanism mediating urate reabsorption can account for the complex manner in which urate excretion is affected by many factors. First, the anion exchanger mediating urate transport is very sensitive to inhibition by probenecid, thereby explaining the uricosuric effect of this drug. Second, increasing the plasma concentrations of endogenous or exogenous organic anions that are accumulated within the cell by Na-cotransport may serve to stimulate urate reabsorption by anion exchange. This may explain the urate retention observed in clinical states in which plasma concentrations of lactate or

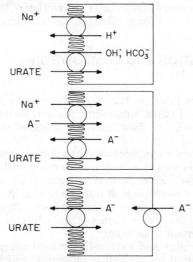

Figure 13. Urate absorption via anion exchange across the luminal membrane of proximal tubular cells. (From Guggino, S. E., Martin, G. J., and Aronson, P. S.: Specificity and modes of the anion exchanger in dog renal microvillus membranes. Am J Physiol 244:F612, 1983.)

ketoacids are elevated. Third, at still higher concentrations such organic anions may compete with intratubular urate for binding to the anion exchanger, thereby promoting urate excretion. This sequence may explain the "paradoxic" effects of drugs such as pyrazinamide and salicylate that reduce urate excretion when given in low doses and increase urate excretion when given in higher doses. In addition to these pharmacologic effects, reabsorption of uric acid may be impaired along with that of other substances in proximal tubular disorders such as the Fanconi syndrome.

ORGANIC CATIONS

A variety of organic cations undergo net secretion in the proximal tubule by a probenecid-insensitive process that is distinct from the secretory system for organic anions. These organic cations are accumulated across the basolateral membrane in response to the interior-negative membrane potential, and then are secreted into the lumen by a mediated process of cation-H^+ exchange. In this way the lumen-to-cell H^+ gradient generated by the tubular acidification process can serve as the driving force for active organic cation secretion. The existence of this transport system has at least two clinical implications: (1) Drugs that share this transport system (e.g., cimetidine and procainamide) may compete for secretion and thereby inhibit the renal excretion of one another. (2) A small component of creatinine excretion results from its secretion by the organic cation system. Under normal conditions the contribution of secretion to creatinine excretion is minor, and the creatinine clearance is a reasonable measure of GFR. However, when the GFR is markedly reduced, the relative contribution of creatinine secretion will be larger. The creatinine clearance may then significantly overestimate the GFR. Moreover, drugs such as cimetidine that compete for the organic cation transport system may inhibit creatinine secretion. Such drugs may cause the plasma creatinine concentration to increase and the creatinine clearance to decrease at a time when the GFR is not actually changing.

Regulation of Volume and Tonicity _____

The regulation of the volume and tonicity of the body fluids is accomplished by two systems that, though interrelated, are best discussed separately. The regulation of volume, particularly of extracellular fluid volume, is a function of sodium balance. The regulation of tonicity, or body fluid osmolality, is a function of water balance. Changes in tonicity may occur independently of changes in volume. It is possible to have, for example, hypotonic extracellular fluid with low, normal, or increased extracellular fluid volume. The renal regulation of sodium balance and water balance will be discussed after a brief description of the normal distribution and composition of the body fluids.

DISTRIBUTION AND COMPOSITION OF BODY FLUIDS

The body fluids, or total body water, may be divided into three distinct subgroups: the intracellular fluid, the extracellular fluid; and the transcellular, or secreted, fluid (Fig. 14).

Total body water accounts for approximately 60 per cent of body weight in humans. Since the water content of fat is far less than that of muscle and other soft tissues, the percentage of total body weight comprised by water falls as fat content increases. Thus, infants have a higher water content than adults, and men a higher content than women.

Intracellular and extracellular fluid compartments are separated by the cell membranes, which, though selective in their permeability to ions and nutrients, are freely permeable to water. Thus, although an ionic gradient may exist across cell membranes, movement of water will establish osmotic equilibrium and the osmotic gradient will be rapidly dissipated.

INTRACELLULAR FLUID VOLUME AND COMPOSITION

Intracellular fluid comprises about 60 per cent of total body water. There is some variation in cellular ionic content from tissue to tissue, but an overall similar pattern can be seen (Fig. 15). The most important cation of the intracellular fluid is potassium, which exists at concentrations of 140 to 150 mEq/l. Potassium is almost entirely within the cells; only 2 to 3 per cent is extracellular. Another cation that is predominantly intracellular is magnesium (present at far lower concentrations than potassium), while, in comparison with the concentration in the extracellular fluid, sodium exists in very low concentrations within the cells. The most important anions of the intracellular fluid are organic phosphate and protein. The intracellular ions are almost certainly compartmentalized among cell organelles, and therefore our discussion of concentrations of ions in cell water is a simplification of the physiologic reality.

EXTRACELLULAR FLUID VOLUME AND COMPOSITION

Extracellular fluid comprises about 35 per cent of total body water (20 per cent of body weight). The extracellular fluid volume is further subdivided by the capillary wall into interstitial fluid (75 per cent) and plasma water (25 per cent). The content of water in dense connective tissue and the inaccessible water in bone matrix do not contribute significantly to fluid and electrolyte pathophysiology and will not be considered further.

The interstitial fluid composition is similar to that of plasma water. However, plasma contains anionic

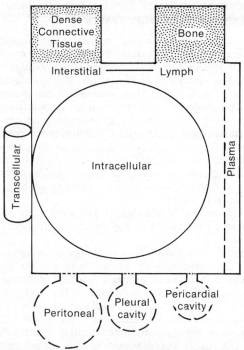

Figure 14. The compartments of total body water. About two-thirds of the body water is intracellular water; the remainder is the water of extracellular fluid. The *dashed line* separating plasma from interstitial fluid represents the capillary membranes. The three cavities drawn with *circular dashed lines* represent potential extracellular spaces that are normally, however, negligible in volume. (From Berliner, R. W., and Giebisch, G. H.: Body fluids and the excretion of urine. In Brobeck, J. R. (ed.): Best and Taylor's Physiological Basis of Medical Practice. 10th ed. Baltimore, Williams and Wilkins Co., 1979, p. 5. Originally from Maffly, R. H.: In Brenner, B. M., and Rector, F. C., Jr. (eds.): The Kidney. Philadelphia, W. B. Saunders Co., 1976, p. 78.)

proteins that are largely confined to the intravascular space. The difference in anionic protein concentration and the free mobility of other ions across the capillary wall establishes a Gibbs-Donnan equilibrium such that the concentration of cations is slightly lower and that of anions slightly higher in the interstitial fluid than in plasma. In both plasma water and interstitial fluid, sodium is the most important cation, and chloride and bicarbonate are the most important anions. Plasma, which contains about 142 mEq/l of sodium, is actually only about 93 per cent water. The additional 7 per cent of plasma volume is protein and lipid. Therefore the concentration of sodium per liter of plasma water is actually higher—that is, 142 mEq/l of plasma divided by 0.93, or 153 mEq/l of plasma water. Since the percentage of plasma as water is relatively constant, the convention is to present sodium concentration as per liter of plasma. Note that if there is pronounced hyperproteinemia or hyperlipemia, the conventional expression of sodium concentration may be falsely low, while the sodium concentration per liter of plasma water is quite normal.

TRANSCELLULAR OR SECRETED FLUID VOLUME AND COMPOSITION

Transcellular fluids are predominantly the products of epithelial cell secretion. The composition of these fluids varies widely according to the cell of origin (Table 1). Under physiologic conditions the secreted fluids tend to be recirculated or reabsorbed. Under pathologic conditions failure to reabsorb continuously secreted fluids may lead to significant losses of volume, as per diarrhea or vomiting. Under these circumstances the specific composition of transcellular fluid will determine the changes in composition of body fluids. Loss of transcellular fluid will be discussed further in

Figure 15. Electrolyte composition of body fluids. *Org. ac.,* organic acids. (From Gamble, J. L.: Chemical Anatomy, Physiology, and Pathology of Extracellular Fluid: A Lecture Syllabus. 6th ed. Cambridge, Mass., Harvard University Press, 1954.)

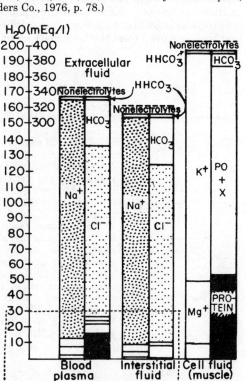

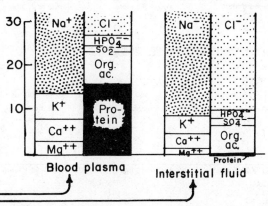

TABLE 1. MEAN ELECTROLYTE CONTENT OF THE TRANSCELLULAR FLUIDS

FLUID	Na$^+$ (mEq/l)	K$^+$ (mEq/l)	Cl$^-$ (mEq/l)	HCO$_3^-$ (mEq/l)
Saliva	33	20	34	0
Gastric juice*	60	9	84	0
Bile	149	5	101	45
Pancreatic juice	141	5	77	92
Ileal fluid	129	11	116	29
Cecal fluid	80	21	48	22
Cerebrospinal fluid	141	3	127	23
Sweat	45	5	58	0

Adapted from Arieff, A.: In Maxwell, M. H., and Kleeman, C. R. (eds.): Clinical Disorders of Fluid and Electrolyte Metabolism. 2nd ed. New York, McGraw-Hill Book Co., 1972.

*The Cl$^-$ concentration exceeds the Na$^+$, K$^+$ concentration by 15 mEq/l in gastric juice. This largely represents the secretion of H$^+$ by the parietal cells.

considering volume contraction, acid-base abnormalities, and potassium depletion.

THE RELATION BETWEEN INTRACELLULAR AND EXTRACELLULAR FLUID SPACES

The high intracellular, relative to extracellular, concentration of potassium and the reverse circumstance for sodium favor movement of potassium out of and sodium into cells. These ionic gradients are not maintained by differing membrane permeabilities but rather by the presence of sodium-potassium pumps and the cell membrane. These pumps extrude sodium from the cell and transport potassium into the cell. They are therefore also critical in protecting cell volume. The high concentration of osmotically active anionic protein within cells relative to the interstitial fluid establishes a Gibbs-Donnan equilibrium that increases the osmotic activity intracellularly. Untoward movement of water into the cell is prevented by the active extrusion of sodium. Interference with the sodium-potassium pump results in cell accumulation of sodium and chloride, loss of potassium, and cell swelling.

DISTRIBUTION OF WATER BETWEEN INTRACELLULAR AND EXTRACELLULAR FLUID SPACES

As noted earlier, water moves freely across cell membranes and an osmotic disequilibrium cannot be sustained. The intracellular and extracellular osmolality must therefore be the same. The distribution of total body water will then depend on the number of active particles in the intracellular versus the extracellular space. Presence of sodium-potassium pumps in cell membranes produces a circumstance in which exchangeable potassium behaves as an obligate intracellular ion and sodium as an obligate extracellular ion. The greater quantity of exchangeable potassium versus sodium results in the majority of body fluid being intracellular.

The following examples of redistribution of body fluids will illustrate the key principles involved (Fig. 16 *A* and *B*).

Example 1. Assume that equilibrium is established under circumstances in which there are 30 liters of intracellular fluid containing 150 mEq/l potassium and 15 liters extracellular fluid containing 150 mEq/l of sodium. The potassium is confined to cells and the sodium to the extracellular fluid. If 4.5 liters of pure water were abruptly removed from the extracellular fluid, the result would appear to be a concentration of the extracellular fluid to 196 mEq/l of sodium. In fact, any increase in sodium concentration in the extracellular fluid would create an osmotic gradient drawing fluid from the intracellular fluid space until osmotic equilibrium was restored. Osmotic equilibrium would be restored when the loss of water from the two compartments was proportional—that is, when 3 liters were lost from the intracellular fluid and 1.5 liters from the extracellular fluid. The result would be a 10 per cent increase in the concentration of sodium (166 mEq/l), rather than the apparent 30 per cent increase initially suggested. Note that the concentration of sodium was modified as though the 4.5 liters of fluid had been removed from the total body water. Note also

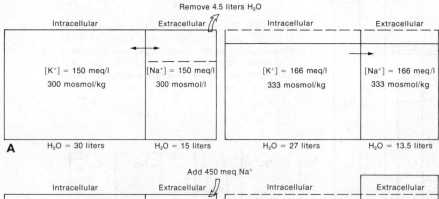

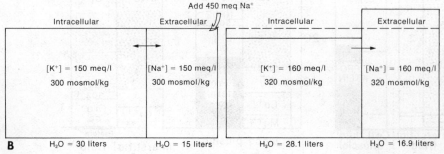

Figure 16. Schematic representation of changes in intracellular and extracellular fluid: *A*, with removal of 4.5 liters of pure water from the extracellular fluid as noted in the *left panel*, resulting in redistribution of fluid and change in osmolality noted in the *right panel; B*, with the addition of 450 mEq of sodium to the extracellular fluid as shown in the left panel, resulting in redistribution of fluid and change in osmolality seen in the right panel. See text for discussion. (Modified from Earley, L. E.: Sodium metabolism. In Maxwell, M. H., and Kleeman, C. R. (eds.): Clinical Disorders of Fluid and Electrolyte Metabolism. 2nd ed. New York, McGraw-Hill Book Co., 1972.)

that the serum sodium concentration rose despite a decrease in extracellular fluid volume.

Example 2. Assume that equilibrium is again established with 30 liters of intracellular fluid with 150 mEq/l of potassium and 15 liters of extracellular fluid with 150 mEq/l of sodium. Now assume that 450 mEq of sodium are added to the extracellular fluid. Though the sodium is confined to the extracellular fluid space, the result would not be a rise of 30 mEq/l of sodium in the extracellular fluid, since that would create an osmotic disequilibrium, drawing fluid from the intracellular to the extracellular fluid space. Fluid would move until the osmotic activity intracellularly equalled that in the extracellular fluid. Equilibrium would occur at a point comparable to what would have been accomplished had the 450 mEq of sodium been distributed in total body water. The actual result would be a rise of ~10 mEq/l of sodium in the extracellular fluid and an expansion of the extracellular fluid at the expense of the intracellular fluid. Note that adding sodium to the extracellular fluid changes sodium concentration as though it has been added to total body water.

These examples illustrate several critical points of fluid distribution: (1) Water added to or removed from any fluid compartment will behave as though it were added to or removed from total body water. (2) Sodium added to or removed from extracellular fluid will alter sodium concentration as though it had been added to or removed from total body water. (3) The change in sodium concentration tells nothing of the changes in extracellular fluid volume. Hypernatremia may exist with low, normal, or increased extracellular fluid. The same is true for hyponatremia or a normal serum sodium concentration. (4) Changes in the volume of the intracellular fluid and extracellular fluid tend to be proportional and in the same direction with gain or loss of water. Intracellular and extracellular fluid volume will change in opposite directions with gains or losses of restricted solutes such as sodium or potassium.

OTHER IMPORTANT SOLUTES

Glucose is primarily an extracellular solute and enters cells slowly, particularly in the absence of insulin. As glucose accumulates in the extracellular fluid, water is drawn from the intracellular space. The addition of water to the extracellular space dilutes the sodium so that apparent hyponatremia is present. The hyponatremia secondary to shifts of fluid produced by hyperglycemia may be misleading in suggesting hypoosmolality. Increased osmolality of the body fluids actually exists.

Urea, as opposed to glucose, crosses cell membranes rapidly and therefore does not produce a sustained redistribution of fluid. Though urea is measured as a contributor to extracellular osmolality, it does not represent effective osmotic activity, which exerts a transmembrane effect.

The osmolality of extracellular and, by inference, of intracellular fluid can be estimated, employing the following assumptions: (1) Sodium is the predominant osmotically active cation of the extracellular fluid. Since sodium will be accompanied by an approximately equal number of osmotically active anions, the ionic contribution to osmolality is two times the concentration of sodium. (2) Glucose will behave as an osmoti-

cally active, predominantly extracellular, solute. Since the molecular weight of glucose is 180, the osmotic contribution of glucose is

$$\frac{[\text{glucose mg/dl}]}{180} \times 10 \; or \; \frac{[\text{glucose mg/dl}]}{18}.$$

(3) Urea will equilibrate rapidly across cell membranes and will not therefore contribute to transmembrane fluid movements. Nonetheless the contribution of urea to osmolality must be calculated. As with glucose, correction is made for the molecular weight of urea (60) or urea nitrogen (28). The contribution of blood urea nitrogen is then $\frac{[\text{BUN mg/dl}]}{2.8}$. The plasma osmolality may now be estimated as

$$2 \times [\text{Na mEq/l}] + \frac{[\text{glucose mg/dl}]}{18} + \frac{[\text{BUN mg/dl}]}{2.8}.$$

The "effective" osmolality, that osmotic activity moving fluid across cell membranes, omits the urea component. Note that in calculating osmotic activity we use mEq/l plasma for sodium and mg/dl plasma for glucose and urea. Osmolality is actually mOsm/kg of water. However, clinically, the estimate described is quite useful, unless a significant quantity of plasma volume is composed of substances other than water. Thus, major discrepancies between the measured osmolality and calculated osmolality usually indicate excessive quantities of protein or lipid in plasma or the presence of an unmeasured solute such as alcohol.

CELLULAR RESPONSE TO REDISTRIBUTION OF FLUID

Avoidance of major swelling or contraction in response to changes in extracellular osmolality is a property of most cells and is absolutely critical for the brain with its attachments within a fixed-size rigid chamber. Examination of the brain's response to hypoosmolar and hyperosmolar changes is instructive.

In hyponatremic states in experimental animals, brain swelling occurs initially but begins to diminish in hours. Correction of swelling is essentially complete at 24 hours. The brain responds to extracellular hypotonicity by losing potassium and chloride and thus reducing its osmotic burden.

Hypernatremic states present a greater spectrum of clinical possibilities and a greater number of potential responses. In experimental animals, hypernatremia leads initially to loss of water and gain of sodium, potassium, and chloride by brain cells. By four hours, increased concentrations of sodium, potassium, and chloride account for only 65 per cent of the increase in brain osmotic activity, and by one week they account for less than 50 per cent. Between four hours and several days, brain water content returns to normal, and increased osmotic activity is sustained largely through the generation or accumulation of organic solutes such as amino acids. Hyperglycemia also causes an acute loss of brain water, which returns to normal levels in a few hours, again because of changes in the concentrations of ions and organic solutes. Urea, which penetrates the brain more slowly than it does other tissues, draws water from the brain for periods of four to six hours but eventually equilibrates with brain water. Exogenous substances such as mannitol and glycerol remove water from the brain and do not result in the generation of new intracellular organic molecules. Therefore their use is not associated with effective regulation of the intracellular volume of the brain, and brain volume decreases.

The volume and composition of body fluid compartments and the interchange between these compartments has been described. General comments on the regulation of cell volume have stressed the importance of sodium-potassium pumps in cell membranes and the adaptive mechanisms displayed by, for example, cells of the brain. We will now examine first the regulation of the extracellular fluid volume and then the regulation of body fluid tonicity.

REGULATION OF VOLUME

Sodium, the dominant cation of the extracellular fluid, is the critical determinant of the extracellular fluid volume. Since sodium behaves as an obligate extracellular cation and, along with its accompanying anions, accounts for the majority of the osmotic activity of the extracellular fluid, it maintains an appropriate proportion of total body water in the extracellular space.

The reabsorption of sodium by the kidney is a finely regulated process that serves primarily to regulate extracellular fluid volume but that is coupled to a series of other tubular functions. For example, sodium reabsorption is related to hydrogen ion secretion for the reclamation of bicarbonate and the ultimate acidification of the urine; it is linked to potassium secretion; it plays a role in the reabsorption of organic molecules; and it plays a critical role in renal concentrating and diluting ability. With all of these linked processes it may be difficult to predict what the renal response will be in any given circumstance. However, under almost all circumstances the kidney will protect extracellular fluid volume at the expense of all other functions. Therefore, by determining what the kidney perceives to be the state of extracellular fluid volume, it will be possible to predict the renal handling of sodium and the processes coupled to sodium transport.

MECHANISMS OF TUBULAR SODIUM TRANSPORT

Perhaps the simplest way to review regulation of sodium excretion is to follow sodium through the nephron, defining the differences in the handling of sodium by each anatomic segment and then noting the control mechanisms that play upon each of these segments.

Sodium is freely filtered at the glomerulus; 60 to 70 per cent of the filtered sodium is reabsorbed in the proximal tubule. Sodium enters the proximal tubular cell via a number of carrier-mediated transport systems in the luminal membrane (e.g., Na-H exchange, Na-glucose cotransport, Na-amino acid cotransport) and possibly also by simple diffusion. Sodium is then pumped actively across the basolateral membrane via the Na-K-ATPase. In the earliest segments of the proximal tubule, the principal anion accompanying transtubular Na reabsorption is bicarbonate, the reabsorption of which results from Na-H exchange (see

below). The ionic current of Na arising from its cotransport with such neutral substances as glucose and alanine is accompanied by passive Cl reabsorption driven by the small lumen-negative potential difference across the tubular wall. Solute reabsorption in the proximal tubule is nearly isosmotic, being accompanied by the reabsorption of water. Consequently the concentration of sodium in the lumen remains almost constant along the length of the proximal tubule. Because there is preferential reabsorption of HCO_3 rather than Cl in the early part of the proximal tubule, the concentration of HCO_3 in the lumen falls and that of Cl rises. The resulting transtubular gradient for Cl directed outward then serves as a driving force for additional passive Cl reabsorption. Whether there is also a component of transcellular Cl transport that is more directly coupled to the transport of Na, as by cotransport or double ion exchange (i.e., Na-H and Cl-HCO_3 exchanges) is unclear.

An important aspect of proximal tubular Na transport is that it functions as a pump-leak system. Recall that proximal tubular cells are joined at their luminal borders by tight junctions. Potential pools of fluid exist in the lateral intercellular spaces between cells (Fig. 17). The net effect of proximal tubular transport processes is to pump Na and accompanying solutes into these lateral intercellular spaces. Water is osmotically drawn into these spaces as well. Sodium and water may now either enter the peritubular capillary, so as to accomplish net reabsorption, or leak back into the lumen across the tight junction. The movement of sodium and water from the intercellular space into the capillary depends on the Starling forces governing bulk fluid movement across the capillary wall, namely, the hydrostatic pressure gradient and the oncotic pressure gradient. The more these forces favor capillary uptake of fluid, the less sodium and water will leak back into the lumen. Conversely, the less favorable the forces are for capillary uptake of fluid, the more sodium and water will leak back into the lumen.

The descending limb of the loop of Henle is permeable to water but less so to Na. In this segment, water

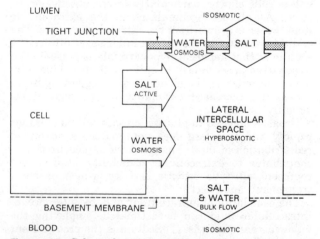

Figure 17. Salt and water transport through the lateral intercellular spaces between proximal tubular cells. (From Burg, M. B.: In Brenner, B. M., and Rector, F. C., Jr. (eds.): The Kidney. 2nd ed. Philadelphia, W. B. Saunders Co., 1981, p. 337.)

is extracted from the tubule into the hyperosmotic medullary interstitium (see below), causing the intratubular NaCl concentration to rise. The thin ascending limb of Henle is impermeable to water but permeable to NaCl. There is passive NaCl reabsorption driven by the outward gradient of NaCl that resulted from water extraction in the descending limb. Clearly, any factor, such as a change in medullary interstitial osmolarity, that alters the amount of descending limb water reabsorption will affect NaCl reabsorption in the thin ascending limb. Active transport of Na appears to be of minor importance in the thin limbs of the loop of Henle.

In contrast, the thick ascending limb of Henle is a major site for active NaCl reabsorption. As shown in Figure 18, there is entry of Na, K, and Cl across the luminal membrane by a cotransport process that is sensitive to inhibition by loop diuretics such as furosemide and bumetanide. The driving force for this process is the inward Na gradient established by the active transport of Na across the basolateral membrane via the Na-K-ATPase. The luminal membrane cotransport system serves to maintain the intracellular concentration of Cl at a sufficiently high level to ensure its passive exit across the basolateral membrane by simple diffusion. The ionic current of Cl across the basolateral membrane helps to establish a lumen-positive transtubular potential difference in this nephron segment. Because the thick ascending limb of Henle is impermeable to water, active reabsorption of NaCl causes the luminal NaCl concentration to fall along this segment. This in turn tends to limit the further net reabsorption of NaCl. In states in which the rate of delivery of NaCl and fluid out of the proximal tubule is enhanced, the absolute amount of NaCl reabsorbed in the thick ascending limb will increase because the luminal NaCl concentration will be maintained at a nonlimiting value over a greater fraction of the tubular length. Thus, while normally some 20 to 25 per cent of filtered Na is reabsorbed in the loop of Henle, this percentage may increase when NaCl delivery to this nephron segment is increased.

The remaining 5 to 10 per cent of filtered Na is reabsorbed by active processes in the distal nephron. Throughout the distal nephron, Na extrusion across the basolateral membrane is via the Na-K-ATPase. In the early distal tubule, recent evidence suggests that a major fraction of Na entry across the luminal membrane occurs via a Na-Cl cotransport system that is

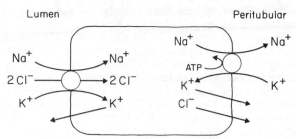

Figure 18. Cotransport of sodium, potassium, and chloride across cell of the thick ascending limb of Henle.

sensitive to inhibition by thiazide diuretics. In the later distal tubule and collecting tubule, the major mechanism for Na entry across the luminal membrane is diffusion through Na-selective channels that are sensitive to inhibition by the diuretics amiloride and triamterene. The ionic current of Na arising from this process helps to generate a lumen-negative transtubular potential difference in these nephron segments, thereby promoting passive Cl reabsorption. Aldosterone, the steroidal hormone produced by the zona glomerulosa of the adrenal gland, stimulates Na reabsorption in the distal tubule and collecting tubule. It appears that the primary effect of this hormone is to increase the number of amiloride-sensitive Na channels in the luminal membrane, and a secondary effect is to increase the number of Na pumps (Na-K-ATPase) in the basolateral membrane.

REGULATION OF RENAL SODIUM EXCRETION

Under normal conditions the renal excretion of Na is regulated so as to match Na intake, thereby maintaining Na balance. A balance study illustrating this point is shown in Figure 19. During the initial three-day period the subject is ingesting 10 mEq Na per day, urinary Na output equals intake, and the subject's weight is constant at 70 kg. Dietary Na intake is then abruptly increased to 150 mEq/day. Urinary Na output begins to rise, but does not equal intake until about five days later. There is thus a temporary period of positive Na balance. The subject drinks sufficient water to keep plasma osmolality and Na concentration unchanged. The period of positive Na balance therefore represents a time during which there is a net gain of isotonic saline, as reflected by a 1.0-kg increase in body weight. It is the resulting expansion of the extra-

Figure 19. Normal sodium balance. (From Reineck, H. J., and Stein, J. H.: In Maxwell, M. H., and Kleeman, C. R. (eds.): Clinical Disorders of Fluid and Electrolyte Metabolism. 3rd ed. New York, McGraw-Hill Book Co., 1979, p. 90.)

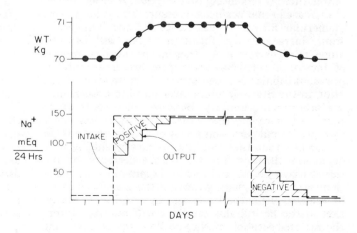

cellular fluid volume that signals the kidney to increase the urinary Na output. Renal Na excretion is not regulated importantly by the plasma Na concentration. Even a hyponatremic expansion would induce an increased Na excretion. When Na intake is reduced there is a period of negative Na balance. The associated contraction of extracellular fluid volume causes urinary Na output to fall until it again equals Na intake. Assuming an extracellular fluid volume of 17 liters in this 70-kg subject, it is apparent that a 6 per cent expansion of the extracellular volume (1 liter) can effect a 15-fold increase in Na excretion. Clearly this is a control system with a very high gain. It should be emphasized that this 1-liter increase in extracellular fluid would be clinically undetectable in a normal individual. It could be detected only by careful, serial measurements of body weight and blood pressure. While blood pressure would increase slightly, it would remain within the normal range. Indeed, in normal individuals Na balance can be maintained by means of a virtually Na-free diet (less than 10 mEq/day), without manifestation of overt signs of extracellular fluid volume depletion, and by means of a high Na diet (over 200 mEq/day), without detectable signs of volume excess. The mechanisms by which an increase in extracellular fluid volume is sensed and stimulates renal Na excretion are summarized as follows:

In the absence of any factors causing abnormal partitioning of fluid between the intravascular and interstitial compartments (see below), any increase in extracellular fluid volume will be accompanied by an increase in plasma volume. Assuming no abnormalities in vascular capacitance or cardiac function, an increase in plasma volume will cause an increase in central venous and cardiac filling that in turn will lead to an increase in cardiac output and arterial pressure. The resulting increase in renal perfusion pressure, however subtle, is probably the most important manifestation of extracellular fluid volume expansion that causes stimulation of renal Na excretion. There are at least four mechanisms by which an increase in renal perfusion pressure stimulates Na excretion.

One important effect of increased renal perfusion pressure is to inhibit renin secretion by the juxtaglomerular cells of the afferent arteriole. The conversion of renin substrate to angiotensin I is therefore reduced, resulting in a decrease in angiotensin II, an important stimulator of aldosterone secretion. A decrease in aldosterone reduces Na reabsorption in the distal nephron, thereby promoting Na excretion. A second effect of increased renal perfusion pressure is to enhance the glomerular filtration rate (GFR). All else being constant, increasing the filtration of Na will help to augment its excretion. Another important consequence of increased renal perfusion pressure is to inhibit proximal tubular Na reabsorption because of an alteration in the Starling forces favoring fluid uptake into the peritubular capillary. Because the GFR is autoregulated more effectively than is renal plasma flow, increased renal perfusion pressure will cause the GFR to rise less than the renal plasma flow, resulting in a decreased filtration fraction. With a decreased filtration fraction the normal rise in the protein concentration in the blood passing through the glomerulus will be reduced. Thus the lesser rise in protein concentration in the peritubular capillary will tend to inhibit the net reabsorption of Na and fluid in the proximal

tubule by mechanisms discussed earlier. In addition, when renal perfusion pressure is increased, the hydrostatic pressure in the peritubular capillary will tend to increase, an effect that will also serve to inhibit proximal tubular Na and fluid reabsorption. A fourth consequence of increased renal perfusion pressure is to enhance medullary blood flow. This tends to wash out the hypertonicity of the medullary interstitium, resulting in decreased water reabsorption in the thin descending limb of Henle. With a decrease in descending limb reabsorption of water the NaCl concentration in the fluid entering the ascending limb will be lower, an effect that will serve to inhibit passive NaCl reabsorption in the thin ascending limb and active NaCl reabsorption in the thick ascending limb.

The subtle changes in central venous and cardiac filling accompanying alterations in extracellular fluid volume are also sensed by volume receptors in the great veins of the thorax and in the cardiac atria. These receptors probably are involved in modulating sympathetic nerve activity in the kidney. High-pressure baroreceptors in the arterial tree may also influence renal sympathetic nerve traffic. Renal sympathetic nerve activity appears to influence tubular Na reabsorption directly and also via changes in intrarenal hemodynamics. The net effect is that renal Na reabsorption is enhanced when sympathetic nerve activity is increased in states of volume contraction. In addition, increased beta-adrenergic stimulation augments renin secretion, an effect that will also enhance Na reabsorption via the action of aldosterone. Conversely, when increased plasma volume is sensed by central volume receptors and baroreceptors, the resulting decline in renal sympathetic activity serves to stimulate Na excretion.

Central volume receptors may also influence the secretion of natriuretic hormones. In fact, an extremely potent natriuretic factor has recently been isolated and purified to homogeneity from cardiac atria. The natriuretic effect of this peptide appears to result principally from an increased GFR due to altered renal hemodynamics. It is not yet known if this substance is secreted into the plasma under physiologically appropriate circumstances. The existence of a different natriuretic factor having the digitalis-like action of inhibiting Na-K-ATPase has also been postulated. This factor is presumed to inhibit tubular Na reabsorption. However, the chemical identity, site of synthesis, and precise physiologic role of this digitalis-like factor is unknown.

The regulation of renal Na excretion is clearly multifactorial, as summarized in Figure 20. With extracellular fluid volume expansion, Na excretion is increased by the processes indicated. With volume contraction these processes are reversed, and sodium is retained by the kidney. In essence, this is a feedback system designed to maintain an adequate "effective" circulating blood volume. From the standpoint of renal Na excretion the most important receptor for sensing the adequacy of effective blood volume is the kidney itself. Subtle alterations in renal perfusion pressure and blood flow directly and indirectly influence Na excretion as discussed. The role of effector mechanisms dependent on sensing of plasma volume by central volume receptors and baroreceptors is somewhat less certain, but probably also of importance.

Because of the multifactorial control of Na excretion, an abnormality of only a single effector mechanism is

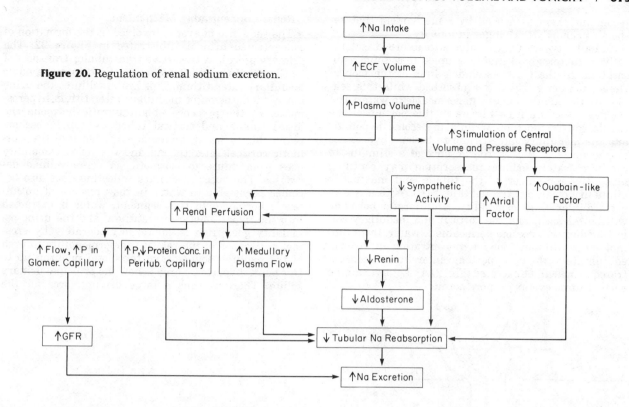

Figure 20. Regulation of renal sodium excretion.

unlikely to cause progressive Na retention. For example, a reduction in GFR should tend to promote Na retention. However, except at severely depressed levels of GFR (i.e., less than 3 to 5 ml/min), Na balance can still be maintained. Presumably as extracellular fluid volume expansion begins to occur secondary to reduction in GFR, the other effector mechanisms illustrated in Figure 20 are recruited to restore Na balance. That is, renin and aldosterone are suppressed, physical forces favoring proximal tubular Na reabsorption are decreased, natriuretic hormones may be secreted, for example. Thus there is "escape" from the salt-retaining effect of a reduction in GFR. The signal for this escape is the modest volume expansion that is commonly manifested by arterial hypertension in patients with chronic renal failure. Similarly, one can escape from the salt-retaining effect of aldosterone. In subjects given mineralocorticoids as part of an experimental protocol, a short period of Na retention occurs, but then urinary Na excretion increases to match intake, and Na balance is restored. The likely explanation for this escape phenomenon is that as volume expansion begins to take place, other effector mechanisms are called into play to promote Na excretion. Thus, GFR tends to increase, physical forces favoring tubular Na reabsorption tend to decrease, natriuretic hormones may be secreted, and so on. Again the signal for this escape is the modest volume expansion that is commonly manifested by arterial hypertension in patients with chronic mineralocorticoid excess, as in cases of aldosterone-secreting adrenal tumors. Finally it should be noted that whereas one can escape from the salt-retaining effect of excessive aldosterone, the converse is not true. Aldosterone is essential for maximal renal conservation of Na. Thus when aldosterone secretion is severely deficient, progressive negative Na balance culminating in hypovolemia and shock occurs in patients ingesting a low salt diet.

REGULATION OF TONICITY

Humans are mobile mammals capable of surviving in a broad spectrum of environments. Intake of sodium and water varies greatly, yet the osmolality of body fluids is maintained remarkably constant at about 290 mOsm/kg of water. This constancy of osmolality is maintained by a two-limbed system: the thirst mechanism and the renal concentrating and diluting mechanisms.

THIRST

The sensation of thirst is governed by cells in the hypothalamus that may anatomically overlap the cells responsible for antidiuretic hormone production. Thirst is triggered by rises in osmolality, falls in perfusion pressure, and probably by angiotensin. Drugs such as chlorpropamide have also been reputed to stimulate thirst. When osmolality rises, thirst is triggered and the person seeks water. When osmolality falls, thirst is inhibited. This thirst mechanism is effective enough to protect osmolality even if the renal mechanisms of concentration and dilution are defective.

RENAL CONCENTRATING AND DILUTING MECHANISMS

The basic problem for renal regulation of tonicity is excretion of either a dilute or concentrated urine as needed. This problem is solved by processes that, in simplest terms, separate solute from solvent and then recombine them as needed by a mechanism that responds primarily to changes in tonicity.

Actually, two-thirds of water is reabsorbed isotonically in the proximal tubule, coupled to sodium reabsorption. In the thick ascending limb of the loop of Henle, sodium chloride is reabsorbed while this segment of the tubule remains impermeable to water. The removal of solute from filtrate in this portion of the tubule causes the tubular fluid to become hypotonic and the medullary interstitium to become hypertonic to plasma (Fig. 21). In the absence of a stimulus to conserve water, sodium reabsorption may continue along the remainder of the tubule and maximally dilute urine can be excreted (Fig. 21B). With a rise in extracellular fluid osmolality, antidiuretic hormone will be released, and the cortical and medullary collecting duct will become permeable to water. Intraluminal water will move down a concentration gradient to equilibrate with the hypertonic interstitium; concentrated urine will be excreted (Fig. 21A). Let us examine each of these events in more detail.

Renal Concentrating Mechanism

The sequence of events involved in the formation of concentrated urine is illustrated in Figure 22. The primary process is the active transtubular transport of NaCl out of the thick ascending limb into the outer medullary interstitium. This process dilutes the urine but renders the outer medullary interstitium hyperosmotic. In the presence of antidiuretic hormone the distal tubule and cortical collecting tubule become permeable to water, water is extracted into the isosmotic cortical interstitium, and the urine osmolality goes from dilute to isosmotic as urine volume decreases. The outer medullary collecting duct also becomes permeable to water in the presence of antidiuretic hormone. In this segment, water is extracted into the hyperosmotic interstitium, and the urine osmolality goes from isosmotic to moderately hyperosmotic. Because of the relative impermeability to urea of the nephron segments of the distal nephron up to this point, hypertonic urea is now the principal urinary solute. There is thus a large driving force for the

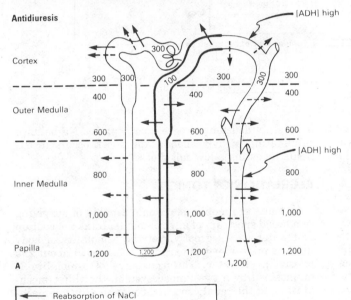

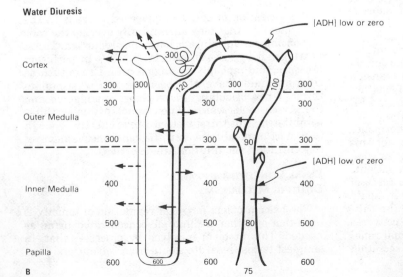

Figure 21. Urine and interstitial osmolality along the nephron during antidiuresis (A) and water diuresis (B). (From Valtin, H.: Renal Function. 2nd ed. Boston, Little, Brown and Co., 1983, p. 162.)

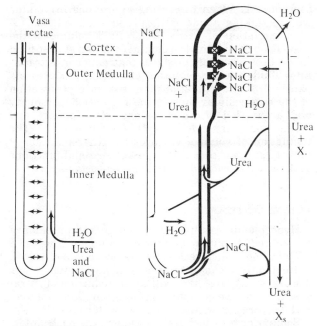

Figure 22. Renal concentrating mechanism. (From Berliner, R. W.: The concentrating mechanism in the renal medulla. Kidney Int 9:216, 1976.)

passive reabsorption of urea in the inner medullary collecting duct, which is permeable to urea. The addition of urea to the inner medullary interstitium increases its osmolality. This facilitates the extraction of water from the thin descending limb of Henle. As discussed earlier, this raises the intratubular NaCl concentration above the interstitial NaCl concentration. The thin ascending limb of Henle has a low permeability to water and a high permeability to NaCl relative to urea. Thus, in this segment passive diffusion of NaCl outward proceeds faster than passive diffusion of urea inward. As a consequence the urine is diluted in the thin ascending limb, and net solute in the form of NaCl is added to the inner medullary interstitium. As a result of the entry of urea from the medullary collecting duct and NaCl from the thin ascending limb of Henle, the inner medullary interstitium has a higher osmolality than the outer medullary interstitium. The inner medullary collecting duct becomes permeable to water in the presence of antidiuretic hormone. Accordingly, in this nephron segment additional water is extracted from the urine, and the urine becomes maximally concentrated (1000 to 1200 mOsm/kg). It should be noted that the countercurrent arrangement of blood flow in the vasa recta serves to minimize washout of solute from the hypertonic medullary interstitium.

Given the above sequence of events, it should be clear that the ability to concentrate the urine maximally requires adequate delivery of NaCl to the thick ascending limb of Henle, active transport of NaCl in this nephron segment, secretion of antidiuretic hormone, responsiveness of the distal tubule and collecting duct to antidiuretic hormone, adequate delivery of urea to the collecting duct, sufficiently slow urine flow through the distal nephron to permit osmotic equilibration, and sufficiently slow blood flow through the vasa recta to minimize washout of medullary hypertonicity. Thus the ability to concentrate the urine

maximally is impaired when NaCl delivery to the loop of Henle is inadequate (e.g., severe extracellular fluid volume contraction), when loop diuretics are administered, when antidiuretic hormone secretion is impaired (e.g., central diabetes insipidus), when the tubular response to antidiuretic hormone is impaired (e.g., nephrogenic diabetes insipidus), when urea excretion is subnormal (e.g., low-protein diet), or when urine flow through the distal nephron and blood flow through the vasa recta are increased (e.g., osmotic diuresis).

Renal Diluting Mechanism

As described earlier, solute reabsorption in the proximal tubule is accompanied by the nearly isosmotic reabsorption of water so that no measurable dilution of the urine takes place in this nephron segment. In fact, the urine is not diluted below the plasma osmolality until it reaches the thick ascending limb and early distal tubule, the major water-impermeable segments of the nephron where active NaCl reabsorption is unaccompanied by water reabsorption. The urine is further diluted (down to 40 to 60 mOsm/kg) along the rest of the distal nephron where active Na reabsorption continues, but the permeability to water is small in the absence of antidiuretic hormone. The ability to excrete large volumes of maximally dilute urine clearly requires adequate delivery of tubular fluid to the ascending limb of Henle, functioning active transport systems in the thick ascending limb and early distal tubule, and the absence of antidiuretic hormone. Thus the ability to excrete water loads maximally is impaired when GFR is decreased, when proximal tubular Na and fluid reabsorption is increased, when loop diuretics or thiazides are administered, or when antidiuretic hormone is not adequately suppressed.

Antidiuretic Hormone

Throughout the discussion of dilution and concentration, mention has been made of antidiuretic hormone. Antidiuretic hormone is an octapeptide produced in the supraoptic and paraventricular nuclei of the hypothalamus. It is transported down the nerves from the hypothalamus to be stored in the posterior hypophysis and to a lesser extent in the median eminence. In response to a variety of stimuli, antidiuretic hormone is released and alters the permeability of the late distal tubule and collecting duct to water. The renal tubule cell contains receptors for antidiuretic hormone. When antidiuretic hormone interacts with the receptor, it activates adenyl cyclase to form cyclic $3',5'$-adenosine monophosphate, the second messenger for increasing luminal membrane permeability to water. It appears likely that water channels are recruited into the luminal membrane by a process of membrane fusion involving a pool of intracellular vesicles whose membranes have a high density of water channels. For the effective action of antidiuretic hormone, it must be produced, stored, released, bound by the tubule cell, and capable of activating the metabolic events that increase water permeability. If all of these events occur, there must still be a hypertonic medullary interstitium, or water reabsorption will not occur.

Factors Releasing Antidiuretic Hormone

The release of antidiuretic hormone is primarily dependent upon changes in osmolality. As little as a 1 to 2 per cent change in osmolality is sufficient to

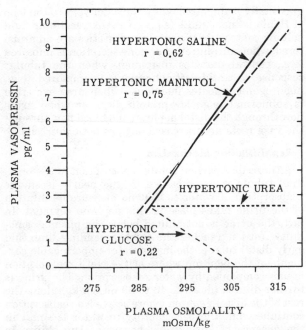

Figure 23. Relationship of plasma vasopressin to osmolality in healthy adults infused intravenously with hypertonic solutions of various solutes. *Lines* and *r values* indicate regression function and correlation coefficient obtained with each type of infusion. (From Robertson, G. L., Athar, S., and Shelton, R. L.: Disturbances in Body Fluid Osmolality. Bethesda, Md., American Physiological Society, 1977, p. 133.)

initiate or inhibit antidiuretic hormone release. Changes in osmolality are sensed in the hypothalamus (osmoreceptors). Actually it is not a change in osmolality of the extracellular fluid per se that is sensed, but either a change in osmoreceptor cell size or a change in the concentration of some intracellular substance. When plasma osmolality is raised by urea, which equilibrates rapidly by entering cells, antidiuretic hormone release is not enhanced. However, when plasma osmolality is increased by sodium chloride, which may enter cells only very slowly, water leaves cells and antidiuretic hormone is released (Fig. 23).

Nonosmolar mechanisms are also capable of releasing antidiuretic hormone. Most nonosmolar stimuli alter baroreceptor tone. These stimuli may be changes in volume or may be pharmacologic. Hypovolemia is the best example of antidiuretic hormone release via baroreceptor stimulation. The release of antidiuretic hormone by hypovolemia is potent enough to override the tonicity regulation of antidiuretic hormone. Severe hypovolemia will stimulate secretion of antidiuretic hormone even in the presence of hypotonicity. However, the extent of hypovolemia necessary to release antidiuretic hormone is proportionally greater than that required of a change in tonicity. While a 1 to 2 per cent change in tonicity is more than sufficient to alter antidiuretic hormone release, a 5 to 10 per cent change in volume of extracellular fluid is required for the same effect.

ABNORMALITIES OF VOLUME AND TONICITY

Analysis of the pathophysiology of altered volume and tonicity is facilitated by recalling a few basic concepts: (1) When discussing alterations in volume we are talking about extracellular fluid volume. (2) The regulation of extracellular fluid volume is the regulation of sodium, the dominant cation of that fluid space. Loss of sodium produces contraction of extracellular fluid volume; retention of sodium produces expansion. (3) The regulation of the sodium concentration of the extracellular fluid is the regulation of tonicity and a function of water balance. (4) Tonicity and volume may vary independently of each other. (5) The regulation of volume will override the regulation of tonicity and, for that matter, all other renal functions such as acid-base and potassium homeostasis.

VOLUME DEPLETION

Hypovolemia results from negative sodium balance or the redistribution of vascular volume. The term *dehydration,* which technically refers to loss of water, is frequently misused to refer to hypovolemia. In our discussion, hypovolemia will mean reduction of intravascular volume or total extracellular fluid volume, and dehydration will refer only to water loss.

Sodium may be lost via the kidney, the gastrointestinal tract, or the skin. Fluid may be distributed out of vascular spaces into compartments within the body that are at least transiently inaccessible to the circulation.

Renal Salt Wasting

The renal tubule operating under the integrated influences of the GFR, aldosterone action, physical forces, and other, less well defined, humoral stimuli should excrete sodium to prevent volume expansion and conserve sodium to prevent hypovolemia. The failure of the kidney to extract sodium to concentrations of less than 10 mEq/l of urine in spite of volume depletion indicates a renal defect.

Tubular salt wasting may occur as the result of injury secondary to endogenous or exogenous agents, as in tubulointerstitial disease; mineralocorticoid deficiency, as in Addison's disease; endogenous osmotic diuresis, as in glycosuria; and as the result of agents such as diuretics. A special case of renal salt wasting is seen in uremia. In the patient who develops renal insufficiency and remains on a fixed salt intake, the fraction of sodium that must be excreted rises progressively as the GFR falls. The mechanism involved in this adjustment to reduced GFR cannot be turned off easily or quickly. Thus, if a regimen of low-sodium intake is begun abruptly in a patient with renal failure, the kidney will continue to excrete a high percentage of the filtered sodium, and clinical salt wasting will ensue. The salt wasting of renal failure will be discussed further in the section on uremia.

Gastrointestinal Loss

The loss of sodium via the gastrointestinal tract is most commonly the result of vomiting or diarrhea. Less commonly, fistulas may form connecting the gastrointestinal tract to the outside of the body. The loss of sodium via the gastrointestinal tract results in a renal response that conserves sodium (urine sodium less than 10 mEq/l) and water (urine osmolality greater than plasma osmolality).

Skin Loss

The loss of sodium via the skin is of importance in burns and in conditions characterized by major desquamation. Sweat losses of sodium are rarely clinically important. When skin loss of sodium is clinically important the renal response will be exactly the same as with gastrointestinal losses and will reflect an attempt to reexpand extracellular fluid volume.

Redistribution of Volume

Clinical hypovolemia, expressed as inadequate circulating blood volume, may result from loss of vascular volume into the interstitial spaces, as would occur with changes in vascular permeability, or into temporarily compartmentalized spaces from which the fluid cannot be rapidly remobilized, as into the retroperitoneum in pancreatitis or into loops of obstructed bowel. It may also result from a collection of blood or edema in areas of trauma.

With redistribution of intravascular volume the kidney responds as to extrarenal causes of sodium loss and retains sodium and water. With redistribution of sodium out of the vascular space, however, estimates of the extent of vascular volume deficiency are difficult, and eventual return of redistributed fluid to the circulating volume may lead to volume overload. The management of volume lost from and returned to vascular spaces from "third spaces" is one of the most difficult problems in clinical fluid management.

Water Loss

Hypovolemia may result from the loss of water alone as in diabetes insipidus or with increased insensible loss. Since water is lost proportionally from intracellular and extracellular fluid volumes, only one-third of pure water loss is from the extracellular fluid and only 25 per cent of the extracellular fluid loss is from the vascular space. Therefore, clinically important losses of vascular volume are rare as a complication of pure water loss. The problem of pure water loss is more likely to be hypernatremia.

Approach to Hypovolemia

The management of hypovolemia depends upon a careful assessment of the route and cause of sodium deficit. Examination of the renal response to volume contraction will define whether the kidney is contributing to the salt wasting or attempting to compensate for the salt loss. Definition of the route of loss directs attention to other therapeutic maneuvers, such as the treatment of hyperglycemia (glycosuria), diarrhea, and so on. Replacement of sodium is required regardless of the route of loss. The concentration of sodium in the replacement fluid—that is, isotonic or hypotonic—and the anion accompanying the sodium are a function of the tonicity and acid-base status of the patient and will be discussed under these sections.

HYPERVOLEMIA

Hypervolemia, the expansion of the extracellular fluid space, is usually manifested as increased interstitial fluid volume—that is, edema—with or without increased intravascular volume. In either event, total body sodium is increased, and the renal sodium excretion mechanism has proved inadequate to protect against the accumulation of excess sodium.

The most obvious case of sodium retention with inadequate renal excretion would be acute renal failure with anuria and continued salt and water intake. The next logical possibility would be a diseased kidney with impaired ability to excrete sodium and an intake of sodium that exceeded the maximum renal excretory capacity.

A more complex situation would exist if otherwise normal kidneys retained sodium in spite of expanded extracellular fluid volume because the kidneys responded as though to hypovolemia. For example, if severe cardiac failure were present, resulting in reduced cardiac output, renal perfusion might be reduced, resulting in the retention of sodium, which would distribute into the venous system and the interstitial fluid of the lungs, or peripheral tissues, or both. Actually, sodium retention may occur in congestive heart failure even before significant reduction in cardiac output can be measured. Numerous suggestions as to the mechanisms involved range from altered mineralocorticoid secretion, to redistribution of renal blood flow, to activation of the sympathetic nervous system, but a satisfactory explanation is not yet in hand.

Renal hypoperfusion with excessive total body sodium might also result from a redistribution of extracellular fluid so that a greater proportion would be in interstitial spaces and less intravascularly. The redistribution might occur if plasma oncotic pressure is reduced by loss of albumin, as in nephrotic syndrome or protein-losing enteropathy, or if albumin synthesis is impaired, as in cirrhosis. With decreased plasma oncotic pressure, fluid would move from vessels into the interstitial space. The intravascular volume would be reduced, and subsequent reduction in renal perfusion would result in sodium retention. The sodium retained would distribute disproportionately into the interstitial space, producing edema as vascular volume gradually was expanded. If vascular permeability were increased, as might occur with severe allergic reaction or diffuse vasculitides, intravascular volume would be lost into the interstitium. The reduced intravascular volume would then result in sodium retention.

Edema

Edema, an increase in interstitial fluid, may be local or generalized. In either case it may be associated with an increased or decreased intravascular volume. Edema results from (1) increased hydrostatic pressure, (2) reduced oncotic pressure, (3) increased capillary permeability, (4) reduced lymphatic drainage, or (5) any combination of these circumstances. The balance between vascular volume and interstitial fluid volume is maintained by the balance between hydrostatic pressure moving fluid out of vessels, oncotic pressure moving fluid into vessels, and vascular permeability, which determines the rate of fluid movement and the size of particles that can leave vessels.

Hydrostatic pressure may be increased locally by venous thrombosis, resulting in edema accumulation in the capillary bed feeding into the occluded venous system. Thrombophlebitis is a prime example of this type of disorder. Hydrostatic pressure may also be increased locally with obstruction to lymphatic flow. A generalized increase in hydrostatic pressure may be seen in congestive heart failure or constrictive pericarditis. The loss of fluid diffusely could reduce intravascular volume; reduce renal perfusion; stimulate renin, angiotensin, and aldosterone; and lead to sodium retention, which would exacerbate the edema. A generalized increase in hydrostatic pressure would also occur whenever sodium intake exceeded the renal capacity to excrete sodium.

Reduced oncotic pressure results from reduced albumin synthesis or increased albumin loss. In either case, reduced plasma oncotic pressure will result in a shift of fluid into interstitial spaces, a reduction in intravascular volume, reduced renal perfusion, and sodium retention. If, in addition to reduced oncotic pressure, there is a change in hydrostatic pressure, as in the increased portal venous pressure of cirrhosis, the hypoalbuminemia may be expressed as localized (ascites) rather than generalized edema.

Increased permeability of the capillaries may occur locally with trauma and inflammation as, for example, in a sprained ankle, or may occur as a generalized process in severe hypersensitivity reactions. The loss of volume from the vascular space leads to the same sequence of events described for reduced oncotic pressure.

The presence of generalized edema does not usually become evident until there is the retention of fluid equal to about 5 to 10 per cent of body weight. Because of the large increase in extracellular fluid volume required to produce generalized edema, body sodium will almost always be increased even if the serum sodium concentration is low.

Assume an extracellular fluid volume of 15 liters at 140 mEq/l of sodium, or 2100 mEq of sodium. Now assume that the extracellular fluid has expanded by 5 liters, resulting in 20 liters of extracellular fluid. If the serum sodium concentration is 125 mEq/l, 2500 mEq of sodium will be present. These calculations assume modest fluid retention and hyponatremia to illustrate that in the presence of generalized edema it is reasonable to assume increased total body sodium. This assumption is important in the discussion of hyponatremia.

HYPERTONICITY

Hypertonicity may result from relative excesses of sodium, glucose, or both. Elevations of tonicity may also be seen in special circumstances from alcohol excess and may be measured with elevated serum urea. In the last circumstance the urea crosses cell membranes so rapidly that no change in cell volume or composition occurs and no physiologic response to altered tonicity is sustained. For our discussion we will focus on hypertonicity associated with increased serum sodium or glucose.

Theoretically an increased sodium concentration could occur as the result of hypertonic sodium intake, increased water loss, a combination of sodium intake and water loss, and a combination of sodium loss and water loss with proportionally more water loss.

Increased Sodium Intake

It is rare to develop more than transient hypernatremia from sodium intake in adults. The usual source of hypertonic sodium intake is the concentrated sodium bicarbonate solution administered to combat severe metabolic acidosis, particularly during cardiopulmonary resuscitation. The usual ampule of sodium bicarbonate contains 1000 mEq/l. A less common source of hypertonic sodium intake is sodium sulfate used for the treatment of hypercalcemia. Since sodium sulfate is Na_2SO_4, isotonic solutions will contain 200 mEq of sodium and 100 mEq of sulfate. Diluting the sodium sulfate so that the sodium concentration is approximately 150 mEq/l will avoid the problem.

In children a number of cases of hypernatremia have occurred as the result of formula mixing errors. When formulas were prepared from raw materials, instances of sodium being added appropriately and added again by mistake in place of sugar resulted in an intake with a higher ratio of sodium to water than infants could excrete. The subsequent sodium overload produced acute shifts of fluid out of brain cells with severe brain injury and frequently death (Fig. 24).

In the event of hypernatremia resulting from exces-

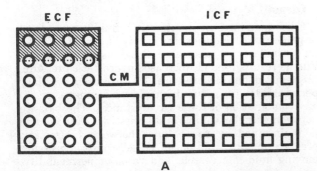

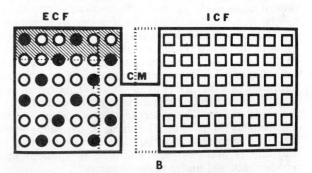

Figure 24. *A,* Normal state of body fluids: In this and subsequent figures, *CM* represents cell membranes and *ECF* and *ICF,* extracellular and intracellular fluid compartments respectively. The *shaded area* denotes the one-fourth of ECF that is intravascular. *Open circles* and *squares* represent the impermeant solutes normally present in the ECF and ICF respectively. The density of symbols reflects solute concentration and their number total solute content in each compartment. ECF volume is half that of ICF because ECF solutes are only half that of ICF and because the CM is freely permeable to water. *B,* Hypertonicity due to ECF impermeant solute gain: New impermeant solutes in ECF *(solid circles)* cause water to shift from ICF to ECF, maintaining solute concentrations in both compartments equal. Therefore, solute concentration of the ICF occurs, the ICF is contracted, and the ECF is expanded. The relative volumes of the two compartments have changed, reflecting their relative solute content. (From Feig, P. U., and McCurdy, D. K.: The hypertonic state. N Engl J Med 297:1444, 1977.)

sive sodium intake, interruption of the sodium intake should suffice if cardiovascular and renal function are intact. Administration of free water may be necessary to prevent marked reduction in brain size and tearing of dural vessels. In the absence of renal function, dialytic treatment may be necessary to correct severe hypernatremia.

Water Loss

Pure water loss may occur as the result of insensible losses or through the kidney in diabetes insipidus (Fig. 25). Pure water loss, occurring particularly in the elderly in hot weather, produces a vicious cycle. A weak individual loses water, becoming dehydrated and somewhat hypernatremic. The dehydration increases the weakness, while the hypernatremia may depress mental functions. The combination produces a situation in which the likelihood is reduced that thirst will be perceived or satisfied. The failure to sense or respond to thirst and the continued insensible loss lead to progressively more severe hypernatremia. The dehydration and hypernatremia lead to reduced renal perfusion and increased antidiuretic hormone secretion. The result is the excretion of small amounts of urine, low in sodium and highly concentrated. Cautious replacement of free water corrects the problem in patients with insensible pure water loss.

In diabetes insipidus the problem of water loss is different. Either because of a central defect in antidiuretic hormone production or release or a renal insensitivity to antidiuretic hormone, water is lost via the kidney. The water loss occurs from the most distal sites in the nephron—that is, beyond the sites of the majority of sodium reabsorption. Therefore it is possible for the patient to retain sodium maximally and still excrete volumes of water equal to 10 to 15 per cent of the GFR. Note that the excretion of 10 to 15 liters of dilute urine may occur with a total sodium excretion of no more than a few milliequivalents. The loss of water in diabetes insipidus results in concentration of plasma and stimulation of the thirst mechanism leading to the ingestion of large quantities of water to replace losses. The clinical picture, then, is one of polyuria and polydipsia. Unfortunately there is a clinical disorder termed psychogenic polydipsia, in which polydipsia and polyuria are also the primary problems. The difficulty facing the physician is to distinguish psychogenic polydipsia from central diabetes insipidus and from nephrogenic diabetes insipidus. This can be done with attention to physiologic principles.

If a patient with increased fluid intake excretes large quantities of dilute urine free of glucose, there are two major possibilities: First, the patient may be primarily ingesting large quantities of fluid, and the diluting mechanisms of the kidney may be operating to protect plasma osmolality by excreting maximally dilute urine. Second, the kidneys may be losing water inappropriately, raising plasma tonicity and stimulating the thirst mechanism to increase water intake. If the first circumstance exists, plasma osmolality would be low normal or low, reducing the stimulus to antidiuretic hormone release. In the second circumstance the plasma osmolality would be high normal or high, stimulating antidiuretic hormone release. In this second circumstance the lack of urine concentration would result from a defect in antidiuretic hormone production or release (central diabetes insipidus), or, if antidiuretic hormone release is adequate, from renal insensitivity to antidiuretic hormone action (nephrogenic diabetes insipidus). The difficulty in distinguishing between psychogenic polydipsia and either form of diabetes insipidus occurs when the plasma osmolality is within the normal range. To differentiate between these conditions the patient should be denied access to water and observed carefully. In the patient with psychogenic polydipsia, water deprivation sufficient to raise the serum osmolality to above normal will release antidiuretic hormone and result in urine more concentrated than the plasma as the kidney responds to the secreted antidiuretic hormone. If the plasma osmolality does not rise to above normal, failure to concentrate the urine may simply reflect inadequate stimulation of antidiuretic hormone release. If the plasma osmolality rises above normal and the urine is not concentrated, the administration of exogenous antidiuretic hormone should result in urinary concentration in patients with central diabetes insipidus but should have little effect if the patient has nephrogenic diabetes insipidus.

The ability to measure plasma concentrations of antidiuretic hormone has improved the diagnostic accuracy of differentiating causes of polyuria. Patients with psychogenic polydipsia will have low plasma concentrations of antidiuretic hormone that can be raised by dehydration. Patients with central diabetes insipidus will have low plasma concentrations of antidiuretic hormone that are not raised by dehydration. Patients with nephrogenic diabetes insipidus will have plasma concentrations of antidiuretic hormone appropriate for the plasma osmolality, but will have an inadequate renal response to the hormone.

States of partial diabetes insipidus exist in which the concentration of the urine to levels equal to or greater than plasma tonicity may occur. In central partial diabetes insipidus, exogenous antidiuretic hormone may produce further concentration of the urine. In patients with central partial diabetes insipidus there may be an initial rise in urine osmolality during dehydration and then a fall as endogenous antidiuretic

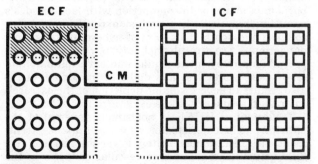

Figure 25. Hypertonicity due to pure water loss. Loss of water concentrates all impermeant solutes. Both ECF and ICF contract, and ECF volume remains half that of ICF because there is no change in solute content of the two compartments. Note that only 1/12 of the total volume loss is incurred by the intravascular compartment. In this and subsequent figures, dotted lines indicate the normal volumes of the body fluid compartments, as shown in Figure 24. (From Feig, P. U., and McCurdy, D. K.: The hypertonic state. N Engl J Med 297:1444, 1977.)

hormone is exhausted and a partial defect becomes expressed as a complete one.

Nephrogenic diabetes insipidus may occur because of inability of the tubule to create or sustain a hypertonic medullary interstitium, or because the collecting duct does not become appropriately permeable to water. The collecting duct may have reduced water permeability because of anatomic lesions such as amyloidosis or sickle cell infarction of the papilla, chemical alterations in permeability such as hypokalemia or hypercalcemia, toxin-induced injuries of the collecting duct such as methoxyflurane or outdated tetracycline, the lack of antidiuretic hormone effect because of a defective antidiuretic hormone receptor as in X-linked nephrogenic diabetes insipidus, or because of interference with the translation of the reception of antidiuretic hormone into the sequence of biochemical events that increase water permeability, as occurs with demeclocycline or lithium.

The treatment of central diabetes insipidus is to replace antidiuretic hormone or, if the defect is partial, to potentiate antidiuretic hormone action pharmacologically, as with chlorpropamide. If the diabetes insipidus is nephrogenic, a search for causes that can be corrected may be followed by a program that reduces the osmotic load to be excreted. A diet relatively low in protein and with limited sodium intake will reduce the osmotic load to be excreted and thereby reduce urine volume. In addition, administration of a diuretic such as thiazide together with a low-salt diet will produce extracellular fluid volume contraction, resulting in enhanced proximal tubular reabsorption of salt and water and thus in reduced urine volume. In essence this program reduces the production of urea for excretion and reduces renal perfusion so that the volume of solute containing fluid reaching the diluting segment of the nephron is reduced. Consequently the volume of free water produced and excreted is reduced.

Sodium Intake with Water Loss

This combination of events occurs rarely and is usually physician induced. It occurs most commonly when a patient with fixed salt and water excretion receives intravenous fluids that have a higher concentration of sodium and less free water than is excreted. The resulting hypernatremia can be corrected by adjusting fluid therapy to provide less sodium and more water.

Water Loss Out of Proportion to Sodium Loss

Water loss disproportionate to sodium loss results in the most dangerous form of hyperosmolality. The pathophysiology can best be illustrated by the syndrome of hyperglycemic, hyperosmotic, nonketotic coma (HHNK) (Fig. 26).

Assume that, because of a deficiency of insulin or its action, glucose behaves as an obligate extracellular molecule. Since less insulin is required to prevent ketosis than to prevent hyperglycemia, the further assumption is that some insulin action is present. However, hyperosmolality itself may inhibit ketone production, and the status of insulin lack remains controversial. In any event, glucose accumulates in the extracellular fluid, shifting water from the intracellular to the extracellular fluid. The initial effect is a fall

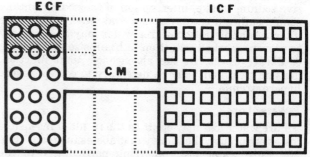

Figure 26. Hypertonicity due to hypotonic loss. Loss of hypotonic fluid from ECF (in this case with about a third of the normal ECF concentration) causes severe ECF and intravascular volume contraction. Note that although the total volume loss is only 50 per cent more than with pure water loss (Fig. 25), ECF and intravascular volume contraction exceed that in Figure 25 by 150 per cent. The ICF volume contraction and the degree of hypertonicity (density of symbols) are identical. (From Feig, P. U., and McCurdy, D. K.: The hypertonic state. N Engl J Med 297:1451, 1977.)

in intracellular fluid volume and a rise in extracellular fluid volume. The glucose concentration in the extracellular fluid is elevated, and the extracellular fluid sodium concentration falls acutely. The acutely expanded extracellular fluid with the elevated glucose concentration delivers a load of glucose for reabsorption to the proximal tubule that exceeds the tubular maximum for glucose and initiates an osmotic diuresis. As will be discussed under diuretics, osmotic diuresis results in the loss of urine, which approaches one-half normal saline (approximately 70 mEq/l of sodium). The urine losses can be conceptualized as equivalent to the loss of equal volumes of isotonic saline and of free water. The loss of isotonic saline will contract the extracellular fluid, and the loss of water will raise the tonicity of the body fluids. As this process proceeds, the initially expanded extracellular fluid is first reduced to normal volume and then becomes absolutely contracted. When the contraction of the extracellular fluid becomes severe enough, the GFR falls and renal losses of glucose are reduced, worsening the hyperglycemia. This vicious cycle of events proceeds until hypovolemia alone, or in conjunction with lactic acidosis resulting from tissue hypoperfusion, results in vascular collapse and death. This form of hypertonicity is most dangerous, since it results not only in water loss shared proportionally by intracellular and extracellular fluid (as in pure water loss and diabetes insipidus), but it also results in severe volume depletion of the extracellular fluid secondary to the osmotic diuresis.

Treatment of HHNK is not simply reversal of the pathophysiologic defects, for, as we will discuss, treatment with insulin may acutely lower the extracellular fluid volume and precipitate vascular collapse. In the patient with severe HHNK and poorly maintained blood pressure, treatment must be directed first at expanding the extracellular fluid and stabilizing the blood pressure. Such treatment would dictate the use of isotonic salt, colloid, or even whole blood rather than the hypotonic salt solution that will ultimately be required for correction of the hypertonicity. In addition, insulin therapy, which is necessary to lower the blood sugar, will facilitate the movement of glucose into cells, where it will be metabolized. Since the osmotically active glucose will be leaving the extracellular fluid and since glucose may be an important contributor to extracellular fluid osmolality and thus volume, shifts of glucose into cells and its ultimate metabolism will result in movement of water from the extracellular fluid into the intracellular fluid and in further contraction of extracellular fluid volume. If insulin is given before volume is expanded, disastrous shifts from extracellular fluid to intracellular fluid may occur. Treatment is directed at stabilizing the extracellular fluid volume and blood pressure, and then lowering plasma glucose while replacing hypotonic salt losses. During the final phases of therapy, adequate quantities of free water must be provided to permit correction of hypernatremia.

HYPONATREMIA

Hyponatremia, as defined by a serum sodium concentration of less than 136 mEq/l, may occur with an increased, decreased, or normal volume of extracellular fluid. Hyponatremia usually indicates decreased body fluid tonicity. However, there are several circumstances in which the low serum sodium concentration is factitious or represents a redistribution of water without a fall in tonicity.

Factitious Hyponatremia

The true concentration of sodium in plasma water is the concentration of sodium per unit volume of plasma divided by the percentage of plasma that is water: approximately 93 per cent. Since the percentage of plasma composed of water varies very little under normal circumstances, sodium concentrations are expressed per liter of plasma or serum without correction. With marked hyperlipidemia or hyperproteinemia, the percentage of plasma volume composed of water falls as does the measured serum sodium concentration. Despite the low concentration of sodium per liter of plasma, the concentration in plasma water is normal, as is plasma osmolality.

Recognition of factitious hyponatremia is aided by observing serum lactescence and by measuring the serum protein concentration. It is confirmed by correcting for the percentage of plasma as water and by determining that plasma osmolality is normal. No treatment is required for the apparent hyponatremia.

TABLE 2. HELPFUL CLINICAL FINDINGS IN THE ASSESSMENT OF THE TOTAL BODY SODIUM CONTENT

VOLUME OVERLOAD	VOLUME CONTRACTION
1. Presence of peripheral edema and/or ascites	1. Absence of peripheral edema and ascites
2. Distended neck veins	2. Collapsed neck veins
3. Normal skin turgor	3. Diminished skin turgor
4. Normal axillary sweat	4. Absence of axillary sweat
5. Signs of congestive heart failure	5. Resting or orthostatic tachycardia and hypotension

From DeFronzo, R. A., and Thier, S. O.: Pathophysiologic approach to hyponatremia. Arch Intern Med 140:900, 1980. Copyright 1980, American Medical Association.

Redistribution of Water

The addition of a non-sodium, osmotically active substance to the extracellular fluid produces an osmotic gradient that favors the movement of water from intracellular fluid to extracellular fluid. As the extracellular fluid volume increases by the addition of water, the serum sodium concentration falls. Despite the fall in the serum sodium concentration, plasma osmolality is normal or slightly increased. In contrast to factitious hyponatremia, however, the true concentration of sodium in plasma water is decreased. The most common causes of redistribution of water are hyperglycemia and the administration of mannitol. Treatment is reduction of the plasma glucose concentration or removal of mannitol.

If hyponatremia is neither factitious nor explained by redistribution of water, it should be defined as existing with hypervolemia, hypovolemia, or euvolemia. The status of the extracellular fluid volume can be assessed by examining the patient for evidence of altered skin turgor, postural hypotension, edema, neck vein distension, axillary sweat, and so on (Table 2). Measurement of urinary osmolality and urine sodium, blood urea nitrogen, and serum creatinine concentrations will provide additional useful information (Table 3).

Increased Extracellular Fluid

The hyponatremia seen with edematous states is almost always associated with increased total body sodium, as well as increased total body water. Congestive heart failure, cirrhosis, and nephrotic syndrome are the most common causes of hyponatremia and

TABLE 3. PATHOPHYSIOLOGIC APPROACH TO THE DIAGNOSIS OF HYPONATREMIA

	URINE SODIUM	URINE OSM	BUN	TREATMENT
I. INCREASED EXTRACELLULAR FLUID (Cirrhosis, Nephrosis, Congestive Heart Failure)	↓	↑ → ISO	N → ↑	Sodium and Water Restriction
II. DECREASED EXTRACELLULAR FLUID				
A. Nonrenal Loss (Gastrointestinal, Skin)	↓	↑ → ISO	N → ↑	
B. Renal Loss (Diuretics, Renal Disease, Addison's Disease)	↑	ISO	N → ↑	Isotonic NaCl
III. NORMAL EXTRACELLULAR FLUID				
A. SIADH	↑	↑	↓	Water Restriction
B. "Reset Osmostat"	Variable	Variable	N	Treat Underlying Disease

From DeFronzo, R. A., and Thier, S. O.: Pathophysiologic approach to hyponatremia. Arch Intern Med 140:899, 1980. Copyright 1980, American Medical Association.

edema. The term *decreased effective circulating plasma volume* has been used to explain the development of hyponatremia and edema. What this term really means is that, despite an expanded extracellular fluid volume, the kidneys behave as though hypoperfused; that is, the kidneys retain sodium and concentrate the urine. With hypoalbuminemia of cirrhosis or the nephrotic syndrome there may be a true contraction of intravascular volume, but that is rarely the case in congestive heart failure. In congestive heart failure, renal perfusion may be altered as the result of diminished cardiac output or of redistribution of renal blood flow.

The result is a urine sodium concentration that is usually less than 10 mEq/l and urine osmolality higher than plasma osmolality. Concentration of the urine is the result of a decreased urine flow rate, increased water reabsorption, and the concentration of urine about nonsodium solute. There may also be excessive release of antidiuretic hormone in response to nonosmolar stimuli.

If renal perfusion falls sufficiently to limit the delivery of sodium chloride to the ascending limb of Henle's loop, the medullary interstitial gradient will be dissipated and isosthenuria will result. The presence of isosthenuria with a low urine sodium concentration implies prolonged or severe renal hypoperfusion and is a warning that acute renal failure may ensue. Interpretation of urinary electrolytes and osmolality requires that the patient not have received diuretics.

Though the blood urea nitrogen concentration may be normal early in the states of hyponatremia and edema, it will rise out of proportion to the serum creatinine concentration with prolonged renal hypoperfusion.

The treatment of hyponatremia and edema is the restriction of salt and water intake, correction of congestive heart failure, stimulation of albumin synthesis, and reduction of albumin loss. If congestive heart failure or hypoalbuminemia cannot be corrected, correction of the serum sodium concentration will have little effect on the long-term clinical course of the patient.

Acute water intoxication is a special circumstance in which hyponatremia with a normal total body sodium content and an expanded intracellular fluid and extracellular fluid volume develop on the basis of water intake. Acute water intoxication occurs when the ingestion of water exceeds the ability of the kidney to excrete free water. This circumstance may occur with only a modest increase in water intake in a patient who has severe chronic renal failure and a GFR that limits water excretion. It can also occur in the presence of a normal GFR if the rate of water ingestion exceeds the normal kidney's ability to produce free water (15 to 20 ml/min). Note that an individual excreting 20 ml/min of water could excrete 1200 ml of free water per hour, or more than 25 liters per day. The capacity to excrete 25 liters of water per day is misleading in discussions of acute water intoxication. If a patient, in fact, ingests several liters in one to two hours, that intake will easily exceed the maximum excretory rate and result in water retention and acute hyponatremia.

Decreased Extracellular Fluid

Hyponatremia may occur with decreased extracellular fluid volume secondary to renal or nonrenal losses of sodium.

The renal losses of sodium most commonly occur as the result of diuretic use. Diuretics may produce impaired free water excretion by several mechanisms. First, diuretics such as furosemide, ethacrynic acid, mercurials, and thiazides interfere with sodium chloride reabsorption in the diluting segments of the tubule, thereby impairing free water production. Second, any diuretic resulting in negative sodium balance produces a contraction of the extracellular fluid volume and renal hypoperfusion. The extracellular fluid volume contraction enhances proximal tubule sodium reabsorption, and decreased quantities of solute and fluid are then delivered to the distal diluting sites. The result is impaired free water production. Third, diuretics that produce severe hypokalemia have been reported to alter osmoreceptor response to changes in the tonicity and to permit release of antidiuretic hormone at inappropriately low serum tonicities. Finally, it is possible that diuretics such as the thiazides may potentiate the action of antidiuretic hormone.

Renal sodium loss is also seen with renal disease, particularly tubulointerstitial diseases. In these patients, impairment of function of the diluting segment of the tubule and disruption of the normal architecture of the medullary interstitium lead to an inability to generate adequate quantities of free water.

Patients with mineralocorticoid deficiency, as in Addison's disease, develop negative sodium balance. The contraction of the extracellular fluid leads to increased reabsorption of sodium chloride in the proximal tubule and is also associated with increased nonosmotic release of antidiuretic hormone. The result is impaired ability to generate free water and antidiuretic hormone-stimulated retention of water. The hyponatremia that is seen with glucocorticoid lack differs from that seen with mineralocorticoid lack in being associated with a normal or slightly increased extracellular fluid volume. The mechanism of glucocorticoid-lack hyponatremia will be discussed in the section on normovolemic hyponatremia.

Hyponatremia may also be associated with nonrenal salt wasting. Sodium may be lost through the gastrointestinal tract, through the skin as in burns, or into loculated internal areas as in pancreatitis, peritonitis, or trauma. Regardless of the route of nonrenal sodium loss, the result is a decrease in extracellular fluid volume and thus renal hypoperfusion. With renal hypoperfusion, proximal tubular sodium reabsorption is enhanced, and there is decreased sodium delivery to the distal diluting sites. If extracellular fluid volume contraction is sufficiently severe, antidiuretic hormone will be released in response to a volume stimulus. The net result will be decreased ability to generate free water and increased reabsorption of free water.

Patients who have hyponatremia with a decreased extracellular fluid volume will have decreased skin turgor, postural hypotension and tachycardia, flat neck veins, and absence of edema. If the route of sodium loss was via the kidneys, the urinary sodium concentration will be high (greater than 20 to 30 mEq/l) and isosthenuria will be present, since the kidney will not be able to generate or maintain a maximally concentrated medullary interstitium. With very severe degrees of volume contraction the urine may actually become somewhat more concentrated than plasma (300 to 450 mOsm/kg). This modest urinary concentration is the result of passive back-diffusion of water with low urine flow rates, and antidiuretic hormone release in response to a hypovolemic stimulus. By the time these mechanisms have led to increased urinary concentration, postural hypotension will almost always be present, and the blood urea nitrogen concentration will likely be elevated out of proportion to the serum creatinine concentration. When the patient has hyponatremia from nonrenal sodium loss, the kidneys will respond appropriately to volume contraction. The urine sodium concentration will be low (less than 10 mEq/l), and the urine osmolality will be high (greater than 400 mOsm/kg). The blood urea nitrogen concentration may be normal initially, but, as with renal sodium losses, the BUN will rise out of proportion to the serum creatinine as renal hypoperfusion becomes more pronounced.

The treatment of hyponatremia with a decreased extracellular fluid is the reexpansion of the extracellular fluid with isotonic salt solutions. The anion accompanying the sodium and the need for potassium will be determined by the clinical setting. Needless to say, the underlying cause of sodium loss must be identified and corrected, or the sodium replacement will have to correct previous deficits and ongoing losses. Note also that when one is correcting hyponatremia due to renal sodium wasting there is potentially less leeway for error than in correcting the hyponatremia of nonrenal sodium loss. Just as the kidney was unable to retain sodium appropriately, it may be unable to excrete excesses of sodium if volume replacement is overly aggressive. The patient who has renal salt wasting should be assumed to be at greater risk for volume overload and should receive more cautious salt replacement.

Normal Extracellular Fluid

By far the most common cause of hyponatremia with a normal extracellular fluid volume is the inappropriate secretion of antidiuretic hormone. By definition, this syndrome exists when an individual with an apparently normal extracellular fluid volume on physical examination has, in spite of plasma hypotonicity, concentrated urine that contains high concentrations of sodium unexplained by renal disease or mineralocorticoid lack. The sequence of events leading to this picture begins with the excessive production and release of antidiuretic hormone activity. In the presence of antidiuretic hormone activity, ingested free water is retained, expanding the extracellular fluid and intracellular fluid volumes slightly and beginning the process of dilution of the serum sodium concentration. The expanded extracellular fluid volume results in an increased GFR and the reduced reabsorption of sodium in the proximal tubule. The extracellular fluid volume expansion also reduces aldosterone secretion so that the increased quantities of sodium delivered out of the proximal tubule escape reabsorption in the distal nephron. The result is natriuresis occurring at the same time that free water is being retained. The net result is the development of severe hyponatremia, while the urine contains large quantities of sodium and is concentrated to levels above plasma osmolality.

An examination of the patient with the syndrome of inappropriate antidiuretic hormone secretion will reveal no obvious changes in extracellular fluid volume status. That the extracellular fluid volume is slightly expanded and that the GFR is elevated is attested to by the fact that the BUN concentration is frequently low (less than 10 mg/dl) and that other materials reabsorbed in the proximal tubule such as uric acid and phosphate are often reduced in concentration in the plasma of these patients. The urinary osmolality of these individuals will almost invariably be higher than the plasma osmolality and will never be maximally diluted. Urinary sodium concentration is elevated during the development of this syndrome and during periods of increased water ingestion. Steady states may develop in patients with the syndrome of inappropriate antidiuretic hormone, during which the urinary sodium excretion will reflect sodium intake and may be low.

Treatment of the syndrome of inappropriate antidiuretic hormone secretion requires definition of the cause of increased antidiuretic hormone activity. Antidiuretic hormone activity may be increased because of (1) excessive production or release of antidiuretic hormone or of an antidiuretic hormone-related material by tumor, (2) the excessive pituitary release of antidiuretic hormone, (3) the potentiation of the action of normal levels of antidiuretic hormone, or (4) the presence of a non-antidiuretic hormone substance that stimulates tubular water reabsorption. If the mechanism underlying the syndrome can be identified and treated, the abnormalities of free water excretion will be corrected. Whether or not the underlying mechanism can be treated, the patient will respond to restriction of free water intake and the administration of salt ad libitum. Recently a series of drugs that interfere with the action of antidiuretic hormone on the collecting duct has been proposed as treatment for the syndrome of inappropriate antidiuretic hormone. Thus, demeclocycline and lithium may produce a nephrogenic diabetes insipidus and inhibit the effect of increased antidiuretic hormone activity on the tubule. Finally, if the degree of hyponatremia is severe enough to produce CNS dysfunction in a patient in whom further extracellular volume expansion is a risk, it may be necessary to administer a diuretic such as furosemide. Furosemide interferes with the production of a concentrated medullary interstitium, thereby limiting free water reabsorption, and additionally enhancing urinary sodium loss. If measured urinary sodium losses are then replaced with hypertonic salt solution, the serum sodium concentration can be raised without risking dangerous expansion of the extracellular fluid.

A similar picture of hyponatremia with normal extracellular fluid volume is seen with glucocorticoid lack. With glucocorticoid lack a pattern of hyponatremia in association with increased urinary sodium concentration and less than maximally dilute urine osmolality is the rule. There is evidence of abnormal release of antidiuretic hormone in patients with glucocorticoid lack. Patients with glucocorticoid lack may appear in every way similar to those patients with the syndrome of inappropriate antidiuretic hormone secretion. The difference is that the administration of glucocorticoid to patients with glucocorticoid lack will result in prompt dilution of the urine and correction of the hyponatremia.

Finally, there is a population of patients with hyponatremia and normal extracellular fluid volume who suffer from chronic debilitating diseases. These patients rarely develop severe degrees of hyponatremia. They behave as do normal individuals in diluting and concentrating urine and in excreting and retaining sodium. The difference is that their serum osmolality seems to be set at a lower level than the normal. These individuals are said to have a reset osmostat. The reset osmostat will improve with correction of the underlying debilitating disease. The level of hyponatremia that develops under these circumstances rarely requires direct treatment.

Acid-Base

Acid-base homeostasis, the regulation of hydrogen ion concentration, is the result of three finely integrated systems: (1) the chemical buffers of the body, (2) the respiratory system, and (3) the kidneys.

Much of the confusion encountered in discussions of acid-base pathophysiology results from the use of different vocabularies to describe normal physiology and particularly to describe clinical acid-base disturbances. To provide a solid foundation for the analysis of the pathophysiology of acid-base disturbances, we will review normal physiology briefly and then develop the terminology for discussion of clinical acid-base disturbances.

HYDROGEN ION CONCENTRATION

Though it would be easier to describe hydrogen ion concentration as nanomoles (nM) per liter, convention dictates the use of pH in discussion of acid-base physiology. The pH is the negative logarithm of the hydrogen ion concentration. Therefore the pH scale is logarithmic and not linear, as would be a scale of hydrogen ion concentration. Hence, minor changes in pH may reflect large changes in hydrogen ion concentration, and equal changes in pH units above and below a mean will not reflect equal changes in hydrogen ion concentration. The normal pH of extracellular fluid ranges from 7.36 (44 nM) to 7.44 (36 nM) with a mean of 7.40 (40 nM). The extremes of pH compatible with survival are 6.80 to 7.80.

Definitions

Acids and bases are defined according to the scheme of Brønsted and Lowry. An acid is a proton donor; a base is a proton acceptor that combines with hydrogen ion to form an acid.

$$\underset{\text{(acid)}}{HA} \leftrightarrows \underset{\text{(proton)}}{H^+} + \underset{\text{(base)}}{A^-}$$

The acid HA is the conjugate acid of A^-, and A^- is the conjugate base of HA.

Origins of Hydrogen Ion

Acidemia, increased hydrogen ion concentration, may be of metabolic or of respiratory origin.

Metabolic Origin

The daily production of hydrogen ion is enormous (10,000 to 15,000 millimoles). However, the vast majority of this hydrogen ion production results from cellular metabolism of carbon-containing compounds to CO_2 and water. Virtually all of this acid is excreted via the lungs, and thus no net acid retention occurs. Balance is maintained since the reaction of the released CO_2 to form hydrogen ion is

$$CO_2 + H_2O \leftrightarrows H_2CO_3 \leftrightarrows H^+ + HCO_3^-.$$

The process is then reversed to form the CO_2 that is excreted by the lungs. As long as the respiratory system is able to maintain a stable P_{CO_2} and thus a constant H_2CO_3 concentration, the rates of hydrogen ion release and fixation will be constant and no net change will occur in acid-base balance.

As most organic compounds are metabolized to CO_2 and water, their metabolism does not alter acid-base status. If, however, the metabolism of an organic compound does not proceed completely to CO_2 and water, excess hydrogen ion may accumulate. This accumulation may occur in at least three ways. First, a metabolic pathway may lead to the production of an organic acid such as lactic acid. Though it might ordinarily be metabolized completely to CO_2 and water, in the presence of hypoxemia lactic acid will accumulate. Second, an organic acid formed as part of a metabolic process may be buffered by sodium bicarbonate, consuming bicarbonate and producing the sodium salt of the acid anion. If the anion of the acid is lost in the urine or stool before it can be metabolized via a pathway that would consume a hydrogen ion, the net result will be equal to the retention of a hydrogen ion. Third, if the organic acid produced is a compound such as uric acid, which is a metabolic cul-de-sac, there is no opportunity for further metabolism, and hydrogen ion accumulates. In the first circumstance, that of the production of lactic acid, ultimate metabolism of the organic compound to CO_2 and water may restore hydrogen ion balance. In the latter two circumstances—that is, the loss of the anion of the acid or the production of an acid in a metabolic cul-de-sac—the net production of acid can be balanced only by hydrogen ion excretion.

Thus, under normal circumstances, metabolism of organic compounds to CO_2 and water produces no net change in hydrogen ion concentration. In disease states, failure to metabolize compounds completely to CO_2 and water or the loss of the anion from incompletely metabolized organic acids may result in large excesses of hydrogen ion.

The acid produced as CO_2 is referred to as volatile acid in that it may be excreted via the lungs. Fixed acid production refers to nonvolatile acids, which must be excreted via the kidneys. The net production of fixed acid is normally about 1 mEq/kg/24 hours. There are three major sources of fixed acid hydrogen ions. First, there is the incomplete metabolism of neutral organic precursors to CO_2 and water, which was discussed above. Second, there is the oxidative catabolism of sulfur-containing amino acids, such as methionine and cysteine, to sulfuric acid. Finally, there is the hydrolysis of phosphate linkages of proteins to phosphoric acid. The last two sources of acid production are the basis of the correct prediction that diets high in protein and clinical processes that are highly catabolic will be acidifying. ·

Respiratory Control of Hydrogen Ion

The respiratory system regulates the partial pressure of CO_2 in body fluids. The amount of CO_2 in solution in blood is calculated by multiplying P_{CO_2} by the solubility coefficient for CO_2 (0.03). This calculation yields the normal dissolved CO_2 concentration of approximately 1.2 mM. The result of hypoventilation from any cause is described by the equation $CO_2 + H_2O \rightarrow H_2CO_3 \rightarrow H^+ + HCO_3^-$. The rise in H_2CO_3 as part of CO_2 retention produces an increase in hydrogen ion concentration.

ORIGINS OF BASE

We have emphasized the production of hydrogen ion from both metabolic and respiratory sources, since acid production under physiologic circumstances is quantitatively much more important than base production. Alkali production will be discussed in greater detail in the section on pathophysiology. However, it is worth noting that when a neutral organic compound is metabolized to a charged anion a hydrogen ion is formed, and when a charged anion is metabolized to CO_2 and water the hydrogen ion is fixed. This latter circumstance predicts that increased quantities of sodium citrate or lactate in the diet may have the effect of adding alkali to the system, that is, the metabolism of citrate or lactate will require that hydrogen ion be removed from solution, leaving behind a hydroxyl ion. This is the same principle that explains why hydrogen ion accumulated as the result of incomplete metabolism of organic compounds will be consumed if those compounds are subsequently completely metabolized to CO_2 and water. It should also be obvious that just as hypoventilation leading to the retention of CO_2 will raise the concentration of carbonic acid, hyperventilation with the excretion of CO_2 will lower carbonic acid and thus hydrogen ion concentration.

BUFFERS

Alterations in hydrogen ion concentration will initially be attenuated by the body buffer systems. These buffer systems will dampen but not prevent a change in pH. The change in pH will trigger subsequent respiratory and renal responses.

A buffer system is a solution of a weak acid and its conjugate base. There are both extracellular and intracellular buffers. The major buffer system of the extracellular fluid is the carbonic acid/bicarbonate system. Lesser contributions to extracellular buffering come from phosphate and protein buffers. Intracellular buffering within the vascular space is predominantly a function of hemoglobin within red cells. The hemoglobin buffers may account for one-third of whole blood buffering. In other cells, phosphate and protein buffers are most important. There is also a large reservoir of

buffering capacity in the crystalline structure of bone. It appears that bone provides an enormous reservoir of buffer that can be used in states of chronic acid retention. Buffering by bone does not play an important role in acute acid-base disturbances.

A discussion of buffer systems requires an understanding of the Henderson-Hasselbalch equation.

According to the law of mass action, for the reaction

$$HA \leftrightarrows H^+ + A^-$$

the relationship exists

$$\frac{[H^+][A^-]}{[HA]} = K.$$

Strong acids are almost completely ionized, weak acids only partially so. Therefore, the greater the concentration of H^+ and A^- necessary to satisfy the equation, the stronger the acid.

The equation can now be rearranged to read

$$[H^+] = K \frac{[HA]}{[A^-]}.$$

This equation would suffice for calculations using hydrogen ion concentration in nanomoles. However, to develop the equation for use of pH we must first take the logarithm of the equation

$$\log[H^+] = \log K + \log \frac{[HA]}{[A^-]}.$$

Multiplying by -1:

$$-\log[H^+] = -\log K + \log \frac{[A^-]}{[HA]}.$$

We have defined pH as the negative logarithm of the hydrogen ion concentration ($-\log[H^+]$). We will define $-\log K$ as the pK. The pK will be seen to equal the pH of a solution in which an acid is 50 per cent ionized. The pK will be characteristic for each acid, and the lower the pK the stronger the acid. By applying our definitions of pH and pK, we now have the Henderson-Hasselbalch equation:

$$pH = pK + \log \frac{[A^-]}{[HA]}.$$

From the Henderson-Hasselbalch equation it should become obvious that buffer systems are most efficient at a pH that equals their pK. When the pH equals the pK, the acid is 50 per cent ionized and $[A^-] = [HA]$. Any addition of H^+ or OH^- will change the ratio of $\frac{[A^-]}{[HA]}$ least when they are at equal concentrations. For example, note what would happen if the concentration of A^- were 50 mM and the concentration of HA were also 50 mM, and we added sufficient hydrogen ion to titrate the concentration of A^- by 10 mM. We would now have 40 mM A^- and 60 mM HA, or a ratio of 0.67 rather than 1.0. The change in pH would be the change from the log of 1.0 to the log of 0.67. If, on the other hand, we started with 20 mM A^- and 80 mM HA, or a ratio of 0.25, and added the same amount of acid, we would have a final concentration of 10 mM A^- and 90 mM HA, or a ratio of approximately 0.11. In the first example, the pH would have fallen 0.18 unit. In the second circumstance the pH would have fallen 0.35 unit for the same amount of acid added. The relationship of the efficiency of a buffer system to the pK of the acid holds for a closed system. A closed system is one in which the addition of hydrogen ion, for example, will raise the concentration of acid and lower the concentration of its conjugate base to exactly the same extent. In an open system the concentration of acid and its conjugate base may be varied independently.

CO_2/Bicarbonate Buffer System

The carbonic acid/bicarbonate buffer system is defined by the Henderson-Hasselbalch equation as

$$pH = 3.5 + \log \frac{[HCO_3^-]}{[H_2CO_3]}.$$

However, H_2CO_3 is in equilibrium with dissolved CO_2, which is in equilibrium with CO_2 gas. Taking these other equilibria into account, a more useful form of the Henderson-Hasselbalch equation to describe the CO_2/bicarbonate buffer system is:

$$pH = 6.1 + \log \frac{[HCO_3^-]}{0.03 \times P_{CO_2}}.$$

If this were a closed system any increase in hydrogen ion would decrease the concentration of bicarbonate, increase the concentration of carbonic acid by a similar amount, and lower pH. As bicarbonate concentration is increased, hydrogen ion would be taken up and pH would rise. These changes are perhaps easier to visualize by returning to the simple equation for hydrogen ion concentration:

$$[H^+] = K \frac{[H_2CO_3]}{[HCO_3^-]}.$$

Clearly an increase in HCO_3^- concentration will result in a lowering of hydrogen ion concentration. The CO_2/bicarbonate buffer system operates to donate a hydrogen ion when hydrogen ion concentration falls and to accept hydrogen ions when the hydrogen ion concentration rises.

Recall that we discussed that a buffer system is most efficient operating at or near its pK. If the CO_2/bicarbonate buffer (pK 6.1) were operating as a closed system, then at the physiologic pH of 7.4 it might buffer acid loads well, but it would be a poor buffer for alkali loads. Fortunately the CO_2/bicarbonate buffer system is an open system; the concentrations of CO_2 and HCO_3^- can be varied independently. CO_2 is regulated by the respiratory system and HCO_3^- by kidneys.

Phosphate and Protein Buffers

The phosphate buffer system potentially has three pK's. For the system utilizing $\frac{H_2PO_4^-}{H_3PO_4}$ the pK is 2, for the $\frac{HPO_4^=}{H_2PO_4^-}$ system the pK is 6.8, and for the $\frac{PO_4^\equiv}{HPO_4^=}$ system the pK is 11.8. Under physiologic conditions

the $\frac{HPO_4^=}{H_2PO_4^-}$ system with a pK of 6.8 is most important. At a pH of 7.4 there will be 4 molecules of $HPO_4^=$ for every molecule of $H_2PO_4^-$. The protein buffers play an important role in the intracellular fluid and a modest role in the extracellular fluid. Proteins may have several dissociating groups on a single molecule, and therefore will have an apparent pK that is a function of all of the pK's of the dissociating groups that operate in the physiologic range.

In biologic fluids, particularly in intracellular fluids, there are numerous buffer systems with varying pK's. The titration of a biologic fluid, then, is a complex titration of numerous buffers simultaneously. Without dissecting the various components of the buffering systems, one refers to the apparent pK of intracellular buffers, for example.

The CO_2/bicarbonate buffer system is by far the most important buffer of the extracellular fluid. Proteins and phosphates are most important in the intracellular fluid. At pH 7.4 approximately 50 per cent of a fixed acid load will be buffered extracellularly and 50 per cent in the intracellular fluid. An alkali load, on the other hand, will be buffered approximately two-thirds in the extracellular fluid and one-third in the intracellular fluid. The more efficient buffering of alkali in the extracellular fluid suggests that the apparent pK of the extracellular fluid buffers is higher than the apparent pK of the intracellular buffers. If this conclusion is correct, progressively higher percentages of acid loads should be buffered intracellularly as the pH of body fluids falls. In fact, progressively larger percentages of an acid load are buffered within cells as the pH falls; intracellular buffers may account for 80 per cent or more of buffering capacity at low pH's.

Buffering of CO_2

The CO_2/bicarbonate buffering system of the extracellular fluid and its related intracellular buffers are the primary buffers of fixed acid and fixed base. They are not very effective in buffering changes originating within the CO_2/bicarbonate system. The major site of buffering of CO_2 is the red blood cell, and its major buffer is hemoglobin. The red cell hemoglobin buffering system is particularly suited to deal with CO_2, since the red cells are highly permeable to CO_2 and contain high concentrations of carbonic anhydrase, the enzyme that hydrates CO_2 to H_2CO_3. CO_2 is buffered by diffusing into red cells, where it is hydrated to H_2CO_3 and then dissociates to H^+ plus HCO_3^-. The H^+ combines with Hb^- to form HHb. The HCO_3^- diffuses out of the cell in exchange for chloride. The result is that retained CO_2 is buffered and bicarbonate is released into the blood in exchange for chloride. Thus, in states of CO_2 retention, both H_2CO_3 and HCO_3^- rise. The reversal of these events occurs with hyperventilation.

Most fixed acids are strong acids; they are essentially completely ionized at body fluid pH and must be buffered immediately to prevent a rapid fall in pH. The total buffer stores available to deal with an acute fixed acid load are only 12 to 15 mEq/kg of body weight. In chronic acidemia the alkaline calcium salts of bone, which represent an enormous reservoir, may be utilized. Skeletal buffers do not play an important role in protecting against an acute acid load. When a fixed acid is buffered in the extracellular fluid, the reaction

$$HA + NaHCO_3 \rightarrow NaA + CO_2 + water$$

takes place, then the CO_2 is excreted by the lungs. This reaction consumes HCO_3^-. The normal daily production of fixed acid would consume the readily available buffer pool in less than two weeks if there were no mechanism for regenerating buffers. The kidneys play the major role in regeneration of buffer stores.

We have now outlined the relations of the key systems in the maintenance of acid-base homeostasis. The buffers mitigate but do not prevent the change in pH. The change in pH that occurs with, for example, an increase in fixed hydrogen ion concentration will stimulate the respiratory center to excrete CO_2 and will initiate the processes of hydrogen ion excretion and bicarbonate regeneration in the kidney.

RESPIRATORY CONTRIBUTION TO ACID-BASE REGULATION

This subject is discussed in far greater detail in the section on the lungs. The essential facts for a discussion of clinical disorders of acid-base homeostasis are the following: When a fixed acid is buffered by bicarbonate in the extracellular fluid, the CO_2 produced will be eliminated by the lungs. An increase in hydrogen ion concentration will reduce the concentration of bicarbonate in the blood, and will stimulate the respiratory center to increase the excretion of CO_2. The respiratory response will lower blood carbonic acid content and partially correct the metabolic acidosis. In states in which the hydrogen ion concentration is lowered and the serum bicarbonate concentration rises, respiration will be depressed and CO_2 will be retained. The retained CO_2 will raise the concentration of carbonic acid and partially correct for the elevated bicarbonate concentration.

The respiratory responses just described are the normal responses to altered pH. The respiratory system may contribute primarily to abnormalities of pH by either failing to excrete CO_2 or excreting CO_2 too rapidly. Hypoventilation will lead to

$$CO_2 + H_2O \rightarrow H_2CO_3 \rightarrow HCO_3^- + H^+.$$

Thus the retention of CO_2 results in a rise in hydrogen ion concentration. During hyperventilation

$$H^+ + HCO_3^- \rightarrow H_2CO_3 \rightarrow H_2O + CO_2.$$

Under these circumstances hydrogen ion is removed from body fluids and excreted via the lungs. Primary respiratory abnormalities of acid-base status are buffered largely by intracellular buffers and trigger renal responses that will be discussed in greater detail under the clinical abnormalities of acid-base balance.

RENAL REGULATION OF HYDROGEN ION SECRETION

The kidneys have the capacity to accomplish the net excretion of hydrogen ions or of bicarbonate as required to return body fluid pH to 7.4 and to regenerate the store of body buffers. Three major processes are involved in renal regulation of hydrogen ion secretion. First is bicarbonate reabsorption, second is the titration of urinary buffers, and third is the excretion of ammonium ion. All three processes result from the

active secretion of H^+, as shown in Figure 27. Whenever an H^+ is secreted from a tubular cell into the urine, an OH^- is formed within the cell. This OH^- combines with CO_2 to form intracellular HCO_3^-, a reaction catalyzed by the intracellular enzyme carbonic anhydrase in both the proximal and distal nephron. Exit of HCO_3^- from the cell across the basolateral membrane ultimately results in the addition of HCO_3^- to the blood. The H^+ secreted from the cell into the tubular fluid has three potential fates.

First (Fig. 27A), secreted H^+ can combine with intratubular HCO_3^- to form H_2CO_3, which dissociates into CO_2 and H_2O, a reaction that can also be catalyzed by carbonic anhydrase, which is present on the luminal membrane in the proximal but not the distal nephron. Thus, for each secreted H^+ combining with an intratubular HCO_3^-, there is the disappearance of one intratubular HCO_3^- and the addition of one HCO_3^- to the blood. The net result of this process is to reabsorb filtered bicarbonate.

Alternatively, secreted H^+ can combine with urinary buffers, of which the principal one is phosphate (Fig. 27B). For each secreted H^+ combining with HPO_4^{-2} to form $H_2PO_4^-$, there is the addition of one HCO_3^- into the peritubular blood. This additional bicarbonate is called new or regenerated bicarbonate, and replaces bicarbonate consumed in buffering fixed acid. Titration of urinary buffers such as phosphate is referred to as the titratable acidity of the urine. The titratable ac-

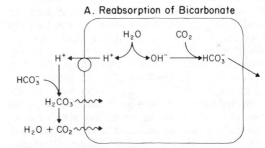

Figure 27. Processes resulting from active H^+ secretion along the nephron.

idity of the urine is measured as the amount of base necessary to return the urine to the pH of the glomerular filtrate (normally 7.4). It is equal to the amount of H^+ that was required to titrate urinary buffers (principally phosphate) from the pH of the glomerular filtrate to the pH in urine.

The third process resulting from H^+ secretion is the secretion of NH_4^+. Ammonia is produced in the cells of the proximal tubule, predominantly by removal of the amide nitrogen of glutamine. Additional ammonia may be derived from the amino group of glutamine, from asparagine, and to a lesser extent from the oxidative deamination of other amino acids. The ammonia produced exists as a nonionized gas, and, according to our earlier definitions, is a base. Ammonia can combine with H^+ to form ammonium according to the equation:

$$NH_3 + H^+ \leftrightarrows NH_4^+$$

The pK for this reaction is 9.3, so that at physiologic pH and below, the NH_4^+ form is favored. The nonionic form, NH_3, diffuses easily across cell membranes. NH_4^+ is far less permeant. Thus, when secreted H^+ combines with intratubular NH_3 to form NH_4^+ (Fig. 27C), it promotes the net secretion of ammonium. At any given rate of NH_3 production, the lower is the intratubular pH, the higher is the rate of NH_4^+ secretion. For each NH_4^+ added to the urine by this mechanism, one new or regenerated HCO_3^- is added to the blood.

Total renal H^+ secretion is the sum of the filtered bicarbonate that is reabsorbed, the titratable acid that is formed, and the NH_4^+ that is secreted. Net acid excretion, which represents the amount of new or regenerated HCO_3^- added to the blood by the kidney, is equal to the sum of the titratable acid and the urinary ammonium less any amount of urinary HCO_3^- that is excreted. Under normal conditions, this net acid excretion balances the loss of blood bicarbonate consumed in buffering fixed acids. Under some conditions the maintenance of acid-base balance requires the net loss of HCO_3^- from the body. Net alkali excretion by the kidney is accomplished to the extent that urinary HCO_3^- exceeds the sum of urinary titratable acid and urinary ammonium. Let us now examine the tubular mechanisms for H^+ and HCO_3^- transport in more detail.

Proximal Tubular H^+ Secretion

The principal mechanism for active H^+ secretion in the proximal tubule is a carrier-mediated process of Na^+ for H^+ exchange across the luminal membrane of the cell (Fig. 28, top). The inward Na gradient across the luminal membrane serves as the driving force for H^+ secretion via this mechanism. There is no direct input of metabolic energy. Thus, H^+ cannot be secreted uphill against a gradient that is any larger than the magnitude of the inward Na gradient. Because the inward Na gradient across the luminal membrane of the proximal tubular cell is probably no greater than 10-fold, at most a 1.0-unit pH gradient can be generated across this barrier.

The most abundant acceptor for secreted H^+ in the proximal tubule is the freely filtered HCO_3^-. Thus the major fraction of H^+ secretion in the proximal tubule is devoted to reabsorbing HCO_3^-. As tubular fluid pH and HCO_3^- concentration decline along the proximal

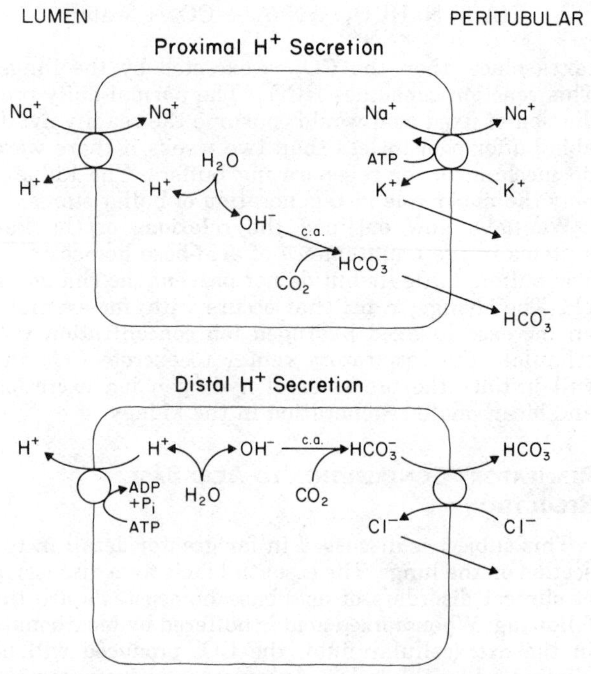

Figure 28. Cellular mechanisms of active H^+ secretion in the proximal and distal nephron.

tubule, the passive back leak of HCO_3^- from the peritubular interstitium into the tubular lumen across the leaky tight junction becomes more and more significant. As a result, the extent of acidification in the proximal tubule is determined by the balance between the process of HCO_3^- reabsorption across the cell and the process of passive HCO_3^- back leak between cells. To understand how proximal tubular HCO_3^- transport is regulated, it is useful to review the factors known to influence the processes of transcellular HCO_3^- reabsorption and paracellular HCO_3^- back leak.

The most important determinant of the rate of luminal membrane Na^+-H^+ exchange is intracellular pH. Intracellular H^+ is both a transportable substrate and an allosteric activator for this transport system. Thus, factors that lower intracellular pH stimulate the rate of proximal tubular HCO_3^- reabsorption, and those that elevate intracellular pH inhibit it. The rate of luminal membrane Na^+-H^+ exchange is also affected by changes in intratubular pH. Because intratubular H^+ acts as a competitive inhibitor of Na^+ binding to this transport system, the rate of H^+ secretion and HCO_3^- reabsorption is depressed when intratubular pH and HCO_3^- concentration are reduced, and stimulated when intratubular pH and HCO_3^- concentration are elevated. In the physiologic range of luminal HCO_3^- concentrations, a true tubular maximum (T_m) for bicarbonate reabsorption is not observed. The back leak of HCO_3^- from peritubular space into the tubular lumen is modulated by the same physical forces that govern the reabsorption of Na and fluid in the proximal tubule: When the Starling forces favoring water and solute uptake into the peritubular capillary are reduced, the back leak of HCO_3^- into the tubular lumen is enhanced; and when the forces favoring capillary uptake of water and solutes are increased, HCO_3^- back leak is inhibited.

With the above considerations in mind, let us briefly review the stimuli that regulate the delivery of HCO_3^-

out of the proximal tubule. When arterial P_{CO_2} is decreased, intracellular CO_2 decreases, intracellular pH increases, the rate of HCO_3^- reabsorption is inhibited, and the delivery of HCO_3^- out of the proximal tubule is enhanced. Conversely, when P_{CO_2} is elevated, proximal tubular excretion of HCO_3^- is depressed.

Raising the plasma HCO_3^- concentration increases the filtered load of HCO_3^-, an effect that stimulates HCO_3^- reabsorption. However, when the HCO_3^- concentration in the peritubular capillary is increased, passive HCO_3^- exit out of the proximal tubular cell is inhibited, and intracellular pH rises. The inhibitory effect of elevated cell pH prevents HCO_3^- reabsorption from rising sufficiently to match the increased filtered load. Thus, raising the plasma HCO_3^- concentration increases the delivery of HCO_3^- out of the proximal tubule, and lowering the plasma HCO_3^- concentration, by a converse series of events, depresses proximal tubular HCO_3^- excretion.

During extracellular fluid volume expansion, the glomerular filtration rate tends to increase, augmenting the filtered load of HCO_3^-. At the same time, the physical forces favoring capillary uptake of water and solutes become less favorable, thereby favoring tubular back leak of HCO_3^-. Accordingly, volume expansion promotes the delivery of HCO_3^- out of the proximal tubule. Conversely, volume contraction depresses HCO_3^- excretion by this nephron segment.

Hypokalemia reduces the delivery of HCO_3^- out of the proximal tubule. When extracellular K^+ concentration is reduced, passive K^+ exit out of the cell is enhanced. It has been suggested that this current of positive ions out of the cell promotes the passive exit of HCO_3^-, thereby lowering intracellular pH and stimulating the rate of H^+ secretion.

Carbonic anhydrase inhibitors such as acetazolamide elevate intracellular pH by blocking the buffering of intracellular OH^- with CO_2, and lower intratubular pH by blocking the disappearance of intratubular H_2CO_3 formed from H^+ and HCO_3^-. As a result, these drugs markedly inhibit HCO_3^- reabsorption and enhance HCO_3^- delivery out of the proximal tubule.

Finally, it should be mentioned that parathyroid hormone modestly increases HCO_3^- excretion by the proximal tubule, an effect due to a reduction in the number or activity of luminal membrane Na^+-H^+ exchangers. Mineralocorticoids have no direct effects on H^+ secretion in this portion of the nephron. There is little evidence to support the suggestion that Cl^- is an important determinant of proximal tubular HCO_3^- reabsorption.

Distal Nephron H$^+$ Secretion

Under normal conditions, the tubular fluid that exits the proximal tubule has a pH of approximately 6.8 and a HCO_3^- concentration of about 5 mM. The sum of the titratable acid and NH_4^+ in the tubular fluid at this point is almost equal to 5 mM. Thus there normally is neither net acid nor alkali excretion in the proximal tubule. In essence, the acidification process in the proximal tubule may be characterized as a large-capacity, small-gradient system whose principal function is to add to the blood the same number of bicarbonate ions as were filtered (about 4500 mEq/day). In contrast, the acidification process in the distal tubule, cortical collecting tubule, and collecting duct—the

other sites of significant H^+ secretion in the nephron—may be characterized as a small-capacity, large-gradient system whose principal function is to add to the blood the number of new bicarbonate ions required to replace those consumed in buffering fixed acid of dietary and metabolic origin (normally 70 to 100 mEq/day).

Acidification in the distal nephron occurs via an adenosine triphosphate (ATP)-driven proton pump (H^+-ATPase) located in the luminal membrane of the acid-secreting cells (Fig. 28, *bottom*). This pump is capable of generating a 3.0-unit pH gradient across the luminal membrane. Thus the minimum urinary pH that can be achieved along the distal nephron is approximately 4.4. For each H^+ secreted across the luminal membrane, an intracellular HCO_3^- is formed by the combination of OH^- with CO_2, a reaction catalyzed by intracellular carbonic anhydrase. Bicarbonate then exits the cell across the basolateral membrane in exchange for Cl^-, which leaks back out across the basolateral membrane passively.

Passive back leak of HCO_3^- into the tubular lumen is negligible along the distal nephron. However, some cells in the distal tubule and cortical collecting tubule have the capacity to secrete HCO_3^- actively. These cells extrude H^+ across the basolateral membrane, thereby forming intracellular HCO_3^-, which exits across the luminal membrane in exchange for intratubular Cl^-. The process of active HCO_3^- secretion is probably of significance only when the plasma HCO_3^- concentration is elevated. Under most circumstances, distal acidification is determined primarily by the rate and extent of active, transcellular H^+ secretion. Let us briefly review the factors known to influence this process.

The number of H^+ pumps in the luminal membrane is regulated by intracellular pH. When intracellular pH falls, H^+ pumps are recruited into the luminal membrane by a process of membrane fusion involving a pool of intracellular vesicles whose membranes have a high density of H^+ pumps. When intracellular pH rises, H^+ pumps are removed from the luminal membrane by an endocytotic process, and the intracellular vesicles form again. In addition, the rate of H^+ secretion via the luminal membrane H^+ pumps is quite sensitive to the electrochemical gradient for H^+ across the luminal membrane; that is, with decreases in intratubular pH, increases in intracellular pH, or decreases in the lumen-negative transtubular potential difference, the rate of active H^+ secretion is inhibited.

In the distal nephron, secreted H^+ may combine with HCO_3^- escaping the proximal tubule, may form titratable acid, and may combine with NH_3 to form NH_4^+. Because H^+ secretion is gradient limited, the presence of titratable buffers and NH_3 is essential for facilitating the secretion of H^+. The greater the amount of buffer or NH_3 available, the greater the number of H^+ that can be secreted into the urine before the limiting pH value of 4.4 is reached. The excretion rate of phosphate, the principal titratable buffer, is regulated by parathyroid hormone as part of the homeostatic mechanism controlling calcium and phosphate balance. From the point of view of acid-base homeostasis, the excretion of phosphate may be considered relatively fixed (usually less than 50 millimoles/day) and serves to limit the amount of titratable acid that can be excreted. In contrast, the renal production rate of ammonia is highly variable and is regulated in response to changes in acid-base balance. In general, factors thought to depress intracellular pH—such as decreases in plasma HCO_3^- concentration, increases in P_{CO_2}, or hypokalemia—stimulate NH_3 production. These adaptive effects on NH_3 production require three to five days to become maximal. With maximal stimulation, NH_4^+ excretion can exceed 500 mEq/day.

Although not directly coupled to the transport of Na as in the proximal tubule, H^+ secretion in the distal nephron is influenced by the rate of Na reabsorption. As discussed earlier, Na reabsorption in this portion of the nephron occurs as an ionic current through Na-selective channels in the luminal membrane. Because the effect of this ionic current is to make the transtubular potential more lumen-negative, it indirectly serves to stimulate the rate of active H^+ secretion, which is sensitive to electrical potentials. Thus, H^+ secretion is stimulated by aldosterone and inhibited by diuretics such as amiloride and triamterene that block the Na^+ channels. In addition, aldosterone stimulates the rate of H^+ secretion in the distal nephron by unknown mechanisms that are independent of its effects on Na transport.

In view of the above considerations, the control of distal nephron H^+ secretion may now be summarized. Net acid secretion is enhanced in states in which intracellular pH is decreased, as when plasma HCO_3^- concentration is reduced, P_{CO_2} is elevated, or plasma K^+ concentration is depressed. Conversely, net acid secretion in the distal nephron is inhibited when plasma HCO_3^- is elevated, P_{CO_2} is reduced, or plasma K^+ is elevated. Moreover, an increased plasma HCO_3^- concentration stimulates HCO_3^- secretion in this portion of the nephron. In states in which aldosterone levels are increased, as during volume contraction, the rate of distal nephron H^+ secretion is enhanced. Distal acidification is reduced by carbonic anhydrase inhibitors, by the Na channel blockers amiloride and triamterene, and by aldosterone deficiency or spironolactone. Finally, recent evidence suggests the presence of Cl^--HCO_3 exchange mechanisms in the distal nephron. As a result, distal HCO_3^- secretion is inhibited and net acid excretion is enhanced under conditions in which the luminal Cl concentration is decreased, as during sodium sulfate infusions and clinical states of chloride depletion.

Concept of the Bicarbonate Tubular Maximum

As discussed above, a true T_m for bicarbonate reabsorption does not exist in the proximal tubule under physiologic conditions. Nevertheless it is useful for approaching clinical disorders of acid-base balance to employ the concept of a whole kidney T_m for bicarbonate. This T_m differs from true tubular maxima that are expressed as filtered loads of milligrams per minute; it is expressed as a concentration. The T_m for bicarbonate in essence represents the threshold for bicarbonate excretion. The bicarbonate T_m is usually about 26 mEq/l under normal conditions. When the serum bicarbonate is greater than 26 mEq/l, bicarbonate is excreted in the urine. When the serum bicarbonate is less than 26 mEq/l, virtually all filtered bicarbonate is reabsorbed and further H^+ secretion results in net acid excretion and the regeneration of bicarbonate buffer.

Of great importance, the T_m for bicarbonate is not a firmly fixed concentration but is influenced by the various factors that affect proximal and distal H^+ secretion. Thus the bicarbonate T_m is elevated by hypercapnea, volume contraction, hypokalemia, chloride depletion, and mineralocorticoid excess. It is depressed by hypocapnea, volume expansion, parathyroid hormone excess, and mineralocorticoid deficiency.

DEFINITIONS OF CLINICAL ACID-BASE DISTURBANCES

An arterial blood pH below 7.36 is defined as acidemia; a pH above 7.44 is alkalemia. Acidosis and alkalosis are disease states that if unopposed or untreated would produce acidemia and alkalemia. Acidosis may exist without acidemia, and alkalosis without alkalemia.

Acidosis and alkalosis are further divided into primary disorders, termed respiratory or metabolic. A respiratory disorder is characterized by a primary rise or fall in arterial P_{CO_2}. The actual value of P_{CO_2} recorded need not lie outside the normal range to indicate a primary disorder. The value for P_{CO_2} need only be inappropriately high or low for the clinical setting. Thus a P_{CO_2} of 40 in the presence of severe metabolic acidosis would be inappropriately elevated and would represent primary respiratory acidosis. A metabolic disorder is characterized by a primary alteration in the arterial bicarbonate concentration. Again, the bicarbonate concentration need not lie outside the normal range to indicate the presence of acidosis or alkalosis. Metabolic acidosis in a patient with an initially elevated bicarbonate concentration might simply lower the bicarbonate concentration into the normal range.

Primary acid-base disorders initiate a series of events that tend to oppose a rise or fall in pH. These events are called compensation and have the dimensions of time and extent. Appropriate compensation is defined as the response expected in 95 per cent of normal individuals in response to a similar primary acid-base disturbance.

In respiratory acidosis, for example, the retention of CO_2 raises the concentration of carbonic acid. H_2CO_3 is buffered largely within red cells, producing a rise in serum bicarbonate of a few milliequivalents per liter. In a normal individual, serum bicarbonate will rise only 3 to 5 mEq/l as P_{CO_2} rises from 40 to 80 mm of mercury. The rise of 3 to 5 mEq/l of bicarbonate is inadequate to prevent a significant fall in arterial pH, but it represents appropriate compensation during the first few hours after an acute rise in P_{CO_2}. It is appropriate because that response is all that could be expected in 95 per cent of normal individuals in the same period. After a few hours the kidneys will increase the excretion of hydrogen ion and generate bicarbonate to raise the serum bicarbonate by as much as 10 to 15 mEq/l, resulting in a further rise in arterial pH. The renal response requires time and represents compensation for more sustained respiratory acidosis. Compensation that was appropriate for acute respiratory acidosis would be inappropriate for chronic respiratory acidosis.

In metabolic acidosis a fall in bicarbonate concentration produced by the retention of fixed acid would represent buffering of the fixed acid by the carbonic acid/bicarbonate system. This buffering would oppose the fall in arterial pH, but some fall would occur and stimulate the respiratory center to increase ventilation, thereby lowering the arterial P_{CO_2}. The ventilatory response occurs within minutes and is predictable. The appropriateness of the response is again defined by the response of 95 per cent of normal individuals to the same acid stimulus.

Compensation should be conceptualized as a secondary event in response to a primary acid-base disturbance; an initiating event is not a compensatory response. Therefore, hyperventilation in response to metabolic acidosis should not be termed compensatory respiratory alkalosis, nor should the rise in bicarbonate in response to respiratory acidosis be termed compensatory metabolic alkalosis. Rather, the term compensated metabolic acidosis should be used to indicate that a patient's ventilatory response is secondary to and appropriate for the degree of acidemia. Referring to compensated respiratory or metabolic acid-base disturbance does not imply that the pH has been returned to normal. It implies only that the extent and rapidity of the compensatory response are appropriate.

We can now describe six primary simple acid-base disturbances on the basis of the initiating event and the extent and timing of the compensatory response. These disturbances are as follows:

(1) Respiratory acidosis, acute: compensated for by buffers

(2) Respiratory acidosis, chronic: compensated for by renal hydrogen ion excretion

(3) Respiratory alkalosis, acute: compensated for by buffers

(4) Respiratory alkalosis, chronic: compensated for by renal bicarbonate excretion early, but ultimately by renal H^+ ion retention

(5) Metabolic acidosis: compensated for by buffers, ventilatory response, and later renal response

(6) Metabolic alkalosis: compensated for by buffers, ventilatory response, and later renal response

Note that we have distinguished acute from chronic respiratory disorders, but not metabolic disorders. This distinction is made because the expected range of compensation in respiratory disorders depends upon the duration of the abnormal P_{CO_2}. The acute response of buffers is modest. The chronic response of renal hydrogen ion secretion corrects pH to a much greater degree. Metabolic disturbances are not divided into acute and chronic, since buffer and respiratory responses are quite rapid. Later changes in renal excretion of hydrogen ion or bicarbonate are important in correcting metabolic acid-base disturbance, but they do not alter the predicted slope of P_{CO_2} response.

Two or more primary acid-base disturbances may exist simultaneously. If a patient is said to have metabolic acidosis and respiratory alkalosis, it means that two separate primary acid-base disorders exist. The patient is said to have a mixed acid-base disturbance. Mixed disturbances may be additive, such as respiratory acidosis and metabolic acidosis. When the disturbances are additive, the pH will invariably be abnormal, as each primary disturbance will interfere with the normal compensatory response to the other. In a mixed disturbance the primary abnormalities may be opposite in direction, such as metabolic acidosis and respiratory alkalosis. When the primary disturbances tend to produce changes in pH in opposite directions, the resultant pH may be high, low, or normal. Therefore, a clinical diagnosis of an acid-base disturbance cannot rest solely on a deviation of pH from normal. The importance of recognizing the presence of a mixed disturbance lies in the suggestion of a previously unsuspected disease state and in the warning that correction of one primary acid-base disturbance may leave an unopposed disorder to produce an even more severe alteration of pH.

The diagnosis of a mixed acid-base disturbance is based primarily on clinical information. If a patient has two disease processes that should produce acid-base disturbances, the presence of a mixed disturbance should be assumed. Therefore, it is likely that a patient with chronic severe renal failure (metabolic acidosis) and severe vomiting from an obstructing duodenal ulcer (metabolic alkalosis) has a mixed acid-base disturbance. There will be times when the clinical picture will be confusing and the laboratory will help. Use of laboratory data to diagnose a mixed acid-base disturbance requires knowledge of normal compensation and recognition of apparently inadequate or excessive responses to primary disturbances. A helpful approach to the analysis of acid-base disorders requires that the following questions be answered:

(1) Is acidemia or alkalemia present?

(2) Is the acid-base disturbance respiratory or metabolic?

(3) If respiratory, is it acute or chronic?

(4) If metabolic acidosis, is it hyperchloremic or anion gap? (This distinction will be discussed in detail in the section on metabolic acidosis.)

(5) If metabolic alkalosis, is urinary chloride present or absent?

(6) Is compensation appropriate?

(7) If compensation is not appropriate, what mixed disturbance exists?

(8) Finally, if neither acidemia nor alkalemia exists, is there evidence of an increased anion gap or an abnormality of P_{CO_2} or bicarbonate to suggest a primary acid-base disturbance? If such evidence exists in spite of a normal pH, what mixed disturbance is present?

CHEMICAL MEASUREMENTS OF ACID-BASE DISTURBANCES

The outline of clinical acid-base disorders that was presented depends on nothing more complicated than the measurement of the components of the Henderson-Hasselbalch equation: pH, P_{CO_2}, and HCO_3^-. Use of pH, P_{CO_2}, and HCO_3^- permits definition of an acid-base disturbance as respiratory or metabolic acidosis or alkalosis, and as compensated or uncompensated. It also indicates a simple or mixed disturbance.

A series of measurements has been developed that attempts to assess the metabolic component of acid-base disturbances. The determinations of whole blood buffer base, standard bicarbonate, and base excess or deficit all depend upon in vitro titrations of whole blood. Whole blood titration by CO_2 does not, however, reproduce whole body responses accurately. In acute circumstances the whole blood will produce a higher bicarbonate concentration for a given P_{CO_2} than will the intact individual (Fig. 29). The reason for this

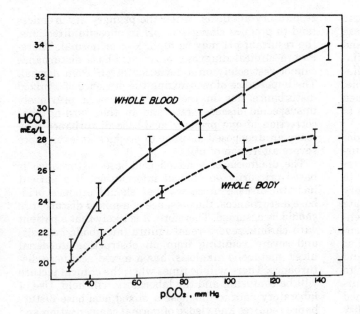

Figure 29. Comparison of carbon dioxide titration curve for whole blood and whole body. The bicarbonate concentrations are significantly different (p <0.01) at carbon dioxide tension of 70 mm Hg and above. (From Rastegar, A., and Thier, S.: Physiologic consequences and bodily adaptations to hyper- and hypocapnia. Chest 62:335, 1972. Originally from Cohen, J. J., Brackett, N. C., and Schwartz, W. B.: The nature of carbon dioxide titration curve in the normal dog. J Clin Invest 43:777, 1964.)

discrepancy is that the red cells of whole blood are better buffers of CO_2 than are other cells of the body. On the other hand, chronic exposure to CO_2 produces a greater bicarbonate response in the intact individual, since renal hydrogen ion secretion adds bicarbonate to the body fluids. The use of in vitro titration curves adds little to the interpretation of acid-base disturbances and may occasionally be misleading. The remainder of this discussion of acid-base disturbances will use only the simple measurements of the components of the Henderson-Hasselbalch equation.

APPROACH TO CLINICAL ACID-BASE ABNORMALITIES

The simplest approach to acid-base abnormalities requires a careful history and physical examination to direct attention to potential primary disturbances. Examination of laboratory data—including the blood count, urinalysis, and chemistries, particularly electrolytes, creatinine, and glucose—will strengthen the impressions gained from the history and physical examination. Measurements of arterial pH, P_{CO_2}, and bicarbonate will confirm the presence of an acid-base disturbance and should allow definition of the appropriateness of compensation. Compensation may be assessed by the use of formulas derived to express normal compensation or by reference to acid-base nomograms that display the expected range for normal compensation. When a nomogram indicates that the data derived from a patient lie outside the range for a compensated primary disturbance, a mixed disturbance is present. If the nomogram indicates, however, that the patient's data are consistent with a single compensated primary disturbance, a mixed disturbance may still exist; if the data suggest a mixed disturbance, one must focus on the clinical picture.

CLINICAL ACID-BASE DISTURBANCES

RESPIRATORY ACIDOSIS

Respiratory acidosis may be acute with compensation derived from cellular buffers, or chronic with compensation dependent upon the renal excretion of hydrogen ion. Respiratory acidosis results from the retention of CO_2. The most common causes of CO_2 retention are primary pulmonary disease, central nervous system depression, acute severe pulmonary edema, and neuromuscular or bony abnormalities of the thorax. The retained CO_2 raises the concentration of carbonic acid and lowers arterial blood pH. The clinical setting and the compensatory responses distinguish between acute and chronic respiratory acidosis.

Acute Respiratory Acidosis

With the development of acute hypercapnia, cellular buffers provide over 95 per cent of the compensatory response to the acidosis. The CO_2/bicarbonate buffer system, which is critical in the defense against metabolic acidosis and alkalosis and which plays a role in the response to chronic respiratory acidosis, has little place in the response to acute respiratory acidosis. The CO_2 retained in acute respiratory acidosis increases the blood carbonic acid concentration and therefore the hydrogen ion activity. Recall that

$$CO_2 + H_2O \leftrightarrows H_2CO_3 \leftrightarrows H^+ + HCO_3^-.$$

The hydrogen ion produced will enter cells in exchange for sodium and potassium and will be buffered by intracellular proteins. The bicarbonate that remains in the extracellular fluid will increase blood bicarbonate and provide a portion of the compensatory response. In addition, CO_2 will diffuse rapidly into red blood cells, where the high intracellular concentration of carbonic anhydrase facilitates hydration to carbonic acid. The H_2CO_3 dissociates into H^+, which is buffered by hemoglobin and HCO_3^-, which leaves the red blood cell in exchange for chloride. The combined acute compensatory increase in bicarbonate in response to a rise in P_{CO_2} from 40 to 80 mm of mercury will be less than 5 mEq/l.

In humans, raising arterial P_{CO_2} from 40 to 80 mm of mercury produces a curvilinear response in serum

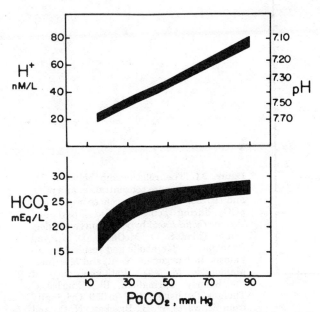

Figure 30. Combined significance band for acute hypocapnia and acute hypercapnia in man. The significance band for H^+ ion concentration is in the upper section of the figure and for bicarbonate concentration in the lower portion. (From Rastegar, A., and Thier, S.: Physiologic consequences and bodily adaptations to hyper- and hypocapnia. Chest 62:325, 1972. Originally from Arbus, G. S., Herbert, L. A., Levesque, P. R., et al.: Characterization and clinical application of the "significance band" for acute respiratory alkalosis. N Engl J Med 280:117, 1969.)

bicarbonate with progressively smaller increments in bicarbonate per increase in P_{CO_2}. For any given increase in P_{CO_2} the serum bicarbonate concentration rises rapidly and begins to plateau in about 10 minutes. Hydrogen ion concentration rises linearly as a function of increasing P_{CO_2} (Fig. 30). The slope of $\frac{\Delta H^+}{\Delta P_{CO_2}}$ in acute respiratory acidosis is 0.78 nM/l/mm of mercury. The linearity of the hydrogen ion response indicates that the defense of hydrogen ion concentration is constant throughout a wide range of P_{CO_2}. Hydrogen ion concentration is never returned to normal by the compensation of acute respiratory acidosis.

Since the compensatory increase in serum bicarbonate in acute respiratory acidosis is small, there is little protection against acidemia. There is also little risk of posthypercapnia alkalosis (see section on chronic respiratory acidosis). Therefore, rapid correction of ventilatory function and adequate oxygenation are the goals of therapy of acute hypercapnia. The hypoxemia that accompanies acute hypercapnia may also produce lactic acidosis.

Chronic Respiratory Acidosis

If hypercapnia is prolonged, cellular buffers will be exhausted. Compensation for chronic respiratory acidosis will therefore depend upon the ability of the kidney to secrete hydrogen ion and to produce and retain increased quantities of bicarbonate.

Most of our knowledge concerning the renal responses to chronic hypercapnia comes from carefully controlled observations of dogs in environmental chambers (Fig. 31). Similar experiments could not be performed with humans, but what observations have been made in man are consistent with the animal studies.

Within the first 24 hours of hypercapnia there is a small rapid rise in serum bicarbonate. This rise in bicarbonate is equal to no more than 50 per cent of the total increase seen at steady state in hypercapnia and occurs without an increase in renal hydrogen ion secretion. Therefore the initial rise in bicarbonate is the response of buffers. The serum bicarbonate level rises progressively for the next three to six days to reach a new steady-state level. This secondary rise in bicarbonate is the result of increased hydrogen ion secretion in the urine in the form of ammonium chloride and titratable acid. The total hydrogen ion secretion is actually sufficient to account for both the initial and the secondary rise in serum bicarbonate, indicating that the buffers used during the first day of hypercapnia were replenished. The increased hydrogen ion secretion by the kidney is facilitated by the elevated arterial P_{CO_2}, which also results in an elevation of the T_m bicarbonate. The elevated T_m bicarbonate permits the maintenance of an elevated serum bicarbonate concentration as long as the CO_2 retention persists.

With all of these compensatory responses, defense of pH is still incomplete. With chronic hypercapnia the serum bicarbonate concentration rises in a curvilinear fashion in response to increasing P_{CO_2} but reaches much higher plateau levels than in acute hypercapnia. The hydrogen ion concentration again rises linearly but with a much less steep slope (0.32 nM/l/mm of mercury) than seen in acute respiratory acidosis.

In chronic respiratory acidosis, compensation produces a much greater rise in serum bicarbonate than is seen in acute respiratory acidosis. If ventilatory function is repaired too rapidly, P_{CO_2} may fall faster than the kidney can correct for the excess serum bicarbonate. Recovery from chronic hypercapnia is characterized by decreased renal net acid excretion as NH_4^+ and titratable acidity. The retained H^+ lowers serum HCO_3^-. What was originally a metabolic compensation of chronic respiratory acidosis may now emerge as metabolic alkalosis; that is, bicarbonate is elevated out of proportion to P_{CO_2}. The fall in P_{CO_2} should permit the gradual excretion of bicarbonate via the kidney. However, if an elevated T_m bicarbonate is maintained by extracellular fluid volume contraction, hypokalemia, or inadequate availability of chloride, the kidney will not excrete bicarbonate and metabolic alkalosis will persist. This posthypercapnic alkalosis may depress ventilatory drive and complicate respiratory care.

RESPIRATORY ALKALOSIS

Acute Respiratory Alkalosis

Acute respiratory alkalosis is the result of hyperventilation. The hyperventilation may result from anxiety, hypoxemia, hypermetabolic states, intrinsic pulmonary disease, hormones and drugs, CNS lesions, or excessive mechanical ventilation.

Acute respiratory alkalosis depends almost entirely on cellular buffers for compensation. The buffer process is the reverse of that described for acute respiratory acidosis: Hydrogen ion is released from cellular buffers and chloride leaves red blood cells in exchange for

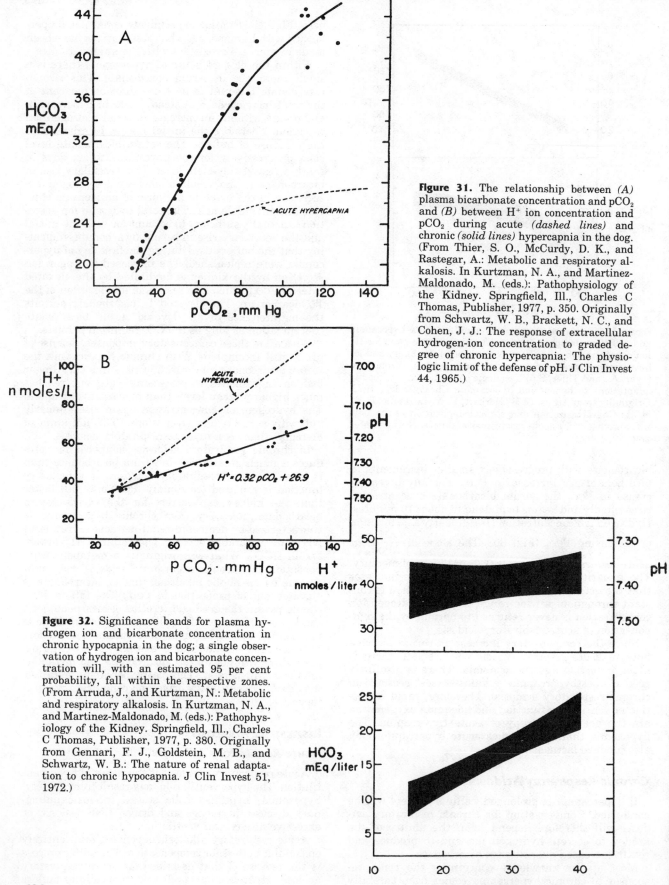

Figure 31. The relationship between *(A)* plasma bicarbonate concentration and pCO₂ and *(B)* between H⁺ ion concentration and pCO₂ during acute *(dashed lines)* and chronic *(solid lines)* hypercapnia in the dog. (From Thier, S. O., McCurdy, D. K., and Rastegar, A.: Metabolic and respiratory alkalosis. In Kurtzman, N. A., and Martinez-Maldonado, M. (eds.): Pathophysiology of the Kidney. Springfield, Ill., Charles C Thomas, Publisher, 1977, p. 350. Originally from Schwartz, W. B., Brackett, N. C., and Cohen, J. J.: The response of extracellular hydrogen-ion concentration to graded degree of chronic hypercapnia: The physiologic limit of the defense of pH. J Clin Invest 44, 1965.)

Figure 32. Significance bands for plasma hydrogen ion and bicarbonate concentration in chronic hypocapnia in the dog; a single observation of hydrogen ion and bicarbonate concentration will, with an estimated 95 per cent probability, fall within the respective zones. (From Arruda, J., and Kurtzman, N.: Metabolic and respiratory alkalosis. In Kurtzman, N. A., and Martinez-Maldonado, M. (eds.): Pathophysiology of the Kidney. Springfield, Ill., Charles C Thomas, Publisher, 1977, p. 380. Originally from Gennari, F. J., Goldstein, M. B., and Schwartz, W. B.: The nature of renal adaptation to chronic hypocapnia. J Clin Invest 51, 1972.)

bicarbonate. The result is a fall in serum bicarbonate of 7 to 8 mEq/l as P_{CO_2} decreases from 40 to 15 mm of mercury. In response to a decrease in P_{CO_2}, a new steady-state bicarbonate level is achieved in approximately 10 minutes. The curve of bicarbonate response to hypocapnia continues a curvilinear relationship and is continuous with the curve for acute hypercapnia. The hydrogen ion response to a reduction in P_{CO_2} is linear and has the same slope from 40 to 15 mm of mercury P_{CO_2} as from 40 to 80 mm of mercury P_{CO_2} (Fig. 30).

Chronic Respiratory Alkalosis

There are very few data on stable hypocapnia that permit the calculation of the slope for hydrogen ion response to decreased P_{CO_2} or a plot of serum bicarbonate against reduced P_{CO_2} levels (Fig. 32). What is known indicates that the response to chronic hypocapnia is biphasic. The initial rapid fall in bicarbonate is associated with a stabilization of pH, usually at above normal levels. The final lowering of the serum bicarbonate concentration is not the result of renal bicarbonate excretion. Rather, there is a reduced net excretion of H^+ or NH_4^+ and titratable acid. The retained H^+ lowers the serum HCO_3^-. The retention of H^+ ion is sufficient to account for the entire fall in serum HCO_3^-, indicating that buffering capacity has been restored. The reduction in the T_m bicarbonate that accompanies reduced P_{CO_2} permits the maintenance of reduced serum HCO_3^-. Recovery from chronic hypocapnia is characterized by increased net acid excretion as NH_4^+ and titratable acid.

Fortunately, chronic respiratory alkalosis is most commonly a physiologic adjustment to high altitudes or a consistent response in pregnancy. In hypocapnia associated with severe anemia, pulmonary disease, and CNS disease, treatment must be directed at the underlying disorder. Rarely, rebreathing procedures will be required to protect the patient from dangerous alkalemia.

METABOLIC ACIDOSIS

The response to acute metabolic acidosis depends upon the nature of the acid load, the buffering capacity available, the respiratory response, and the renal response. In metabolic acidosis the rapid respiratory response sustains life until virtually all of the acutely available buffers are exhausted. The respiratory response to metabolic acidosis results from changes in the pH of arterial blood, sensed by the aortic and carotid bodies and from changes in the cerebrospinal fluid pH. Usually, metabolic acidosis develops slowly enough so that the modest lag in reaching full ventilatory response seen with sudden development of acidemia is not observed. The ventilatory response to a lowering of pH is predictable enough to be described by a formula:

$$P_{CO_2} = 1.5\ (HCO_3^-) + 8.4 \pm 1.1\ \text{(Fig. 33)}.$$

This formula describes normal compensation accurately enough to suggest that a patient with a higher than predicted P_{CO_2} has primary respiratory acidosis, while a patient with a lower than predicted P_{CO_2} has primary respiratory alkalosis.

As mentioned above, there may be a slight lag in the respiratory response to acute acidemia. Therefore the equation should be held to suggest primary respiratory acidosis only if there has been time for a full respiratory response (a few hours). The disequilibrium in the ventilatory response is much more striking as acidemia is corrected. As alkali is given to correct acidemia, hyperventilation may persist for as much as 24 hours after the correction of the arterial pH. This lag is due to a slower rate of rise in CSF pH as compared with arterial pH.

In response to a challenge with metabolic acid the kidneys will reabsorb filtered bicarbonate completely within two hours of the challenge. The urine will become maximally acid (pH < 5.3). There will be a small rise in urinary titratable acidity and ammonium excretion, probably attributable to the fall in urine

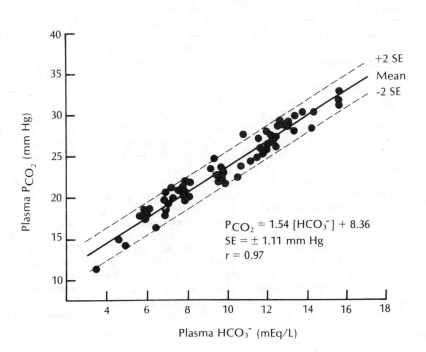

Figure 33. Respiratory response to decreased plasma bicarbonate level induced by metabolic acidosis. *SE,* standard error. (From Wilson, D. M.: In Knox, F. G. (ed.): Textbook of Renal Pathophysiology. Hagerstown, Md., Harper and Row, Publishers, Copyright 1978 by Mayo Clinic/Foundation. Originally from Albert, M. S., Dill, R. B., and Winters, R. W.: Quantitative displacement of acid-base equilibrium in metabolic acidosis. Ann Intern Med 66:312, 1967.)

$P_{CO_2} = 1.54\ [HCO_3^-] + 8.36$
$SE = \pm 1.11\ \text{mm Hg}$
$r = 0.97$

pH. If the acid challenge is continued, the urine pH will remain low and hydrogen ion excretion as titratable acid will rise modestly. The most impressive change over the next three to five days will be a rise in ammonium excretion to levels of as high as 300 to 500 mEq/day. This rise in ammonium excretion will permit a marked increase in hydrogen ion secretion and may allow the reestablishment of acid-base balance notwithstanding a continuing acid challenge.

Classification of Metabolic Acidosis

Metabolic acidosis may be conceptualized as follows:

(1) If the rate of production of acid exceeds the normal hydrogen ion excretory capacity, acidemia will occur. For example, if the metabolism of lactic acid is interrupted by hypoxemia, the lactic acid may accumulate faster than the kidney can excrete the retained hydrogen ion. The hydrogen will be buffered by bicarbonate and the respiratory response by hyperventilation will lower the Pco_2. Nonetheless, if acid production is rapid enough, severe acidemia will result.

(2) If the rate of acid production is normal but there is impaired ability of the kidney to excrete the normal quantity of hydrogen ion, net acid retention will occur; this is the situation in renal failure. The accumulation of hydrogen ion will titrate bicarbonate buffers and stimulate a ventilatory response. However, as long as renal excretion of acid is less than the daily fixed acid production, acidemia will occur.

(3) If bicarbonate or an incompletely metabolized anion of an organic acid is lost in excess quantities in the urine or stool, the result will be net retention of hydrogen ion. If the rate of base loss exceeds the capacity of compensatory mechanisms to correct for the hydrogen ion retention, acidemia will ensue (Table 4).

Though conceptualizing the development of metabolic acidosis in terms of increased acid production, decreased acid excretion, and increased base loss is physiologically sound, there is a more clinically useful framework within which to discuss metabolic acidosis. This latter classification utilizes the serum electrolytes and divides metabolic acidoses into hyperchloremic and anion gap varieties. The anion gap is defined as the difference between the serum sodium concentration and the sum of the serum chloride and bicarbonate concentrations. For example, if the serum sodium concentration is 140 mEq/l, and the serum chloride and bicarbonate concentrations are 105 and 25 mEq/l respectively, the anion gap would be 10. The normal anion gap is 10 to 12 mEq/l and reflects unmeasured anions in the serum. As metabolic acidosis develops and bicarbonate is consumed in the process of buffering hydrogen ion, two possibilities exist: (1) The acid retained is equivalent to hydrochloric acid, and the serum chloride concentration will rise in an amount equivalent to the fall in bicarbonate. Under these circumstances there will be hyperchloremia and no change in the anion gap: hyperchloremic metabolic acidosis. (2) If, on the other hand, bicarbonate is consumed in buffering an organic acid, the anion of which remains in the serum, the bicarbonate concentration will fall and the unmeasured anions of the organic acid will accumulate. The anion gap will rise above the normal 10 to 12 mEq/l, and when it exceeds 14 mEq/l an anion gap acidosis is said to exist. Cal-

TABLE 4. CAUSES OF METABOLIC ACIDOSIS

Decreased H^+ Excretion
Uremia
Renal tubular acidosis
Ureteroenterostomy
Adrenal insufficiency

Increased H^+ Production
Loss of potential alkali
  diarrhea
  $CaCl_2$ digestion
  biliary or pancreatic fistulae
Ingestion of potential acid
  NH_4Cl
  arginine HCl
  H^+ exchange resin
  methionine
  hyperalimentation
Metabolic abnormalities
  Ketosis
    insulin lack
    starvation
    alcohol ingestion
  Lactic acidosis
    tissue hypoxia
    toxins
  Miscellaneous
    salicylates
    ethylene glycol
    methanol
    paraldehyde

From Thier, S. O., McCurdy, D. K., and Rastegar, A.: Metabolic and respiratory acidosis. In Kurtzman, N. A., and Martinez-Maldonado, M. (eds.): Pathophysiology of the Kidney. Springfield, Ill., Charles C Thomas, Publisher, 1977, p. 342.

culation of the anion gap or delta, as it is also called, is an important part of the evaluation of a patient's acid-base status. Usually, evaluation of the electrolytes will confirm clinical impressions of the existence of an acid-base disturbance; occasionally, such an evaluation is the first clue to the presence of a disturbance.

Hyperchloremic Metabolic Acidosis

The causes of hyperchloremic metabolic acidosis can be considered in three categories (Table 5): those induced by acidifying drugs, those resulting from primary renal dysfunction, and those related to the gastrointestinal tract.

Acidifying salts such as ammonium chloride may induce hyperchloremic metabolic acidosis. When ammonium chloride is administered, ammonia is metabolized via amino acids to urea. The removal of ammonia from ammonium chloride will leave hydrochloric acid in the body. The hydrochloric acid reacts with sodium bicarbonate to form sodium chloride, CO_2, and water. The result is a rise in serum chloride and a fall in serum bicarbonate concentration. Under these circumstances the urine is maximally acid (pH < 5.3).

Carbonic anhydrase inhibitors such as acetazolamide may also induce hyperchloremic metabolic acidosis. With the administration of a carbonic anhydrase inhibitor, sodium bicarbonate is lost in the urine. The loss of sodium bicarbonate results in a rise in chloride concentration via the retention of dietary sodium chloride and contraction of the extracellular fluid volume around the normal or slightly increased quantity of chloride. The result is a fall in serum bicarbonate

TABLE 5. CLASSIFICATION OF METABOLIC ACIDOSIS BY ELECTROLYTE PATTERN

Hyperchloremic Acidosis
1. Acidifying drugs
   NH_4Cl
   $CaCl_2$
   Lysine HCl
   Acetazolamide
2. Renal dysfunction
   Interstitial nephritis (mild-moderate azotemia)
   Renal tubular acidosis (proximal, distal, and hyperkalemic)
3. Gastrointestinal origin
   Diarrhea
   Ureteroenterostomy

Increased Anion Gap Acidosis
1. Renal failure
2. Diabetic ketoacidosis
3. Lactic acidosis
4. Ingestion of drugs or toxins
   Methanol
   Ethylene glycol
   Salicylate
   Paraldehyde

From Thier, S. O., McCurdy, D. K., and Rastegar, A.: Metabolic and respiratory acidosis. In Kurtzman, N. A., and Martinez-Maldonado, M. (eds.): Pathophysiology of the Kidney. Springfield, Ill., Charles C Thomas, Publisher, 1977, p. 342.

concentration and a rise in serum chloride concentration. The urine under these circumstances contains increased quantities of bicarbonate and is not maximally acid in spite of acidosis (pH > 5.3).

The hyperchloremic metabolic acidosis produced by renal dysfunction will either result from diminished ability to produce ammonia or from inability to acidify the urine maximally. With mild to moderate degrees of renal insufficiency, particularly in association with interstitial nephritis and reduced renal tubular cell mass, the production of ammonia is impaired. A reduced capacity to produce and excrete ammonia has predictable pathophysiologic consequences.

Consider that the 70 mEq of fixed acid produced daily will be buffered such that:

$$HA + NaHCO_3 \rightarrow NaA + H_2O + CO_2.$$

The NaA is filtered at the glomerulus. The tubule must reabsorb the sodium and secrete hydrogen ion, the A^- remaining in the urine to combine with secreted hydrogen ion to re-form HA. Recall that each time a hydrogen ion is secreted, a bicarbonate ion is available for return to the blood. The excretion of hydrogen ion and the reabsorption of sodium thus re-forms HA in the urine and returns sodium bicarbonate to the blood.

The result is that acid is formed but does not circulate freely in body fluids because it is buffered by sodium bicarbonate. The result of the buffering is the formation of a neutral salt NaA. The kidney then reabsorbs the sodium of the NaA as sodium bicarbonate while re-forming the acid HA in the urine for excretion.

Unfortunately the A^- of HA may be the anion of a strong acid. If, for example, the anion were chloride, the secretion of hydrogen ion into the urine would form hydrochloric acid. Since hydrochloric acid is completely dissociated and since hydrogen ion secretion is gradient limited at a urine pH of 4.5, very little hydrogen ion would be excreted before the urine pH

limited further secretion. Under normal circumstances ammonia would be present in adequate quantities to form ammonium chloride from the hydrochloric acid in the urine, thereby preventing a precipitous fall in urine pH and allowing the secretion of retained acid.

If, as in interstitial nephritis, ammonia production is reduced, the following sequence of events occurs: When all available ammonia has been used to accept secreted hydrogen ion, the urine pH will fall to maximally acid levels and limit further hydrogen ion secretion. If hydrogen ion secretion ceases before all of the sodium in NaA has been reabsorbed as sodium bicarbonate, NaA will be lost in the urine. Since the NaA was derived from sodium bicarbonate, its loss in the urine will result in a fall in serum bicarbonate concentration and the retention of hydrogen ion. The loss of the sodium of NaA in the urine will lead to a mild contraction of the extracellular fluid and stimulation of the renin-aldosterone pathway. Sodium will then be retained as the most available form in the diet (NaCl), raising the serum chloride concentration. Sodium will also be retained in exchange for potassium under the influence of aldosterone. The result will be hyperchloremic acidosis with a relatively low serum potassium concentration for the degree of acidemia, and the urine will be maximally acid. This sequence of events occurs with mild to moderate renal insufficiency. As renal insufficiency progresses, the unmeasured anions such as phosphate and sulfate are retained and an increased anion gap develops.

Renal tubular acidosis (RTA) is a syndrome characterized by hypokalemic-hyperchloremic metabolic acidosis in association with urine that is less than maximally acid (pH > 5.3). All forms of RTA have some degree of renal bicarbonate wasting: The higher the urine pH the greater the bicarbonate concentration. Clinically, RTA may occur as muscle weakness or paralysis, bone pain, kidney stones, or nephrocalcinosis. At least three major categories of RTA have been defined: distal (classic), proximal, and hyperkalemic. The first two categories indicate the tubular site at which a definite defect of hydrogen ion secretion and bicarbonate reabsorption exists. They should not be interpreted to mean that only the indicated site is involved.

Distal (Classic) Renal Tubular Acidosis

Distal RTA is characterized by a defect in the secretion of hydrogen ion by the distal tubule such that urine cannot be maximally acidified regardless of how acidemic the patient may become. Defective acidification of distal tubule fluid could occur as the result of decreased electrogenic hydrogen ion secretion; increased hydrogen, H_2CO_3, or CO_2 diffusion back from the lumen; decreased electrogenic sodium reabsorption; decreased intracellular bicarbonate production (via carbonic anhydrase); or a decreased bicarbonate exit across the basolateral membrane, perhaps because of a defective HCO_3^--Cl^- exchange system.

When bicarbonate infusion results in increased distal delivery, the secretion of hydrogen ion generates increased luminal P_{CO_2}. A primary defect in electrogenic hydrogen ion secretion would result in reduced generation of urine P_{CO_2} when bicarbonate is infused. Such a reduction in P_{CO_2} has been reported in RTA, but could also result from increased back diffusion of

H^+, H_2CO_3, or CO_2 due to increased distal tubule permeability. Another approach to defining the pathophysiology of distal RTA depends upon the infusion of Na_2SO_4, which normally enhances both H^+ and K^+ secretion. In some patients with distal RTA, only H^+ secretion is impaired during Na_2SO_4 infusion, suggesting an isolated H^+ secretory defect. In other patients an impaired K^+ as well as H^+ secretory response to Na_2SO_4 indicates that a more generalized distal tubule defect must be present, and this will be discussed with hyperkalemic renal tubular acidosis. Back diffusion of H^+, H_2CO_3, or CO_2 may occur in distal RTA, but is difficult to document. Impaired HCO_3^- formation may occur with carbonic anhydrase inhibition, but is not a clinically important cause of RTA. Little evidence exists concerning defective HCO_3^--Cl^- exchange. Regardless of the mechanism involved, what is clear is that distal tubule pH cannot be lowered below 5.3. With impaired distal hydrogen ion secretion a predictable series of events follows. Just as in the case of the hyperchloremic acidosis of renal insufficiency, fixed acid (HA) reacts with sodium bicarbonate to form the salt NaA. In the distal tubule, secretion of hydrogen ion and reabsorption of sodium results in the formation of HA in the urine and the addition of sodium bicarbonate to the blood. If hydrogen ion secretion is defective, NaA will be lost in urine that is less than maximally acid. Since the NaA was derived from sodium bicarbonate, its loss in the urine will reduce serum bicarbonate. In addition, the higher the urine pH the more sodium bicarbonate will appear in the urine. The loss of NaA and sodium bicarbonate will also contract the extracellular fluid and stimulate aldosterone secretion. Sodium will be retained as sodium chloride, producing hyperchloremia, and will be exchanged for potassium, producing hypokalemia. If the hypokalemia is severe enough, muscle weakness or paralysis may appear. The persistent retention of hydrogen ion will eventually call bone buffers into play. During the buffering process bone calcium will be mobilized, demineralizing bone and producing pain. The calcium will be delivered to the kidney where it will be excreted in increased quantities in the urine. In addition, patients with distal RTA excrete less than normal quantities of citrate in the urine. It appears that the citrate is reabsorbed more actively in the proximal tubule, owing to intracellular acidosis. The excretion of increased quantities of calcium in urine that is less than maximally acid and contains inadequate quantities of citrate results in an increased incidence of calcium deposition as stones and as nephrocalcinosis.

The sequence of events that occurs in distal RTA is summarized in Figure 34. Note that all of the clinical manifestations of distal RTA can be traced to a single defect in hydrogen ion secretion.

The diagnosis of distal RTA depends upon demonstrating that the urine pH does not fall below 5.3 in response to acidemia. If, in the patient's steady-state condition, the degree of acidemia is minimal, an exogenous acid challenge may be required to document a failure to acidify the urine. There is a variant of distal RTA called incomplete RTA in which acidemia does not develop despite inability to acidify the urine maximally. In patients with incomplete RTA it appears that the excretion of hydrogen ion as ammonium ion is sufficient to compensate for the mild bicarbonate leak and mild reduction in titratable acid excretion.

The treatment of distal RTA requires an attempt to identify the underlying cause. If a cause can be identified, it should be treated. In any event, the metabolic acidosis and hypokalemia require treatment with potassium replacement and bicarbonate. In the section on potassium homeostasis we will discuss the fact that acidemia shifts potassium out of cells and alkalemia shifts it into cells. The administration of alkali to an individual who is hypokalemic may lower serum potassium still further and produce dangerous muscle weakness or arrhythmias. Therefore, in treating a patient with a hypokalemic-hyperchloremic acidosis such as distal RTA, it is important to begin correcting the hypokalemia before administering bicarbonate.

Proximal Renal Tubular Acidosis

The proximal tubule is the site of reabsorption of 85 to 90 per cent of filtered bicarbonate. If a defect develops in proximal tubular bicarbonate reabsorption the following sequence of events will occur: First, sodium bicarbonate will be lost in the urine, reducing the serum bicarbonate concentration and producing acidemia. The loss of sodium bicarbonate will also produce extracellular fluid volume contraction and will thus stimulate aldosterone secretion. Delivery of large quantities of sodium and the poorly reabsorbed anion bicarbonate (resulting in a lowered luminal chloride concentration) to the distal nephron despite increased aldosterone secretion results in severe renal potassium wasting and hypokalemia. At the onset of proximal RTA the delivery of sodium bicarbonate out of the proximal tubule may overwhelm the distal capacity to reabsorb bicarbonate. Under these circumstances sodium bicarbonate will be present in high concentrations in the urine, which will be far less than maximally acid. As systemic acidemia develops the serum

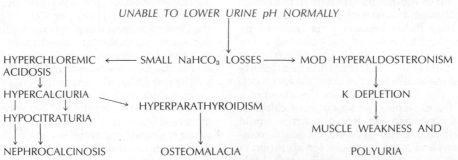

Figure 34. Complications of distal RTA. (From Stanbury, J. B., Wyngaarden, J. B., and Fredrickson, D. S.: The Metabolic Basis of Inherited Disease. New York, McGraw-Hill Book Co., 1978.)

bicarbonate concentration and the filtered load of bicarbonate will fall to a point where the proximal tubule can again reabsorb 85 to 90 per cent of what is filtered. At this point, delivery of bicarbonate to the distal nephron will be diminished, and if the distal mechanisms are intact the urine will become maximally acid with a pH significantly below 5.3.

The proximal tubular reabsorptive defect may extend to other substances such as glucose, amino acids, and phosphate. If large quantities of calcium and phosphorus are lost in the urine, the secretion of parathyroid hormone will be stimulated. Increased quantities of parathyroid hormone and hypophosphatemia both reduce the T_m bicarbonate and may aggravate the defect in proximal RTA. The defect in proximal tubular function has at least one benefit: Citrate is usually not well reabsorbed in the proximal tubule and is excreted in relatively large quantities in the urine of patients with proximal RTA. For this reason apparently, renal calculi and nephrocalcinosis are distinctly uncommon in proximal RTA.

The treatment of proximal RTA again requires a search for an underlying cause that can be corrected. Treatment of the acidemia and hypokalemia is required as in distal RTA. In proximal RTA, however, the administration of sodium bicarbonate usually results in a marked increase in urinary bicarbonate. With treatment, increased delivery of sodium bicarbonate out of the proximal tubule potentiates the potassium wasting state. Therefore, hypokalemia is likely to be a more persistent problem in proximal RTA. Attempts have been made to raise the T_m for bicarbonate by producing extracellular fluid volume contraction with diuretics and by inhibiting parathyroid hormone when it is increased.

Hyperkalemic Renal Tubular Acidosis

Hyperkalemic-hyperchloremic metabolic acidosis is the most common form of RTA in adults. It may result from inadequate aldosterone secretion or responsiveness, or from impairment of aldosterone–independent distal H^+ and K^+ secretion. The effect of aldosterone on the distal nephron is to enhance sodium reabsorption and thereby enhance the K^+ and H^+ gradients that can be achieved. For example, aldosterone may increase the maximal lumen-to-plasma potassium gradient three- to fivefold. K excretion may be adequate to maintain balance even in the absence of aldosterone, if urine flow rate is high enough so that a maximum urine-to-plasma gradient is not necessary to excrete the required quantity of potassium. With renal insufficiency or with reduced urine flow rates, aldosterone becomes critical.

Aldosterone deficiency may be primary (idiopathic hypoaldosteronism, congenital enzymatic defects, Addison's disease) or secondary to hyporeninemia. In the latter case it has been postulated that a primary defect in renin production results in inadequate aldosterone secretion and subsequent H^+ and K^+ retention. Patients typically have mild renal insufficiency, and many have diabetes mellitus. While the majority of patients with hyporeninemia and hypoaldosteronism may have the pathophysiology just described, other sequences of events could produce the same picture. For example, patients with a primary reduction in aldosterone secretion might become hyperkalemic, and

the hyperkalemia could then suppress renin production. Still another sequence of events has both the hyporeninemia and hypoaldosteronism secondary to enhanced distal chloride reabsorption. The chloride reabsorption accompanied by sodium would expand the ECF, suppressing renin and aldosterone secretion. Further, the reduced luminal negativity associated with the chloride reabsorptive shunt would impair K^+ and H^+ secretion.

Aldosterone may also be present in normal or increased concentrations, but the distal nephron may be functionally, anatomically, or pharmacologically (spirolactone) unable to respond. Finally the pathways of distal H^+ and K^+ secretion may also be primarily dysfunctional or may be inhibited by drugs such as triamterene and amiloride. One of the most common causes of hyperkalemic-hyperchloremic metabolic acidosis is obstructive uropathy. Under these circumstances both aldosterone responsiveness and the secretory mechanisms for K^+ and H^+ are impaired.

Obviously, hyperkalemic-hyperchloremic metabolic acidosis represents a heterogeneous group of disorders. They are characterized by K^+ and H^+ retention, but not necessarily by inability to acidify the urine pH. Proper treatment depends upon a correct definition of the pathophysiology. The hyperchloremic metabolic acidosis resulting from loss of renal tubular mass and reduced NH_4^+ production is commonly discussed with this group of disorders. However, as discussed earlier, the pathophysiology of the acidosis associated with decreased NH_4^+ production leads to potassium loss with serum K increased as a result of redistribution rather than retention.

Gastrointestinal Causes of Hyperchloremic Acidosis

Loss of Alkali in the Stool. Diarrhea commonly produces hyperchloremic acidosis despite the fact that the pH and bicarbonate concentration of stool are below that of blood. The reason for the development of the acidosis is that organic anions such as citrate, which would have been metabolized to CO_2 and water, consuming a hydrogen ion in the process, are lost in the stool. To produce an acidifying effect the organic anion would have to have been lost with sodium that originated from sodium bicarbonate or with potassium. The sequence of events, then, would be the formation of an organic acid that would be buffered to a sodium salt, and the sodium salt would then be lost in the stool. The result would be the consumption of sodium bicarbonate and the retention of hydrogen ion. Stool losses usually include high concentrations of potassium, resulting ultimately in a chemical picture of hypokalemic-hyperchloremic acidosis.

Ureteral Reimplantation. When ureters are reimplanted into bowel, the urine produced by the kidneys must come in contact with intestinal mucosa before being excreted from the body. If the contact time between urine and intestinal mucosa is sufficiently long, chloride will be reabsorbed and bicarbonate secreted. The result will be a hyperchloremic metabolic acidosis.

Summary

We have described hyperchloremic metabolic acidosis in three categories: that arising from drugs, that arising from renal defects, and that arising from gastrointestinal causes. Among the drug causes there were acidifying salts that resulted in maximally acid urine and carbonic anhydrase inhibitors that resulted in impaired urinary acidification. Among renal defects there was renal insufficiency, characterized by defective ammonia production and maximally acid urine; and there was renal tubular acidosis, characterized by inadequately acid urine. Finally, there were the gastrointestinal causes, predominantly diarrheal states and rarely circumstances of ureteral reimplantation into bowel. It should now be possible to distinguish between most forms of hyperchloremic acidosis by taking a careful history, making a physical examination, measuring the serum electrolytes, and checking the urine pH.

Anion Gap Acidosis

The major causes of anion gap acidosis are listed in Table 5. They include uremic metabolic acidosis, diabetic ketoacidosis, lactic acidosis, and a series of ingestions, most of which are associated with some degree of lactic acidosis. These causes of anion gap acidosis might also be conceptualized as being due to decreased excretion of an acid other than hydrochloric acid or the increased production of organic acids.

Uremic Metabolic Acidosis

The acidosis of uremia develops in a predictable fashion as renal function deteriorates. As discussed with hyperchloremic acidosis, a reduction in renal mass is accompanied by a reduction in ammonium production. Whereas ammonium accounts for two-thirds of the net acid excretion per day in normal individuals, it accounts for less than half of the hydrogen ion secreted in patients with more than a 50 per cent reduction in glomerular filtration rate. The reduction in ammonium excretion is a function of decreased ammonia production and not of decreased acidification of the urine. In fact, in patients with as little as 30 per cent of normal renal function the urine may still be maximally acidified. The ability to acidify the urine maximally does not indicate normal bicarbonate reabsorption, however. Acidification does not occur until bicarbonate levels are significantly below normal. If the serum bicarbonate level is raised to normal levels, the kidneys will waste bicarbonate until acidemia reemerges. Among the reasons for the increased bicarbonate wasting at normal serum bicarbonate concentrations in uremia are the reduced T_m bicarbonate resulting from volume expansion, increased parathyroid hormone levels, and perhaps natriuretic substances (see Uremia).

When renal failure progresses to glomerular filtration rates below 20 per cent of normal, the undetermined anions in the plasma increase to produce an anion gap. The anion gap of uremia is usually 15 to 20 mEq/l and rarely more than 25 mEq/l. The increased anion gap includes retained phosphate and sulfate and almost certainly contains increased quantities of organic anions.

The serum potassium concentration is variable in uremic acidosis and depends upon the rapidity of onset of the acidemia, the presence of aldosterone, the presence of insulin, sympathetic tone, and tubular function.

These factors will be discussed in more detail in the section on hyperkalemia. In general, the more rapid the onset of acidemia, the higher the serum potassium concentration; the less available aldosterone, insulin, or beta catechol stimulation, the greater the hyperkalemia; and the more extensive the tubulointerstitial disease, the more severe the hyperkalemia.

In patients with chronic uremic metabolic acidosis, bone buffering of hydrogen ion is important, maintaining the serum bicarbonate concentration stable despite net hydrogen ion retention. The treatment of uremic acidosis is directed at correcting the numerous metabolic effects of acidemia. The most important acute abnormalities are decreased myocardial contractility and hyperkalemia. A longer-term goal of therapy is the reduction of bone dissolution, which accompanies the buffering process. Acidemia can be corrected with the use of sodium bicarbonate. When renal failure is severe, the ability to excrete excess sodium may be impaired, and sodium bicarbonate must be administered with great care. If the patient has severe acidemia and sodium retention with oliguric renal failure, dialysis is indicated.

Diabetic Ketoacidosis

Diabetic ketoacidosis results from the increased production of organic acids. The clinical syndrome is characterized by hyperglycemia, acidosis, hypertonic dehydration, and deficits of potassium and phosphate. Fortunately the metabolic defect that produces diabetic ketoacidosis can be corrected specifically with the use of insulin (see Section VI).

In the absence of insulin, glucose accumulates in the extracellular fluid, drawing water from the intracellular fluid space. The increased filtered load of glucose produces osmotic diuresis that results in the loss of hypotonic salt and potassium in the urine. The result is a contraction of extracellular fluid volume and an elevation of extracellular fluid osmolality. The rise in extracellular fluid osmolality stimulates thirst, and the patient will usually seek water if possible. The results of decreased glucose uptake into cells will be hyperglycemia, a variable sodium concentration depending upon whether the patient was able to drink water, and a reduction in serum potassium concentration.

In addition to producing hyperglycemic osmotic diuresis, insulin lack results in the mobilization of increased quantities of free fatty acids from adipose tissue. The free fatty acids are converted to the ketoacids, beta-hydroxybutyric acid, and acetoacetic acid in the liver. At the pH of body fluids, ketoacids are fully ionized. In diabetic ketoacidosis the ketoacids may be produced at a rate of up to 7 mmoles/min. At this rate of acid production the body buffers and the renal ability to excrete hydrogen ion may be overwhelmed, and severe acidemia will ensue. The acidemia may produce a rise in serum potassium, which will result in a normal or even elevated serum potassium concentration, even in the presence of total body potassium depletion.

The presenting picture of a patient with diabetic ketoacidosis is generally one of a dehydrated individual who is hyperventilating in respiratory compensation for metabolic acidemia. Hyperglycemia is typically present but may on occasion be minimized if the patient has been fasting for a prolonged period. Typically, blood and urine will have strongly positive tests for ketones. Remember, however, that the nitroprusside reagent that tests for ketones reacts with acetoacetate and not with beta-hydroxybutyrate. Whereas the ratio of beta-hydroxybutyrate to acetoacetate is about 3:1 in diabetic ketoacidosis, in circumstances of altered redox potential such as lactic acidosis, the ratio shifts even more dramatically toward beta-hydroxybutyrate. Under these circumstances, large quantities of ketones may give only a weak nitroprusside reaction.

The treatment of diabetic ketoacidosis should correct the hyperglycemia, acidosis, hypertonic dehydration, and deficits of potassium and phosphate. The administration of insulin will halt the generation of ketoacids and may increase their rate of metabolism. The insulin will also facilitate the movement of glucose into cells, where it may be metabolized. Thus, insulin administration will treat both the acidosis and the hyperglycemia. Hypertonic dehydration is treated by the administration of hypotonic salt solutions. If volume depletion is severe when the patient is first seen, isotonic salt solutions may be given until the patient's blood pressure is stabilized, following which hypotonic solutions are administered. Expansion of the extracellular fluid with sodium chloride solutions during continued urinary loss of the sodium salts of ketoacids frequently results in hyperchloremic acidosis during the recovery from diabetic ketoacidosis. Potassium should be administered when the serum potassium concentration is anything but distinctly elevated. Since phosphate depletion may also play an important role in diabetic ketoacidosis, the administration of potassium phosphate may be beneficial, but only rarely. The routine administration of phosphate in diabetic ketoacidosis has not been shown to be beneficial. Phosphate should be administered with great attention to the serum calcium concentration. The administration of phosphate can precipitate hypocalcemia. The administration of alkali for the treatment of diabetic ketoacidosis is rarely necessary, but should be used if buffer stores are almost completely depleted when the patient is first seen. It is important to recognize that there is commonly a precipitating event, such as infection, underlying the development of diabetic ketoacidosis. It is essential that any precipitating event be identified and treated.

Lactic Acidosis

Lactic acid is produced from pyruvic acid as the last step in anaerobic glycolysis. The conversion of pyruvate to lactate provides a means of regenerating nicotinamide-adenine dinucleotide (NAD) in the face of hypoxia. Once lactate has been formed, it can be metabolized only by being reoxidized to pyruvate in the liver. These brief comments on lactate production and metabolism are sufficient to predict that lactic acidosis is most likely to occur in the face of tissue hypoxia, liver disease, decreased hepatic perfusion, and decreased available NAD. Frequently several of these factors occur in concert, permitting the development of lactic acidosis when none of the contributing factors alone would have produced the disorder. There is also a state of lactic acidosis that has been termed spontaneous, since none of the identifiable underlying processes favoring lactate production can be identified.

Lactic acidosis is also a common complication of the ingestion of a number of toxins. Thus, intoxication with methanol, ethanol, ethylene glycol, and salicylate as well as the ingestion of phenformin will produce lactic acidosis. Lactic acid may be produced at rates of up to 10 mmoles/min; emergency treatment is required. Though acute treatment involves the administration of bicarbonate in large quantities, little will be accomplished if efforts to interrupt the production of lactic acid are not successful. The quantity of sodium bicarbonate required simply to keep arterial pH at 7.2 or above may be in the range of 1000 mEq or more. The administration of this much sodium may produce extracellular fluid volume overload, leading to pulmonary congestion, hypoxemia, and worsening of the lactic acidosis. If the quantities of sodium bicarbonate that must be administered to protect pH produce extracellular fluid volume overload, dialysis should be instituted. During the time that bicarbonate is being administered, steps should be taken to correct tissue hypoxia. Bicarbonate therapy will produce only a transient improvement in acid-base status. It will stimulate further lactic acid production and may make the lactic acidosis worse if the underlying cause cannot be corrected. Therefore adequate oxygen supply must be guaranteed, anemia should be corrected, and shock of cardiac, hypovolemic, and septic origin should be treated. If the ingestion of a medication or toxin may be contributing to the lactic acidosis, the offending substance should be removed from the body if possible. Dichloroacetate can also reduce lactic acid levels transiently and may be associated with an improved blood pressure. It has not yet, however, been shown to improve mortality. Finally, other sources of acid production, such as diabetic ketoacidosis, should be sought and treated.

If the cause of lactic acidosis can be identified and treated, the production of lactate may be interrupted. With the cessation of lactate production, the risk of developing severe alkalemia emerges. Alkalemia may result from a combination of persistent hyperventilation in association with aggressive alkali therapy, or it may result from the ultimate metabolism of the retained lactate ion. What happens in the latter circumstance is that lactic acid is produced and buffered by the body's bicarbonate stores. During the initial phase of treatment of lactic acidosis, bicarbonate is infused in large quantities. When lactate production is halted, the accumulated lactate will be metabolized. During the process of metabolism of lactate, one hydrogen ion will be fixed for each lactate molecule metabolized to CO_2 and water. The removal of hydrogen ion from solution increases hydroxyl ion, which in combination with CO_2 generates bicarbonate. The bicarbonate that was consumed in buffering lactic acid is now restored by the metabolism of lactate, and the patient has also received exogenous bicarbonate, infused during the state of severe acidemia. Therefore an alkaline overshoot should be anticipated in the treatment of lactic acidosis and can be blunted by the administration of adequate amounts of chloride to permit the excretion of bicarbonate.

METABOLIC ALKALOSIS

The development of metabolic alkalosis can be analyzed in terms of those factors that initiate the alkalosis and those that sustain it. The circumstances that would induce metabolic alkalosis, such as the ingestion of alkali or the net loss of acid, would raise the serum bicarbonate concentration. However, the kidney has an enormous capacity to excrete bicarbonate and, unless the T_m bicarbonate were elevated, the acutely elevated bicarbonate concentration would return to normal. We must then recall that the factors that elevate the T_m bicarbonate are those that enhance sodium reabsorption, such as volume contraction, and those that facilitate secretion of hydrogen ion, such as the elevation of P_{CO_2}, the depletion of total body potassium, mineralocorticoid excess, and the hypochloremic state. In any circumstance of metabolic alkalosis, attention must be directed at correcting the initiating events producing the alkalosis and at correcting the factors sustaining it.

Ingestion of Alkali

The ingestion of alkali alone is rarely a cause of clinically important metabolic alkalosis. The quantities of alkali that must be ingested to produce metabolic alkalosis are no longer prescribed. At the present time the ingestion of alkali is important as a contributor to other causes of metabolic alkalosis and not as a primary cause.

Loss of Hydrochloric Acid

Gastric Losses. In the process of vomiting an individual loses both hydrochloric acid and sodium chloride. During the process of the secretion of hydrogen ion to form the hydrochloric acid, bicarbonate is returned to the blood just as it is during hydrogen ion secretion in the renal tubule. Therefore the loss of hydrochloric acid results in a rise in the serum bicarbonate concentration. Acutely, the elevated serum bicarbonate concentration exceeds the T_m for bicarbonate, leading to the delivery of increased quantities of sodium bicarbonate to the distal tubule and into the urine. The loss of sodium bicarbonate in the urine and of sodium chloride in the vomitus produces extracellular fluid volume contraction that stimulates the release of renin to generate angiotensin, and thus to stimulate the secretion of aldosterone. The increased delivery of sodium bicarbonate to the distal tubule occurs in the presence of mild alkalemia, which shifts potassium into distal tubular cells, and hyperaldosteronism, which stimulates the distal reabsorption of sodium and secretion of potassium and hydrogen. The net result is that alkalemia is generated by the loss of hydrochloric acid. The alkalemia is sustained by an elevation of the T_m bicarbonate. The T_m bicarbonate elevation is sustained by contraction of the extracellular fluid volume, hypochloremia, hyperaldosteronism, and hypokalemia. If the alkalemia becomes severe enough it will depress respiration, leading to retention of CO_2. The elevated P_{CO_2} will also contribute to the elevated T_m bicarbonate. As long as vomiting persists, and adequate replacement of sodium and potassium chloride is not undertaken, the hypokalemic-hypochloremic metabolic alkalosis of vomiting will persist (Fig. 35).

Renal Loss. Perhaps the most common cause of metabolic alkalosis is the use of diuretics. Diuretics, particularly those that interfere with sodium chloride reabsorption in the ascending limb of the loop of Henle and early distal tubule, characteristically produce hy-

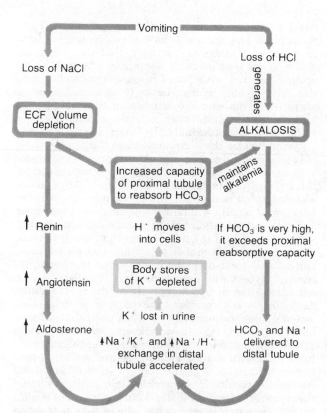

Figure 35. The sequence of events in vomiting, leading to the generation and maintenance of metabolic alkalosis. Metabolic alkalosis may occur after prolonged vomiting by the sequence of electrolyte disturbances due to loss of NaCl (left) and loss of HCl (right). Potassium loss in vomitus is not significant (usually <15 mEq/liter). The loss of HCl is associated with a rise in serum bicarbonate concentration that transiently exceeds proximal tubular reabsorptive capacity. Sodium bicarbonate is delivered to the distal nephron, increasing potassium as well as sodium excretion. (From Giebisch, G. H., and Thier, S. O.: Potassium: Physiological and Clinical Importance. A monograph. Somerville, N. J., Hoechst-Roussel Pharmaceuticals, Inc., 1977, p. 43. Originally from Giebisch, G. H.: The sea within us: A clinical guide to fluid and electrolyte balances. Copyright 1975, G. D. Searle & Co., Prepared by Science and Medicine Publishing Co., Inc.)

pokalemic metabolic alkalosis. These diuretics are usually administered in edematous states, characterized by high levels of aldosterone secretion. When the diuretic action leads to the delivery of increased quantities of sodium chloride to the aldosterone-stimulated distal nephron, sodium reabsorption is enhanced, and the secretion of potassium, hydrogen, and ammonium ions is facilitated. The resulting increased hydrogen ion secretion generates an increase in serum bicarbonate concentration. In the presence of the sodium avidity of edematous states, hypochloremia induced by the diuretics, secondary hyperaldosteronism, and potassium depletion also induced by the diuretics, the T_m bicarbonate will be elevated. With an elevated T_m bicarbonate, elevation of serum bicarbonate will be maintained and may induce the retention of CO_2. The elevated P_{CO_2} will again contribute to bicarbonate retention.

When diuretics are used for the treatment of nonedematous states (see section on diuretics), they may produce extracellular fluid volume contraction and stimulate aldosterone. The delivery of sodium chloride to the aldosterone-stimulated distal nephron will reproduce the same sequence of events seen in the edematous patient and again result in metabolic alkalosis. Diuretic-induced metabolic alkalosis can be corrected by the administration of potassium chloride.

The Role of Mineralocorticoids in Metabolic Alkalosis

It has been difficult to demonstrate a role for mineralocorticoid excess in the generation of metabolic alkalosis in humans. In carefully controlled studies the administration of mineralocorticoids for up to three months failed to induce metabolic alkalosis, and led to the suggestion that mineralocorticoids were more important in sustaining alkalosis than in generating it. Nonetheless, the incidence of metabolic alkalosis in patients with spontaneous or iatrogenic excesses of mineralocorticoids is so great that it seems possible that the reported studies simply fail to demonstrate the developing pathophysiology. From animal studies it appears that the administration of mineralocorticoids leads to retention of sodium in the distal nephron. The retained sodium expands the extracellular fluid, depressing proximal tubular reabsorption of sodium. The increased sodium delivery to the distal nephron in the presence of excess mineralocorticoid results in the retention of sodium and the stimulation of hydrogen, ammonium, and potassium excretion. Metabolic alkalosis is generated by the increased acid excretion sustained by the hypokalemia, hypochloremia, and mineralocorticoid excess.

Removal or antagonism of mineralocorticoid excess is the treatment of choice for mineralocorticoid-induced metabolic alkalosis. Potassium chloride should be administered.

Unusual Causes of Metabolic Alkalosis

(1) Salt wasting states. In patients who have a defect in sodium reabsorption in either the proximal tubule or the loop of Henle, the delivery of excess quantities of sodium to the distal nephron may result in some salt wasting, producing extracellular fluid volume contraction and aldosterone stimulation. The poorly reabsorbed sodium is now delivered to the distal nephron where stimulation by aldosterone enhances the secretion of potassium, hydrogen, and ammonium ions. The result is the development of metabolic alkalosis as has been described for diuretics.

(2) Hypercalcemia. Hypercalcemia acutely stimulates the secretion of hydrogen ion in both the stomach and kidney, leading to an alkalemic state. If the hypercalcemia is not caused by hyperparathyroidism, it will suppress parathyroid hormone. The reduced parathyroid hormone activity permits elevation of the T_m bicarbonate and contributes to sustained metabolic alkalosis.

(3) Chloride loss in the stool. There is a congenital defect in the exchange of bicarbonate and chloride in the ileum. The result is the loss of excessive quantities of chloride in the stool and the retention of bicarbonate in the blood. There are also acquired forms of severe chloride loss in the stool that may be associated with volume contraction, hyperaldosteronism, and metabolic alkalosis.

(4) Contraction alkalosis. It has been suggested that the loss of sodium chloride without proportional loss of sodium bicarbonate or the loss of large quantities of water will result in a relative concentration of bicarbonate in the extracellular fluid. This relative increase in bicarbonate concentration is referred to as contraction alkalosis. It seems likely that the extracellular fluid volume contraction of contraction alkalosis contributes a component of secondary hyperaldosteronism to the development and maintenance of the alkalosis.

(5) Posthypercapneic metabolic alkalosis. This was described in the section on chronic pulmonary acidosis.

Metabolic alkalosis has also been categorized as saline dependent or saline resistant. In saline-dependent metabolic alkalosis the administration of chloride in any form will correct the alkalosis; that is, despite the persistence of hypokalemia, the administration of sodium chloride will lead to correction of the alkalosis. Saline-dependent metabolic alkalosis is characterized by absence of chloride in the urine during steady-state alkalosis. It is important to add that though the alkalosis can be corrected without potassium, it is essential to treat these patients with potassium when they are hypokalemic. There is another population of patients whose metabolic alkalosis is not corrected by the administration of saline, but rather requires large quantities of potassium chloride. This form of metabolic alkalosis, termed saline resistant, is characterized by the presence of chloride in the urine during steady-state alkalosis. Saline-dependent alkalosis is seen with vomiting and with diuretic use, circumstances in which there is avidity for sodium retention. Saline-resistant alkalosis is most commonly seen with mineralocorticoid excess, a circumstance in which there is extracellular fluid volume expansion and reduced proximal sodium reabsorption.

Potassium

Potassium, the most plentiful cation in the body, is largely restricted to the intracellular fluid. Of the approximately 50 mEq of potassium per kilogram of wet weight in the body, over 97 per cent is in the intracellular fluid at concentrations of approximately 150 mEq/l, while the less than 3 per cent present in the extracellular fluid is normally maintained between 3.5 and 5.0 mEq/l. Thus a concentration gradient from intracellular fluid to extracellular fluid favors the loss of potassium from cells. This is the reverse of the situation for sodium, in which a high concentration in the extracellular fluid and low concentration intracellularly favors diffusion into cells. The maintenance of high intracellular potassium and high extracellular sodium concentrations is accomplished through the function of ion exchange pumps in the cell membrane that extrude sodium and move potassium back into cells. These pumps, which play a key role in maintaining cell volume and electrical activity, depend on the sodium-potassium-adenosinetriphosphatase (ATPase) system. The high intracellular concentration of potassium is critical in regulating a host of biologic processes, including cell volume, acid-base status, electrophysiologic properties of cells, and synthesis of RNA, protein, and glycogen. The importance of these processes predicts that altered potassium metabolism will have profound clinical effects.

A discussion of the pathophysiology of altered potassium metabolism will be facilitated by a review of (1) normal potassium balance and distribution, and (2) pathophysiology of potassium metabolism, including: (a) mechanisms contributing to the development of hypokalemia and hyperkalemia, (b) the clinical manifestations of hypokalemia and hyperkalemia, and (c) the treatment of hypokalemia and hyperkalemia.

NORMAL POTASSIUM BALANCE AND DISTRIBUTION

The normal total body potassium content is determined by the balance between intake and excretion. Of equal importance to the total quantity of potassium in the body is the distribution of potassium between the intracellular and extracellular fluid compartments.

Intake

The average North American diet contains 60 to 100 mEq of potassium per day, the majority of which is absorbed in the small intestine. Although the large intestine can excrete potassium, under ordinary circumstances it makes a small contribution to potassium

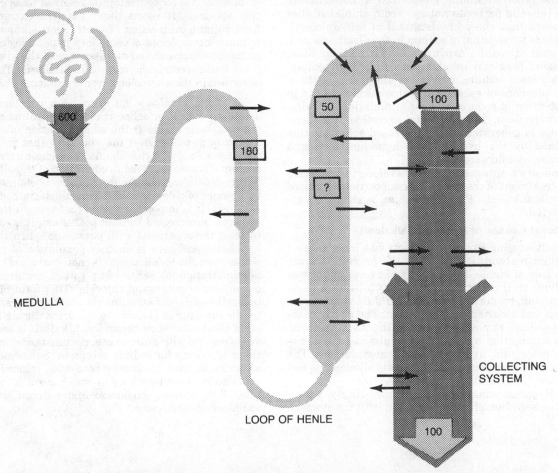

Figure 36. Main sites of tubular potassium transport. Schematic nephron consisting of glomerulus, proximal tubule, loop of Henle, distal tubule, and collecting duct system. In a healthy adult about 100 mEq of potassium are ingested daily, and some 600 mEq are filtered. In metabolic balance, roughly 100 mEq of potassium are excreted by the kidneys, neglecting here the relatively small amounts excreted by extrarenal routes. The direction of the arrows across the tubular epithelium indicates the direction of net transport of potassium. Of the 600 mEq filtered, some 180 mEq remain two-thirds of the way down the proximal tubule. Probably most of this potassium is reabsorbed in the loop of Henle. Along the distal tubule and the collecting duct system, net potassium secretion dominates, so that most of the potassium appearing in the final urine is derived by tubular secretion. *Double arrows* across the distal tubule and collecting duct system indicate the capacity of these tubular segments to either reabsorb or secrete potassium. (From Giebisch, G. H., and Thier, S. O.: Potassium: Physiological and Clinical Importance. Somerville, N. J., Hoechst-Roussel Pharmaceuticals, 1977, p. 31. Originally from Grantham, J. J.: In Brenner, B. M., and Rector, F. C., Jr. (eds.): The Kidney. Philadelphia, W. B. Saunders Co., 1976, p. 299.)

balance. However, since the colon is responsive to aldosterone, it may have an important excretory function in the pathologic states.

Excretion

Net potassium balance is primarily determined by renal excretion (Fig. 36). Our present concepts of the normal renal handling of potassium are derived from micropuncture studies in animals and have been extrapolated to man. Potassium is freely filtered at the glomerulus, with the concentration of potassium in glomerular ultrafiltrate equal to that in plasma. Regardless of potassium intake, reabsorption of filtered potassium in superficial nephrons is nearly complete after passage through the proximal tubule and loop of Henle; approximately 5 per cent of filtered potassium is delivered to the early distal tubule. In animals maintained with a low potassium intake, the distal nephron continues to reabsorb potassium, and less than 1 per cent of the filtered potassium is ultimately excreted in the urine. With normal or high potassium intake, the proximal tubule and the loop of Henle continue to reabsorb approximately 95 per cent of filtered potassium. Despite this nearly complete reabsorption of potassium in the proximal portions of the nephron, final urine contains quantities of potassium equivalent to 10 to 20 per cent of the filtered load. Since only 5 per cent of filtered potassium reaches the distal nephron, it follows that the distal nephron adds potassium to the final urine. Addition of potassium to the urine appears to be a function of connecting tubule cells and principal cells of the collecting tubule. Intercalated cells in both segments appear to play a role in potassium reabsorption. The factors affecting secretion of potassium by the distal tubule and collecting duct are well defined and represent the focus for an analysis of renal potassium wasting or retention.

Distal tubular potassium secretion depends upon (1) potassium intake, (2) renal tubular cell potassium concentration, (3) delivery of sodium and the rate of urine flow to the distal nephron, (4) the anion accompanying sodium delivered to the distal nephron, (5) the level of mineralocorticoid and glucocorticoid activity, (6) beta$_2$-catechol activity, and (7) the functional integrity of the distal tubule cells (Fig. 37).

There is growing evidence that the deep nephrons behave differently from the superficial nephrons. In the deep nephrons, reabsorption of potassium in the medullary collecting duct results in recycling of potassium into the descending limb of Henle's loop. There is clear evidence that the potassium delivered to the end of the descending limb may exceed filtered potassium and is a function of urinary potassium concentration. The recycling of potassium in the deep nephrons provides a potential means of enhancing tubular response to extremes of potassium challenge, but the actual physiologic contribution of this mechanism is unknown.

(1) Potassium intake: There is an adaptation to a chronic increase in potassium intake that permits a person to excrete quantities of potassium that would produce hyperkalemia if administered without an adequate adaptive period. This adaptive mechanism correlates with an increase in sodium-potassium-adenosinetriphosphatase activity in cells of the distal nephron and is similar to the adaptation that allows

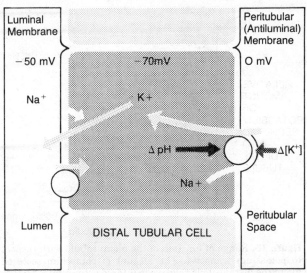

Figure 37. Elements of potassium transport system. A hypothetical secretory distal tubular cell is shown. As discussed, the cellular potassium concentration of tubular secretory cells is maintained at a high level by a peritubular sodium-potassium exchange pump. The activity of this pump is regulated by the extracellular potassium concentration and by changes in cellular pH. Electrical polarization is asymmetrical, and the smaller luminal potential difference allows for some potassium leakage into the lumen. Thus, across the luminal cell membrane, potassium ions diffuse from cell into the lumen, but it is not certain whether this process is supported by an active pump. Some exchange of potassium for sodium may also occur, particularly at the level of the collecting tubule epithelium. In conditions of a low potassium intake, one can also demonstrate the presence of an active potassium reabsorptive pump at the luminal cell membrane. Sodium ions normally diffuse into the cell across the luminal membrane and stimulate peritubular sodium-potassium exchange. (From Giebisch, G. H., and Thier, S. O.: Potassium: Physiological and Clinical Importance. Somerville, N. J., Hoechst-Roussel Pharmaceuticals, 1977, p. 35. Originally from Giebisch, G.: Renal potassium excretion. In Rouiller, C., and Muller, A. F. (eds.): The Kidney: Morphology, Biochemistry, Physiology. Vol. 3. New York, Academic Press, 1971.)

the person with decreasing renal function to excrete increasing amounts of potassium per remaining nephron mass (Fig. 38). The stimulation of aldosterone by prolonged increased intake of potassium may also contribute to the adaptive mechanism. Though the presence of chronic adaptation to increased potassium intake is well recognized, the cellular events controlling this adaptation are still a subject of debate. The intracellular concentration of potassium almost certainly plays a role.

(2) Renal tubular cell potassium concentration: The amount of potassium that can be secreted by the distal tubule cell is dependent upon the cellular potassium rather than on the serum potassium concentration. Thus when serum and cellular potassium are increased by potassium loading, potassium excretion rises. When serum potassium is lowered and cellular potassium increased by either respiratory or metabolic alkalemia, potassium excretion rises. During acute acidemia, which raises serum potassium and lowers cellular potassium, there is a reduction in potassium excretion. The situation is more complicated in chronic acidemia, which may be associated with potassium wasting. The

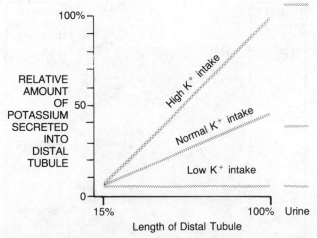

Figure 38. Range of function of the distal tubule with respect to potassium transport. The amount of potassium secreted along the distal tubule relative to filtered potassium is plotted as a function of distal tubular length. 100 per cent of the ordinate in each case equals an amount of potassium equal to that filtered into the glomerulus. Three metabolic situations are shown: high, normal, and low potassium intake. Note that the amount of potassium secreted at any given point along the distal tubule is a direct function of potassium intake and the distance along the distal tubule. Horizontal bars on the far right indicate amount of potassium in the final urine and reflect effect of the collecting duct in modifying urine leaving the distal tubule. (From Giebisch, G. H., and Thier, S. O.: Potassium: Physiological and Clinical Importance. Somerville, N. J., Hoechst-Roussel Pharmaceuticals, 1977, p. 32. Originally from Giebisch, G.: Renal potassium excretion. In Rouiller, C., and Muller, A. F. (eds.): The Kidney: Morphology, Biochemistry, Physiology. Vol. 3. New York, Academic Press, 1971.)

mechanisms by which acidemia converts from a potassium-retaining to a potassium-wasting state are not well understood, but may reflect a change in the delivery of sodium to the distal nephron.

(3) Delivery of sodium and the urine flow rate to the distal nephron: The amount of sodium and fluid delivered to the distal nephron is critical in determining potassium excretion. When the positively charged sodium ion is actively reabsorbed in the distal nephron, an anion lags behind in the tubular lumen, producing an electrical potential difference across the tubule with the lumen negative. This electrical gradient facilitates the movement of positively charged potassium from cell to lumen. The relationship between sodium delivery and potassium excretion will be a variable one, since, in addition to sodium delivery, the avidity of the tubule for sodium (that is, the need to conserve sodium), the cellular potassium concentration, and the permeance of the anion accompanying sodium will all affect this relationship. Potassium uptake from blood into cell occurs by a direct sodium-for-potassium exchange. The rate of delivery of urine to the distal nephron (independent of sodium content) also regulates potassium secretion; the greater the rate of delivery, the greater the rate of secretion.

(4) Anion accompanying sodium: Theoretically the more impermeant the anion accompanying sodium to the distal nephron, the greater will be the electrical gradient generated by sodium reabsorption. In other words, as sodium is reabsorbed, the lumen will become more negative if sodium is accompanied by a relatively nonreabsorbable anion such as bicarbonate rather than by a more readily reabsorbable anion such as chloride. The increased gradient would favor potassium secretion. In fact, it now appears that as chloride concentration per se falls in the distal tubule fluid, potassium secretion is stimulated independent of voltage changes. The lowered chloride concentration may favor potassium secretion via a coupled K-Cl transport mechanism.

(5) Mineralocorticoid and glucocorticoid effect: Aldosterone secretion is controlled by two major factors: the renin-angiotensin system and potassium. Once secreted, aldosterone binds to the nuclei of the distal tubular cells and, by a sequence of steps that are dependent upon protein synthesis, stimulates the reabsorption of sodium by increasing the number of amiloride-sensitive channels in the luminal membrane of the distal tubular cell. Thus, for any given quantity of sodium delivered to the distal nephron, reabsorption is greater in the presence of aldosterone. Although the distal nephron is capable of aldosterone-independent sodium reabsorption and potassium secretion, aldosterone plays an important role in protecting against hyperkalemia during periods of volume contraction or potassium loading or both. Aldosterone is the primary mineralocorticoid affecting the distal nephron, but there are other substances that have mineralocorticoid-like effects (desoxycorticosterone, 18 hydroxycorticosterone, licorice extract). Glucocorticoids are capable of modest binding to aldosterone receptors at concentrations achievable physiologically. Dexamethasone can enhance potassium secretion but the effect is more likely due to an enhancement of urine flow rate.

(6) Beta$_2$-catechols: Increased quantities of beta$_2$-catechols will inhibit net secretion of potassium in the distal tubule. Whether the mechanism of action is inhibition of secretion or enhancement of reabsorption is not known.

(7) Functional integrity of the distal tubule cell: Finally, even if there is adequate potassium intake, adequate delivery of sodium and fluid to the distal nephron, and adequate aldosterone, there must be an adequate number of functioning intact distal tubule cells to reabsorb sodium and excrete potassium. Diseases capable of producing interstitial nephritis can alter function of the distal tubular cell.

Distribution

The distribution of potassium between intracellular and extracellular fluid is maintained via membrane-situated ion exchange pumps. Seventy-five per cent or more of total body potassium is in muscle cells, where it exists at concentrations as high as 150 mEq/l. Intracellular potassium concentration may vary somewhat from tissue to tissue, but is invariably manyfold higher than the extracellular concentration.

The distribution of potassium across the cell membrane may be modified by a number of factors that would therefore change the serum potassium concentration without affecting total body potassium content. The most important factors modifying distribution are (1) cellular integrity, (2) acid-base status, (3) hormonal effects, and (4) drugs.

If the integrity of the cell membrane is interrupted, as when red cells are hemolyzed or tissue is crushed by injury, potassium is released from cells into the extracellular fluid. If the extent of cell injury is sufficient, serum potassium may rise into the lethal range. Acute serum hypertonicity, without cell injury, may lead to a shift of potassium out of cells.

A major proportion of excess hydrogen ion resulting from either metabolic or respiratory acidosis is buffered intracellularly (see section on acid-base metabolism). When hydrogen ions enter cells to be buffered, potassium leaves. Thus, acidemia would be expected to raise the potassium concentration in the extracellular fluid. When alkali is added to the body, hydrogen ions leave cells to buffer the alkali, and potassium replaces hydrogen in the cell. Thus, acute alkalemia would be expected to reduce the concentration of potassium in the extracellular fluid. The effects of pH are more complex than originally anticipated. It is now evident that metabolic derangements cause greater potassium shifts than respiratory abnormalities. Of the causes of metabolic acidosis, those associated with hyperchloremia cause greater potassium shifts than organic acidoses, an observation that may be due to a greater proportion of organic acid entering the cell intact, while chloride confined largely to the extracellular space requires that a cation (K^+) exit from the cell as H^+ enters to be buffered.

Insulin is capable of redistributing potassium into cells, a fact that has been useful in the treatment of hyperkalemia. The interaction between potassium and insulin has now been defined as a major acute adaptive mechanism preventing hyperkalemia and one in which there is feedback control. In other words, the infusion of potassium into an animal stimulates the release of insulin, which enhances potassium uptake primarily by muscle and liver cells. Potassium infusion into subjects with an intact insulin secretory mechanism leads to only very minor elevations in serum potassium. However, the same potassium infusion into subjects with impaired insulin secretion may lead to striking hyperkalemia. The role of insulin in preventing hyperkalemia will be discussed subsequently.

A second critical hormone that regulates and is regulated by potassium is aldosterone. In the discussion of the volume and composition of the body fluids, the renin-angiotensin system was noted to be primarily responsive to changes in volume of the extracellular fluid. A second regulator of aldosterone synthesis and release is potassium. Elevations in serum potassium as small as 0.2 to 0.3 mEq/l result in a prompt increase in aldosterone secretion, while reductions in potassium inhibit it. Increased circulating aldosterone in turn enhances potassium movement into cells and increases gastrointestinal potassium secretion, but more importantly increases the renal excretion of potassium. This is a rather simplified description of the interaction between potassium and aldosterone. In fact, potassium also affects renin production, elevations of potassium inhibiting renin release. Potassium would therefore modulate aldosterone secretion directly by acting on the adrenal to stimulate secretion and indirectly via the kidney to inhibit secretion by inhibiting renin release. Pharmacologic doses of glucocorticoids acting via aldosterone receptors may also shift potassium into cells.

Epinephrine causes a fall in plasma potassium at the same time that it produces a fall in urinary potassium excretion. Since the plasma potassium falls without concomitant loss from the body, epinephrine must shift potassium intracellularly. It is now clear that the effect is specific for beta$_2$ stimulation. Beta$_1$ stimulation does not affect plasma potassium concentration. Selective beta$_2$ stimulation lowers and selective inhibition raises plasma potassium concentration. Patients on a regimen of beta$_2$ or nonselective beta blockers have slightly higher serum potassium levels when taking the drugs than when not taking them. When other mechanisms protecting serum potassium concentration are impaired, beta$_2$ blockade may be dangerous. Alpha catechol stimulation raises serum potassium, an effect that is inhibited by alpha catechol blockers.

There are a host of drugs that affect potassium distribution. Digitalis, by inhibiting membrane ion-exchange pumps, may produce hyperkalemia when ingested in toxic quantities. Succinylcholine, a depolarizer of cell membranes, permits greater potassium exit from cells and can produce hyperkalemia. Nonsteroidal anti-inflammatory agents inhibit prostaglandin synthesis and its subsequent stimulation of the renin-aldosterone system. The reduction of aldosterone production may result in hyperkalemia.

All states of hypokalemia or hyperkalemia may now be analyzed in terms of potassium intake, excretion, and distribution.

HYPOKALEMIA

Hypokalemia (Table 6), a serum potassium less than 3.5 mEq/l, can occur because of decreased dietary intake, redistribution of potassium from extracellular to intracellular fluid, or true loss of potassium from the body. Inadequate dietary potassium intake is rarely a clinically important cause of hypokalemia. Redistribution of potassium from extracellular to intracellular fluid does occur in response to excessive insulin, acute alkalemia, and as a part of hypokalemic periodic paralysis, but is a far less common cause of hypokalemia than is true depletion of body potassium.

Loss of Potassium

Loss of potassium from the body can occur by one of three potential routes: (1) skin, (2) the kidneys, and (3) the gastrointestinal tract.

Skin Loss. The loss of potassium through the skin is rarely an important cause of hypokalemia. Though sweat may contain high concentrations of potassium, the volume of sweat is usually insufficient to account for significant potassium losses. Furthermore, with sweating and depletion of extracellular fluid volume, stimulation of aldosterone is likely to produce renal potassium wasting that will be at least as significant as the sweat potassium loss.

Kidney Loss. Potassium depletion in the adult most commonly occurs secondary to renal losses of potassium, and these losses are most often diuretic induced. Potassium wasting via the kidney may occur as the result of increased potassium secretion, decreased potassium reabsorption, or both. Increased potassium secretion should be anticipated whenever there is (1) increased intracellular potassium, (2) increased delivery of fluid and sodium to the distal nephron, (3) decreased delivery of chloride to the distal secretory site, or (4) stimulation of sodium reabsorption and

TABLE 6. HYPOKALEMIA

Redistribution
  Insulin
  Alkalemia
  Periodic paralysis

Loss From Body
  Renal
    Normotensive
      Diuretics
      Renal tubular dysfunction (RTA, Fanconi syndrome, etc.)
      Bartter's syndrome
      Welt's syndrome
      Magnesium deficiency
    Hypertensive
      High renin—high aldosterone
        Renovascular hypertension
        Malignant hypertension
        Renin-secreting tumor
      Low renin—high aldosterone
        Adrenal adenoma
        Adrenal hyperplasia
          Microadenomata
          Dexamethasone suppressible
          Congenital hyperaldosteronism
      Low renin—low aldosterone
        Liddle syndrome
        Licorice ingestion
        Excess DOCA, corticosterone
        Congenital hyperplasia
          17-Hydroxylase deficiency
          11-Hydroxylase deficiency
      Low renin—variable aldosterone
        Cushing syndrome
        ACTH excess
  Gastrointestinal
    Vomiting (loss is renal)
    Diarrhea (and cathartics)
    Villous adenoma
    Fistulae
  Skin
    Sweat
    Burns

From Giebisch, G. H., and Thier, S. O.: Potassium: Physiological and Clinical Importance. Somerville, N. J., Hoechst-Roussel Pharmaceuticals, 1977, p. 41.

potassium secretion via aldosterone or via aldosterone-insensitive pathways in the distal nephron.

The physiologic mechanisms involved in renal potassium wasting form the basis of understanding a practical clinical scheme that divides renal potassium wasters into normotensive and hypertensive groups and then further subdivides the hypertensive groups on the basis of the secretion of renin and aldosterone.

Renal potassium wasting in the normotensive pattern. Patients with renal potassium wasting in the absence of hypertension must have acquired or congenital tubular dysfunction or both. The most common cause of acquired renal tubular potassium wasting is the administration of diuretics (see section on diuretics). All diuretics that inhibit sodium reabsorption proximal to the potassium secretory site would be expected to increase sodium and fluid delivery to that site and to facilitate potassium excretion. Thus, diuretics working in the proximal tubule, loop of Henle, and early distal convoluted tubule will all increase sodium delivery to the potassium excretory site and produce kaliuresis. The kaliuresis would predictably be increased if the sodium delivery were associated with delivery of de-

creased chloride concentration. Decreased chloride concentration would occur predictably with the use of carbonic anhydrase inhibitors such as acetazolamide or in association with the alkalosis produced by ethacrynic acid, furosemide, bumetanide, the organomercurials, and the thiazides. A third mechanism by which diuretics may produce renal potassium wasting is the direct inhibition of potassium reabsorption coupled to sodium chloride reabsorption as occurs in the loop of Henle with ethacrynic acid, furosemide, and bumetanide. Finally, all diuretics have the potential to produce extracellular fluid volume contraction and thus secondary hyperaldosteronism, which accentuates renal potassium loss. It follows that all diuretics that do not specifically interfere with potassium secretion (for example, spironolactone, amiloride, triamterene) may produce potassium depletion. The extent of potassium depletion will be a complex function of the potency of the diuretic, the dose and frequency of administration, the patient's acid-base status, the intrinsic rate of sodium delivery to the distal nephron, and the level of aldosterone.

While diuretics produce potassium wasting as a function of their intended mechanism of action, other drugs may produce kaliuresis as a result of their nephrotoxicity. Several nephrotoxins, both exogenous and endogenous, are capable of producing a generalized tubular dysfunction known as the Fanconi syndrome. The Fanconi syndrome is characterized by a generalized proximal tubular dysfunction affecting the reabsorption of sugar, amino acids, uric acid, phosphate, and bicarbonate. While there may be reduced potassium reabsorption, it is more likely that potassium wasting in the Fanconi syndrome is secondary to reduced proximal reabsorption of sodium bicarbonate with increased delivery of sodium and the impermeant anion bicarbonate as well as a decreased concentration of chloride to the distal nephron. The capacity of the distal nephron to reabsorb sodium bicarbonate is exceeded with a resulting loss of sodium and bicarbonate in the urine. The combination of sodium bicarbonate loss that results in volume contraction and aldosterone stimulation together with increased delivery of sodium bicarbonate to the distal tubule produces marked kaliuresis and severe potassium depletion.

Potassium wasting by mechanisms similar to those described for the Fanconi syndrome may occur with an isolated defect in proximal tubular bicarbonate reabsorption referred to as proximal renal tubular acidosis. Both proximal and distal renal tubular acidosis, which were discussed in detail in the section on metabolic acidosis, are associated with marked potassium wasting in association with sodium avidity of the distal tubule and a high aldosterone level.

Renal potassium wasting might conceivably result from specific tubular dysfunctions such as proximal sodium wasting or decreased potassium reabsorption, but reports of such disorders are few and unconvincing. Bartter's syndrome, hypokalemia in association with hyperaldosteronism but without hypertension, seems to result from a primary defect in chloride reabsorption. Magnesium depletion has been used experimentally to produce renal potassium wasting; Welt's syndrome is the clinical counterpart of hypomagnesemia with hypokalemia.

Renal potassium wasting in the hypertensive patient.

Virtually all patients with hypertension and renal potassium wasting have an excess of mineralocorticoid activity. Logically these patients may be divided into those in whom mineralocorticoid is stimulated by excessive renin levels and those in whom mineralocorticoid activity is primary and renin is suppressed.

High renin activity occurs characteristically in patients with renal arterial disease and in patients with malignant hypertension. There are isolated instances of cysts or other forms of unilateral renal disease resulting in increased renin production, but almost all of these circumstances can be ascribed to relative renal ischemia stimulating renin release. There are rare patients with renin-secreting tumors.

Patients with primary excesses of mineralocorticoid activity (and therefore low renin levels) can be subdivided into those in whom the mineralocorticoid is aldosterone and those who have increases of other compounds with mineralocorticoid activity. Primary elevations of aldosterone levels are associated with adrenal adenomas or with diffuse adrenal hyperplasia. Those patients with low aldosterone levels and low renin levels may have (1) increases of substances with mineralocorticoid activity (licorice ingestion), (2) increases of a nonaldosterone mineralocorticoid substance, or (3) rarely stimulation of aldosterone-independent potassium secretion (Liddle's syndrome). The last group of patients, those with variable levels of aldosterone and low renin levels, may have Cushing's syndrome or ectopic ACTH production from tumor.

Gastrointestinal Loss. While the kidney is the major route of potassium depletion in adults, the gastrointestinal tract is the most important route of potassium depletion in children. Most hypokalemia from gastrointestinal loss is the result of diarrhea. The potassium appearing in the stool may be the result of decreased small-intestinal potassium absorption or secretion of potassium via the colon. Recall that the colon is responsive to aldosterone. Therefore, diarrhea with its initial loss of potassium and sodium will be associated with extracellular fluid volume contraction, which will stimulate aldosterone secretion. The aldosterone will stimulate colonic potassium secretion and, in addition, will increase renal potassium excretion.

Though vomiting is frequently associated with hypokalemia, it is not the potassium loss in the vomitus that accounts for the potassium depletion. The potassium concentration in gastric contents is relatively low, in the range of 10 to 15 mEq/l. Yet patients who develop hypokalemia are likely to be depleted of several hundred milliequivalents of potassium. The magnitude of potassium depletion would require the loss of more than 10 liters of vomitus, a circumstance that would be distinctly unusual. What actually occurs is the loss of hydrochloric acid and sodium in the vomitus, resulting in transient metabolic alkalemia and some degree of extracellular fluid volume contraction. The concentration of bicarbonate in plasma rises, and when filtered at the glomerulus, the bicarbonate exceeds the proximal tubular capacity of reabsorbing bicarbonate. Sodium bicarbonate is then delivered in increased quantities to the distal nephron, which, because of the concomitant sodium loss in the vomitus, is being stimulated by aldosterone. The combination of increased delivery of sodium bicarbonate with a concomitant fall in chloride concentration and increased aldosterone stimulation leads to marked increases in renal potassium wasting and the potassium depletion of vomiting.

While vomiting may be associated with hypochloremic-hypokalemic metabolic alkalosis, most gastrointestinal potassium wasting is associated with metabolic acidosis. Since the extent of potassium depletion at any given serum potassium concentration is greater in acidemia than in alkalemia, correction of diarrhea-induced hypokalemia is likely to require greater quantities of potassium.

CLINICAL MANIFESTATIONS OF HYPOKALEMIA

Recalling the critical cellular functions that depend upon potassium allows the prediction that depletion of this cation will produce multiple clinical abnormalities. A survey of the effects of potassium depletion on major organ systems and on general cell metabolism will put the problem in perspective.

Cardiovascular System

By far the most dangerous complication of hypokalemia is the development of cardiac arrhythmias. Virtually any arrhythmia may be encountered. Of particular concern is hypokalemia developing in the patient who is taking digitalis. One of the important actions of digitalis is to inhibit the sodium-potassium-ATPase of cardiac muscle membrane, reducing the cellular reuptake of potassium. Digitalis would aggravate intracellular potassium depletion, a situation that would be additive with digitalis in producing rapid spontaneous diastolic depolarization and increasing the automaticity of cardiac muscle cells. Severe hypokalemia is also capable of reducing peripheral vascular resistance, thus lowering blood pressure.

Neuromuscular System

As the degree of hypokalemia progresses from modest to severe, patients may experience initial muscle weakness that can progress to loss of reflexes and ultimately to paralysis with apnea as a terminal event. In addition to the effect on neuromuscular membrane function, hypokalemia is also capable of reducing muscle perfusion. Vigorous muscle exercise in the presence of hypokalemia can produce relative ischemia of muscle and rhabdomyolysis. If hypokalemia is severe enough, rhabdomyolysis may occur even in the absence of exercise.

Renal System

The most important effect of hypokalemia on renal function is loss of concentrating ability and reduced responsiveness to antidiuretic hormone. In this condition, pathologic studies in man do not demonstrate changes in either the collecting duct or the ascending limb of the loop of Henle, but rather demonstrate vacuolation of proximal tubular cells. Hypokalemia is also predictably associated with a shift of hydrogen ions into tubular cells, facilitating the excretion of acid and favoring production and maintenance of metabolic alkalosis. A less predictable effect on renal function is interference with the excretion of a sodium load. The resulting edema will clear on replacement of potassium. Finally, though the major effects of hypokalemia are on tubular function, there may also be an associated mild reduction of glomerular filtration rate with BUN rarely exceeding 40 to 50 mg/dl.

Gastrointestinal System

The primary effect of hypokalemia on the bowel is production of ileus and, occasionally, severe colonic distension.

Endocrine System

Potassium depletion is associated with reduced pancreatic release of insulin in response to hyperglycemia. The resulting decreased glucose tolerance can be corrected by replenishing potassium stores. Hypokalemia might also be expected to reduce aldosterone synthesis and release, but this effect will not override the aldosterone stimulation produced by volume contraction.

General Metabolic Effects

The best-defined abnormality in metabolism associated with hypokalemia is a negative nitrogen balance resulting from impaired protein synthesis. The additional effects of hypokalemia on metabolic processes such as impairment of energy production from the hydrolysis of ATP undoubtedly contribute to the clinical picture of severe hypokalemia, but cannot presently be dissected out as independent events.

TREATMENT OF HYPOKALEMIA

The correction of hypokalemia depends on defining the mechanism of hypokalemia and the extent of the potassium deficit if one is present. Determining the extent of potassium deficit is an indirect process in clinical medicine. What can be measured is the serum potassium concentration, which must then be correlated with cellular potassium content. Correlations of serum potassium concentrations with total body potassium content must take cognizance of the patient's acid-base status. At pH 7.4, empiric observations have determined that a potassium concentration greater than 3.5 mEq/l indicates no more than a 10 per cent depletion in total body potassium. Potassium concentrations of 2.5 mEq/l are associated with reductions of up to 20 per cent of total body potassium and, as the serum potassium concentration falls still further, there are progressively larger increments in potassium depletion for each decrement in serum potassium. Acidemia will produce a higher and alkalemia a lower serum potassium concentration for any given deficit of total body potassium.

Unless the basic mechanism by which potassium depletion has occurred is identified and treated, therapy will have to replace not only the potassium deficit but an ongoing loss. The rate of potassium replacement should be a function of the clinical manifestations of hypokalemia, the cause of the potassium loss, and the extent of the potassium deficit. The presence of cardiac arrhythmias or severe muscle paralysis dictates more rapid intravenous replacement of potassium deficits. Hypokalemia associated with alkalosis dictates that the potassium replacement be in the form of potassium chloride. Hypokalemia in the presence of metabolic acidosis dictates that the potassium must eventually be given as potassium bicarbonate or an equivalent salt. The word *eventually* is key. If bicarbonate is given early in the therapy of hypokalemia and acidosis, it may result in the shift of potassium into cells and worsening of the hypokalemia. Therefore it is reasonable to initiate therapy with potassium chloride and

to shift to potassium bicarbonate as a rise in serum potassium is documented.

HYPERKALEMIA

Hyperkalemia (Table 7) is defined as a serum potassium greater than 5.0 mEq/l. While hypokalemia is rarely, if ever, seen as an artifact of the laboratory determination of potassium, hyperkalemia may be factitious. Hemolysis of the blood sample with release of potassium from red cells or the release of potassium from increased numbers of white cells or platelets during clotting will result in the report of hyperkalemia by the laboratory. A heparinized sample of blood, drawn without a tourniquet, should yield a normal potassium measurement. Because of the lethal potential of hyperkalemia, the results of the redrawn blood test should not be awaited, but rather the characteristic ECG changes of hyperkalemia should be sought and treatment initiated if necessary.

If true hyperkalemia is indeed present, it may be caused by increased intake, decreased excretion, or redistribution of potassium from cells into extracellular fluid. Increased intake of potassium alone will rarely produce hyperkalemia. Even if intake of potassium is increased, the development of hyperkalemia should suggest impaired excretion or redistribution of potassium or both. Defective renal excretion of potassium can occur (1) as the result of reduced delivery of sodium and fluid to the distal nephron, (2) from damage to the distal tubular cell, (3) from a deficiency of aldosterone, or (4) from administration of the diuretics spironolactone, triamterene, or amiloride.

In circumstances in which delivery of sodium to the distal nephron is limited by either a marked reduction in glomerular filtration rate or an increase in proximal reabsorption of sodium, there may be inadequate distal sodium reabsorption to permit potassium secretion. If there is adequate delivery of sodium and volume

TABLE 7. HYPERKALEMIA

Pseudohyperkalemia
  Hemolysis in test tube
  Platelet release
  WBC release

Retention in Body
  Increased intake—diet, meds
  Decreased excretion: renal
    Oligoanuria
    ↓ GFR
    ↓ Tubular secretion
    1° Structural or functional disease
    ↓ Aldosterone
      Decreased production (renin normal or ↑)
      Decreased stimulation (hyporeninemic states)
      Antagonism of activity (spironolactone)
    Meds—Triamterene

Excessive Tissue Release or Redistribution
  Hemolysis
  Tissue necrosis
  Acidemia
  ↓ Insulin
  Periodic paralysis—Gamstorp's disease

From Giebisch, G. H., and Thier, S. O.: Potassium: Physiological and Clinical Importance. Somerville, N. J., Hoechst-Roussel Pharmaceuticals, 1977, p. 29.

to the distal nephron, inability to excrete potassium can result from damage to the distal tubular cell, as in interstitial nephritis.

If there is adequate delivery of sodium and volume and an intact distal tubular cell, there still is a requirement for aldosterone to respond to changes in potassium intake by increasing potassium excretion. Therefore, hyperkalemia may result from a deficiency of aldosterone. Such a deficiency may occur as part of a generalized loss of adrenal cortical mass in Addison's disease, as an isolated deficiency in the production or release of aldosterone, or as the result of reduced stimulation of aldosterone by a hyporeninemic state. Hyporeninemic-hypoaldosteronism has been reported with increased frequency in patients with diabetes mellitus and interstitial nephritis. This population of patients may be particularly sensitive to the development of hyperkalemia if they are also insulin deficient. Ordinarily in patients with renal failure, insulin and aldosterone will suffice to regulate serum potassium. If a patient lacks only insulin, aldosterone, though less effective than insulin in protecting against hyperkalemia, will remain as the last defense against life-threatening hyperkalemia. Interference with the action of aldosterone, as might occur with the administration of the diuretic spironolactone, would then precipitate severe hyperkalemia. Another cause of hyperkalemia has been described with increased distal tubular chloride reabsorption. This "chloride shunt" is associated with extracellular fluid volume expansion and reduced renin-stimulated aldosterone production. The chloride shunt has also been postulated to reduce luminal negativity and thereby potassium secretion.

Finally, if adequate amounts of sodium and volume are delivered to the distal nephron, if the distal tubular cells are intact, and if mineralocorticoid is present, potassium excretion may still be impaired by administration of the diuretics spironolactone, triamterene, or amiloride.

Redistribution of potassium, as occurs with chronic acidemia in uremia, may result in elevated serum potassium levels while total body potassium stores are reduced. Aside from acidemia, the most important cause of redistribution of potassium is cell injury (hemolysis or tissue necrosis).

CLINICAL MANIFESTATIONS OF HYPERKALEMIA

Electrophysiologic effects of hyperkalemia are so lethal that only two clinical manifestations need be mentioned. First and most important is the effect of hyperkalemia on the heart. Although the electrical effects of hyperkalemia do not correlate well with the serum potassium concentration, the progression of hyperkalemic effects on the electrocardiogram is reasonably predictable within a given individual. Initially there is peaking of the T waves, which is followed by lengthening of the PR interval, loss of the P wave, widening of the QRS complex, and ultimately ventricular fibrillation or standstill. Obviously hyperkalemia is a medical emergency. The other clinical manifestation of hyperkalemia is muscle weakness and, occasionally, muscle paralysis. These neuromuscular complications are usually of secondary importance to the cardiac events.

TREATMENT OF HYPERKALEMIA

The treatment of hyperkalemia can be directed at antagonizing effects of potassium on the electrophysiologic events in cardiac muscle by giving calcium, or at redistributing potassium into the cell by giving insulin and glucose or an alkalinizing solution such as sodium bicarbonate. None of these forms of therapy alters the total body potassium load. Total body potassium can be reduced by use of resins that exchange sodium for potassium in the bowel or by use of dialysis.

If hyperkalemia is chronic, efforts must be directed at correcting the patient's acid-base status, ensuring the delivery of adequate quantities of sodium to the distal nephron, and ensuring adequate levels of mineralocorticoid. If hyperkalemia persists, dietary restriction of potassium and the judicious use of potassium exchange resins may permit control of the hyperkalemia.

Calcium, Magnesium, and Phosphate _____

Calcium, magnesium, and phosphate are major components of bone and muscle. The homeostasis of these minerals depends upon intestinal absorption, equilibrium with bone stores, and renal excretion. These processes are regulated by parathyroid hormone, calcitonin, and vitamin D_3 and its active metabolites. The physiology and pathophysiology of these hormones has been covered in detail in the section on endocrinology. We will discuss the renal handling of calcium, magnesium, and phosphate and the effects of these ions on the kidney.

CALCIUM

Calcium is present in plasma at a concentration of 9.5 ± 1.0 mg/dl. Plasma calcium is 50 per cent ionized, about 40 per cent protein bound (predominantly to albumin), and about 10 per cent complexed with substances such as citrate. The 60 per cent of serum calcium that is non-protein bound is ultrafiltered at the glomerulus and 98 to 99 per cent reabsorbed during passage through the nephron (Fig. 39). The reabsorption of calcium in the proximal tubule occurs by both passive and active processes. The transtubular permeability to calcium in this segment is high. The process of fluid reabsorption along the proximal tubule tends to elevate the intratubular calcium concentration slightly above the peritubular concentration, thereby providing a driving force for passive calcium reabsorption. The reabsorption of calcium in the proximal tubule therefore closely parallels the reabsorption of sodium and water. Factors that inhibit proximal tubular sodium reabsorption—such as volume expansion,

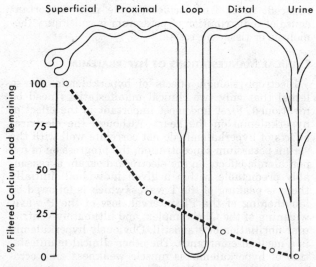

Figure 39. Calcium reabsorption along the nephron. (From Sutton, R. A. L., and Dirks, J. H.: Renal handling of calcium, phosphate, and magnesium. In Brenner, B. M., and Rector, F. C., Jr. (eds.): The Kidney. 2nd ed. Philadelphia, W. B. Saunders Co., 1981, p. 561.)

parathyroid hormone, proximal diuretics—also inhibit calcium reabsorption. Active transport makes at least a small contribution to calcium reabsorption in the proximal tubule. Calcium ions passively diffuse across the luminal membrane down a steep electrochemical gradient. Two mechanisms have been identified for then pumping calcium uphill across the basolateral membrane. One is an adenosine triphosphate (ATP)-driven calcium pump (Ca-ATPase). The other is a carrier system facilitating the exchange of intracellular calcium with extracellular sodium, so that the inward sodium gradient across the basolateral membrane provides the driving force for uphill calcium extrusion. The relative contributions of ATP-driven calcium transport and Na-Ca exchange to calcium reabsorption in the proximal tubule are not known.

In the thick ascending limb of Henle the process of active NaCl reabsorption generates a lumen-positive transtubular potential, as discussed earlier. This lumen-positive potential provides the driving force for passive reabsorption of calcium in this nephron segment that has appreciable transtubular calcium permeability. Thus, calcium reabsorption in the thick ascending limb is inhibited by agents such as loop diuretics that block Na-K-Cl cotransport. Parathyroid hormone increases calcium reabsorption in the thick ascending limb by enhancing the permeability to calcium.

Calcium reabsorption in the distal tubule occurs predominantly by active transport. The relative contributions of ATP-driven calcium transport and Ca-Na exchange are not known. Of note is that thiazide diuretics stimulate calcium reabsorption in the distal tubule. It is possible that by blocking sodium entry across the luminal membrane, thiazides reduce intracellular sodium and thereby increase the driving force for active calcium extrusion via Na-Ca exchange across the basolateral membrane. Calcium reabsorption in the distal nephron is stimulated by parathyroid hor-

mone and by metabolic alkalosis and is inhibited by metabolic acidosis.

The factors modifying calcium excretion are hormones, extracellular fluid volume, acid-base status, and physical activity.

The hormones that alter calcium excretion are parathyroid hormone, calcitonin, and vitamin D. Parathyroid hormone inhibits the reabsorption of calcium in the proximal tubule but enhances it in the loop of Henle and the distal tubule. The enhancement of distal calcium reabsorption is sufficient such that the net result is decreased urinary calcium. The increased urinary calcium excretion seen with hyperparathyroidism results from the combination of increased intestinal absorption and bone resorption, producing an increased filtered load of calcium that overrides the increased distal tubule calcium reabsorption. However, for any given degree of hypercalcemia the extent of hypercalciuria will be less with increased parathyroid hormone activity than with any other cause of hypercalcemia. Calcitonin has a small and clinically unimportant action of increasing the urinary calcium. Vitamin D_3 and its active metabolites directly enhance tubular calcium reabsorption. However, they also stimulate intestinal calcium absorption and facilitate bone resorption so that the net effect of increased quantities of vitamin D_3 is almost invariably increased calciuria.

Extracellular fluid volume expansion that depresses tubular sodium reabsorption affects calcium similarly and produces an increase in urinary calcium excretion.

Diuretics that alter proximal and loop sodium reabsorption are also calciuric agents. Thiazides stimulate calcium reabsorption and reduce calcium excretion.

Acidemia increases bone mobilization of calcium and decreases tubular reabsorption of calcium. The result is increased calciuria. Alkalemia has less predictable effects.

Physical immobilization with prolonged bed rest results in increased mobilization of calcium from bone and an increase in calciuria. If the physical immobilization is associated with a disease that produces increased bone turnover, such as Paget's disease, hypercalcemia may also occur.

Finally, calcium excretion displays a diurnal variation with highest excretion at about midday.

Hypercalcemia produces functional and anatomic injury to the kidney. As the plasma calcium concentration rises, a loss of renal concentrating ability is demonstrable. Impaired concentrating ability results from interference with sodium chloride reabsorption in the loop of Henle (decreasing the medullary interstitial osmotic gradient), and from direct interference with the action of antidiuretic hormone. With higher filtered loads of calcium, sodium reabsorption is inhibited throughout the tubule. The ensuing natriuresis results in a profound extracellular fluid volume contraction. Extracellular fluid volume contraction stimulates the renin-aldosterone axis, which, in the face of increased delivery of sodium to the distal nephron, results in hypokalemia. Acute hypercalcemia stimulates hydrogen ion secretion and produces acute alkalemia. Hypercalcemia will also cause constriction of afferent glomerular arterioles, producing a further decrease in the glomerular filtration rate. The results of the impaired renal function initiated by hypercalcemia are polyuria, polydipsia, hypokalemia, marked extracellular fluid volume contraction, and azotemia. The volume contraction may be sufficient to produce vascular collapse. Alkalemia may occur but is usually transient.

Anatomic injury secondary to hypercalcemia usually begins in the collecting ducts and medullary loops of Henle, where calcium concentration is greatest. Deposition of calcium with cell injury leads to sloughing of cellular debris into tubules. The cellular debris obstructs tubules and erodes into the medullary interstitium, where the precipitated calcium initiates a process of scarring. The scarring may progress to chronic renal failure and is not always corrected by correction of hypercalcemia. With anatomic injury an acidifying defect is more commonly seen and a picture of distal renal tubular acidosis may emerge. Diminished ammonia production may also contribute to the decreased ability to excrete hydrogen ion. The clinical picture of chronic hypercalcemic injury adds chronic renal failure and acidosis to the functional defects seen with acute hypercalcemia.

Treatment of hypercalcemia has been discussed in detail elsewhere (Section VIII). From the renal standpoint, expansion of the extracellular fluid volume with saline usually supplemented with potassium is essential. If extracellular fluid volume expansion and adequate urine flow are established, a diuretic such as furosemide, which inhibits loop sodium chloride and calcium reabsorption, will enhance calciuria and aid in the treatment of hypercalcemia. If furosemide is used for treatment of hypercalcemia, it is critical that the infusion of saline maintain extracellular fluid volume expansion. If extracellular fluid volume contraction occurs, proximal calcium reabsorption will be enhanced and hypercalcemia will be potentiated.

MAGNESIUM

Magnesium is present in plasma at a concentration of 2.0 ± 0.5 mEq/l. About 30 per cent of magnesium is protein bound (largely to albumin). The majority of magnesium is ionized and a small fraction is complexed, as is calcium. Ultrafiltered magnesium is reabsorbed in the proximal tubule and the ascending limb of Henle (Fig. 40). The molecular mechanisms of magnesium reabsorption are not known. In both tubular segments, magnesium reabsorption is proportional to its intratubular concentration. Thus, in states with reduced proximal tubular sodium and water reabsorption, such as volume expansion, the intratubular concentration of magnesium rises less than otherwise, magnesium reabsorption is depressed, and magnesium excretion is increased. Magnesium reabsorption in the loop of Henle is enhanced during hypomagnesemia or hypocalcemia and is reduced during hypermagnesemia or hypercalcemia. Changes in plasma magnesium or calcium concentration have similar but smaller effects on magnesium reabsorption in the proximal tubule. Parathyroid hormone has the direct effect of enhancing magnesium reabsorption. However, hyperparathyroidism is usually associated with increased urinary excretion of magnesium. The explanation for this apparent paradox is that in hyperparathyroidism there is hypercalcemia, which produces increased magnesium excretion sufficient to override any direct effect of

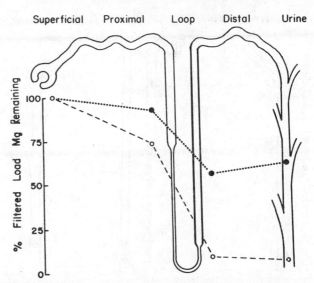

Figure 40. Magnesium reabsorption along the nephron under normal conditions *(open circles)* and after magnesium loading *(closed circles).* (From Sutton, R. A. L., and Dirks, J. H.: Renal handling of calcium, phosphate, and magnesium. In Brenner, B. M., and Rector, F. C., Jr. (eds.): The Kidney. 2nd ed. Philadelphia, W. B. Saunders Co., 1981, p. 597.)

parathyroid hormone on magnesium reabsorption. Calcitonin increases urinary magnesium excretion, while vitamin D has little effect. Diuretics affect magnesium excretion in a manner comparable to their effect on calcium excretion.

There are instances of renal magnesium wasting occurring as a genetic defect and occurring as the result of nephrotoxic injury (aminoglycosides).

The effects of hypermagnesemia are predominantly neurologic, depressing neural function. Hypomagnesemia, however, does affect the kidney. With prolonged hypomagnesemia there is deposition of calcium in the medullary interstitium and shortly thereafter microliths containing calcium appear within the lumens of the loops of Henle. The calcium-containing stones may then erode through into the cells of the loop of Henle and into the medullary interstitium, setting up a process of interstitial scarring. These anatomic findings are the most striking evidence of hypomagnesemic injury to the kidney. In addition, hypomagnesemia is associated with kaliuresis and may induce hypokalemia. Additional reports have documented that hypomagnesemia may be associated with reductions in glomerular filtration rate, impairment of concentrating ability, aminoaciduria, and so on. None of these functional impairments, other than hypokalemia, have been demonstrated to be of importance clinically in humans.

The approach to hypomagnesemia includes identification and treatment of the cause of magnesium loss and the replacement of magnesium deficits.

PHOSPHATE

Phosphate is normally present in plasma at a concentration of 4 ± 1.0 mg/dl. It is largely in ionized form and is almost completely ultrafiltered at the

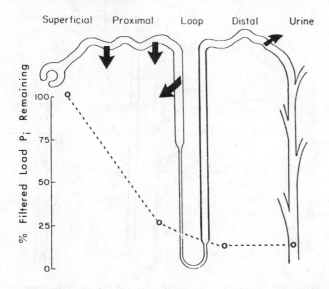

Figure 41. Phosphate reabsorption along the nephron. (From Sutton, R. A. L., and Dirks, J. H.: Renal handling of calcium, phosphate, and magnesium. In Brenner, B. M., and Rector, F. C., Jr. (eds.): The Kidney. 2nd ed. Philadelphia, W. B. Saunders Co., 1981, p. 579.)

glomerulus. The majority of phosphate (70 to 90 per cent) is reabsorbed in the convoluted and straight portions of the proximal tubule (Fig. 41). At these sites, phosphate is reabsorbed by a process of sodium cotransport across the luminal membrane, followed by downhill exit across the basolateral membrane. Phosphate thus shares a common driving force—namely, the electrochemical sodium gradient across the luminal membrane—with many other solutes reabsorbed in the proximal tubule. This probably accounts for the observation that when the filtered load of one or more of these other solutes is increased, as during hyperglycemia, phosphate reabsorption is depressed and phosphate excretion is enhanced. Presumably an increase in the amount of glucose reabsorbed across the luminal membrane via cotransport with sodium decreases the sodium gradient available to drive phosphate reabsorption. The mechanism of phosphate transport at its distal reabsorptive site (Fig. 41) is not known.

An important factor regulating renal phosphate transport is parathyroid hormone. Parathyroid hormone inhibits phosphate reabsorption in both the proximal and distal nephron, resulting in phosphaturia and a fall in serum phosphate concentration. In the proximal tubule, parathyroid hormone binds to its receptor on the basolateral membrane and thereby stimulates the production of cyclic $3'5'$-adenosine monophosphate (cAMP). It is believed that the activity of the sodium-phosphate cotransport system in the luminal membrane is inhibited as the result of phosphorylation by a cyclic AMP-stimulated protein kinase. The molecular mechanism for parathyroid hormone action in the distal nephron is not known, but is likely also to be cyclic AMP-mediated inasmuch as a parathyroid hormone–sensitive adenylate cyclase is present along distal portions of the nephron.

Volume expansion inhibits phosphate reabsorption in the proximal tubule but not in the distal nephron. When parathyroid hormone is absent the increased load of phosphate delivered out of the proximal tubule is reabsorbed distally, and significant phosphaturia does not occur.

There are complex interactions between acid-base homeostasis and renal phosphate handling. In general, increases in plasma HCO_3^- concentration or P_{CO_2} inhibit phosphate reabsorption and promote phosphaturia. Carbonic anhydrase inhibitors such as acetazolamide are also phosphaturic.

Tubular phosphate reabsorption demonstrates a remarkable adaptation to dietary phosphate intake that is independent of any associated changes in parathyroid hormone. In particular, low phosphate intake markedly stimulates phosphate reabsorption because of an increased number or activity of Na-phosphate cotransport carriers on the luminal membrane of proximal tubular cells. In fact, phosphate reabsorption is so avid during phosphate deprivation that there is resistance to such normally phosphaturic stimuli as parathyroid hormone and bicarbonate infusions. Adequate levels of active metabolites of vitamin D are required for this renal adaptation to low-phosphate diets to take place. Indeed, deficiency of or insensitivity to vitamin D may result in phosphate wasting. Phosphate wasting associated with reduced vitamin D activity plays an important role in several disorders, such as vitamin D-resistant rickets and vitamin D-dependent rickets.

VITAMIN D-RESISTANT RICKETS

Vitamin D-resistant rickets (VDRR), or hypophosphatemic rickets as it is also known, is a disorder inherited as an X-linked dominant trait. It is characterized by osteomalacia, hypophosphatemia, normal or low-normal serum calcium concentration, normal to low urine calcium excretion, diminished intestinal absorption of phosphate and calcium, a tubular defect characterized by a reduced tubular maximum for phosphate, reduced levels of 1,25-dihydroxycholecalciferol, and resistance to large doses of vitamin D. At present it is difficult to distinguish between two schools of thought as to the basic defect in VDRR. One school holds that there is increased sensitivity to parathyroid hormone or to some other phosphaturic substance. The second school holds that there is a primary renal tubular defect in phosphate transport. There are data supporting both postulates, but there is no definitive answer. Patients with VDRR respond to large doses of vitamin D and phosphate replacement therapy. A form of VDRR, biochemically indistinguishable from the hereditary disorder, occurs rarely with malignant disease and remits with removal of the tumor.

VITAMIN D-DEPENDENT RICKETS

Vitamin D-dependent rickets (VDDR), inherited as an autosomal recessive trait, is characterized by hypophosphatemia and severe osteomalacia. It is also characterized by significant hypocalcemia and by response to large doses of vitamin D. There are at least two broad groups of patients with VDDR. The first group includes individuals who are more responsive to vitamin D than are those patients with VDRR. The defect in this first group with VDDR is defective conversion of 25-hydroxyvitamin D_3 to 1,25-dihydroxyvitamin D_3. Because of the inadequate quantity of active vitamin D, calcium absorption from the intestine is impaired, resulting in a reduced serum calcium concentration and the stimulation of parathyroid hormone release. The release of parathyroid hormone produces phosphaturia and aminoaciduria in these patients. It can be shown that the phosphaturia and aminoaciduria respond to an inhibition of parathyroid hormone release or to extirpation of the parathyroid glands. The second group with VDDR has normal or elevated levels of 1,25-dihydroxyvitamin D_3. They have a heterogeneous set of receptor and postreceptor defects for 1,25-dihydroxyvitamin D_3 action. The subsequent pathophysiology of this resistance to vitamin D is similar to that in patients with inadequate vitamin production.

In summary, phosphate depletion may occur as a primary tubular defect in the disease VDRR. In VDDR, however, the hypophosphatemia appears to result from the compensatory responses initiated by insufficient active vitamin D production or tissue response (receptor and postreceptor defects), leading to inadequate calcium absorption and secondary stimulation of parathyroid hormone release. These related diseases are presented as examples of (1) a primary tubular defect (VDRR) and (2) a defect that, though initially indistinguishable from that of VDRR, is clearly a secondary phenomenon (VDDR).

Diuretics

Diuretics are pharmacologic agents designed to produce negative sodium balance. They affect different mechanisms of sodium reabsorption at various sites along the length of the tubule. While interfering with sodium reabsorption, the diuretics also have important effects on body fluid tonicity, acid-base regulation, potassium balance, calcium balance, renal blood flow, and the action of hormones. Because diuretics may produce negative sodium balance and may also affect a number of other important renal processes, they are considered for use in edematous and nonedematous states. Use in edematous states is directed at reducing total body sodium as a primary objective. Use in nonedematous states is directed at the predictable modifications in body chemistry that occur with specific diuretics.

Diuretics should be used only after the physician has mastered the following information: (1) the mechanism and site of action of the diuretics, (2) the potency and pharmacokinetics of each of the diuretics, (3) the toxicity of the diuretics, (4) the reasons for refractoriness to diuretics, (5) the rationale of combining diuretics for therapeutic use, (6) the indications for the use of the diuretics, and (7) an understanding of the means of monitoring diuretic action.

MECHANISM AND SITE OF DIURETIC ACTION

A discussion of the mechanism and site of diuretic action requires a review of the physiology of volume and tonicity regulation (see section beginning on p. 666). A few simple concepts will help in this analysis of diuretic action. First, when a diuretic works to interfere with sodium reabsorption at any site in the nephron it will interfere not only with the reabsorption of sodium but with all other processes coupled to sodium reabsorption at that site. In addition, interfering with sodium reabsorption at one site will lead to the increased delivery of sodium downstream along the nephron to all more distal sites of reabsorption. The increased delivery of sodium will enhance the effect of sodium reabsorption at all of the more distal sites.

Thus one might reason that a diuretic that interfered with proximal tubular sodium reabsorption (sites 1 and 2, Fig. 42) would enhance the delivery of sodium and water to the ascending limb of the loop of Henle and the more distal nephron. The increased delivery of sodium chloride and water will result in the transport of more sodium chloride from the ascending limb into the medullary interstitium. Since the ascending limb is impermeable to water, greater quantities of the free water will be produced as sodium chloride is reabsorbed. If antidiuretic hormone is absent, the increased quantities of free water will be excreted. If antidiuretic hormone is present, the increased osmotic activity of the medullary interstitium will result in greater reabsorption of free water. The delivery of increased quantities of sodium and water out of the proximal tubule therefore creates the possibility of either increased free water production or reabsorption.

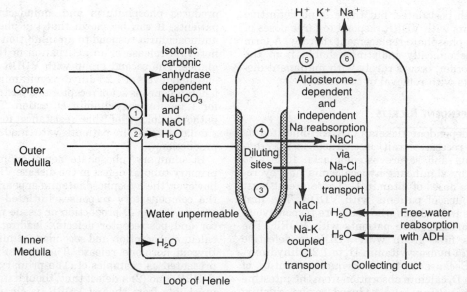

Figure 42. The nephron, indicating functional areas involved in salt and water regulation. (From Brater, D. C., and Thier, S. O.: Renal disorders. In Melmon, K. L., and Morrelli, H. F. (eds.): Clinical Pharmacology, Basic Principles in Therapeutics. 2nd ed. New York, Macmillan Co., 1978, p. 352.)

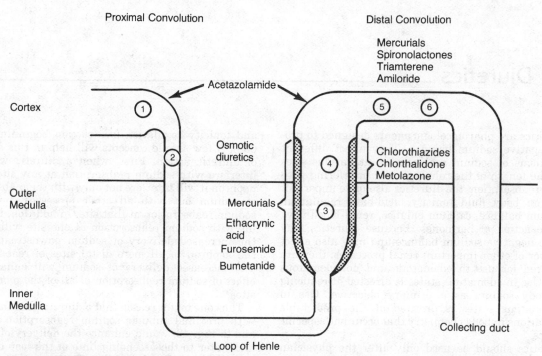

Figure 43. Sites of diuretic action.

Site 1. Proximal tubule. Sensitive to inhibitors of carbonic anhydrase. A diuretic acting at this site produces *increased* free-water production or reabsorption and *increased* potassium loss.

Site 2. Proximal tubule. An osmotic diuretic would act at this site and produce *increased* free-water production or reabsorption and *increased* potassium loss.

Site 3. Medullary diluting segment of ascending limb. A diuretic action at this site produces *decreased* free-water production or reabsorption and *increased* potassium loss.

Site 4. Cortical diluting segment of ascending limb. A diuretic acting at this site produces *decreased* free-water production, does not affect free-water absorption, and *increases* potassium loss.

Site 5. Aldosterone-sensitive portion of distal tubule: A diuretic acting at this site produces *decreased* potassium loss, but acts only in the presence of aldosterone.

Site 6. Aldosterone-insensitive portion of distal tubule. A diuretic acting at this site produces *decreased* potassium loss. (From Brater, D. C., and Thier, S. O.: Renal disorders. In Melmon, K. L., and Morrelli, H. F. (eds.): Clinical Pharmacology, Basic Principles in Therapeutics. 2nd ed. New York. Macmillan Co., 1978, p. 366.)

The continued flow of salt and water to the more distal nephron will result in increased secretion of potassium.

The net result of the use of a proximal-acting diuretic would be increased excretion of sodium in the urine, an increased capability for free water production or reabsorption, and increased excretion of potassium. If the urine also contained increased quantities of bicarbonate, the proximal process affected would be the reabsorption of sodium bicarbonate (site 1). If the urine did not contain increased bicarbonate, the process affected would be the proximal reabsorption of sodium chloride (site 2).

If a diuretic acted in the ascending limb of the loop of Henle (site 3), it would interfere with the reabsorption of sodium-potassium–coupled chloride at a site that would reduce the creation of free water. At the same time it would reduce delivery of osmotically active material into the medullary interstitium, thereby reducing the capability for reabsorbing free water if antidiuretic hormone were present. The delivery of sodium and water to the more distal areas of the nephron would result in the excretion of increased quantities of potassium.

It is possible for a diuretic to work only in the cortical segment of the thick ascending limb of Henle's loop and early distal tubule (site 4), thereby interfering with coupled sodium-chloride reabsorption in a segment of the tubule that produces free water. Free water production would therefore be inhibited. However, the cortical diluting segment transports sodium chloride into an interstitial area with high blood flow and no vasa recta. Thus, no significant interstitial gradient is created and the interference with sodium chloride reabsorption into this area has no effect on the ability to reabsorb free water. The delivery of sodium chloride beyond the cortical diluting segment of the ascending limb would also result in increased urinary potassium excretion.

Finally, if a diuretic interfered with the reabsorption of sodium in the distal tubule and collecting duct, where potassium excretion is coupled to sodium reabsorption, there would be a reduction in potassium excretion. If the diuretic acted only by antagonizing the effect of aldosterone, it would act only in the presence of aldosterone (site 5). It is also possible to reduce sodium reabsorption in the distal nephron by a diuretic acting directly on the apical sodium channels (site 6).

By observing the pattern of electrolyte excretion, the ability to create and reabsorb free water, and the effect on potassium excretion, it is possible to pinpoint the site of action and in many instances the mechanism of action of each of the diuretics (Fig. 43).

A diuretic will be effective only if sodium is delivered to the site of the diuretic action. Since with extracellular fluid volume contraction more of sodium is reabsorbed proximally and less is delivered to the distal nephron, the more distal-acting diuretics will lose their effectiveness. On the other hand, the loop is capable of reabsorbing large quantities of sodium and undoing the effect of proximal-acting diuretics during states of sodium avidity. It should also be obvious that diuretics acting at different sites of the nephron or acting at the same site through different mechanisms may be additive in their effects. This concept of combining diuretics based on sound physiologic and pharmacologic principles will be discussed in detail later.

OSMOTIC DIURETICS

The action of osmotic diuretics is based on two important physiologic concepts. First, the proximal tubule is incapable of reabsorbing sodium against a steep concentration gradient. Therefore, if water is obligated to remain in the lumen of the proximal tubule, sodium reabsorption will be impaired. Second, though increased delivery of sodium chloride to the thick ascending limb of Henle's loop results in progressive increases in sodium reabsorption by mechanisms that are not saturable under physiologic conditions, these mechanisms are gradient limited; that is, if the concentration of sodium chloride in the fluid entering the thick ascending limb is low enough to produce a steep gradient for transport from lumen to interstitium, the transport of sodium chloride will be impaired.

Osmotic diuretics act as nonreabsorbable substances that obligate water to the proximal tubule and thereby interfere with sodium reabsorption. The increased water retained in the proximal tubule, together with the progressively increased percentage of total osmolality contributed by the osmotic diuretic, results in the delivery of luminal fluid with a progressively lower concentration of sodium chloride to the thick ascending limb of the loop of Henle. The lowered concentration of sodium chloride results in the need to transport sodium chloride against a concentration gradient that is ultimately limiting and results in reduced ascending limb sodium chloride reabsorption. The result is the delivery of increased quantities of water, osmotically active material, and sodium chloride out of both the proximal tubule and ascending limb of Henle's loop. The net result is negative sodium balance under circumstances in which free water production may be increased in the absence of antidiuretic hormone and in which potassium excretion is increased.

Exogenous substances that are osmotic diuretics include mannitol and glycerol. Endogenous osmotically active materials include glucose and urea. Note that osmotic diuretics are not only active within the kidney but have important effects on the distribution of body fluids as well. Exogenous osmotically active materials are confined to the extracellular fluid space and are capable of producing important extracellular fluid volume expansion. Osmotic diuretics are indicated under circumstances in which maintenance of extracellular fluid volume and renal perfusion are critical.

CARBONIC ANHYDRASE INHIBITORS

Carbonic anhydrase inhibitors, of which acetazolamide is a prime example, are a group of compounds that have an important proximal and lesser distal tubular site of action. By interfering with carbonic anhydrase, this group of diuretics impairs proximal hydrogen ion secretion and its coupled sodium reabsorption. The failure of hydrogen ion to be secreted proximally impairs proximal bicarbonate reabsorption, leading to increased delivery of bicarbonate out of the proximal tubule. The interference with isotonic sodium bicarbonate reabsorption in the earliest portion of the proximal convoluted tubule may dampen the rise in chloride concentration, along the remainder of the proximal convolution. Failure of the chloride concentration to rise will blunt the development of a chloride concentration gradient from lumen to blood and impair sodium chloride reabsorption. The delivery of increased quantities of sodium bicarbonate and sodium chloride out of the proximal tubule results in an enhanced ability of the nephron to generate free water and under appropriate circumstances to reabsorb free water. The sodium chloride delivered from the proximal tubule is usually reabsorbed in the ascending limb, but since sodium bicarbonate is not effectively reabsorbed at this site, the sodium bicarbonate will be delivered to the distal nephron. Potassium excretion will be increased on the basis of increased sodium delivery, reduced chloride concentration, and possibly because bicarbonate acts as a relatively nonreabsorbable anion, increasing the luminal negativity of the distal nephron and thereby enhancing potassium secretion. It has also been suggested that inhibition of carbonic anhydrase in the distal tubule will produce an intracellular deficit of hydrogen ions, which will be replaced by potassium. The higher intracellular potassium concentration will also facilitate potassium secretion.

Carbonic anhydrase inhibitors used alone are of limited clinical usefulness. Their dominant proximal action is usually undone to a great extent by the ascending limb of the loop of Henle, which reabsorbs much of the delivered sodium. The development of mild acidemia ultimately provides adequate hydrogen ions to bypass the need for carbonic anhydrase for hydrogen ion secretion. Once this latter circumstance occurs, carbonic anhydrase inhibitors are ineffective.

ETHACRYNIC ACID, FUROSEMIDE, AND BUMETANIDE

These drugs, which act in the ascending limb of Henle's loop, are the most potent diuretics presently available. A portion of their diuretic action has been suggested to be due to redistribution of blood flow from juxtamedullary to cortical areas. This is the reversal of the distribution seen during most salt-retaining states. Whether the changes in blood flow are primary or secondary events in producing sodium diuresis is not really known. These diuretics do impair sodium-potassium–coupled chloride reabsorption in the ascending limb of the loop of Henle and thereby interfere with sodium reabsorption. Furosemide also has a carbonic anhydrase inhibitory action at very high doses. The effect of ethacrynic acid, furosemide, and bumetanide is to interfere with the creation of free water and, by inhibiting the transport of sodium, potassium, and chloride into the medullary interstitium, to interfere with free water reabsorption. All three diuretics deliver increased quantities of sodium to the potassium excretory sites and thereby enhance potassium excretion. They may also block potassium reabsorption directly in the thick ascending limb of Henle's loop.

THE THIAZIDES, CHLORTHALIDONE, AND METOLAZONE

These diuretics act on coupled sodium-chloride reabsorption in a portion of the tubule that is important for the creation of free water but unimportant for the reabsorption of free water: the cortical diluting segment of the thick ascending limb of Henle's loop and probably the early distal convoluted tubule. Since this site of action is proximal to the potassium excretory site, the use of these diuretics is associated with significant potassium wasting. Indapamide, an indoline diuretic, appears to work in the cortical diluting segment. Its cellular mechanism of action has not been elucidated.

ANTAGONISTS OF ALDOSTERONE

The only clinically useful aldosterone antagonists are the spironolactones. These drugs are competitive inhibitors of the action of aldosterone on the tubule. They impair sodium reabsorption and inhibit potassium and hydrogen ion secretion in states of hyperaldosteronism. In the absence of aldosterone these drugs are without significant effect. The spironolactones act at a site in the nephron beyond which free water is created and increased medullary interstitial tonicity is generated. Therefore they are without effect on free water production or reabsorption.

Theoretically the effect of aldosterone could be antagonized by interfering with aldosterone synthesis. Heparin is capable of inhibiting aldosterone synthesis and occasionally of producing hyperkalemia. To date there have been no antagonists of aldosterone synthesis that have found use as diuretic agents.

TRIAMTERENE AND AMILORIDE

These diuretics act in the distal nephron. By blocking the sodium entry channel they interfere with the entry of sodium from the lumen into the tubular cells. Interference with sodium reabsorption at these distal sites in the nephron reduces available sodium for use by the sodium-potassium pumps in the basolateral membrane, thereby impairing potassium secretion. The reduced sodium reabsorption also results in a less negative lumen potential and thus inhibits potassium and hydrogen secretion. The use of these diuretics results in the excretion of sodium and the retention of potassium and hydrogen ion. They have no effect on free water production or reabsorption.

OTHER DIURETICS

The organomercurial compounds that interfere with sodium reabsorption throughout the ascending limb of Henle's loop and the distal tubule have effects that are a combination of the diuretics such as furosemide plus those drugs acting at the sodium-potassium exchange area. With the availability of ethacrynic acid, furosemide, and bumetanide, these drugs have fallen out of clinical use and are most important now in a historical context. The same may be said for ammonium chloride and other acidifying salts that were used in their own right or as an adjunct to mercurial therapy. They are no longer used as primary diuretic agents and will not be discussed further.

TABLE 8. EFFECTS OF DIURETICS ON ELECTROLYTE EXCRETION

AGENT	CHANGES IN URINARY ELECTROLYTES				MAXIMAL FRACTIONAL EXCRETION OF SODIUM	INHIBITORY FACTORS		SITE OF ACTION (See Figure 43 for Site Numbers)
	Na^+	K^+	Cl^-	HCO_3^-	%	Acidosis	Alkalosis	
Weak Diuretics								
Acetazolamide	↑	↑	↓	↑	~4	+		1
Spironolactone	↑	↓	↑	↑	~2			5
Triamterene	↑	↓	↑	↑	~2			6
Amiloride	↑	↓	↑	↑	~2			6
Moderately Effective Diuretics								
Thiazide compounds (Chlorthalidone Metolazone)	↑	↑	↑	↑	~8			4
Potent Diuretics								
Organomercurials	↑	↑	↑		~20		+	3, 4
Furosemide	↑	↑	↑		~23			3, 4
Ethacrynic acid	↑	↑	↑		~23			3, 4 (? 5, 6)
Bumetanide	↑	↑	↑		~23			3, 4 (? 2)

Modified from Brater, D. C., and Thier, S. O.: Renal disorders. In Melmon, K. L., and Morrelli, H. F. (eds.): Clinical Pharmacology, Basic Principles in Therapeutics. 2nd ed. New York, Macmillan Co., 1978, p. 371. Originally from Goldberg, M.: The physiology and pathophysiology of diuretic agents. In Fulton, W. F. M. (ed.): Modern Trends in Pharmacology and Therapeutics. London, Butterworth & Co., 1967.

NEWER DIURETICS

There will undoubtedly be a series of newer diuretics developed over the years. A thiazide-like diuretic with uricosuric properties is being introduced in some countries. As this and other new diuretics are introduced, their site and mechanism of action can be analyzed according to the principles already presented for the existing diuretics.

POTENCY AND PHARMACOKINETICS

Having determined site of action and mechanism of action of any diuretic, it is important to know the potency of the agent before prescribing it. The potency of diuretics is usually defined by their ability to increase the fractional excretion of sodium. Ordinarily some 99 per cent of filtered sodium is reabsorbed during its passage through the tubule, leaving something in the range of 1 per cent of filtered sodium for excretion. The 1 per cent of filtered sodium excreted in the urine is termed the fractional excretion. The fractional excretion of sodium produced by diuretics is a measure of their relative potency (Table 8). Note that when diuretics are tested, what is reported is the maximal fractional excretion of sodium achieved. This figure represents the highest fractional excretion achieved under carefully controlled experimental conditions and does not represent the average fraction of filtered sodium excreted during the use of the diuretic. Thus the maximal fractional excretion of sodium achieved by distal diuretics such as triamterene and spironolactone is about 2 per cent, while acetazolamide achieves a maximal fractional excretion of 4 per cent. Thiazide diuretics and related compounds are capable of producing just under 10 per cent maximal fractional excretion, while those diuretics acting predominantly throughout the ascending limb of Henle's loop are capable of producing maximal fractional excretions of

20 to 25 per cent. Knowledge of the maximal fractional excretion of sodium produced by each diuretic and knowledge of its site of action will permit the physician to judge the potency of the diuretic and to predict the effects of the drug on electrolyte excretion and water balance. A detailed discussion of the pharmacokinetics of diuretics is beyond the scope of this chapter, but suffice it to say that a diuretic should be used at the lowest dose that will be effective, administered as infrequently as possible, and administered by a route that will achieve the onset of action desired.

TOXICITY

Most of the toxic effects of the diuretics are predictable on the basis of their mechanisms and sites of action.

Hypovolemia

If, by definition, all diuretics produce negative sodium balance, excessive sodium depletion may be a complication of any of these drugs. Obviously, the more potent the diuretic the more likely it is to produce hypovolemia.

Hyponatremia

Diuretics may produce hyponatremia by increasing sodium loss in a patient who continues to ingest water, by inhibiting the formation and excretion of free water by the renal tubule, by enhancing antidiuretic hormone release, and by potentiating antidiuretic hormone action. Those diuretics acting in the diluting segments of the nephron are most likely to produce hyponatremia.

Hypokalemia

Any diuretic acting proximal to the sodium-potassium exchange area of the distal nephron is capable of producing hypokalemia. Therefore all diuretics acting in the proximal tubule, the ascending limb of the loop of Henle, or in the cortical diluting segment and early distal tubule may produce hypokalemia.

Hyperkalemia

Those diuretics that interfere with sodium reabsorption in the distal nephron are capable of producing hyperkalemia. They are also capable of producing some degree of acidemia, which will lead to shifts of potassium from cells to extracellular fluid, increasing the level of hyperkalemia.

Alkalemia

Those diuretics that interfere with sodium-potassium–dependent or sodium-coupled chloride reabsorption act in the ascending limb of the loop of Henle and the distal tubule. These diuretics are all capable of producing chloride depletion, potassium depletion, volume contraction, and the stimulation of aldosterone. This series of events generates and sustains metabolic alkalosis.

Acidemia

Diuretics that produce bicarbonate wasting, such as the carbonic anhydrase inhibitors, and those diuretics that interfere with hydrogen ion secretion, such as spironolactone, triamterene, and amiloride, are all capable of producing metabolic acidosis.

Hyperuricemia

Elevation of the serum uric acid may be associated with any diuretic capable of producing volume depletion. The production of volume depletion leads to increased reabsorption of virtually all substances reabsorbed in the proximal tubule, including uric acid. Reexpansion of the extracellular fluid in individuals who have developed hyperuricemia while taking diuretics will significantly reduce the degree of hyperuricemia. Most of the diuretics are also organic acids secreted by the renal tubule. It is possible that these organic acids affect uric acid excretion by other mechanisms.

Glucose Intolerance

Glucose intolerance is seen with those diuretics that produce prolonged hypokalemia. Intracellular potassium is necessary for the synthesis and release of insulin; in states of potassium depletion, glucose intolerance occurs on the basis of insulin deficiency.

Common toxic effects are described in Table 9, and, of course, any drug is capable of producing an idiosyncratic reaction.

REFRACTORINESS TO DIURETICS

Unresponsiveness to diuretics may result from incorrect administration or from a series of pathophysiologic events blunting their effectiveness. Obviously a diuretic must be given in the appropriate dose and by the appropriate route to be effective. When a diuretic is given in an appropriate fashion and without effect, the most likely reason is that there is inadequate sodium being delivered to the site of diuretic action. Any circumstance that reduces renal perfusion and urine flow will obviate diuretic effectiveness. Thus, congestive heart failure, hepatic failure, and hypovolemia will all impair diuretic action. Renal failure per se also predicts that diuretics will be unlikely to act effectively and that toxic effects of the diuretic acting directly on nonrenal tissues will be increased.

There are also pathophysiologic changes that interfere with diuretic action. For example, the development of acidemia would bypass the action of carbonic anhydrase inhibitors and render them ineffective.

STRATEGY OF COMBINING DIURETICS

Two or more diuretics may be combined either (1) to counterbalance undesirable effects, or (2) to have additive diuretic actions.

The combination of diuretics to avoid undesirable side effects is best illustrated by the use of a thiazide diuretic that will produce adequate diuresis but persistent hypokalemia, with a spironolactone that will produce only a small increment in diuretic action but will blunt the hypokalemic effect of the thiazide. When diuretics are used in this fashion it may not be assumed that average doses will counterbalance each other, but rather the diuretics must be titrated one against the other to achieve the desired balance.

Diuretics may also be combined to take advantage of different sites of action or of different mechanisms of action at the same site. A carbonic anhydrase inhibitor might have effects that would be additive to loop diuretics such as furosemide, and an additional boost might be obtained by the addition of a potassium-sparing diuretic such as a spironolactone. In choosing such combinations, the diuretics should act at different sites so that the effect of one diuretic will be potentiated as sodium is delivered to its site of action by the effect of a more proximally acting drug.

Though it is only of theoretic interest at the moment, the use of two diuretics that act at the same site but by different mechanisms is possible. Spironolactone and triamterene both impair potassium secretion and inhibit sodium reabsorption in the distal tubule. Spironolactones require the presence of aldosterone, while triamterene does not. Their actions may be additive. Though there is little reason at present to combine these two diuretics, the theoretic considerations that indicate that they would be additive may ultimately be applied to diuretics working by different mechanisms in more important sites such as the loop of Henle or the proximal tubule.

PATHOPHYSIOLOGIC INDICATIONS FOR THE USE OF DIURETICS

EDEMATOUS STATES

As mentioned earlier, the diuretics may be used to treat edematous or nonedematous states. For the treat-

TABLE 9. COMPLICATIONS OF USE OF DIURETICS

DIURETIC	HYPER-URICEMIA	HYPO K$^+$	HYPER K$^+$	ACIDOSIS	ALKALOSIS	OTHER
Osmotic	−	+	−	−	+ contraction	Hyper- or hypo-osmolality
Acid-forming salts	−	+	−	+	−	
Organomercurials	−	+	+ (rare, acute)	−	+	Tubular necrosis, hypersensitivity reactions
Acetazolamide	?	+	−	+	−	Urinary tract calculi, hepatic coma
Thiazides (Chlorthalidone / Metolazone)	+	+	−	−	+	Cutaneous vasculitis, agranulocytosis, thrombocytopenia, anemia, pancreatitis, glucose intolerance, hepatic coma
Ethacrynic acid	+	+	−	−	+	Hyper- and hypoglycemia, gastrointestinal bleeding, deafness, hepatic coma
Furosemide	+	+	−	−	+	Glucose intolerance, deafness, hepatic coma
Bumetanide	+	+	−	−	+	Ototoxicity, hepatic coma, ? glucose intolerance
Spironolactone	−	−	+	−	−	Gynecomastia
Triamterene	−	−	+	+	−	Azotemia, muscle cramps
Amiloride	−	−	+	+	−	Azotemia

Modified from Brater, D. C., and Thier, S. O.: Renal disorders. In Melmon, K. L., and Morrelli, H. F. (eds.): Clinical Pharmacology, Basic Principles in Therapeutics. 2nd ed. New York, Macmillan Co., 1978, p. 372.

ment of edematous states it is important to define the pathophysiology carefully before choosing a diuretic. Note that in states of localized edema or under circumstances in which the edema is part of a compensatory mechanism that attempts to expand a contracted intravascular volume, as in states of low plasma albumin concentration, the use of diuretics may produce further intravascular volume contraction. They should be used in these circumstances only with a clear knowledge of this potential hazard and the positive decision that this risk is necessary to treat whatever may be the edematous circumstance.

In states in which volume overload includes an expanded intravascular volume, as in congestive heart failure, the administration of a diuretic to reduce intravascular volume is usually a sound decision.

NONEDEMATOUS STATES

By now it is clear that diuretics have many actions besides producing negative sodium balance in the treatment of volume overexpansion. In nonedematous states, diuretics are quite effective in a number of clinical settings:

(1) Diuretics are antihypertensive agents that reduce intravascular volume, not from above normal to normal but rather from normal to somewhat contracted.

(2) Diuretics cause contraction of vascular volume to below normal levels, thereby enhancing salt and water reabsorption in the proximal tubule. The effect of increased sodium and water reabsorption is used in the treatment of nephrogenic diabetes insipidus or to enhance the reabsorption of sodium bicarbonate in the treatment of proximal renal tubular acidosis.

(3) Diuretics facilitate the treatment of hyponatremia in the syndrome of the inappropriate secretion of antidiuretic hormone. Under circumstances in which volume overload is considered dangerous, furosemide may be given to reduce the reabsorption of free water and to increase sodium diuresis. Measurement of urinary sodium and then under-replacement with hypertonic saline will result in a rise in serum sodium without extracellular fluid volume expansion.

(4) Hypernatremia on rare occasions may require the use of a diuretic and replacement of free water.

(5) Hyperkalemia and hypokalemia may be treated with potassium wasting and potassium sparing diuretics, respectively.

(6) Acidemia, particularly in association with extracellular fluid volume overload, may be treated effectively with the use of a chloruretic diuretic, and bicarbonate replacement. Alkalemia may be treated with a carbonic anhydrase inhibitor.

(7) Hypercalcemia may be treated by the use of furosemide, which interferes with calcium reabsorption in the ascending limb of the loop of Henle. For effective therapy, saline must also be administered to prevent the diuretic-induced volume contraction from enhancing proximal calcium reabsorption.

(8) Calcium stone disease may be treated with thiazide diuretics to produce volume contraction, enhancing proximal calcium reabsorption. Thiazides also enhance distal calcium reabsorption. This therapy is useful for idiopathic hypercalciuria. For uric acid and cystine stones the administration of a carbonic anhydrase inhibitor plus sodium bicarbonate will alkalinize the urine and prevent stone precipitation. Drug excretion may be enhanced by modifying urine pH. Thus salicylate or barbiturate intoxication may be treated with acetazolamide and sodium bicarbonate.

These uses of diuretics in nonedematous states represent the application of pharmacologic and physiologic observations to the clinical situation. There may be many more uses of diuretics that the imaginative physician can design in an attempt to correct fluid and electrolyte abnormalities.

ASSESSMENT OF THE EFFECTIVENESS OF THE DIURETIC PROGRAM

The use of potent agents such as the diuretics requires that the physician define the goals of diuretic therapy and identify the potential side effects of the diuretic program to be used. The use of the diuretics should then be coupled to the establishment of clear therapeutic end points in terms of change in volume, blood pressure, serum chemistries, and urine composition, so that the diuretic program can be modified or terminated as necessary.

In summary, diuretics are a potent group of drugs capable of modifying a variety of renal tubular functions by acting to inhibit sodium reabsorption at various sites along the nephron. By their actions they produce a series of associated fluid and electrolyte changes that may represent unwanted side effects but may also be useful therapeutic maneuvers. The physician should know the site of action, potency, appropriate routes, and dosage schedules of administration of the diuretics and the expected side effects. After careful consideration of the clinical indications for the use of a diuretic, the least potent drug necessary to accomplish the desired end point should be chosen and used as infrequently as possible. Frequency of administration and dosage can be increased as necessary. If a drug is no longer effective, a more potent diuretic may be used. Ultimately it may be necessary to combine diuretics to achieve the desired action; combinations of diuretics may also be used to avoid undesirable side effects. Each modification of a diuretic program requires careful assessment of the effects of diuresis and care in looking for untoward side effects. If the patient proves refractory to the diuretics, mechanisms producing refractoriness should be checked. Finally the diuretics should be considered pharmacologic agents capable of broad use and not simply agents to produce negative sodium balance. When viewed in the broader context, their strength as therapeutic approaches to a whole variety of fluid and electrolyte and renal abnormalities becomes evident.

Glomerulonephritis

When strictly applied, the term *glomerulonephritis* refers to inflammation of the glomerular tuft. In general usage, however, it refers to a group of diseases in which glomerular pathology is dominant but in which interstitial disease exists as well. This group of diseases also includes some that are better termed glomerulopathies, since the glomerulus is the most prominent site of pathology but inflammation per se is absent.

PATHOLOGIC TERMINOLOGY

Glomerulonephritis is described as focal or diffuse. The term *focal* indicates that glomerular involvement is spotty; *diffuse* indicates that all glomeruli are involved. Focal lesions may be further subdivided into those that are segmental, involving only individual tufts of glomeruli, and those that uniformly affect the involved glomeruli.

The lesions are further described as minimal change, sclerotic, proliferative, and membranous.

Minimal change lesions do not appear unusual on light microscopy, but may show swelling of the epithelial foot processes on electron microscopy.

Sclerotic lesions refer to glomeruli that show sclerotic and hyalinizing changes.

Proliferative changes may be endothelial, epithelial, or mesangial. When the proliferation involves mesangial and endothelial cells, it is termed endocapillary (Fig. 44); when it involves the lining cells of Bowman's capsule, proliferation is referred to as epithelial cell crescents (Fig. 45). Membranoproliferative changes refer to the proliferation of mesangial cells whose cytoplasm may become interposed between the basement membrane and the endothelial cell, giving a duplicated or split appearance to the capillary wall. Increased mesangial matrix produces a lobular pattern in some glomeruli with membranoproliferative changes.

Membranous change refers to thickening of capillary walls seen on light microscopy and a series of changes on electron microscopy, which will be discussed in more detail later. Membranous glomerulopathy is characterized by absence of inflammation (Fig. 46).

PATHOGENESIS

A host of pathogenetic mechanisms have been proposed to explain the development of glomerulonephritis. The most extensively discussed of these mechanisms are (1) the presence of antibody directed against and interacting with the glomerular basement membrane; (2) the presence of antibody-antigen complexes that are trapped in the glomerulus; (3) the formation of immune deposits by the binding of immunoglobulin to antigens normally present or antigens previously localized in the glomerulus—this in situ formation of immune complexes is the only mechanism that has been demonstrated to form subepithelial deposits; and (4) the activation of the alternate complement pathway. Though these most commonly discussed mechanisms all involve immunologic processes, it is also likely that there are pathogenetic mechanisms for the production of glomerulonephritis that are nonimmunologic.

ANTIGLOMERULAR BASEMENT MEMBRANE DISEASE

In an experimental model, antiglomerular basement membrane disease can be produced by injecting prep-

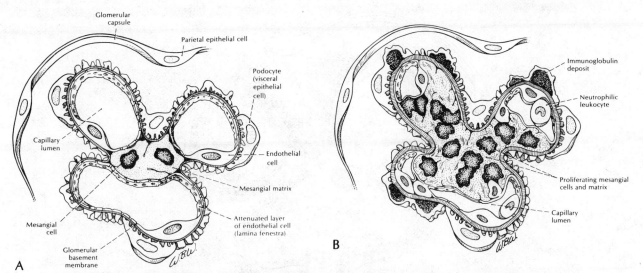

Figure 44. Acute serum sickness nephritis. After a single injection of bovine serum albumin, rabbits show acute intracapillary proliferative glomerulonephritis involving primarily mesangial cells; also, there is swelling of endothelial cells and localization of neutrophilic leukocytes in capillary lumina. Immune deposits are scattered along glomerular basement membrane in the subepithelial location. *A*, Normal glomerular lobule. *B*, Intracapillary proliferative lesion of acute serum sickness nephritis involving a glomerular lobule. Glomerular lesion develops at time of immune phase of antigen disappearance, soon after first antibody to injected antigen is synthesized by host, and combines with antigen to form soluble immune complexes. Antigen, rabbit IgG, and complement are localized in the glomerular capillary walls by immunofluorescence. (From Donadio, J. V., Jr.: Glomerular Disease—Mediation of Injury. In Knox, F. G. (ed.): Textbook of Renal Pathophysiology. Hagerstown, Md., Harper and Row, Publishers. Copyright 1978 by Mayo Clinic/Foundation.)

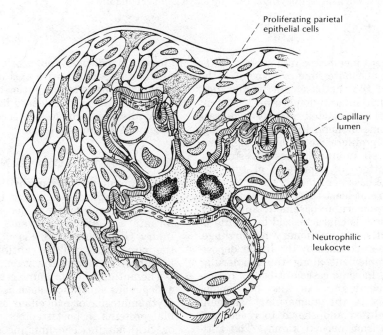

Figure 45. Anti-glomerular basement membrane (GBM) nephritis. After injection of heterologous or homologous GBM in adjuvant, rabbits or sheep show severe, extracapillary proliferative glomerulonephritis with associated necrosis of glomerular tufts and localization of neutrophilic leukocytes. No immune deposits are found. Shown is an extracapillary proliferative lesion of anti-GBM nephritis, involving glomerular lobule. The glomerular lesion develops within days after a single injection of GBM. Rabbit or sheep IgG and complement are located in the glomerular basement membrane by immunofluorescence. (From Donadio, J. V., Jr.: Glomerular Disease—Mediation of Injury. In Knox, F. G. (ed.): Textbook of Renal Pathophysiology. Hagerstown, Md., Harper and Row, Publishers. Copyright 1978 by Mayo Clinic/Foundation.)

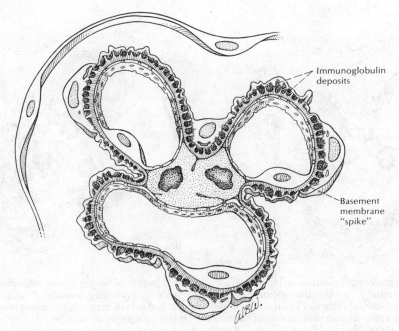

Immunoglobulin
deposits

Basement
membrane
"spike"

Figure 46. Autologous immune complex nephritis. After injection with homologous renal antigen in adjuvant, rats show a form of chronic nephritis, called membranous glomerulonephritis or nephropathy, in which there is thickening of glomerular capillary walls but no proliferation or localization of neutrophilic leukocytes. Immune deposits are found in a subepithelial location along all of the glomerular capillaries, and deposits are interspersed by projections of glomerular basement membrane (also called spikes). A membranous lesion of autologous immune complex nephritis involving a glomerular lobule is shown. The glomerular lesion develops weeks after a single injection of renal antigen. Antigen, rat IgG, and complement are localized in glomerular capillary walls by immunofluorescence. (From Donadio, J. V., Jr.: Glomerular Disease—Mediation of Injury. In Knox, F. G. (ed.): Textbook of Renal Pathophysiology. Hagerstown, Md., Harper and Row, Publishers. Copyright 1978 by Mayo Clinic/Foundation.)

arations of rat basement membrane into rabbits. After the rabbits have had adequate time to respond to the antigenic stimulus of the rat basement membranes, the rabbit serum, rich in antiglomerular basement membrane antibodies, is reinjected into rats. The rats will then develop glomerulonephritis, termed Masugi nephritis, which is a proliferative lesion on light microscopy and which on immunofluorescent staining presents a linear pattern of deposition of IgG and complement along the basement membrane.

In humans there are at least three clinical pictures associated with antiglomerular basement antibodies. Goodpasture's syndrome is characterized by proliferative glomerulonephritis and pulmonary hemorrhage. The disease is also characterized by the linear deposition of IgG and complement along the glomerular basement membrane. In some cases antibodies to pulmonary basement membrane can also be demonstrated. The antibody to the glomerular basement membranes can be eluted and shown to react with basement membrane from normal kidney. The antibody can also be concentrated and injected into squirrel monkeys, where it produces glomerulonephritis. Thus the antibody to glomerular basement membrane seems to be of pathogenetic importance in both animal models and human disease. It is important to note that antiglomerular basement membrane is not specific for Goodpasture's syndrome but is also involved in other glomerulonephritic states such as rapidly progressive

glomerulonephritis and acceleration of loss of renal function in patients with existing renal disease. In the latter circumstance, formation of antibody to basement membrane antigen, released as a part of the primary renal disease, produces a secondary antiglomerular basement membrane lesion.

ANTIBODY-ANTIGEN COMPLEX NEPHRITIS

In immune complex nephritis, circulating antibody-antigen complexes that need have no relationship to glomerular antigens are deposited in glomeruli and initiate a sequence of events leading to glomerular injury. Glomerular injury is most likely to result when the circulating soluble antibody-antigen complexes have been formed in the state of antigen excess.

The antigens for immune complex nephritis may be endogenous substances such as DNA in systemic lupus erythematosus, or exogenous materials such as microbial proteins in poststreptococcal glomerulonephritis, or viral agents. The immune complexes may deposit in the subepithelial or subendothelial regions of the glomerulus, or they may appear within the glomerular basement membrane. The subepithelial complexes are most likely formed in situ, while complexes in other locations may be formed in situ or filtered from the circulation.

The type of glomerular lesion seen in immune complex deposition varies with the size of the complexes

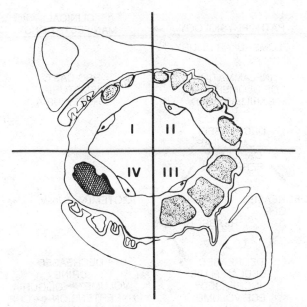

Figure 47. Schematic presentation of four types of membranous nephropathy. See text for explanation. (From Kashgarian, M., Hayslett, J. P., and Spargo, B. H.: Renal Disease. Kalamazoo, Mich., The Upjohn Company. Copyright 1974, Universities Associated for Research and Education in Pathology, Inc.)

and the duration and intensity of the antigenic stimulus. In classic poststreptococcal glomerulonephritis, subepithelial deposits are associated with proliferative glomerulonephritis, while in some forms of lupus erythematosus nephritis, large subendothelial deposits are associated with severe proliferative glomerulonephritis. On the other hand, prolonged low-level antigenic stimulation may produce the classic changes of membranous glomerulopathy (Fig. 47). In this last case, immune complexes appear in the subepithelial area (I). They appear to become embedded in the epithelial surface of the glomerular basement membrane, producing a spike-and-dome picture on light microscopy, utilizing silver stains (II). The immune complexes may appear within the glomerular basement membrane (III), or they may disappear, leaving a hole in the glomerular basement membrane that produces a moth-eaten appearance (IV). This entire spectrum of changes in membranous glomerulopathy occurs without inflammatory response (Fig. 47).

ALTERNATE COMPLEMENT PATHWAY

The precise pathogenetic role of activation of the alternate complement pathway in the production of glomerulonephritis is not known, nor is it known what factor or factors activate the alternate complement pathway in patients who do develop glomerulonephritis. Nonetheless there is a population of patients with apparent activation of the properdin or alternate complement pathway who have depressed levels of C3–C9 with well-maintained concentrations of C1, C2, and C4. Some of the patients have a factor (C3 nephritic factor) in their blood that is capable of activating a substance in normal serum that will break down C3 in vitro. There is also evidence that these patients have a defect in their complement system that results

in a lack of feedback inhibition of C3 consumption. In any event, patients with hypocomplementemia associated with alternate pathway activation are more likely to develop membranoproliferative glomerulonephritis.

PATHOGENESIS OF THE CLINICAL MANIFESTATIONS OF GLOMERULONEPHRITIS

Proteinuria

Proteinuria is the most important evidence of clinically significant glomerular injury. Recall that the healthy glomerular apparatus is a very selective ultrafilter that allows almost no protein to enter Bowman's space. However, if as little as 1 mg of protein per deciliter of glomerular filtrate appeared in Bowman's space, the filtered load of protein per 24 hours would be in excess of 1 g. Since the normal excretion of protein is less than 150 mg/24 hours, it follows that protein must be reabsorbed, catabolized, or both by the tubule. The most likely route for protein reabsorption is pinocytosis of the protein by the proximal tubular cells. The protein ordinarily excreted by normal individuals is composed of approximately 25 per cent albumin, and the remainder is globulin. Of the globulin present in the urine, perhaps 30 per cent is Tamm-Horsfall protein, a large-molecular-weight globulin that is produced in the loop of Henle and distal nephron.

With glomerular injury the glomerular apparatus becomes more permeable to proteins. The increased glomerular permeability is almost always associated with pathologic changes in the glomerular basement membrane or the foot processes of the epithelial cells or both. It has also been suggested that a change in the polyanionic character of the glomerular supporting matrix reduces the barrier to the passage of anionic proteins. The proteinuria of glomerular injury is predominantly an albuminuria. The markedly increased ratio of albumin excretion to the excretion of globulins is typical of glomerular injury and differentiates this form of proteinuria from that seen with predominantly tubular injury, where globulin excretion is more striking. The degree of albuminuria as well as its presence is of importance. In individuals excreting more than 3.5 g of protein in the urine per day, a clinical picture termed the nephrotic syndrome is likely to develop if the proteinuria persists for prolonged periods. Importance has also been attached to the selectivity of the proteinuria seen in glomerular injury. The assumption is that as glomerular injury proceeds from mild to severe, permeability to progressively larger protein molecules will increase. Thus, a measurement of the ratio of the excretion of albumin to the excretion of the larger gamma globulin IgG should be a measure of the selectivity of the glomerular leak. The higher the ratio, the more selective the leak; the lower the ratio, the less selective.

Hematuria

The presence of red blood cells in the urinary sediment may result from bleeding anywhere in the urinary tract. When the red blood cells originate from the glomerulus and must traverse the length of the nephron, particularly in conjunction with large quantities of protein, they may be entrapped in casts. The presence of red blood cell casts is excellent presumptive evidence of glomerular origin of the hematuria. The red blood cells enter the tubule as a result of damage to the glomerular capillary endothelial wall.

Pyuria

The presence of white blood cells in the urine is usually associated with tubulo-interstitial more than with glomerular disease. However, reviewing the pathology of the glomerulus in proliferative glomerulonephritis, one is struck by the large number of infiltrating polymorphonuclear cells. The passage of these polymorphonuclear cells through the damaged glomerular capillary endothelial cells accounts for their presence in the urine and the characteristic increase in pyuria seen during acute proliferative glomerulonephritis.

Oliguria

If glomerular injury is severe enough to reduce glomerular filtration rate, oliguria may result. Acutely, the fall in glomerular filtration rate seen with acute glomerulonephritis occurs in the presence of a still functioning tubule that is capable of increasing the reabsorption of salt and water and thus reducing further the volume of urine excreted.

Edema

Edema may result from the retention of salt and water seen as part of the process that in its extreme leads to oliguria. Edema may also be associated with the hypoalbuminemia that develops as the result of glomerular protein wasting. The latter circumstance will be discussed in detail under the nephrotic syndrome.

Hypertension

The retention of salt and water, expanding the intravascular and total extracellular fluid volume, may produce a rise in blood pressure. If these volume changes are coupled with increased release of renin, increased resistance in the arterial system will contribute to the hypertension.

Azotemia

If the glomerular filtration rate falls sufficiently there will be reduced filtration of urea and other waste products. In addition, the passive reabsorption of the urea that is filtered will be increased during the process of increased proximal reabsorption of salt and water that accompanies renal hypoperfusion. The combination of decreased filtration and increased reabsorption of urea will produce azotemia.

The composite clinical picture of glomerulonephritis will therefore depend upon the type and extent of glomerular injury. If the injury is minimal, proteinuria alone may be present. If proliferative changes are present, red blood cells, red blood cell casts, and white blood cells may appear. If the proliferative changes are extensive, diminished glomerular filtration rate may result in fluid retention and edema, oliguria, azotemia, and possibly hypertension—the picture of acute glo-

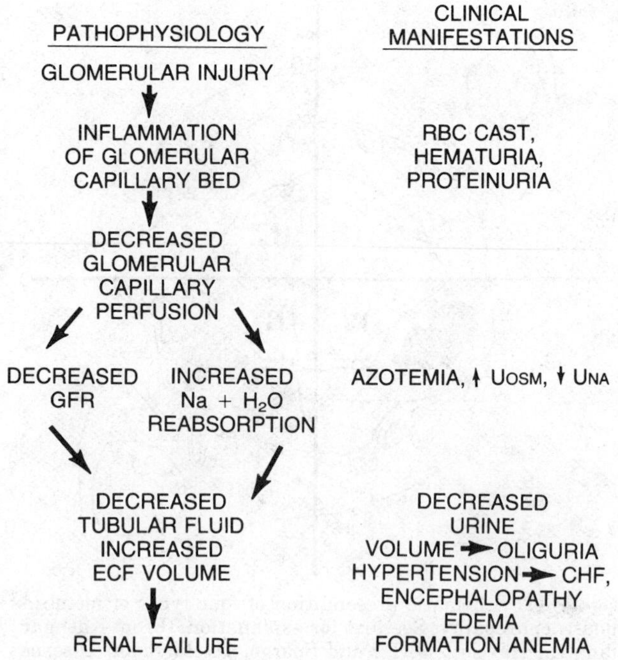

Figure 48. Sequence of events in acute glomerulonephritis. (Kindly provided by Norman Siegel.)

merulonephritis (Fig. 48). After an initial injury to the glomerulus it is possible for complete healing to occur. However, the glomerular injury may progress from an initial insult either rapidly to renal failure in a matter of 6 to 18 months—the picture of rapidly progressive glomerulonephritis—or it may progress gradually over years to chronic renal failure—the picture of chronic glomerulonephritis. Though chronic renal failure as a result of chronic glomerulonephritis may appear after a clinically quiescent period, proteinuria, as evidence of continuing renal damage, would likely have been present throughout the entire course of the illness. Throughout the spectrum of acute glomerulonephritis, rapidly progressive glomerulonephritis, and chronic glomerulonephritis, the clinical syndrome of nephrotic syndrome may appear if proteinuria is severe enough.

NEPHROTIC SYNDROME

Nephrotic syndrome is defined as the excretion of greater than 3.5 g of protein in the urine per 24 hours and hypoalbuminemia, with hyperlipemia, lipiduria, and edema frequently associated. An analysis of the pathophysiology of nephrotic syndrome will indicate that proteinuria is the critical defect for the development of the syndrome (Fig. 49).

PROTEINURIA

Recall that the normal urinary protein excretion is less than 150 mg/24 hours and that the nephrotic syndrome is defined as the excretion of greater than 3.5 g of protein, predominantly albumin, per 24 hours. Increased protein excretion could result from increased filtration of protein, decreased tubular reabsorption of protein, or increased tubular leak of protein. The latter two possibilities can be dealt with rather easily. There is little to suggest a tubular origin of the proteinuria

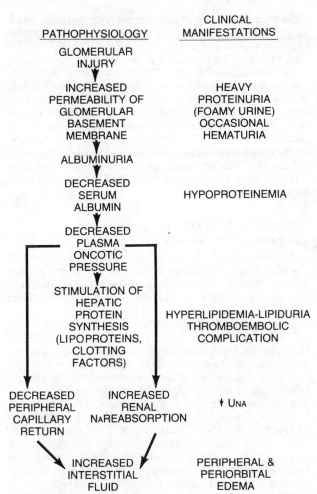

PATHOPHYSIOLOGY

CLINICAL
MANIFESTATIONS

GLOMERULAR
INJURY

INCREASED
PERMEABILITY OF
GLOMERULAR
BASEMENT
MEMBRANE

HEAVY
PROTEINURIA
(FOAMY URINE)
OCCASIONAL
HEMATURIA

ALBUMINURIA

DECREASED
SERUM
ALBUMIN

HYPOPROTEINEMIA

DECREASED
PLASMA
ONCOTIC
PRESSURE

STIMULATION OF
HEPATIC
PROTEIN
SYNTHESIS
(LIPOPROTEINS,
CLOTTING
FACTORS)

HYPERLIPIDEMIA-LIPIDURIA
THROMBOEMBOLIC
COMPLICATION

DECREASED
PERIPHERAL
CAPILLARY
RETURN

INCREASED
RENAL
Na REABSORPTION

↓ U$_{Na}$

INCREASED
INTERSTITIAL
FLUID

PERIPHERAL &
PERIORBITAL
EDEMA

Figure 49. Sequence of events in the nephrotic syndrome. (Kindly provided by Norman Siegel.)

in nephrotic syndrome. The pattern of protein excretion does not resemble that seen in any form of tubular injury, and the extent of proteinuria in terms of grams excreted for 24 hours far exceeds anything seen in the most severe forms of tubular injury. Decreased tubular reabsorption of protein is also unlikely as a sole cause of the proteinuria. The extent of proteinuria in nephrotic syndrome may far exceed any quantity that could be provided by a combination of normal filtered protein and total lack of tubular reabsorption; that is, if the normal kidney filtered somewhere between 1 and 10 g of protein per day and the tubule failed to reabsorb all of the filtered protein, it would still be impossible to account for excretions of protein that may reach 20-g levels in the nephrotic syndrome. Therefore it is most likely that the proteinuria of nephrotic syndrome is a result of glomerular leakage. Consistent with this concept is the observation that in every patient with nephrotic syndrome there are changes in the glomerulus, with at least swelling of the epithelial foot processes being universally found. Second, the proteinuria is predominantly albuminuria with relatively less globulin loss, which is consistent with the change in the permeability of the ultrafiltering apparatus. Finally, in animal models it is possible to show that the glomerulus is the source of protein leak in experimental nephrotic syndrome.

Though the protein excreted is predominantly albumin, larger proteins such as the immune globulins and clotting factors may also be lost in the urine. The pattern and extent of protein loss are reflected in the plasma.

HYPOALBUMINEMIA

In the nephrotic syndrome the plasma albumin concentration is reduced to less than 3.5 and occasionally to less than 2 g/dl. At least one important factor controlling hepatic protein synthesis appears to be the oncotic pressure of the plasma perfusing the liver. Thus hypoalbuminemia results in a nonspecific increase in hepatic protein synthesis. The resulting plasma protein pattern represents the balance between increased loss of protein in the urine and increased hepatic synthesis. If protein loss exceeds synthesis, the plasma concentration will fall. If synthesis exceeds loss, plasma concentration will rise. Eventually loss and synthesis will achieve a new steady state. The classic pattern that results is that of a low albumin level, because the initial loss exceeds production; increased alpha$_2$-globulin, because production exceeds urinary loss of this very large molecule; and a variable concentration of IgG, because the balance between production and loss may be tipped in either direction. The roles of altered protein synthesis and catabolism in nephrotic syndrome remain unclear. Though the normal liver, which produces 12 to 15 g/day of protein, can increase production by more than 2 g/day, synthesis does not increase adequately to prevent hypoalbuminemia in patients losing as little as 3.5 g of urinary protein daily. No specific defect in synthesis has been demonstrated. In some individuals with nephrotic syndrome, increased catabolism of proteins has been demonstrated, but this is by no means a uniform finding.

HYPERLIPIDEMIA

Hypoalbuminemia is also related to the production of a hyperlipidemic state. The exact cause and effect relationship between hypoalbuminemia and hyperlipidemia is not clear. However, the following observations are worthy of note: (1) Raising the oncotic pressure of plasma by the infusion of either albumin or dextran will reduce the hyperlipidemia in experimental animals. (2) The rate of synthesis of lipoproteins is increased in states of hypoalbuminemia, as is the synthesis of other proteins. (3) Albumin may be required for the normal process of metabolism of lipoproteins. In any event, the result is typically an increase of cholesterol and triglycerides.

LIPIDURIA

In any patient with a sufficient degree of glomerular proteinuria there will be some loss of beta lipoprotein, and hence associated cholesterol, into the urine. The proximal tubule cells pinocytose the lipoprotein-cholesterol complex and then split the beta lipoprotein from the cholesterol, allowing the precipitation of the liquid crystal of cholesterol within the cell. Proximal tubular cells laden with liquid crystals of cholesterol may slough into the urine and become the oval fat bodies seen in nephrotic syndrome. These cells may disintegrate to release lipid droplets, or they may become incorporated into fatty casts. In oval fat bodies, lipid droplets, and fatty casts, the crystals of cholesterol ester may be seen by polarizing light as birefringent Maltese crosses.

EDEMA

The loss of albumin with inadequate hepatic synthesis to maintain plasma levels within the normal range results in a fall in plasma oncotic pressure and a loss of intravascular volume into the interstitium. The decreased intravascular volume is associated with decreased renal perfusion and increased secretion of renin, which ultimately results in increased secretion of aldosterone. Sodium is retained avidly by the kidney not only proximally and in the distal convoluted tubule as has long been believed but, importantly, in the collecting duct as well, at least in animal models. The retained sodium and water in the presence of decreased oncotic pressure distribute disproportionately between the vascular and extravascular space, favoring the latter, and producing edema.

The clinical picture of nephrotic syndrome is predictable on the basis of the pathophysiology. Patients will have edema, usually dependent in location; that is, the edema will be pedal when the patient is sitting or standing and periorbital when the patient has been lying flat. Postural hypotension may be present if the degree of hypoalbuminemia is extreme and the vascular volume is markedly reduced. If, however, the glomerular injury is associated with increased renin production, hypertension may be present even with reduced intravascular volume. Patients with nephrotic syndrome are susceptible to infection, probably as a result of impaired local defense mechanisms in edematous tissue and ascitic fluid, and due also to a reduced concentration of plasma IgG. Typically, infections occur with gram-positive organisms; pneumococcal peritonitis has been a classically described complication. Thromboembolic phenomena occur with increased frequency in association with reduced intravascular volume and increased clotting factors, including fibrinogen. The increase in clotting factors occurs as a result of the increased protein synthesis resulting from hypoalbuminemia. Thromboembolic complications may include renal vein thrombosis, which would then accelerate the deterioration of renal function. Less commonly the balance between the increased loss of proteins in urine and the increased production of protein by the liver will result in a reduction in clotting factors and a bleeding tendency. Finally, prolonged existence of the nephrotic syndrome and its associated hyperlipidemia have been associated with acceleration of atherosclerotic processes.

SPECIFIC FORMS OF GLOMERULONEPHRITIS

A discussion of the clinical aspects and treatment of the glomerulonephritides is beyond the scope of this section. Rather, we will outline the types of glomerulonephritis in light of the previous pathophysiologic discussion (Table 10).

Treatment of the glomerulonephritides depends upon an understanding of their pathogenesis. Treatment of infection for control of the glomerular lesions of infective endocarditis or secondary amyloidosis is well established. Reduction of the antigenic stimulus via the treatment of streptococcal pharyngitis and erysipelas has not been shown to prevent glomerulonephritis, but is logical. Control of the abnormal glucose metabolism of the diabetic state is also logical, but similarly has not been shown to prevent or reverse the glomerular lesions. Beyond these proven or logical approaches to the treatment of glomerulopathies lies the majority of present therapy of glomerulonephritis. Treatment is based on the assumption that there is an immunologic origin to most glomerulonephritides and that the process of leukocyte attraction and activation and of activation of clotting factors contributes to glomerular

TABLE 10. OUTLINE OF CLINICAL GLOMERULOPATHIES

CATEGORY	TYPICAL CLINICAL PICTURE			
	Hypertension	Hematuria	Nephritic Picture	Nephrotic Syndrome
I. Primary glomerular				
A. Minimal lesion	–	–	–	+
B. Focal and segmental sclerosis	–	±	–	+
C. Proliferative				
1. Focal (IgA; Henoch-Schönlein)	–	+	±	±
2. Diffuse (Postinfectious)	+	+	+	±
3. Membranoproliferative (Type I, II, III—Mesangiocapillary)	+	+	+	+
4. Mesangioproliferative (Focal or diffuse proliferative—see 1 and 2)				
5. Crescentic (Goodpasture's; rapidly progressive glomerulonephritis)	+	+	+	+
D. Membranous	±	–	–	+
II. Systemic Diseases				
A. Diabetic glomerulosclerosis	+	±	–	+
B. Amyloidosis	±	–	–	+
C. Vasculitis (SLE)	+	+	+	+
D. Malignancy associated (Minimal lesion, proliferative-membranoproliferative, membranous—see 1 and 3 and D above)				
E. Infective endocarditis (Focal or diffuse proliferative disease—see 1 and 2)				

injury. Thus, treatment has been directed at reducing inflammation (glucocorticoids), reducing antibody formation (glucocorticoids, immunosuppressive agents), removing antibodies or immune complexes (plasmapheresis), and preventing fibrin deposition (heparin). Many of these therapeutic methods have been used in combination. Interestingly, the most successful therapy for the treatment of glomerulonephritides has been the use of glucocorticoids for the treatment of lipoid

nephrosis, particularly in children. Recall that in lipoid nephrosis there is evidence of neither immunologic activity nor inflammation. This final point is meant to remind the reader that despite the enormous number of observations on the pathology of glomerulonephritis and our ability to correlate pathologic with clinical events, our understanding of the pathogenesis of the glomerulonephritides is incomplete and sketchy at best.

Tubulo-Interstitial Diseases

The division of renal disorders into tubulo-interstitial and glomerular diseases indicates the site of the primary or predominant pathologic process. It does not mean that the tubules and interstitium are unaffected in the glomerulopathies or that the glomeruli are spared in the tubulo-interstitial diseases. When we talk about tubulo-interstitial disease, we are referring to disorders characterized by anatomic lesions. The purely functional tubular abnormalities will be discussed separately.

Since the tubulo-interstitial diseases produce a predominantly tubular dysfunction, the pathophysiologic results can be predicted. Proteinuria (usually the result of glomerular injury) is absent or modest. Urinary protein is usually less than 1 g/24 hours and rarely more than 2 g/24 hours. Urinary dilution and concentration that require the highest degree of integration of structure and function are most commonly impaired. Some degree of salt wasting is also common. Reduction in tubular mass is associated with a reduction in ammonia production in the development of hyperchloremic metabolic acidosis. Impaired secretion of hydrogen ion and bicarbonate reabsorption may add to the acidosis. Potassium excretion will be variable, but may be severely impaired in disorders such as sickle cell disease or amyloidosis. It has been suggested that prolonged periods of insufficient production of 1,25-dihydroxyvitamin D_3 are more likely to occur with diseases affecting the renal tubule, which is the site of production of the active vitamin. Eventually, if the process of tubular interstitial damage is extensive enough, glomerular filtration rate falls and uremia occurs.

Tubulo-interstitial diseases will be presented briefly. The discussion will focus on the different mechanisms that may produce tubulo-interstitial injury. No attempt will be made to discuss the disease entities in detail (Table 11).

Tubulo-interstitial diseases may be congenital or acquired. The congenital disorders are primarily the cystic diseases of the kidney: juvenile and adult polycystic disease, medullary cystic disease, and medullary sponge kidney (see Hereditary Renal Diseases). Hereditary nephritis with deafness, which has a noncystic tubulo-interstitial component, also has a prominent glomerular component.

In the polycystic diseases the cysts are composed of portions of the renal tubules. Enlargement of the cysts ultimately leads to compression of normally functioning renal tissue and development of uremia. Medullary

TABLE 11. TUBULO-INTERSTITIAL DISEASE

Congenital—Primarily Structural Defects
  Juvenile polycystic disease
  Adult polycystic disease
  Medullary sponge kidney
    Primarily functional defects (see Hereditary Renal Diseases)

Acquired
  Infection
  Toxins—endogenous
         exogenous
  Immunologic injury
  Mechanical injury—obstruction
  Physical injury—radiation
  Ischemia
  Infiltrative diseases—amyloid

cystic disease is characterized either by cystic changes or predominantly by fibrosis in the medullary interstitium. The result is progressive destruction of the medullary interstitium, again producing uremia. With severe medullary interstitial disarray there is early loss of diluting and concentrating ability and a prominent component of salt wasting. Medullary sponge kidney is a more benign lesion characterized predominantly by x-ray findings of dilatation and cystic changes in the region of the large papillary collecting ducts. The disease would be an anatomic curiosity were it not for a high incidence of calcium oxalate and calcium phosphate stone formation. In some patients with medullary sponge kidney, a degree of renal tubular acidosis may contribute to the formation of stones. (See Table 12 for a comparison of renal cystic diseases.)

Acquired tubulo-interstitial disease may result from infection, toxins, immunologic injury, mechanical injury, physical injury, ischemic disease, and infiltrative diseases.

Infection

Pyelonephritis refers to infection of the kidney. The route of renal infection may be hematogenous or by ascent from the bladder. In humans, pyelonephritis is commonly associated with bladder infection, and evidence favors an ascending route of infection as the cause of the majority of cases of pyelonephritis. Acute pyelonephritis is characterized by the presence of bacteria and an acute inflammatory reaction in the interstitial region of the kidney. The infection tends to be focal and confined to wedge-shaped segments. Involvement of glomeruli is extremely rare. More diffuse renal

TABLE 12. CYSTIC DISEASES OF THE KIDNEY

	MEDULLARY CYSTIC	POLYCYSTIC	SPONGE KIDNEY
Flank pain	No	Yes	Occasionally
High BP	No*	Yes	No
Hematuria	No	Yes	Occ. (stone)
Azotemia	Yes	Yes (30–40)	No
Age at death	Younger (20–30)	40–50	Normal
X-ray	Normal or small	Large	Normal—fan pattern
Stones	No	No	Yes

From Gardner, K. D., Jr.: Cystic Diseases of the Kidney. New York. John Wiley and Sons, 1976, p. 182. Originally from The New England Journal of Medicine 274:983, 1966.

*Hypertension may be seen early in the course of medullary cystic diseases, but is usually seen prior to the onset of salt wasting and major renal insufficiency.

involvement may occur and is typically associated with mechanical abnormalities of the urinary tract. With time or treatment the acute inflammation in the renal interstitium gives way to a more chronic mononuclear cell infiltrate and ultimately to the deposition of fibrous tissue and scar. The extent of scarring is usually minimal. Unless there is mechanical obstruction, reflux, a foreign body in the urinary tract, or an impairment of host defenses, acute pyelonephritis is unlikely to produce sufficient renal injury to result in uremia.

The involvement of the renal interstitium by bacteria exposes the body's defense mechanisms to the bacterial antigens. Antibodies are formed to the invading bacteria. The presence of antibody-coated bacteria in the urine is accepted as evidence that renal parenchyma has been invaded. Urinary tract infection localized to the bladder is not associated with antibody-coated bacteria. Invasion of the renal interstitium is also associated with an impairment of renal concentrating ability. Thus, the failure to concentrate the urine in a patient with urinary tract infection is taken as evidence of upper urinary tract involvement.

The urine of an individual with acute pyelonephritis usually contains bacteria in sufficient quantities to be seen in sediment from an uncentrifuged sample. In addition, white cells and white cell casts may be present. A urine culture revealing the presence of more than 10^5 organisms should confirm the diagnosis of acute urinary tract infection. Bacterial counts of less than 10^5 may be significant if the same species is isolated repeatedly or if the urine is obtained by catheterization or by suprapubic aspiration.

Chronic pyelonephritis is typically associated with the development of asymmetric renal scarring. The difficulty in assessing the clinical importance of chronic pyelonephritis is that a number of processes are capable of producing an indistinguishable pathologic picture without infection. For example, reflux nephropathy and ischemic renal injury may produce a picture of chronic pyelonephritis. To complicate the matter further, those processes that produce a pathologic picture of chronic tubulo-interstitial nephritis may be associated with a higher incidence of infection. It is probably safest to assume that chronic pyelonephritis from recurrent infection is unusual in the absence of some abnormality of urinary drainage. If no functional or mechanical impairment of urinary drainage can be discerned, a careful search for other causes of tubulo-interstitial injury is warranted.

Toxins

Toxins may be endogenous or exogenous. Endogenous toxins include calcium (hypercalcemia), uric acid (hyperuricemia), light chains (multiple myeloma), and so on. Endogenous toxins may injure renal tubular cells directly, as in the case of light chains, or they may precipitate in the medullary interstitium and initiate a process of fibrosis and scarring, as in the case of sodium urate.

Exogenous toxins include heavy metals, aminoglycoside antibiotics, phenacetin, and so on. Perhaps the most important exogenous toxins are the aminoglycoside antibiotics, which are associated with a large number of cases of acute tubular necrosis (see section on Acute Tubular Necrosis). Acute renal failure is being recognized with increasing frequency in patients taking nonsteroidal anti-inflammatory agents. The injury produced by these drugs is mediated at least in part by inhibition of the synthesis of vasodilatory prostaglandins. This inhibition in the presence of causes of renal vasoconstriction is particularly likely to produce renal injury (see p. 656–657). There is also interstitial nephritis, which may or may not be associated with nephrotic syndrome produced by nonsteroidal anti-inflammatory agents. This latter form of injury may be mediated through T cells. Phenacetin, however, has received the greatest attention as a cause of exogenous tubulo-interstitial toxicity. Phenacetin, when ingested in large quantities over a prolonged time (and perhaps potentiated by aspirin), is capable of producing severe interstitial nephritis and papillary necrosis. Experimental evidence suggests that phenacetin or its metabolites are concentrated in the medullary interstitium. In that location they produce an oxidant type of injury to the membranes of the tubules. This oxidant injury is potentiated by the presence of aspirin. The result is injury to the loops of Henle and the collecting ducts, with the ultimate production of sufficient interstitial fibrosis and scarring to produce papillary necrosis. During the development of phenacetin-induced nephritis, concentrating ability is lost initially and uremia is produced ultimately. There is evidence to suggest that if phenacetin can be identified as a potential cause of tubulo-interstitial injury, discontinuation of the phenacetin may permit stabilization or even improvement in renal function.

Immunologic Injury

A form of hypersensitivity interstitial nephritis has been reported in association with the ingestion of a large number of medications. A classic example of drug-induced hypersensitivity interstitial nephritis is methicillin nephritis. Large doses of methicillin have been associated with the development of interstitial nephritis characterized by the presence of large numbers of mononuclear cells and eosinophils. The extent of injury may be sufficient to produce a picture of acute tubular necrosis. Microscopic hematuria and eosinophiluria are commonly seen. This clinical and pathologic picture has now been reported with a large number of other antibiotics, diuretics, anticonvulsants, and so on. It is probably safest to assume that virtually any drug can induce hypersensitivity interstitial nephritis. Further evidence of an immunologic origin of the renal injury has been obtained in a few patients who demonstrate the deposition of IgG along the tubular basement membranes and the presence of circulating antibodies to tubular basement membrane antigen. Patients with this form of tubulo-interstitial disease will usually respond to withdrawal of the offending agent.

Mechanical Injury

Obstruction to urinary tract flow from any cause and vesicoureteral reflux have been associated with tubulo-interstitial injury. The functional correlates of urinary tract obstruction and the release of obstruction are discussed in detail in the section on acute renal failure. Vesicoureteral reflux has been well documented to produce tubulo-interstitial injury in the absence of infection. It is worth noting, however, that infection per se can produce vesicoureteral reflux, and, before a diagnosis of primary vesicoureteral reflux can be made, infection should be eradicated and the extent of vesicoureteral reflux reassessed.

Physical Injury

Radiation to the kidney at cumulative doses of greater than 2500 R can produce tubulo-interstitial injury. Once radiation therapy has been initiated, tubulo-interstitial disease may progress with or without accelerated hypertension to produce chronic renal failure.

Ischemic Disease

In hypertension, renal vascular changes may be associated with a pattern of tubulo-interstitial injury. Similar changes may occur in kidneys affected by cholesterol embolization and most dramatically in patients who have sickle cell disease. In patients with sickle cell disease, microscopic thrombi involving the vasa recta may result in ischemic injury to the medullary interstitium and ultimately in the development of papillary necrosis. In patients with sickle cell disease, renal concentrating ability is lost, and there is now evidence that renal potassium secretion is markedly impaired. As discussed earlier, renal injury caused by nonsteroidal anti-inflammatory agents is at least in part ischemic injury.

Infiltrative Diseases

Amyloidosis, which classically affects the glomeruli and produces the nephrotic syndrome, may also occur as peritubular deposition in the region of the collecting duct. Interference with tubular function at this site results in nephrogenic diabetes insipidus and in impaired secretion of hydrogen ion and potassium.

This brief survey of the mechanisms by which tubulo-interstitial disease may be produced is meant to provide perspective on the complex etiology of tubulo-interstitial damage. Just a few years ago all tubulo-interstitial disease was diagnosed as pyelonephritis. It should now be clear that tubulo-interstitial nephritis is simply a pathologic end point that can be reached via a spectrum of causes. The diagnosis of tubulo-interstitial nephritis is never complete until each of the causes has been considered.

Hereditary Renal Diseases

There are a large number of inherited renal diseases, many of which are rare. Rather than catalog heritable renal diseases, we will examine examples of the mechanisms by which these disorders alter physiology.

The general categories of pathophysiology of inherited renal disease are (1) a primary anatomic defect, (2) an anatomic defect secondary to a primary metabolic defect, (3) a generalized functional abnormality secondary to a metabolic defect, and (4) a primary specific functional defect. Within these categories there may be subgroups defining more specific pathophysiologic mechanisms. This discussion of the potential mechanisms for the expression of inherited renal disease should develop a framework into which all other presently recognized and yet to be described disorders will fit.

PRIMARY ANATOMIC DEFECT

Primary anatomic diseases may be predominantly tubulo-interstitial, as in adult and juvenile polycystic disease, medullary cystic disease, and medullary sponge kidney. They may also be predominantly glomerular, albeit with a significant tubulo-interstitial component, as in hereditary nephritis with deafness or hereditary nephrotic syndrome. Anatomic lesions may be inherited as autosomal dominant, autosomal recessive, or sex-linked traits. These disorders may be expressed as anatomic lesions confined to the kidney, as in medullary cystic disease, or involving the kidney plus other organs, as in the hepatic fibrosis of juvenile polycystic diseases.

With the exception of medullary sponge kidney, all of the inherited anatomic defects presented typically produce chronic renal failure and uremia. The approach to the disorder involves the management of uremia and appropriate genetic counseling (Table 13).

ANATOMIC DEFECTS SECONDARY TO METABOLIC DEFECTS

An inherited metabolic defect can result in the accumulation of a nephrotoxin. The nephrotoxin may be the immediate result of the metabolic defect, as in

TABLE 13. PRIMARY STRUCTURAL ABNORMALITIES

TUBULAR-INTERSTITIAL	CLINICAL MANIFESTATIONS

Polycystic disease
  Adult
  Juvenile
Medullary cystic disease
	} Uremia

Medullary sponge kidney	Stones, infection
Glomerular (with or without interstitial disease)	
Hereditary nephritis and deafness Hereditary nephrotic syndrome	} Uremia

From Thier, S. O.: Medical management of hereditary renal diseases. In Papadatos, C. J., and Bartsocas, C. S. (eds.): The Management of Genetic Disorders. New York, Alan R. Liss, Inc., 1979, p. 283.

Fabry's disease, or it may accumulate secondary to the deficiency of a protein that would otherwise bind or facilitate the excretion of the toxic substance, as copper accumulates in Wilson's disease. A nephrotoxin may also accumulate as the result of normal production and excessive storage, as in cystinosis. Theoretically, cellular damage might result from the loss of a critical metabolite, but as yet there is no good example of a clinical renal disease resulting from this mechanism (Table 14).

The general principles governing the approach to metabolic defects producing anatomic renal lesions are: (1) correct the defect by correcting the metabolic lesion (that is, replace an enzyme), (2) reduce the intake of an accumulating toxin or its precursor, (3) remove an accumulating toxin by chelation, for example, and (4) replace the genetically defective kidney with a normal kidney in circumstances in which toxin accumulation can be controlled. If the accumulation of toxin cannot be controlled, the transplanted kidney will suffer the same injury as the original. Finally, if a deficiency of a critical substance could be shown to be responsible for the renal injury, replacement of that substance would be in order.

GENERALIZED FUNCTIONAL ABNORMALITY SECONDARY TO A METABOLIC DEFECT

The same theoretic considerations that applied to the category of anatomic damage secondary to a metabolic defect apply to this category. The only difference is that the accumulating toxin alters tubular function but does not produce anatomic damage. The classic examples of this type of disorder are galactosemia, in which a deficiency of galactose 1-phosphate uridyl transferase results in the cellular accumulation of galactolol and galactose 1-phosphate; and hereditary fructose intolerance, in which a deficiency of fructose 1-phosphate aldolase leads to the accumulation of fructose 1-phosphate. The result in both cases is Fanconi syndrome. Since the involved enzymes cannot be replaced, restriction of the precursors of the toxins—that is, galactose and fructose—is the treatment of choice (Table 15).

FANCONI SYNDROME

The generalized tubular dysfunction seen with Wilson's disease, cystinosis, and a host of other nephrotoxic stimuli is termed Fanconi syndrome. This syndrome results from a generalized proximal tubular dysfunction and is usually associated with light or electron microscopic changes in the cells of the proximal tubule. Disruption of the endoplasmic reticulum and changes in mitochondria have been described after exposure to nephrotoxins that produce the Fanconi syndrome. Two theories have been proposed to explain the findings of the Fanconi syndrome. The first holds that there is reduced proximal tubular reabsorption of all substances due to anatomic damage or to inhibition of energy available for transport. The second theory suggests that reabsorption is intact, but that there is increased back leakage of reabsorbate into the proximal tubule. According to this second theory, the substances that leak back in the proximal tubule (glucose, amino acids, phosphate, and so on) are then delivered

TABLE 14. METABOLIC DEFECT PRODUCING STRUCTURAL DEFECT

DISEASE	DEFECT RESULTING IN TOXIC INJURY	TOXIN	TREATMENT
Fabry	Enzyme defect (α-galactosidase A)	Ceramide Di- and trihexose	Enzyme replacement (transplant)
Wilson	?Protein deficiency (ceruloplasmin) ?Decreased capacity for hepatic copper excretion	Copper	Reduce copper intake Remove copper (D-penicillamine)
Cystinosis	Probable lysosomal defect	Cystine	Replace defective kidney with one unaffected by defect (transplant)

From Thier, S. O.: Medical management of hereditary renal diseases. In Papadatos, C. J., and Bartsocas, C. S. (eds.): The Management of Genetic Disorders. New York, Alan R. Liss, Inc., 1979, p. 287.

TABLE 15. METABOLIC DEFECT PRODUCING GENERALIZED FUNCTION DEFECT

DISEASE	DEFECT	TOXIN	TREATMENT
Galactosemia	Enzyme deficiency (galactose-1-phosphate uridyl transferase)	Galactilol, galactose-1-PO$_4$	Restrict galactose intake
Hereditary fructose intolerance	Enzyme deficiency (fructose-1-phosphate aldolase)	Fructose-1-PO$_4$	Restrict fructose intake

From Thier, S. O.: Medical management of hereditary renal diseases. In Papadatos, C. J., and Bartsocas, C. S. (eds.): The Management of Genetic Disorders. New York, Alan R. Liss, Inc., 1979, p. 289.

to the distal nephron, where they are normally minimally reabsorbed and therefore appear in the urine. In any event, the picture in Fanconi syndrome is one of aminoaciduria, phosphaturia, glycosuria, uricosuria, calcium wasting, and bicarbonate wasting. Renal potassium wasting may be a secondary phenomenon resulting from the increased delivery of sodium bicarbonate to the distal nephron. The clinical picture is one of osteomalacia, growth retardation, chronic metabolic acidosis, and weakness from hypokalemia.

PRIMARY SPECIFIC TUBULAR DYSFUNCTION

Specific disorders of tubular function may result from impaired reabsorption, impaired secretion, or lack of tubular response to a hormone.

Reabsorptive defects may result in the loss of a substance in the urine with no clinical manifestations (renal glycosuria), the loss of a substance in the urine that is a critical nutrient (Hartnup disease), the loss of a substance in the urine that initiates a series of compensatory responses that produce clinical disease (hypophosphatemic rickets), and the loss of a substance that by its presence in increased quantities in the urine produces disease (cystinuria) (Table 16).

In renal glycosuria glucose appears in the urine at low or normal filtered loads. The curve of glucose reabsorption as a function of glucose load demonstrates increased splay and may show a reduced T_m for glucose. This disorder, inherited as an autosomal dominant trait, produces no clinical disease. It is dangerous only if diabetes mellitus is misdiagnosed and treatment is begun inappropriately.

Hartnup disease appears clinically as a pellagra-like illness. This disorder of neutral amino acid transport in kidney and intestine is transmitted as an autosomal recessive trait. Tryptophan, one of the poorly transported amino acids, is normally metabolized to nicotinamide. In Hartnup disease the failure to absorb tryptophan from the gut and the loss of tryptophan in the urine leads to a deficiency of nicotinamide and produces a pellagra-like illness. Treatment would include the provision of adequate quantities of tryptophan or nicotinamide in the diet.

Hypophosphatemic rickets, an X-linked trait, may result from a reduction in the T_m phosphate leading to phosphate depletion and the development of osteomalacia. A coexistent insensitivity to vitamin D contributes to the bone disease of this sex-linked disorder. Replacement of adequate quantities of phosphate and large doses of vitamin D will improve the osteomalacia (see section on Vitamin D-Resistant Rickets, p. 714).

Cystinuria, to be discussed in detail in the section on urinary tract calculi, is an example of a clinical disease produced by an excess in the urine of a substance that is inadequately reabsorbed from the glomerular filtrate. Since the disease results not from the loss of cystine but rather from its presence in the urine, treatment must be directed at reducing urinary cystine (see section on Urinary Tract Calculi, p. 734).

Defects in secretion are best exemplified by the syndrome of renal tubular acidosis (Table 17). This syndrome was discussed in detail in the section on acid-base pathophysiology.

Finally, renal tubular dysfunction may occur as the result of an insensitivity to a hormone. The classic example of this type of inherited disorder is nephrogenic diabetes insipidus. This disorder is a sex-linked trait expressed as a failure to concentrate the urine. The strategy for distinguishing between the causes of polyuria is discussed in the section on Volume and Tonicity (pp. 679–680).

In summary, specific functional disorders of the tubule can result from altered kinetics of reabsorption, as in renal glycosuria; reduced reabsorptive capacity

TABLE 16. SPECIFIC DISORDERS OF TUBULAR FUNCTION (REABSORPTIVE)

DISEASE	DEFECT	CLINICAL	TREATMENT
Renal glycosuria	Abnormal kinetics of glucose reabsorption: splay or reduced T_m glucose	Glycosuria	None
Hartnup	Defective neutral amino acid transport in gut and kidney	Pellagra-like illness	Tryptophan and/or nicotinamide
Hypophosphatemic rickets	Reduced T_m PO_4, vitamin D resistance	Rickets	Vitamin D and phosphate
Cystinuria	Defective dibasic amino acid and cystine transport in gut and kidney	Urinary calculi	Fluid, alkalinization, D-penicillamine, mercaptopropionyl glycine

From Thier, S. O.: Medical management of hereditary renal diseases. In Papadatos, C. J., and Bartsocas, C. S. (eds.): The Management of Genetic Disorders. New York, Alan R. Liss, Inc., 1979, p. 291.

TABLE 17. SPECIFIC DISORDERS OF TUBULAR FUNCTION

DISEASE	DEFECT	CLINICAL	TREATMENT
Renal Tubular Acidosis			
Classic	Gradient limited H^+ secretion	Nephrocalcinosis, urinary stones, osteomalacia, paralysis (hypokalemia)	Bicarbonate, phosphate, and potassium
"Proximal"	Reduced T_m HCO_3^-	Paralysis (hypokalemia)	Bicarbonate, potassium, thiazides, and sodium restriction
Nephrogenic diabetes insipidus	Tubular unresponsiveness to antidiuretic hormone	Diabetes insipidus	Thiazides and sodium restriction

From Thier, S. O.: Medical management of hereditary renal diseases. In Papadatos, C. J., and Bartsocas, C. S. (eds.): The Management of Genetic Disorders: New York, Alan R. Liss, Inc., 1979, p. 293.

TABLE 18. PRINCIPLES OF TREATMENT OF HEREDITARY RENAL DISEASES

Correct the genetic defect	Avoid loss of critical substances
Avoid accumulation of toxic substances	Provide adequate intake of substance lost
In tissue	Modify renal excretion to reduce loss of critical substance
Reduce intake of toxins or their precursors	Decrease filtered load
Facilitate removal of toxins	Increase reabsorption
In urine	Decrease secretion
Reduce intake of toxins or their precursors	Provide medical support for loss of all renal function
Reduce the concentration of the toxin in urine	Medical management of uremia
Decrease filtered load	Provide surgical treatment for loss of all renal function
Increase reabsorption	Renal transplantation with kidney unaffected by the
Decrease secretion	genetic defect
Increase urine volume	Do not treat the genetic disease unless clinically indicated

From Thier, S. O.: Medical management of hereditary renal diseases. In Papadatos, C. J., and Bartsocas, C. S. (eds.): The Management of Genetic Disorders. New York, Alan R. Liss, Inc., 1979, p. 282.

for a substance, as in hypophosphatemic rickets; a defect in a stereospecific transport mechanism, as in the aminoacidurias, Hartnup disease, and cystinuria; a defect in secretion, as in renal tubular acidosis; and insensitivity to hormone, as in nephrogenic diabetes insipidus.

A general approach to the management of hereditary renal diseases is presented in Table 18.

Urinary Tract Calculi

A urinary tract calculus will form when the concentration of its component crystal-forming substance exceeds solubility. However, crystal-forming substances may remain in solution in urine at concentrations that would exceed their solubility in water. In urine, solubility is affected not only by the concentration of the stone-forming substance, but by the salt content of the urine, the urinary pH, the concentration of inhibitors of crystallization in the urine, obstruction to urine flow, infection, and the presence of potentiators of crystallization such as scar tissue. The approach to urinary tract stone disease is to define the cause of the disease and to treat the primary process if possible. In addition, mechanical abnormalities of the urinary tract and infection must be sought and treated. The quantity of stone-forming substance in the urine may be reduced by reducing the filtered load, enhancing tubular reabsorption, or converting the substance to a more soluble form. The concentration of stone-forming substance should be reduced by increasing fluid intake. Finally, the physical chemistry of the urine should be modified by altering pH or by increasing the concentration of inhibitors of crystallization, such as pyrophosphate or magnesium.

There are distinct areas in the world in which the incidence of stone disease is markedly increased. The factors contributing to this increased incidence are as follows: (1) Genetic. The more inbred a society, the more likely it is that metabolic stone disease of genetic origin will appear. (2) Climate. The hotter and drier the climate, the more likely it is that individuals will have persistently concentrated urine and be prone to stone formation. In areas where exposure to sunlight is prolonged and intense, an increased production of vitamin D in the population may result in increased calcium absorption and excretion. (3) Unusual diet or mineral content of water may also contribute to an increased incidence of stone formation.

The volume of urine (amount of urine water) is of obvious importance in determining the concentration of stone-forming constituents. Antidiuretic hormone is released in response to an increase in serum tonicity, resulting either from decreased water intake or increased insensible loss. The rise in plasma tonicity will also trigger the thirst mechanism. Concentration of the urine will also occur with or without excess antidiuretic hormone if renal perfusion falls. Water intake, which the patient may correlate with thirst, should be gauged to prevent urinary concentration. Therefore, if the patient is drinking fluids in volumes and at a frequency sufficient to prevent thirst, it is likely that the urine will be dilute. Second, the patient must drink adequate fluid to maintain a urine output during the night hours, since renal perfusion falls during sleep. If the patient is not drinking enough fluid to induce nocturia, and does not drink water at the time of voiding, it is likely that the urine will become concentrated during the night. It is important to prevent even brief periods of excessive urinary concentration, since crystal formation, once initiated, is difficult to reverse. The optimal use of water in the therapy of stone disease does not rest solely with defining a volume of water that must be ingested. The patient must drink the water as evenly as practical throughout the day and night. If the patient experiences thirst, or sleeps through the night, then the volume and pattern of water intake are probably not adequate to prevent concentration of the urine. This attention to the physiology of dilution and concentration can make water intake a powerful tool in the treatment of stone disease.

In addition to the general principles of the treatment of urinary calculi, there are specific forms of urinary tract stone disease that can be treated not only by recalling these principles, but by a series of more direct attacks upon the defined pathophysiology.

CYSTINURIA

Cystinuria, inherited as an autosomal recessive trait, is a disorder of amino acid transport expressed in the mucosa of the renal tubule and the small intestine. The transport of the structurally related amino acids cystine, lysine, arginine, and ornithine is defective. Cystine, the least soluble naturally occurring amino acid, precipitates particularly in acid urine, forming stones that account for the clinical presentation of the disease.

Most of the cystine circulating in plasma originates from the metabolism of methionine via the trans-sulfuration pathway. Cystine and the dibasic amino acids lysine, arginine, and ornithine are freely filtered and normally are almost completely reabsorbed in the proximal convoluted tubule by transport mechanisms that are saturable and energy dependent. The mechanisms for reabsorption of these amino acids display striking stereospecificity; that is, only cystine and the dibasic amino acids share the reabsorptive mechanism, and they compete with each other for reabsorption; other amino acids are not reabsorbed by this mechanism. In cystinuria, only the reabsorption of cystine and dibasic amino acids is affected; the reabsorption of all other amino acids proceeds normally.

In cystinuria the plasma concentration of cystine is normal or low and the GFR is usually well maintained. Thus the filtered load of cystine is either normal or low. The inability of the tubule to reabsorb a low or normal filtered load of cystine localizes the clinically important lesion in cystinuria to the kidney. Additional observations indicate that there is a defect in the brush border of kidney tubules and of intestinal mucosa that is reflected by partial or total inability to transport cystine and the dibasic amino acids actively. This transport system shared by cystine and the dibasic amino acids cannot be demonstrated in other tissues or in the basal lateral membrane of the renal tubule cells. The transport mechanism for cystine in the basal lateral renal cell membrane is independent of that for the transport of the dibasic amino acids and is not

$$CS\text{-}SC + PSH \longleftrightarrow CS\text{-}SP + CSH$$
$$PS\text{-}SP + CSH \longleftrightarrow CS\text{-}SP + PSH$$
$$CS\text{-}SC + PS\text{-}SP \longleftrightarrow 2\,CS\text{-}SP$$

Figure 51. Penicillamine therapy.

abnormal in cystinuria. Thus, renal tubule cells may accumulate cystine normally from the basal lateral surface, while reabsorption from the lumen is impaired by a defect in the brush border. The cystine accumulated within the renal tubule cell may leak or be transported into the tubular lumen. If the cystine that enters the lumen cannot be reabsorbed because of a defect in the brush border, apparent secretion of cystine will occur; that is, both the filtered cystine plus the cystine moving from cell to lumen will appear in the urine, producing cystine clearance in excess of the clearance of inulin. Studies in humans and dogs with cystinuria have in fact documented cystine secretion. The schema of this proposed pathophysiologic outline is presented in Figure 50.

Based on the pathophysiology of cystinuria one would reason that the disease should be treated by reducing cystine excretion. Dietary restriction of methionine reduces cystine production and therefore excretion, but only to a modest degree. There has until recently been no effective means of enhancing cystine reabsorption. Observations as to whether glutamine stimulates cystine reabsorption have been conflicting. Presently, cystine excretion is reduced by converting the cystine to a more soluble mixed disulfide by the use of D-penicillamine (Fig. 51) or mercaptopropionyl glycine.

The concentration of cystine in the urine is reduced by increasing fluid intake according to the principles already discussed, and the physical chemistry of the urine is modified to increase solubility primarily by raising the urine pH to 7.5 or greater if possible.

URIC ACID STONE DISEASE

Uric acid is the metabolic end-product of purine degradation. In most animals the enzyme uricase metabolizes uric acid to the more soluble allantoin. This enzyme has been lost with the evolutionary advance to the primates. Man and other primates must therefore excrete the relatively insoluble uric acid in the urine (see section on Disorders of Metabolism).

Uric acid is freely filtered through the glomerulus and is both reabsorbed and secreted by the proximal tubule. The quantity of uric acid excreted is usually far less than the filtered load, indicating net reabsorption. However, under specific experimental conditions secretion of uric acid can be demonstrated. Measurements of the differences in urinary excretion of uric acid before and after the inhibition of secretion by pyrazinamide were taken to be measurements of the quantitative component of secretion. If secretion all occurred distal to reabsorption, then the estimate would be valid. However, it now appears that the quantity of uric acid that the proximal tubule can secrete may exceed the filtered load. When secretion exceeds filtered load, net reabsorption can occur only if there is postsecretory reabsorption. A picture is now

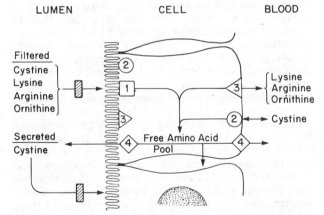

Figure 50. The renal tubular cell showing, at the luminal surface *(1)* a shared pathway for cystine and the dibasic amino acids (this pathway is defective in cystinuria); *(2)* a pathway for cystine transport independent of the shared pathway; and *(3)* a pathway for the dibasic amino acids lysine, arginine, and ornithine, independent of the shared pathway. Transport mechanisms similar and if not identical to 2 and 3 are present in the basolateral membrane as well. Uptake of cystine from the basolateral membrane with transfer into the lumen may result in secretion. *(4)*. (From Thier, S. O.: Dibasic amino acid transport: Lessons from human disease. Trans Am Clin Climatol Assoc 95:134, 1983.)

emerging of a proximal tubule with both secretion and reabsorption along its length. Clearly, reabsorption must still be quantitatively more important than secretion.

Uric acid stone formation occurs most commonly on the basis of anatomic defects or dehydration, and not as a function of altered excretion. A higher incidence of uric acid stone formation occurs when the urine is persistently acid. This circumstance occurs in that subpopulation of patients with gout who have normal 24-hour excretion rates for uric acid in the presence of elevated serum uric acid concentrations. A still higher incidence of uric acid stones will be seen in patients who excrete excess quantities of uric acid per 24 hours. Patients may either excrete uric acid at an increased rate while maintaining serum uric acid in the normal range, or they may overproduce uric acid to an extent that elevates the serum uric acid and the urinary uric acid excretion rate. The latter circumstance describes a smaller subpopulation of patients with gout who clearly overproduce uric acid and also describes a group of patients who have increased uric acid production, frequently as a result of myeloproliferative disorders.

The approach to the treatment of uric acid stone disease would be first to examine the patient for anatomic abnormalities of the urinary tract. A high fluid intake would be of benefit in all circumstances. Alkalinization of the urine could change the solubility of uric acid from 15 mg/dl at pH 5 to 200 mg/dl at pH 7. Finally, uric acid excretion could be reduced either by reducing the intake of purines, which is not very effective, or by interfering with the enzymatic production of uric acid through the use of allopurinol. Allopurinol is a competitive inhibitor of the enzyme xanthine oxidase. Xanthine oxidase catalyzes the conversion of hypoxanthine to xanthine, and xanthine to uric acid. Thus, allopurinol would directly reduce uric acid production. In addition, allopurinol is metabolized to oxypurinol, which is a more long-acting competitive inhibitor of xanthine oxidase. Allopurinol is also metabolized to a nucleotide, consuming 5-phosphoribosylpyrophosphate. The allopurinol nucleotide and the reduction of 5-phosphoribosylpyrophosphate levels could inhibit de novo purine synthesis and reduce uric acid production (Fig. 52). However, it is more likely that hypoxanthine that accumulates is recycled

via hypoxanthine-guanine phosphoribosyltransferase and reduces the need for de novo synthesis. In addition to its direct role in the formation of urinary tract calculi, uric acid may also play a role in the formation of calcium oxalate stones. This will be discussed further in the section on calcium stones.

CALCIUM STONE DISEASE

The majority of all urinary tract calculi are composed of calcium, and the majority of calcium stones are calcium oxalate. The pathophysiology of calcium stone formation under most circumstances is not known. There are risk factors that increase the likelihood of calcium stone disease. These include (1) a positive family history for nephrolithiasis, (2) a very low fluid intake, (3) ingestion of drugs such as acetazolamide, vitamins A or D, or ascorbic acid, (4) hyperoxaluria, (5) hyperuricosuria, and (6) hypercalciuria. There are also populations of calcium stone formers in whom the pathophysiology of calcium precipitation can be defined. By examining the mechanisms of stone formation in these patients we may develop insights that can be generalized to the remainder of patients.

HYPEROXALURIA

Oxalic acid is the final product in the metabolism of glyoxylic acid and ascorbic acid in man. Oxalate in combination with calcium forms a compound that is insoluble in aqueous solution. Hyperoxaluria, the excretion of greater than 40 to 60 mg of oxalate in the urine per 24 hours, may occur as the result of abnormal metabolism, increased intake of oxalate or its precursors, and increased intestinal absorption.

There are rare autosomal recessive traits that in the homozygous state produce diseases termed glycolic aciduria and L-glyceric aciduria. Under these circumstances marked increased production of oxalate leads to hyperoxaluria in an extremely virulent form of calcium oxalate stone formation (Fig. 53). Dietary intake of oxalate may be increased by ingesting large quantities of cocoa, tea, parsley, rhubarb, spinach, pepper, and nuts. The ingestion of large quantities of ascorbic acid, which is metabolized to oxalate, will also increase urinary oxalate excretion. Increased intestinal oxalate absorption is perhaps the most important source of hyperoxaluria in clinical practice. Normally, oxalate is absorbed from the large intestine by passive diffusion. The presence of calcium in the intestinal lumen leads to formation of the insoluble salt calcium oxalate, thereby reducing oxalate absorption and therefore its renal excretion. A number of gastrointestinal disorders characterized by some degree of malabsorption are associated with hyperoxaluria. In these disorders the degree of steatorrhea correlates well with the degree of oxalate hyperabsorption from the colon, and ultimate hyperoxaluria. There have been two explanations proffered for the hyperoxaluria seen with intestinal disorders. The first, the solubility theory, suggests that the unabsorbed fatty acids form complexes with calcium in the intestinal lumen. The calcium association with fatty acids permits formation of the more soluble sodium oxalate and free oxalate for passive absorption via the colon. The second, the permeability theory, holds that the delivery of in-

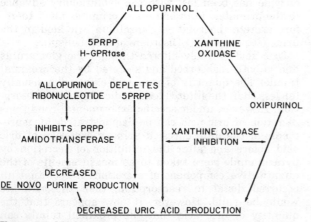

Figure 52. Mechanism of action of allopurinol. (From Thier, S. O.: The physiologic approach to hyperuricemia. Physiology in medicine. N Engl J Med 286:5, 1972.)

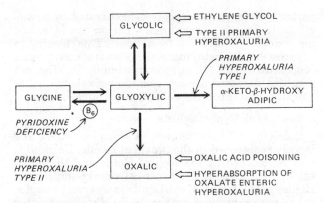

Figure 53. Disorders of oxalate metabolism in man. *Open arrows* indicate exogenous causes of hyperoxaluria. *Closed arrows* indicate the known acquired and hereditary enzyme defects of mechanisms leading to hyperoxaluria. (From Williams, H. E., and Smith, L. H., Jr.: Disorders of oxalate metabolism. Am J Med 145:729, 1968.)

creased quantities of fatty acids and bile salts to the colon injures the colonic mucosal barrier, increasing the permeability of the colon to oxalate. It is likely that components of both theories contribute to the increased absorption of oxalate. If the intake of oxalate is reduced or if the oxalate is complexed in insoluble form in the intestinal lumen, oxalate hyperabsorption will be reduced.

The treatment of hyperoxaluria, then, has focused on approaches to the metabolic pathways producing oxalate. The use of pyridoxine to shift glyoxylate metabolism away from oxalate may reduce oxalate excretion 50 per cent in some patients, and should be tried in all cases. None of the other approaches to altering the metabolism of oxalate production have been successful. Dietary oxalate intake should be reduced in states of hyperoxaluria. Finally, in states of intestinal dysfunction, oxalate may be bound in the intestine by the use of resins such as cholestyramine. Cholestyramine may also bind bile acids and fatty acids, freeing calcium to form insoluble salts with oxalate. Under carefully monitored circumstances it may also be possible to reduce oxalate absorption by administering calcium by mouth to precipitate the calcium oxalate within the lumen. Calcium should be used primarily in individuals who are not hypercalciuric.

HYPERURICOSURIA

A number of patients with calcium oxalate stone formation have been found to have hyperuricosuria with or without hyperuricemia. There have been two major explanations for the increased incidence of calcium oxalate stone formation in the presence of hyperuricosuria. The first is that a crystal of monosodium urate may act as a nidus for calcium stone formation. The second, more attractive, theory is that precipitated uric acid presents a crystalline structure similar enough in configuration to that of calcium oxalate to allow growth of calcium oxalate crystal on the uric acid crystalline foundation. This process is called epitaxial crystal growth. If, as has been noted in preliminary observations, in the majority of patients with hyperuricosuria and calcium oxalate stone formation the urine pH is in the 5.0 to 5.5 range (at which uric acid is the predominant form) then the theory of epitaxial crystal growth would offer the best explanation of the association of hyperuricosuria and calcium oxalate stone formation. Whatever the mechanism, reduction of uric acid excretion via the use of allopurinol would be effective.

HYPERCALCIURIA

Urinary calcium excretion is a function of the dietary intake and absorption of calcium, the equilibrium between bone and plasma, and the renal excretion of calcium. Increased calcium excretion then, could occur as a result of increased calcium absorption, increased net bone resorption, and decreased renal reabsorption of calcium. These potential mechanisms of hypercalciuria are summarized in Table 19.

Absorptive Hypercalciuria

In absorptive hypercalciuria the final common pathway leading to hypercalciuria is increased intestinal absorption of calcium. Several pathophysiologic sequences could explain this increased absorption. For example, a primary increase in intestinal transport could lead to an increased calcium pool, depressed parathyroid function, a normal or high serum phosphorus level, and normal or low concentrations of 1,25-dihydroxyvitamin D_3. Since the latter two chemistries are atypical, primary hyperabsorption seems highly unlikely. A renal phosphate leak would lead to an increase in 1,25-dihydroxyvitamin D_3 and increased

TABLE 19. PATHOPHYSIOLOGIC FEATURES OF FOUR CATEGORIES OF HYPERCALCIURIA

	CALCIUM ABSORPTION	BONE RESORPTION	EXTRACELLULAR CALCIUM	PT FUNCTION	CALCIUM EXCRETION FL	CALCIUM EXCRETION Reab	1,25 (OH)$_2$ D$_3$	SERUM P$_i$
Absorptive HC	↑ *	N, ↑	N, ↑	N, ↓	↑	↓	N, ↑	N, ↓
Renal HC	↑	N, ↑	N, ↓	↑	↓	↓	↑	N, ↓
Subtle 1° HPT	↑	↑	N, ↑	↑	↑	↑	↑	N, ↓
Resorptive HC	↓	↑	N, ↑	↓	↑	↓	↓	N, ↑

From Broadus, A. E.: In Felig, P., Baxter, J. D., Broadus, A. E., and Frohman, L. A. (eds.): Endocrinology and Metabolism. New York, McGraw-Hill Book Co., 1981, p. 1150.

*Features in rectangles in each category denote the known or postulated primary defect.

HC = hypercalciuria; 1° HPT = primary hyperparathyroidism, parathyroid; FL = filtered load; Reab = tubular calcium reabsorption; Pi = inorganic phosphorus.

calcium absorption and depressed parathyroid activity. This sequence of events probably occurs in a subset of patients with absorptive hypercalciuria. The majority of patients, however, do not have a reduced T_m phosphate or serum phosphate, but almost all have an elevated concentration of 1,25-dihydroxyvitamin D_3. Therefore, increased production of 1,25-dihydroxyvitamin D_3, which has, in fact, been demonstrated, would explain increased calcium absorption and decreased parathyroid activity, but would not account for the reduced serum phosphate concentration seen in perhaps one-third of patients. The conclusion at present must be that there are subpopulations of patients with absorptive hypercalciuria and that no single defect can yet account for the entire group. Reduced parathyroid activity is a uniform consequence of increased calcium absorption. The result of parathyroid suppression is decreased tubular reabsorption of calcium resulting in increased fractional excretion, even in the fasting state.

The picture of absorptive hypercalciuria is associated with the idiopathic form of the disease, vitamin D intoxication, and sarcoidosis (which probably represents increased sensitivity to vitamin D).

Hyperparathyroidism

Primary hyperparathyroidism may be thought of as the prototype disorder of resorptive hypercalciuria. Excessive parathyroid hormone stimulates the release of calcium from bone and inhibits resorption of phosphate in the proximal renal tubule. The combination of increased parathyroid hormone and reduced phosphate stimulates the production of 1,25-dihydroxyvitamin D_3 by the kidney. The increased dihydroxyvitamin D_3 concentration leads to an increase in intestinal calcium absorption. The increased calcium absorption and increased mobilization of calcium from the bone elevates the serum calcium concentration and increases filtered calcium. Parathyroid hormone stimulates the reabsorption of calcium in the distal nephron. However, the balance between increased filtration and increased reabsorption would be presumed to favor increased excretion of calcium in the urine. Patients with hyperparathyroidism need not have strikingly elevated serum calcium levels. In fact, many patients will have only high-normal levels on most determinations. In these individuals it is likely that the serum levels of ionized calcium are persistently elevated, and when they are challenged with an increased calcium intake they almost invariably demonstrate increases in serum calcium levels to above the normal range.

There is reason to believe that patients with subtle hyperparathyroidism who form stones more commonly have an absorptive form of hypercalciuria. Virtually all such patients have elevated plasma concentrations of 1,25-dihydroxyvitamin D_3 and increased intestinal absorption of calcium. The degree of hypercalciuria correlates better with the concentration of 1,25-dihydroxyvitamin D_3 than with parathyroid activity. Although primary hyperparathyroidism may produce resorptive hypercalciuria, it is more clearly seen in association with (1) malignant disease either as the result of direct bony invasion or as the result of humoral hypercalcemia (for example, prostaglandins), (2) hyperthyroidism, and (3) renal tubular acidosis. The clearest case of resorptive hypercalciuria and its

pathophysiology, however, is demonstrated by immobilization. When immobilized, a person has increased net release of calcium from bone. This results in suppression of parathyroid activity and reduced plasma concentration of 1,25-dihydroxyvitamin D_3. The net result is increased urinary excretion of calcium, without increased intestinal calcium absorption.

Renal Leak Hypercalciuria

Calcium is freely filtered at the glomerulus and largely reabsorbed in the proximal tubule. Calcium is also reabsorbed in the loop of Henle and the distal tubule. Throughout the proximal tubule and loop of Henle, reabsorption of calcium is inseparably coupled to the reabsorption of sodium. In the distal convoluted tubule the reabsorption of calcium is stimulated by parathyroid hormone, and that stimulated reabsorption may be independent of sodium reabsorption. In renal leak hypercalciuria a defect in calcium reabsorption at an as yet undefined site in the tubule leads to calcium loss in the urine. The persistent loss of calcium lowers the total body pool of calcium and at least transiently lowers serum calcium. The fall in serum calcium stimulates the secretion of parathyroid hormone, which increases bone calcium mobilization and stimulates reabsorption of calcium in the distal nephron. It also leads to increased urinary excretion of phosphate. The combination of parathyroid hormone excess and phosphate loss stimulates production of 1,25-dihydroxyvitamin D_3, which in turn stimulates intestinal calcium absorption. Thus far, all patients with renal calcium leak hypercalciuria fall into the category of having an idiopathic illness.

At least three major pathophysiologic categories for the development of idiopathic hypercalciuria have been described above. If one considers primary hyperparathyroidism separately, there are four categories (Table 19). Though the sequence of events for each of the categories is clear in a theoretic sense, clinically it may be difficult to define which mechanism is operating in a given patient. The problem arises from two important observations. First, by the time the patient is seen with any of these mechanisms, except true resorptive hypercalciuria, there will be increased absorption of calcium from the intestine. Second, the variations in parathyroid hormone function that may contribute to distinguishing among the three categories are difficult to measure. Immunoassays for plasma parathyroid hormone measure a family of molecular species representing both active and inactive hormone. In fact, most of the antigen measured seems to be the inactive C-terminal peptide, which has a comparatively long half-life. Thus it is difficult to perform physiologic manipulations of parathyroid hormone and to measure the results. The measurement of nephrogenous cyclic $3',5'$-adenosine monophosphate (cAMP) has proved to be a sensitive and rapidly responsive means of determining the action of parathyroid hormone on the kidney. Normally, filtered cyclic AMP is completely excreted in the urine. Cyclic AMP appearing in the urine at levels above the filtered load represents nephrogenous cyclic AMP. Nephrogenous cyclic AMP is produced rapidly and in large quantities in response to parathyroid hormone. Thus it is possible to measure nephrogenous cyclic AMP as a rapid sensitive indicator of parathyroid function.

The separation of patients with hypercalciuria into those with absorptive versus those with renal leak versus those with resorptive versus those with hypercalciuria associated with hyperparathyroidism can now be accomplished using our understanding of the pathophysiology of each. If patients are given a large calcium challenge by mouth, all groups except the patients with resorptive hypercalciuria will evidence increased absorption of calcium. This last group of patients also has low concentrations of parathyroid hormone and of 1,25-dihydroxyvitamin D_3. They are easily separated from patients with increased calcium absorption. With the increased absorption of calcium, the serum calcium will rise from the normal to the high-normal range in patients with absorptive hypercalciuria. In patients with renal leak hypercalciuria who tend to have low-normal serum calcium concentrations, the calcium will rise only modestly and still remain in the low-normal range. This failure of the calcium level to rise is a function of the persistent renal leak. In patients with primary hyperparathyroidism the serum calcium will rise from the normal range to above normal in almost

all circumstances. With the rise in serum calcium to the high-normal range, patients with absorptive hypercalciuria will evidence suppression of 50 per cent or more of their originally normal levels of nephrogenous cyclic AMP. Patients with renal leak hypercalciuria will have elevated levels of nephrogenous cyclic AMP, because the parathyroid glands are persistently stimulated by the fall in serum calcium that accompanies the renal calcium leak. With an oral calcium challenge, serum calcium levels in patients with renal hypercalciuria do not rise adequately to suppress nephrogenous cyclic AMP. It is likely, though not proved, that if the serum calcium levels are raised to high-normal or above, these patients would evidence suppression of nephrogenous cyclic AMP. In patients with primary hyperparathyroidism, the elevated levels of nephrogenous cyclic AMP remain elevated even after a rise in the serum calcium to above the normal level. Thus, by documenting that individuals with hypercalciuria have increased absorption of an oral calcium load and then observing the changes in serum calcium concentrations and nephrogenous cyclic AMP

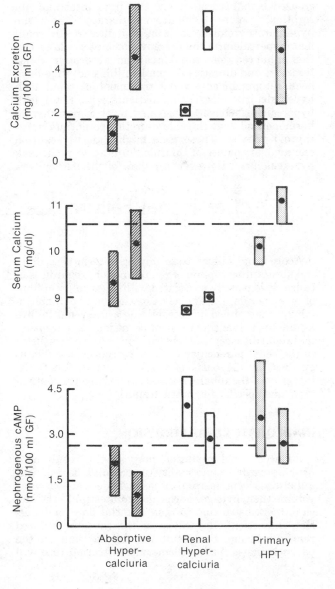

Figure 54. Results of oral calcium tolerance test in 25 patients with absorptive hypercalciuria *(crosshatched bars),* two patients with renal hypercalciuria *(open bars)* and 10 patients with subtle primary hyperparathyroidism *(strippled bars).* For each patient subgroup, the bar to the left corresponds to the control period, and the bar to the right to the experimental period after oral administration of calcium. The *solid dots* represent mean values, and the *vertical height of the bars* the range of values. The *dashed lines* denote the upper limit of normal ±2 S.D. at baseline conditions. The patients were referred for treatment from a biased population, and the size of each group may not represent the incidence of these disorders in patients with hypercalciuria. (From Broadus, A. E., and Thier, S. O.: Metabolic basis of renal stone disease. N Engl J Med 300:844, 1979.)

excretion, it is possible to distinguish between the forms of hypercalciuria associated with increased calcium absorption. These findings are summarized in Figure 54.

The implications of distinguishing among the various pathophysiologic mechanisms for hypercalciuria become evident in planning therapy. If a patient has absorptive hypercalciuria, he or she may be treated by reducing dietary calcium or by binding calcium in the intestine. These patients may also be treated with thiazide diuretics, which stimulate distal calcium reabsorption and, by producing extracellular fluid volume contraction, will enhance the reabsorption of sodium and calcium in the proximal tubule. Thiazide diuretics potentiate the action of parathyroid hormone, but that should not be an issue in the treatment of absorptive hypercalciuria. In patients with hypercalciuria as the result of primary hyperparathyroidism, thiazide diuretics may be potentially dangerous. With hyperparathyroidism, however, restriction of dietary calcium and the binding of calcium in the gut may reduce hypercalciuria. However, in cases in which a significant degree of the hypercalciuria results from increased bone resorption and not from intestinal absorption, more definitive therapy of the hyperparathyroidism is usually indicated. In renal leak hypercalciuria the therapy of choice would be one that enhanced renal tubular calcium absorption. Since thiazides and diuretics accomplish this end, they have been recommended for the treatment of renal leak hypercalciuria. Recall that patients with renal leak hypercalciuria have an elevated level of parathyroid hormone and that thiazide diuretics potentiate parathyroid activity. These facts might initially caution one against the use of thiazide diuretics in renal leak hypercalciuria. However, a review of the pathophysiology of renal leak hypercalciuria indicates that increased parathyroid activity results from a lowered serum calcium level. As the serum calcium level rises with increased calcium retention, parathyroid hormone activity may be suppressed. The treatment for resorptive hypercalciuria is treatment of the underlying disease and, when appropriate, mobilization of the patient.

In addition to attending to abnormalities in oxalate metabolism, uric acid metabolism, and calcium metabolism, the physician treating calcium stone disease must also encourage increased fluid intake and should consider modifying the physical chemistry of the urine to prevent calcium crystallization. Both pyrophosphate and magnesium have been shown to be inhibitors of calcium-containing crystal formation in the urine. They are used on the basis of these observations, but their clinical efficacy is not firmly established. Alteration of the urine pH has been suggested to prevent calcium stone formation. While it is true that acidification of the urine inhibits the crystallization of calcium phosphate, it is also true that at urine pH between 4.5 and 8.0, calcium oxalate solubility is hardly altered. In fact, acidification of the urine, which usually is accomplished at the expense of some degree of systemic acidification, results in increased urinary calcium and decreased urinary citrate excretion. These latter events may enhance crystal formation. Before using acidification of the urine for the treatment of calcium phosphate stones, one should note that a large number of pure calcium phosphate stones occur in patients with renal tubular acidosis, who would be harmed by acidification, and in patients with primary hyperparathyroidism, in whom more definitive therapy is indicated.

Acute Renal Failure

Acute renal failure is an imprecise term describing the abrupt interruption of renal function, regardless of cause. It is usually associated with oliguria (< 400 ml of urine per day) or anuria. A discussion of pathophysiology is simplified by categorizing acute renal failure as due to (1) inadequate renal perfusion, (2) parenchymal renal disease, or (3) obstruction to urine flow distal to the renal parenchyma. These categories are distinguished on the basis of clinical setting, functional integrity of the tubule, response to therapeutic maneuvers, and specific diagnostic tests.

INADEQUATE RENAL PERFUSION

Reduced renal perfusion may be the result of a primary cardiac abnormality (myocardial disease, valvular disease, pericardial disease), inadequate vascular volume (hemorrhage, burns, gastrointestinal loss, and so on), or obstruction to renal arterial flow (embolus, clot, dissection). Regardless of the cause of reduced renal perfusion, the result will be the same if the parenchyma is intact. Glomerular filtration rate will fall, but less than total renal plasma flow. The resulting increased filtration fraction will produce a relative increase in intratubular hydrostatic pressure, a decrease in postglomerular hydrostatic pressure, and an increase in postglomerular oncotic pressure; all three changes favor proximal tubule sodium reabsorption. The increased proximal sodium and water reabsorption will elevate the intraluminal urea concentration and slow the flow of urine along the tubule; both changes favor urea reabsorption but have no effect on creatinine reabsorption. The reduced renal perfusion will stimulate renin release and thereby aldosterone secretion, leading to enhanced distal tubule sodium reabsorption. Finally a reduced urine flow rate will favor water reabsorption in the collecting duct, even in the absence of antidiuretic hormone. If intravascular volume is sufficiently contracted or cardiac output sufficiently reduced, nonosmotic stimulation of antidiuretic hormone release will cause still greater distal water reabsorption. It is also possible that redistribution of blood flow from the outer to inner cortex will facilitate salt and water retention.

Decreased renal perfusion will therefore result in

reduced urine volume and a urine sodium concentration that is usually less than 10 mEq/l. The urine will be more concentrated than plasma. The blood urea nitrogen will rise at a proportionally greater rate than the serum creatinine. Urinalysis will reveal no significant proteinuria, and the urine sediment will not be unusual. If renal perfusion falls sufficiently so that increased proximal reabsorption limits the delivery of sodium chloride to the ascending limb of Henle's loop, concentrating ability will be impaired and isosthenuria will result.

During hypoperfusion the kidney responds as though there were an inadequate vascular volume, and it functions to expand extracellular fluid volume. The treatment of acute renal failure secondary to hypoperfusion requires that the specific cause be sought and corrected With return of adequate perfusion the physiologic events described above are reversed; urine volume will rise, urine will become less concentrated and contain greater concentrations of sodium, and the blood urea nitrogen and serum creatinine will decrease.

PARENCHYMAL DAMAGE

Acute renal failure may result from glomerular injury (see Glomerulonephritis), tubulo-interstitial injury (see Tubulo-Interstitial Diseases), or a combination of the two. We will limit the discussion of acute parenchymal renal failure to a consideration of the syndrome termed acute tubular necrosis.

Acute tubular necrosis most commonly results from ischemic injury or exposure to nephrotoxins. In either case, anatomic injury and dysfunction may appear along the entire tubule. With ischemic injury the tubular basement membrane is frequently fragmented, particularly in the S_3 segment.

Oliguria is usually present despite renal blood flow that may be one-third or more of normal. Though urine output is reduced, the urine is not concentrated and contains sodium at concentrations significantly above those seen with hypoperfusion. The blood urea nitrogen and serum creatinine rise in parallel. Urinalysis may reveal mild to moderate proteinuria, renal tubular cells, granular casts, and, with ischemic injury, even red cells or rarely red cell casts.

Although the mechanism is not known by which oliguria develops in the presence of rates of renal blood flow adequate to maintain good urine output in chronic renal failure, several possibilities have been suggested. The suggestions can be divided into those that hold that there is primarily an abnormality of glomerular filtration and those that suggest primary tubular dysfunction (Fig. 55).

A primary reduction in afferent arteriolar flow or glomerular permeability would account for a reduced glomerular filtration rate. Though changes in glomerular ultrastructure and function have been demonstrated in some experimental models, they are not uniform findings in acute tubular necrosis. Glomerular filtration rate would be reduced if renal blood flow were redistributed away from the outer cortex, which contains the majority of glomeruli, to the inner cortex and medulla. At least some radionuclide blood flow studies are consistent with this possibility. Though redistribution of blood flow could account for a reduced glomerular filtration rate with well-maintained renal blood flow, the mechanisms by which the redistribution is initiated and is reversed with recovery from acute tubular necrosis are not known.

Oliguria, initiated by primarily tubular events, may occur as the result of local production of renin and angiotensin, release of adenosine, obstruction to urine flow, and back leak of filtrate.

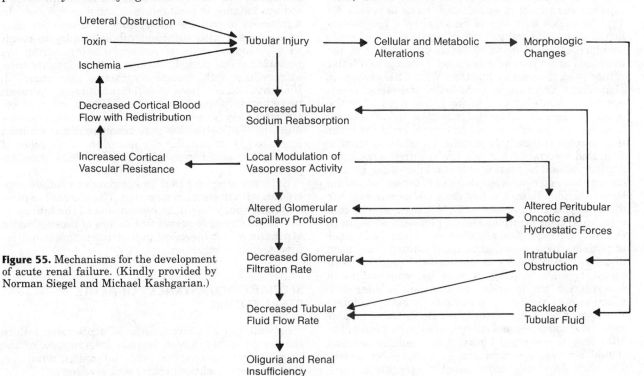

Figure 55. Mechanisms for the development of acute renal failure. (Kindly provided by Norman Siegel and Michael Kashgarian.)

A primary abnormality of tubular function results in the delivery of increased quantities of sodium chloride to the macula densa, and, if the macula densa function is intact, renin will be released. Individual nephrons contain sufficient substrate, renin, and converting enzyme to produce enough angiotensin II locally to reduce their own glomerular filtration rate. For this mechanism to apply requires that the cells of the macula densa remain functional while other tubular cells are injured. Adenosine has also been implicated as a mediator of reduced glomerular filtration. Experimental evidence suggests, however, that adenosine could account for a fall of no more than 50 per cent in glomerular filtration rate.

Since acute tubular necrosis is almost always associated with the deposition of cellular debris in the renal tubules, tubular obstruction has been postulated to occur and to reduce urine output. Local production of angiotensin has again been invoked to account for the reduced glomerular perfusion.

It is also possible for ultrafiltrate to form at rates adequate to produce urine volumes in excess of 400 ml/day but for leakage of the filtrate out of the tubule to result in oliguria. Consistent with this postulate is the finding of tubular injury on microscopic examination, and the evidence that the tubule has increased permeability to inulin in acute tubular necrosis.

An additional postulate is that in acute renal failure the metabolism of the renal cell is impaired (perhaps by increased influx of calcium) and recovery will not occur until its metabolic processes can regenerate the intracellular nucleotide pool.

Clearly, no single mechanism fully explains acute tubular necrosis. Perhaps we simply have not discovered the correct explanation, or perhaps the correct explanation involves a series of events that includes several of those described above. In any event, acute tubular necrosis, once established, tends to persist for days to weeks. Recovery is heralded by a progressive increase in urine volume: the diuretic phase of acute tubular necrosis. During the early diuretic phase, the increased urine volume may reflect a change in tubular rather than glomerular function. With little change in glomerular filtration rate, the BUN and serum creatinine may continue to rise for a few days after the onset of diuresis. With the increased urine volume, however, the loss of sodium and potassium in the urine may become clinically important. Careful attention to fluid and electrolyte balance are required during the diuretic phase to prevent extracellular fluid volume contraction and dangerous changes in serum potassium concentration. Within a few days of the onset of the diuretic phase the blood urea nitrogen and serum creatinine concentrations should plateau and begin to fall as the glomerular filtration rate rises. A number of patients have nonoliguric renal failure. This form of acute renal failure is particularly common with aminoglycoside toxicity. It may be more subtle in presentation but is easier to manage. Tubular dysfunction may persist for prolonged periods. Complete recovery of renal function is the rule in acute tubular necrosis, though some dysfunction may be permanent after very severe renal injury. Acute tubular necrosis should always be approached as a reversible lesion. The mortality with acute tubular necrosis is more closely related to the cause of the renal failure than to the renal failure per se. Thus the mortality with acute tubular necrosis occurring in an otherwise healthy pregnant woman who suffers an episode of hypotension is minimal, whereas the majority of patients who develop acute tubular necrosis after rupture of an aortic aneurysm may die.

OBSTRUCTION TO URINE FLOW

Obstruction to the flow of urine at any point from the late collecting duct to the urethra may produce oliguria or anuria. A pattern of periods of anuria alternating with bursts of diuresis is said to be characteristic of obstruction.

With the acute onset of obstruction, the kidney responds as to a fall in arterial perfusion. Glomerular filtration rate falls, sodium is reabsorbed avidly, and the urine becomes concentrated. With time or with the more gradual onset of obstruction, tubular function becomes impaired, urine sodium concentration rises, and isosthenuria develops. The urinalysis reveals minimal proteinuria. The urine sediment may not be unusual or may reveal evidence of the cause of obstruction: white blood cells and tissue with papillary necrosis, red blood cells and crystals with urinary calculi, and so on. Acute renal failure secondary to obstruction is usually reversible with prompt relief of the obstruction. In the absence of infection, complete recovery is possible, even after complete obstruction for four to seven days.

With relief of obstruction postobstructive diuresis may occur. The postobstructive diuresis has three possible components: (1) There is the diuresis of sodium. In most patients the onset of obstruction is associated with sodium retention. Relief of obstruction is then associated with excretion of the retained sodium. When sodium balance is reestablished, the diuresis ends. In a minority of patients the episode of obstruction may be associated with sufficient tubular injury to result in a prolonged state of sodium wasting during the postobstructive period. In this latter circumstance, extracellular fluid volume contraction may occur. (2) If obstruction has been of sufficient duration to result in retention of large quantities of urea, relief of obstruction may be associated with urea-induced osmotic diuresis. (3) Obstruction may result in distal nephron insensitivity to antidiuretic hormone. With relief of obstruction nephrogenic diabetes insipidus may appear.

Evidence suggests that prostaglandin synthesis increases with ureteral obstruction. The increase in prostaglandins may facilitate reperfusion of the kidney in the postobstructive period. Inhibitors of prostaglandin synthesis might therefore impair renal functional recovery after obstruction.

SPECIAL CIRCUMSTANCES OF ACUTE RENAL FAILURE

Several special circumstances of acute renal failure require comment. These include interruption of the urinary drainage system, renal infarction, renal cortical necrosis, and the hepatorenal syndrome.

The drainage of urine may be diverted as the result

of trauma or, more rarely, as a complication of surgery. The urine may then drain into tissue, from which it is reabsorbed. Though the kidneys function normally, the urine is, in effect, recycled, resulting in azotemia, acidemia, and hyperkalemia. Since the urine does not drain to the outside of the body, anuria or oliguria is observed. As renal function is intact, recognition of the anatomic lesion and reestablishment of adequate drainage completely reverse the "renal failure."

Renal cortical necrosis may occur in a variety of circumstances, most of which are characterized by disseminated intravascular coagulation. Cortical necrosis is more likely to produce complete anuria than is the syndrome of acute tubular necrosis. In addition, cortical necrosis is much more likely to result in some degree of permanent renal insufficiency.

Renal infarction may occur with acute interruption of arterial perfusion of the kidney or with acute complete renal venous thrombosis. Complete renal infarction is associated with anuria. The development of acute anuria following an event capable of occluding renal arterial blood supply, such as an embolus to the renal artery or trauma producing clot in the renal artery, should not be taken to indicate irreversible renal damage. Recovery of sufficient renal function to sustain life has been reported after renal arterial occlusion of several days' duration. It is likely in those individuals who recovered renal function that the kidneys were protected by collateral circulation through capsular blood vessels. Capsular vessels may provide adequate blood flow to ensure some viability of tissue but inadequate blood flow to maintain urine output.

Hepatorenal syndrome is a term applied to the development of progressive oliguria and azotemia in patients with severe hepatic dysfunction. These patients are usually severely jaundiced and have ascites. They are not hypotensive and have no other evident cause for renal failure. The impairment of renal function is not explicable on the basis of an anatomic lesion. Rather, tubular function is maintained until the latest stages of the syndrome. The oliguria results from a reduced glomerular filtration rate, which may be associated with redistribution of renal blood flow. Sodium is avidly reabsorbed from the filtrate, and the urine is concentrated. The blood urea nitrogen rises out of proportion to the serum creatinine, and the findings of urinalysis are not unusual. Late in the syndrome, with severe reduction in renal perfusion, concentrating ability may be lost. The renal damage is reversible, as is evident from the rare observations of spontaneous recovery, the reports of recovery after portal systemic shunts, and the striking observation that the kidney from a patient dying with hepatorenal syndrome will function normally when transplanted into a recipient with uncomplicated chronic renal failure. There is no adequate explanation for the development of the hepatorenal syndrome, though humoral, neural, and circulatory mechanisms have all been invoked.

APPROACH TO THE PATIENT WITH ACUTE RENAL FAILURE

Evaluation of acute renal failure begins with a careful assessment of the clinical setting. A history of trauma, hypotension, exposure to toxins, urinary tract calculi, and so on is critical. Evidence of hypotension, reduced skin turgor, congestive heart failure, atrial fibrillation, and so on must be sought on physical examination.

While accumulating the data from a careful history and physical examination, the physician should establish an adequate vascular volume, blood pressure, and cardiac output. With adequate cardiac output, persistent oliguria usually indicates parenchymal damage or obstruction. Obviously, lesions of the aorta or renal arteries could still account for renal hypoperfusion, but, in the absence of history or physical findings suggestive of these possibilities, they need not be pursued at this point.

Obstruction to urine flow producing acute renal failure in a patient with two kidneys is usually at the level of the bladder outlet. Rectal examination for prostatic enlargement in men and pelvic examination for mass lesions in women should precede straight catheterization of the bladder. If there is no obstruction at the level of the bladder outlet, oliguria or anuria could occur only if both kidneys were simultaneously obstructed or if there were only a single functioning kidney that was obstructed. If there are two normal-sized kidneys, it is necessary to prove only that one is unobstructed but not functioning to confirm parenchymal disease.

After establishing adequate cardiac output and ruling out bladder outlet obstruction, the physician should examine the urine before performing any further diagnostic or therapeutic maneuvers (Table 20). Note that many maneuvers, such as the administration of diuretics or mannitol, will modify the urine composition and impair its diagnostic value. If the urine has a sodium concentration less than 10 mEq/l and an osmolality significantly above that of plasma, and if the urine sediment is not unusual, it is likely that the kidneys are still being inadequately perfused. If the same urine findings are present with a urine sediment demonstrating many crystals and perhaps red cells and white cells, obstruction above the level of the bladder should be suspected. If the urine electrolyte findings are again the same but the urine now shows excessive protein, red cells, and red cell casts, it is likely that the patient has early acute glomerulonephritis. If there is isosthenuria and the urine contains increased quantities of sodium (more than 20 mEq/l), it is likely that parenchymal renal injury is present. With isosthenuria and increased urinary sodium concentration, the presence of renal tubular cells, red cells, and white cells is consistent with acute tubular necrosis. The additional presence of occasional red cell casts may be consistent with an ischemic origin of acute tubular necrosis or with a later stage of acute glomerulonephritis. It may be necessary to perform a renal biopsy to distinguish between the last two possibilities.

This brief discussion of the evaluation of acute renal failure presents only the characteristic findings of each of the categories. There is, in fact, enormous variation, particularly in urine volume and composition, within each of the categories. Therefore the physician should constantly reassess the patient's status and use the natural history of the renal failure to support initial diagnostic impressions. Thus the patient with acute

TABLE 20. URINE FINDINGS IN PRERENAL AZOTEMIA AND ACUTE RENAL FAILURE

LABORATORY TEST	PRERENAL AZOTEMIA	ACUTE RENAL FAILURE
Urine sodium concentration (mEq/l)	<10	>20
Urine to plasma creatinine ratio	>14 to 1	<14 to 1
Urine to plasma urea ratio	>14 to 1	<14 to 1
Urine osmolality	>100 mOsm above plasma osmolality	Equal to or less than plasma osmolality
Urinary sediment	Normal	Casts, cellular debris

From Schrier, R. W., and Conger, J. D.: Acute renal failure: Pathogenesis, diagnosis, and management. In Schrier, R. W. (ed.): Renal and Electrolyte Disorders. Boston, Little, Brown and Co., 1976, p. 308.

renal failure on the basis of hypoperfusion should have a prompt increase in urine volume with reduction in blood urea nitrogen and serum creatinine concentrations following improved perfusion. The patient with obstruction should have a prompt increase in urine volume with relief of obstruction, and the increased urine volume should be associated with a prompt reduction in blood urea nitrogen and creatinine. On the other hand, the patient with acute tubular necrosis will more typically have an increase in urine volume with the onset of the diuretic phase but will have a continuing increase or plateauing of the blood urea nitrogen and creatinine. The blood urea nitrogen and creatinine levels begin to fall only after several days of diuresis.

MANAGEMENT OF ACUTE RENAL FAILURE

A discussion of the management of acute renal failure is beyond the scope of this text. The establishment of adequate renal perfusion and the relief of obstruction are obviously essential. This brief discussion will focus on the management of the syndrome of acute tubular necrosis. The principles involved are simple and require that the physician provide for the loss of the key renal functions.

As the kidney can no longer excrete nitrogenous waste products, treatment is directed at reducing the production of these substances. Protein intake is limited both absolutely and to foods containing high proportions of essential amino acids. Caloric intake is maintained as high as possible to prevent endogenous protein breakdown. The increased catabolism of febrile states may be treated by controlling sepsis and lowering temperature as necessary. Antianabolic drugs such as tetracycline and catabolic drugs such as glucocorticoids are avoided.

Sodium balance is maintained by restricting sodium intake to provide only enough sodium to replace that lost in urine and through drainage sites.

Water intake should be adequate to replace measured water loss plus insensible loss. Insensible loss is usually 300 to 400 ml/day but may be higher in a febrile patient and lower in a patient using a respirator. In patients in whom sodium loss is minimal, the adequacy of water replacement can be assessed by following the serum sodium concentration. If the serum sodium concentration rises above normal, water replacement is inadequate. If it falls to hyponatremic levels, water replacement is excessive.

Acid-base abnormalities may occur during acute renal failure, with metabolic acidemia the most common abnormality. The degree of acidemia frequently requires no treatment. If treatment is required, sodium bicarbonate may be given as tolerated by the patient's volume status. If acidemia becomes severe and sodium bicarbonate cannot be administered because of hypervolemia, dialysis is required.

Hyperkalemia is an extremely dangerous complication of acute renal failure. All potassium intake should be avoided and, if necessary, potassium may be removed from the body by the use of exchange resins, dialysis, or both.

Abnormalities of calcium, phosphorus, and magnesium metabolism are usually not problems during acute renal failure. However, hypermagnesemia may develop if patients are given magnesium-containing antacids.

Since the kidney plays a major role in determining the pharmacokinetics of many drugs, it is essential to review all medications that the patient is receiving and to modify the drug dose or form appropriately.

In a patient who is awake and has no abnormality of the urinary drainage system, it is unnecessary and unwise to maintain continuous bladder drainage once it is established that oliguria exists. It is far better to allow the patient to void spontaneously even if only every two or three days and to perform straight catheterization intermittently to be assured that no significant residual urine volume has accumulated.

Finally, even with the most careful attention to all of the principles of therapy, renal failure may persist sufficiently long to produce uremia. Development of the uremic state should be anticipated, and dialysis should be used before clinical symptoms develop.

The same principles that apply to the oliguric state in acute renal failure may be applied to the diuretic phase. The major differences during the diuretic phase are that there is sodium wasting rather than sodium retention, that potassium wasting may occur, and that the patient will now tolerate greater volumes of administered fluid, facilitating management of the electrolyte status. In addition, doses of medications that were effective during the oliguric phase may have to be increased during the diuretic phase.

Chronic Renal Failure

Chronic renal failure is the result of prolonged reduction of renal function regardless of cause. As renal function decreases, clinical disease develops from retention of substances normally excreted by the kidneys, loss of substances normally retained by the kidneys, and the compensatory responses to lost function. The clinical picture of renal failure is termed uremia and can be re-created by examining the effects of the loss of each of the key renal functions individually and as they affect each of the major organ systems.

EXCRETION OF WASTE PRODUCTS

The excretion of nitrogenous waste products occurs primarily by glomerular filtration. Urea and creatinine are most commonly measured as indices of nitrogenous waste product retention. Recall that urea is freely filtered and reabsorbed primarily by passive diffusion, a process that depends on the urine flow rate. The slower the urine flow rate, the greater the reabsorption of urea. Therefore, with renal hypoperfusion or obstruction to urine flow, the blood urea nitrogen concentration will rise proportionally more rapidly than the glomerular filtration rate falls. The blood urea nitrogen is also affected by nonrenal factors; for example, dietary protein, blood in the gastrointestinal tract, and increased tissue breakdown will all elevate the blood urea nitrogen. Similarly, catabolic drugs (glucocorticoids) and antianabolic drugs (tetracycline) will raise the blood urea nitrogen level. Extrarenal factors may produce an increase in blood urea nitrogen that does not represent a fall in glomerular filtration rate. Creatinine clearance is a more reliable means of assessing glomerular filtration rate. The creatinine produced and excreted each day is a function of muscle mass. If muscle mass is stable, creatinine excretion will be constant under steady-state conditions. If creatinine excretion is to remain constant as glomerular filtration rate falls, the serum creatinine concentration must rise proportionally to the fall in glomerular filtration rate; that is, the product of glomerular filtration rate times serum creatinine is constant, and a plot of glomerular filtration rate versus serum creatinine is a hyperbola (Fig. 56). At very high serum concentrations there may be some secretion of creatinine. Thus, at very high serum creatinine concentrations, measurements of glomerular filtration rate may be falsely elevated, though the absolute value of the glomerular filtration rate will be very low.

In practice, both the blood urea nitrogen and the serum creatinine concentrations are measured simultaneously. If the normal blood urea nitrogen:creatinine ratio of approximately 10:1 to 12:1 is markedly altered, extrarenal factors affecting urea production and excretion are suggested. A disproportionate rise in blood urea nitrogen versus creatinine may be the earliest clue to gastrointestinal bleeding, hypovolemia, and so on (Table 21).

Retention of nitrogenous waste products is associated with headache, nausea, vomiting, uremic frost (the precipitation of urea crystals on the skin as sweat evaporates), impaired platelet function, depressed red blood cell production and survival, serositis, neuropathy, and abnormal endocrine function. Though high concentrations of urea per se may produce clinical symptoms, an elevated blood urea nitrogen value is more likely a correlate of the retention of numerous toxic substances. Intermediate-sized peptides in the range of molecular weight 500 to 5000, termed middle molecules, have been assigned an important role in uremic toxicity, as have substances such as guanidinosuccinic acid. No best candidate for the uremic toxin has yet emerged, and it is likely that several substances contribute to the clinical picture. It is also likely that compensatory responses to reduced renal function such as the production of supraphysiologic concentrations of hormones contribute to "uremic" symptoms.

Nitrogenous metabolic products may also bind to proteins, displacing drugs. The result is an increased

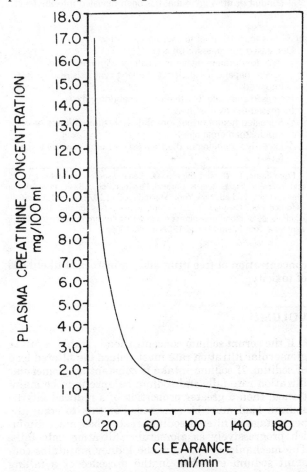

Figure 56. Relationship between serum creatinine and creatinine clearance. (From Alfrey, A. C.: Chronic renal failure: Manifestations and pathogenesis. In Schrier, R. W. (ed.): Renal and Electrolyte Disorders. Boston, Little, Brown and Co., 1976, p. 326. Originally from Doolan, P. D., Alpen, E. L., and Theil, G. B.: A clinical appraisal of the plasma concentration and endogenous clearance of creatinine. Am J Med 32:65, 1962.)

TABLE 21. ASSESSING THE BUN:CREATININE RATIO

Normal: 10:1

BUN more than 10 times serum creatinine
  Increased substrate: increased protein delivery for breakdown to urea nitrogen
    Excess protein ingestion when renal function depressed
    Presence of blood in the intestine when renal function depressed
    Excessive tissue catabolism
      Burns
      High fever
      Corticosteroids
      Rapid wasting states
    Antianabolic agents: tetracyclines
  Increased renal reabsorption of urea nitrogen
    Prerenal causes of underperfusion
      Dehydration
      Congestive heart failure
      Bilateral renal ischemia
      Hepatorenal syndrome if the liver has adequate function to form urea
    Glomerulonephritides
    Obstruction
    Bypass procedures in which urea is reabsorbed by an ileal conduit or from urine that has been deviated into the fecal stream

BUN less than 10 times the serum creatinine
  Decreased substrate for urea
    Very low protein intake in a patient with renal disease
    Severe hepatic insufficiency: hepatic synthesis of urea is impaired
  Increased substrate for creatinine, rhabdomyolysis
  Increased removal of urea
    Repeated hemo- or peritoneal dialysis (urea diffuses more rapidly than creatinine)
    Excessive vomiting or diarrhea (loss of urea in vomitus or feces)

From Brater, D. C., and Thier, S. O.: Renal disorders. In Melmon, K. L., and Morrelli, H. F. (eds.): Clinical Pharmacology, Basic Principles in Therapeutics. 2nd ed. New York, Macmillan Co., 1978, p. 374. Originally modified from Dossetor, J. B.: Creatininemia versus uremia. The relative significance of blood urea nitrogen and serum creatinine concentrations in azotemia. Ann Intern Med 65:1287–1299, 1966.

concentration of free drug and an increased likelihood of toxicity.

VOLUME

If the serum sodium concentration is stable, a fall in glomerular filtration rate must reduce the filtered load of sodium. If sodium intake is constant as glomerular filtration rate falls and sodium balance is to be maintained, then a greater proportion of a reduced filtered sodium load must be excreted. For this to occur the percentage of filtered sodium reabsorbed must diminish progressively as glomerular filtration rate falls. The mechanisms by which the kidney maintains constant sodium excretion in the presence of a falling glomerular filtration rate are complex. They likely include progressive osmotic diuresis through the remaining functioning nephrons, in part as the result of higher concentrations of filtered urea. The changes in physical factors associated with "hyperperfusion" of the remaining nephrons would favor increased fractional excretion of sodium. There is also evidence that

a natriuretic substance, possibly a small peptide, is present in increased quantities in patients with chronic renal failure. Whatever the mechanisms involved, they represent a gradual adjustment to the loss of renal function and can be reversed only gradually. In renal failure, excretion of a given sodium intake requires that the renal tubule function at near-maximal sodium excretory capacity with each decrement in glomerular filtration rate. Any rapid increase in sodium intake will result in retention and expansion of the extracellular fluid volume. Conversely, a high proportion of filtered sodium will be excreted for some time after sodium intake is reduced. The result will be a salt-wasting state. Therefore the kidney in renal failure cannot respond rapidly to increases or decreases in sodium intake and behaves as though maximum excretory capacity is limited and as though there is an obligatory rate of sodium excretion that cannot be acutely lowered. Actually, if sodium intake is gradually reduced over weeks or months, the mechanisms that led to the reduced reabsorption of filtered sodium at the higher intake readjust and the individual can tolerate sodium restriction, which would earlier have produced negative sodium balance.

TONICITY

In a kidney undergoing osmotic diuresis with urea and with a limited capacity to reabsorb sodium chloride, the medullary interstitial gradient will be reduced. Free water production and reabsorption will be impaired, and isosthenuria will result. Excessive intake or severe restriction of water may result in hypoosmotic or hyperosmotic states. If, however, the thirst mechanism is intact, osmolality may be regulated adequately during renal failure. Nothing need be done about tonicity regulation unless there is evidence that the thirst mechanism is not protecting the patient or unless the patient requires intravenous fluids or tube feedings. Under the latter circumstances, free water intake must be titrated against the serum sodium concentration.

POTASSIUM

Though the most common problem of potassium metabolism in chronic renal failure is the development of hyperkalemia, some patients may manifest potassium wasting. With the development of chronic renal failure the renal handling of potassium is analogous to that for sodium in that the capacity to excrete or retain potassium maximally is blunted. In considering the analogy, one must remember that sodium excretion is dependent on filtration and reabsorption, while potassium excretion is dependent on reabsorption and secretion. As progressively smaller quantities of potassium are delivered to the kidney, the percentage of delivered potassium that is excreted increases. Abrupt increases in potassium intake exceed excretory capacity and produce hyperkalemia. The mechanisms that permit a greater proportion of potassium delivered to the kidney to be excreted during chronic renal failure also impair the ability of the kidney to retain potassium maximally during periods of severe potassium restriction. Therefore patients who are placed on a regimen of severe potassium restriction may develop negative potassium balance. In chronic renal failure, extrarenal mechanisms of potassium disposal play an important protective role. There is gradual adjustment in the intestines' ability to secrete potassium during chronic renal failure. For detailed discussion of hyperkalemia and hypokalemia see section beginning on page 703.

ACID-BASE

In chronic renal failure a reduced capacity for the production of ammonia, inability to increase titratable acid excretion, and some impairment of bicarbonate reabsorption all contribute to an inability to excrete the net acid produced each day. The retained hydrogen ion titrates the buffers of the extracellular fluid and cells and stimulates increased pulmonary excretion of CO_2. These events might predictably lead to a progressive fall in the serum bicarbonate concentration and eventual exhaustion of buffering capacity. However, in chronic renal failure the buffering capacity of bone comes into play. The bone buffers result in apparent stabilization of the serum bicarbonate concentration and gradual demineralization of bone. The enormous buffer reserves of bone permit a positive hydrogen ion balance to persist for months or years, without totally exhausting the buffers required for response to acute acid-base disturbances.

CALCIUM, PHOSPHORUS, AND VITAMIN D

The retention of phosphate in chronic renal failure reduces the concentration of serum ionized calcium, thereby stimulating the release of parathyroid hormone. The parathyroid hormone increases renal phosphate excretion and stimulates calcium release from bone and renal calcium reabsorption. The result is that the serum phosphate concentration is lowered and the serum ionized calcium concentration rises. This sequence of events permits serum calcium and phosphorus concentrations to be maintained within the normal range until the glomerular filtration rate falls to as low as 20 per cent of normal. However, serum levels of calcium and phosphorus are maintained at the cost of striking increases in circulating parathyroid hormone. The parathyroid hormone contributes importantly to the development of renal osteodystrophy and to the pruritus of chronic renal failure. Excessive parathyroid hormone may reduce proximal tubule bicarbonate reabsorption and contribute to the acidosis of uremia.

In addition, as renal disease progresses, the production of 1,25-dihydroxyvitamin D_3 that occurs in renal tubular cells is reduced. As the concentration of the active form of vitamin D_3 falls, the absorption of calcium from the gut diminishes. The result is negative calcium balance, further stimulation of parathyroid hormone, and increased likelihood of renal osteodystrophy.

The net effect of these abnormalities is a gradually diminishing serum calcium concentration; a rising serum phosphate concentration; secondary hyperparathyroidism, producing some degree of osteitis fibrosa cystica; and inadequate quantities of 1,25-dihydroxyvitamin D_3, contributing to osteomalacia.

MAGNESIUM

The excretion of magnesium by the kidney is usually reduced in chronic renal failure. Rarely, in forms of renal disease characterized by severe polyuria, magnesium depletion may occur. The importance of magnesium retention is that it produces depression of the central nervous system. Therefore in individuals who have chronic renal failure, magnesium-containing medications are to be avoided.

HORMONES

The kidney is the source of erythropoietin, renin, and prostaglandins. Erythropoietin is produced in progressively smaller quantities as chronic renal failure progresses. The loss of erythropoietin stimulation contributes to the anemia of chronic renal failure. Even the small quantities of erythropoietin produced by chronically shrunken and failing kidneys contribute to the maintenance of red blood cell mass. Therefore, in a patient whose renal function will not maintain life without dialysis, bilateral nephrectomy will still result in a worsening of the anemia.

Renin, which is ultimately converted to angiotensin II, is produced in the kidney. Chronic renal failure may be associated with increases of renin release and renin-dependent hypertension. Most forms of hypertension seen with chronic renal failure, however, do not depend on elevated renin concentrations; the hypertension is more commonly volume dependent.

The role of altered prostaglandin production in chronic renal failure is not known.

THE ORGAN SYSTEM EFFECTS OF CHRONIC RENAL FAILURE

HEMATOPOIETIC

As renal mass is lost, erythropoietin production falls. The lack of erythropoietin stimulation reduces red blood cell production. In addition, uremic toxins depress red blood cell production directly and also shorten red blood cell survival.

Although platelet counts are usually well maintained, platelet function is impaired by uremic toxins. The abnormal platelet function may contribute to bleeding problems, which in turn complicate the anemia of chronic renal failure.

The anemia of chronic renal failure is usually normochromic normocytic anemia, but may become hypochromic and microcytic if there is an important degree of blood loss.

CARDIOVASCULAR

Hypertension is a common complication of chronic renal failure. Though it may result from excessive renin production, hypervolemia is a more important factor in the majority of patients. The presence of hypertension as well as an increased incidence of hypertriglyceridemia contributes to acceleration of atherosclerosis. The hypertriglyceridemia or type 4 hyperlipoproteinemia results from impaired removal of triglycerides from the circulation. The combination of hypertension, hypervolemia, anemia, and myocardial ischemia commonly results in congestive heart failure.

In addition, pericarditis, a form of serositis, is classically a fibrinous process that produces a loud pericardial friction rub. The pericarditis may be painful. In the minority of patients it may result in effusions severe enough to produce cardiac tamponade.

NEUROLOGIC

Both central nervous system dysfunction and peripheral neuropathy occur. These complications respond to vigorous dialysis and are thus assumed to be due to uremic toxins rather than to the loss of essential nutrients.

MUSCULOSKELETAL

Renal osteodystrophy refers to the bony abnormalities in chronic renal failure. These abnormalities include osteitis fibrosa generalisata, as a result of secondary hyperparathyroidism; osteomalacia, as the result of inadequate production of 1,25-dihydroxyvitamin D_3; osteosclerosis, particularly of the axial skeleton for unexplained reasons; and retardation of growth, in part resulting from net positive hydrogen ion balance.

Numerous articular and periarticular symptoms develop with chronic renal insufficiency. The best-defined abnormalities are gout and pseudogout (the precipitation of calcium pyrophosphate crystals). In patients with severe degrees of phosphate retention, metastatic calcification of soft tissue may occur.

ENDOCRINE

The most important endocrine dysfunction other than secondary hyperparathyroidism is the development of carbohydrate intolerance. Carbohydrate intolerance is the result of increased resistance of peripheral tissues to the action of insulin and of increased concentration of plasma glucagon. Peripheral sensitivity to insulin is enhanced by dialysis, and resistance is therefore assumed to result from retention of a uremic toxin. Patients with diabetes mellitus may actually require less insulin with the development of chronic renal failure, since there is also an impairment of insulin degradation in association with uremia.

Unexplained hypergastrinemia increases the likelihood of peptic ulcer disease, and fertility may be reduced in both men and women. Although abnormal levels of growth hormone, thyroid hormone, and adrenal steroids have been recorded in patients with uremia, there does not seem to be any clinically important dysfunction of these organs in chronic renal failure.

GASTROINTESTINAL

Nausea and vomiting are common in chronic renal failure. Peptic ulcers and colonic ulceration (uremic colitis) may bleed and contribute to the anemia of renal failure. Pancreatitis has also been reported in higher frequency in patients with uremia.

IMMUNOLOGIC

There is a reduced delayed hypersensitivity response in patients with uremia. This impaired cellular immunity may in part be reversed by dialysis.

PULMONARY

A form of serositis may develop in the pleura during uremia. Uremic pleuritis may be hemorrhagic and occurs with or without pericarditis. A form of pulmonary edema termed uremic pneumonitis has been reported. It is very difficult to distinguish what has been described from pulmonary edema due to volume overload or cardiac dysfunction.

SKIN

The skin of patients with chronic renal failure is typically hyperpigmented. The mechanisms leading to the increased melanin production are not known. In addition, pruritus is a troublesome complication of renal failure. It may result in part from the deposition of urea crystals in skin follicles, and in part from secondary hyperparathyroidism.

THE CLINICAL PICTURE OF UREMIA

On the basis of the previous discussion, one would predict that the uremic patient would appear sallow from anemia, hyperpigmented, and might show evidence of skin excoriation as a response to pruritus. The patient would likely be hypertensive and, depending upon recent sodium intake, might evidence hypervolemia or hypovolemia. Examination of the heart might reveal cardiac enlargement, an S4 gallop, and possibly a pericardial friction rub. Examination of the lungs might show a pleural friction rub and the presence of some pleural effusion. Neurologic examination might reveal a positive Chvostek or Trousseau sign resulting from hypocalcemia, and, in addition, peripheral neuropathy might be present.

On questioning, the patient would likely complain of weakness, headache, and nausea and vomiting. Complaints about lower gastrointestinal function would be far less common. Bone and joint pain might well be problems.

Laboratory examination would indicate anemia, elevated blood urea nitrogen and serum creatinine concentrations, a low serum calcium concentration, and a high serum phosphate concentration. Serum sodium concentration would likely be normal unless the thirst mechanism had been impaired. The serum potassium concentration might be high, normal, or low. Serum bicarbonate concentration would probably be reduced, and some evidence of an anion gap metabolic acidosis would be present.

All of the abnormalities of physical examination, clinical history, and laboratory evaluation are predictable results of the loss of renal function.

TREATMENT OF UREMIA

A discussion of the treatment of uremia is well beyond the scope of this text. However, principles of treatment that are derived from an understanding of the pathophysiology will be reviewed briefly.

The retention of nitrogenous waste products can be reduced in chronic renal failure by reducing the quantity of protein ingested in the diet and by ensuring that ingested protein is high in its content of essential amino acids. There is growing evidence that a reduction in protein intake may retard the rate of fall of the glomerular filtration rate in chronic renal failure (see p. 662). The use of alpha keto acids of branched-chain amino acids to enhance protein anabolism while lowering the blood urea nitrogen is still experimental. Adequate caloric intake is also important in preventing protein catabolism.

The intake of sodium should be adequate to maintain maximum intravascular volume short of volume overload. Rapid increases or decreases in sodium intake should be avoided. When ideal body weight and extracellular fluid volume have been achieved, sodium intake should be modified to maintain that ideal weight. The intake of fluids should be regulated by the patient's thirst mechanism. In the absence of hyponatremia or hypernatremia, the physician need not set specific levels of fluid intake. At very late stages of renal failure and in patients undergoing dialysis, limits of water intake may have to be established. When a patient requires intravenous fluids, those fluids should contain adequate sodium to replace losses and adequate water to maintain the serum sodium concentration in the physiologic range.

It is safest to err on the side of potassium restriction. Foods or medications high in potassium content should be avoided. In the later phases of chronic renal failure it may be necessary to remove potassium from the body by means of exchange resins.

The patient's acid-base status can usually be regulated by the judicious use of sodium bicarbonate. The serum bicarbonate concentration may safely be maintained in the range of 16 to 20 mEq/l. Efforts to raise the serum bicarbonate concentration to 25 or 26 mEq/l may result in serious overcorrection and the precipitation of tetany. If the patient cannot tolerate sodium bicarbonate because of volume expansion, dialysis may be required.

Serum phosphate may be lowered by using phosphate binders, such as aluminum hydroxide gels. Once the serum phosphate has been lowered to 6 mg/dl or less, vitamin D and calcium supplementation may be initiated. If vitamin D and calcium are given in association with severely elevated serum phosphate concentrations, metastatic calcifications may occur. The active dihydroxyvitamin D_3 is now widely available and is the drug of choice. When dihydroxyvitamin D_3 is not available, vitamin D_3 in very large doses will be effective.

The use of magnesium-containing antacids or cathartics should be avoided.

The anemia of chronic renal failure may respond to the use of androgens and will be helped by the administration of iron in cases of iron deficiency. Some improvement in red cell production and in red cell survival may be achieved by the initiation of dialysis.

Platelet dysfunction will be improved by dialysis. Careful attention to the control of hypertension and hypervolemia will provide some degree of protection for the cardiovascular system. Unfortunately, serositis, neuropathy, gastrointestinal symptoms, glucose intolerance, and depression of delayed hypersensitivity respond only to dialysis or transplantation.

The principles for the management of chronic renal failure should be followed to prevent complications and to keep the patient as comfortable as possible until dialysis is initiated or transplantation undertaken. In those countries in which dialysis and transplantation are not readily available, the principles of conservative management outlined will provide the longest possible symptom-free period for the patient developing uremia.

REFERENCES

Barger, A. C., and Herd, J. A.: The renal circulation. N Engl J Med 284:482, 1971:

Brenner, B. M., Ichikawa, I., and Deen, W. M.: Glomerular filtration. In Brenner, B. M., and Rector, F. C., Jr. (eds.): The Kidney. 3rd ed. Philadelphia, W. B. Saunders Co., 1985.

Burkholder, P. M.: Functions and pathophysiology of the glomerular mesangium (editorial). Lab Invest 46:239–241, 1982.

Clive, D. M., and Stoff, J. S.: Renal syndromes associated with nonsteroidal antiinflammatory drugs. N Engl J Med 310:563–572, 1984.

Osathanondh, V., and Potter, E. L.: Development of human kidney as shown by microdissection. I. Preparation of tissue with reasons for possible misinterpretations of observations. II. Renal pelvis, calyces, and papillae. III. Formation and interrelationship of collecting tubules and nephrons. Arch Pathol 76:271–276, 277–289, 290–302, 1963.

Thornburn, G. D., Kopald, H. H., Herd, J. A., Hollenberg, M., O'Morchue, C. C., and Barger, A. C.: Intrarenal distribution of nutrient blood flow determined with krypton[85] in unanesthetized dog. Circ Res 13:290–307, 1963.

Tischer, C. C.: Anatomy of the kidney. In Brenner, B. M., and Rector, F. C., Jr. (eds.): The Kidney. 3rd ed. Philadelphia, W. B. Saunders Co., 1985.

Regulation of Volume and Tonicity

Arieff, A. I., and Guisado, R.: Effects on the central nervous system of hypernatremic and hyponatremic states. Kidney Int 10:104–116, 1976.

Berl, T., Anderson, R. J., McDonald, K. M., and Schrier, R. W.: Clinical disorders of water metabolism. Kidney Int 10:117–132, 1976.

Berliner, R. W.: The concentrating mechanism in the renal medulla. Kidney Int 9:214–222, 1976.

Burg, M. B.: Renal handling of sodium, chloride, water, amino acids, and glucose. In Brenner, B. M., and Rector, F. C., Jr. (eds.): The Kidney. 3rd ed. Philadelphia, W. B. Saunders Co., 1985.

DeFronzo, R. A., and Thier, S. O.: Fluid and electrolyte disturbances: Hypo- and hypernatremia. In Martinez-Maldonado, M. (ed.): Manual of Renal Therapeutics. New York, Plenum Press, 1983, pp. 1–23.

DeWardener, H. E.: The control of sodium excretion. In Orloff, J., Berliner, R. W., and Geiger, S. R. (eds.): Handbook of Physiology. Section 8, Renal Physiology. Washington, D.C., American Physiological Society, 1973, pp. 677–720.

DeWardener, H. E.: The control of sodium excretion. Am J Physiol 4:F163–F173, 1978.

Dunn, M. J.: Nonsteroidal antiinflammatory drugs and renal function. Ann Rev Med 35:411–428, 1984.

Feig, P. U., and McCurdy, D. K.: The hypertonic state. N Engl J Med 297:1444–1454, 1977.

Grantham, J. J., and Edwards, R. M.: Natriuretic hormones: At last, bottled in bond? J Lab Clin Med 103:333–336, 1984.

Harrington, J. T., and Cohen, J. J.: Measurement of urinary electrolytes—indications and limitations. N Engl J Med 293:1241–1243, 1975.

Jamison, R. L.: Urine concentration and dilution. In Brenner, B. M., and Rector, F. C., Jr. (eds.): The Kidney. 3rd ed. Philadelphia, W. B. Saunders Co., 1985.

Robertson, G. L., Shelton, R. L., and Athar, S.: The osmoregulation of vasopressin. Kidney Int 10:25–37, 1976.

Seely, J. F., and Levy, M.: Control of extracellular fluid volume. In Brenner, B. M., and Rector, F. C., Jr. (eds.): The Kidney. 3rd ed. Philadelphia, W. B. Saunders Co., 1985.

Skorecki, K. L., and Brenner, B. M.: Body fluid homeostasis in man. Am J Med 70:77–88, 1981.

Acid-Base

Aronson, P. S.: Mechanism of active H^+ secretion in the proximal tubule. Am J Physiol 245:F647–F659, 1983.

Arruda, J. A. L., and Kurtzman, N. A.: Metabolic and respiratory alkalosis. In Kurtzman, N. A., and Martinez-Maldonado, M. (eds.): Pathophysiology of the Kidney. Springfield, Ill., Charles C Thomas, 1977, pp. 356–388.

Batlle, D.: Renal tubular acidosis. Med Clin North Am 67:859–878, 1983.

Cogan, M. G., Rector, F. C., and Seldin, D. W.: Acid-base disorders. In Brenner, B. M., and Rector, F. C., Jr. (eds.): The Kidney. 3rd ed. Philadelphia, W. B. Saunders Co., 1985.

Garella, S., Dana, C. L., and Chazan, J. A.: Severity of metabolic acidosis as a determinant of bicarbonate requirements. N Engl J Med 289:121–126, 1973.

Good, D. W., and Burg, M. B.: Ammonia production by individual segments of the rat nephron. J Clin Invest 73:602–610, 1984.

Jacobson, H. R., and Seldin, D. W.: On the generation, maintenance, and correction of metabolic alkalosis. Am J Physiol 245:F425–F432, 1983.

Koeppen, B. M., and Steinmetz, P. R.: Basic mechanisms of urinary acidification. Med Clin North Am 67:753–770, 1983.

Martinez-Maldonado, M., and Sanches-Montserrat, R.: Respiratory acidosis and alkalosis. Clin Nephrol 7:191–200, 1977.

McCurdy, D. K.: Mixed metabolic and respiratory acid-base disturbances: Diagnosis and treatment. Chest 62:35S–44S, 1972.

Narins, R. G., and Emmett, M.: Simple and mixed acid-base disorders: A practical approach. Medicine 59:161–187, 1980.

Oliva, P. B.: Lactic acidosis. Am J Med 48:209–225, 1970.

Seldin, D. W., and Rector, F. C., Jr.: The generation and maintenance of metabolic alkalosis. Kidney Int 1:306–321, 1972.

Tannen, R. L.: Ammonia and acid-base homeostasis. Med Clin North Am 67:781–798, 1983.

Thier, S. O., McCurdy, D. K., and Rastegar, A.: Metabolic and respiratory acidosis. In Kurtzman, N. A., and Martinez-Maldonado, M. (eds.): Pathophysiology of the Kidney. Springfield, Ill., Charles C Thomas, 1977, pp. 335–355.

Warnock, D. G., and Rector, F. C., Jr.: Renal acidification mechanisms. In Brenner, B. M., and Rector, F. C., Jr. (eds.): The Kidney. 3rd ed. Philadelphia, W. B. Saunders Co., 1985.

Potassium

Bia, M. J., and DeFronzo, R. A.: Extrarenal potassium homeostasis (editorial review). Am J Physiol 240:F257–F268, 1981.

DeFronzo, R. A., Bia, M., and Smith, D.: Clinical disorders of hyperkalemia. Ann Rev Med 33:521–554, 1982.

DeFronzo, R. A., and Thier, S. O.: Fluid and electrolyte disturbances. Hypo- and hyperkalemia. In Martinez-Maldonado, M. (ed.): Manual of Renal Therapeutics. New York, Plenum Press, 1983, pp. 25–55.

Epstein, F. H., and Rosa, R. M.: Adrenergic control of serum potassium. N Engl J Med 309:1450–1451, 1983.

Gennari, F. J., and Cohen, J. J.: Role of the kidney in potassium homeostasis: Lessons from acid-base disturbances. Kidney Int 8:1–5, 1975.

Giebisch, G.: Renal potassium excretion. In Rouiller, C., and Muller, A. F. (eds.): The Kidney: Morphology, Biochemistry, Physiology. New York, Academic Press, 1971, vol. 3, p. 329.

Giebisch, G., Malnic, G., and Berliner, R. W.: Renal transport and control of potassium excretion. In Brenner, B. M., and Rector, F. C., Jr. (eds.): The Kidney. 3rd ed. Philadelphia, W. B. Saunders Co., 1985.

Calcium, Magnesium, and Phosphate

Avioli, L. V., and Haddad, J. G.: The vitamin D family revisited (editorial retrospective). N Engl J Med 311:47–49, 1984.

DeFronzo, R. A., and Thier, S. O.: Inherited disorders of renal tubular function. In Brenner, B. M., and Rector, F. C., Jr. (eds.): The Kidney. 3rd ed. Philadelphia, W. B. Saunders Co., 1985.

DeLuca, H. F.: The kidney as an endocrine organ involved in the function of vitamin D. Am J Med 58:39–47, 1975.

Dirks, J. H.: The kidney and magnesium regulation. Kidney Int 23:771–777, 1983.

Fraser, D., and Scriver, C. R.: Familial forms of vitamin D-resistant rickets revisited. X-linked hypophosphatemia and autosomal recessive vitamin D dependency. Am J Clin Nutr 29:1315–1329, 1976.

Knochel, J. P.: Fluid and electrolyte disturbances: Treatment of hypophosphatemia and phosphate depletion. In Martinez-Maldonado, M. (ed.): Manual of Renal Therapeutics. New York, Plenum Press, 1983, pp. 93–114.

Massry, S. G., and Seelig, M. S.: Hypomagnesemia and hypermagnesemia. Clin Nephrol 7:147–153, 1977.

Mundy, G. R., and Martin, T. J.: The hypercalcemia of malignancy: Pathogenesis and management. Metabolism 12:1247–1277, 1982.

Slatopolsky, E., Rutherford, W. E., Rosenbaum, R., Martin, K., and Hruska, K.: Hyperphosphatemia. Clin Nephrol 7:138–146, 1977.

Stoff, J. S.: Phosphate homeostasis and hypophosphatemia. Am J Med 72:489–495, 1982.

Sutton, A. L., and Dirks, J. H.: Renal handling of calcium, phosphate, and magnesium. In Brenner, B. M., and Rector, F. C., Jr. (eds.): The Kidney. 3rd ed. Philadelphia, W. B. Saunders Co., 1985.

Diuretics

Brater, D. C., and Thier, S. O.: Renal disorders. In Melmon, K. L., and Morrelli, H. F. (eds.): Clinical Pharmacology, Basic Principles in Therapeutics. 2nd ed. New York, Macmillan Co., 1978, pp. 349–387.

Gennari, F. J., and Kassirer, J. P.: Osmotic diuresis. N Engl J Med 291:714–720, 1974.

Goldberg, M.: The renal physiology of diuretics. In Orloff, J., and Berliner, R. W. (eds.): Handbook of Physiology. Section 8, Renal Physiology. Washington, D.C., American Physiological Society, 1973.

Martinez-Maldonado, M., Eknoyan, G., and Suki, W. N.: Diuretics in nonedematous states. Physiological basis for their clinical use. Arch Intern Med 131:797, 1973.

Reineck, H. J., and Stein, J. H.: Mechanisms of action and clinical uses of diuretics. In Brenner, B. M., and Rector, F. C., Jr. (eds.): The Kidney. 3rd ed. Philadelphia, W. B. Saunders Co., 1985.

Seely, J. F., and Dirks, J. H.: Site of action of diuretic drugs. Kidney Int 11:1–8, 1977.

Glomerulonephritis

Coggins, C. H.: Management of glomerulonephritis and nephrotic syndrome. In Martinez-Maldonado, M. (ed.): Manual of Renal Therapeutics. New York, Plenum Press, 1983, pp. 173–190.

Couser, W. G., and Salant, D. J.: In situ immune complex formation and glomerular injury (editorial review). Kidney Int 17:1–13, 1980.

Fauci, A. S., Haynes, B. F., and Katz, P.: The spectrum of vasculitis: Clinical, pathologic, immunologic, and therapeutic considerations. Ann Intern Med 89:660–676, 1978.

Glasscock, R. J., Cohen, A. H., Bennett, C. M., and Martinez-Maldonado, M.: Primary glomerular diseases. In Brenner, B. M., and Rector, F. C., Jr. (eds.): The Kidney. 3rd ed. Philadelphia, W. B. Saunders Co., 1985.

Glasscock, R. J., and Cohen, A. H.: Secondary glomerular diseases. In Brenner, B. M., and Rector, F. C., Jr. (eds.): The Kidney. 3rd ed. Philadelphia, W. B. Saunders Co., 1985.

Row, P. G., Cameron, J. S., Turner, D. R., et al.: Membranous nephropathy. Long term follow-up and association with neoplasia. QJ Med 44:207–239, 1975.

Wilson, C. B.: Recent advances in the immunological aspects of renal disease. Fed Proc 36:2171–2175, 1977.

Tubulo-interstitial Diseases

Andres, G. A., and McCluskey, R. T.: Tubular and interstitial disease due to immunologic mechanisms. Kidney Int 7:271–289, 1975.

Cotran, R.: Tubulointerstitial disease. In Brenner, B. M., and Rector, F. C., Jr. (eds.): The Kidney. 3rd ed. Philadelphia, W. B. Saunders Co., 1985.

Gardner, K. D., Jr. (ed.): Cystic Diseases of the Kidney. New York, John Wiley and Sons, 1976.

Heptinstall, R. H.: Interstitial nephritis. A brief review. Am J Pathol 83:214–236, 1976.

Murray, T., and Goldberg, M.: Chronic interstitial nephritis: Etiological factors. Ann Intern Med 82:453, 1975.

Salvatierra, O., and Tanagho, E. A.: Reflux as a cause of end stage kidney disease: Report of 32 cases. J Urol 117:441–443, 1977.

Wilson, D. R.: Renal function during and following obstruction. Ann Rev Med 28:329, 1977.

Hereditary Renal Diseases

Andreoli, T. E., and Schafer, J. A.: Nephrogenic diabetes insipidus. In Stanbury, J. B., Wyngaarden, J. B., and Fredrickson, D. S. (eds.): The Metabolic Basis of Inherited Disease. New York, McGraw-Hill Book Co., 1974, p. 1634.

Culpepper, R. M., Hebert, S. C., and Andreoli, T. E.: Nephrogenic diabetes insipidus. In Stanbury, J. B., Wyngaarden, J. B., Fredrickson, D. S., Goldstein, J. L., and Brown, M. D. (eds.): The Metabolic Basis of Inherited Disease. 5th ed. New York, McGraw-Hill Book Co., 1983, pp. 1867–1888.

DeFronzo, R. A., and Thier, S. O.: Renal tubular defects in phosphate and amino acid transport. In Andreoli, T. E., Hoffman, J. F., and Fanestil (eds.): Physiology of Membrane Disorders. New York, Plenum Press, 1985.

Desnick, R. J., Klionsky, B., and Sweeley, C. C.: Fabry's disease (α-galactosidase A deficiency). In Stanbury, J. B., Wyngaarden, J. B., and Fredrickson, D. S. (eds.): The Metabolic Basis of Inherited Disease. New York, McGraw-Hill Book Co., 1974, p. 810.

Desnick, R. J., and Sweeley, C. C.: Fabry's disease: Alpha-galactosidase A deficiency. In Stanbury, J. B., Wyngaarden, J. B., Fredrickson, D. S., Goldstein, J. L., and Brown, M. D. (eds.): The Metabolic Basis of Inherited Disease. 5th ed. New York, McGraw-Hill Book Co., 1983, pp. 906–944.

Froesch, E. R.: Essential fructosuria, hereditary fructose intolerance, and fructose-1,6-diphosphatase deficiency. In Stanbury, J. B., Wyngaarden, J. B., and Fredrickson, D. S. (eds.): The Metabolic Basis of Inherited Disease. New York, McGraw-Hill Book Co., 1974, p. 121.

Gitzelmann, R., Steinmann, B., and Van Den Berghe, G.: Essential fructosuria, hereditary fructose intolerance, and fructose-1,6-diphosphatase deficiency. In Stanbury, J. B., Wyngaarden, J. B., Fredrickson, D. S., Goldstein, J. L., and Brown, M. D. (eds.): The Metabolic Basis of Inherited Disease. 5th ed. New York, McGraw-Hill Book Co., 1983, pp. 118–140.

Krane, S. M.: Renal glycosuria. In Stanbury, J. B., Wyngaarden, J. B., and Fredrickson, D. S. (eds.): The Metabolic Basis of Inherited Disease. New York, McGraw-Hill Book Co., 1974, p. 1607.

Rosenberg, L. E., and Scriver, C. R.: Disorders of amino acid metabolism. In Bondy, P., and Rosenberg, L. E. (eds.): Metabolic Control and Disease. Philadelphia, W. B. Saunders Co., 1980, p. 583.

Sass-Kortsak, A., and Bearn, A. G.: Hereditary disorders of copper metabolism: [Wilson's disease (hepatolenticular degeneration) and Menkes' disease (kinky-hair or steely-hair syndrome)]. In Rosenberg, op. cit. p. 1098.

Scriver, C. R.: Hartnup disease: A genetic modification of intestinal and renal transport of certain neutral alpha-amino acids. N Engl J Med 273:530, 1965.

Segal, S., and Thier, S.: Cystinuria. In Stanbury, J. B., Wyngaarden, J. B., Fredrickson, D. S., Goldstein, J. L., and Brown, M. D. (eds.): The Metabolic Basis of Inherited Disease. 5th ed. New York, McGraw-Hill Book Co., 1983, pp. 1774–1791.

Thier, S. O.: Medical management of hereditary renal diseases. In Papadatos, C. J., and Bartsocas, C. S. (eds.): The Management of Genetic Disorders. New York, Alan R. Liss, Inc., 1979, pp. 281–297.

Urinary Tract Calculi

Broadus, A. E., Dominguez, M., and Bartter, F. C.: Pathophysiologic studies in hypercalciuria: Use of an oral calcium tolerance test to characterize distinctive hypercalciuric subgroups. J Clin Endocrinol Metab 47:751–760, 1978.

Broadus, A. E., and Thier, S. O.: Metabolic basis of renalstone disease. N Engl J Med 300:839–845, 1979.

Coe, F. L. (guest editor): Nephrolithiasis. Volume 5 of Contemporary Issues in Nephrology, a series edited by B. M. Brenner and J. H. Stein. New York, Churchill Livingstone, 1980.

Coe, F. L., and Favus, M. J.: Disorders of stone formation. In Brenner, B. M., and Rector, F. C., Jr. (eds.): The Kidney. 3rd ed. Philadelphia, W. B. Saunders Co., 1985.

Coe, F. L., and Kavalach, A. G.: Hypercalciuria and hyperuricosuria in patients with calcium nephrolithiasis. N Engl J Med 291:1344–1350, 1974.

Rieselbach, R. E., and Steele, T. H.: Influence of the kidney upon urate homeostasis in health and disease. Am J Med 56:665–675, 1974.

Segal, S., and Thier, S.: Cystinuria. In Stanbury, J. B., Wyngaarden, J. B., Fredrickson, D. S., Goldstein, J. L., and Brown, M. D. (eds.): The Metabolic Basis of Inherited Disease. 5th ed. New York, McGraw-Hill Book Co., 1983, pp. 1774–1791.

Williams, H. E., and Smith, L. H., Jr.: Primary hyperoxaluria. In Stanbury, J. B., Wyngaarden, J. B., Fredrickson, D. S., Goldstein, J. L., and Brown, M. D. (eds.): The Metabolic Basis of Inherited Disease. 5th ed. New York, McGraw-Hill Book Co., 1983, pp. 204–230.

Acute Renal Failure

Anderson, R. J., Linas, S. L., Berns, A. S., et al.: Nonoliguric acute renal failure. N Engl J Med 296:1134–1138, 1977.

Levinsky, N. G.: Pathophysiology of acute renal failure. N Engl J Med 296:1453–1458, 1977.

Levinsky, N. G., Alexander, E. A., and Venkatachalam, M. A.: Acute renal failure. In Brenner, B. M., and Rector, F. C., Jr. (eds.): The Kidney. 3rd ed. Philadelphia, W. B. Saunders Co., 1985.

Schrier, R. W., and Conger, J. D.: Acute renal failure: Pathogenesis, diagnosis, and management. In Schrier, R. W. (ed.): Renal and Electrolyte Disorders. 2nd ed. Boston, Little, Brown and Co., 1980, pp. 375–408.

Chronic Renal Failure

Bennett, W. M., Singer, I., Golper, T., Feig, P., and Coggins, C. J.: Guidelines for drug therapy in renal failure. Ann Intern Med 87:754–783, 1977.

Brater, D. C.: Drugs and the kidney: Adjusting drug regimens in patients with renal disease. In Martinez-Maldonado, M. (ed.): Manual of Renal Therapeutics. New York, Plenum Press, 1983, pp. 207–225.

Bricker, N. W.: On the pathogenesis of the uremic state: An exposition of the "trade-off hypothesis." N Engl J Med 286:1093–1099, 1977.

David, D. S.: Calcium metabolism in renal failure. Am J Med 58:48–56, 1975.

Dossetor, J. B.: Creatinemia versus uremia. The relative significance of blood urea nitrogen and serum creatinine concentrations in azotemia. Ann Intern Med 65:1287–1299, 1966.

Knochel, J. P., and Seldin, D. W.: The pathophysiology of uremia. In Brenner, B. M., and Rector, F. C., Jr. (eds.): The Kidney. 3rd ed. Philadelphia, W. B. Saunders Co., 1985.

Maher, J. F., Bryan, C. W., and Ahearn, D. J.: Prognosis of chronic renal failure. II. Factors affecting survival. Arch Intern Med 135:273–278, 1975.

Rutherford, W. E., Blondin, J., Miller, J. P., Greenwalt, A. S., and Vavra, J. D.: Chronic progressive renal disease: Rate of change of serum creatinine concentration. Kidney Int 11:62–70, 1977.

Stein, J. H., Lifschitz, M. D., and Barnes, L. D.: Current concepts on the pathophysiology of acute renal failure (editorial review). Am J Physiol 234:F171–F181, 1978.

RESPIRATION

JOHN F. MURRAY, M.D.

Structural Components of the Respiratory System

GENERAL CONSIDERATIONS

Respiration can be defined as those processes that contribute to gas exchange. Occasionally, a distinction is made between *internal* respiration, the gas exchange between cells and blood or within cells, and *external* respiration, the gas exchange between the surrounding environment, whether water or air, and the body. Now the unqualified term respiration, when used in a medical context, means external respiration and refers to the uptake of O_2 and the elimination of CO_2 between ambient air and blood in pulmonary capillaries. Furthermore, the *respiratory system* includes all the organs that participate in the exchange of O_2 and CO_2. In addition to the lungs, the nasopharynx and upper air passages, the thoracic cage, the muscles involved in breathing, and the portions of the brain and nervous system concerned with the regulation of breathing all contribute to respiration. Thus respiratory diseases are

a large group of afflictions that affect one or more of the organs of respiration. Although extremely diverse, respiratory diseases have one important feature in common: when severe, they may produce *respiratory failure*—in other words, an abnormality of gas exchange characterized by an excess of CO_2 and/or a deficiency of O_2 in the bloodstream.

The discussion of respiration will be divided into three sections. In the first section, the structural components of the normal respiratory system are reviewed. The second section includes the physiologic basis of respiration in healthy persons, and the third section describes the pathophysiologic abnormalities that characterize various respiratory diseases.

Definitions

The tracheobronchial system can be divided into two types of airways: cartilaginous airways, or *bronchi,* and membranous (noncartilaginous) airways, or *bron-*

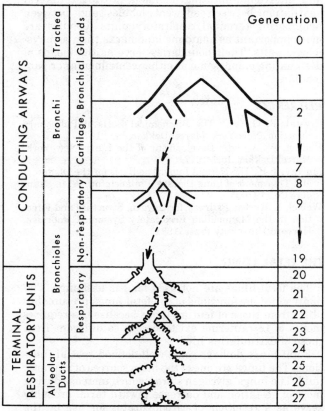

Figure 1. Schematic representation of the conducting airways and terminal respiratory units, with nomenclature of components and generation number. Note that trachea is generation number 0 and main bronchi generation number 1. (Adapted from Weibel, E. R.: Morphometry of the Human Lung. Berlin, Springer-Verlag, 1963, p. 111; reprinted by permission of the author and publisher.)

753

chioles. The only respiratory function of bronchi, as distinguished from their nonrespiratory role (for example, clearance of particles), is to serve as conductors of air between the external environment and the distal sites of gas exchange. Bronchioles, however, are further subdivided to designate their distinctive functions. *Nonrespiratory bronchioles,* including *terminal bronchioles,* serve as conductors of inspired and expired air, whereas *respiratory bronchioles* serve as sites of gas exchange. Conventionally, the definition of *conducting airways* includes the trachea, the bronchi, and the nonrespiratory bronchioles, including terminal bronchioles.

Distal to the ends of the terminal bronchioles are the *terminal respiratory units,* including several branches of respiratory bronchioles and *alveolar ducts* and, finally, the *alveolar sacs* and *alveoli.* Collectively, the gas-exchanging portion of the lung is sometimes referred to as the parenchyma, which means the essential functional elements of an organ, as distinct from its framework or stroma. Conducting airways receive their blood supply from branches of the bronchial arteries while terminal respiratory units receive theirs from branches of the pulmonary arteries. Particles and other materials that deposit on the surface of the conducting airways are removed by mucociliary clearance; in contrast, clearance from the terminal respiratory units is mainly by alveolar macrophages. The subdivisions of airways and terminal respiratory units are shown schematically in Figure 1.

A cluster of three to five terminal bronchioles, each with its appended terminal respiratory unit, is usually referred to as a pulmonary lobule. Contiguous lobules are incompletely delimited by connective tissue septa, and intercommunicating channels provide collateral ventilation between adjacent lobules and between neighboring terminal respiratory units. Lobules are more important as anatomic landmarks than as physiologic units. Their boundaries serve as the means of designating emphysema as either centrilobular or panlobular.

REFERENCES

Crystal, R. G. (ed.): The Biochemical Basis of Pulmonary Function. New York, Marcel Dekker, Inc., 1976.

Hodson, W. A. (ed.): Development of the Lung. New York, Marcel Dekker, Inc., 1977.

Murray, J. F.: The Normal Lung: The Basis for the Diagnosis and Treatment of Lung Disease. Philadelphia, W. B. Saunders Co., 1976.

Weibel, E. R.: The Pathway for Oxygen: Structure and Function in the Mammalian Respiratory System. Cambridge, Harvard University Press, 1984.

THE FETAL LUNG

The fetal lungs are not used for gas exchange. The nonrespiratory functions of the fetal lungs presumably differ from those of mature lungs because the requirements of intrauterine existence are so different from those of extrauterine life.

Fetal lungs do have some well-defined special functions. The lungs are one of the main sources of amniotic fluid. The lungs' glycogen stores, which increase during most of gestation and decrease toward term, probably serve as a reservoir of carbohydrates for use by the rest of the growing organism and by the lungs' own cells to meet their energy requirements. Furthermore, the lungs certainly serve as the site of production of surface-active materials (*surfactant*) that are crucial to ventilatory function, beginning with the first postnatal breath and continuing for the rest of life.

Surfactant Synthesis and Release

Type II epithelial cells (granular pneumocytes) (Fig. 2) appear in the fetal alveolar epithelium in a sequence temporally related to the appearance of surface-active substances in the lungs and amniotic fluid. If the production of surface-active substances is faulty or delayed or if the baby is born prematurely before adequate amounts have been synthesized and released, neonatal respiratory distress (hyaline membrane disease) is likely to develop. The amount of pulmonary surface-active material in amniotic fluid has a high predictive value for the neonatal respiratory distress syndrome and is of considerable assistance in timing elective deliveries, in applying vigorous preventive therapeutic maneuvers to the newborn infant, and in deciding whether or not to treat the mother before delivery with a corticosteroid to accelerate functional maturation of the fetal surfactant-producing system.

Toward the end of gestation, the concentrations of endogenous circulating corticosteroids rise and cause an increase in surfactant production in exactly the same way as do exogenously administered steroids. This response can be explained by the presence of high-affinity cytoplasmic receptors for glucocorticoids in type II cells; after binding has occurred, a series of reactions takes place that culminates in increased synthesis of one of the key lipid constituents of surface-active material. Other hormones (thyroxin, estradiol, insulin) also affect surfactant production, but their

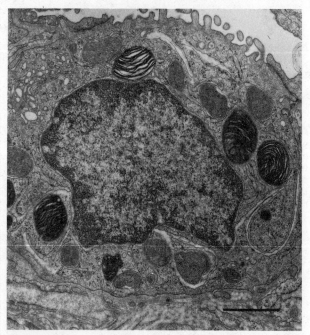

Figure 2. Electron photomicrograph of a type II alveolar epithelial cell showing characteristic lamellar inclusion bodies and microvilli; horizontal bar = 1 μm. (Courtesy of Dr. Mary Williams.)

TABLE 1. COMPOSITION OF PULMONARY SURFACE-ACTIVE MATERIAL*

CHEMICAL COMPONENTS (%)		LIPID FRACTIONS (%)		PHOSPHATIDYLCHOLINE FATTY ACID COMPONENTS (%)	
Lipid	85	Phosphatidylcholine	75	Palmitate (16:0)	71
Protein	13	Neutral lipid	9.1	Myristate (14:0)	6.1
Hexose	<1.7	Cholesterol	6.6	Stearate (18:0)	3.6
Nucleic acid	<0.7	Phosphatidylethanolamine	6.3	Palmitoleate (16:1)	11
		Sphingomyelin	2.1	Oleate (18:1)	3.9
Hexosamine	<0.5	Lysolecithin	0.9	Unidentified	3.6

physiologic role is less certain than that of corticosteroids.

The pathophysiologic mechanisms concerned with surfactant synthesis and release are poorly understood. Direct neural control is unlikely because the type II cells do not appear to be innervated. There is evidence that increased ventilatory activity leads to increased production of surfactant and that the metabolic events controlling this response may involve a complex interplay among beta-adrenergic agonists, acetylcholine, and prostaglandins.

Pulmonary surface-active material is a complex mixture composed chiefly of lipids and several proteins, one of which, the surfactant apoprotein, appears to be unique to the lung (Table 1). Although surface-active material is rich in dipalmitoyl lecithin (DPL), the principal ingredient of phosphatidylcholine, surfactant and DPL are not synonymous and much more than just DPL is required to produce all of the surface-active properties found in normal lungs.

Also listed in Table 1 are the fatty acid components of phosphatidylcholine from adult lungs. There appears to be a developmental sequence of incorporation of different fatty acids into surface-active material during fetal maturation such that the presence of "immature" fatty acids correlates with the presence of hyaline membrane disease.

The sequence of intracellular storage and the subsequent release of surface-active material and its movement to the surface film is shown schematically in Figure 3. Surfactant is formed in the cytoplasm of type II epithelial cells and stored as folded layers in the lamellar bodies (Fig. 2). How the newly synthesized phospholipid is transported to the lamellar bodies is unknown. After formation of a lamellar body is completed, it migrates to the apical surface of the cell and is released, presumably by membrane fusion and exocytosis, into the overlying liquid hypophase. After extrusion, many of the lamellar bodies seem to unravel and are transformed into a second form of surfactant, *tubular myelin*. How tubular myelin and other precursors are finally incorporated into the monomolecular surface film is uncertain. Similarly, it is not known what happens to effete or inactivated surfactant; some can be found phagocytosed by alveolar macrophages, and some may be recycled by type II cells.

Physiologic Role of Surfactant

Surface tension exists at any air-liquid interface, and the lungs are no exception. Thus the surface tension of the monomolecular film that covers the alveolar surface has considerable influence on the mechanical behavior of the lungs and is one of the two principal determinants of their elastic recoil (to be

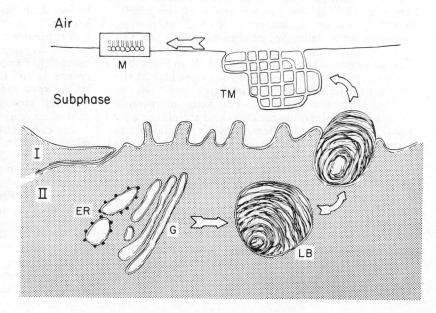

Figure 3. Presumed pathway of lung surfactant formation, storage, and distribution. Synthesis occurs within type II cell, beginning in the endoplasmic reticulum *(ER)* and progressing through the Golgi *(G)* to the lamellar bodies *(LB)* where it is stored. The lamellar bodies migrate to the apical surface of the cell and are ejected into the alveolar subphase, where they expand into tubular myelin *(TM)* figures, which, in turn, spread as a monolayer *(M)* at the air-liquid interface. (From Goerke, J.: Biochim Biophys Acta 344:241, 1974; reprinted by permission of the author and publisher.)

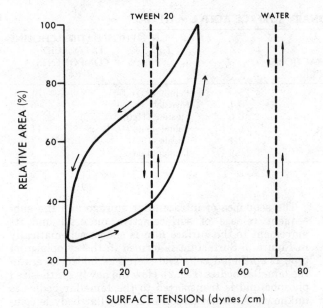

Figure 4. Surface area–surface tension relationships for lung washings containing normal surfactant (solid lines) and for Tween 20 (a detergent) and H_2O (dashed lines). Note that when the surface film containing surfactant is reduced in area, its surface tension decreases nearly to 0 dynes/cm. The *arrows* indicate expansion (upward) or compression (downward) of the material. (Adapted from Clements, J. A., and Tierney, D. F.: Handbook of Physiology. Section 3, Respiration. Vol. II. Washington, D.C., American Physiological Society, 1965, p. 1565; reprinted by permission of the authors and publisher.)

discussed later). Two special characteristics of pulmonary surface-active material deserve emphasis. (1) The surface tension of the film is area dependent and differs depending on whether the film is being expanded (inflation of the lung) or contracted (deflation of the lung). The difference in surface area–surface tension relationships during expansion and compression is a form of *hysteresis* (Fig. 4) and presumably accounts for the hysteresis observed in the volume-pressure relationships of normal lungs during inflation and deflation (see Fig. 16). (2) The surface tension of the film is relatively low throughout expansion and contraction, compared with water, but reaches extremely low values when the area of the film is decreased (Fig. 4). This same phenomenon stabilizes alveoli and serves to prevent atelectasis. If surface tension were high at the alveolar air-liquid interface, the lungs would tend to collapse at the end of each breath; infants' lungs would be especially vulnerable because their alveoli are very small and the physical forces favoring collapse are thereby amplified. The presence of normal surface-active material with its extremely low surface tension offsets this collapsing tendency; hence its absence in premature and other newborn babies often leads to the respiratory distress syndrome.

Surfactant is essential not only for providing mechanical stability to the alveoli once they become air-filled but also for decreasing interstitial and pulmonary capillary pressures; by this means the removal of lung liquid and the lowering of pulmonary vascular resistance are enhanced during the critical first minutes after delivery.

REFERENCES

Ballard, P. L.: Hormonal influences during fetal development. Ciba Found Symp 78:251, 1980.

Clements, J. A.: Functions of the alveolar lining. Am Rev Respir Dis 115 (part 2):67, 1977.

King, R. J.: Pulmonary surfactant. J Appl Physiol 53:1, 1982.

Oyarzum, M. J., and Clements, J. A.: Control of lung surfactant by ventilation, adrenergic mediators, and prostaglandins in the rabbit. Am Rev Respir Dis 117:879, 1978.

STRUCTURE OF THE MATURE LUNG

Neonatal lungs undergo remarkable functional changes during the first few minutes of life that enable them to maintain adequate pressures of O_2 (Po_2 = 62 mm Hg) and CO_2 (Pco_2 = 38 mm Hg) in the arterial bloodstream. Gas exchange, however, is carried out in the lungs that obviously still retain their fetal structure, although some morphologic changes can be recognized in the caliber of the newborn's pulmonary blood vessels and the geometry of its saccules that are presumably related to inflation. Development of the human lungs to their adult state continues long after birth; however, the rate at which the different structural components of the lungs mature during this period varies considerably.

Airways

The number of bronchial divisions varies markedly *within* the lungs, depending on the length of pathways from segmental bronchi to the various gas exchange units throughout the lung. For example, only 10 bronchial branches may be present between a segmental bronchus and terminal respiratory units near the hilum, whereas more than 25 branches may exist between a segmental bronchus and terminal units in the most distal parts of the lung.

As the tracheobronchial system branches, the diameter of each new generation of airways decreases progressively from the trachea outward (Fig. 5). However, the change in caliber is such that the cross-sectional area of the airway lumen steadily increases at each successive level throughout the system. This is especially marked from the bronchioles outward because branching of these segments is accompanied by practically no decrease in diameter of new generations. The progressive increase in cross-sectional area means that the velocity of airflow must steadily decrease as the airstream moves peripherally through the airways and that the resistance to airflow imposed by small airways must be only a small proportion of that of large airways.

The conducting airways are not rigid tubes through which air flows between the oropharynx and the terminal respiratory units; they are flexible structures that dilate and contract passively, in response to influences such as lung inflation, and actively, in response to a variety of neurohumoral and chemical stimuli; in addition, they have secretory capabilities. The active reactions are mediated by the elements that compose the walls of airways: epithelium, smooth muscles, glands, nerves, and mast cells, which are capable of releasing potent pharmacologic substances; all of these components may contribute to bronchial reactivity under special conditions.

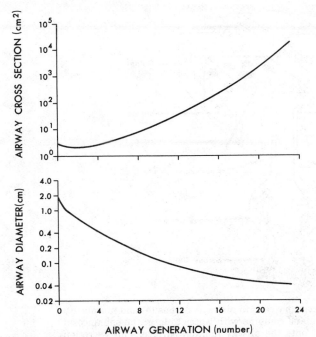

Figure 5. Semilogarithmic plot of the relationship between average diameter and cross-sectional area of airways as airway generation increases. The trachea is generation 0, the main bronchi generation 1, and so on, as shown in Figure 1. (Adapted from Weibel, E. R.: Morphometry of the Human Lung. Berlin, Springer-Verlag, 1963, p. 111; reprinted by permission of the author and publisher.)

Bronchial Epithelium. The entire system of airways, from the trachea to the respiratory bronchioles, is covered with an epithelial lining that rests on a thin basement membrane overlying the lamina propria—a loose network of fibers that contains cells, a rich capillary plexus, and unmyelinated nerves. In large airways, the epithelium is of the ciliated pseudo-stratified columnar type; however, the thickness of the lining layer gradually decreases in height as the airways become smaller so that in the terminal bronchioles the epithelium consists of a single layer of ciliated cells that are more cuboidal than columnar, and in the respiratory bronchioles the epithelial cells become even flatter.

The pseudostratified columnar epithelium of bronchi is now known to contain eight different types of cells. *Ciliated cells,* the dominant cells of the epithelial layer, are present throughout all conducting airways and extend into respiratory bronchioles. The coordinated, sweeping motion of the cilia impels the superficial layer of secretions (the "mucous blanket") along its journey from peripheral airways into the pharynx. This so-called mucociliary escalator is an important natural defense mechanism because it is the chief pathway for removing inhaled particles deposited on the surface of the mucous blanket of the airways.

Several types of secretory cells are present in the respiratory epithelium. The two most prominent are *mucous cells* called *goblet cells* because of their characteristic swollen appearance and *serous cells* (particularly in the newborn). Both epithelial mucous and serous cells have their greatest number in the trachea and large bronchi and become infrequent in bronchioles. Mucous (goblet) cells increase in number

throughout the airways of smokers and can even be found in terminal bronchioles where they are normally sparse.

The *Clara cell* is the main secretory cell of the terminal and respiratory bronchiolar epithelium. Some Clara cells have conspicuous plump protoplasmic extensions that protrude into the lumen of the air passage and are thus readily recognizable. In respiratory bronchioles, the epithelium between the interstices of the outpouching alveoli consists of low cuboidal cells with diminutive cilia and nonciliated Clara cells. Clara cells are thought to have a secretory function because they are furnished with strong-reacting oxidative enzymes. It is possible that Clara cells are one of the sources of the extracellular surface lining of terminal bronchioles in which glands are absent and goblet and serous cells are scanty.

Basal cells differentiate as needed to replace superficial ciliated and goblet cells. Thus they constitute a reserve population of cells that replenishes the surface epithelium.

Brush cells are rare and their function remains unknown. They have microvilli and other structures that are similar to those of the brush cells of the epithelium of the gastrointestinal tract, suggesting that they may have a similar role in liquid absorption.

Argyrophil or Kulchitsky-like cells, much more impressive in the epithelium of newborns than in that of adults, have a characteristic ultrastructure and may be innervated. The function of these cells is unknown, but they are believed to be the precursors of oat cell carcinomas.

Clumps of 10 to 30 serotonin-containing and argyrophilic cells called *neuroepithelial bodies* are found in the bronchial, bronchiolar, and even alveolar epithelium. These heavily innervated structures are of considerable interest because of their strategic location; this has suggested to some that they may regulate airway and/or pulmonary blood vessel caliber, but their physiologic function, if any, is unknown.

Bronchial Glands. The bronchial glands are found in the submucosal layer beneath the lamina propria of bronchi; they are especially numerous in medium-sized bronchi, less prevalent in smaller bronchi, and absent in bronchioles. Glands are simple tubuloalveolar structures composed of four distinct regions (Fig. 6): (1) a short, funnel-shaped, ciliated duct that is a continuation of the surface epithelium; (2) a nonciliated collecting duct; (3) mucous tubules, lined with mucus-secreting cells, opening into the collecting duct; and (4) serous tubules lined with serum-secreting cells, opening into mucous tubules.

Bronchial glands are innervated by parasympathetic postganglionic efferent fibers. The question of direct sympathetic regulation of bronchial glands is unsettled. Parasympathetic agonists or nervous activity stimulates glycoprotein secretion by individual cells and causes the glands to discharge their contents. Secretion by bronchial glands is part of a reflex response to stimulation of rapidly adapting irritant receptors in large bronchi. The reflex pathways (Fig. 6) have both afferent and efferent fibers in the vagus nerve. In addition to mucous secretion, stimulation of irritant receptors causes cough, which, by the phenomenon of dynamic compression, narrows large airways. Evolutionary design seems to have purposely located

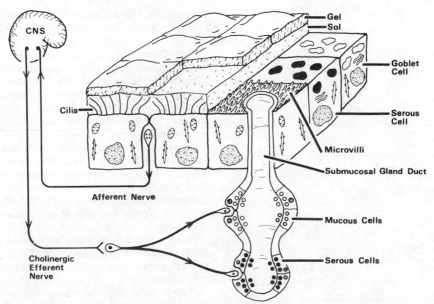

Figure 6. Schematic illustration of bronchial gland and secretory cells in airways. Serous (●) and mucous (○) secretions from the appropriate cells in the submucosal gland combine with water to form the submucosal gland secretion, which is discharged via the gland duct onto the airway luminal surface. This secretion mixes with the mucous and serous secretions from the epithelial goblet and serous cells to coat the epithelial surface with an upper gel and a lower more fluid sol in which the cilia beat and propel the gel toward the mouth. The apical surfaces of some cells are covered by microvilli whose function is unknown. Golgi apparatus (≋) of the secretory epithelial cells, and nuclei (◔), endoplasmic reticulum (↕), and mitochondria (⬭) in the other surface cells are shown. Endings of cholinergic afferent nerves in the lateral intercellular spaces close to the junctions between epithelial cells send impulses to the central nervous system and reflexly stimulate secretion from the serous and mucous cells of the submucosal glands via cholinergic efferent nerves. (From Nadel, J. A., Davis, B., and Phipps, R. J.: Annu Rev Physiol 41:369, 1979; reprinted by permission of the authors and publisher.)

irritant receptors, bronchial glands, and sites of airway narrowing during cough within the same airways.

Mucous cells, and probably serous cells, seem to produce secretory granules continuously but release them into the glandular lumen intermittently. The chemical composition of their respective secretions is unknown. The material that reaches the airway lumen, therefore, represents a mixture of the products of both cell types and any chemical reactions that result from the combinations. (There is a possibility that secretions from serous cells may be enzymatic and alter the physical properties of secretions from mucous cells.) Secretory activity may be stimulated by parasympathomimetic drugs and depressed by parasympatholytic drugs.

Mast cells, which closely resemble circulating basophilic leukocytes, are found in many tissues, including the submucosa and connective tissues of the lungs. Human mast cells are believed to contain heparin, histamine, slow-reacting substances, eosinophil chemotactic substance, proteolytic enzymes, dopamine, and serotonin. On the basis of their in vitro and in vivo activity, circulating basophils and mast cells have been implicated in the pathogenesis of atopic (extrinsic) asthma and other immediate (type I) hypersensitivity responses.

Smooth Muscle. The location of smooth muscle in the walls of the tracheobronchial tree varies in airways of different sizes. In the trachea and main bronchi, the only muscle fibers are located in the posterior muscle bundle. Medium and small bronchi have a distinct muscle layer with a helical orientation of fibers spiral-

ing in both directions and criss-crossing in the walls. Thus the effect of muscle contraction depends on the location and density of the fibers. In the large airways, muscle shortening serves to oppose or even overlap the tips of the U-shaped cartilages. In medium and small bronchi, due to the geodesic distribution of muscle elements, contraction decreases both the caliber and length of the bronchus.

Smooth muscle does not end in the terminal bronchioles, but spirals of muscle form part of the walls of respiratory bronchioles, and bands of muscle have been identified in the openings of alveolar ducts; contraction of these elements decreases the distensibility of the terminal respiratory units. In contrast, contraction of smooth muscles in conducting airways increases resistance to airflow.

Connective Tissue. Cartilaginous airways and large pulmonary arteries, which travel side by side throughout the substance of the lung, are surrounded by a sleeve of loose connective tissue, the bronchovascular sheath, that contains lymphatic vessels and an interstitial space in which fluid may accumulate (see section on Liquid and Solute Exchange). In contrast to bronchioles, which are firmly attached to the adjacent lung parenchyma, small arteries carry their sheaths into the terminal respiratory units.

Terminal Respiratory Units

Terminal respiratory units contain a characteristically variable branching pattern. There are usually two to five orders of respiratory bronchioles (indicated by Roman numerals in Fig. 7), the last of which leads

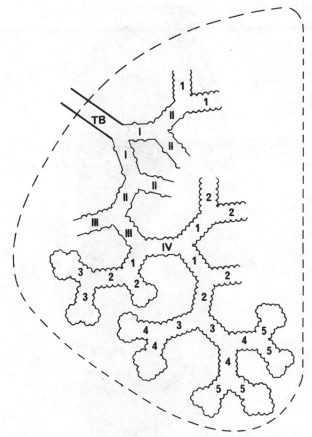

Figure 7. Schematic representation of the anatomic subdivisions in a single plane through a terminal respiratory unit (that is, those structures distal to a terminal bronchiole, *TB*). Roman numerals indicate respiratory bronchioles; arabic numerals indicate alveolar ducts. The entire unit can be visualized by rotating the structures within the hatched boundary through 360 degrees. (From Murray, J. F.: The Normal Lung. Philadelphia, W. B. Saunders Co., 1976, p. 43.)

into the first of two to five orders of alveolar ducts (indicated by Arabic numerals). Alveolar ducts are relatively short (with lengths only one to one and one half times their diameter) and they branch in rapid sequence; each duct has openings for 10 to 16 alveoli. The last in the series of alveolar ducts empties into one to three dome-shaped alveolar sacs from which the terminal alveoli project.

The extent of alveolarization of respiratory bronchioles increases, proceeding from the terminal bronchiole toward the periphery. The chief difference between alveolar ducts and respiratory bronchioles is that the ducts are completely alveolarized and ciliated respiratory epithelium is absent (Fig. 8). Alveolar ducts can be viewed mainly as a supporting framework of delicate connective tissue fibers and slender smooth muscle cells interspersed between the succession of alveoli that emerge from them. The three-dimensional latticework of connective tissue fibers that support alveoli is continuous throughout the lung parenchyma and is anchored peripherally and centrally, through a system of fibers connected to the visceral pleura and through an axial fiber system that is a continuation of the fibrous sheath of conducting airways, respectively. When the lungs are inflated, the elastic fiber network, which is fastened at the hilum and pleural surface, is stretched; this provides firm support for the terminal respiratory units and contributes to the tendency of the lungs to recoil inward.

Alveoli. The lungs contain approximately 20 to 25 million saccules at birth and several hundred million alveoli when they are fully grown. New alveoli are formed by alveolarization of originally nonrespiratory bronchioles and by multiplication. Alveolar multiplication is most rapid during the first three to four years of life, but ceases before somatic growth is complete; thereafter, while the thorax continues to enlarge, alveoli must increase in size. Alveoli of a human adult are about 250 μm in diameter and relatively uniform in size. The number of alveoli per person varies with

Figure 8. Scanning electron photomicrograph of a normal human lung showing two alveolar ducts and some of the numerous alveoli arising from them. The vertical tissue layer on the left is part of the interlobular septum that separates the terminal respiratory unit shown from its neighbors. (Courtesy of Dr. Jacob Bastacky.)

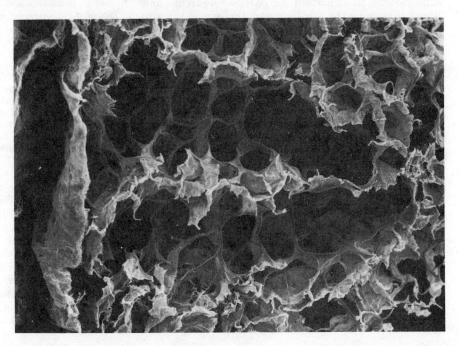

body height; 300,000,000 is the conventional number but over 500,000,000 were estimated in one person.

The total alveolar surface area is about 140 m², of which nearly 85 to 95 per cent is covered with pulmonary capillaries. Thus the alveolar-capillary interface has a surface area of approximately 125 m² and provides an area of contact between the body and its external environment that is more than 70 times greater than that via the skin. To protect themselves and the rest of the body from the numerous potentially harmful substances and infectious agents that may be inhaled and deposited within the lungs, the airways and alveolar surfaces are equipped with elaborate defense mechanisms that are considered in the section Normal Physiology of the Respiratory System.

Alveolar-Capillary Membrane. The alveolar-capillary membrane (Fig. 9) consists of several layers: (1) alveolar epithelium, (2) capillary endothelium, (3) contiguous tissue elements in the intercalated interstitial space, and (4) surfactant lining.

The *alveolar epithelium* consists of a continuous layer of tissue made up of two principal cell types: type I cells, or *squamous pneumocytes*, cover 95 per cent of the alveolar surface. Cytoplasmic organelles, such as mitochondria, are rare and are usually located in the surrounding cytoplasm near the nucleus. Type II cells, or *granular pneumocytes*, are more numerous than type I cells, but owing to their cuboidal shape they occupy less than 5 per cent of the alveolar surface. Type II cells have microvilli and osmiophilic lamellated inclusion bodies (Fig. 2) and are the source of surface-active material. They are also the principal cells involved in the repair of the alveolar surface after a variety of injuries to type I cells. The basic process is rapid hyperplasia of type II cells to restore a protective surface layer; subsequently, the proliferated type II cells differentiate into type I cells and a normal epithelial surface is restored.

The *capillary endothelium* is composed chiefly of the cytoplasmic extensions of endothelial cells, which by their contiguous arrangement form a thin capillary tube. Besides its important but passive role in gas and liquid exchange, the capillary endothelium is the site of active biochemical processes, such as the conversion and inactivation of polypeptides, prostaglandins, nucleotides, and amines, that have important physiologic functions (see section on Biochemical Transformations). The endothelium of other pulmonary blood vessels may also be the site of similar events, but the large surface area of the capillary bed makes it the predominant locus of these activities.

The alveolar epithelium and the capillary endothelium both rest on separate basement membranes; however, because of important anatomic and functional differences the alveolar-capillary membrane has been subdivided into two separate regions. (1) The "thin portion" of the interalveolar septum, or *air-blood barrier,* occurs over the convex half of the capillary surface that appears to bulge into the alveolus and over which the two basement membranes are fused (Fig. 9). Because the quantity of gas, including O_2 and CO_2, that diffuses across a membrane in a given time is inversely related to the thickness of the membrane, the thin portion is the predominant site of gas exchange. (2) The "thick portion" is found where the two basement membranes are separated by an interstitial space con-

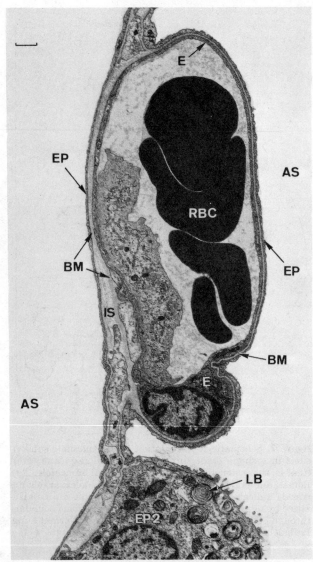

Figure 9. Electron photomicrograph of a transverse section through a capillary in the interalveolar septum of a normal human lung. The surface of the septum facing the two alveolar spaces *(AS)* is mainly lined by thin squamous extensions of type I epithelial cells *(EP)*. The lower right-hand portion of the septum is covered by a type II epithelial cell *(EP2)* containing osmiophilic lamellar bodies *(LB)*. The capillary, containing red blood cells *(RBC)*, is lined by endothelium *(E)*. Both epithelium and endothelium rest on basement membranes *(BM)* that are fused over the "thin" portion of the septum and that are separated by an interstitial space *(IS)* over the "thick" portion of the septum. Horizontal bar = 1 μm. (Courtesy of Dr. Ewald R. Weibel.)

taining fine elastic fibers, small bundles of collagen fibrils, and a few fibroblasts. The thick portion is the site of continuous liquid filtration from pulmonary capillaries into the interstitial space. Pulmonary capillaries weave their way back and forth through the interstitial space of the interalveolar septum, first presenting their thin portion to the alveolus on one side and then to the alveolus on the other side. Thus the interstitial space is perforated by capillaries and should be viewed as a communicating meshwork and not as a continuous sheet. The interstitial space of the interalveolar septum connects directly with the interstitial space surrounding airways and blood vessels. The alveolar epithelium is covered by an irregular layer of fluid (the hypophase) on top of which lies the monomolecular film of surface-active material (Fig. 3).

Alveolar macrophages (Fig. 10) are phagocytic cells that are found in varying numbers submerged in the extracellular lining of the alveolar surface. They originate from stem cell precursors in the bone marrow and reach the lung through the bloodstream, presumably as circulating monocytes. However, because the enzyme content of alveolar macrophages differs considerably from that of monocytes, the macrophages presumably do not migrate directly from bloodstream to alveolus. Transformation of blood monocytes to alveolar macrophages is believed to occur within a population of proliferating interstitial cells. Alveolar macrophages probably replicate within the lungs and may maintain a substantial population by this means. Alveolar macrophages constitute the chief mechanism of clearance of bacteria and other particles that are deposited on the surface of the terminal respiratory units. Deficiencies in their function undoubtedly contribute to the pathogenesis of pulmonary infections.

Intercommunicating Channels. At least three types of intercommunicating channels are known to exist: alveolar pores of Kohn, canals of Lambert, and other, unnamed, pathways. These channels serve as important pathways for collateral ventilation in the presence of airways obstruction and thus affect gas exchange and tend to prevent atelectasis.

Pulmonary Arteries

During gestation, all branches of the pulmonary arterial system are relatively thick walled owing to their medial layer of smooth muscle. Soon after birth, however, the vessels rapidly become thinner, so that by four months of age they show nearly the same relationship between wall thickness and external diameter as that found in adult lungs. The postnatal

evolution of both the abundant elastic elements in elastic arteries and the thick layer of smooth muscle in muscular arteries to their final adult structure can proceed only if pulmonary arterial pressure falls to the normal low values found in infants living near sea level. If pulmonary hypertension is maintained after birth, for example, either because of hypoxia from residence at high altitude or because of congenital cardiac anomalies such as a large ventricular septal defect or truncus arteriosus, then thinning and/or atrophy of the muscular and elastic elements fails to occur.

Branches of conducting airways and arteries, but not of pulmonary veins, maintain an intimate partnership as they course from hilum to terminal respiratory unit. Factors that affect the regional distribution of ventilation will therefore also affect the distribution of blood flow to the same region, and vice versa. When both ventilation and blood flow are impaired similarly, compared with disproportionate involvement of one or the other, optimum conditions for gas exchange are maintained (see section on Gas Exchange).

Thin-walled muscular arteries and arterioles within lobules are directly exposed to the gas tensions in the alveolar spaces. This presumably explains why pulmonary arterial vasoconstriction occurs in response to alveolar hypoxia. It is not known whether hypoxia causes smooth muscle constriction itself or if secondary mediators are involved. Intact neural pathways to the central nervous system are not required. Pulmonary arterial vasoconstriction in response to alveolar hypoxia is an important compensatory mechanism that is actuated in many pathologic conditions, such as bronchial asthma and chronic bronchitis, and may play a major role in the pathogenesis of pulmonary arterial hypertension and cor pulmonale (see below).

Pulmonary Veins

There are more pulmonary veins than arteries, and because the number of conventional branches of both systems is equal, there is an increased density of veins

Figure 10. Scanning electron photomicrograph of a normal human lung showing an alveolar macrophage *(Ma)* attached to the epithelium partly by filopodia *(FP)* and forming an undulating membrane *(U)* in the direction of forward movement toward the left. Several capillaries *(C)* are evident and a type II epithelial cell *(EP2)* can be seen in the background. (Original magnification ×3700). (From Gehr, P., Bachofen, M., and Weibel, E. R.: Respir Physiol 32:121, 1978; reprinted with permission of the authors and publisher.)

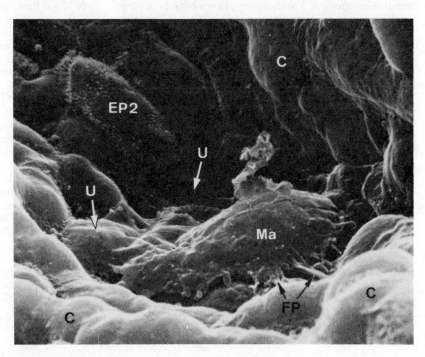

per unit area of lung. Except during gestation, veins have a thinner muscular layer in their walls than arteries. In patients with congenital or acquired heart disease the thickness of the smooth muscle layer of pulmonary arteries and veins varies with corresponding changes in intravascular pressures; thus medial hypertrophy of the walls of veins is pathognomonic for pulmonary venous hypertension. Because of a larger cross-sectional area of the pulmonary veins, resistance to blood flow on the venous side of the pulmonary circulation is less than that on the arterial side.

Pulmonary veins serve, with the left atrium, as a reservoir of blood for the left ventricle. Thus if pulmonary arterial inflow is suddenly interrupted, the left ventricle continues to fill with blood from pulmonary veins and to eject a substantial stroke volume for several beats. Prolonged disturbances in right ventricular output are ultimately reflected in left ventricular output, but minor variations, such as might occur during respiration, are probably partially buffered by the pulmonary venous reservoir.

Bronchial Circulation

The lungs receive blood from two different vascular systems, the pulmonary circulation and the bronchial circulation. There are important differences in the amount of blood flow, the composition of the blood, and the tissues supplied by these two sources. The pulmonary circulation consists of virtually the entire cardiac output; it contains mixed venous blood, and the oxygenation of this blood is essential for life. In contrast, blood flow through the bronchial circulation consists of only a small proportion (less than 1 to 2 per cent) of the cardiac output; incoming bronchial arterial blood is of systemic origin, and normal adult lungs remain viable without it. However, this statement oversimplifies the role of the bronchial circulation because it does not acknowledge the probable value of bronchial blood flow to the developing fetal lungs and its crucial contributions to gas exchange in various congenital cardiac anomalies. Furthermore, there may be a striking increase in the size and number of bronchial arteries in certain kinds of lung disease, especially chronic inflammation and neoplasms.

The bronchial arteries in the human adult vary considerably in number and origin. There is often a single artery to the right lung that arises from an upper right intercostal artery or from the right subclavian or internal mammary artery. The two arteries supplying the left lung usually arise as direct branches from the upper thoracic aorta. As soon as the bronchial arteries enter the lungs, they begin to branch. Two or three bronchial arterial branches, which anastomose with each other to form a peribronchial plexus with an elongated and irregular mesh, accompany each subdivision in the conducting airways.

The bronchial arteries are the principal source of nutrient blood to (1) the conducting airways from the main bronchi to the terminal bronchioles, (2) the pulmonary nerves and ganglia, (3) the elastic and some muscular pulmonary arteries and veins, (4) the lymph nodes and lymph tissue, (5) the visceral pleura, and (6) the connective tissue septa. Near the end of the terminal bronchioles, the bronchial arterioles terminate in a network of capillaries that anastomose extensively with the capillary plexus in the alveoli of the adjoining respiratory bronchioles. Because respiratory bronchioles are supplied by branches of the pulmonary artery, communication between the pulmonary circulation and the bronchial circulation occurs at the junction of the conducting airways and the terminal respiratory units.

Two different venous pathways conduct blood from capillaries supplied by bronchial arteries to either the right or left atrium (Fig. 11). True *bronchial veins,* which are found only near the hilum, empty into the azygos, hemiazygos, or intercostal veins, carrying this part of bronchial blood into the right atrium. Veins that originate from bronchial capillaries within the lung unite to form venous tributaries (sometimes called *bronchopulmonary veins*) that join the pulmonary vein. Blood leaving the capillary bed around terminal bronchioles flows through anastomoses with the alveolar capillaries, and the mixture of blood returns to the left atrium through pulmonary veins.

Blood flow to the lungs through its two circulations is balanced, even though the amount supplied by each differs markedly. If the perfusing pressure in one system increases or decreases, the amount of blood supplied by the other system changes in the opposite direction. This means that if pressure falls in part of the pulmonary arterial circulation (for example, distal to the site of a pulmonary embolus), blood flow to that part of the lung through the bronchial circulation increases. Conversely, if pressure in the bronchial system falls (for example, in autotransplantation, which deprives the lung of all its bronchial blood flow), blood flow in the pulmonary circulation increases to supply those tissues that formerly received blood from the bronchial circulation.

This reciprocal relationship is obviously of great benefit in preserving viability of pulmonary structures when one or the other circulation is impaired. The adequacy of the mechanism depends on the presence of functioning anastomoses between the two circulations that are capable of accommodating an increase in blood flow. When the increase in collateral flow does not occur, lung damage develops: pulmonary infarction may follow pulmonary embolism when the bronchial circulation is compromised, or necrosis of the airways may accompany bronchial transection when the pulmonary circulation is affected.

Nerve Supply

Surprisingly few detailed anatomic studies have been conducted on the afferent and efferent nerve supply of normal human lungs. The subsequent discussion summarizes available information, but the conclusions must be regarded as tentative and likely to be modified.

Afferent and Efferent Pathways. Human lungs are innervated by branches from the right and left vagus nerves and the upper four or five thoracic sympathetic ganglia, all of which contribute fibers to the anterior and posterior pulmonary plexuses at the hilum of each lung. As the bronchi, arteries, and veins enter the lungs, they carry with them extensions of the plexus. Ramifying nerve fibers continue to invest airways and blood vessels as they subdivide within the lungs.

A schematic summary of the presumed innervation of the human airways is presented in Figure 12.

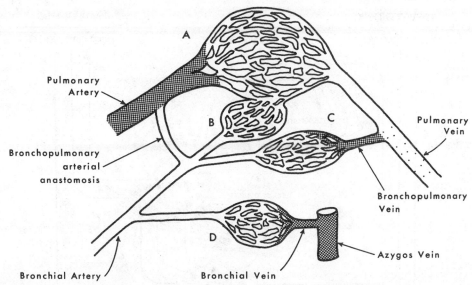

Figure 11. Schematic representation of the relationships between the bronchial and pulmonary circulations. The pulmonary artery supplies the pulmonary capillary network A. The bronchial artery supplies capillary networks B, C, and D. Network B represents the bronchial capillary supply to bronchioles that anastomoses with pulmonary capillaries and drains through pulmonary veins. Network C represents the bronchial capillary supply to most bronchi; these vessels form bronchopulmonary veins that empty into pulmonary veins. Network D represents the bronchial capillary supply to lobar and segmental bronchi; these vessels form true bronchial veins that drain into the azygos, hemiazygos, or intercostal veins. (From Murray, J. F.: The Normal Lung. Philadelphia, W. B. Saunders Co., 1976, p. 42.)

Preganglionic parasympathetic fibers, which descend in the vagus nerves and travel through the pulmonary plexus, terminate in ganglia situated along the course of conducting airways. The ganglia are composed of excitatory cholinergic neurons and inhibitory nonadrenergic neurons. Other neurons with an integrative function are probably also present as well as glial cells. Postganglionic fibers to the smooth muscle cells are either excitatory or inhibitory. Nonmyelinated efferent fibers have been followed to the smooth musculature of all divisions of conducting airways and respiratory bronchioles and even to alveolar ducts in which the filaments terminate in a small band of smooth muscle. Excitatory fibers seem also to terminate in the glands to cause discharge of their contents. Sympathetic postganglionic fibers also terminate on the ganglia, the smooth muscle mass, and probably the glands. Parasympathetic innervation seems to predominate over sympathetic innervation.

Sensory afferent endings are present within the epithelium and the underlying collection of smooth muscle cells; neurons associated with these endings may lie in the vagus nerve itself or the vagal nuclei. The smooth muscle cells (Fig. 12) may be connected by low resistance junctions, such as the nexus, that allow the muscle mass to function in concert like a syncytium.

Nerve fibers that appear to be of sympathetic origin lie within the walls of pulmonary artery branches, including arterioles as small as 30 μm and, in rare instances, even pulmonary capillaries. These fibers presumably do not innervate endothelial cells but may form connections with adjacent pericytes. The arrangement of parasympathetic nerves within the pulmonary circulation is even less well known and probably less extensive. It has not been possible to demonstrate any influences mediated by the autonomic nervous system on the pulmonary circulation of spontaneously breathing, normal human adults.

Postganglionic nerves control the caliber of the conducting airways, the volume of terminal respiratory units, the activity of bronchial glands, and the tone and diameter of pulmonary blood vessels. Thus, efferent fibers mediate vital responses that may affect the adequacy of gas exchange by regulating the distribution of ventilation and perfusion and contribute to the defense of the lungs and body against injury from inhaled substances.

A third member of the autonomic nervous system, besides its sympathetic and parasympathetic components, is known as the nonadrenergic, or purinergic, nervous system. The lungs are supplied with purinergic nerve fibers although the extent of the distribution is not known. Activation of purinergic pathways seems to cause smooth muscle spasm, but the contribution of this response to the regulation of airway and vascular tone in humans is not known.

Receptors. The role of pulmonary-based reflexes in the normal control of breathing is considered in the section Normal Physiology of the Respiratory System; their contributions to abnormal breathing patterns and sensations are included in the discussions of various disorders in the section Pathophysiology of the Respiratory System.

STRETCH RECEPTORS. Filaments of myelinated nerves that lie in close association with smooth muscle cells in the walls of airways presumably serve as slowly adapting stretch receptors. When deformed by mechanical changes in airway caliber, activation of these receptors initiates the Hering-Breuer reflex and affects the pattern of breathing.

IRRITANT RECEPTORS. Fine nerve fibers have been observed between superficial cells of the epithelium of large, mainly extrapulmonary, airways. These fila-

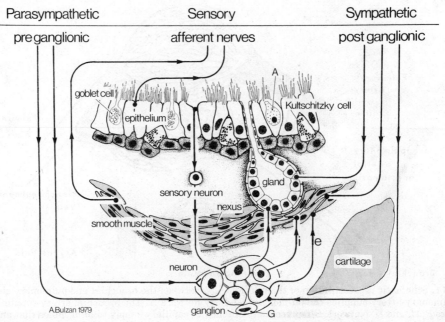

Figure 12. Schematic summary of the innervation of the airways. In the human lung, parasympathetic preganglionic fibers descend into the vagus and terminate in the ganglia. The ganglia contain excitatory neurons that are cholinergic and inhibitory neurons that are nonadrenergic. Other neurons with an integrative function are probably also present. Glial cells (G) are present in the ganglia. Blood vessels and collagen are excluded from the neuropile. Postganglionic fibers to the smooth muscle are excitatory (e) or inhibitory (i). Excitatory fibers may also terminate in the glands. Sensory afferent endings are present in the epithelium and the smooth muscle. The neurons associated with these endings may be in the vagus nerve or in the vagal nuclei. Sensory neurons may also be present in the mucosa, and fibers from these neurons may terminate in the ganglia, as in the gastrointestinal tract. Sympathetic postganglionic fibers terminate on the ganglia in humans and in other species, but adrenergic fibers to the glands or smooth muscle have not been demonstrated in humans although they have been found in some mammals.

In the epithelium, there are cells, such as the Kulchitsky cell and the granular cell (A), which is found only in the chicken, whose functions are unknown. Nerves may be related to these cells. The human airway smooth muscle cells are connected by low resistance junctions, such as the nexus, and these connections may permit the muscle mass to act as a syncytium. (From Richardson, J. B.: Am Rev Respir Dis 119:785, 1979; reprinted by permission of the author and publisher.)

ments are believed to be the rapidly adapting receptors that respond to irritative mechanical and chemical stimuli by producing cough, bronchospasm, and discharge by mucous glands.

C FIBERS. A vast network of unmyelinated nerves, the so-called C fibers, exists in airways and blood vessels in the lungs and other intrathoracic structures. The entire C fiber network responds mainly to chemical stimuli and to some extent to lung inflation by causing bronchial and tracheal constriction, rapid shallow breathing, and a decrease in heart rate.

Virtually all afferent nerve fibers to the central nervous system from receptors in the lungs and airways travel in the vagus nerve. Numerous other signals that affect respiration are transmitted to the central nervous system via afferent nerves that serve extrapulmonary receptors. The structure and function of the most important of these, the chemoreceptors and skeletal muscle proprioceptors, are considered later in the discussion of the Control of Breathing.

Muscles of Respiration

The final effectors of breathing are the muscles of respiration. Contraction of certain muscle groups enlarges the thorax, whereas contraction of other groups compresses it. The thorax is that part of the body between the neck and abdomen and includes the proximal parts of the shoulders as well as the bones and soft tissues of the chest wall that overlie the lungs; expansion and compression of the thoracic cavity normally cause air to flow into and out of the lungs. The thorax is encased by a bony framework of ribs that is shaped like a truncated cone.

Diaphragm. The diaphragm separates the thoracic cavity from the abdominal cavity and is the main source of inspiratory muscle force. Its muscle fibers vary in length; they are longest in the posterolateral portion, where the greatest muscular excursion takes place. The diaphragm is normally perforated near its center by separate openings, each called a hiatus, for the aorta, inferior vena cava, and esophagus. Each of these areas of potential weakness can be the site of a hernia of abdominal contents into the thorax.

The phrenic nerve, the sole motor nerve to the diaphragm, arises in the neck from the fourth cervical nerve and is joined by branches from the third and often from the fifth cervical segments. The phrenic nerves pierce the diaphragm and send the terminal branches to its inferior surface.

The sensory innervation of the diaphragm is chiefly by the two phrenic nerves, except for the outermost perimeter, which is supplied by branches from the sixth to twelfth thoracic segmental nerves. Free sensory endings and pacinian corpuscles have been identified throughout the diaphragm. In contrast to the intercostal muscles, however, the concentration of muscle spindles and tendon organs in the diaphragm is very low.

Intercostal and Accessory Muscles. Between the ribs lie two bands of muscles, the external and internal intercostal muscles. The external intercostal muscles extend from the articulations between the ribs and vertebral bodies to the origin of the costal cartilages. In contrast, the internal intercostal muscles extend from the sternum to the angles of the ribs. Whether the external intercostal muscles and the internal intercostal muscles have selective inspiratory and expiratory functions, respectively, or whether all the intercostal muscles are inspiratory at low and mid lung volumes and all become expiratory at high lung volumes has not been finally established.

Internal and external intercostal muscles receive their motor and sensory innervation from the intercostal nerves, which arise from the first to twelfth thoracic segmental nerves. The lower intercostal nerves, which receive a few sensory branches from the diaphragm, also supply the abdominal muscles. The intercostal muscles are richly supplied with proprioceptors. These receptors are believed to exert an important influence on respiratory muscle activity, which is described in the section on Control of Breathing.

The scalene and sternomastoid muscles are important accessory muscles of inspiration in humans. The scalene muscles, which elevate or fix the first two ribs, are recruited at approximately the same time during inspiration as the intercostal muscles; thus, they may be used at rest and are active during relatively quiet breathing. In contrast, the sternomastoids, which elevate the sternum, are utilized only during strenuous breathing.

Abdominal Muscles. Several muscles of the abdominal wall play a role in breathing. Of these, the rectus, external and internal obliques, and transverse abdominal muscles are the most important; as a group they are considered expiratory.

Breathing

Normal breathing at rest is performed by contraction of the muscles of inspiration, chiefly the diaphragm; when the person is supine, expiration is passive, but when sitting or erect, there is often slight expiratory (abdominal) muscle contribution. As the demands for breathing progressively increase (e.g., during exercise), additional muscles are recruited, both inspiratory (intercostal and accessory muscles) and expiratory (abdominal). In contrast, patients with various lung diseases, in whom the work of breathing may be remarkably increased, often must use their accessory and expiratory muscles at low levels of exercise or even at rest.

Lymphatic Vessels and Lymph Nodes

The lungs are richly supplied with lymphatic capillaries, contain aggregates of lymphocytes located in the bronchioles, and have numerous lymph nodes situated near the hila. The lymphatic system of the lungs plays a vital role in liquid and solute exchange and defense mechanisms of healthy persons. Pulmonary edema and certain pulmonary infections or occupational disorders occur because of failure of or overwhelming of normal lymphatic function.

Lymphatic Vessels. The pulmonary lymphatic system in adult humans consists of two networks: the "superficial" or pleural plexus located within the connective tissue layer of the visceral pleura and the "deep" or peribronchovascular lymphatic plexus surrounding the airways, arteries, and veins and contained within interlobular connective tissue (Fig. 13). Valves are numerous in all lymph channels. The bicuspid valves are placed so that their leaflets direct flow for variable distances on the surface of the lungs in pleural lymphatics, but ultimately most branches enter the lungs, and the bulk of the flow proceeds toward the hilum through interlobular and peribronchovascular vessels.

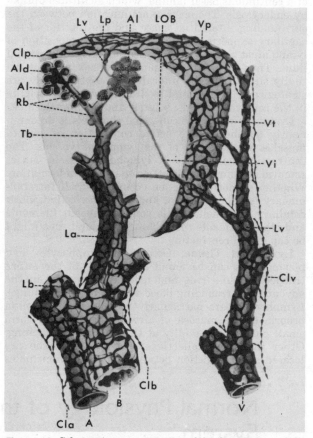

Figure 13. Schematic representation of the distribution of the pulmonary lymphatics. A = pulmonary artery; Al = alveolus; Ald = alveolar duct; B = bronchus; Cla = collecting lymph vessel accompanying pulmonary artery; Clb = collecting lymph vessel accompanying bronchus; Clp = subpleural collecting lymph vessel; Clv = collecting lymph vessel accompanying pulmonary vein; La = periarterial lymphatic plexus; Lb = peribronchial lymphatic plexus; LOB = lobule; Lp = subpleural lymph vessel; Lv = perivenous lymphatic plexus; Rb = respiratory bronchiole; Tb = terminal bronchiole; V = pulmonary vein; Vi = intralobular branch of pulmonary vein; Vp = subpleural branch of pulmonary vein; and Vt = interlobular branch of pulmonary vein. (From Nagaishi, C.: Functional Anatomy and Histology of the Lung. Baltimore, University Park Press, 1972, p. 148; reprinted by permission of the author and publisher.)

Lymphatic capillaries do not exist in the lung parenchyma within the interalveolar septum. However, typical lymphatic channels have been observed *between* adjacent terminal respiratory units, where there is connective tissue, and within the interlobular, pleural, and peribronchovascular connective tissue sheaths. All pulmonary capillaries within the interalveolar septum, from which liquid and solute filtration occurs, are probably within a few 100 μm or, at most, 1 mm of the nearest juxta-alveolar lymphatic. The pulmonary lymphatic capillaries contain numerous anchoring filaments between the external surface of the endothelium and the surrounding interstitium. Adjacent endothelial cell margins overlap extensively with intercellular clefts of varying widths in between. Interstitial liquid presumably enters lymphatic channels through these clefts; another reason that lymphatics are so effective in absorbing liquid may be their lack of a continuous basal lamina, which facilitates uptake by endocytosis. The open communication between the surrounding interstitial space and the interior of the capillary supports the notion that the composition of lymph must be virtually identical to that of interstitial fluid. Thus, although lymphatic vessels are not actually situated in the interalveolar septum, they are strategically located and well designed to participate in the removal of fluids, solutes, and macromolecules.

Lymph flow in large collecting channels is predominantly attributable to active contraction of smooth muscles in the walls of the lymphatic vessels. The contractile mechanism in lymphatic vessels causes removal of lymph in proportion to its rate of formation. Whether or not contraction occurs in small intrapulmonary lymphatics is not known; however, lymphatic capillary endothelial cells contain myosin filaments and other filaments resembling actin, and thus might be capable of contracting.

Lymphoid Tissue. Occasional lymphocytes and plasma cells can be found in the wall of the entire tracheobronchial tree and to a lesser extent in the adventitia surrounding blood vessels in normal lungs. Lymphocytes are particularly notable in the lamina propria of the mucosa of airways, where they form small clusters, especially at the points of branching. Other important collections of lymphoid tissue are located at the junction between terminal bronchioles and respiratory bronchioles. It is believed that the islands of lymphoepithelium in the mucous membrane of conducting airways, the so-called bronchus-associated lymphoid tissue, probably make an important contribution to both antibody-mediated and cell-mediated pulmonary immune responses. These lymphatic aggregations are situated where they appear to favor the traffic of alveolar macrophages during their journeys between interstitial tissue and airway lumen.

Lymph Nodes. Intrapulmonary lymph nodes drain into extrapulmonary nodes in the hilum and along the mediastinum. The patterns of extrapulmonary lymph drainage are complex and occur through a variable maze of interconnecting mediastinal, paratracheal, and subdiaphragmatic lymph channels and nodes.

REFERENCES

Bienenstock, J., McDermott, M. R., and Befus, A. D.: The significance of bronchus-associated lymphoid tissue. Bull Eur Physiopathol Respir 18:153, 1982.

Breeze, R. G., and Wheeldon, E. B.: The cells of the pulmonary airways. Am Rev Respir Dis 116:705, 1977.

Comparative Biology of the Lung. Am Rev Respir Dis 128(Suppl):S1, 1983.

Crapo, J. D., Barry, B. E., Czehr, P., Bachofen, M., and Weibel, E. R.: Cell number and cell characteristics of the normal human being. Am Rev Respir Dis 126:332, 1982.

Gail, D. B., and Lenfant, C. J. M.: Cells of the lung: Biology and clinical implications. Am Rev Respir Dis 127:366, 1983.

Leak, L. V.: Structure of the blood and lymphatic vascular system in the lung. In Witchi, H., and Nettesheim, P. (eds.): Mechanisms in Respiratory Toxicology. Boca Raton, FL, CRC Press, 1981, p. 77.

Murray, J. F.: The Normal Lung: The Basis for the Diagnosis and Treatment of Pulmonary Disease. Philadelphia, W. B. Saunders Co., 1976.

Polgar, G., and Weng, T. R.: The functional development of the respiratory system from the period of gestation to adulthood. Am Rev Respir Dis 120:625–695, 1979.

Richardson, J.: State of the art: Nerve supply to the lungs. Am Rev Respir Dis 119:785–802, 1979.

Thurlbeck, W. M.: Postnatal growth and development of the lung. Am Rev Respir Dis 111:803, 1975.

Weibel, E. R.: Is the lung built reasonably? Am Rev Respir Dis 128:752, 1983.

Weibel, E. R.: The Pathway for Oxygen: Structure and Function in the Mammalian Respiratory System. Cambridge, Harvard University Press, 1984.

Normal Physiology of the Respiratory System

GENERAL CONSIDERATIONS

Respiration was defined earlier as "those processes concerned with gas exchange between an organism and its environment." This definition applies to *all* members of the animal kingdom. The first lungs were merely primitive air sacs with a few blood vessels in the walls that served as accessory organs of gas exchange to supplement the gills. Eons later, as animals grew accustomed to a solely terrestrial life, the lungs became highly compartmentalized to provide the vast air-blood surface necessary for O_2 uptake and CO_2 elimination, and a respiratory control system developed to regulate breathing in accordance with metabolic demands and other needs. The lungs also assumed a variety of other specialized functions to maintain homeostasis, such as the biochemical transformation of circulating substances and the defense of the body, that have little or no connection with gas exchange.

Definitions

The basic processes leading to the uptake of O_2 and the elimination of CO_2 by human beings are usually separated into four functional subdivisions.

Ventilation: The movement of air from outside to inside the body and its distribution within the tracheobronchial system to the gas exchange units of the lungs.

Diffusion: The movement of O_2 and CO_2 across the alveolar-capillary membrane between the gas in alveolar spaces and the blood in pulmonary capillaries.

Blood flow: The movement of mixed venous blood through the pulmonary arterial circulation, its distribution to the capillaries of the gas exchange units, and its removal from the lungs through pulmonary veins.

Control of breathing: The regulation of ventilation to maintain adequate gas exchange, usually in accordance with changing metabolic demands or other special needs.

The first three of these processes are obviously interdependent and their relationship can be understood by remembering that *ventilation* delivers fresh air, and that *blood flow* delivers unoxygenated, CO_2-rich blood to the gas exchange units, where O_2 uptake and CO_2 elimination take place by *diffusion*. The *control of breathing* ensures that normal levels of O_2 and CO_2 are maintained in the bloodstream despite constantly changing metabolic needs.

The mechanisms that contribute to each of these processes and how they are integrated to maintain normal gas exchange are discussed in this section. It is now possible by means of specialized tests of respiratory function to measure the adequacy of the various components of respiration. The most important of these tests, which are referred to in the section on the Pathophysiology of Respiratory Diseases, will be briefly described. Because the lungs have vital physiologic functions besides gas exchange, this section includes discussions about nonrespiratory activities such as liquid and solute exchange, biochemical transformations, and defense mechanisms.

REFERENCES

Bates, D. V., Macklem, P. T., and Christie, R. V.: Respiratory Function in Disease: An Introduction to the Integrated Study of the Lung. 2nd ed. Philadelphia, W. B. Saunders Co., 1971.

Comroe, J. H., Jr., Forster, R. E., II, DuBois, A. B., Briscoe, W. A., and Carlsen, E.: The Lung: Clinical Physiology and Pulmonary Function Tests. 2nd ed. Chicago, Year Book Medical Publishers, 1962.

Comroe, J. H., Jr.: Physiology of Respiration: An Introductory Text. 2nd ed. Chicago, Year Book Medical Publishers, 1974.

Cotes, J.: Lung Function: Assessment and Application in Medicine. 3rd ed. Oxford, Blackwell Scientific Publications, 1975.

Murray, J. F.: The Normal Lung: The Basis for Diagnosis and Treatment of Pulmonary Disease. Philadelphia, W. B. Saunders Co., 1976.

West, J. B.: Respiratory Physiology—The Essentials. Baltimore, Williams and Wilkins, 1974.

VENTILATION

To move air from outside the body into the gas exchange units of the lungs, sufficient force must be exerted to expand the lungs and chest wall and to overcome the resistance and inertia in the system so that air will flow through the tracheobronchial tree. Normally, this force is generated by contraction of the muscles of respiration, but occasionally the force is provided by a mechanical ventilator. In either case, the volume of gas that reaches the individual gas exchange units is determined by the mechanical properties of the lung parenchyma, airways, and chest wall.

Static Properties

Both the lungs and chest wall are distensible structures with elastic properties. They can be viewed as behaving like balloons, because it takes a force to expand them, and when the force is removed, they recoil back to their original volumes. Although the lungs and chest wall are similar in that both are elastic organs, they differ considerably in their resting volumes when there is no expanding force. This means that the lungs and chest wall have different volume-pressure relationships and, conversely, that the volume-pressure relationships of each structure can be used to describe its individual elastic properties. Furthermore, the volume-pressure relationships of the lungs and chest wall account for normal lung volumes in healthy persons as well as abnormal volumes in patients with various respiratory disorders. The subdivisions and terminology used to describe different lung volumes are shown in Figure 14. The most important of these are the following.

Vital capacity (VC): the volume of gas that can be exhaled after a maximal inspiration.

Residual volume (RV): the volume of gas remaining in the lungs at the end of a maximal expiration.

Total lung capacity (TLC): the volume of gas contained in the lungs at the end of a maximal inspiration.

Functional residual capacity (FRC): the volume of gas remaining in the lungs at resting end-expiratory position of the lungs and chest wall.

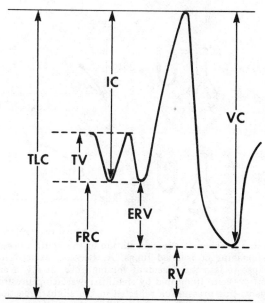

Figure 14. Representative spirometric tracing showing subdivisions of static lung volumes: *TLC* = total lung capacity; *IC* = inspiratory capacity; *TV* = tidal volume; *FRC* = functional residual capacity; *ERV* = expiratory reserve volume; *RV* = residual volume; *VC* = vital capacity. (From Hinshaw, H. C., and Murray, J. F.: Diseases of the Chest. Philadelphia, W. B. Saunders Co., 1979, p. 77.)

Tidal volume (TV): the volume of gas inspired or exhaled during each breath.

Lungs. The static properties of the isolated lungs are shown schematically in Figure 15, in which the lungs are depicted as two collapsible balloons supported by a rigid Y-shaped tube. Because the lungs collapse almost completely, a small amount of pressure is required to expand them with the amount of gas normally present at RV (Fig. 15A). To inflate them further (Fig. 15B), a small amount of additional pressure is required, and the curve describing the volume-pressure relationships (solid line) is relatively steep. Finally, at TLC the lungs are maximally inflated and the volume-pressure curve has flattened. It can be appreciated from the diagrams that the pressure required to inflate the lungs from RV to TLC must be sufficient to overcome the increasing recoil pressure generated by the progressively increasing elastic forces within the stretched components of the lungs.

The total force causing the inflated human lung to recoil inward originates from two quite different sources: part arises from the lung tissue itself and part arises from the film of surface-active material that lines the terminal respiratory units. The two components of elastic recoil can be demonstrated by comparing the volume-pressure relationship of the air-filled lungs with those of the saline-filled lungs. Less pressure is required to inflate the lungs to a given volume, and hysteresis, the difference between the inspiratory

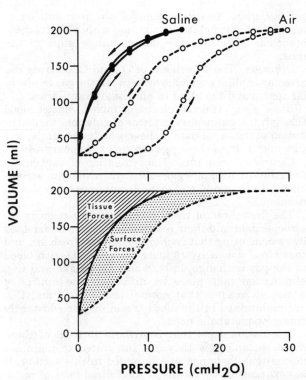

Figure 16. Volume-pressure curves of lungs filled with saline and with air *(upper panel)*. The use of saline eliminates the effect of surface forces at the air-liquid interface and allows subdivision of the total pressure required to inflate the lung into the amounts necessary to overcome tissue forces and surface forces *(lower panel)*. The arrows indicate whether the lung is being inflated or deflated; note that when using saline, hysteresis (that is, the difference between inflation and deflation limbs of the curve) is virtually eliminated. (Adapted from Clements, J. A., and Tierney, D. F.: Handbook of Physiology. Section 3, Respiration. Vol. II. Washington, D.C., American Physiologic Society, 1965, p. 1565; reprinted by permission of the authors and publisher.)

and expiratory curves, is nearly absent when saline is used instead of air (Fig. 16). Filling the lungs with saline eliminates the effect of surface forces at the air-liquid interfaces in the lungs so that the pressure required to inflate the lungs is only that necessary to overcome the tissue forces. The influence of isolated surface-active material on the surface area–surface tension relationships, which are equivalent to volume-pressure relationships, was discussed previously (Fig. 4). A comparison of Figures 16 and 4 also helps to illustrate the contribution of surface forces to the elastic recoil of the lungs.

The elastic fibers are probably responsible for the tissue recoil at low lung volumes and midlung volumes; the flat portion of the volume-pressure curve at high lung volumes is determined by collagen fibers reaching the limits of their distensibility.

Thus the elastic recoil properties of the lungs govern their distensibility or *compliance*. The compliance of the lungs (C_L) is the change in volume (ΔV) produced by a change in distending pressure (ΔP), or

$$C_L = \frac{\Delta V}{\Delta P}.$$

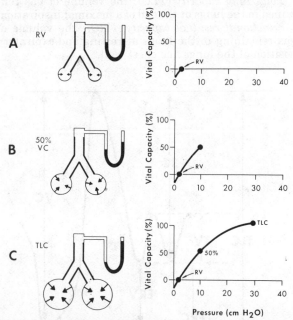

Figure 15. Schematic representation of the volume-pressure relationships of isolated lungs. *A,* Because excised lungs collapse to less than residual volume *(RV)*, at *RV* a small recoil pressure (indicated by small arrows facing inward) is evident; this pressure is reflected in the slight deflection of the column in the manometer and the value on the horizontal (pressure) axis. *B,* At 50 per cent vital capacity *(VC)*, the recoil pressure is increased (more and larger arrows than in *A*); thus more pressure is reflected in the manometer and on the horizontal axis. *C,* At total lung capacity *(TLC),* recoil pressure is maximal (normally about 30 cm H_2O). (From Murray, J. F.: The Normal Lung. Philadelphia, W. B. Saunders Co., 1976, p. 81.)

This relationship means that compliance is also the slope of the volume-pressure curve, which changes as the lungs are inflated (Fig. 15). Compliance is highest near RV, where the volume-pressure curve is steepest, and then progressively decreases because the curve flattens as the lungs are inflated to TLC. To measure compliance, it is necessary to know the distending pressure, known as the *transpulmonary pressure*, "across" the lungs; the transpulmonary pressure is the difference between alveolar pressure, which is the same as atmospheric pressure (or 0 cm H_2O) when a subject holds his breath with his glottis open, and pleural pressure. It is now relatively easy to estimate pleural pressure by measuring pressure in the esophagus through a small catheter with a balloon near its tip that is passed through the nose or mouth. Because the esophagus is located between the two pleural spaces, esophageal pressure measurements provide a close approximation of pleural pressure at the level of the balloon in the thorax. Static volume-pressure (elastic recoil) curves of the lungs are determined by recording esophageal pressure and lung volume while the subject holds his breath at different lung volumes with his glottis open to eliminate the effect of changes in alveolar pressure. Measurements are made first at full inspiration and then at successively decreasing lung volumes to FRC to provide a deflation volume-pressure curve; studies between FRC and residual volume are less reliable because of inaccuracies in the measurement of esophageal pressure at low lung volumes.

Chest Wall. The static properties of the isolated chest wall (including the diaphragm and abdominal contents that must be displaced during breathing) are shown in Figure 17. The chest wall is a compressible and distensible structure that contains an appreciable volume in its resting state. To decrease the volume of the thorax, an increasing force must be applied to overcome the increasing tendency of the chest wall to resist compression and recoil back to its resting position. Conversely, to increase the volume of the thorax, the applied force must overcome the elastic forces in the chest wall that cause it to recoil inward and return to its resting position.

Respiratory System. It is useful to consider the behavior of the lungs and chest wall separately, but obviously they function in concert. Their action is coupled by the pleural pressure that keeps the lungs expanded against the chest wall; in the absence of shifts of blood into and out of the thorax, the lungs and chest wall must each change their volume by exactly the same amount. Thus the pressures required to inflate and deflate the respiratory system (or lungs and chest wall combined) can be derived, as shown in Figure 18, by simply finding on each curve in Figures 15 and 17 the pressures required to achieve a given volume and then adding the pressures together. The solid line in Figure 18 indicates the pressure that must be applied by contraction of the respiratory muscles to change the volume of the thoracic structures from their resting position; in other words, to inflate or deflate the respiratory system, a force must be generated to offset the elastic recoil pressures of both the lungs and chest wall at whatever new volume is achieved.

The concepts concerning recoil are useful because, as will be shown, they explain the origin of lung volumes in healthy subjects and the abnormalities that are found in patients with disease that affects the lungs and/or the chest wall. In addition, the concepts are applied daily in the management of patients with mechanically assisted ventilation. The pressure generated by a ventilator to cause a given volume of gas

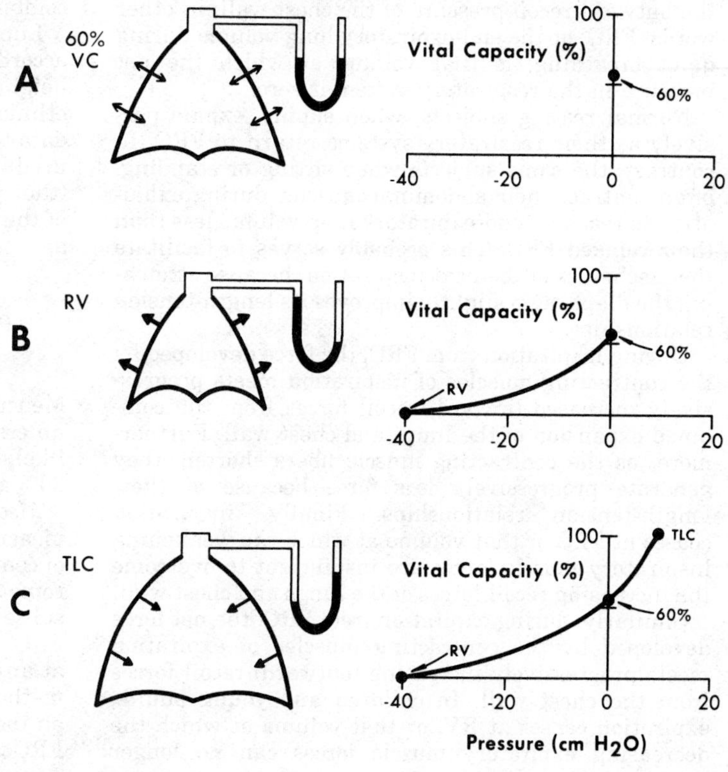

Figure 17. Schematic representation of the volume-pressure relationships of the isolated chest wall. *A,* The chest wall in the relaxed position (zero pressure) has a volume approximately 60 per cent of vital capacity *(VC). B,* When the chest wall is compressed to residual volume *(RV),* it tends to recoil outward to its resting position and thus generates the negative pressure shown on the manometer and horizontal axis. *C,* When the chest wall is expanded to total lung capacity *(TLC),* the chest wall tends to recoil inward and thereby generates the positive pressure shown on the manometer and horizontal axis. (From Murray, J. F.: The Normal Lung. Philadelphia, W. B. Saunders Co., 1976, p. 86.)

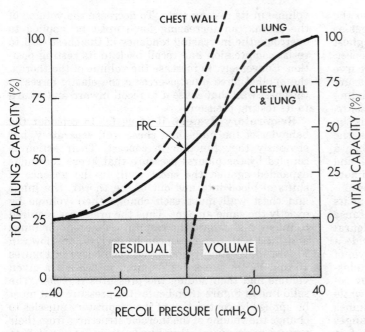

Figure 18. Volume-pressure relationships of the respiratory system (solid line) obtained by adding the recoil pressures of the lungs (hatched line) from Figure 15 and the chest wall (hatched line) from Figure 17. Lung volumes are expressed as per cent of total lung capacity or per cent of vital capacity. FRC = functional residual capacity.

to enter the lungs must be sufficient to overcome the recoil properties of the lungs and chest wall combined. It is now possible with most ventilators to measure the volume being delivered and the pressures at end-inspiration and end-expiration so that respiratory system compliance can be derived; these values, which are discussed more fully in the section on Respiratory Failure, are helpful in adjusting ventilators and in following the course of seriously ill patients.

Lung Volumes. Figure 18 illustrates that FRC occurs at the volume of the system at which the inward recoil pressure of the lungs is equal and opposite to the outward recoil pressure of the chest wall; in other words, FRC, or the end-expiratory lung volume during quiet breathing, is that volume at which the net pressure in the respiratory system is zero.

Normal resting subjects, when supine, exhale passively so their respiratory systems return to FRC. In contrast, the same subjects when sitting or standing, often contract their abdominal muscles during exhalation to reach an end-expiratory lung volume less than their relaxed FRC. This probably serves to facilitate the mechanics of the next inspiration, because stretching the diaphragm slightly improves its length-tension relationships.

During inspiration from FRC, the force developed by the contracting muscles of inspiration meets progressively increased (inward) recoil forces from the combined expansion of the lungs and chest wall. Furthermore, as the contracting muscle fibers shorten, they generate progressively less force because of their length-tension relationships. Finally, inspiration ceases at TLC or that volume at which the weakening inspiratory muscle forces are insufficient to overcome the increasing recoil forces of the lungs and chest wall.

Similarly, during expiration from FRC, the net force developed by the contracting muscles of expiration meets progressively increasing (outward) recoil forces from the chest wall. In children and young adults, expiration ceases at RV, or that volume at which the decreasing expiratory muscle forces can no longer overcome the increasing forces required to compress

the chest wall. In older persons, RV is governed increasingly by factors that regulate the caliber and patency of peripheral airways; thus, even though the expiratory muscles are capable of compressing the chest wall and emptying the lungs more completely, they are prevented from doing so by airway closure and trapping of gas in the lungs.

The VC, or volume between maximum inspiration and expiration, is determined by the factors that influence TLC and RV—in other words, the balance of forces generated by the muscles of respiration and the mechanical properties of the lungs and chest wall combined.

Lung volumes also vary among healthy persons according to age, sex, and body build (especially height). Because body build varies slightly from one ethnic group to another, it is important to have normal data that relate to the population being studied. Measured values are usually expressed as both the observed (that is, actually measured) volume and the per cent of the predicted value for a normal subject of the same age, sex, and height.

$$\text{Per cent predicted} = \frac{\text{Observed value}}{\text{Predicted value}} \times 100$$

Measured values should not be considered abnormal unless they are clearly outside the range of values likely to be found in normal persons (VC = 100 ± 20% and TLC, RV, FRC = 100 ± 25%).

Measurement of lung volumes: the VC is easily measured by means of a spirometer or one of a variety of commercially available recording systems. Most spirometers can also be used to obtain airflow rates (see subsequent discussion), but they do not measure RV, FRC, or TLC. To measure *all* of the gas in the lungs at any of these volumes, one of two basically different methods must be used: either dilution or washout of an inert gas or whole-body plethysmography. Usually, FRC is determined because it is the normal end-expiratory lung volume and an easy volume for a subject to maintain during a test requiring multiple breaths. When FRC is measured, RV is derived by subtracting expiratory reserve volume, and TLC is obtained by adding VC to RV.

(1) Gas dilution or washout involves measurements of the volume and concentration of an inert gas like nitrogen (N_2), neon (Ne), or helium (He). With these methods, just the amount of gas in free communication with the airways during the breathing maneuver is measured; dilution or washout techniques do not detect gas trapped beyond closed (or very narrowed) airways or in poorly communicating regions like bullae.

(2) Another method of measuring FRC is with a body plethysmograph, which is a large, air-tight box resembling a telephone booth. The subject sits in the plethysmograph and breathes through a mouthpiece in which a shutter can be closed to stop the flow of air. When the subject attempts to inhale against the closed shutter, the volume of the thorax changes and expands the gas in the lungs; this lowers the pressure measured inside the mouthpiece. The expansion of the thorax also raises the pressure in the box by compressing the gas surrounding the subject. By applying Boyle's law, which states that the pressure times the volume of a gas is constant if temperature remains the same, FRC can be calculated. The body plethysmograph measures the *total* volume of gas in the thorax during the breathing maneuver, whether in contact with the tracheobronchial system or not, including any gas that may be trapped behind closed airways, sequestered in poorly communicating bullae, or in other spaces (for example, a pneumothorax). Plethysmographs are also used, as described subsequently, to measure airways resistance.

In normal subjects, FRC or TLC measurements by dilution and plethysmographic techniques are virtually identical. In contrast, in patients with obstructed airways or bullous disease, the communicating volume may be considerably less than the plethysmographic volume, and the difference is a measure of the noncommunicating (sometimes called trapped) volume.

Dynamic Properties

To cause air to flow from outside the body into the gas exchange units, a muscular (or other mechanical) force must be exerted to overcome not only the elastic recoil properties of the lungs and chest wall but also their resistive and inertial properties. In contrast to the distensibility of the lungs and chest wall, which are not affected by movement and are measured under static conditions, the forces required to offset resistance and inertia are markedly influenced by the velocity of airflow and hence are dynamic properties. Under normal circumstances, inertial forces are small and usually ignored, but in some patients discussed in the next section (for example, those with obesity-hypoventilation), inertial forces are physiologically important.

Airways Resistance. The resistance (R) to a fluid, either gas or liquid, flowing through a set of tubes like the tracheobronchial tree depends on the pressure difference between the beginning and the end of the tubes (ΔP) and the flow ($\dot{Q}$) through the system, so that

$$R = \frac{\Delta P}{\dot{Q}}.$$

By measuring the appropriate pressure differences with suitable techniques, the resistances of the airways, lungs, lung tissue, and chest wall can all be determined. Of these, airways resistance is most commonly measured, and, according to the above equation, the test requires simultaneous measurements of the flow in the tracheobronchial system and the pressure difference between the mouth and alveolar spaces. Measurements of airflow and mouth pressure are easy to perform; alveolar pressure can be determined by studying patients in a body plethysmograph. Isolated measurements of airways resistance have limited clinical usefulness, but detailed experimental studies have provided valuable pathophysiologic concepts concerning the behavior of the lungs in various disorders. Fortunately, the important dynamic properties of the respiratory system can be assessed by several different tests of airways function, some of which are simple and readily available.

Factors Affecting Airways Resistance. Airways resistance depends on the number, length, and cross-sectional area of the conducting airways. The length of airways varies considerably from person to person, depending on age and body size; airways length also varies within an individual person, depending on the phase of ventilation, lengthening during inspiration as lung volume increases and shortening during expiration. Because resistance to airflow in a given airway changes according to the fourth power of the radius of the airway, the cross-sectional area within the tracheobronchial tree is by far the most important as well as potentially the most variable determinant of airways resistance.

The cross-sectional area of any given intrathoracic airway must be determined by the balance between those forces tending to contract the walls, primarily tension of airway smooth muscle and elastic elements, and those forces providing outward traction on the walls, either from the attached lung parenchyma, in the case of bronchioles, or from pleural pressure, in the case of bronchi. Airways resistance is significantly influenced by the following variables.

Lung Volume. Airways resistance can be shown to vary with changes in lung volume according to the relationship shown in Figure 19 (*top panel*); changes in lung volume above FRC have little effect on airways resistance, but between FRC and RV airways resistance increases rapidly and becomes infinite at RV. The curvilinear relationship between changes in airways resistance and lung volume can be transformed into a nearly linear diagram by plotting the reciprocal of airways resistance, *airways conductance* (Caw = 1/Raw), against lung volume (Fig. 19, *lower panel*). Furthermore, the marked variations in individual values of airways resistance and conductance among children and adults of both sexes, primarily the result of differences in body size, can be reduced if conductance is related to lung volume. This relationship has led to the use of the term *specific airways conductance,* or airways conductance divided by the lung volume at which it was measured. Although it is useful to relate measurements of airways conductance to those of lung volume, the determinant of the relationship between lung volume and airways resistance is the elastic recoil at the given lung volume. Elastic recoil provides the principal distending force that governs airway caliber.

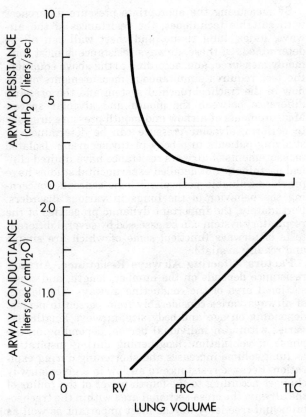

Figure 19. Schematic illustrations of the relationship between airway resistance *(top panel)* and airway conductance *(lower panel)* and lung volume. The hyperbolic resistance-volume curve converts to a straight line when the same data are expressed as conductance-volume.

ELASTIC RECOIL. The elastic recoil properties of the lungs affect airways resistance by influencing the diameter of both bronchioles and bronchi; first, by providing radial traction on bronchioles through direct attachments between the walls and adjacent lung parenchyma; and, second, by being one of the two determinants (alveolar pressure being the other) of intrapleural pressure, which provides the distending pressure surrounding airways enclosed within the bronchovascular sheath. Elastic recoil not only affects the geometry of airways but also provides the driving pressure that governs maximal velocity of airflow.

GEOMETRY OF AIRWAYS. Changes in the geometry of normal bronchi depend not only on the transmural pressure across their walls but also on the distensibility and thickness of the elements composing the walls. Both small and large bronchi increase their diameter about 60 per cent and their length about 40 per cent during inflation from the airless state to TLC. In the absence of smooth muscle tone, virtually all the increase in bronchial diameter is achieved by the time distending pressures of 6 to 10 cm H_2O are reached; higher pressures do not cause much more dilatation. In contrast, bronchial length continues to increase throughout inflation. This means that there is a considerable difference between the volume-pressure relationships of the lungs and the diameter-pressure relationships of the airways. The consequences of this difference are that airways enlarge early during the course of lung inflation and are nearly completely distended at about FRC; thereafter, airways change mainly in length while the lung expands to TLC. This behavior accounts for the flattening of the airways resistance versus lung volume curve (Fig. 19) at volumes above FRC.

There is a small amount of resting smooth muscle tone in the walls of normal airways that serves to narrow their lumen and decrease their distensibility. Administration of bronchodilator drugs to normal subjects causes slight relaxation of bronchial smooth muscle and a corresponding decrease in airways resistance. An increase in smooth muscle tone (that is, bronchospasm) not only narrows the lumen of the airway but also decreases the distensibility of the walls. In addition to bronchospasm, a variety of other pathologic processes can cause substantial narrowing of airways by thickening the walls from cellular infiltration or edema, by secretions in the lumen, or by external compression.

Of all the factors affecting resistance to airflow, the most important is the caliber of the airways. As shown previously in Figure 5, although the diameters of successive generations of airways decrease, their total cross-sectional area increases progressively throughout the tracheobronchial tree from the main bronchi to the peripheral airways. This means that airways resistance steadily decreases from central to peripheral airways and, correspondingly, that most of the resistance of the human tracheobronchial tree resides in large airways. About two thirds of total airways resistance originates in airways *greater than* 2 mm in diameter, so that pathologic processes can decrease the caliber of the small peripheral airways without affecting total airways resistance very much. Hence, these airways have been called the lungs' "quiet zone." Because they are frequently involved early in the evolution of clinically important lung disease, tests have been devised to examine their functional behavior, such as maximal expiratory flow-volume curves breathing air and a mixture of He and O_2 and closing volume (both discussed subsequently).

Tests of Airways Function. Several tests reflect the resistance to airflow within airways. One of the simplest, and certainly the most widely used, is the forced expiratory volume in one second (FEV_1) expressed as a ratio of the forced vital capacity (FVC), or FEV_1/FVC (Fig. 20). To perform the FVC maneuver, the subject inspires maximally and then exhales as rapidly and completely as possible. In normal persons, the FVC equals the VC from a slow or nonexpulsive maneuver, but in patients with airways obstruction, vigorous expiration may cause airways to narrow or close so that the FVC may be less than the VC; the magnitude of the difference between values is a measure of the severity of the phenomenon known as air trapping. The FEV_1/FVC decreases with age in normal persons after reaching adulthood and is usually higher in women than in men.

Additional indexes of airways resistance besides the FEV_1 can also be obtained from the recording of an FVC maneuver (Fig. 20). Several derivatives of time, such as (1) the $FEV_{0.5}$ and FEV_3 (the subscript denoting the number of seconds at which the expired volume is measured) and (2) the maximal mid-expiratory flow rate (MMFR or often $MMFR_{25-75\%}$ to indicate that the

Figure 20. Schematic representation of a normal forced vital capacity *(FVC)* maneuver (expired volume against time, heavy line) and the derivation of several variables commonly used to evaluate airway obstruction. $MEFR_{200-1200}$ = maximal expiratory flow rate, measured between expired volumes of 200 and 1200 ml; $MMFR_{25-75}$ = maximal mid-expiratory flow rate, measured between 25 per cent and 75 per cent of the total *FVC*; FEV_1 = forced expiratory volume in 1 second, expressed as percentage of total FVC; and FEV_3 = forced expiratory volume in 3 seconds expressed as percentage of total FVC. (From Murray, J. F.: Respiratory structure and function. In Wyngaarden, J. B., and Smith, L. H., Jr. (eds.): Cecil Textbook of Medicine. 17th ed. Philadelphia, W. B. Saunders Co., 1985, p. 374.)

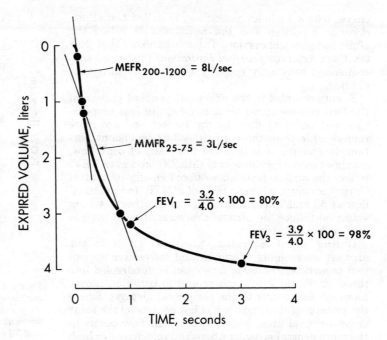

rate was measured between expired volumes of 25 and 75 per cent of the FVC), are used. None of these has any particular advantage over the FEV_1, which is by far the most widely used, except that the MMFR, for reasons to be described, is less dependent on the effort exerted by the subject than the other variables and reflects the behavior of small as well as large airways.

Another way of recording the events during an FVC maneuver is to plot flow against expired volume to provide a maximal expiratory flow-volume curve (Fig. 21). From these records, peak flow and maximal flow rates at any given expired volume, usually 50 per cent ($\dot{V}max_{50}$) or 75 per cent ($\dot{V}max_{75}$), can be determined and reported as the percentage of the predicted values

for a subject of the same age, sex, and body size. Flow-volume curves can also be used to demonstrate the effect of changes in expiratory effort on expiratory flow rates (Fig. 22). If the subject makes a weak effort, the curve shown by dashed line A in Figure 22 is produced; progressively increasing efforts result in curves B and C, respectively. Finally, a maximal effort produces the curve shown by the solid line (Fig. 22). The family of curves demonstrates two important consequences of the behavior of airways: (1) increasing expiratory efforts cause progressively higher peak flows early in expiration, and (2) despite increasing efforts, the flow rates late in expiration are all the same. Thus the early segment of the maximal expiratory flow-volume

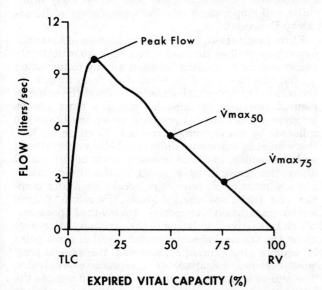

Figure 21. Representative forced expiratory flow-volume tracing of a normal adult man showing points of peak flow, maximal flow at 50 per cent expired vital capacity *($\dot{V}max_{50}$)*, and maximal flow at 75 per cent expired vital capacity *($\dot{V}max_{75}$)*. *TLC* = total lung capacity; *RV* = residual volume.

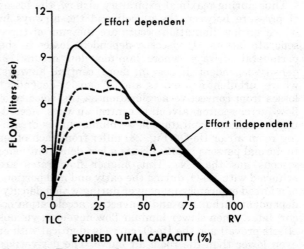

Figure 22. Expiratory flow-volume curves demonstrating the effect of varying degrees of effort: dashed lines *A, B,* and *C* represent increasing efforts; solid outer line represents maximal effort. The early effort-dependent and later effort-independent segments are shown. *TLC* = total lung capacity; *RV* = residual volume. (From Hinshaw, H. C., and Murray, J. F.: Diseases of the Chest. Philadelphia, W. B. Saunders Co., 1979, p. 87.)

curve, which includes peak flow, is called the effort-*dependent* portion and the remainder is called the effort-*independent* portion. The mechanisms that govern these expiratory *airflow limitations* (discussed subsequently) have only recently been satisfactorily explained.

Events recorded in the effort-independent portion of the flow-volume curve obviously require less cooperation and understanding by the subject and are more reproducible than those in the effort-dependent portion. In general, it is believed that tests of peak flow, maximal expiratory flow rate (MEFR), and even FEV_1 reflect the airflow resistance offered chiefly by central "large" airways, whereas tests of MMFR and maximal flow at 50 and 75 per cent of VC (or at other low lung volumes) reflect the airflow characteristics of peripheral or "small" airways.

During forced expiration, pressure is lost in the airways overcoming frictional and convective opposition to airflow. *Frictional losses* can be subdivided into those attributable to laminar and to turbulent flows. Laminar flow occurs in the peripheral airways, where the velocity of the airstream is low because of the large cross-sectional area, whereas turbulent flow occurs in the more central airways where the velocities are high because the cross-sectional area is small. Losses of pressure in laminar flow are independent of the density but dependent on the viscosity of the gas. In contrast, losses of pressure in turbulent flow are dependent on the density and largely independent of the viscosity of the gas being breathed. *Convective acceleration* refers to the acceleration of gas molecules as they flow from the peripheral branches of the tracheobronchial tree, in which the total cross-sectional area is large and the velocity is low, through the more central airways, where the cross-sectional area is much smaller and the velocity considerably higher. The pressure losses required to produce convective acceleration are, like losses from turbulence, dependent on the density, not the viscosity, of the gas involved.

Thus during maximal expiratory airflow, the losses of pressure between the alveoli and the airways in which airflow limitation occurs are the sum of three separate factors: (1) viscosity-dependent losses in the peripheral airways, where laminar flow occurs; (2) density-dependent losses in more central airways, where turbulent flow exists; and (3) density-dependent losses from convective acceleration as the velocity of flow increases from alveoli to central airways. Accordingly, maximal expiratory flow-volume curves breathing room air or He-O_2 (Fig. 23) differ from each other in normal persons because He is a less dense but more viscous gas than N_2. Thus higher flow rates are achieved with He-O_2 during the early and mid portions of a forced expiratory maneuver during which density-dependent turbulence and convective acceleration occur; later, when slower laminar flow develops, viscous effects prevail and the He-O_2 curve is identical with or even lower than the room air curve. The derivatives that are used to compare He-O_2 with room air maximal expiratory flow-volume curves are also shown in Figure 23. Normally, as indicated, flow rates are higher breathing He-O_2 than room air throughout most of expiration; differences in flows are measured at 50 per cent ($\Delta \dot{V}max_{50}$) and 75 per cent ($\Delta \dot{V}max_{75}$) of expired

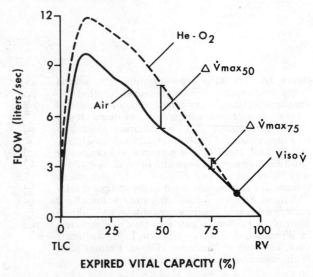

Figure 23. Forced expiratory flow-volume curves from a normal subject breathing air (solid line) and 79 per cent He and 21 per cent O_2 (He-O_2, dashed line). The difference in maximal flows at expired vital capacity values of 50 per cent ($\Delta \dot{V}max_{50}$) and 75 per cent ($\Delta \dot{V}max_{75}$) and the volume at which the curves converge ($Viso_{\dot{v}}$) are shown. TLC = total lung capacity; RV = residual volume. (From Hinshaw, H. C., and Murray, J. F.: Diseases of the Chest. Philadelphia, W. B. Saunders Co., 1979, p. 88.)

VC. The volume at which the two curves intersect is the $Viso_{\dot{v}}$.

In the presence of narrowing of peripheral airways, turbulence and convective acceleration are less prominent so the He-O_2 curve is closer to the room air curve than it should be; this means that $\Delta \dot{V}max_{50}$ and $\Delta \dot{V} max_{75}$ decrease and $Viso_{\dot{v}}$ increases. Comparison of He-O_2 and room air maximal expiratory flow-volume curves may be a useful test for evaluating residual abnormalities in asymptomatic patients with bronchial asthma and for detecting the presence of early bronchitis and emphysema (see Pathophysiology of Respiratory Diseases).

Flow Limitation. The basic mechanism of maximal expiratory airflow limitation has been quantitatively recognized as a coupling between airway compression on the one hand, and pressure drop from airflow on the other. Peribronchial pressure is about the same as pleural pressure, but alveolar pressure must always be greater than pleural pressure (when the lungs are inflated) by elastic recoil pressure. To cause airflow, there must be a pressure difference between the alveoli and the mouth, and this pressure must be dissipated along the airways as a result of the three factors already mentioned: convective acceleration and laminar and turbulent energy losses. Therefore, during forced expiration, bronchial *transmural* pressure, which is positive or dilating in the periphery, decreases along the tracheobronchial system until at some point it becomes zero; thereafter, bronchial transmural pressure becomes negative—or compressive—centrally. The site at which the pressures inside and outside the airway are the same is the equal pressure point, shown schematically in Figure 24. The explanation for flow limitation is that any effort-induced increase in pleural pressure decreases bronchial transmural pressure and

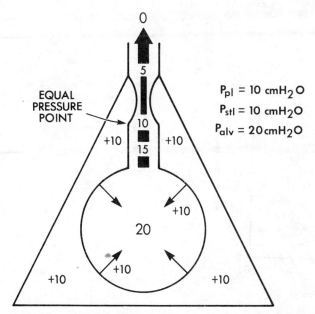

$P_{pl} = 10 \text{ cmH}_2\text{O}$

$P_{stl} = 10 \text{ cmH}_2\text{O}$

$P_{alv} = 20 \text{ cmH}_2\text{O}$

Figure 24. Schematic diagram of the equal pressure point concept. At a particular lung volume during forced expiration, pleural pressure *(Ppl)* = 10 cm H_2O and static recoil pressure *(Pstl)* = 10 cm H_2O; the sum of these pressures, alveolar pressure *(Palv)* = 20 cm H_2O, is the driving pressure that is dissipated as air flows along the airway to the mouth, where the pressure is zero. Accordingly, there must be a point along the airway at which the pressures inside and outside the wall are the same—the equal pressure point. Downstream (toward the mouth) from the equal pressure point, the airway is compressed because the pressure surrounding it is greater than the pressure in the lumen.

airway cross-sectional area just enough to compensate for the increased pressure difference driving the flow.

A major step toward defining the physical forces that govern airflow limitation was introduced by examining how the variables that affect wave speed apply to the respiratory system. The wave speed theory states that the airways, like other systems, cannot accommodate an airflow faster than the speed at which pressures will propagate along the airways. The velocity at which pressures will propagate in a given system is called the wave speed. The pertinent wave speed is that at which a small disturbance travels in a compliant tube filled with fluid. In the circulation, this is the speed at which the pulse propagates in arteries. In the airways, wave speed is faster than in the circulation because air is less dense than blood. In addition to the density of the fluid, wave speed depends on the cross-sectional area of the tubes and the compliance of their walls.

At low expiratory airflows, wave speed is high (cross-sectional area is great and the airways are stiff); as airflow increases, wave speed decreases because cross-sectional area decreases and compliance increases. Finally, an airflow is reached that equals the local wave speed, and flow limitation occurs; the location at which limitation occurs is called the choke point. Further increases in driving pressure serve only to narrow the airways downstream (i.e., toward the mouth) from the choke point and thus have no influence on the velocity of airflow.

When these considerations are used to model the behavior of the respiratory system, maximal expiratory

airflow limitation can be described quite accurately, especially at high and mid lung volumes. At low lung volumes, predicted airflow velocities are higher than those observed, presumably because viscosity-dependent forces begin to prevail over density-dependent forces.

Distribution of Ventilation

An essential corollary to the bulk movement of air from outside the body into the lungs is the partition of the airstream as it moves through the tracheobronchial system to the terminal respiratory units where gas exchange takes place. Inspired air and incoming pulmonary capillary blood must both be distributed in relation to each other for optimal gas exchange to occur. However, ventilation is not distributed uniformly even in normal lungs, and marked derangements may develop in the presence of lung disease.

The unevenness of ventilation in healthy persons occurs because of the vertical gradient of pleural pressure that exists between the uppermost and lowermost regions of the lungs. The origins of the vertical gradient are complex and include the weight of the lung, its attachments at the hilum, and the shape and effects of the chest wall and abdominal contents. Among the consequences of the gradient are differences in the size of alveoli throughout the lungs (larger at the top than at the bottom) and regional differences in the distribution of inspired ventilation (Fig. 25).

When a person breathes normally from FRC in the upright position, more inspired air is distributed to the basilar portions of the lungs than to the apexes. This occurs because the regional differences in pleural pressure cause the apex and base to function on different segments of the same volume-pressure curve (Fig. 25A). Because the *change* in intrapleural pressure during quiet breathing is the same throughout the pleural space, the lower regions inflate more than the upper because they are operating on a steeper part of the curve. When inspiration continues to TLC, alveoli at the top and bottom of the lung are inflated to nearly the same size because, even though the pleural pressure difference persists, both regions are now functioning on the flat portion of the volume-pressure curve (middle panel). During expiration from FRC to RV (lower panel), pleural pressure surrounding the most dependent portion of the lung becomes positive and this causes airways in that region to close. As exhalation continues, closure moves progressively up the lung and involves more and more airways.

Closing Volume. Regional differences in filling and emptying underlie the test of closing volume, which also examines the adequacy of the distribution of ventilation. The test for closing volume is carried out by labeling alveolar gas by one of two methods: bolus or resident gas techniques. With either technique, alveoli in the uppermost regions contain a higher concentration of the label than those in the lowermost regions. With the most commonly used method, the subject inhales a single breath of 100 per cent O_2 from RV to TLC. Because alveoli at the top of the lungs are larger than those at the bottom at RV and because both fill to nearly the same volume at TLC (Fig. 25), the resident N_2 within alveoli at the beginning of the breath is diluted with varying amounts of O_2 such that the concentration of N_2 at the end of the breath is

FUNCTIONAL RESIDUAL CAPACITY

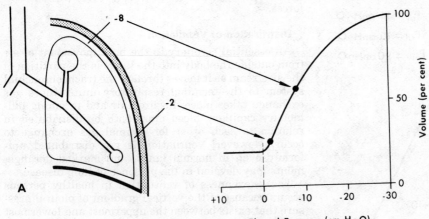

A

TOTAL LUNG CAPACITY

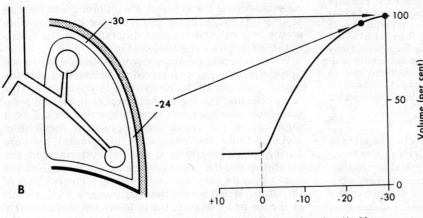

B

RESIDUAL VOLUME

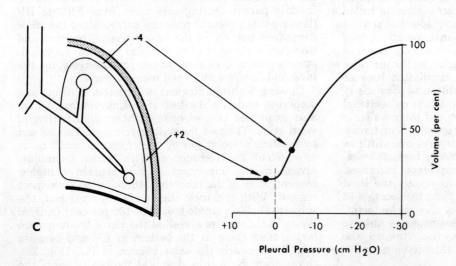

C

Figure 25. Schematic representation of the effects of the pleural pressure gradient on alveolar size and airways caliber at functional residual capacity *(A)*, total lung capacity *(B)*, and residual volume *(C)*. The right portion of each panel shows a normal volume-pressure curve and the positions on the curve at which the various lung units are operating. For further discussion, see text. (From Hinshaw, H. C., and Murray, J. F.: Diseases of the Chest. Philadelphia, W. B. Saunders Co., 1979, p. 90.)

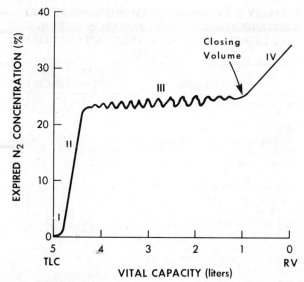

Figure 26. Representative tracing of the measurement of closing volume by the single-breath oxygen (resident gas) method. Measurement of expired N_2 concentration at the mouth during exhalation from total lung capacity *(TLC)* to residual volume *(RV)* yields a tracing with four phases (I to IV) described in text. Closing volume is in the junction of phases III and IV. Cardiogenic oscillations are shown during phase III (the alveolar plateau).

higher at the top than at the bottom. Accordingly, a recording of the N_2 concentration, measured at the mouth during a slow exhalation back to RV, should resemble the tracing shown in Figure 26. The changing N_2 concentrations demonstrate four phases of emptying: Phase I reflects the composition of gas from the tracheobronchial system and contains only O_2 and no N_2; the concentration of N_2 rapidly rises during phase II because airway and alveolar gases are mixing; a near-plateau with cardiogenic oscillations is evident in phase III as alveoli throughout the lung empty; finally, the plateau is abruptly terminated by a steep rise in concentration during phase IV. Closing volume is the junction between phases III and IV and is that volume at which airways in the dependent regions of the lungs are believed to close so that the concentration of the test gas in the expirate indicates the progressively increasing contributions of the preferentially labeled alveoli in the upper regions of the lungs.

Closing volume may be expressed as per cent of measured VC or, if RV is known, as *closing capacity* in liters; closing capacity equals closing volume plus RV. Of the two, closing capacity seems to be the more sensitive method for the early detection of pathologic abnormalities.

Because an increase in closing volume or closing capacity reflects premature closure of pathologically narrowed airways, increased values occur, as expected, in patients with lung disorders in which the patency of peripheral airways is compromised by either decreased elastic recoil (for example, in emphysema) or abnormalities of the airways themselves (for example, in bronchitis or asthma). Furthermore, changes in closing volume have been observed as an early manifestation of lung disease in asymptomatic patients. In addition, the slope of phase III is also useful in the

early detection of lung disease because it provides a sensitive measure of the evenness of the distribution of ventilation. Well-ventilated units fill and empty more completely and rapidly than poorly ventilated units; this means that the concentration of N_2 will be lower in the better ventilated regions that empty earlier during exhalation than poorly ventilated regions. Thus the more uneven the distribution of ventilation within the lungs, the steeper is the slope of phase III.

Single-Breath O_2 Test. The factors that govern the slope of phase III are basically the same as those that underlie the single-breath O_2 test for the distribution of ventilation. In the single-breath O_2 test, the slope of the alveolar plateau between expired volumes of 750 ml and 1250 ml is measured from the tracing and reported as the increase in N_2 concentration, expressed as per cent. Normal values are less than 2.5 per cent.

Tests Using Radioactive Gases. Other tests of the distribution of ventilation take advantage of the gamma ray–emitting properties of certain radioactive gases, chiefly ^{133}Xe, that are nontoxic and can be detected by external counters. The distribution of ventilation can be assessed in two different ways: by counting the isotope distributed over the lungs during a breath hold at end-inspiration after inhaling a single breath containing ^{133}Xe or by counting the isotope distributed over the lungs at intervals during the elimination of ^{133}Xe through quiet breathing of room air after the lungs are initially labeled uniformly by rebreathing the isotope from a closed system.

REFERENCES

Bachofen, H., Gehr, P., and Weibel, E. R.: Alterations of mechanical properties and morphology in excised rabbit lungs rinsed with a detergent. J Appl Physiol 47:1002–1010, 1979.

Gil, J., Bachofen, H., Gehr, P., and Weibel, E. R.: Alveolar volume-surface area relation in air- and saline-filled lungs fixed by vascular perfusion. J Appl Physiol 47:990–1001, 1979.

Hoppin, F. G., Green, M., and Morgan, M. S.: Relationship of central and peripheral airway resistance to lung volume in dogs. J Appl Physiol 44:728, 1978.

Hyatt, R. E.: Expiratory flow limitation. J Appl Physiol 55:1, 1983.

Macklem, P. T.: Respiratory mechanics. Annu Rev Physiol 40:157, 1978.

McCarthy, D. S., Spencer, R., Green, R., and Milic-Emili, J.: Measurement of "closing volume" as a simple and sensitive test for early detection of small airway disease. Am J Med 52:747, 1972.

Menkes, H. A., and Traystman, R. J.: Collateral ventilation. Am Rev Respir Dis 116:287, 1977.

West, J. B. (ed.): Regional Differences in the Lung. New York, Academic Press, 1977.

PULMONARY BLOOD FLOW

The chief function of the pulmonary circulation is to deliver blood in a thin film to the gas exchange units so that O_2 uptake and CO_2 elimination can occur. The physiologic determinants of pulmonary blood flow are analogous to those of ventilation in that regulating mechanisms govern the total volumes of both ventilation and blood flow to meet metabolic needs and that the distribution of ventilation and blood flow within the lungs is such that proportionate amounts of inspired fresh air and incoming mixed venous blood are delivered to individual gas exchange units. Ventilatory volume is controlled by the factors that regulate breathing (see subsequent discussion), whereas the volume of blood flowing through the lungs is determined mainly by the extrapulmonary mechanisms that govern cardiac output.

Ventilation is distributed within the lungs, as just described, by regional differences of pleural pressure and by local factors affecting airways resistance and parenchymal distensibility. Although the distribution of ventilation in normal persons is uneven in that there is more ventilation to the dependent than the superior regions, the distribution of perfusion is even more nonuniform. Regional blood flow is determined chiefly by the vertical gradient of pulmonary arterial pressure, which varies considerably, whereas regional ventilation is determined by the vertical gradient of pleural pressure, which also varies but not nearly as much.

Pulmonary Hemodynamics

The lungs normally "accept" the entire output of blood from the right ventricle, exchange CO_2 and O_2 between blood and alveolar gas, and return the "arterialized" blood to the left ventricle for distribution to the rest of the body. Although blood flow to the lungs is higher than that to any other organ, the pressure within the pulmonary circulation is low; pulmonary arterial pressure is approximately one fifth that within systemic arteries. Not only is the pulmonary circulation a high flow–low pressure system at rest, but it can also accommodate increases in cardiac output during exercise up to several times resting values with only a small increase in pulmonary arterial pressure. This means that pulmonary vascular resistance is low to begin with and decreases even further when pulmonary blood flow increases. A comparison of the pulmonary and systemic circulations in a normal subject at rest and during exercise is presented in Table 2.

By means of a small flexible catheter with a balloon at its tip (Swan-Ganz catheter), one can measure pressure in the pulmonary artery and obtain an estimate of the pressure in the left atrium (the "wedge" pressure). This method has proved of great value in studying patients in pulmonary function laboratories and in monitoring seriously ill patients in critical care units. Cardiac output can be measured relatively easily, either by applying the Fick principle or by the indicator dilution technique, and, when combined with measurements of pulmonary vascular pressures, the total resistance to blood flow in the pulmonary circulation can be calculated. Vascular resistance is determined from the same general equation used to compute airflow resistance ($R = \Delta P \div \dot{Q}$); in the case of pulmonary vascular resistance (PVR), inflow and outflow pressures are pulmonary arterial (PPA) and left atrial (PLA) pressures, respectively, and flow through the system is cardiac output ($\dot{Q}$):

$$PVR = \frac{P_{PA} - P_{LA}}{\dot{Q}}.$$

TABLE 2. COMPARISON OF PULMONARY AND SYSTEMIC HEMODYNAMIC VARIABLES DURING REST AND EXERCISE OF MODERATE SEVERITY IN NORMAL ADULT MAN*

CONDITION	REST (SITTING)	EXERCISE (BICYCLING)
Oxygen consumption, ml/min	300	2000
Blood flow		
Cardiac output, liters/min	6.3	16.2
Heart rate, beats/min	70	135
Stroke volume, ml/beat	90	120
Intravascular pressures		
Pulmonary arterial pressure, mm Hg	20/10	30/11
Mean, mm Hg	14	20
Left atrial pressure (mean), mm Hg	8	10
Brachial arterial pressure, mm Hg	120/70	155/78
Mean, mm Hg	88	112
Right atrial pressure (mean), mm Hg	5	1
Resistances		
Pulmonary vascular resistance, units†	0.95	0.62
Systemic vascular resistance, units†	13.2	6.9

*From Murray, J. F.: The Normal Lung. Philadelphia, W. B. Saunders Co., 1976.
†Units = mm Hg/liters/min.

Pulmonary vascular resistance may be increased or decreased by either "passive" or "active" factors that affect the caliber of blood vessels (Table 3). These are important in the pathogenesis of pulmonary hypertension and cor pulmonale (see Pathophysiology of Respiratory Disease).

Changes in pressures within or surrounding pulmonary blood vessels, shifts of blood into and out of the lungs, and changes in whole blood viscosity all cause *passive* changes in pulmonary vascular resistance; the word passive is used to indicate that the change in caliber of the vessels is not caused by active contraction or relaxation of the smooth muscles. Pulmonary arteries and veins contain smooth muscles, and *active* vasoconstriction or vasodilatation may occur under the influence of neurogenic activity, humoral substances, or chemical stimuli. Undoubtedly, the most important of the active stimuli that cause pulmonary arterial vasoconstriction is alveolar hypoxia. This mechanism provides a useful compensatory response to the presence of local disorders (for example, airway narrowing from bronchospasm or secretions) that impair ventilation to a given region of the lung. When ventilation is decreased, alveolar hypoxia results, which, in turn, causes pulmonary arterial vasoconstriction; by this means, blood flow is shifted away from less well ventilated to better ventilated regions of the lungs, and the overall matching of ventilation and perfusion is restored toward normal. The result of this compensatory mechanism is an improvement in gas exchange.

Distribution of Pulmonary Blood Flow

In normal persons blood flow is greatest to the dependent regions of the lung, where pulmonary arterial pressure is highest, and conversely, blood flow is least to the superior regions, where pulmonary

TABLE 3. PASSIVE AND ACTIVE FACTORS THAT AFFECT PULMONARY VASCULAR RESISTANCE (PVR) AND THE DIRECTION OF THE RESPONSES

	RESPONSE
Passive Factors	
Pulmonary arterial pressure (PPA)	Increasing PPA decreases PVR
Left atrial pressure (PLA)	Increasing PLA decreases PVR
Perivascular interstitial pressure (PIS)	Increasing PIS increases PVR
Lung volume	Increasing or decreasing lung volume from FRC increases PVR*
Pulmonary blood volume	Shifting blood from systemic to pulmonary vessels decreases PVR
Whole blood viscosity	Increasing viscosity increases PVR
Active Factors	
Neurogenic stimuli	
Sympathetic activity	Increases PVR in experimental animals; no effect in man
Parasympathetic activity	No effect
Humoral substances	
Catecholamines, histamine, angiotensin, serotonin, prostaglandin F	Increase PVR
Acetylcholine, bradykinin, prostaglandin E, phentolamine	Decrease PVR
Chemical stimuli	
Alveolar hypoxia	Increases PVR
Acidemia	Increases PVR
Alveolar hypercapnia	Increases PVR in experimental animals; no effect in man

*FRC = functional residual capacity.

arterial pressure is lowest. In upright lungs under resting conditions the apexes are barely perfused, and there is considerably more blood flow per unit lung volume to the lower than to the upper regions. The presence of nonuniform blood flow, which is not matched by comparable changes in the distribution of ventilation, leads to important differences between regions of the lung in their defense capabilities and adequacy of gas exchange.

A model of the lung (Fig. 27) has been developed that accounts for the pattern of the distribution of blood flow. The lung can be divided into zones according to the relationships among alveolar pressure (Palv), pulmonary arterial pressure (PPA), and pulmonary

venous (PPV) or left atrial pressure. In Figure 27, pulmonary arterial pressure is insufficient to raise blood high enough to perfuse the uppermost region of the lung; furthermore, pulmonary capillaries are depicted as being collapsed because the alveolar pressure surrounding them exceeds both pulmonary arterial and venous pressures (Palv > PPA > PPV). These conditions define zone 1, the region of no blood flow.

Blood flow begins in zone 2 at the level at which the hydrostatic effect of the pressure in the pulmonary artery is first "felt"; blood flow increases steadily below this level because pulmonary arterial pressure increases progressively. Thus the conditions in zone 2, which have been likened to a waterfall, are that

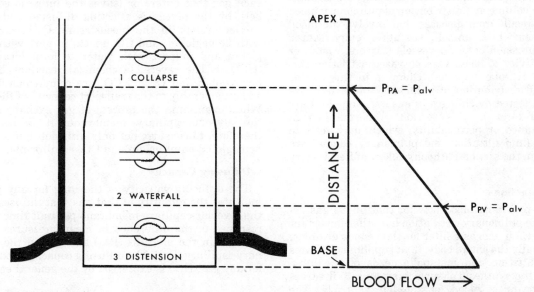

Figure 27. Schematic representation of the three zones of the lung in which different hemodynamic conditions govern blood flow. Alveolar pressure *(Palv)* is assumed to be 0; the heights of the columns on the left and right of the lung represent the magnitude of pulmonary arterial (PPA) and pulmonary venous (PPV) pressures, respectively. See text for discussion. (Modified from West, J. B., Dollery, C. T., and Naimark, A.: J Appl Physiol 19:713, 1964; reprinted by permission of the authors and publisher.)

pulmonary arterial pressure exceeds alveolar pressure but that alveolar pressure exceeds venous pressure ($Ppa > Palv > Ppv$). Because the effect of venous pressure is not transmitted to zone 2, the driving pressure for blood flow through the zone is determined by the difference between pulmonary arterial and alveolar pressures.

Zone 3 begins at the level at which the effect of venous pressure is "felt." In zone 3, therefore, the conditions are that both pulmonary arterial and venous pressures exceed alveolar pressure ($Ppa > Ppv > Palv$), and the driving pressure for blood flow is determined by the customary pressure difference from pulmonary artery to pulmonary vein.

In healthy subjects in the upright position, most of the lung is in zone 3; there is usually a small zone 2 toward the apex and no zone 1 at all. It is obvious that changing the hydrostatic pressures relative to the height of the lung must affect the distribution of blood flow. Accordingly, pulmonary blood flow is more uniform in the supine than in the upright position because the vertical height of the lung is decreased and the pressures are relatively constant. Similarly, exercise in the upright position raises pulmonary arterial and venous pressures (Table 2) so that blood flow to the upper regions improves and overall perfusion becomes more uniform than at rest.

Distribution of pulmonary blood flow can readily be measured by radioactive substances, such as ^{99m}Tc albumin aggregates or ^{133}Xe dissolved in saline, that can be detected by external counters after intravenous injection. Although these studies are usually performed for diagnostic purposes in patients with suspected pulmonary emboli, they also provide useful clinical information in selected patients with bronchogenic carcinoma or giant bullous lesions who are being evaluated for possible lung surgery. Furthermore, the results of studies on the distribution of pulmonary blood flow have provided important insights into the pathophysiology of various lung diseases. Abnormalities in the volume and distribution of pulmonary blood flow may result from diseases that involve the blood vessels themselves (emboli, vasculitis, emphysema), from compression of blood vessels (tumors, cysts), or from reactivity of blood vessels (vasoconstriction secondary to alveolar hypoxia). Changes in the cardiac output and distribution of pulmonary blood flow are usually reflected by changes in gas exchange and are considered later in this section. Abnormalities in hemodynamics or permeability, which may lead to increased fluid filtration and pulmonary edema, are discussed in the section Pathophysiology of Respiratory Diseases.

Other Functions

Besides providing blood flow for continuous gas exchange, the pulmonary circulation has other important functions: (1) it acts as a filter for the venous drainage from virtually the entire body; (2) it supplies substrates for the nutrition and metabolic needs of the lung, including the synthesis of surfactant; and (3) it serves as a reservoir of blood for the left ventricle. The important roles of the pulmonary circulation in providing a large surface area for the absorption and filtration of liquids and solutes and in modifying the pharmacologic properties of a variety of circulating substances by biochemical transformation are considered in more detail later in this section.

REFERENCES

Bergofsky, E. H.: Humoral control of the pulmonary circulation. Annu Rev Physiol 42:221, 1980.

Fishman, A. P.: Vasomotor regulation of the pulmonary circulation. Annu Rev Physiol 42:211, 1980.

Fung, Y. B., and Sobin, S. S.: Pulmonary alveolar blood flow. In West, J. B. (ed.): Bioengineering Aspects of the Lung. New York, Marcel Dekker, Inc., 1977.

Harris, P., and Heath, D.: The Human Pulmonary Circulation. Its Form and Function in Health and Disease. 2nd ed. Edinburgh, Churchill Livingstone, 1977.

Hughes, J. M. B.: Local control of blood flow and ventilation. In West, J. B. (ed.): Regional Differences in the Lung. New York, Academic Press, Inc., 1977, p. 420.

West, J. B.: Blood flow. In West, J. B. (ed.): Regional Differences in the Lung. New York, Academic Press, Inc., 1977, p. 86.

DIFFUSION, OXYHEMOGLOBIN EQUILIBRIUM, AND CARBON DIOXIDE EQUILIBRIUM

The pulmonary circulation continuously delivers mixed venous blood to the capillaries of the lungs, and ventilation ensures periodic delivery of fresh air to the alveolar spaces. As soon as a new increment of incoming blood arrives in the arterial end of a capillary, it is exposed to a mixture of gases on the other side of the alveolar-capillary membrane that is composed of gas remaining from the previous breath enriched by gas from the latest breath. At this instant, because of concentration—or pressure—differences of O_2 and CO_2 between pulmonary capillary blood and alveolar gas, diffusion of both gases begins. Thus diffusion is the essential process by which O_2 is taken into the body and CO_2 is eliminated from it. The actual quantity of each gas that enters or leaves the lungs is governed both by the processes affecting diffusion and by the carrier system in the bloodstream: O_2 reacts solely with hemoglobin, and CO_2 reacts in part with hemoglobin and in part with water to form bicarbonate (HCO_3^-). The reversible chemical reactions between hemoglobin and O_2 and CO_2 are complementary and add considerably to the transport capacity of the blood. When examining the process of gas exchange across the alveolar-capillary membrane, it is necessary, therefore, to consider not only diffusion but also oxyhemoglobin equilibrium and CO_2 equilibrium.

Diffusing Capacity

The diffusing capacity of the lung for any gas (G) indicates the quantity of that gas that diffuses across the alveolar-capillary membrane per unit time ($\dot{V}G$) in response to the difference in mean pressures of that gas within the alveolus ($P\bar{A}_G$) and within the pulmonary capillary ($P\bar{c}_G$). The diffusing capacity of the lungs for any gas (DL_G) is expressed by the general equation:

$$DL_G = \frac{\dot{V}G}{P\bar{A}_G - P\bar{c}_G}.$$

Most inert gases (for example, N_2) diffuse across the air-blood barrier extremely rapidly so that the amount taken up by the lung is not detectably limited by the diffusibility of the gas and the properties of the lungs and blood, but is determined solely by the solubility of the gas and the volume of tissue and blood into which it can dissolve. This phenomenon is taken advantage of by using highly soluble gases like acetylene, dimethyl ether, and nitrous oxide to measure lung tissue volume and pulmonary capillary blood flow.

The only two gases that can be used to measure the diffusing capacity of the lungs are O_2 and CO; these are suitable because of their unique ability to combine chemically with hemoglobin. Thus both have to diffuse across the alveolar-capillary membrane in such large quantities in order to saturate the available hemoglobin at the gas pressure prevailing in the alveoli that it may not be possible for complete equilibrium to occur before the hemoglobin-containing red blood cells leave the pulmonary capillaries and gas transfer ceases. Of the two gases, CO is much more widely used for the measurement of diffusing capacity than O_2 because of the ease and convenience of applying the various CO tests and because O_2 uptake is not limited by diffusion (in other words, it is not a test of diffusing capacity) in normal subjects except during heavy exercise or while breathing low concentrations of O_2.

Two general types of tests for measuring diffusing capacity of the lung are available that involve either a breath-holding maneuver (single breath) or continuous rebreathing (steady-state) methods. (1) The single-breath test for the measurement of pulmonary diffusing capacity is noninvasive, easy for the subject to perform, rapid, and safe. Accordingly, it is widely used not only in pulmonary function laboratories but also as a screening method for the early detection of lung disease. The major disadvantage of the test, apart from the cost and complexity of the apparatus, is that it requires a 10-second breath hold, which is difficult for normal subjects to perform during exercise and may be impossible for patients with severe dyspnea to endure at rest. (2) All six steady-state methods involve the continuous breathing or rebreathing of a gas mixture containing a small amount of CO, but each has a different approach to the derivation of mean alveolar CO pressure. Steady-state methods take longer to perform than the single-breath method and most, but not all, are noninvasive; nonuniformity of ventilation and blood flow probably affect the results of steady-state methods more than those of the single-breath technique, but steady-state methods are easier to use during exercise than a test requiring a 10-second breath hold maneuver.

Factors Affecting CO-Diffusing Capacity. The quantity of CO that will diffuse in a known period from alveolar gas into capillary blood and combine with hemoglobin in response to a given pressure difference between gas and blood is determined by (1) the solubility and diffusibility of CO in each of the layers of the air-blood barrier, (2) the surface area and thickness of the barrier, and (3) the rate of chemical reaction between CO and hemoglobin within red blood cells. The anatomic pathway and site of reactions for diffusion are illustrated in Figure 28. Because the solubility and diffusibility of CO are physical characteristics that presumably do not change under ordinary circumstances, the two chief components of diffusing capacity in healthy persons and patients are the area and thickness of the alveolar-capillary membrane available for diffusion (DM) and the pulmonary capillary blood volume (Vc), which incorporates the reservoir of hemoglobin with which the CO combines at a finite rate (Θ).

It is possible to subdivide values for overall diffusing capacity (DL) into its components (DM and Vc) by performing several measurements of DL_{CO} with the subject breathing gas mixtures of different concentrations of CO and O_2. Because CO and O_2 compete with each other for available positions on the hemoglobin molecule, changing the O_2 concentration changes the rate with which CO reacts with hemoglobin (in other words, Θ) and thus affects DL_{CO}. The values from a series of tests can be plotted as shown in Figure 29 and solved graphically for DM and Vc according to the following equation:

$$\frac{1}{DL} = \frac{1}{DM} + \frac{1}{\Theta Vc}.$$

About half of the total resistance to the diffusion of CO from alveolar gas to capillary blood resides in the membrane component and the other half in the chemical reaction that takes place in the pulmonary capillary blood volume. Accordingly, changes in the hemoglobin concentration have a calculable effect on total CO diffusion that should be taken into account when establishing the predicted "normal" value for a patient with anemia or polycythemia.

Normal values for CO-diffusing capacity depend chiefly on the person's lung volume and therefore are closely correlated with body size, especially height. Because single-breath and steady-state methods yield different results in the same subject, suitable regression equations for the particular tests being used must be solved to obtain predicted normal values for a given subject.

Diffusing capacity is normally higher in the supine than in the erect posture because position changes Vc. When blood flow to the lungs and pulmonary arterial pressure increase as in muscular exercise, Vc increases through recruitment of previously nonperfused capillaries and dilatation of others; these phenomena account for the progressive increases in DL_{CO} during increasingly strenuous exercise. Similarly, the elevated pulmonary arterial pressures encountered in residents of high altitude also recruit capillaries and increase Vc and cause an increase in "normal" DL_{CO}. For unexplained reasons (possibly related to changes in lung structure), natives of high altitude have higher DL_{CO} values than sojourners fully acclimatized to the same altitude.

Abnormalities of CO-Diffusing Capacity. DL_{CO} may increase or decrease in patients with various cardiopulmonary disorders that affect Vc, DM, or both. When tests of diffusing capacity were first applied to the study of patients who had disturbances of gas exchange, it was assumed that a major abnormality was thickening of the air-blood barrier by a pathologic process that lengthened the pathway for diffusion of gases, i.e., an *alveolar-capillary block syndrome*. The "block" meant that the distance O_2 molecules had to traverse between gas and blood was increased and, in turn, that extra time was required for diffusion to reach equilibration across the air-blood barrier. Accordingly, in the presence of a block, diffusion might be limited and there would be a difference in P_{O_2}

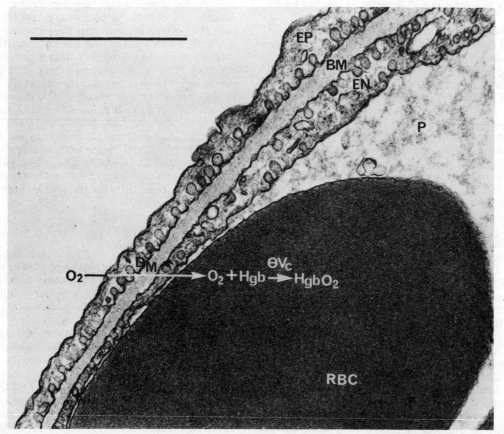

Figure 28. Electron photomicrograph showing the pathway for O_2 diffusion across the air-blood barrier in a human lung. An O_2 molecule must cross the epithelium *(EP)*, basement membrane *(BM)*, endothelium *(EN)*, plasma layer *(P)*, and red blood cell *(RBC)* membrane; resistance to movement through these barriers comprises the membrane component *(DM)* of the total resistance to diffusion. After entering the red blood cell, O_2 must combine chemically with hemoglobin *(Hgb)*; this reaction comprises the resistance imposed by the capillary blood volume *(Vc)* and rate of chemical combination (Θ). Horizontal bar = 1 μm. (Courtesy of Dr. Ewald R. Weibel.)

between gas in the alveolus and in the bloodstream at the end of the journey of red blood cells through pulmonary capillaries. The importance of alveolar-capillary block has been greatly exaggerated because (1) arterial hypoxia at rest in patients with decreased diffusing capacities is usually not caused by the diffusion abnormality per se but by ventilation-perfusion inequalities (see subsequent discussion on Gas Exchange), and (2) decreases in DL from changes in DM, such as would occur with a "block," are rare, whereas decreases in DL from changes in Vc are common.

Oxyhemoglobin Equilibrium

The initial movement of O_2 across the air-blood barrier takes place between alveolar gas and plasma, but as soon as O_2 molecules enter and begin to accumulate in plasma, a new concentration difference is established between O_2 in the plasma and that in the interior of neighboring red blood cells. This difference causes O_2 to diffuse into the cells, where most of it combines chemically with hemoglobin. Each 1.0 g of hemoglobin can react with and serve as the carrier for as much as 1.34 ml O_2. Thus the O_2 *capacity* of the blood is determined by the concentration of "active" hemoglobin (that is, the hemoglobin that is chemically

able to combine with O_2 in the blood) and can be computed according to the following equation:

$$O_2 \text{ capacity, ml/dl} = \text{hemoglobin, g/dl,} \times 1.34, \text{ml/g.}$$

Almost all O_2 molecules react with hemoglobin, but an additional small quantity of O_2 is present in physical solution in the bloodstream (O_2 dissolved), according to the solubility (α) of O_2 (αO_2 = 0.003 ml/dl plasma/mm Hg) and the partial pressure of O_2 in the plasma. The O_2 *content* of the blood is the total amount of O_2 present in the blood, both chemically combined with hemoglobin and dissolved in plasma.

The relationship between the actual amount of O_2 combined with the hemoglobin contained in a given amount of blood and the O_2 capacity of that quantity of hemoglobin determines the *per cent saturation of hemoglobin* (So_2):

$$So_2, \% = \frac{O_2 \text{ content} - O_2 \text{ dissolved}}{O_2 \text{ capacity}} \times 100.$$

Per cent saturation of hemoglobin is seldom obtained by separately measuring O_2 content and O_2 capacity but instead is determined directly from spectrophotometric analysis of blood or is derived indirectly by

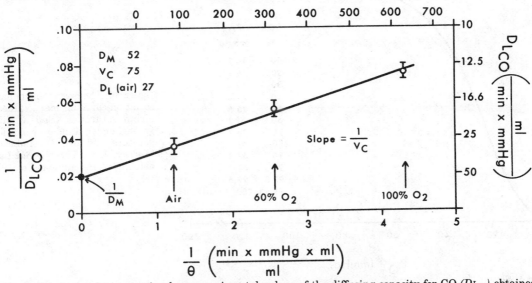

Figure 29. A plot demonstrating how experimental values of the diffusing capacity for CO (DL_{CO}) obtained at different alveolar Po_2 values can be analyzed mathematically to obtain the subdivisions of total diffusing capacity: diffusing capacity of the membrane (DM) and pulmonary capillary blood volume (Vc). Changing alveolar Po_2 changes the reaction coefficient (Θ) and allows $1/DL$ to be plotted against $1/\Theta$. Under these conditions, DM is derived from the value of the Y-intercept and Vc from the slope of the line. (From Murray, J. F.: The Normal Lung. Philadelphia, W. B. Saunders Co., 1976, p. 157.)

calculations from simple measurements of Po_2, pH, and temperature.

Values for arterial and mixed venous blood composition in normal adults are given in Table 4. About 65 times more O_2 is carried in arterial blood combined with hemoglobin than is dissolved in plasma and cells, thus emphasizing the importance of hemoglobin as an O_2 carrier.

Affinity Between Oxygen and Hemoglobin. The reversible chemical reaction between O_2 and hemoglobin is defined by the oxyhemoglobin equilibrium curve (Fig. 30), which relates the per cent saturation of hemoglobin to the Po_2. The characteristic feature of the O_2 equilibrium curves of most mammalian hemoglobins is their sigmoid shape, a configuration that indicates that the *affinity* for O_2 progressively increases as successive molecules of O_2 combine with hemoglobin. The sigmoid shape of the curves is physiologically advantageous because the flat upper portion allows arterial O_2 content to remain high and virtually constant despite fluctuations in arterial Po_2 and the middle steep segment enables large quantities of O_2 to be released at the Po_2 prevailing in the peripheral capillaries. The affinity between O_2 and hemoglobin is conventionally expressed as the Po_2 at which the available hemoglobin is half saturated (P_{50}) under standard conditions of temperature (37°C) and pH (7.40).

The P_{50} of human blood is normally 26.6 mm Hg, but this value is known to vary considerably both in normal subjects under certain conditions and in patients with a variety of diseases. The effects of shifts in the position of the oxyhemoglobin equilibrium curve are depicted schematically in Figure 31; note that hemoglobin concentration has been arbitrarily set at 14.9 g/dl so that O_2 capacity (that is, 100 per cent saturation) is 20.0 ml/dl and arteriovenous (or tissue) O_2 differences can be derived easily. When the affinity of hemoglobin for O_2 increases (curve B in Fig. 31), O_2 is taken up more readily and released less readily at any given Po_2; under these circumstances, the equilibrium curve is shifted to the left of the normal curve (curve A) and the P_{50} is lower than usual ($P_{50} = 22.6$ mm Hg). When the affinity of hemoglobin for O_2 decreases, the new curve is shifted to the right (curve C) of the normal one and the P_{50} increases ($P_{50} = 30.6$ mm Hg). When arterial Po_2 is normal, shifts in the

TABLE 4. NORMAL VALUES FOR ARTERIAL AND MIXED VENOUS BLOOD IN A 25-YEAR-OLD PERSON AT REST*

VARIABLE	ARTERIAL BLOOD	MIXED VENOUS BLOOD
Po_2, mm Hg	95	40
Pco_2, mm Hg	40	46
pH, units	7.40	7.36
Temperature, °C	37.0	37.0
Hemoglobin, g/dl	14.9	14.9
O_2 capacity, ml/dl	20.0	20.0
O_2 content, ml/dl	19.79	14.62
Combined with hemoglobin	19.50	14.50
Dissolved O_2	0.29	0.12
Hemoglobin saturation, %	97.5	72.5
CO_2 content, ml/dl	49.0	53.1
Carbamino CO_2	2.2	3.1
Bicarbonate CO_2	44.2	47.0
Dissolved CO_2	2.6	3.0

*Data in part from Severinghaus, J. W. In Altman, P. C., and Dittner, D. S. (eds.): Respiration and Circulation. Federation of American Societies for Experimental Biology, 1971; and Singer, R. B., same publication.

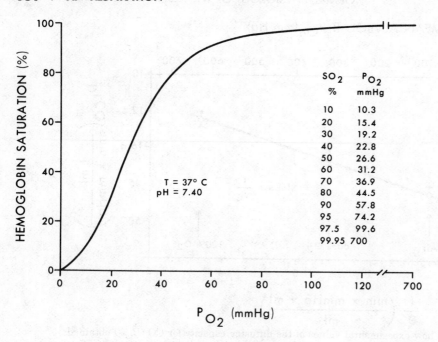

Figure 30. The normal oxyhemoglobin dissociation curve for man. Values for hemoglobin saturation (So_2) at different Po_2 values, under standard conditions of temperature and pH, are indicated. (From Murray, J. F.: The Normal Lung. Philadelphia, W. B. Saunders Co., 1976, p. 162.)

| SO_2 | P_{O_2} |
%	mmHg
10	10.3
20	15.4
30	19.2
40	22.8
50	26.6
60	31.2
70	36.9
80	44.5
90	57.8
95	74.2
97.5	99.6
99.95	700

curves in either direction influence the release of O_2 in the tissues considerably more than the uptake of O_2 in the lungs. This phenomenon is also depicted in Figure 31 by the convergence of the flat portions (exaggerated for schematic effect) and the separation of the steep segments of the three curves. A decrease in O_2 affinity is physiologically useful because it increases the amount of O_2 released at the tissues, where Po_2 is 40 mm Hg, by 1.6 ml/dl. In other words, the shift from curve A to curve C increases O_2 release from 4.5 to 6.1 ml/dl. In contrast, an increased O_2 affinity (curve B) is disadvantageous because it reduces the amount normally available to the tissues by 1.6 ml/dl, or from 4.5 to 2.9 ml/dl. When arterial Po_2 is low, as in the hypoxia occurring at high altitude and in severe pulmonary diseases, an increase in P_{50} is not physiologically useful because it impairs O_2 uptake by arterial blood as much as or even more than it facilitates O_2 release by capillary blood.

Factors Affecting Oxyhemoglobin Affinity. Several commonly encountered factors in every-day clinical situations affect oxyhemoglobin affinity. Affinity is *increased* by hypothermia, alkalemia, hypocapnia, and decreased concentration within red blood cells of certain organic phosphates, particularly 2,3-diphosphoglycerate, and by the presence of CO-hemoglobin, sulfhemoglobin, or methemoglobin. Affinity is *decreased* by fever, acidemia, hypercapnia, and increased 2,3-diphosphoglycerate. A variety of genetically determined abnormalities of the amino acid composition of hemoglobin have been described that either increase or decrease affinity for O_2. All of these are rare, but they provide interesting examples of how the body adapts to life-long changes in oxyhemoglobin affinity.

The effect of changes in intracellular pH, from reciprocal changes in hydrogen ion concentration (symbolized [H+]), is known as the *Bohr effect*. In the lungs, [H+] decreases as CO_2 is eliminated from pulmonary

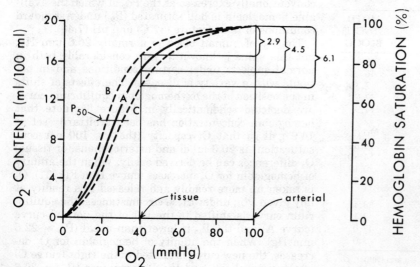

Figure 31. Schematic diagram showing the effects of increases and decreases in O_2 affinity on the amount of O_2 available at the Po_2 values prevailing in arterial blood and at the tissues. P_{50} = Po_2 at which hemoglobin saturation is 50 per cent. Hemoglobin concentration is assumed for convenience to be 14.9 g/dl; therefore, O_2 content at 100 per cent saturation is 20 ml/dl. *Curve A* = normal blood; *curve B* = blood with increased affinity (decreased P_{50}); *curve C* = blood with decreased affinity (increased P_{50}). (From Murray, J. F.: The Normal Lung. Philadelphia, W. B. Saunders Co., 1976, p. 163.)

capillary blood and oxyhemoglobin affinity is increased; in the peripheral capillaries, CO_2 is added to the bloodstream causing $[H^+]$ to increase and O_2 affinity to decrease. The combined effect is physiologically favorable because it enhances both O_2 uptake in the lungs and O_2 release to the tissues.

Carbon Dioxide Equilibrium

The CO_2 produced by the aerobic metabolic processes that consume O_2 diffuses from cells into tissue capillaries and undergoes a series of chemical reactions at the beginning of its journey to the lungs. Once the blood is exposed to alveolar gas containing inspired fresh air, the chemical reactions reverse and some of the CO_2 evolves into the gas phase. Transport of CO_2 differs from that of O_2 because CO_2 is carried in three forms instead of two: dissolved, as bicarbonate, and in combination with hemoglobin as carbamino compounds (Table 4). The quantity of CO_2 transported in the bloodstream depends on the amounts present in each form, which are determined, like O_2, on the pressure of the gas (Pco_2) and the quantity of hemoglobin with which they can react.

(1) Some CO_2, like O_2, dissolves in the plasma in proportion to its gas pressure, but because CO_2 is more than 20 times more soluble than O_2 (αCO_2 = 0.068 ml/dl plasma/mm Hg) an appreciable amount (about 5 per cent) of the total CO_2 content of arterial blood is transported in solution.

(2) As soon as CO_2 diffuses from around tissue capillaries into the bloodstream, most of it enters red blood cells, where it is hydrated to form carbonic acid (H_2CO_3), which then dissociates to form hydrogen ion (H^+) and bicarbonate ion (HCO_3^-):

$$CO_2 + H_2O \overset{CA}{\rightleftharpoons} H_2CO_3 \rightleftharpoons H^+ + HCO_3^-.$$

The first hydration reaction is of the molecular type and thus tends to proceed slowly; however, the rate is increased several hundred times by the enzyme carbonic anhydrase (CA), which is present within red blood cells. The second reaction is of the ionic type and thus occurs rapidly without an enzyme. Some of the newly produced H^+ and HCO_3^- remain within red blood cells, but some of the HCO_3^- diffuses into the plasma because cell membranes are much more permeable to negatively charged anions (such as HCO_3^- and Cl^-) than to positively charged cations (such as K^+ and H^+). The movement of HCO_3^- tends to create an electrostatic difference across the cell membrane that is neutralized by the movement of Cl^- into the red blood cell (the "chloride shift").

In the lungs these reactions proceed in the reverse direction to liberate CO_2. Carbonic anhydrase also plays an important role in the dehydration of H_2CO_3, because without it the release of CO_2 would not be completed during the brief time that red blood cells spend traversing pulmonary capillaries.

(3) A small amount of the CO_2 that enters red blood cells combines reversibly with hemoglobin to form carbamino compounds. Although only about 5 per cent of the total CO_2 content is in the form of carbamino compounds, they provide about 30 per cent of the CO_2 that evolves in the lungs from red blood cells flowing through the pulmonary capillaries.

The CO_2 equilibrium curves of oxygenated and deox-

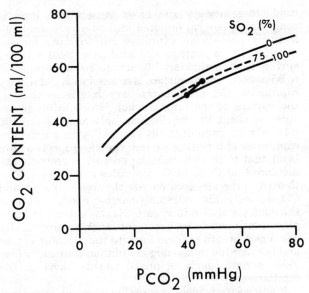

Figure 32. Normal CO_2 equilibration (dissociation) curves for whole blood at 0, 75, and 100 per cent oxyhemoglobin saturation (So_2). The heavy line connecting the two points shows the usual extent of the Haldane effect in arterial and venous blood. (From Murray, J. F.: The Normal Lung. Philadelphia, W. B. Saunders Co., 1976, p. 168.)

ygenated blood are shown in Figure 32. The curves are nearly linear in the physiologic range (Pco_2 40 to 50 mm Hg), and considerably more CO_2, about 6 ml/dl, is bound within this range by unsaturated rather than fully saturated hemoglobin. The shift from the well-oxygenated (lower) curve to the less well oxygenated (middle) curve occurs as O_2 is extracted from blood in peripheral capillaries. This enhances CO_2 uptake and transport by the blood and is known as the *Haldane effect*. Physiologically, the Haldane effect is of far greater importance to CO_2 transport than is the Bohr effect to O_2 transport. The Haldane effect is accounted for by the enhanced ability of unoxygenated hemoglobin to combine with (that is, buffer) the H^+ ions released in the dissociation of H_2CO_3 and to form carbamino compounds.

REFERENCES

Grant, B. J. B.: Influence of Bohr-Haldane effect on steady state gas exchange. J Appl Physiol 52:1330, 1982.

Hill, E. P., Power, G. G., and Longo, L. D.: Kinetics of O_2 and CO_2 exchange. In West, J. B. (ed.): Bioengineering Aspects of the Lung. New York, Marcel Dekker, Inc., 1977.

Perutz, M. F.: Structure and mechanism of hemoglobin. Br Med Bull 32:195, 1976.

Rose, G. L., Cassidy, S. S., and Johnson, R. L., Jr.: Diffusing capacity at different lung volumes during breath holding and rebreathing. J Appl Physiol 47:32, 1979.

Thomas, H. M., III, Lefrak, S. S., Irwin, R. S., Fritts, H. W., Jr., and Caldwell, P. R. B.: The oxyhemoglobin dissociation curve in health and disease. Role of 2,3-diphosphoglycerate. Am J Med 57:331, 1974.

Wagner, P. D.: Diffusion and chemical reaction in pulmonary gas exchange. Physiol Rev 57:257, 1977.

GAS EXCHANGE

The anatomic organization of the lungs is designed chiefly for the purpose of gas exchange. In addition to conducting airways and blood vessels, the lung is composed of several hundred million alveoli that collectively provide an extensive surface area for gas transfer. In an average size adult, the total alveolar surface is approximately 140 m²; moreover, because 85 to 95 per cent of this surface is covered with pulmonary capillaries, the alveolar-capillary interface—that is, the surface of the lung through which diffusion occurs—is about 125 m². Because only about 70 to 100 ml of blood is present at any moment in the pulmonary capillaries of a resting subject, the blood forms a thin layer that facilitates diffusion because it restricts the distance that O_2 and CO_2 molecules must travel. Furthermore, the air-blood barrier through which O_2 and CO_2 diffuse is also extremely narrow, about 0.5 μm in the example shown in Figure 28. Gas exchange takes place continuously because ventilation intermittently delivers a breath of fresh air into the alveolar spaces and because the pulmonary circulation constantly provides a new supply of mixed venous blood in the capillaries.

It follows that "ideal" gas exchange occurs when just the right amounts of blood and inspired air are brought together at the air-blood barrier to oxygenate the blood fully and to eliminate all of its excess CO_2. The performance of the normal lung is not quite perfect, but it is close enough that an introduction to gas exchange can begin by considering an ideal system.

"Ideal" Relationships

Understanding of gas exchange has been greatly enhanced by the use of the simple two-compartment lung model shown in Figure 33. In this and subsequent figures, the hemoglobin concentration of the blood is assumed to be 15.0 g/dl, and the arteriovenous difference for O_2 is 4.6 ml/dl and for CO_2 3.7 ml/dl. The large double-pointed arrows indicate both the magnitude and the distribution of ventilation. The small arrows indicate diffusion of O_2 and CO_2 between alveolar gas and pulmonary capillary blood. The "arterialization" of blood is signified by the change in shading from black (mixed venous blood) to light gray (arterial blood).

The stippled area indicates the "dead space" of the respiratory tract; it can be appreciated from the illustration that the amount of air required to fill the dead space is "wasted" with respect to gas exchange. Thus each breath, or the amount of air breathed per minute, can be subdivided into two fractions depending on whether or not they contribute to gas exchange: *wasted ventilation* and *alveolar ventilation*. The fraction of wasted ventilation (V_D) can be measured easily from the CO_2 pressures of simultaneously collected samples

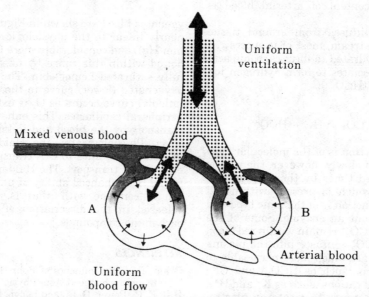

Uniform ventilation

Mixed venous blood

A

B

Arterial blood

Uniform blood flow

Figure 33. Schematic representation of gas exchange in an idealized two-compartment model of the lung in which there is uniform distribution of ventilation and blood flow. (Adapted from Comroe, J. H., Jr., Forster, R. E., II, Dubois, A. B., Briscoe, W. A., and Carlsen, E.: The Lung. Clinical Physiology and Pulmonary Function Tests. 2nd ed. Chicago, Year Book Medical Publishers, Inc., 1962, p. 89; reprinted by permission of the authors and publisher.)

	A	B	A + B	Units
Alveolar ventilation	2.4	2.4	4.8	liter/min
Pulmonary blood flow	3.0	3.0	6.0	liter/min
Ventilation-perfusion ratio	0.8	0.8	0.8	
Mixed venous P_{O_2}	40	40	40	mm Hg
Mixed venous S_{O_2}	75	75	75	per cent
Mixed venous P_{CO_2}	46	46	46	mm Hg
Alveolar P_{O_2}	101	101	101	mm Hg
Arterial P_{O_2}	101	101	101	mm Hg
Arterial S_{O_2}	97.5	97.5	97.5	per cent
Arterial P_{CO_2}	40	40	40	mm Hg
(Alveolar-arterial) P_{O_2}	0	0	0	mm Hg

of expired air (PE_{CO_2}) and arterial blood (Pa_{CO_2}) by means of the modified Bohr equation:

$$V_D = \frac{Pa_{CO_2} - PE_{CO_2}}{Pa_{CO_2}}.$$

Alveolar ventilation cannot be measured directly but is derived by subtracting wasted ventilation from the minute volume of ventilation, which is easily determined by measuring the total volume of air breathed in or out of the mouth.

The effectiveness of gas exchange by the lungs is commonly assessed by measurements of PO_2 and PCO_2 in arterial blood. However, additional important information about the mechanisms that underlie any abnormality (if present) is obtained from the PO_2 values in simultaneous blood and mean alveolar gas specimens to derive the alveolar-arterial PO_2 difference. It is difficult to measure mean alveolar PO_2 (PA_{O_2}) satisfactorily, but it can be calculated with reasonable accuracy using the standard alveolar air equation:

$$PA_{O_2} = PI_{O_2} - PA_{CO_2} \left[FI_{O_2} + \frac{1 - FI_{O_2}}{R} \right]$$

where $PI_{O_2} = PO_2$ of inspired gas, PA_{CO_2} = alveolar PCO_2 (usually assumed to equal arterial PCO_2), FI_{O_2} = fractional concentration of O_2 in inspired gas, and R = respiratory exchange ratio (normally 0.8).

In Figure 33, alveolar ventilation and blood flow are distributed uniformly to the two gas exchange units; normally, as shown, there is less alveolar ventilation than pulmonary blood flow and the overall *ventilation:perfusion* ratio of the lung is 0.8. Because diffusion equilibrium is attained between the blood and gas phases, the values for both PO_2 and PCO_2 are the same in alveolar gas and end-capillary blood. Furthermore, because ventilation and blood flow are proportionately equal in the two units, there is no alveolar-arterial PO_2 difference.

Normal Gas Exchange

Normal values for the gas pressures of O_2, CO_2, N_2, and H_2O at sea level (barometric pressure 760 mm Hg) in ambient air, conducting airways (that is, the dead space), gas exchange units, and arterial and mixed venous blood are provided in Table 5. Ambient air consists primarily of N_2 and O_2 with varying amounts of water vapor. As air is inhaled, it is warmed to the subject's body temperature and fully saturated with water vapor (PH_2O at 37° C = 47 mm Hg); the addition of water vapor in effect dilutes the inspired mixture of N_2 and O_2 and reduces their respective pressures pro-

portionately. After the inspirate reaches alveoli, gas exchange takes place. More O_2 is removed than CO_2 is added; this causes the volume of each unit to decrease slightly and raises the concentration and pressure of N_2 within the gas phase slightly.

The values given in Table 5 indicate that gas exchange in the healthy lung, in contrast to the ideal lung, is not perfect because there is a small (6 mm Hg) alveolar-arterial PO_2 difference. The difference occurs because of the normal presence of slight mismatching of ventilation with respect to perfusion and a small right-to-left shunt. It should also be noted (Table 5) that the sum of the individual gases in mixed venous blood is less than the total atmospheric pressure. Because the tissue and spaces of the body are in approximate equilibrium with venous blood, these structures are also subatmospheric. The "suction" effect helps to keep the lung expanded against the chest wall and also causes the reabsorption of gas from a pneumothorax or pneumomediastinum once the leak has sealed.

Measurements of arterial PO_2 and PCO_2 and calculations of alveolar-arterial PO_2 differences are reliable guides to the overall adequacy of respiration. Normal values for PO_2, but not for PCO_2, vary with age, and both PO_2 and PCO_2 are influenced by the altitude at which the subject is living and whether or not acclimatization to recent changes in altitude has occurred.

Arterial *hypoxia*, defined as a decrease below normal of arterial PO_2, can be caused by five different physiologic abnormalities: (1) hypoventilation, (2) impaired diffusion, (3) ventilation-perfusion mismatching, (4) right-to-left shunting, and (5) breathing air (or a gas mixture) with a low PO_2. Two or more of these may coexist in patients with respiratory disease; however, by employing the concepts described in the section on Pathophysiology of Respiratory Diseases, the contribution of each mechanism to a given patient's hypoxia can be inferred from results of routine blood gas analysis and, when necessary, the value of PO_2 attained when the subject breathes 100 per cent O_2. Knowledge of the mechanism(s) at fault provides considerable insight into the pathophysiology of a patient's lung disease that leads to appropriate therapeutic decisions.

Hypoventilation

The simplest disturbance of gas exchange occurs when not enough fresh air is breathed into alveolar spaces to allow pulmonary capillary PO_2 to increase to normal levels and to enable CO_2 to leave the bloodstream. This condition, called *hypoventilation*, is shown schematically in Figure 34. During hypoventilation the PCO_2 must increase. The increase in arterial PCO_2

TABLE 5. NORMAL GAS PRESSURES (IN MM HG) DURING INSPIRATION IN AMBIENT AIR, CONDUCTING AIRWAYS, TERMINAL UNITS (ALVEOLI), AND ARTERIAL AND MIXED VENOUS BLOOD*

GAS PRESSURE	AMBIENT AIR	CONDUCTING AIRWAYS	TERMINAL UNITS	ARTERIAL BLOOD	MIXED VENOUS BLOOD
PO_2	156	149	101	95	40
PCO_2	0	0	40	40	46
PH_2O	15†	47	47	47	47
PN_2	589	564	572	573	573
P_{TOTAL}	760	760	760	755	706

*Modified from Murray, J. F.: The Normal Lung. Philadelphia, W. B. Saunders Co., 1976.
†PH_2O varies according to humidity and has a proportionate effect on PO_2 and PN_2.

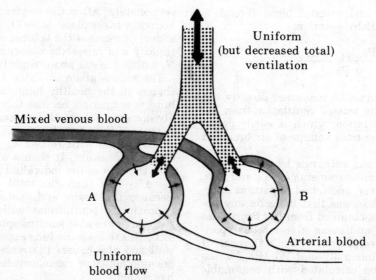

Uniform
(but decreased total)
ventilation

Mixed venous blood

A

B

Arterial blood

Uniform
blood flow

Figure 34. Schematic representation of the effects of hypoventilation on gas exchange. Alveolar ventilation is one half that in Figure 33. (Adapted from Comroe, J. H., Jr., Forster, R. E., II, Dubois, A. B., Briscoe, W. A., and Carlsen, E.: The Lung. Clinical Physiology and Pulmonary Function Tests. 2nd ed. Chicago, Year Book Medical Publishers, Inc., 1962, p. 216; reprinted by permission of the authors and publisher.)

	A	B	A + B	Units
Alveolar ventilation	1.2	1.2	2.4	liter/min
Pulmonary blood flow	3.0	3.0	6.0	liter/min
Ventilation-perfusion ratio	0.4	0.4	0.4	
Mixed venous P_{O_2}	34	34	34	mm Hg
Mixed venous S_{O_2}	64.3	64.3	64.3	per cent
Mixed venous P_{CO_2}	90	90	90	mm Hg
Alveolar P_{O_2}	53	53	53	mm Hg
Arterial P_{O_2}	53	53	53	mm Hg
Arterial S_{O_2}	87.2	87.2	87.2	per cent
Arterial P_{CO_2}	80	80	80	mm Hg
(Alveolar-arterial) P_{O_2}	0	0	0	mm Hg

(Pa_{CO_2}) is the hallmark of hypoventilation because of the relationship between CO_2 production (Vco_2) and alveolar ventilation (V_A):

$$Pa_{CO_2} = K \frac{\dot{V}_{CO_2}}{\dot{V}_A}$$

where K is a constant. This equation indicates that if alveolar ventilation is halved, arterial P_{CO_2} will double (assuming CO_2 production is unchanged). Although arterial P_{CO_2} may theoretically increase in other disturbances of gas exchange (ventilation-perfusion abnormalities and right-to-left shunts), for clinical purposes an elevated value should be interpreted as indicating alveolar hypoventilation.

Pure hypoventilation is a relatively uncommon clinical event. It may be caused by diseases that affect the respiratory centers in the brain, by depression of the central nervous system from anesthetic agents or other sedative drugs, by neuromuscular disorders that impair respiratory muscle function, by thoracic cage injuries, and by severe disease of the lung parenchyma or airways. The alveolar-arterial P_{O_2} difference is not increased in pure hypoventilation. More commonly, hypoventilation is found in association with other disturbances of gas exchange. When these coexist, they can be recognized by the fact that the decrease in arterial P_{O_2} is more than can be accounted for by the increase in arterial P_{CO_2}, and the alveolar-arterial P_{O_2} difference therefore increases.

Alveolar *hyperventilation,* the converse of hypoventilation, means that ventilation is in excess of CO_2 production. Hyperventilation is often caused by fever, drugs, central nervous system disorders, or psychogenic influences. Accordingly (see above equation), arterial P_{CO_2} must decrease. *Hyperpnea* means increased breathing that may or may not be related to metabolism, and hence the term carries no implication about the value of arterial P_{CO_2}.

Diffusion Abnormalities

O_2 uptake is not limited by diffusion in healthy subjects except when they breathe air or gas mixtures containing a low P_{O_2} (as at high altitudes) or when they are exercising strenuously. The reason normal persons are not diffusion-limited is shown in Figure 35, which depicts the time course of the diffusion-dependent changes in P_{O_2} in pulmonary capillaries. Mixed venous blood with a P_{O_2} of 40 mm Hg reaches the beginning of the pulmonary capillary at time zero; calculations indicate that red blood cells spend about 0.75 second traversing the capillaries of a resting subject but that O_2 uptake reaches equilibration in less than 0.25 second. This means that the velocity of blood flow can at least triple during exercise or other stresses without causing detectable alveolar–end-capillary P_{O_2}

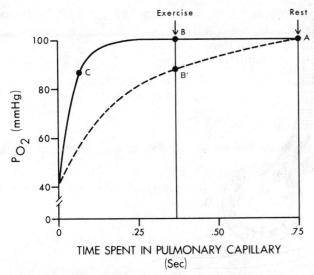

Figure 35. Schematic diagram showing the time course of changes in P_{O_2} and P_{CO_2} at rest and during exercise in normal subjects and in patients with decreased diffusing capacities from thickened alveolar-capillary membranes and decreased pulmonary capillary blood volumes. At rest, equilibration occurs between the pressures in the blood and gas phases (point A) in both normal subjects *(solid line)* and patients with decreased diffusing capacities from a thickened air-blood barrier *(dashed line)*; during exercise, because the time available for gas exchange is shortened, equilibration occurs in normal subjects *(point B)* but not in patients with alveolar-capillary block *(point B')*. When the capillary bed is destroyed or obstructed, the velocity of blood flow increases in the remaining vessels under resting conditions *(point B)*; during exercise, equilibration is no longer possible *(point C)*.

differences. In contrast, in patients with decreased diffusing capacities, equilibrium across the air-blood barrier can also be reached while the patient is resting, but alveolar–end-capillary differences are likely to occur during exercise.

Impaired diffusion from thickening of the alveolar-capillary membrane in Figure 35 (dashed line) differs from normal diffusion (solid line) in that more time is required for O_2 to achieve equilibrium across the thickened membrane. In patients at rest, blood flow is sufficiently slow that equilibrium (point A) may be attained even when diffusing capacity is reduced substantially. However, an increase in the velocity of blood flow shortens the exposure time of red blood cells to alveolar P_{O_2}, which causes alveolar–end-capillary P_{O_2} differences (point B') to develop. In patients whose decreased diffusing capacities are caused by a decrease in capillary blood volume, the mechanism of arterial hypoxia during exercise is different from that in alveolar-capillary block; this process is also displayed in Figure 35. As capillaries are progressively obliterated or destroyed, previously unperfused capillaries are recruited until finally the velocity of blood flow in the remaining vessels increases. When the disease process is advanced, the time available for gas exchange in these patients at rest may be as short as it is in normal subjects during exercise (point B); consequently, during exercise the short pulmonary capillary transit time becomes even shorter and blood fails to equilibrate (point C).

Ventilation-Perfusion Mismatching

In contrast to the ideal conditions that served to introduce the subject of gas exchange, the distributions of inspired air and pulmonary blood flow in normal subjects are neither uniform nor proportionate to each other. Thus a slight ventilation-perfusion imbalance exists in healthy persons. Furthermore, increased (above normal) mismatching of ventilation and perfusion is by far the most common cause of arterial hypoxia encountered clinically. Virtually all forms of lung disease are associated with a detectable ventilation-perfusion abnormality.

The two-compartment model used to depict ideal gas exchange has been modified to that shown in Figure 36. The composition of mixed venous blood, the total blood flow, and the distribution of blood flow are the same as in Figure 33. However, the same total alveolar ventilation is now distributed unevenly between the two gas exchange units so that unit A receives three times more inspired air than unit B. Because blood flow is equally distributed to the two units, the *ventilation:perfusion ratios* differ and, in turn, cause the alveolar and end-capillary gas compositions to vary. The O_2 and CO_2 contents of the end-capillary blood from each alveolus are determined by gas pressures in the alveoli, which are the same as those in end-capillary blood, and by the respective hemoglobin dissociation curves for the two gases. The final composition of arterial blood depends on the actual O_2 and CO_2 contents (or saturations) in the two pathways. Mixing of the pathways establishes the arterial O_2 and CO_2 contents from which the respective P_{O_2} and P_{CO_2} values can be derived. It is impossible to determine the final composition of arterial blood from the end-capillary P_{O_2} and P_{CO_2} values alone, without taking into account the actual contents, because of the alinear characteristics of both equilibrium curves.

The final composition of mixed alveolar gas can be computed by allowing for the differences in ventilation to the two units. (In Fig. 36, [3(114) + 77]/4 = 105) for mean alveolar P_{O_2}.) An important consequence of a ventilation-perfusion imbalance is evident even in this simplified diagram (Fig. 36) and analysis: *there must be a difference between the O_2 and CO_2 pressures in mixed alveolar gas and arterial blood.* Alveolar-arterial differences occur because the relative overventilation of one unit does not fully compensate, by adding O_2 or eliminating CO_2, for the disturbances created by underventilating the other unit. The failure to compensate is greater in the case of O_2 than CO_2 owing to the flatness of the oxyhemoglobin equilibrium curve compared with the CO_2 equilibrium curve (Fig. 36). Increasing ventilation to unit A increases alveolar P_{O_2} but adds only a trivial amount of O_2 to the bloodstream because the events are in accordance with the relationships on the flat part of the oxyhemoglobin equilibrium curve. In contrast, when ventilation to unit A is increased, the steeper slope of the CO_2 curve allows for extra CO_2 output, which slightly overcompensates for the failure to eliminate CO_2 in unit B.

The values in Figure 36 are useful conceptually but are not completely accurate because mixed venous blood composition is held constant and is not affected, as it would be in vivo, by the circulation of arterial blood with reduced O_2 and increased CO_2 through the tissues of the body. These complexities and other

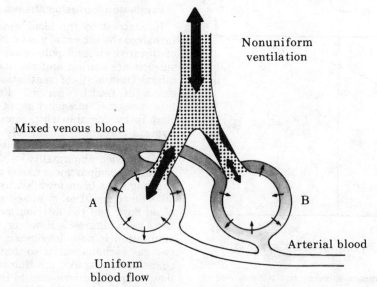

Figure 36. Schematic representation of the effects of a ventilation-perfusion abnormality on gas exchange. (Adapted from Comroe, J. H., Jr., Forster, R. E., II, Dubois, A. B., Briscoe, W. A., and Carlsen, E.: The Lung. Clinical Physiology and Pulmonary Function Tests. 2nd ed. Chicago, Year Book Medical Publishers, Inc., 1962, p. 95; reprinted by permission of the authors and publisher.)

	A	B	A + B	Units
Alveolar ventilation	3.6	1.2	4.8	liter/min
Pulmonary blood flow	3.0	3.0	6.0	liter/min
Ventilation-perfusion ratio	1.2	0.4	0.8	
Mixed venous P_{O_2}	40	40	40	mm Hg
Mixed venous S_{O_2}	75	75	75	per cent
Mixed venous P_{CO_2}	46	46	46	mm Hg
Alveolar P_{O_2}	114	77	105	mm Hg
Arterial P_{O_2}	114	77	89	mm Hg
Arterial S_{O_2}	98.2	95.4	96.8	per cent
Arterial P_{CO_2}	36	45	38	mm Hg
(Alveolar-arterial) P_{O_2}	0	0	16	mm Hg

refinements have been taken into account by a computer analysis of the effects of increasing ventilation-perfusion inequality on arterial P_{O_2} and P_{CO_2} (Fig. 37). As the inequality increases, arterial P_{O_2} falls continuously and precipitously, and arterial P_{CO_2} rises gradually at first and then more markedly. This means, contrary to the usual teaching, the ventilation-perfusion imbalance can be an important cause of CO_2 retention in patients with pulmonary disease. This statement at first glance may appear to conflict with the common clinical observations that many patients with various pulmonary diseases (for example, emphysema and bronchial asthma) have arterial hypoxia resulting from ventilation-perfusion abnormalities, but they also have arterial P_{CO_2} values that are within or, at times, even below the normal range. This apparent discrepancy is explained by the fact that these patients are ventilating in excess of normal, and, owing to the respective shapes and positions of the equilibrium curves for O_2 and CO_2, hyperventilation of the ventilatable units increases CO_2 elimination but does not increase O_2 uptake; thus increasing alveolar ventilation "corrects" the CO_2 retention that would otherwise occur, but arterial hypoxia persists. This underscores the clinical axiom mentioned earlier that for practical purposes an increased arterial P_{CO_2} indicates alveolar hypoventilation.

Right-to-Left Shunts

Another departure from ideal gas exchange is caused by right-to-left shunts of blood in, around, or distal to the lungs; these are found to a slight degree in normal subjects and may be of considerable magnitude in patients with pulmonary disease. A schematic representation of the effects of a right-to-left shunt upon gas exchange is shown in Figure 38. Alveolar ventilation and its distribution are the same as they were under ideal conditions, but distribution of cardiac output is different. Total blood flow remains the same (6 liters/min), but only 2 liters/min each, instead of 3 liters/min each, reaches units A and B; the remaining 2 liters/min flows through the shunt pathway. Expressed quantitatively, there is a right-to-left shunt of one third of the total cardiac output.

Gas exchange in units A and B is unimpaired; in fact, because the individual ventilation:perfusion ratios are slightly higher than normal, a little extra O_2 is taken up and more CO_2 is eliminated than would occur if the ratios were normal. However, this slight augmentation of gas exchange does not nearly compensate for the deleterious effect on overall oxygenation of the continuous flow of mixed venous blood through the shunt. The net result from the mixing of blood from the normal and shunt pathways is analogous to the effects of a ventilation-perfusion inequality: an

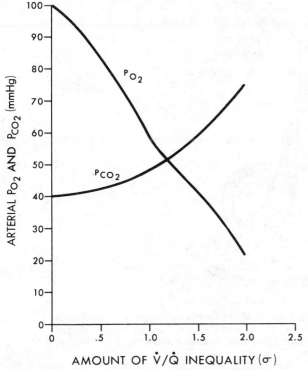

Figure 37. Effect of increasing ventilation:perfusion ratio $(\dot{V}/\dot{Q})$ inequality on arterial P_{O_2} and P_{CO_2} in a lung model in which O_2 uptake and CO_2 output are kept constant at 300 and 240 ml/min, respectively. (Adapted from West, J. B.: Respir Physiol 7:88, 1969; reprinted by permission of the author and publisher.)

inevitable reduction of arterial P_{O_2}, an increase in arterial P_{CO_2}, and the development of alveolar-arterial differences for the two gases. The consequences of a right-to-left shunt are similar to those of a ventilation-perfusion imbalance owing to basic similarities between the two disturbances; a shunt can be viewed as an extreme ventilation-perfusion abnormality, one in which there is perfusion but *no* ventilation at all. It is impossible to differentiate between a ventilation-perfusion disturbance and a right-to-left shunt while a person is breathing ambient air; therefore, the effects of both are combined and designated as *venous admixture* or a shunt-like effect.

Effects of Breathing 100 Per Cent O_2. Arterial hypoxia from a right-to-left shunt can be separated from that caused by a ventilation-perfusion inequality by having the subject breathe 100 per cent O_2, in the laboratory or at the bedside, and measuring arterial P_{O_2}. Table 6 shows how this distinction can be made from examination of the alveolar and arterial P_{O_2} values that result when ideal lungs and lungs with either a ventilation-perfusion abnormality or right-to-left shunt breathe 100 per cent O_2; all of the N_2 is ultimately washed out and replaced by O_2 in ventilatable units. When this occurs only O_2, CO_2, and H_2O are left, so that

$$PA_{O_2} = PA_{TOTAL} - PA_{CO_2} - PA_{H_2O}.$$

Because the total pressure and H_2O vapor pressure are the same in all communicating lung units, alveolar P_{O_2} differs from unit to unit only according to any

corresponding differences in alveolar P_{CO_2}. Blood perfusing each unit equilibrates at the high alveolar P_{O_2} so that blood leaving ideal lungs and lungs with a ventilation-perfusion abnormality also contains a high P_{O_2} value. By this mechanism, the administration of 100 per cent O_2 is said to "correct" a ventilation-perfusion disturbance. Because some lung units may be ventilated extremely poorly through collateral pathways or only intermittently at high lung volumes when the subject takes a deep breath, it is obviously important to allow enough time and to insist that the subject take occasional deep breaths to ensure complete N_2 washout and replacement by O_2 when performing the 100 per cent O_2 test.

In lungs with a right-to-left shunt, N_2 is also eliminated from the ventilated alveoli, and hence blood perfusing these units equilibrates at the increased alveolar P_{O_2}. The problem in oxygenation is not corrected, however, because mixed venous blood continues to flow through the shunt pathway(s) and to mix with blood that has perfused normal units. The poorly oxygenated blood from the shunt lowers the P_{O_2} of the resulting arterial blood and increases the alveolar-arterial P_{O_2} difference, compared with the value obtained while breathing room air. An increased (above normal limits) alveolar-arterial P_{O_2} difference during a properly conducted 100 per cent O_2 study signifies the presence of an excessive right-to-left shunt, and the magnitude of the difference between the P_{O_2} value obtained and the normal value can be used to quantify the proportion of cardiac output that is shunted by using the so-called shunt equation:

$$\frac{\dot{Q}_S}{\dot{Q}_T} = \frac{Cc' - Ca}{Cc' - C\bar{v}}$$

where $\dot{Q}_S/\dot{Q}_T$ is the proportion of total cardiac output $(\dot{Q}_T)$ that is shunted $(\dot{Q}_S)$, and Cc', Ca, and $C\bar{v}$ are the O_2 contents of end-capillary, arterial, and mixed venous bloods, respectively. The Cc' and Ca are derived from alveolar and arterial P_{O_2} values, which are used to compute dissolved O_2 and per cent saturation, and the subject's hemoglobin concentration. Arterial P_{O_2} is measured directly, and alveolar P_{O_2} is computed using the equation previously described for determining the value when breathing 100 per cent O_2. For maximal accuracy, mixed venous O_2 content should be measured directly; however, if appropriate samples cannot be obtained, it is often estimated by assuming an arteriovenous O_2 difference of 4.5 to 5.0 ml/dl. As a rough clinical guide, an alveolar-arterial P_{O_2} difference of 15 mm Hg while breathing 100 per cent O_2 indicates a right-to-left shunt of approximately 1 per cent of the cardiac output.

Sites of Right-to-Left Shunting. When a normal young subject breathes 100 per cent O_2, an alveolar-arterial P_{O_2} difference of between 30 and 50 mm Hg can customarily be detected by the methods described in the previous paragraphs. This demonstrates the presence of a right-to-left shunt of approximately 2 to 3 per cent of the cardiac output. The normal shunt pathways are not around alveoli as shown schematically in Figure 38 but develop by admixture from other sources of unoxygenated blood such as the bronchial veins and the mediastinal veins that empty into pulmonary veins, and the thebesian vessels of the left

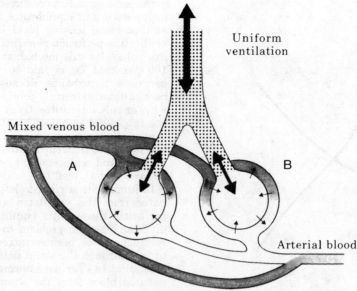

Uniform ventilation

Mixed venous blood

A   B

Arterial blood

Right to Left shunt

Figure 38. Schematic representation of the effects of a right-to-left shunt on gas exchange. (Adapted from Comroe, J. H., Jr., Forster, R. E., II, Dubois, A. B., Briscoe, W. A., and Carlsen, E.: The Lung. Clinical Physiology and Pulmonary Function Tests. 2nd ed. Chicago, Year Book Medical Publishers, Inc., 1962, p. 245; reprinted by permission of the authors and publisher.)

	A + B	Shunt	A + B + Shunt	Units
Alveolar ventilation	4.8	0	4.8	liter/min
Pulmonary blood flow	4.0	2.0	6.0	liter/min
Ventilation-perfusion ratio	1.2	0	0.8	
Mixed venous P_{O_2}	40	40	40	mm Hg
Mixed venous S_{O_2}	75	75	75	per cent
Mixed venous P_{CO_2}	46	46	46	mm Hg
Alveolar P_{O_2}	114	—	114	mm Hg
Arterial P_{O_2}	114	—	59	mm Hg
Arterial S_{O_2}	98.2	—	90.5	per cent
Arterial P_{CO_2}	36	—	39	mm Hg
(Alveolar-arterial) P_{O_2}	0	—	55	mm Hg

ventricular myocardium that empty directly into the left ventricular cavity. However, the diagram in Figure 38 is not purely schematic but accurately depicts the pattern of blood flow for shunts in many pathologic conditions. In some instances, a discrete abnormal anatomic pathway does exist (for example, intracardiac communications, pulmonary arteriovenous fistulas), but in most other instances shunts occur through normal vessels perfusing regions of lung that are not ventilated at all because the alveoli are filled or closed or the airways leading to the terminal units are completely obstructed (for example, pneumonia, pulmonary edema, atelectasis). As shown by the examples in the section on Pathophysiology of Respiratory Diseases, most right-to-left shunts in patients with pulmonary disease are accounted for by the perfusion of nonventilated lung through relatively normal vascular channels.

TABLE 6. EFFECT OF BREATHING 21 PER CENT AND 100 PER CENT O_2 ON MEAN P_{O_2} VALUES IN ALVEOLAR GAS AND ARTERIAL AND MIXED VENOUS BLOOD IN TWO-COMPARTMENT LUNG MODELS WITH IDEAL GAS EXCHANGE (FIG. 33), A VENTILATION-PERFUSION ABNORMALITY (FIG. 36), AND A RIGHT-TO-LEFT SHUNT (FIG. 38)*

SOURCE	IDEAL		VENTILATION-PERFUSION ABNORMALITY		RIGHT-TO-LEFT SHUNT	
	21%	100%	21%	100%	21%	100%
Mixed venous P_{O_2}, mm Hg	40	51	40	51	40	42
Alveolar P_{O_2}, mm Hg	101	673	105	675	114	677
Arterial P_{O_2}, mm Hg	101	673	89	675	59	125
Alveolar-arterial P_{O_2} difference, mm Hg	0	0	16	2	55	552

*Modified from Murray, J. F.: The Normal Lung. Philadelphia, W. B. Saunders Co., 1976.

REFERENCES

Filley, G. F.: Acid-Base and Blood Gas Regulation. 2nd ed. Philadelphia, Lea and Febiger, 1972.

Hughes, J. M. B.: Editorial review: Pulmonary gas exchange. Clin Sci 58:119, 1980.

Wagner, P. D.: Ventilation-perfusion relationships. Annu Rev Physiol 42:235, 1980.

West, J. B.: Causes of carbon dioxide retention in lung disease. N Engl J Med 284:1232, 1971.

West, J. B.: Ventilation/Blood Flow and Gas Exchange. 3rd ed. Philadelphia, Blackwell Scientific Publications, Ltd., 1977.

West, J. B., and Wagner, P. D.: Pulmonary gas exchange. In West, J. B. (ed.): Bioengineering Aspects of the Lung. New York, Marcel Dekker, Inc., 1977.

OXYGEN TRANSPORT

Oxygen must be supplied continuously to all cells of the body to enable them to carry out their normal metabolic activities; this is true regardless of the specialized function of different cell types, although some cells require more O_2 than others. Without a supply of O_2 to the brain, a human being will lose consciousness in about 20 to 30 seconds and will die in a few minutes. The O_2 demands of a rigorous physical and metabolic existence are met by the integrated responses of the three components of the O_2 transport system: (1) the lungs, which transfer O_2 from environmental air into blood; (2) the heart and blood vessels, which circulate oxygenated blood throughout the body; and (3) the red blood cells, which provide the reservoir of hemoglobin to carry O_2.

Systemic O_2 transport (SO_2T), or the amount of O_2 delivered to the tissues of the body per unit time, can be calculated from the cardiac output ($\dot{Q}$) and the arterial O_2 content (aO_2) according to the formula:

$$SO_2T, \text{ ml/mm} = \dot{Q}, \text{ liters/min}, \times aO_2, \text{ ml/liters}$$

Because the arterial O_2 content is determined by the concentration of hemoglobin available for combination with O_2 and the per cent saturation of hemoglobin, the above equation can be rewritten as follows:

$$SO_2T = \dot{Q} \times (\text{hemoglobin concentration} \times 1.34)$$
$$\times \frac{\text{per cent saturation}}{100},$$

or, because per cent saturation is a function of Po_2 according to the relationship defined by the oxyhemoglobin dissociation curve (Fig. 30),

$$SO_2T = \dot{Q}$$
circulatory component

$$\times (\text{hemoglobin concentration} \times 1.34)$$
erythropoietic component

$$\times f(Po_2).$$
respiratory component

Determinants of O_2 Transport

The subtitles in the previous equation identify the contributions to total O_2 transport of the three organ systems involved: the *circulatory system* determines cardiac output and peripheral blood flow, the *erythropoietic system* determines red blood cell mass and hemoglobin concentration, and the *respiratory system*

TABLE 7. OXYGEN UPTAKE, CONSUMPTION, AND DELIVERY AND THE COMPONENTS OF THE DELIVERY SYSTEM AT REST AND DURING EXERCISE

VARIABLE	REST	EXERCISE
O_2 uptake:consumption	250	4000 ml/min
O_2 delivery	1000	5000 ml/min
Cardiac output	5	25 liters/min
Hemoglobin concentration	15	15 g/dl
Arterial blood Po_2	95	95 mm Hg
Arterial blood O_2 content	200	200 ml/liter
Venous blood Po_2	40	15 mm Hg
Venous blood O_2 content	150	40 ml/liter

determines arterial Po_2. In a normal adult at rest, substantially more O_2 is delivered to the tissues than is used by them (Table 7). Although at first glance the difference between the O_2 supplied and the O_2 consumed may appear to be an unwarranted luxury, this is not true in the case of individual organs (for example, the heart, which uses virtually all the O_2 it receives), and the excess provides some leeway during sudden emergencies when additional O_2 is needed immediately by certain tissues.

Oxygen transport is an important physiologic variable because it sets the upper limit for the quantity of O_2 available to meet the total metabolic needs of the body. Oxygen utilization cannot exceed the supply of O_2 for very long; if it does, the deprived cells must shift from aerobic to anaerobic metabolic pathways to supply their energy needs. One of the consequences of anaerobic metabolism is the production of excess lactic acid. If not relieved, progressive acidosis ultimately disrupts intracellular metabolism and may cause cellular death. Under ordinary circumstances, O_2 transport is always higher than O_2 consumption except in severe exercise, in which a temporary O_2 debt is tolerated.

Adequacy of O_2 Transport

As shown in Table 7, the relationship between O_2 delivery and O_2 uptake-consumption is considerably different during exercise compared with rest. Uptake-consumption increases 16-fold while delivery increases only five-fold. The discrepancy is accounted for by the decrease in venous blood Po_2 and O_2 content; this indicates that substantially more O_2 has been extracted from blood perfusing the exercising muscles. Note that values for hemoglobin concentration and for arterial blood Po_2 and O_2 content are the same during rest and exercise. Thus the changed balance between O_2 delivery and consumption is reflected in new values in the venous blood but not in the arterial circulation.

In pathologic conditions, narrowing of the margin between O_2 supply and demand can develop in several ways: if the demand increases, if the transport system itself is deficient, or if both occur. As is the case during exercise, the balance between O_2 supply and utilization is reflected in the composition of mixed venous blood. A decrease in O_2 delivery or an increase in O_2 consumption means that more O_2 will be extracted from the available arterial blood and that venous Po_2 must decrease. There are, however, some shortcomings in placing full reliance on mixed venous P_{O_2} values as a guide to tissue oxygenation that are discussed in the subsequent section on Respiratory Failure.

REFERENCES

Grote, J., Reneau, D., and Thews, G. (eds.): Oxygen Transport to Tissue II. New York, Plenum Press, 1976.

Finch, C. A., and Lenfant, C.: Oxygen transport in man. N Engl J Med 286:407, 1972.

Klocke, R. A.: Oxygen transport and 2,3-diphosphoglycerate (DPG). Chest 62 (Suppl. Pt. 2):79S, 1972.

Sandoval, J., Long, G. R., Skoog, C., Wood, L. D. H., and Oppenheimer, L.: Independent influence of blood flow rate and mixed venous P_{O_2} on shunt fraction. J Appl Physiol 55:1183, 1983.

Tenney, S. M.: A theoretical analysis of the relationship between venous blood and mean tissue oxygen pressure. Respir Physiol 20:283, 1974.

CONTROL OF BREATHING

The demands of the body for uptake of O_2 and elimination of CO_2 vary considerably in normal persons during their usual daily life; O_2 consumption may increase more than 20-fold in a well-trained athlete from a "basal" level while asleep to a maximal level during strenuous exercise. Remarkably, over this entire range, arterial P_{O_2} changes very little, a few millimeters of mercury at most. This constancy is made possible by a series of control mechanisms that regulate ventilation in accordance with metabolic demands and roughly in proportion to associated increases in cardiac output.

Respiration is also governed by increases or decreases in the concentration of nonvolatile acids in the blood; the changes in ventilation that occur under these conditions serve to restore arterial pH toward a more normal value and are one of the principal means by which the body compensates for nonrespiratory acid-base imbalances. Hyperventilation occurs in normal persons upon ascent to high altitudes, in patients with various pulmonary diseases, and in patients with a variety of common clinical disorders, such as sepsis, metabolic diseases, and psychiatric disturbances. Besides the changes in the pattern of ventilation that occur in response to clinical abnormalities or environmental circumstances, specially coordinated respiratory movements are required for talking, singing, sniffing, coughing, hiccuping, sneezing, vomiting, and breath holding.

The general pattern of organization of the neurologic respiratory control system is shown schematically in Figure 39. Basically, the system consists of a group of *sensors,* which monitor the adequacy of respiration, a *controller,* which integrates afferent information from the sensors with signals of its own, and a group of *effectors,* which respond to commands from the controller. The control of normal breathing will be discussed in the following order: central organization, sensors, effectors, and integrated responses. When appropriate, the reader will be referred to other sections of this chapter for additional information about respiratory control in normal persons and in patients with disease.

Central Organization

Control of respiration by the central nervous system is functionally and anatomically partitioned: the brain stem regulates automatic respiration, whereas the cerebral cortex effects voluntary respiration. Integrating neurons in the spinal cord process efferent information from both respiratory centers in the brain with afferent information from peripheral proprioceptors and send the final signals to the muscles of respiration. Efferent autonomic impulses also travel in the vagus nerves

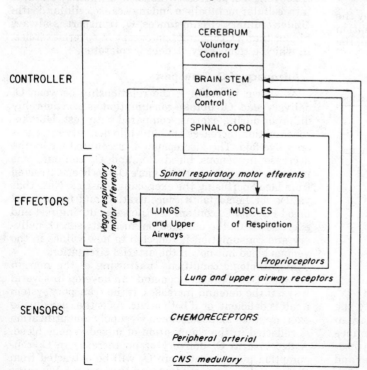

Figure 39. Schematic representation of the respiratory control system showing the interrelationships among the central nervous system controller, effectors, and sensors and also the connections between these elements. (From Berger, A. J., Mitchell, R. A., and Severinghaus, J. W.: N Engl J Med 297:92, 138, 194, 1977; reprinted by permission of the authors and publisher.)

from the central nervous system to the airways and lung parenchyma.

Medulla. The medulla appears to be the headquarters for spontaneous respiration: (1) Rhythmic respiration continues, although the pattern of breathing is likely to change, following transection of the brain at the pontomedullary junction; this indicates that higher centers are not necessary to maintain automatic ventilatory efforts. Moreover, transection below the medulla eliminates respiratory movements. (2) Most of the neurons that demonstrate respiratory periodicity are located in the medulla. The details of the origin of ventilatory oscillations remain uncertain.

The medullary respiratory groups are two bilateral aggregations of respiratory neurons (Fig. 40). The *dorsal respiratory group* (DRG) situated in the ventrolateral portion of the nucleus of the tractus solitarius, which appeared with the evolution to air breathing, consists chiefly of inspiratory neurons. The *ventral respiratory group* (VRG), which is the more primitive of the two groups, located in the nucleus ambiguus and nucleus retroambiguus contains both inspiratory and expiratory neurons.

The location of the DRG within the tractus solitarius, which is the recipient of incoming visceral afferent information in the ninth and tenth cranial nerves, suggests that the DRG serves to process afferent signals into a respiratory motor response. The primary site of automatic respiratory oscillations is in or extremely close to the DRG. Axons from the DRG project to inspiratory spinal motoneurons, principally the phrenic motoneurons. Neurons of the DRG project to the VRG and affect its function, but not vice versa. Axons from the VRG, which is driven by the DRG, project either to certain spinal respiratory motoneurons (chiefly intercostal and abdominal) or by the way of the vagus to muscles of the larynx as well as to airway parasympathetic ganglia that, in turn, inner-

vate airway smooth muscle. However, destruction of the DRG does not cause cessation of rhythmic breathing, suggesting that central respiratory pattern generators are associated with both the DRG and VRG.

Pons. Neurons with respiratory activity have been identified in the pons as well as in the medulla. Pontine neurons exhibit both inspiratory and expiratory (phase-spanning) activity; they may serve to smooth the transition from one phase of respiration to the next.

The pons also contains two important regulatory centers: the *apneustic center* and the *pneumotaxic center*. These aggregates of neurons, presumably located in the lower and upper pons, respectively, act on medullary centers and thus modulate respiratory activity. The pneumotaxic center is believed to act as a fine tuner of the pattern of breathing by influencing the response to afferent stimuli generated during hypoxia, hypercapnia, and lung inflation. The apneustic center appears to contain the normal inspiratory inhibitory mechanism. When this cutoff switch is faulty, apneusis, or prolonged inspiration, results from unrestrained activity of the medullary inspiratory neurons.

Higher Centers. Voluntary, or behavior-related, control of breathing resides in the cerebral cortex, although the exact sites of activity are not completely known. Stimulation of some parts of the cortex inhibits respiratory movements, whereas stimulation of other parts increases respiratory frequency. Pathways from the cerebral cortex to the origin of respiratory muscle motoneurons in the spinal cord are distinct from those tracts concerned with automatic respiration.

The importance of the voluntary control system should not be underestimated. Frequent behavior-related activities involving breathing, such as talking, crying, swallowing, and laughing, cause marked changes in ventilation that may override completely the automatic controls, which respond chiefly to chem-

Figure 40. Schematic representation of the medullary respiratory neuronal groups, cell types, and suggested interconnections. The dorsal respiratory group *(DRG)* located in the ventrolateral nucleus of the tractus solitarius *(NTS)* is where vagal sensory information is first incorporated into a respiratory motor response. The *DRG* drives the ventral respiratory group *(VRG)* and some spinal inspiratory motoneurons. The VRG is composed of nucleus ambiguus *(NA)* and nucleus retroambiguus *(NRA)*. Vagal respiratory motoneurons arise from NA. Axons from NRA project to some spinal inspiratory and probably all spinal expiratory motoneurons. Inspiratory cells are indicated by open circles, and expiratory by hatched circles. Dashed lines indicate some of the proposed intramedullary neural interconnections. *CI* = first cervical dorsal root; α, β, γ, δ subscripts = inspiratory cell subtype designations. (From Berger, A. J., Mitchell, R. A., and Severinghaus, J. W.: N Engl J Med 297:92, 138, 194, 1977; reprinted by permission of the authors and publisher.)

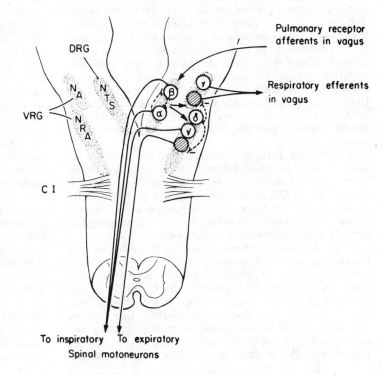

ical stimuli. For example, during phonation, sensitivity to CO_2 decreases dramatically and the subject tolerates considerably higher arterial P_{CO_2} values than when quiet.

Another behavior-related drive to breathing is created by the state of wakefulness, which, in turn, is a reflection of respiratory excitation by the reticular-activating system. These neurons are located in the reticular formation, which extends from the upper cervical cord through the brain stem into the diencephalon.

Sensors

The brain constantly receives a multitude of messages from a variety of sensory receptors. Vision, sound, smell, and touch create an awareness of the external environment; proprioceptive impulses define the relationship of the body to that environment. In addition, most autonomic functions—including respiration—are governed by neural mechanisms that contain components designed to evaluate the performance of the particular function and to change activity when adverse conditions are encountered.

Peripheral Chemoreceptors. Hyperventilation is one of the principal compensatory responses to sudden hypoxemia. This reaction depends on specialized chemoreceptors that monitor the chemical composition of arterial blood: the carotid and aortic bodies.

The carotid bodies are nestled in the bifurcation of the common carotid arteries. They are extremely well vascularized and their blood flow is high relative to their size. The carotid bodies contain two main cell types—type I cells (also called glomus cells, chief cells, or enclosed cells) and type II cells (also called supporting cells, sheath cells, enclosing cells, or sustentacular cells)—that are interspersed among numerous axons and their terminals and abundant blood vessels. Virtually all of the nerve endings in contact with glomus cells are probably axons of afferent sensory nerves that travel in a branch of the carotid sinus nerve and reach the brain in the glossopharyngeal (ninth cranial) nerve. The few terminals on glomus cells that appear to be efferent (5 per cent of the total) are from sympathetic fibers that reach the carotid body from the superior cervical ganglion. Other sympathetic nerves from the same source innervate blood vessels within the carotid body. The only efferent nerves that travel with the afferent axons in the sinus nerve are preganglionic parasympathetic fibers that innervate blood vessels.

Remarkably little is known about the location of aortic bodies in man. Afferent nerve impulses from aortic chemoreceptors travel to the brain in the vagus nerves. Since the ventilatory response to hypoxia in man is abolished by carotid body resection or denervation, it has been concluded that the chemoreceptor activity of aortic bodies is slight or nil.

PHYSIOLOGIC FUNCTIONS. A plot of the relationship between carotid chemoreceptor nerve activity and arterial P_{O_2} shows a progressive increase in impulse traffic as P_{O_2} decreases below 500 mm Hg with a sharp increase in activity when P_{O_2} goes below 100 mm Hg. Below 30 mm Hg, the initial marked increase in impulse activity is not sustained and gradually declines. Whereas the chemoreceptor response to changing arterial P_{O_2} is strikingly alinear, the response to

changing P_{CO_2} from 20 to 60 mm Hg and pH from 7.20 and 7.60 is nearly linear. When two stimuli affect the peripheral chemoreceptors simultaneously, the effects are synergistic; in other words, the resulting increase in nerve activity is greater than the sum of the two separate responses. Besides responding to changes in P_{O_2}, P_{CO_2}, and pH, chemoreceptor activity is provoked by decreases in blood flow, such as may occur when systemic blood pressure falls or when sympathetic activity provokes vasoconstriction of vessels in the carotid bodies.

The actual chemosensitive elements within the carotid bodies are thought to be the afferent nerve terminals with their activity modulated through the presence of reciprocal synapses with the glomus cells. Glomus cells are believed to contain catecholamines, especially dopamine, which serve as the neurotransmitter.

HYPOXIA RESPONSE TESTS. When a normal subject breathes a low concentration of O_2, the resulting decrease in arterial P_{O_2} of the blood flowing through the carotid bodies stimulates an increased frequency of impulses in the sinus nerve. After central processing, the signals actuate an effector response consisting of increased ventilation, cardiac output, and blood pressure. By gradually decreasing the concentration of O_2 in the inspired mixture and measuring corresponding changes in ventilation, it is possible to evaluate a subject's response to hypoxia. The relationship between arterial P_{O_2} and ventilation (Fig. 41, *left*) is hyperbolic and differs according to whether arterial P_{CO_2} is allowed to fall, as it normally does when ventilation increases, or is held constant by adding CO_2 to the inspired mixture, as is the case when performing an isocapnic hypoxia response test. Because hyperbolic curves are cumbersome to analyze, the response to hypoxia is now often expressed as the relationship between expired ventilation and arterial O_2 saturation, monitored with an ear oximeter (Fig. 41, *right*). Under these circumstances, hypoxic sensitivity is reported as the slope of the line ($\Delta \dot{V}/1$ per cent desaturation). Ventilatory responses to isocapnic hypoxia vary widely, with nearly a 10-fold variation in $\Delta \dot{V}/1$ per cent desaturation having been observed in normal subjects. Hypoxic sensitivity decreases with increasing age and is characteristically depressed or even absent in long-term residents of high altitudes (discussed subsequently). Blunted responses to hypoxia contribute to the pathophysiologic abnormalities of patients with severe chronic bronchitis or massive obesity and after the administration of opiates and other sedative drugs.

Central Chemoreceptors. Total denervation of the peripheral chemoreceptors abolishes the hyperpnea of acutely induced hypoxia but does not eliminate, although it reduces slightly, the ventilatory responses to increases in arterial P_{CO_2}. This early demonstration of the existence of respiratory chemoreceptors that are anatomically distinct from the carotid and aortic bodies initiated a number of ingenious experiments that have established the location of chemosensitive regions within the central nervous system and the way in which these neurons respond to certain chemical changes in their environment.

Changes in the composition of an artificial cerebrospinal fluid (CSF) used to perfuse the brain from the third or lateral cerebral ventricles to the cisterna

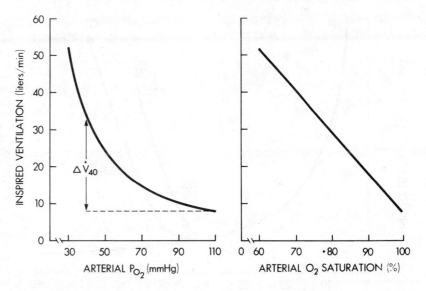

Figure 41. Typical hypoxic response curves of a normal person at sea level, at standard constant arterial P_{CO_2}. *Left panel* shows curvilinear relationship between inspired ventilation and arterial P_{O_2}; also indicated in the hypoxic sensitivity index. *Right panel* shows linear relationship between inspired ventilation and increasing arterial desaturation. (Modified from Berger, A. J., Mitchell, R. A., and Severinghaus, J. W.: N Engl J Med 297:92, 138, 194, 1977; reprinted by permission of the authors and publisher.)

magna can be shown to have a marked influence on ventilation; increasing [H^+] stimulates ventilation, whereas lowering [H^+] depresses it. The chemosensitive elements of the central nervous system seem therefore to be within "reach" of the CSF.

Three bilateral areas in the medulla are involved in central chemosensitivity: (1) a chemosensitive region on the ventrolateral medullary surface lateral to the pyramids and medial to the roots of the seventh through tenth cranial nerves; (2) a chemosensitive area caudal to the first one, lateral to the pyramids, but medial to the root of the twelfth nerve, (3) a third region, which is not itself chemosensitive, located between the other two. The importance of this area can be demonstrated by the nearly complete loss of CO_2-induced ventilatory responses when it is electrocoagulated; this observation has led to the conclusion that afferent fibers from the two chemosensitive regions enter the middle region from which they then project to the respiratory integrating sites elsewhere in the medulla.

PHYSIOLOGIC FUNCTIONS. Intravenous administration of HCl causes hyperpnea, and although blood pH decreases, CSF pH increases. Similarly, administration of $NaHCO_3$ increases arterial pH but decreases CSF pH. The changes in CSF and arterial pH in *opposite* directions during infusion of nonvolatile acids or bases differ strikingly from the fact that pH values in both CSF and blood change in the *same* direction when P_{CO_2} is altered. These observations indicate that the ventilatory responses in patients with acute nonrespiratory acidosis or alkalosis are not mediated by central chemoreceptors, because changes in CSF pH are in the wrong direction, and therefore must be attributed to chemosensitive mechanisms located elsewhere, presumably the carotid bodies.

These paradoxic phenomena are explained by the relative diffusibilities of CO_2, H^+, and HCO_3^- across biologic membranes. CO_2 diffuses readily across cell membranes and, consequently, a change in blood P_{CO_2} immediately affects intracellular pH throughout the body. In contrast, because H^+ and HCO_3^- are poorly diffusible ions, adding them to the bloodstream has only a small immediate effect on intracellular pH. The

rapid diffusion of CO_2 and slow diffusion of H^+ and HCO_3^- account for the different acute ventilatory stimuli that reach central chemoreceptors in patients with respiratory and nonrespiratory acid-base disorders. Even though CSF is an extracellular fluid, it is separated from the bloodstream by an important biologic membrane: the blood-brain barrier. Thus CO_2 has rapid access to CSF and affects its pH, but H^+ and HCO_3^- are excluded temporarily.

CARBON DIOXIDE RESPONSE TESTS. The ideal test of central chemoreceptor sensitivity would measure the changes in ventilation that result from a given change in pH within the chemosensitive cells, but there are many theoretic and practical reasons why such a test cannot be designed. One approach to the problem has been through the use of CO_2 response curves; although these have proved useful, they have certain limitations. (1) The stimulus cannot be quantified precisely because it is impossible to measure pH in or even near the central receptors; (2) the peripheral chemoreceptors and other CO_2-sensitive sites as well as the central chemoreceptors are stimulated by the pH effects of breathing CO_2; (3) there is a wide range of "normality"; and (4) the response is modified, and thus difficult to interpret, by changes in the mechanics of breathing.

Two types of CO_2 response tests are available: the steady-state method, now largely abandoned, and the quicker, easier rebreathing method, in which the subject breathes from a bag prefilled with 7 to 8 per cent CO_2 and excess O_2 (40 to 93 per cent) while ventilatory volume and end-tidal CO_2 concentration are recorded continuously.

A plot of the relationships between ventilation and end-tidal P_{CO_2} obtained by the steady-state and rebreathing techniques is shown in Figure 42. After a few breaths, the rebreathing curve is parallel to the steady-state curve but displaced about 8 mm Hg to the right. The CO_2 sensitivity is reported as the slope of the curve ($\Delta \dot{V}$/mm Hg). Normal values in healthy adults range from 2 to 5 liters/min/mm Hg.

The ventilatory response to CO_2 decreases with age, but not as much as the response to hypoxia. Sensitivity to CO_2 is also blunted in certain endurance athletes and can be severely depressed by a variety of sedatives,

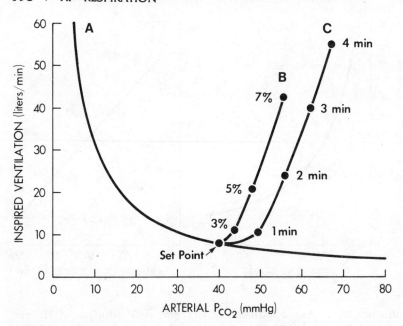

Figure 42. Three CO_2 response curves relating inspired ventilation *(BTPS)* to arterial P_{CO_2} of a normal person at sea level. Curve A approximates the metabolic hyperbola, a reciprocal relation between alveolar P_{CO_2} and alveolar ventilation when inspired gas contains no CO_2. Curve A assumes that dead space is 30 per cent of the total ventilation. Curve B is the steady-state ventilatory response to elevated arterial P_{CO_2}, obtained by breathing CO_2 mixtures (for example, 3 per cent, 5 per cent, and 7 per cent) for at least 10 minutes each. Curve C is the rebreathing CO_2 response, obtained by rebreathing from a bag of 5 to 7 liters prefilled with 7 per cent CO_2 in 40 to 93 per cent O_2 for about 4 minutes. The overall "gain" of the respiratory control system is the ratio of the slope of B to A at the set point, which is about -10. (From Berger, A. J., Mitchell, R. A., and Severinghaus, J. W.: N Engl J Med 297:92, 138, 194, 1977; reprinted by permission of the authors and publisher.)

narcotics, and anesthetic agents. As discussed in the section on Pathophysiology of Respiratory Diseases, important differences in CO_2 sensitivity can be demonstrated among patients with obstructive pulmonary diseases, such as chronic bronchitis and emphysema.

Intrapulmonary Receptors. Activation of receptors located in the nose, oropharynx, and larynx can cause apnea, bradycardia, and sneezing and can trigger the diving and the sniff or aspiration reflexes. Although these effects may be dramatic and profound, stimulation of these extrathoracic receptors elicits protective responses and thus the receptors do not exert continuous control over natural breathing. In contrast, the activity of intrathoracic receptors affects the normal pattern of breathing in most mammals in which it has been studied.

The physiologic effects of stimulation of the three best characterized tracheobronchial and parenchymal receptors, which have their afferent pathways in the vagus nerves, are listed in Table 8. Vagally mediated effects on breathing appear to be substantially weaker in man than in other mammals, but stretch reflexes are active in newborn infants and can be demonstrated with large breaths in healthy adults. In pathologic conditions, however, activation of these receptors is believed to account for the abnormal breathing patterns in patients with many common forms of lung disease discussed in the section on Pathophysiology of Respiratory Diseases (asthma, pulmonary embolism, and pulmonary edema).

Proprioceptors. Both the intercostal muscles and the diaphragm are furnished with proprioceptors, although there are far more muscle spindles in the former than in the latter. Information from these sensors, as described in more detail subsequently, is mainly integrated at the segmental level to influence agonist-antagonist muscle relationships. However, some proprioceptive impulses travel in ascending spinal and sensory tracts to the brain where they may affect the pattern of breathing and, it has been postu-

TABLE 8. CHARACTERISTICS OF THE THREE PULMONARY VAGAL SENSORY REFLEXES*

RECEPTOR	LOCATION	FIBER TYPE	STIMULUS	RESPONSES
Pulmonary stretch, slowly adapting	Associated with smooth muscle of intrapulmonary airways	Medullated	1. Lung inflation 2. Increased transpulmonary pressure	1. Hering-Breuer inflation reflex 2. Bronchodilatation 3. Increased heart rate 4. Decreased peripheral vascular resistance
Irritant, rapidly adapting	Epithelium of (mainly) extrapulmonary airways	Medullated	1. Irritants 2. Mechanical stimulation 3. Anaphylaxis 4. Pneumothorax 5. Hyperpnea 6. Pulmonary congestion	1. Bronchoconstriction 2. Hyperpnea 3. Expiratory constriction of larynx 4. Cough
C fibers	"Pulmonary" (lung parenchyma) and "bronchial" (airways and blood vessels)	Nonmedullated	1. Chemical injury 2. Lung inflation 3. Increased interstitial volume (congestion) 4. Microembolism	1. Rapid shallow breathing 2. Expiratory constriction of larynx, trachea, and bronchi 3. Hypotension, bradycardia

*From Murray, J. F.: The Normal Lung. Philadelphia, W. B. Saunders Co., 1976.

lated, reach conscious level. Thus an imbalance between the neural output of muscle spindles from the intercostal muscles and the mechanical load placed on the muscles is believed to cause dyspnea in certain disorders (see section on Pathophysiology of Respiratory Diseases).

Effectors

Efferent impulses from the brain travel to respiratory motoneurons in the spinal cord and also to the tracheobronchial system and larynx in the vagus nerves (Fig. 40). Efferent vagal fibers complete the reflex arcs of those responses listed in Table 8 that involve bronchial constriction or dilatation and/or laryngeal constriction.

Innervation. The innervation of skeletal muscle, including respiratory muscles, is shown schematically in Figure 43. The efferent motor nerve contains two types of axons: the main muscle fibers are innervated by *alpha motoneurons* and the muscle fibers within the muscle spindles are innervated by *gamma motoneurons*. The signals transmitted along motoneurons to the muscles involved in ventilatory movements, agonist and antagonist groups, are the final integrated product of all the impulses that originate in the brain and descend in the spinal cord plus those that originate from segmental sensory stimuli.

Stretching a muscle causes its muscle spindles to discharge and send afferent signals to the cord; these, in turn, stimulate the alpha motoneuron and cause the main muscle to contract, which counteracts further stretch. Similarly, because the afferent signals from muscle spindles are widely distributed to other spinal segments, synergistic muscle groups are activated and antagonist groups are inhibited. All of these events increase opposition to the stretch that actuated the response in the first place.

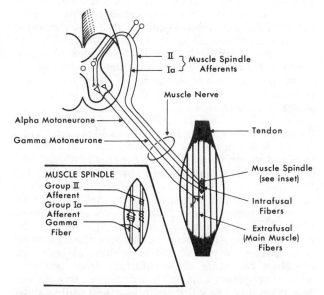

Figure 43. Schematic representation of the proprioceptive and motor innervation of skeletal muscle. See text for discussion. (Adapted from Campbell, E. J. M., Agostoni, E., and Davis, J. N.: The Respiratory Muscles: Mechanics and Neural Control. 2nd ed. London, Lloyd-Luke Medical Books Inc., 1970; reprinted by permission of the authors and publisher.)

Although the precise role of muscle spindles in the regulation of breathing is not certain, studies following deafferentation in man and other animals by dorsal root section clearly establish their contribution to normal ventilation. The function of muscle spindles may be to provide a mechanism by which the main muscle mass compensates, by adjusting its force of contraction, to changes in the load upon it. In addition, impulses may contribute to the fast component of increased ventilation at the onset of exercise.

Mechanical Behavior. The strength of contraction of respiratory muscles, like other muscles, depends on the interaction of extrinsic and intrinsic factors. The summation of the factors can be measured during maximal inspiratory and expiratory efforts by having the subject breathe forcefully through a tube, which can be intermittently occluded and in which pressure can be measured. In young adult men maximal static inspiratory pressure is approximately -125 cm H_2O and maximal static expiratory pressure is approximately $+230$ cm H_2O. The extrinsic factors that affect these values are age, sex, and general muscular development. Women generate about 70 per cent of the values found in men, and there is a decline after 20 years of age of approximately 0.5 cm H_2O/year in maximal inspiratory and expiratory pressures in both sexes.

The two intrinsic factors that affect the strength of respiratory muscle contraction are their length-tension and force-velocity relationships. The length-tension relationship dictates that maximal tension is generated when contraction occurs in a muscle that is slightly stretched above its resting length and that after shortening begins tension decreases rapidly. This explains why maximal static expiratory force is generated at TLC, the volume at which expiratory muscles are most stretched before contraction, and, for similar reasons, why maximal static inspiratory force is achieved at RV. The relationships among maximal static inspiratory and expiratory efforts, lung volume, and recoil of the respiratory system are shown in Figure 44. The force-velocity relationships may limit maximal velocity of airflow during strenuous exercise and during forced breathing maneuvers.

The respiratory muscles are capable of sustaining mild to moderate levels of contractile effort throughout a person's lifetime, but they may fatigue rapidly during maximal efforts. Fatigue occurs rapidly when contractile effort exceeds a certain threshold value, which appears to be approximately 40 to 50 per cent of maximal effort, depending on how performance is monitored. Normal persons can increase the strength and endurance of their respiratory muscles by special exercises; accordingly, respiratory muscle training is now being incorporated into rehabilitation programs of patients with chronic lung diseases such as emphysema and cystic fibrosis.

Tests of Ventilatory Drive. The tests of ventilatory responses to hypoxia and CO_2, although useful and informative, are influenced by mechanical abnormalities of the chest wall, lung parenchyma, and airways. Alternate tests, such as measurements of mechanical work, O_2 cost of breathing, and diaphragmatic electromyographic activity, have been used to differentiate patients with impaired ventilatory drive from those with abnormal mechanics of breathing, but these tests

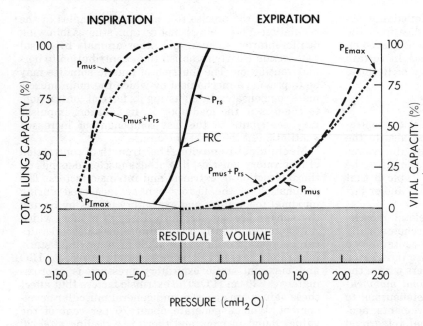

Figure 44. Volume-pressure diagram of the respiratory system (*Prs* same as Figure 18) showing the pressures generated by the respiratory muscles (*Pmus*) and the muscles plus the recoil of the respiratory system (*Pmus* + *Prs*) during inspiration and expiration. *FRC* = functional residual capacity; PI_{max} = maximal inspiratory pressure; PE_{max} = maximal expiratory pressure.

are technically demanding and require considerable patient cooperation. A relatively new test involving occlusion pressure to measure respiratory center output is being increasingly used because it eliminates many of the problems inherent in other methods.

The test is performed by having the subject breathe through a mouthpiece with separate inspiratory and expiratory valves. During expiration at a time unknown to the subject, the operator closes the inspiratory valve, so that the subject begins the next breath in the usual way, unaware that the airway has been occluded. Instead of inhaling air, negative pressure is generated in the mouthpiece until the subject notices that the airway is occluded and makes conscious efforts to resist. However, the pressure generated during the initial 0.2 to 0.3 second of occlusion represents the force developed by the inspiratory muscles in response to the same total respiratory neural drive as in a normal breath. Because there is no flow of gas and because lung volume scarcely changes during inspiration against an occlusion, the pressure generated is virtually unaffected by the mechanical properties of the respiratory system and by the force-velocity relationships of the muscles. However, because of the length-tension relationship of the respiratory muscles, the measurements are influenced by changes in lung volume, and thus serial studies must be made at the same volume, preferably with the subject in the supine position.

The pressure developed during the first 0.1 second after occlusion, often called the $P_{0.1}$, reflects both the neuronal drive to the muscles of inspiration and the contractile capabilities of these muscles. Additional information can be obtained by performing a series of occlusion pressure measurements while CO_2 is added to the inspired gas. From these observations the relationship between changes in $P_{0.1}$ and alveolar (actually end-tidal) PCO_2 can be derived ($\Delta P_{0.1}/\Delta PA_{CO_2}$). For these reasons, occlusion pressure appears to be a useful way of assessing the effector components of the respiratory control system.

Integrated Responses

Certain abnormalities of the respiratory system are discussed in the section on Pathophysiology of Respiratory Diseases. The most commonly observed physiologic adjustments to the control of breathing in normal persons occur during sleep and exercise; both will be reviewed briefly.

Sleep. Recent investigations of respiratory control during sleep have shown striking differences from the awake state. The changes observed differ among the various phases of sleep. Sleep is not a uniform state but a recurring cyclic pattern of sequential stages with a periodicity in adults of approximately 90 minutes. Two distinct sleep states have been defined on the basis of behavioral, electroencephalographic, electromyographic, and electro-oculographic criteria: rapid eye movement (REM) or active sleep and nonREM or quiet sleep. NonREM sleep is subdivided into four stages of progressively deepening sleep, the deepest of which (3 and 4) are often called slow wave sleep because of the characteristic electroencephalographic pattern that develops.

During the lighter stages (1 and 2) of nonREM sleep, the pattern of breathing is irregular and periodic. Tidal volume and respiratory rate vary, and there may be brief episodes of apnea (Cheyne-Stokes breathing). The changes in breathing pattern correspond to fluctuations between wakefulness and sleep. The extent of periodic breathing varies in normal subjects but increases in persons older than 40 years and is almost invariable at high altitudes. Breathing becomes regular during slow wave sleep, but because the component of ventilatory drive related to behavioral activities, including the state of wakefulness from reticular-activating system stimuli, is withdrawn, minute volume is usually 1 to 2 liters/min less than while quietly awake. Accordingly, arterial PCO_2 increases 4 to 8 mm Hg, PO_2 decreases 3 to 10 mm Hg, and pH decreases 0.03 to 0.05 unit. Furthermore, during nonREM sleep, ventilatory responses to classic respiratory stimuli (hypoxia, hypercapnia, and lung inflation) are preserved, which indicates that dominant control during these stages is by automatic components and that breathing demands are dictated by metabolic needs.

Breathing during REM sleep is characteristically irregular but not periodic, with brief periods of apnea up to 15 and sometimes 20 seconds or even longer in normal adults and children and 10 seconds in infants. Irregular breathing often coincides with bursts of REM and other muscle activity. At other times, chest wall motion is paradoxic and there are marked fluctuations in the smooth muscle tone of airways, because of the great variation in the concentrations of O_2 and CO_2 in the airstream.

In contrast to nonREM sleep, breathing during REM sleep is much less dependent on chemical stimuli; responses to CO_2 are profoundly blunted or even absent, although responsiveness to hypoxia is retained. The origin of the respiratory drive during REM sleep is unknown, but it does not appear to depend on metabolic (chemical) stimuli. Breathing during this phase of sleep may relate to the neural activity inherent in the REM state itself in much the same way that activity of the reticular-activating system augments breathing during wakefulness.

Exercise. As O_2 consumption increases during mild and moderate exercise, defined as below the anaerobic threshold, ventilation increases proportionately and both arterial Po_2 and Pco_2 remain constant. The control of breathing during these kinds of exercise is thought to include a rapid or *neural component* and a slow or *humoral component*. During exercise above the anaerobic threshold, the formation of lactate and the presence of acidemia add another stimulus to ventilation to those already present, and arterial Pco_2 decreases.

The neural component is believed to cause the immediate increase in ventilation that accompanies the onset of exercise. It is conceivable that some of the early increase in breathing is a conditioned, or learned, response, but considerable evidence points to the role of proprioceptive impulses arising from the exercising muscles as providing the necessary drive.

For 20 to 30 seconds after the onset of exercise, the newly increased level of ventilation remains relatively constant. Thereafter, ventilation gradually increases until it reaches a new steady state, which depends on the severity of the exercise being performed. The delayed ventilatory response is attributable to the slow appearance of a humoral substance that is not a hormone but the addition of CO_2 to the bloodstream. The generation of CO_2 by the exercising muscles and the stimulating effects of CO_2 on peripheral and central chemoreceptors appear to be the sole and adequate explanation for the humoral component. Much more controversy concerns the cause, magnitude, and even presence of the neural drive to breathing during exercise.

REFERENCES

Berger, A. J., Mitchell, R. A., and Severinghaus, J. W.: Regulation of respiration. N Engl J Med 297:92, 138, 194, 1977.

Clark, F. J., and von Euler, C.: On the regulation of depth and rate of breathing. J Physiol (London), 222:267, 1972.

Derenne, J. P., Macklem, P. T., and Roussos, C.: The respiratory muscles: Mechanics, control, and pathophysiology. Am Rev Respir Dis 118:119, 373, 581, 1978.

Gautier, H.: Control of the pattern of breathing (editorial review). Clin Sci 58:343, 1980.

Leith, D. E., and Bradley, M.: Ventilatory muscle strength and endurance training. J Appl Physiol 41:508, 1976.

Milic-Emili, J., Whitelaw, W. A., and Derenne, J. P.: Occlusion pressure—a simple measure of the respiratory center's output. N Engl J Med 293:1029, 1975.

Mitchell, R. A., and Berger, A. J.: Neural regulation of respiration, respiratory control and clinical applications. In Hornbein, T. F. (ed.): Lung Biology in Health and Disease. New York, Marcel Dekker, Inc., 1981, vol. 17, pt. I, pp. 541–620.

Phillipson, E. A.: Respiratory adaptations in sleep. Annu Rev Physiol 40:133, 1978.

LIQUID AND SOLUTE MOVEMENT

The dynamics of liquid and solute movement in the lungs has been one of the most active subjects of anatomic and physiologic experimentation during the last 15 years. The major new clinicophysiologic concepts that have emerged are that (1) the lungs are not "dry" organs, as was formerly believed, but are the sites of constant liquid filtration and removal at rates that are at least as great as those in most other organs and (2) when the rate of liquid filtration in the lungs exceeds the rate of its removal, pulmonary edema begins to form and thereafter follows an orderly and reproducible sequence. The first concept will be reviewed here, the second in the section on Pathophysiology of Respiratory Diseases (Pulmonary Vascular Disorders).

Formation of Liquid

The factors that determine the rate of liquid filtration across semipermeable membranes in the body are defined by the Starling equation. Thus the forces operating on the pulmonary capillary endothelium, which is clearly the major site of filtration in the lungs, can be expressed as follows:

$$\dot{Q}_f = K_f \left[(Pmv - Ppmv) - \sigma \left(\pi mv - \pi pmv \right) \right]$$

where $\dot{Q}_f$ = the net liquid filtration across the endothelial surface, K_f = the filtration coefficient (an expression of the leakiness of the membrane), Pmv = the hydrostatic pressure within the microvascular lumen, $Ppmv$ = the hydrostatic pressure within the perimicrovascular interstitial space, πmv = the colloid (or protein) osmotic pressure within the bloodsteam, πpmv = the colloid osmotic pressure within the perimicrovascular interstitial space, and σ = the reflection coefficient. The Starling equation explains two important aspects of liquid filtration across the pulmonary endothelial surface: (1) that three important factors regulate the movement of fluid—the permeability of the membrane (K) and the opposing forces offered by the hydrostatic pressure ($Pmv - Ppmv$) and the colloid osmotic pressure ($\pi pmv - \pi mv$)—and (2) that the net hydrostatic and colloid osmotic forces are determined by the intravascular (Pmv and πmv) and extravascular ($Ppmv$ and πpmv) pressures—in other words, the pressures operating *across* the endothelial surface and not just those within the capillary. The difference between intravascular and extravascular pressures is often referred to as the transmural or transmicrovascular pressure. The quantities designated in the equation and the discussion about them indicate that filtration of liquid occurs across the endothelium of small pulmonary blood vessels. Under ordinary conditions, about 66 per cent of net liquid filtration is from the capillaries, 27 per cent from venules, and 7 per cent from arterioles. Presumed values for the pressures that determine the direction and magnitude of liquid movement in the normal human lung are shown in Figure 45; the derivation of these values will be discussed subsequently.

Hydrostatic Forces. The hydrostatic pressures of importance in regulating filtration of liquid in the lungs are the pressure within the pulmonary microcirculation and the interstitial pressure surrounding the vessels. The exact values for these pressures are not known, but some reasonable approximations can be made. The pressure within the capillaries must lie between the mean pressures known to exist in the pulmonary veins (5 mm Hg) and in the pulmonary arteries (14 mm Hg). Judging from information about the uneven distribution of resistances to blood flow through various segments of the circulation, pressure in the capillaries is believed to be closer to that in the veins than in the arteries and has been assigned a value of 8 mm Hg. Interstitial, or pericapillary, pressure is more difficult to deduce. Intuitively, interstitial pressure is probably close to alveolar pressure, which is atmospheric or 0 mm Hg, because the two spaces are separated by only a thin membrane composed of the alveolar epithelium and its overlying layer of surfactant; neither of these delicate structures seems capable of preventing virtually full transmission of pressure from the alveolar space into the interstitium. However, the surface film does have slight recoil properties that "use up" some of the alveolar pressure; thus the pressure in the interstitial space across the membrane from the alveolus must be subatmospheric. The exact value depends on the surface tension at the air-liquid interface and the radius of the curvature of the surface; calculations and experimental approximations suggest values ranging from −2 to −17 mm Hg. Given the dimensions of the alveoli and the characteristics of the surface-active material, a value of −2 mm Hg has been used in this analysis, but it is possible that it is lower. Assuming that these values are correct, the net transmural hydrostatic pressure difference is 10 mm Hg (8 mm Hg intravascular minus −2 mm Hg interstitial).

Colloid Osmotic Forces. The microvascular endothelium is not freely permeable to all molecules present in the bloodstream. Low molecular weight substances, including most solutes and electrolytes, move readily across the membrane and are present in approximately equal concentrations in plasma and interstitial liquid. The passage of larger molecules is restricted, however, creating concentration differences across the membrane that in turn create osmotic pressure differences. Nearly all of the transcapillary osmotic pressure difference, which depends on the number of molecules and is independent of the kind of molecules, is attributable to differences in protein concentration.

Thus it is necessary either to know the protein composition, from which oncotic pressure can be calculated, or to measure the oncotic pressure directly in specimens of plasma and interstitial liquid. It is easy to obtain plasma and to determine its oncotic pressure, which averages 24 mm Hg in normal persons, but no one has succeeded in obtaining a sample of interstitial liquid. The best approximation of the composition of interstitial liquid has been derived by analyzing lymph from the lungs; this approximation rests on the experimental evidence that the protein concentration in pulmonary lymph is nearly identical to that in the liquid in interstitial spaces. Analysis of lung lymph from several mammalian species, including man, has revealed a substantial protein content and a colloid osmotic pressure of approximately 19 mm Hg. Thus the calculated transmural colloid osmotic pressure difference is only 6 mm Hg (25 mm Hg intravascular minus 19 mm Hg interstitial). Therefore the balance between the hydrostatic pressure (an outward force of 10 mm Hg) and protein osmotic pressure (an inward force of 6 mm Hg) in the Starling formulation is such that there is a net outward filtration pressure of 4 mm Hg acting across the microvascular endothelium.

Permeability of the Alveolar-Capillary Membrane. Permeability in biologic systems denotes the ease with which substances cross membranes, including the pulmonary microvascular endothelium and the alveolar epithelium. All molecules do not move across pulmonary capillaries with equal freedom; some are more selectively retained within the bloodstream than others. In general, low molecular weight substances cross more readily than those with high molecular weights, but lipid solubility, electrical charge, and molecular orientation are also important. In the Starling equation, the permeability coefficient describes the porosity, or leakiness, of the microvascular endothelium for water. When the permeability of the membrane increases, more liquid is filtered at any given balance of forces across the membrane, and large molecules in the blood have freer access to the inter-

NORMAL

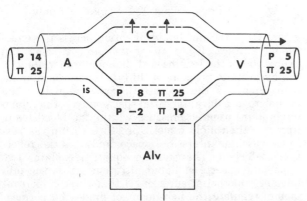

Figure 45. Schematic diagram of the normal pulmonary circulation showing pulmonary artery (*A*) giving off two capillaries (*C*) that lead to a pulmonary vein (*V*). The vessels are surrounded by an interstitial space (*is*) contiguous to an alveolar space (*Alv*). The prevailing normal intracapillary and interstitial hydrostatic (*P*) and protein osmotic (Π) pressures are shown. The *arrows* indicate the direction and magnitude of liquid movement. (From Hinshaw, H. C., and Murray, J. F.: Diseases of the Chest. Philadelphia, W. B. Saunders Co., 1979, p. 630.)

stitial space than when permeability is normal. The alveolar epithelium is normally much less permeable than the microvascular endothelium; this arrangement prevents the constant flow of liquid from capillaries into the interstitial space from continuing into the alveolar space.

The differences in permeability of the two membranes may be explained by the more complicated junctions between adjacent epithelial cells. Pulmonary capillary endothelial junctions are composed of one or sometimes two strands, which may have a beaded appearance in some regions and are discontinuous in other regions (Fig. 46, *top panel*). In contrast, epithelial cell junctions are considerably more complex and consist of an intricate network of interconnecting junctional strands (Fig. 46, *bottom panel*). The junctions form a continuous belt-like region surrounding both type I and type II epithelial cells and resemble those described in other "tight" epithelial barriers.

The different rates of movement of small and large molecules through membranes can be accounted for by assuming that pores with varying dimensions exist; however, the anatomic counterparts of the postulated pores system in the alveolar-capillary membrane are not known. It is generally believed that liquid and solutes pass across interendothelial junctions, which restrict the passage of protein-sized lipid-insoluble molecules; liquid is prevented from entering the alveoli by the presence of complex interepithelial junctions. Macromolecules may be transported bidirectionally in pinocytic vesicles in both endothelial and epithelial cells, but how the protein molecules normally found in interstitial liquid got there is not known.

Once filtered, liquid does not accumulate in the perimicrovascular interstitial space of the interalveolar septum. Instead, liquid moves into the interstitial spaces surrounding airways and blood vessels where the lymphatic capillaries are located, through which the liquid is removed from the lungs. The continuity between the perimicrovascular and peribronchovascular interstitial spaces provides the necessary pathway for the movement of filtered liquid from its site of formation to its site of removal from the lungs in the pulmonary lymphatics and also, under certain conditions, back into the bloodstream. The driving force is created by the difference in pressure in the two inter-

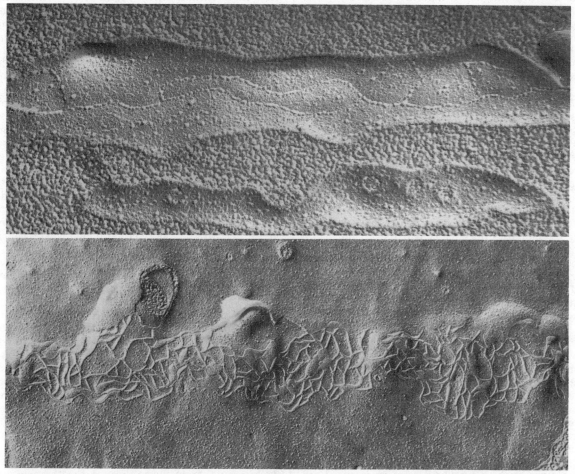

Figure 46. Freeze fracture studies of the intercellular junctions between pulmonary capillary endothelial cells *(top panel,* original magnification ×118,000) and alveolar epithelial cells *(bottom panel,* original magnification ×48,000). Note that the endothelial junction consists of one or two beaded strands, whereas the epithelial junction is composed of numerous connected continuous strands. The complexity of the junctions reflects, and may determine, the relative permeabilities of the two cellular barriers to liquid and solute movement. (Courtesy of Dr. E. Schneeberger.)

stitial spaces: the pressure in the perimicrovascular interstitium is slightly subatmospheric (-2 mm Hg), whereas that in the peribronchovascular interstitium is slightly more negative than pleural pressure (-5 mm Hg). Thus there is a built-in pathway and constant pressure difference that keeps the interalveolar septum from filling with liquid.

Removal of Liquid

The only way that a positive net transcapillary liquid exchange can be sustained without finally filling the interstitial spaces and flooding the alveolar spaces is through an efficient system for removing substances filtered from the vascular compartment. The lymph capillaries of the lungs provide the chief disposal mechanism for much of the liquid, all of the proteins and macromolecules, and, at times, even particles.

The interstitial liquid that reaches the peribronchial interstitial space probably has access to the lumen of the lymphatic capillaries through openings in the thin, discontinuous basal lamina and gaps between adjacent cells. As liquid accumulates in the interstitium and distends the space, the lymph channels are pulled open, not collapsed as might be expected because of their delicate structure, by the tension that develops on tethers that connect the lymphatics to the surrounding bronchovascular sheath.

Pulmonary lymph flows toward the hilum because of the pressure generated by rhythmic contractions of the smooth muscles in the walls of lymphatic vessels and the pressure gradient that exists between the periphery and the hilum. Undoubtedly, ventilatory movements and circulatory pulsations contribute to the propulsive forces, but lymphatic contraction seems to be the more important. The bicuspid funnel-shaped valves throughout the lymphatic microcirculation ensure a one-way flow of lymph into collecting channels. When liquid filtration increases, so do both the strength and frequency of lymphatic pulsations. Lymphatic removal capacity can probably increase at least five-fold to ten-fold above basal rates. Thus the pulmonary lymphatics must be considered an important and responsive system that protects the lung against pulmonary edema. Abnormal accumulation of water occurs *only* when the rate of filtration of liquid from blood vessels exceeds the rate of removal of liquid through the lymphatics.

Measurement of Lung Water Content

Several different approaches are being explored to measure lung water content or alveolar-capillary membrane permeability, but none has reached the stage of routine clinical application. The most widely used of these methods are: (1) the multiple indicator dilution technique, which measures extravascular water as the difference in the volumes of distribution of a diffusible and nondiffusible indicator; (2) the soluble gas method, which measures lung tissue volume by the uptake of a soluble gas, such as acetylene, from an inspired gas mixture; and (3) measurement of rates of movement of isotopically labeled substances from the alveolar space to the bloodstream, or vice versa, which assesses the permeability characteristics of the intervening alveolar-capillary membrane.

REFERENCES

Bhattacharya, J., and Staub, N. C.: Direct measurement of microvascular pressures in the isolated perfused dog lung. Science 210:327, 1980.
Ciba Foundation Symposium 38 (new series): Lung Liquids. Amsterdam, Elsevier Co., 1976.
Crandall, E. D., Staub, N. C., Goldberg, H. S., and Effros, R. M.: Recent developments in pulmonary edema. Ann Intern Med 99:808, 1983.
Pietra, G. G.: The basis of pulmonary edema with emphasis on ultrastructure. In Thurlbeck, W. M., and Abell, M. R. (eds.): The Lung: Structure, Function and Disease. Baltimore, Williams and Wilkins, 1978.
Schneaberger, E. E.: Structural basis for some permeability properties of the air-blood barrier. Fed Proc 37:2471, 1978.
Staub, N. C.: Pulmonary edema. Physiol Rev 54:678, 1974.
Staub, N. C. (ed.): Lung Water and Solute Exchange. New York, Marcel Dekker, Inc., 1978.
Staub, N. C.: The pathogenesis of pulmonary edema. Prog Cardiovasc Dis 23:53, 1980.

BIOCHEMICAL TRANSFORMATIONS

The actual work involved in gas exchange is performed chiefly by the respiratory muscles, which provide the mechanical force required for ventilation, and by the heart, which pumps blood through the pulmonary circulation. Because gas exchange by diffusion is a passive process that does not require energy, virtually the entire metabolic cost of respiration is borne by organs other than the lungs. However, the lungs are metabolically active and have an O_2 consumption that at times may be appreciable, especially when lung disease is present. The metabolic needs of normal human lungs are probably of the order of 1 to 2 per cent of resting whole body O_2 consumption. Some of the O_2 utilized by the lung is for processes related to respiration, such as the syntheses of surfactant, collagen, and elastin; some is used to satisfy the metabolic requirements of the approximately 40 different cell types that compose the lungs; and the remainder is spent by cells performing nonrespiratory functions, such as phagocytosis and the synthesis, storage, release, activation, and inactivation of a variety of chemical substances.

Many of the nonrespiratory activities performed by the lungs can also be carried out in other organs of the body. However, the lungs are unique in that they receive the entire cardiac output and are interspersed between the gastrointestinal tract and the systemic circulation. Thus the lungs are strategically located to alter the composition of blood before it flows to the rest of the body. Because of the lungs' ability to transform circulating chemical substances, the concentrations of chylomicrons, clotting factors, prostaglandins, biogenic amines, nucleotides, kinins, and angiotensins are different in systemic arterial blood than in mixed venous blood.

Chylomicrons and Lipids

Lymph, rich in chylomicrons absorbed from the gastrointestinal tract, flows through the thoracic duct to the systemic venous system and then to the right side of the heart and to the lungs. Isolated lungs are known to clear fatty acids from the blood, and after absorption of fatty foods from the intestines there is a measurable increase in the lipid content of the lungs. Uptake and metabolism of chylomicrons appear to reside in the pulmonary endothelial cells, whose ability to process lipids differs only quantitatively from that of lactating mammary glands. Metabolism of chylomicrons is probably facilitated by the presence in the lungs of the enzyme lipoprotein lipase; in addition, an esterase believed to be involved in lipid metabolism has been found on the luminal surface of pulmonary endothelial cells.

Clotting Factors

One of the several nonrespiratory functions of the lungs is that of serving as a filter of venous blood from the entire body. In keeping with the notion that some clotting occurs continuously, even in healthy persons, lungs are furnished with a fibrinolytic system to break down small clots and aggregates of platelets and fibrin formed during "normal" intravascular coagulation. Factors capable of promoting fibrinolysis, such as *plasminogen activator,* have been identified in endothelial cells of the entire pulmonary circulation. The efficiency of this removal system can be appreciated by recognizing that the lungs can completely clear pathologic pulmonary emboli that are orders of magnitude larger than the spontaneously occurring clots. In addition to its fibrinolytic mechanisms, the lung appears to be guarded against local clotting by stores of the potent anticoagulant *heparin.*

Paradoxically, the lungs also contain substances that can initiate coagulation. A tissue factor, or *thromboplastin,* has been found on the plasma membranes of endothelial cells of the pulmonary artery and its vasa vasorum. The contribution, if any, of the lung's coagulation system to normal homeostasis remains mysterious. It has been speculated that in certain forms of diffuse lung injury, local release of thromboplastin from the damaged lung parenchyma may cause both the formation of the small vessel thrombi that are virtually always found and the disseminated intravascular coagulation that occasionally complicates these disorders.

Prostaglandins

The ubiquitous prostaglandins are not stored in the lung, unlike many other compounds; rather they are synthesized and released on demand. Most newly formed endogenous prostaglandins exert their physiologic effects locally rather than systemically, largely because of the remarkably efficient inactivation system in the lungs. During a single passage through the lungs, 60 to 90 per cent of prostaglandins of the E and F series are taken up and degraded, which prevents them from accumulating in the blood. Thus these compounds are viewed as *local* hormones rather than the traditional *circulating* hormones. Prostaglandins of the A series, which are inactivated in some species (guinea pig and rabbit) but not in others (dog and cat), and prostacyclin, which is not inactivated, may serve as circulating hormones in certain mammals. A major unresolved question concerns the possibility that the inactivation of prostaglandins is less efficient in the presence of pulmonary disease and that, under these circumstances, they may exert potent systemic effects. To date, there are no data to substantiate or refute this statement.

Clearance of prostaglandins of the E and F series from circulating blood requires cellular uptake through an active transport system on or near the luminal surface of pulmonary endothelial cells. The sites of intracellular degradation have not been identified. In addition to being the chief sites of the uptake of prostaglandins from circulating blood, pulmonary endothelial cells are also involved in the synthesis and release of these substances; once prostaglandins are released in the lungs, a variety of bronchomotor and/or vasomotor responses can occur, depending on which compound predominates.

In general, prostaglandins of the E series are dilators and those of the F series are constrictors of the pulmonary vasculature and airways. Other prostaglandins, and the related thromboxanes and endoperoxides, also appear to exert a direct effect on smooth muscle cells. Prostaglandins may play a role in the vasoconstriction induced by hypoxia, the pathophysiology of asthma and other anaphylactic disorders, and the responses initiated by pulmonary embolism and mechanical stresses of the lungs. The synthesis and release by the lungs of prostacyclin is of considerable interest, because this substance is a strong vasodilator and is the most potent endogenous inhibitor of platelet aggregation known.

Biogenic Amines

The processing of biogenic amines by the lungs is remarkably selective. *Serotonin* is efficiently cleared in a single passage, whereas *histamine* is not taken up at all. Similarly, circulating *norepinephrine* is removed by the lungs, whereas its precursor, *dopamine,* and its end-product, *epinephrine,* are not affected.

Both serotonin and norepinephrine are removed from the circulation by pulmonary endothelial cells. Some of these amines are stored intact within the cells and some are degraded; subsequently, both the intact substance and its metabolic products are returned to the bloodstream. Although there are qualitative similarities in the handling of serotonin and norepinephrine, the sites of metabolic activity and the pathways involved are not fully defined and may not be the same. Both processes appear to be saturable so that when high concentrations of either substance occur in venous blood, the excess can "spill over" into the systemic arterial circulation.

Nucleotides

Adenosine 5'-triphosphate (ATP) and *adenosine 5'-monophosphate* (AMP) are cleared from the pulmonary circulation during a single passage by means of degradation effected by phosphate esterase enzymes. The physiologic importance of the clearance of circulating nucleotides is unknown. It is speculated that the system serves to prevent the entry of adenine, a potent vasodilator that may be released from muscles during strenuous exercise and crush injuries, into the systemic circulation.

Kinins and Angiotensins

The lungs process circulating vasoactive polypeptide hormones of presumed physiologic and pathophysiologic importance, the most carefully studied of which are *bradykinin,* a potent endogenous vasodilator, and the *angiotensins,* a group of polypeptides involved in blood pressure and sodium regulation. Angiotensin I, a relatively inactive decapeptide, is formed in the blood from an α2-globulin precursor by the enzymatic action of renin and in turn is converted to the highly active octapeptide angiotensin II during passage through the lungs. One of the metabolic products of angiotensin I is also transformed in the lungs to angiotensin III, a compound that is more potent in stimulating the release of aldosterone but less active in constricting blood vessels than angiotensin II.

The same enzyme—*angiotensin-converting enzyme*—cleaves both bradykinin and angiotensin I. Angiotensin-converting enzyme has also been identified within cells of blood vessels from other organs. In contrast, the enzyme that inactivates angiotensin II is not present in the lungs but is found in other organs. The implications of these differences in the location of the two enzymes are clear. First, the presence of an enzyme capable of degrading a vasodilator and forming a vasoconstrictor on the surface of pulmonary endothelial cells, where it has access to the whole cardiac output, governs the vasomotor properties of blood flowing to the entire body. Second, the location of the angiotensin II–metabolizing enzyme everywhere but the lungs and the predominantly intracellular rather than surface location of the angiotensin I–converting enzyme both suggest that peripheral tissues are more concerned with the destruction and not the formation of angiotensin II and can use this process to regulate their own blood flow.

Angiotensin-converting enzyme has been shown to be increased in patients with certain pulmonary diseases, particularly active sarcoidosis. However, the clinical significance of these observations, such as the influence on blood pressure regulation or sodium homeostasis, is not at all apparent.

REFERENCES

Bakhle, Y. S., and Vane, J. R. (eds.): Metabolic Functions of the Lung. New York, Marcel Dekker, Inc., 1977.

Gail, D. B., and Lenfant, C. J. M.: Cells of the lung: Biology and clinical implications. Am Rev Respir Dis 125:366, 1983.

Hyman, A. L., Spannhake, E. W., and Kadowitz, P. J.: Prostaglandins and the lung. Am Rev Respir Dis 117:111, 1978.

Mellins, R. B.: Metabolic functions of the lung and their clinical relevance. Am J Roentgenol 138:999, 1982.

DEFENSE MECHANISMS

The body is in direct contact with its external environment not only on the skin but also in the lungs. In fact, the internal surface area of the lungs is more than 70 times greater than the external surface of the skin. Each day the lungs of a normal person are exposed to more than 10,000 liters of inhaled ambient air that may contain hazardous dusts, toxic chemicals, or infectious microorganisms. Thus it is no wonder that the respiratory tract is elaborately equipped with a variety of defense mechanisms (Table 9) to protect it and the rest of the body from injury and the introduction of disease.

The lungs, like other organs, are under the protective influence of certain generalized defense mechanisms, such as blood-borne and resident phagocytic cells, immune surveillance cells, and antibodies and antimicrobial substances present in the bloodstream and in

TABLE 9. MECHANISMS THAT CONTRIBUTE TO THE DEFENSE OF THE RESPIRATORY TRACT*

Nonspecific defense mechanisms
  Clearance
    Nasal clearance
    Tracheobronchial clearance
    Alveolar clearance
  Secretions
    Tracheobronchial lining (mucus)
    Alveolar lining (surfactant)
    Lysozyme
    Interferon
    Complement
  Cellular defenses
    Nonphagocytic
      Airway epithelium
      Terminal respiratory epithelium
    Phagocytic
      Blood phagocytes (polymorphonuclear, neutrophilic leukocytes, monocytes)
      Tissue phagocytes (alveolar macrophages)

Specific defense (immunologic) mechanisms
  Antibody-mediated (B lymphocyte-dependent) immunologic responses
    Serum immunoglobulins
    Secretory immunoglobulins
  Cell-mediated (T lymphocyte-dependent) immunologic responses
    Lymphokine mediated
    Direct cellular cytotoxicity

*From Murray, J. F.: The Normal Lung. Philadelphia, W. B. Saunders Co., 1976.

secretions, including respiratory tract fluids. In addition to systemic defense mechanisms, the respiratory tract has its own indigenous anatomic features that affect the deposition of particles and gases and also a specialized system for removing substances after they are deposited. Once injury has occurred, the lungs depend on certain systemic mechanisms to control the inflammatory response. These processes are essential in maintaining the normal physiologic integrity of the lungs; conversely, disruptions in the system are closely linked to the pathophysiology of disease.

Deposition of Particles

The term *aerosol* is used to describe any system of liquid droplets or solid particles dispersed in air (or some other gas) that remains airborne for a reasonable time. The essential requirements of an aerosol are that the particles be sufficiently small so they settle slowly and that the aerial suspension be stable. Because large particles tend to settle rapidly, clinically important aerosols, whether industrial, natural, or therapeutic, are composed mainly of particles less than 10 μm in diameter.

Particles are removed from the airstream the instant they contact any portion of the lining of the respiratory tract. Furthermore, once a particle has touched the luminal surface, it ordinarily is not resuspended in the airstream and therefore must be cleared from the body by some other means. Three different physical forces govern the deposition of particles within the respiratory system: inertia, sedimentation, and diffusion.

Inertia. Particles inhaled in the airstream are forced to change direction repeatedly as they travel through the numerous curves and branches in the nasopharynx and tracheobronchial tree. However, once in motion, a particle tends to move in the same direction because of its inertial forces. This means that if a particle continues in its original direction when it should turn, it will touch and hence be deposited upon the luminal surface. Because inertial forces increase with air velocity, inertial deposition of particles is greater in the upper than in the lower airways and is enhanced by increased frequency of breathing.

Sedimentation. Although an aerosol is a reasonably stable suspension, the particles are under the influence of gravity and will settle if given enough time. Deposition by sedimentation occurs more readily in relatively still air and thus is greater near to and within the terminal respiratory units than in the conducting airways. For similar reasons, at a given minute volume, sedimentation is augmented by breathing slowly and deeply. The speed of settling is determined by the density of the particle and the square of its diameter; accordingly, a silica particle settles faster than a grain of pollen the same size.

Diffusion. Aerosol particles may demonstrate random (brownian) motion if the particles are small enough to be influenced by the continuous bombardment of the surrounding gas molecules. Consequently, deposition by diffusion is negligible for particles larger than 0.5 μm and is important only in the terminal respiratory units, where the mass movement of air is trivial. Diffusion of gas molecules, not bulk flow, causes mixing of newly inspired fresh air with gas remaining from the previous breath in the terminal respiratory units. However, owing to differences in size, the diffusion of gas molecules is orders of magnitude faster than the diffusion of particles.

These theoretic considerations and experimental observations have led to the following conclusions about the distribution of spherical particles of unit density contained in "idealized aerosols" within the human respiratory system.

(1) Almost all particles larger than 10 μm are deposited in the nasal passages and hence do not penetrate as far as the tracheobronchial tree. Conversely, the efficiency of nasopharyngeal filtering decreases as particle size decreases, becoming negligible at about 1 μm.

(2) The percentage of particles that penetrate into the terminal respiratory units increases from essentially zero with particles 10 μm and above to a maximum with particles 1 μm and below.

(3) Particles approximately 2 μm in aerodynamic diameter demonstrate a peak of deposition on the alveolar surface; larger particles are trapped in the airways, and smaller particle retention decreases because impaction in alveoli decreases down to a particle size of about 0.5 μm.

(4) Particles smaller than 0.5 μm are also retained in considerable numbers owing to a relative increase in the force of impaction by diffusion with decreasing particle size.

When one is considering the distribution and retention behavior of irregularly shaped materials of varying densities, appropriate corrections must be introduced.

Deposition of Gases

Gases are classified into three main groups: *therapeutic, inert,* and *toxic*. Therapeutic gases include O_2 and inhalation anesthetics. Inert gases are normally of no physiologic consequence, but they are used in the laboratory to study various aspects of respiratory function. Toxic gases produce an undesirable physiologic effect that is usually accompanied by a pathologic response. Sometimes gases must be classified in more than one category; for example, O_2, a commonly used therapeutic gas, may be toxic when administered in high concentrations for several days.

The penetration into and retention within the respiratory tract of toxic gases is exceedingly variable and depends on the physical properties of the gas, its concentration in the inspired air, and the rate and depth of ventilation. Inhalation of a noxious gas usually has an immediate and profound effect on the pattern of breathing. Reflexes are triggered by chemical stimulation of receptors located in the nose (sneezing, laryngeal closure), larynx (coughing, laryngeal closure, slowing of breathing), airways (coughing, laryngeal narrowing, hyperpnea, bronchoconstriction), and lung parenchyma (rapid, shallow breathing).

In contrast to inhaled particles, which may or may not touch the luminal surface, part of the airstream containing an inhaled toxic gas is always in contact with the moist epithelial lining of the nasopharynx, conducting airways, and distal airspaces. Therefore, some of the foreign gas is absorbed as the inspirate flows through the air passages, and the amount removed varies according to the solubility of the gas. Highly water-soluble gases like SO_2, when present in low concentrations, are completely extracted by the nose in healthy subjects during brief exposures; in contrast, insoluble gases like phosgene and chlorine are removed much less completely in the upper airways and hence penetrate more deeply into the respiratory tract. The amount of water-soluble gas that can be contained in tissues is limited, and saturation occurs quickly unless the amount already dissolved is removed by blood flow or chemical degradation. This means that if a highly soluble gas is present in high concentration, the absorptive capacity of the proximal surfaces becomes overwhelmed and the gas penetrates more deeply into the tracheobronchial tree. Less soluble gases that are poorly extracted in the conducting airways reach and mix with the air contained in distal respiratory units and a fraction of the foreign gas is absorbed immediately. The amount taken up is proportional not only to the solubility and alveolar concentration of the foreign gas but also to the volume of tissue to which the gas is exposed. Because the alveolar surface is so extensive, large amounts of a toxic gas may be extracted by the lung even though the solubility of the gas is relatively low.

Clearance of Particles

Almost all of the solid particles that impact in the airways and on the alveolar surface are ultimately eliminated from the body. However, the mechanisms involved and the time required for complete removal vary greatly, depending on the chemical properties of the particles and how far into the respiratory tract they penetrate before impacting. There are two interdigitating clearance systems that serve to remove particles deposited in different locations: clearance from the nasopharynx and tracheobronchial tree is achieved by *mucociliary transport* and clearance from terminal respiratory units by *macrophage transport*. The efficacy of these processes is demonstrated by the fact that residents of most North American cities inhale several hundred grams of mineral particles during their lifetimes but only a few grams can be recovered from their lungs post mortem.

Nasal Clearance. The nose is structured anatomically so that most of the particulate matter that is inhaled through it impacts near the front on nonciliated epithelium, where the passages are narrow and tortuous and where hairs are located; deposition of particles anteriorly facilitates their removal by nose blowing and sneezing. Particles deposited more posteriorly are swept backward over the mucus-lined, ciliated epithelium to the nasopharynx, where they are swallowed.

Tracheobronchial Clearance. As in the posterior nasopharynx, removal of particles from all the conducting airways and possibly the proximal respiratory bronchioles as well is carried out by mucociliary clearance. Efficient removal depends on proper functioning of the two main components of the mucociliary system: the ciliated cells of the tracheobronchial epithelium and the double-layered film of mucus that covers the luminal surface.

Human ciliated cells have approximately 200 cilia and contain numerous mitochondria clustered beneath the basal bodies of the cilia, presumably to provide the chief sources of energy for ciliary activity. A cilium is a complex structure that contains several pairs of separate filaments, each surrounded by a membrane. The cilia of a single cell and those of continuous, but not anatomically connected, cells appear to be coordinated so that a wave of effective surface motion spreads in a proximal direction. Cilia beat rapidly with a characteristic biphasic stroke—a fast forward flick followed by a slow backward movement.

The mucous lining throughout most of the airways is composed of a double (sol-gel) layer on the surface of the bronchial epithelium, depicted in Figure 47. The inner layer, in which the cilia beat, is the liquid or sol phase of the transport medium, and the outer layer is the viscous or gel phase. The viscous layer is formed of discontinuous plates of mucus that are nonabsorbent to water and thus help to protect the sol phase from desiccation; moreover, the tips of the beating cilia just strike the innermost part of the gel covering them, facilitating proximal movement of the layer. Thus, any particles that deposit on the surface of the mucus are carried along with it to the oropharynx, where they are swallowed or expectorated.

Mucociliary clearance is usually measured by cinefluoroscopic or bronchoscopic monitoring of the rate of motion of discs placed on the luminal surface and external detection by gamma cameras of the rate of disappearance of inhaled aerosolized radioisotopes. The results vary widely, even among apparently healthy people.

Alveolar Clearance. The disposition of solid particles that settle on the alveolar surface differs from that of particles deposited on the airway surface in that participation by the alveolar macrophage is required. Alveolar macrophages must (1) locate the particle, (2) phagocytize it, and (3) find their way out of the labyrinthine terminal respiratory unit to the beginning of the mucociliary escalator. Thereafter, particles ascend to the pharynx and are swallowed. Most of the particulate load deposited on the alveolar surface is eliminated by the mechanism just described. However, other pathways may be utilized, depending on the quantity of dust to be disposed of (the "dust burden"), the physicochemical composition of the particles, and the reactivity of the subject to them (the "host factor").

As an alternative route, instead of moving along the surface of the terminal respiratory unit the particle-laden macrophage can move through the interstitial space of the interalveolar septum until it reenters the lumen of the air spaces. Presumably, this occurs at the

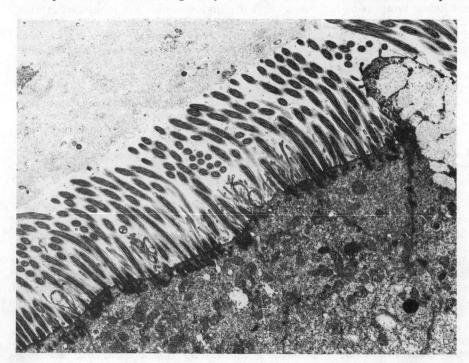

Figure 47. Electron photomicrograph of a portion of the mucociliary apparatus. The tips of the cilia touch the base of the mucous layer. Note the similarity between the appearances of the mucous layer and the secretory granules of the epithelial mucous (goblet) cell. (Uranyl acetate and lead citrate; original magnification ×6600.) (From Yoneda, K.: Am Rev Respir Dis 114:837, 1976; reprinted by permission of the author and publisher.)

site of, or actually through, the lymphatic aggregates at the junctions of respiratory and terminal bronchioles, where traffic of cells is favored. Septal transport represents a "shortcut" from alveolus to terminal bronchiole compared with surface transport but takes longer to traverse.

Some of the particles that reach the interstitial space enter lymphatic capillaries instead of reentering bronchioles. If the particle successfully navigates more centrally located lymph channels and lymph nodes, it reaches the bloodstream and may circulate anywhere in the body.

Unless the particle load is heavy and macrophage transport is overwhelmed, little, if any, of the inhaled material reaches the hilar lymph nodes or bloodstream. However, with increasing exposure and saturation of phagocytic capacity, more and more particles can be found in regional lymph nodes and elsewhere in the body.

Bioactive particles, such as those that cause a fibrogenic or immunologic reaction, may be sequestered in the lung parenchyma by inflammatory response after the particles have been carried into the interstitial spaces and then released by alveolar macrophages. This reaction is complex, and many details about its mechanisms are lacking; however, the cytotoxicity of the inhaled substance and host responsiveness are clearly important factors that contribute to the outcome.

Protease Inhibition

In any inflammatory response, regardless of whether it is of infectious, physicochemical, or immunologic origin, *proteases* are released by leukocytes, macrophages, and other cells that participate in the reaction. These enzymes, including elastase and collagenase, probably are major contributors to tissue destruction caused by inflammation. *Protease inhibitors* are also present in inflammatory exudates, presumably serving to restrain the exuberance of inflammatory reactions by deactivating newly released proteases.

Alpha₁-antitrypsin is the circulating human protease inhibitor that has attracted the most attention because of the diseases that are found in association with its deficiency, most notably pulmonary emphysema. Models of this form of emphysema have been produced by injecting the plant enzyme papain and, subsequently, enzymes obtained from mammalian leukocytes and macrophages into the lungs of experimental animals. All of these enzymes digest lung tissue and cause typical emphysematous lesions. Emphysema presumably develops in patients with a genetically determined decrease in serum levels of α_1-antitrypsin because of the unrestrained digestive activity of proteases released in their lungs. A similar imbalance, but in this instance excessive protease activity relative to available inhibitor capacity, may cause the type of emphysema that is found in heavy smokers.

α_1-Antitrypsin and other antiproteases also inhibit several other enzymes, including plasmin, plasma thromboplastin antecedent, and kallikrein, that are integral parts of interrelated, cascading enzyme systems that affect coagulation, vascular permeability, kinin generation, fibrinolysis, and complement formation. Thus a deficiency of one or more protease inhibitors could cause emphysema by a variety of indirect mechanisms. Whether α_1-antitrypsin and other protease inhibitors act directly or indirectly, it is clear that they should be regarded as systemic determinants of the structure and function of the lungs.

Oxidant Inhibition

In addition to attack by endogenous proteolytic enzymes, the lungs are subject to injury through the local production of powerful oxidants such as superoxide anion, hydrogen peroxide, and the product of these reactants, hydroxyl radical. Oxidants may be generated in the lungs by two distinct mechanisms: (1) polymorphonuclear leukocytes and other cells involved in local inflammatory reactions and (2) the direct effects on lung tissue of high concentrations of inhaled O_2 or toxic substances like paraquat. In either case the liberated oxidants have potent cytotoxic effects on lung parenchymal cells, although there are variations in susceptibility among different cells. Production of oxidants by the cellular constituents of inflammatory reactions serves as a double-edged sword; one edge is the direct cytotoxicity of the reactants, and the other, equally sharp, is their ability to inactivate α_1-antitrypsin. Inactivation of the lungs' major defense against proteolysis allows unrestrained activity of neutrophil elastase and other proteolytic enzymes that are also released during inflammation; this sequence is believed to compound lung damage in inflammatory disorders such as adult respiratory distress syndrome (described subsequently). To combat the effects of locally generated oxidants, the lungs are equipped with several intracellular and extracellular protective mechanisms, including the antioxidant enzyme systems—superoxide dismutase, catalase, glutathione peroxidase, NADPH, and cytochrome c reductase—and the oxidant-free radical scavengers, alpha-tocopherol and ascorbic acid.

REFERENCES

Brain, J. D., Proctor, D. F., and Reid, L. M. (eds.): Respiratory Defense Mechanisms, Parts 1 and 2. New York, Marcel Dekker, Inc., 1977.

Brain, J. D., and Valberg, P. A.: Deposition of aerosol in the respiratory tract. Am Rev Respir Dis 120:1352, 1979.

Green, G. M., Jakob, G. J., Low, R. B., and Davis, G. S.: Defense mechanisms of the respiratory membrane. Am Rev Respir Dis 115:479, 1977.

Martin, W. J., Gadek, J. E., Hunninghake, G. W., and Crystal, R. G.: Oxidant injury to lung parenchymal cells. J Clin Invest 68:1277, 1981.

Wanner, A.: Clinical aspects of mucociliary transport. Am Rev Respir Dis 116:73, 1977.

Pathophysiology of Respiratory Diseases _____

GENERAL CONSIDERATIONS

Pathophysiology is the study of disordered function, the processes that create abnormalities and the responses to them. Sometimes the reaction to a pathologic process is similar to that provoked by a normal process: the hyperpnea in response to fever can be explained in large part by the same metabolic (chemical) stimuli that cause hyperpnea during exercise. Sometimes, however, the reaction to disease is unique: the astonishingly marked and rapid changes in the mechanical properties of the lungs and chest wall during an asthmatic attack have never been observed in a normal person.

TABLE 10. EXPLANATION OF ABBREVIATIONS DEFINED EARLIER AND USED IN THIS SECTION

Lung Volumes	
TLC	total lung capacity
VC	vital capacity
FRC	functional residual capacity
RV	residual volume
Mechanics	
FEV_1	forced expiratory volume in 1 second
FVC	forced expiratory VC
FEV_1/FVC	ratio of FEV_1 to FVC
$\Delta\dot{V}max_{50}$	difference between maximal expiratory flow rates at 50 per cent expired FVC breathing room air and a mixture of O_2 and helium
$\Delta\dot{V}max_{75}$	difference between maximal expiratory flow rates at 75 per cent expired FVC breathing room air and a mixture of O_2 and helium
$Viso_{\dot{V}}$	volume at which maximal expiratory flow-volume curves breathing room air and a mixture of O_2 and helium converge
Gas Exchange	
O_2	oxygen
CO_2	carbon dioxide
CO	carbon monoxide
N_2	nitrogen
He	helium
P_G	partial pressure of a gas (e.g., P_{O_2} = partial pressure of O_2)
DL_{CO}	diffusing capacity for CO
P_{50}	the P_{O_2} at which hemoglobin is 50 per cent saturated
Acid-base	
H^+	hydrogen ion
$[H^+]$	concentration of H^+
pH	negative logarithm of H^+ activity
HCO_3^-	bicarbonate
$[HCO_3^-]$	concentration of HCO_3^-
Control of Breathing	
$P_{0.1}$	pressure generated in the first 0.1 second when inhaling from FRC against an occluded airway
CSF	cerebrospinal fluid

Organization

The section on Normal Physiology of the Respiratory System dealt with the physiology of normal respiration including gas exchange, O_2 transport, the control of breathing, and the physiology of the major nonrespiratory functions of the lung, including liquid and solute exchange, biochemical transformations, and defense mechanisms. This section deals with the pathophysiologic counterparts of most of these processes. Abnormalities of pulmonary defenses, particularly infections, are reviewed elsewhere.

The two types of disorders of ventilation, restrictive and obstructive, are considered in separate subsections because they are so different. Abnormalities of blood flow are discussed under the general heading of circulatory disorders to enable inclusion of pulmonary edema, pulmonary hypertension, and cor pulmonale. Disorders of gas exchange and control of breathing are discussed, and two new subjects are introduced: disorders of the pleura, which may have a profound effect on respiration, and respiratory failure, the pathophysiologic state that represents the culmination of abnormalities affecting any of the organs of respiration.

Because it is clearly impossible to discuss the physiologic responses to all possible respiratory diseases, certain arbitrary selections have been made. Examples were chosen primarily to demonstrate general pathophysiologic principles. For the most part, the diseases being considered are common and important medical problems. For convenience, abbreviations of certain physiologic terms, which were introduced and defined earlier and which will be used in this section and the next, are listed in Table 10.

REFERENCES

Bates, D. V., Macklem, P. T., and Christie, R. V.: Respiratory Function in Disease: An Introduction to the Integrated Study of the Lung. 2nd ed. Philadelphia, W. B. Saunders Co. 1971.

Cherniak, R. M., and Cherniak, L.: Respiration in Health and Disease. 3rd ed. Philadelphia, W. B. Saunders Co. 1983.

Fraser, R. G., and Paré, J. A. P.: Synopsis of Diseases of the Chest. Philadelphia, W. B. Saunders Co., 1983.

Saunders, K. B.: Clinical Physiology of the Lung. Oxford, Blackwell Scientific Publications, 1977.

West, J. B.: Pulmonary Pathophysiology—The Essentials. Baltimore, Williams and Wilkins, 1977.

RESTRICTIVE VENTILATORY DISORDERS

The restrictive ventilatory disorders are a group of pulmonary and extrapulmonary diseases that all share the common physiologic abnormalities of decreased lung volumes, particularly VC and TLC. Because VC is also decreased in obstructive ventilatory disorders (discussed next), it is necessary to demonstrate both the absence of obstruction to air flow and the presence of a decreased TLC to document that pure restriction exists. There may be other important associated abnormalities in patients with restrictive disorders, such as decreased DL_{CO}, maldistribution of inspired air, and disturbances of gas exchange, but none of these is essential for the diagnosis, and whether or not they are present depends on the type of underlying disease, its severity, and its extent. Thus, restrictive ventilatory disorders are not a specific clinical entity but a characteristic pattern of changes in lung volumes that may be produced by many different diseases.

Lung volumes are determined, as explained in the section on Normal Physiology of the Respiratory System, by the mechanical properties of the lungs and chest wall and by the force that can be generated by the muscles of respiration to overcome the recoil characteristics of the respiratory system (Fig. 18). Restrictive ventilatory disorders can be caused by diseases that affect either the distensibility characteristics of the lungs or chest wall, which includes the maximal volume they are able to contain, or the strength of the respiratory muscles. A classification that utilizes these principles is presented in Table 11. Disorders of the chest wall, pleura, and respiratory muscles are often referred to as *extrapulmonary* causes of restrictive ventilatory defects, in contrast to intrinsic diseases of the lungs that cause *pulmonary* restriction.

Disorders of the Chest Wall

The chest wall can be viewed as the container for the lungs and as the structure that must be expanded and contracted by the action of the respiratory muscles for normal breathing to occur. Disorders of the chest wall can cause restrictive lung disease if its size is too small to contain a normal volume of air and/or the structure is so stiff that the force developed by the respiratory muscles fails to cause normal expansion. In Table 11, scoliosis is cited as an example of increased stiffness and thoracoplasty as an example of decreased volume; neither is entirely true, although these are the predominant abnormalities, because both stiffness and size are affected in the two conditions. The deformed chest cage in patients with severe scoliosis is smaller than that in normal persons, and the compliance of the chest wall after thoracoplasty is decreased.

Patients with severe scoliosis will serve as a focus for discussion, although the abnormalities are representative of those in other patients with disorders of the chest wall. In general, the severity of the pathophysiologic abnormalities in patients with scoliosis correlates well with the extent of the deformity. Thoracic spinal angulation greater than 70° places the person at risk of developing respiratory failure sometime during his or her lifetime; an angle greater than 100° is usually associated with effort intolerance and one greater than 120° with hypercapnia.

TABLE 11. CAUSES AND EXAMPLES OF RESTRICTIVE VENTILATORY DISORDERS

Disorders of the chest wall
  Increased stiffness—scoliosis
  Decreased volume—thoracoplasty
Disorders of the pleura
  Increased stiffness—fibrothorax
  Decreased volume—pneumothorax
Disorders of the respiratory muscles
  Decreased strength—amyotrophic lateral sclerosis
Disorders of the lungs
  Increased stiffness—diffuse interstitial fibrosis
  Decreased volume—pneumonectomy

Lung Volumes. By applying the same concepts that led to an understanding of the determinants of lung volumes in normal subjects, the reasons for the changes observed in patients with scoliosis become apparent. The chief abnormality is a marked change in the position and slope of the volume-pressure curve of the chest wall. The resting volume of the chest wall (alone) is decreased and its volume-pressure curve is shifted downward and considerably flattened; this means that the chest wall is extremely stiff. These changes alone account for most of the decrease in TLC, VC, and FRC and the relatively well-preserved RV. The volume-pressure curve of the lungs is also abnormal, but this is believed to be a secondary change. Because of the deformed thorax, the lungs are small and it is impossible for them to undergo the periodic hyperinflations that are necessary for the maintenance of normal surface activity at the air-liquid interface. In the absence of intermittent deep breaths, surface forces increase and alveoli collapse. In patients with scoliosis the use of forced inflations with intermittent positive pressure, for example, causes an increase in VC, presumably from opening of collapsed units. Because pulmonary compliance increases proportionately more than VC, a redeployment of surface forces probably also occurs.

Mechanics of Ventilation. The effects of scoliosis on the mechanics of ventilation are predictable from knowledge of the elastic recoil of the lungs and the caliber of the tracheobronchial system. In the absence of intrinsic disease of the airways, FEV_1/FVC is in the high normal range because the volume of air to be expelled is low and the cross-sectional area of the airways is at least what it should be at a given lung volume throughout the FVC maneuver. The situation is analogous to a normal subject inflating his or her lungs to the same lung volume as the TLC of a patient of the same age, sex, and predicted height with severe scoliosis and then both persons making forced expiratory maneuvers. The resulting "partial" maximal expiratory flow-volume curve of the normal subject and the "complete" curve of the scoliotic patient are superimposable (Fig. 48). Thus the air flow rates in patients with scoliosis are consistent with the elastic recoil generated by normal lungs operating at a decreased volume.

Gas Exchange. Patients with severe scoliosis ultimately develop marked hypoxia and hypercapnia. The multiple pathophysiologic mechanisms that contribute to these abnormalities of gas exchange have been partially clarified, although some basic questions remain unanswered.

Diffusing capacity of the lungs, corrected for lung volume, is within the normal range in patients with mild to moderately severe scoliosis but is decreased in those with advanced disease. The reason for this reduction is not known, and it is possible that it is related to errors in predicting what the value ought to be in the presence of a marked skeletal deformity with resulting decrease in TLC. Furthermore, the presence of maldistribution of inspired air, which is usually present, may cause spurious results. If the DL_{CO} is truly decreased, the explanation must lie in some unknown effect of scoliosis on the alveolar-capillary membrane or the pulmonary capillary blood volume.

The severe hypoxia of scoliosis is caused by ventila-

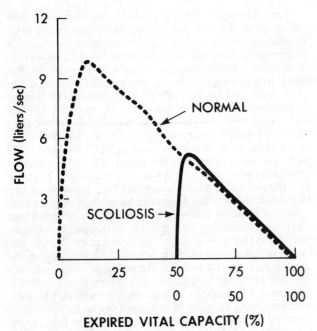

Figure 48. Representative forced expiratory flow-volume tracings of a normal adult (dotted line, from Figure 21) and a patient with severe scoliosis (solid line). Note that the vital capacity of the patient with scoliosis is smaller than normal but that the maximal airflow achieved during exhalation is normal at that reduced lung volume.

tion-perfusion mismatching. At very low lung volumes, much of the parenchyma lies behind closed or narrowed airways and thus is perfused but poorly ventilated. Ventilation-perfusion abnormalities also develop in normal persons who breathe well below their FRC values and, more pertinently, below their closing capacities.

The problem of gas exchange is worsened by the previously mentioned tendency for lung units to collapse because of the inability of scoliotic patients to take deep breaths periodically and redistribute surfactant. Furthermore, the severity of hypoxia in these patients is augmented because of their abnormal pattern of breathing. For reasons that are not understood, patients with chest deformities breathe with small tidal volumes, which increases the fraction of wasted ventilation with each breath, and with normal or low minute volumes. Because this combination decreases alveolar ventilation, arterial P_{CO_2} must rise and the decreased P_{O_2} from ventilation-perfusion mismatching is worsened. These findings should be contrasted with those in patients with diffuse interstitial fibrosis, discussed subsequently, who also have ventilation-perfusion abnormalities and arterial hypoxia but who maintain normal or usually low P_{CO_2} values by hyperventilating. The presence of hypercapnia and hypocapnia in these two groups of patients, both of whom have restrictive ventilatory disorders, is best explained by differences in the control of breathing. The efferent ventilatory responses in patients with scoliosis are limited by the mechanical abnormalities of the chest wall; in contrast, the afferent drive is increased from stimulation of intrapulmonary receptors in patients with infiltrative diseases whose chest walls are capable of responding to the increased drive to breathe.

Pleural Restriction

Disorders of the pleura can produce restrictive ventilatory disorders in two ways: (1) by filling the pleural space and compressing the lung on the affected side and (2) by forming a thick constricting layer on the surface of the lung. In either case, because the involved lung is smaller than normal at FRC and cannot inflate to its usual TLC, a restrictive ventilatory defect is present.

In patients with pathologic conditions the pleural space can be filled with air (pneumothorax) or liquids, such as pus (empyema), blood (hemothorax), or undifferentiated liquid (pleural effusion). The pathophysiologic factors leading to and resulting from pneumothorax and pleural effusion are considered later in this section. The lung volumes in patients with these disorders demonstrate typical restriction. The present discussion will consider the pathophysiologic consequences of a fibrothorax, which usually results from the organization of an inflammatory exudate or, sometimes, a hemothorax.

Lung Volumes. A fibrothorax obliterates the pleural space and leaves a thick fibrous layer, which may calcify, on the surface of the affected lung. Although the lung underneath may be perfectly normal, the constricting, poorly distensible shell decreases resting lung volume and prevents full inflation of the affected side. Thus FRC, VC, and TLC are decreased and RV is low-normal or slightly decreased. However, these abnormalities are usually more severe than can be accounted for by involvement of only one lung. Accordingly, even though clinical, roentgenographic, and sometimes pathologic evidence indicates unilateral pleuritis, the expandability of the contralateral lung is also impaired. This is not an unreasonable finding because it simply means that the two hemithoraxes do not behave independently of each other. The thoracic cage, which obviously surrounds both hemithoraxes, probably serves as the coupling force in that it transmits the effects of a local disturbance, which reduces the volume and limits the expansion of one lung, from the affected side to the other side.

Mechanics of Ventilation. Changes in FEV_1/FVC and expiratory air flow rates in patients with fibrothorax are typical of those in patients with other forms of restrictive ventilatory defects: normal or supernormal FEV_1/FVC values and well-preserved maximal expiratory flow rates during forced expiration. As in patients with scoliosis discussed previously, and for similar reasons, the elastic recoil of the lungs in patients with fibrothorax is normal or slightly increased at the reduced range of VC available.

Gas Exchange. In patients with unilateral pleuritis, blood flow to and ventilation in the lung with pleural disease is reduced, especially at the base, but ventilation is reduced more than perfusion. In the contralateral normal lung, expansion is limited and blood flow is also redistributed away from the base. The redistribution of blood flow away from the bases is undoubtedly a consequence of the effects of lung volume on pulmonary vascular resistance. In the upright position lung expansion is less at the bases than at the apex because of both the effects of the gradient of pleural pressure (discussed in the section on Normal Physiology of the Respiratory System) and the location of the pleuritis. Accordingly, pulmonary vascular resistance is abnormally increased at the base and blood flow is redistributed upward.

Studies with ^{133}Xe demonstrate regional changes in the distributions of ventilation. Decreased arterial P_{O_2} values and increased alveolar-arterial P_{O_2} differences found in these studies are presumably caused by the resulting ventilation-perfusion mismatching.

Muscle Weakness

Severe weakness of the inspiratory muscles should cause a restrictive ventilatory defect when it is impossible to inflate the lungs completely. Obviously, failure to reach full inflation must decrease both VC and TLC, which satisfies the definition of restriction. Weakness of the expiratory muscle groups may prevent full expiration and thus increase RV. Expiratory muscle weakness might also be expected to impair maximal expiratory flow rates, especially during the early effort-dependent portion of the forced expiratory maneuver. There is enormous variation, however, in the results of respiratory function testing in patients with various neurologic diseases. The differences depend on the type and severity of underlying disease and, in particular, on which muscle groups are impaired. Furthermore, although careful neurologic examination provides a useful profile of a given patient's muscle strength, it is not a good predictor of possible pulmonary function abnormalities.

Lung Volumes. A true restrictive ventilatory defect with decreased VC and TLC is found only when the diaphragm is markedly weakened. This presumably is because the diaphragm has considerable reserve as a pressure generator and its function must be severely impaired before its ability to expand the thorax is limited. When maximal static inspiratory pressure, mainly diaphragmatic in origin, is decreased to approximately 60 per cent of normal, values of TLC are still within normal limits. Values of RV increase when exhalation is incomplete and there is a rough correlation between the maximal static expiratory pressure generated at TLC, a measure of the total expiratory force that can be generated, and an increase in RV (provided that the pressure developed is less than 50 per cent of the predicted value). Thus it seems that there is considerable reserve inherent in the expiratory muscle groups as well as the inspiratory muscle groups and that substantial impairment, which may be selective or involve both groups, must occur before lung volumes are affected.

In some patients with respiratory muscle weakness values of FRC are in the upper limits of the normal range. This may result from an upward shift of the volume-pressure curve of the chest wall, but the finding of a normal rather than an increased transpulmonary pressure at FRC argues against this possibility. A more likely explanation is that a decreased tone of the abdominal muscles allows passive descent of the diaphragm, which enlarges the chest wall configuration at FRC. When substantial losses of lung volumes occur from atelectasis and/or increased surface forces, FRC is likely to decrease.

Mechanics of Ventilation. As is the case with other types of restrictive ventilatory defects, patients with muscle weakness have normal or supernormal values for FEV₁/FVC because their lungs are small but air empties through normal-sized airways. Maximal ex-

piratory flow-volume curves in patients with severe muscle weakness reveal that (1) in some patients flow rates are greater than predicted at the lung volumes available to the patient and (2) in others peak flow is decreased, the maximal expiratory flow-volume envelope is reached, and then flow abruptly drops away from the envelope as RV is approached (Fig. 49). The physiologic explanation for the first type must lie either in increased elastic recoil of the lungs, possibly related to increased surface forces, or in patchy atelectasis in which the caliber of conducting airways is better preserved than the number of participating air spaces. The mechanism for the second type of abnormal maximal expiratory flow-volume curve is related to decreased expiratory muscle force. Insufficient pressure is generated by the weakened muscles to produce normal peak flows and to empty the lungs completely to ordinary RV, and the weaker the expiratory muscles are, the lower the peak flow and the higher the RV.

It is probable that other physiologic aspects of muscle function, such as the rate of fatigue, which is not assessed by measuring static pressures or even single-breath maneuvers, may contribute to time-dependent pulmonary function abnormalities. These are likely to be extremely important clinically, both during exercise and in dealing with respiratory complications such as infections.

Gas Exchange. Arterial P_{O_2} and P_{CO_2} are well maintained in patients with muscle weakness until extremely advanced disease is present. Furthermore, when hypercapnia occurs it appears to be specifically

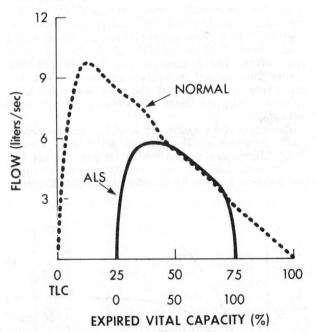

Figure 49. Representative forced expiratory flow-volume tracings of a normal adult (dotted line, from Figure 21) and a patient with severe amyotrophic lateral sclerosis (solid line, *ALS*). Note that the vital capacity in ALS is limited because the patient is too weak to inhale to normal total lung capacity *(TLC)*. During forced expiration, the normal flow-limiting segment is reached temporarily, but then maximal airflow decreases and residual volume increases because the expiratory muscles are too weak to exhale completely.

related to failure of the diaphragm. Because the volume-pressure characteristics of the chest wall and lungs are presumably normal in most patients with muscle weakness, FRC is also normal and, as mentioned, may be within the upper limits of the normal range. Breathing from a normal or slightly increased FRC tends to ensure distribution of air to all regions and to prevent the ventilation-perfusion abnormalities that develop at low lung volumes (see discussion of scoliosis). If atelectasis supervenes, arterial Po_2 decreases from increased venous admixture.

Diffuse Infiltrative Diseases

Although extrapulmonary diseases are important causes of restrictive ventilatory disorders, the classic and most common causes are diffuse infiltrative pulmonary diseases, such as sarcoidosis, lymphangitic carcinomatosis, asbestosis, and other similar conditions. Of these, the prototype intrapulmonary disorder that will be discussed is diffuse interstitial fibrosis, a process that may be associated with collagen-vascular diseases, occupational exposure, and other known lung injuries, but it is often of unknown origin.

Lung Volumes. In patients with diffuse interstitial fibrosis of the lung parenchyma, there is a tendency for the chest cage, respiratory muscles, and airways to be relatively unaffected and to retain the capabilities appropriate for the original size of the (unaffected) lungs. This means that the abnormalities of lung volumes in this disorder must be explainable mainly by alterations in the volume-pressure characteristics of the lungs. This appears to be the case, as shown in Figure 50 (*left panel*). Because of the shift downward of the volume-pressure curve, TLC and VC are decreased considerably and FRC and RV are decreased slightly. Note that the recoil pressures of the diseased lungs toward TLC are substantially higher than normal values. The respiratory muscles can generate higher than normal inspiratory pressure at TLC because they are working at a shorter length (because volume is less) and hence at an improved mechanical advantage.

There are two possible explanations for the abnormally increased recoil pressures of the lungs toward TLC: (1) increased stiffness of functioning alveoli and (2) complete loss of some units with overdistension of the remaining normally functioning alveoli. Evidence for or against these possibilities can be obtained by replotting the volume-pressure curve of the lungs in terms of per cent of *observed* VC instead of *predicted* VC (or TLC). When this is carried out (Fig. 50, *right panel*), the data fall within the normal range, indicating that alveoli in the shrunken lungs are, for the most part, behaving normally. Data from other patients, however, do not transpose to the normal range, indicating that their functioning units are abnormally stiff. Thus there is direct support for both patterns of involvement, although no information is available about morphologic-physiologic correlates of the two types.

The measurement of elastic recoil pressure at TLC has been recommended as a means of differentiating patients with extrapulmonary causes of restriction, in whom recoil pressure may be low because of atelectasis, from patients with intrapulmonary cases of restriction, in whom recoil pressure is high. If recoil pressure is decreased, the presence of extrapulmonary restriction may be inferred. However, this distinction is not always possible because, as indicated previously, the value can be surprisingly high in some patients with respiratory muscle weakness and other extrapulmonary disorders resulting from increased surface forces.

Mechanics of Ventilation. The FEV_1/FVC and specific airways conductance, which reflect mainly the resistance to airflow in large- and medium-sized airways, are at normal or high normal levels in patients with diffuse interstitial fibrosis. Maximal expiratory flow-volume curves usually show well-preserved flows at available lung volumes, but in contrast to patients with extrapulmonary causes of restriction, when plotted against static elastic recoil pressure at those volumes, flow rates may be normal or, in many instances, abnormally decreased. Low maximal expiratory flow at a particular recoil pressure means that the resistance of peripheral small airways is increased. (See discussion of Obstructive Ventilatory Disorders for further explanation.) This kind of analysis from direct measurements of maximal expiratory flow-volume and static volume-pressure relationships led to the expectation that small airways are narrowed in many patients with diffuse interstitial fibrosis, a prediction that has now been substantiated by morphologic evidence. Furthermore, the presence of frequency dependence of compliance, another test of small airways

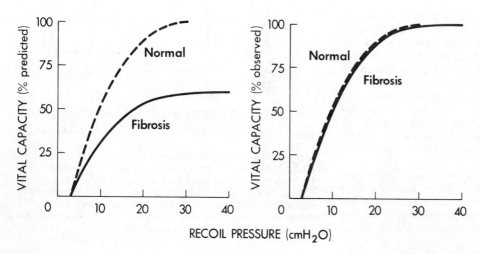

Figure 50. Representative volume-pressure curves of a normal adult (dotted line, from Figure 15) and a patient with diffuse interstitial fibrosis (solid line). When vital capacity is plotted as per cent predicted, the curve in fibrosis is shifted down and rightward of the normal curve; when plotted as per cent of observed vital capacity, the curves superimpose.

behavior, proved to be the best predictor of the presence of narrowing of small airways from peribronchiolar fibrosis or inflammation, or both, in lung biopsy specimens. So the concept of what was regarded originally as exclusively a parenchymal pathophysiologic disturbance has been broadened to include involvement of small airways secondary to extension of the interstitial process into peribronchiolar tissues.

Gas Exchange. Typical findings in patients with diffuse interstitial fibrosis include a decreased arterial PO_2, increased alveolar-arterial PO_2 difference, compensated respiratory alkalosis, a markedly decreased diffusing capacity, and increased wasted ventilation. The presence of both arterial hypoxia and decreased diffusing capacity led to the formulation of the "alveolar-capillary block syndrome," a pathophysiologic concept in which arterial PO_2 was believed to be decreased because the increased pathway for diffusion created alveolar–end-capillary PO_2 differences. However, as discussed previously (Fig. 35), such differences are not likely to be present or of substantial magnitude in patients with decreased diffusing capacities at rest. During exercise, such a barrier to diffusion might become physiologically meaningful.

The lack of importance of alveolar-capillary block has been reinforced by two kinds of studies: (1) the first provided an alternate explanation for the arterial hypoxia observed in patients with decreased diffusing capacities by showing that ventilation-perfusion abnormalities were the mechanisms responsible; (2) the second, a detailed investigation of the distribution of ventilation:perfusion ratios in patients with interstitial lung disease and low diffusing capacities, demonstrated substantial venous admixture from blood flow to regions with extremely low ventilation:perfusion ratios or right-to-left shunts, or both. Moreover, calculated arterial PO_2 values based on these abnormalities accounted for the measured PO_2 values; these observations excluded a contribution of diffusion limitation to hypoxia in these patients at rest. In contrast, in the same patients during exercise, predictions of arterial PO_2 from the distributions of ventilation:perfusion ratios overestimated measured values by 10 mm Hg, suggesting that diffusion impairment was contributing to the hypoxia. But even though diffusion limitation of O_2 became discernible during exercise, ventilation-perfusion mismatching was still the more important cause of hypoxia.

The chronic (compensated) respiratory alkalosis found in these patients is usually mild, with PCO_2 values averaging approximately 35 mm Hg. The increased neural drive to breathe, which has been demonstrated by measurements of $P_{0.1}$, cannot be explained by a peripheral chemoreceptor response to hypoxia and is attributed to central nervous system stimulation by intrapulmonary reflexes. Which receptors are involved is not known, but the pulmonary C fibers (J receptors), which are situated along with the pathologic infiltrations in the interstitium of the lung parenchyma, are likely candidates.

The typical rapid and shallow pattern of breathing in patients with diffuse interstitial fibrosis is probably also reflex in origin. This is an inefficient way to breathe because it increases the fraction of each breath that does not contribute to gas exchange (wasted ventilation). Thus, sufficient ventilation to lower PCO_2 values in the presence of increased wasted ventilation requires a considerably increased minute volume. During exercise, wasted ventilation in patients with interstitial fibrosis either increases above values found at rest or does not decrease normally; this response, which probably reflects uneven distribution of inspired air, simulates that found in patients with pulmonary vascular occlusive disorders (discussed subsequently) and must be kept in mind when interpreting the results of respiratory function studies.

REFERENCES

Disorders of the Chest Wall

Bergofsky, E. H.: Respiratory failure in disorders of the thoracic cage. Am Rev Respir Dis 119:643, 1979.

Kafer, E.: Idiopathic scoliosis. Gas exchange and the age dependence of arterial blood gases. J Clin Invest 58:825, 1976.

Olgiati, R., Levine, D., Smith, J. P., Briscoe, W. A., and King, T. K. C.: Diffusing capacity in idiopathic scoliosis and its interpretation regarding alveolar development. Am Rev Respir Dis 126:229, 1982.

Sinha, R., and Bergofsky, E. H.: Prolonged alteration of lung mechanics in kyphoscoliosis by positive pressure hyperinflation. Am Rev Respir Dis 106:47, 1972.

Pleural Restriction

Colp, C., Reichel, J., and Park, S. S.: Severe pleural restriction: The maximum static pulmonary recoil pressure as an aid in diagnosis. Chest 67:658, 1975.

Davidson, F. F., and Glazier, J. B.: Unilateral pleuritis and regional lung function. Ann Intern Med 77:37, 1972.

Sonnenblick, M., Melzer, E., and Rosin, A. J.: Body positional effect in unilateral pleural effusion. Chest 83:784, 1983.

Muscle Weakness

Gibson, G. J., Pride, N. B., Newsom Davis, J., and Loh, L. C.: Pulmonary mechanics in patients with respiratory muscle weakness. Am Rev Respir Dis 115:389, 1977.

Gross, D., Ladd, H. W., Riley, E. J., Macklem, P. T., and Grassino, A.: The effect of training on strength and endurance of the diaphragm in quadriplegia. Am J Med 68:27–35, 1980.

Kreitzer, S. M., Feldman, N. T., Saunders, N. A., and Ingram, R. H., Jr.: Bilateral diaphragmatic paralysis with hypercapnic respiratory failure. A physiologic assessment. Am J Med 65:89, 1978.

Diffuse Infiltrative Diseases

Crystal, R. G., Bitterman, P. B., Rennard, S. I., Hance, A. J., and Keogh, B. A.: Interstitial lung diseases of unknown cause: Disorders characterized by chronic inflammation of the lower respiratory tract. N Engl J Med 310:154, 235, 1984.

DiMarco, A. F., Kelsen, S. G., Cherniack, N. S., and Gothe, B.: Occlusion pressure and breathing pattern in patients with interstitial lung disease. Am Rev Respir Dis 127:425, 1983.

Fulmer, J. D., Roberts, W. C., von Gal, E. R., and Crystal, R. G.: Small airways in idiopathic fibrosis: Comparison of morphologic and physiologic observations. J Clin Invest 60:595, 1977.

Gibson, G. J., and Pride, N. B.: Pulmonary mechanics in fibrosing alveolitis. The effects of lung shrinkage. Am Rev Respir Dis 116:637, 1977.

Luce, J. M.: Interstitial lung disease. Hosp Pract 18:173, 1983.

OBSTRUCTIVE VENTILATORY DISORDERS

The "classic" obstructive ventilatory disorders are asthma, emphysema, chronic bronchitis, and (occasionally) bronchiectasis. These diseases share the common characteristic of causing enough narrowing within the tracheobronchial tree to increase resistance to the flow of air. The term *obstructive* was originally employed to indicate that the results of spirometry, the only test routinely available at the time, revealed a decreased FEV_1/FVC. Because it was not possible to differentiate among the different entities capable of decreasing FEV_1/FVC values, they were lumped together in the nonspecific category of *chronic obstructive pulmonary disease,* or COPD. Now, however, it is possible by means of specialized tests to identify additional physiologic abnormalities and to sort out the various diseases that cause airways obstruction even when they coexist. The similarities and differences among asthma, emphysema, and chronic bronchitis are discussed subsequently.

In general, the cross-sectional area must decrease 50 to 60 per cent at some level within the system of airways before resistance to airflow increases sufficiently to be detectable as an abnormality of FEV_1/FVC. Because of the branching pattern of the tracheobronchial tree, thousands of peripheral airways finally emerge from a few central airways. Thus extremely widespread disease of bronchioles must be present to cause obstruction equal in severity to that resulting from disease of a few central bronchi. The importance of peripheral airways as the sites of early involvement in several major diseases has led to the development of tests to examine their physiologic behavior. Application of these tests has revealed several physiologic disturbances, which will be reviewed next, in asymptomatic persons. Another recent practical application of pulmonary function tests has been to evaluate patients with central (that is, laryngotracheal) airway obstruction resulting from prolonged endotracheal intubation or other abnormalities.

The behavior of airways can be measured as airways resistance during submaximal flows or during maximal forced expiratory maneuvers. The types of results obtained from each type of test have certain advantages and disadvantages. Measurements of airways resistance are influenced to some extent by the dimensions of all the air passages between the alveoli and the mouth. Resistance varies inversely with lung volume, approaching infinity near RV and reaching a minimum near TLC; this hyperbolic relationship between airways resistance and lung volume can be made linear by converting resistance to its reciprocal conductance (see Fig. 19). To correct for the effect of the lung volume at which measurements were made, resistance is usually reported as the conductance:volume ratio or specific conductance. This test, which is rapidly and easily performed, is chiefly a test of the caliber of large central airways; however, it does not differentiate between obstruction of intrathoracic and extrathoracic airways and it may be abnormal in the presence of severe narrowing of small peripheral airways. Because of the relative nonspecificity of the results, tests of airways resistance have been largely replaced by the more useful tests of maximal forced expiratory airflow.

Measurements of maximal airflow during an FVC maneuver, which can be performed rapidly and easily, reflect the properties of both the lung parenchyma and the tracheobronchial system. The determinants of maximal flow and the mechanisms causing airflow

limitation in normal persons were reviewed in the section on Normal Physiology of the Respiratory System. During the early part of a maximal forced expiration, or effort-dependent portion, the rate of airflow is governed by the strength and rapidity of expiratory muscle contraction, the high elastic recoil pressure of the fully inflated lungs, and the caliber of the trachea and large central bronchi. In contrast, during the latter two thirds of an FVC maneuver, the rate of airflow is effort independent and is determined by the elastic recoil of the lungs and by the resistance of airways between the alveoli and the choke point. Furthermore, the driving pressure for airflow (that is, elastic recoil) is sufficient to overcome losses of pressure from turbulence and convective acceleration. Thus the rate of flow is dependent on the density of the gas being breathed, and the velocity of airflow can be increased by breathing a low-density gas mixture such as He-O_2. In the presence of the obstructive diseases discussed subsequently, the elastic recoil of the lungs and/or the caliber of the airways is abnormal. Depending on the sites and magnitude of involvement, characteristic abnormalities of maximal expiratory flow-volume relationships can be determined while breathing air and He-O_2 and are useful diagnostically and prognostically.

Peripheral Airways Obstruction

The small peripheral airways of the lungs are believed to be the first sites of pathologic involvement in patients with chronic bronchitis, emphysema, and (possibly) certain occupational diseases. If detected at a time when lesions are confined to small airways, these disorders may be reversible. Thus cessation of smoking, use of bronchodilators, and avoidance of further exposure to smoke and fine dust allows healing to occur and prevents progression to the incurable, disabling, advanced state of the disease that would otherwise occur. There is some evidence to support this optimistic hypothesis, but many important questions remain to be answered before it can be considered established.

The problem in assessing the physiologic function of small airways stems from the anatomic considerations reviewed earlier (Fig. 5). Because of the pattern of airways branching, the sum of the diameters of the pair of daughter branches exceeds the diameter of the parent branch. Accordingly, the cross-sectional area of the tracheobronchial system steadily increases from central to peripheral airways such that the sum of the cross-sectional areas of airways smaller than 2 mm in diameter is almost 1000 times greater than the area of the trachea. The two chief physiologic consequences of this anatomic pattern are that the velocity of inspired airflow progressively decreases as the airstream moves peripherally and that small airways contribute only a relatively small portion, approximately 33 per cent, to total airways resistance. For this reason, peripheral airways have been called the lungs' quiet zone, and special tests of pulmonary function (Table 12) are required to examine their behavior. There is no rigid anatomic separation between the continuum of large-to-small airways that compose the tracheobronchial tree. Chiefly because of the types of direct measurements that have been carried out, small airways are usually referred to as those less than 2 to 3 mm in diameter and large airways as those greater than 2 to 3 mm in diameter.

TABLE 12. TESTS OF SMALL PERIPHERAL AIRWAYS OBSTRUCTION THAT MAY BE ABNORMAL IN PATIENTS WHOSE LUNG VOLUMES AND FEV$_1$/FVC ARE NORMAL*

Frequency dependence of compliance
Distribution of ventilation and perfusion
Closing volume
Slope of phase III
Viso$_V$
$\Delta \dot{V}max_{50}$
$\Delta \dot{V}max_{75}$

*For definitions of abbreviations, see Table 10.

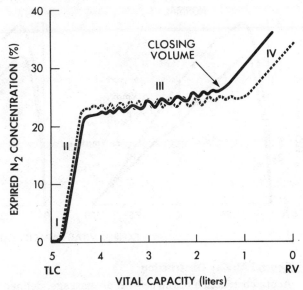

Figure 51. Representative tracings of the measurement of closing volume by the single-breath oxygen method in a normal subject (dotted line, from Figure 26) and a patient with early peripheral (small) airways disease (solid line). Note that the presence of airways disease is reflected by a steeper than normal slope of phase III and a shift of the junction of phases III and IV (the closing volume) to a higher than normal lung volume. TLC = total lung capacity; RV = residual volume.

Simple inexpensive tests of peripheral airways function are available. Of these, derivatives of the test of closing volume and the maximal expiratory flow-volume curves correlate best with pathologic evidence of peripheral airways disease; the use of He-O$_2$ flow-volume curves improved discrimination in some but not all studies. More complex studies, such as measurement of frequency dependence of compliance, are usually confined to research laboratories.

Closing Volume. As discussed in the section on Normal Physiology of the Respiratory System, the normal presence of a vertical gradient of pleural pressure means that alveoli at the top and bottom of the lungs are different in size at RV and FRC, but not at TLC, and that they inflate and deflate nonuniformly because their compliance is different (that is, their behavior is determined by flat and steep segments, respectively, of the same volume-pressure curve). During the test for closing volume, the lung is labeled from top to bottom by inhaling a bolus of some identifiable inert gas or, more commonly, by a breath of 100 per cent O$_2$. The sudden increase in concentration of the label during the subsequent exhalation from TLC to RV defines the closing volume and is believed to reflect the onset of closure of small peripheral airways in the dependent portions of the lungs. Closing capacity is the closing volume plus RV.

The determinants of airways closure are (1) the stability and intrinsic caliber of peripheral airways, which depend in turn on smooth muscle tone, thickness of the wall, mechanical properties of the surface film, and secretions in the lumen, and (2) the tethering effect of attachments of the surrounding lung parenchyma, which is determined by the elastic recoil of the lungs. Thus it can be appreciated that narrowing of peripheral airways from intrinsic pathologic changes or from loss of elastic recoil, or both, would increase closing volume and closing capacity (Fig. 51). Physiologic and pathologic correlations indicate that structural abnormalities of airways in the absence of emphysema and decreased recoil are associated with increased closing capacity. These observations are consistent with evidence that the physiologic and presumably the structural disturbances are reversible after cessation of smoking. This would not occur if emphysema caused closing volume to increase.

Slope of Phase III. The slope of phase III of the tracing recorded during the closing volume maneuver reflects the evenness of the distribution of ventilation. Thus abnormalities of small airways cause both maldistribution of inspired gas, so that the lungs are not

normally labeled, and uneven emptying of the lungs with delayed appearance of the label from alveoli served by narrowed airways or by collateral pathways (Fig. 51). The slope of phase III is one of the best tests for the presence of small airways disease. The results of the test correlate well with pathologic observations, and abnormalities are frequently observed when other tests of pulmonary function (except Viso$_V$) show no abnormalities.

Volume of Isoflow (Viso$_V$). A detailed explanation for the effects of breathing a less dense but slightly more viscous gas like He-O$_2$, compared with air, on maximal expiratory flow-volume curves is provided in the section on Normal Physiology of the Respiratory System. To summarize the concepts, the driving pressure from the alveoli to the choke points during forced expiration in normal subjects is dissipated in three different ways: (1) causing viscosity-dependent laminar flow in peripheral airways; (2) causing density-dependent turbulent flow in more central airways; and (3) causing density-dependent convective acceleration as the velocity of flow increases from alveoli to central airways.

In patients with disease of peripheral airways, more pressure than normal is dissipated overcoming resistance in those airways in which flow is laminar and viscosity dependent (density independent). This means that less pressure is "left over" to cause turbulence and convective acceleration. Accordingly, the Viso$_V$ increases and $\Delta \dot{V}max_{50}$ and $\Delta \dot{V}max_{75}$ should decrease (Fig. 52). Of these, changes in Viso$_V$ have been shown to correlate with pathologic abnormalities in peripheral airways. Furthermore, as is the case with the slope of phase III, changes in Viso$_V$ have been shown to be reversible after cessation of smoking.

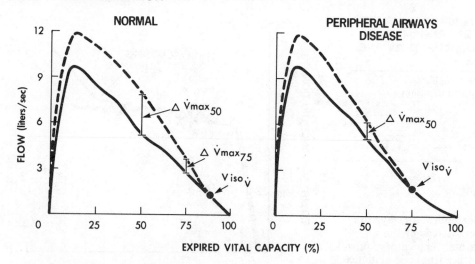

NORMAL

PERIPHERAL AIRWAYS DISEASE

FLOW (liters/sec)

EXPIRED VITAL CAPACITY (%)

Figure 52. Representative tracings of forced expiratory flow-volume curves breathing air (solid lines) and 79 per cent He and 21 per cent O_2 (He-O_2, dashed lines). The patient with peripheral airways disease *(right panel)* differs from normal *(left panel*, from Figure 23) in that the He-O_2 curve is depressed; this decreases the difference between maximal flows breathing He-O_2 and air at 50 per cent and 75 per cent expired vital capacity ($\Delta\dot{V}max_{50}$ and $\Delta\dot{V}max_{75}$) and increases the lung volume at which the curves converge ($Viso_{\dot{v}}$).

Central Airway Obstruction

Acute obstruction of the central air passage, defined as the airway between the glottis and the carina, is usually a dramatic and life-threatening event that does not allow time for physiologic studies. In contrast, chronic obstruction develops slowly and permits detailed investigation of the ensuing abnormalities. Although such lesions were uncommon in the past, consisting mainly of rare tumors of the trachea, chronic obstruction of the central airway is now being encountered increasingly as a complication of prolonged intubation from either an endotracheal tube or a tracheostomy.

In general, there are two types of obstruction from disease of the central airway: (1) fixed narrowing or stenosis, which results from dense scars in the wall, infiltrating tumors, or external compression, and (2) variable narrowing or tracheomalacia, which occurs when the cartilaginous support is lost from erosion or inflammation and the airway becomes floppy. The physiologic abnormalities differ in the two kinds of obstruction and are also influenced by whether the obstruction is located in the airway inside or outside the thorax.

There are several characteristic patterns of abnormal pulmonary function tests that help to define the location of the obstruction and its magnitude. Lung volumes, diffusing capacity, and arterial blood gas values are within normal limits in patients with "pure" laryngotracheal obstruction. The FEV_1/FVC test is relatively insensitive to localized obstruction of the upper airway because substantial narrowing must occur before the result becomes abnormal. When normal subjects breathe through restricted orifices, their FEV_1/FVC remains above 90 per cent of control values until a 6-mm diameter orifice is used. Similarly, because the lesion is centrally located, tests of peripheral airways obstruction such as closing volume and distribution of ventilation (slope of phase III) are within the normal range.

The most useful test result in the assessment of patients with obstruction of the upper airway is the maximal inspiratory and expiratory flow-volume curve (Fig. 53). The determinants of the effort-dependent and effort-independent segments of the expiratory portion of the curve are discussed in detail in the section on Normal Physiology of the Respiratory System. In contrast to the expiratory limb, the inspiratory limb is completely effort dependent. In normal subjects (Fig. 53A), the expiratory flow:inspiratory flow ratio at mid-

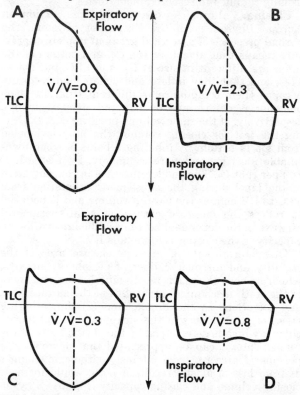

Figure 53. Representative tracings of maximum inspiratory and expiratory flow-volume curves showing the effects of tracheal narrowing of different types and at different locations. *A,* Normal tracing; the ratio of maximum expiratory to inspiratory flow ($\dot{V}/\dot{V}$) at 50 per cent vital capacity (vertical dashed line) = 0.9. *B,* Variable extrathoracic obstruction; $\dot{V}/\dot{V}$ = 2.3. The reason inspiratory flow does not increase is explained in Figure 54. *C,* Variable intrathoracic obstruction; $\dot{V}/\dot{V}$ = 0.3, The reason expiratory flow does not increase is explained in Figure 55. *D,* Fixed inspiratory or expiratory obstruction, $\dot{V}/\dot{V}$ = 0.8, a normal value, but contour of tracing is diagnostic. *TLC* = total lung capacity, *RV* = residual volume. (From Hinshaw, H. C., and Murray, J. F.: Diseases of the Chest. Philadelphia, W. B. Saunders Co., 1979, p. 621.)

VC is approximately 0.9. Inspiratory flow exceeds expiratory flow because the entire tracheobronchial system is maximally dilated during most of inspiration, whereas compression of central segments occurs during most of expiration. In patients with variable *extra*thoracic obstruction (Fig. 53*B*), the narrowing worsens during inspiration because the drop in pressure as air flows across the lesion causes the atmospheric pressure surrounding the airway to exceed the negative pressure in the lumen (Fig. 54); during expiration, the site of obstruction dilates because the positive pressure inside the airway exceeds the pressure outside it. Accordingly, the expiratory flow:inspiratory flow ratio at 50 per cent VC is greater than 2. In patients with variable *intra*thoracic obstruction (Fig. 53*C*), the negative pleural pressure generated during inspiration dilates the site of narrowing and relieves the obstruction. In contrast, the narrowing worsens during forced expiration because the positive pleural pressure exceeds the pressure in the lumen of the airway as pressure is dissipated, causing air to flow across the obstruction (Fig. 55). Thus the mid-VC expiratory flow:inspiratory flow ratio is about 0.3. When the obstruction is fixed (that is, cannot be enlarged or narrowed further) or located at the thoracic inlet, flow is similarly decreased during most of inspiration and expiration so that the ratio at 50 per cent VC is approximately 1.0 (Fig. 53*D*). The maximal flows achieved by patients with a fixed central airway obstruction can be simulated by normal subjects breathing through a fixed orifice of known diameter. Accordingly, data from healthy persons can be used to predict with reasonable accuracy the cross-sectional area at the site of involvement in patients. As indicated previously, because maximal air flow in the larynx and trachea is turbulent and hence density dependent, breathing a less dense gas than air, such as He-O_2, results in increased flows in patients with central airway obstruction.

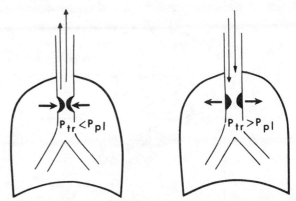

Figure 55. Effect of the phase of respiration on an intrathoracic variable obstruction. Direction of airflow is indicated by long, thin arrows. During forced expiration (left) the pleural pressure *(Ppl)* surrounding the trachea may be greater than the intratracheal pressure *(Ptr)*, causing the intrathoracic obstruction to increase *(horizontal arrows)* and limiting maximal airflow. During forced inspiration *(right)*, Ppl is greater than Ptr so the trachea dilates *(arrows)*, thus decreasing the obstruction and allowing airflow to increase. (From Kryer, M., Bode, F., Antic, R., and Anthonisen, N., Am J Med 61:85, 1976; reprinted with permission of the authors and publisher.)

Asthma

To most persons, asthma means wheezing, regardless of its cause. However, the term *asthma* has a much more specific medical connotation and is used to describe a distinct pathophysiologic entity. A committee of the American Thoracic Society defined asthma as ". . . a disease characterized by an increased responsiveness of the trachea and bronchi to various stimuli, and manifested by widespread narrowing of the airways that changes in severity either spontaneously or as a result of treatment." Essentially, asthma is reversible airways obstruction. The person who is asthma prone, often called an "asthmatic," differs from healthy subjects by reacting in an exaggerated manner to a wide variety of stimuli. Thus asthmatics are characterized as having a peculiar hyperresponsiveness of the airways that causes them to react to stimuli that would not affect the airways of normal persons. When stimulated, a patient with asthma may develop bronchospasm, hypersecretion, infiltration with inflammatory cells, and edema; these cause diffuse narrowing of the tracheobronchial system and obstruction to airflow. The nonasthmatic may respond in a manner similar to the asthmatic but only to much greater, much more intense, and often qualitatively different stimuli to the air passages.

The pathogenesis of asthma is complex and poorly understood. It seems clear that no single factor causes the clinical syndrome; allergic, infectious, occupational, environmental, physical, and psychologic disturbances have all been implicated. As mentioned, however, airways hyperresponsiveness is common to all asthmatics; this reactivity can be provoked by specific stimulants such as inhaled antigens to which the person is sensitized, cholinergic drugs, or histamine or by nonspecific stimuli such as exercise and numerous inhaled, irritating (but nonantigenic) substances. With the use of specific allergens, the decrease in FEV_1/FVC may be immediate, delayed, or both (Fig. 56).

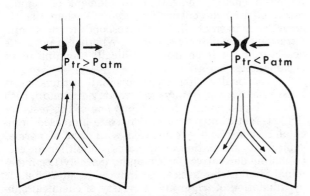

Figure 54. Effect of the phase of respiration on an extrathoracic variable obstruction. Direction of airflow is indicated by long, thin arrows. During forced expiration *(left)* the positive intratracheal pressure *(Ptr)* exceeds atmospheric pressure *(Patm)* so that the variable extrathoracic obstruction dilates *(horizontal arrows)* and there is no obstruction to airflow. During forced inspiration *(right)*, Ptr is less than Patm so the obstruction narrows further *(arrows)* and maximal airflow is limited. (From Kryer, M., Bode, F., Antic, R., Anthonisen, N.: Am J Med 61:85, 1976; reprinted with permission of the authors and publisher.)

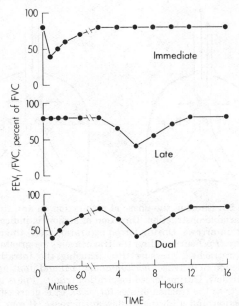

Figure 56. Reactions to bronchial provocation. Schematic diagram showing the time course of serial measurements of FEV_1/FVC, expressed as per cent of FVC, after bronchial provocation in a susceptible person. Three types of reactions are illustrated: immediate, late, and dual. (From Hinshaw, H. C., and Murray, J. F.: Diseases of the Chest. Philadelphia, W. B. Saunders Co., 1980, p. 749.)

To accommodate these diverse features, two hypotheses about the pathophysiology of asthma are being investigated: (1) bronchial obstruction is caused by the action of specific chemical mediators, such as histamine, leukotrienes including slow-reacting substance of anaphylaxis, prostaglandins, and other substances, released during anaphylaxis and during the response to nonspecific stimuli and (2) bronchial narrowing is caused by an abnormality in the neural regulation of airway smooth muscle tone, such as an imbalance either between parasympathetic (constrictor) and sympathetic (dilator) activity or between noncholinergic and nonadrenergic pathways that influence airway caliber. These are not mutually exclusive possibilities and they have been combined into a third theory that postulates that reflex events, triggered by release of mediators, interact with the chemicals to augment the ensuing bronchoconstriction.

Bronchial obstruction during an asthmatic attack is not solely caused by bronchoconstriction. Edema and inflammatory infiltration of the mucosa and secretions in the lumen all contribute to the narrowing of airways. These are much more difficult to treat than bronchospasm and are responsible for much of the morbidity and virtually all of the mortality associated with acute attacks. Given the interplay of factors affecting the caliber of airways in asthmatics, it is not surprising that there are striking differences in the physiologic abnormalities encountered in asthmatics during symptom-free intervals between attacks, during episodes of exercise-induced asthma, and during severe attacks. The ventilatory disturbances of each of these will be discussed briefly. Because abnormalities of oxygenation and CO_2 elimination in asthmatics do not correlate well with abnormalities of ventilation, gas exchange is discussed separately.

Pathophysiology Between Asthmatic Attacks. Asthma is, by definition, a reversible disorder. Yet, nearly all asthmatics, including those who are asymptomatic and have no wheezes detectable by auscultation of the chest, have abnormal results of tests of ventilatory function between attacks. Even when spirometry was the only method widely used for measuring pulmonary function, abnormalities of FEV_1/FVC were commonly observed in asymptomatic asthmatics. These results were interpreted as indicating that residual airways obstruction existed between attacks. Now, using more sensitive tests, many asthmatics have been identified who have normal values for FEV_1/FVC but who have increased closing volumes, maldistribution of inspired air, abnormal maximal expiratory flow-volume curves breathing room air and He-O_2, and frequency-dependent changes in compliance. These abnormalities all point to the presence of widespread narrowing in small peripheral airways.

Not all asthmatics are asymptomatic between attacks, and many patients demonstrate persistent decreases in FEV_1/FVC, maximal expiratory flow rates, and specific conductance. When these patients are given He-O_2 to breathe, some—the "responders" —demonstrate an increase in their maximal expiratory flow-volume curves, whereas others—the "nonresponders"—do not. These different responses indicate that the sites of obstruction are located in different-sized airways in the two groups. The improvement in expiratory flow rates in the responders means that the obstruction must be sufficiently central, presumably in large airways, for convective acceleration and turbulent flow regimens to have developed. In contrast, the lack of improvement in the nonresponders means that only fully developed laminar flow has evolved and that the obstruction must be in small peripheral airways. Additional studies in related but not the same patient groups revealed that (1) when the obstruction is in large airways, as shown by improvement in expiratory flow rates when breathing He-O_2, the bronchial narrowing can be relieved (in part) by parasympatholytic drugs, indicating an element of vagally mediated bronchoconstriction, and (2) when the obstruction is in small airways, it responds to the administration of sympatholytic agents. Whether or not these observations will be useful clinically remains to be documented.

The particular characteristic of all asthmatics is hyperreactivity of airways to a variety of stimuli, both antigenic and nonantigenic. Thus one of the tests for the asthmatic state is to demonstrate increased bronchial responsiveness, compared with that of normal subjects, to inhalation of an aerosol of either an acetylcholine derivative (for example, mecholyl) or histamine. Similar changes can be induced in an asthmatic by inhalation of frigid air, a variety of chemical substances, and even a deep breath. Because the bronchoconstriction provoked by these maneuvers is, in general, blocked by atropine, parasympathetic (vagal) efferent pathways are presumably involved. A transient state of bronchial hyperreactivity has been shown to develop after a viral infection of the upper respiratory tract in otherwise healthy persons and to be inducible in normal subjects by exposure to low concentrations of ozone or sulfur dioxide. These responses apparently involve both sensitization of irritant receptors in the upper airways (larynx, trachea, main bronchi) and afferent and efferent vagal impulses. Based on these observations, it has been postulated that intrinsic asthma may develop in some patients as a result of permanent sensitization of these receptors or of vagally mediated bronchoconstrictor overactivity, or of both.

Exercise-Induced Asthma. As indicated in the previous discussion, patients with asthma are susceptible to acute attacks provoked by a variety of nonantigenic stimuli. One of the most common and important of these stimuli is exercise. In fact, the nearly invariable association between (extrinsic) asthma and demonstrable exercise-induced bronchoconstriction has caused some experts to believe that the absence of inducible bronchospasm precludes the diagnosis of the underlying disease. Furthermore, the association can be used diagnostically in patients in whom asthma is suspected; a history of exercise-induced wheezing or the provocation of such an episode in the laboratory strongly supports the diagnosis.

Under ordinary conditions of ambient temperature and humidity, the severity of exercise-induced bronchoconstriction is directly related to the intensity and duration of the work being performed. In general, maximal worsening of expiratory airflow occurs when the work load reaches 60 to 80 per cent of maximal predicted O_2 consumption for six to eight minutes. However, attacks may occur at much lower work loads in a cold or dry environment, or both, and even can be reproduced by voluntary hyperventilation without exercise. These observations have found a common denominator in the magnitude of respiratory heat losses during exercise or hyperventilation and the onset of asthma in susceptible persons. The colder or drier the ambient air and the more vigorous the breathing maneuver, the greater will be the demands for heat and water exchange by the respiratory tract and the deeper will the inspired airstream penetrate into the tracheobronchial system before it is warmed to body temperature and fully humidified; as a consequence, the respiratory mucosa of central airways can become extremely cool.

Proximal large airways contain numerous rapidly acting irritant receptors that, when stimulated, may cause bronchoconstriction; thus, it is possible that these receptors are stimulated by cooling and provoke the attacks. But there is also pharmacologic evidence that chemical mediators are involved in the pathogenesis of exercise-induced asthma, an association that was considerably strengthened by finding a marked increase in circulating neutrophil chemotactic activity that accompanied the decrease in FEV_1/FVC after exercise in susceptible persons. This observation is also consistent with the results of other studies that increasingly suggest that the polymorphonuclear leukocyte plays an important role in the pathogenesis of asthma. It is now known that a substantial proportion of children who develop acute asthmatic attacks after exercise will also develop delayed reactions several hours later; these are apt to be more variable in time of onset and severity than the acute attacks, but they are also associated with an increase in circulating neutrophil chemotactic activity.

Pathophysiology During Severe Asthma. During a severe asthmatic attack, resistance to airflow is even more increased than during exercise-induced asthma because the presence of inflammation and secretions compounds the effect of bronchospasm. The only way that markedly narrowed airways can be held sufficiently open to permit ventilation is for patients to breathe at extremely high lung volumes. The increased elastic recoil at high lung volumes pulls airways open and thus counteracts their tendency to close. Thus, during a severe asthmatic attack, the VC progressively decreases and finally approximates tidal volume, and both FRC and RV increase substantially. This means that, although premature closure of airways is the principal pathologic feature of severe asthma, many of the physiologic consequences derive from the requirement of breathing at extremely high lung volumes.

The work of breathing is markedly increased (1) because the necessity of breathing from an increased FRC demands an increase in inspiratory muscle force to overcome the increased recoil of lungs and chest wall at that volume and (2) because of the necessity of generating increased muscle forces during inspiration to overcome the increased resistance to airflow through narrowed airways. Although resistance to expiration is greater than to inspiration, expiration is mainly passive in asthmatics because the increased recoil of the hyperinflated respiratory system is adequate to expel air and to cause deflation to the new FRC, which is the volume at which the narrowed airways close. Augmenting expiratory force does not increase the rate of airflow and would further narrow air passages. Consequently, and in contrast to prevailing beliefs, pleural pressures, which reach high negative values during inspiration (-30 cm H_2O), do not increase much above normal values during expiration and seldom exceed positive values of a few cm H_2O (Fig. 57).

The potentially devasting consequences of these mechanical disturbances are respiratory or circulatory failure or both. If the inspiratory muscles are unable to generate sufficient force to reach a high enough lung volume to allow adequate breathing, CO_2 retention, severe hypoxia, and even complete apnea occur. Similarly, if the inspiratory muscles are unable to sustain the requisite hyperinflation of the respiratory system for the duration of the attack, muscle fatigue develops quickly and leads to rapidly progressive respiratory failure.

Hyperinflation and its accompanying increased negativity of mean pleural pressure during an asthmatic attack also create profound cardiovascular disturbances. When severe, these abnormalities can cause acute cor pulmonale and right-sided heart failure (see also subsequent discussion of this subject in this section).

One of the consequences of hyperinflation is that pulmonary vascular resistance must rise. It was pointed out earlier (Table 3) that as lung volume increases above FRC, so does pulmonary vascular resistance. This occurs because the effects of inflating the lungs on capillaries and possibly other small "alveolar" vessels, whose resistance increases as they are lengthened and flattened, outweighs the effects on larger "extra-alveolar" vessels, whose resistance decreases as they are distended. Marked increases in pulmonary vascular resistance during inspiration probably account for the presence of pulsus paradoxus during severe asthmatic attacks. Another consequence

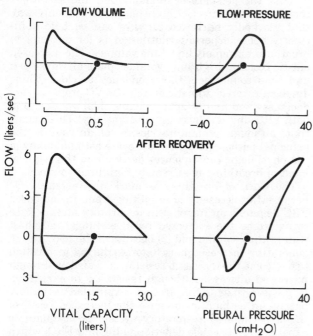

Figure 57. Representative tracings of flow-volume (maximal inspiratory and expiratory flow versus vital capacity) and flow-pressure (maximal flows versus pleural pressure) tracings of a subject with asthma during an acute attack *(upper two tracings)* and after recovery *(lower two tracings)*. Note the change in flow and vital capacity calibrations in the two tracings. (Modified from Stalcup, S. A., and Mellins, R. B.: N Engl J Med 297:592, 1977; reprinted with permission of the authors and publisher.)

of the increased negativity of pleural pressure is that the performance of both the right and left ventricles may be impaired by what amounts to an increase in their afterloads. In other words, to maintain the same levels of pulmonary arterial pressure and systemic arterial pressure—relative to pleural pressure—that existed before the attack, the work of the heart must increase. The circulatory disturbances are compounded by the demands of increased O_2 consumption related to increased work of breathing and the effects of anxiety, release of endogenous catecholamines, and administration of sympathomimetic, theophylline, or other cadiac-stimulating drugs.

Gas Exchange Abnormalities. A wide spectrum of arterial Po_2 and Pco_2 values has been reported in patients with asthma, both during and between attacks. In general, these results do not correlate particularly well with conventional tests of airways obstruction, like the FEV_1/FVC. This is not surprising when it is remembered that values for the FEV_1/FVC maneuver reflect mainly the behavior of large central airways, whereas the degree of obstruction in peripheral airways, which affects the matching of ventilation and perfusion in terminal respiratory units, is of greater importance in determining values for Po_2 and Pco_2.

Typical findings of arterial blood analysis during an acute asthmatic episode are $Po_2 = 55$ mm Hg, $Pco_2 = 32$ mm Hg, and pH = 7.46, indicating hypoxia, hypocapnia, and acute respiratory alkalosis. It has long

been assumed that these abnormalities are caused by a ventilation-perfusion disturbance with accompanying hyperventilation, which decreases Pco_2 but does not correct the hypoxia. This notion has been confirmed by recent studies of gas exchange in asthmatics using the method of infusing six inert gases of varying solubilities and measuring their retention and excretion. From these data, curves showing the distributions of ventilation and perfusion to regions of differing ventilation:perfusion ratios can be constructed. Although not many asthmatics have been studied by this method, the most striking findings in those that have been are (1) a normal distribution of ventilation, (2) a bimodal distribution of perfusion such that a large proportion of the cardiac output (up to 50 per cent) is distributed to regions with very low ventilation:perfusion ratios, and (3) a decrease in arterial Po_2 values that is entirely accounted for by the large blood flow to regions with low ventilation:perfusion ratios. The most likely explanation for these observations is the presence of diffusely distributed obstruction of peripheral airways, presumably by mucous plugs, to large regions of lung in which collateral ventilation from relatively unaffected neighboring units prevents atelectasis and shunting of blood.

The familiar finding that the administration of isoproterenol worsens gas exchange further and causes arterial Po_2 to decrease from its initially low value was also confirmed by the six-gas method. The mechanism appears to be drug-induced release of vasoconstriction in the regions with low ventilation:perfusion ratios so that the proportion of cardiac output they receive increases. Because isoproterenol also increases cardiac output, effects on mixed venous Po_2 tend to offset, in part, the increase in perfusion to low ventilation-perfusion regions. In other words, if cardiac output did not increase, the drug-induced redistribution of blood flow to regions with poor gas exchange would decrease arterial Po_2 substantially more than it does. Surprisingly, breathing 100 per cent O_2 did not increase blood flow to low ventilation-perfusion regions, indicating that the pulmonary arterial vasoconstriction released by isoproterenol was not secondary to alveolar hypoxia.

Asymptomatic patients with asthma who had only slight impairment of their FEV_1/FVC values also had bimodal distributions of perfusion. These results suggest that asthmatics who are asymptomatic and who have minimal disturbances of FEV_1/FVC tests and only moderately increased alveolar-arterial Po_2 differences may have as much as one half of their lung units situated behind completely obstructed peripheral airways and thus are ventilated solely through collateral pathways. Another observation in asymptomatic asthmatics is that they tend to hyperventilate; thus low arterial Pco_2 values are often encountered between attacks.

Emphysema

Emphysema is a term of Greek origin meaning inflation; medically, the word means a pathologic accumulation of air in tissues or organs, such as occurs in patients with subcutaneous emphysema, mediastinal emphysema, and interstitial (peribronchial) emphysema. The pathologic accumulation of air in patients with pulmonary emphysema was originally

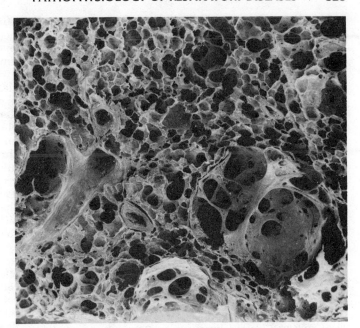

Figure 58. Scanning electron photomicrograph of the lung of an adult man showing the contrast between normal lung parenchyma and alveolar spaces and emphysematous regions where the alveoli have coalesced and there are large fenestrae in the remaining walls. (Courtesy of Dr. Janice Nowell.)

taken to mean overdistension of air spaces, but this definition is no longer applicable. Although lung tissue involved by emphysema is frequently overinflated, the essential criterion for the diagnosis of pulmonary emphysema is destruction of the interalveolar septa (Fig. 58).

In contrast to chronic bronchitis, which is defined in functional terms, emphysema is defined in anatomic terms as follows: an abnormal permanent enlargement of the air spaces distal to the terminal nonrespiratory bronchiole accompanied by destruction of their walls. Emphysema is, therefore, a disease of the terminal respiratory units. However, the eventual consequences of emphysema extend beyond the terminal respiratory units. The destructive process involves not only the lung parenchyma but also the conducting airways. There are different kinds of emphysema—centrilobular, panlobular, paraseptal, and irregular—but all include destruction of alveolar walls.

To simplify this presentation, the unqualified term *emphysema* is used to signify *pulmonary emphysema*. Furthermore, the physiologic disturbances that characterize emphysema (Table 13) will be related chiefly to the destruction of lung parenchyma and consequent decrease in the elastic recoil of the lungs. In addition, it is assumed, as is usually the case, that the destructive process has caused loss of support of the tracheobronchial system. Although this model is realistic and instructive, the physiologic abnormalities in patients with emphysema vary greatly depending on the type, location, and extent of the destructive process. From a clinical point of view, pure emphysema hardly ever exists alone; virtually all patients have associated chronic bronchitis and sometimes asthma and/or bronchiectasis.

Lung Volumes. The changes in lung volumes in pure emphysema can be explained solely by the effects of loss of elastic recoil of the diseased lungs. As shown in Figure 59, this is indeed the case. The volume-pressure diagram of the chest wall is that of a normal person and is the same as that shown in Figure 18,

but the volume-pressure diagram for the lungs is shifted upward and to the left, signifying marked loss of elastic recoil. Therefore, the static mechanical properties of the respiratory system differ from those of normal subjects: (1) TLC is increased, because the usual inspiratory muscle force causes the weakened lungs to contain a larger than normal volume; (2) FRC is increased, because the loss of inward recoil in the lungs offers less opposition to the outward recoil of the chest wall; (3) RV is increased, because the loss of recoil and tethering of airways cause them to close prematurely; and (4) VC is nearly normal, because the increase in RV is partially offset by the increase in TLC.

Mechanics of Ventilation. The important determinants of flow are the elastic recoil of the lungs, which supplies the driving pressure, and the cross-

TABLE 13. PULMONARY FUNCTION ABNORMALITIES IN PATIENTS WITH SEVERE "PURE" EMPHYSEMA*

TEST	RESULT
Lung volumes	
Vital capacity	Normal or decreased
Total lung capacity	Increased
Functional residual capacity	Increased
Residual volume	Increased
Mechanics of ventilation	
FEV_1/FVC	Markedly decreased
Maximal expiratory flow	Markedly decreased
Specific airways conductance	Decreased
Distribution of ventilation	Marked abnormality
Diffusing capacity	Markedly decreased
Gas exchange	
P_{O_2}	Slightly decreased
P_{CO_2}	Normal
pH	Normal
(Alveolar-arterial) P_{O_2}	Slightly increased
Right-to-left shunt	Absent
Wasted ventilation	Markedly increased

*For definitions of abbreviations, see Table 10.

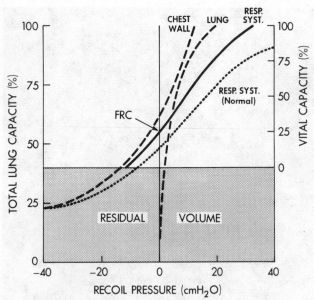

Figure 59. Representative volume-pressure curves of the chest wall and lung (dashed lines) and respiratory system (solid line) of a patient with emphysema. For comparison, the volume-pressure curve of the respiratory system *(resp. syst.)* of a normal adult (dotted line, from Figure 18) is shown. See text for further discussion. FRC = functional residual capacity.

sectional area of the (upstream) airways between the alveoli and the choke point, which determines the resistance to airflow. By obtaining the pressures at several lung volumes less than 75 per cent of VC from a static volume-pressure curve, and relating these pressures to the flow rates achieved at the same lung volumes from a maximal expiratory flow-volume curve, it is possible to construct a flow-pressure curve (Fig.

60). The resulting diagram defines the relationship in healthy persons between static elastic recoil and the maximal expiratory flow rates generated by that amount of recoil through normally patent upstream airways. This analysis makes it possible to differentiate the mechanisms of airways obstruction when it is caused purely by decreased elastic recoil on the one hand or by narrowed airways on the other hand. When elastic recoil pressure is decreased, as in patients with emphysema, maximal flow is necessarily limited throughout expiration because recoil is decreased at all lung volumes (Fig. 60). Maximal flow is also decreased in patients with chronic bronchitis, but, as shown in Figure 60, the mechanism is different from that in emphysema: elastic recoil is normal throughout VC but airflow is reduced because airways are narrowed from intrinsic disease (Fig. 60D, open symbols).

Thus the chief mechanism of expiratory obstruction in pure emphysema is directly attributable to the effects of lung destruction on elastic recoil. Increased collapsibility of airways may also contribute to expiratory airflow limitation. In dogs when the trachea is softened by enzymatic digestion, maximal expiratory flow rates decrease even though elastic recoil and upstream resistance are unchanged. The extent to which this occurs in patients with emphysema is unknown, but studies of the kind plotted in Figure 60 suggest that loss of recoil is more important, because if increased compressibility had occurred, the points would lie below the normal line.

Gas Exchange. Accompanying the destruction of intra-alveolar septa is loss of the alveolar-capillary surface for gas exchange. This is reflected by a decrease in the diffusing capacities of the lungs for both O_2 and CO. Because not all pulmonary capillaries are perfused in normal persons, under resting conditions extra pathways are ordinarily present that can accommodate increased blood flow during exercise and are available

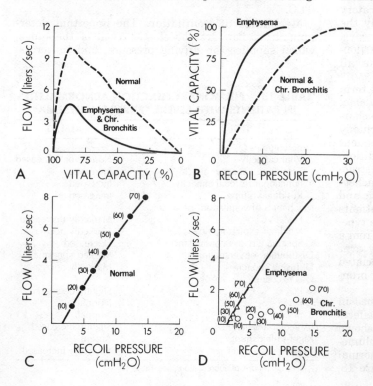

Figure 60. *A*, Representative forced expiratory flow-volume tracings from a normal subject (dashed line, from Figure 21) and two patients with chronic airflow obstruction, one with emphysema and the other with chronic *(chr)* bronchitis (single solid line, curves are superimposable). *B*, Volume-pressure tracings of the same three persons showing that the curve of the patient with emphysema (solid line) is shifted to the left of those of the normal subject and the patient with chronic bronchitis (single dashed line, curves are superimposable). *C* and *D*, From the tracings in the top two panels it is possible to construct flow-pressure curves for the three situations. The relationship in the normal person is shown by the solid line in both panels and the solid circles in the left panel. The lung volumes at which the comparisons were made are shown in parentheses. Note that the reduced airflow rates in emphysema *(open triangles)* fall along the normal line, whereas those in chronic bronchitis *(open circles)* are shifted far to the right.

in case some channels are destroyed or obstructed. Thus it can be inferred that a certain amount of emphysema can occur without affecting measurements of DL_{CO} at rest because blood flow simply shifts from the obliterated to other available capillaries. However, during exercise in the presence of emphysema, DL_{CO} would not increase as much as it does normally because the spare pathways are already used up. Such appears to be the case, although the quantitative relationships between lung destruction and decrease in DL_{CO} need to be investigated further.

A decreased DL_{CO} is usually not associated with an increased alveolar-arterial PO_2 difference, especially if measurements are made at rest. This concept has been substantiated by measuring the excretion and retention of six gases of varying solubilities in patients with advanced chronic obstructive pulmonary disease characterized as mainly emphysematous in origin. This method provides data concerning the distributions of ventilation and perfusion and the magnitudes of right-to-left shunt flow and wasted ventilation. From this information and direct measurements of arterial PO_2, the importance of diffusion abnormalities can be assessed.

Patients with severe emphysema typically are found to have the gas exchange abnormalities listed in Table 13. The slightly decreased PO_2 (60 to 70 mm Hg) occurs because most of the cardiac output is distributed to units with slightly lower (0.6) than normal (0.8) ventilation:perfusion ratios. There is essentially no blood flow to units of very low ventilation:perfusion ratios or to right-to-left shunts. In contrast to the pattern of the distribution of blood flow, a large fraction of ventilation is distributed to regions with high ventilation:perfusion ratios. This is consistent with the pathologic hallmark of emphysema—destruction of the lung parenchyma. The decrease in elastic recoil makes involved units more ventilable, whereas the loss of capillaries decreases their perfusion.

The single breath O_2 test is markedly abnormal in patients with emphysema, signifying uneven distribution of inspired air. This observation, however, carries no implication concerning the adequacy of gas exchange (for example, if perfusion were also uneven but in proportion to ventilation, gas exchange would not be impaired). A considerable amount of the total ventilation, regardless of how the various units fill and empty, is distributed to regions that are poorly perfused. Arterial PCO_2 values are usually normal in patients with emphysema, even in the advanced stages, a finding that may seem surprising in the presence of severe obstruction to airflow. However, the observation is readily explained by the fact that there is some CO_2 elimination from the regions that are well ventilated but poorly perfused. This effect is sufficient to offset the mild tendency for PCO_2 to increase from the extensive perfusion of regions with slightly lower than normal ventilation:perfusion ratios. The price that these patients must pay to maintain arterial PCO_2 within the normal range is, obviously, an increased minute volume of ventilation to make up for the large amount of wasted ventilation, which contributes little or nothing to gas exchange.

Predictions of arterial PO_2 values from the observed distributions of ventilation and blood flow agree extremely well with direct measurements of PO_2. The agreement reinforces previous statements that despite severe decreases in diffusing capacity, limitation of diffusion is not an important cause of arterial hypoxia in these or other patients at rest.

During exercise, arterial PO_2 decreases in patients with severe emphysema. Even this decrease is not caused by failure of diffusion equilibration to occur, as is theoretically possible (Fig. 35), because measured arterial PO_2 values during exercise agree well with those predicted from the observed distributions of ventilation and perfusion. The distributions during exercise are virtually the same as those at rest. Therefore, because the decrease in arterial PO_2 during exercise cannot be explained by either diffusion limitation or worsened ventilation-perfusion mismatching, it must be attributable to a decrease in mixed venous PO_2. This, in turn, implies that O_2 consumption during exercise increases proportionately more than cardiac output and that the arteriovenous O_2 difference widens. As discussed more thoroughly later in this section (Respiratory Failure), in the presence of a certain fixed pattern of ventilation-perfusion imbalance, decreasing cardiac output and mixed venous O_2 content causes arterial PO_2 to decrease.

It is possible to predict what must happen to lung volumes and the mechanics of ventilation when elastic recoil decreases. However, although there is a general correspondence between worsening emphysema and increasing loss of recoil, the relationship is far from perfect. Theoretic analysis of gas exchange abnormalities in patients with emphysema is even more tenuous than estimates of mechanical disturbances because so much depends on the matching of ventilation and perfusion in the remaining (not destroyed) terminal respiratory units, a consequence that is completely unpredictable. Thus the present understanding of gas exchange must rest on direct observations in patients characterized as having "mainly" emphysema. These studies are useful, and the findings contrast with those from patients believed to have "mainly" chronic bronchitis (discussed subsequently). However, in nearly all cases, the coexistence of emphysema and chronic bronchitis prevents sorting out the pure effects of each condition.

Control of Breathing. The influence of emphysema on the control of breathing also must be assessed by direct measurements in patients because there is no inherent reason why destruction of the lung parenchyma should affect regulatory mechanisms. These studies suffer from the same limitations as those of gas exchange in that they depend on clinical and physiologic, and not on morphologic, characterization of patients. Nevertheless, from among all patients with chronic obstructive pulmonary disease, two groups have been identified that can be viewed as representing the ends of the continuum of pathophysiologic findings. (1) Patients with type A disease in whom slight arterial hypoxia is usually present but PO_2 is reasonably well maintained and the PCO_2 is normal; these are the so-called pink puffers or fighters because they increase their ventilation, regardless of the extra work involved, to prevent hypercapnia. (2) Patients with type B disease, the so-called blue bloaters or nonfighters, in whom obstruction to airflow is equal in severity to that of the type A group, but PO_2 is severely decreased and PCO_2 is increased. It is often inferred that type A and type B patients have emphysema and chronic bronchitis, respectively, but there is little pathologic evidence to support such an absolute differentiation.

Both type A and type B patients have decreased responses to inhaled CO_2. Presumably, this is, in part, attributable to the presence of airflow obstruction, because similar decreases can be produced in normal persons by having them breathe through an obstructed airway. The two important differences between eucapnic and hypercapnic patients with obstructive pulmonary disease are that the former have greater increases in both diaphragmatic electrical activity and $P_{0.1}$ values during CO_2 breathing than the latter. The increased drive to breathe and increased respiratory muscle activity undoubtedly help the pink puffer maintain normal arterial P_{CO_2} values. The fascinating reasons why the blue bloaters fail to respond similarly are considered in the next subsection.

Chronic Bronchitis

Chronic bronchitis is defined in clinical terms, although its pathology is now well documented. The essential component of all definitions is excessive production of mucus, usually with recurrent cough and expectoration. The American Thoracic Society further specifies that these symptoms must be present on most days for at least three months per year during a period of two successive years or more. Other causes of cough and sputum, such as tuberculosis or bronchiectasis, must be excluded. Chronic bronchitis means, therefore, production of excess respiratory secretions, mainly recognized by the presence of cough. However, the term does not describe the severity of the pathophysiologic consequences, which may vary enormously. At one end of the continuum of chronic bronchitis are patients with a morning cigarette cough productive of small amounts of mucus who are otherwise asymptomatic and whose only physiologic abnormalities are related to obstruction in small airways. At the other end of the continuum are patients with a severe disabling condition accompanied by increased resistance to airflow, hypoxia, and often hypercapnia and cor pulmonale. The qualifiers "simple" and "obstructive" have been used to designate these two extremes of the spectrum of chronic bronchitis, but the terms have not been quantified and the transition between them is uncertain. The pulmonary function abnormalities of the extremely common milder form of simple chronic bronchitis have been described previously in the discussion of peripheral airways obstruction. The less common but much more dramatic manifestations of narrowing of the bronchial system are listed in Table 14 and described in the following pages.

Lung Volumes. The presence of disease in and around small peripheral airways that decreases their cross-sectional area accounts for the changes in lung volumes in patients with chronic bronchitis. As expected, the major abnormality is an increased RV, which reflects premature closure of the narrowed airways during expiration. If the cross-sectional area is compromised sufficiently that airways would close at normal FRC, the lungs would be held at an increased volume, presumably by augmented effort of inspiratory muscles. This situation is analogous, in part, to that in patients with asthma in whom airways close prematurely. Similarly, as in patients with asthma, the

TABLE 14. PULMONARY FUNCTION ABNORMALITIES IN PATIENTS WITH SEVERE "OBSTRUCTIVE" BRONCHITIS*

TEST	RESULT
Lung volumes	
Vital capacity	Markedly decreased
Total lung capacity	Normal
Functional residual capacity	Increased
Residual volume	Markedly increased
Mechanics of ventilation	
FEV_1/FVC	Markedly decreased
Maximal expiratory flow	Markedly decreased
Specific airways conductance	Decreased
Distribution of ventilation	Markedly abnormal
Diffusing capacity	Normal
Gas exchange	
P_{O_2}	Markedly decreased
P_{CO_2}	Increased
pH	Decreased
(Alveolar-arterial) P_{O_2}	Markedly increased
Right-to-left shunt	Absent
Wasted ventilation	Slightly increased

*For definitions of abbreviations, see Table 10.

recoil of the lungs and chest wall appears to be normal in patients with chronic bronchitis; thus TLC is also normal because the fundamental pathologic abnormalities—widespread and severe narrowing of airways—are comparable in both these clinical types of airways obstruction.

Mechanics of Ventilation. Utilizing the same concepts that were developed in the previous discussion about the volume-pressure, flow-volume, and flow-pressure relationships in normal subjects and patients with emphysema (Fig. 60), the mechanisms of airflow obstruction in patients with chronic bronchitis can be explained. In these patients, whose pulmonary elastic recoil is normal, the sole cause for limitation of maximal expiratory flow must be increased resistance in the peripheral airways. This agrees nicely with pathologic findings of inflammation, fibrous thickening, squamous metaplasia, and secretions in bronchioles and small bronchi in heavy cigarette smokers with chronic bronchitis. Because the sites of limitation of flow are located in peripheral airways, where laminar flow is fully developed, patients with severe chronic bronchitis do not increase maximal expiratory flow after breathing $He-O_2$ and values of $Viso_V$ are abnormally high.

Because the pathologic abnormalities of the conducting bronchioles and bronchi in patients with chronic bronchitis are neither uniformly located within certain airways nor equal in the narrowing that is produced, the effects on local resistance to airflow vary widely. This explains one of the characteristic pulmonary function findings in patients with bronchitis—markedly abnormal distribution of inspired air.

Gas Exchange. As stated in the previous discussion of control of breathing in emphysema, two groups of patients with chronic obstructive airways disease can be identified on the basis of their blood gas data: those with relatively well maintained arterial P_{O_2} values and no CO_2 retention and those with severe hypoxia and hypercapnia. The former findings occur in a reasonably homogeneous group of type A patients who appear to have mainly emphysema. In contrast, type

B patients with severe hypoxia and hypercapnia are a much more heterogeneous group clinically, functionally, and pathologically, and it is a mistake to regard them all as having mainly chronic bronchitis. Nevertheless, it is possible to examine a subset of patients with severe narrowing of conducting airways and minimal emphysema to discover what effect chronic bronchitis has on gas exchange.

The first important observation is that these patients have normal diffusing capacities. Although diffusing capacity is to some extent influenced by maldistribution of inspired air, which is an important consequence of chronic bronchitis, the normal values for single breath DL_{CO} correlate well with the fact that in this disease the alveolar-capillary surface for gas exchange is intact.

The characteristically low values of arterial PO_2 in patients with chronic bronchitis can be explained by ventilation-perfusion abnormalities. A large fraction of the cardiac output is distributed to regions with low ventilation:perfusion ratios, thus accounting for the hypoxia; right-to-left shunting of blood is absent or trivial. The remainder of the blood flow and virtually all of the ventilation is distributed to regions with slightly higher than normal (1 to 10) ventilation:perfusion ratios. Alveolar ventilation, however, is insufficient to offset the effect on CO_2 elimination of the large amount of blood flow to regions with low ventilation:perfusion ratios. Thus the presence of hypercapnia can be regarded as a failure of the ventilatory control system, which normally increases breathing in response to increases in arterial PCO_2, to respond appropriately. (See subsequent discussion of control of breathing.)

When patients with chronic bronchitis breathe 100 per cent O_2 for 30 minutes, there is no change in the pattern of the distributions of ventilation and perfusion, and, particularly, right-to-left shunts do not develop. The pattern of distributions might be expected to change because it is frequently stated that blood flow is redistributed away from lung units in which there is alveolar hypoxia. Severe alveolar hypoxia must be present in patients with chronic bronchitis in those regions with low ventilation:perfusion ratios, yet relief of the alveolar hypoxia by breathing O_2 does not alter the amount of blood flow to these regions. Thus the hypoxia-vasoconstrictor mechanism is inoperative or overwhelmed in these patients. When patients with acute respiratory failure and comparably low ventilation:perfusion ratios from disease of the lung parenchyma breathe 100 per cent O_2, right-to-left shunts develop from (presumably) closure of air spaces. That this phenomenon does not occur in patients with chronic bronchitis suggests that different mechanisms are involved, probably the presence of sufficient pathways of collateral ventilation to prevent alveolar collapse.

Control of Breathing. The ventilatory response to induced hypercapnia (CO_2-response test) is decreased in nearly all patients with chronic obstructive pulmonary disease. This uniform observation clearly does not distinguish those patients who cannot breathe because of mechanical limitation from those who do not breathe because of decreased ventilatory drive. The results of studies of mouth occlusion pressure ($P_{0.1}$) in hypercapneic and eucapneic patients with COPD re-

vealed that both groups had significantly greater values than normal subjects, indicating an increased neural drive to breathe, but that the two groups did not differ from each other. The main functional feature that distinguished patients who were hypercapneic from those who were not was that the former breathed more rapidly and shallowly. The low tidal volumes and, particularly, short inspiration, indicate faulty respiratory timing, perhaps from abnormal respiratory muscle function or reflex control.

REFERENCES

Peripheral Airways Obstruction

Berend, N., and Thurlbeck, W. M.: Correlations of maximum expiratory flow with small airway dimensions and pathology. J Appl Physiol 52:346, 1982.

Cosio, M., Ghezzo, H., Hogg, J. C., Corbin, R., Loveland, M., Dosman, J., and Macklem, P. T.: The relations between structural changes in small airways and pulmonary-function tests. N Engl J Med 298:1277, 1978.

Rodarte, J. R., Hyatt, R. E., Rehder, K., and Marsh, H. M.: New tests for the detection of obstructive pulmonary disease. Chest 72:762, 1977.

Wright, J. L., Lawson, L. M., Pare, P. D., et al.: Morphology of peripheral airways in current smokers and ex-smokers. Am Rev Respir Dis 127:474, 1983.

Central Airway Obstruction

Harrison, B. D. W.: Upper airway obstruction—a report on sixteen patients. Q J Med 45:625, 1975.

Kryer, M., Bode, F., Antic, R., and Anthoniesen, N.: Diagnosis of obstruction of the upper and central airways. Am J Med 61:85, 1976.

Miller, R. D., and Hyatt, R. E.: Evaluation of obstructing lesions of the trachea and larynx by flow-volume loops. Am Rev Respir Dis 108:475, 1973.

Asthma

Boushey, H. A., Holtzman, M. J., Sheller, J. R., and Nadel, J. A.: Bronchial hyperreactivity: State of the art. Am Rev Respir Dis 121:389–413, 1980.

Lee, T. H., Assoufi, B. K., and Kay, A. B.: The link between exercise, respiratory heat exchange, and the mast cell in bronchial asthma. Lancet 1:520, 1983.

Lee, T. H., Nagy, L., Nagakura, T., Walport, M. J., and Kay, A. B.: Identification and partial characterization of an exercise-induced neutrophil chemotactic factor in bronchial asthma. J Clin Invest 69:889, 1982.

McFadden, E. R., Jr.: Respiratory heat and water exchange: Physiological and clinical implications. J Appl Physiol 54:331, 1983.

Rodenstein, D., and Stanescu, D. C.: Elastic properties of the lung in acute induced asthma. J Appl Physiol 54:152, 1983.

Wagner, P. D., Dantzker, D. R., Iacovoni, V. E., Tomlin, W. C., and West, J. B.: Ventilation-perfusion inequality in asymptomatic asthma. Am Rev Respir Dis 118:511, 1978.

Emphysema and Chronic Bronchitis

Altose, M. D., McCauley, W. C., Kelsen, S. G., and Cherniack, N. S.: Effects of hypercapnia and inspiratory flow-resistive loading on respiratory activity in chronic airways obstruction. J Clin Invest 59:500, 1977.

Hogg, J. C., Macklem, P. T., and Thurlbeck, W. M.: Site and nature of airway obstruction in chronic obstructive lung disease. N Engl J Med 278:1355, 1968.

Matsuba, K., and Thurlbeck, W. M.: Disease of the small airways in chronic bronchitis. Am Rev Respir Dis 107:552, 1973.

Oliver, A., Kelsen, S. G., Deal, E. C., and Cherniack, N. S.: Mechanisms underlying CO_2 retention during flow-resistive loading in patients with chronic obstructive pulmonary disease. J Clin Invest 71:1442, 1983.

Sorli, J., Grassino, A., Lorange, G., and Milic-Emili, J.: Control of breathing in patients with chronic obstructive lung disease. Clin Sci 54:295, 1978.

Thurlbeck. W. M.: Chronic Airflow Obstruction in Lung Disease. Philadelphia, W. B. Saunders Co., 1976.

Thurlbeck. W. M., Henderson, J. A., Fraser, R. G., and Bates, D. V.: Chronic obstructive lung disease. A comparison between clinical, roentgenologic, functional and morphologic criteria in chronic bronchitis, emphysema, asthma and bronchiectasis. Medicine 49:81, 1970.

PULMONARY VASCULAR DISORDERS

The blood vessels of the lungs are directly or indirectly affected by many common and important respiratory disorders. Moreover, the pathophysiologic manifestations of this involvement vary considerably, ranging from severe disturbances of gas exchange on the one hand to circulatory failure on the other. There is no satisfactory classification of the various pulmonary vascular disorders, but two general types of involvement are recognized—primary and secondary. Primary diseases originate within blood vessels of the lungs and the pathologic process may or may not extend into the neighboring parenchyma and/or airways; examples of primary vascular disease, such as primary pulmonary hypertension and pulmonary veno-occlusive disease, are rare. Secondary disorders begin elsewhere in the lungs or even in other organs, but the consequences of the extravascular process impair the functional capabilities of the pulmonary circulation; disturbances of function may occur either in association with morphologic abnormalities or in blood vessels that are anatomically intact. Secondary involvement of the pulmonary circulation is extremely common. Examples of the type with pathologic findings include the destruction of blood vessels by advancing emphysema, obliteration of capillaries by progressive interstitial fibrosis, and the occlusion of arteries by pulmonary emboli. Examples of extravascular processes that affect the function of normal vessels by causing them to narrow or exposing them to excess pressure are the pulmonary hypertension of asthma or of alveolar hypoxia and the pulmonary edema of left heart failure.

It is obvious that the pathophysiologic alterations leading to and resulting from disorders of the pulmonary circulation can be extremely variable. To cover the usual spectrum of abnormalities, this discussion includes pulmonary edema, pulmonary embolism, pulmonary hypertension, and cor pulmonale.

Pulmonary Edema

There is no completely satisfactory definition of pulmonary edema. Usually, pulmonary edema means an abnormal accumulation of liquid in the lungs, but strictly speaking that definition includes pneumonia and other forms of inflammatory exudates, which are excluded from the ensuing discussion. The physiologic factors that normally control the filtration and removal of liquid and solutes in the lungs are considered in the section on Normal Physiology of the Respiratory System, and normal values for the hydrostatic and protein osmotic forces operating across the capillary endothelium are illustrated in Figure 45. The lungs cannot

become edematous until the rate of fluid filtration exceeds the rate of fluid removal. Thus pulmonary edema develops only when one or more of the intravascular or extravascular forces governing filtration of liquid changes by a sufficient amount, when the permeability of the pulmonary capillary endothelium increases, and/or when lymphatic drainage is impaired. In most kinds of pulmonary edema, regardless of origin, the sequence of accumulation of liquid appears to be the same; furthermore, the location and magnitude of the excess water within the lungs determine the severity of abnormalities of respiratory function.

Sequence of Formation of Pulmonary Edema. When filtration across the pulmonary capillary endothelium increases, the excess water appears first in the pericapillary interstitial space. However, only a small amount of liquid is accommodated in the interalveolar septum because of the ease with which water moves from the pericapillary into the peribronchovascular interstitial space. The extra liquid in the interalveolar septum cannot be recognized by light microscopy and accounts for a gain in weight of the lung of only a slight percentage. In contrast, substantial volumes of pulmonary edema can accumulate in the peribronchovascular interstitial space when the rate of filtration exceeds the rate of removal. This process produces the "cuffs" that are visible by light microscopy

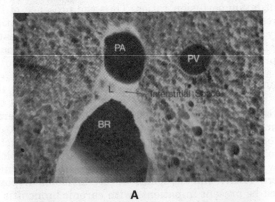

A

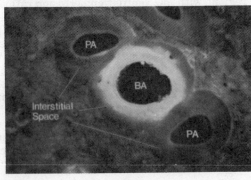

B

Figure 61. Frozen specimen of normal *(A)* and edematous *(B)* sheep lungs. Small bronchus *(BR)*, pulmonary artery *(PA)*, and vein *(PV)* are identified. In the normal lung the only visible interstitial space lies between the bronchus and artery and contains two lymphatics *(L)*. In the edematous lung marked expansion of the peribronchovascular space is evident. Alveolar flooding is also present. (From Staub, N. C.: Am Rev Respir Dis 109:358, 1974; reprinted with permission of the authors and publisher.)

(Fig. 61). The bronchovascular space can accommodate an increase in weight of up to 30 to 35 per cent of the lung, which in the normal human adult represents 200 to 300 ml of liquid.

Alveolar flooding occurs after both the pericapillary and bronchovascular interstitial spaces are filled and the rate of filtration continues to exceed that of removal. However, the actual site of the leak that allows interstitial liquid to enter alveoli is not known. What is known is that alveoli are completely filled with either liquid or air (Fig. 62); partial filling and gas trapping are never prominent in histologic studies of edematous lungs. The most likely pathway for alveolar flooding is between or across epithelial cells, but no breaks in the continuity of the normally tight membrane can be demonstrated by ultrastructural studies. It has been speculated that the liquid flows peripherally from a leak or from some site of communication proximal to alveoli, but this theory needs confirmation. Foam clearly means that air and liquid have intermixed, probably in airways. The tiny stable bubbles observed in specimens of pulmonary edema are due to the presence of surfactant with its remarkably low surface tension. In some forms of pulmonary edema, particularly those of cardiac origin, blood-tinged foam is often present. This does not mean that the permeability of the alveolar-capillary membrane is sufficiently increased to enable passage of particles as large as red blood cells; in fact, the permeability characteristics in patients with cardiogenic pulmonary edema are apparently normal. Instead, the copious pink frothy secretions produced by some patients with pulmonary edema consist of a mixture of small quantities of blood from a relatively few ruptured vessels, presumably as a result of the increased hydrostatic pressure in the dependent regions of the lungs and clear liquid from the remainder. The presence of alveolar flooding with foam represents the *last stage* in the sequence of pathophysiologic events culminating in clinically apparent pulmonary edema. Accumulation of substantial excess interstitial liquid precedes alveolar flooding and can be used to detect early pulmonary edema.

Increased Hydrostatic Forces. An increase in the transmural hydrostatic pressure difference across the pulmonary capillary endothelium is the most clear-cut cause of increased filtration of liquid in the lungs. However, the process itself initiates compensatory changes that tend to offset the effect of the increase in pressure. Furthermore, an increase in transmural pressure difference can result from either an increase in the pressure within the microcirculation (intravascular pressure) or a decrease in pressure surrounding the vessels (perimicrovascular interstitial pressure).

Pulmonary edema is frequently said to be cardiogenic or noncardiogenic in origin. The association of cardiac disease with increased pulmonary microvascular pressure is clear, and thus the term *cardiogenic* has pathophysiologic meaning. However, the term *noncardiogenic pulmonary edema* literally includes all other forms of pulmonary edema, of which there are many, and the term is often used incorrectly to indicate edema from increased permeability of the alveolar-capillary membrane. Because the term *noncardiogenic* has no pathophysiologic connotation, it should be abandoned.

CARDIOGENIC PULMONARY EDEMA. Pulmonary capillary pressure increases (1) when left ventricular end-diastolic filling pressure increases (for example, aortic

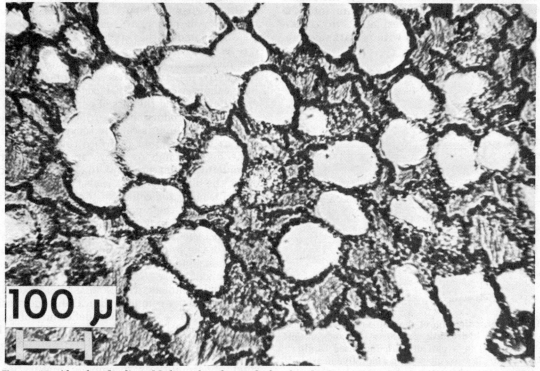

Figure 62. Alveolar flooding. Moderately advanced alveolar flooding in frozen specimen of dog lung. The striking all-or-none filling of alveolar edema is evident. (From Staub, N. C.: Human Pathol 1:419, 1970; reprinted with permission of the authors and publisher.)

valve disease, hypertensive or coronary arterial heart disease, or myocardiopathies), (2) when left atrial pressure increases (for example, mitral valve disease or left atrial myxoma), and (3) when pulmonary venous pressure increases. When microvascular hydrostatic pressure increases, the resultant increase in filtration of liquid causes secondary consequences (Fig. 63). Because permeability does not change, the fluid that leaks is essentially a low-protein ultrafiltrate of plasma; this liquid dilutes or washes out the proteins already present in the interstitial space and thereby decreases the interstitial protein osmotic pressure and increases the net transmural osmotic pressure. For every 2-mm Hg increase in microvascular hydrostatic pressure there is approximately a 1-mm decrease in interstitial protein osmotic pressure. By this means, 50 per cent of the initial increase in hydrostatic pressure is nullified. No one knows what happens to pericapillary hydrostatic pressure when the interstitial space becomes edematous; there are reasons why pressure could change in either direction, but because the changes are probably small, if they occur at all, the normal value is used in Figure 63. The dilution of interstitial liquid protein in patients with cardiogenic pulmonary edema is reflected in measurements of protein concentration in samples of liquid aspirated from their airways: both albumin and total protein concentrations in edema fluid are decreased relative to the amounts in serum so that the edema fluid:serum ratios of albumin and total protein concentrations are decreased, usually to less than 0.6.

If intravascular hydrostatic pressure were suddenly decreased back to a normal value of 8 mm Hg, the transmural protein osmotic force (14 mm Hg), shown in Figure 63, would exceed the restored transmural hydrostatic force (10 mm Hg) and some of the edema would move back across the endothelium into the bloodstream. This mechanism explains why cardiogenic pulmonary edema clears with remarkable rapidity in some patients. For exactly the same reasons, cardiogenic pulmonary edema also is probably cleared to some extent by the bloodstream as low-protein liquid begins to collect in the peribronchovascular interstitial space. Reabsorption should occur because the space is drained by bronchial capillaries and veins, in which the hydrostatic pressure might be substantially lower than in the pulmonary microcirculation.

HIGH ALTITUDE PULMONARY EDEMA. The abnormal mechanisms that produce high altitude pulmonary edema are unclear. It is known that pulmonary venous (that is, wedge) pressure remains within normal limits, but pulmonary arterial pressure increases. This combination implies an increase in pulmonary arterial resistance, presumably from vasoconstriction of arterioles or some other reactive site in the pulmonary circulation, between large arteries and capillaries. Patients who have had an episode of high altitude pulmonary edema have a greater pulmonary arterial pressor response than normal persons when both groups are given low concentrations of O_2 to breathe. The presence of hyperactive pulmonary arteries per se does not account for the presence of edema unless either the vasoconstriction is nonuniform, in which case some pulmonary capillaries would not be protected by proximal vasoconstriction and filtration pressure would increase, or the edema results from filtration through the walls of arteries proximal to the sites of vasoconstriction.

REEXPANSION PULMONARY EDEMA. A rare but striking form of pulmonary edema occurs in some patients shortly after rapid expansion of a lung by evacuating a large pleural effusion or a pneumothorax; in most instances, the lung has been collapsed for several days before reexpansion. The astonishing feature of reexpansion pulmonary edema is that the edema is confined to the reexpanded lung. The mechanisms underlying this form of pulmonary edema are unknown. It is classified among the kinds of edema caused by increased hydrostatic forces because there are reasons perimicrovascular interstitial pressure might become unusually negative in these circumstances. After a lung collapses completely, blood is redistributed to the opposite side, and the loss of perfusion on the affected side causes production of surfactant to cease. When the collapsed lung is rapidly reexpanded, surface tension at the air-liquid interface could conceivably become high enough to create an extremely negative perimicrovascular pressure that would "suck" liquid out of the blood vessels. It is also possible that the lack of perfusion of the collapsed lung damages capillaries and increases their permeability so that the vessels leak after the lung is expanded and blood flow is restored. The results of the few available measurements of the protein concentration of the edema fluid in humans and experimental animals favor the second mechanism.

OTHER DISORDERS WITH INCREASED SURFACE TENSION. There are many common clinical disorders associated with a known or presumed deficiency of surfactant and/or increased surface forces in the lungs. The prototype disorder is the neonatal respiratory distress syndrome, a complication of prematurity in which the chief abnormality is incomplete maturation of the surfactant-producing system. Therefore, the lack of the normal presence of low surface tension at the air-liquid

INCREASED CAPILLARY HYDROSTATIC PRESSURE

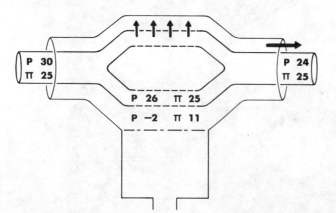

Figure 63. Schematic diagram of the pulmonary circulation and the prevailing hydrostatic pressures *(P)* and protein osmotic pressure (Π) in a patient with increased capillary hydrostatic pressure (for example, from congestive heart failure). For explanation of anatomy and normal values, see Figure 45. (From Hinshaw, H. C., and Murray, J. F.: Diseases of the Chest, Philadelphia, W. B. Saunders Co., 1979, p. 636.)

interface of the premature infant contributes not only to the development of atelectasis but also to an increased filtration of liquid in the lungs. This explains the frequency with which pulmonary edema is found post mortem in babies who die of the neonatal respiratory distress syndrome and also the value of diuretics in the treatment of this disorder.

Alterations in the function of type II cells and inactivation of surfactant by extravasation of plasma into alveolar spaces are presumed to increase surface tension in patients with the adult respiratory distress syndrome (see subsequent discussion). Because this must decrease perimicrovascular interstitial pressure, the resulting increase in transcapillary hydrostatic forces probably augments the leak of liquid that is already present owing to the increase in permeability that characterizes these disorders.

Decreased Protein Osmotic Forces. Most clinicians have seen patients with extremely low serum albumin concentrations (1 g/dl or even less); these patients nearly always have massive anasarca, ascites, and bilateral pleural effusions, but they do not have pulmonary edema. This simple observation illustrates the fact that the mechanisms that govern the formation of pleural fluid are influenced by systemic factors and thus are different from those that cause pulmonary edema. (Further information about the forces controlling the formation and removal of pleural fluid is provided subsequently in this section.) It is clear that when the concentration of protein in serum decreases, the concentration in interstitial liquid also decreases. However, the exact relationship between the protein osmotic pressure values in the bloodstream and the interstitium is still the source of considerable controversy. Figure 64 indicates a proportionate change (60 per cent) in the two values and demonstrates that the transmural pressure difference also decreases by 60 per cent (from a normal value of 6 to 2 mm Hg). If the hydrostatic forces and permeability are unchanged,

DECREASED PLASMA ONCOTIC PRESSURE

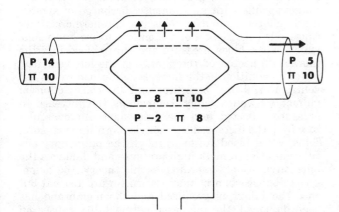

Figure 64. Schematic diagram of the pulmonary circulation and the prevailing hydrostatic pressures *(P)* and protein osmotic pressure (II) in a patient with decreased plasma oncotic pressure (for example, from the nephrotic syndrome). For explanation of anatomy and normal values, see Figure 45. (From Hinshaw, H. C., and Murray, J. F.: Diseases of the Chest. Philadelphia, W. B. Saunders Co., 1979, p. 639.)

INCREASED MEMBRANE PERMEABILITY

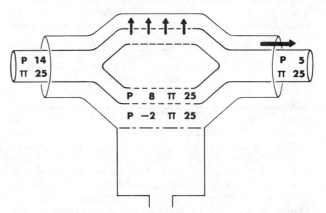

Figure 65. Schematic diagram of the pulmonary circulation and the prevailing hydrostatic pressures *(P)* and protein osmotic pressure (II) in a patient with increased permeability of the alveolar-capillary membrane (for example, inhalation of corrosive chemicals). For explanation of anatomy and normal values, see Figure 45. (From Hinshaw, H. C., and Murray, J. F.: Diseases of the Chest. Philadelphia, W. B. Saunders Co., 1979, p. 640.)

filtration must increase. The reason florid pulmonary edema does not develop under these circumstances is presumably that lymphatic removal increases to keep pace with the augmented rate of liquid formation. However, one consequence of decreasing the protective transmural protein osmotic pressure difference is that pulmonary edema occurs at a lower hydrostatic pressure difference than when protein concentrations are within normal limits.

Increased Permeability. Water, solutes, and even high molecular weight protein molecules cross the pulmonary microvascular endothelium from the bloodstream into the interstitial liquid, but the routes they travel are not known with certainty. Physiologists refer to pores of various sizes to describe the available pathways for movement of molecules across membranes, but the anatomic counterparts of these channels have not been convincingly established. Nevertheless, permeability is an extremely important quality of biologic membranes, including the pulmonary microvascular endothelium and alveolar epithelium.

If intravascular hydrostatic and protein osmotic forces are constant, an increase in permeability of the pulmonary microcirculation means that more liquid will be filtered: the greater the increase in permeability, the greater the leak of liquid across the endothelium. One obvious consequence of an increase in pulmonary microvascular permeability is shown in Figure 65; virtually pure plasma leaks into the interstitium and raises the interstitial protein osmotic pressure to equal that of plasma. Thus the protective effect of the normal transmural osmotic pressure difference is lost. Another consequence of increased permeability of the alveolar-capillary membrane and the extravasation of plasma is that the concentrations of protein in liquid obtained from the lower respiratory tract and that of a simultaneously obtained blood specimen are the same. These findings contrast with those of cardiogenic pulmonary edema, in which protein concentration is lower in edema fluid than in blood; measurements of this type can be used clinically, when alveolar fluid is available for sampling, to differentiate pulmonary edema resulting from increased hydrostatic forces from that caused by increased permeability.

ADULT RESPIRATORY DISTRESS SYNDROME. Many kinds of diffuse injury to the alveolar-capillary membrane increase its permeability and lead to pulmonary edema. The adult respiratory distress syndrome is a term used to describe the clinical, roentgenographic, physiologic, and pathologic consequences of widespread damage to the lung parenchyma. The syndrome occurs most often in patients hospitalized for a serious medical or surgical problem that does not involve the lungs directly (for example, shock of any cause, sepsis, severe burns, acute hemorrhagic pancreatitis, and multiple traumatic injuries). It may also develop in patients whose lungs *may* be injured but the extent of the damage is not fully developed when they are first seen (for example, after inhalation of smoke or corrosive chemicals, near-drowning, and aspiration of gastric contents). After an initial period in which evidence of pulmonary involvement may be minimal or even absent, progressive physiologic abnormalities develop: arterial hypoxia from right-to-left shunting of blood and decreased lung compliance. Roentgenograms reveal extensive diffuse consolidation of air spaces without enlargement of the heart. Pathologic findings in the acute stage are marked hemorrhagic pulmonary edema and, often, hyaline membranes.

The sequence of events that characterizes the adult respiratory distress syndrome has been associated with an extraordinarily diverse group of underlying disorders, and the list is steadily growing. The unifying aspect of these multiple conditions is that they all cause diffuse injury to the alveolar-capillary membrane, which initiates a similar series of subsequent reactions (Fig. 66). Damage to endothelial and type I epithelial cells increases their permeability and allows plasma to leak into the interstitial and alveolar spaces. The presence of protein, especially fibrin, in alveoli inactivates the surfactant layer at the air-liquid interface and increases its surface tension; this, in turn, promotes alveolar instability and increases the hydrostatic forces, causing filtration by making perimicrovascular pressure more negative. The combination of these processes results in lungs that are filled with a protein-rich edema fluid that often contains numerous red blood cells, a constellation of abnormalities that is referred to as congestive atelectasis.

The organization of intra-alveolar proteinaceous material produces hyaline membranes. As shown in Figure 66, the effects of treatment are apt to worsen the underlying abnormalities: (1) administration of O_2 in high concentrations for more than a few days has a direct toxic effect on endothelial and epithelial cells; (2) excessive hydration, which inadvertently results from efforts to control blood pressure, augments filtration by increasing intracapillary hydrostatic pressure; and (3) repeated overinflation of lung units, particularly if carried out from a low end-expiratory lung volume, recruits reserve surfactant molecules into the surface film and subsequently dislodges them when the film collapses at end-expiration. Although this massaging effect and depletion of the surface film has

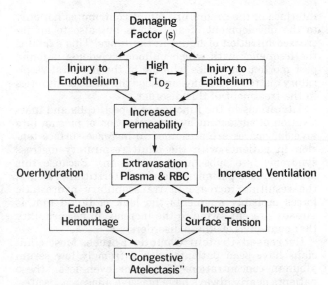

Figure 66. Schematic representation of the proposed pathogenetic sequence in patients with the adult respiratory distress syndrome (within rectangles). The mechanisms of action of iatrogenic factors that worsen the process are also indicated. See text for complete discussion.

been demonstrated only in experimental animals, it is likely that a similar process occurs in patients with adult respiratory distress syndrome.

NEUROGENIC PULMONARY EDEMA. The precise abnormalities that underlie what is called neurogenic pulmonary edema are poorly characterized. It is possible that increases in permeability or the presence of hemodynamic abnormalities, or both, which may accompany severe neurologic disorders, are responsible. Systemic blood pressure increases as intracerebral pressure increases (Cushing reflex), and this may be accompanied by increases in left atrial and pulmonary microvascular pressure. Thus, many cases of neurogenic pulmonary edema are probably hydrostatic in origin.

It has been postulated that various insults to the brain (for example, trauma, seizures, vascular accidents, hypotension) produce hypoxia of the midbrain that responds with an immense discharge of sympathetic efferent impulses. Massive adrenergic activity causes (1) constriction of systemic arteries and veins, which raises blood pressure and shifts blood into the thorax, (2) decreased compliance of the left ventricle, which in addition to the increased afterload raises left ventricular filling pressure, and (3) constriction of pulmonary veins, which compounds the increase in pressure reflected into the pulmonary microvasculature from the increased left ventricular filling pressure. Thus, extra blood surges through the pulmonary circulation at extremely high pressure and damages the microcirculation. According to this theory, the hemodynamic disturbances may return toward normal but once the injury is produced and the membrane has been damaged, the increased permeability causes an excessive leak of liquid that culminates in pulmonary edema. This sequence may explain the findings of nearly normal values of pulmonary arterial and wedge pressures and high concentrations of protein in pulmonary edema fluid from patients with neurogenic pulmonary edema.

There is, however, only scanty clinical evidence to support this proposed mechanism. Furthermore, the results of most experimental studies indicate that the pulmonary edema that occurs during various neurologic insults probably has a hemodynamic basis.

DRUG-INDUCED PULMONARY EDEMA. Several drugs are known to increase permeability of the alveolar-capillary membrane and produce acute pulmonary edema. Heroin is the most common drug associated with pulmonary edema, but the disorder may occur from both the intravenous and oral administration of methadone. Whether the injury in opiate-induced pulmonary edema is related to the drug itself or to a contaminant is unknown; the process cannot be reproduced in laboratory models. Pulmonary edema is also associated with excessive drug overdose (usually in suicide attempts) with salicylates, ethchlorvynol, and propoxyphene. Large intravenous doses of acetylsalicylic acid and ethchlorvynol have been shown experimentally to increase the permeability of the alveolar-capillary membrane, and it is likely that they have a similar effect in human beings. Other drugs (nitrofurantoin and sulfonamides) can produce acute pulmonary edema, usually with fever and eosinophilia, presumably as a hypersensitivity phenomenon.

Decreased Lymphatic Drainage. The pulmonary lymphatics play a major role in the normal handling of liquid in the lung by providing an important system through which water, solutes, and protein are removed from the lungs. As long as lymphatic drainage keeps pace with filtration, excessive accumulation cannot occur. Thus, developing pulmonary edema can be viewed as a state in which lymphatic removal cannot keep up with filtration. It follows that if the normal capacity of the pulmonary lymphatics to accommodate liquid were compromised by disease, pulmonary edema would occur at a lower rate of filtration than usual and might even occur in the absence of an increase in filtration. This concept appears to be true, but its application to clinical situations is limited.

Removing a lung from an experimental animal and then replacing it by reanastomosing the blood vessels and bronchus (autotransplantation) completely disrupts the lymphatic channels on that side of the thorax. Because the autotransplanted lung has no drainage pathways for the liquid that continues to be formed, the lung gains weight for a few days after the operation, and interstitial pulmonary edema develops. However, within three or four days, before alveolar flooding occurs, continuity of lymphatic channels is restored by reanastomosis and formation of new vessels; drainage then resumes and the weight of the lung returns toward normal. The capacity to develop collateral pathways presumably explains the failure of pulmonary edema to occur in patients with disorders in which massive obliteration of pulmonary lymphatics is known to occur (for example, silicosis and lymphangitic carcinomatosis); however, it is likely that the threshold for pulmonary edema formation is changed in patients with these diseases. The closest condition to "elephantiasis" of the lungs in adults occurs in some patients with lymphangiomyoangiomatosis (a rare disorder of young women that is associated with stasis of lymphatic drainage and episodes of interstitial pulmonary edema) and in infants with congenital lymphangiec-tasis (a rare disorder that may be associated with pulmonary edema).

Pulmonary Function Abnormalities. Given the enormous variation in the amount of liquid that accumulates in the lungs during the evolution of pulmonary edema, it is apparent that a wide variety of pulmonary physiologic abnormalities is likely to result. Many of these changes are well documented, but their relationship to the amount and localization of the edema is not known. However, certain reasonable inferences about the findings in patients with cardiogenic pulmonary edema are possible, as shown in Table 15.

An increase in left ventricular filling pressure raises pressures throughout the pulmonary circulation and causes pulmonary vascular congestion. Because of the increased pulmonary capillary blood volume, $D_{L_{CO}}$ also increases, and because the increased pulmonary arterial pressure makes the distribution of blood flow more uniform than normal with respect to perfusion, arterial P_{O_2} increases slightly.

During the stage of interstitial edema, the accumulation of liquid in bronchovascular spaces and possibly the bronchial walls narrows the caliber of airways, causing them to close prematurely, which increases closing volume. Although there may be some narrowing of blood vessels at this time, the process affects the distribution of ventilation more than the distribution of perfusion so that a ventilation-perfusion inequality develops and arterial P_{O_2} values decrease. Interstitial edema per se causes little or no change in lung volumes and the mechanics of ventilation.

When alveolar flooding occurs, VC and other lung volumes decrease, pulmonary compliance decreases, chiefly from loss of ventilable units, and arterial P_{O_2} worsens. However, the mechanism causing hypoxia shifts from a ventilation-perfusion abnormality, from narrowing of airways, to a right-to-left shunt, from perfusion of unventilable liquid-filled alveoli.

Arterial P_{CO_2} may be decreased, normal, or increased, and the mechanisms underlying these changes have not been clarified. Hyperventilation presumably occurs from stimulation by excess liquid of the pulmonary C fibers located in the lung parenchyma. Hypoventilation implies a breakdown in the control of breathing, but it is uncertain which step is involved.

TABLE 15. RELATIONSHIPS BETWEEN PROGRESSIVE STAGES OF CARDIOGENIC PULMONARY EDEMA AND PULMONARY FUNCTION ABNORMALITIES*

STAGE	ABNORMALITY
Pulmonary vascular congestion	Increased $D_{L_{CO}}$ Increased arterial P_{O_2} (slight)
Interstitial pulmonary edema	Increased closing volume Decreased arterial P_{O_2} from ventilation-perfusion mismatching
Alveolar flooding	Decreased vital capacity Decreased compliance Decreased arterial P_{O_2} from right-to-left shunt

*For definitions of abbreviations, see Table 10.

Pulmonary Embolism

The term *embolus* literally means a plug, and the term *embolism* refers to the sudden obstruction of a vessel by a plug that has traveled through the bloodstream to its site of impaction. Emboli can form in veins or enter the venous circulation in a variety of ways; the plugs are then carried with the venous blood through the right atrium and ventricle and into the pulmonary arterial circulation where, if they are large enough (>10 to 20 μm), they lodge. Of the many possible sources of emboli, blood clots outweigh all others by far in their clinical importance. Thus ordinary pulmonary embolism is not a primary disease but a consequence of venous thrombosis, a disorder arising in organs other than the lungs. The factors promoting venous thrombosis are discussed elsewhere in this book.

The pathophysiologic consequences of pulmonary embolism are well documented because of the clinical frequency with which the process occurs. However, the mechanisms underlying these changes are in some instances controversial and in other instances unknown. This discussion will review the prevailing theories concerning the pathophysiologic origin of some of the commonly observed manifestations of pulmonary embolism; dyspnea, undoubtedly the most common symptom, is considered later in this section (Disorders of the Control of Breathing).

Hyperventilation. The episodic bouts of dyspnea accompanying pulmonary embolism are often associated with hyperventilation. The breathing pattern is usually rapid and shallow, an inefficient combination because it increases the fraction of each breath that is considered wasted ventilation because it does not contribute to O_2 uptake or CO_2 elimination. However, as implied by the term *hyperventilation,* arterial P_{CO_2} is decreased and thus minute volume must increase substantially. The change in breathing pattern cannot be related to alterations in blood gases and is believed to be reflex in origin. The receptors and neural pathways involved have not been identified in humans, but the pulmonary C fibers situated in the lung parenchyma, whose afferent pathways are in the vagus nerves, are likely candidates because, when stimulated by microembolism in experimental animals, they cause comparable tachypnea.

Hypoxia. Pulmonary embolism is associated with characteristic—but nonspecific—changes in arterial blood gases and pH. Arterial blood analysis reveals decrease in P_{O_2} below 80 mm Hg in 90 per cent of patients with angiographically proven embolism, a decrease in P_{CO_2}, and an increase in pH. Because of the hyperventilation, O_2 exchange is even worse than the arterial P_{O_2} value indicates and is better estimated by measurements of the alveolar-arterial P_{O_2} difference.

The P_{CO_2} and pH values indicate hyperventilation and acute respiratory alkalosis, abnormalities that are an obvious consequence of the increased ventilatory drive already mentioned. The mechanism underlying the decreased arterial P_{O_2} is puzzling and appears to differ in humans and experimental animals. An excellent study in patients with proven pulmonary embolism demonstrated that right-to-left shunting of blood was the major abnormality that contributed to the observed hypoxia. Although the sites of the shunt are not definitely known, it was postulated that they occurred through regions of microatelectasis because the magnitude of the shunt decreased when the patients took deep breaths. In contrast, studies in dogs using sophisticated methods for evaluating gas exchange have revealed mainly ventilation-perfusion disturbances and little shunting after induced pulmonary embolism. It is obvious that neither shunts nor ventilation-perfusion mismatching can develop *distal* to the embolus if the obstruction is complete because pulmonary arterial blood flow to the involved lung ceases. The presence of arterial hypoxia is one of the clearest indications that secondary changes, presumably neurohumoral in origin, take place in uninvolved regions of the lungs.

Pulmonary Arterial Pressure. The impaction of a clot in the pulmonary arterial circulation may or may not be associated with an increase in pulmonary arterial pressure. When pulmonary hypertension occurs, multiple and/or massive embolism is nearly always present. Two mechanisms have been advanced to account for pulmonary hypertension resulting from embolization. The first is simple mechanical obliteration of large segments of the circulation by one or more emboli, and the second is active vasoconstriction from neurohumoral stimuli, which compounds the effects of whatever mechanical narrowing exists. Because pulmonary arterial pressure correlated well with angiographic estimates of the extent of occlusion of the pulmonary circulation in one study, the increased pressure in patients with previously normal hearts and lungs has been explained solely by mechanical obstruction. However, these patients all survived long enough to be hospitalized and catheterized; accordingly, the data do not exclude an important role for neurohumorally mediated vasoconstriction as a contributor to some of the early sudden deaths from pulmonary embolism. Catheterization studies have shown that the right ventricle is incapable of withstanding a sudden pressure increase of greater than 40 to 50 mm Hg. Furthermore, more than half of the cross-sectional area of the pulmonary circulation must be obliterated before pulmonary arterial pressure begins to rise. Thus it follows that pulmonary hypertension occurs when just the right amount of the circulation is occluded—that is, enough to cause the pressure to increase but not enough to cause acute right ventricular failure and death.

Pulmonary Infarction. Myocardial infarction and cerebral infarction are widely understood and appropriately used terms that mean death and necrosis of the myocardium and cerebrum, respectively. In contrast, the term *pulmonary infarction,* which means death and necrosis of part of the lungs, is often loosely and incorrectly applied. Confusion exists because the presence of pleuritic pain, hemoptysis, and parenchymal infiltrations in chest roentgenograms, all common features of pulmonary embolism, may indicate that infarction has occurred but are more likely to indicate that hemorrhage from ischemia (not death) of cells is present. True infarction after pulmonary embolism is uncommon, and the incidence is probably much less than the usually quoted figure of 10 per cent because so many emboli go undiagnosed.

Because the lungs have a dual blood supply, whether

or not infarction occurs depends on the interaction between two phenomena: the extent of occlusion of the pulmonary arterial circulation and the capacity of the bronchial arterial system to provide O_2 and metabolic substrates to the involved lung parenchyma. Thus pulmonary infarction is likely to develop when arterial obstruction is complete rather than partial and when the bronchial circulation is compromised and blood flow through it cannot increase. The importance of the bronchial circulation explains why pulmonary infarctions occur in patients with one or more of the following clinical conditions: (1) congestive heart failure, in which there is reduced blood flow through the bronchial circulation; (2) chronic pulmonary disease, in which there may be loss of or other structural changes in bronchial arteries; and (3) prolonged shock, in which bronchial blood flow is impaired because of the low systemic arterial pressure.

Pulmonary Hypertension

The pulmonary circulation of normal persons is characterized as a high flow–low pressure system; this means that resistance to blood flow through the lungs is low. Furthermore, during exercise vascular resistance decreases even further so that blood flow increases substantially but pulmonary arterial pressure increases only slightly (see Table 2). The ability to accommodate a large increase in flow with a small change in pressure means that the cross-sectional area of the vascular pathways must increase considerably. This is effected by recruitment of blood vessels that were not perfused at rest and by dilatation of the entire circulatory bed. It follows that any process that narrows the cross-sectional area of the pulmonary circulation will progressively impair the ability of the vascular bed to expand and its resistance to decrease during exercise. This phenomenon explains why the diagnosis of *early* vascular involvement can be established only by measuring pulmonary arterial pressure while the patient exercises (Fig. 67). By the time clinically recognizable pulmonary hypertension is present at rest, the process is usually severe and often irreversible.

Pulmonary arterial hypertension in patients with respiratory disorders occurs in response to a reduction of the cross-sectional area of the pulmonary vascular bed, either by vasoconstriction or structural changes (obliteration or occlusion) of the blood vessels, or both. Initially, these two processes occur quite independently of each other. Later, regardless of the cause of pulmonary hypertension, secondary anatomic changes ensue that narrow the vascular bed further and aggravate the condition. Pulmonary arterial pressure must increase when pulmonary venous pressure increases; this sequence is common in patients with left-sided heart disease but occurs only rarely in patients with occlusive diseases of their pulmonary veins. Pulmonary arterial hypertension also occurs in patients with excessive amounts of blood flowing through the lungs (for example, interatrial septal defect) and in patients with abnormal communications between the systemic and pulmonary circulations (for example, Eisenmenger's syndrome). The pathophysiology of these cardiac abnormalities is considered elsewhere in this book.

Vasoconstriction. The pulmonary blood vessels, particularly arteries, have an abundant nerve supply. Most of the fibers appear to be of sympathetic origin,

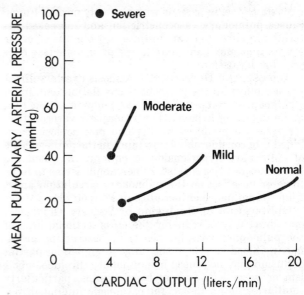

Figure 67. Schematic representation of the relationships between mean pulmonary arterial pressure and cardiac output in normal subjects and in patients with mild, moderate, and severe pulmonary hypertension. *Solid circles* are values at rest. Note that as the process worsens, resting pressure increases, resting output decreases, and an increase in output causes progressively steeper increases in pressure.

which leads to the expectation of some degree of neural control of the caliber of pulmonary blood vessels. Although it is possible under rigorous laboratory conditions to demonstrate sympathetic vasoconstrictor responses in experimental animals, adrenergic activity in man is trivial or even absent. Similarly, the adult human pulmonary circulation responds weakly or not at all to naturally occurring humoral substances (for example, serotonin and histamine) and to pharmacologic vasoactive agents (for example, isoproterenol and phenoxybenzamine). Several prostaglandins and their derivatives have pulmonary vasoactivity in experimental animals, and prostaglandin F is a vasoconstrictor in humans.

HYPOXIA. The most important pulmonary arterial vasoconstrictor by far is hypoxia. How hypoxia causes pulmonary arteries to constrict is not known, but there are two major theories: (1) constriction is an indirect response to alveolar hypoxia mediated by chemical substances, and (2) constriction is a direct effect of hypoxia on pulmonary arterial smooth muscle. Vasoconstriction from alveolar hypoxia is mainly a local phenomenon because it occurs in isolated and perfused lungs with no nerve supply; however, it is also possible that neurohumoral responses in otherwise healthy persons may augment whatever local reaction occurs.

Persons born and raised at high altitudes have pulmonary hypertension and abundant smooth muscle in the walls of their pulmonary arteries. Infants have a greater amount of pulmonary smooth muscle and a greater vasoconstrictor response to hypoxia than adults. Some persons are known to hyperreact to a given hypoxic challenge and appear to be susceptible to high altitude pulmonary edema. Although hyperreactivity or excess vascular smooth muscle, or both, may favor the development of pulmonary hypertension, hypoxia per se, in persons with perfectly normal lungs, causes pulmonary vasoconstriction and increased arterial pressure and can initiate a sequence of other events that may culminate in cor pulmonale (see subsequent discussion).

Acidosis and Hypercapnia. Acidosis exerts a direct pressor effect on the pulmonary circulation and, more significantly, compounds the vasomotor reaction to a given degree of hypoxia. The synergistic vasoconstrictor response produced by hypoxia and acidosis combined is of considerable importance in the pathogenesis of pulmonary hypertension in patients in whom the two abnormalities coexist. Hypercapnia seems to have little or no effect on the pulmonary circulation apart from the influence of increases in P_{CO_2} on pH.

Obliteration or Occlusion of Vessels. Obviously, one direct way of reducing the cross-sectional area of the pulmonary vascular bed is by obstructing or removing blood vessels in the lungs. Complete or partial occlusion may be caused by pulmonary thromboembolism or vasculitis. Loss of blood vessels, particularly capillaries, is an important pathologic finding in patients with emphysema and interstitial fibrosis and is a consequence of pulmonary resection. Because the cross-sectional area of the pulmonary vascular system increases progressively from central pulmonary arteries to capillaries, the effect of an obstructive or obliterative process on pulmonary vascular resistance depends on the location of the abnormality. Millions of capillaries need to be destroyed to equal the effect of occluding one lobar artery.

Secondary Changes. Once pulmonary hypertension occurs, regardless of its cause, secondary changes occur in the walls of pulmonary arteries that produce further narrowing. The earliest abnormality is hypertrophy of smooth muscle in the media of small arteries. Later in sequence, a cascade of reactions leads to increased deposition of elastin, intimal proliferation, and formation of atheromatous plaques. At times, fibrinoid necrosis develops, which predisposes to thrombosis in situ. Finally, aneurysmal and angiomatoid changes occur. The effect of these reactions is to reduce an already restricted vascular bed. The progressively worsening vicious circle is shown in Figure 68; because the rate of development and the extent of the tissue reactions are directly related to the severity of the pulmonary hypertension, once set in motion the process is self-perpetuating and steadily accelerating.

The effects of pulmonary hypertension per se on lung volumes, mechanics of ventilation, and gas exchange are frequently misunderstood. There is no pathophysiologic reason why intrinsic narrowing of the cross-sectional area of the pulmonary circulation, especially on the arterial side, should affect lung volumes or mechanics in any way. Similarly, arterial hypoxia should not occur because a reduction in blood flow to gas exchange units means that ventilation:perfusion ratios *increase*, and arterial P_{O_2}, if anything, should also increase. These generalities are true in patients with primary pulmonary hypertension and vasculitis, even when pulmonary arterial pressure is considerably elevated. Of course if pulmonary hypertension is secondary to airway, parenchymal, or neuromuscular disease, characteristic abnormalities of volumes, mechanics, and arterial P_{O_2} are evident.

Pulmonary hypertension is associated with certain

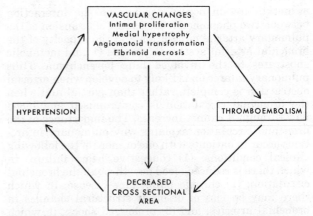

Figure 68. Schematic diagram showing how pulmonary hypertension, once established from any cause, is compounded by secondary structural changes that predispose to thromboembolic narrowing, both of which further decrease the cross-sectional area of the pulmonary vascular pathways, which worsens the hypertension. (From Hinshaw, H. C., and Murray, J. F.: Diseases of the Chest. Philadelphia, W. B. Saunders Co., 1979, p. 687.)

functional disturbances: (1) Arterial P_{CO_2} is chronically decreased, presumably from reflex ventilatory drive; which receptors are stimulated is unclear, but distortion of mechanoreceptors in dilated pulmonary arteries may be involved. (2) Wasted ventilation, which may be normal during rest, increases during exercise because the effects of taking deep breaths overcome the compensatory redistribution of ventilation away from poorly perfused regions. Increased wasted ventilation is the pathophysiologic hallmark of pulmonary vascular occlusive diseases because the abnormality represents ventilation to regions where there is little or no perfusion. Maintaining a lower than normal arterial P_{CO_2} in the face of increased wasted ventilation means that minute volume must increase considerably. This may account, in part, for the dyspnea that is the chief early symptom of patients with pulmonary vascular occlusive disease. Diffusing capacity is normal in these patients unless pulmonary capillaries are involved in the pathologic process.

Late in the course of evolution of pulmonary hypertension from vascular obliteration, arterial hypoxia from right-to-left shunting of blood may supervene. In some instances the shunt develops through a patent foramen ovale as right ventricular end-diastolic and right atrial pressures increase. In other instances the shunt appears to be through pathways in the lungs. Possible sites include arteriovenous communications in previously existing but functionless vessels or angiomatoid malformations; either of these might develop as a response to sustained and severe hypertension.

Cor Pulmonale

Cor pulmonale, defined as hypertrophy and/or dilatation of the right ventricle secondary to some form of respiratory disease, is invariably associated with pulmonary hypertension; *respiratory disease* is a better term than *pulmonary disease* because, as will be shown, organs besides the lungs are involved in the pathogenesis of cor pulmonale. Implicit in both the definition and the clinical diagnosis of cor pulmonale is the exclusion of congenital and acquired forms of heart disease as causes of the pulmonary arterial hypertension.

Although obviously a continuum, the abnormal processes leading to cor pulmonale can be viewed as occurring in two stages: first, the onset of pulmonary hypertension as a result of narrowing of the vascular bed, and second, the development of right ventricular hypertrophy or dilatation, or both, in response to the increased pulmonary arterial pressure. Cor pulmonale causes signs of right ventricular failure when pulmonary hypertension is severe and usually long lasting. Thus patients with cor pulmonale *always* have pulmonary arterial hypertension but may or may not have right ventricular failure.

Acute cor pulmonale is relatively uncommon. The most common cause is acute pulmonary embolism, but, as mentioned, pulmonary arterial pressure does not increase substantially until 50 to 60 per cent of the cross-sectional area of the circulation is obstructed and the right ventricle cannot maintain a sudden increase in pulmonary arterial pressure of greater than 40 to 50 mm Hg. For reasons discussed previously, acute cor pulmonale can complicate the course of a severe asthmatic attack.

Chronic cor pulmonale is much more common than the acute variety. Pulmonary hypertension usually develops slowly, which allows time for the right ventricle to enlarge. There are two basically different pathophysiologic sequences that can each culminate in chronic cor pulmonale; in many patients both pathways are involved.

Pulmonary Vascular Occlusion. The sequence of events leading to cor pulmonale in patients with pulmonary vascular occlusive disease is straightforward (Fig. 69). Gradual narrowing of the arterial circulation, from whatever cause, leads to a slow increase in pulmonary arterial pressure that evokes a corresponding increase in right ventricular muscle mass. In patients with obliterative vascular diseases, pulmonary arterial pressures may reach systemic levels and cause conspicuous right ventricular hypertrophy. Because of the self-perpetuating cycle of progressive vascular narrowing (Fig. 68) or because of an additional

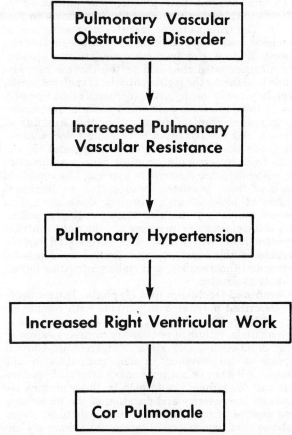

Figure 69. Schematic representation of the pathogenetic sequence leading from pulmonary vascular obstruction, regardless of cause, to cor pulmonale. Contrast this straightforward pathway with the sequence shown in Figure 70. (From Hinshaw, H. C., and Murray, J. F.: Diseases of the Chest. Philadelphia, W. B. Saunders Co., 1979, p. 698.)

resistive load from an acute complication, the hemodynamic burden on the right ventricle ultimately becomes excessive and failure occurs.

Hypoxia. The sequence of mechanisms in response

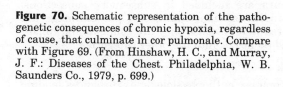

Figure 70. Schematic representation of the pathogenetic consequences of chronic hypoxia, regardless of cause, that culminate in cor pulmonale. Compare with Figure 69. (From Hinshaw, H. C., and Murray, J. F.: Diseases of the Chest. Philadelphia, W. B. Saunders Co., 1979, p. 699.)

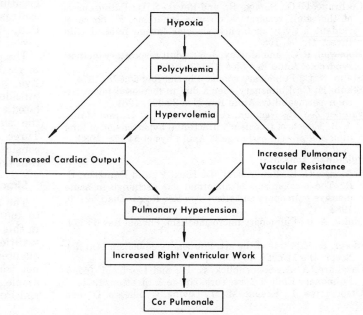

to chronic hypoxia that produces cor pulmonale in patients with perfectly normal lungs is shown in Figure 70. The chief cause of vascular narrowing and of increased pulmonary vascular resistance is arterial vasoconstriction. However, other mechanisms are usually also activated that add to the chronic hemodynamic load facing the right ventricle: (1) polycythemia, secondary to chronic hypoxia, increases blood viscosity and, in turn, increases pulmonary vascular resistance; (2) increased cardiac output, from the stimulus of hypoxia and the increased circulating blood volume, augments blood flow through the lungs; and (3) acidosis, from hypercapnia or other causes, compounds the vasoconstrictor response to hypoxia. The combined result of these processes ensures that an increased volume of blood of high viscosity flows through a reduced pulmonary vascular bed; accordingly, pulmonary arterial pressure increases and the right ventricle hypertrophies. When hypoxia is severe, the responsiveness of the heart becomes limited by depressed myocardial contractility, and right ventricular failure is likely to develop.

Combined Occlusion and Hypoxia. The sequence just described may occur in patients with completely normal lungs whose hypoxia results from residence at high altitude, failure of ventilatory control, neuromuscular disease, or upper airways obstruction. Chronic hypoxia is also prominent in many patients with lung disease. Whether or not pulmonary arterial hypertension and cor pulmonale develop in these persons depends on the severity and duration of the underlying lung disease. If there are associated structural abnormalities that narrow or obliterate the pulmonary circulation, hemodynamic complications are more likely to occur than if the lungs are normal. Thus loss of vessels from interstitial fibrosis and emphysema in patients with hypoxia from chronic bronchitis augments their tendency to develop cor pulmonale.

REFERENCES

Pulmonary Edema

Cochrane, C. G., Spragg, R., and Revak, S. D.: Pathogenesis of the adult respiratory distress syndrome. Evidence of oxidant activity in bronchoalveolar lavage fluid. J Clin Invest 71:754, 1983.

Hopewell, P. C., and Murray, J. F.: Adult respiratory distress syndrome. Annu Rev Med 27:343, 1976.

Staub, N. C.: Pulmonary edema. Physiol Rev 54:678, 1974.

Staub, N. C.: Pulmonary edema due to increased microvascular permeability. Annu Rev Med 32:291, 1981.

van der Zee, H., Neuman, P. H., Minnear, F. L., and Malik, A. B.: Effects of transient intracranial hypertension of lung fluid and protein exchange. J Appl Physiol 54:178, 1983.

Pulmonary Embolism

D'Alonzo, G. E., Bower, J. S., De Hart, P., and Dantzker, D. R.: The mechanisms of abnormal gas exchange in acute massive pulmonary embolism. Am Rev Respir Dis 128:170, 1983.

Malik, A. B.: Pulmonary microembolism. Physiol Rev 63:114, 1983.

Moser, K. M.: State of the art. Pulmonary embolism. Am Rev Respir Dis 115:829, 1977.

Sasahara, A. A., Sonnenblick, E. H., and Lesch, M. (eds.): Pulmonary Emboli. New York, Grune & Stratton, 1975.

Utsonomiya, T., Krausz, M. M., Levine, L., Shepro, D., and

Hechtman, H. B.: Thromboxane mediation of cardiopulmonary effects of embolism. J Clin Invest 70:361, 1982.

Pulmonary Hypertension

Ahmed, T., Oliver, W., Frank, B. L., and Robinson, M. J.: Hypoxic pulmonary vasoconstriction in conscious sheep. Am Rev Respir Dis 126:291, 1982.

Fishman, A. P.: Hypoxia on the pulmonary circulation: How and where it acts. Circ Res 38:221, 1976.

Hermiller, J. B., Bambach, D., Thompson, M. J., et al.: Vasodilators and prostaglandin inhibitors in primary pulmonary hypertension. Ann Intern Med 97:480, 1982.

Nadel, J. A., Gold, W. M., and Burgess, J. H.: Early diagnosis of chronic pulmonary vascular obstruction. Value of pulmonary function tests. Am J Med 44:16, 1968.

Cor Pulmonale

Bergofsky, E. H.: Tissue oxygen delivery and cor pulmonale in chronic obstructive pulmonary disease. N Engl J Med 308:1092, 1983.

Ferrer, M. I.: Cor pulmonale (pulmonary heart disease): Present-day status. Am Heart J 89:657, 1975.

Fishman, A. P.: State of the art. Chronic cor pulmonale. Am Rev Respir Dis 114:775, 1976.

Slutsky, R. A., Ackerman, W., Karliner, J. S., Ashburn, W. L., and Moser, K.: Right and left ventricular dysfunction in patients with chronic obstructive lung disease. Assessment by first-pass radionuclide angiography. Am J Med 68:197, 1980.

GAS EXCHANGE ABNORMALITIES

In human beings respiration has been subdivided into four functional processes: ventilation, diffusion, blood flow, and control of breathing. Each of these contributes uniquely to the maintenance of normal values of P_{O_2} and P_{CO_2} in arterial blood. Impairment in any one of the processes, if sufficiently severe, often leads to an abnormality of gas exchange; furthermore, such a disturbance tends to be reflected in arterial P_{O_2} and P_{CO_2} values because available compensatory mechanisms are usually incapable of restoring normal conditions.

Five mechanisms may lead to decreased arterial P_{O_2}—hypoventilation, diffusion limitation, ventilation-perfusion mismatching, right-to-left shunts, and breathing a gas mixture with a low inspired P_{O_2}; in contrast, there is only one cause of increased arterial P_{CO_2}—hypoventilation. In many respiratory disorders, two or more of these abnormal mechanisms coexist.

The pathophysiologic abnormalities of gas exchange in patients with various types of restrictive, obstructive, and pulmonary vascular disorders have been considered previously. Gas exchange disturbances related to abnormalities of the control of breathing and the pleura are included in subsequent subsections. Three additional abnormalities of gas exchange are considered here because they are common and important and do not fit into the other categories.

Shock

The complex pathophysiologic disturbances leading to and resulting from shock are dealt with elsewhere in this book. This discussion considers only the abnormalities of gas exchange that are secondary consequences of a marked decrease in blood pressure and not from intrinsic pulmonary complications (for example, "shock lung"). The presence of decreased arterial P_{O_2} in patients with perfectly normal lungs demonstrates dramatically the effect on oxygenation of decreases in cardiac output; arterial P_{CO_2} may be increased or decreased depending on the amount of CO_2 being produced and the ventilatory response.

Ordinarily, slight decreases in cardiac output and mixed venous O_2 content have only a trivial influence on arterial P_{O_2} because there is so little venous admixture (from ventilation-perfusion mismatching and right-to-left shunts combined) in normal lungs. However, when cardiac output is profoundly decreased, as may occur in some forms of shock, the effect of perfusing poorly or nonventilated pathways with blood containing an extremely low O_2 content becomes evident as a decrease in arterial P_{O_2} (see subsequent section).

Systemic hypotension with its attendant poor perfusion of tissues leads to anaerobic metabolism and the generation of lactic acid. Acidemia stimulates the peripheral chemoreceptors and, if the respiratory system is capable of responding, causes hyperventilation; thus the typical finding in patients in shock is a decreased arterial P_{CO_2}. (Hyperventilation is also observed in some patients with gram-negative bacteremia before they are hypotensive and acidemic; this presumably reflects increased drive to breathe, but the stimulus and where it is acting are unknown.) However, several factors can interact to modify this response. (1) The sudden production and/or release into the circulation of large quantities of lactic acid makes H^+ available, which reacts with plasma HCO_3^- to generate H_2CO_3 and increase P_{CO_2}; when this process evolves CO_2 faster than the lungs remove it, P_{CO_2} increases. The resulting hypercapnia is usually transient if the patient is able to hyperventilate. (2) Patients who are being mechanically ventilated with a constant minute volume and cannot increase their ventilation thus are more likely to become hypercapnic than patients breathing spontaneously. Furthermore, patients receiving assisted ventilation may develop another abnormality that, by itself, can also cause hypercapnia. (3) If the fall in cardiac output is accompanied by a decrease in pulmonary arterial pressure, blood flow to the most superior regions of the lungs decreases and wasted ventilation increases; any increase in wasted ventilation when minute volume is constant, as is the case when patients are being mechanically ventilated, occurs at the expense of alveolar ventilation, which must decrease CO_2 elimination and increase arterial P_{CO_2} levels.

That adverse physiologic consequences of mechanical ventilation may occur does not mean that use of ventilators is contraindicated in patients with shock. Just the reverse seems to be true. The work of breathing may be considerably increased during hypotension; this means that the respiratory muscles need more O_2 than usual at a time when there is much less O_2 available. Under these conditions, ventilatory failure from respiratory muscle fatigue can occur, and mechanical ventilation is mandatory. Moreover, *early* introduction of assisted ventilation during shock, by putting the respiratory muscles to rest, would liberate the O_2 that they would otherwise consume for use by other organs.

Atelectasis

When a bronchus to a region of the lung is completely occluded, atelectasis may or may not develop. The determining factor is whether or not pathways are available to allow sufficient collateral ventilation to keep the lung inflated. Because there are numerous collateral channels toward the periphery, atelectasis usually follows obstruction of large central bronchi. In this circumstance, gas is reabsorbed from the distal lung in much the same manner as from a pneumothorax space (see subsequent discussion) and the involved portion collapses.

Any residual blood flow to the atelectatic lung, which is completely nonventilated, constitutes a right-to-left shunt. However, this effect is minimized by two factors that cause a local increase in pulmonary vascular resistance that, in turn, serves to redistribute blood away from the airless region. The shortening and tortuosity of the blood vessels, referred to as gnarled, in the collapsed lung decrease their cross-sectional area, which increases their resistance and shifts blood flow to more normal regions. Alveolar hypoxia in the involved region also causes local pulmonary arterial vasoconstriction and an increase in vascular resistance. Thus the magnitude of the right-to-left shunt in atelectasis is usually less than the volume of involved lung would suggest. However, the severity of the arterial hypoxia can be augmented under three circumstances: (1) when there is sufficient disease in the remaining lung to prevent the redistribution in blood flow from occurring; (2) when there is a decrease in cardiac output and the O_2 content of blood in the shunt pathways decreases; and (3) when vascular resistance in the unaffected lung is increased by hyperinflation and blood flow is redistributed back to the nonventilated lung; this can occur when positive pressure is used in vigorous efforts to inflate the collapsed region.

Atelectasis may be caused by abnormalities of gas exchange as well as contribute to them. This special circumstance occurs in patients with certain forms of acute respiratory failure in whom there are regions with very low ventilation:perfusion ratios. When these patients are given 100 per cent O_2 to breathe, the units become atelectatic because once the N_2 is replaced by O_2, the O_2 in the alveoli can diffuse into capillary blood faster than it can be replaced through the narrowed air passages. Thus, units that were being ventilated, albeit poorly, and that had low ventilation:perfusion ratios to begin with are converted to nonventilated units that are the sites of right-to-left shunts. This phenomenon occurs only with administration of 100 per cent O_2; breathing lower concentrations does not wash out all the N_2, so the units cannot close. This has led to the belief that N_2 has a "splinting" effect and that the test for right-to-left shunts should be carried out with 95 per cent instead of 100 per cent O_2.

Carbon Monoxide Poisoning

Incomplete combustion of organic materials produces CO, an odorless, tasteless, and colorless gas. Poisoning from the inhalation of CO is included in the subsection on abnormalities of gas exchange because the remarkable affinity of CO for hemoglobin impairs O_2 transport and release.

Both O_2 and CO compete for the same binding sites on hemoglobin molecules. However, because the affinity of CO for hemoglobin is 210 times greater than that of O_2, low concentrations of CO occupy numerous binding sites and prevent those sites from combining

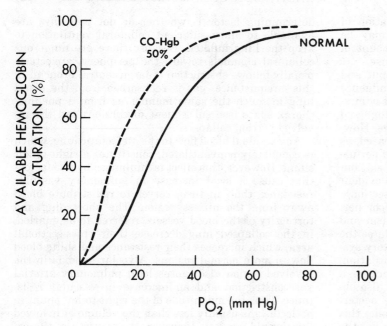

Figure 71. Oxyhemoglobin equilibrium curves of available (active) hemoglobin in the presence of 50 per cent CO-hemoglobin (50 per cent CO-Hgb) and of normal blood (0 per cent CO-Hgb, from Figure 30). Note that the 50 per cent CO-Hgb curve is shifted to the left of the normal curve, indicating that affinity for O_2 is increased and that release of O_2 at any prevailing tissue Po_2 is decreased. (From Hinshaw, H. C., and Murray, J. F.: Diseases of the Chest. Philadelphia, W. B. Saunders Co., 1979, p. 767.)

with O_2. In other words, as the concentration of CO-hemoglobin in the bloodstream increases, the O_2-carrying capacity steadily decreases. For example, if the total hemoglobin concentration of the blood is 15 g/dl and the CO-hemoglobin concentration is 50 per cent, only 7.5 g/dl of hemoglobin is available to combine with O_2.

Tissue oxygenation of a patient with 50 per cent circulating CO-hemoglobin is much more severely compromised than that of a patient with an anemia of 7.5 g/dl because of another pathophysiologic consequence of the presence of CO: The oxyhemoglobin equilibrium curve of the hemoglobin available to combine with O_2 shifts progressively leftward as CO-hemoglobin concentration increases (Fig. 71). Thus, not only does CO decrease the O_2-carrying capacity by combining with hemoglobin, but it shifts the oxyhemoglobin curve for the *remaining* hemoglobin to the left. Although it may seem paradoxical, a secondary and extremely important consequence of the increased affinity of CO for hemoglobin is to increase the affinity of O_2 for the remaining binding sites.

Cellular hypoxia results because, at the prevailing capillary and extracellular Po_2, less O_2 is released by the unusually avid hemoglobin. This causes tissue Po_2 to decrease, and a little more O_2 is released. Finally, a new equilibrium value is reached but one that may be too low to cause diffusion of a sufficient amount of O_2 from the capillaries into the neighboring cells to sustain aerobic metabolism. This deficiency is especially critical in organs like the brain that have a high rate of oxidative metabolism and cannot sustain substantial anaerobic metabolism.

It is not always appreciated that arterial Po_2 is within normal limits in patients with CO poisoning; this must be the case if the lungs are also normal because arterial Po_2 is, for practical purposes, independent of the amount and kind of hemoglobin in the bloodstream. Thus CO poisoning illustrates four important pathophysiologic principles: (1) O_2 *transport* capacity is decreased through loss of available binding sites by hemoglobin for O_2; (2) O_2 *availability* is decreased because of the leftward shift of the oxyhemoglobin-dissociation curve, and venous Po_2 decreases; (3) *arterial* Po_2 is unaffected by the presence of abnormal hemoglobin because, with the single exception of intracardiac right-to-left shunts, Po_2 is determined by the adequacy of respiration; and (4) *ventilation* does not increase despite marked reductions in arterial O_2 content because the O_2 needs of the peripheral chemoreceptors are satisfied by the small amount of O_2 dissolved in plasma.

REFERENCES

Shock

Aubier, M., Trippenbach, T., and Roussos, C.: Respiratory muscle fatigue during cardiogenic shock. J Appl Physiol 51:499, 1981.

Roussos, C., and Macklem, P. T.: The respiratory muscles. N Engl J Med 307:786, 1982.

Atelectasis

Dantzker, D. R., Wagner, P. D., and West, J. B.: Instability of lung units with low VA/Q ratios during O_2 breathing. J Appl Physiol 38:886, 1975.

Ford, G. T., Bradley, C. A., and Anthonisen, N. R.: Forces involved in lobar atelectasis in intact dogs. J Appl Physiol 48:29–33, 1980.

Thomas, H. M., and Garrett, R. C.: Strength of hypoxic vasoconstriction determines shunt fraction in dogs with atelectasis. J Appl Physiol 53:44, 1982.

Carbon Monoxide Poisoning

Astrup, P.: Some physiological and pathological effects of moderate carbon monoxide exposure. Br Med J 4:447, 1972.

Lahiri, S., Mulligan, E., Nishino, T., Mokashi, A., and Davis, R. O.: Relative responses of aortic body and carotid body chemoreceptors to carboxyhemoglobinemia. J Appl Physiol 50:580, 1981.

DISORDERS OF THE CONTROL OF BREATHING

The anatomic and physiologic organization of the peripheral and central structures concerned with normal control of breathing are described in the section on Normal Physiology of the Respiratory System. The medulla serves as the integrative focus of nerve traffic from higher centers in the brain and from peripheral receptors in the carotid bodies and lungs; the medulla is also the source of rhythmic respiratory oscillations, although centers in the pons are necessary for smooth regular breathing. Nerve impulses from the brain descend in the spinal cord to the segmental level, where the supraspinal messages are integrated with additional afferent information arising from proprioceptors in the respiratory muscles. The outcome of all these processes is a signal to respiratory muscles through their alpha motoneurons and a relaying of the message to synergistic and antagonistic muscle groups.

Given the number of different structures involved and the complexity of the system, it is obvious that a variety of neurologic disorders can affect the control of breathing. Many of these are considered elsewhere in this book and will not be reviewed here. The purpose of this subsection is to describe the pathophysiologic mechanisms that underlie the sleep-apnea syndromes, the obesity-hypoventilation syndrome, the hyperventilation syndromes, the ventilatory responses to non-respiratory (metabolic) acidemia and alkalemia, and the symptoms of breathlessness and dyspnea.

Sleep-Apnea Syndromes

The striking but similar clinical and laboratory features of a wide variety of disparate disorders, including sudden infant death syndrome, brain stem and upper cervical cord lesions, primary (idiopathic) hypoventilation syndrome, obesity-hypoventilation syndrome, adenotonsillar enlargement, and structural abnormalities of the chin, have been linked to a common pathophysiologic sequence called the sleep-apnea syndrome. The syndrome is usually defined as the occurrence of more than 30 apneic spells of greater than 15 seconds during a night's sleep associated with frequent arousals and often with a deficiency of slow wave sleep. Apneic pauses are usually 15 to 120 seconds in duration, but episodes as long as 3 minutes have been observed; the cycle of apnea, asphyxia, awakening, and resumption of breathing may be repeated several hundred times each night with as much as 50 per cent of a night's sleep spent while apneic. Although apnea is the central pathophysiologic feature of the sleep-apnea syndromes, from which numerous consequences derive, two quite different mechanisms may cause the episodes: central apnea and obstructive apnea.

Central Apnea. The presence of central apnea is signified not only by absence of airflow but also by simultaneous cessation of respiratory efforts as demonstrated by recording of esophageal pressure or of diaphragmatic electromyography. This combination suggests that there is a primary disorder of respiratory rhythm generation, a notion that is consistent with the observation that central apnea often occurs in patients with neurologic lesions involving the brain stem and/or upper cervical cord.

Obstructive Apnea. Apnea from obstruction differs from the central variety in that respiratory efforts are maintained, and may even be vigorous, but there is no airflow. This combination indicates complete closure of the airway, although the precise site of obstruction is unknown. Obstructive sleep apneas typically occur in persons whose upper air passage is compromised to begin with from obesity, enlarged tonsils and adenoids or tongue, or micrognathia. But anatomic narrowing by itself is insufficient to cause apnea, and closure of the airway is caused by abnormal relaxation during sleep of the several muscles that normally function actively to maintain patency of the upper airway. Electromyographic recordings from the genioglossus, an important muscle that contracts during each inspiration to pull the tongue forward and to open the upper airway, are abnormally silent in patients during sleep apnea from obstruction. This observation explains why relaxation of the supporting muscles occurs, but the origin of the abnormally decreased electromyographic activity is a mystery.

Physiologic Consequences. Evidence of profound physiologic disturbances is found in patients with the typical sleep-apnea syndrome. During an apneic pause, there is progressive hypoxia, hypercapnia, increases in pulmonary and systemic arterial pressures, and sinus bradycardia or other cardiac arrhythmias. As expected, the pathophysiologic consequences depend on the duration and frequency of apneic episodes, severity of changes in P_{O_2} and P_{CO_2}, and extent of nocturnal sleep disruption. However, the manifestations also depend, in part, on whether the apnea is central or obstructive in origin.

Patients with central apnea often complain of nocturnal insomnia, which may be misdiagnosed as anxiety or depression, whereas patients with obstructive apnea nearly always have pathologic daytime somnolence, which may be incorrectly regarded as narcolepsy. Two of the striking features of obstructive apnea are (1) the stupendous snoring that antedates the full-blown syndrome by years and that develops a cyclic periodicity during apnea when silence occurs, and (2) the abnormal sleep behavior with frequent and often noisy awakenings. The hypersomnolence is believed related to chronic sleep deprivation, particularly of the deeper stages of nonREM sleep; especially serious consequences of sleep withdrawal are severe personality disorders and intellectual deterioration.

Acute pulmonary hypertension during sleep apnea results from pulmonary arterial vasoconstriction secondary to alveolar hypoxia; acute systemic hypertension during the episodes can be explained by adrenergic activity secondary to the hypoxemia. It is not known, however, how the acute nocturnal increases in pulmonary and systemic arterial pressures are converted to sustained daytime elevations in the pressures. Bradycardia during apnea is accounted for by the effects of hypoxic stimulation of peripheral chemoreceptors without the influence of hyperventilation, the event that normally causes tachycardia. Profound hypoxemia causes secondary polycythemia by the elaboration of erythropoietin in the kidney, which stimulates the bone marrow.

The combination of these effects leads to cor pulmonale by the sequence described previously and illustrated in Figure 70. Thus the pathophysiologic consequences of severe sleep-apnea syndromes present an excellent example of how cor pulmonale can develop in patients whose lungs are perfectly normal.

Obesity-Hypoventilation Syndrome

The case of an obese poker player who was dealt a full house but then fell asleep without capitalizing on it led to investigations that culminated in a case report with the subtitle "a Pickwickian Syndrome." (Pickwickian is used to refer to Joe, the fat boy in Charles Dickens' book *The Posthumous Papers of the Pickwick Club,* commonly called the "Pickwick Papers.") Additional reports, both before and since, have led to a thorough description of what is more aptly called the *obesity-hypoventilation syndrome.* However, there are now reasons to believe that the obesity-hypoventilation syndrome should be classified as another member of the family of sleep-apnea syndromes just described. But, because there are several respiratory pathophysiologic abnormalities associated with massive obesity that are not found in other causes of sleep apneas, the obesity-hypoventilation syndrome is discussed separately.

The obesity-hypoventilation syndrome is characterized clinically by extreme obesity, somnolence, plethora, cardiac enlargement, and edema. Laboratory findings include polycythemia and the abnormalities of respiratory function tests listed in Table 16. Although massive obesity is an essential feature of the syndrome, only a small proportion of massively obese patients develop hypoventilation and its systemic consequences. Thus it is important not only to examine the pathophysiologic sequence by which obesity leads to abnormalities of gas exchange and cor pulmonale but also to consider why these complications develop in only some obese patients. The terms *simple obesity* and *obesity-hypoventilation* are used to differentiate between these two conditions.

Lung Volumes and Mechanics. The abnormalities in lung volumes and mechanics of ventilation that characterize the obesity-hypoventilation syndrome are explained chiefly by the effects of massive obesity on

the chest wall; the abnormalities of gas exchange are attributable both to disturbances arising within the lungs and to failure of central regulation of breathing.

Massive obesity decreases the distensibility of the chest wall (including both the thorax and abdomen), which has the secondary effect of decreasing the compliance of the underlying lungs. The shifts to the right in the volume-pressure curves of the lungs and chest wall mean that FRC decreases; because RV does not change or may even increase because of premature airway closure, FRC and RV approach each other. One of the most distinctive features of obesity is the striking decrease or virtual absence of expiratory reserve volume, the difference between FRC and RV. This abnormality is not specific for obesity, however, but is found in other conditions in which the compliance of the chest wall is similarly decreased (for example, pregnancy and ascites).

The effects of obesity on VC depend on (1) the net reduction in overall compliance of the respiratory system and (2) the inspiratory muscle strength. In patients with simple obesity, the decreased compliance of the respiratory system can largely be overcome by generating normal inspiratory muscle force so that VC is only slightly decreased. It is possible that some obese persons respond to the chronic respiratory work load by muscle hypertrophy, in which case inspiratory pressures are supernormal and VC may be within normal limits. Patients with obesity-hypoventilation usually have substantially decreased VC values because their respiratory system compliance and/or their inspiratory muscle strength is more impaired than in simple obesity.

Breathing at lower than normal FRC means that the caliber of airways is decreased and that resistance to airflow is increased. However, this effect is small, and FEV_1/FVC values are within the normal range in obese persons unless coexisting (unrelated) disease is present. The most important mechanical impairment is the increased work of breathing from the combined effects of decreased compliance and increased resistance or increased impedance of the chest wall. There is a general inverse correlation among obese patients between the work of breathing and arterial P_{CO_2} values, which has led to the speculation that the mechanical abnormalities might contribute to the hypoventilation. (The decrease in CO_2 responsiveness in normal subjects induced by mechanical loading has already been mentioned.)

Gas Exchange. As FRC decreases and approaches RV, airways in the dependent regions of the lungs narrow and may even close. This means that ventilation to these regions becomes progressively less and finally stops. Blood flow, however, is well maintained in dependent regions because of the effects of gravity on pulmonary arterial pressure (Fig. 27). Reduction of ventilation but preservation of perfusion creates a ventilation-perfusion imbalance that, when extreme, becomes a right-to-left shunt (perfusion but no ventilation at all). Thus arterial hypoxia from increased venous admixture inevitably occurs in massively obese patients. Although the syndrome is designated obesity-*hypoventilation,* the abnormalities of gas exchange are characterized by severe hypoxia and only mild or moderate hypercapnia.

Hypoxia is mild and hypercapnia is absent in simple

TABLE 16. PULMONARY FUNCTION ABNORMALITIES IN PATIENTS WITH OBESITY-HYPOVENTILATION*

TEST	RESULT
Lung volumes	
Vital capacity	Decreased
Total lung capacity	Decreased
Functional residual capacity	Decreased
Residual volume	Normal
Expiratory reserve volume	Nearly absent
Mechanics of ventilation	
FEV_1/FVC	Normal
Maximal expiratory flow	Normal
Specific airways conductance	Normal
Distribution of ventilation	Normal
Diffusing capacity	Normal
Gas exchange	
P_{O_2}	Markedly decreased
P_{CO_2}	Increased
pH	Decreased
(Alveolar-arterial) P_{O_2}	Markedly increased
Right-to-left shunt	Increased
Wasted ventilation	Slightly increased

*For definitions of abbreviations, see Table 10.

obesity. In contrast, in obesity-hypoventilation, abnormalities of gas exchange are much worse. Clearly, factors other than the effects of excess weight on ventilation-perfusion relationships are involved, and a disturbance in the control of breathing must be present. For example, patients with simple obesity have increased values of $P_{0.1}$ compared to normal subjects, whereas $P_{0.1}$ values in patients with the obesity-hypoventilation syndrome are decreased. In patients with simple obesity, these results indicate that arterial P_{CO_2} is maintained in the normal range by increased neural drive to breathe and, conversely, in those patients whose neural drive is blunted, that P_{CO_2} increases. But the cause of the decreased drive and whether it is innate or acquired are not known.

Another reason obese patients may develop the obesity-hypoventilation syndrome seems to lie in the presence of associated sleep apnea. Several studies have documented the presence of both obstructive and central apnea, particularly the former, in patients with obesity-hypoventilation syndrome. Numerous apneic episodes undoubtedly cause the hypersomnolence, which is usually a striking feature of the obesity-hypoventilation syndrome, through the mechanism of frequent arousals and sleep deprivation already described.

Thus the pathophysiologic abnormalities of the sleep-apnea syndromes become superimposed on the mechanical and gas exchange abnormalities of obesity, and the florid obesity-hypoventilation syndrome results. This concept accounts for many previously unanswered questions about the pathogenesis of obesity-hypoventilation, but it creates another, as yet unsolved, mystery: Why does sleep apnea develop in only some patients with massive obesity?

Hyperventilation Syndromes

Considerable attention is usually devoted to the pathophysiologic mechanisms responsible for hypoventilation and hypercapnia when, in fact, hyperventilation and hypocapnia are much more common. The difference in concern probably is that because hypercapnia is accompanied by hypoxia, unless O_2 is being breathed, it often occurs in patients with obviously severe underlying disease. In contrast, hyperventilation may occur in apparently healthy persons, and because it provokes secondary responses in many organs, attention may be directed to these manifestations rather than to the primary cause. A distinction must be made between the terms *hyperpnea,* which indicates increased minute volume of ventilation but which carries no implication concerning the resulting arterial P_{CO_2}, and *hyperventilation,* which means alveolar ventilation in excess of CO_2 production so that arterial P_{CO_2} must be decreased.

Hyperventilation is always associated with a decreased arterial P_{CO_2}, but the effects on pH vary with the time course, the extent of renal compensation (discussed more fully in the subsection on Respiratory Failure), and the presence of coexisting nonrespiratory (metabolic) acid-base abnormalities. The far-reaching consequences of acute hyperventilation with hypocapnic alkalosis are listed in Table 17. The major pathophysiologic consequences involve the heart (decreased blood flow because of coronary vasoconstriction and arrhythmias) and the brain (decreased blood flow

TABLE 17. SOME IMPORTANT PATHOPHYSIOLOGIC CONSEQUENCES OF ACUTE HYPERVENTILATION AND HYPOCAPNIC ALKALOSIS

Cardiac output	Decreased
Stroke volume	Decreased
Coronary blood flow	Decreased
Repolarization of heart	Impaired
Oxyhemoglobin affinity	Increased
Cerebral blood flow	Decreased
Muscle contraction	Carpopedal spasm and tetany
Serum potassium	Decreased

because of cerebral vasoconstriction). The transport of O_2 to all organs is decreased because of the decrease in cardiac output, and the availability of O_2 is compromised because the alkalosis increases O_2 affinity, which shifts the oxyhemoglobin equilibrium curve to the left.

Voluntary hyperventilation is often followed by a period of posthyperventilation apnea, which may have severe consequences, and many deaths have occurred in underwater swimmers who hyperventilated before submerging in an effort to prolong their time under water. Involuntary hyperventilation can occur in perfectly healthy persons or in patients with a variety of underlying disorders.

Assisted ventilation, either by a hand-actuated bag or a mechanical ventilator, is often excessive as judged by the frequency with which decreases in arterial P_{CO_2} are observed. Hyperventilation may be impossible to avoid unless end-tidal CO_2 concentration is continuously monitored; even this approach has its shortcomings because end-tidal P_{CO_2} does not indicate corresponding arterial values when increased wasted ventilation is present.

Hyperventilation occurs in patients with a variety of pulmonary diseases, including severe obstructive ventilatory disorders. Patients with asthma, chronic infiltrative lung diseases, pulmonary edema, and pulmonary embolism are apt to have low arterial P_{CO_2} values. The common mechanism responsible in each of these conditions is stimulation of receptors with resulting increased drive to breathe. However, it is likely that different receptors and neural pathways are involved in various diseases. The peripheral chemoreceptors are activated by acute hypoxemia, whereas the airway and parenchymal receptors are activated by mechanical deformation, irritation, congestion, inflammation, and other stimuli associated with bronchopulmonary disease. The receptors and stimuli in patients with diseases of the pulmonary circulation are not known, but hyperventilation is characteristic of both acute and chronic occlusive vascular disorders.

Maternal hyperventilation, probably mediated by the central nervous system effects of progestational hormones, begins approximately three weeks after fertilization, lasts the duration of pregnancy, and continues for three weeks after delivery. Hyperventilation in excess of metabolic needs is observed during fever and sepsis and in severe liver disease in the absence of fever; in these conditions, increased drive to breathe must be present, but the stimuli and responding centers are unknown.

Many diseases of the central nervous system, such as strokes, meningitis, and tumors, are associated with hyperventilation, but the increased breathing can be related to metabolic stimuli. Pure central hyperventilation, presumably by an irritative effect on respiratory centers in the absence of other stimuli, is rare. However, a variety of drugs, especially salicylates, cause hyperventilation by stimulating respiratory centers in the brain.

Anxiety and other psychogenic influences can initiate acute or chronic hyperventilation. There is, however, an unfortunate tendency to regard hyperventilation of unknown cause as psychogenic in origin in all patients. This overlooks some of the subtle diseases associated with hyperventilation, especially early pulmonary vascular occlusive diseases and infiltrative diseases of the lungs.

Metabolic Acid-Base Adjustments

Nonrespiratory (metabolic) acidosis occurs when there is an increase in nonvolatile acids or a decrease in bases, and nonrespiratory alkalosis occurs where there is an excessive loss of acids or an accumulation of bases. In either case, the resulting change in [H$^+$] causes acidemia or alkalemia, which both affects [HCO$_3^-$] and initiates secondary ventilatory adjustments. Strictly speaking, these responses do not represent disorders of the control of breathing; however, they are included in this section because the time course and magnitude of the ventilatory adjustments vary considerably and the changes can be misinterpreted as an abnormality of respiration.

An acute increase in [H$^+$] causes [HCO$_3^-$] to decrease and ventilation to increase through stimulation of the peripheral chemoreceptors; however, as P$_{CO_2}$ decreases, the central chemoreceptors become depressed, which offsets part of the peripheral drive to breathe. After one or two days, the [HCO$_3^-$] of cerebrospinal fluid decreases and the offsetting mechanism is removed; this allows ventilation to increase further and restores pH more toward normal values.

Once cerebrospinal fluid adjustments are complete (24 to 48 hours), ventilation tends to be reset at the increased level; thus even if the initial stimulus is corrected and blood pH becomes normal (as in the treatment of diabetic ketoacidosis or renal acidosis), hyperventilation persists until new changes in cerebrospinal fluid [HCO$_3^-$] have taken place. In the event that hyperventilation cannot occur, the acidemia from a given decrease in [HCO$_3^-$] is more severe than when P$_{CO_2}$ is able to decrease.

All of the various kinds of nonrespiratory alkalosis are associated with an increase in [HCO$_3^-$], but the extent of respiratory compensation, if any, depends on the underlying cause of the alkalosis. Under some circumstances, such as the administration of HCO$_3^-$ or other buffers, P$_{CO_2}$ rises, which minimizes the pH change at any given level of [HCO$_3^-$]. In contrast, there is less predictable respiratory compensation in the presence of alkalosis resulting from either the administration of diuretics or hyperaldosteronism.

Breathlessness

Dyspnea is one of the most important symptoms encountered in medical practice, yet its pathophysiology is very poorly understood. Broadly defined, dyspnea means uncomfortable or difficult breathing. Breathlessness is sometimes used synonymously with dyspnea but can be said to have even broader generic implications and to mean simply an awareness of breathing. Ventilation is ordinarily performed imperceptibly, but even perfectly healthy persons experience breathlessness during strenuous exercise. This transient but normal sensation means that symptoms related to breathing must be evaluated in the context of the circumstances under which they are encountered. Used in a clinical context, dyspnea refers to a pathologic symptom that is usually a disagreeable perception of breathing under conditions in which sensations are neither quantitatively nor qualitatively the same as usual. Studies of dyspnea are hampered by this (or any) definition because the subject or patient must feel and recount the sensation, and as such it is impossible to quantify. Furthermore, like the symptom pain, some persons suffer a lot from apparently little provocation; in contrast, others complain little from what is judged to be substantial stimulation.

Several different sensations, which may be in part interrelated, provide some insight into the pathophysiologic mechanisms of breathlessness: (1) breath holding, (2) inhalation of CO$_2$, (3) tracheobronchial irritation, (4) obstruction to breathing, and (5) dyspnea itself.

Sensations During Breath Holding. Normal subjects can hold their breath for about a minute and with training this can be increased to several minutes; but sooner or later the urge to inspire can no longer be resisted. The demand to breathe is not chemical in origin because it is completely relieved during the first inspiration even when a gas mixture is inhaled that is more hypoxic and hypercapnic than the gas in the lungs of the subject at the time. The sensation that develops and progressively increases with time during breath holding coincides with the onset and increasing strength and frequency of diaphragmatic contractions. The sensation of breath holding is abolished by local anesthesia of both vagal nerves in the neck, which interrupts afferent impulses from the lungs, and by complete muscle paralysis with curare; in contrast, the sensation is not affected by spinal anesthesia up to the first thoracic segment. Breath-holding time is increased by bilateral phrenic nerve block and by bilateral carotid body denervation. These observations and studies in patients with various neurologic lesions suggest that during breath holding afferent impulses from the lungs and carotid bodies generate a stimulus to diaphragmatic contraction; this activates receptors in the diaphragm, possibly tendon receptors, such that phrenic afferent impulses ultimately reach higher centers in the brain, where they are translated to unpleasant sensations.

Sensations During Inhalation of CO$_2$. Inhalation of CO$_2$ has been used extensively to test CO$_2$ responsiveness in both normal subjects and patients with lung disease. The sensation experienced during the test is typically described as not being able to breathe deeply enough, despite a striking increase in both tidal volume and respiratory frequency. Studies using local nerve blocks, spinal anesthesia, and curare have led to the conclusion that the disagreeable sensation perceived while breathing CO$_2$ depends mainly on diaphragmatic contraction and that vagal and glossopharyngeal afferent impulses are unimportant.

Sensations from Tracheobronchial Irritation. Most persons have experienced a dull achy sensation in the anterior part of the chest or lower part of the neck that creates an awareness of breathing, especially during deep inspiration. This symptom occurs during influenzal tracheobronchitis and episodes of air pollution and can be reproduced by inhalation of irritant gases. Bilateral vagal blockade in the neck and local anesthetics administered as aerosols abolish the sensation. Thus tracheobronchial receptors, possibly the rapidly adapting irritant receptor with afferent pathways in the vagus nerves, are presumably involved.

Sensation of Obstruction to Breathing. When healthy subjects breathe through their mouths, addition of small elastic or resistive loads produces a sensation that enables the subject to recognize that a change has occurred in the mechanics of ventilation. It is now known that much of the awareness of mechanical loads is perceived in the mouth and pharynx. Evidence in favor of a contributing role of receptors in the chest wall, tracheobronchial system, or lung parenchyma is incomplete.

Dyspnea. The previous paragraphs have described how breathlessness, or an awareness of breathing, can occur in circumstances in which the term dyspnea is not ordinarily used. However, certainly some of the receptors and neural pathways already considered may be involved in the symptom of dyspnea. In most pathophysiologic conditions, especially cardiorespiratory disorders, dyspnea occurs when the stimulus for ventilation exceeds the patient's ability to respond to that stimulus: (1) An increased drive to ventilation can result from hypoxia, hypercapnia, or acidemia; from increased afferent impulses arising in the lungs, upper airways, thoracic cage, and diaphragm; and possibly from direct central nervous system stimulation. (2) An inability to respond to the prevailing drive to breathe occurs in patients with mechanical abnormalities of their lungs and/or chest wall. In many situations both increased drive and impaired ventilatory mechanics are apparently present; the results of a limited number of studies involving nerve or receptor blockade suggest that of the two mechanisms, increased drive plus the abnormal breathing pattern that often results is the more important.

REFERENCES

Sleep-Apnea Syndromes

Fletcher, E. C., Gray, B. A., and Levin, D. C.: Nonapneic mechanisms of arterial oxygen desaturation during rapid-eye-movement sleep. J Appl Physiol 54:632, 1983.
Guilleminault, C., and Dement, W. C.: Sleep Apnea Syndromes. New York, Alan R. Liss, Inc., 1978.
Phillipson, E. A.: Respiratory adaptations in sleep. Annu Rev Physiol 40:133, 1978.
Remmers, J. E., deGroot, W. J., Sauerland, E. K., and Anch, A. M.: Pathogenesis of upper airway occlusion during sleep. J Appl Physiol 44:931, 1978.
Tilkian, A. G., Guilleminault, C., Schroeder, J. S., Lehrman, K. L., Simmons, F. B., and Dement, W. C.: Hemodynamics in sleep induced apnea. Studies during wakefulness and sleep. Ann Intern Med 85:714, 1976.

Obesity-Hypoventilation

Boushey, H. A.: The pickwickian syndrome—Medical Staff Conference. West J Med 127:24, 1977.
Sampson, M. G., and Grassino, A.: Neuro-mechanical properties in obese patients during carbon dioxide rebreathing. Am J Med 75:81, 1983.

Hyperventilation Syndromes

Plum, F.: Hyperpnea, hyperventilation and brain dysfunction. Ann Intern Med 76:328, 1972.
Waites, T. F.: Hyperventilation—chronic and acute. Arch Intern Med 138:1700, 1978.
Zwillich, C. W., Pierson, D. J., Creagh, E. M., and Weil, J. V.: Effects of hypocapnia and hypocapneic alkalosis on cardiovascular function. J Appl Physiol 40:333, 1976.

Metabolic Acid-Base Adjustments

Adrogue, H. J., Breusilver, J., Cohen, J. J., and Madias, N. E.: Influence of steady-state alterations in acid-base equilibrium on the fate of administered bicarbonate in the dog. J Clin Invest 71:867, 1983.
Fend, W., Vale, J. R., and Broch, J. A.: Respiration and cerebral blood flow in metabolic acidosis and alkalosis in humans. J Appl Physiol 27:67, 1976.

Breathlessness

Burki, N. K.: Dyspnea. Clin Chest Med 1:47, 1980.
Guz, A.: Respiratory sensations in man. Br Med Bull 33:175, 1977.
Killian, K. J., and Campbell, E. J. M.: Dyspnea and exercise. Annu Rev Physiol 45:465, 1983.

DISORDERS OF THE PLEURA

The inside of each hemithorax, including the surfaces presented by the rib cage, diaphragm, and mediastinum, is covered by a layer of mesenchymal cells called the *parietal pleura*. The entire outer surface of each lobe of both lungs is also covered by a mesothelial layer called the *visceral pleura*. These two surfaces fuse and thus are continuous with each other at the hilum of the lungs. Although both pleural surfaces are similar in being composed of a single layer of mesothelial cells that lie on an underlying network of connective tissue containing blood and lymphatic vessels, there are important differences between the parietal and visceral pleuras. The parietal pleura is loosely attached to the chest wall and is innervated with sensory receptors and nerves. In contrast, the visceral pleura adheres to the underlying lung, is more richly vascularized, and is insensitive to pain, touch, and temperature. The blood supply to the visceral pleura varies among species; in humans it is from the bronchial circulation, and in dogs, the blood supply is from the pulmonary circulation. The chief distinguishing features between the parietal and visceral pleuras in most species are that the parietal surfaces have a greater number of lymphatics and also contain stomata, large direct openings that lead into underlying lymphatic channels.

The pleura may be the site of a variety of infectious, inflammatory, and neoplastic diseases. Each of these may produce a cellular protein-rich exudate that can organize into a constricting and poorly distensible layer that decreases the volume of the underlying lung. Thus one of the pathophysiologic consequences of pleural disease is a restrictive ventilatory disorder of the type described earlier in this section. Pneumothorax and pleural effusion, the two disorders discussed here, are analogous to fibrothorax in that each may cause similar decreases in lung volumes, but the pathophysiologic abnormalities that cause the conditions differ in many respects.

Pneumothorax

The term *pneumothorax* denotes the presence of gas in the pleural space. There are only three ways that air or some other gas can gain access to the pleural space: (1) Injuries such as penetrating wounds of the chest wall, perforation of the diaphragm, and rupture of the esophagus through the mediastinal pleura can enable gas to enter through the parietal pleura covering one of the structures that forms the boundaries of a hemithorax; (2) rupture of a bleb or a subpleural abscess can cause gas to enter through a rent in the visceral pleura covering the lungs; (3) certain gas-forming microorganisms can generate gas within the pleural space. Before describing how gas leaves the pleural space once it has entered, it is necessary to discuss why no gas is present in the space under normal conditions.

Factors Holding the Lung Against the Chest Wall. At FRC the elastic recoil forces of the lungs and chest wall are equal in magnitude but opposite in direction (Fig. 18). These opposing forces tend to separate the visceral and parietal pleuras and to create a space that, if present, would need to be filled with either liquid or gas. However, the lungs and chest wall do not separate from each other but remain continuously apposed under normal conditions because of the mechanisms that prevent gas and liquid from collecting in the pleural space. Furthermore, the same factors serve to remove gas from a pneumothorax or liquid from a pleural effusion when either occurs as part of a pathologic process.

Each pleural space, although an anatomically delimited cavity, is otherwise analogous to a tissue space and thus is governed by the mechanisms that regulate tissue pressures everywhere in the body. The net result of the uptake and consumption of O_2 and the formation and release of CO_2 within cells is that the sum of the partial pressures of all the gases at the end of the capillaries and in venous blood is approximately 706 mm Hg (Table 5). This means that the tissues are exposed to a gas pressure that is substantially less than atmospheric pressure ($706 - 760 = -54$ mm Hg). This high negative pressure creates a suction force that keeps the pleural space free of gas and causes the reabsorption of gases if they gain entrance to the pleural cavity or any other tissue space.

Pathophysiologic Consequences. In the presence of a pneumothorax, the lung on the affected side is partially or completely collapsed. Depending on the extent of the decrease in lung volume, which depends in turn on how much gas has entered the pleural cavity and the collapsibility of the lung, there will be a corresponding loss of pulmonary elastic recoil. Because of the decreased inward recoil of the lung, the tendency of the chest wall to recoil outwardly has less opposition and the thorax assumes a larger than normal resting volume. The expandability of the involved lung is decreased by the presence of the pneumothorax. Thus TLC, VC, FRC, and RV are proportionately decreased; the decreased RV stands in contrast to other forms of nonatelectatic restrictive disorders in which RV tends to be relatively better preserved than VC and TLC.

Hyperventilation nearly always accompanies pneumothorax, especially at its onset, presumably from a reflex activation of stretch or other vagally mediated receptors in the collapsed lung. Similarly, tachycardia, also of reflex origin, is a common finding.

When gas accumulates under greater than atmospheric pressure and a *tension pneumothorax* develops, not only does the lung collapse as completely as it can on the affected side, but also there is a shift of the mediastinum into the contralateral hemithorax, which decreases the volume of the uninvolved lung. The results of short periods (30 minutes) of tension pneumothorax in experimental animals indicated that only a small proportion of the increased pressure in the pleural space on the side of the collapsed lung was transmitted to the contralateral lung, and that cardiac output was well maintained by an increase in heart rate. However, the extent to which these findings apply to the human counterpart is not known. There is no doubt that humans can die from tension pneumothorax, but whether death occurs from acute circulatory or respiratory failure is uncertain. In either situation, prompt decompression of the involved hemithorax is curative.

Mechanisms of Gas Reabsorption. When a mixture of gases enters the pleural space, it does so at approximately atmospheric pressure (total) and at different concentrations than exist in the pleural capillaries. Even in cases of tension pneumothorax, the excess pressure (10 to 30 mm Hg) is only a small fraction of total atmospheric pressure (760 mm Hg).

The concentration differences cause gases to diffuse from the region of higher to lower partial pressure. Because the pressures of a mixture of gases in the pleural space can never be the same as that in the bloodstream, reabsorption occurs until it is complete and the lung is fully expanded.

For example, during a spontaneous pneumothorax, humidified room air ($P_{O_2} = 149$, $P_{N_2} = 564$, $P_{H_2O} = 47$ mm Hg) enters the pleural cavity. Some reabsorption of gases starts immediately, but the lung cannot expand until the leak in the pleura has sealed. Once this occurs, expansion begins because O_2 (chiefly) and N_2 diffuse from the pleural space into the bloodstream, and CO_2 diffuses in the opposite direction, because of the prevailing concentration differences. Because more O_2 is absorbed than CO_2 is added to the pneumothorax, the volume of the space decreases; this in turn has the effect of increasing the concentration of the remaining gases and creating new pressure differences that cause gases to diffuse out of the pleural space. This process, although continuous, can be viewed as occurring in increments: The initial concentration difference causes a decrease in volume; this causes an increase in concentrations, which causes a new decrease in volume; and so on, until the space is empty.

Pleural Effusion

The generic term *pleural effusion* simply means a collection of liquid in the pleural space but does not indicate either what kind or how much is present. The liquid is usually characterized as blood, chyle, or pus, or, when nondistinctive, as plain effusions. The presence of blood, chyle, or pus is attributable to some specific pathogenetic abnormality and will not be considered further. Plain effusions are differentiated into transudates and exudates depending on the amounts of protein and lactic dehydrogenase in the liquid relative to the amounts in the serum. Transudates differ from exudates in having less protein and lactic dehydrogenase, a difference that, as will be explained, relates to how the underlying disease affects the factors that regulate liquid formation into and removal from the pleural space.

Mechanisms of Liquid Accumulation. Like pulmonary edema, with which it has many similarities, pleural effusion can occur only when the rate of formation of liquid exceeds the rate of removal. Thus, when the pathophysiology of pleural effusion is examined, its presence must be accounted for by an imbalance of the transpleural hydrostatic or protein osmotic forces, a change in permeability of the membrane, a decrease in the rate of reabsorption, or various combinations of these mechanisms.

Normal Liquid Exchange in the Pleural Space. Normally, there is only a small amount of liquid in each pleural cavity; the exact volume has never been measured accurately in healthy persons but is probably less than about 3 to 7 ml. This liquid forms a thin film between the parietal and visceral pleural surfaces that allows them to slide easily over each other. The liquid also transmits forces that are applied to the chest wall directly to the underlying lung.

The factors that govern the movement of liquid into and out of the pleural cavities are not completely understood at present. Judging from preliminary studies in sheep, which have a pleural blood supply similar to that in humans, under normal conditions, pleural liquid is formed mainly by the parietal pleura and perhaps to a slight extent by the visceral pleura. Once formed, liquid is reabsorbed primarily into lymphatics located in proximity to the parietal pleura. Cells and particles appear to be removed through preformed stomata within the parietal pleura that connect the pleura and lymphatic spaces (Fig. 72).

Pathophysiologic Consequences. There are many specific causes of pleural effusion and many possible ways of classifying the various underlying conditions. Effusions are often subdivided into transudates (an ultrafiltrate of plasma with a low concentration of protein) and exudates (a "weeping" of plasma with a high protein concentration); traditionally, a pleural liquid protein concentration of 3.0 g/dl has been used to differentiate transudates and exudates. Because some misclassification results from the use of protein values alone, additional studies are recommended to improve the distinction. The following three criteria

are widely used to define an exudate: (1) a pleural fluid:serum ratio of total protein of 0.5 or greater, (2) a pleural fluid lactic dehydrogenase activity of 200 IU or greater, and (3) a pleural fluid:serum ratio of lactic dehydrogenase activity of 0.6 or greater. Regardless of the character of the liquid, provided it has not organized and formed a fibrothorax, similar abnormalities in respiratory function are observed.

Lung volumes, particularly VC and TLC, are reduced from the space-occupying effects of the liquid. Although observations are limited, gas exchange, at least as reflected in arterial P_{O_2} and P_{CO_2} values, is well maintained. The vertical gradient of pleural pressure in normal lungs has been estimated as approximately 0.25 cm H_2O per cm distance; recent data suggest it may be twice this value. It might be anticipated that when the pleural space is filled with liquid, the pressure gradient would increase to 1 cm H_2O per cm; this in effect would add considerable weight to the dependent region of the lungs and might close airways, affect expansion of the basilar regions, and cause redistribution of inspired gas away from the bases. However, none of these predictions can be validated. Studies of regional lung function with ^{133}Xe in patients with pleural effusion revealed some displacement of the lung under the liquid, but regional lung volumes and lung expansion were not decreased and the distribution of gas inhaled slowly from RV showed no abnormalities. Thus it appears that the effective static pleural pressure applied to both lungs was the same despite the presence of liquid in one pleural cavity. There was, however, impaired washout of gas from the region underlying the effusion, suggesting that the swings in dynamic pressure applied to the region are decreased by the presence of the liquid.

REFERENCES

Pneumothorax

Agostoni, E.: Mechanics of the pleural space. Physiol Rev 52:57, 1972.

Gustman, P., Yerger, L., and Wanner, A.: Immediate cardiovascular effects of tension pneumothorax. Am Rev Respir Dis 127:171, 1983.

Pleural Effusion

Anthonisen, N. R., and Martin, R. R.: Regional lung function in pleural effusion. Am Rev Respir Dis 116:201, 1977.

Kinasewitz, G. T., Groome, L. J., Marshall, R. P., and Diana, J. N.: Permeability of the canine visceral pleural. J Appl Physiol 55:121, 1983.

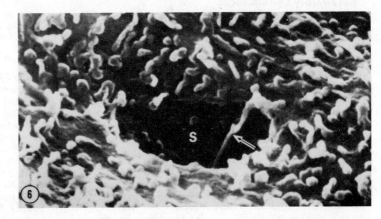

Figure 72. High power scanning electron micrograph of a stoma *(S)*. The stomata occur with the mesothelial cells, which have few, stubby microvilli. A cellular bridge *(arrow)* crosses this stoma. (Original magnification ×14820.) (From Albertine, K. H., Wiener-Kronish, J. P., and Staub, N. C.: Anat Rec 208:401, 1984; reprinted by permission of the authors and publisher.)

RESPIRATORY FAILURE

Respiration has been defined as "those processes concerned with gas exchange between an organism and its environment." It follows that *respiratory failure* is associated with disturbances in the uptake of O_2 or the elimination of CO_2 and that these abnormalities must be reflected by changes in the partial pressures of these gases in arterial blood. Thus the measurement of arterial blood gas pressures provides the basis for a definition of respiratory failure that is both precise and clinically applicable: *a condition in which arterial Po_2 is below the range of normal values* (excluding intracardiac right-to-left shunts) *or arterial Pco_2 is above the range of normal values* (excluding respiratory compensation for metabolic alkalosis). This definition underscores the fact that respiratory failure is a laboratory and not a clinical diagnosis.

Understanding what is meant by a normal range of values is important because arterial Po_2 varies in persons with age, and both arterial Po_2 and Pco_2 vary with ascending altitude. The normal range includes the biologic variabilities among individual subjects and the analytic variations inherent in the measurements. Because the presence of respiratory failure is established in the laboratory, not at the bedside, the physician's ability to diagnose the condition depends on the accuracy of the laboratory tests used to measure Po_2 and Pco_2. With properly calibrated electrodes, results should be accurate to ± 2 mm Hg. Normal mean arterial $Po_2(Pa_{O_2})$ values in subjects 20 years of age or older can be calculated from the following regression equation:

$$Pa_{O_2} = 100 - 0.32 \text{ (age)}.$$

The normal range of variation is ± 5 mm Hg from the mean value. Arterial Pco_2 does not vary with age and is normally within the range of 40 ± 5 mm Hg in healthy persons at sea level.

Respiratory failure is not a disease but a disorder of function that can be caused by a variety of conditions that directly or indirectly affect the lungs; in some circumstances, the lungs are completely normal (for example, in patients who have taken an overdose of sedative drugs). Respiratory failure is analogous to heart failure, renal failure, and liver failure, each of which represents the functional consequences of numerous disparate diseases.

Respiratory Disturbances

A decrease in arterial Po_2 can result only from one or more of the following five mechanisms: hypoventilation, limitation of diffusion, ventilation-perfusion mismatching, right-to-left shunting of blood, or breathing gas with a low Po_2. The unlikely contribution of impairment of diffusion to decreased arterial Po_2 values is ignored. The effects of breathing air with a decreased Po_2 at high altitude are accounted for in the definition of normal arterial Po_2 values. Pathologic hypoxia from breathing low concentrations of O_2 is uncommon but may occur in situations in which the O_2 is diluted by accumulation of some other gas (for example, in smoke-filled rooms or in mines where pockets of CO_2 or methane may develop) or in which the O_2 is consumed (for example, by fire). These effects must be transient for the victim to survive, so by the time an arterial

blood specimen is obtained the patient must be breathing ordinary air or enriched gas, and thus the Po_2 value will not reveal the extent of the hypoxia that may have been present. Accordingly, when interpreting the results of a given patient's arterial blood Po_2 and Pco_2 values, the possible causes of abnormalities reduce to hypoventilation, ventilation-perfusion imbalance, or right-to-left shunts. Because arterial Po_2 and Pco_2 change in opposite directions by nearly the same amount during hypoventilation, the contribution of hypoventilation to the patient's arterial hypoxia can be readily assessed. For example, if $Po_2 = 50$ mm Hg and $Pco_2 = 80$ mm Hg in a 30-year-old man, both have changed from their normal values by the same amount (40 mm Hg) and "pure" hypoventilation is present; in contrast, if $Po_2 = 30$ mm Hg and $Pco_2 = 80$ mm Hg in the same patient, the change in Pco_2 from normal does not account for the entire change in Po_2, so that hypoventilation *plus* either ventilation-perfusion abnormalities or shunts must be present. These can be distinguished by examination of two arterial blood samples, one obtained while the patient breathes room air and the other while he or she breathes enriched gas, usually 100 per cent O_2 (Table 6). The importance of breathing high concentrations of O_2 is shown in Figure 73. In the presence of a severe ventilation-perfusion abnormality ($\sigma = 2.0$), arterial Po_2 values are relatively unaffected (that is, the response is similar to that of a true shunt) until greater

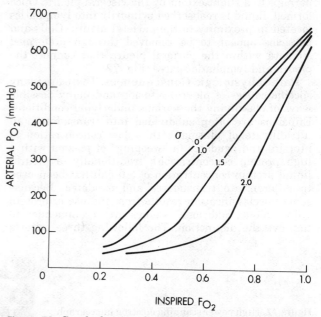

Figure 73. Graph showing the effects of changing inspired O_2 concentration (F_{O_2}) on arterial Po_2 in the presence of varying amounts of ventilation-perfusion inequality. When ventilation and perfusion are evenly matched ($\sigma = 0$), the relationship between inspired F_{O_2}, from 21 to 100 per cent, is linear. As ventilation-perfusion inequalities worsen ($\sigma = 1.0$ to 2.0), the effect of breathing a given F_{O_2} is progressively less. Note that when the ventilation-perfusion abnormality is severe ($\sigma = 2.0$), breathing gas with an F_{O_2} as high as 0.7 has little effect on arterial Po_2. (Modified from West, J. B., and Wagner, P. D.: Bioengineering Aspects of the Lung. New York, Marcel Dekker, Inc., 1977; reprinted with permission of the authors and publisher.)

than 70 per cent O_2 is breathed; even then, normal arterial Po_2 values do not occur unless 95 or 100 per cent O_2 is breathed.

The importance of identifying the mechanism(s) of each patient's hypoxia is underscored by appreciating that different causes have different pathogenetic and therapeutic connotations. (1) Hypoventilation implies failure of neural or muscular control of breathing and is treated by vigorous efforts to improve alveolar ventilation; when these are unsuccessful, intubation and mechanically assisted ventilation are often required. (2) Ventilation-perfusion mismatching usually denotes a disorder involving airways (for example, secretions, mucosal edema, and/or bronchospasm) such that the distribution of inspired air to affected regions is decreased more than their blood flow; this condition is treated by means of respiratory physical therapy, bronchodilators, and (possibly) corticosteroids. (3) Right-to-left shunts, or perfusion of nonventilated regions, nearly always indicate closure of terminal respiratory units by microatelectasis or macroatelectasis or filling of units by blood, pus, or other liquids (for example, pneumonia or pulmonary edema); these conditions are treated with antimicrobial drugs, diuretics, and end-expiratory pressure. Thus the pathophysiologic evidence from blood gas analysis helps to determine if the disease involves the neuromuscular system, airways, and/or lung parenchyma.

In addition to abnormalities in arterial Pco_2 and/or Po_2, which by definition must be present, most patients with respiratory failure have substantial alterations in the mechanical properties of their respiratory system. The only regular exceptions to this generality are certain patients with neuromuscular disorders, including drug overdosage, in whom the lungs and thorax may be completely normal, and patients with pulmonary vascular diseases that customarily spare the airways and parenchyma. When present, pathologic changes in either the lungs or chest wall (sometimes both) usually affect the compliance, resistance, or impedance of the respiratory system. These changes mean that a greater than normal force, manifested as a higher pressure, must be generated by the respiratory muscles or by a mechanical ventilator to achieve a given tidal volume. In patients receiving assisted ventilation, these pressures can be measured so that the mechanical properties of the lungs and chest wall *combined* can be assessed if tidal volume is also known.

Normally, a tidal volume of 750 ml is achieved by generating a pressure across the lungs and chest wall of 10 cm H_2O; thus the compliance of the respiratory system of a healthy adult breathing from FRC is 75 ml/cm H_2O. A decrease in compliance of either the lungs or the chest wall affects the distensibility of the whole system such that higher inspiratory pressures are needed to produce the same tidal volume. Thus, information concerning changes in the distensibility of the respiratory system can be obtained in patients being ventilated if end-inspiratory and end-expiratory pressures are measured under static conditions and tidal volume is known. It is essential that pressures be determined when there is no airflow; this is seldom a problem at end-expiration, and many ventilators are equipped with a plateau or end-inspiratory hold device to allow measurement of static end-inspiratory pressure. Serial studies of respiratory system compliance provide useful information about changing mechanical properties that reflect worsening or improvement of the underlying disease. When resistance to airflow is increased, a higher than usual peak pressure is required to cause air to flow past the extra resistance; end-expiratory pressure may be normal or decreased depending on the compliance of the respiratory system. By comparing *peak*-inspiratory pressure with *end*-inspiratory pressure, some insight can be gained into the flow-resistive properties of the respiratory system; if the two pressures are similar, resistance effects are small. There are limits to this information, however, because resistive phenomena are markedly influenced by small changes in inspiratory flow rates, which makes it difficult to obtain serial observations under identical conditions.

The normal metabolic cost of breathing is small: approximately 0.5 ml of O_2/liter of ventilation, or only 1 to 3 per cent of the total O_2 consumed at rest. Decreasing respiratory system compliance or increasing resistance or impedance may increase the O_2 cost (work) of breathing considerably. Under extreme conditions, increasing ventilation uses up more O_2 than is added to the bloodstream by the augmented minute volume; when this occurs in patients at rest, mechanically assisted ventilation or supplementary O_2 is usually required.

When the mechanical demands imposed on the respiratory muscles are great and prolonged, or the availability of O_2 and energy supplies to the muscles is limited, or when both occur, fatigue develops that may cause inadequate ventilation. There is increasing evidence that this sequence may lead to respiratory failure and is often responsible for episodes of prolonged ventilator dependency (failure to wean).

Circulatory Disturbances

Acute left heart failure, such as occurs after a severe myocardial infarction, can cause pulmonary edema and acute respiratory failure. Conversely, acute respiratory failure can cause acute right heart failure (acute cor pulmonale). Unless enlarged, the right ventricle is incapable of dealing with sudden pressure loads above 40 to 50 mm Hg and fails. Thus, acute right heart failure may occur in any condition in which pulmonary vascular resistance increases abruptly. This happens most commonly in patients with pulmonary emboli of sufficient size or number to obstruct a large proportion of the pulmonary vascular bed (usually more than 50 to 60 per cent of the cross-sectional area). At times, acute cor pulmonale develops in patients with severe bronchial asthma or bronchiolitis because of marked overinflation of the lungs and the effects of increasingly negative pleural pressure on right ventricular afterload.

Acute right heart failure may also occur in patients with chronic lung disease during an episode of superimposed acute respiratory failure. Most of these patients have some degree of chronic cor pulmonale to begin with, and the worsening of a subclinical or stable condition is provoked by the added effects of the superimposed acute lung disease. The most common precipitating causes are bouts of bronchitis or pneumonia but may include pneumothorax, pulmonary embolism, excessive sedation, surgical procedures, or trauma. In these patients, resistance to blood flow through the lungs increases acutely above its previous value because (1) alveolar hypoxia and acidemia cause pulmonary arterial vasoconstriction, (2) certain lung diseases (for example, pulmonary embolism) may further reduce the cross-sectional area of the pulmonary vascular bed, (3) hyperinflation of the lungs increases pulmonary vascular resistance, and (4) arterial hypoxia may depress myocardial contractility. These factors are important to recognize because they are reversible and in many instances treatable.

Decreases in cardiac output have a secondary pathophysiologic consequence in patients with lung disease. Although arterial P_{O_2} has been viewed as being determined solely by the processes involved in respiration, changing cardiac output influences these events by affecting the composition of mixed venous blood. Increases in mixed venous P_{O_2} and P_{CO_2} usually have little effect on arterial P_{O_2} and P_{CO_2} *in persons with normal lungs* because the amount of venous admixture is small except when cardiac output is extremely low, as in patients in shock. However, in the presence of lung disease with a substantial amount of venous admixture, resulting from either a marked ventilation-perfusion abnormality or a large right-to-left shunt (or both), mixed venous O_2 content has a considerable effect on the ultimate composition of arterial blood. Figure 74 illustrates the interacting effects on arterial P_{O_2} of increasing venous admixture, shown as ventilation-perfusion mismatching of worsening severity, and of changing cardiac output: for a given amount of

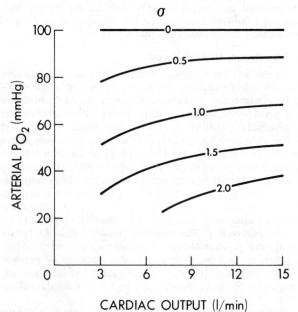

Figure 74. Schematic representation of the effects of changing cardiac output on arterial P_{O_2} in presence of varying amounts of ventilation-perfusion inequality. When ventilation and perfusion are evenly matched ($\sigma = 0$), changing cardiac output has no effect on arterial P_{O_2}. As ventilation-perfusion inequalities worsen ($\sigma = 0.5$ to 2.0), arterial P_{O_2} decreases at any given cardiac output, and increasing cardiac output increases P_{O_2}. (Modified from West, J. B., and Wagner, P. D.: Bioengineering Aspects of the Lung. New York, Marcel Dekker, Inc., 1977; reprinted with permission of the authors and publisher.)

ventilation-perfusion imbalance, the lower the cardiac output, the lower the arterial P_{O_2}.

Because of the relationships among O_2 consumption ($\dot{V}_{O_2}$), cardiac output ($\dot{Q}$), and arterial and mixed venous O_2 contents (Ca_{O_2} and $C\bar{v}_{O_2}$) expressed by the Fick equation,

$$\dot{Q} = \frac{\dot{V}_{O_2}}{Ca_{O_2} - C_{O_2}^-}$$

it has been customary to use mixed venous P_{O_2} as a guide to the adequacy of systemic O_2 transport in seriously ill patients (see previous section for further details). This holds over a wide range of cardiac output because O_2 consumption is an independent variable that reflects the metabolic needs of the body and is not dependent on O_2 delivery. In certain conditions, such as sepsis and adult respiratory distress syndrome, this correspondence no longer prevails. In sepsis, peripheral arteriovenous anastomoses appear to open; certainly they become functionally apparent; in adult respiratory distress syndrome O_2 consumption seems to be determined by O_2 delivery, a most unusual linkage. In either case, mixed venous P_{O_2} cannot be relied upon as a guide to satisfactory O_2 delivery.

At times, it may be difficult to differentiate disease that is primarily cardiac in origin, with secondary pulmonary complications, from that which is primarily respiratory in origin. This is particularly the case in patients with pulmonary edema that might be caused by either an increase in alveolar capillary-membrane permeability or an increase in pulmonary capillary pressure, or both. Given the pathophysiologic conditions reviewed previously (see Pulmonary Vascular Disorders), the contribution of possible increases in pulmonary capillary hydrostatic pressure from left ventricular failure can be assessed by measuring pulmonary arterial wedge pressure with a flow-directed catheter, and the role of changes in permeability from injury to the lungs can be assessed by measuring the concentrations of protein in simultaneously obtained specimens of pulmonary edema fluid (when available) and serum.

The therapeutic implications of whether or not alveolar-capillary membrane permeability has been increased are shown in Figure 75. When permeability is normal, pulmonary capillary pressure, as reflected in measurements of wedge pressure through a flow-directed catheter, can be increased considerably more than when permeability is increased. Persons with normal permeability and protein osmotic pressure can tolerate increases in their wedge pressures to 25 mm Hg before pulmonary edema begins to occur; when the protein osmotic pressure of the bloodstream is reduced, the threshold for fluid retention is decreased. In contrast (Fig. 75), when permeability is increased, slight increases in wedge pressure may be associated with the rapid development of pulmonary edema. Some patients with substantial damage to their membranes can have severe pulmonary edema when the wedge pressure is abnormally low (shown by the asterisk in Fig. 75); these patients have effectively extravasated into their lungs and become hypovolemic. This underscores the importance of fluid restriction in patients whose alveolar-capillary membranes are damaged.

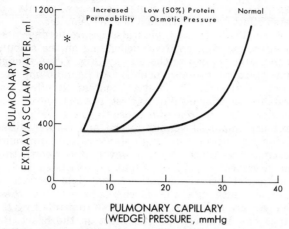

Figure 75. Schematic diagram showing the effect of changing pulmonary capillary (wedge) pressure on the quantity of extravascular water in the lungs. See text for complete discussion.

Acid-Base Disturbances

Changes in ventilation affect the P_{CO_2} and H_2CO_3 content of the blood, which in turn changes its pH. Figure 76 shows the effects of acute and chronic increases or decreases in arterial P_{CO_2} on plasma $[HCO_3^-]$ and blood pH. Acute hypoventilation and CO_2 retention (line A) are associated with an immediate increase in $[HCO_3^-]$ of approximately 1 mEq/liter for each 10 mm Hg. During the next one to three days, renal compensation serves to diminish the severity of

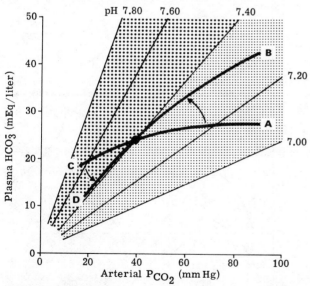

Figure 76. Pooled results from several studies of the effects of acute and chronic variations in arterial P_{CO_2} on plasma HCO_3^- and pH. When P_{CO_2} is raised acutely (acute respiratory acidosis), HCO_3^- and pH values lie along line A. After compensation by retention of HCO_3^- is complete (chronic respiratory acidosis), values lie along line B. When P_{CO_2} is lowered acutely (acute respiratory alkalosis), resulting HCO_3^- and pH values lie along line C. After compensation by rejection of HCO_3^- is complete (chronic respiratory alkalosis), values lie along line D. (From Murray, J. F.: The Normal Lung. Philadelphia, W. B. Saunders Co., 1976, p. 215.)

the acidemia (line B); for each 10 mm Hg increase in P_{CO_2}, renal retention of HCO_3^- adds a further 2 mEq/ liter to a total of approximately 3 mEq/liter. However, these two mechanisms do not restore pH to normal and respiratory acidosis is never fully compensated.

The responses to hyperventilation and a lowering of P_{CO_2} are opposite in direction but greater in magnitude than those of hypoventilation. The response in the blood to acute hyperventilation (line C) is an immediate decrease of $[HCO_3^-]$, 1.5 mEq/liter for each 10 mm Hg decrease in P_{CO_2}, from buffering and generation of lactic acid. Subsequently, renal compensation causes an additional decrease of 3 mEq/liter, or a total of 4.5 mEq/liter, for each 10 mm Hg decrease in P_{CO_2}. These three mechanisms are usually adequate to restore pH to the normal (line D) or upper limits of the normal range.

Many patients with respiratory failure have mixed respiratory and nonrespiratory acid-base disturbances. In addition, there may be associated or coexisting electrolyte abnormalities. The pathophysiologic mechanisms that underlie these changes are discussed elsewhere in this book.

Mechanical Ventilation

The indications for mechanically assisted ventilation derive from the pathophysiologic mechanisms that cause respiratory failure in the first place: lack of ventilatory drive, mechanical abnormalities of the lung parenchyma, airways, or chest wall, and occasionally, severe hypoxia that is unresponsive to conventional O_2 therapy. Two types of mechanical ventilators can be used to provide assisted ventilation; pressure ventilators, in which a certain (adjustable) airway pressure is generated by the machine during each breathing cycle, and volume ventilators, in which a constant (adjustable) tidal volume is delivered to the patient during each breath. Most commercially available ventilators of both types can be set either to cycle automatically or to assist breathing once it is initiated by the patient. Most devices also provide means of controlling inspiratory and expiratory flow rates. During the last 20 years, there has been a gradual shift from pressure to volume ventilators because of the latter's greater flexibility and reliability.

Several variations in breathing patterns besides intermittent positive pressure ventilation are possible with many commercially available ventilators or by simple adaptations of breathing circuits. These include application of positive end-expiratory pressure to achieve continuous positive pressure ventilation, continuous positive airway pressure, and intermittent mandatory ventilation. Definitions of these terms are provided in Table 18 and illustrations of the effects of different breathing patterns on airway and pleural pressures are shown in Figure 77.

End-Expiratory Pressure. Both pressure- and volume-cycled ventilators increase airway pressure during inspiration but ordinarily allow it to fall to zero (atmospheric) pressure during expiration; this pattern of assisted ventilation is known as intermittent positive pressure ventilation, or IPPV. At times, it is desirable to add positive pressure to the airway during expiration (positive end-expiratory pressure; PEEP) as well as during inspiration to hold the lungs at a higher end-expiratory volume than the FRC that would occur

TABLE 18. LIST OF COMMON ABBREVIATIONS APPLIED TO MECHANICAL VENTILATION AND THEIR DEFINITIONS

IPPV: Intermittent Positive Pressure Ventilation. The intermittent (cyclic) application of positive pressure to the airway, either automatically or when breathing is initiated by the patient, to expand the lungs and chest wall. Used to ventilate patients continuously.

IPPB: Intermittent Positive Pressure Breathing. The intermittent (cyclic) application of positive pressure to the airway to enhance breathing and/or to deliver a nebulized solution to a patient who is spontaneously breathing. Used to treat patients intermittently.

PEEP: Positive End-Expiratory Pressure. The application of positive pressure to the airways to increase pressure above atmospheric at end-expiration.

CPPV: Continuous Positive Pressure Ventilation. The application of continuous positive pressure to the airways throughout inspiration, produced by mechanically assisted ventilation (IPPV) and end-expiratory pressure (PEEP). Used to ventilate patients continuously.

CPAP: Continuous Positive Airway Pressure. The application of continuous positive pressure to the airway throughout the respiratory cycle in patients who are breathing spontaneously. Used to treat patients continuously.

IMV: Intermittent Mandatory Ventilation. The application of positive pressure to the airway at preset intervals to deliver an assisted breath intermittently to patients who are otherwise breathing spontaneously.

at zero end-expiratory pressure; this pattern of assisted ventilation (IPPV with PEEP) is known as continuous positive pressure ventilation, or CPPV.

The chief physiologic effects of PEEP derive from the increase in FRC, which depends, in turn, on the compliance of the respiratory system and the amount of PEEP applied to it. Keeping the lungs at a high lung volume in patients with certain diseases (1) prevents closure of alveoli and airways during expiration and often considerably improves gas exchange by decreasing right-to-left shunting and improving the matching of ventilation and perfusion, (2) increases pulmonary compliance by recruitment of alveoli, and (3) probably prevents depletion of the film of surfactant, a well-documented phenomenon in animal studies, and thus preserves alveolar stability. A corollary benefit of the improvement in oxygenation is the ability to decrease inspired O_2 concentration, thus decreasing the potential for the development of O_2 toxicity.

Contrary to many published statements, the use of PEEP does not dam fluid back in pulmonary capillaries and decrease the rate of fluid filtration in conditions associated with pulmonary edema. The effects of PEEP on the pathophysiologic manifestations of pulmonary edema are complex; however, judging from the results of several clinical and experimental studies, it can be concluded that PEEP does not affect the rate of fluid filtration but does improve the abnormalities in pulmonary function resulting from the accumulation of a given amount of excess water in the lungs. The improvement in gas exchange when PEEP is used in patients with pulmonary edema is related not only to the increase in end-expiratory lung volume noted above but also to a redistribution of the edema fluid within the lungs: from the alveolar spaces to the

expanded peribronchovascular spaces, where its adverse effect on gas exchange is much smaller.

When PEEP is used, pleural pressure becomes less negative (or even positive) depending on the amount of pressure applied to the airway (Fig. 77). Although end-expiratory pressure usually results in an improvement in arterial Po_2 and O_2 content, it often also decreases cardiac output. At first, it was believed that cardiac output decreased because the increased pleural pressure impaired venous return and cardiac filling and/or the increase in lung volume raised pulmonary vascular resistance. Now, however, it is known that the decrease in cardiac output is associated with a substantial decrease in both left and right ventricular volumes; although the mechanisms causing these changes are unknown, it is possible that inflating the lungs has a tamponade-like effect on the heart. Because of the variable and unpredictable effects of PEEP on cardiac output and O_2 content, O_2 transport (the product of cardiac output and O_2 content) may increase or decrease depending on whether the adverse circulatory or the beneficial gas exchange consequences predominate.

Continuous Positive Airway Pressure. Another method of maintaining a larger lung volume than would otherwise occur is with a continuous positive airway pressure breathing system, or CPAP (Fig. 78). This technique can be used only by patients who are breathing spontaneously. Humidified air, with or without supplemental O_2, is supplied through the inlet side

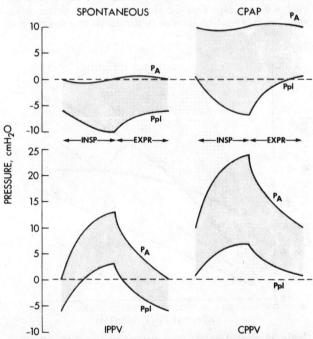

Figure 77. Schematic diagram showing the relationships between alveolar pressure *(PA)* and pleural pressure *(Ppl)* during inspiration *(insp)* and expiration *(expr)* during spontaneous breathing and breathing with continuous positive airway pressure *(CPAP)*, intermittent positive pressure ventilation *(IPPV)*, and continuous positive pressure ventilation *(CPPV)*. The mechanical properties of the lungs and chest wall are assumed to be normal; tidal volume = 1 liter. (From Hinshaw, H. C., and Murray, J. F.: Diseases of the Chest. Philadelphia, W. B. Saunders Co., 1979, p. 989.)

CPAP SYSTEM

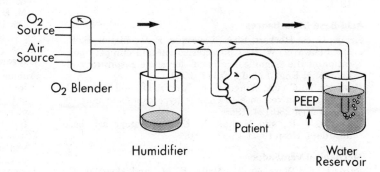

Figure 78. Schematic diagram of system to provide continuous positive airway pressure *(CPAP)* in a spontaneously breathing person. Airway and alveolar pressures throughout the respiratory cycle are set by submerging the expiratory tube in a water reservoir to achieve the desired amount of positive end-expiratory pressure *(PEEP)*. (From Hinshaw, H. C., and Murray, J. F.: Diseases of the Chest. Philadelphia, W. B. Saunders Co., 1979, p. 991.)

of the apparatus at a rate substantially higher than the patient's minute volume; a pressure is established throughout the system by an arrangement of valves or by submerging the outlet limb beneath the surface in a water bottle (as shown in the figure) to achieve the desired value of PEEP. The application of CPAP increases lung volumes throughout the respiratory cycle: during expiration by preventing airway pressure from returning to atmospheric level and during inspiration by supplementing whatever inspiratory muscle force is developed. Thus the physiologic effects of CPAP with spontaneous ventilation and of PEEP with mechanical ventilation are similar at the end of *expiration* and the beginning of inspiration but differ during the remainder of the breathing cycle because pleural pressure changes in opposite directions, becoming more negative during spontaneous breathing but less negative (or even positive) during assisted breathing (compare the two wave forms in Figure 77). These differences are accompanied by circulatory changes such that the decrease in cardiac output with CPAP is less than that produced by CPPV.

Intermittent Mandatory Ventilation. A mixed breathing pattern in which spontaneous breaths are interspersed with occasional assisted breaths at a preset frequency is referred to as intermittent mandatory ventilation, or IMV. The circulatory consequences of IMV are usually negligible but depend on the frequency of assisted breaths and the pressure applied to the lungs.

Oxygenation

Respiratory failure cannot occur without arterial hypoxia. Occasional patients are observed with normal or even high arterial P_{O_2} values and with hypercapnia; these patients are hypoventilating but must also be receiving supplementary O_2, which prevents the usual decrease in arterial P_{O_2} from occurring. The effects of hypoventilation on arterial P_{O_2} are easy to correct by adding small amounts of O_2 to the patient's inspired air. In contrast, the response of arterial P_{O_2} to the administration of low or moderate concentrations of O_2 is variable in patients with ventilation-perfusion abnormalities and poor in patients with right-to-left shunts (see Fig. 74). As ventilation-perfusion mismatching worsens, the effect of a given inspired O_2 concentration on arterial P_{O_2} progressively decreases. In patients with severe ventilation-perfusion abnormalities ($\sigma = 2.0$), breathing O_2 concentrations as high as 50 or 60 per cent has a trivial effect on arterial P_{O_2}.

In the presence of right-to-left shunts, arterial P_{O_2} fails to reach normal values (>550 mm Hg) even with 100 per cent O_2.

O_2 transport depends on the interaction among the cardiac output, the amount of hemoglobin available to combine with O_2, and the arterial P_{O_2}. Tissue oxygenation is determined by O_2 transport, the release of O_2, which is governed by the affinity between O_2 and hemoglobin, and tissue O_2 metabolism. The balance between O_2 supply and demand is reflected in the P_{O_2} of venous blood leaving various organs. Thus, oxygenation of the whole body is indicated by the composition of mixed venous blood, subject to the constraints noted previously in the discussion of circulatory disturbances.

Administration of O_2 increases arterial P_{O_2}, which has two desirable therapeutic consequences: (1) The saturation of hemoglobin with O_2 may increase up to 100 per cent, and (2) progressively more O_2 dissolves in plasma. But there are limits to these gains and it is dangerous to breathe 100 per cent O_2 for more than 24 to 48 hours. Other methods of increasing tissue oxygenation are available that depend on increasing O_2 delivery by means of augmenting cardiac output or hemoglobin concentration. The results of measurements of mixed venous P_{O_2} provide the best available assessment not only of overall oxygenation in patients with disorders involving any component of the O_2 delivery system but also of the response to therapy.

REFERENCES

Respiratory Disturbances

Macklem, P. T.: Respiratory muscles: The vital pump. Chest 78:753, 1980.
Pontoppidan, H., Geffin, B., and Lowenstein, E.: Acute respiratory failure in the adult. N Engl J Med 287:743, 760, 799, 1972.
Sykes, M. K., McNicol, M. W., and Campbell, E. J. M.: Respiratory Failure. 2nd ed. Oxford, Blackwell Scientific Publications, 1976.
West, J. B.: Ventilation/Blood Flow and Gas Exchange. 3rd ed. Oxford, Blackwell Scientific Publications, 1977.

Circulatory Disturbances

Conway, C. M.: Haemodynamic effects of pulmonary ventilation. Br J Anaesth 47:761, 1975.
Unger, K. M., Shibel, E. M., and Moser, K. M.: Detection of left ventricular failure in patients with adult respiratory distress syndrome. Chest 67:8, 1975.

Zapol, W. M., and Snider, M. T.: Pulmonary hypertension in severe acute respiratory failure. N Engl J Med 296:476, 1977.

Acid-Base Disturbances

Arbus, G. S., Herbert, L. A., Levesque, P. R., Etsten, B. E., and Schwartz, W. B.: Characterization and clinical application of the "significance band" for acute respiratory alkalosis. N Engl J Med 280:117, 1969.

Brackett, N. C., Jr., Wingo, C. F., Muren, O., and Solano, J. T.: Acid-base response to chronic hypercapnia in man. N Engl J Med 280:124, 1969.

Kassirer, J. P., and Madias, N. E.: Respiratory acid-base disorders. Hosp Pract 15:57, 1980.

Mechanical Ventilation

Pare, P. D., Warriner, B., Baile, E. M., and Hogg, J. C.: Redistribution of pulmonary extravascular water with positive end-expiratory pressure in canine pulmonary edema. Am Rev Respir Dis 127:590, 1983.

Pontoppidan, H., Wilson, R. S., Rie, M. A., and Schneider, R. C.: Respiratory intensive care. Anesthesiology 47:96, 1977.

Weissman, I. M., Ranaldo, J. E., Rogers, R. M., and Sanders, M. H.: Intermittent mandatory ventilation. Am Rev Respir Dis 127:641, 1983.

Oxygenation

Aubier, M., Murciano, D., Milic-Emili, J., Daghfous, J., Pariente, R., and Derenne, J. P.: Effects of the administration of O_2 on ventilation and blood gases in patients with chronic obstructive pulmonary disease during acute respiratory failure. Am Rev Resp Dis 122:747, 1980.

Lutch, J. S., and Murray, J. F.: Continuous positive-pressure ventilation: Effects on systemic oxygen transport and tissue oxygenation. Ann Intern Med 76:193, 1972.

Tenney, S. M., and Mithoefer, J. C.: The relationship of mixed venous oxygenation to oxygen transport: With special reference to adaptations to high altitude and pulmonary disease. Am Rev Respir Dis 125:474, 1982.

PATHOPHYSIOLOGY OF CARDIOVASCULAR DISEASE

ANDREW G. WALLACE, M.D.,
and ROBERT A. WAUGH, M.D.

Introduction

Pathophysiology focuses on the functional alterations produced by disease. It attempts to integrate and relate mechanisms of disease and their functional consequences. Pathophysiology should provide students with an understanding of symptoms and signs of disease and of the logic that underlies treatment choices directed at correcting abnormal function and its clinical consequences. The early chapters in this section focus on normal structure and function of components of the cardiovascular system. A second group of chapters concerns mechanisms responsible for cardiovascular diseases and their structural characteristics. A third group is devoted to the functional consequences of cardiovascular disease and to the physiological basis of symptoms and signs of those diseases.

Each component of the cardiovascular system has certain intrinsic functional characteristics. Each component of the system is coupled to one or more other components so that the function of one can modify the function of others. Furthermore, there is an elaborate control system through which neural, chemical, and humoral mechanisms can modify the intrinsic behavior of each component. Systems analysis is a branch of engineering science in which the behavior of complex systems can be predicted and understood by quantifying the function of each component and the relation between parts of the system. The application of these concepts to the function of the cardiovascular system is developed in the discussion of Mechanisms of Cardiovascular Control (p. 893). Diseases may attack one or a few components of the system, but understanding the consequences of disease at a systems level is just as important as understanding the effects of the disease on the component primarily affected.

A chapter of this section is devoted to the cardiovascular responses to exercise (p. 905), a topic of particular interest because exercise uniquely stresses the ability of the normal cardiovascular system to adapt appropriately to widely ranging metabolic demands that at a regional level are widely discordant. Because of the magnitude and the discordant nature of these demands, exercise also highlights the capacity of cardiovascular control systems to regulate and integrate total and regional perfusion in a manner that is advantageous to the organism. Disorders of cardiovascular function manifest their earliest effects on system performance when the system is stressed maximally. Cardiovascular functions are frequently normal at rest during early stages of disease, and inadequate function is evident only during a stress such as exercise. Symptoms and signs of cardiovascular disease may be evident only during exercise, or if present at rest they are exaggerated by exercise.

The circulation delivers components necessary for cellular function to the cells and transports products of cellular metabolism away from those cells to other sites responsible for their modification or elimination. Most forms of cardiovascular disease ultimately produce their important effects by limiting perfusion and hence transport, either at rest or during activities that enhance the demand for perfusion. In some cases, reduced perfusion is at a local or regional level. In others, cardiac output and its ability to increase are limited by inadequate blood volume, valvular or congenital diseases, alterations of rhythm, myocardial disease, or pericardial disease. Heart failure and shock represent pathophysiological states that are a consequence of reduced perfusion. The clinical picture of these states reflects both the effects of reduced perfusion per se and the cardiovascular adjustments in an effort to restore perfusion. Nothing highlights the need for an integrated understanding of physiology, pathology, and control more than the manifestations of circulatory failure.

The Circulation

The structural integrity and function of all cells of the body depend upon an adequate delivery of oxygen and substrates. The human organism has well-developed mechanisms that permit it to adapt to stimuli calling for varying metabolic activity, whether those stimuli originate outside the body, or as a result of one organ placing a greater demand on another, or as a compensation for disease of a part of any given organ.

Thus, arterial blood flow is adjusted to meet basal functions, but total perfusion and its distribution can be altered to meet changes in the metabolic requirements. The fundamental function of the circulation, therefore, is to serve as a perfusion system.

A simplified first approximation of the circulatory perfusion system is shown in Figure 1. In this model the heart is viewed as a pump that supplies a certain volume of blood (the cardiac output) to the arteries. The system of arteries appears as a conduit through which blood pumped by the heart reaches peripheral arterioles and capillaries. Arterioles are small vessels with a muscular media; the resistance offered by them determines the volume of blood that leaves the arterial system to supply a capillary bed. Because of their small size and very thin walls capillaries are the principal site for exchange of oxygen, substrates, and metabolites, a process referred to as transcapillary exchange. Having traversed the capillaries, blood is reaccumulated by various tributaries into central venous channels, which again are depicted as conduits through which blood returns to the heart. In any steady-state condition, the volume of blood that leaves the arterial system will return to the venous system and the heart will transfer into the arterial system all of the blood returned to it from the veins.

Movement of blood through arteries, arterioles, capillaries, and veins is the consequence of a pressure gradient between arteries and veins that is created by the pumping action of the heart, a mechanical event in which heart muscle converts chemical energy to mechanical energy through the act of shortening. As a starting point for understanding circulatory function, one can visualize an equilibrium state in which the heart is arrested and blood has been moved from the arterial system to the venous system such that the pressure everywhere in the circulation is equal. This pressure is referred to as the mean circulatory filling pressure (MCFP), which is determined solely by the volume of blood within the circulatory system and the net compliance of the system. In normal animals and in man it has been estimated that MCFP is approximately 7 mm Hg.

When normal rhythmic contraction of the heart is restored after determining MCFP, a new steady state is rapidly reached in which the heart pumps blood into the arterial reservoir and the arterial pressure is determined by the relation between blood flow and resistance. In this new steady state a simple but fundamental expression describes the condition:

$$\text{Flow (Q)} = \frac{P_A - P_{RA}}{\text{Resistance}}$$

where Flow (Q) = cardiac output in liters/minute, P_A = the mean arterial pressure in mm Hg, P_{RA} = the mean right atrial pressure, and Resistance is a derived parameter representing the forces that impede flow from the arterial conduit to the right atrium.

CARDIAC OUTPUT

The properties of the systemic circulation could be discussed with equal logic by starting with cardiac output, arterial blood pressure, or arterial resistance.

It seems appropriate, however, to discuss cardiac output first, since perfusion of the capillary bed is perhaps the most important role of the circulation. Cardiac output is defined as the quantity of blood pumped by the left ventricle into the aorta each minute. During any steady state, cardiac output is also equivalent to the volume of blood pumped by the right ventricle into the pulmonary artery, and it is equivalent to the blood flowing from systemic veins into the right atrium or from pulmonary veins into the left atrium. In normal adults, cardiac output under basal conditions is approximately 5 liters/minute. Normally, cardiac output varies in direct proportion to body size, so that it is customary when comparing individuals of different size to normalize cardiac output by dividing it by body surface area in square meters. The normal cardiac index for male and female adults is approximately 3 liters/minute/square meter.

Cardiac output is equal to the volume of blood ejected by the right or left ventricle per beat (stroke volume) multiplied by the number of beats per minute (the heart rate).

The major determinant of cardiac output is the

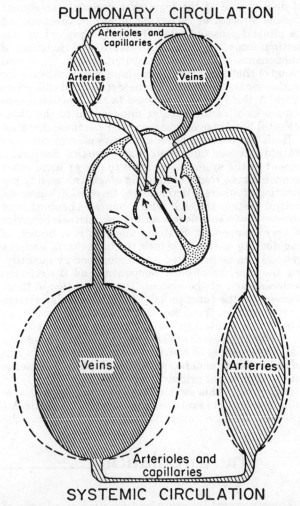

PULMONARY CIRCULATION

Arterioles and capillaries

Arteries Veins

Veins Arteries

Arterioles and capillaries

SYSTEMIC CIRCULATION

Figure 1. Schematic representation of the circulation, showing both the distensible and the resistive portions of the systemic and pulmonary circulations. (With permission from Guyton, A. C.: Textbook of Medical Physiology. 5th ed. Philadelphia, W. B. Saunders Co., 1976, p. 223.)

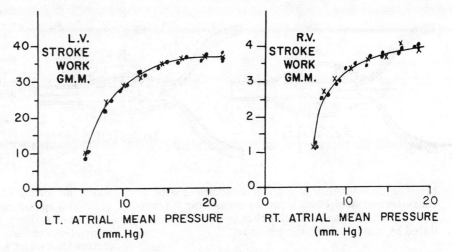

Figure 2. Right and left ventricular function curves in a dog, depicting ventricular stroke work output as a function of the respective right and left mean atrial pressures. (With permission from Guyton, A. C., Jones, C. E., and Coleman, T. G.: Cardiac Output and Its Regulation. Philadelphia, W. B. Saunders Co., 1973, p. 151.)

metabolic rate of the body as reflected by total oxygen consumption per minute. When oxygen consumption of the body increases above basal levels cardiac output increases. This change in cardiac output is accomplished by an increase in heart rate with relatively small changes in stroke volume. In the intact organism a number of factors come into play that determine the manner in which the heart adjusts cardiac output to meet peripheral metabolic demands, and some of these factors operate through changes in heart rate. The heart also has the intrinsic ability to adjust its output (for example, an isolated heart) even under conditions in which heart rate is not allowed to change (for example, during pacing at a constant rate). This in-

trinsic ability of the heart, upon which all other mechanisms are superimposed, is referred to as the law of the heart, or Starling's law (Fig. 2). Operationally, this law states that within limits the ventricle will pump whatever volume of blood is returned to it from the venous system. (See The Heart as a Pump, p. 881.)

THE ARTERIAL CONDUITS

The aorta and its major branches serve as conduits for the transfer of blood from the heart to the peripheral arterioles and capillaries. Unlike metal pipes or glass tubes, arterial conduits are elastic and distensi-

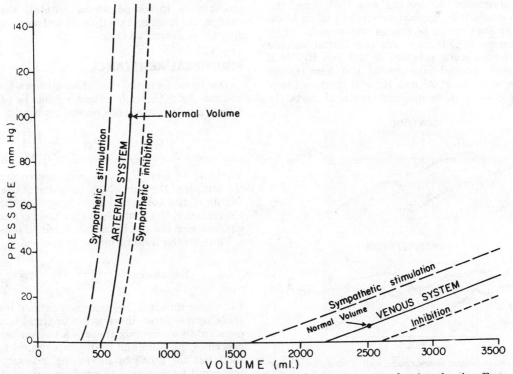

Figure 3. Pressure-volume curves of the systemic arterial and venous systems, showing also the effects of sympathetic stimulation and sympathetic inhibition which respectively decrease and increase compliance. (With permission from Guyton, A. C.: Textbook of Medical Physiology. 5th ed. Philadelphia, W. B. Saunders Co., 1976, p. 233.)

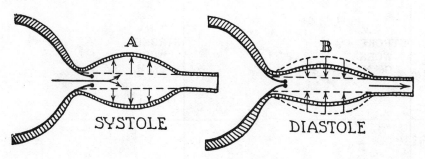

Figure 4. Diagram to illustrate role of elastic walls of aorta in maintenance of circulation. *A*, Walls are distended as ventricular contents enter aorta. *B*, Following closure of aortic valves, elastic recoil of walls drives blood peripherally. Elastic walls serve to store energy during systole and to release it during diastole. (With permission from Barron, D. H.: The pressure gradient and pulse in the vascular system. In Ruch, T. C., and Fulton, J. F. (eds.): Medical Physiology and Biophysics. 18th ed. Philadelphia, W. B. Saunders Co., 1960, p. 668.)

ble. The distensibility of a given structure is usually characterized in physical terms by measuring its compliance, which represents the change in volume produced by a given change in pressure.

$$\text{Compliance} = \frac{\text{increase in volume}}{\text{increase in pressure}}$$

Thus, for a given length of aorta the increase in volume for, say, a 50 mm Hg increase in pressure (that is, its compliance) may be significantly greater than the increase in volume of an equal length of femoral artery. The compliance of any given vessel is also related to the initial volume and pressure within the vessel. Thus, the change in volume produced by a 50 mm Hg change in pressure is greater if the pressure change is from 25 to 75 mm Hg than if the pressure change is from 75 to 125 mm Hg. The usual method of determining the compliance of a structure is to determine its static pressure-volume relation; for an artery such as the aorta this is done with both ends and all branches obstructed to prevent any leak from the system. It would take approximately 500 ml of blood to fill the entire arterial system at zero pressure (Fig. 3). An increase of 250 ml above this initial volume would produce a static pressure of 100 mm Hg. At a normal mean arterial pressure of 100 mm Hg an increase or decrease of 25 mm Hg will produce about a 0.75 ml change in volume/cm length of aorta. In

short, the aorta is distensible. Its distensibility is small at normal operating pressures and decreases with age.

When the heart is beating, the compliance of the arterial system and stroke volume are the principal factors that affect pulse pressure at a given arteriolar resistance. During ventricular ejection, the work done by ventricular muscle is liberated as energy in the form of pressure. Part of that energy is used to move blood in the aortic arch forward, part is used to accelerate the blood, and part is used to distend the aorta and enlarge its volume (Fig. 4). This latter component of the energy liberated by the heart is stored in elastic fibers of the aorta and subsequently liberated during diastole as elastic recoil, which effectively moves blood peripherally even after the heart has ceased its contraction.

Changes in pressure and cross-sectional area of the ascending aorta in man are nearly in phase with one another (Fig. 5). At normal mean aortic pressure the change in cross-sectional area during the cardiac cycle averages 11 per cent of the diastolic value. When mean pressure is increased above normal, the per cent change in cross-sectional area between systole and diastole is decreased (Fig. 5).

PERIPHERAL RESISTANCE

The basic formula that characterizes the flow of a viscous fluid through a small tube is described by Hagen's modification of Poiseuille's law:

$$Q = P_A - P_B \left(\frac{\pi}{8} \cdot \frac{1}{N} \cdot \frac{R^4}{L} \right)$$

where Q = flow, $P_A - P_B$ = pressure gradient over the length of the tube, N = viscosity of the fluid, R = radius of the tube, and L = length of the tube. For convenience, the term resistance has been employed to characterize the net force that tends to impede flow.

Thus, in the fluid formula:

$$\text{Resistance} = \frac{P_A - P_B}{\text{Flow}} \text{ or } \frac{8}{\pi} \cdot N \cdot \frac{L}{R^4}$$

In this formulation, resistance is defined in relation to three terms. First, there is a numerical term that is a constant $(8/\pi)$. Second, there is a viscous term (N) that describes the fluid and that, simply put, expresses the fact that for fluids of increasing viscosity a greater force will be required to produce any given flow. Finally, there is a geometric term (L/R^4) that expresses the fact that for any given fluid the forces that tend to impede the flow of the fluid are directly proportional

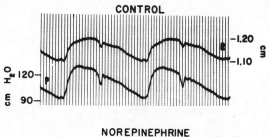

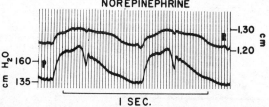

Figure 5. Curve of lateral pressure and radius obtained during the control state and following administration of 1.0 µg of *l*-norepinephrine. Relation between pressure and diameter in the ascending aorta of man. (With permission from Greenfield, J. C., Jr., and Patel, D. J.: Circ Res 10: 779, 1962.)

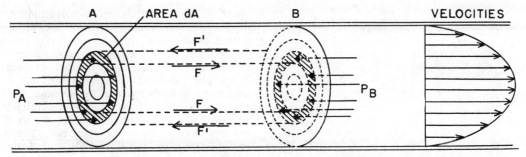

Figure 6. Diagram of flow of viscous fluid through a tube in concentric cylindric laminae, showing parabolic distribution of velocities. Pressure force $(P_A - P_B)$ dA is balanced by difference between shear force, F and F^1. F^1 is greater than F because velocity gradient is increased closer to wall. (With permission from Burton, A. C.: Hemodynamics and physics of the circulation. In Ruch, T. C., and Fulton, J. F. (eds.): Medical Physiology and Biophysics. 18th ed. Philadelphia, W. B. Saunders Co., 1960, p. 648.)

to the length of the tube and inversely proportional to the fourth power of the radius.

Thus, the major factor that determines the resistance of flow of blood from a major artery into any given capillary bed is the caliber or radius of the arteriole. In the aorta and large arteries high flow rates are maintained with very little pressure gradient, while in smaller vessels the flow rate is much lower despite a large pressure gradient. The dependence of resistance on the fourth power of the radius has another very important physiological consequence. The structure of the arterial system is such that the resistance of each organ is arranged effectively in parallel with all other organs. Thus, distribution of the total flow through an arterial perfusion system is regulated by the relative resistance offered by each vascular bed.

It is often erroneously considered that resistance or the impediment to flow through a vessel can be equated with energy lost as heat owing to friction between the blood and walls of vessels. In fact, it is the friction within the blood itself that offers resistance to flow. There is a cohesive force between a liquid and any surface that it wets, such that even when the liquid flows through a vessel there is a very thin layer of liquid in contact with the wall, which has zero velocity. The next layer of liquid, nearer to the axis of the stream, has a small velocity, and each subsequent layer has a greater velocity until maximal velocity is encountered at the center or axis of the stream. The velocity profile is parabolic (Fig. 6). It is zero at the wall, it increases by a decreasing amount per unit distance from the wall to the axis, and it is maximal at the axis. The velocity gradient between adjacent layers of the flowing stream produces a shear force. An intrinsic property of any fluid is that it resists shear stress (or rate of change of shear). In this analysis, then, energy lost from the vascular system exists only when fluid is moving; resistance is not related to friction, but for a vessel of any given caliber it is determined by viscosity and by the velocity gradient across the vessel.

ARTERIAL PRESSURE

The high pressure in systemic arteries represents a form of stored or potential energy that is originally derived from contraction of the heart and is available to cause blood flow against the resistance offered by peripheral arterioles. If a needle is placed into an artery and connected to a column, blood will rise in the column to a height equivalent to the blood pressure. By custom, however, blood pressure is expressed in millimeters of mercury (mm Hg)—that is, the height to which a column of mercury (rather than blood) would be raised if the force in the arterial system were applied directly to a mercury column. Since the density of mercury is 13.6 relative to water (or blood), 1 mm Hg is equivalent to 1.36 cm of blood. Mean arterial pressure is the average of all instantaneous pressure over an interval of time equivalent to at least one cardiac cycle. Normal resting mean arterial pressure increases with age, ranging from 70 to 80 mm Hg in children and from 80 to 100 mm Hg in adults.

The laws of hydrostatics define fluid pressure as a force (dynes) exerted by the fluid on a plane of unit area (cm^2). In a fluid at rest under the influence of gravity, pressure increases with depth according to the following equation:

$$Pressure = pgh$$

where:

p = density of the fluid (gm/cm^3)
g = acceleration of gravity (980 cm/sec/sec)
h = depth in cm

According to this formula:
1 mm Hg = 13.6 (density) × 980 (acceleration of gravity) × 0.1 (depth) = 1330 dynes/cm^2.

When arterial pressure is accurately measured just above the aortic valve, the pressure pulse has a typical contour (Fig. 7). At the onset of ejection, pressure and the rate of change of pressure increase rapidly, corresponding to the rapid acceleration of ejection. Following the abrupt rise in pressure, a relative plateau occurs, corresponding to a phase during which the ventricle continues to eject at a relatively constant velocity. During the later phase of systole, aortic pressure decreases rapidly as blood flow decelerates. The end of systole is marked by an incisura, or notch, that corresponds to aortic valve closure. This notch is created when the falling aortic pressure is transiently interrupted by a brief low amplitude rise or reflected wave from aortic valve closure. After the incisura aortic pressure declines more slowly toward its minimum diastolic value. The peak systolic pressure, the rate of rise of aortic pressure, and the pulse pressure will be determined by stroke volume, the velocity of ventricular ejection, and the compliance of the aorta.

The heart is a pulsatile pump in which the volume of blood ejected per beat requires 40 per cent or less of the total duration of the cardiac cycle. In very small

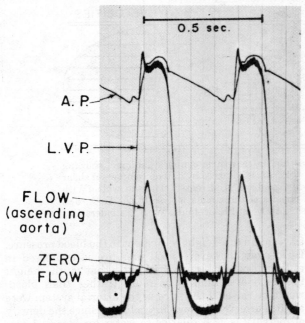

Figure 7. Contours and time relationships of aortic pressure (A. P.) and left ventricular pressure (L. V. P.), and the ascending aorta flow. (Superimposed tracings.) (With permission from Spencer, M. P., and Greiss, F. C.: Dynamics of ventricular ejection. Circ Res 10:275, 1962.)

peripheral vessels, however, flow is nearly continuous, and we are used to thinking of a steady rate of flow, in which a large pressure gradient is needed to overcome a resistance dominated by the dimensional term in the Poiseuille-Hagen equation. In the aorta, where flow is discontinuous, the geometric factor is very small because the radius is large and flow is dominated by inertia. Inertia is that property of mass (in this case the blood in the aorta) that resists change in movement. Thus, in the proximal aorta the pressure gradient created by ventricular contraction is used primarily to cause acceleration of the aortic blood mass.

At the aortic valve, arterial pressure rises rapidly as blood is transferred from the ventricle into the proximal aorta. However, because of the compliance of the proximal aorta the energy of the cardiac impulse is used partially to distend the vessel and not entirely to accelerate the blood mass. The pressure rise in the proximal aorta is transmitted rapidly to the periphery because blood is noncompressible and because the arterial conduits are relatively nondistensible. The velocity of transmission of the pressure pulse is influenced primarily by the characteristics of the arterial wall; it increases toward the periphery because compliance decreases in moving from the aorta to distal vessels. Even though velocity of transmission of the pressure pulse increases down the aorta, the pressure gradient and flow velocity are remarkably constant as one moves toward the periphery. The amplitude and velocity of pulse wave transmission increase with age because the arterial system becomes stiffer.

CAPILLARY DYNAMICS

The primary goal of the circulatory system is to ensure a constant and appropriately composed environ-

ment in the interstitial space surrounding cells. This objective is achieved by perfusion of capillary beds and by the exchange of fluid and material across the capillary walls. As a consequence substances utilized by the tissue are replaced and products of cellular metabolism are removed. An understanding of capillary dynamics depends upon an understanding of four general concepts: (1) those aspects of capillary structure uniquely related to function, (2) the nature of perfusion through a capillary or capillary bed, (3) the exchange of fluid across the capillary wall, and (4) the exchange of solutes across the capillary wall.

Capillaries are small conduits each having an internal radius of 5 to 10 microns and a length estimated at 0.4 to 0.7 mm. They can be distinguished not only on the basis of size, but also by the absence of smooth muscle within their walls. Capillaries are of two general types, one in which the endothelial cells and basement membrane are continuous over the length of the capillary (continuous) and a second type in which there are gaps or fenestrations between endothial cells and through the basement (fenestrated) membrane (Fig. 8). The former are typically found in skeletal and heart muscle and the latter in intestine, in parts of the kidney, and in specialized areas such as the choroid plexus. In cross section a capillary is composed of three layers, the endothelial cell, basement membrane, and adventitia. Endothelial cells have many plasmalemmal vesicles, and there is ample evidence of pinocytosis on both the luminal and external sides of the cell. Basement membrane is a matted substance of poorly resolvable overlapping filaments resembling collagen embedded in a matrix that is rich in glycoproteins. Adventitia is composed of pericytes, fibroblasts, some collagen, and elastic fibers.

At the junction between endothelial cells of continuous capillaries there are clefts. These clefts are about 40 Å in width at the lumen and 200 Å in width at the basement membrane side. Most, but not all, clefts appear under the electron microscope to be occluded by fusion or near fusion of adjacent endothelial membranes in the zonula occludens. Although still controversial, the most widely held view is that unoccluded clefts represent small pores through the endothelial barrier, that these pores constitute perhaps 0.1 per cent of the capillary surface area, and that they are approximately 40 Å in size, allowing transcapillary movement of molecules with a molecular weight of up to 80,000 and a molecular radius of less than 40 Å. Finally, pores are plastic in the sense that certain agents—for example, heat or histamine—may enhance pore size and hence capillary permeability. The pinocytotic vesicles of endothelial cells are prolific in number and appear to play a major role in transcapillary transport of molecules of molecular weight of 100,000 or greater, such as proteins and hormones.

Capillaries arise from very small arterioles referred to as metarterioles or terminal arterioles. The junction between the capillary and arteriole has a smooth muscle cuff or sphincter. Distal to these sphincters many capillaries interconnect to form a complex network that ultimately forms tributaries to collecting venules. The precapillary cuffs or sphincters undergo rhythmic contraction and relaxation, producing either a flow state or no-flow state in any given capillary. Despite the intermittence of flow in single capillaries,

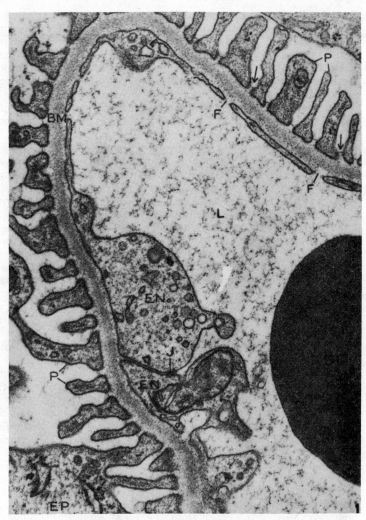

Figure 8. Peripheral area of a glomerular capillary from a normal rat. The capillary wall is composed of three distinct layers: the endothelium (EN) with its periodic interruptions or fenestrae (F); the basement membrane (BM), which is a continuous layer, 0.1 to 0.15 μ in thickness; and the foot process (P) of the epithelium (EP). In a number of places (arrows) a thin line or "slit membrane" can be seen in the urinary slits bridging the narrow (~ 250 Å) gap between foot processes. (Specimen fixed in osmium tetroxide and embedded in Epon. Section stained with lead hydroxide.) RBC = red blood cell. J = junction between two endothelial cells. (Original magnification × 40,000.) (With permission from Farquhar, M. G.: Glomerular permeability investigated by electron microscopy. In Siperstein, M. D., Colwell, A. R., and Meyer, K. (eds.): Small Blood Vessel Involvement in Diabetes Mellitus. American Institute of Biological Sciences, 1964, Plate I, p. 382.)

there are so many capillaries in a given bed that the net effect is continuous flow (Fig. 9). The total cross-sectional area of the capillary bed has been estimated at 2500 sq cm or about 100 times that of the aorta. Since for a given volume of flow, velocity is directly related to cross-sectional area, blood flows through the capillaries at a velocity of only 0.3 mm/second compared to a velocity of 30 to 33 cm/second in the aorta. The relatively slow flow facilitates diffusion across the walls of individual capillaries whose lengths average only about 0.5 mm.

The movement of fluid (filtration) across the capil-

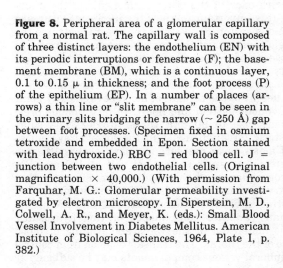

Figure 9. Overall structure of a capillary bed. (With permission from Guyton, A. C.: Textbook of Medical Physiology. 5th ed. Philadelphia, W. B. Saunders Co., 1976, p. 251.)

lary wall is governed by four major factors in addition to permeability of the wall: capillary pressure (Pc), interstitial fluid pressure (Pisf), plasma osmotic pressure (Πp), and interstitial oncotic pressure (Πist). At the arteriolar end of an open capillary, Pc equals 25 mm Hg, while at the venular end Pc = 10 mm Hg. Throughout the capillary, Pisf equals −6.3 mm Hg, Πp = 28 mm Hg, and Πist = 5 mm Hg. Thus, at the arteriolar end of the capillary there is outward filtration caused by a force of 8.3 mm Hg, and at the venular end of the capillary there is inward filtration caused by a force of 6.7 mm Hg. These forces are sufficiently great that there is a continuous movement of water from capillaries to tissue and back to capillaries. A most impressive view of this exchange rate is the calculation that all of the water within the blood compartment exchanges with the interstitial compartment once every minute.

The capillary is for all practical purposes infinitely permeable to water, and water movement is hence governed principally by hydrodynamic forces. Quite a different situation applies to the movement of materials of varying size dissolved within the plasma and interstitial water. These materials move through the capillary wall according to the laws of diffusion across a lipid membrane. At one extreme are lipid-soluble substances that can diffuse rapidly through the endothelial cells at a rate governed almost exclusively by the concentration gradient between the capillary and interstitial fluid. This is the manner of transport of solutes such as oxygen and carbon dioxide in the form of H_2CO_3.

At the other extreme are very large molecules, such as proteins and hormones, that move principally by vesicular transport. It has been estimated that a single vesicle requires 300 seconds to make the transit across an endothelial cell and that the net rate of movement for a substance dependent on vesicular transport is 10^7 slower than water. Thus, albumin and similar sized materials are essentially confined to the vascular compartment and under normal conditions exchange between the blood and tissues is extraordinarily slow.

Between these two extremes is a large class of materials, such as electrolytes, urea, and glucose. These water-soluble but lipid-insoluble substances move largely through pores, and net movement is governed by capillary perfusion (that is, flow), by the concentration difference between the capillary and interstitium, and by the permeability surface area product.

THE VENOUS SYSTEM

The system of veins between distal capillary beds and the right atrium fulfills two primary functions: (1) to act as a conduit through which blood is transferred back to the heart, and (2) to act as a reservoir that contains up to 65 per cent of the blood volume at any point in time. The venous system has a compliance approximately 24 times that of the arterial system (see Fig. 3), a consequence of an eightfold greater intrinsic distensibility and a threefold greater volume. The venous system is not, however, simply a passive series of conduits with a relatively large volume for storage purposes. Most veins other than the large conduits within the thoracic and abdominal cavities are equipped with valves that allow flow only toward the heart. The deep veins pass through large compartments containing skeletal muscles that contract intermittently in all but the supine or stationary standing positions. With every voluntary movement requiring muscular contraction, the veins are compressed, flow toward the heart is facilitated, and venous pressure is maintained lower than would be the case if gravity alone were allowed to influence peripheral venous pressure. Veins also have a muscular media that is innervated by the sympathetic nervous system. The contraction of this muscular coat can drastically change the compliance of the veins and hence of the volume or reservoir function.

In a normal man in the supine position the pressure in very small peripheral veins is approximately 10 mm Hg, whereas the mean pressure in the right atrium is approximately 5 mm Hg. Thus, the pressure gradient that promotes flow is about 5 mm Hg. This force is derived from left ventricular contraction and represents a residual force after energy is dissipated in putting blood through the resistance offered by the arterioles and capillaries. The pressure gradient between small peripheral veins and the right atrium is small relative to that in the arterial system because of the large cross-sectional area of major veins and be-

cause venous flow is nearly continuous and does not require instantaneous increases to accelerate flow. Peripheral venous pressure will increase passively by an amount approximately equal to the rise in right atrial pressure whenever blood volume is expanded or when the impedance to flow into the right heart is increased. Finally, if there is contraction of the venous system in response to neurogenic or humoral agents, venous pressure will rise.

As with each of the other components of the circulation, it is important to know the intrinsic features of the venous system. The stress that best illustrates the intrinsic functions of the venous system is gravity. In the absence of reflex adjustments and skeletal muscle activity, a person who assumes the standing posture will create a hydrostatic force in the veins equivalent to the height of the column of blood between any point in the venous system and heart. In fact, venous pressure may rise to 90 mm Hg or higher. The same hydrostatic force will exist in the arterial system so that if mean aorta pressure at heart level is 100 mm Hg, arterial pressure in the feet will be 190 mm Hg. One consequence of this hydrostatic effect is that capillary pressure in the feet will increase markedly, promoting interstitial edema. Because veins are highly compliant, another consequence of this hydrostatic force is distention of the veins and pooling of blood outside of the thorax. The transfer of blood from central to peripheral venous compartments may be sufficiently great to cause a striking reduction in cardiac output and fainting. These hydrostatic effects of stationary standing can be completely abolished if the individual stands in a pool of water where water level is equal to heart level. The protective effect of standing in water occurs because the water outside the body exerts a hydrostatic force on the tissue and hence on the veins that is equal in magnitude but opposite in direction to that within the veins. Were it not for compensatory mechanisms, the intrinsic features of the venous system would render the human organism extraordinarily vulnerable to hydrostatic effects of gravity whenever the upright position was assumed. Except for those rare activities undertaken in water, the venous valves, the pumping effect of skeletal muscle activity, and reflexly mediated venoconstriction are critically important to maintenance of an adequate central volume and hence of cardiac output.

THE PULMONARY CIRCULATION

The lung provides an interface at which the entire cardiac output can be brought into gaseous equilibrium with alveolar air. Thus, the pulmonary circulation exists for the purpose of perfusion, but, unlike any component of the systemic circulation, pulmonary perfusion plays little or no nutritive role. The critical unit within the lung for gaseous exchange is the alveolar-capillary membrane. Each alveolus is an epithelium-lined air sac, 200 to 250 μ in diameter; there are about 300 million alveoli in the normal adult human lung. The total surface area of these alveolar sacs is in the range of 70 to 80 square meters. Precapillary vessels lead to a dense network of capillaries, each of which is 10 to 14 μ in length and 7 to 9 μ in diameter. The total surface area of these capillaries is 50 to 90 square meters. Each capillary is eccentrically incorporated into a septum, dividing alveoli so that one side of the capillary projects into the alveolus; the alveolar-capillary barrier is thin and adapted for gas exchange with alveolar air. The other side of the capillary is incorporated into an alveolar septum and the ultrastructure of this interface is thickened by a larger interstitial space, collagen, and elastic fibers. The thick side is now thought to be adapted principally for support and for water exchange between the capillary and interstitial space. The structure and function of the pulmonary circulation are described in greater detail in Section XI.

In the absence of intracardiac or extracardiac communications between the pulmonary and systemic circulations, pulmonary blood flow is equivalent to cardiac output. The driving force causing blood to flow through the lung is the pressure gradient between the pulmonary artery and the left atrium. Under normal resting conditions the mean pulmonary artery pressure is 12 to 15 mm Hg and mean left atrial pressure is 4 to 5 mm Hg. Simple inspection of these numbers reveals that the pressure gradient required to move the cardiac output through a normal lung is small when compared with the gradient required to move the cardiac output through the systemic vascular bed. Application of Poiseuille's law provides an estimate of the pulmonary vascular resistance of 200 to 400 dynes, whereas a similar calculation of systemic vascular resistance yields a value of 1000 to 1500 dynes. It is now generally believed that the low resistance to flow offered by the pulmonary circulation is attributable to its structure: small arterioles relatively devoid of a muscular media, a ratio of thickness to lumen size smaller than in systemic vessels, and absent precapillary sphincters. Hence, in the systemic circulation the pressure drop from artery to capillary is large and occurs predominantly at the arteriolar and precapillary level. In the lung, the pressure drop is small and is distributed more evenly along the vascular tree. Capillary flow in the systemic bed is nearly continuous; pulmonary capillary flow is clearly pulsatile.

Because the pulmonary circulation is a low pressure system, regional perfusion is susceptible to the influence of gravity. In the upright subject pulmonary blood flow is greatest at the bases of the lung and least at the apex. In this posture, the effect of gravity produces a relative increase in arterial and venous pressure at the base and causes dilatation of the vessels because of the increased transmural pressure (vascular-alveolar). At the apices gravity has the opposite effect, tending to reduce transmural pressure even to the point that vessels may collapse and flow cease. It follows that any influence that raises left atrial or pulmonary artery pressure (other than intrapulmonary obstruction) will reduce the degree to which pulmonary perfusion is nonuniform.

The pulmonary arteries, capillaries, and veins are highly distensible. Furthermore, in the normal state the pulmonary circulation operates at a low pressure, and at a relatively low point on its pressure-volume curve. The distensible nature of the pulmonary arteries enables these conduit vessels to accept the right ventricular stroke volume with a relatively small increase in pressure (that is, the pulse pressure is approximately 12 to 15 mm Hg). An increase in pulmonary blood flow causes a comparatively small increase in pulmonary arterial pressure, even during exercise or the large left-to-right shunts in atrial septal defect. When a major branch of the pulmonary artery is obstructed acutely pulmonary artery pressure rises only slightly, again because the resistance in remaining open channels decreases in response to the increase in flow. The effectiveness with which changes in transmural pressure can influence vascular resistance drops with inspiration and increases with expiration.

The volume of blood contained within the lung is normally about 270 ml/M² (body surface area) or approximately 10 per cent of the total blood volume. However, because of the variable capacitance of this highly distensible system, pulmonary blood volume can vary significantly in response to changes of posture, to changes of cardiac output, with expansion or contraction of total blood volume, and with positive or negative pressure breathing.

It would appear that the pulmonary circulation is in a vulnerable position, because it is in series between two pressure pumps, because it is a low pressure system and hence subject to external forces, and because of the large opportunity even under normal circumstances for mismatching of ventilation and perfusion. The fact is that the system operates with remarkable efficiency. Gaseous equilibrium between alveolar air and pulmonary capillary blood is achieved, or nearly so, the alveolar-arterial gradient for CO_2 being only 1 to 2 mm Hg and that for O_2 being only 5 to 10 mm Hg breathing ambient air at rest. Furthermore, these gradients do not increase significantly during exercise, which greatly enhances pulmonary blood flow, oxygen uptake, and CO_2 production. In essence, gaseous equilibrium is attributable largely to the fact that the lung has highly effective mechanisms for diverting flow away from alveoli that are underventilated, and to a very large capacity for alveolar-capillary exchange of CO_2 and O_2 in normally ventilated air spaces. To the extent that the alveolar ventilation-perfusion ratios are perturbed in one direction in any given zone of the lung, intrinsic control mechanisms tend to produce an equal but opposite exchange in other zones. The consequence is that the system is to a large extent self-correcting and in the absence of disease maintains alveolar-capillary gas equilibrium over a wide range of conditions.

THE CORONARY CIRCULATION

In the normal human heart there are two primary coronary arteries, the left and right, which arise from their respective sinuses of Valsalva. The left main coronary artery is usually 5 to 8 mm in diameter and varies in length from 1 to 2 mm to 1 to 1.5 cm. The left main coronary artery divides into two or three major branches: the anterior descending artery, which courses down the anterior interventricular groove, and the circumflex artery, which ascends in the left atrioventricular sulcus to the acute margin of the heart where it then descends over the left ventricle toward the apex; diagonal branches course over the left ventricle between the anterior descending and circumflex arteries. The right coronary artery descends in the right atrioventricular groove to the acute margin and in 90 per cent of cases continues around the acute margin to the crux and divides usually into two branches, which descend in the posterior interventricular groove toward the apex. Each major coronary artery gives rise to several epicardial branches. The anterior descending artery normally curves around the apex of the heart and is met in the lower third of the posterior interventricular groove by the posterior descending branch(es) of the right coronary artery.

The large epicardial vessels and their branches lead to other vessels that arise at right angles from the parent conduits and penetrate the ventricular walls. These penetrating arteries rapidly divide into two classes: those that quickly branch into a network that provides nutrient flow to the outer 60 to 70 per cent of the wall, and those that course through the wall to the endocardium with little or no change in diameter where they subdivide to form a looping arcade of anastomotic channels, the subendocardial plexus. The nutrient vessels to the subendocardial muscle—that is, the inner 20 to 30 per cent of the wall—arise from these arcades. These anatomical considerations are important because of the following: (a) there is a potential for interarterial anastomoses between epicardial arteries; (b) epicardial coronary arteries are essentially conduits; (c) perfusion of the outer two thirds and the inner one third of the ventricular wall arises from different branches of the epicardial vessels; (d) endocardial flow is derived from vessels that must course through the wall of the heart where they are subjected to intramural forces; and (e) within the subendocardium there is a second system, which provides the structure for interarterial anastomoses.

Three methods have thus far been employed in man to estimate total myocardial blood flow (that is, coronary artery flow). These include the nitrous oxide method, the isotope washout method, and continuous thermal dilution for measurement of blood flow in the coronary sinus. All three techniques have shown normal resting coronary blood flows in man of 70 to 100 ml/min/100 grams with an average of about 80 ml/min/100 grams of tissue. Since the normal weight of the heart in an average sized adult is 300 grams, total coronary blood flow is about 250 ml/min, or approximately 5 per cent of normal cardiac output.

Coronary artery blood flow decreases markedly, often approaching zero, during the isovolumic period of ventricular contraction. Flow increases abruptly but transiently with the onset of ventricular ejection and then plateaus or diminishes during the remainder of cardiac systole. With closure of the aortic valve coronary flow rises again to its maximum and then decreases gradually throughout the diastolic interval, generally paralleling the diastolic pressure in the aortic root. Under normal resting conditions, about 80 per cent of the total flow occurs during diastole and about 20 per cent during systole. The fact that blood flow is so much less during systole indicates that the intensity and duration of ventricular contraction have a marked effect on coronary flow.

The factors that are known to influence coronary blood flow and its distribution can be conveniently viewed under four major headings: (1) autoregulatory, (2) metabolic, (3) physical, and (4) neural. When coronary artery perfusion pressure is abruptly changed in either direction, there is a sudden increase or decrease in coronary flow that is roughly proportional to the change in pressure. When this new pressure is maintained, flow gradually returns toward normal. This phenomenon is referred to as *autoregulation,* and the net consequence is that the steady-state pressure-flow relationship is nearly flat in the range of perfusion pressures from 60 to 120 mm Hg. The precise mechanisms responsible for autoregulation are unknown.

The *metabolic activity of the heart* is the most important determinant of coronary blood flow of the normal heart. When myocardial work or contractility is varied over wide ranges (by changing stroke volume, heart rate, aortic pressure, or cardiac sympathetic tone), the relation between coronary blood flow (ml/100 grams/min) and myocardial oxygen consumption (ml/100 grams/min) is nearly linear (Fig. 10). Whether the final determinant of coronary vascular resistance is pO_2 per se or some other agent related to the pO_2, it is clear that coupling between coronary flow and myocardial metabolic activity involves tissue pO_2. At normal oxygen tensions changes in wall tension, the rate of development of wall tension, and heart rate dominate in the control of coronary vascular resistance. Adenosine, formed by the hydrolysis of cyclic AMP, is a potent coronary vasodilator and plays an important role in the coronary vasodilatation induced by hypoxia or brief periods of coronary occlusion and reperfusion (that is, reactive hyperemia).

Physical forces play an important role in coronary regulation because of the penetrating transmural coronary blood vessels. During systole, wall stress exceeds cavity pressure and impedes flow in transmural arteries. The coronary flow that does occur in systole is confined to the epicardial layers, where wall stress is the least. In diastole, the stress acting on the penetrating arteries is removed, coronary perfusion pressure exceeds wall stress, and flow reaches a maximal value. Since total flow to epicardial and endocardial zones is nearly equal, resistance in endocardial vessels must be lower than in vessels supplying the epicardium in diastole. However, when diastolic wall stress is enhanced—for example, in severe aortic insufficiency or aortic stenosis with marked hypertrophy—the effect of this stress on transmural vessels may exceed the dilating capacity of endocardial vessels and a state of endocardial underperfusion develops. This situation is exaggerated by tachycardia, which shortens the diastolic interval per beat. Thus, physical factors may become dominant in determining endocardial flow and the endocardial:epicardial flow ratio. In the chapter on coronary heart disease these considerations are discussed in greater detail.

Neural mechanisms also influence the coronary arterial bed. Sympathetic nerve activity has been demonstrated to cause coronary vasoconstriction through an alpha receptor mechanism. There is also a sympathetic coronary vasodilator mechanism mediated through beta receptors. These mechanisms are to a large degree overshadowed by the effects of sympathetic nerve activity on myocardial function and oxygen consumption. Thus, stimulation of sympathetic nerves to the intact working heart may increase coronary blood flow and decrease coronary resistance through a mechanism discussed above whereby flow is coupled to metabolic activity. In paced, fibrillating, or arrested hearts, stimulation of cardiac vagal afferent

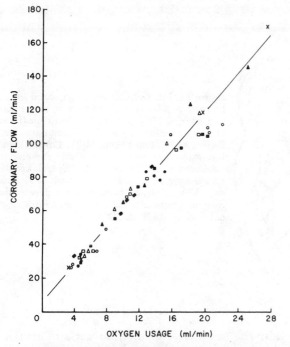
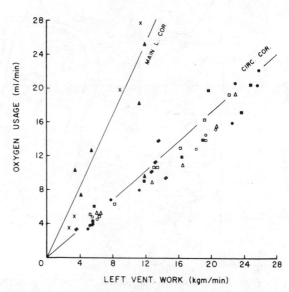

Figure 10. Graphs showing the relationship of coronary flow to oxygen usage (left), and the relationship of oxygen usage to left ventricular work (right). (With permission from Khouri, E. M., Gregg, D. E., and Rayford, C. R.: Effect of exercise on cardiac output, left coronary flow and myocardial metabolism in the unanesthetized dog. Circ Res 17:436, 1965.)

nerves increases coronary blood flow and decreases coronary vascular resistance. This vasodilatation is cholinergically mediated and can be blocked with atropine. Despite this indisputable evidence of neural innervation of the coronary circulation, its role in modulating coronary flow in the intact animal and man is uncertain and there is currently little, if any, clear evidence that alterations in innervation of the coronary vessels play a role in human disease.

REFERENCES

Berne, R. M., and Rubio, R.: Coronary circulation. In Berne, R. M., Sperelakis, N., and Geiger, S. R. (eds.): Handbook of Physiology. Vol. I, Heart. Section 2, Cardiovascular System. Bethesda, Md., American Physiological Society, 1979, p. 873.

Cobb, F. R., Bache, R. J., and Greenfield, J. C., Jr.: Regional myocardial blood flow in awake dogs. J Clin Invest 53:1618, 1974.

Downey, J. M., Downey, H. F., and Kirk, E. S.: Effects of myocardial strains on coronary blood flow. Circ Res 34:286, 1974.

Fishman, A. P.: Dynamics of the pulmonary circulation. In Hamilton and Dow (eds.): Handbook of Physiology. Section 2, Circulation, Vol. II, Bethesda, Md., American Physiological Society, 1963, p. 1667.

Garlick, D. G., and Renkin, E. M.: Transport of large molecules from plasma to interstitial fluid and lymph in dogs. Am J Physiol 219:1595, 1970.

McDonald, D. A.: Blood Flow in Arteries. Baltimore, Williams and Wilkins Co., 1960.

Spencer, M. P., and Greiss, F. C.: Dynamics of ventricular ejection. Circ Res 10:274, 1962.

Excitation of the Heart

Although the function of the normal heart is influenced by neurogenic and other external factors, a heart that has been separated completely from these influences continues to beat in a regular, rhythmic, and coordinated manner. From an electrophysiological point of view, therefore, the fundamental properties of excitability, impulse initiation, and propagation are intrinsic characteristics of cardiac tissues. The heart is composed of several types of tissues, and although they possess many similarities, there are important structural and functional differences. The cells of the heart can be divided into two general subgroups: the first, ordinary working myocardium responsible for the pumping action of the heart; the second, specialized tissues responsible for initiating the cardiac impulse and determining the sequence of excitation of working muscle (Fig. 11).

The property of spontaneous impulse formation is referred to as *automaticity*. Numerous regions throughout the specialized conduction system are capable of automatic behavior under normal physiological conditions. However, the frequency of impulse formation is

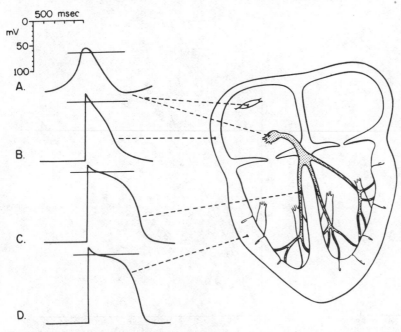

Figure 11. Intracellular action potential shapes at various sites in the heart. A = Sinus node and AV node; B = atrium; C = Purkinje tissue; D = ventricular muscle. (With permission from Scher, A. M., and Spach, M. S.: Cardiac depolarization and repolarization and the electrocardiogram. In Berne, R. M., Sperelakis, N., and Geiger, S. R. (eds.): Handbook of Physiology. Vol. 1, Heart. Section 2, Cardiovascular System. Bethesda, Md., American Physiological Society, 1979, p. 358.)

greatest in the region of the sinoatrial node, and for this reason the sinus node normally functions as the pacemaker of the heart.

In the ventricles, specialized cells called *Purkinje fibers* are organized into a system that programs the sequence of activation of working muscle. Purkinje cells and their organization confer upon the system the property of high conduction velocity. The Purkinje system rapidly distributes the electrical impulse to endocardial shells of both ventricles, and subsequent activation of the large mass of working ventricular muscle is responsible for generating the QRS complex on the surface electrocardiogram (Fig. 12). In general, the form of the QRS complex is determined by the sequence of ventricular activation and by the respective mass of the two ventricles.

The atrial chambers are thin-walled and contain orifices for the entrance of systemic and pulmonary veins. Specialized fibers resembling Purkinje cells are found in the atria, but they are not organized into specialized tracts or bundles to the extent observed

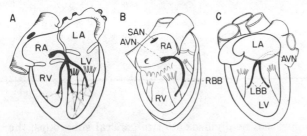

Figure 12. Distribution of the AV conduction system in the heart. SAN = Sinoatrial node; AVN = AV node; RBB = right bundle branch; LBB = left bundle branch; RA = right atrium; LA = left atrium; RV = right ventricle; LV = left ventricle. *A,* Frontal view. *B,* View from right. *C,* View from left. (With permission from Scher, A. M., and Spach, M. S.: Cardiac depolarization and repolarization and the electrocardiogram. In Berne, R. M., Sperelakis, N., and Geiger, S. R. (eds.): Handbook of Physiology. Vol. 1, Heart. Section 2, Cardiovascular System. Bethesda, Md., American Physiological Society, 1979, p. 358.)

within the ventricles. Rather, in certain locations working atrial musculature becomes more densely packed and longitudinally oriented, creating routes of preferential impulse propagation at a velocity greater than observed in thinner, less organized parts of the atrial chambers. The velocity of conduction over these preferred routes does not approach that in the Purkinje system of the ventricles. Activation of the atrial musculature is responsible for the P wave on the surface electrocardiogram. The morphology of the P wave is determined by the sequence of atrial activation, which in turn is determined primarily by the site of impulse formation within the sinoatrial (SA) node located in the right atrium. A second factor in the morphology of the P wave is the relative mass of the two atria. Finally, the preferential routes of atrial propagation play an important role in intra-atrial conduction, influencing the conduction time from sinus node to atrioventricular (AV) node and from sinus node to left atrium.

The *atrioventricular node* is the only normal avenue over which an impulse can be transmitted from atrium to ventricle. In addition, it has a number of unique structural and functional properties, the most important of which is its exceedingly slow conduction velocity. The long time required for conduction through the atrioventricular node is responsible for the delay between atrial and ventricular activation, the P-R interval of the electrocardiogram (Fig. 13).

CELLULAR PHYSIOLOGY

In nearly all cells of the body there is a difference in the electrical voltage between the inside and outside of the cell, the so-called membrane potential. In excitable cells, an appropriate stimulus leads to a change in membrane properties as a consequence of which ions flow across the membrane and elicit an action potential. When excitable cells are connected by couplings that offer a low resistance to the flow of current, an action potential elicited in one cell is capable of

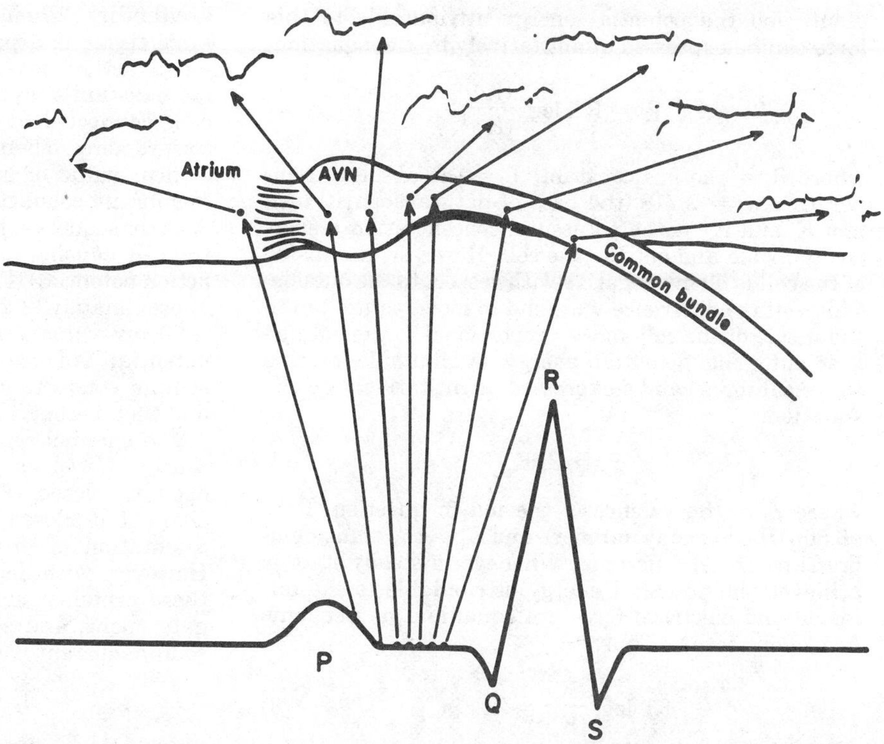

Figure 13. Excitation sequence of the lower atrium, AV node (AVN), and common bundle within the P-R segment of the surface electrocardiogram. (With permission from Scher, A. M., and Spach, M. S.: Cardiac depolarization and repolarization and the electrocardiogram. In Berne, R. M., Sperelakis, N., and Geiger, S. R. (eds.): Handbook of Physiology. Vol. 1, Heart. Section 2, Cardiovascular System. Bethesda, Md., American Physiological Society, 1979, p. 363.)

being transmitted to another and to another—that is, conducted. Nerve and heart are examples of excitable cells over which impulse conduction can occur. To appreciate the basis for excitation of the heart and for functional differences between ordinary working myocardium and the specialized conduction system, it is essential to have a working concept of the electrophysiology of the cardiac cell. This concept is in turn based upon an understanding of the electrical properties of the membrane that separates the inside and outside of the cell, the forces that influence the distribution of ions across the cell membrane, and the changes in the properties of the membrane that develop when it is excited.

Each myocardial cell is surrounded by an envelope referred to as the sarcolemma, composed of its unit membrane (the plasmalemma) and its basement membrane (the glycocalyx). The basement membrane is 400 to 500 Å in thickness and contains principally negatively charged glycoproteins. The unit membrane consists of a lipid bilayer matrix 50 to 100 Å in thickness and contains protein molecules embedded in this matrix. Some of these proteins protrude through the entire bilayer and are associated with channels through which ions move during an action potential, and with membrane activities such as the Na^+-K^+–linked ion pump. Other proteins are located principally on the inner surface of the bilayer, protrude only partially into the lipid bilayer, and are associated with specific enzyme activities such as adenylate cyclase. Still other proteins are located on the outside of the membrane, project partially into the lipid bilayer, and serve as receptor sites for various transmitters, hormones, and drugs. The lipid bilayer is in a fluid state that allows the membrane proteins to move or float from one area to another, and together the components of the unit membrane represent the boundary or site of polarization between the inside and outside of the resting cardiac cell.

A difference in the concentration of ions between the inside and outside of resting cardiac cell is created by an energy-dependent active ion transport mechanism. The major ion pump transports sodium out of the cell linked with an obligatory transport of potassium into the cell. The disequilibrium of ions that is known to exist between the inside and outside of the cell has two principal features. First, there are large differences in the concentration of ions across the membrane; second, there is a transmembrane difference in electrical potential.

Ions in solution tend to migrate from regions of higher concentration to regions of lower concentration. Hence, differences in ionic concentration represent a passive diffusion force that will tend to promote ionic movement. The magnitude of this force is proportional to the concentration gradient. For ionized particles, movement is also affected by electrical forces. In a resting cardiac cell, the intracellular space has a negative potential of approximately 90 mv relative to the extracellular space. This difference in electrical potential acts as a second passive force so that positively charged ions tend to migrate to the inside of the cell and negatively charged ions are repelled from the inside. The potential energy of any given ion on either the inside or outside of the cell membrane is the result of diffusion and electrical forces. When the potential energy with respect to a given ion is the same inside and outside the cell, no net movement will occur and the inside and outside of the cell are said to be in a steady state with respect to the ion in question. The transmembrane potential that would exactly counteract a diffusion force attributable to a difference in concentration across the membrane during steady state is referred to as the equilibrium potential for that ion.

Potassium exists at a concentration 30 times greater on the inside of the sarcolemma than on the outside. The diffusion force tending to move potassium out of the cell (P_c) is proportional to the concentration gradient, and the potential energy attributable to this force can be expressed quantitatively by the equation:

$$P_c = RT \log_e \frac{(K_i)}{(K_o)} \qquad (1)$$

where R = the gas constant, T = the absolute temperature, e = 2.718 (the base of natural logarithms), and K_i and K_o = the potassium concentration respectively inside and outside the cell. However, the inside of the cell is 90 mv negative with respect to the outside. This voltage difference will tend to move potassium to the inside of the cell and is proportional to the voltage gradient. The potential energy attributable to this electrical force can be expressed quantitatively by the equation:

$$P_e = ZFE_m \qquad (2)$$

where Z = the valence of the ion in question, F = 96,500 (the Faraday number), and E_m = the transmembrane potential difference. Whenever a steady state is achieved the potential energy attributable to the diffusion and electrical force are equal and no net ionic movement occurs. Thus:

$$RT \log_e \frac{(K_i)}{(K_o)} = ZFE_m \qquad (3)$$

or at 37° C:

$$E_k = 61.5 \log_{10} \frac{(K_i)}{(K_o)} \qquad (4)$$

This is the Nernst equation, which describes the membrane potential that must exist for potassium to be in equilibrium across the membrane of a resting cardiac cell. Whenever membrane potential is constant the sum of all ionic currents across the membrane must equal zero. Furthermore, ionic movement across the cell membrane is related not only to the concentration gradient but also to the permeability of the membrane to the ion in question. These considerations lead to a more general description of membrane voltage, the Hodgkin and Katz modification of Goldman's constant field equation, where:

$$V_m = \frac{RT}{F} \log \left(\frac{P_K K_i + P_{Na} Na_i + P_{Cl} Cl_o \dots}{P_K K_o + P_{Na} Na_o + P_{Cl} Cl_i \dots} \right) \qquad (5)$$

When equation 4 is solved using known values for intracellular and extracellular K^+ concentration, E_K = −90 mv, which is nearly identical to the observed membrane potential across the resting cell. These observations suggest that the potassium equilibrium potential is the major factor responsible for resting transmembrane potential. If equation 4 is solved for the sodium equilibrium potential, a value of +50 mv is obtained. Since this is oppositely directed and far from the observed resting membrane potential it is very unlikely that the Na potential contributes to resting potential. The explanation lies in equation 5 if we assume that the resting membrane is permeable to potassium but less permeable to sodium. Solution of equation 5 gives a V_m of −90 mv — that is, the equilibrium potential for K^+.

An important characteristic of heart cells is their excitability. When a local area of myocardium or Purkinje tissue is depolarized (by a stimulus or a propagated action potential), the membrane potential at more distant sites within the same cell and in adjacent cells connected by low resistance couplings is moved toward zero. When the membrane potential reaches a critical value of approximately −65 mv (threshold), membrane conductance to sodium increases abruptly. As a consequence, positively charged sodium ions enter the cell, causing further depolarization (phase 0 of the action potential) (Fig. 14). Membrane potential reaches approximately +20 mv, but never quite equals the +50 mv value predicted by the sodium equilibrium potential. This is because activation of the channel for sodium conductances lasts only a millisecond or two and then becomes at least partially inactivated.

The channel regulating sodium conductance is currently viewed as regulated by a "gate" that can be open or closed (Fig. 14, lower panel). The sodium channel is closed in the resting fiber owing to the orientation of proteins that make up the channel. However, with depolarization to the threshold value, these proteins undergo a conformational change, the gate opens, and sodium rapidly enters the cell. The sodium current is described by the equation:

$$I_{Na} = gNa (V_M - V_{Na})$$

where gNa = the sodium conductance of the channel and V_m and V_{Na} = the membrane potential and the sodium equilibrium potential, respectively. The actual sodium current at any time is governed by the variable parameter gNa, which according to the Hodgkin-Huxley model is described by the equation:

$$gNa = \bar{g} Na\ m^3 h$$

This latter equation expresses the idea that sodium conductance is determined by two channel properties: $\bar{g}Na$, the maximal conductance when all channels are open; and m^3h, which is a kinetic term describing the gating mechanism or the probability that a channel will be open at a particular membrane potential and time. In the kinetic term m^3 represents the voltage-dependent activation of sodium conductance (opening the gate) and h is the voltage- and time-dependent inactivation of sodium conductance (i.e., closing the gate).

Assume, for illustrative purposes, that at a resting potential of −90 mv, h = 1 (open) and m = 0 (closed). With depolarization m changes very rapidly to 1 and the channel is maximally open. Once the cell is depolarized h changes more slowly from 1 to 0, reducing the value m^3 h and hence gNa.

There is a second and much more slowly inactivated inward current that appears to contribute to the plateau of the action potential in cardiac fibers. Recent evidence suggests that this inward current develops about 20 msec after phase 0 of the action potential and is attributable largely to movements of calcium ions and perhaps to a lesser extent to additional inward sodium movements. Abnormal action potentials arising solely from this second slow inward current can be observed in Purkinje and muscle fibers after depolarization to levels of −65 to −75 mv (which inactivates the fast sodium channel) or in fibers in which the fast sodium channel has been blocked specifically by an

Figure 14. A schematic diagram of a cardiac action potential is shown at top, and the events that determine the time voltage course of the action potential are shown in the lower diagram. When the cell is quiescent (phase 4), its membrane is much more permeable to potassium than any other ion, so that its resting transmembrane voltage is near the potassium equilibrium potential (V_k). At excitation (O), the cell membrane suddenly becomes permeable to sodium; the intense inward sodium current carries sufficient positive charge into the cell to carry the transmembrane voltage to a value near the sodium equilibrium potential (V_{Na}). In the several phases of repolarization (1 through 3), changes in transmembrane action potential initially reflect the decreasing sodium conductance and subsequently the marked increase from outside to inside is controlled by a two component sodium channel, m and h, which appear to work in opposition to each other. With sufficient depolarization, activation of the m site permits rapid influx of sodium. In succeeding phases of the depolarization-repolarization cycle, sodium conductance is decreased by closure of the h site; in phase 4 the sodium-carrying system is again available and awaiting activation. (With permission from Bigger, J. T.: Antiarrhythmic drugs in ischemic heart disease. In Braunwald, E. (ed.): The Myocardium: Failure and Infarction. New York, HP Publishing Co., Inc., 1974, p. 296.)

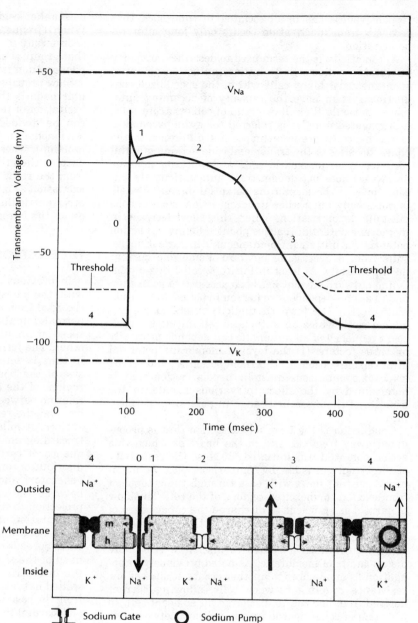

agent such as tetrodotoxin (TTX). Catecholamines are known to facilitate calcium entry and to augment the slow inward current, whereas specific slow channel blocking drugs attenuate inward calcium movement and the slow current. An important difference between sinus and atrioventricular node cells on the one hand, and working muscle and Purkinje cells on the other, may be a relative or absolute absence of rapid sodium channels in the former. Such an absence could account for certain of the characteristics of the action potential in sinoatrial and atrioventricular node cells, their insensitivity to TTX and their sensitivity to agents thought to block the slow channel selectively.

Following the plateau of the action potential, potassium conductance, which had been reduced by depolarization and remained low during the plateau, returns to its higher level. This rising potassium conductance allows potassium to move out of the cell ($I_K = gK [V_m - V_K]$) and as a consequence of the egress of positively charged K^+, the cell repolarizes.

Recall that the variables m and h, which determine rapid sodium conductance, were reversed from their normal values as a consequence of depolarization, and that the membrane is unresponsive during the plateau. As the membrane repolarizes, the values of m and h, which are dependent on membrane potential and time, return to the levels that existed before depolarization. These variables follow membrane potential closely, but that recovery of h is probably dependent on both V_m and time. Under normal circumstances, recovery of the sodium-carrying system is closely coupled to repolarization. However, under the influence of a number of agents, including reduced temperature and drugs that alter the kinetics of h, repolarization and recovery of responsiveness can be dissociated in time such that recovery from inactivation occurs only long after repolarization.

Automaticity is the term used to describe a property of certain cardiac cells to initiate an action potential spontaneously. Many cells within the specialized conducting system have the capacity of becoming automatic, but only the cell or group of cells that initiates a propagated impulse is referred to as the pacemaker of the heart. There is an important difference in the characteristics of the transmembrane action potential recorded from automatic cells and working myocardium that does not demonstrate automaticity. In automatic cells the membrane potential during diastole is not steady but rather undergoes slow spontaneous diastolic depolarization. When this slow decrease in membrane potential reaches about -60 mv, an action potential is initiated. Spontaneous depolarization results from a decreasing outward membrane current during diastole. At least in Purkinje cells, this diminishing outward current has been ascribed to potassium and to a time-dependent reduction in potassium permeability (gK). The term rhythmicity refers to the frequency with which an automatic cell initiates impulses. Frequency of an automatic cell depends primarily on three factors: (1) the level of membrane potential after repolarization, (2) threshold potential, and (3) the slope of spontaneous diastolic depolarization that is determined by the effects of various agents on the kinetics of the diastolic change in potassium permeability.

Conduction is the term for excitation that is propagated away from the site in the heart at which this action potential was initiated. Because the resistivity of the cytoplasm is low by comparison with the membrane, current flows with ease through the cytoplasm from excited to unexcited regions of the cell. This flow of current is sufficient to discharge the capacitance of distal membrane and hence to bring the membrane to threshold, where its resistance drops, allowing more inward current as a source to discharge still more distant units of membrane. As noted previously, propagation from one fiber to another occurs at sites of low resistance coupling between cells, allowing current derived from one cell to discharge an adjacent cell. In a system of cells, the conduction velocity between two points in the system will be influenced by the dimension and geometry of the cells, by the nature and frequency of connections, by the passive or cable properties of the fiber, by the threshold potential, and by the amplitude and velocity of phase 0 of the action potential. Assuming that the individual cells that make up a system are normal, a strong case has been made for the fact that differences in apparent conduction velocity in different regions of the heart are attributable primarily to geometry and to the nature and frequency of intercellular connections.

During normal rhythm, impulse formation takes place in the sinoatrial node. For several reasons, the sinus node acts as the pacemaker, dominating other potentially automatic regions of the specialized conduction system. One reason for this dominance is that impulses formed in the sinus node are initiated at a greater frequency than other latent pacemakers and spread of the impulse from the node discharges these other latent pacemaker cells before their own inherent charge. A second factor is the interaction between pacemaker regions of different inherent rhythmicity. When a frequency of excitation greater than that which is inherent to one group of cells is superimposed on that group, their own rate of firing is suppressed. This phenomenon is referred to as overdrive suppression.

Slow propagation of the impulse at the atrioventricular node is the basis for the normal delay between excitation of the atria and of the ventricles. The node can be divided functionally into three regions: AN (atrionodal junction), N (nodal), and NH (nodal-His junction). These regions progress from superficial to deep as the atrioventricular junctional zone is viewed from the right atrium; they represent the sequence of excitation as a normal impulse propagates through the atrioventricular junction. Conduction velocity is slowest in the N region.

THE ELECTROCARDIOGRAM

In previous sections of this chapter we have dealt with the physiological basis of the action potential recorded from single cardiac cells, with mechanisms of normal impulse formation, and determinants of the speed of impulse propagation from one region to another. The form of the electrocardiogram at any point in time is determined by the location, geometry, and size of the boundary between excited and unexcited regions of the heart and the factors that influence the relation between the potential difference at this boundary and the resulting potential at points on the body surface. It follows that an understanding of the electrocardiogram depends upon a knowledge of the sequence of cardiac excitation, the resulting potential distribution on the surface of the heart (that is, the generator), and the factors that determine the relation between the epicardial potential distribution and its projection to the body surface.

Excitation of the atrium begins in the region of the sinus node high in the right atrium. The excitation wave spreads outward over the right atrium, from the head of the sinus node into the left atrium, and down the interatrial septum (Fig. 15). Because of the thin-walled nature of all three of these structures, the wave front is best viewed as a surface phenomenon, with endocardial to epicardial spread an insignificant factor in determining P wave morphology. As noted previously, there are areas of preferential impulse propagation in the atrial walls and septum. Hence, the advancing wave front on any one of these surfaces is irregular, with projecting pseudopods of early activity and valleys of delayed trailing excitation. However, because of the location of the sinus node the overall direction of the wave front is downward and from right to left. During the earliest portions of the P wave the dominant wave front is advancing down the right atrial wall along the sulcus terminalis. Very shortly thereafter, two widely separate activation fronts develop, one in the lower portion of the right atrial free wall and the second in the upper portion of the left atrium near the entrance of the pulmonary veins. While these two excitation waves persist, activity begins in the central portion of the atrial septum spreading toward the region of the atrioventricular node. Finally, the terminal portion of the P wave is attributable to complex and colliding wave fronts in the posterior and inferior regions of the left atrium.

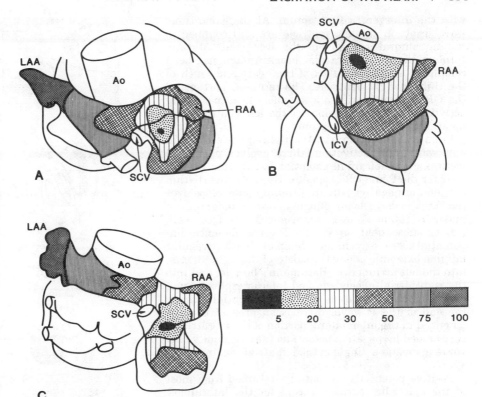

Figure 15. Normal activation sequence of the human atrium. *A*, Superior view of the right atrium and the interatrial band. *B*, Posterior view of the right atrium. *C*, The right atrium and interatrial band of a second heart. (Adapted from Durrer, D., Dam, R. T. van, Freud, G. E., Janse, M. J., Meijler, F. L., and Arzbaecher, R. C.: Total excitation of the isolated human heart. Circulation 41:908, 1970.)

Ventricular activation proceeds in an orderly sequence (from apex to base) as might be expected from the anatomic distribution of the Purkinje system (Fig. 16). Initial excitation begins on the left surface of the septum near the apex, producing a wave front directed from left to right and from posterior to anterior in the chest because of the plane of the septum. This is followed within a few milliseconds by activation of the endocardial surface of the right ventricle near the apex. Within 5 to 10 msec of the onset of the QRS complex the impulse has spread rapidly over the Purkinje network, and there are shells of depolarized endocardial muscle that encircle the cavities of both right and left ventricles. These shells are closed near the apex, but they are open posteriorly and near the base. Fusion of these shells progresses up the septum from apex to base, which actively spreads in an endocardial or epicardial direction in the free wall of each ventricle. By 10 to 15 msec, excitation reaches the epicardial surface of the anterior right ventricle at its margin

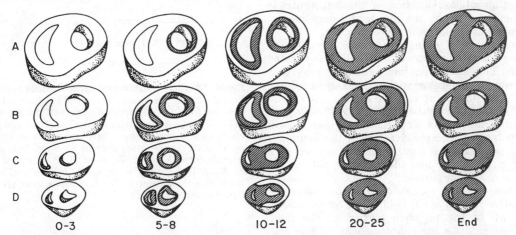

Figure 16. A map of the sequence of ventricular activation in the dog. Activation is depicted for four sections of the heart from base to apex (A to D) and at five periods between the onset (0 to 3) and the end (End) of activation. The cavity of the right ventricle is shown on the left of each section, and the cavity of the left ventricle is shown on the right of each section. The boundary between excited tissue and tissue not yet excited is depicted by a heavy line. The volume of muscle already excited at the end of each period is depicted by the cross-hatched areas. Note the initial activity along the left septal surface and the endocardial surface of the right ventricle in 0 to 3 (C and D). The last area to be excited is at the posterior aspect of the base of the intraventricular septum in (End-A). (With permission from Wallace, A. G.: Electrophysiology of the myocardium. In Gordon, B. L., Carleton, R. A., and Faber, L. P. (eds.): Clinical Cardiopulmonary Physiology. 3rd ed. New York, Grune and Stratton, 1969, p. 181.)

with the interventricular septum. At the same time, wave fronts in the left ventricle are still confined to the intramural portions of the free wall. Midway through the QRS, epicardial breakthrough has been completed around the apex of the heart and much of the thinner right ventricle. The terminal portions of the QRS complex arise almost solely from persisting activity in the basal regions of the left ventricle and upper interventricular septum.

From these considerations of the sequence of atrial and ventricular activation, there evolves a general picture of the epicardial potential distribution responsible for the P and QRS complex. During sinus rhythm a region of negative potential (minima) develops over the sinus node with surrounding positive potentials of maximal intensity over the right atrial free wall. During subsequent parts of the P wave the epicardial potentials are exceedingly complex, with irregular minima extending along the sulcus of the right atrium, into the left atrium over Bachmann's bundle, and into the right atrial appendage and inferior right atrium, each surrounded by areas of positive potential. During the end of the P wave, there is an area of positive potential in the inferolateral portion of the left atrium, surrounded by negative potentials that gradually converge upon and extinguish the left atrial maxima (Fig. 17).

Positive potentials are initially recorded from most of the epicardial surface (except for the lateral left ventricle) during ventricular activation. The maximal positive potential (maxima) is over the anterior right ventricle. With the onset of epicardial breakthrough over the right ventricle, negative potentials are recorded from the surface of the right ventricle and positive potentials from the left ventricle, and the maxima is on the diaphragmatic surface of the left ventricle. The area of negative potential then expands over both ventricles, generally from apex to base, leaving a positive potential only over the lateral left ventricle. Finally, a positive potential maxima over the posterolateral-basal portion of the left ventricle becomes extinguished by the converging negative potentials owing to epicardial breakthrough.

Whenever areas of voltage difference exist on the epicardial surface, an electrical field will be generated in the body. The heart, therefore, can be considered as a current source (generator) within the body (a volume conductor). At any point in time during activation, regions of epicardium not yet depolarized have a positive potential and areas already depolarized have a negative potential. The positive side of the boundary separating polarized and depolarized regions acts as a source for current flow and the negative side of the boundary is a sink for current.

On the body surface, regions close to the source are in the positive portion of the field, while areas close to the sink are in the negative portion of the field. Because the body is a three-dimensional volume conductor rather than a plane, all points of equal potential on the surface of the volume describe an equipotential surface. The regions of maximal positive potential at any instant are opposite the source, and the regions of maximal negative potential are opposite the sink. Surrounding these maxima and minima are concentric regions of equal potential, but as the distance from source and sink respectively increases, the current

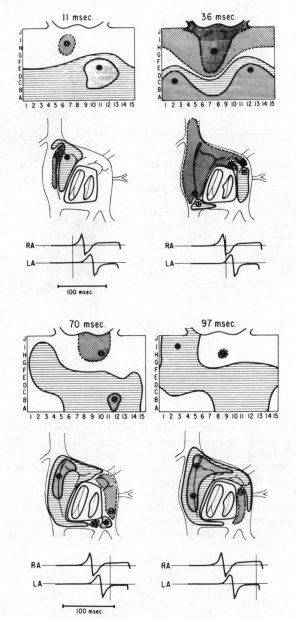

Figure 17. Body surface and atrial surface potential distributions during the sequence of atrial excitation (P wave). The data are from a dog heart during normal sinus rhythm. Upper panel includes body surface, atrial surface, and RA and LA electrograms at 11 msec (left) and 36 msec (right). Lower panel contains the same data at 70 msec (left) and 97 msec (right). (From King, T. D., Barr, R. C., Herman-Giddens, G. S., Boaz, D. E., and Spach, M. S.: Isopotential body surface maps and their relationship to atrial potentials in the dog. Circ Res 30:396, 1972.)

density and hence the magnitude of the potential decreases toward zero. Because the location of maxima and minima on the epicardium changes during the process of excitation, and they also change in size, the field created in the volume conductor changes in strength and in position. Accordingly, at a point on the body surface, the potential with respect to any other point varies in sign and amplitude throughout excitation. The sign of the potential will be positive if the recording point faces the source, and negative if it faces the sink. The amplitude of the potential, positive or negative, will be determined by the distance of the recording point from the source or sink and the conductivity of the tissues between the electrode and the source of potential.

In general, because atrial activation starts in the sinus node and progresses over the atria and septum toward the atrioventricular valves, the sinoatrial node region is a sink and the atrial margins of the atrioventricular rings act as a source. Hence, the right shoulder tends to be in the negative portion of the field throughout most of atrial activation, and the left lower chest is in the positive portion of the field (Fig. 17). Hence, the P wave is upright in electrocardiographic leads I, II, III, AVF, and V2-V6.

With ventricular activation the initial situation is one of left-to-right activation in the septum, producing positive potentials over the right anterior chest and negative potentials over the left shoulder and back. Subsequently, with epicardial breakthrough over the right ventricle, the maximum positive potentials move to the left side of the chest and negative potentials develop over the right arm and right anterior chest. Finally, as epicardial breakthrough develops over the apex of the left ventricle, the lower chest develops negative potentials and maximum positive potentials shift to the left shoulder and back. This sequence produces a QRS complex that is predominantly positive in leads II, III, AVF, and V4-V6, and predominantly negative in AVR and V1. The alterations of P or of QRS as a consequence of disease reflect primarily changes in the orientation and/or strength of the electrical field on the body surface, secondary to either delayed activation or hypertrophy of individual cardiac chambers. Lastly, because of the sequence of excitation, it is not surprising that specific delays or hypertrophy of individual chambers typically alter either the initial or terminal portions of P and QRS.

In ventricular muscle, the action potential has a duration of 250 to 300 msec and a plateau phase during which membrane potential is relatively stable in a depolarized state. Yet, the entire process of ventricular activation and inscription of the QRS complex is completed in 80 to 90 msec. As a consequence, there is an interval of time after the QRS when nearly all myocardial cells are in the same state of depolarization, when the difference in potential between regions of the heart is negligible, and no appreciable electrical field is created; hence there is little or no recordable potential difference between recording sites on the body surface. This interval corresponds to the relatively isoelectric period (the ST segment) on the EKG separating the end of QRS and the onset of T. When individual cells enter the phase of rapid repolarization (phase 3 of the action potential) a situation again exists in which regions of the heart in different stages of repolarization create boundaries of potential difference; a consequent electrical field in the volume conductor and resulting potential difference recorded during the repolarization process is referred to as the T wave. Generally, the amplitude of the T wave is less than that of QRS because the strength of the boundary

potential is always somewhat less than during excitation, where inactive cells are at -90 mv and depolarized cells are at $+10$ to 20 mv. The duration of the T wave is greater than that of QRS because repolarization is of much longer duration than depolarization and because the process of repolarization does not appear to be propagated; hence, cells repolarize at their own intrinsic rate. An interesting feature of repolarization is that the process seems to start later and last longer in endocardial than in epicardial muscle. As a consequence, the sequence of recovery is more or less opposite to the sequence of excitation. If the sequence of repolarization were the same as depolarization one would expect the T wave to be directed opposite to QRS in most EKG leads. The fact that the sequence of repolarization is actually the reverse of excitation is felt to explain the characteristic feature of the normal EKG, in which the polarity of QRS and T is the same in most leads. Recent studies have shown that during repolarization a maxima of positive potential develops early in the T wave over the anterior right ventricle with negativity recorded over the atria and only the posterior base of the left ventricle. Positive potentials persist over the anterior surface of right and left ventricles throughout the T wave with the maxima moving superiorly and then simply collapsing at the end of T as surrounding areas drop toward zero potential and engulf the maxima. Just as changes in the sequence of excitation will cause changes in the morphology of the QRS complex, changes in the sequence of recovery will account for changes in the morphology of the T wave. Drugs and electrolyte changes have their principal effect on the T wave.

REFERENCES

Bigger, J. T., Jr.: Electrical properties of cardiac muscle and possible causes of cardiac arrhythmias. In Dreifus, L. S., and Likoff, W. (eds): Cardiac Arrhythmias. Hahnemann Symposium #25. New York, Grune and Stratton, 1973, p. 13.

Carmeliet, E., and Vereecke, J.: Electrogenesis of the action potential and automaticity. In Berne, R. M., Sperelakis, N., and Geiger, S. R. (eds.): Handbook of Physiology. Vol. 1, Heart. Section 2, Cardiovascular System. Bethesda, Md., American Physiological Society, 1979, p. 269.

Durrer, D., van Dam, R. T., Freud, G. E., Janse, M. J., Meijler, F. L., and Arzbaecher, R. C.: Total excitation of the isolated human heart. Circulation 41:899, 1970.

Lieberman, M., Kootsey, J. M., Johnson, E. A., and Sawanobori, T.: Slow conduction in cardiac muscle. Biophys J 13:37, 1973.

Noble, D.: The Initiation of the Heart Beat. Oxford, England, Clarendon Press, 1975.

Spach, M. S., Barr, R. C., Lanning, C. F., and Tucek, P. C.: Origin of body surface QRS and T wave potentials from epicardial potential distributions in the intact chimpanzee. Circulation 55:268, 1977.

Sperelakis, N.: Origin of the cardiac resting potential. In Berne, R. M., Sperelakis, N., and Geiger, S. R., (eds.): Handbook of Physiology. Vol. 1, Heart. Section 2, Cardiovascular System. Bethesda, Md., American Physiological Society, 1979, p. 187.

Trautwein, W.: Membrane currents in cardiac muscle fibers. Physiol Rev 53:793, 1973.

Wallace, A. G.: Electrophysiology of the Myocardium. In Gordon, B. L. (ed.): Clinical Cardiopulmonary Physiology. New York, Grune and Stratton, 1969, p. 171.

Myocardial Contraction _____

STRUCTURE CONSIDERATIONS

The ventricular myocardium is composed of muscle cells, arranged more or less in parallel. These cells connect end-to-end as well as side-to-side, giving any given sample the appearance of a syncytium. Each cell is fully enclosed by the *sarcolemma*: the plasma or unit membrane plus its basement membrane. A typical myocardial cell is approximately 100 μ in length and 15 to 20 μ in diameter. At regular intervals in working muscle cells there are invaginations of sarcolemma that traverse the cell at right angles to the sarcomeres (Fig. 18). These transverse (T) tubules range in diameter from 100 to 1000 Å and are continuous with the extracellular space. T tubules typically intersect each sarcomere at the Z line (Fig. 18). The sarcoplasmic reticulum (SR) is an intracellular system of tubules that is generally arranged parallel to sarcomere orientation and forms an extensive intracellular network surrounding the contractile proteins of each sarcomere. Couplings refer to the special arrangements at sites of close opposition between the SR and the sarcolemma. Couplings that occur at the cell surface are referred to as peripheral and those between SR and transverse tubules as interior couplings. The most important functions of the sarcolemma, transverse tubules, and

SR are discussed under the sections on excitation and excitation-contraction coupling.

Within each myocardial cell, approximately 85 per cent of the intracellular volume is occupied by myofibrils (contractile machinery) and by mitochondria (units responsible for production of energy). In this section we will deal principally with the contractile properties of the myofibrils and in the section on myocardial metabolism with the processes of energy supply, which are largely a mitochondrial function.

Myofibrils are striated, exhibiting a characteristic and repeating pattern of light and dark bands. The light bands are more isotropic and are referred to as I bands. The darkly staining bands are birefringent under polarized light (anisotropic) and are thus referred to as A bands. Each I band is divided in half by a Z line and the region between two Z lines is the fundamental structural or contractile unit of muscle, the sarcomere (Fig. 19).

From each Z line thin filaments composed almost entirely of actin project toward the center of the sarcomere. Within the A band there is a second type of filament, the thick filament, composed of myosin. Actin and myosin filaments overlap in the region of the A band, but only actin filaments are found in the I band. When a sarcomere is viewed in cross section, at the

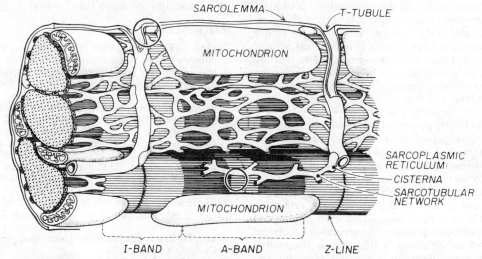

Figure 18. Ultrastructure of the working myocardial cell. Contractile proteins are arranged in a regular array of thick and thin filaments (seen in cross section at the left). The A-band represents the region of the sarcomere occupied by the thick filaments into which thin filaments extend from either side. The I-band is the region of the sarcomere occupied by thin filaments; these extend toward the center of the sarcomere from the Z-lines, which bisect each I-band. The sarcomere, the functional unit of the contractile apparatus, is the region between each pair of Z-lines; it contains two half I-bands and one A-band. The sarcoplasmic reticulum, a membrane network that surrounds the contractile proteins, consists of the sarcotubular network at the center of the sarcomere and the cisternae, which abut on the t-tubules and the sarcolemma. The transverse tubular system (t-tubule) is lined by a membrane that extends from the sarcolemma and carries the extracellular space into the myocardial cell. In contrast to the t-tubules of skeletal muscle, those of the myocardium can run in a longitudinal as well as a transverse direction. Mitochondria are shown in the central sarcomere and in cross section at the left. (With permission from Katz, A. M.: Physiology of the Heart. New York, Raven Press, 1977, p. 9.)

Figure 19. Myocardial structure, as seen under the light and electron microscopes, is schematized. Top drawing shows section of myocardium as it would appear under light microscope, with interconnecting fibers or cells attached end-to-end and delimited by modified cell membranes called intercalated disks. Ultrastructural schematization (center drawing) illustrates the division of the fiber longitudinally into rodlike fibrils, in turn composed of sarcomeres, the basic contractile units. Within the sarcomeres, thick filaments of myosin, confined to the central dark A band, alternate with thin filaments of actin that extend from the A lines (delimiting the sarcomere) through the I band and into the A band, where they overlap the myosin filaments. These landmarks are seen in detailed drawings (bottom). (With permission from Sonnenblick, E. H.: Myocardial ultrastructure in the normal and failing heart. In Braunwald, E. (ed.): The Myocardium: Failure and Infarction. New York, HP Publishing Co., Inc., 1974, p. 4.)

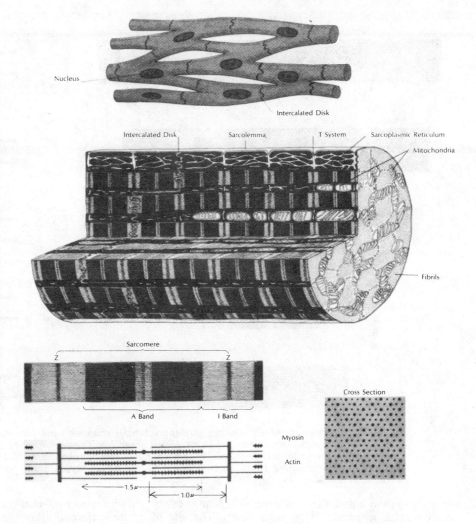

level of the A band each thick filament is surrounded by a hexagonal array of thin filaments. In the I band, where thick filaments are absent, the thin filaments are less highly ordered in their arrangements (Fig. 19).

Muscle contraction is based upon sarcomere shortening. When the sarcomere shortens, the lengths of the actin and myosin filaments remain constant, but they slide past each other so that each thin filament is pulled toward the center of a sarcomere. The distance between Z lines is reduced and the width of the I band is reduced in direct proportion to the extent of sarcomere shortening (Fig. 20).

Each thick filament is composed of an aggregation of myosin molecules. A myosin molecule is composed of an elongated tail consisting of two heavy polypeptide chains wound around each other to form an α helix. At the end of each chain, the chain takes on a globular structure to form a "head" owing to the addition of four (two pairs) light polypeptides (Fig. 21). The myosin molecule has a length of 1600 Å and a molecular weight of 480,000. Each molecule has a tail (the helically wound heavy chains) and two heads. Within each filament, myosin molecules are oriented with their

heads toward one end of the filament and their tails projecting toward the center of the filament. Thus, each thick filament is studded with heads that project from the filament (Fig. 22).

Furthermore, the junction between each head and its filamentous tail appears to be a point of physical flexibility. Myosin heads have potent ATPase activity and hence the capacity to liberate chemical energy. They also have the ability to bind the actin.

Thin filaments consist of two identical actin strands wound together as a double-stranded helix like two strands of pearls (Fig. 23). In the groove between actin chains there is a second protein, tropomyosin, itself consisting of two coiled polypeptide chains. The molecular weight of each tropomyosin molecule is 68,000 and the length of each molecule is approximately 395 Å. A third protein within the thin filament, troponin (Fig. 24) (or more accurately troponin complex) consists of three subunits or proteins. One of these proteins, troponin T, serves to bind the complex to tropomyosin. A second component, troponin I, appears to inhibit the potential site of actin-myosin binding. The third component, troponin C, contains high and low affinity binding sites of calcium. Troponin complex is bound to

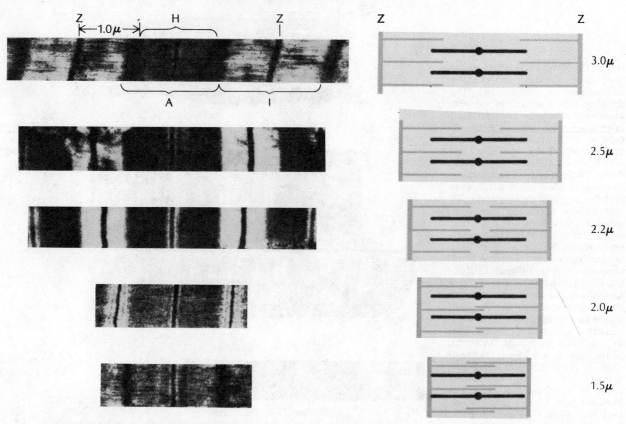

Figure 20. The way in which altering sarcomere length changes band pattern is shown in actual frog sartorius muscle sarcomeres (left) and in correlated diagrams. The sarcomere at 2.2 μ is at Lmax, at which maximum contractile force is produced. (With permission from Sonnenblick, E. H.: Myocardial ultrastructure in the normal and failing heart. In Braunwald, E. (ed.): The Myocardium: Failure and Infarction. New York, HP Publishing Co., Inc., 1974, p. 7.)

tropomyosin at a periodicity of every 400 Å or at every eighth actin monomer of an actin chain. The site of this troponin complex also corresponds to the ends of each tropomyosin molecule.

A rise in intracellular free Ca^{++} ion concentration triggers the contractile event. When the calcium concentration rises to a sufficient level within the vicinity of the contractile proteins, Ca^{++} binds to troponin C, which may effect a change in the affinity of troponin I for actin and allow the entire tropomyosin molecule to shift from the periphery to the center of the groove between actin strands (Fig. 25). This shift of tropomyosin, which in the resting state inhibits the potential sites of actin-myosin interaction, exposes these sites on each actin monomer. Exposure of the myosin binding site on each actin monomer is accompanied by

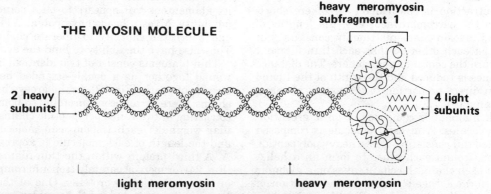

Figure 21. Myosin molecule. Myosin is an elongated molecule consisting of a "tail" (left) and a "head" (right). The tail consists of a coil (composed of two α-helical chains wound around each other) that extends into the paired globular head of the molecule. The latter contains, in addition, four light subunits. Enzymatic cleavage at the point indicated by the lower arrow produces heavy and light meromyosins, while enzymatic cleavage of heavy meromyosin at the point indicated by the upper arrow yields heavy meromyosin subfragment 1. (With permission from Katz, A. M.: Physiology of the Heart. New York, Raven Press, 1977, p. 91.)

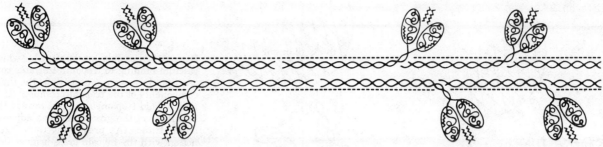

Figure 22. Organization of individual myosin molecules in the thick filament. The "backbone" of the thick filament is delineated by dashed lines. Individual myosin molecules have opposite polarities in the two halves of the sarcomere (right and left). The bare area in the center of the thick filament is a region devoid of cross-bridges, which can be seen to arise from the "tail-to-tail" organization of myosin molecules unique to the center of the thick filament. The cross-bridges represent the "heads" of the individual myosin molecules, which project at right angles to the long axis of the thick filament. (With permission from Katz, A. M.: Physiology of the Heart. New York, Raven Press, 1977, p. 93.)

tropomyosin

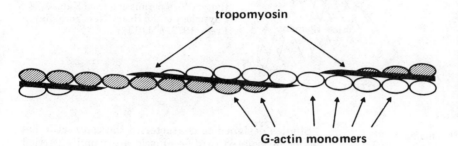

G-actin monomers

Figure 23. Tropomyosin is found along with actin in the thin filament, where it is located in the "groove" between the two strands of G-actin monomers. (With permission from Katz, A. M.: Physiology of the Heart. New York, Raven Press, 1977, p. 99.)

Figure 24. Troponin complexes are found along with actin and tropomyosin in the thin filament. The troponin complexes are bound to tropomyosin at approximately 400-Å intervals along the thin filament. (With permission from Katz, A. M.: Physiology of the Heart. New York, Raven Press, 1977, p. 100.)

$\sim$ 400 Å

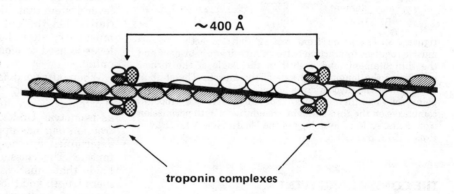

troponin complexes

a strong binding interaction between actin and the myosin heads. At least initially, this binding does not result in the release of energy or a shift in the orientation of the actin-myosin cross-bridge. However, in the presence of Ca^{++}, actin is a potent activator of myosin ATPase. The energy subsequently released by hydrolysis of ATP causes the myosin head to bend at its flexible junction with the tail and, by a mechanism analogous to the rowing action of a crew, pulls the thin filaments toward the center of each sarcomere (Fig. 26). Once this pull or stroke is completed, the binding of ATP to myosin causes the actin-myosin bridge to break, and each myosin head returns to

perpendicular orientation and is ready for another interaction with an upstream actin monomer. Thus, during each contraction, the sequence of making a bridge-tilt of the myosin head, pulling on the actin filament, and breaking of bridges is repeated many times, as long as there are sequential bridges to be made, the Ca^{++} ion concentration is high enough to promote bridges, and ATP is present in excess of demand. Relaxation ensues when the pumping capacity of the sarcoplasmic reticulum reduces the free Ca^{++} concentration, which was initially raised as a consequence of the action potential, to a level below the threshold for binding to troponin C.

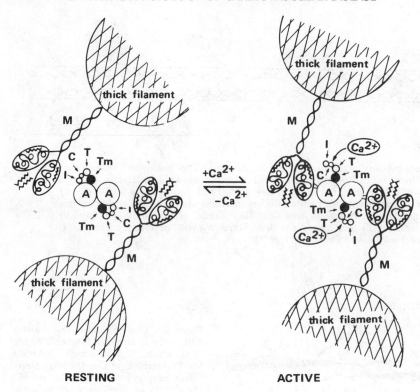

RESTING

ACTIVE

Figure 25. Possible mechanism by which calcium binding to troponin initiates contraction. In resting muscle (left) the three components of the troponin complex (I, C, and T) hold tropomyosin (Tm) toward the periphery of the groove between adjacent actin strands (A), preventing their interaction with the myosin cross-bridges (M). Binding of Ca^{2+} to troponin C (right) sets into motion a series of cooperative interactions between the proteins of the thin filament that reduces the affinity between troponin I and actin. The resulting detachment of bonds between troponin I and actin causes tropomyosin to shift its position toward the center of the groove between the actin strands, allowing the latter to interact with the myosin cross-bridges and thereby initiate muscular activity. (With permission from Katz, A. M.: Physiology of the Heart. New York, Raven Press, 1977, p. 110.)

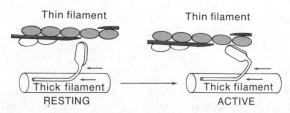

RESTING

ACTIVE

Figure 26. Transition from resting (left) to active (right) muscle requires interaction between myosin cross-bridges and the thin filament, and a shift in the angle of the former relative to the longitudinal axis of the muscle. The shift in the angle of the myosin cross-bridges appears to involve two points of flexibility (arrows). For simplicity, the troponin complexes on the thin filament are omitted. (With permission from Katz, A. M.: Physiology of the Heart. New York, Raven Press, 1977, p. 112.)

THE CONTRACTING EVENT

The sliding filament hypothesis focuses on the mechanism of actin-myosin interaction as the basis for understanding the behavior of the contractile element in cardiac muscle. That hypothesis predicts that, were it possible to tetanize a strand of cardiac muscle, the maximal tension developed by the strand would be proportional to the number of potential sites for actin-myosin interaction, which in turn would be related to sarcomere length and the extent of overlap between thick and thin filaments. On the other hand, if muscle could be stimulated to shorten without carrying any load, the maximal velocity of shortening should be proportional to the velocity at which cross-bridges can be made, broken, and remade.

Studies designed to characterize the contractile behavior of isolated cardiac muscle are usually carried out on strands, strips, or papillary muscles of sufficiently small size to reduce problems related to diffusion of oxygen and substrate. One end of the muscle is attached to a tension transducer and the other to a lever system that allows the investigator to set preload (initial length) and afterload (the weight the muscle must carry after shortening begins). Movement of the lever is used to monitor the extent and rate of shortening.

When afterload is set at a level higher than the maximal capacity of the muscle to create tension, shortening is precluded and the twitch is referred to as isometric. Under such conditions the force of contraction depends upon initial muscle length, which is determined by the diastolic load or preload on the muscle. The classic explanation of this relationship holds that muscle length determines average sarcomere length and that sarcomere length determines the extent of overlap between thick and thin filaments, and hence the number of potential cross-bridges.

When initial muscle length is fixed, and afterload is set at values less than the maximal capacity of the muscle to create tension, shortening occurs. The extent of shortening and peak velocity vary inversely with afterload. A plot of the relation between afterload and velocity of shortening describes a force-velocity curve (Fig. 27). From the force-velocity curve, parameters such as work and power can be derived. The force-velocity relation is of interest because it suggests two basic and independent mechanisms by which the performance of cardiac muscle is altered. When initial length is increased, peak force development and the rate of shortening at any given load are augmented,

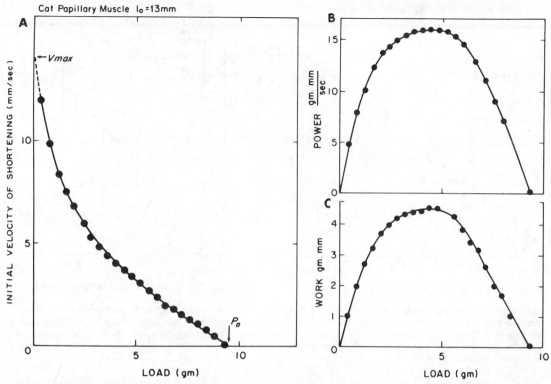

Figure 27. Force-velocity relation of the cat papillary muscle. On the right, power (force × velocity of shortening) and work (force [or load] × displacement [△L]) are given as functions of load. (With permission from Sonnenblick, E. H.: The mechanics of myocardial contraction. In Briller, S. A., and Conn, H. L., Jr. (eds.): The Myocardial Cell: Structure, Function and Modification by Cardiac Drugs. Philadelphia, University of Pennsylvania Press, 1966, p. 187.)

while the peak velocity of shortening at a muscle load equivalent to only the preload changes little or not at all. In contrast, inotropic interventions that augment the contractility of heart muscle shift the force-velocity curve upward and to the right at any given preload. These interventions increase peak force development, peak velocity of shortening, and the velocity of shortening at all levels of afterload. From these observations it has been hypothesized that inotropic influences modulate the degree, the rate, or both, of formation of bridges between actin and myosin.

Cardiac muscle is more complex than skeletal muscle. Conclusions about the behavior of the sarcomere based upon studies of whole muscle preparations are fraught with interpretive problems. For one thing, cardiac muscle cannot be tetanized. The active state of cardiac muscle that is related to intracellular calcium concentration turns on slowly following depolarization, falls before the muscle regains responsiveness to another stimulus, and is never constant. Thus, peak tension on any given twitch is related to the duration of the active state on that twitch and is always less than would be the case if intracellular calcium concentration were not time-dependent. There are problems in trying to determine the force on the sarcomere from measurements of tension on the whole muscle and in determining the velocity and extent of changes in sarcomere length from measurements of the whole muscle. In brief, it is probably unjustified to draw conclusions about the relationship between length, tension, and shortening velocity of the sarcomere from

studies of the mechanics of strips or segments of cardiac muscle.

Recent studies have used optical techniques to follow sarcomere length throughout a contraction. When a papillary muscle was held at constant length (that is, isometric) during contraction, the sarcomeres shortened and extended the damaged ends of the muscle. Thus, the sarcomeres were not isometric and the large apparent compliance in series with the contractile element was artifactually large and attributable to the damaged ends of the muscle. When contractions were initiated and sarcomere length was held constant (optical feedback), peak force and the rate of force development were much greater than in muscles in which muscle length but not sarcomere length was controlled. In support of the sliding filament hypothesis, peak developed isometric force was found to be linearly related to sarcomere length over the range of sarcomere lengths from 1.6 to 2.1 μ. Similar techniques were used to study the velocity of shortening of unloaded contractions. At any given initial sarcomere length, peak shortening velocity was achieved early in the contraction. Peak velocity was a function of initial sarcomere length but, regardless of initial length, shortening velocity at any given sarcomere length was similar. The range of sarcomere lengths over which shortening velocity was proportional to length was 1.6 to 2.0 μ (Fig. 28). An important conclusion from these observations is that shortening velocity at any given load is related to instantaneous sarcomere length during a twitch and is not predetermined by initial length.

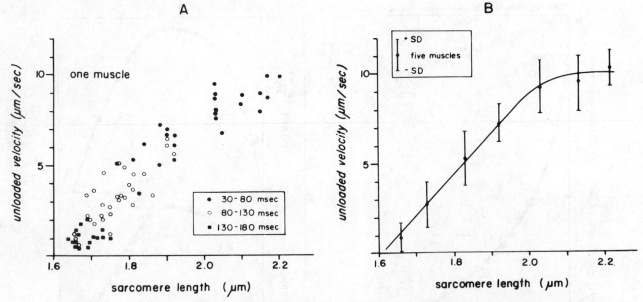

Figure 28. *A*, Unloaded velocity as function of instantaneous sarcomere length. Velocities are obtained at various times during contraction from contractions initiated at different sarcomere lengths. All data points appear to fall on same curve. *B*, Similar to *A*, except data are for five muscles. (With permission from Pollack, G. H., and Krueger, J. W.: Sarcomere dynamics in intact cardiac muscle. Eur J Cardiol 4(Supplement):61, 1976.)

A second important conclusion is that peak velocity of shortening is related to initial sarcomere length over the range from 1.6 to 2.0 μ rather than being independent of length as had been suggested from force-velocity studies of papillary muscles. The intensity of the active state, which is presumed to reflect the amount of calcium bound to troponin (that is, activation), depends on sarcomere length. It follows that if the inotropic state or contractility of cardiac muscle is equated at a molecular level with the degree of activation of contractile elements, then a change in sarcomere length must be regarded as an inotropic intervention.

The discussion in this section on myocardial contraction has focused on the morphological characteristics of the contractile unit of heart muscle (the sarcomere) and on data from which investigators have attempted to derive a functional understanding of factors that determine the nature of the contractile event. The picture is necessarily incomplete. Efforts to

understand sarcomere dynamics will continue because of interest in this important biological phenomenon and disorders of heart muscle function in man.

REFERENCES

Jewell, B. R.: A reexamination of the influence of muscle length on myocardial performance. Circ Res 40:221, 1977.

Johnson, E. A., and Manring, A.: Cardiac muscle mechanics now and then. J Mol Cell Cardiol 9:1, 1977.

Julian, F. J., and Moss, R. L.: The concept of active state in striated muscle. Circ Res 38:53, 1976.

Nassar, R., Manring, A., and Johnson, E. A.: Light diffraction of cardiac muscle: Sarcomere motion during contraction. In The Physiological Basis of Starling's Law of the Heart. Ciba Foundation Symposium #24. North Holland, Amsterdam, Elsevier-Excerpta Medica, 1974, p. 57.

Noble, M. I. M., and Pollack, G. H.: Molecular mechanisms of contraction. Circ Res 40:333, 1977.

Pollack, G. H., and Krueger, J. W.: Sarcomere dynamics in intact cardiac muscle. Europ J Cardiol 4(Suppl.):53, 1976.

Excitation Contraction Coupling

An abrupt rise in intracellular (Ca^{++}) ion concentration is responsible for activating cross-bridge formation between actin and myosin and hence for initiating contraction of muscle. In relaxed cardiac muscle during diastole, the concentration of free Ca^{++} in the myoplasm is around 0.2 μM. At this concentration the Ca^{++} regulatory sites on troponin are largely unoccupied, and tropomyosin inhibits the actin-myosin interaction. The threshold for just detectable tension in cardiac muscle is a Ca^{++} concentration around 0.3 to 0.6 μM. The Ca^{++} concentration rises to a maximum of 4 μM during the most forceful contraction, a concentration considerably less than that required to produce full activation of the myofilaments (12.5 μM). The resulting tension corresponds to about 70 per cent of that maximally possible. It has been calculated that approximately 30 μmoles of Ca^{++} per ml of cytoplasm must be released to fill 90 per cent of the binding sites on troponin, so that somewhat less than this amount must be released in the most forceful contraction.

The action potential of the cardiac cell propagates along the surface sarcolemma and invades the T tubules, which are simply intracellular invaginations of sarcolemma that provide a mechanism for impulse transmission into the depths of the cell (see Fig. 19). The resulting depolarization leads to an influx of Ca^{++} into the cytoplasm through the sarcolemma by either or both of two mechanisms, a membrane-potential gated Ca^{++} channel and a Na^{+}/Ca^{++} exchange mechanism. This influx is thought to act as a "trigger," causing the release of Ca^{++} from specialized sections of the sarcoplasmic reticulum (the junctional SR) that are closely apposed to the undersurface of the sarcolemma. At this time it is not known how much of the calcium needed for contraction is derived from intracellular versus extracellular sites. Contraction strength on any given beat appears to be determined by the sum of activator calcium made available from two sources, the junctional SR and sarcolemmal influx. The amplitude of a given contraction, and presumably the contribution from each of these two sources, is a complex function of the history of the rate and pattern of stimulation of the muscle.

A calcium pump in the SR appears to play the major role in relaxation, by actively sequestering Ca^{++} from the myoplasm and thereby reducing the free Ca^{++} concentration below that at which binding to troponin occurs. This causes the cross-bridges to break and the muscle to relax. This uptake of Ca^{++} by the SR is an energy-dependent process involving the transport of two Ca^{++} from the cytoplasm into the lumen of the SR for every molecule of ATP hydrolyzed. There the Ca^{++} is largely bound to the protein calsequestrin, located in the junctional SR where the total concentration (bound and free) is approximately 60 mM, the free concentration being estimated to be 3 to 5 mM. The Ca^{++} that enters the cell from the extracellular space is extruded from the cell by two sarcolemmal mechanisms, an ATP-driven Ca^{++} pump and the Na^{+}/Ca^{++} exchanger. The picture that emerges, therefore, is one of an internal recirculation of calcium involving release from junctional SR binding to troponin binding and uptake by longitudinal SR, and a return to junctional SR. This sequence is initiated by depolarization and repolarization on any given action potential. The amount of Ca^{++} available to this internal recirculation system is in turn influenced by the amount of Ca^{++} entering the cell from extracellular fluid, which is a function of action potential duration, as well as the rate and pattern of excitation.

REFERENCES

Fabiato, A.: Myoplasmic free calcium concentration reached during the twitch of an intact isolated cardiac cell and during calcium-induced release of calcium from the sarcoplasmic reticulum of a skinned cardiac cell from the adult rat or rabbit ventricle. J Gen Physiol 78:457, 1981.

Gibbs, C., and Chapman, J. B.: Cardiac energetics. In Berne, R. M., Sperelakis, N., and Geiger, S. R. (eds.): The Handbook of Physiology. The Cardiovascular System, Vol. I, The Heart. Bethesda, Md., American Physiological Society, 1979, p. 775.

Johnson, E. A.: Force-interval relationship of cardiac muscle. In Berne, R. M., Sperelakis, N., and Geiger, S. R. (eds.): The Handbook of Physiology. The Cardiovascular System, Vol. I, The Heart. Bethesda, Md., American Physiological Society, 1979, p. 475.

Morad, M., and Goldman, Y.: Excitation-contraction coupling in heart muscle: Membrane control of development of tension. Progr Biophys Mol Biol 27:257, 1973.

Robertson, S. P., Johnson, J. D., and Potter, J. D.: The time course of Ca^{2+} exchange with calmodulin, troponin, parvalbumin, and myosin in response to transient increases in Ca^{2+}. Biophys J 34:559, 1981.

Winegrad, S.: Electromechanical coupling in heart muscle. In Berne, R. M., Sperelakis, N., and Geiger, S. R. (eds.): The Handbook of Physiology. The Cardiovascular System, Vol. I, The Heart. Bethesda, Md., American Physiological Society, 1979, p. 393.

The Heart as a Pump

GENERAL CONCEPTS

The heart is a pump whose capacity to propel blood through the body has fascinated investigators and students since William Harvey's "discovery" of the circulation, published in 1628. The era of classical cardiac physiology began in the nineteenth century with efforts to characterize the pumping ability of the heart and the factors that control cardiac output. Although methods have changed, the hydraulic approach to cardiac function continues today. In the middle of the twentieth century two independent developments converged to form a new basis of analysis of cardiac pump function. One of these was the development of cardiac catheterization and angiographic techniques that made it possible to apply hydraulic studies to man. The other was the extension to heart muscle of techniques and concepts previously applied to skeletal muscle in an effort to understand the mechanics of muscle in terms of its structural components. The coupling of hydraulics and mechanics brought to the circulatory field the talents and disciplines of physics and engineering. For the physician, the insights brought by these disciplines are focused on understanding normal cardiac function as a basis for appreciating the nature, location, and extent of deranged function in human disease. These concepts also provide the basis for identifying and evaluating potential forms of therapy aimed at improving the pump function of diseased hearts.

The normal cardiac cycle can be viewed as a sequence of changes in pressure, volume, and flow (Fig. 29). We will describe here only the events of the left side of the heart, but qualitatively similar changes occur in the right heart. At end diastole, the left atrial and left ventricular pressures approach equilibrium and left

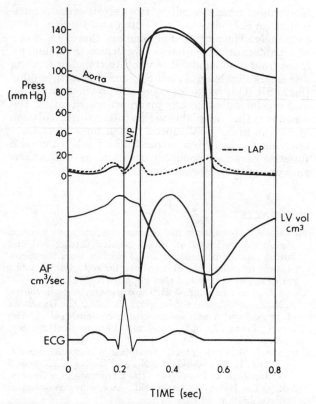

Figure 29. Pressure-volume-flow relations during the normal cardiac cycle. Aorta = aortic pressure; LVP = left ventricular pressure; LAP = left atrial pressure; LV vol = left ventricular volume; AF = aortic flow recorded with electromagnetic flow meter; ECG = electrocardiogram. Time in seconds is on the horizontal axis.

ventricular volume is maximum. With the onset of ventricular contraction, the mitral valve closes and during an interval of approximately 60 msec ventricular cavity pressure rises rapidly because of the tension exerted on the endocardial surface by the contracting muscle. During this interval, ventricular volume is constant and the interval is thus referred to as the isovolumic phase. When ventricular pressure exceeds that in the aorta, the aortic valve opens and the ejection phase begins. Flow velocity in cm/sec (as measured by flow probes around the ascending aorta) reaches its peak very early in systole, declines gradually throughout the midphase of ejection, and then declines rapidly in the last third of ejection. During the initial phase of ejection, when there is acceleration of the ejection velocity, left ventricular pressure continues to exceed aortic pressure. During the later stages of ejection, as flow decelerates aortic pressure exceeds left ventricular pressure, although forward flow continues until the aortic valve closes. The duration of the normal ejection phase is 250 to 300 msec.

When the cross-sectional area beneath a flow probe is known, velocity can be converted to flow (cm³/sec) and the integral of this curve is a measure of stroke output. During ejection, the volume of blood propelled into the aorta per unit time is precisely equal to the volume of blood that leaves the ventricle. It follows that the time integral of aortic flow will be related to a corresponding but inverse change in ventricular volume. The time course of change in ventricular volume can be calculated from left ventricular cinean-

giograms with the difference between end-diastolic and end-systolic ventricular volumes accurately reflecting stroke volume. Stroke volume can therefore be quantitated independently by aortic flow measurements and angiography.

At the onset of myocardial relaxation the tension exerted by the muscle on the endocardium drops precipitously, and ventricular pressure falls rapidly. The aortic valve is closed by the large pressure gradient between the aorta and the ventricle and for a period of 40 to 50 msec the ventricle continues to relax at a constant volume. This period is referred to as the isovolumic relaxation phase and ends when ventricular pressure falls below atrial pressure and the mitral valve opens.

When the mitral valve opens, the pressure gradient between the atrium and ventricle is maximal and flow into the ventricle accelerates. The ventricle fills initially at a rapid rate and then more slowly, reaching a near plateau during the last third of diastole at normal heart rates of 60 to 70 beats per minute. Atrial contraction produces a transient late rise in the atrioventricular pressure gradient and ejects an additional volume of blood into the ventricle (perhaps 10 to 20 per cent of the subsequent stroke volume). With atrial relaxation, a ventriculoatrial pressure gradient develops that tends to close the mitral valve just before the next ventricular contraction. The atrial contraction and its contribution to ventricular filling have been likened to a booster pump, the consequence of which is that the left ventricular end-diastolic volume and pressure are higher for any given mean atrial pressure than would be the case in the absence of this atrial booster pump function.

CLINICAL CORRELATIONS OF PUMP FUNCTION

Before proceeding to more detailed analyses of how the heart functions as a pump, a brief discussion of how activation and relaxation of the heart relate to phasic alterations in venous, arterial, and precordial wave forms as well as heart sounds and murmurs is in order. Once this normal bedside clinical physiology is understood, the various perturbations induced by disease processes become more easily understood.

As the jugular venous valves are either rudimentary or nonoperative under normal conditions of venous flow, the jugular veins and particularly the internal jugular system accurately reflect certain right-sided events (Fig. 30—Jugular Venous Pulse). With right atrial systole, right atrial pressure rises, propelling blood into the right ventricle and also causing a retrograde positive venous wave (the A wave), which normally occurs just before the carotid pulse. The right atrium then relaxes and, in concert with systolic descent of the heart, causes a negative wave or collapse of the venous pulse, the X descent. Following atrial relaxation, continuing venous inflow fills the right atrium, causing the onset of a second, smaller positive wave—the V wave. Following pulmonary valve closure, right ventricular pressure falls and the tricuspid valve opens, yielding a second, small negative wave—the Y descent—a reflection of right ventricular filling. (The C wave reflects a positive wave from closure and billowing of the tricuspid valve and/or a

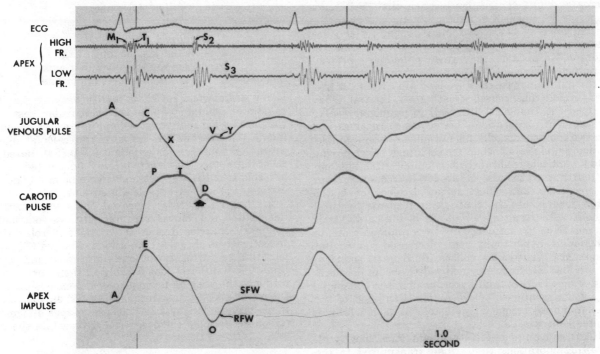

Figure 30. A simultaneous recording in a normal subject of the electrocardiogram, a high and low frequency heart sound recording at the apex, the jugular venous pulse, the carotid pulse, and the apex impulse. The physiological significance of these various wave forms and the abbreviations used are discussed in the text.

transmitted arterial wave. It is frequently recorded but usually is not of much clinical significance.)

During left ventricular ejection, blood flows into the aorta, producing a transmitted pulse that is subsequently appreciated clinically in the carotid, brachial, femoral, and other arterial pulses (Fig. 30—Carotid Pulse). The normal carotid arterial pulse rises to a single, early systolic peak (the percussion wave). A second, smaller wave (the tidal wave) reflects a combination of continuing ejection of blood and a retrograde wave reflected from the upper body's peripheral arterial tree. Following aortic valve closure (solid arrow), a third wave, the dicrotic wave (D), occurs and is due to a reflected positive wave from the lower body's peripheral arterial tree. Normally, only the initial upstroke and systolic peak are appreciated clinically in the central arterial pulse.

With left atrial systole, blood enters the left ventricle, causing it to distend, and this may be recorded over the area of the left ventricular apex (Fig. 30—Apex Impulse) as a small presystolic positive wave (or A wave). This wave normally is not palpable, but under certain conditions in which the force of left atrial systole is augmented (e.g., as in a stiff, noncompliant left ventricle) it may become palpable. With the onset of isovolumic systole, the apex of the heart moves toward the chest wall, where it is appreciated as a small (less than quarter-sized), brief (less than one third of the systolic cycle) impulse. With the onset of ejection (E point), the heart becomes smaller and rotates away from the chest wall. Following aortic valve closure, when left ventricular pressure falls below left atrial pressure, the mitral valve opens (O point) and blood begins to flow into the left ventricle, at first rapidly (producing the rapid filling wave—RFW) and then more slowly (slow filling

wave—SFW). Under some normal conditions (e.g., the child or young adult), this early diastolic filling is rapid and large enough to cause a brief, palpable impulse as the blood flowing into the ventricle is decelerated abruptly by the walls of the ventricular chamber and the mitral valve apparatus. This impulse is the palpable equivalent of a physiological ventricular gallop (S_3 or third heart sound—vide infra).

Heart sounds (Fig. 30—Apex) are created by the acceleration and/or deceleration of blood with resultant vibration of the blood and cardiac structures (Rushmer's cardiohemic system). The first heart sound is due to atrioventricular valve coaptation or closure and the resulting abrupt deceleration of blood that had been set into motion by ventricular contraction. The normal first heart sound is split by approximately 30 milliseconds because of asynchronous mitral (M_1) and then tricuspid (T_1) valve closure, which, in turn, is due to asynchronous electrical activation of the two ventricular chambers. The second heart sound (S_2) reflects semilunar valve coaptation or closure and the resultant abrupt deceleration of blood in the central systemic and pulmonary arterial vascular trunks, with resulting vibration of the cardiohemic system. During expiration, valve closure is usually synchronous, producing a single heart sound, but with inspiration the second heart sound splits into aortic and pulmonic components. This splitting is due, in part, to earlier aortic valve closure that, in turn, is due to trapping of blood in the pulmonary venous tree, a smaller left ventricular stroke volume, and a shortened left ventricular ejection time. The majority of the inspiratory splitting, however, is due to delayed pulmonary valve closure that is, in turn, due to the inspiration-induced filling of the right ventricle and a larger right ventricular stroke volume. This larger stroke volume variably increases right ventricular ejection time but, more importantly, imparts a greater kinetic energy to the ejected mass of blood that takes longer for the low resistance pulmonary vascular circuit to overcome. In addition, inspiration may raise pulmonary arterial compliance. Thus, blood continues to move antegrade in the pulmonary vasculature long after right ventricular systole has ceased creating an inertial delay (termed the "hangout" interval) in pulmonary valve closure. With expiration, this sequence reverses and the two components of S_2 narrow and/or become single. Gallop sounds result when the column of blood moving into a ventricle is abruptly decelerated. Atrial gallops (or fourth heart sounds—S_4) are low in frequency, occur in presystole, and reflect abrupt deceleration of the blood flowing into the ventricle in response to atrial systole, with resulting vibrations of the cardiohemic system. Such abrupt deceleration is commonly due to ventricular hypertrophy with decreased ventricular compliance. Ventricular gallops (third heart sounds—S_3) are also low frequency and reflect abrupt deceleration of blood either from hyperdynamic early diastolic filling (as mentioned above in the discussion of the apex impulse) or from early diastolic filling of a failing, dilated ventricle.

Heart murmurs reflect turbulent blood flow with resulting vibrations that, when transmitted to the chest wall, are of sufficient magnitude to be appreciated by the exploring stethoscope (or hand, where the vibrations are termed "thrills"). Such turbulence may occur with "increased" or hyperdynamic flow through anatomically normal structures, as in the example of the innocent murmur that arises from the ventricular outflow tracts of young people. Turbulence also results when normal blood flow occurs through anatomically distorted structures. The characteristics of these "pathological" murmurs (timing, frequency or pitch, shape, location on the chest wall, and loudness) will vary according to the site and severity of the disease process. For example, stenotic aortic and regurgitant mitral valves both produce systolic murmurs, while regurgitant aortic and stenotic mitral valves both produce diastolic murmurs (see discussion of valvular heart disease).

GEOMETRIC AND MECHANICAL FACTORS

The heart is an organ that has a geometric configuration different from any pump encountered outside of a living organism. The geometry of this pump is important because it forms the basis for many of the calculations of chamber volume and flow used in clinical studies. In addition, the geometry is important for the calculation of wall tension and stress from measurements of pressure and volume and it is the necessary link to understanding the translation of the mechanics of heart muscle into the hydraulic phenomena of pressure and flow. Furthermore, the geometry of the heart changes in specific ways in human disease, and our knowledge of the pathophysiology of those diseases would be incomplete in the absence of an understanding of this altered geometry.

The configuration of clay casts of the left ventricular chamber approximates that of an ellipsoid. The formula for the volume of an ellipsoid is:

$$V = 4/3 \, \pi \, abc$$

where:

V = volume (cm^3)
a = ½ the long or major axis
b = ½ of the longest minor axis
c = ½ of the shortest minor axis

Using postmortem hearts of widely varying size, the calculated volume of the left ventricular cast was compared with the actual volume (by water displacement). The correlation between the calculated and estimated volumes was excellent ($r = 0.993$). Based on these data the left ventricle may be treated as an ellipsoid to calculate ventricular volume and to derive estimates of wall stress and dimensions.

In the living state, however, it is important to understand and characterize precisely how ventricular geometry changes during activation and relaxation. Investigations of cavity dimensional changes (Fig. 31), particularly during isovolumic contraction and relaxation, have differed considerably in their conclusions owing to the varying technologies and models used. In the closed-chest, awake animal (Fig. 32) during isovolumic (pre-ejection) systole, the base-to-apex dimension (L_1 or major axis) increases modestly, while the two

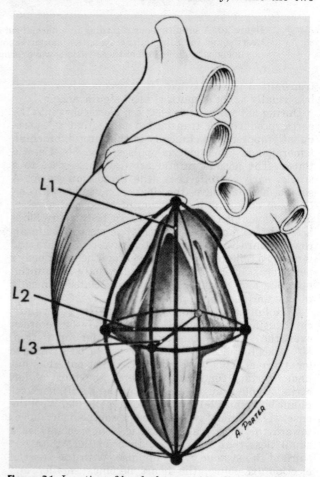

Figure 31. Location of beads demarcating ellipsoidal shell of cardiac muscles. (With permission from Mitchell, J. H., and Mullias, C. B.: Dimensional analysis of left ventricular function. In Tanz, R. D., Kavaler, F., and Roberts, J. (eds.): Factors Influencing Myocardial Contractility. New York, Academic Press, 1967, p. 178.)

A   B

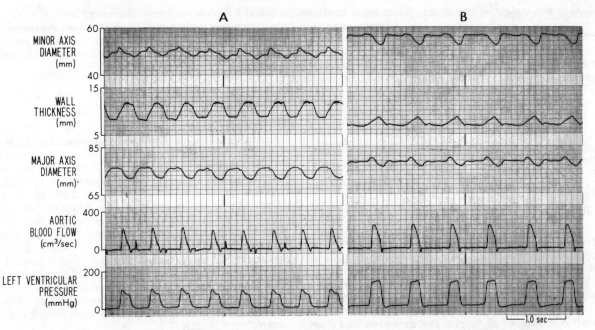

MINOR AXIS DIAMETER (mm)

WALL THICKNESS (mm)

MAJOR AXIS DIAMETER (mm)

AORTIC BLOOD FLOW (cm³/sec)

LEFT VENTRICULAR PRESSURE (mmHg)

1.0 sec

Figure 32. Dimensional characteristics of the left ventricle in the open chest, anesthetized state (Panel *A*) and in the same dog one week later in the closed chest, conscious state (Panel *B*). Note that in Panel *A*, during isovolumic contraction, the minor axis dimension increases while the major axis dimension decreases slightly. In Panel *B*, during isovolumic contraction, the minor axis dimension decreases slightly while the major axis dimension increases. These changes reflect isovolumic sphericalization and ellipticalization, respectively, reflecting the differing experimental conditions. In the closed chest, awake preparation, occlusion of the vena cava (with dramatic decrease in pre-load) caused sphericalization of isovolumic systole. (With permission from Rankin, J. S., McHale, P. A., Arentzen, C. E., Ling, D., Greenfield, J. C., Jr., and Anderson, R. W.: The three dimensional dynamic geometry of the left ventricle in the conscious dog. Circ Res 39:311, 1976.)

minor axis dimensions (L_2 and L_3) decrease slightly, all consequent to the ventricle's assuming a more elliptical shape. Also contributing to the decrease in minor axis dimensions is modest systolic wall thickening. When the volume of the heart is diminished by vena caval occlusion or by thoracotomy, isovolumic wall thickening is greater and the changes in dimension are directionally opposite owing to the ventricle's assuming a more spherical shape.

With the onset of ejection, all three cavity dimensions decrease and the wall thickens even further throughout ejection. The relative contribution of length and circumferential shortening to ejection varies somewhat with the loading conditions (initial volume and aortic pressure), but under most normal conditions the per cent change in the circumferential dimension is much greater than the change in apex-to-base length.

Left ventricular wall thickness changes during systole are impressive. During the isovolumic phase there is an increase in thickness of about 10 per cent of the end-diastolic value. During the ejection phase thickness increases further by another 10 to 15 per cent, reaching its maximal value at the end of ejection (Fig. 32).

The concept of wall stress is also important in understanding certain features of the cardiac pump. While stress has the same units as pressure (force per unit area) in a chamber of any given geometry, wall stress is not equivalent to cavity pressure. Furthermore, the heart is a contractile muscle, not an inert material: systolic wall stress is generated by the con-

tractile event, which causes cavity pressure to rise. Systolic wall stress is important because this force determines the extent and velocity of fiber shortening according to the force-velocity relation. Systolic wall stress is also the principal determinant of oxygen consumption by the heart. In diastole, the heart behaves as an elastic material and the relation between wall stress and strain determines the diastolic pressure-volume relationship and hence sarcomere length at the onset of the next contraction.

The pressure in a ventricle at any point during the cardiac cycle is a measure of the force acting on the wall in a direction perpendicular to the wall. It is equally valid for the heart to consider that the pressure in the cavity, at least during systole, is a consequence of the force generated by the wall on the volume of blood contained within the chamber. By convention, pressure in the cardiovascular system is expressed in mm Hg, where 1 mm Hg is equivalent to a force of 1330 dynes/cm². The dyne is a standard force unit equivalent to the force that will impart an acceleration of 1 cm/sec/sec to a 1-gram mass.

Newton's third law of physics states that whenever one body exerts a force on another, the second always exerts on the first a force that is equal in magnitude but oppositely directed. In its simplest form this law is illustrated by hanging a weight on a string. The weight represents a force in the direction of the earth's center (as a consequence of gravity) and it is opposed by a force in the opposite direction, the tension in the string. In this simple system, tension in the string is equal to the weight of the object. When some medium (for example, blood) is enclosed by a membrane (for example, the endocardium) and there is a higher pressure within the membrane than on the outside, tension or force exists within the membrane. The force within the membrane can be calculated from the law of LaPlace:

$$P = T \frac{1}{R_1} + \frac{1}{R_2}$$

where:

P = the pressure difference across the membrane;
T = the tension (dynes/cm²); and
R_1 and R_2 = radii of curvature.

Hence, if a slit were made in the membrane, tension in dynes/cm² would be the force tending to pull the edges of the slit apart.

When a medium under pressure is enclosed by a membrane that has thickness (for example, the ventricular wall), the force within the wall is more appropriately expressed as tension per unit area in a direction parallel to the wall. It should be noted that although pressure and wall stress have the same units, they are not quantitatively the same; for any given pressure, average wall stress is related to the geometry of the chamber; and stress will be maximal at the endocardium and will approach zero at the epicardium. Finally, to the extent that a ventricle thickens in response to elevated pressure or volume (hypertrophy), an increase in thickness will distribute the resulting wall stress over a larger area, tending to reduce (or normalize) the stress per unit of thickness.

When left ventricular wall stress is measured directly and wall thickness is measured simultaneously in dogs (Fig. 33) peak wall stress occurs approximately 65 msec after the onset of left ventricular contraction (very shortly after aortic valve opening) and then decreases throughout the ejection phase. These same studies showed that vasodilatation induced by nitroglycerin decreased wall stress, vasoconstriction induced by phenylephrine increased wall stress, and a positive inotropic agent (isoproterenol) decreased wall stress principally as a consequence of more rapid systolic emptying of the ventricle, despite an increase in peak aortic systolic pressure.

CONTRACTILE MECHANICS

A major impetus to define the geometry of the heart throughout the cardiac cycle has been the hope that when muscle length and stress could be estimated with accuracy it would be possible to describe the contractile effort in terms of basic muscle mechanics. In hydraulic terms, Starling's law of the heart describes a fundamental property of heart muscle: when aortic pressure is held constant, stroke volume varies directly with ventricular end-diastolic volume. This law has its counterpart in muscle physiology, where developed tension and the extent of shortening of a muscle vary directly with its initial length. As noted in the chapter on muscle contractility, these concepts have now been extended to the cellular level, where force development and extent of shortening have been correlated with sarcomere length.

Part of the increase in force-generating capacity of heart muscle as sarcomere length is extended can be ascribed to the sarcomere structure where at an optimal length (approximately 2.2 μ) the overlap between actin and myosin filaments juxtaposes and aligns a maximal number of active, cross-bridge–making sites. Length-dependent changes in the contractile state may also involve achieving an optimal angle between the force-generating sites as well as a length-dependent effect on the calcium release mechanism and hence on the intensity of the active state per se (see Myocardial Contraction, p. 874).

According to classic concepts, active cardiac muscle can be illustrated using a model composed of three functionally discrete components: (1) the contractile element (CE), which is responsible for generating force and shortening; (2) a series elastic element (SE), which couples the contractile element to the ends of muscle; and (3) a parallel elastic element (PE), which plays

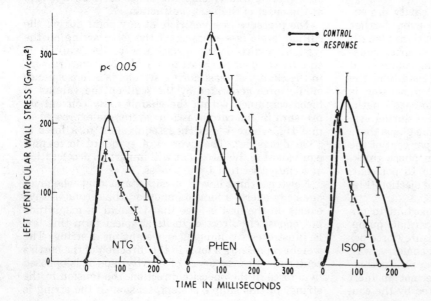

Figure 33. Measured left ventricular circumferential wall stress data during control (solid circles and solid lines) and in response (open circles and broken lines) to nitroglycerin (NTG), phenylephrine (PHEN), and isoproterenol (ISOP). Data are plotted as means ± SE. (With permission from McHale, P. A., and Greenfield, J. C., Jr.: Evaluation of several geometric models for estimation of left ventricular circumferential wall stress. Circ Res 33: 308, 1973.)

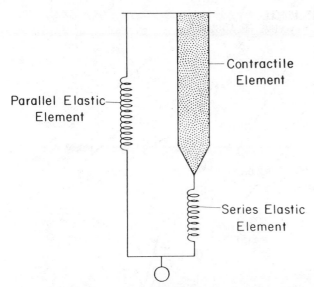

Figure 34. The Hill model for muscle, 1938. (With permission from Powell, W. J., Jr.: Basic concepts in cardiovascular physiology as applied to clinical medicine. In Willerson, J. T., and Sanders, C. A. (eds.): Clinical Cardiology. New York, Grune and Stratton, 1977, p. 24.)

relatively little role during contraction but bears most of the stress on the muscle during diastole—that is, at rest. The components are depicted for a muscle in Figure 34 and for a circumferential slice of the left ventricle in Figure 35.

First we will consider the interaction of the CE and the SE during contraction. From Figure 35 we can see that contractile elements are coupled to each other in sequence around the circumference of the ventricle. The couplings are depicted as springs and represent the SE elements. The activation of the CE creates a force within the wall and that force or stress (dynes/cm²) is borne by both the CE and the SE. Force develops rapidly during contraction of isolated muscle at constant length, or of the heart during the isovolumic phase. To the extent that the SE element is compliant, it is possible for the contractile element to shorten by extending the SE with no overall change

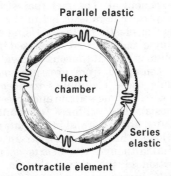

Figure 35. Mathematical model of heart according to A. V. Hill's skeletal muscle mode. (With permission from Fry, D. L., Griggs, D. M., Jr., and Greenfield, J. C., Jr.: Myocardial mechanics: Tension velocity-length relationships of heart muscle. Circ Res 14:73, 1964.)

in muscle length. The compliance of the SE element is a current subject of debate, but recent evidence suggests that the SE element is quite stiff; it changes in length probably no more than 1 to 2 per cent over stress levels ranging from zero to the maximal stress during a truly isometric contraction.

Based on such a model, examination of the force-velocity relationship in the intact heart demonstrates that at any given volume there is an inverse relationship between wall stress and circumferential fiber shortening rate. Furthermore, for any given wall stress, fiber shortening rate is greater at longer fiber lengths. Therefore, cardiac muscle in the intact heart appears to follow the force-velocity relationship. The fact that velocity of shortening at any given stress and stress at any given velocity both increase with length is entirely consistent with Starling's law (Fig. 36).

If the SE component of heart muscle is very stiff, the value of the force-velocity relation is enhanced because wall stress at any length and velocity of shortening at any stress closely approximate the behavior of the contractile element and hence the actin-myosin interaction.

At the level of the sarcomere, the force-velocity-length relationships state the following: (1) the extent of sarcomere shortening at any given load will increase with an increase in initial sarcomere length, (2) the capacity for force development will increase with increases of initial sarcomere length, and (3) the extent and rate of shortening at any given load will increase with a positive inotropic influence. When these concepts are extended to the intact beating heart, statement 1 forms the basis of Starling's law; that is, stroke volume at any given aortic pressure is related to end-diastolic volume. Statement 2 predicts that the peak left ventricular pressure during an isovolumic contraction will increase with increases of end-diastolic volume. The force-velocity relation also implies that for any given contractile state and end-diastolic volume, stroke volume will vary inversely with aortic pressure. Statement 3 predicts that a positive inotropic influence will increase stroke volume and the velocity of ejection for any given initial volume and aortic pressure. In assessing the applicability of the force-velocity relation to the intact heart, however, its geometry must be considered. Hence, instantaneous wall stress is a more accurate reflection of force than is pressure alone, and fiber length and shortening rate are more accurate reflections of changes of muscle length than are stroke volume and the ejection rate.

The attractiveness of the force-velocity relation to those who are interested in defining the contractility of heart muscle in vivo is dampened by two major obstacles. The first of these is pragmatic. Simultaneous measurement of instantaneous pressure and volume with the accuracy needed requires methods that are not standard in the usual diagnostic catheterization laboratory. A related problem is that assumptions involved in estimating instantaneous wall stress-length and fiber shortening rate are considerable and of unestablished validity, particularly in the diseased heart. The calculations are also laborious and time consuming. An assumption of perhaps even greater importance is that estimates of contractility derived from the force-velocity relation are based on the concept that contractility is independent of muscle length

HEART MUSCLE
TENSION–VELOCITY–VOLUME RELATIONSHIPS

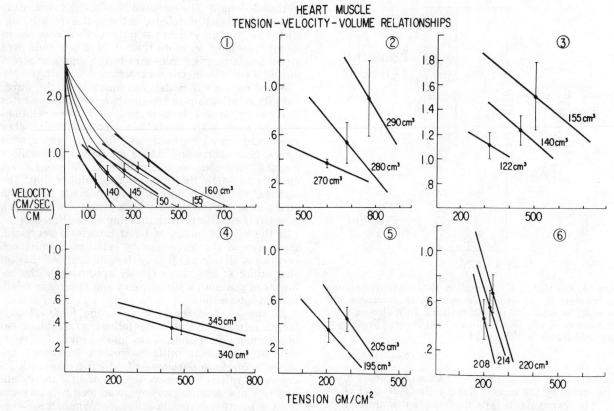

Figure 36. Summary of tension-velocity regression lines from data from six dogs. The length of the vertical bars drawn through the grand mean of each curve represents twice the standard error of estimate. In the plot for dog No. 1 light curves are sketched through the regression lines to suggest a possible similarity of these data for the intact heart to that shown by Sonnenblick for the papillary muscle preparation. (With permission from Fry, D. L., Griggs, D. M., Jr., and Greenfield, J. C., Jr.: Myocardial mechanics: Tension-velocity-length relationships of heart muscle. Circ Res 14:78,1964.)

and that estimates can be compared across individuals with hearts of varying size and initial volume. The current view is that contractility is length-dependent. If this view proves correct then diastolic volume and inotropic state cannot be regarded as independent mechanisms that regulate ventricular performance.

During diastole, the stress-strain relationship can be used to assess stiffness of the muscle and a related parameter, the compliance of the chamber. In terms of hydraulics, this relationship is significant because it will determine the end-diastolic pressure that is required to achieve any given end-diastolic volume. In terms of muscle mechanics the relationship is important because end-diastolic stress will determine sarcomere length and hence the force generated on the subsequent contraction. Our initial consideration will focus on the diastolic properties of normal cardiac muscle and normal ventricles. Subsequently we will consider changes of the stress-strain relationship in certain pathological conditions.

Analysis of the stiffness of cardiac muscle, in terms of the stress-strain relationship, stems from the application of engineering principles to physiology. In engineering, the stress-strain relation is a way to characterize a material (steel, concrete, rubber, and so on) in terms of changes in shape or dimension when a force is applied to the material. Stress is defined as a force per unit area that tends to deform the material

from its natural unstressed dimensions. Strain is a dimensionless term that refers to the relative change in dimension that occurs when a stress is applied to the material.

For certain materials the relation between strain (ϵ) and stress (σ) is linear, and the material is said to obey Hooke's law. For biological materials the relation between strain and stress is nonlinear. Fortunately, over the normal working range of diastolic volumes the stress-strain relationship of cardiac muscle is very nearly an exponential. The fact that stiffness varies with length in cardiac muscle led to the introduction of the concept of elastic stiffness. Using this concept, pressure-volume curves were analyzed over a wide range of volumes. Instantaneous midwall stress and strain were computed from pressure and geometric data. Applying these techniques to normal subjects, and to those with chronic volume and pressure overload (aortic stenosis), the stiffness constant was only slightly elevated above normal in patients with chronic volume overload. Thus, the stress-strain relation was nearly normal although the hearts operated on an elevated portion of the curve—that is, at elevated stiffness levels. In patients with significant aortic stenosis the stiffness constant was more than twice normal, implying that the hypertrophied muscle was stiffer. It is of interest that these conclusions are in qualitative agreement with studies of the passive length-stress relation of papillary muscles removed from animals with experimentally induced chronic volume and pressure overload.

REFERENCES

Dodge, H.T., Sandler, H., Ballew, D. W., and Lord, J. D., Jr.: The use of biplane angiocardiography for the measurement of left ventricular volume in man. Am Heart J 60:762, 1960.

Fry, D. L., Griggs, D. M., Jr., and Greenfield, J. C., Jr.: Myocardial mechanics: Tension-velocity-length relationships of heart muscle. Circ Res 14:73, 1964.

Jewell, B. R.: A reexamination of the influence of muscle length on myocardial performance. Circ Res 40:221, 1977.

McDonald, I. G.: The shape and movements of the human left ventricle during systole. Am J Cardiol 26:221, 1970.

McHale, P. A., and Greenfield, J. C., Jr.: An evaluation of several geometric models for estimation of left ventricular circumferential wall stress. Circ Res 33:303, 1973.

Mirsky, I.: Assessment of passive elastic stiffness of cardiac muscle: Mathematical concepts, physiologic and clinical considerations, directions of future research. Prog Cardiovasc Dis 18:277, 1976.

Mitchell, J. H., and Mullins, C. B.: Dimensional analysis of left ventricular function. In Tanz, R. D., Kavaler, F., and Roberts, J. (eds.): Factors Influencing Myocardial Contractility. New York, Academic Press, 1967, p. 177.

Pollack, G. H., and Krueger, J. W.: Sarcomere dynamics in intact cardiac muscle. Europ J Cardiol 4(Suppl.):53, 1976.

Rankin, J. S., McHale, P. A., Arentzen, C. E., Ling, D., Greenfield, J. C., Jr., and Anderson, R. W.: The three dimensional dynamic geometry of the left ventricle in the conscious dog. Circ Res 39:304, 1976.

Rushmer, R. F.: Cardiovascular dynamics. 4th ed. Philadelphia, W. B. Saunders Co., 1976.

Cardiac Metabolism

The concept has been developed that myocardial contraction results from the sliding together of actin and myosin filaments, a process that depends upon the creation of bridges or chemical bonds between actin and myosin. This process requires energy and results in shortening of the sarcomere. The primary source for this energy is the hydrolysis of ATP to ADP and P_i and the liberation of energy from the high energy bond that couples ADP and P_i. This hydrolysis is catalyzed by myosin ATPase.

There are three known mechanisms (Fig. 37) available to muscle for the synthesis of ATP, the ultimate source of energy required for muscle contraction and for the basal energy requirements of muscle: these are oxidative phosphorylation, anaerobic glycolysis, and transfer of a high-energy phosphate bond from creatine phosphate (CP) to ADP. Mitochondrial oxidative phosphorylation is the dominant mechanism used by heart muscle to generate ATP. This mitochondrial ATP, in turn, is used to phosphorylate creatine to form creatine

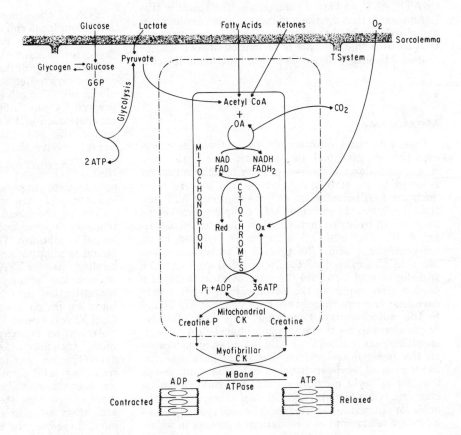

Figure 37. Metabolic pathways for energy (ATP) production including the creatine phosphate shuttle. OA = Oxaloacetate; NAD = nicotinamide adenine nucleotide; FAD = flavin adenine dinucleotide; NADH = reduced NAD; $FADH_2$ = reduced FAD; Ox = oxidation; Red = reduction; G-6-P = glucose-6-phosphate; P_1 = inorganic phosphate. (Modified from Mason, D. T., Zeli, R., Amsterdam, E., and Massami, R. A.: Mechanism of cardiac contraction: Structural, biochemical, and functional relations in the normal and diseased heart. In Sodeman, W. A., Jr., and Sodeman, W. A. (eds.): Pathologic Physiology—Mechanisms of Disease. 5th ed. Philadelphia, W. B. Saunders Co., 1974, p. 213, and from Bessman, S. P., and Geiger, P. J.: Transport of energy in muscle: The phosphorylcreatine shuttle. Science 211:448, 1981.)

phosphate. CP, in turn, is used as a high-energy phosphate bond carrier from mitochondrial ATP to myofibrillar ATP, the primary source of energy for muscle contraction (Fig. 37). The dynamic balance of this CP shuttle between the myofibrils and mitochondria explains why anoxia causes muscle contraction to cease rapidly. Since oxidative phosphorylation is almost exclusively aerobic, anoxia causes ATP and, ultimately, CP production to fall rapidly, eliminating the high-energy bond carrier for myofibrillar ATP production. In this regard, cardiac muscle resembles red skeletal muscle fibers, which have abundant mitochondria and are principally aerobic; lipid, in the form of fatty acids, serves as the major substrate. These characteristics of cardiac and red skeletal muscle are in contrast to white or "fast" skeletal muscle fibers where metabolic pathways for anaerobic production of ATP and stores of CP are abundant, carbohydrate rather than lipid is the principal substrate, mitochondria are sparse, and contraction is, ultimately, much less dependent on oxygen.

The purpose of this chapter is to review the most significant steps in cardiac metabolism. These include the uptake of fatty acids and glucose, their conversion to acetate, the conversion of acetate to carbon dioxide and hydrogen atoms, the transfer of electrons from hydrogen to oxygen with the formation of water, and the trapping of large amounts of that energy in the form of ATP. At each step in this metabolic chain important control mechanisms exist that help to explain the preferential use of fatty acids as a substrate for cardiac metabolism and the dependence of the system on oxygen. A second important feature of these control mechanisms is their sensitivity to regulation by ATP, ADP, and other compounds. The result of this regulation is that uptake and metabolism of substrates are closely coupled to energy utilization in a manner that assures that the rate of formation of ATP will be matched to energy demands for the function of the cell.

FAT

METABOLISM

Following entry into the cell, free fatty acids represent the principal fuel for the heart. The initial step in intracellular metabolism of fatty acids is a process referred to as activation. During this process fatty acids are first bound to an enzyme requiring ATP and then the fatty-acid–enzyme–AMP complex is converted to acyl-CoA by a step involving the substitution of CoA for AMP. The acyl-CoA complex is referred to as activated fatty acid. The process of activation takes place in the cytosol of the myocardial cell and the transfer of acyl-CoA into the mitochondria involves a carrier step requiring the seven-carbon organic acid carnitine and two transferase enzymes that are bound to the mitochondrial membrane. The first of these enzymes catalyzes the conversion of acyl-CoA to acyl-carnitine plus reduced CoA. The second enzyme located on the inner mitochondrial membrane catalyzes the conversion of acyl-carnitine to acyl-CoA, and hence transfer of acyl-CoA from outside to inside the mitochondria is completed. The final step in preparing fatty acids for entry into the tricarboxylic acid cycle involves a process referred to as β-oxidation, a process in which

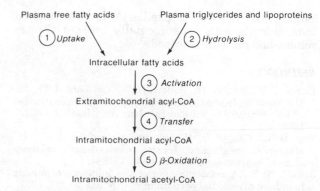

Figure 38. Overall scheme of fatty acid metabolism. The conversion of circulating lipids to the 2-carbon fragments that are oxidized within the cell involves five key reactions: (1) uptake of plasma free fatty acids; (2) liberation of esterified fatty acids by hydrolysis of plasma triglycerides and lipoproteins; (3) fatty acid activation—i.e., binding to CoA; (4) transfer of activated fatty acids (acyl CoA) from the cytosol to the mitochondrial matrix; and (5) β-oxidation to yield the 2-carbon fragment acetyl-CoA. (With permission from Katz, A. M.: Physiology of the Heart. New York, Raven Press, 1977, p. 52.)

two carbon fragments are split from acyl-CoA and then coupled to CoA in the form of acetyl CoA. This process of β-oxidation involves four discrete steps, and in the process FAD is reduced to $FADH_2$ and NAD is reduced to NADH. Acetyl CoA formed by the intramitochondrial process is identical to the acetyl CoA formed from aerobic glycolysis of glucose (Fig. 38).

CONTROL

Each of the steps necessary for the production of ATP from fat is subject to controlling forces. Free fatty acids are soluble in the lipid of the sarcolemma of myocytes. Because this uptake occurs largely, if not exclusively, by diffusion, it is proportional to the concentration gradient between the outside and the inside of the cell. The concentration gradient for diffusion is favored by any influence that increases the plasma concentration of FFA or enhances utilization of FFA within the cell. One such influence is sympathetic nerve activity that increases both the plasma FFA concentration and myocardial utilization of FFA. (Note that utilization of FFA is absolutely dependent upon an adequate supply of oxygen.)

Fatty acids are insoluble in water and are transported in the blood, either esterified to glycerol as triglyceride, or as nonesterified charged free fatty acids bound to albumin. The majority of free fatty acids are bound to albumin and there are at least two classes of binding sites for FFA, one with a high affinity and one with a low affinity. Thus, when the plasma FFA concentration rises the high-affinity binding sites become saturated and an increasing proportion of the total FFA is bound to low affinity sites.

Activation of intracellular fatty acids involves an initial transformation to the corresponding acyl-CoA derivative, a step involving acyl-CoA synthesis and requiring ATP. The activity of acyl-CoA synthetase has been shown to be inhibited by adenosine. Furthermore, since this step requires ATP, the process of activation ultimately depends on oxygen. At least in part, therefore, the failure to utilize FFA under conditions of hypoxia can be accounted for by the inhibitory effects of a lack of oxygen (less ATP and more adenosine) on the process of activation.

The transport of activated fatty acids from the cytosol to the inside of mitochondria involves the carrier carnitine and two acyl-CoA transferases. Transferase I is soluble, located between the inner and outer mitochondrial membranes, and is now thought to transfer acyl units from coenzyme A to carnitine. Transferase II is found on the inner mitochondrial membrane and functions to transfer acyl units from carnitine to coenzyme A within the mitochondria. At present there are few data concerning the factors that regulate the transferase enzymes. It is known that in the heart, transfer of acyl units from the cytosol to mitochondria depends upon carnitine; it is also known that carnitine levels can change dramatically and rapidly—for example, in response to glucagon.

Since acyl-CoA is transferred into mitochondria, its ultimate use in the Krebs cycle depends upon a final step referred to as β-oxidation with CoA. This process involves four steps: (1) acyl dehydrogenase, which requires FAD; (2) hydration of the double bond by enol hydrolase to form the beta hydroxyacyl derivative; (3) a second dehydrogenase step that requires NAD; and (4) reaction of the beta keto acyl-CoA with another CoA to yield acetyl CoA and an acyl-CoA that is shorter by two carbon atoms than the original fatty acid. This last reaction is catalyzed by thiolase. In the overall process of β-oxidation, the availability of FAD and NAD appear to be rate-limiting. Because these cofactors must be in an oxidized state, the process depends upon an adequate oxygen supply. Furthermore, because FAD is also used in the conversion of succinate to fumarate within the Krebs cycle, it is apparent that any influence that enhances glycolytic flux through the Krebs cycle will tend to inhibit fatty acid oxidation.

GLUCOSE

METABOLISM

Glycolysis is the process by which glucose is converted to pyruvic acid. The latter compound is then decarboxylated to form the two-carbon fragment acetate, which is coupled to CoA before entry into the tricarboxylic acid cycle. Glucose enters the myocardial cell from the blood by a carrier-mediated but non–energy-requiring process of transport. Glucose transport is accelerated by insulin but is not insulin-dependent. The process of conversion of intracellular glucose to pyruvic acid involves ten steps, all of which take place outside the mitochondria. The first step in glycolysis is the phosphorylation of glucose by ATP, a step catalyzed by the enzyme hexokinase. Glucose-6-phosphate formed by this reaction is then converted to fructose-6-phosphate, which in turn is phosphorylated by ATP to form fructose 1,6 diphosphate, which is split into dihydroxyacetone phosphate and two molecules of glyceraldehyde-3-phosphate. This last compound is oxidized in the presence of NAD and a dehydrogenase enzyme to form 1,3-diphosphoglycerate. In a series of four non–rate-limiting steps, 1,3-diphosphoglycerate is converted to pyruvate (for further details, see Section VI Fig. 7 and pp. 326–327).

Pyruvate, formed from the metabolism of glucose,

has two possible fates. One of these is conversion to lactic acid by a process of reduction catalyzed by lactic acid dehydrogenase and using NADH as a hydrogen donor. The alternative fate of pyruvate is conversion to acetyl CoA. This latter process is a complicated series of reactions involving pyruvate dehydrogenase, reduced CoA, lipoic acid, thiamine, and ATP. In the process, NAD is converted to NADH. At least two important factors favor the process of conversion of pyruvate to acetyl CoA rather than to lactic acid. One of these is the high affinity of the myocardial LDH isoenzyme for lactate and its low affinity for pyruvate. As a consequence lactate is consumed rather than produced by the heart, unless hypoxia leads to an accumulation of pyruvate owing to breakdown of its metabolism by the tricarboxylic acid cycle. A second factor in the preferential conversion of pyruvate to acetyl CoA rather than to lactate is also a consequence of the high oxygen availability to the normal heart. In the presence of oxygen, any NADH formed within the cytosol is rapidly transferred into the mitochondria and converted to NAD; NAD is then transferred back into the cytosol. Since the conversion of pyruvate to lactate occurs only in the cytosol and depends on NADH, this reaction is curtailed by the relative lack of NADH in the cytosol under conditions of adequate oxygenation.

CONTROL

Within the glycolytic pathway there are multiple sites for control of glycolytic flux. Glucose transport can be facilitated by insulin and by epinephrine. The hexokinase reaction exhibits end product inhibition by glucose-6-phosphate, but the extent of that inhibition is modulated to a significant extent by relative concentrations of ATP and ADP. As a consequence, physiological activities that utilize ATP and increase the concentration of ADP effectively remove the brake on the hexokinase reaction. By far the most important and the rate-limiting control point is the phosphofructokinase step. The activity of this enzyme is inhibited potently by ATP and by creatine phosphate, the principal high-energy stores within the myocardial cell. Conversely, the activity of the enzyme is greatly enhanced by ADP (the product of physiological activity) and by cyclic AMP, which increases in response to beta-adrenergic agonists. An increase in hydrogen ion and associated acidosis inhibit the enzyme. The net consequence of these controls is a system in which glycolytic flux can be substantially augmented during an increase in myocardial work, whether that increase in work is the result of an imposed hydraulic stress or a consequence of beta-adrenergic stimulation. It is important to note, however, that the magnitude of the increase in glycolytic flux with activity is related importantly to substrate availability. When glucose is the only available substrate, glucose utilization is within limits, proportional to the increase in cardiac work. However, when fatty acids are provided in the coronary perfusate, fat is used in preference to glucose, and the increase in substrate utilization that accompanies an increase in work is derived predominantly from fat.

The reason for preferential use of fat rather than glucose by the working heart is explained largely by the factors that control pyruvate dehydrogenase, the enzyme responsible for converting pyruvate to acetyl CoA. As noted previously, pyruvate dehydrogenase is a multienzyme complex. The reactions promoted by this enzyme complex are strongly inhibited by acetyl CoA and very possibly by other factors. The result is that when fat is available, beta oxidation of fat to acetyl CoA inhibits the conversion of pyruvate to acetyl CoA. In isolated preparations in which pyruvate is the only available substrate, approximately 60 per cent of the enzyme pyruvate dehydrogenase is in an active form. However, when fatty acids are provided, only about 5 per cent of pyruvate dehydrogenase is in an active form. Thus, not only are there internal control mechanisms that regulate glycolytic flux, but in addition the rate of glycolysis is regulated by the availability of fat. Fat is used preferentially and this is explained, at least in part, by the ability of acetyl CoA resulting from fat metabolism to inhibit utilization of pyruvate.

ACETATE

METABOLISM

The final step in the formation of acetyl CoA, whether derived from pyruvate or from beta oxidation of fatty acids, takes place within mitochondria. The subsequent oxidation of acetyl CoA to carbon dioxide and water occurs within the mitochondria and is referred to as the Krebs cycle or the tricarboxylic acid cycle (refer to Section VI Fig. 10 and pp. 329–332). The initial step in the Krebs cycle is the condensation of acetyl CoA (two-carbon acetate fragment) with oxaloacetate (four carbons) to form citrate (six carbons). In the process coenzyme A is released for reutilization. In a subsequent chain of nine reactions each mole of citrate is converted to oxaloacetate yielding two molecules of carbon dioxide, one mole of ATP (at the succinyl CoA to succinate step), and eight hydrogen atoms. At each step in the Krebs cycle, in which hydrogen is released, the release is catalyzed by a substrate-specific dehydrogenase and the hydrogen is released in packets of two atoms. Of the eight hydrogens released, three are transferred to NAD in the form of NADH, two are transferred to FAD in the form of $FADH_2$, and the remaining three are passed directly from the dehydrogenase to the oxidative process. The process of oxidative phosphorylation, by which electrons derived from hydrogen atoms are passed along the respiratory chain with the production of ATP and H_2O, will be discussed in the next section. It should be noted, however, that the oxidation of each molecule of acetyl CoA yields 12 moles of ATP. Furthermore, the operation of the Krebs cycle uses one molecule of oxaloacetate to oxidize each mole of acetyl CoA, and in the process regenerates one mole of oxaloacetate. The facts that the Krebs cycle is regenerative, that it is the most efficient source for generating ATP, that it can operate using either glucose or fat as a substrate, and that its operation ultimately depends upon oxygen, all contribute to its central and predominant role in providing fuel for cardiac metabolic activity.

CONTROL

The rate of turnover of the Krebs cycle is related to the availability of its substrate, acetyl CoA, to the availability of oxidized NAD and FAD, and to the regulatory influence of several compounds on the velocity of enzymatically mediated steps in the cycle. Most current evidence points to the conversion of isocitrate to α keto glutarate, a step catalyzed by the enzyme isocitric dehydrogenase, as the rate-limiting step in the Krebs cycle. This step, like two others in the Krebs cycle, utilizes NAD as a hydrogen acceptor, and therefore depends on oxidized NAD as a cofactor, which in turn depends on the availability of oxygen. Furthermore, isocitric dehydrogenase exists in an inactive and an active form. Conversion from its inactive form is stimulated by ADP and inhibited by ATP. Enzyme activity is therefore proportional to the ratio of ADP:ATP. The actions of ADP and of ATP on enzyme activity are thought to occur through an allosteric effect that influences the affinity of the enzyme for isocitrate. Thus, when acetyl CoA is available in excess, the rate of turnover of the Krebs cycle is determined by the ADP:ATP ratio. This ratio in turn is influenced by the activities of the cell that utilize ATP as an energy source and produce ADP. In this way, the oxidation of acetyl CoA within mitochondria is governed by the energy requirements of the heart. Furthermore, an accumulation of NADH and depletion of NAD in the absence of adequate oxygen has the capacity to turn off the oxidation of isocitrate and slow the rate of turnover of the Krebs cycle.

There are other points in the Krebs cycle in which the opportunity for control exists. For example, the condensation of acetyl CoA and oxaloacetate to form citrate is catalyzed by an enzyme, citrate synthase, the activity of which is inhibited by ATP and by NADH. While the net effects of ATP and NADH at this step are similar to their actions on isocitric dehydrogenase, the focus of control is on the latter enzyme, which catalyzes the rate-limiting step in the Krebs cycle.

OXIDATIVE PHOSPHORYLATION

The products of the Krebs cycle include CO_2, H_2O, and H atoms. Each atom of hydrogen represents a hydrogen ion (H^+) plus an electron (e^-). The operation of the respiratory chain is best understood as a system in which the electron from a hydrogen atom is passed along the components of the respiratory chain and ultimately transferred to molecular oxygen. In the process, a hydrogen ion (H^+) is produced. For each two hydrogen atoms converted to hydrogen ions, two electrons are transferred to oxygen, yielding O^{2-}. The combination of two H^+ ions with one O^{2-} then yields H_2O.

The successive transfer of electrons have hydrogen along the respiratory chain to oxygen involves a series of oxidation and reduction steps. In the initial stages involving NAD, FAD, and LipoQ the electron is carried within an organic ring structure. In the second group of five stages, the electron is carried within the heme ring of the cytochrome system, wherein the iron-porphyrin groups undergo reversible oxidation and reduction. In the final step, the electron is passed to oxygen ($\frac{1}{2}O_2$), each oxygen atom accepting two electrons. Finally $2H^+$ ions combine with O^{2-} yielding H_2O.

At three steps in the respiratory chain, the transfer of electrons from one component to the next in the chain is accompanied by the release of very large amounts of energy and the formation of ATP. These steps are indicated in Section VI Figure 11, pp. 329–331, and occur when the electron is transferred (1) from NAD to flavoprotein; (2) from cytochrome b to cytochrome c; and (3) from cytochrome a to molecular oxygen. This process is referred to as oxidative phosphorylation and is now thought to involve a chemiosmotic process in which the energy released from electron transfer is initially used to establish a concentration gradient across the inner mitochondrial membrane, and this potential energy in the form of a charge gradient is then used to form ATP. Recent evidence that ionophores that render the mitochondrial membrane permeable to certain cations are capable of uncoupling respiration from ATP formation is consistent with the chemiosmotic hypothesis.

CONTROL

The discussion above has focused on that generation of ATP as a consequence of the operation of a respiratory chain that enables electrons to be passed from either NADH or $FADH_2$ to oxygen. In this process, referred to as electron transfer, large amounts of energy (about 51,000 cal) per mole of NADH oxidized are released. Coupled to the electron transfer chain is the process of oxidative phosphorylation, in which about 21,000 cal of this energy (or 40 to 50 per cent) is captured in the form of high-energy bonds of three moles of ATP formed from the coupling of three moles of ADP and P_i. When isolated mitochondria are incubated in the presence of high levels of substrate and oxygen, the rate of respiration (O_2 consumed or ATP formed) is determined by the availability for ADP. When ADP is low, respiration is slow. When ADP is high, respiration is fast. Under conditions in which ATP formation is proportional to ADP availability, and when three moles of ATP are formed per mole of oxygen consumed, the mitochondria, or, more aptly, electron transfer and phosphorylation, are described as tightly coupled. Many agents are now available that have the capacity to either block electron transfer at specific sites in the chain or uncouple electron transfer and phosphorylation of ADP. These tools are of tremendous experimental value and may have importance in understanding certain disease states. In the normal heart, however, it is evident that cellular respiration is controlled by ADP. As a consequence, any influence that increases the metabolic requirements of the heart results in utilization of ATP; ADP is formed and in turn stimulates respiration to form more ATP. In its simplest form, therefore, the beauty of the system is that the energy needed for physiological functions is provided as a consequence of those functions as long as oxygen and substrates are available.

In summary, the mechanical activity of heart muscle requires large amounts of energy, which are provided to the contractile proteins by myosin ATP with CP as the high-energy phosphate bond carrier (or shuttle) between contractile protein ATP utilization and mitochondrial ATP generation sites (see Fig. 38). Thus, although phosphorylation of ADP by CP is an important source of ATP at the myofibrillar level, this CP is ultimately derived from ATP generated by mitochondrial oxidative phosphorylation. Although there are other mechanisms available to heart muscle for generating limited amounts of ATP, by far the most important source is mitochondrial oxidative phosphorylation. Oxidation phosphorylation is coupled to a process of electron transfer in which hydrogen atoms derived from oxidation of acetyl CoA are converted to hydrogen ions, the electrons are transferred to oxygen, and water is produced. Acetyl CoA is derived either from pyruvate or from beta-oxidation of fatty acids. Pyruvate is derived either from glucose or from extraction of lactate from the blood, and fatty acids enter the cell by diffusion in proportion to the concentration gradient between the blood and the cell. Glycogen can be synthesized and stored by myocytes and then used as a reserve for glucose-6-phosphate. However, utilization of glycogen to form ATP is relatively minor in the heart. The preferential use of fatty acids by the heart is normal and is enhanced by increased contractile activity. This preference is best explained by the fact that acetyl CoA derived from fat inhibits pyruvate dehydrogenase. Phosphofructokinase appears to be the rate-limiting step in the Krebs cycle. The fact that the activity of both of these enzymes is regulated by the ADP:ATP ratio provides a mechanism whereby the flux of substrates is closely controlled by energy-consuming activities of heart muscle. Because heart muscle is so dependent on aerobic metabolism, ischemia due to interruption of coronary blood leads within seconds to a rapid decline of contractile function and within minutes to loss of cell viability.

REFERENCES

Bessman, S. P., and Geiger, P. J.: Transport of energy in muscle: The phosphorylcreatine shuttle. Science 211:448, 1981.
Randle, P. J.: Regulation of glycolysis and pyruvate oxidation in cardiac muscle. Circ Res 38(Suppl. I) 8, 1976.
Rovetto, M. J.: Myocardial metabolism. In Wilkerson, R. D. (ed.): Cardiac Pharmacology. New York, Academic Press, 1981, p. 335.
Vary, T. C., Reibel, D. K., and Neely, J. R.: Control of energy metabolism of heart muscle. Annu Rev Physiol 43:419, 1981.

Mechanisms of Cardiovascular Control

The structural integrity and function of cells throughout the body depend upon delivery of oxygen and other substrates for metabolism. Thus, the ultimate goal of the circulation is tissue perfusion. The requirements for perfusion of any given organ or tissue may vary widely between the extreme characteristics of resting, or basal, function and maximal activity. Whether the organism is basal or active or in transition between these two states, the circulation as a whole must be capable of adapting to the stress of gravity. This stress is encountered daily in making the transition from the supine to the erect posture. It is maximized, for example, when pilots encounter the considerable G forces associated with acceleration or deceleration, on the one hand, and weightlessness on the other. Under any given condition the need for perfusion in one organ or area may greatly exceed the needs in other areas. Hence, the circulation must be capable of distributing increased perfusion to some areas while maintaining a constant or reduced perfusion to other areas. To ensure that these roles are performed, the circulation is endowed with an elaborate control system. The purpose of this chapter is to develop a conceptual framework of overall circulatory regulation and to consider in appropriate detail the functional characteristics of the more important components of this system. As we discuss various disease processes in subsequent chapters, it will become apparent that diseases affect primarily one or more of the components of this scheme, and that manifestations of disease reflect either normal or abnormal compensatory reponses to such disturbances.

In a classic paper on systems analysis of circulatory control, Guyton and his colleagues have identified about 400 basic physiological phenomena and their interrelationships that describe circulatory function and control. Their model predicts with remarkable accuracy both the short-term and long-term adaptations to perturbations of components of the system. The circulatory control system appears to be geared toward ensuring adequate oxygen delivery to cells. Although the extraction of oxygen and of other substrates from arterial blood may increase in response to an increase in metabolic activity of the tissue in question, most studies indicate that transport of oxygen is flow-limited, and that an increase in oxygen uptake is met primarily by an increase in local perfusion. Because flow to any organ depends upon arterial blood pressure and the vascular resistance of that organ, factors that influence systemic pressure and local vascular resistance form the basis of an understanding of overall circulatory control. Local factors that regulate vascular resistance in response to changing metabolic activity are of central importance.

Arterial blood pressure is a major determinant of organ perfusion. Yet, arterial blood pressure is itself determined by cardiac output and the impedance to flow that is in large part due to net or total vascular resistance. Several mechanisms, largely neural and humoral, have the capacity to modulate vascular resistance independent of local control and to influence the mechanisms by which cardiac output is adjusted to meet peripheral metabolic demands.

The evidence strongly indicates that cardiac output is determined mainly by peripheral factors. One of these is peripheral vascular resistance. Cardiac output will increase and remain elevated with a major drop in total peripheral resistance, such as occurs with creation of an arteriovenous fistula. The second determinant of cardiac output is venous return. The latter is related to blood volume and to the capacitance of the systemic venous system. Thus, cardiac output may be limited by an inadequate blood volume—for example, after hemorrhage—or by standing after the administration of agents that reduce venous tone and increase the capacitance of the systemic venous bed. It follows that a third level of understanding of circulatory control involves these factors that regulate venous tone and, even more importantly, factors that control blood volume.

LOCAL CONTROL

In many organs and tissues, particularly those with a high and variable capacity for metabolic activity, blood flow is dominantly controlled by local factors and regulated in proportion to metabolic needs of the organ (Fig. 39). Muscle is perhaps the best example of such a tissue. At rest, skeletal muscle blood flow is approximately 5 ml/100 grams/min, but can increase to 50 to 75 ml/100 grams/min during active exercise. The concentration of oxygen in the tissue, either directly or indirectly, through the release of vasodilator substances, appears to be the most important factor in regulating muscle blood flow. Furthermore, while neural and humoral factors have the ability to modulate muscle blood flow to an important extent at rest, these factors have less effect during muscular activity and almost no effect at maximal metabolic activity. The heart resembles exercising skeletal muscle. Coronary blood flow is 70 to 100 ml/100 grams/min in resting subjects and increases in direct proportion to myocardial activity and oxygen requirements.

At an opposite extreme are organs such as the kidney. Under basal conditions, the kidneys receive 1000 to 1400 ml/min of arterial flow, or nearly 22 per cent of the cardiac output. Renal blood flow far exceeds the requirements for delivery of nutrients, including oxygen. Hence the arteriovenous oxygen difference is extremely narrow. It is not surprising, therefore, that no relationship has been established between the met-

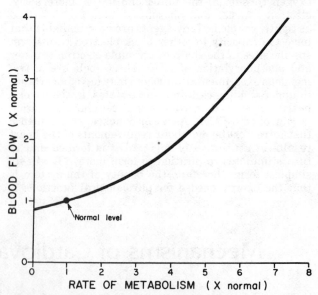

Figure 39. Effect of increasing rate of metabolism on tissue blood flow. (With permission from Guyton, A. C.: Textbook of Medical Physiology. 5th ed. Philadelphia, W. B. Saunders Co., 1976, p. 252.)

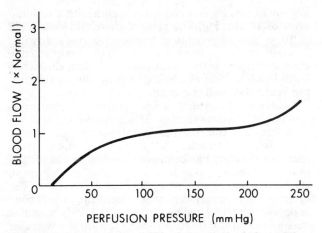

Figure 40. Autoregulation of blood flow in the kidney. When the perfusion pressure to the kidney is increased, the relation between perfusion pressure and flow is not linear. In the range of perfusion pressures between 100 and 200 mm Hg, blood flow increases very little. The phenomenon of autoregulation appears to result from vasoconstriction in response to an increase in perfusion pressure, and vasodilation in response to a decrease in perfusion pressure.

abolic activity of the kidney and its blood flow. In essence, the architecture of the renal circulation is adapted to serve the primary role of filtering a very large proportion of the cardiac output on a continuous basis. Total renal blood flow is high because the net vascular resistance of the kidney is extremely low. The glomerular capillary bed receives nearly all of the renal blood flow through low-resistance afferent arterioles. Blood egresses from the glomerulus through efferent arterioles, which offer the principal resistance to flow, and as a result glomerular capillary pressure is high (approximately 60 mm Hg). Beyond the efferent arteriole, the largest portion of renal blood flow enters cortical veins to leave the kidney. A small proportion perfuses the metabolically active peritibular capillary bed.

Studies of the renal circulation have served to highlight a second important mechanism of local vascular control, namely autoregulation (Fig. 40). When arterial pressure is raised acutely from 100 to 200 mm Hg, a 100 per cent increase, there is an increase of only approximately 7 per cent in renal blood flow. This phenomenon occurs in other vascular beds but is uniquely well developed in the kidney. The phenomenon of autoregulation in the kidney results from active vasoconstriction of the afferent arteriole in response to an increase in renal perfusion pressure. Details of autoregulatory phenomena will be developed in other sections of this text; suffice it to say that the proximity of the distal nephron to the afferent arteriole, the location of the juxtaglomerular apparatus, and the fact that an increase in fluid flow through the distal nephron causes afferent arteriolar constriction all imply local feedback control systems.

NEURAL CONTROL

Superimposed on local mechanisms that modulate arterial vascular resistance, and hence perfusion of individual organs, is a neural mechanism. By far the most important of these is the control of peripheral sympathetic nerve activity which has the important capacity to influence arterial resistance, the tone of venous capacitance vessels, and the pumping ability of the heart at any given level of venous pressure.

Sympathetic nerve activity originates within the reticular formation of the lower third of the pons and the upper medulla from regions that are represented bilaterally. Together, these areas are referred to as the vasomotor center. The vasomotor center transmits sympathetic impulses in a tonic or intrinsic fashion, and this rate of intrinsic activity is in turn modulated by neural input from other regions. These regions include an inhibitory center that is centrally located in the vasomotor region of the medulla, numerous reflexogenic areas of the cardiovascular system, and higher levels of the central nervous system. For many years it was felt that the output of sympathetic nerve impulses from the vasomotor center was uniform; that is, impulse traffic in all efferent sympathetic nerves was thought to be equal and the level of activity was modulated by the vasomotor center. While many circumstances exist in which a more or less uniform output is observed, recent studies strongly indicate that efferent activity is targeted to specific organs, to specific vascular beds, and even to specific segments of a given vascular bed. Thus, the potential for a differential rather than a uniform output of sympathetic impulses clearly exists. Closely coupled to the concept of a differential output from the vasomotor center is the recognition that different parts of the circulation have different functions. Hence, the overall cardiovascular change will differ in response to stimuli that elicit an increase in sympathetic activity preferentially to the heart, to arterial resistance vessels, or to large capacitance veins. Finally, the distribution of adrenergic nerves to various segments of the circulation is not uniform and the number and type of adrenergic receptors in these segments also varies.

The neurons of the vasomotor center are under the constant influence of afferent impulses that originate from mechanoreceptors located within the heart, lungs, and arteries; from chemoreceptors located in skeletal muscle; from thermoreceptors; and from other regions of the central nervous system. Each source of afferent input to the vasomotor center produces a characteristic pattern of efferent neural output. Yet the net response to a complex input from more than one source is an even more complex result of integration of afferent signals within the vasomotor region.

Each efferent sympathetic nerve pathway is composed of a preganglionic neuron and a postganglionic neuron. The cell bodies of the preganglionic fibers lie within the thoracic and upper lumbar spinal cord. These fibers pass from the cord via anterior roots of each spinal nerve and then via the white ramus to synapse with postganglionic cell bodies located within the ganglia of the sympathetic chains. From these ganglia, postganglionic sympathetic nerves pass to their effector organ by one of two routes: (1) through peripheral sympathetic nerves, or (2) returning to the spinal nerve via a grey ramus.

Probably the most extensively studied of the neural mechanisms for cardiovascular control is the baroreceptor reflex. Baroreceptors are a special class of mechanoreceptors of which the carotid sinus is the most noteworthy. The carotid sinus is a focal area at the origin of the internal carotid, containing both diffuse and "glomerular-like" nerve endings that respond to stretch and to rate of stretch by initiating afferent nerve impulses that pass over the sinus nerve to the glossopharyngeal nerve and hence to the vasomotor center. Impulse traffic over the sinus nerve has been shown by numerous investigators to be intermittent, synchronous with the rise in arterial pressure, and quantitatively (impulses/sec) related to mean arterial pressure and the rate of rise of arterial pressure during the systolic pressure pulse. An increase in arterial pressure leads to an increase of impulse traffic over the sinus nerve (Fig. 41), which in turn inhibits the output of sympathetic efferent impulses arising from the vasomotor centers. The consequence is a decrease in sympathetic vasoconstrictor tone, a decrease in sympathetic tone to the heart, and a decrease in sympathetic tone to capacitance veins. The net result is a tendency for arterial pressure to fall, or at least to return toward the level that existed before carotid arterial pressure was increased. Conversely, a drop of pressure within a baroreceptor region diminishes impulse frequency over the sinus nerve, removes the inhibitory influence on the vasomotor center, and leads to an increase in sympathetic efferent activity and to arterial constriction, an increase in venous tone, an increased rate and contractility of the heart, and a restoration of blood pressure.

The baroreceptor reflex functions as a negative feedback loop in which a rise of pressure within the baroreceptor leads to a series of effects that tend to reduce pressure toward its initial level. The baroreflex is regarded as a rapid feedback loop because the reflex becomes maximally active within a period of seconds (10 to 30). It is also regarded as a powerful reflex. For example, if the arterial pressure is increased from 100 to 180 mm Hg suddenly, the baroreceptor reflex will return the pressure to approximately 110 mm Hg.

Thus a 70 mm Hg compensation occurs with a residual error of 10 mm Hg. The ratio of these two values (70 ÷ 10, or 7) is referred to as feedback gain of the reflex. In addition to the carotid sinus, other important mechanoreceptors with operationally similar characteristics but less gain are located within the aortic arch, the ventricles, and the atria.

A second important reflex control mechanism is typified by chemoreceptors. The carotid body is a minute structure composed essentially of vascular tissue, which is a conglomerate AV fistula. The blood flow to each carotid body has been estimated to be 200 ml/100 grams of tissue, which is the highest of any organ in the body when expressed as flow per unit weight. The arteriovenous oxygen difference across the carotid body is approximately 1 vol%. Within this highly vascular tissue are epithelial cells oriented toward the vascular surface and densely innervated with sensory nerve fibers that respond to changes in pO_2. The principal role of the chemoreceptor is to induce an increase in ventilation when the pO_2 of arterial blood drops. However, the chemoreceptor also responds to changes in arterial blood pressure, presumably because a drop in local tissue pO_2 occurs when perfusion pressure is reduced. Stimulation of the carotid body leads to a relatively selective increase in vascular resistance in skeletal muscle, and to bradycardia due to vagal nerve enhancement. From the point of view of its cardiovascular effects, the chemoreflex, like the baroreflex, is rapid in its onset. When the chemoreflex is initiated by a change in blood pressure, the gain of the reflex is approximately 4 and hence significantly less potent than the baroreflex.

HUMORAL CONROL

In addition to the mechanisms for cardiovascular control, generally defined as neural-reflex controls, humoral mechanisms play an important role in blood pressure regulation. Prominent among these is the renin-angiotensin system, which primarily affects arterial resistance vessels, with little or no direct effect on the heart or on veins. A decrease in arterial blood pressure causes the kidney to release renin. Renin is synthesized by juxtaglomerular cells in the macula densa and released into the renal venous effluent. The rate of renin release by juxtaglomerular cells can be affected by pressure in the afferent arteriole (a baromechanism), by the concentration of sodium within the macula densa, by the activity of renal sympathetic nerves, and by other factors such as the plasma potassium concentration. Renin is a proteolytic enzyme with a molecular weight of approximately 35,000. Renin splits a circulating alpha globulin called angiotensinogen to form a decapeptide, angiotensin I. Angiotensin I is then converted to an octapeptide (angiotensin II) within the pulmonary circulation. Angiotensin II is a potent constrictor of arterial resistance vessels, where it acts by first binding to an angiotensin receptor. Plasma levels of angiotensin are relatively low and are thought to have little or no direct role in the control of vascular resistance in physiological states. A proposed indirect role maintains that angiotensin traverses the blood-brain barrier and modifies the response of the medullary vasomotor center to baro-

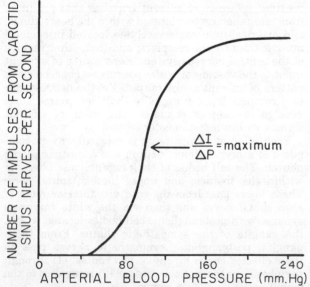

Figure 41. Response of the baroreceptors at different levels of arterial pressure. (With permission from Guyton, A. C.: Textbook of Medical Physiology. 5th ed. Philadelphia, W. B. Saunders Co., 1976, p. 269.)

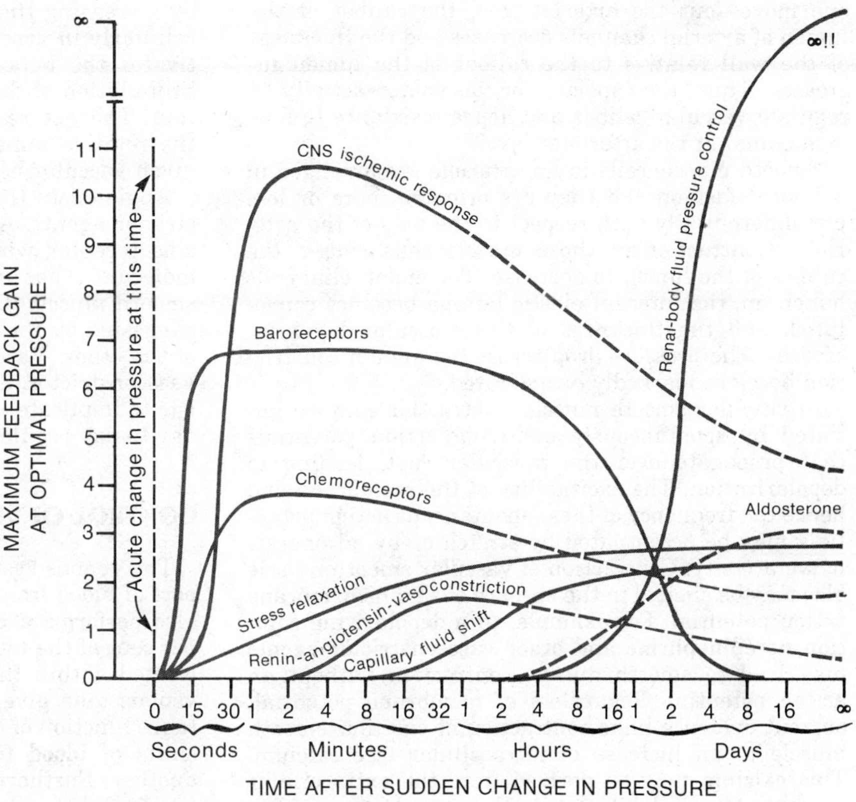

Figure 42. Response times of the major arterial blood pressure regulating mechanisms. This figure also shows approximate feedback gains of these mechanisms at different times after the responses have been initiated. Note especially the infinite gain that occurs in the renal–body fluid pressure control mechanism at infinite time. (With permission from Guyton, A. C.: Integrative hemodynamics. In Sodeman, W. A., Jr., and Sodeman, W. A. (eds.): Pathologic Physiology—Mechanisms of Disease. 5th ed. Philadelphia, W. B. Saunders Co., 1974, p. 160.)

receptor input. Others have demonstrated that angiotensin accumulates at binding sites on the arterial wall and that local concentrations can mediate vasoconstriction despite relatively low plasma concentration.

It should be noted that the renin-angiotensin-vasoconstrictor system also functions as a negative feedback loop. A decrease in arterial pressure activates the system, which in turn causes blood pressure to rise. In contrast to the carotid sinus baroreflex, where the response time is maximal within seconds, the renin-angiotensin system has a response time of 20 to 30 minutes. Furthermore, the gain of the renin-angiotensin feedback is approximately 2 (Fig. 42). It follows from these considerations that the renin-angiotensin system is intrinsically less potent than the baroreflex, and because of its response time is less likely to play a significant role in acute changes of blood pressure. It is important to note, however, that the renin-angiotensin system is coupled to the faster neural system, since increased sympathetic activity is a potent cause of renin release. Furthermore, the renin-angiotensin system is coupled to an even longer-range blood pressure control mechanism (to blood volume control), since angiotensin II is a potent stimulator of aldosterone release from the adrenal cortex.

In general, adrenal medullary secretion of catecholamines can be viewed as a component of the neural reflex mechanism of blood pressure control. It is of interest, however, that the pattern of secretion of norepinephrine and epinephrine exemplifies an earlier point regarding the selectivity of sympathetic output in response to specific stimuli. For example, acute psychological stress causing anxiety leads to a predominant release of epinephine with associated vasodilatation. Other forms of stress that provoke a competitive response elicit a predominant release of norepinephrine.

CONTROL OF RESISTANCE VESSELS

In a typical microvascular circuit, blood enters the circuit through an arteriole and exits through a venule. Beyond the heavily muscled arteriole, flow divides into several branches referred to as metarterioles, which are characterized by a much less dense muscular media. From these metarterioles, numerous capillaries arise that fall into two distinct classes. One group, the AV capillaries, course directly from the metarteriole to the venule and retain a diffusely distributed muscular coat. True capillaries, on the other hand, have no muscular coat and form interconnecting networks before rejoining the AV capillary to enter the venule. The origin of each capillary from its parent metarteriole is surrounded by a sphincter of smooth muscle capable of maintaining the distal capillary bed open or closed. Arterioles and venules have a dense sympathetic nerve innervation, but metarterioles and precapillary sphincters are only sparsely innervated, if at all. The picture that emerges is one in which local factors operate to control the resistance of arterioles and metarterioles, while neural input modulates the tone of arterioles and only indirectly modulates the flow through more distal segments of the microvascular circuit.

The resistance to flow offered by a microvascular circuit is primarily a function of vascular caliber. As one moves out the arterial tree, the caliber of the lumen of arterial channels decreases and the thickness of the wall relative to the caliber of the lumen increases. Thus, the capacity for vasomotor activity to regulate vascular caliber and hence resistance to flow is maximal at the arteriolar level.

Smooth muscle cells in an arteriole are arranged in a helical fashion and they are oriented more or less circumferentially with respect to the axis of the arteriole. Contraction of these muscle cells causes the caliber of the lumen to decrease. The endothelial cells bunch up, the internal elastic lamina becomes convoluted, and the thickness of the muscular layer increases. The pressure drop across the area of constriction becomes markedly exaggerated.

In vascular smooth muscle, contraction may be initiated by spontaneously occurring action potentials that propagate over the muscular coat, leading to depolarization. The excitability of the membrane and hence the frequency of these spontaneous action potentials may be accentuated by stretch or by adrenergic nerve activity. Contraction of vascular smooth muscle also may be elicited in the absence of a transmembrane action potential. For example, in a depolarizing solution norepinephrine and other vasoconstrictor agents may lead to smooth muscle contraction without an action potential. Regardless of membrane potential, current evidence links contraction of vascular smooth muscle to an increase of intracellular free calcium. This calcium may be derived from the extracellular space or from a labile intracellular pool. As in other muscle, a rise in free calcium above some threshold value promotes actin-myosin interaction by removing the inhibitory effect of troponin on actomyosin ATPase.

Prominent among factors that regulate the caliber and resistance of arterioles is the phenomenon of autoregulation. Different vascular beds differ markedly in their ability to maintain a relatively constant flow over widely ranging perfusion pressures. The renal and cerebral beds are particularly noteworthy in this regard. One theory of autoregulation holds that the frequency of spontaneous smooth muscle action potentials increases with stretch. The effect would be an increased vasomotor tone in response to stretch, which would tend to restore vessel caliber to that which prevailed before the increase in distending pressure. Another theory is that pO_2 regulates vascular vasomotor tone and leads to vasoconstriction with increased pO_2 and vasodilatation with decreased pO_2. A third theory is that increased perfusion pressure causes transudation of fluid into the extravascular space, which then leads mechanically to a reduction in vascular caliber by extravascular compression. Despite attractive features to each theory, proof of the mechanism of autoregulation remains to be established.

Also within the general purview of local factors that regulate blood vessel caliber and resistance are changes of tissue pO_2, pH, potassium, adenosine, and so on. These are discussed at length in the chapter on exercise physiology. Suffice it to say that, by whatever mechanism, tissues have a pronounced ability to regulate their own arterial resistance in response to local changes in metabolic activity.

Arterial resistance vessels contain either alpha receptors, beta-2 receptors, or both. Norepinephrine activates the alpha receptor and leads to vasoconstriction by increasing the concentration of free calcium intracellularly in vascular smooth muscle. Epinephrine activates the beta-2 receptor and the alpha receptor. Stimulation of the beta-2 receptor leads to vasodilatation. The net response to epinephrine depends upon the relative number of each type of receptor in any given vascular bed.

Angiotensin II is the most potent of known vasoconstrictor agents. Angiotensin acts by binding to a specific receptor with high affinity for the angiotensin molecule. That its mechanism of action on vascular smooth muscle differs from that of norepinephrine is suggested by the fact that each potentiates the action of the other. Vasopressin is another potential arterial vasoconstrictor, although little evidence currently exists to implicate a physiological role for vasopressin in day-to-day regulation of arteriolar resistance.

CONTROL OF VEINS

The venous system provides a conduit for the transport of blood from distal vascular beds to the heart. It also performs a capacitance function, since about 65 per cent of the total blood volume at any given time is located within the venous compartment. Changes in venous tone give a dynamic character to the capacitance function of the system capable of producing large shifts of blood from one segment of the system to another. Furthermore, because systemic veins are interposed between the capillary bed and the heart, changes of venous tone have both upstream and downstream effects. Constriction of the venous system will raise central venous pressure and hence cardiac output by the Starling effect. Venoconstriction also raises capillary hydrostatic pressure and hence the rate of capillary filtration of fluid, a consequence of which is regulation of the ratio of extravascular to intravascular fluid volume.

In contrast to arterial resistance vessels, veins are directly affected very little by pO_2, pCO_2, or other metabolic factors in surrounding tissue or in the blood passing through the vein. Veins are affected to an important extent by alterations in sympathetic nerve activity and by certain circulating vasoactive substances. With regard to their innervation, cutaneous veins, splanchnic veins, and some of the large tributaries, such as the cephalic vein, are richly innervated with sympathetic efferent nerve fibers and they contain a predominance of alpha receptors and a paucity of beta-2 (dilator) receptors. In these vascular beds, an increase in sympathetic nerve activity leads to prominent venoconstriction. In other vascular beds, the most noteworthy of which is skeletal muscle, sympathetic nerves and alpha receptors are infrequent or absent in the veins and venoconstriction does not occur in response to stimuli that activate the sympathetic nervous system. In skeletal muscle, venous volume is controlled principally by muscle activity and the mechanical effect of that activity on neighboring veins (the muscle pump).

It was noted previously that the sympathetic nervous system has the capacity for differential output. Venous responses to different stimuli illustrate this capacity. Mental stimulation, in the form of a requirement to perform mental arithmetic, or the response to immersion of one limb in cold water, elicits prompt and significant constriction of cutaneous veins with little or no change in splanchnic venous volume. In contrast, tilting to the erect position causes tachycardia, increased arterial resistance, and splanchnic venoconstriction, but has little or no effect on cutaneous venous tone. These observations are consistent with the view that autonomic control of different organs is selective.

Cutaneous veins are also an integral component of the thermoregulatory system of the body. A reduction in body temperature causes cutaneous venoconstriction and body heating causes venodilatation. These changes are mediated by sympathetic efferents coupled to the thermoregulatory center in the brain. Cutaneous venous tone aids in temperature control by altering the vascular surface available for heat transfer between the skin and the environment and by altering the velocity of flow through this surface and hence the time available for heat transfer to occur. It is also of interest that cold potentiates and heat attenuates the responsiveness of the cutaneous venous vessels to adrenergic agents.

In summary, from these considerations it follows that control of the venous system is principally a consequence of central modulation of efferent adrenergic nerve activity acting through changes in venous tone. The effects of changes of adrenergic efferent activity on veins are in part related to the distribution of efferent nerves and to the distribution of receptors responsive to the adrenergic neurotransmitter norepinephrine. Venous responses are also determined by the nature of the stimulus that causes an increased sympathetic nerve activity. Some stimuli principally cause a change in cutaneous venomotor tone, others affect mainly the splanchnic capacitance vessels, and still others alter both venous regions. The capacity for differential changes in venous tone is clearly evident although the central mechanisms that determine this differential output of efferent neural impulses is unclear. It is apparent that changes in venous tone are coupled to other aspects of circulatory function and control. Changes in venous tone can affect central venous pressure and hence cardiac output, they can affect peripheral venous pressure and hence capillary filtration and blood volume, and they can affect cutaneous venous vascular surface area and consequently the rate of loss of heat from the body.

CONTROL OF BLOOD VOLUME

A third important component of the cardiovascular control system is the renal–body fluid system for the regulation of blood volume. Like the neural reflex system and the renin-angiotensin system, this control mechanism operates by negative feedback and is ultimately geared to maintain a normal arterial blood pressure. Central to an understanding of this control mechanism is the knowledge that urinary output of water and electrolytes is related to arterial blood pressure (Fig. 43). When arterial perfusion pressure is increased urinary output increases, and when arterial pressure is decreased urinary output decreases. At its most basic level this relationship is a simple hydrodynamic consequence of the effect of renal arterial perfusion pressure on glomerular filtration rate. Other

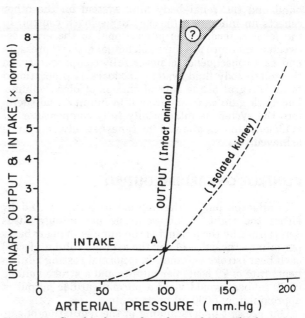

Figure 43. Graphical procedure for analyzing the long-term level of arterial pressure, based on the renal–body fluid mechanisms for pressure control. The steep solid curve is the normal urinary output curve in an intact animal. (With permission from Guyton, A. C.: Textbook of Medical Physiology. 5th ed. Philadelphia, W. B. Saunders Co., 1976, p. 282.)

important factors come into play and will be discussed subsequently. Blood volume is determined primarily by body fluid balance, which in turn is related to a summation of the rates of intake, nonrenal loss, and urinary output of sodium and water. Feedback in this control loop is provided by the fact that blood volume is an important determinant of arterial pressure, which in turn influences urine output, thereby completing the loop. In descriptive terms, if blood pressure is reduced—for example, by hemorrhage—renal output of sodium and water is reduced. If fluid intake is maintained constant, fluid balance will become positive and blood volume will increase until it becomes sufficient to restore blood pressure to the level that existed prior to hemorrhage. There are two important differences between the renal–body fluid control system and those discussed previously. First, this system takes a very long time to correct blood pressure (Fig. 42). In the absence of other control mechanisms, days or even weeks would be required to correct a major change in blood pressure induced by transfusion or by hemorrhage. A second and more significant difference is the gain of this system. In previous sections dealing with the baroreflex and the renin-angiotensin systems we have noted that the gains of these control mechanisms were approximately 7 and 2, respectively. Again, let us define gain as the ratio of compensation to residual error after the feedback system has operated to achieve a new steady state. With the renal–body fluid system, the capacity for gain is infinite. Descriptively, infinite gain means that, assuming a normal kidney, the system will continue to function until blood pressure returns to precisely the reference level or until the residual error is zero. This difference between the neural reflex or renin-angiotensin system on the one hand and the renal–body fluid system on the other reflects an inherent difference in feedback control. In the former, feedback is proportional to the error between a reference pressure and actual arterial pressure and as a consequence is never fully compensatory. In the renal–body fluid system, feedback is proportional to an integral of the rate of change of blood volume. Feedback gain can vary from 0 to infinity, and therefore the system is intrinsically fully compensatory if sufficient time is allowed for a new steady rate to be achieved.

CONTROL OF CARDIAC OUTPUT

Cardiac output is the volume of blood ejected by either the right or left ventricle per minute. It is determined by the product of the number of heart beats per minute (heart rate) and the average volume ejected each beat (stroke volume). In a normal resting adult a heart rate of 70 beats per minute and a stroke volume of 70 ml/beat would yield a normal cardiac output of approximately 5000 ml per minute.

Our present understanding of the regulation of cardiac output has come from three separate but ultimately converging lines of investigation. One approach has focused on the heart and on highly controlled experimental conditions in which heart rate, venous return, and aortic pressure can be individually controlled and manipulated. An important outcome of these studies was the elucidation of "the law of the heart," described in detail in a previous chapter. This law, Starling's law, simply stated, is that within limits, the heart will eject whatever volume of blood is returned to it. The capacity of the heart to vary its output in response to changes in venous return requires no reflex or humoral adjustments and no change in heart rate. It is a consequence of ventricular dilatation and a resulting increase in the force of contraction of each myocardial element (Fig. 44). An increase in heart rate at constant venous pressure will increase cardiac output, and a decrease in vascular resistance at constant venous pressure and heart rate will increase cardiac output.

A second line of investigation in recent years has utilized technological advances that enable investigators to record continuously cardiac output, vascular pressures, heart rate, and cardiac dimensions in intact animals and man. These observations have now been made in normal and pathological conditions at rest and during widely different activities, including exercise. Probably the most important concept derived from these studies is that cardiac output is regulated in proportion to the metabolic needs of the body. When the rate of metabolism increases, as reflected by total body oxygen uptake, there is a parallel increase in cardiac output (Fig. 45). We have noted previously that an increase in the oxygen requirements by any given organ leads to local vasodilatation and a drop in arterial resistance. A decrease in arterial resistance leads to an increase in venous return to the heart, and both lead to an increase in cardiac output. In a very

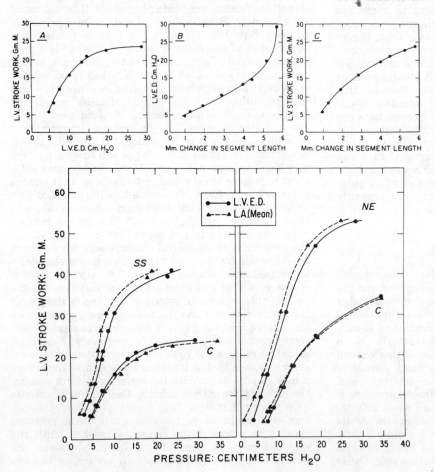

Figure 44. Panel *A* shows the relation between left ventricular end-diastolic pressure and stroke work. Panel *B* shows the relation between changes in end-diastolic myocardial segment length and left ventricular end-diastolic pressure. Panel *C* shows the relation between changes in left ventricular end-diastolic myocardial segment length and stroke work. Lower left panel, dashed lines show relation between mean left atrial pressure and left ventricular stroke work during control period (C) and during stellate stimulation (SS). Solid lines show relation between left ventricular end-diastolic pressure and stroke work during control period (C) and during stellate stimulation (SS). Bilateral cervical vagotomy; right stellate intact. Heart rate constant at 171 per minute. Lower right panel, symbols same as at left except that a continuous infusion of 0.36 gamma per minute of norepinephrine base was administered during curve marked (NE) after control curve (C) was obtained. Bilateral cervical vagotomy; right stellate intact. Heart rate constant at 140 per minute. (With permission from Sarnoff, S. J., and Mitchell, J. H.: The regulation of the performance of the heart. Am J Med 30:749, 1961.)

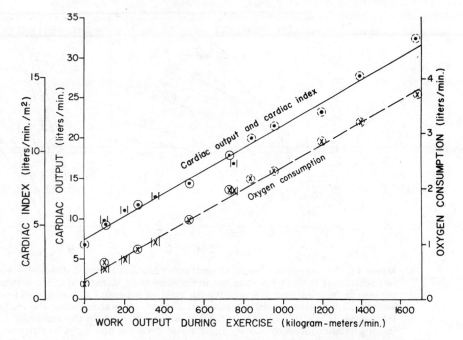

Figure 45. Relationship between cardiac output and work output (solid curve) and between oxygen consumption and work output (dashed curve) during exercise. (With permission from Guyton, A. C., Jones, C. E., and Coleman, T. G.: Cardiac Output and Its Regulation. Philadelphia, W. B. Saunders Co., 1973, p. 5.)

important sense, arterial resistance controls cardiac output. A striking example of this is the very large increase in cardiac output that accompanies the opening of a fistula between the arterial and venous systems (Fig. 46). Although reflex changes participate in the net cardiovascular adjustment to such a condition, they are not necessary for an increase in cardiac output to occur. Similarly, although reflex changes participate in the normal response of the heart to augmented peripheral demands such as exercise, they are not necessary to observe an increase in cardiac output during physical activity. An example is the fact that cardiac output increases in a nearly normal manner in animals with denervated hearts or in patients with transplanted and denervated hearts during moderate exercise. Together, these lines of investigation indicate the dominant role of peripheral resistance and venous return in the control of cardiac output.

A third line of investigation has focused on changes of the heart other than those attributable to an in-crease in venous return, when cardiac output varies to meet alterations in the peripheral demand for oxygen delivery and blood flow. When peripheral resistance drops—for example, during exercise—the baroreceptors are activated to restore blood pressure toward normal. The resulting baroreflex leads to an inhibition of vagal tone to the heart and to an increase in sympathetic tone. Because vagal efferent nerve activity has a negative chronotropic and inotropic effect on the atria and ventricles, while sympathetic activity has a positive chronotropic and inotropic effect, the consequence of the baroreflex adjustment is to increase heart rate and contractile performance.

As indicated above, heart rate per se can lead to changes of cardiac output at any given venous pressure. A positive inotropic effect on the atria leads to a decrease in venous pressure at any given rate of venous return, because the atria are interposed between the central veins and their respective ventricles and function as booster pumps. The booster pump function of

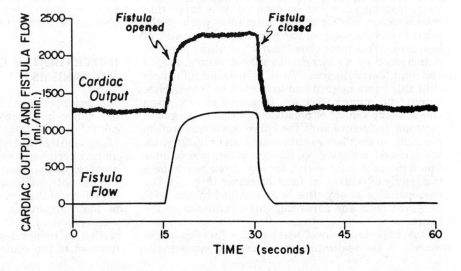

Figure 46. Effect of suddenly opening and suddenly closing an AV fistula, showing changes in fistula flow and cardiac output. (With permission from Guyton, A. C.: Textbook of Medical Physiology. 5th ed. Philadelphia, W. B. Saunders Co., 1976, p. 299.)

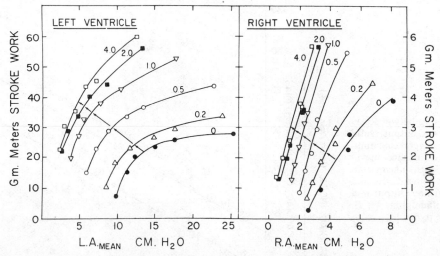

Figure 47. The concept of a family of ventricular function curves. Left panel: LA = mean left atrial pressure, left ventricular stroke work increases in response to an increase in filling pressure. Six ventricular function curves are depicted, each representing the relation between LA pressure and stroke work in the absence of electrical stimulation of stellate ganglion (o), and while stimulating the stellate ganglion at 6 volts and frequencies of 0.2, 0.5, 1.0, 2.0, and 4.0 stimuli per second. In the right panel, similar data are presented for the relation between RA = right atrial pressure and right ventricular stroke work. Sympathetic stimulation shifts the function curve of both ventricles upward and to the left; that is, the work performed at any given filling pressure is increased and for any given work, the filling pressure is lower as a consequence of sympathetic stimulation. (With permission from Sarnoff, S. J., and Mitchell, J. H.: The regulation of the performance of the heart. Am J Med 30:756, 1961.)

the atria influences cardiac output not only by ejecting more or less blood into the ventricles with each atrial contraction but also by regulating mean atrial pressure relative to any given ventricular end-diastolic volume and thereby favoring or impeding venous return to the heart.

Sympathetic and, to a lesser extent, parasympathetic influences also modulate ventricular contractility through their respective neurotransmitters—norepinephrine (positive inotropic action) and acetylcholine (negative inotropic action). A positive inotropic action on the ventricles leads to more complete systolic emptying and to a lower end-diastolic volume and pressure at any given heart rate and venous return. Perhaps a more useful view of inotropic influences on the ventricle is embodied in the ventricular function curve concept proposed by Sarnoff. According to this view, Starling's law can be depicted as a curve that relates either cardiac output or minute work of the heart to end-diastolic volume or pressure at a constant heart rate. This curve shows that when filling pressure is increased by an increase in venous return, output and minute work increase. Positive inotropic influences shift this curve upward and to the left so that cardiac output and minute work are increased at any given end-diastolic volume or pressure. Conversely, negative inotropic influences shift the curve downward and to the right so that less cardiac output and minute work are derived from any given filling pressure and volume. The important point is that for any given heart there is a family of ventricular function curves (Fig. 47). The one operative at any time is determined by the level of sympathetic and parasympathetic influence on the heart.

One important consequence of the function curve concept is the realization that increased sympathetic and decreased parasympathetic activity provides the heart with a much higher maximal pumping capability than would be true in the absence of such neural input. A second important corollary to the concept of a family of curves is that under the influence of varying neural input, the heart is capable of maintaining widely different levels of cardiac output at correspondingly different levels of venous return, and with little or no change in central and pulmonary venous pressures. Most forms of myocardial disease depress the intrinsic function curve of the ventricle and diminish the range over which normal reflex adjustments can modulate cardiac output at any given end-diastolic volume. As myocardial disease progresses the heart is forced to rely on dilatation (the Starling mechanism) and on changes of heart rate to meet varying peripheral demands. At the extreme of heart failure, changes of cardiac output become dependent almost solely on changes of heart rate.

INTEGRATION OF CIRCULATORY CONTROL MECHANISMS

In prior sections of this chapter we have discussed the major important components of the circulatory control system: local factors that determine local perfusion, central and neural reflex mechanisms for modulating peripheral vascular tone and cardiac function, humoral mechanisms, and the renal–body fluid system for the control of blood volume. We have also discussed the effects of these components separately with respect to their actions on arterial resistance vessels, the venous system, and the heart. The purpose of this section is to develop further the concept of overall function of the control system, since the behavior of

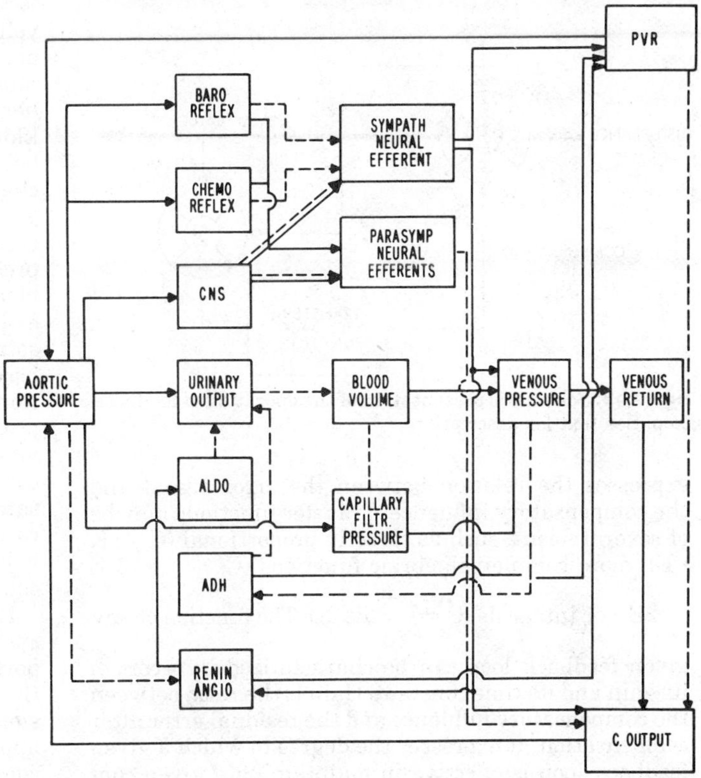

Figure 48. Schematic diagram of the relationships among several of the factors that are known to influence arterial blood pressure. CNS = Central nervous system; ALDO = aldosterone; ADH = antidiuretic hormone; PVR = peripheral arterial vascular resistance; C output = cardiac output. Solid lines indicate that an increase of the variable in one block increases the value of the variable in the second block. Dashed lines indicate that an increase of the variable in the first block decreases the value of the variable in the second block. See text for details.

the system involves an understanding not only of its parts, but also of the coupling of these parts into an integrated scheme of cardiovascular regulation.

Figure 48 shows the relation between some of the more important components believed to play a role in blood pressure regulation. No effort has been made to show all of the known components or the subsystems within each component. For such a detailed analysis the reader is referred to the articles by Guyton noted in the bibliography. For the purpose of this discussion we have included factors already mentioned in this chapter. In this diagram a solid arrow connecting two blocks indicates that an increase in the original factor (first block) causes an increase in the subsequent factor (second block). A broken arrow between blocks indicates a negative influence of one factor on the other. The diagram depicts an overall feedback system in which arterial blood pressure ultimately influences factors that determine either peripheral arterial resistance, or cardiac output, or both. Cardiac output, in turn, determines arterial blood pressure. In general, the upper part of the diagram refers to neural and reflex components of the feedback loop, the middle of the diagram refers to the renal–body fluid system for feedback control of blood volume, and the lower part of the diagram refers to humoral components of the feedback loop.

Even this simplified diagram reveals many important features of the system for cardiovascular control. First, the system is composed of multiple components. A second important feature is illustrated by starting with arterial pressure, and following the arrows over any path back to arterial pressure. In so doing one or more broken lines are encountered, indicating that all of the loops operate with negative feedback (that is, a rise in arterial pressure will lead to an event or chain

of events that will tend to restore blood pressure to its starting value). A third feature of the diagram is that many of the components affect more than one subsequent event. For example, sympathetic activity affects peripheral resistance, the heart, renin secretion, and many other components. The renin-angiotensin system affects peripheral resistance and aldosterone secretion. Not only do many components of the system have the capacity to affect more than one subsequent event, but each component itself is more often than not influenced by two or even more elements of preceding components of the chain. Hence the behavior of any given component reflects an integration of the inputs from preceding elements in the chain.

Figure 49 illustrates the general form of a feedback loop. The heavy arrow depicts the variable being controlled by the feedback system and could represent any controlled variable (for example, blood pressure, the level of the blood sugar, arterial pO_2, and so on). The summing circuit on the left shows that the actual value of the variable at any time will be influenced by the normal or reference level to which the system stabilizes or settles in the absence of any disturbing influence. A second factor that influences the actual level of the variable is any disturbance or perturbing force. A third factor is the compensatory influence that results from operation of the feedback system. The feedback loop of a controlled system always involves a sensor (for example, the carotid sinus) that responds to the variable being controlled. The output of the sensor is related to the difference between the actual level of the controlled variable and the normal or reference level of that variable. This difference can be viewed as an error and has both sign (above and below normal level) and a magnitude. The transfer function for the feedback loop is a mathematical function that

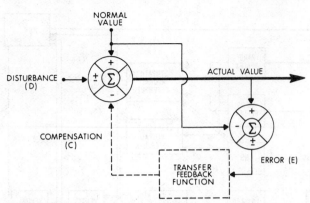

Figure 49. Schematic presentation of the operation of feedback loop. See text for description.

expresses the relation between the error signal and the compensatory influence. Transfer functions may be of several forms, such as directly proportional ($C = K \cdot E$), more complex algebraic functions ($C = 1 + 3E + 2E^2$) or integrals ($C = \int_0^{\pm} de/dt$). The function of any given feedback loop can be characterized in terms of its gain and its time constant. Gain is the ratio between the compensatory influence and the residual error after compensation. It expresses the degree to which a given feedback loop is effective in maintaining a given controlled variable at its normal level. When a controlled variable is changed instantaneously from its normal value to some new value and the disturbing influence is then maintained, the compensatory influence changes over time from its normal value to a new steady-state value. The time required for compensation to reach 50 per cent of its new value is referred to as the time constant of the feedback loop. The time constant of the baroreflex is a matter of seconds, for the renin-angiotensin system a matter of minutes to an hour, and for the renal–body fluid system a matter of days.

The baroreflex is an example of a proportional feedback system. In this system, arterial pressure determines the number of neural impulses originating from the carotid and aortic baroreceptors, which in turn modulate the output of sympathetic and vagal nerve impulses from the vasomotor center. The latter, in turn, influence peripheral resistance, heart rate, myocardial contractility, and hence arterial pressure. When the blood pressure is normal (that is, no disturbing force), the compensation is zero. When a disturbance causes the blood pressure to change by a quantity (D), compensation occurs, but in a proportional system the change is always less than D. In a proportional system the gain is always more than 0 but less than infinity. For the carotid sinus reflex the gain is approximately 7 and the time constant five to ten seconds. Proportional feedback systems act relatively quickly but are always less than fully compensatory.

The renal–body fluid system is an example of an integral feedback system. In this system arterial pressure determines the rate of urinary output. The rate of urine output, the rate of nonrenal fluid loss from the vascular space, and the rate of fluid intake all act to determine the rate of change of extracellular fluid volume. The integral of this rate of change over time is then added to or subtracted from the normal blood volume to determine the actual blood volume. In the absence of other control systems, blood volume determines central venous pressure, cardiac output, and hence blood pressure. In this integral system, the kidney will either retain or excrete fluid at a rate below or above fluid intake. The corresponding rate of change of extracellular fluid volume will be integrated over time until the blood volume reaches a level that restores blood pressure to its normal value. When blood pressure is normal the compensation is zero. When the blood pressure is changed by a disturbance (D) (for example, withdrawal of 500 ml of blood), the compensation changes from zero to a value that over time becomes equivalent to D. At this point the compensation is equivalent to D, the residual error in blood pressure is zero, and the gain of the system can be viewed as infinity. Thus, integral systems have the capacity for infinite gain, and they are fully compensatory. Because compensation is a time integral of the rate of change of some variable (in this case blood volume), integral systems are intrinsically slow (time constants of days).

Returning to Figure 48, we can see that the overall system for cardiovascular control is composed of proportional and integral feedback loops. With respect to the control of blood pressure and hence tissue perfusion, the baroreflex and chemoreflex have gains of approximately 4 and 7, respectively. They have time constants of 5 to 15 seconds and operate principally through sympathetic and parasympathetic neural efferents to effect changes in arterial resistance, venous tone, heart rate, and cardiac output. These proportional feedback loops are rapidly responsive and highly effective although not completely so in compensating for a change in blood pressure. They are ideally suited to responding to acute events, such as a change in posture or exercise. The renal–body fluid feedback has infinite gain, but a time constant of four to five days. This integral system is ultimately completely effective in compensating for a change in blood pressure that would otherwise occur—for example, with a significant and sustained alteration of the intake of salt and water in the diet. This system will ultimately correct the blood volume deficit following a hemorrhage, but the acute mechanism for restoring blood pressure following a hemorrhage will depend more on the baroreflex.

Between the extremes represented by the baroreflex and the renal–body fluid system, there are a group of proportional feedback loops, operating principally through humoral or hormonal mechanisms. These loops are intermediate in the sense that their intrinsic time constants are in minutes or hours. They include the secretion of aldosterone by the adrenal cortex, the secretion of ADH by the pituitary and the secretion of renin by the kidney with subsequent formation of angiotensin II. In general, the gain of these feedback loops is approximately 1 to 3. The response time of these feedback loops is intrinsically slow, but can be accelerated by their interaction with a more rapid acting proportional control system. For example, a drop in arterial pressure also activates the baroreflex, which causes an increase in sympathetic neural efferent activity. Enhanced sympathetic activity to the kidney, even in the absence of a drop in renal artery perfusion pressure, causes a prompt and substantial release of renin. The release of renin leads to formation of angiotensin II, which itself is a vasoconstrictor and also augments the response of peripheral resistance vessels to sympathetic neural efferent activity. Finally, angiotensin also causes the release of aldosterone from the adrenal, which shifts the relation between arterial pressure and urinary output by promoting tubular reabsorption of sodium and water. Multiple interactions of this type between the components of the cardiovascular control system provide (a) backup, should one component fail or malfunction, (b) a mechanism for ensuring that over minutes, hours, or days the burden of sustaining an adequate perfusion pressure is shared by components, and (c) a smoothly operating and stable system for blood pressure control that is also capable of rapidly adjusting to a major disturbance that would otherwise seriously perturb tissue perfusion and its distribution.

REFERENCES

Abboud, F. M., Heistad, D. D., Mark, A. L., and Schmid, P. G.: Reflex control of the peripheral circulation. Prog Cardiovasc Dis 18:371, 1976.

Abboud, F. M., Mark, A. L., Heistad, D. D., Schmid, P. G., and Barnes, R. W.: The venous system. In Levine, H. J. (ed.): Clinical Cardiovascular Physiology. New York, Grune and Stratton, 1976, p. 207.

Berne, R. M., and Rubio, R.: Coronary circulation. In Berne, R. M., Sperelakis, N., and Geiger, S. R. (eds.): Handbook of Physiology. Section 2, The Cardiovascular System. Baltimore, Williams and Wilkins, 1979, p. 873.

Dustan, H. P., Tarazi, R., and Bravo, E. L.: Physiological characteristics of hypertension. Am J Med 52:610, 1972.

Guyton, A. C., Coleman, T. G., Cowley, A. W., Jr., Manning, R. D., Jr., Norman, R. A., Jr., and Ferguson, J. D.: A systems analysis approach to understanding long-range arterial blood pressure control and hypertension. Circ Res 35:159, 1974.

Lefkowitz, R. J., and Limbird, L. E.: Techniques for the study of biochemical basis of drug action. Prog Cardiovasc Dis 18:309, 1975.

Linden, R. J.: Reflexes from the heart. Prog Cardiovasc Dis 18:201, 1975.

Zitnik, R. S., and Shepherd, J. T.: Control of the venous system in man. In Yu, P. N., and Goodwin, J. F. (eds.): Progress in Cardiology. Philadelphia, Lea and Febiger, 1972, p. 185.

Cardiovascular Adaptations to Exercise

The architecture of the circulation and its control are designed to enable the human organism to perform work over a wide range of energy expenditure. During activity muscle functions as a machine, converting chemical energy into mechanical work and heat. There is now considerable evidence that the transport function of the circulation is matched closely to the level of exercise, and that circulatory factors limit the maximal capacity of muscle to perform work over any extended period of time. One corollary of this fact is that most forms of cardiovascular disease are first manifested by impairment in the maximal capacity for exercise. A second important corollary is that symptoms attributable to cardiovascular disease are evident during exercise long before they are evident at rest. It follows from these observations that an understanding of exercise physiology plays a central role in the interpretation of symptoms and signs in cardiac patients.

SKELETAL MUSCLE

Skeletal muscle consists of many individual fibers arranged in parallel. Each fiber is made up of a number of internally parallel elements called myofibrils and each of these elements is composed of sarcomeres arranged in series over the length of the myofibril. The sarcomere is the basic contractile unit of muscle. (Structure, function, and energetics of muscle are covered on pages 874–880.)

ATP appears to be the only direct source of energy for making and breaking cross-bridges during contraction of sarcomeres. During maximal exercise, skeletal muscle uses as much as 1×10^{-3} moles of ATP/gram

of muscle/min. This rate of ATP consumption is at least 100 times and perhaps in some muscles as much as 1000 times the rate of ATP consumption of resting muscle. Since the amount of ATP stored in muscle at rest is only approximately 5×10^{-6} moles/gram, it is evident that ATP would be depleted in less than a second were it not for the availability of mechanisms for ATP generation of considerable capacity and speed.

The potential sources to meet the large demand for ATP during exercise include the following: (a) utilization of existing ATP stored within the cell, (b) conversion of high-energy stores in the form of phosphocreatine to ATP by a reaction referred to as phosphate transfer ($C - P_i + ADP \rightarrow ATP + creatine$), (c) generation of ATP through anaerobic glycolysis, and (d) oxidative metabolism of acetyl CoA. As noted above, the ATP stored within the muscle cell is insufficient to meet the demands of exercise. Thus, ATP generated and stored prior to the onset of exercise does not represent a significant reservoir of energy for mechanical work. With the onset of exercise of moderate to high intensity, phosphate transfer and anaerobic glycolysis represent initial sources of fuel for replenishing consumed ATP. Glycogen levels and phosphocreatine levels drop precipitously, and lactate concentrations within the cell and in venous effluent from exercising muscles rise. This initial use of creatine phosphate and of anaerobic glycolysis in preference to oxidative metabolism is related in part to the rate of the reactions for ATP production (that is, oxidative metabolism is much slower) and in part to the time lag between the onset of exercise and the increased uptake of substrate and oxygen, both of which require an increase in blood flow. Once blood flow has increased and a new steady state is reached, muscle metabolism is almost entirely aerobic and ATP generation can be accounted for nearly completely by oxygen and substrate uptake from the blood.

Even at rest, skeletal muscle utilizes fatty acids as its major source of fuel for aerobic metabolism. During steady-state exercise the uptake of glucose and fat by working muscle increases. However, the CO_2 production attributable to metabolism of fat increases more than that produced from glucose. At moderate levels of exercise, up to 90 per cent of CO_2 production can be accounted for by utilization of fat. Utilization of glycogen continues at a low rate during submaximal exercise, most of the glycogen being converted to pyruvate, which enters the Krebs cycle. At very high levels of activity approaching maximal oxygen uptake the rate of glycogen depletion is enhanced, lactate production increases, and the amount of ATP generated through anaerobic glycolysis contributes importantly to energy sources available for mechanical work. Thus, for skeletal muscle of any given aerobic capacity, transport of oxygen and substrate (chiefly FFA) limits the level of performance of submaximal work of any significant duration. Circulatory adaptations to increased activity are thus of central importance as determinants of exercise performance under aerobic conditions.

CIRCULATORY ADJUSTMENTS TO EXERCISE

An understanding of circulatory adjustments that occur as a consequence of increased mechanical and metabolic activity in skeletal muscle involves (a) local changes in the exercising muscles; (b) changes of blood pressure, cardiac output, and the distribution of cardiac output; (c) adjustments related to the need to eliminate as efficiently as possible the energy not utilized for mechanical work but released as heat by the exercising muscle; and (d) the role of the nervous system in helping to mediate these adjustments. It is also important to recognize that while the intensity of exercise is an important determinant of quantitative aspects of the response, the type of exercise (that is, dynamic versus static) is characterized by qualitative, interesting, and clinically relevant differences. Furthermore, there are both quantitative and qualitative differences in the cardiovascular response of trained versus sedentary individuals that deserve mention because of their role in exercise physiology as well as their potentially important therapeutic role.

The earliest and most prominent component of the circulatory response to dynamic exercise is a large reduction in the net resistance offered by nutrient blood vessels in working musculature. Blood flow to resting muscle averages 4 to 7 ml/100 grams of tissue. This flow rate may increase to 50 to 75 ml/100 grams during maximal dynamic activity (Fig. 50). The increase in flow is mediated largely by opening of capillary beds that are not open at rest and occurs despite the fact that during activity blood flow decreases with each contraction as a result of the extravascular compressive forces exerted by contracting muscles. Although sympathetic vasodilator fibers have been demonstrated in some species, current data indicate that in most mammals, including man, the drop in local vascular resistance during muscular exercise is caused by the aggregate influence of a drop in tissue pO_2 and perhaps by the release of vasodilator agents, including potassium, acetylcholine, adenosine, lactic acid, and carbon dioxide. At present, it is impossible to say which of these potential factors predominates in local control of vascular resistance during exercise.

During sustained exercise the metabolism of muscle is principally aerobic up to work loads that represent 60 to 80 per cent of maximal oxygen consumption. ATP generation is accomplished by a corresponding increase in the uptake of oxygen and substrate (largely FFA); lactate levels in arterial blood are low and stable. At higher work loads anaerobic metabolism contributes to ATP production, glucose uptake increases relative to fat, and production of lactate increases its concentration in arterial blood.

During strenuous exertion the total oxygen uptake of an individual may increase by a factor of 10, or perhaps even 20 in well-trained athletes. It is clear that if a large drop in vascular resistance of exercising muscle is not met by an appropriate increase in cardiac output and in the vascular resistance of nonexercising areas, blood pressure would drop to levels incompatible with continued effort and the perfusion requirements of active muscles would not be met.

Most investigators have reported a nearly linear relation between $\dot{V}O_2$ (oxygen uptake) and cardiac output (Q) during exercise. One group reported this relation ($Q = 7.03 + 0.0058\ \dot{V}O_2$) in 92 subjects (Fig. 51). The linear relation between $\dot{V}O_2$ and Q during exercise is nearly paralleled by the linear relation between $\dot{V}O_2$ and heart rate, suggesting that the change in heart rate is predominant in increasing the cardiac output. Changes of stroke volume during exercise vary from individual to individual, are more prominent with erect exercise than with exercise in the supine position, and are more evident at the transition from rest to mild exercise than they are with continued stepwise increases in work load and $\dot{V}O_2$.

From the above equation relating $\dot{V}O_2$ and Q during activity it should be clear that while the relation is nearly linear, for any given increase in work the increase in cardiac output is less than the increase in oxygen uptake. Thus, with increasing oxygen demand as reflected by $\dot{V}O_2$, oxygen uptake is met not only by an increase in cardiac output, but also to an important extent by an increase in the arteriovenous oxygen difference—that is, by an increase in oxygen extraction. This relation is shown in Figure 52.

The mechanisms that enable a heart to pump five or more times the resting cardiac output during exercise are dominated by the increase in heart rate that is most closely related to the increase in flow. During maximal effort, however, changes in heart rate alone are not sufficient to account for the increase in the output of the heart. Dimensional studies in animals and man have shown that stroke volume is augmented and that this augmentation is caused by an increased systolic emptying of the ventricle from the same or a slightly increased left ventricular end-diastolic volume and pressure. Thus, while heart rate increases per se play a predominant role in the augmentation of flow in response to exercise, the inotropic effect of increased sympathetic nervous activity and, to a lesser extent, Starling forces also play a role.

Characteristic features of the cardiovascular re-

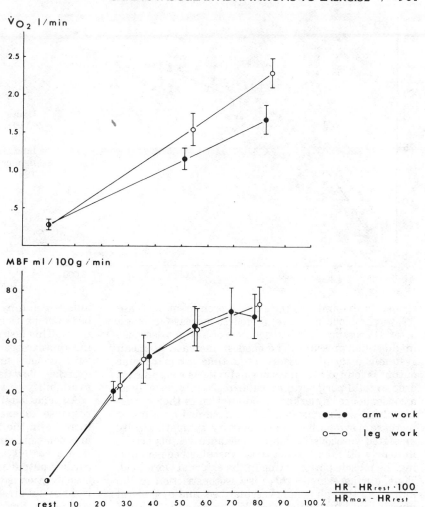

Figure 50. Oxygen uptake ($\dot{V}O_2$) (upper panel) and muscle blood flow (MBF) (lower panel) measured by the ^{133}Xe-clearance method in m. biceps brachi during arm exercise (arm-cranking) and in m. vastus lateralis during leg exercise (bicycling). Both $\dot{V}O_2$ and MBF are related to the relative work load expressed as heart rate (HR) in per cent of the total range between resting and maximal HR. It should be noted that MBF per unit tissue is the same during arm exercise as during leg exercise at the same relative work load, whereas absolute $\dot{V}O_2$ is higher during leg exercise. (With permission from Clausen, J. P.: Muscle blood flow during exercise and its significance for maximal performance. In Keul J. (ed.): Limiting Factors of Physical Performance. Stuttgart, Georg Thieme, 1973, p. 253.)

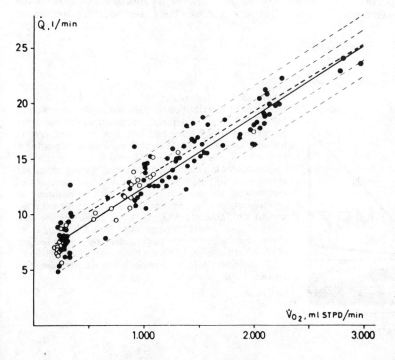

Figure 51. Relationship between cardiac output (Q) and oxygen uptake at rest and during supine exercise in healthy young men and women. Solid symbols indicate men; open symbols women. Full heavy line indicates linear regression line, including all data; heavy broken line indicates linear regression of exercise data only. Thin broken lines indicate SD of all data. (With permission from Ekelund, L. G., and Holmgren, A.: Central hemodynamics during exercise. Circ Res 20 + 21:I-33, 1967.)

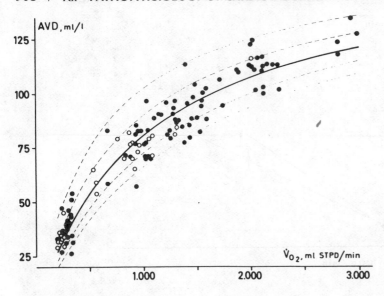

Figure 52. Arterio–mixed venous O_2 difference (AVD) in ml/l in relation to oxygen uptake at rest and during exercise. (With permission from Ekelund, L. G., and Holmgren, A., Central hemodynamics during exercise. Circ Res 20 + 21:I-36, 1967.)

sponse to dynamic exercise are a prominent increase in systolic blood pressure, a modest increase in mean arterial pressure, and little change or a slight decrease in diastolic pressure. The modest increase of mean systemic arterial pressure at a time when cardiac output is four to five times normal reflects a significant drop in total peripheral vascular resistance, largely as a consequence of marked vasodilatation in the exercising muscles. Exercise also is accompanied by a major increase of sympathetic nerve activity: sympathetically mediated vasoconstriction of resistance vessels occurs in nearly all areas except those vascular beds supplying the muscle participating in the external work load. Thus, during exercise there is vasoconstriction in the kidney, in the splanchnic vascular bed, and in skeletal muscle that is not doing work. Viewed as an integrated system, therefore, the transport of oxygen and substrate during exercise is facilitated by the increase in cardiac output, by an increase in arterial perfusion pressure, by a local drop of resistance in exercising

muscles, and by an increase in resistance in vascular beds not participating in the increased metabolic activity. This last response plays a major role in sustaining the necessary increase in arterial perfusion pressure. Besides an increase in total blood flow during exercise, flow is redistributed to optimize substrate availability to working muscle (Fig. 53).

An additional feature of the integrated circulatory response to exercise is a sympathetically mediated increase in the tone of large veins both in exercising and nonexercising parts. This increased tone of capacitance vessels allows the venous system to regulate cardiac output more efficiently. The net effect of venoconstriction is to enhance venous return at any given right atrial pressure and to ensure that cardiac output will not be limited by an inadequate return of blood.

The energy released by chemical transformations in the body is ultimately derived from oxidation of substrate and appears either as mechanical work or as heat. During exercise body temperature increases

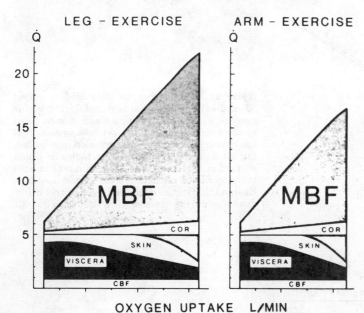

Figure 53. Cardiac output ($\dot{Q}$) in l/min and estimates of its regional distribution in relation to the oxygen uptake ($\dot{V}O_2$) at rest and during submaximal and maximal leg exercise (bicycling) and arm exercise (arm cranking). At any $\dot{V}O_2$ values apply to the situation after 5 to 7 min of exercise when $\dot{V}O_2$ and $\dot{Q}$ have reached a steady state. It should be noted that during maximal exercise as well as at any relative $\dot{V}O_2$ the perfusion of nonworking tissues and the heart can be assumed to be the same during arm exercise as during leg exercise and at any absolute $\dot{V}O_2$, Q is the same for the two types of exercise. (With permission from Clausen, J. P.: Circulatory adjustments to dynamic exercise and effect of physical training in normal subjects and in patients with coronary artery disease. Prog Cardiovasc Dis 18:462, 1976.)

gradually because of the tremendous heat load generated by metabolic activity of exercising muscle that has a maximal efficiency of approximately 25 per cent (that is, the conversion of chemical energy into external work). Heat loss occurs almost entirely through the skin; the mechanisms of this heat transfer include radiation, conduction, convection, and evaporation. Radiation that involves electromagnetic energy in the infrared range of wave lengths accounts for a large percentage of resting heat loss from a nude person in a cool room. However, heat loss through radiation is quantitatively related to the fourth power of the difference between body temperature and the temperature of the environment. During exercise this mechanism becomes progressively less prominent, and it is even less of a factor in settings where the environmental temperature approaches that of the body. Heat loss through conduction, representing the actual transfer of heat from the body to the environment, accounts for only 10 to 12 per cent of resting heat loss, but becomes a very significant factor when an individual performs exercise in water that is cooler than body temperature. Water has several thousand times the specific heat of air and can thus absorb very large amounts of heat. When water or air flow past the body, heat transfer is further augmented by the mechanism of convection. Finally, when water evaporates, 0.58 calories/gram of H_2O are lost. With maximal sweating an individual can dissipate 3 to 3.5 liters per hour, or approximately 1500 calories, through evaporation. The most important factor in the control of body temperature during exercise, however, is the ability of the circulation to carry heat from its source (exercising muscle) to its site of dissipation (skin). Furthermore, as the heat load that must be dissipated increases, cutaneous vasodilatation and an increase of blood volume contained within the skin occur. With exercise of moderate to high intensity and of long duration, the requirements for cutaneous vasodilatation become prominent, and a circulatory adjustment referred to as drift develops. Drift is characterized by a further increase in heart rate, a drop in venous pressure and stroke volume, and a decrease in arterial pressure. These changes appear to be accounted for in large part by the drop in cutaneous vascular resistance and venous tone, which minimize the increase in body temperature that would otherwise occur.

Exercise generally can be of two types: dynamic (or isotonic), in which muscle contraction leads principally to a change in length; and static (or isometric), in which contraction results in tension development with little change in length. Recognizing that most forms of activity involve both types of effort, there are certain interesting quantitative and qualitative differences in the circulatory adaptation to these forms of effort. Dynamic exercise is met by a large increase in cardiac output and heart rate with only a modest elevation of blood pressure and a net reduction of peripheral vascular resistance. These circulatory changes are related closely to the increase in $\dot{V}O_2$ required by the exercising muscle mass. In contrast, static exercise leads to a marked increase of blood pressure and vascular resistance. The increase in cardiac output is only modest and is due almost entirely to an increase in heart rate. Furthermore, the degree of circulatory adaptation to static exercise relates not only to $\dot{V}O_2$, but also to the percentage of maximal tension development. Hence, substantial cardiovascular responses can be elicited by a near maximal isometric contraction of even very small muscle groups. The fact that static exercise principally places an afterload (pressure) stress on the heart while dynamic exercise represents a volume (preload) and rate stress has an important bearing on understanding factors that precipitate symptoms in patients with cardiac disease. This knowledge also has been used extensively in physical diagnosis to evaluate the cause of murmurs and to assess left ventricular function and certain structural abnormalities.

Physiological studies of static exercise have demonstrated that muscle afferent nerve feedback represents an important component of the system for cardiovascular control during exercise, a system that must integrate a hydraulic component, a cortical component, a humoral component, and feedback from traditional baroreceptors. Certainly the manner in which these varied inputs are integrated so that cardiovascular adjustments to exercise are matched to metabolic requirements is one of the most challenging and as yet unanswered features in biosystems control analysis.

EFFECTS OF DYNAMIC EXERCISE TRAINING

Finally, it seems appropriate to comment on aspects of training, or the conditioning effect. The ability to enhance performance through training has been known for years. This fact plays a prominent role in sports medicine and has a scientific basis that has been elucidated in recent years. Only very recently, however, has the focus of the cardiologist been addressed to this phenomenon as an instrument of potential value both in prevention of vascular disease and in treatment of patients with existing disease.

In the broadest sense, training involves enhancement of skill, strength, and endurance. Only the last of these will be dealt with here. Previous sections of this chapter have dealt with the characteristic changes in peripheral muscles and cardiovascular function when an individual makes the transition from the resting state to a new steady state of either submaximal or maximal dynamic exercise. This section deals with adjustments of muscle and cardiovascular function that develop over time (weeks or months) when a previously sedentary individual engages in a dynamic exercise training program of sufficient intensity, duration, and frequency to lead to the training effect. This effect is characterized by important changes not only in the capacity for maximal sustained effort but also by changes at any given level of submaximal effort and at rest. Endurance training increases maximal aerobic capacity—that is, maximal oxygen uptake. Since maximal oxygen uptake defines the functional capacity of the cardiovascular system and reflects the product of cardiac output and arteriovenous oxygen difference, it follows that a change in $\dot{V}O_2$ max must reflect a corresponding change in either maximal cardiac output or maximal extraction of oxygen by the periphery or both. The extent to which $\dot{V}O_2$ max increases with training is related to (a) the baseline conditions of fitness, (b) the presence of structural disease, and (c) the intensity of the training effort. For any given increase in $\dot{V}O_2$ max due to conditioning, however, about half of the effect is attributable to a peripheral component—that is, increased capacity for aerobic metabolism and hence extraction of substrate and oxygen from arterial blood, and about half of the effect is due to increased perfusion—that is, cardiac output at maximal effort. The peripheral component of this effect involves changes of skeletal muscle structure and metabolism. Numerous studies have shown that training increases the size and number of mitochondria per gram of muscle; the level of mitochondrial enzyme activity per gram of mitochondrial protein; the capacity of muscle to oxidize fat, carbohydrate, and ketones; myoglobin levels; and the capacity to generate ATP. The net effect of these changes in muscle is an increase in the capacity for peripheral oxygen extraction (widened AV O_2 difference) and a decrease in lactate production (that is, increased aerobic capacity) at any given work load.

The cardiovascular component of the training effect is characterized by a reduction in heart rate and blood pressure and an increase in stroke volume at any given submaximal workload. With maximal effort, heart rate is unaltered by training, stroke volume is enhanced, maximal AV O_2 difference is enhanced, and the increased oxygen uptake is attributable almost equally to a widened AV O_2 difference and an increase in cardiac output. The therapeutic benefits of training are found not so much in maximal aerobic capacity, but rather in the fact that at submaximal work loads heart rate and blood pressure are less for any given workload, sympathetic discharge is less, total peripheral vascular resistance is less, and the substrate needs of exercising muscle are met to a greater extent by extraction than by increased perfusion and perfusion pressure. Thus, the oxygen requirements of the heart are less at any given workload because heart rate, afterload, extent of shortening, and velocity of shortening are all less. This interpretation of the physiological data regarding training is compatible with the view that (a) maximal $\dot{V}O_2$ is a valid measure of circulatory functional capacity, (b) the oxygen transport capacity of the circulation is the limiting factor in endurance exercise by muscle of any given aerobic capability, and (c) training increases performance and maximal $\dot{V}O_2$ through both a peripheral and a central effect. The therapeutic effects of training reflect the fact that enhanced peripheral mechanisms for oxygen and substrate extraction reduce the stress on the circulation and, in turn, on the heart at any submaximal level of effort.

REFERENCES

Barnard, R. J., Edgerton, V. R., and Peter, J. B.: Effects of exercise on skeletal muscle. II. Contractile properties. J Appl Physiol 28:767, 1970.

Chapman, C. B.: Physiology of muscular exercise; a symposium. Circ Res 20(Suppl. 1):1, 1967.

Gollnick, P. D., Ianuzzo, C. D., and King, D. W.: Ultrastructural and enzyme changes in muscle with exercise. Adv Exp Med Biol 11:69, 1971.

Gollnick, P. D., Armstrong, R. B., Saltin, B., Saubert, C. W., IV, Sembrowich, W. L., and Shepherd, R. E.: Effect of training on enzyme activity and fiber composition of human skeletal muscle. J Appl Physiol 34:107, 1973.

Havel, R. J.: Influence of intensity and duration of exercise on supply and use of fuels. Adv Exp Med Biol 11:315, 1971.

Holloszy, J. O.: Adaptations of muscular tissue to training. Prog Cardiovasc Dis 18:445, 1976.

Huxley, H. E.: The mechanism of muscular contraction. Sci Am 213:18, 1965.

Mitchell, J. H., and Wildenthal, K.: Static (isometric) exercise and the heart: Physiological and clinical consideration. Annu Rev Med 25:369, 1974.

Rowell, L. B.: Human cardiovascular adjustments to exercise and thermal stress. Physiol Rev 54:75, 1974.

Saltin, B., and Karlsson, J.: Muscle glycogen utilization during work of different intensities. Adv Exp Med Biol 11:289, 1971.

Smith, E. E., Guyton, A. C., Manning, R. D., and White, R. J.: Integrated mechanisms of cardiovascular response and control during exercise in the normal human. Prog Cardiovasc Dis 18:421, 1976.

Wasserman, K., and Whipp, B. J.: Exercise physiology in health and disease. Am Rev Resp Dis 112:219, 1975.

Zierler, K. L., Maseri, A., Klassen, G., Rabinowitz, D., and Burgess, J.: Muscle metabolism during exercise in man. Trans Assoc Am Physicians 81:266, 1968.

Embryological Defects and Malformations _____

By the time a human fetus is 3 to 3.5 cm in crown-to-rump length, seven to eight weeks after fertilization of the egg, the heart has achieved its definitive four-chambered configuration and propels blood through the fetal circulation and placenta at a sufficient rate to maintain viability and growth of the fetus. Congenital malformations of the heart result from errors in this developmental process, and the resulting defects therefore have an embryological basis. The purpose of this chapter is to review the normal development of the heart, the embryological basis for common congenital cardiac malformations, and the evidence, albeit sketchy, of how genetic and environmental factors may lead to these malformations.

Most accounts of human cardiogenesis relate the landmarks of cardiac development to each other (that is, as a sequence) and to time (that is, days since fertilization or stages of embryological development). According to this scheme, primordial cardiac cells can be detected within the mesodermal layer of the embryo as early as stage 8, corresponding to the 18th day following fertilization of the egg. At that stage, heart cells are not organized into any identifiable structure and histological features do not identify them as cardiac primordiae. Rather, they are identified by their capacity to differentiate into cardiac muscle when removed from the embryo and supported in tissue culture in vitro. The cells that form these early origins of the heart are bilaterally represented but are joined just rostal to the prechordal plate to form a crescent (Fig. 54). Subsequently there are four principal steps involved in the gross development of the heart:

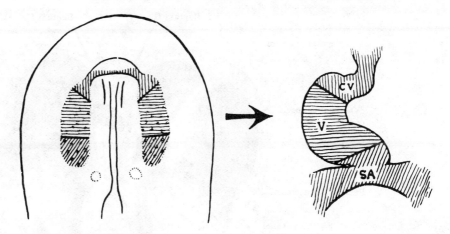

Figure 54. Embryonic fate of the precardiac mesoderm, by regions. CV = Conoven-tricular tissue; V = ventricles; SA = atrial and sinoatrial tissues. Sinoatrial material at this stage is also represented by the bilateral areas of undifferentiated mesoderm at the posterior end of the heart. (Adapted from DeHaan, R. L.: Development of pacemaker tissue in the embryonic heart. Ann NY Acad Sci 127:7, 1965.)

(1) formation of the heart tube, (2) looping of this tube, (3) separation into discrete chambers and vessels, and (4) development of the heart valves.

By the 20th day, or the 9th embryological stage, the splanchnic and somatic mesoderm separate to form two amniocardiac vesicles. The primordial heart cells separate, with the splanchnic layer forming separate but joined bands that subsequently thicken and form troughs and eventually tubes. Along these tubes sulci are evident even at this early stage, which provide evidence of longitudinal segmentation of the tubes into regions that ultimately will form the conus, ventricles, and atrial chambers. By the 22nd day, or the 10th embryological stage, these tubes that earlier were joined only by a few cells fuse over the extent of the conotruncal and ventricular segments to form the primitive single heart tube. This tube is continuous at its cephalic end with the sinus of the ventral aortae, and at its caudal end with the primitive right and left atrial chambers. During stage 10 and continuing into stage 11 the length of the cardiac tube more than doubles. This change in length, together with asymmetrical growth of the right ventricle and the left side of the left ventricle causes the tube to loop upon itself and to the right (like an S on its side). Also during stage 11 (day 24) the primitive atria fuse and the common atrial chamber ascends behind the ventricles to its final location behind the conotruncal segment. At this stage looping is complete, and the heart is divisible into conotruncal, ventricular, and atrial segments. These segments are continuous and septation has not begun (Fig. 55).

By stage 12, the 26th day, a sulcus between the atrium and ventricle is evident externally, and its internal manifestation, the atrioventricular (AV) canal, can be seen migrating to the right of the longitudinal axis of the heart. Endocardial cushions, posterior and anterior, are seen within the AV canal (Fig.

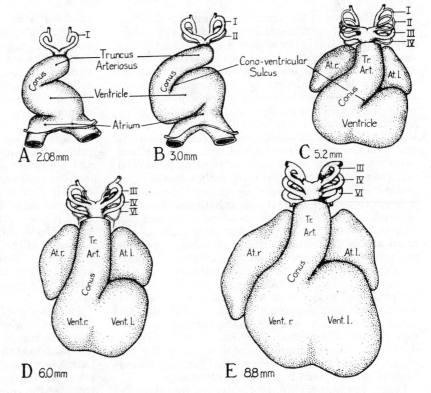

Figure 55. Ventral views of reconstructions of the hearts of young embryos showing the shift in the position of the truncus toward the midline and the reduction of the conoventricular sulcus. Slight modifications in the redrawing have been made in order to bring the various models into comparable orientation. (With permission from Kramer, T. C.: The partitioning of the truncus and conus and the formation of the membranous portion of the interventricular septum in the human heart. Am J Anat 71:348, 1942.)

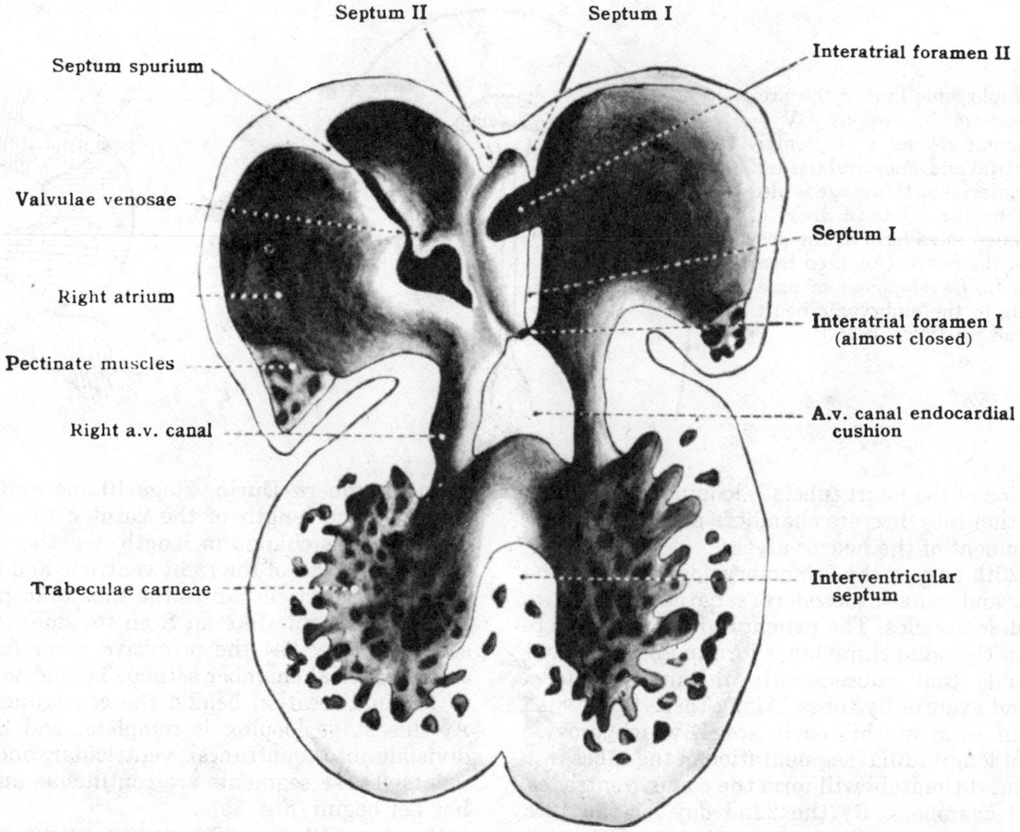

Figure 56. Semischematic drawing of interior of heart to show start of interatrial septum secundum and appearance of interatrial foramen secundum in septum primum. Based on original reconstructions of the heart of a 9.4-mm pig embryo and on Tandler's reconstruction of the heart of human embryos in the seventh week. (With permission from Patten, B. M.: Human Embryology. 2nd ed. New York, McGraw-Hill Book Co., 1953, p. 662.)

56). At the level of the ventricles, a sulcus separating right from left ventricle is evident externally, while internally the trabeculated portions of the ventricular cavities enlarge rapidly like two diverticuli of the endocardium. In the interventricular canal, however, the tissue is not trabeculated; it grows more slowly and as a consequence a septum is formed between the enlarging ventricular cavities, with the residual interventricular canal forming an orifice between the ventricular chambers. In the atrium, the sinus venosus is now well-defined, receiving blood from the umbilical veins, the cardinal veins, and the vitelline plexi. The sinus venosus has migrated principally into the right atrium, and a septum (septum primum) appears as a crescent ridge on the dorsal and cephalic portion of the common atrium. Finally, the conotruncal region has migrated to the left of the longitudinal axis of the heart and by the 28th day (stage 13) ridges appear in the conotruncal segment that will eventually divide the truncus into the aorta and main pulmonary artery. In summary, by this stage fusion and looping are complete and evidence of early but still incomplete septation is seen between the atria, within the AV canal and ventricle, and within the truncus. In addition, the initially common pulmonary vein has developed as an outpouching of the atrium just to the left of the septum primum. Beyond the truncus, paired ventral aortae extend in a cephalic direction.

Stages 14 through 18 (day 32 to day 44) are primarily involved with the completion or near completion of processes already initiated that result in septation of the various segments of the embryonic heart (Fig. 57). By the 16th stage the endocardial cushions have fused to divide the atrioventricular canal into right and left orifices, and tricuspid and mitral valve tissue is seen. Within the atrium, the crescent-shaped septum primum grows rapidly toward the AV cushions, gradually extinguishing the opening (ostium primum) between the left and right atrial cavities. Just as the septum primum is about to fuse with the endocardial cushion and obliterate the ostium, a second orifice develops (ostium secundum) owing to necrosis of cells in the cephalic portion of the septum. Almost simultaneously a second ridge develops on the atrial roof just to the right of the septum primum. This ridge grows rapidly in an inferior direction, again in the form of a crescent. The peak of the crescent forms a flap over the ostium secundum, leaving an oval aperture (the foramen ovale) between the atria. The limbs of the crescent fuse with the septum primum in the floor of the right atrium.

To this point, we have referred to the longitudinal segments of a developing heart as atrial, ventricular, and conotruncal segments. To understand the process of septation of the truncus into the definitive aorta and pulmonary artery and the events that ultimately obliterate the interventricular foramen, it is necessary to consider the conotruncal segment as composed of two components. The first of these is the distal or true truncus arteriosus, which extends from the level of the semilunar valves to the fourth aortic arch; the second is the conus or conus cordis, which lies below the semilunar valves and ultimately forms the infundibulum of the right ventricle. At the cephalic end of the truncus, the fourth aortic arch arises anteriorly, while the sixth aortic arches (pulmonary arteries) arise posteriorly. Septation of the truncus begins at this level with bulky ridges forming on the right and left sides of the truncus, which, when fused, separate the aorta and pulmonary arteries, with the former in an anterior position and the latter posterior. As these ridges descend down the truncus the ridge that started on the left moves anteriorly and eventually to the right side, while the ridge that started on the right moves poste-

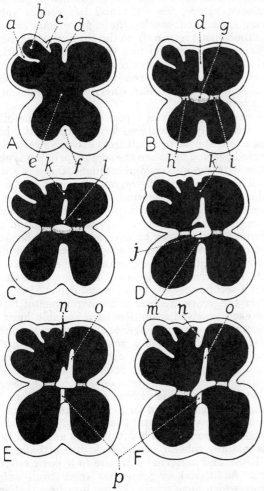

Figure 57. Schematic representation in frontal sections of the developing heart, showing successive stages in the septation processes. a indicates the right venous valve, b the sinus venosus, c the left venous valve, d the septum primum, e the common atrioventricular canal, f the interventricular septum, g the posterior endocardial cushion, h the right atrioventricular orifice, i the left atrioventricular orifice, j the septum intermedium, k the foramen secundum, l the foramen primum (subseptals), m the interventricular foramen, n the septum secundum, o the valve of the foramen ovale, and p the pars membranacea septi. (With permission from Jackson, B. T.: The pathogenesis of congenital cardiovascular anomalies. N Engl J Med 279 (Part 1):85, 1968.)

riorly and eventually to the left. This clockwise rotation, as viewed from above, results from earlier dextral looping of the heart tube. The septum formed by fusion of these ridges within the truncus undergoes a nearly 180-degree spiral, producing an aortic channel that is posterior at the level of the semilunar valves and a pulmonary channel that is anterior at the level of the conus. The truncal ridges extend below the semilunar valves into the conus, where they are more appropriately termed conal ridges. Fusion of the conal ridges produces a short conal septum, and forms the roof of the interventricular foramen, which is bordered posteriorly by the fused AV endocardial cushions and anteriorly by the crest of the interventricular septum. The interventricular foramen is then closed by contributions from the conal system, the endocardial cushions, and the crest of the interventricular septum. The interventricular foramen is then closed by contributions from the conal system, the endocardial cushions, and the crest of the interventricular septum—the resulting closure forming the membranous part of the interventricular septum. At the line of demarcation between the conus and the truncus the semilunar valves form. Within the aortic and pulmonary channels three pads of connective tissue normally extend into each lumen, two arising from truncal ridge tissue and one from independent growth centers on the walls of the aorta and pulmonary trunk. Thus, each semilunar valve is normally tricuspid.

Most investigators believe that congenital malformations of the heart have an embryological basis. At a cellular level cardiogenesis involves growth, differentiation, and morphogenesis. In a general sense, growth of the embryonic heart involves a gain in size due to cell replication. We have seen already that in the developing heart there is a precisely timed sequence to the appearance of each cardiac structure as well as a precisely ordered sequence to bursts of cell replication that cause one structure to grow at one time and another at a different time. Differentiation of cellular components within the developing heart produces connective tissue elements (the AV rings and valves), working myocardium with its full complement of contractile proteins, and specialized tissue capable of impulse formation and rapid conduction. Each of these differentiations leads to altered cellular characteristics and behavior that are essential to the normal function of the developed heart. The processes of morphogenesis include the ability of growing cells to migrate in an apparently directed fashion, and the development of adhesiveness, which allows structures of different origins to fuse with each other. Finally, we see that some structures form but serve only a temporary purpose and then degenerate or become destroyed. From these considerations it follows that congenital malformations of the heart result from developmental errors. These errors include (1) abnormal growth (aplasia, hypoplasia, or dysplasia), (2) failure or partial failure of differentiation, (3) failure or abnormalities of fusion, (4) inadequate or excessive resorption, and (5) abnormal persistence of certain structures. The nature, sites, and timing of the errors determine the malformation that is evident in later fetal and postnatal life.

It is not within the scope of this chapter to review the anatomy of all forms of congenital heart disease or the embryological basis for each. Indeed, the embryological causes for most malformations of the heart are speculative and based largely on extrapolation from what is known about normal development to the structure of abnormally developed hearts. Several examples will suffice to illustrate the major points.

First, let us consider some of the consequences of abnormal growth. At a very early phase of development (stage 10) the heart tube is fused over the length of the conotruncal and ventricular segments. Shortly thereafter the tube curves out to the right and this loop rotates posteriorly. The dextral curvature and rotation have been definitively related to more rapid growth and enhanced mitotic activity of cells on the greater curvature of the loop relative to those on the lesser curvature. A reversal in the pattern of early differential growth rates would lead to a leftward loop and levorotation yielding dextrocardia, a condition in which the heart and great vessels occupy a position in the right chest that is the mirror image of normal anatomy.

In the canal between the atrium and ventricle early evidence of both the anterior and posterior endocardial cushions is seen around the 12th stage, or 26th day, of embryonic life. These cushions undergo rapid growth during the next week and normally fuse by stage 16. Hypoplasia of the endocardial cushions is thought to account for a group of developmental errors, referred to as endocardial cushion defects. Fusion of the cushions normally separates the AV canal into mitral and tricuspid orifices. The cushions also contribute to closure of the ostium primum in septum primum, to closure of the interventricular foramen, and to the formation of the septal or anterior leaflet of the mitral valve and the medial leaflet of the tricuspid valve. In its most severe form, complete AV canal, the cushions fail to meet and fuse and thus the mitral and tricuspid orifices communicate with each other. Above the cushions there is a defect in the lower atrial septum that communicates with a defect below the cushions in the interventricular septum. Both the septal leaflet of the mitral valve and the medial leaflet of the tricuspid valve contain large clefts. Partial AV canal or endocardial cushion defects reflect a situation in which the cushions meet and fuse but fail to obliterate either ostium primum (leaving an atrial septal defect, commonly associated with a cleft anterior mitral leaflet) or fail to obliterate the interventricular foramen (leaving a posterior ventricular septal defect, commonly associated with a defective or cleft medial tricuspid leaflet).

Abnormalities of growth during later phases of cardiac development involve, for example, failure or aplasia of the conotruncal septum leading to a persistent truncus arteriosus. While at least four types of persistent truncus arteriosus have been identified, each is characterized by a large single vessel (the truncus) arising from a single semilunar valve situated above a ventricular septal defect. If present, the pulmonary arteries arise from the truncus. Aplasia of the truncal portion of the conotruncal septum results in the single receiving vessel above the heart from which the pulmonary arteries (sixth aortic arches) arise. Aplasia of the conal part of the conotruncal septum denies the contribution of this septum to ultimate closure of the interventricular foramen and hence a ventricular septal defect. At even a later stage in development aplasia may lead to semilunar valve abnormalities, such as a bicuspid aortic or pulmonary valve. Ebstein's malformation of the tricuspid valve is an example of dysplasia of one of the AV valves.

There are a number of examples of either inadequate or excessive resorption of structures that play an important role at early stages of embryonic development but that regress totally or resorb partially. At approximately stage 12, the AV canal and the sinus venosus appear to migrate to the right, principally because of rapid enlargement of the primitive left atrium. The sinus venosus opens entirely then into the primitive right atrium to the right of the developing septum primum. The orifice of the sinus venosus takes on a nearly vertical orientation and is guarded by two well-developed valves, the right and left venous valves. During subsequent weeks, the right venous valve directs the venous return (from the sinus venosus) across the interatrial foramen into the left atrium. In later fetal life this venous valve regresses to a considerable extent, but inadequate resorption leaves a series of bands or a network (Chiari's network) attached to the crista terminalis.

Secundum type atrial septal defects are one of the more commonly encountered forms of congenital heart disease and appear to result from excessive resorption. As noted previously, when the septum primum is about to fuse with the endocardial cushions, there is a wave of cell necrosis and subsequent resorption in the cephalic portion of the septum, creating a foramen between the right and left atrium (the ostium secundum). If this process is excessive, a very large ostium may be formed that cannot be covered by the subsequent development of the crescent-shaped septum secundum. A persisting interatrial communication results that, if small, is referred to as a patent foramen ovale and, if large, a secundum type atrial septal defect.

Over the years, genetic and environmental factors have each received attention as a possible basis for understanding the pathogenesis of errors in cardiac development. Support of a genetic hypothesis can be found in numerous reports documenting the familial nature of congenital heart disease, its occurrence in identical twins, and its prevalence in certain diseases caused by identifiable chromosomal aberrations (for example, mongolism and Turner's syndrome). Evidence favoring an environmental basis includes the association between congenital heart diseases and viral infections (notably rubella), teratogenic drugs (thalidomide and LAS), and maternal exposure to hypoxic environments. Additional evidence has come from animal studies, which have shown (1) that breeding of affected animals with certain forms of congenital heart disease produces offspring with a high prevalence of the disease and (2) that exposure of animals to teratogenic agents increases by as much as tenfold the incidence of heart malformations in offspring. Yet despite these accounts, no clear-cut basis for congenital heart disease is evident in over 90 per cent of the cases that present to a physician.

Because of this dilemma recent attention has focused on a possible interaction between genetic and environmental influences with much more promising results.

The most critical review and support of this concept is provided in the reference by Nora. In developing a multifactorial hypothesis for the etiology of congenital heart disease, Nora reviewed the world literature as well as his own large experience. A hypothesis that there was no genetic basis for congenital heart disease was rejected when 34 per cent of randomly selected cases of congenital heart disease gave a positive and documented history of one or more relatives with congenital heart disease. In a matched control group without congenital heart disease only 9 per cent of families gave a positive history. This difference was significant, as was the difference in the prevalence of congenital heart disease in first order relatives of affected and control subjects. An additional basis for rejecting the hypothesis resulted from a study of twin births. In conditions that have a genetic basis, both members of an identical pair will be affected more often than both members of a nonidentical pair. With respect to congenital heart disease concordance was observed in 46 per cent of identical pairs and in only 4.2 per cent of nonidentical pairs.

In considering the mechanism of this apparent genetic basis of congenital heart disease three possibilities were evaluated. First, the possibility that a single mutant gene might be held accountable was investigated. When large samples of cases of specific cardiac malformations such as atrial septal defect were considered, the data in families of these cases were not consistent with either a dominant or recessive mode of inheritance, even though 32 per cent of the families had a positive history for congenital heart disease. A second hypothesis considered was that of a gross chromosomal aberration. Except for those very rare instances of syndromes accompanied by congenital heart diseases (Down's syndrome, Turner's syndrome, and D and E trisomies) chromosomal karyotypes on patients with congenital heart diseases were characteristically normal. While these observations do not exclude a submicroscopic chromosomal abnormality, no evidence for an abnormality was observed.

The final hypothesis tested by Nora was a multifactorial etiology that encompassed both genetic and environmental factors. Since a very strong case for either a genetic or environmental factor can be made in some cases of congenital heart disease, this hypothesis seems attractive. Twin studies to test the genetic hypothesis provide additional support for Nora's hypothesis. When a twin is identified with a particular cardiac manifestation it can be concluded that if the other member of an identical pair is not affected by the same condition 100 per cent of the time, environmental factors must be at play. As noted before, concordance was observed in only 46 per cent of identical pairs in which one member of the pair had a congenital cardiac lesion. The genetic model for a disease inherited through a

multifactorial mode predicts that such diseases will be relatively common, show familial aggregation, recur at a rate of 1 to 5 per cent in siblings, occur more frequently in identical twins than in nonidentical twins (but not 100 per cent of the time), and will be susceptible to environmental influence. The data concerning congenital heart disease satisfy all of these criteria. From this model has evolved a working concept that genetic factors predispose an individual to one or more developmental errors in which a process or processes essential to normal development are controlled by more than one gene. Among the genetically predisposed, an environmental influence is usually, but not always, necessary to cause the malformation, and that influence must not only be capable of affecting the process but must occur at a time when the process is active and susceptible to error. This concept allows for those infrequent instances in which a mutant gene or chromosomal aberration is sufficient alone. It is also compatible with the observation that a potent teratogenic agent delivered at the appropriate time does not lead to a cardiac malformation in all offspring. Finally, it allows for the fact that environmental influence may be a relatively major or minor factor in influencing the expression of a condition that is essentially determined by the genetic factor.

REFERENCES

Benjamin, T. J.: The pathogenesis of congenital cardiovascular anomalies. N Engl J Med 279:25, 80, 1968.

DeHaan, R. L.: Development of form in the embryonic heart; an experimental approach. Circulation 35:821, 1967.

Emerit, I., DeGrouchy, J., Vernant, P., and Corone, P.: Chromosomal abnormalities and congenital heart disease. Circulation 36:886, 1967.

Goor, D. A., Lillehei, C. W., Rees, R., and Edwards, J. E.: Isolated ventricular septal defect: Developmental basis for various types and presentation of classification. Chest 58:468, 1970.

Kalter, H., and Warkany, J.: Congenital malformations: Etiologic factors and their role in prevention. N Engl J Med 308:424, 1983.

McKusick, V. A.: A genetical view of cardiovascular disease. Circulation 30:326, 1964.

Nora, J. J.: Multifactorial inheritance hypothesis for the etiology of congenital heart disease: A genetic-environmental interaction. Circulation 38:604, 1968.

O'Rahilly, R.: The timing and sequence of events in human cardiogenesis. Acta Anat 79:70, 1971.

Van Mierop, L. H. S.: Morphological development of the heart. In Berne, R. M., Sperelakis, N., and Geiger, S. R. (eds.): Handbook of Physiology. Section 2, The Cardiovascular System. Bethesda, Md., American Physiological Society, 1979, p. 1.

Van Mierop, L. H. S., and Gessner, I. H.: Pathogenetic mechanisms in congenital cardiovascular malformations. Prog Cardiovasc Dis 15:67, 1972.

Hypertension

Studies of large populations throughout the world have shown that systolic and diastolic arterial blood pressures are distributed over a rather wide range. One typical study reported that for women aged 30 to

39 systolic blood pressure ranged from 85 to 160 mm Hg (mean for the group 122 mm Hg). In the same population, diastolic blood pressure ranged from 62 to 100 mm Hg with a mean of 82 mm Hg. We also know

that blood pressure tends to increase with age, that the rise in systolic pressure with age is greater than the rise in diastolic pressure, and that during at least the first four decades of life blood pressure is higher in men than in women and higher in blacks than in whites.

There is an understandable resistance among physicians to set an arbitrary blood pressure for the purpose of defining the presence or absence of hypertension. Nonetheless, many studies in children have shown that individuals with blood pressures above the 90th percentile for their age are at increased risk for developing complications of hypertension in adult life. Similar studies in young adults document that 20 to 40 per cent of subjects with resting blood pressures intermittently above 150/90 mm Hg subsequently develop sustained hypertension. Finally, above a diastolic pressure of 80 mm Hg, a relation has been established between the level of diastolic pressure and the incidence of atherosclerotic disease. As a practical matter, therefore, the physician should become concerned about the blood pressure when it reaches a level that has been shown to increase the risk of sustained hypertension, complications of hypertensive vascular disease, or accelerated atherosclerosis. The most common definition of this threshold for concern is a blood pressure above the 90th percentile for age and sex, or greater than 130/80 (for individuals under 15 years), greater than 135/90 (for individuals 15 to 45 years), and greater than 140/95 (for individuals above 45 years in age).

We will define hypertension as a condition (regardless of cause) in which the arterial pressure is elevated above a specified level for age and sex (the 90th or 95th percentile may be chosen). The presence of hypertension, however, delineates a very nonhomogeneous population of patients, and accordingly various classification schemes have been proposed. One such scheme is based on the pattern of blood pressure over time (hours or days) and classifies patients as having either labile or sustained hypertension. A second scheme is based on the level of blood pressure and leads to subgroups such as borderline, mild, moderate, and severe. A very important classification with respect to prognosis and treatment is the distinction between benign and malignant hypertension. Malignant hypertension is characterized by fibrinoid necrosis of arterial walls and rapidly progressive deterioration of renal, mental, and visual function related to these changes. When left untreated, malignant hypertension is uniformly fatal. Treated properly it is a reversible phase in the natural course of some hypertensive patients.

The most useful classification from the point of view of pathophysiology is based on etiology. Secondary hypertension is a condition in which the blood pressure is elevated as a result of a specific disease or disorder, generally affecting one of the components of the normal blood pressure control system. In these cases hypertension is an important, but not the only, manifestation of the disease, and there is at least a partial understanding of mechanisms that initiate and then sustain the elevated blood pressure. The other broad category within an etiologic scheme of classification is primary, or so-called essential, hypertension. In these cases blood pressure is elevated, often to a severe level, yet the basic cause eludes definition by currently available tests.

It is important to realize that no form of hypertension can be assumed to be benign or without consequence. By similar reasoning, the term essential is a poor choice of a word to describe primary hypertension. According to our present perspective, hypertension is not essential in the sense that it is idiopathic. History has shown that what is included under essential or primary hypertension today will probably be recognized as a secondary form of hypertension tomorrow. It seems very probable that all forms of hypertension will ultimately be shown to reflect a disorder (genetic or acquired) of one or more of the normal components of the blood pressure regulatory system. It is the complexity of the system and the interaction between its components that make definition of cause difficult in some patients—not the absence of a cause as implied by the terms primary and essential.

The level of arterial blood pressure at any time is determined by the relation between cardiac output and the net resistance to flow offered by the peripheral arterial bed. In a previous chapter we presented many of the known features of an elaborate system for blood pressure control and discussed the nature of components of that system and their interactions (Fig. 50). In the final analysis these components act either directly or indirectly to modify cardiac output, peripheral arterial resistance, or both.

Our current view of hypertension is that elevation of arterial blood pressure is a consequence of some disorder of the blood pressure regulatory system. Although there are many components to the system, they can be conveniently grouped into three major categories based upon the interval between activation of the mechanism and its subsequent effect on blood pressure. One such category consists of the control mechanisms that have the capacity to change blood pressure within seconds. These are referred to as rapidly acting mechanisms; they operate principally through components of the nervous system and affect blood pressure primarily through changes in efferent sympathetic nerve activity. A second category of control mechanisms is intermediate in its course of action, requiring minutes or hours to effect a substantial change in blood pressure. Included in this group are the renin-angiotensin system and possibly other circulating vasoactive agents that act principally on the tone of arterial resistance vessels. Also included in this category are influences that lead to shifts in the distribution of extracellular fluid between the intravascular and extravascular compartments. Finally, there is a group of long-range control systems in which the effect on blood pressure takes hours or days to develop fully. These mechanisms act principally through modifications of blood volume and include among others the relation between arterial blood pressure and renal excretion of salt and water, and modifications of that relationship through the actions of aldosterone and other mineralocorticoids.

An analysis of the system for blood pressure control reveals multiple sites for interaction between components. For example, sympathetic nerve activity can modify renin release by the kidney, conversion of renin to angiotensin leads to aldosterone release by the adrenal, and aldosterone modified the ability of the kidney to excrete salt and water, and hence influences blood volume. It should be apparent from this simple example that regardless of the mechanism that leads to hypertension, secondary changes in other components of the blood pressure control system are the rule rather than the exception.

It is evident from a systems approach to blood pressure control that for the level of arterial pressure to remain elevated (sustained hypertension) there is a failure of the long-term blood pressure control system. Guyton and his colleagues have argued that in all forms of hypertension there must be a shift to the right of the normal curve that relates arterial pressure to renal excretion of salt and water (Fig. 58). In their view, regardless of the factor that initiates a blood pressure rise, sustained hypertension is characterized by a urinary output of sodium and water that is less than would be the case if a comparable blood pressure was induced in a subject without hypertension. Such a point of view is generally compatible with the observation that hypertension is for all practical purposes not found in populations who eat a diet extremely low in salt. It is also compatible with the view that in nearly all hypertensive states, regardless of cause, agents that promote the excretion of salt and water will either lower blood pressure themselves or augment the antihypertensive action of agents that act primarily on other components of the blood pressure control system.

The link between the kidney and hypertension is perhaps best illustrated by the fact that even today renal diseases constitute the most frequently recognized cause of secondary hypertension. An association between acute glomerulonephritis and blood pressure

elevation was noted in the late 1800s. Subsequent studies served to differentiate the hypertensive conditions associated with renal disease into at least two physiologically distinct groups. In one, there is activation of a pressor mechanism, which leads to an increase in peripheral vascular resistance and hence in blood pressure. The most noteworthy example of such a condition is stenosis of a renal artery accompanied by a plasma renin concentration in the venous effluent of the involved kidney that is at least 50 per cent greater than that obtained from the opposite kidney. The second general mechanism by which renal disease may play a role in the etiology of hypertension is related to loss of renal substance and a reduced ability of the kidneys to excrete salt and water. The purest example of this form of hypertension is that which accompanies the anephric state, so-called renoprival hypertension. A more common example is represented by most cases of chronic renal failure. In these latter conditions, plasma renin activity may not be elevated, plasma volume and cardiac output are increased, and peripheral arterial resistance is normal or even reduced. This second form of renal hypertension is also marked by a positive correlation between blood volume and arterial pressure, and a favorable response of the blood pressure to agents that restore plasma volume to the normal range (Fig. 59).

Counterparts of these two forms of renal hypertension have been established in experimental animals. Clamping of the renal artery in dogs leads to hypertension and to an increase in plasma renin activity. Studies have shown that blood pressure may be normalized in such animals without change of blood volume by administration of 1-SAR-8-ala-angiotensin (Saralasin), which is a competitive antagonist of angiotensin II at the arteriolar level.

In a similar way, experimental studies have been performed after both kidneys have been removed. Most of the evidence from such animals and from anephric patients indicates that hypertension will develop if fluid volume is expanded, and that volume expansion is the most likely cause of the increased blood pressure in the renoprival state. Others have argued that a normal kidney may elaborate a vasodepressor substance, the absence of which in the anephric state might contribute to hypertension.

A second important step in our understanding of the mechanisms of hypertension occurred in 1929 when an epinephrine-like substance was identified in a chromaffin tumor of the adrenal removed from a patient with paroxysmal hypertension. Similar tumors had been described pathologically as early as 1886, and Cannon observed in 1921 that a pressor substance was released by the liver upon stimulation of hepatic sympathetic nerves. It was not until 1949, however, that excess norepinephrine production by chromaffin tumor cells was identified as the basis for hypertension in patients with pheochromocytoma. These tumors originate typically from the adrenal medulla. The chromaffin cells of the adrenal medulla synthesize catecholamines from the amino acid tyrosine. In contrast to chromaffin cells located in sympathetic ganglia, adrenal medullary cells also have the capacity to convert norepinephrine to epinephrine, a process requiring the enzyme phenethanolamine-N-methyltransferase. Most adrenal medullary pheochromocytomas secrete a large

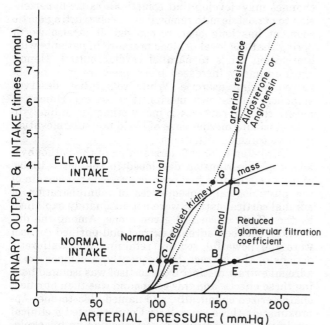

Figure 58. Abnormal urinary output curves and graphical analysis of the long-term level of arterial pressure in various hypertensive states caused by the abnormal renal function. (With permission from Guyton, A. C.: Textbook of Medical Physiology. 5th ed. Philadelphia, W. B. Saunders Co., 1976, p. 286.)

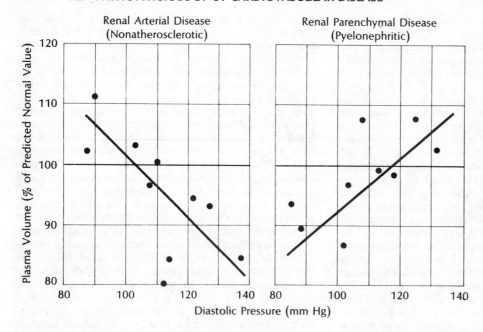

Figure 59. In renovascular hypertension, plasma volume proved inversely related to diastolic pressure (left); in contrast, volume proved directly dependent on pressure in renal parenchymal disease (right), implicating a significant volume component in the latter. (With permission from Frohlich, E. D.: Hemodynamic concepts in hypertension. Hosp Pract 9 (Part 2):11, 1974.)

amount of norepinephrine, but in addition some epinephrine. The symptoms in patients with pheochromocytoma result from release of catecholamines by the tumor, causing a rapid rise in blood pressure, tachycardia, sweating, anxiety, headache, nausea, and vague chest pain. Hypertension in patients with pheochromocytoma may be persistent. However, paroxysms of sudden elevation of arterial pressure are usually evident whether the basal pressure is normal or elevated. Suppression of pancreatic insulin release by norepinephrine (via alpha receptor stimulation) is also evident in these patients and contributes importantly to glucose intolerance associated with pheochromocytoma. Persistent elevation of the plasma norepinephrine level leads to plasma volume contraction. Although surgical removal of a tumor is the definitive treatment, the role of norepinephrine in the pathophysiology of the condition is reflected by the fact that dibenzyline, a specific alpha-adrenergic antagonist, will restore blood pressure, plasma volume, and the plasma insulin responsiveness to normal. Beta-adrenergic blockers such as propranolol effectively control cardiac and other manifestations of the action of norepinephrine on beta receptors.

Among secondary forms of hypertension, aortic coarctation receives justified emphasis, in part because of fascination with its unique features on physical examination, but more importantly because it is a cause of hypertension in which the elevated blood pressure and its consequences can be ameliorated if recognized early. From a physiological point of view the hypertension that accompanies aortic coarctation is evident only in the upper extremities, which are fed by arteries that arise between the aortic valve and the site of coarctation. The hypertension is principally systolic, although diastolic levels may be elevated to a modest degree. The level of systolic hypertension correlates roughly with the severity of aortic obstruction and is attributable to rapid ejection of the stroke volume into a proximal arterial system, the capacitance of which is reduced by exclusion of a major

segment of the aorta distal to the coarctation. Diastolic pressure, on the other hand, is determined principally by the arterial resistance offered by branches of the aorta arising above the coarctation, an important component of which is the size and number of collateral channels through which the aortic chambers above and below the coarctation communicate. Despite many efforts to implicate neurogenic factors and the renin-angiotensin system, most current data indicate that the hypertension of coarctation of the aorta arises principally on a mechanical basis. That secondary changes may develop that sometimes cause hypertension to persist despite removal of the obstructing aortic segment has long been recognized. It is also worth noting that the level of blood pressure in patients with coarctation tends to parallel cardiac output. Hence, extraordinarily increased blood pressure may be observed during exercise. While coarctation deserves emphasis on its own merits, it is an experiment of nature that, in contrast to many others, is unlikely to help elucidate mechanisms of blood pressure elevation in more common situations.

A third step in our understanding of the pathophysiology of hypertension developed in the early 1950s. Many investigators had been impressed that certain of the physiological consequences of administration of adrenal cortical extract were not adequately explained by the effects of cortisol given alone. Among the differences between adrenal extract and purified cortisol were the powerful sodium retaining and kaliuretic actions of the extract. Subsequently, a component of adrenal extract distinct from cortisol was isolated having these effects, and this compound was then purified, characterized chemically, and named aldosterone. Approximately three years later Conn reported a clinical syndrome of hypertension, accompanied by hypokalemia and excess aldosterone in the urine due to a functioning adrenal cortical adenoma. The syndrome was called primary aldosteronism.

Many reports of this syndrome have appeared subsequently in the literature. Hypertension of mild to moderate degree is present in nearly all patients. The majority of patients with primary aldosteronism have an adrenal adenoma, although it has been recognized that bilateral adrenal hyperplasia without an adenoma can simulate both the clinical syndrome and its accompanying biochemical alterations. Virtually all of the clinical features of this syndrome can be ascribed to the action of aldosterone, causing conservation of sodium and excretion of potassium and hydrogen by the kidney. Aldosterone is normally secreted by the zona glomerulosa of the adrenal cortex. The secretory rate of aldosterone is influenced by angiotensin and by potassium. In primary aldosteronism the secretory rate becomes increased and autonomous. Aldosterone acts on epithelial cells of sweat glands, the intestinal tract, and most notably the distal nephron as a consequence of binding to specific nuclear receptors. The response to aldosterone by all of these tissues is sodium retention and loss of potassium and hydrogen ion. Retention of sodium by the kidney leads to expansion of plasma volume, hypertension, and reduced plasma renin concentrations. Potassium loss leads to hypokalemia, muscular weakness, diminished ability of the kidney to concentrate urine, polyuria, and altered glucose tolerance due to diminished insulin production and release. The level of blood pressure that accompanies primary aldosteronism has been correlated with plasma volume. Furthermore, in 80 to 90 per cent of patients with hypertension due to primary aldosteronism plasma volume and blood pressure can be restored to normal or near normal levels by administration of spironolactone, an analog of aldosterone that competitively blocks but does not stimulate the aldosterone binding receptor of epithelial cells (Fig. 60). As noted above, plasma renin activity is depressed in patients with autonomous and excessive secretion of aldosterone. Not only is plasma renin depressed, but the increase in plasma renin concentration that normally accompanies head uptilt or sodium depletion by dietary restriction or loop diuretics is also suppressed.

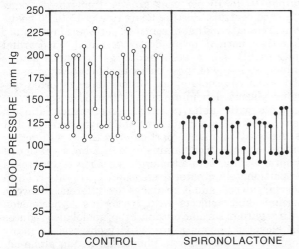

Figure 60. Effect of spironolactone, 400 mg daily for five weeks, on the blood pressure in patients with primary aldosteronism. Each circle with connecting line represents the average systolic and diastolic pressure of a single patient. The order of patients coincides in each half of the figure. (With permission from Spark, R. F., and Melky, J. C.: Aldosteronism in hypertension: The spironolactone response test. Ann Intern Med 69:686, 1968.)

Steroid hormones that have a mineralocorticoid effect, other than aldosterone, have been implicated as the cause of hypertension in at least three other forms of adrenal disease. Hypertension is a common finding in patients with Cushing's syndrome, whether the syndrome results from autonomous secretion of excess quantities of cortisol by adrenal tumors or in response to pituitary or nonpituitary tumors that secrete ACTH and thereby promote adrenal cortical hypersecretion of cortisol. At least two forms of congenital adrenal hyperplasia are accompanied by mineralocorticoid excess and hypertension. In one of these, C-11 hydrolase deficiency, the defect in steroidogenesis prevents the conversion of 11-deoxycorticosterone (DOC) to corticosterone. The resulting deficiency of cortisol production leads to a compensatory release of ACTH and excessive adrenal production of DOC. The mineralocorticoid effect of DOC, although less potent than aldosterone, leads to volume expansion and hypertension. A second hypertensive form of congenital adrenal hyperplasia is C-17 hydrolase deficiency. In this deficiency, cortisol synthesis is impaired at the step where progesterone is converted to 17-alpha-hydroxyprogesterone. Subnormal cortisol production again leads to a compensatory increase of ACTH, which in turn increases the production of 17-deoxycorticosteroids and DOC, which promote sodium retention, potassium loss, volume expansion, and hypertension. All of these forms of adrenal cortical hyperfunction illustrate the potential of mineralocorticoid excess to induce hypertension that, at least initially, is attributable to plasma volume expansion.

From the discussions outlined above, several important generalizations can be drawn. First, the currently recognized forms of secondary hypertension can be related to disturbed function of one of the components of the normal system involved in blood pressure regulation (neurogenic, renal pressor, renoprival, adrenomedullary, adrenocortical). A second observation is that at least initially most of these secondary forms of hypertension result either from an influence that causes peripheral vascular constriction and secondary plasma volume contraction or from primary plasma volume expansion with little or no change in vascular resistance. Third, the blood pressure control mechanisms are coupled together so that in some instances activation of one pressor mechanism leads to activation of a second (for example, increased sympathetic nerve discharge leads to renin release by the kidney, and angiotension II formation from renin leads to aldosterone release). In other instances, these control mechanisms are coupled by negative feedback (for example, volume expansion induced by mineralocorticoid excess inhibits renin release). A fourth important concept is that, regardless of the mechanism that initiates the rise in blood pressure, the ability of the kidney to regulate urinary output of sodium and water in response to changes of arterial perfusion pressure is altered in most forms of persistent hypertension. It follows that whether plasma volume is expanded, normal, or contracted, all forms of persistent hypertension, with the possible exception of aortic coarctation, are characterized by plasma expansion relative to the plasma volume that would prevail if the normal kidney excreted salt and water as it would in response to an increased perfusion pressure and if it were removed from humoral factors that modulate that ability. Finally, it is apparent that certain forms of hypertension reflect the aggregate influence of more than one factor; for example, certain forms of renal disease are characterized by both a renal pressor (renin) and renoprival (volume expansion) component. When hypertension of any specific mechanism is allowed to persist, pathological alterations of the peripheral resistance vessels, including the kidney, may lead to a situation in which removal of the initiating mechanism fails to eliminate hypertension because another adequate cause for blood pressure elevation now dominates.

With this background let us now consider the subject of primary or essential hypertension. Nearly all investigators agree that genetic influences play a role at least as a predisposing factor in the development of hypertension. Essential hypertension appears to cluster within families. For example, if both parents have hypertension the prevalence of hypertension among their offspring is 1 in 2; if only one parent has hypertension the prevalence among offspring is 1 in 3; and if neither parent has hypertension the prevalence among their offspring is only 1 in 20. Other observations also support the importance of genetic factors. For example, two genetically distinct strains of rats have been produced, one that consistently develops hypertension when exposed to a high sodium intake and a second that is resistant to the hypertensive effects of sodium loading. In the sensitive strain of rats and in patients with salt-sensitive hypertension, the ability of the kidney to excrete a sodium load is reduced. Acute salt loading produces an increase in arterial vascular resistance rather than the decrease typically seen in normotensive subjects. The hypertensive rat and most patients with primary hypertension demonstrate an abnormally high intracellular concentration of sodium and calcium in vascular smooth muscle cells. This accumulation of sodium and calcium increases resting vascular smooth muscle tone and leads to an augmented vasoconstrictor response to catecholamines. These abnormalities may result from a genetically transmitted deficiency of a cell membrane component responsible for Na^+-K^+ cotransport that is separate from the membrane Na^+-K^+ ATPase. This defect has been demonstrated in erythrocytes from patients with primary hypertension, in about half of their offspring, and in groups of blacks prone to develop hypertension. It is still premature to conclude that a specific primary genetic defect has been established as a cause for essential hypertension. However, the observations are consistent with the established link between sodium intake and hypertension, the clustering of primary hypertension in families, and the apparent genetic determination in animals and man of the capacity of the kidney to excrete a sodium load.

Another clue to a pathophysiological mechanism potentially responsible for blood pressure elevation in some subjects with primary hypertension comes from hemodynamic studies. Of particular importance are those observations that have been made in patients with hypertension of relatively recent onset not complicated by some of the known consequences of long-standing hypertension regardless of its cause.

It would appear that among patients with essential hypertension there is a subset whose blood pressures are labile, averaging 150–160/90–100 but intermit-

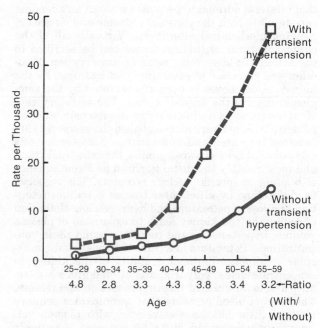

Figure 61. Prevalence of future sustained hypertension in normotensive subjects and patients who initially had transient (borderline) hypertension. Each cohort was followed for five years. (With permission from Julius, S., and Esler, M.: Autonomic nervous cardiovascular regulation in borderline hypertension. Am J Cardiol 36:686, 1975.)

tently within the normal range. A high percentage of these patients subsequently develop sustained hypertension with pressures consistently above 150/90 in the absence of treatment (Fig. 61). On the whole, subjects with borderline hypertension have a cardiac output 10 to 15 per cent greater than that of age-matched controls. Resting heart rate is 15 to 20 beats/min greater than that of controls, peripheral resistance is either normal or modestly elevated, myocardial contractility is enhanced, and forearm venous tone is enhanced. Many of these patients show elevated levels of plasma catecholamines. Others have reported elevated plasma dopamine beta hydroxylase activity in patients with labile essential hypertension. Plasma renin activity is variable in labile hypertensives but is elevated in many, particularly those with other indications of catecholamine excess. Administration of propranolol (a beta-adrenergic antagonist) causes a proportionately greater decrease in heart rate than in normal subjects and it abolishes the difference between normals and subjects with borderline hypertension with regard to cardiac output. Propranolol also reduces the elevated plasma renin activity observed in many borderline hypertensives. Phentolamine (an alpha-adrenergic antagonist) produces an immediate reduction in peripheral vascular resistance in patients with borderline hypertension and elevated renin levels but no change in normal subjects or in hypertensives with low plasma renin. The picture that emerges from these studies is one of a subset of early essential hypertension characterized by lability of blood pressure, a

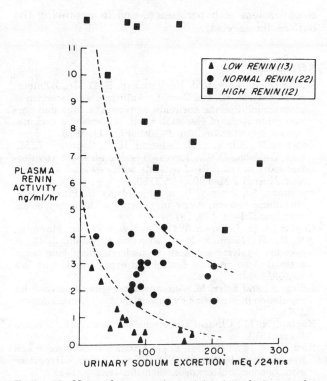

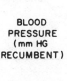

Figure 62. Noon plasma renin activity in relation to the concurrent daily rate of sodium excretion in 47 hypertensive patients. Samples were collected after all antihypertension drugs had been discontinued for at least three weeks. (With permission from Bühler, F. R., Laragh, J. H., Baer, L., Vaughn, E. D., Jr., and Brunner, H. R.: Propranolol inhibition of renin secretion—a specific approach to diagnosis and treatment of renin-dependent hypertensive disease. N Engl J Med 287(Part 2):1211, 1972.)

Figure 63. Effects of spironolactone on blood pressures of patients with "low-renin essential hypertension." (With permission from Liddle, G. W.: Is hypertension essential? Trans Assoc Am Phys 88:61, 1975.)

hyperkinetic circulatory state, evidence of increased sympathetic nerve activity, and a favorable therapeutic response to agents that inhibit sympathetic activity. In these patients elevated plasma renin activity is a biochemical marker of enhanced sympathetic activity and does not seem to imply intrinsic renal disease.

The widespread evidence of altered autonomic activity in this subset of patients suggests strongly a change in the central integrative functions of blood pressure control, functions normally carried out in areas of the medulla oblongata. Pharmacological evidence suggests a central adrenergic mechanism that could reduce blood pressure; the antihypertensive effects of clonidine act through this central mechanism by stimulating central alpha-adrenergic receptors. The evidence currently available favors the view that at least one subset of essential hypertension is on a neurogenic basis. The fault leading to this condition appears to be located in the central nervous system component of the blood pressure regulatory system. The manifestations of this form of essential hypertension are initially attributable to enhanced sympathetic nerve activity. The most effective therapeutic approaches are aimed at interrupting or blocking the effects of augmented sympathetic nerve discharge.

Another approach to subgrouping of patients with uncomplicated essential hypertension has been advocated by Laragh and his colleagues from New York. Subgrouping has been based on measurement of plasma renin activity under standardized conditions. Many factors are known to influence the secretion of renin by the juxtaglomerular cells of the kidney. However, in the absence of medication and under conditions of electrolyte balance, plasma renin activity has been shown to correlate inversely with urinary sodium excretion (Fig. 62). The New York group has observed

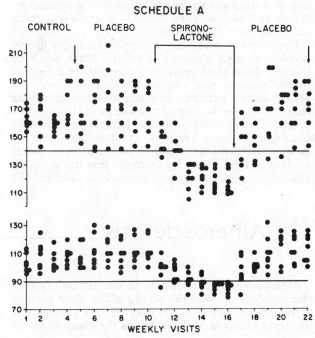

that while plasma renin activity relative to sodium excretion in essential hypertension may overlap with normal subjects, there is an important subgroup in whom plasma renin is suppressed. This low renin group has received particular attention, in part because renin levels not only are suppressed under basal conditions, but also because they fail to increase in a normal manner during various provocative tests. Another reason for special interest in this group is the absence of evidence of sympathetic overactivity, and contrasting hemodynamic findings relative to the high renin essential hypertensives described above. The prevalence of low renin hypertension increases with age but has been estimated to constitute 20 to 25 per cent of essential hypertension in the 30- to 50-year-old group. It appears more prevalent in blacks than in whites.

Of the known causes of secondary hypertension, all of those conditions primarily attributable to mineralocorticoid excess (typified by primary aldosteronism) are characterized by low levels of plasma renin activity and attenuated responsiveness of the renin system to maneuvers that normally increase renin secretion. So far it has not been possible to demonstrate either excessive excretion or secretion or diminished clearance of a specific mineralocorticoid in low renin primary hypertension. However, in most of these patients blood pressures were normalized either by giving agents that inhibited mineralocorticoid synthesis or by giving spironolactone, which inhibited the actions of mineralocorticoids on renal transport of sodium. Subsequent clinical studies have supported the view that adequate doses of spironolactone will generally normalize the blood pressure in low renin essential hypertension (Fig. 63). This is in contrast to the absence of any sustained antihypertensive effect of spironolactone in patients with high renin essential hypertension. What emerges from these studies is the possibility that a significant proportion of patients with essential hypertension and reduced plasma levels of renin have a defect in the control of adrenal steroid production and as a consequence secrete at least in a semiautonomous manner excessive amounts of a mineralocorticoid other than aldosterone.

Hypertension continues to represent a major health problem in most segments of society. Much has been learned about blood pressure control, about defects of control systems that can lead to hypertension, and about dietary patterns and pharmacological agents that can modify the control mechanisms. Although the precise factors responsible for hypertension remain unknown in many patients, the interplay between genetic predisposition and environmental influences is evident in most cases. Fortunately, therapy is highly effective in controlling blood pressure, in reducing the complications of hypertension, and in improving the outlook for survival.

REFERENCES

Bühler, F. R., Laragh, J. H., Vaughan, E. D., Jr., Brunner, H. R., Gavras, H., and Baer, L.: Antihypertensive action of propranolol: Specific antirenin responses in high and normal renin forms of essential, renal, renovascular and malignant hypertension. Am J Cardiol 32:511, 1973.

Canessa, M., Adragna, N., Solomon, H. S., Connolly, T. M., and Tosteson, D. C.: Increased sodium-lithium countertransport in red cells of patients with essential hypertension. N Engl J Med 302:772, 1980.

Engelman, K., Portnoy, B., and Sjoerdsma, S.: Plasma catecholamine concentrations in patients with hypertension. Circ Res 27:I-14, 170, 1970.

Guyton, A. C., Coleman, T. G., Cowley, A. W., Jr., Manning, R. D., Jr., Norman, R. A., Jr., and Ferguson, J. D.: A systems analysis approach to understanding long-range arterial blood pressure control and hypertension. Circ Res 35:159, 1974.

Julius, S., and Esler, M.: Autonomic nervous cardiovascular regulation in borderline hypertension. Am J Cardiol 36:685, 1975.

Kaplan, N. M.: Clinical Hypertension. New York, Medcom Press, 1973.

Kater, C. E., and Biglieri, E. G.: Adrenocortical disease and hypertension. In Sleight, P., and Freis, E. (eds.): Hypertension. London, Butterworth Scientific, 1982, p. 135.

Korner, P. I.: Circulatory regulation in hypertension. Br J Clin Pharmacol 13:95, 1982.

Korner, P. I., and Fletcher, P. J.: Role of the heart in causing and maintaining hypertension. Cardiovasc Med 2:139, 1977.

Liddle, G. W.: Is hypertension essential? In Transactions of the Association of American Physicians, 88th Session. Collingdale, Pa., William J. Dornan, Inc., 1975, p. 55.

Mark, A. L., Gordon, F. J., and Takeshita, A. T.: Sodium, vascular resistance and genetic hypertension. In Brenner, B. M., and Stein, J. H. (eds.): Hypertension. New York, Churchill Livingstone, 1981, p. 21.

Myer, P.: Pathogenesis of primary hypertension: The role of changes in Na^+ transport in cell membranes in the pathogenesis of primary hypertension. In Amergy, A., Fagard, R., Lijnen, P., and Staessen, J. (eds.): Hypertensive Cardiovascular Disease: Pathophysiology and Treatment. The Hague, Martinus Nijhoff. Publishers, 1982, p. 154.

Page, I. H., and McCubbin, J. W.: The physiology of arterial hypertension. In Hamilton, W. F., and Dow, P. (eds.): The Handbook of Physiology, Vol. III. Bethesda, Md., American Physiological Society, 1965, p. 2163.

Sjoerdsma, S., Engelman, K., Waldman, T. A., Cooperman, L. H., and Hammond, W. G.: Pheochromocytoma: Current concepts of diagnosis and treatment. Ann Intern Med 65:1302, 1966.

Stone, R. A., Gunnells, J. C., Robinson, R. R., Schanberg, S. M., and Kirshner, N.: Dopamine-B-hydroxylase in primary and secondary hypertension. Circ Res 34:I-47, 1974.

Atherosclerosis

Atherosclerosis is a disease of the arterial system characterized by focal thickening of the inner portion of the arterial wall. Foci are referred to as plaques and the term atherosclerosis describes the composition of an advanced plaque—athero referring to its lipid or fat content and sclerosis referring to fibrous proteins such as collagen and resulting scar formation.

Normal arteries are composed of three morphologi-

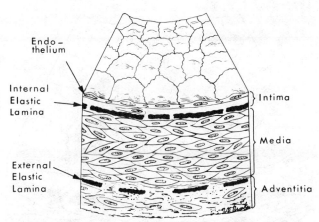

Figure 64. Structure of normal muscular artery. (With permission from Ross, R., and Glomset, J. A.: The pathogenesis of atherosclerosis. N Engl J Med 295:370, 1976.)

cally distinct layers: the intima, the media, and the adventitia (Fig. 64). The intima is composed of a single layer of endothelial cells that lines the lumen of the vessel. This endothelial cell lining rests on its basement membrane and in turn on a sheet of organized elastic fibers referred to as the internal elastic lamina. At birth, the intima is very thin with little or no material in the subendothelial space between endothelial cells and internal elastic lamina. With age the intima thickens concentrically owing principally to the deposition of collagen, elastic fibers, and other connective tissue matrix. The media of an artery is composed of densely packed and highly ordered smooth muscle cells surrounded by small amounts of loosely organized connective tissue elements. There are no fibroblasts in the mammalian media and, in contrast to the intima, the media undergoes very little change with age per se. At the outer zones of the media, elastic fibers take on a more organized sheet-like appearance, the external elastic lamina, which separates the media from the adventitia. Adventitia is a loosely arranged layer consisting of smooth muscle cells, fibroblasts, collagen, some elastic fibers, and mucopolysaccharides referred to as glycosaminoglycans.

Atherosclerosis primarily affects large and medium sized arteries—for example, the aorta, iliac and femoral arteries, coronary and renal arteries, carotids, and other major branches of the aorta. Smaller arteries, while susceptible to the uniform and concentric intimal thickening characteristic of hypertension, are relatively spared by the focal, characteristically eccentric atherosclerotic process.

The earliest evidence of atherosclerosis probably consists of small fatty streaks in which lipid is seen within the intima and inner media and within smooth muscle cells and also in association with extracellular fibrous proteins. These fatty streaks are found commonly within the first decade of life, do not obstruct blood flow, and usually advance little, if at all, for many years. Some investigators feel that fatty streaks are a manifestation of altered endothelial permeability but are not precursors of an atherosclerotic lesion. Others feel that, later in life, lesions that start as a fatty streak may advance to a complicated plaque consisting of a lipid-filled necrotic center, a fibrous cap,

and often calcification. This more advanced lesion by itself or by a superimposed thrombus may eventually occlude the lumen. The consequences of the atherosclerotic process are only in part accounted for by occlusion of involved arteries. Occlusion with subsequent ischemia of the distal vascular system is frequent in the coronary artery tree. At other sites the fibrous cap may be extruded, leaving an ulcerated base upon which platelet aggregates and thrombi form and then subsequently are dislodged to embolize the distal vascular bed. This event commonly occurs in atherosclerosis involving the carotid vessels. Finally, the atherosclerotic process may weaken the structural support of the involved artery and in association with hydraulic forces lead to subsequent aneurysm formation. The latter typically involves the aorta or its major branches.

A layer of endothelial cells normally separates the blood vessel from the circulating blood elements by forming a selectively permeable barrier between the blood and the intima of an artery. This barrier depends upon intact junctions between the endothelial cells and conveys upon the artery the property of being essentially impenetrable to most circulating proteins. The dynamics of the endothelial barrier have been studied extensively. On the basis of tracer studies it appears that those materials that gain access to the underlying intima do so by transport across the endothelial cell by pinocytotic vesicles that function as large pores (250 to 1000 Å in diameter). These data suggest that transport through the large pore system is the sole mechanism for normal passage of molecules with diameters greater than 100 Å, which includes most of the plasma lipoproteins. The concentration of plasma proteins within the arterial wall is about one tenth of that within the blood. Hence, the endothelial lining has come to be viewed as a barrier, protecting the constituents of the intima and media from exposure to high concentrations of circulating plasma components.

The integrity of the endothelial barrier can be disturbed by a number of influences. In the early stages of experimental hypertension tracer molecules enter the aortic intima at an accelerated rate. This increased flux includes molecules the size of plasma lipoproteins; studies indicate that the increased permeability of the endothelium is related to enhanced physiological transport through pores rather than to formation of gaps between the endothelial cells. Other influences that have been shown to increase the permeability of the intima include mechanical injury and distortion of the endothelial architecture from shear forces and turbulence, from vasoactive hormones such as catecholamines, from toxic injury by compounds such as carbon monoxide, and from viral or immunological injury. Any functional or structural insult that injures the endothelium and leads to enhanced permeability may be the event that initiates that atherosclerotic process.

For many years the arterial wall was regarded as a passive participant in the atherosclerotic process, reflecting simply the balance between influx and efflux of plasma constituents across the endothelial barrier. During the past decade one of the most important contributions to atherosclerotic research has been a recognition of the active role the vessel wall plays in the pathogenesis of the lesion. For example, the luminal surface of the endothelial monolayer has been shown to contain low density lipoprotein (LDL) receptors and to synthesize and secrete thromboresistant compounds, which include heparin-like proteoglycans, prostacyclin (PGI$_2$), and plasminogen activator.

According to the response to injury hypothesis, the three major steps in the formation of a plaque in the vessel wall include the following: (1) migration and proliferation of smooth muscle cells; (2) synthesis of new connective tissue elements; and (3) accumulation intracellularly and extracellularly of plasma lipoproteins and other materials.

Smooth muscle cell proliferation in regions of subsequent plaque formation is an early feature of experimental atherosclerosis. In vitro studies in which medial smooth muscle cells derived from the aorta have been grown in tissue culture show that once the cells enter a stationary phase, it is possible to stimulate logarithmic growth again by adding serum. However, serum from which all the low-density lipoprotein has been removed supports a lower rate of cell growth than whole serum. Thus, LDL has been shown to have a growth-promoting effect that is concentration-dependent within the concentration range typically observed in plasma. Platelets also contain a potent smooth muscle mitogenic factor (Fig. 65), that factor being released by platelets when they aggregate over a denuded portion of the vascular tree. According to current views, then, local injury to the endothelium increases the permeability of the endothelial surface and leads to an increase in the local concentration of plasma proteins in the vicinity of medial smooth mus-

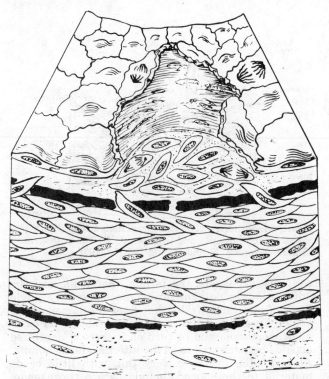

Figure 66. Smooth-muscle cells migrating from the media into the intima through fenestrae in the internal elastic lamina and actively multiplying within the intima. Endothelial cells regenerate in an attempt to recover the exposed intima, which thickens rapidly owing to smooth-muscle proliferation and formation of new connective tissue. (With permission from Ross, R., and Glomset, J. A.: The pathogenesis of atherosclerosis. N Engl J Med 295:421, 1976.)

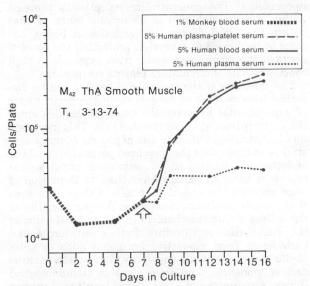

Figure 65. The accumulation of arterial smooth muscle cells in the presence of whole blood serum, platelet-poor plasma serum, or platelet-poor plasma serum plus platelet factor is plotted as a function of time. Initially, 3×10^4 cells were plated in 35-mm dishes in 1 per cent, whole blood serum medium and refed every 48 hours. At day seven, the appropriate test media were added and daily counts were made from triplicate dishes. Variation among dishes averaged less than 10 per cent. (Adapted from Rutherford, R. B., and Ross, R.: Platelet factors stimulate fibroblasts and smooth muscle cells quiescent in plasma serum to proliferate. J Cell Biol 69:199, 1976.)

cle cells. Injury also causes the adherence and aggregation of platelets, which form a carpet over the denuded portion of the vessel: platelet growth-promoting factor is released and permeates the underlying arterial wall. In response to these proteins, smooth muscle cells first migrate into the intima and then proliferate (Fig. 66). Low density lipoproteins may be a cofactor in plasma necessary for cell growth and proliferation but not themselves the mitogenic factor. Rather, platelet growth factor and perhaps mitogens derived from other components, including endothelial cells and macrophages, are responsible for initiating DNA synthesis. Once DNA synthesis is initiated, LDL and perhaps other plasma components, including hormones, are necessary for the smooth muscle cells to traverse the cell cycle.

If injury to the endothelium is transient and followed by subsequent restoration of endothelial integrity, the lesion is self-limited and may even regress. However, this usually self-limited process may progress further in either of two circumstances: first, if the original mechanism that led to endothelial injury persists; or, second, if coexistent hypercholesterolemia causes proliferating smooth muscle cells to become filled with lipid as well as allowing extracellular lipid accumulation. Both factors seem, by an unknown mechanism, to interfere with the subsidence of the lesion. Hypercholesterolemia may alter cell-to-cell relationships in the endothelium and can lead to desquamation of endothelial cells at selected sites in the arterial system. Thus, hypercholesterolemia is not only a source of increased LDL to cells, but also a cause of injury capable of initiating the sequence of events noted above.

The atherosclerotic plaque, particularly in its advanced stages, contains an appreciable amount of connective tissue. Collagen comprises 30 per cent or more of the weight of a plaque and 50 per cent or more of plaque protein. There is also evidence of enhanced synthesis of collagen, elastin, and glycosaminoglycans even in early atherosclerotic lesions. Medial smooth muscle cells are present within the atherosclerotic plaque, prompting the initial speculation that the smooth muscle cell might be responsible for the production of connective tissue components; that is, that it was a multifunctional mesenchymal cell capable of synthesis of fibrous proteins just like the fibroblast. These speculations were supported when tissue culture of vascular smooth muscle showed that these cells in fact incorporated lysine into soluble elastin, proline into procollagen, and sulfate into glycosaminoglycans.

The accumulation of these fibrous proteins within an atherosclerotic plaque is of interest in itself. It is of further interest because at least two of these elastin and one glycosaminoglycan, dermatan sulfate, have a particularly strong affinity for binding low density lipoprotein to form highly stable insoluble extracellular complexes. This is an important observation because evidence from several sources indicates that the low density lipoprotein, alone among the plasma lipoproteins, is selectively bound or trapped within the intima and media subsequent to interventions that enhance the influx of all lipoprotein classes into the arterial wall. With respect to collagen there is yet another observation of interest, but as yet of uncertain significance. There are four genetically distinct types of collagen found in human tissue. Type I collagen is the typical form found in bone and tendon, while Type III is the principal form found in skin and normal blood vessels. Interestingly, the collagen found in human atherosclerotic plaques is almost exclusively Type I with very little Type III present. This observation has suggested to some a fundamental alteration of the metabolism of the smooth muscle cell involving the rates of translation of genes coding alpha I (III), alpha I (I), and alpha II chains or alternatively that the cells of the plaque represent selective proliferation of a genetically distinct subpopulation of cells. Using cell markers for isoenzymes of glucose-6-phosphate dehydrogenase in female heterozygotes (that is, the cell population was a mosaic), it was shown that the cells of a single lesion were either positive or negative for the marker, suggesting monoclonal cell proliferation within an atherosclerotic plaque. It is not necessary, however, to invoke transformation to a neoplastic state; rather the monoclonal character of the lesions could be explained by a polyclonal mechanism in which

certain cells have a selective advantage at proliferation.

The third factor in plaque formation (in addition to cell proliferation and synthesis of fibrous proteins) is the mechanism of lipid accumulation and deposition. A prominent feature of atherosclerosis, even in the early stages of fatty streaks, is an excessive accumulation of cholesterol, mainly in the form of cholesterol esters, within the smooth muscle cells and macrophages. Normal lipid metabolism and the relation of abnormalities in lipid metabolism to atherogenesis are discussed in detail in Section VI.

From the above considerations we are now in better position to understand why most physicians regard atherosclerosis as a multifactorial disease. Serum lipid concentration, factors that influence the permeability of the endothelium, and determinants of the response of vascular smooth muscle to an increase in the concentration of lipoproteins and other growth-promoting factors each have a role. Hormonal and genetic factors have been identified that are capable of acting at one or more sites in this scheme. The process may have its onset early or late in life and may be stationary for long times or rapidly progressive. Finally, it may be focal or diffuse. The tragedy of atherosclerosis is the clinical silence of most of the factors that contribute to its development. Indeed, the consequences of atherosclerosis are themselves silent until arterial obstruction, embolism, or aneurysm precipitates symptoms, which usually indicate far advanced disease.

REFERENCES

Goldstein, J. L., and Brown, M. S.: Lipoprotein receptors, cholesterol metabolism and atherosclerosis. Arch Pathol 99:181, 1975.

Goldstein, J. L., Ho, Y. K., Basu, S. K., and Brown, M. S.: Binding site on macrophages that mediates uptake and degradation of acetylated LDL producing massive cholesterol deposition. Proc Natl Acad Sci USA 76(Part I):333, 1979.

McCullagh, K. A., and Bailian, G.: Collagen characterization and cell transformation in human atherosclerosis. Nature 258:73, 1975.

McCullagh, K. G., and Ehrhart, L. A.: Increased arterial collagen synthesis in experimental canine atherosclerosis. Atherosclerosis 19:13, 1974.

Ross, R.: Atherosclerosis: A problem of the biology of arterial wall cells and their interactions with blood components. Arteriosclerosis 1:293, 1981.

Rutherford, R. B., and Ross, R.: Platelet factors stimulate fibroblasts and smooth muscle cells quiescent in plasma serum to proliferate. J Cell Biol 69:196, 1976.

Shecter, I., Fogelman, A. M., Haberland, M. E., Seager, J., Hokom, M., and Edwards, P. A.: The metabolism of native and malondialdehyde-altered LDL by human monocyte-macrophages. J Lipid Res 22(Part I):63, 1981.

Wissler, R. W.: Development of the atherosclerotic plaque. Hosp Prac 8 (No. 3):61, 1973.

Wolinsky, H.: A new look at atherosclerosis. Cardiovasc Med 1:41, 1976.

Heart Muscle Disease: The Cardiomyopathies

Definitions

The term cardiomyopathy has become widely accepted as a designation for diseases of diverse and often unknown etiology that involve heart muscle. These disease processes may be acute, subacute, or chronic, and the disordered function of the heart muscle may be acute or chronic, stable or progressive, reversible or irreversible. Most investigators have restricted the term cardiomyopathy to diseases in which disordered function of heart muscle is the sole or principal cardiac manifestation of the disease. According to this view, alterations of heart muscle structure and function that result from coronary atherosclerosis, hypertensive vascular disease, and chronic valvular or congenital malformations fall outside the category "cardiomyopathy." In a sense, these arbitrary deletions seem unfortunate because ischemia is a legitimate and obvious member of the class of agents that can lead to myocardial dysfunction or death. Similarly, chronic hemodynamic overload (volume or pressure) may lead to dilatation, hypertrophy, and abnormal myocardial function that persists after correction of the cause; this would seem to qualify hydraulic stress as an equally legitimate mechanism leading to cardiomyopathy. In short, while there may be a pragmatic reason for a restrictive use of the term cardiomyopathy at this stage in our understanding of pathogenesis and pathophysiology, it would seem more appropriate to keep an open mind regarding the potential mechanisms of myocardial injury and the potential consequences of reaction to such injury.

Classification

Etiology. Whether a restricted definition is used or not, cardiomyopathies are a major problem throughout the world. In an effort to create some order out of the chaos and uncertainty that surrounds these conditions, cardiologists have devised a scheme for classifying the cardiomyopathies based upon etiology with two major categories, primary and secondary. Secondary cardiomyopathies are those in which the heart is involved either by an identifiable agent or disease or as a part of a systemic disease (acquired or inherited) in which there is at least a partial understanding of the pathogenesis. Primary cardiomyopathies are those in which the heart is involved without apparent disease elsewhere in the body and in which the pathogenesis of the cardiomyopathy is currently not understood. Primary cardiomyopathy is sometimes referred to as idiopathic myocardial hypertrophy (IMH) or hypertrophic cardiomyopathy.

Anatomical/Histological. Among the secondary cardiomyopathies, cardiac involvement sufficiently unique to be typical of the basic disease is observed in infiltrative diseases such as sarcoidosis or primary amyloid disease, in certain inborn errors of metabolism leading to accumulation of specific metabolic products such as Pompe's disease, in connective tissue diseases such as systemic lupus erythematosus and scleroderma, in inflammatory diseases such as coxsackie viral myocarditis, and the cardiomyopathy associated with *Trypanosoma cruzi* infection (Chagas' disease). Primary cardiomyopathies are divisible into three major groups: (1) those with striking and visible fibrosis or fibroelastosis of the endocardium, (2) those with very striking concentric or asymmetric hypertrophy, and (3) those characterized by flabby, massively dilated hearts, usually with an increase in mass but a relatively normal thickness of the right and left ventricular walls. With a few exceptions there is little of a specific or diagnostic nature observed in these hearts by either light- or electron-microscopic study.

Physiological. Finally, cardiomyopathies may be classified into three major groups based upon their clinical and physiological presentation. These include congestive cardiomyopathy, hypertrophic cardiomyopathy, and restrictive cardiomyopathy.

In this chapter we will discuss these three physiologically distinct states of heart muscle disease with an example of each. Myocardial injury or disease can occur from many other factors or conditions such as ischemia, chronic hydraulic stress, inflammatory myocarditis, infiltrative diseases, inborn errors of metabolism, nutritional deficiency or excess, and toxic substances. The physiological manifestations of these broadly ranging conditions, however, still fall within one of the three major physiological subgroups. Thus, a specific etiology for heart muscle disease is rarely evident from hemodynamic or angiographic study of the patient and depends in the last analysis either on evidence outside the heart indicative of a disease state known to affect the heart muscle or on morphological evidence obtained at autopsy. Even the latter evidence is frequently nonspecific, since the morphological manifestations of reaction to injury are fewer than the known agents that can provoke a reaction and hence lead to a cardiomyopathy.

CONGESTIVE CARDIOMYOPATHY

At a clinical level, congestive cardiomyopathies are characterized by marked cardiac dilatation, by early symptoms of heart failure, and by hemodynamic and angiographic evidence of a diffusely inadequate contractile state of the myocardium. The decrease in contractile performance always involves the left ventricle, but contractile dysfunction of the right ventricle and both atria is also evident when appropriate studies are performed. Cardiac output is generally reduced at rest and increases less than normal during exercise. Arteriovenous oxygen difference is widened at rest and widens even further with exertion. The poor contractile state of the ventricle is evident from a markedly reduced systolic ejection fraction noted on angiographic study (Fig. 67). Pressures in the heart generally par-

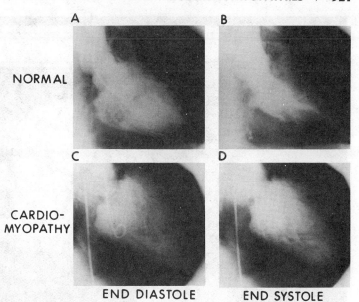

Figure 67. Panels *A* and *B* are end-diastolic and end-systolic left ventriculograms, respectively, taken from a patient with normal left ventricular function (ejection fraction 72 per cent). Panels *C* and *D* are end-diastolic and end-systolic left ventriculograms taken from a patient with a dilated congestive cardiomyopathy and extremely poor left ventricular function (ejection fraction 19 per cent). Note the larger size of the cardiomyopathic ventricle in addition to the diffuse hypocontractility. All angiograms were performed in the right anterior oblique projection.

allel the volume status of the patient and are elevated when heart failure leads to volume expansion. On the other hand, these pressures may be nearly normal or normal when blood volume is restored to normal by diuresis. In later stages of the disease mitral and/or tricuspid regurgitation secondary to ventricular dilatation may develop (see pp. 945–949). This hemodynamic picture is typically found in ischemic cardiomyopathy, in alcoholic cardiomyopathy, in Chagas' disease, in chronic viral myocarditis, in certain patients with systemic lupus erythematosus, and following toxic Adriamycin (doxorubicin) or radiation injury to the heart.

When all known causes of congestive cardiomyopathy have been excluded, a small number of patients remain who have primary myocardial disease of uncertain cause. The heart is large and flabby. Mural thrombi and a history of embolization are common. Although there is hypertrophy, dilatation is always the dominant picture. The histological features are nonspecific, with evidence of degeneration of myocytes, scattered fibrosis, patchy thickening of the endocardium, and myocardial edema. Similarly, the findings by electron microscopy are nonspecific; myocytes vary in size; intracellular vacuoles often contain increased lipid; mitochondria are enlarged with fragmented cristae; the sarcoplasmic reticulum is dilated; and at least in some cases there is found an accumulation of fibrous structures presumed to be mucopolysaccharide on the basis of staining characteristics.

The familial occurrence of cardiomyopathy in some human cases has stimulated great interest in an inbred strain (BIO 14.6) of the Syrian Golden Hamster, in which a cardiomyopathy is transmitted as an autosomal recessive trait. This strain of hamsters (in which there is also skeletal muscle involvement) shows a consistent course characterized by a prenecrotic stage in which cardiac function and structure appear normal, a stage of necrosis during the 10th to 30th day of life, and a terminal stage with fibrosis, hypertrophy, and progressive dilatation with death due to heart failure. At autopsy, mural thrombi are frequent. Although this genetic model of cardiomyopathy has been studied

extensively, the precise nature of the genetic fault and how it is translated into a myopathic picture remain to be clarified. It is mentioned as an example of an animal model of a hereditary cardiomyopathy that has many parallels to human disease, including the occurrence of cardiomyopathy in some patients with skeletal muscle disease.

HYPERTROPHIC CARDIOMYOPATHY

The anatomic and hemodynamic picture in patients with hypertrophic cardiomyopathy contrasts markedly with that of congestive myopathies. The anatomic hallmark of hypertrophic cardiomyopathy is a very marked increase in thickness of the ventricular walls either symmetrically or, when hypertrophy of the septum dominates, in an asymmetric distribution with a cavity volume that is usually normal although sometimes less than normal and only rarely increased (Fig. 68). Hemodynamically, systolic function is well maintained (and even increased). Systolic ventricular emptying is rapid, with 80 to 85 per cent of the stroke volume ejected in the first half of systole as compared to the 45 to 50 per cent ejection of the stroke volume occurring in the first half of systole in normals (Fig. 69). Ejection fractions greater than 75 per cent are usual, and cardiac output, at least at rest, is normal. Another typical systolic hemodynamic feature is obstruction to ventricular outflow at a site beneath the aortic valve. Such obstruction may occur at rest or only with provocative maneuvers (vide infra) and may be seen with concentric (or symmetric) hypertrophy but is more likely when there is dominant septal hypertrophy. On the left side of the heart, obstruction results from an abnormal systolic anterior motion of the anterior leaflet of the mitral valve, bringing the tip of this leaflet into apposition with the hypertrophied septum that bulges into the outflow tract of the left ventricle. Abnormal systolic anterior mitral movement (SAM) is a uniform finding by echocardiography and during left ventricular cineangiography in patients with hypertrophic obstructive cardiomyopathy. The

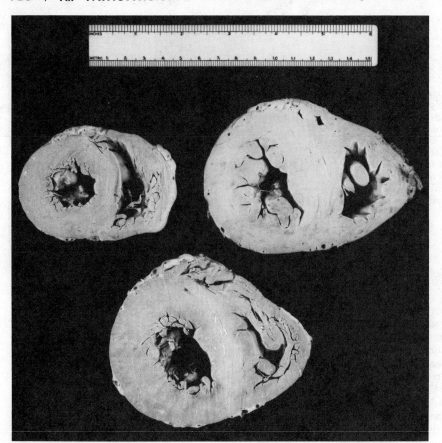

Figure 68. These cross-sectional slices of three different hearts were taken from just beneath the level of the mitral valve and are oriented so that the inferior surface of the slice is being viewed with the smaller right ventricle oriented to the right. The interventricular septum lies between the cavities of the two ventricles. The upper left specimen is a normal heart. Note its smaller overall size and the symmetrically normal septal and posterior wall thickness. The upper right specimen is from a patient with hypertrophic cardiomyopathy and demonstrates marked asymmetrical thickening of the interventricular septum (approximately 3.0 cm) in comparison to the posterior wall (approximately 1.5 cm). The bottom specimen is from a patient with severe calcific aortic stenosis and shows symmetric hypertrophy of both the septum and posterior left ventricular free wall (approximately 2.0 cm each). (These specimens were provided by Donald Hackel, M.D., Duke University Medical Center.)

mechanism for this SAM of the mitral valve is controversial. It may reflect abnormal traction on the leaflet because of the hypertrophied septum and small end-systolic volume. Alternatively, obstruction may not be an important primary event and the leaflet may be drawn into the left ventricular outflow tract by a Venturi effect, in turn created by the distortion in outflow tract hemodynamics due to septal hypertrophy. That both the hypertrophied septum and mitral leaflet participate in left ventricular outflow obstruction is evident from surgical results in which either a septal myotomy alone or mitral valve replacement alone relieves the obstruction. On the right side of the heart, obstruction may also be observed and results from systolic constriction of the outflow tract and the enlarged septum independent of either pulmonary or tricuspid function.

The dynamic nature of the obstructive phenomenon in hypertrophic cardiomyopathy is evident from provocative maneuvers that may dramatically alter the outflow tract gradient. In general, any influence that increases myocardial contractility (catecholamines or postextrasystolic potentiation), reduces end-diastolic volume, or reduces peripheral arterial resistance (amyl nitrite) will enhance obstruction. Conversely, negative inotropic influences (beta blockade), expansion of end-diastolic volume (transfusion, supine posture, or slow heart rate), and peripheral vasoconstriction (methoxamine) will diminish or abolish obstruction. While such obstruction is a dramatic part of the disease spectrum, recent studies have revived the concept that obstruction may have little or nothing to do with the pathogenesis of hypertrophic cardiomyopathy: ejection is

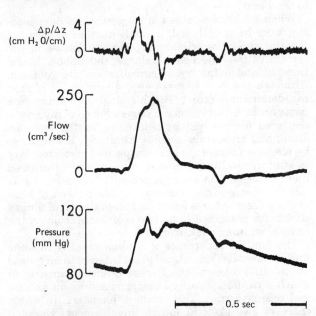

Figure 69. Pulsatile pressure and flow in a patient with hypertrophic subaortic stenosis. From the top down: the pressure difference ($\Delta p/\Delta z$), ascending aortic blood flow, and pressure. The ejection proceeds normally during the first half of systole, but during the latter half flow is markedly attenuated so that 80 to 85 per cent of the total volume occurs during the first half of systole as contrasted to approximately 50 to 55 per cent in normal patients. (With permission from Hernandez, R. R., Greenfield, J. C., Jr., and McCall, B. W.: Pressure-flow studies in hypertrophic subaortic stenosis. J Clin Invest 43:401, 1964.)

completed earlier than normal and independent of any measured gradients. These data would fit with the observed lack of any correlation between the gradient and symptomatology, progression and/or syncope/sudden death as well as the loss of gradients in some patients with disease progression.

The principal hemodynamic abnormality in hypertrophic cardiomyopathy occurs in diastole, wherein the hypertrophic process markedly reduces left ventricular compliance with resistance to diastolic filling and as a consequence ventricular end-diastolic pressures are increased, the "a" wave in the atrial and ventricular pressure tracings is exaggerated, and the rate of decline of atrial pressure after opening of the AV valves, the "Y" descent, is diminished. The hemodynamic abnormalities are most striking on the left side of the heart, but bilateral involvement is common.

These anatomic and hemodynamic abnormalities explain the clinical presentation of hypertrophic cardiomyopathy. The abnormal compliance and elevated left ventricular end-diastolic pressures with or without mitral regurgitation cause dyspnea due to pulmonary congestion. Chest pain, in the absence of coronary artery disease, is explained by subendocardial ischemia due to intramyocardial shunting of blood in combination with the massive hypertrophy; this situation is analogous to that observed in aortic stenosis (see p. 949). Syncope and sudden death are common but the responsible mechanism is controversial, with ventricular arrhythmias and acute reduction in cardiac output the leading suspects. On physical examination, the early and abrupt ejection of blood from the left ventricle causes the arterial pressure pulse to demonstrate a brisk upstroke, in marked contrast to the situation with fixed aortic outflow tract obstruction (e.g., valvular aortic stenosis). The onset of obstruction in later systole plus an exaggerated reflected wave from the periphery may lead to a second palpable wave producing a bifid systolic pulse (termed "spike and dome" to differentiate it from the bisferious pulse of aortic re-

gurgitation). The apex impulse is enlarged and sustained, and augmented left atrial systole (occurring in response to the decreased left ventricular compliance) produces a palpable presystolic A wave as well as an atrial gallop sound on auscultation. Additional auscultatory findings include a mid to late harsh, diamond-shaped systolic murmur reflecting outflow tract turbulence and obstruction. With obstructive cardiomyopathy, mid to late mitral regurgitation (occurring because of the altered mitral coaptation pattern due to SAM) may be noted as a murmur at the apex that is longer than the outflow murmur noted over the base of the heart. The presence or absence and loudness of these murmurs are altered by the same maneuvers that alter the degree of obstruction (p. 928) and in a parallel manner (greater obstruction causes louder and longer murmurs and vice versa).

A familial incidence of hypertrophic cardiomyopathy was noted in 25 to 37 per cent of the early reported series. In subsequent studies it has been reported that asymmetric septal hypertrophy (a common finding in hypertrophic cardiomyopathy with or without obstruction) is nearly always familial and transmitted by an autosomal dominant trait with a high degree of penetration. Morphologic studies have shown a characteristic microscopic picture of ventricular muscle removed from the septum in nearly all patients with asymmetric hypertrophy (Fig. 70). Myocytes show great variation in size with diameters ranging from 10 to 70 μ. The normal parallel arrangement of cells is markedly disordered, with cells arranged obliquely or perpendicular to one another. Each cell has multiple rather than two intercellular junctions corresponding to intercalated disks, and these junctions show an exaggerated convoluted pattern. Electron microscopy shows a variety of nonspecific findings including disarray of myofilaments within cells, widened and spreading Z bands, dilated T tubules, mitochondrial swelling, and an increased number of ribosomes. This histological picture was initially felt to be a unique characteristic of

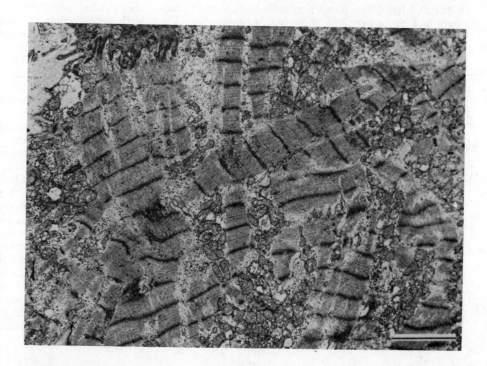

Figure 70. Electron micrograph of part of a cardiac muscle cell showing an area of myofibrillar disarray. (With permission from Maron, B. J., Ferrans, V. J., Henry, W. L., Clark, C. E., Redwood, D. R., Roberts, W. C., Morrow, A. G., and Epstein, S. E.: Differences in distribution of myocardial abnormalities in patients with obstructive and nonobstructive asymmetric septal hypertrophy (ASH): Light and electron microscopic findings. Circulation 50:443, 1974.)

asymmetric septal hypertrophy. This disarray is absent in approximately 5 per cent of patients with typical asymmetric septal hypertrophy, and it occurs in a wide variety of congenital and acquired heart disease (in the absence of cardiomyopathy) as well as in fetal hearts. Thus, the absence of myofiber disarray does not exclude hypertrophic cardiomyopathy, and its presence is not a pathognomonic finding. The extent of disarray, however, may be a more valid marker. Quantitative histological techniques in hypertrophic cardiomyopathy have documented that 25 per cent or more of the septal area shows disarray in approximately half such patients, whereas this degree of disarray rarely occurs in nonhypertrophic controls. The distribution of myofiber disarray is also distinctive and in patients with outflow obstruction, the bizarre histology is most extensive in the septum, and hypertrophy of the free right and left ventricular walls is similar to that developing in any other form of chronic ventricular systolic pressure overload. In patients with asymmetric septal hypertrophy without obstruction, this bizarre histological pattern is distributed widely throughout both the free walls of the ventricles and the septum. A case can be made for the fact that this is a single genetic fault in the control of cell growth, dominant in the septum in those with obstruction and involving the entire ventricular myocardium in those without obstruction. It is also possible that it is a secondary response to some other, as yet unidentified, nongenetic factor.

RESTRICTIVE CARDIOMYOPATHY

In rare instances, patients may present with a clinical picture that resembles constrictive pericarditis, yet with a normal pericardium. Pressure recordings from the ventricles show a moderate elevation of end-diastolic pressure (right, left, or both) with a characteristic early diastolic dip to or near zero followed by a plateau at the elevated end-diastolic pressure level. Right and left atrial mean pressures are elevated and there is a prominent "A" wave with exaggerated "X" and "Y" descents. Right atrial pressure may increase paradoxically during inspiration (Kussmaul's sign, see p. 980). Cardiac output is usually reduced and the peripheral AV oxygen difference is widened. Ventricular volume is normal or only minimally increased; ejection fraction is normal or only modestly reduced. All of these findings resemble those of constrictive pericarditis, yet there is no evidence of pericardial thickening. In constrictive pericarditis, however, the left ventricular end-diastolic pressure, mean left atrial pressure, pulmonary artery diastolic pressure, right ventricular end-diastolic pressure, and mean right atrial pressure are nearly equal (see p. 980). In restrictive disease, on the other hand, diastolic pressures are elevated to a greater extent on one side of the heart than on the other in most cases.

Restrictive cardiomyopathy is rare. In most parts of the world it is reported most often in association with infiltrative diseases: amyloidosis, lymphomas, leukemias, and Whipple's disease. Primary endocardial fibroelastosis, which presents in infants and causes death before 12 months of life, generally presents a restrictive pattern.

Endomyocardial fibrosis leads all causes of organic heart disease in Uganda other than hypertensive and rheumatic. If is frequently encountered in Tanzania, Kenya, Sudan, Nigeria, and those countries formerly known as French West Africa. It primarily affects children and young adults and presents with heart failure and a restrictive hemodynamic picture. Pathologically it is characterized by prominent fibrosis of the endocardium of the inflow tract and apical regions of either the right or left ventricle or both. The outflow tracts are generally spared. Small intramyocardial arteries are frequently occluded by endothelial proliferation. Mural thrombi are frequent. Changes in the ventricular myocardium are minimal, but the atria are dilated and hypertrophied and presumably because of reduced compliance of the ventricular chambers. The pathogenesis of endomyocardial fibrosis is unknown, although the pattern is compatible with the consequences of an organized mural thrombus. In this regard Connor has observed in early cases a marked increase of acid mucopolysaccharides in the endocardium and evidence of collagen necrosis. The geographic distribution of the disease and its occurrence in different ethnic groups are most compatible with an environmental influence.

OTHER CARDIOMYOPATHIES

A wide variety of additional stresses are capable of inducing depressed cardiac function that persists even after the stress is corrected or removed. Common examples are outlined in Table 1 along with some highlights of what is known and/or postulated concerning pathogenesis and the typical clinical manifestations. While these various entities will not all be discussed in detail individually, we will highlight the common as well as the unique pathophysiological characteristics among the various causes and use individual examples to illustrate basic principles.

Each condition varies in the extent to which myofiber (myocardial cell) involvement occurs in comparison with involvement of other heart tissues such as the valves (e.g., mucopolysaccharidoses), the coronary arteries (e.g., certain inborn errors of lipid metabolism), and the conduction system (e.g., Chagas' disease and diphtheritic myocarditis). The degree of myofiber involvement is also quite variable, both within the same etiology and among the different etiologies. Myocardial involvement may remain subclinical (e.g., a mild viral myocarditis) or be associated with fulminant, fatal congestive heart failure (e.g., doxorubicin toxicity). In general, for a given degree of involvement, all chambers are equally affected, but it is not unusual for the initial clinical presentation to be predominantly right-sided or left-sided. With the inborn errors of metabolism, the pathophysiology is usually apparent, with infiltration of a defined biochemical substance causing malfunction of one or more areas of the heart. For example, mucopolysaccharides may infiltrate the coronary arteries and cause ischemic heart disease, the valves and cause regurgitation, or the myocardium and cause significant depression in cardiac function through loss of contractile elements. In many of the other cardiomyopathies, although the etiological stress is obvious (e.g., alcoholic cardiomyopathy), the precise biochemical pathway leading to altered cardiac function is more controversial. With Chagas' disease and viral myocarditis, there may be altered antigenicity (either through exposure to viral envelope proteins, through unmasking of previously "occult" myocardial proteins, or through altered or new proteins resulting from the viral infection) that stimulates cytotoxic T lymphocytes to interact with cell receptors, resulting in cellular swelling, lysis, and death. It is of some interest in this regard that anti–T lymphocyte serum has no effect on the early infection and replication of the virus within myocardial cells but greatly reduces subsequent cell lysis and inflammation. In Chagas' disease, the T lymphocyte becomes cytotoxic because of its effect either directly on the parasite or on the parasitized host cell. The cardiomyopathy of chronic alcohol ingestion has been intensively studied and, although acetaldehyde appears to be the biochemical culprit, the explanation for the variable effects of alcohol in one patient compared to another despite comparable levels of intake remains unexplained. It has been unequivocally shown that it is not due to a concomitant nutritional factor. At a biochemical level, acetaldehyde is apparently toxic to mitochondria and diminishes their ability to oxidize fatty acids and acetaldehyde. Thus, while alcoholic cardiomyopathy is a distinct entity probably related to the metabolic and morphological consequences of chronically elevated acetaldehyde levels, the exact mechanism of toxicity and the variability from one patient to the next remain unexplained.

Pathologically, a feature common to most of these cardiomyopathies is the nonspecific loss of myofibers and their replacement by fibrous scar tissue. With the exception of the inborn errors of metabolism where infiltration by a biochemically unique substance is identifiable, there are usually no diagnostic gross, microscopic, or ultrastructural findings. Grossly, the heart is usually markedly enlarged and pale with hypertrophy and dilatation of all four chambers. Mural thrombi are common. The coronary arteries are normal unless the cardiomyopathy is ischemic. The valves are normal unless the cardiomyopathy is due to end-stage valvular heart disease or involved as part of the primary disease. Microscopically, there is myofiber hypertrophy and variable fibrosis and replacement of myofibers by connective tissue. The cells may be swollen, on electromicroscopy mitochondria show loss of cristae and swollen sarcoplasmic reticulum, and there may be selective loss of myosin filaments. Not uncommonly, particularly with hypertrophy due to valvular heart disease, the Z band substance is streaked and variable thickening of the basement membranes is present (Fig. 71).

The clinical picture is usually that of congestive heart failure that, in its initial presentation, may be primarily right-sided with edema or left-sided with dyspnea but within a year is typically biventricular and is accompanied by symptoms of a low cardiac output including fatigue, a rising blood urea nitrogen, and a fall in urinary output. In some of the inborn errors of metabolism, the patient's general appearance

Figure 71. *A*, Electron micrograph with high magnification showing part of a degenerated cardiac muscle cell. Z band material (Z) shows marked streaking and clumping. Thick myofilaments (arrowheads) are greatly reduced in number. Large numbers of thin myofilaments are present throughout. (×42,000) *B*, Marked proliferation of Z band material occupying the area of one entire sarcomere. Adjacent sarcomeres show lysis of some thick myofilaments (arrowheads). Other Z bands (Z) show less severe thickening. (×20,900) *C*, An elongated accumulation of Z band material adjacent to the sarcolemma. Thick myofilaments have undergone lysis in some areas (arrowheads). (×30,000) (With permission from Maron, B. J., Ferrans, V. J., and Roberts, W. C.: Myocardial ultrastructure in patients with chronic aortic valve disease. Am J Cardiol 35:731, 1975.)

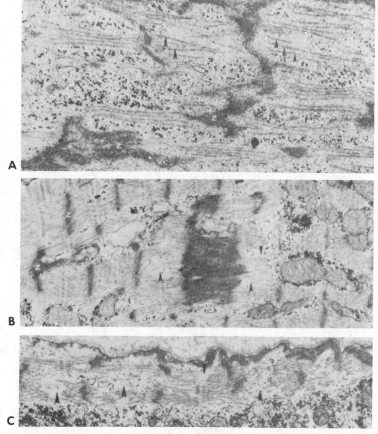

TABLE 1. OTHER CARDIOMYOPATHIES

ETIOLOGY	SPECIFIC EXAMPLES	PATHOGENESIS	PHYSIOLOGICAL MANIFESTATIONS
Pressure and/or Volume Overload Lesions	Systemic hypertension, tetralogy of Fallot, atrial septal defect, ventricular septal defect, patent ductus arteriosus, semilunar valve stenosis or regurgitation, atrioventricular valve regurgitation	When longstanding, the "third stage" of hypertrophy is reached in which the reparative processes become exhausted, leading to a loss of myofibers with cell death and fibrosis	Congestive failure of the chamber subjected to the abnormal load with variable dyspnea, edema, and chamber dilatation
Infectious			
RNA Virus	Coxsackie virus A and B, echovirus	Hematogenous spread to heart with penetration of and replication within myocytes, leading eventually to new antigenic components (viral envelope proteins, "unmasking" of myocardial cell proteins, or newly produced viral proteins) which cause the production of cytotoxic effector T lymphocytes, leading to cell lysis through cell-mediated immunity	Acutely, myocarditis may vary from subclinical to frank biventricular congestive heart failure. Chronically, it may progress to frank biventricular congestive heart failure. (See section on congestive cardiomyopathies.)
Protozoan	Trypanosomiasis (Chagas' disease)	Insect vector leads to hematogenous spread to the heart, with intracellular replication of *Trypanosoma cruzi* leading to acute myocarditis. Chronically, cell-mediated autoimmune destruction of parasitized myocytes by cytotoxic T lymphocytes	Acutely, varies from subclinical myocarditis to severe myocarditis with heart failure. Chronically, arrhythmias, conduction disturbances, and/or congestive heart failure
Inborn Errors of Metabolism			
Glycogenoses	Pompe's disease (Type II glycogenosis)	Absence of lysosomal 1,4-glucosidase with accumulation of glycogen in the heart	Marked cardiomegaly and congestive heart failure
	Cori's disease (Type III glycogenosis)	Absence of amylo 1,6-glucosidase with glycogen accumulation in the heart	Moderate cardiomegaly; heart failure uncommon in infancy
	Andersen's disease (Type IV glycogenosis)	Minor cardiac accumulation of abnormal glycogen due to deficiency of branching enzyme	Heart commonly involved; most deaths are due to cirrhosis
	McArdle's disease (Type V glycogenosis)	Deficiency of muscle phosphorylase with glycogen accumulation	Heart disease reported but usually subclinical
	Hers' disease (Type VI glycogenosis)	Deficiency of liver phosphorylase (heart usually spared)	
Mucopoly-saccharidoses	Hurler's syndrome	Accumulation of mucopolysaccharides in the valves, muscles, and occasionally the coronary arteries due to deficiency of lysosomal alpha-L-iduronidase	Marked cardiac enlargement with mitral and aortic regurgitation producing congestive heart failure and death before the age of 10

TABLE 1. OTHER CARDIOMYOPATHIES (*Continued*)

ETIOLOGY	SPECIFIC EXAMPLES	PATHOGENESIS	PHYSIOLOGICAL MANIFESTATIONS
	Hunter's syndrome	Accumulation of mucopolysaccharides due to deficiency of sulfoiduronate sulfatase	Similar to Hurler's syndrome but less severe
Nutritional	Beriberi heart disease	Dietary deficiency in thiamine (vitamin B_1) causes a deficiency of thiamine pyrophosphate, a cofactor in the decarboxylation of pyruvate to acetyl CoA and of alpha-ketoglutarate to succinyl CoA, all possibly affecting the heart by vasodilatation with a chronic high output state	Heart failure with dyspnea, elevated venous pressure but with warm skin and bounding pulses. Cardiac output typically elevated and contractile performance normal or only mildly impaired; degree of hypertrophy comparable to that with other high output states (e.g., AV fistula)
Toxic	Alcoholic cardiomyopathy	Alcohol dehydrogenase in the liver catalyzes the oxidation of alcohol to acetaldehyde, which the heart can oxidize to acetate. Continued elevated acetaldehyde levels, however, are toxic to mitochondria (mechanism unknown), diminishing their ability to oxidize fatty acids and acetaldehyde and to synthesize protein	Biventricular congestive heart failure with edema, dyspnea, cardiac enlargement, and arrhythmias (see congestive cardiomyopathies)
	Diphtheritic myocarditis	Beta phage lysogenization of *Corynebacterium diphtheriae* causes production of an exotoxin (Mol. wt. 7200 daltons) which: 1. Impairs oxidative phosphorylation by action on cytochrome b 2. Inhibits protein synthesis by inactivation of transferase II (an enzyme responsible for the transfer of amino acids to growing polypeptide chains on ribosomes)	Slowing of pacemaker activity, atrioventricular and intraventricular block, and acute heart failure that carries a high mortality rate
	Doxorubicin (Adriamycin) therapy for neoplastic diseases	The drug affixes itself between adjacent base pairs in the DNA helix and, by preventing normal coiling/folding of the DNA strands, sterically inhibits DNA-dependent RNA polymerase activity	Biventricular congestive heart failure with cardiac dilatation, edema, and low cardiac output. This is particularly likely to occur at doses above 600 mg/M^2; the cardiac toxicity is cumulative, suggesting an irreversible drug-binding step

is virtually diagnostic of the underlying disease process (e.g., Hurler's syndrome or gargoylism). While both Chagas' disease and diptheritic involvement of the heart may be associated with a severe congestive cardiomyopathy, on occasion cardiac function is well preserved and the predominant clinical presentation is that of an intraventricular conduction disturbance with bundle branch block and advanced atrioventricular block. On other occasions, the degree of myocardial functional depression is mild or subclinical and the patient's presentation is that of a significant ventricular arrhythmia with palpitations and neurological symptoms. In the cardiomyopathy of beriberi heart disease wherein the clinical features of congestive heart failure are present (edema, dyspnea, gallop rhythm, and elevated venous pressure), the thiamine deficiency causes vasodilation and the patient's extremities and skin are warm and the arterial pulses are bounding. The cardiac output may actually measure several times above normal and there is some controversy as to whether there is any alteration in myocardial function in this entity—or whether it may be the response of the heart to longstanding vasodilation and an increased cardiac output.

REFERENCES

Bajusz, E., Rona, G., Brink, A. J., and Lockner, A. (eds.): Recent advances in studies on cardiac structure and metabolism. Vol. II, Cardiomyopathies. Baltimore, University Park Press, 1971.

Blieden, L. C., and Moller, J. H.: Cardiac involvement in inherited disorders of metabolism. Prog Cardiovasc Dis 16:615, 1974.

Jones, M., and Ferrans, V. J.: Myocardial degeneration in congenital heart disease. Comparison of morphologic findings in young and old patients with congenital heart disease associated with muscular obstruction to right ventricular outflow. Am J Cardiol 39:1051, 1977.

Maron, B. J., and Epstein, S. E.: Hypertrophic cardiomyopathy. Recent observations regarding the specificity of three hallmarks of the disease: Asymmetric septal hypertrophy, septal disorganization and systolic anterior motion of the anterior mitral leaflet. Am J Cardiol 45:141, 1980.

Maron, B. J., Ferrans, V. J., Henry, W. L., Clark, C. E., Redwood, D. R., Roberts, W. C., Morrow, A. G., and Epstein, S. E.: Differences in distribution of myocardial abnormalities in patients with obstructive and nonobstructive asymmetric septal hypertrophy (ASH): Light and electron microscopic findings. Circulation 50:436, 1974.

Murgo, J. P., Alter, B. R., Dorethy, J. F., Altobelli, S. A., and McGranahan, G. M., Jr.: Dynamics of left ventricular ejection in obstructive and nonobstructive hypertrophic cardiomyopathy. J Clin Invest 66:1369, 1980.

Pathophysiology of Shunts

The physiological consequences of intracardiac and extracardiac shunts have traditionally been interpreted in the context of the postnatal circulatory changes that result from these communications. It is now recognized, however, that not only do faults in normal embryological development lead to physiological changes, but also that abnormal physiology in fetal and postnatal life produces alterations in structure. To perceive adequately this interplay between structure and function in the developing heart, it is important to understand the normal fetal circulation and the important alterations that occur at birth.

THE FETAL CIRCULATION

The pattern of blood flow in the fetus is illustrated in Figure 72. In contrast to the adult, in which the great vessels and cardiac chambers are arranged in series, in the fetus the pulmonary and systemic circulations are arranged in parallel. This parallelism is a consequence of large open communications between the left and right heart at the atrial level and between the aorta and pulmonary artery at the level of the ductus arteriosus. Although the right and left ventricles are separated by an intact septum, they receive blood from a functionally common atrial reservoir and they eject blood into a common receiving chamber (the joined aorta and pulmonary artery). Because of this arrangement, cardiac output in the fetus is best viewed as the combined output of the right and left ventricles.

Oxygenated blood from the placenta enters the fetal body through the umbilical veins that drain into the portal venous system. Most of this blood traverses the hepatic microcirculation and courses through the hepatic veins into the inferior vena cava. The remainder of placental venous return bypasses the liver by way of the ductus venosus and empties directly into the inferior vena cava.

Upon entering the right atrium, about half of the inferior vena cava blood streams across the valve of the foramen ovale into the left atrium. This streaming is facilitated by close proximity of the foramen ovale to the entrance of the inferior vena cava as well as partitioning of the vena cava by the crista dividens, which directs the flow to the left and posteriorly, across the foramen ovale. We will comment subsequently about the factors responsible for the distribution of blood pumped by the right ventricle. Only 10 to 15 per cent of the right ventricular output is pumped through the lungs and returns to the left atrium through pulmonary veins. As a consequence, most of the left atrial blood is derived from the placenta. It contains a relatively high oxygen saturation and after flowing into the left ventricle is pumped into the aorta and preferentially to the head and coronary arteries.

The portion of inferior vena caval blood that is not directed across the foramen ovale and nearly all of the superior vena caval blood and coronary sinus return, which are relatively oxygen desaturated, pass into the right ventricle. Morphologically and physiologically, the right ventricle is the dominant pumping chamber of the fetal heart. About 65 per cent of the combined output of the fetal heart is handled by the right ventricle. Virtually all (80 to 90 per cent) of this right ventricular output reaches the descending aorta by way of the ductus arteriosus; the remainder traverses the lung. This arrangement ensures that a large proportion of the desaturated blood returning to the heart from fetal organs with a high oxygen uptake (brain

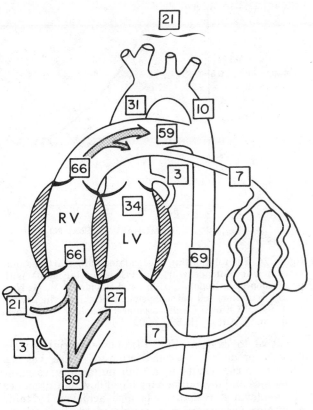

Figure 72. The percentages of the combined left and right ventricular outputs (C. V. O.) that flow through the major vessels and shunts in the fetal heart are shown in the squares. RV = Right ventricle; LV = left ventricle. (With permission from Rudolph, A. M., and Heymann, M. A.: Neonatal circulation and pathophysiology of shunts. In Levine, H. J. (ed.): Clinical Cardiovascular Physiology. New York, Grune and Stratton, 1976, p. 598.)

and heart) will be directed toward the placenta for reoxygenation.

The selective channeling of blood through the ductus is governed by the extremely high pulmonary vascular resistance in the fetus. Since the ductus is approximately the same caliber as the descending aorta, there is equalization of pressures in the pulmonary trunk, aorta, and ventricles. Consequently, the distribution of blood flow from the right ventricle becomes dependent upon the relative vascular resistance offered by the lungs and the systemic bed. Since vascular resistance is extremely high in the pulmonary circuit, while that imposed by the placenta is relatively low, flow is preferentially directed through the ductus from the pulmonary artery to the descending aorta. The modulating influence of resistance upon blood flow is reflected by the fact that 40 per cent of the cardiac output is supplied to the placenta.

POSTNATAL CIRCULATORY CHANGES

The initial alterations that occur at birth are (1) an obliteration of the low resistance placental circulation and (2) ventilation of the lungs with air. When the umbilical vessels are clamped and cut there is an abrupt and substantial increase in systemic vascular resistance, principally in the resistance offered by the lower half of the body. Also, with the first breath by the newborn infant there is a very marked decrease in the resistance to flow offered by the lungs. As a consequence of these marked and discordant changes in systemic and pulmonary vascular resistance, there is a striking reorientation of distribution of the combined ventricular output. When the placental vessels are clamped, the increase in systemic vascular resistance increases left ventricular work and hence left atrial pressure. Concomitantly, venous return to the right atrium, and hence right atrial pressure, drops. The pressure gradient between the left and right atria closes the valve covering the foramen ovale and eliminates the streaming of right atrial blood into the left atrium. When ventilation by the newborn begins, there is a prompt rise in pulmonary venous blood flow, pulmonary venous pO_2, and arterial pO_2. These changes cause powerful constriction of the ductus arteriosus and markedly reduce the shunt of pulmonary arterial flow into the descending aorta. The diminution of this shunt is also aided by the drop in pulmonary vascular resistance. The consequences of these changes are to obliterate the structural communications between the right and left heart and between the pulmonary artery and aorta, to reverse the relation between pulmonary and systemic vascular resistance that obtained in utero, and to convert the circulation into one in which the pulmonary and systemic vascular beds are in series rather than in parallel. Let us now consider the events in this transformation in greater detail and certain consequences of failure of these normal mechanisms.

FORAMEN OVALE CLOSURE

In the fetus, streaming of inferior vena caval blood directly into the left atrium maintains patency of the foramen ovale. At birth there is a rapid decrease in venous return due to loss of the placental circulation. Consequently, right atrial pressure falls. Simultaneous ventilation of the lungs produces a diminution in pulmonary vascular resistance. Pulmonary blood flow increases as does venous return to the left atrium and left atrial pressure. Ultimately, left atrial pressure exceeds that in the right atrium and functional closure of the valve of the foramen ovale against the septum secundum occurs. Valve closure occasionally may be delayed for several months, in which case a small left-to-right shunt will be present. Twenty per cent of adults have a probe-patent foramen without evidence of shunting. Shunting through a patent foramen is sometimes the only means of infant survival as evidenced by right-to-left shunting in tricuspid or pulmonic atresia with an intact ventricular septum. A similar beneficial effect occurs in transposition of the great vessels with an intact ventricular septum in which bidirectional shunting through an interatrial communication helps support oxygenation of peripheral tissues.

DUCTUS ARTERIOSUS CLOSURE

The ductus arteriosus contains a large amount of smooth muscle in its media. Patency in the fetus is both chemically and mechanically mediated. Prostaglandins E_1 and E_2, which are released in the wall of the ductus, have a smooth muscle vasodilator effect that can be inhibited by indomethacin. The same vasodilatory influence has been shown with lowered oxygen tensions and with acetylcholine. Patency of the ductus is further promoted by the large volume and pressure of right ventricular output, which is directed through this channel into the aorta. After birth, the ductus constricts rapidly initially at its pulmonary end. The ductus is functionally closed by 10 to 15 hours. During this period there is bidirectional flow, but as pulmonary resistance falls and systemic resistance rises, a transient left-to-right shunt is created. Permanent anatomic closure is effected in one to three weeks by a process of intimal proliferation, thrombosis, and fibrosis.

The probable mechanism behind closure of the ductus at birth is exposure to increased oxygen tension (Fig. 73). Oxygen has been observed to produce constriction of smooth muscle in the ductus wall either by a direct effect or by means of a chemical mediator. In fetal lamb studies the more premature the animal, the less well developed is this constrictor mechanism. Furthermore, ductal constriction can be reversed and patency reestablished as late as three days after birth by continuous exposure to low oxygen gas mixtures. These findings may well explain the high incidence of persistent ductus in premature infants, especially those born at high altitude. It may also explain the frequent persistence of congenital cardiac malformation associated with severe hypoxemia. Inhibition of prostaglandin synthesis with aspirin or indomethacin constricts the ductus and can be used to promote closure in premature infants.

CHANGES IN PULMONARY CIRCULATION

The medial smooth muscle of precapillary pulmonary arterioles in the fetus is quite thick and extremely

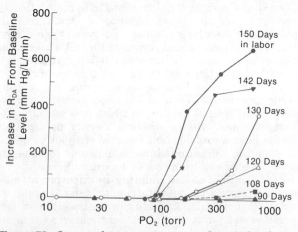

Figure 73. Oxygen dose-response curves from isolated, perfused fetal lamb ductus arteriosus of increasing gestational ages. Constriction of ductus arteriosus is shown as an increase in resistance (RDA) across ductus arteriosus. (With permission from McMurphy, D. M., Heymann, M. A., Rudolph, A. M., and Melmon, K. L.: Developmental changes in constriction of the ductus arteriosus: Responses to oxygen and vasoactive agents in the isolated ductus arteriosus of the fetal lamb. Pediatric Res 6:235, 1972.)

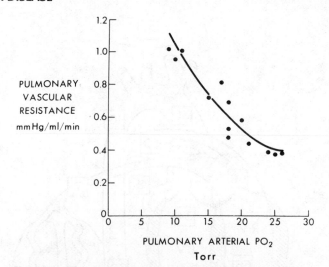

Figure 74. The relationship of calculated pulmonary vascular resistance to pulmonary arterial PO_2 in a fetal lamb. (With permission from Rudolph, A. M., and Heymann, M. A.: Neonatal circulation and pathophysiology of shunts. In Levine, H. J. (eds.): Clinical Cardiovascular Physiology. New York, Grune and Stratton, 1976, p. 600.)

sensitive to oxygen (Fig. 74). Low arterial oxygen tension produces vasoconstriction of these vessels. This, in turn, results in a high pulmonary vascular resistance and low pulmonary blood flow. Maintenance of an elevated resistance is also achieved by tonic arteriolar vasoconstriction regulated by sympathetic nerves as well as by tortuosity and kinking of these vessels in the collapsed lung. Coincident with ventilation of the lungs at birth, pulmonary resistance falls dramatically. Pulmonary blood flow increases tenfold in the first ten minutes after birth. This rise in flow is partly attributed to mechanical expansion of the lungs with gas, which may distend small vessels in the interalveolar spaces. The most significant factor leading to a decline in pulmonary vascular resistance is increased oxygen tension. The elevation of pO_2 is thought to produce a direct local vasodilatory response in pulmonary arteriolar smooth muscle. In addition, the increase in oxygen tension activates a chemoreflex involving bradykinin, which fosters vasodilatation. Hence, the abrupt decline in pulmonary vascular resistance that is most striking in the two to three days after birth is related to release from pulmonary arteriolar constriction and possibly to active vasodilatation. The subsequent fall in pulmonary vascular resistance and drop in pulmonary arterial pressure to adult levels is paralleled by a thinning of the medial smooth muscle and an increase in lumen size. By six to eight weeks of life the pulmonary circuit is transformed from a high pressure, high resistance, low flow system with a small cross-sectional area to a low pressure, low resistance, high flow bed with a large cross-sectional area (Fig. 75).

The involution of pulmonary arterioles and the resulting decrease in pulmonary vascular resistance after birth can be retarded by several factors. One of these is arterial hypoxia. High altitude, intrinsic lung disease, and congenital cardiac malformations associated with cyanosis may either delay or prevent the normal thinning of the medial smooth muscle layer of pulmonary arterioles. Failure of pulmonary vascular resistance to regress after birth is also seen in situa-

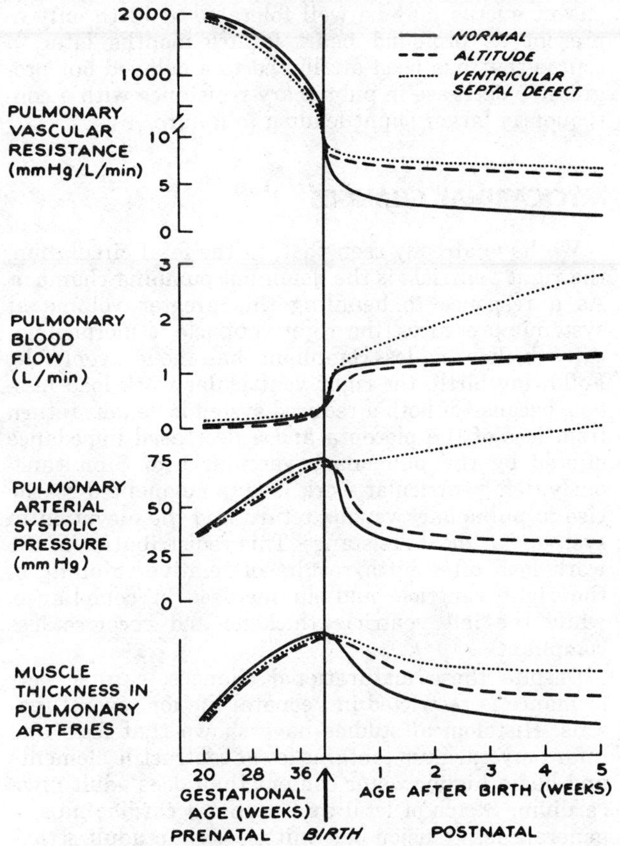

Figure 75. Schematic representation of fetal and postnatal changes in pulmonary vascular resistance, pulmonary blood flow, pulmonary arterial systolic pressure, and thickness of smooth muscle in medial layer of pulmonary arterioles. Postnatally, the pulmonary vascular resistance falls more slowly in infants born at high altitude or with a ventricular septal defect of large size. Pulmonary blood flow increases rapidly at birth in the normal infant and probably at the same rate at high altitude. In the presence of a ventricular septal defect, pulmonary blood flow increases as pulmonary vascular resistance falls. Pulmonary arterial pressure normally falls rapidly after birth; the fall is delayed at high altitude and pressure remains slightly elevated. Pulmonary arterial pressure does not fall when a large ventricular septal defect is present, and it increases as systemic arterial pressure rises. The muscle in the pulmonary arterioles does not regress as rapidly as normal in infants at high altitudes. In infants with ventricular septal defect, the muscle does not regress normally and soon after birth increases in amount. (With permission from Rudolph, A. M.: The changes in the circulation after birth: Their importance in congenital heart disease. Circulation 41:345, 1970.)

tions in which abnormally high pulmonary artery flow rates or pulmonary venous obstruction maintain a hydraulic stress on the arterioles. One such circumstance often accompanied by a persistently high pulmonary resistance is obstructive lesions on the left side of the heart, such as mitral atresia or hypoplastic left heart. Delayed regression of the pulmonary vascular resistance is observed in infants with large ventricular septal defects (Fig. 75). In such cases and in patients with widely patent ductus arteriosus, failure

of pulmonary vascular resistance to decrease after birth may actually be beneficial: the higher than normal pulmonary resistance reduces the magnitude of the left-to-right shunt and lessens the likelihood of heart failure in infancy. Vogel has reported that infants with ventricular septal defects born at high altitude have a lower pulmonary blood flow and a much lower incidence of congestive heart failure than infants with structurally similar defects who are born at sea level. Conversely, large ventricular defects and

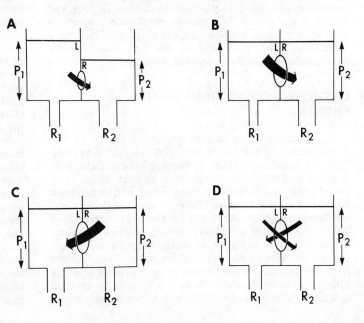

Figure 76. Diagrammatic representation of the factors controlling shunting between two chambers. (Arrows indicate direction of shunt.) P_1 = Pressure in left-sided chamber; L = left-sided chamber; R_1 = outflow resistance of left-sided chamber; P_2 = pressure in right-sided chamber; R = right-sided chamber; R_2 = outflow resistance at right-sided chamber. (With permission from Rudolph, A. M., and Heymann, M. A.: Neonatal circulation and pathophysiology of shunts. In Levine, H. J. (ed.): Clinical Cardiovascular Physiology. New York, Grune and Stratton, 1976, p. 603.)

patent ductus may be well tolerated at birth only to present as profound heart failure months later, a course that has been attributed to a delayed but progressive decrease in pulmonary resistance with a consequently larger shunt leading to failure.

MYOCARDIAL CHANGES

We have already seen that, in the fetal circulation, the right ventricle is the dominant pumping chamber. As a response to handling this greater volume at systemic pressures, the right ventricle is morphologically thicker and less compliant than the left ventricle. Following birth, the right ventricular work load lessens, because of both a reduced systemic venous return from loss of the placenta and a decreased impedance offered by the pulmonary vascular bed. Simultaneously, left ventricular work load is augmented by the rise in pulmonary venous return and the elevation in systemic arterial resistance. This redistribution of the work load after birth results in relative thinning of the right ventricle and an increase in compliance, while the left ventricle thickens and becomes less compliant.

Despite these maturational changes, cardiac performance is restricted in neonatal life for several reasons. Histological studies have shown that fetal and infant myocardium contains fewer contractile elements and has a higher water content than does adult myocardium. Strips of fetal and neonatal cardiac muscle generate less tension per unit mass than adult strips. It has further been noted that cardiac sympathetic innervation may be incompletely developed at birth, thereby limiting the inotropic response to conditions that result in increased sympathetic nerve activity. The inference from these observations, which have been confirmed experimentally, is that the ability of the fetal and neonatal myocardium to enhance stroke volume is impaired; changes of cardiac output are mediated almost solely by changes of heart rate. Circulatory shunts that impose a large volume overload on the myocardium at birth, especially on the left ventricle, are likely to precipitate cardiac failure and death of the infant. In contrast, conditions characterized by a volume overload on the right ventricle or a gradually developing load on the left ventricle are better tolerated and compatible with survival.

LEFT-TO-RIGHT AND RIGHT-TO-LEFT SHUNTS

As a consequence of embryological faults in the development of the heart and great vessels it is common for communications to persist between the pulmonary and systemic circulations and for blood to be shunted in one direction or the other and sometimes in both directions across these communications. Connections can occur either within the heart (atrial and ventricular septal defects) or outside the heart (anomalous return of systemic or pulmonary veins, patent ductus arteriosus, and so on). By convention, shunts from the arterial to the venous system are regarded as left-to-right, while those from the venous to arterial circuit are designated right-to-left. In the former group

oxygenated blood will bypass the peripheral arterial circulation and reenter the systemic venous system, while in the latter situation venous blood will pass into the systemic arterial tree without being oxygenated in the lungs.

There are three interrelated factors that determine the size and direction of circulatory shunts (Fig. 76): (1) the size of the communication between involved vessels or chambers; (2) the pressure difference between the involved vessels or chambers; (3) the outflow resistances from the chambers. In the face of a small communication between chambers, the pressure difference becomes the predominant force that regulates the magnitude and direction of the shunt (Fig. 76A). Outflow resistances do not primarily influence the shunt, but rather exert their effect by altering the pressure levels in the involved compartments. This situation is illustrated by a small ventricular septal defect. In contrast, with a large communication, equalization of pressure in the chambers on either side of the abnormal connection is the rule, and outflow resistances become the primary determinant of shunt direction and volume (Fig. 76B). This is the case with either a large persistent ductus arteriosus or a large ventricular septal defect. Shunts may be unidirectional if resistances and pressures differ (Fig. 76C), or bidirectional if these variables are essentially the same (Fig. 76D).

Circulatory shunts may also be influenced by the structural development of the ventricles. For example, the magnitude and direction of shunting with a large atrial septal defect are functions of the relative distensibility of the ventricles, since pressures in both atria are equivalent. If right ventricular compliance is higher than that of the left ventricle, as is normally the case, then a left-to-right shunt occurs. However, if right ventricular compliance becomes reduced as a consequence of hypertrophy and is less than that of the left ventricle, a right-to-left shunt may result.

With respect to left-to-right shunts, it is useful to classify the anatomic conditions into two broad physiological groups, regardless of the site of the communication (see Table 2). The first group is referred to as dependent shunts in which the shunt channel is sufficiently large for equalization of pressure across the channel. The dynamics of this type of shunt depend chiefly on the ratio between the pulmonary and systemic vascular resistances. Because the rate of change of pulmonary vascular resistance after birth is much greater than that of systemic resistance, pulmonary resistance becomes the critical variable affecting the pattern of blood flow and clinical course of infants with these lesions. Although alterations in ventricular compliance or concomitant valvular or subvalvular obstructive lesions play a role in controlling shunt flow, they are usually of secondary importance. The second class of left-to-right shunts is referred to as obligatory. The characteristic feature of these defects is that there is a connection between a high pressure and a low pressure chamber or vessel as exemplified by a systemic arteriovenous fistula. The pressure gradient and the size of the communication, rather than pulmonary resistance, are the principal determinants of shunt magnitude and direction. In contrast to dependent shunts in which pulmonary vascular resistance regulates pulmonary blood flow, obligatory shunts are marked by a high pulmonary blood flow that in turn

TABLE 2. CLASSIFICATION OF LEFT-TO-RIGHT SHUNTS

DEPENDENT
  Aorta to Pulmonary Artery
    Patent ductus arteriosus
    Truncus arteriosus communis
    Aortopulmonary fenestration
    Anomalous origin of coronary artery
    Hemitruncus arteriosus
    Pulmonary lobular sequestration
  Aorta to Right Ventricle
    Sinus of Valsalva fistula
    Coronary arteriovenous fistula
  Left Ventricle to Right Ventricle
    Ventricular septal defect
    Endocardial cushion defect
  Left Atrium or Pulmonary Veins to Right Atrium
    Atrial septal defects: incompetent foramen ovale, primum,
      secondum, and sinus venosus
    Partial anomalous pulmonary venous connection

OBLIGATORY
  Aorta to Right Atrium or Systemic Vein
    Systemic arteriovenous fistula
    Sinus of Valsalva fistula
    Coronary arteriovenous fistula
  Left Ventricle to Right Atrium
    Left ventricular—right atrial communication
    Endocardial cushion defect

modifies pulmonary resistance. In the case of an atrioventricular canal defect, obligatory and dependent shunting may coexist.

Even though patent ductus arteriosus is classified as a dependent shunt, the physiology of the condition is determined mostly by the size of the communication. Furthermore, depending upon the size of the communication, the pressure gradient, pulmonary vascular resistance, and ventricular compliance may each play an important role in the pathophysiology. An examination of these relationships in patent ductus arteriosus is useful, and similar considerations apply to other dependent shunts—for example, ventricular septal defects, where the size of the communication may also vary. In the case of a small ductus, the right-to-left shunt flow that was present in the fetus ceases in the immediate postnatal period. Shortly thereafter, when systemic resistance rises and pulmonary resistance falls toward normal levels, a continuous pressure gradient between the aorta and pulmonary artery develops. Nonetheless, flow through the ductus in this situation is generally low, pulmonary artery pressure remains normal, and the volume overload on the left ventricle is only modest. With communications of larger size, pulmonary blood flow and the venous return to the left heart rise. Expansion of left atrial and left ventricular volumes is seen, the work load on the left ventricle increases, and the large left ventricular stroke volume is maintained in part by the Starling mechanism and in part by hypertrophy. As long as these compensatory mechanisms are adequate, cardiac output is maintained, the resistance in the pulmonary bed is generally normal, and pulmonary artery pressure is normal or only moderately elevated in relation to the increased flow.

In the setting of a large ductus, mean aortic and pulmonary artery pressures equalize at the systemic level. This equalization of pressures results because a large ductus fails to offer significant resistance to flow between the aorta and pulmonary artery, and hence little or no pressure gradient exists. In this situation the direction and magnitude of the resulting shunt will depend on the ratio of pulmonary to systemic vascular resistance. If pulmonary resistance drops, then a very large left-to-right shunt will occur with marked elevations in pulmonary blood flow and pulmonary venous return. Overloading of the left atrium and left ventricle takes place, and because the neonatal myocardium is unable to handle this large volume stress, cardiac failure follows, usually within the first month of life. On the other hand, if pulmonary resistance remains high, pulmonary blood flow and venous return are less, the left heart is protected from a large volume overload, and cardiac failure is less likely.

The circumstance of a large ductus with relatively high pulmonary vascular resistance and equalization of mean aortic and pulmonary artery pressures produces a situation of bidirectional shunting. During ventricular systole pulmonary artery pressure may rise more rapidly than aortic pressure, a pulmonary-to-aortic pressure gradient is produced, and shunting is transiently right-to-left. Late in systole and throughout diastole pulmonary artery pressure drops more rapidly than aortic pressure, the pressure gradient reverses, and the shunt is left-to-right. In this situation the net shunt is usually left-to-right and it is of interest that most of the diastolic left-to-right flow across the ductus is derived from the descending aorta.

When pulmonary artery pressure remains at systemic levels for months or years due to a large nonobstructing ductus, changes in the pulmonary vessels may ensue that increase pulmonary vascular resistance. These changes include medial hypertrophy and intimal proliferation. A level of pulmonary vascular resistance is finally attained at which left-to-right shunting is abolished and is replaced by right-to-left flow. Right ventricular pressure overload, right ventricular hypertrophy, and cyanosis then occur.

We have seen that a small patent ductus arteriosus functions as an obligatory shunt, while a large ductus functions as a dependent shunt. We have also seen in the case of a large ductus with an initially dependent left-to-right shunt, that over years as a consequence of elevated pulmonary artery pressure, pulmonary vascular changes may ensue that cause the shunt to reverse and become right-to-left. In the older terminology, this chain of events was referred to as the Eisenmenger reaction. The most important general point, however, is that for dependent left-to-right shunts, regardless of the site of the communication, pulmonary vascular resistance and its changes over time are the most critical factors in determining the clinical course of the patient.

In obligatory shunts it is the level of pulmonary blood flow rather than resistance that is the major determinant of circulatory hemodynamics. The case of a large congenital systemic arteriovenous fistula will illustrate this concept. These fistulae are frequently located in the hepatic or cerebral circulations. An immediate consequence of shunting from a high pressure artery to a lower pressure vein is that arterial flow distal to the shunt site is decreased. Systemic resistance is low as a consequence of the fistula; in order to maintain cardiac output and tissue perfusion the myocardium compensates by an increase in heart rate and stroke volume. The fistula places a volume overload on both the right and left heart that is proportional to the flow through the fistula. The large venous return from a peripheral fistula engenders a correspondingly high and "obligatory" increase in pulmonary blood flow. The size of the shunt and the magnitude of pulmonary blood flow are independent of pulmonary vascular resistance. This is in contrast to dependent shunts. Other examples of shunts in which the left and right heart participate in the volume overload and the shunt is obligatory include sinus of Valsalva aneurysms in which rupture has occurred into the right heart, coronary AV fistulae, and left ventricular–right atrial communications. Experimental studies have shown that in these obligatory shunts, all of which are associated with an elevated pulmonary blood flow, the normal regression of pulmonary vascular resistance after birth may be delayed or impaired. Continued exposure of the lung to a massive pulmonary blood flow may lead to secondary changes in the pulmonary arterioles with the development of an increase in pulmonary vascular resistance and pulmonary hypertension in later life. These changes do not lead to right-to-left shunting or cyanosis, however, unless the condition is accompanied by an independent anatomic fault such as an atrial septal defect, which provides a separate channel for right-to-left shunting secondary to right ventricular hypertrophy and reduced right ventricular compliance.

In congenital heart lesions that involve right-to-left shunting, we are confronted with a wide and complex array of structural abnormalities. Some observers have categorized these malformations according to anatomical considerations; however, a classification based upon physiological alterations provides a more useful point of departure for pathophysiological understanding. The hallmark of right-to-left shunts is that deoxygenated blood enters the systemic arterial circulation. The degree of arterial desaturation that results is a function of the ratio between normally oxygenated pulmonary venous return and deoxygenated shunt flow, which mix on the arterial side of the circulation. With any given shunt, the volume of blood traversing the defect has been shown to fluctuate to a lesser extent than the volume of pulmonary blood flow, regardless of the size and location of the channel. Thus, pulmonary blood flow is the primary factor determining arterial oxygen tension. Palliative operations are therefore designed to either restrict or enhance pulmonary blood flow rather than to eliminate the abnormal communication.

We can define two major classes of right-to-left shunts, based upon the volume of pulmonary blood flow (Table 3): those conditions in which pulmonary blood flow is increased above normal and those in which pulmonary blood flow is diminished below normal. The two groups represent simply opposite extremes of a continuum in which there is always a right-to-left shunt, but pulmonary flow may be increased, nearly normal, or reduced.

The most common right-to-left shunt lesion during infancy associated with increased pulmonary blood flow is complete transposition of the great vessels. In this anomaly, the aorta arises from the right ventricle and the pulmonary artery arises from the left ventricle.

TABLE 3. CLASSIFICATION OF COMMON RIGHT-TO-LEFT SHUNTS

Increased Pulmonary Blood Flow
  Complete transposition of the great vessels
  Taussig-Bing anomaly
  Truncus arteriosus
  Total anomalous pulmonary venous connection
  Single ventricle with low pulmonary resistance and no
    pulmonic stenosis
  Hypoplastic left ventricle
  Common atrium

Decreased Pulmonary Blood Flow
  Tetralogy of Fallot
  Pulmonic stenosis with intact ventricular septum and patent
    foramen ovale or atrial septal defect
  Tricuspid atresia or stenosis
  Ebstein's anomaly
  Eisenmenger syndrome
  Anomalous systemic venous return to the left atrium

The position of the AV valves and relationship of the atria to the ventricles are normal. Systemic venous and pulmonary venous blood return to the right atrium and left atrium, respectively. Two parallel but separate circuits exist. For viability to be maintained, there must be a shunt channel to permit oxygenated and deoxygenated blood to mix. During intrauterine life, the foramen ovale and the ductus arteriosus fulfill this requirement and fetal development and survival are usually ensured. At birth, normal physiological closure of the ductus and the foramen ovale precipitate profound cyanosis and hypoxia because of the independence of the two circulations, and heart failure develops because the myocardium is perfused with desaturated blood returning to the right heart and pumped into the aorta and coronary arteries. Heart failure and death are avoided when a communication between the two circulations persists. In descending order of frequency, these have been observed at the atrial, pulmonary, and ventricular levels. Survival of the infant is possible when desaturated blood returning to the right atrium gains access to the lung either by crossing an atrial septal defect to the left atrium, left ventricle, and pulmonary artery; or by crossing a ventricular septal defect to the left ventricle and pulmonary artery; or by crossing a patent ductus to the pulmonary artery. In each case, pulmonary blood flow is increased. For survival, it is also essential that some oxygenated pulmonary venous blood return to the systemic circulation. This is accomplished in transposition by bidirectional shunting at whatever level a communication persists between the pulmonary and systemic circulations. In transposition, left-to-right shunting refers to the volume of blood passing across an atrial defect, ventricular defect, or ductus into the right side of the heart, which, if it were not for the transposition, would recirculate to the lung. Because of the transposed aorta and pulmonary artery, this blood does not recirculate to the lung but enters the systemic circulation. In transposition, the anatomic right-to-left shunt refers to the volume of blood shunted from the right atrium, right ventricle, or aorta to the lung. However, the physiological or functional right-to-left shunt refers to the volume of systemic venous return that does not cross the anatomical shunt and hence recirculates to the systemic arteries without passing through the lung to become oxygenated.

The most common right-to-left shunt associated with a decreased pulmonary blood flow is tetralogy of Fallot. The anatomical features of this anomaly are right ventricular outflow tract stenosis, right ventricular hypertrophy, dextroposition of the aorta, and a ventricular septal defect. The primary site of obstruction is either at the pulmonary valve or at the infundibulum, which may be stenotic or atretic. The greater the obstruction to right ventricular outflow, the greater the reduction in pulmonary blood flow and pressure. During intrauterine life, this low pressure–flow state may lead to underdevelopment and hypoplasia of the main and branch pulmonary arteries. To sustain flow to the placenta, blood that would normally be channeled through the pulmonary trunk and across the ductus to the descending aorta instead is handled by the left ventricle and is pumped into the ascending aorta and aortic isthmus. Pathological studies have demonstrated that the aortic arch of an infant with tetralogy is increased in diameter as a response to this volume load. The low pressure and flow in the pulmonary tree may foster retrograde left-to-right flow in the ductus.

Following birth, the ductus arteriosus closes. In the face of right ventricular outflow tract obstruction, viability of the infant is maintained by a communication at the ventricular level, which allows shunting of blood across the ventricular septal defect in a right-to-left direction. The ventricular defect is usually large and peak systolic pressures in the two ventricles and aorta are equal. The circulatory dynamics of this lesion will depend primarily on the volume of pulmonary blood flow that is related to the severity of right ventricular outflow tract obstruction. Of secondary importance are the outflow resistances of the systemic and pulmonary vascular beds and the quantity of systemic blood that enters the pulmonary tree from bronchial arteries or a persistent ductus arteriosus.

In the context of neonatal circulatory development, one can readily appreciate that the normal thinning and compliance changes of the right ventricle are impaired in tetralogy of Fallot. Outflow obstruction raises the pressure in the right ventricle and compensatory hypertrophy is seen. Rather than diminishing in a normal manner, pulmonary vascular resistance may remain elevated in patients with tetralogy, since the oxygen tension of blood distal to the outflow obstruction is diminished, and normal maturation of medial smooth muscle in the arterioles is retarded. With less severe obstruction to right ventricular outflow, the normal reduction in pulmonary vascular resistance occurs after birth, pulmonary blood flow is higher, and systemic arterial desaturation and cyanosis are less marked. Conversely, if outflow obstruction is enhanced by hypertrophy the magnitude of the right-to-left shunt will increase, and cyanosis may become more evident with age. In this latter situation, pulmonary nutritional flow and left atrial return may be principally derived from collateral bronchial arterial flow.

As hypoxemia progresses with greater right-to-left shunting, secondary polycythemia occurs. Any arteriolar intimal damage from pulmonary flow or hypoxemia will be aggravated by this increase in blood viscosity, which stimulates a self-perpetuating rise in pulmonary outflow resistance. Longevity in patients with tetralogy of Fallot depends primarily upon sufficient pulmonary flow to sustain an adequate arterial oxygen tension. It is the level of systemic arterial hypoxemia consequent to a low pulmonary flow that is the critical factor affecting the clinical course. This is in contrast to right-to-left shunts with a higher pulmonary flow (that is, ventricular septal defect) in which prognosis relates more to the response of the pulmonary vessels and the left ventricle to chronic volume overload.

SHUNT CALCULATION AND DETECTION

There are a number of simple methods for detecting shunts, particularly left-to-right shunts, at the bedside. These include changes in the electrical potential at the end of a platinum-tipped electrode following inhalation of hydrogen gas (a reducing agent), indicator dilution curves using cold saline and a thermistor-tipped catheter, radionuclide injections with precordial and head counting, and, more recently, echocardiography with injections of saline that produce microcavitations (bubbles) that can be tracked through the heart. More precise localization and quantitation of shunts may be achieved in the catheterization laboratory by indicator dye-dilution curves and by detecting the site and magnitude of oxygen step-ups. Of these, the Fick expression, which is based upon oxygen step-ups, is the most widely used approach, particularly when quantitation of shunt flow is desired.

REFERENCES

Burchell, H. B.: Dependent and obligatory intracardiac shunts in congenital heart disease. Circulation 41:177, 1970.

Dalen, J. E.: Shunt detection and measurement. In Grossman, W. (ed.): Cardiac Catheterization and Angiography. Philadelphia, Lea and Febiger, 1974, p. 96.

Engle, M. A.: Cyanotic congenital heart disease. Am J Cardiol 37:283, 1976.

Friedman, W. F., Hirschklau, M. J., Printz, M. P., Pitlick, P. T., and Kirkpatrick, S. E.: Pharmacologic closure of patent ductus arteriosus in the premature infant. N Engl J Med 295:526, 1976.

Heymann, M. A., and Rudolph, A. M.: Control of the ductus arteriosus. Physiol Rev 55:62, 1975.

Heymann, M. A., and Rudolph, A. M.: Effects of congenital heart disease on fetal and neonatal circulations. Prog Cardiovasc Dis 15:115, 1972.

Nadas, A., and Fyler, D.: General principles of shunts. In Pediatric Cardiology. Philadelphia, W. B. Saunders Co., 1972, p. 301.

Rudolph, A. M.: The changes in the circulation after birth: Their importance in congenital heart disease. Circulation 41:343, 1970.

Rudolph, A. M.: The effects of postnatal circulatory adjustments in congenital heart disease. Pediatrics 36:763, 1965.

Rudolph, A. M., and Heymann, M. A.: Neonatal circulation and pathophysiology of shunts. In Levine, H. (ed.): Clinical Cardiovascular Physiology. New York, Grune and Stratton, 1976, p. 597.

Rudolph, A. M., and Heymann, M. A.: The fetal circulation. Annu Rev Med 19:195, 1968.

Spach, M. S., Serwer, G. A., Anderson, P. A. W., Canent, R. V., Jr., and Levin, A. R.: Pulsatile aortopulmonary pressure flow dynamics of patent ductus arteriosus in patients with various hemodynamic states. Circulation 61:110, 1980.

Valvular Heart Disease

Nowhere in the field of cardiovascular pathophysiology is the complex interplay among various adaptive mechanisms better illustrated and understood than in the study of valvular heart disease. The following section will deal with each of the four classic left heart valvular lesions (mitral stenosis, mitral regurgitation, aortic stenosis, and aortic regurgitation), discussing in sequence the etiology, pathophysiology, clinical features (symptoms and physical examination), and common laboratory findings (chest x-ray, EKG, and echocardiogram).

MITRAL STENOSIS

Etiology. Mitral stenosis is almost exclusively rheumatic and (with or without regurgitation) is the most frequent late consequence of rheumatic endocarditis. The valve leaflets and chordae tendineae become diffusely thickened as a consequence of the addition of either fibrous tissue, calcium, or both. The valve leaflets become fused along at least a part of their commissural margins, and chordae become shortened and sometimes fused as well. The chordae may retract to an extreme degree so that at surgery or autopsy the mitral leaflets appear to insert directly into the papillary muscles. The amount of calcification of the mitral apparatus varies but generally is more prominent in men and in older patients. In diastole, the stenotic mitral valve has the appearance of a funnel or of an inverted bishop's hat or miter. Thus, in the open position the valve has a primary orifice reflecting the cross-sectional area at the level of the anulus, and a secondary orifice representing the area that separates the leaflets near the apex of the funnel (Fig. 77). In rheumatic mitral stenosis, thickening of the leaflets, commissural fusion, and shortening of chordae each contributes to a reduction in the size of the secondary orifice. Quite commonly the leaflet bellies are thin, freely mobile, and relatively uninvolved.

Pathophysiology. Normally, in early diastole, when left ventricular pressure falls below the left atrial pressure, blood flows rapidly from the left atrium into the left ventricle, separating widely the anterior and posterior mitral valve leaflets. This sequence of left atrial emptying and left ventricular filling leads to a mid-diastolic reversal in the LA-LV pressures that floats the anterior and posterior mitral valve leaflets toward each other to a nearly closed position. With atrial systole, the leaflets are again widely separated, followed by final closure that is initiated by a combination of left atrial relaxation plus the passive rise in left ventricular pressure resulting from the atrial booster pump function and finished by the onset of active left ventricular systole and pressure development. In mitral stenosis, the continuing LA-LV diastolic pressure gradient and restricted emptying of the left atrium cause the anterior and posterior mitral leaflets to remain widely opened throughout diastole, with no mid-diastolic closure of the leaflets. In nearly all cases, the normal mirror image motion of the anterior leaflet relative to the posterior leaflet is abol-

ished so that in diastole, the posterior leaflet is pulled anteriorly by anterior leaflet opening.

The distinguishing characteristic of mitral stenosis is diastolic obstruction to blood flow. The cause of this obstruction is a decrease in mitral valve diastolic orifice area. In 1951, Gorlin and Gorlin introduced a hydraulic formula for calculation of the cross-sectional area of the mitral valve using data obtained at cardiac catheterization. The formula as currently used in most hemodynamic laboratories is:

$$MVA = \frac{MVF}{K \cdot 44.5 \sqrt{MVG}}$$

where:

  MVA = mitral valve area in cm²
  MVF = mitral valve flow in ml/sec
   K = orifice constant for mitral valve (typically 0.85)
  MVG = mean diastolic pressure gradient from left atrium to left ventricle

and where:

$$MVF = \frac{CO}{heart\ rate \times DFP}$$

where:

  CO = cardiac output in ml/min
  DFP = diastolic filling period in sec/beat

Normal individuals have a mitral valve area of 4 to 6 cm² and a negligible mean diastolic gradient across the mitral valve. Mitral stenosis seldom produces symptoms even with exercise until the mitral valve area is reduced to less than 2.5 cm². A mitral valve area less than 1.5 cm² is regarded as significant stenosis and an area of less than 1.0 cm² is regarded as severe stenosis. The pressure gradient across the mitral valve is related not only to mitral valve area but also to mean diastolic flow rate across the valve, and hence to cardiac output. This relationship is depicted in Figure 78. In severe mitral stenosis, left atrial pressure sometimes exceeds 30 mm Hg and the mean mitral valve gradient is 25 mm Hg or more.

In most patients with rheumatic mitral stenosis, the valve orifice narrows progressively with age. Hemodynamic findings reflect the time of observation during the long natural history of the disease, the severity of mitral stenosis as reflected by mitral valve area, and whether or not the patient is studied under basal conditions or during some stress such as exercise. In at least some patients with mitral stenosis, alterations of left ventricular function, pulmonary dynamics, cardiac rhythm, right ventricular function, and tricuspid valve function may contribute to the hemodynamic picture and to clinical symptoms and signs. Initially and particularly in younger patients, cardiac output is maintained by progressive elevations in left atrial pressure with a large gradient across the mitral valve. With chronicity and particularly as the mitral valve area falls below 1.5 cm², cadiac output decreases, lessening the left atrial pressure with a fall in the diastolic mitral valve gradient. Over a range of left atrial pressures from 5 to approximately 20 mm Hg, left atrial pressure is passively transmitted through the

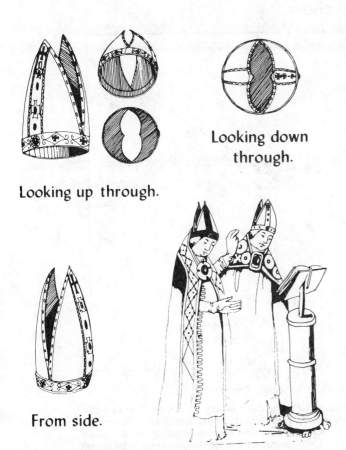

Looking up through.

Looking down through.

From side.

Figure 77. The miter of the mitral valve. The term "mitral" is derived from the Latin term "matra," meaning cap, which in turn was derived from the Greek word "mitra," meaning turban or headdress. Bishops of the Christian Church wore headdresses, which they called "miters," fashioned after those of ancient Hebrew high priests. Vesalius is recorded as having compared the shape of the bishops's miter with that of the mitral valve. (With permission from Roberts, W. C., and Perloff, J. K.: Mitral valvular disease: A clinicopathologic survey of the conditions causing the mitral valve to function abnormally. Ann Intern Med 77:940, 1972.)

pulmonary vascular bed to the pulmonary artery. In this situation pulmonary vascular resistance remains normal and the pressure gradient across the lungs is normal.

The changes in the pulmonary circulation of patients with mitral stenosis were studied by Friedman and Braunwald utilizing iodine-131 labeled microaggregates of albumin to obtain lung scans and to characterize the distribution of pulmonary blood flow of patients with mitral stenosis in the erect position. In normal subjects blood flow to the lower third of the lungs greatly exceeded that to the upper third, producing an upper-to-lower flow ratio of 0.4. In patients with mitral valve disease this ratio varied from 0.4 to 1.8 with a mean of 1.0. Furthermore, there was a direct relation between left atrial pressure and the upper to lower blood flow ratio with an r value of +0.91 (Fig. 79).

Pulmonary vascular changes, including intimal and medial thickening, occur in patients with mitral stenosis but do not correlate well with average pulmonary vascular resistance found at catheterization. In all likelihood this reflects, at least in part, the nonuniform

distribution of the arterial changes that are typically most marked at the base of the lung. In addition, there is evidence of functional pulmonary vasoconstriction at the lung bases in mitral stenosis. Pulmonary venous pressure and hence pulmonary capillary pressure are influenced by gravity and are always higher in dependent parts of the lung. When capillary pressure is sufficiently high to cause transudation of fluid into the interstitial space in excess of that which can be removed by regional lymphatics, there is a local decrease in lung compliance, a reduction in regional ventilation:perfusion ratio, and pulmonary venous hypoxemia that initiates reflex pulmonary arteriolar constriction, diverting pulmonary blood flow away from the lung bases to the apices. Functional pulmonary vasoconstriction is indicated by the substantial fall in pulmonary artery pressure and pulmonary vascular resistance in patients with pulmonary hypertension and mitral stenosis that follows inhalation of oxygen or infusion of acetylcholine or hexamethonium, agents known to cause pulmonary arteriolar vasodilatation. In most patients, pulmonary hypertension is relieved by successful mitral valve surgery. When pulmonary hypertension is disproportionate to the elevated left atrial pressure, and pulmonary artery pressure does not fall to normal after surgical correction, recurrent pulmonary emboli, irreversible pulmonary vascular changes, or pulmonary vascular changes associated with accompanying obstructive airway disease are probably at fault.

With significant mitral stenosis, regardless of the

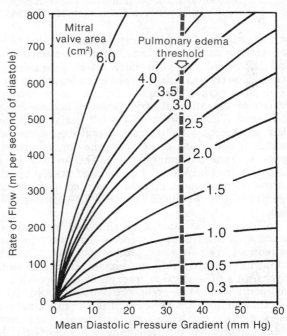

Figure 78. Chart illustrating the relation between mean diastolic gradient across the mitral valve and rate of flow across the mitral valve per second of diastole, as predicted by the Gorlin and Gorlin formula. Note that when the mitral valve area is 1.0 cm² or less, very little additional flow can be achieved by an increased pressure gradient. (With permission from Schlant, R. C.: Altered cardiovascular function of rheumatic heart disease and other acquired valvular disease. In Hurst, J. W., Logue, R. B., Schlant, R. C., and Wenger, N. K. (eds.): The Heart, Arteries and Veins. 3rd ed. New York, McGraw-Hill Book Co., 1974, p. 816.)

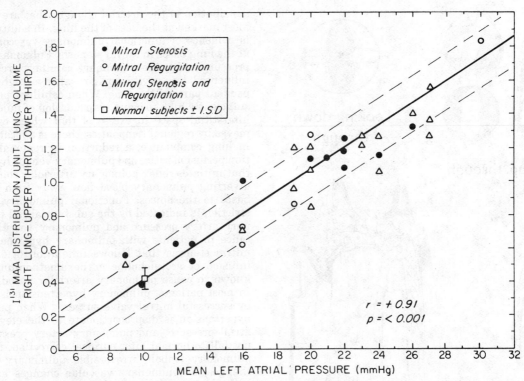

Figure 79. Relationship between the ratio of upper third to lower third pulmonary blood flow and the mean left atrial pressure. The diagonal solid and broken lines represent the regression line ± SD. (With permission from Friedman, W. F., and Braunwald, E.: Alterations in regional pulmonary blood flow in mitral valve disease studied by radioisotope scanning: A simple nontraumatic technique for estimation of left atrial pressure. Circulation 34:371, 1966.)

severity of hemodynamic changes at basal states, physical activity exaggerates the abnormal hemodynamics and left atrial and pulmonary artery pressures increase. The rise in cardiac output is inadequate to meet peripheral oxygen demands and may even decrease despite an elevated left atrial pressure because of the shortened diastolic interval for left atrial emptying that accompanies tachycardia. Resulting pulmonary venous hypertension leads to dyspnea or, in extreme cases, to frank pulmonary edema. The limited rise in cardiac output is reflected by a reduced oxygen uptake during exercise and a markedly reduced maximal oxygen uptake and reduced tolerance for vigorous exercise.

Left ventricular function is abnormal in many patients with severe mitral stenosis. The ventricle may be reduced in size in some, presumably from disuse, or it may be enlarged mildly, presumably from rheumatic myocarditis. The ejection fraction of the ventricle is commonly reduced on preoperative angiographic studies; this finding of a myocardial factor in mitral stenosis, perhaps combined with the reduced compliance of the atrophic left ventricle, may well account for the failure of adequate mitral valve surgery to restore cardiac function and hemodynamics to normal in some patients.

Clinical Features. In patients with significant mitral stenosis the earliest symptom is usually dyspnea on exertion, which correlates with the rise in pulmonary venous pressure. In part, dyspnea is attributable to activation of pulmonary venous "J receptors" and in part to the increased work of breathing, which accompanies the decrease in lung compliance. Approximately one third of patients with mitral stenosis will experience hemoptysis. Hemoptysis results from rupture of bronchial venous varices, which can be seen on bronchoscopy. These varices develop because of bronchopulmonary venous connections that allow left atrial pressure to be transmitted not only to the pulmonary veins, but also to bronchial veins. It is of interest that hemoptysis related to bronchial venous rupture is a relatively early symptom in patients with mitral stenosis. In fact, its incidence correlates inversely with pulmonary vascular resistance. This observation suggests that rupture occurs when pulmonary venous pressure rises abruptly. Patients in whom pulmonary arteriolar resistance is increased or in whom bronchopulmonary venous vessels have had time to hypertrophy are protected from this consequence of mitral stenosis.

Systemic emboli, arising from the left atrium, occur with an average incidence of 2 to 3 per cent per year in patients with mitral stenosis. The incidence may be as high as 4 to 5 per cent per year in those with atrial fibrillation and less than 1 per cent per year in those with normal rhythm. Embolization does not correlate well with mitral valve area or the level of left atrial pressure.

Findings on physical examination depend upon severity. With moderate stenosis, pulmonary venous and arterial hypertension cause right ventricular hypertrophy and ultimately an increase in central venous pressure. The neck veins may therefore become abnormally distended and a large (or giant) A wave due to augmented right atrial systole may occur. With more severe pulmonary hypertension and right ventricular dilatation, tricuspid regurgitation may develop producing a systolic wave ("S" or "CV" wave) in the venous pulse that obliterates the normal "X" descent. When the stenosis is severe and the cardiac output is diminished, the arterial pulse may be small and difficult to feel. Palpation of the precordium may reveal a sustained systolic impulse at the lower left sternal edge due to contraction of the hypertrophied right ventricle. The left ventricular impulse is small and very brief and, with progressive right ventricular enlargement and displacement of the left ventricle away from the chest wall, may not be palpable at all. On auscultation, the first heart sound is loud and snapping, both because of the rheumatic changes in the texture of the leaflets and because the elevated left atrial pressure causes a delay in mitral valve closure such that leaflet coaptation occurs when the rate of rise in left ventricular pressure is well developed, leading to a greater deceleration of blood and vibration of the "cardiohemic system." A second auscultatory feature is an opening snap, a high frequency sound 30 to 130 milliseconds after the aortic component of the second heart sound due to abrupt deceleration of blood (with vibrations) as the stenotic valve is snapped open in early diastole and reaches the limits of diastolic excursion imposed by the rheumatic valvular changes. This snap is coincident with maximal diastolic distention of the mitral valve funnel. The higher the left atrial pressure, the sooner the mitral valve is snapped open in diastole and the shorter the A_2-OS interval. The third classic feature is a murmur due to turbulent blood flow across the mitral valve in diastole. This murmur is typically low frequency or rumbling in quality, and its intensity correlates with mital valve flow rate, although mitral valve configuration and texture may modify the intensity of the murmur at any given flow rate. The longer the duration of the murmur, the more likely the LA-LV gradient is to be high and persistent throughout diastole. The murmur of mitral stenosis typically increases just before the first heart sound, and there is now convincing evidence that this accentuation results from progressive narrowing of the mitral orifice due to ventricular systole. Flow across the valve continues despite the onset of ventricular activation as a consequence of a high LA to LV pressure gradient, accentuated by atrial systole. The other auscultatory findings in isolated mitral stenosis reflect the level of pulmonary artery pressure and may include the murmurs of tricuspid and/or pulmonary regurgitation. It is noteworthy that the most extreme cases of mitral stenosis may be silent because the mitral valve may become truly rigid, with a soft first heart sound, an absent opening snap, and a mitral flow rate insufficient to produce a diastolic rumble.

Laboratory Findings. The chest x-ray is a remarkably accurate reflection of the pathophysiology of mitral stenosis. The left atrium is enlarged in all but the mildest cases. The pulmonary vascular pattern reflects an upward redistribution of blood flow. The main pulmonary artery is dilated and peripheral branches taper off rapidly as pulmonary pressure increases. Pulmonary lymphatic markings become exaggerated particularly at the bases. Right ventricular hypertrophy and a normal or reduced left ventricular size create a typical contour of the heart on posteroanterior views, and the enlarged right ventricle encroaches on the normal retrosternal space. Calcium may be seen, particularly in the mitral valve, with or occasionally without image intensification fluoroscopy. The EKG shows evidence of left atrial enlargement and signs of right ventricular hypertrophy, which correlate roughly with the level of pulmonary artery pressure. Atrial fibrillation is a common arrhythmia.

The echocardiogram shows thickening of the mitral leaflets, a loss of mid-diastolic closure, a small atrial wave, and congruent movement of the anterior and posterior mitral valve leaflets (instead of the normal mirror image pattern). Two-dimensional echocardiography can accurately image the tip of the funnel, allowing a measurement of the orifice area that correlates well with the area found at catheterization.

MITRAL REGURGITATION

Etiology. In recent years a number of authors have drawn attention to the fact that the mitral valve leaflets are but one component of a more complex unit, the mitral apparatus. The functional competence of this unit depends upon the integrity of each of its components. From a functional point of view the mitral apparatus consists of the posterior left atrial wall, the anulus of the mitral valve, the anterior and posterior leaflets, the chordae tendineae, and the papillary muscles as well as their base of support within the left ventricular wall (Fig. 80). Structural changes in one or more of these components may impair normal closure of the entire unit and lead to regurgitation.

Early hemodynamic studies in normal animals showed that, subsequent to atrial contraction and relaxation, a pressure gradient exists between the left atrium and left ventricle that is sufficient to cause approximation or near approximation of the mitral leaflets before the onset of ventricular systole. Minor degrees of early systolic mitral regurgitation may be observed in the absence of either an effective or properly timed atrial contraction. The papillary muscles contract very early in the course of normal ventricular contraction. Because of the funnel shape of the normal mitral valve, papillary muscle contraction exerts a vertical force on the mitral apparatus and causes the leaflets to move toward a position of apposition. More will be said later about the role of pathological changes of the papillary muscles in the genesis of mitral regurgitation. Even when the papillary muscles are normal, however, mild to moderate degrees of mitral regurgitation can be observed when the sequence of ventricular excitation is altered—for example, on spontaneous or induced premature ventricular beats.

Common causes of significant mitral regurgitation involve pathological alterations of the anulus, the leaflets, the chordae tendineae, and the papillary muscles. The anulus of the mitral valve is normally a tough but pliable unit to which the leaflets are attached. A reduction in the size of the anulus (the primary mitral orifice) is a normal event in systole. A reduction of 20 to 50 per cent in the cross-sectional area of the orifice must be bridged by the opposed leaflets when the mitral valve closes. Dilatation or calcification and loss of pliability of the anulus, without

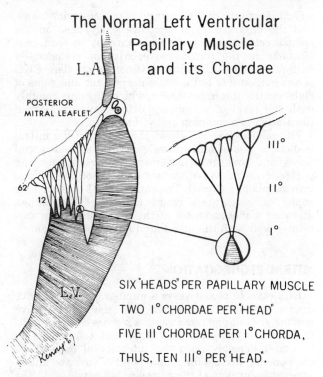

The Normal Left Ventricular Papillary Muscle and its Chordae

L.A.

POSTERIOR
MITRAL LEAFLET

62

12

L.V.

III°

II°

I°

SIX "HEADS" PER PAPILLARY MUSCLE

TWO I° CHORDAE PER "HEAD"

FIVE III° CHORDAE PER I° CHORDA,

THUS, TEN III° PER "HEAD".

Figure 80. Diagram of the average number of chordae tendineae normally originating from each ventricular papillary muscle. Although great variation exists, each left ventricular papillary muscle contains about six "heads," each of which contains two primary, or first-order, chordae tendineae. Each primary cord subdivides into two secondary chordae, each of which divides into two or three tertiary, or third-order, chordae. The number of chordae attached to each left ventricular papillary muscle thus averages 12, and the number of chordae inserting directly into the mitral leaflets from a single papillary muscle averages 62. (These numbers were found by counting chordae and papillary muscle heads in 12 normal hearts.) LA = Left atrium; LV = left ventricle. (With permission from Roberts, W. C., and Perloff, J. K.: Mitral valvular disease: A clinicopathologic survey of the conditions causing the mitral valve to function abnormally. Ann Intern Med 77:942 1972.)

involvement of the leaflets per se, may oppose the normal sphincter-like constriction of the anulus and contribute to mitral regurgitation. Congenital or acquired abnormalities of one or both leaflets may lead either to deficient or excessive leaflet tissue or to restricted mobility of normal-sized leaflets. Rheumatic endocarditis typically causes scarring, contracture, and reduced mobility of one or both leaflets. Excessive leaflet tissue is observed in many patients with Marfan's syndrome and even more commonly in Barlow's syndrome (the click-murmur syndrome). In some of the latter cases the leaflets consist of normal but redundant tissue and in others there is a marked degree of fibromyxomatous change. Generally, the posterior leaflet is involved more than the anterior, but redundancy of both leaflets may occur. The abnormality results in prolapse of a part of one or both leaflets into the left atrium during systole. The amount and timing of the onset of mitral regurgitation are both highly variable in these patients. Prolapse may occur with no regurgitation, with minor regurgitation confined to the latter half of systole, or with massive regurgitation

throughout systole. A congenitally cleft mitral valve due to abnormal development of the endocardial cushions may also lead to mitral regurgitation.

Chordae tendineae represent struts that connect the margins of the leaflets to the heads of papillary muscles. Chordae may be abnormally long or short, may insert ectopically and/or may rupture. Rupture may occur spontaneously without apparent cause, because of infectious endocarditis, or as a consequence of degenerative changes in association with the prolapsing mitral valve syndrome. Primary chordal shortening may occur as a consequence of rheumatic endocarditis and scarring. Chordae tendineae arise from the heads of papillary muscles and divide many times, with secondary, tertiary, and even more branches before inserting into a leaflet (Fig. 82). As a consequence, the amount of mitral regurgitation will depend upon the amount and level of chordal involvement and whether it is due to abnormalities of length, insertion, or rupture.

Normal closure of the mitral apparatus is critically determined by the structural and functional integrity of the papillary muscles. Papillary muscle dysfunction is usually a consequence of coronary disease and is a common cause of mitral regurgitation. Papillary muscle infarction leads to fibrosis and retraction and very often there is associated infarction of the left ventricular wall that supports the papillary muscle, with reduced (hypokinesia to akinesia) or paradoxical (systolic bulging or dyskinesia) wall motion. The syndrome of mitral regurgitation resulting from ischemic heart disease varies. At one extreme, mitral regurgitation may develop only during episodes of angina. Stable mitral regurgitation of mild to moderate amounts may result from scarring of the papillary muscle or a related portion of the ventricular wall. Acute and often fatal mitral regurgitation occurs after rupture of the belly of a papillary muscle in the setting of myocardial infarction. It has been proposed that abnormal alignment of the papillary muscles and/or dilatation of the mitral anulus may cause mitral insufficiency in any condition characterized by marked dilatation of the left ventricle.

Finally, it is appropriate to consider the role of the posterior left atrial wall in mitral insufficiency. The anterior leaflet of the mitral valve is attached to the anulus of the aortic valve and is not affected per se by left atrial enlargement. The posterior mitral leaflet, however, is continuous with the endocardium of the left atrial wall. Furthermore, while the surface areas of the leaflets are nearly identical, the base–to–free edge length of the posterior leaflet is approximately one half that of the anterior leaflet. As a consequence, the anterior leaflet is normally much more mobile than the posterior leaflet. When the left atrium becomes dilated, regardless of cause, the posterior mitral leaflet becomes increasingly tethered and even less mobile. This tethering of the posterior leaflet reduces the contribution of the leaflet to valve coaptation during systole. Thus, left atrial dilatation may cause mitral regurgitation. Because the left atrium dilates in response to mitral regurgitation, and because dilatation further augments regurgitation, mitral regurgitation itself tends to promote further regurgitation.

Pathophysiology. The fundamental hemodynamic alteration in patients with significant mitral regurgitation is incompetence of the mitral valve during ventricular systole. As a consequence, a portion of left ventricular stroke volume on each beat regurgitates into the left atrium. Total left ventricular volume change during systole can be determined from angiographic studies in which left ventricular end-diastolic and end-systolic volume are calculated from the angiogram (see p. 884). Forward stroke volume (cardiac output divided by heart rate) can be calculated either from dye-dilution curves or by the Fick principle. The difference between total stroke volume and forward stroke volume is the regurgitant volume, which can also be expressed as a percentage of the total stroke volume (that is, the regurgitant fraction). Regurgitant fractions of 30 to 80 per cent are commonly observed in patients with symptomatic mitral insufficiency.

The hydraulic effects of mitral regurgitation have important consequences on the dynamics of left ventricular contraction and on the left atrium. The left ventricle becomes dilated in mitral regurgitation. The increase in end-diastolic volume correlates with the degree of mitral regurgitation as reflected by the regurgitant volume. This change in end-diastolic volume appears to represent a normal compensatory mechanism (the Starling effect) by which the left ventricle adapts to the increased volume load presented by the incompetent valve. Ventricular hypertrophy also develops, but the increase in left ventricular mass occurs with little or no change in wall thickness.

In the normal heart, the systolic phase of ventricular contraction is divided into two periods, the isovolumic phase and the ejection phase. During isovolumic contraction pressure rises in the ventricle without a volume change. Peak wall stress occurs very near the onset of ejection and then diminishes during the ejection phase, reaching about 50 per cent of the peak value by the end of ejection. In mitral regurgitation, up to one half of the regurgitant volume is ejected into the left atrium prior to aortic valve opening. Thus, the preejection period is not isovolumic, and wall stress, which is proportional to ventricular pressure and internal radius, increases during the preejection period less than would be predicted if internal radius did not diminish consequent to regurgitation. Estimates of peak left ventricular wall stress in mitral regurgitation are only moderately higher than normal. In short, the ventricle unloads before it ejects.

The forward cardiac output is maintained near normal, at least at rest, in patients with mild to moderate mitral regurgitation. To an important extent the effect of any given regurgitant fraction on forward cardiac output depends upon the cause of mitral regurgitation. When abnormal valve function is attributable to diseases of the leaflets or chordae tendineae and left ventricular function is normal, cardiac output is well maintained for long periods of time. On the other hand, when mitral regurgitation is a consequence of papillary muscle dysfunction or of diseases (ischemic or otherwise) that impair myocardial contractility, forward output is less well maintained.

The left atrium is always enlarged in patients with chronic mitral regurgitation. Recordings of left atrial pressure show a typical alteration of the atrial pressure pulse in which the normal decline of atrial pressure after mitral valve closure is abolished and left atrial pressure typically rises throughout ventricular systole as a consequence of the regurgitation of left ventricular blood into the left atrium, producing a regurgitant or "CV" wave. The peak left atrial pressure during the CV wave may reach 50 to 75 mm Hg and is determined by the regurgitant volume, the size of the left atrium at the onset of regurgitation, and left atrial compliance (Fig. 81). In some patients with mitral regurgitation, the left atrium may become massively dilated (giant left atrium). In these patients, left atrial pressure may be nearly normal despite very large regurgitant volumes.

Pulmonary artery pressure and the response of the pulmonary circulation to mitral regurgitation are a function of the left atrial pressure and are therefore similar to those in mitral stenosis. In chronic mitral regurgitation with progressive left atrial dilatation and minimally elevated mean left atrial pressures, however, the pulmonary vasculature may remain "protected" from hypertension until late in the patient's course. As in mitral stenosis, however, there are some patients in whom the rise in pulmonary artery pressure exceeds that which can be accounted for by passive transmission of the left atrial pressure. In these patients, pulmonary vascular resistance is elevated, reflecting a structural change in the pulmonary arterioles as well as a vasoconstrictive element in some.

Clinical Features. The clinical picture of mitral regurgitation is determined predominantly by the amount of mitral regurgitation and the rapidity with which the regurgitation develops. In addition, certain findings characterize mitral regurgitation produced by any one of these several structural faults in the mitral apparatus.

For many years the focus of clinical interest in mitral regurgitation was directed at the patient with rheumatic endocarditis. Clinicians were impressed that mild to moderate mitral regurgitation was tolerated well for many years without symptoms. Hemodynamic studies in these relatively asymptomatic individuals revealed widely ranging regurgitant volumes, yet for-

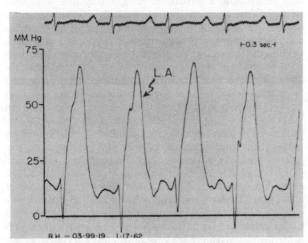

Figure 81. Left atrial (LA) pressure pulse obtained from a 23-year-old woman who suddenly developed mitral regurgitation two months before these studies during the course of acute bacterial endocarditis. Note the elevated left atrial pressure with particularly tall V waves. (With permission from Braunwald, E, and Awe, W. C.: The syndrome of severe mitral regurgitation with normal left atrial pressures. Circulation 27:33, 1963.)

ward cardiac output was maintained at least at rest and the increase in left atrial volume was sufficient to prevent an excessive rise in left atrial pressure of significant pulmonary hypertension. Symptoms that relate to forward heart failure or to pulmonary hypertension were typically absent. When symptoms did appear (frequently 15 to 25 years after detection of the murmur) fatigue, particularly on exertion, was prominent and was related to a reduced cardiac output and other clinical and hemodynamic evidence of left ventricular failure. In these patients pulmonary hypertension was only moderate.

A very different clinical picture is observed when mitral regurgitation develops acutely—for example, as a consequence of a ruptured chorda tendinea or a ruptured head of a papillary muscle. In these patients the left atrium is hardly enlarged. As a consequence, regurgitant volumes of only modest amounts may greatly increase left atrial pressure, producing CV waves of 50 mm Hg or more, an elevated mean left atrial pressure, and acute pulmonary venous hypertension and congestion. Symptoms are prominent and of relatively abrupt onset. Dyspnea on exertion, or even at rest, is evident. An extreme example is the acute mitral insufficiency produced by a ruptured papillary muscle in the setting of acute myocardial infarction. This condition is frequently accompanied by acute pulmonary edema and is fatal within 24 hours in a high percentage of patients in the absence of surgical intervention. On physical examination, the findings reflect the amount of regurgitation and its cause.

As noted previously, significant mitral regurgitation leads to an increase in left ventricular volume, and with chronicity, the left ventricular apex impulse is displaced to the left, is enlarged, and is sustained in contour. Because the left atrium is dilated, fibrotic, and thin-walled, atrial systole (for the minority of patients remaining in sinus rhythm) is ineffective and palpable A waves are unusual. In patients with papillary muscle dysfunction due to anterolateral myocardial infarction, a sustained ectopic impulse (typically in the third or even the second left intercostal space above the area of the normal apex impulse) may be felt. More commonly, regardless of the papillary muscle involved, the infarction also includes the apex, leading to a sustained, enlarged apical impulse that may be laterally displaced. In both instances, and in contrast to a primarily valvular regurgitation, augmented A waves due to a more forceful left atrial contraction (in response to a less compliant ventricle) commonly impart a bifid character to the impulse. A characteristic midsystolic retraction of the left ventricular apex impulse coincides with the click in some patients with Barlow's syndrome. A prominent early systolic thrust along the left sternal border indicates the presence of right ventricular hypertrophy secondary to pulmonary hypertension. A smaller and delayed left parasternal lift is observed in patients with severe mitral regurgitation but without serious pulmonary hypertension, and has been ascribed to anterior displacement of the right ventricle as the left atrium and pulmonary veins are expanded by the regurgitant volume in concert with limitation of posterior expansion by the spine and ribs. On auscultation, an apical systolic murmur is evident in nearly all patients. The classic murmur in rheumatic mitral regurgitation is a high frequency (or blowing) pansystolic murmur, maximal at the apex and radiating to the axilla and to the back. Rapid ventricular filling during early diastole produces a prominent S_3 and with very severe regurgitation a diastolic flow rumble due to markedly increased diastolic blood flow across the valve follows the S_3. With rupture of chordae tendineae, the murmur is usually pansystolic, but frequently has a musical quality presumably due to vibrations of a pure frequency involving some part of the mitral apparatus. Ruptured chordae most frequently involve the posterior leaflet. The resulting regurgitant jet is directed toward the atrial septum and left atrial wall that is contiguous with the aortic root. The resulting murmur may radiate to the upper right sternal edge and simulate aortic stenosis. With rupture of anterior chordae the jet is directed posteriorly and the pansystolic murmur radiates loudly to the back and sometimes up the spine to the head. When papillary muscles become scarred consequent to ischemic heart disease and mitral regurgitation develops, the left ventricular wall is also usually either hypokinetic, akinetic, or frankly aneurysmal. The murmur may be pansystolic and similar to that of rheumatic heart disease. Typically, however, the onset of regurgitation is delayed so that the murmur begins after S_1 (and is therefore not pansystolic) and has a crescendo quality.

The most common example of delayed mitral regurgitation and a delayed murmur is observed in Barlow's syndrome, also referred to as the prolapsing mitral valve syndrome. Echocardiographic studies show that in this condition the valve closes only to reopen in later systole as a consequence of prolapse of one or both leaflets into the left atrium. The resulting murmur is delayed and typically follows a systolic click. Echocardiographic studies have shown that the click correlates with the parachute-like billowing of redundant valve tissue. An important feature of the click-murmur syndrome is the variability in timing and intensity of the click and murmur. The condition may be thought of as a situation in which the mitral valve apparatus is too large for the ventricle. Maneuvers that diminish heart size, such as standing (with decreased venous return), performing a Valsalva maneuver (raising intrathoracic pressure by expiring against fixed resistance and thereby decreasing venous return), or afterload reduction with amyl nitrite (an arteriolar vasodilator), make the click and murmur earlier. Maneuvers that enlarge diastolic heart size, such as the supine position and/or elevation of the legs (maneuvers that augment venous return), make the click and murmur later. Maneuvers that increase afterload (squatting, phenylephrine infusion) also make the heart larger and move the click and murmur later but, because of the increased intraventricular pressure, may make both louder. Regardless of cause, the intensity of the murmur in mitral regurgitation correlates poorly with the regurgitant volume.

Laboratory Findings. Radiographic findings also reflect the severity and chronicity of mitral regurgitation. In acute mitral regurgitation, the left ventricle and left atrium are minimally enlarged and the x-ray changes are confined to pulmonary venous distention, interstitial edema, or frank pulmonary edema. In chronic mitral regurgitation the x-ray changes parallel the severity of regurgitation with left ventricular enlargement and left atrial enlargement. Sometimes the left atrium is massively dilated with a volume to 300 to 600 ml. The changes attributable to pulmonary hypertension and to right ventricular hypertrophy are typically later in onset but when they occur are basically similar to those observed in mitral stenosis. The EKG is typically normal or shows only nonspecific ST-T wave changes in the click-murmur syndrome. In longstanding mitral regurgitation there is left ventricular hypertrophy, sometimes right ventricular hypertrophy, and atrial fibrillation in 50 to 75 per cent of patients. In acute mitral regurgitation, the EKG usually does not show left ventricular hypertrophy, the rhythm is sinus, and in those patients with ischemic disease leading to papillary muscle dysfunction, the EKG may show signs of prior myocardial infarction. In rheumatic mitral regurgitation, the echo typically shows changes similar to those seen in mitral stenosis (p. 945) even if regurgitation is dominant. With ruptured chordae tendineae, echo may reveal a flail leaflet and/or the torn chordae themselves. In endocarditis, vegetations may be seen with or without evidence of valvular dysfunction. In the click-murmur syndrome the echo typically shows elongated leaflets that coapt normally at the onset of systole but then one or both leaflets subsequently prolapse into the atrium, with

the timing of the onset of the prolapse a function of its severity and varying from early (with severe regurgitation) to late (with mild regurgitation) systole.

AORTIC STENOSIS

Etiology. In contrast to mitral stenosis, isolated stenosis of the aortic valve is almost always nonrheumatic. Thus, when aortic stenosis is due to rheumatic carditis it is nearly always accompanied by anatomic involvement of the mitral valve. The structural basis for isolated aortic stenosis varies greatly with the age of the patient. In children less than 15 years of age, approximately 60 per cent of the cases of aortic stenosis result from a congenital unicuspid valve in which the orifice is either a centrally located hole in a domed, commissural valve or is eccentrically located, producing the appearance of unicommissural valve (Fig. 82). In the age group from 15 to 65, approximately 60 per cent of the cases of aortic stenosis are superimposed upon a congenitally bicuspid valve, in which stenosis of the orifice develops with age (the remainder are either rheumatic or due to degenerative calcification). In patients over 65 years of age, isolated aortic stenosis develops on a tricuspid valve (over 90 per cent). In

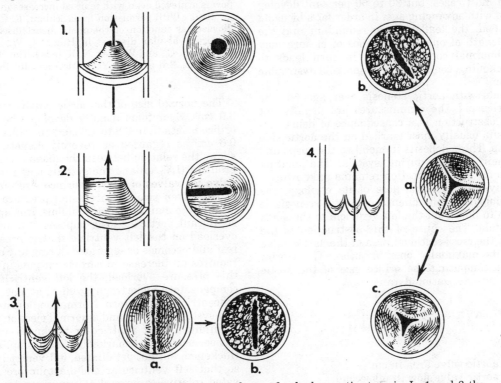

Figure 82. Diagram illustrating the various forms of valvular aortic stenosis. In 1 and 2 the stenosis is produced by dome-shaped valves. Each of these valves is intrinsically stenotic. In 1 the valve has no lateral attachments to the wall of the ascending aorta. The orifice is centrally located. In 2 the valve has one lateral attachment (commissure) and its orifice is eccentrically located. In 3 a congenitally bicuspid valve is shown. This bicuspid semilunar valve is not intrinsically stenotic but becomes stenotic only as it becomes calcified. The calcification in this instance is usually uniformly distributed. In 4 a tricuspid aortic valve is shown (a). When rheumatic fever attacks this valve, one of the commissures is usually fused, and the valve becomes bicuspid. Later, calcium deposition occurs and stenosis appears (b). Rarely, all three commissures are fused (c) and the valve becomes stenotic in the absence of calcium deposition. (With permission from Braunwald, E., Roberts, W. C., Goldblatt, A., Aygen, M. M., Rockoff, S. D., and Gilbert, J. W.: Aortic stenosis: Physiological, pathological, and clinical concepts. Ann Intern Med 58:496, 1963.)

these latter patients, the cusps are heavily calcified, but commissural fusion is absent. Calcium deposits in the mitral anulus with otherwise normal mitral leaflets are observed in approximately 75 per cent of these cases. Thus, the pathology indicates that aortic stenosis is congenital in most cases before age 15, acquired on a congenitally deformed but nonstenotic valve in those 15 to 65, and probably a degenerative change of a previously normal valve in those over age 65.

In congenital aortic stenosis, obstruction is present at birth. Because the orifice size is fixed, the gradient across the valve increases with age in proportion to the increase in cardiac output. Left ventricular hypertrophy of a marked degree is often complicated by endocardial fibrosis, fibrosis and atrophy of papillary muscles, and resulting mitral insufficiency. The aortic valve is thickened and occasionally the anulus of the valve is hypoplastic.

In a bicuspid aortic valve approximately 50 per cent of the time the cusps are oriented right and left with one coronary ostium arising from behind each cusp. In the remaining cases the cusps are anterior and posterior with both coronary ostia arising behind the anterior cusp. Congenitally bicuspid valves are extremely common, occurring in approximately 2 per cent of births. Obstruction is presumably absent or minimal at birth in most cases, but 30 to 50 per cent develop obstruction with advancing age. In order for a bicuspid valve to open, the leaflet(s) are redundant and the excessive length of one or both lines of closure may produce abnormal contact, which in turn leads to fibrous thickening, commissural fusion, and dystrophic calcification.

In patients with aortic stenosis over age 65, the valve is tricuspid, the commissures are usually not fused, and obstruction is a consequence of dense calcium deposits usually most marked on the aortic side of each cusp. These deposits immobilize the cusps and prevent their opening during systole. The inciting mechanism for this calcification remains unknown.

Pathophysiology. Regardless of its etiology, the basic physiological consequence of aortic stenosis is obstruction to flow from the left ventricle to the aorta during systole. The cause of this obstruction is the decrease in the cross-sectional area of the aortic valve orifice in its maximally open position. The Gorlin formula for computing the orifice size of the aortic valve from catheterization data is:

$$AVA = \frac{AVF}{K \cdot 44.5 \sqrt{AVG}}$$

where:

AVA = aortic valve area in cm²
AVF = aortic valve flow in ml/second
K = orifice constant for aortic valve (typically 1.0)
AVG = mean systolic pressure gradient (LV-Ao)

and where:

$$AVF = \frac{CO}{heart\ rate \times SEP}$$

where:
CO = cardiac output in ml/min
SEP = systolic ejection period in sec/beat

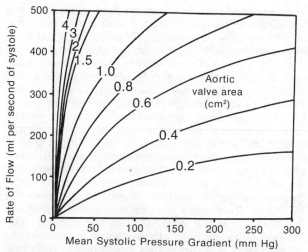

Figure 83. Chart illustrating the relation between mean systolic pressure gradient across the aortic valve and the rate of flow across the aortic valve per second of systole, as predicted by the Gorlin and Gorlin formula. Although the effective area of the aortic valve in the adult is about 2.6 to 3.5 cm², there is relatively little obstruction to blood flow until the area is markedly reduced. At the "critical" valve area, about 0.5 to 0.7 cm², relatively little further increase in flow is achieved even with marked increases in mean systolic gradient. (With permission from Schlant, R. C.: Altered cardiovascular function of rheumatic heart disease and other acquired valvular disease. In Hurst, J. W., Logue, R. B., Schlant, R. C., and Wenger, N. K. (eds.): The Heart, Arteries and Veins. 3rd ed. New York, McGraw-Hill Book Co., 1974, p. 811.)

The normal size of the aortic valve orifice is 2.5 to 3.0 cm². Symptoms usually develop when the aortic orifice is less than 0.8 to 1.0 cm²; an orifice of less than 0.6 cm² is regarded as severely stenotic. Figure 83 shows the relation between the mean systolic pressure gradient (LV-Ao) and the systolic flow rate across the valve for valves of varying orifice size. For an orifice of any given size an increasing pressure gradient is required to maintain a normal flow. It is apparent that significant aortic stenosis imposes a systolic pressure overload on the left ventricle that is present even at rest and becomes exaggerated during any activity that requires an increase in cardiac output. In response to this pressure overload, the left ventricle undergoes compensatory hypertrophy, which, at least initially, is concentric in its pattern. Normal end-diastolic volume, end-systolic volume, and a normal ejection fraction are maintained. Left ventricular thickness and mass increase, sometimes markedly. The compliance of the thickened, but not yet dilated, left ventricle is reduced so that left ventricular end-diastolic pressure is elevated relative to normal at any given cavity volume. Furthermore, during atrial systole the "A" wave in the left atrial pressure pulse and its reflection in the left ventricular pressure pulse are exaggerated. These changes reflect principally the diminished compliance of the left ventricle at end-diastole.

Significant aortic valve obstruction not only produces a systolic pressure gradient from left ventricle to aorta, but also leads to characteristic changes in the arterial pressure pulse recorded distal to the aortic valve. Because of obstruction, the time required for left ventricular ejection is prolonged. The velocity of left ventricular emptying particularly in the first third of systole is reduced. These changes are reflected in a diminished pulse pressure, a reduced rate of rise of pressure (dp/dt) in early systole, and a delay in the time between the onset of ejection and achievement of peak aortic pressure. The high frequency components of the jet across the stenotic orifice cause fatigue of structural components in the ascending aortic wall. As a consequence, the aortic wall loses its ability to resume a normal diameter in diastole and becomes progressively distended, a phenomenon referred to as post-stenotic dilatation.

Clinical Features. The symptoms produced by aortic stenosis develop in a remarkably predictable sequence, particularly in younger patients. The most frequent early symptom is anginal type chest pain; the second is dizziness or frank syncope, particularly during exertion. Last to develop are symptoms attributable to heart failure. Fallen and his colleagues studied a series of patients with aortic stenosis without demonstrable coronary artery disease. In those with aortic stenosis but without a history of angina, coronary blood flow increased normally, the extraction coefficient of oxygen across the coronary vascular bed diminished, and coronary vascular resistance diminished during isoproterenol infusions. Only one of seven patients showed evidence of lactate production, an index of anaerobic glycolysis, during the infusion. In contrast, in patients with angina, the increase in coronary blood flow and the decrease in coronary vascular resistance in response to isoproterenol were markedly attenuated and the coefficient of oxygen extraction increased in all. Most showed evidence of abnormal lactate metabolism compatible with ischemia. From these and other studies on the determinants of coronary blood flow and its distribution it seems probable that total coronary blood flow, which is greatly augmented even at rest in aortic stenosis, is unable to increase adequately during stress. Under these conditions, the distribution of wall tension, particularly in diastole, will determine the transmural distribution of a relatively fixed total coronary flow. In laboratory animals, when total coronary flow is near maximal an increase in wall stress redistributes coronary flow preferentially to the epicardial layers at the expense of endocardial layers. The resulting subendocardial ischemia would seem to be sufficient to account for the development of ischemic pain. Thus, the most probable explanation for angina on effort in patients with aortic stenosis and no coronary artery disease is an intramyocardial redistribution of the available total flow, the latter being near maximal even at rest.

Syncope in patients with aortic stenosis very probably has more than one cause. In some patients, transient rhythm disturbances (atrial fibrillation or ventricular tachycardia) lead to a sudden decrease in cardiac output and cerebral perfusion pressure with resultant syncope. The left ventricle in aortic stenosis is very dependent upon adequate diastolic filling to generate the pressure gradient necessary to achieve a normal stroke volume during systole. Any rhythm disturbance that involves diastolic filling, either because of a shortened diastolic interval or the absence of an appropriately timed atrial systole, will reduce forward cardiac output. If such a disturbance is sustained for more than a few consecutive heartbeats,

aortic and cerebral perfusion pressure can drop precipitously.

Perhaps the most intriguing explanation for syncope in aortic stenosis is the evidence of an abnormal peripheral vascular response to exercise. Normally the forearm vascular bed constricts during leg exercise. Patients with aortic stenosis show either a failure of forearm vasoconstriction or actual vasodilatation during leg exercise. In these patients, forearm vasodilatation is associated with a marked rise in left ventricular end-diastolic pressure during exercise. Following aortic valve replacement these patients demonstrated a normal vasoconstrictor response to exercise. These observations are most compatible with activation of a reflex vasodilator mechanism in response to stimulation of left ventricular baroreceptors during exercise in patients with aortic stenosis. Syncope would then result from failure of a normal peripheral mechanism to maintain blood pressure during exercise, perhaps exaggerated by the extent to which aortic stenosis might limit the normal increase in cardiac output accompanying physical effort. A decrease, rather than the expected increase, of aortic systolic pressure during exercise is a frequent finding in patients with significant aortic stenosis.

The severity of aortic stenosis is best assessed on physical examination by its downstream (aortic pressure pulse) and upstream (left ventricular) consequences. Severe aortic stenosis reduces the rate of rise of aortic pressure and delays the attainment of peak pressure. These changes can be noted on palpation and quantitated by physiological records of the carotid artery pressure pulse. Severe aortic stenosis also produces concentric, often severe hypertrophy of the left ventricle. The left ventricular impulse in concentric hypertrophy is therefore forceful and sustained. It is neither displaced to the left nor diffuse unless left ventricular dilatation has developed. A prominent and palpable S_4 due to left atrial systole reflects the reduced compliance of a thickened left ventricle.

Aortic stenosis produces a harsh systolic heart murmur that begins with aortic ejection (after S_1), ends before aortic valve closure (before S_2), and is diamond-shaped or crescendo-decrescendo in contour. These features define an ejection type murmur. The murmur is loudest over the aortic area (upper right sternal edge) and radiates to neck vessels and to the left ventricular apex. It is frequently accompanied by a palpable thrill over the aortic area. The peak intensity of the murmur tends to be relatively early in mild aortic stenosis and relatively late in severe aortic stenosis. The occurrence of the peak is related to the time at which maximal ejection velocity (and hence turbulence) is achieved. In congenital aortic stenosis, the valve orifice is reduced, but the leaflet tissue is still pliable and mobile. With tensing of this dome in early systole a click (or ejection sound) is produced. An ejection sound is typically absent in conditions associated with thickened, calcified, or immobile leaflets. Similarly, the aortic component of S_2 is reduced or absent in thickened calcified valves, but preserved in congenital dome-shaped valves. When significant obstruction is present, aortic closure may be so delayed that it follows pulmonary closure. When the aortic component is audible, this causes a second heart sound that is single on inspiration and split on expiration—paradoxical splitting.

Laboratory Findings. Radiographic studies may show calcium in the aortic valve. Concentric left ventricular hypertrophy without dilatation is frequently best appreciated by posterior displacement of the ventricle behind the inferior vena caval shadow on lateral films. Post-stenotic dilatation of the ascending aorta produces an exaggerated rightward aortic bulge on anterior x-ray views of the heart. The electrocardiogram shows left ventricular and left atrial hypertrophy. The quantitative evidence of ventricular hypertrophy on EKG correlates roughly with the severity of stenosis. Echocardiography frequently reveals evidence of thickened and immobile aortic leaflets, but the appearance of the aortic valve does not accurately portray the severity of stenosis.

AORTIC REGURGITATION

Etiology. Rheumatic fever continues to be the major etiological factor in aortic regurgitation, although there are many other important causes. In acute rheumatic fever, the murmur of aortic regurgitation is second only to mitral regurgitation in frequency as a manifestation of endocarditis. Furthermore, when a murmur of aortic regurgitation develops in the setting of acute rheumatic fever it rarely disappears. Many of the large series dealing with the natural history of aortic regurgitation were based on clinics that specialized in the treatment of rheumatic fever and thus regarded rheumatic endocarditis as by far the most common cause. In his text on diseases of the heart, Wood regarded rheumatic endocarditis with thickening, retraction, and distortion of the cusps as responsible for 60 to 70 per cent of all cases of aortic regurgitation.

Prior to World War II and the development of penicillin, syphilis was the second leading cause of aortic regurgitation. Aortitis is a tertiary manifestation of luetic disease. The initial lesion is an endarteritis involving the vasa vasorum with a focal granulomatous response that spreads into the medial layer of the aorta, causing necrosis, atrophy, and scarring of smooth muscle and elastic tissue. Aneurysmal dilatation of the involved aorta is a consequence leading to dilatation of the aortic anulus and separation of the cusps at their commissural margins. The hemodynamic consequences of aortic regurgitation may lead to rolling under and thickening of the cusp margins, but obstruction to aortic outflow is not produced.

Another view of aortic regurgitation has been offered by Roberts, who reviewed 400 autopsied patients with significant valvular heart disease. Of those patients with pure aortic regurgitation and no clinical or pathological evidence of mitral valve disease, over 90 per cent had nonrheumatic aortic regurgitation. Conversely, of those with aortic regurgitation and pathological evidence of additional mitral valve disease, over 95 per cent were attributed to rheumatic fever. It follows from these considerations that while rheumatic fever is still a common cause of aortic regurgitation, other etiologies will be found in about 50 per cent of all patients, and in even a higher percentage of those in whom aortic regurgitation is the sole valvular lesion. In addition to syphilis, the other common nonrheumatic causes of aortic regurgitation may be categorized as due to a primary leaflet abnormality

(bicuspid valve, rheumatic fever, prolapse, endocarditis, trauma), loss of support for leaflet insertion (high ventricular septal defects), or dilatation of the root and separation of commissural margins (aneurysms, syphilis, rheumatoid spondylitis).

Sinus of Valsalva aneurysms are a rare and interesting cause of aortic insufficiency. Most current evidence suggests that these patients are born with a fault in the aortic media of one sinus of Valsalva. The aneurysm is not present at birth but develops later in life. In order of frequency these aneurysms involve the right sinus, the noncoronary sinus, and the left sinus. The aneurysm may grow to sufficient size to distort the anulus of the aortic valve leading to typical aortic regurgitation, or the aneurysm may rupture into one of the cardiac chambers. Aneurysms of the right sinus of Valsalva usually rupture into the right ventricle, while those of the noncoronary cusp usually rupture into the right atrium. These latter conditions are unique because the rupture produces all the classic peripheral findings of aortic regurgitation, plus those of a left-to-right shunt.

Pathophysiology. The basic hemodynamic fault in patients with aortic regurgitation is retrograde flow from the ascending aorta into the left ventricle (or rarely into the right atrium or right ventricle). When an electromagnetic flowmeter is placed around the ascending aorta at the time of surgery the pattern and amount of forward and retrograde flow throughout the cardiac cycle can be monitored (Fig. 84). During diastole, the flow is retrograde (Ao to LV). The peak retrograde flow velocity occurs shortly after the second heart sound. Retrograde flow decreases over time, but persists throughout the diastolic interval. The integral of the retrograde velocity curve can be used to quantitate regurgitant volume accurately when the internal diameter of the flow probe is known. During systole, flow is in an antegrade direction and the total stroke volume ejected by the left ventricle equals the sum of the forward stroke volume and the regurgitant volume. The ratio between the regurgitant volume and total forward stroke volume is referred to as the regurgitant fraction. Regurgitant volume and regurgitant fraction can also be estimated at the time of cardiac catheteri-

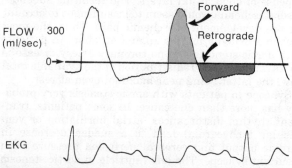

Figure 84. Flowmeter recording of phasic aortic flow of patient with moderately severe aortic regurgitation. Forward stroke volume (light stippled area above the base line) was measured as 100 ml/systole. Retrograde flow (dark stippled area below the base line) was 60 ml/diastole. Thus, retrograde flow was 60 per cent of forward flow. (With permission from Mennel, R. G., Joyner, C. R., Thompson, P. D., Pyle, R. R., and MacVaugh, H.: The preoperative and operative assessment of aortic regurgitation. Am J Cardiol 29:363, 1972.)

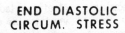

END DIASTOLIC
CIRCUM. STRESS

END DIASTOLIC
LOAD

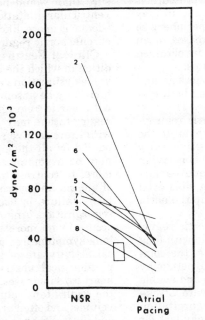

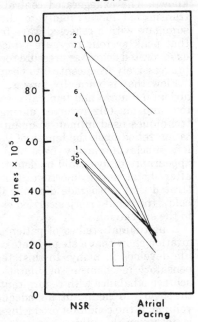

Figure 85. The effects of increasing heart rate by atrial pacing on left ventricular end-diastolic wall stress, and left ventricular end-diastolic load (the product of left ventricular pressure and the internal left ventricular surface area) in patients with aortic insufficiency. A marked reduction of both parameters is seen at higher heart rates. Small squares include the normal range. (With permission from Judge, T. P., Kennedy, J. W., Bennett, L. J., Wills, R. E., Murray, J. A., and Blackman, J. R.: Quantitative hemodynamic effects of heart rate in aortic regurgitation. Circulation 44:364, 1971.)

zation using the difference between stroke volumes measured by Fick or dye techniques and angiographic techniques. Using these techniques, regurgitant volumes of 20 to 80 ml per beat and occasionally as high as 200 ml per beat have been recorded.

From many recent reports it is evident that the regurgitant volume per beat depends greatly on hemodynamic variables other than the effective orifice size of the incompetent valve during diastole. Heart rate, because of its effect on the length of the diastolic period, is a major determinant of regurgitant volume. In aortic regurgitation, as heart rate was increased by pacing from 70 to 104 beats/min, the average duration of diastole decreased from 540 to 340 msec/beat and regurgitant flow decreased from 111 to 73 ml/beat. Similarly, pharmacological agents that enhance peripheral vascular resistance markedly increase the regurgitant flow per beat. Thus, influences that either slow the heart or augment peripheral vascular resistance enhance the diastolic volume of the left ventricle and the wall stress that must be developed during a subsequent systole in order to maintain a normal net forward stroke volume. Conversely, influences that either speed the heart and/or reduce peripheral resistance will diminish the regurgitant volume, diminish the diastolic stress of the left ventricle, and diminish the wall tension that must be developed during systole (Fig. 85).

Significant aortic regurgitation imposes a volume overload on the left ventricle that leads to left ventricular dilatation. Several investigators have reported a good correlation between regurgitant volume (the amount of aortic leak) and left ventricular end-diastolic volume. Together with the increase in end-diastolic volume, left ventricular end-diastolic pressure is also generally increased. The magnitude of this increase reflects the degree of regurgitation and the compliance of the dilated left ventricle. End-diastolic wall stress computed from end-diastolic pressure, cavity dimen-

sions, and wall thickness is always increased. The left ventricular pressure curve during systole is not grossly altered from normal in patients with aortic regurgitation, although peak left ventricular pressure may be moderately increased. The left ventricular volume at any level of developed pressure, however, is greatly exaggerated. Thus, stroke work is enhanced in proportion to the increase in total stroke volume, and the wall tension or stress that must be developed to generate that work is very greatly exaggerated.

Compare this situation to that in mitral regurgitation, wherein left ventricular volume diminishes greatly during the preejection period because of regurgitation into the low pressure left atrium. As a consequence left ventricular volume is reduced from its end-diastolic value when pressure equivalent to that in the aorta is reached. As a result, wall stress is relatively low. In aortic regurgitation, left ventricular volume remains large during the preejection period and throughout the ejection phase when pressure equivalent to that in the aorta is generated. Thus, aortic regurgitation of any given volume is a much greater stimulus to left ventricular hypertrophy than a comparable volume of mitral regurgitation. It is also not surprising to note that aortic regurgitation places a greater energy demand on the left ventricle during systole and requires a greater total oxygen consumption than does mitral regurgitation.

The increased stroke volume of the left ventricle and the diastolic leak in aortic regurgitation produce important changes in the aortic pressure pulse, pulse transmission, and patterns of flow in the aorta and its major branches. The aortic pressure pulse is greatly widened owing to an increase in peak systolic pressure, the rate of rise of systolic pressure (dp/dt), and a fall in pressure during diastole because of retrograde flow into the ventricle. The duration of left ventricular ejection is prolonged because of the increased total forward stroke volume although this increase may be blunted somewhat by a fall in peripheral vascular resistance, the mechanism for which remains unknown. The exaggerated central arterial pressure is transmitted more rapidly to the periphery. It may summate with a reflected wave from the periphery so that peak systolic pressure typically increases to an exaggerated degree as pressure recordings are obtained progressively from central to peripheral sites.

Flow that is normally forward in the thoracic and abdominal aorta and femoral vessels during both systole and diastole reverses during diastole. The first techniques used in man to quantitate aortic regurgitation relied upon the length of the aorta distal to the left subclavian artery from which a positive early appearance of dye could be detected in the subclavian after distal aortic injection. This technique demonstrated that retrograde diastolic flow from sites even below the renal arteries carried dye back up the aorta to the subclavian.

Longitudinal studies of patients with aortic regurgitation show that a steady state compatible with long life develops in many. In this steady state, the compensatory mechanisms of dilatation and hypertrophy achieve a balance with regurgitant volume and enable the heart to maintain an adequate forward stroke volume. If the condition producing aortic regurgitation is not progressive this compensated state may last for many years. Deterioration occurs if the aortic valve becomes less competent over time, if some superimposed condition such as hypertensive disease augments the amount of regurgitation, or if myocardial function deteriorates as a consequence of either coronary artery disease or progressive left ventricular hypertrophy. When deterioration develops, hemodynamic studies show that end-systolic as well as end-diastolic left ventricular volumes increase, ejection fraction declines, and mitral regurgitation may develop. The lack of an adequate forward cardiac output leads to the clinical syndrome of congestive heart failure.

At least a brief comment should be made about the condition of aortic regurgitation in which the diastolic run-off is not into the left ventricle but rather into either the right ventricle or right atrium. This situation occurs after rupture of a sinus of Valsalva aneurysm and occasionally as a consequence of bacterial endocarditis involving the sinuses of Valsalva. The peripheral signs are identical to those of typical aortic insufficiency. Furthermore, the left-to-right shunt resulting from the aortic leak is carried to the left ventricle so that a comparable volume overload on the left ventricle and resulting left ventricular hypertrophy occur. The major difference between aortic regurgitation with right ventricular run-off and left ventricular run-off is the participation of the right ventricle and pulmonary circuit in the former. As a consequence, right as well as left ventricular dilatation and hypertrophy occur, the x-ray shows evidence of increased pulmonary blood flow, and catheter studies show evidence of a left-to-right shunt. The site of this shunt can be determined by angiographic studies after injection of a contrast agent into the root of the aorta.

Acute aortic regurgitation is less well tolerated than gradually developing aortic regurgitation. In part this is because the left ventricle, which has not had time to dilate and hypertrophy, is less able to maintain an adequate forward stroke volume. Acute aortic regurgitation also produces a more marked elevation of left ventricular end-diastolic pressure and left atrial pressure than would be true if there had been time for ventricular dilatation to occur. As a result, pulmonary edema is more likely to occur with acute than with chronic aortic regurgitation.

Clinical Features. Like any cardiac valvular condition in which the hydraulic abnormality produced by valve dysfunction varies from trivial to extreme, symptoms may be absent or of varying severity in patients with aortic regurgitation. Mild to moderate aortic regurgitation may produce no symptoms at rest or with exercise. Even severe aortic regurgitation accompanied by all the signs of a large regurgitant volume may be asymptomatic and tolerated for a decade or more. In contrast to aortic stenosis, where symptoms of angina and syncope usually antedate heart failure, heart failure is usually the first symptom in aortic regurgitation. Angina is a late symptom and syncope occurs in no more than 10 per cent of patients. The long symptom-free period and the tolerance for physical activity are of great interest with respect to the physiological observations concerning the effects of heart rate increases. An increase in heart rate reduces the regurgitant volume per beat, reduces end-diastolic volume, and often dramatically reduces left ventricular end-diastolic pressure. When patients with mild or moderate aortic insufficiency exercise, heart rate increases and exercise also leads to peripheral vasodilatation. Both of these changes favorably affect left ventricular end-diastolic volume and pressure and produce either no change or a decrease in systolic wall stress per beat. These favorable effects of left ventricular function contrast with the hemodynamic changes that accompany exercise in most other valvular conditions—that is, mitral stenosis, mitral regurgitation, and aortic stenosis, where the demand for an increase in cardiac output is usually accompanied by a rise in left atrial pressure and by pulmonary congestion.

When angina develops in patients with aortic regurgitation, the regurgitant volume is usually very large. Hypertrophy, which is usually prominent in these patients, markedly increases the need for coronary blood flow. This need is further augmented by the high wall stress that must be developed by the dilated ventricle to maintain a normal aortic pressure and enhanced total forward stroke volume. The reduction of aortic diastolic pressure and the increased diastolic wall stress both contribute to a reduction in the pressure gradient needed to provide coronary perfusion to the hypertrophied left ventricle. Clinical investigators for years have noted that angina in aortic regurgitation is often atypical: it occurs frequently at rest, in the recumbent position, and very often during sleep. This anomalous situation again raises the question of whether the unusual hemodynamic response of recumbency—that is, bradycardia, increased regurgitant fraction, increased ventricular volume and wall stress, and reduced diastolic aortic pressure—may not cause subendocardial ischemia on a purely hydraulic basis.

Syncope in aortic regurgitation has been correlated with the presence of ventricular ectopic activity and is presumed to reflect transient arrhythmias. Syncope is sufficiently infrequent, however, and studies of this phenomenon are so few that a definitive statement regarding its mechanism cannot be made.

Premature ventricular contractions are common and because the first beat after the compensatory pause has a greater stroke volume, patients may sense a "hard beat" or "thumping" sensation, particularly when supine and lying on the left side.

The most reliable signs of severe aortic regurgitation are noted on examination of the arterial pressure pulse. The augmented stroke volume produces a prominent and rapid rise of the arterial pressure pulse while the subsequent diastolic collapse of the pulse relates to regurgitation per se. The waterhammer pulse (a slapping peripheral pulse), audible pistol shots (explosive sounds synchronous with systole noted on auscultation over the femoral arteries), alternating pallor/rubor of the nail beds (capillary pulse), and the bobbing of the head synchronous with the heartbeat are all a consequence of the altered arterial pressure pulse. The prominent and rapidly rising arterial pressure pulse sometimes produces a very marked reflected wave in late systole, which at the brachial or carotid arteries may be felt as a double systolic pulse or bisferious pulse. When a stethoscope is placed over the femoral arteries and compressed to indent the artery, turbulence is created and heard as an audible systolic murmur. When aortic regurgitation is severe, diastolic retrograde flow in the femoral artery can be very prominent and with proper pressure by the stethoscope not only is a systolic murmur heard, but also a separate diastolic murmur (Duroziez's sign). The apical impulse in severe aortic regurgitation is typically enlarged, laterally displaced, and hyperdynamic, rolling briskly under the examiner's palpating fingers.

Auscultation in patients with aortic regurgitation is dominated by the finding of an aortic diastolic murmur. The typical murmur is a diastolic high frequency (or blowing) murmur best heard along the left sternal border and radiating to the apex. The murmur is created by the diastolic jet through the incompetent valve. Occasionally, the murmur has a musical, cooing, or so-called sea gull character reflecting a pure frequency component usually related to vibrations of a ruptured, everted, or prolapsed semilunar cusp. When the murmur of aortic regurgitation is best heard along the right sternal border, aneurysmal dilatation of the aorta should be suspected.

Rapid filling of the left ventricle in aortic regurgitation commonly produces a loud S_3. In mid or late diastole left ventricular pressure rises to near that in the left atrium and tends to appose the leaflets of the mitral valve. The Austin-Flint murmur (a mid-diastolic and/or presystolic rumble) in aortic regurgitation has been ascribed to continuing flow from left atrium to left ventricle across a partially closed mitral valve. Strong evidence in support of this view has been provided by correlations between mitral valve movement assessed by echocardiography and the Austin-Flint murmur as recorded by phonocardiography. In general, the Austin-Flint murmur indicates at least moderate, if not severe, aortic regurgitation.

Laboratory Findings. The radiographic features of aortic regurgitation reflect the consequences of relatively marked and isolated left ventricular dilatation and hypertrophy. The entire thoracic aorta is also typically dilated. Aortic regurgitation is best seen by fluoroscopy, in which the left ventricle is dilated and hyperdynamic pulsations of the aorta are evident. The EKG shows signs of left ventricular hypertrophy. Left atrial hypertrophy occurs when left ventricular end-diastolic pressure and hence mean left atrial pressure are increased. The most typical echocardiographic finding in aortic regurgitation is a fluttering movement of the anterior mitral leaflet in diastole produced by the regurgitant jet. In the young, an eccentrically located leaflet within the aortic root may reveal a bicuspid leaflet. Frequently, the aortic valve leaflets do not show gross deformity by echo, although flail leaflets, prolapsing leaflets, aortic dissections, aortic root dilatation, and the vegetations of bacterial endocarditis have been noted.

REFERENCES

Braunwald, E.: Mitral regurgitation: Physiological, clinical and surgical considerations. N Engl J Med 281:425, 1969.

Braunwald, E., Roberts, W. C., Goldblatt, A., Aygen, M. M., Rockoff, S. D., and Gilbert, J. W.: Aortic stenosis: Physiological, pathological and clinical concepts. Ann Intern Med 58:494, 1963.

Dalen, J. E., and Alpert, J. S. (eds.): Valvular Heart Disease. Boston, Little, Brown and Company, 1981.

Dodge, H. T., Kennedy, J. W., and Petersen, J. L.: Quantitative angiographic methods in the evaluation of valvular heart disease. Prog Cardiovasc Dis 16:1, 1973.

Friedman, W. F., and Braunwald, E.: Alterations in regional pulmonary blood flow in mitral valve disease studied by radioisotope scanning: A simple nontraumatic technique for estimation of left atrial pressure. Circulation 34:363, 1966.

Goldschlager, N., Pfeifer, J., Cohn, K., Popper, R., and Selzer, A.: The natural history of aortic regurgitation: A clinical and hemodynamic study. Am J Med 54:577, 1973.

Judge, T. P., Kennedy, J. W., Bennett, L. J., Willis, R. E., Murray, J. A., and Blackmon, J. R.: Quantitative hemodynamic effects of heart rate in aortic regurgitation. Circulation 44:355, 1971.

Mark, A. L., Kioschos, J. M., Abboud, F. W., Heistad, D. D., and Schmid, P. G.: Abnormal vascular responses to exercise in patients with aortic stenosis. J Clin Invest 52:1138, 1973.

Nichol, P. M., Gilbert, B. W., and Kisslo, J. A.: Two-dimensional echocardiographic assessment of mitral stenosis. Circulation 55:120, 1977.

Perloff, J. K., and Roberts, W. C.: The mitral apparatus: Functional anatomy of mitral regurgitation. Circulation 46:227, 1972.

Roberts, W. C.: Anatomically isolated aortic valvular disease: The case against its being of rheumatic etiology. Am J Med 49:151, 1970.

Vincent, W. R., Buckberg, G. D., and Hoffman, J. I. E.: Left ventricular subendocardial ischemia in severe valvar and supravalvar aortic stenosis: A common mechanism. Circulation 49:326, 1974.

Wood, P.: An appreciation of mitral stenosis. Br Med J 1:1051, II: 1113, 1954.

Myocardial Hypertrophy

Myocardial hypertrophy is defined as a condition in which the cardiac mass is greater than normal relative to the size of the organism whose circulation must be sustained. Hypertrophy is a response to increased work whether that work reflects a demand for increased volume of blood flow (as in anemia, exercise, or valvular regurgitation) or increased resistance to the flow of a normal volume (obstruction at the pulmonic or aortic valve or increased resistance of the pulmonary or systemic arterial beds). Hypertrophy occurs in any part of the heart that participates in increased work, and hence may involve one or more chambers.

Nearly all organs in the body grow during the course of normal maturation. This growth involves one of two fundamental processes. One of these is hyperplasia, the process by which cells multiply by mitotic division. The other process is hypertrophy of a fixed number of cells due to synthesis of additional cellular components but without replication of the cell through mitotic division. Normal growth of the heart falls into the hypertrophic category, there being no evidence that cardiac muscle cells divide after birth. The concept that myocardial hypertrophy is an extension of normal growth and does not involve hyperplasia of muscle cells is fundamental. One corollary to this fact is that muscle cells have the genetic capacity to direct the synthesis and assembly of cellular components over a wide continuum of cell size, ranging from that which is characteristic of the neonatal heart, to normal adult size (approximately 15 to 20 μ cell diameter), to that of extreme hypertrophy, which may be 15 to 30 μ. A second corollary is that synthesis and degradation of cellular components must be controlled and coupled by some mechanism to the work load or physiological stress placed on the myofibers.

To understand the functional consequences of hypertrophy it is useful to approach the problem from several points of view. The first involves a structural or morphometric analysis of the participation of various intracellular organelles in the growth process, and the alterations that seem to distinguish normal or adaptive growth on the one hand from pathological enlargement on the other. A second point of view recognizes that the components of a muscle cell, with the exception of its nucleus, are in a constant and rapid state of turnover. Thus, to understand the process by which a cardiac cell grows from its normal size to some larger size requires insight into the biochemical mechanisms involved in the synthesis and degradation of proteins.

The physiological consequences of growth can be appreciated only if we understand certain behavioral characteristics of cellular organelles, such as the contractile proteins and mitochondria of hypertrophied cells, the mechanics of hypertrophied muscle, and the physiological alterations at an organ level, which may not be obvious from studies of isolated muscle. Finally, while hypertrophy can be regarded as adaptive and compensatory up to a point, there is clearly a limit to this process beyond which function, whether evaluated at the level of the organ, the muscle, or the cell or its organelles, deteriorates. Hence, at one extreme we have the problem of distinguishing normal growth from pathological hypertrophy and at the other extreme pathological hypertrophy from decompensation.

During morphometric and stereological studies of normal postnatal growth of heart cells, while weight increased by a factor of three, there was no evidence of an increase in the number of myocytes. Rather, cell dimensions and the volume of individual cells increased in proportion to total heart weight and to body weight. With the increase in cell volume there was an apparent decrease in cell surface membranes in proportion to cell volume. This conclusion was based upon calculations in which external cell surface area was derived from surface sarcolemma alone. Subsequently, when it became evident that transverse tubules (T tubules) were invaginations of surface sarcolemma and participated in cell growth, recalculations of cell surface area that include the composite surface (external sarcolemma plus T tubules) yielded surface-to-volume ratios that changed very little during normal growth (Fig. 86). The percentage of cell volume occupied by myofibrils and by mitochondria remained relatively constant (approximately 45 per cent and 35 per cent respectively). Myofibrillar proteins, mitochondria, and cell volume therefore increased by approximately equal proportions during normal growth. Furthermore, the ratio of sarcoplasmic reticulum to myofibrillar volume remains constant during normal growth, indicating that the sarcoplasmic reticulum also participates in cell growth. The picture that emerges is one in which surface membrane, contractile proteins, sarcoplasmic

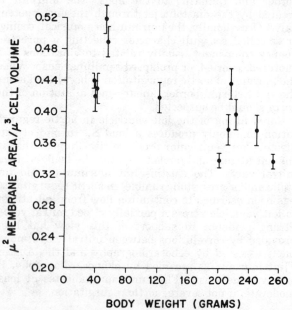

Figure 86. Composite surface:volume ratio (membrane area of external sarcolemma + T-system/unit cell volume) as a function of body weight during normal growth. (With permission from Page, E., Earley, J., and Power, B.: Normal growth of ultrastructures in rat left ventricular myocardial cells. Circ Res 34 + 35:II-15, 1974.)

reticulum, and mitochondria all increase in a relatively uniform manner during normal growth. In contrast, the size of the nucleus in cardiac myocytes remains relatively constant through growth, and hence nuclear volume in proportion to cell volume diminishes progressively as heart weight and body weight increase. This observation implies that there is a substantial reserve capacity for the DNA content of the nucleus to synthesize the increased amounts of messenger RNA needed to direct normal growth. Even in normal cardiac muscle the nuclei are hyperchromatic and contain polyploid amounts of DNA.

A variety of experimental procedures have been developed that produce a comparable increase in cardiac mass. In some, the work overload is induced by an increase in pressure produced by the ventricle (aortic constriction), in others by a volume stimulus (AV fistula or exercise) and in still others by a hormonal stimulus, such as excessive thyroid hormone. In each form of resulting hypertrophy, the increase in mass is principally due to an increase in muscle cell size and to a lesser extent hyperplasia of connective tissue elements. The extent to which connective tissue participates in hypertrophy is variable, being maximal with a pressure stress and least with exercise.

Regardless of the stimulus that elicits hypertrophy, the myocytes appear to increase in length, in diameter, and in volume. However, the pattern of accumulation of intracellular components differs with the stimulus. With a pressure stress, myofibrillar volume and mitochondrial volume both increase, but the increase in myofibrillar protein is much greater than the increase in mitochondrial volume. With exercise or a volume overload the increase in myofibrils and mitochondria is proportional. With excessive thyroid hromone myofibrillar and mitochondrial volume both increase, but the increase in mitochondria is much greater. In all of these states, the accumulation of sarcoplasmic reticulum tends to parallel the increase in contractile proteins, and a normal ratio of composite membrane surface area to cell volume is maintained.

With any given stimulus to heart growth, the pattern of intracellular components varies with time and with the stage of hypertrophy. An increase in mitochondrial volume appears to be the earliest morphometric change in developing hypertrophy, followed by synthesis of new myofibrillar proteins. Similarly, the proliferation of connective tissue cells appears early and is followed by enhanced collagen synthesis. Stable compensated hypertrophy is characterized by an increase in cell size, a pattern of intracellular components consistent with the stimulus leading to hypertrophy, and a new steady state with respect to the reactions responsible for synthesis and degradation of cellular components. After months or years of stable hyperfunction of the hypertrophied heart, heart failure generally ensues. During this late stage the capacity for protein synthesis diminishes, mitochondrial volume diminishes, and mitochondrial structure is altered. Large numbers of myocytes develop vacuolization, fat accumulation, and atrophy; and additional collagen is deposited in the interstitial space leading to progressive cardiofibrosis.

Much of the published work on biochemical changes associated with hypertrophy has focused on the synthesis and turnover of myofibrillar proteins and on mitochondria, since these components are known to increase in hypertrophy and are ultimately responsible for the capacity of the sarcomere to contract and to provide the energy necessary to contract. Myofibrillar proteins (actin, myosin, troponin, and tropomyosin) are synthesized on polyribosomes located within the cytosol of the cell. Messenger RNA is transcribed from nuclear genetic material (DNA) within the nucleus. Messenger RNA passes out of the nucleus into the cytosol carrying the genetic code and attaches to ribosomes. Amino acids enter the cytosol from blood, become activated in the presence of ATP and enzyme, and then in the presence of aminoacyl tRNA synthetase are coupled to tRNA. Each type of tRNA appears capable of binding a specific amino acid, and the mid portion of the tRNA polynucleotide contains a specific site (the anticodon) that attaches to mRNA at a specific site (the codon). In this manner, amino acids are lined up on the ribosome in a sequence determined by the sequence of codon words in mRNA. The polypeptide generated on the ribosome is formed by peptide bonds between adjacent amino acids and the simultaneous separation of the polypeptide chain from mRNA. The length of the polypeptide chain is determined by code words on mRNA that start (initiate) and stop (terminate) the formation of a chain.

During the developing phase of experimental cardiac hypertrophy, there is an increase in amino acid transport into the heart, an increase in both ribosomal and transfer RNA, and increased incorporation of C^{14} labeled amino acids into myofibrillar protein. Despite this evidence favoring increased synthesis as a basis for the accumulation of myofibrillar protein, precise measurement of the rates of synthesis of myosin and other contractile proteins has been difficult because of problems in estimating the specific activity of direct protein precursors.

Because myofibrillar proteins are in a continuous state of turnover, a decrease in the degradation rate of these proteins is an equally tenable hypothesis for their accumulation during developing hypertrophy. During the development of hypertrophy, both synthesis and degradation of protein are accelerated. However, rates of synthesis appear to exceed rates of degradation until a new steady state is achieved at the larger stable mass.

Assembly of mitochondria is apparently more complex than that of myofibrillar proteins because this organelle is itself composed of more components and because synthesis of these components involves two genetically separate subsystems. Mitochondria contain DNA, messenger and transfer RNA, ribosomes, and amino acids. Isolated mitochondria are endowed with the machinery for and capability of synthesizing up to 10 per cent of their own protein. Other mitochondrial proteins are synthesized on cytoplasmic ribosomes under nuclear genetic control and then transported into the mitochondrion for incorporation into mitochondrial components. Following aortic constriction, mitochondrial mass increases, the activity of mitochondrial respiratory enzymes increases, and the incorporation of labeled amino acid precursors into mitochondrial proteins increases. On the other hand, the specific activity of labeled enzymes within purified mitochondria does not increase. These data have been interpreted as evidence in favor of synthesis of additional mitochondrial mass. In the normal heart, turnover of mitochondria and of mitochondrial proteins such as cytochrome C labeled with a nonreusable precursor (aminolevulinic acid) is approximately 5.5 days. Following aortic constriction the amount of cytochrome C increases to higher levels than in sham-operated animals, and during the early phase of developing hypertrophy its half-life is prolonged, indicating a decreased rate of degradation. It seems reasonable to conclude that the increase in mitochondrial mass following a stimulus that produces hypertrophy involves both an increased rate of synthesis and a decreased rate of degradation.

Although a substantial amount of information has accrued in recent years regarding the morphology and biochemical characteristics of hypertrophied cardiac cells, relatively little is understood about the biochemical signal that couples an increased workload to muscle growth. One popular hypothesis states that the level of high energy phosphate stores influences the rate of protein synthesis and/or degradation within the cell. This hypothesis attaches particular significance to the ADP:ATP ratio, the so-called phosphorylation potential, in regulating the rates of protein synthesis. According to this proposal, increased work would result in increased utilization of ATP and higher levels of ADP. The altered ADP:ATP ratio would then stimulate protein synthesis. An increase in contractile proteins would distribute the increased work over a larger number of sarcomeres and an increase in the number and size of mitochondria would provide greater capacity for ATP generation. Once this capacity restores a normal ADP:ATP ratio, the stimulus for continued growth would be negated. In the chapter dealing with normal metabolism of the heart we have seen important examples in which enzyme activity is regulated by high energy phosphates and their derivatives. Other hypotheses regarding the coupling of work and growth include the possibility (1) that products of cell metabolism other than ADP and creatine may induce or derepress protein synthesis, (2) that cyclic AMP may regulate protein synthesis at the level of RNA transcription, and (3) that products of metabolism and hormones may influence the activity of degradative enzymes.

In recent years a number of investigators have attempted to gain insight into the function of the hypertrophied heart through studies of the mechanics of muscle isolated from preparations in which cardiac hypertrophy was induced experimentally. Recall that the response of the heart to stresses that induce hypertrophy is variable. The extent to which connective tissue hyperplasia and collagen synthesis participate in the increased myocardial mass differs with the stimulus causing hypertrophy and the duration of the stimulus. At an ultrastructural level, an increase in both myofibrillar and mitochondrial volume contributes to enlargement of myocardial cells, but the extent of this participation of subcellular organelles is not always parallel. It is not surprising that the functional consequences of hypertrophy are also variable, and relate, at least in part, to the stimulus causing the increased myocardial mass.

Most investigators regard cardiac hypertrophy as a fundamental response to hyperfunction, and they view the associated increase in muscle mass as compensatory in the sense that an increase in the number of sarcomeres may provide the contractile units necessary to sustain an increased work load. The question of whether or not hypertrophy is beneficial can be addressed in two ways. First, is the hypertrophied heart capable of performing more work than normal? Second, what are the contractile characteristics of hypertrophied muscle per unit of mass?

The answer to the first question is fairly straightforward. When the heart is subjected to moderate stress (increased preload, increased afterload, or exercise) and a sufficient period of time is allowed for stable hyperfunction and hypertrophy to develop, the heart is capable of performing more than normal work. The preparations in which this increased capacity for pump performance have been observed include the following: (1) AV fistula, (2) banding of the pulmonary artery, (3) banding of the aorta, and (4) chronic exercise conditioning. The evidence of an increased work capacity of the heart in these preparations includes the following: (1) a higher maximal cardiac output during volume loading of the hypertrophied ventricle and (2) a higher peak systolic pressure developed during isovolumic contraction at any given initial volume. Studies of the temporal sequence of these changes indicate that the increase in the capacity for pump performance parallels the increase in myocardial mass.

The answer to the second question is more complex.

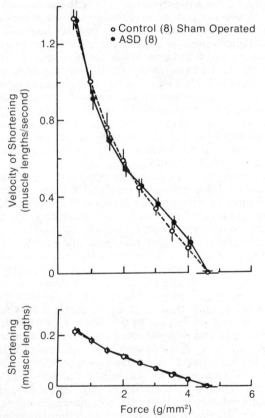

Figure 87. Top: Average force-velocity values ± 1 SE for papillary muscles from eight sham-operated control cats and eight atrial septal defect (ASD) cats. Bottom: Extent of shortening vs force. (With permission from Cooper, G., Puga, F. J., Zujko, K. J., Harrison, C. E., and Coleman, H. N.: Normal myocardial function and energetics in volume-overload hypertrophy in the cat. Circ Res 32:143, 1973.)

When right ventricular hypertrophy was produced in cats by creating an atrial septal defect (volume overload), there was a nearly twofold increase in right ventricular weight and in the size of right ventricular papillary muscles. To compare muscles of different sizes, results were normalized in terms of muscle length and cross-sectional area. The curve that related developed tension (grams/mm²) to length, the force velocity curve, and the oxygen consumption per milligram of tissue at any given load were all superimposable when hypertrophied and normal muscle were compared (Figs. 87 and 88). It was concluded that contractility and energetics in volume overload hypertrophy without failure were normal per unit of muscle mass. Comparable results have been reported for exercise-induced hypertrophy. Contrasting results were reported when right ventricular hypertrophy was induced in cats by pulmonary artery banding. The degree of increase in right ventricular mass in these animals was nearly identical (twofold increase) to those with volume overload, but peak isometric tension at any given length and the velocity of shortening at any given load were substantially depressed when hypertrophied muscles were compared with normal (Fig. 89). This decrease in contractile function per unit mass following pressure-induced hypertrophy develops in the absence of clinical or hemodynamic evidence of heart failure.

Because of the known relation between myosin ATPase activity and the intrinsic velocity of muscle shortening, it is understandable that the changes in muscle shortening velocity in different forms of myocardial hypertrophy led a number of investigators to characterize this enzymatic activity of cardiac myosin in pathological states. While it is premature to draw a general picture of myosin ATPase activity in all forms and degrees of hypertrophy, several interesting observations are of note. Myosin ATPase activity has been shown to increase in cardiac hypertrophy that accompanies exercise or thyrotoxicosis and to decrease in chronic pressure overload hypertrophy and heart failure. A correlation between myosin ATPase activity and contractile function in these forms of hypertrophy has been established. The possibility that depressed or enhanced ATPase activity represents a consequence of synthesis of myosin of a different primary structure is

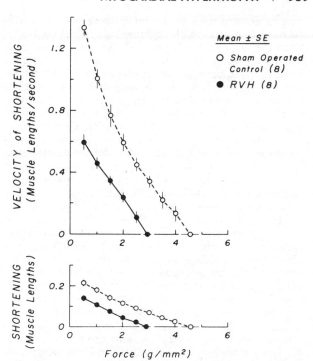

Figure 89. Top: Average force-velocity values ± SE for papillary muscles from eight sham-operated control cats and eight RVH cats. Bottom: Extent of shortening vs total applied force (load). (With permission from Cooper, G., Satava, R. M., Harrison, C. E., and Coleman, H. N.: Mechanism for the abnormal energetics of pressure-induced hypertrophy of cat myocardium. Circ Res 33:216, 1973.)

an area of investigation of potentially great significance.

In addition to the contractile differences between volume- and pressure-overload ventricles, there also appear to be significant differences in diastolic properties. In hypertrophy due to a pressure overload, the pressure-volume curve of the involved ventricle is shifted to the left and is steeper. Not only is the ventricle stiffer, but the passive stiffness of muscle removed from these ventricles is also increased. With chronic volume overload, the pressure-volume curve is shifted to the right (that is, lower pressure at any given volume). The relation between wall stress and stiffness of these ventricles indicates a slightly enhanced compliance.

Our knowledge of the functional consequences of cardiac hypertrophy in man have been greatly aided by the development of angiographic techniques to estimate the dimensions of the ventricle, its volume, thickness, and mass. The majority of such studies have focused on the left ventricle, because it is more often evaluated in acquired heart disease and its geometry is better defined. In general, patients have been divided into those with chronic volume and chronic pressure overload states. It is pertinent in either state to separate patients into those with compensated hypertrophy (normal cardiac index and ejection fraction) and those with decompensation (reduced cardiac index and ejection fraction).

In patients with compensated left ventricular hypertrophy due to volume overload (that is, aortic and mitral regurgitation), the increase in total stroke vol-

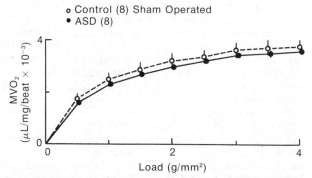

Figure 88. Average oxygen consumption values ± 1 SE for the muscles depicted in Figure 87. MVO₂ = Myocardial oxygen consumption. (With permission from Cooper, G., Puga, F. J., Kujko, K. J., Harrison, C. E., and Coleman, H. N.: Normal myocardial function and energetics in volume-overload hypertrophy in the cat. Circ Res 32:144, 1973.)

ume is accompanied by an increase in both the end-diastolic and end-systolic volumes of the left ventricle. However, the relation between stroke volume and end-diastolic volume is such that the ejection fraction remains near normal (two thirds of the end-diastolic volume) and forward cardiac output, at least at rest, is normal. Cardiac mass increases with chronic volume overload, but the cardiac size is due principally to an expanded chamber volume with only a modest increase in wall thickness. With compensated chronic pressure overloads, end-diastolic and end-systolic volumes, ejection fraction, and stroke volume are all nearly normal. The left ventricular mass increases, principally as the result of an increase in wall thickness.

Most investigators regard the energy requirements of increased contractile work to be the signal that causes hypertrophy. There is an excellent correlation between left ventricular stroke work and left ventricular mass regardless of the valvular condition that produced the hypertrophy (Fig. 90). This observation led Dodge to speculate that the extent of hypertrophy was closely coupled to the stimulus for energy requiring contractile activity—namely, stroke work.

The correlation between left ventricular mass and stroke work is improved if patients are subgrouped on the basis of their ejection fraction. An important result of studying subgroups was the finding that as ejection fraction fell below normal, reflecting decompensation, the mass for any given external stroke work became greater. This observation led to the conclusion that not only is hypertrophy a response to increased work load, but hypertrophy is also an attempt to compensate for deteriorating myocardial function at the end-stage of either chronic volume- or pressure-overloaded states. This conclusion is consistent with the observation that

hypertrophy may be a consequence of primary or of secondary myocardial disease, such as coronary disease. In the first, the initial event is a diminished contractile function, while in the second diminished performance results from deletion of contractile units as a consequence of necrosis or infarction.

The concept that hypertrophy is a compensatory response originated with Linzbach, who postulated that an increase in sarcomeres and in wall thickness provided the ventricle with a mechanism by which the increase in wall stress could be distributed over a larger surface and hence restore the stress per unit of cross-section to normal. The most widely accepted formula for calculating average circumferential wall stress at the equator of the left ventricle is:

$$\text{Stress } (\sigma) = \frac{P \cdot r_m}{h}\left[1 - \frac{r_m^3}{a^2(2\,r_m + h)} \right]$$

Where:

σ = wall stress
P = left ventricular pressure
r_m = mid-wall radius
h = thickness
a = base-to-apex length

From this formula it is apparent that stress will increase with an increase in left ventricular pressure or with an increase in volume, resulting in an increase in r_m. On the other hand, an increase in thickness (h) will tend to diminish stress at any given pressure and volume.

Ventricular wall stress in a large number of patients with compensated volume and pressure overloads was evaluated and compared with wall stress in normal subjects. Peak wall stress was not significantly different from normal in either form of hypertrophy. An increase in wall thickness consequent to hypertrophy tends to normalize wall stress and is consistent with the view that hypertrophy is compensatory in the sense that it maintains a nearly normal work requirement for each sarcomere.

We have noted before that with decompensation, the left ventricular ejection fraction falls. The heart dilates and the mass increases out of proportion to the external work load. In patients with decompensation due to either a volume or pressure overload, peak systolic wall stress is greater than normal. In man and in nearly all experimental models of hypertrophy, decompensation is accompanied by a marked decrease in any index of myocardial contractile function. This mechanical defect has been correlated with a decrease in myosin ATPase activity. Tissues removed from decompensated hearts demonstrate a diminished capacity of sarcoplasmic reticulum for binding calcium, and mitochondria are defective with respect to respiratory control and calcium accumulation. The oxygen consumption per gram of hypertrophied muscle is either normal or increased at any given work level, despite the decrease in contractility and myosin ATPase activity. Whether this apparent change in the efficiency of hypertrophied muscle is due to an increase in nonphosphorylating respiratory activities of the cell or to the partitioning of energy expenditure between mechanical function and heat production has not been resolved. The most important conclusion from these studies is that hypertrophy is compensatory in that it

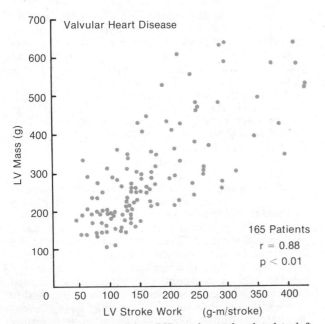

Figure 90. Left ventricular (LV) stroke work related to left ventricular mass in 165 subjects with various types of valvular lesions, many of which impose pressure and/or volume overloads on the left ventricle. (With permission from Dodge, H. T., Frimer, M., and Stewart, D. K.: Functional evaluation of hypertrophied heart in man. Circ Res 34 + 35:II-123, 1974.)

permits the heart to meet increased demands for work. But hypertrophy is not without cost. Advanced hypertrophy, regardless of cause, leads to a decrease in contractile function, a decrease in myosin ATPase activity, and alterations in the energetics of the muscle. Muscle removed from hypertrophied and decompensated hearts demonstrated an exaggeration of these abnormalities.

REFERENCES

Alpert, N. R., and Mulieri, L. A.: The partitioning of altered mechanics in hypertrophied heart muscle between the sarcoplasmic reticulum and the contractile apparatus by means of myothermal measurements. Basic Res Cardiol 72:153, 1977.

Cooper, G., IV, Puga, F. J., Zujko, K. J., Harrison, C. E., and Coleman, H. N., III: Normal myocardial function and energetics in volume-overload hypertrophy in the cat. Circ Res 32:140, 1973.

Cooper, G., IV, Satava, R. M., Jr., Harrison, C. E., and Coleman, H. N., III: Mechanism of the abnormal energetics of pressure-induced hypertrophy of cat myocardium. Circ Res 33:213, 1973.

Dodge, H. T., Frimer, M., and Stewart, D. K.: Functional evaluation of hypertrophied heart in man. Circ Res 34–35:II–122, 1974.

Everett, A. W., and Zak, R.: Problems and interpretations of techniques used in studies of protein turnover. In Wildenthal, K. (ed.): Degradative Processes in Heart and Skeletal Muscle. Amsterdam, Elsevier Press, 1980, p. 31.

Hamrell, B. B., and Alpert, N. R.: The mechanical characteristics of hypertrophied rabbit cardiac muscle in the absence of congestive heart failure. Circ Res 40:20, 1977.

Hood, W. P., Jr., Rackley, C. E., and Rolett, E. L.: Wall stress in the normal and hypertrophied human left ventricle. Am J Cardiol 22:550, 1968.

Martin, A. F., Rabinowitz, M., Blough, R., Prior, G., and Zak, R.: Measurements of half-life of rat cardiac myosin heavy chains with leucyl-tRNA as a precursor pool. J Biol Chem 252:3422, 1977.

Meerson, F. A.: The myocardium in hyperfunction, hypertrophy and heart failure. Circ Res 25:II–1, 1969.

Morgan, H. E., Rannels, D. E., and McKee, E. E.: Protein metabolism of the heart. In Berne, R. M., Sperelakis, N., and Geiger, S. R. (eds.): Handbook of Physiology. Section 2, The Cardiovascular System. Vol. I, The Heart. Bethesda, Md., American Physiological Society, 1979, p. 845.

Morkin, E., Kimata, S., and Skillman, J. J.: Myosin synthesis and degradation during development of cardiac hypertrophy in the rabbit. Circ Res 30:690, 1972.

Page, E., Polimeni, P. I., Zak, R., Earley, J., and Johnson, M.: Myofibrillar mass in rat and rabbit heart muscle: Correlation of microchemical and stereological measurements in normal and hypertrophic hearts. Circ Res 30:430, 1972.

Coronary Heart Disease

Atherosclerosis of the coronary arteries is by far the most common cause of myocardial ischemia. Its ultimate consequence, myocardial infarction, is the single most common cause of death among adults in Western cultures. Autopsies in large communities reveal coronary atherosclerosis in 70 to 75 per cent of all cases; at least half of American military casualties during the Korean conflict (mean age in the twenties) had evidence of this disease. Hence, coronary atherosclerosis is extremely prevalent and has its origins in early life (see chapter on atherosclerosis).

ANATOMIC CONSIDERATIONS

When coronary atherosclerosis has reached the stage of producing ischemia, the disease is usually extensive (Fig. 91). In a study of 107 cases of fatal myocardial infarction, coronary arteries were examined in great detail (a minimum of two cross sections every 5 mm of the left main, anterior descending, circumflex, and right arteries). Although the degree of luminal narrowing varied, only four of several thousand cross sections were free of disease. One might argue logically that autopsy material in fatal infarction would provide an overly biased estimate of the extent of disease in symptomatic living patients. While it is clear that angina pectoris and other manifestations of coronary artery disease occur in some patients with focal, as opposed to diffuse, disease, the burden of evidence still indicates that the extramural coronary arteries are extensively involved in most patients when symptoms present. Extensive disease is also found at autopsy

when sudden death is the initial clinical manifestation of coronary disease. A second line of evidence is that coronary arteriography, which typically underestimates the amount of disease, commonly shows at least

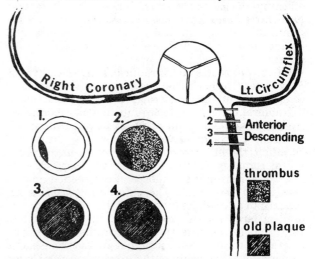

Figure 91. Diagram illustrating the diffuse nature of coronary atherosclerosis and the usual status of a vessel at and distal to a thrombus. At level 2 in the anterior descending artery the lumen is obstructed primarily by a thrombus. At level 3, however, the major per cent of narrowing is the result of old atherosclerotic plaquing, and just distal to the thrombus the lumen is severely narrowed (more than 75 per cent) or totally obstructed by old plaque only. (With permission from Roberts, W. C., and Buja, L. M.: The frequency and significance of coronary arterial thrombi and other observations in fatal acute myocardial infarction. Am J Med 52:430, 1972.)

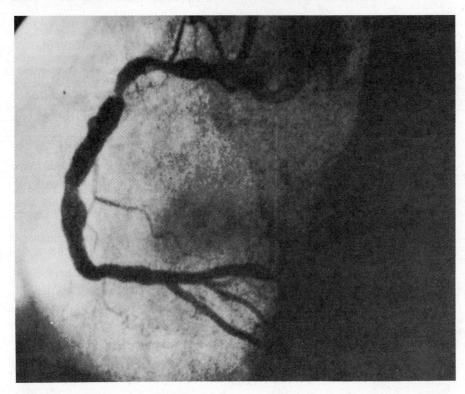

Figure 92. Right coronary artery, LAO projectional. Note multiple areas of ectasia throughout and two zones of moderate narrowing in the proximal portion of the vessel. (With permission from Gensini, G. G.: Coronary Arteriography. Mt. Kisco, N.Y., Futura Publishing Co., 1975, p. 245.)

minor involvement of all three coronary arteries in patients with angina. Finally, when surgical approaches are used to bypass high grade proximal obstructions in the major coronary vessels, these high grade obstructions, while relatively focal, are contiguous with areas of less severe distal disease (Fig. 92).

It is extremely important to make a distinction between atherosclerosis, which is a diffuse process affecting the coronary arterial tree but which may have little or no physiological consequence, and hydraulically significant lesions that compromise flow during situations of high myocardial demand or even at rest.

What constitutes a hydraulically significant coronary artery lesion? The answer to this question is complex. First, under normal conditions the major extramural coronary arteries function as conduits between the aorta and an array of intramural vessels that supply blood to the ventricular wall. In the normal situation, the major resistance to flow is in the intramural coronary vessels, and this resistance changes phasically during the sequence of contraction and relaxation of the heart. The extramural arteries are referred to as conduits (a) because their cross-sectional area is large relative to normally encountered flow rates and (b) because there is a negligible pressure drop along these arteries such that pressures measured in very distal segments of the extramural vessels are essentially identical to aortic pressure. When the lumen of an extramural coronary artery is narrowed, the lesion is defined as hydraulically significant when a pressure gradient is produced across the constricted segment. The magnitude of this pressure gradient for any given degree of constriction will vary with the flow rate through the vessel. The flow rate will be determined by aortic perfusion pressure and the total coronary resistance—that is, the sum of resistances at the

level of the constriction and at the level of the intramural and nutrient vessels. Hence, when total coronary resistance is high due to a large intramural resistance, flow rate will be low and an 80 to 90 per cent reduction in the lumen of an epicardial vessel will produce a minimal drop in distal coronary perfusion pressure. On the other hand, if intramural resistance is small and coronary flow rate is high, a much smaller reduction in the caliber of an epicardial vessel will result in a pressure gradient and a consequent reduction in coronary perfusion pressure.

Whenever a lesion in an extramural vessel is sufficient to produce a pressure drop in the distal coronary artery, the distribution of flow in the vascular bed perfused by that artery is altered. When the circumflex coronary artery is narrowed to a degree that drops distal coronary pressure from 122/84 (average aortic pressure) to 80/35 mm Hg, total flow through the circumflex artery is unaltered. However, even this small gradient reduced the ratio of endocardial to epicardial flow from a control value of 1.12 to 0.6—that is, a situation of marked subendocardial underperfusion.

In evaluating the significance of a coronary atherosclerotic lesion, the lesion must be considered in terms of its physiological consequence—namely, whether or not it produces a significant drop in distal coronary perfusion pressure and if so under what circumstances (for example, myocardial work level). A lesion that compromises the lumen will be more significant in a vessel with a large distal vascular bed than the same lesion in a vessel with a smaller distal vascular bed. In general, the significance of any given degree of luminal reduction will be proportional to the diameter of the involved artery.

Returning to the pathology of coronary atherosclerosis, at least three additional points are worthy of note. Atherosclerosis is a disease principally, if not solely, of the extramural coronary arteries. A second important point regarding the topography of coronary atherosclerosis is that severe disease—that is, 70 per cent or greater narrowing of the lumen—occurs much more frequently in the proximal half than in the distal half of any extramural artery. Furthermore, the high-grade obstructive lesions tend to be short (2 to 5 mm). In order of frequency, such lesions involve the anterior descending (43 per cent) more frequently than the right coronary (28 per cent) and the circumflex (23 per cent) and only rarely the left main coronary artery (5 to 6 per cent). The proximal location of high grade obstructions and their short length are the anatomic features that make surgical bypass and restoration of distal coronary artery perfusion pressure a feasible approach to selected patients with symptomatic coronary artery disease (Fig. 93).

CORONARY PERFUSION AND ISCHEMIA

Events that occur in patients with coronary atherosclerosis and that are attributable to obstructive coronary artery disease are best viewed as a consequence of ischemia. Ischemia is a state in which arterial flow is inadequate to meet the oxygen requirements of myocardial cells. The transition from a state in which arterial perfusion is adequate to one in which perfusion is insufficient may develop as a consequence of either a reduction in flow or an increase in flow that is inadequate to meet the demands of myocardial cells. When ischemia is present there is a prompt shift from aerobic to anaerobic metabolism. Accompanying this shift in metabolism are changes in the specialized functions (mechanical and electrical) of the myocardial cell. These functional changes can be viewed as being due to cell injury, and cell injury can be regarded as reversible or irreversible.

It has long been known that atherosclerotic narrowing of coronary arteries is uneven in its extent and that infarction is localized to regions supplied by the involved artery or arteries. Furthermore, ischemic necrosis may be confined to or be predominantly in the subendocardial muscle with at least relative sparing of an epicardial muscle overlying the infarct. More recent studies in living patients and animals using isotopic tracer techniques have demonstrated the dynamic nature of ischemia. Events that provoke ischemia result in relative flow deficits to regions supplied by significantly diseased arteries, and in ischemic regions the available flow is maldistributed across the wall.

Thallium-201 is a radioisotope with biological activity similar to potassium. When thallium is injected intravenously it becomes evenly mixed in blood ejected by the left ventricle and is subsequently extracted by the heart in proportion to regional myocardial blood flow. Imaging of the heart with a gamma scintillation camera after injection yields a picture that portrays the distribution of the isotope and reveals areas of relative perfusion deficit. When patients with a documented prior myocardial infarction are scanned using these techniques, there is typically an area of reduced perfusion even at rest corresponding to the region of the myocardial scar. In patients with angina pectoris, but without prior infarction, scans at rest are typically normal. However, when thallium is administered during exercise that is sufficient to induce angina, one or more zones of relative perfusion deficit are noted (Fig. 94). When these studies are carried out in conjunction with coronary arteriography, there is generally good agreement between the location of zones of new perfusion deficit by thallium and the location of significant obstruction lesions in the coronary arteries. Such studies in man document both the dynamic nature of ischemia and its regional distribution.

As noted above, the histological changes of infarction in patients with coronary artery disease have suggested that ischemia and the extent of resulting infarction frequently are more severe in subendocardial than in subepicardial layers within the zone of is-

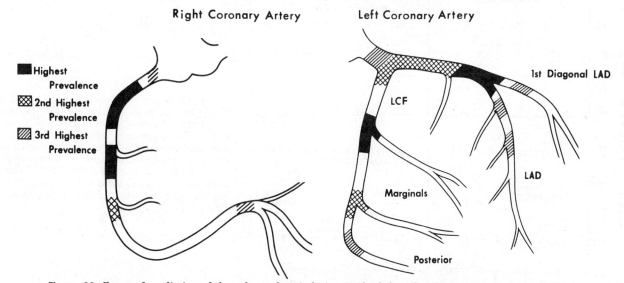

Figure 93. Zones of prediction of the atherosclerotic lesion in the left and right coronary arteries. LAD = left anterior descending artery; LCF = left circumflex artery. (With permission from Gorlin, R.: Coronary Artery Disease. Philadelphia. W. B. Saunders Co., 1976, p. 57.)

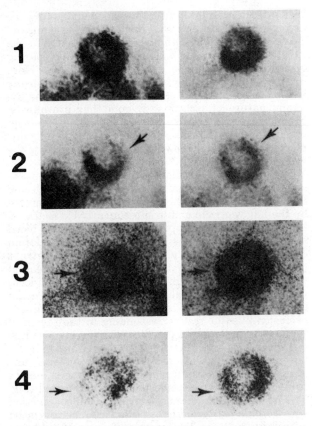

Figure 94. Thallium-201 images during (left) and four hours after (right) cold pressor stress test. *1,* Normal subject. *2,* Single vessel coronary disease. *3,* Double vessel coronary disease. *4,* Triple vessel coronary disease. Arrows point to transient perfusion defects that clear four hours after stress. (From Ahmed, M., Dubiel, J. P., and Haibach, H.: Cold pressor thallium-201 scintigraphy in the diagnosis of coronary artery disease. Am J Cardiol 50:1255, 1982.)

chemia. Another indication that ischemia is not uniform across the thickness of the ventricular wall is the observation that changes of the ST segment during exercise-induced angina are usually those that are characteristic of subendocardial rather than transmural ischemia. To examine the possibility that the transmural distribution of myocardial blood flow distal to a partially occluded coronary artery is uneven, regional coronary perfusion was measured at rest and during exercise in dogs with a coronary occlusion that was not sufficient to alter resting total coronary inflow but that limited the increase in total flow that occurred with exercise. At rest, these studies showed that mean myocardial blood flow was 0.94 ± 0.06 ml/gram/min and increased to 2.45 ± 0.15 ml with exercise in the absence of coronary occlusion. Distribution of flow across the left ventricular wall was uniform (Fig. 95). When the circumflex coronary artery was occluded to a degree that did not alter resting flow or its distribution but that limited the increase in total flow during exercise to 44 per cent of that which occurred normally, there was marked maldistribution of flow across the wall during exercise. Within the distribution of the circumflex artery, flow to epicardial layers increased from normal resting values to 1.96 ± 0.16 ml/gram/min with exercise, while the flow to endocardial layers decreased from normal to 0.34 ± 0.09 ml/gram/min. In the posterior papillary muscle region, endocardial to epicardial flow ratios decreased from 1.08 at rest to 0.22 during exercise in animals with coronary constriction (Fig. 96). These and other studies extend the important concept of the regional nature of ischemia in patients with coronary artery disease. Ischemia is regional in the sense that zones distal to obstructive lesions become ischemic relative to other parts of the same ventricle. In addition, within the ischemic zone decreased perfusion may be confined to subendocardial layers and is nearly always more severe in the subendocardial than in the subepicardial layers.

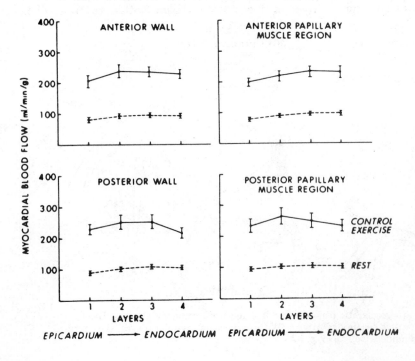

Figure 95. Mean left ventricular myocardial blood flow (ml/min per g) ± SEM to four transmural layers of anterior free wall, anterior papillary muscle region, posterior free wall, and posterior papillary muscle region at rest and during control exercise. (With permission from Ball, R. M., and Bache, R. J.: Distribution of myocardial blood flow in the exercising dog with restricted coronary artery inflow. Circ Res 38:63, 1976.)

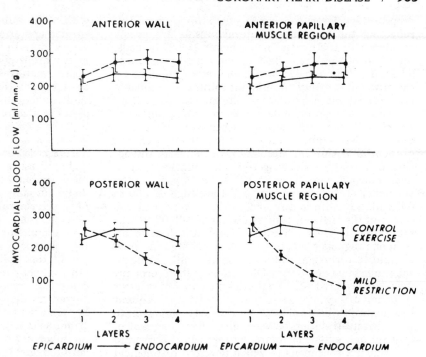

Figure 96. Mean left ventricular myocardial blood flow (ml/min per g) ± SEM to four transmural layers of the anterior free wall, anterior papillary muscle region, posterior free wall, and posterior papillary muscle region during control exercise and exercise with mild restriction of coronary inflow. (With permission from Ball, R. M., and Bache, R. J.: Distribution of myocardial blood blow in the exercising dog with restricted coronary artery inflow. Circ Res 38:63, 1976.)

The observations cited above have focused on factors that influence flow and flow distribution beyond a partially occluded coronary artery. These data highlight the dynamic nature of ischemia and the regional distribution of the transient perfusion deficit when myocardial demands are elevated in the presence of a flow-limiting stenosis. When a previously patent coronary artery is completely and permanently obstructed,

ischemia leads to infarction, unless collaterals are sufficiently well developed to prevent a marked drop in distal coronary perfusion pressure.

Several recent reports have described the temporal sequence of changes in regional myocardial blood flow and its transmural distribution following abrupt, total, and permanent coronary artery occlusion. With such occlusions, the pressure in the distal coronary artery

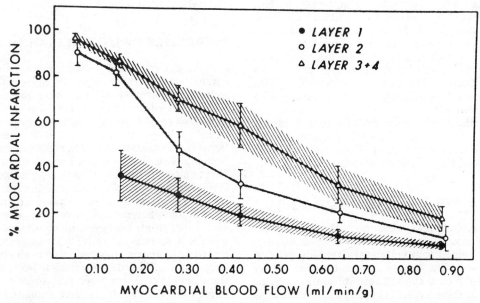

Figure 97. The per cent myocardial infarction ± SEM in myocardial samples from transmural layers 1, 2, and 3 plus 4 are plotted as a function of myocardial blood flow two hours after coronary occlusion. Layer 1 = Endocardium; Layer 2 = mid wall; Layers 3-4 = epicardium. (With permission from Rivas, F., Cobb, F. R., Bache, R. J., and Greenfield, J. C., Jr.: Relationship between blood flow to ischemic regions and extent of myocardial infarction: Serial measurement of blood flow to ischemic regions in dogs. Circ Res 38:445, 1976.)

drops to levels in the range of 15 to 20 mm Hg, reflecting the fact that collateral vessels are poorly developed in the normal nonischemic heart. In dogs, occlusion of the circumflex coronary artery produces an abrupt drop in blood flow to the region supplied by the circumflex artery. Within one minute of occlusion, the average blood flow in the circumflex distribution decreased to approximately 0.25 ml/gram/min compared with flow in regions perfused by the patent anterior descending, which average about 1.18 ml/gram/min. Within the circumflex distribution, the degree of initially reduced perfusion is markedly nonhomogeneous with flows in epicardial layers at the periphery of the ischemic zone in the range of 0.50 to 0.60 ml/gram/min and in endocardial layers near the center of the ischemic zone in the range of 0.02 to 0.10 ml/gram/min. Over a period of 24 hours, flow to all ischemic regions tends to increase despite maintained circumflex occlusion, this increase generally being in the range of a two- to threefold change. When coronary flow is measured at 15 minutes to two hours after coronary artery occlusion and related to subsequent histological evidence of infarction (six days later), there is an inverse relation between blood flow (per cent of control) and extent of infarction (per cent necrosis in the regional specimens in which flow and histological change are compared). Furthermore, for any given reduction in blood flow, the per cent of muscle infarcted is greater in subendocardial layers than in subepicardial layers. Finally, necrosis is absent or minimal in zones where the blood flow reduction at 15 minutes to two hours is not less than 50 per cent of the control flow (Fig. 97). These data illustrate that after abrupt and total coronary occlusion, blood flow reduction in the distal vascular bed is nonhomogeneous, the degree of reduction is greater in subendocardial than subepicardial layers of any given transmural specimen, necrosis is rare in zones where flow is decreased by less than 50 per cent of the control flow, and for any given reduction in flow below 50 per cent of control the extent of necrosis is greater in subendocardial than in subepicardial layers. The latter findings are compatible with the fact that systolic wall stress is greater at the endocardium than at the epicardium for any given level of developed ventricular pressure. Hence, the oxygen requirements of the endocardial muscle are greater than those of the epicardium and it is not surprising that the per cent infarction of subendocardial muscle is greater than that of epicardial muscle for any degree of blood flow reduction.

COLLATERALS AND COLLATERAL FLOW

In a previous chapter, dealing with the normal anatomy and function of the coronary circulation, evidence was presented that collateral channels exist in the normal heart but simply do not function under normal hydraulic conditions. These collaterals appear to be of at least three types: (1) epicardial connections between branches of the major extramural vessels; (2) septal connections that course through the interventricular septum to connect the anterior and posterior descending coronary arteries; and (3) a subendocardial network of collaterals that connect perforating branches of the same or adjacent extramural vessels

within the subendocardium. In patients undergoing cardiac operations for conditions other than coronary artery disease, occlusion of the left main coronary artery drops peripheral coronary arterial pressure to approximately 15 mm Hg, and retrograde flow from the left main coronary is less than 3 ml/min, or essentially negligible. On the other hand, coronary pressure distal to a chronically obstructed coronary artery may be 25 to 40 mm Hg, and retrograde flow, although well below normal, may be substantial. In animal studies, abrupt coronary occlusion produces a marked drop in distal pressure with negligible retrograde flow, while more gradual occlusion over weeks yields much higher distal coronary pressures and retrograde flows. Coronary arteriograms in normal man rarely show collateral channels, but they are evident and sometimes very prominent in patients with chronic coronary artery obstructive disease. From these studies it is apparent that collateral channels are present normally but that they must enlarge to be of functional significance. Enlargement of these channels takes time, and current evidence suggests that a major pressure drop between the two ends of the collateral is the principal stimulus to enlargement. Collaterals undoubtedly play an important role in maintaining the viability of myocardium distal to a major occlusion. The functional significance of collaterals is evident from the fact that some patients with even total occlusion of a coronary artery may be asymptomatic and show no evidence of myocardial scar. On the other hand, evidence that nutrient flow beyond an occluded artery is less than normal even at rest in some symptomatic patients, and the observation that coronary pressure and retrograde flow are nearly always reduced beyond an obstruction in patients who require coronary surgery, both indicate that collaterals, even when fully developed, may be inadequate to compensate for a high grade proximal coronary obstruction.

METABOLIC CONSEQUENCES OF ISCHEMIA

Metabolic studies of ischemic myocardium have been carried out in three types of preparations. In one, individual coronary arteries have been occluded and metabolism of the ischemic zone assessed by cannulating veins that drain the ischemic area and by measuring coronary arteriovenous differences of oxygen, lactate, substrates, and other components across the ischemic vascular bed. Other studies have isolated the heart and controlled total coronary perfusion at various levels, producing global rather than regional ischemia. In both types of studies, biopsies at various periods after inducing ischemia have been used to measure substrates, high energy compounds, and products of metabolic activity. Finally, the metabolic function and activity of various enzymes have been studied in specimens and subcellular fractions of specimens obtained from ischemic hearts. Each preparation has its advantages and disadvantages, but from the aggregate of these studies a reasonably clear picture has emerged of the metabolic changes that accompany myocardial ischemia, their basis, and the sequence of changes that lead to cell death if ischemia is severe and maintained.

Because of the high metabolic rate of working myocardium, a reduction in coronary perfusion is followed almost instantaneously by a decline in tissue oxygen tension; the extent of this decrease parallels the degree of blood flow reduction. The metabolism of glucose and of fat produces reducing equivalents that in the presence of oxygen are normally transferred to the pyridine nucleotides NAD and FAD, and hence by the electron transport system to oxygen, yielding water. In the absence of oxygen, the pyridine nucleotides accumulate in their reduced state (NADH and $FADH_2$) and there is a buildup of reducing equivalents and a rapid development of intracellular acidosis. As noted in the section on cardiac metabolism, pyruvate formed from glucose has two possible fates: conversion to acetyl CoA, which requires NAD, or conversion to lactic acid, which uses NADH. Because NADH accumulates rapidly in the face of oxygen lack, lactate rather than acetyl CoA is formed from pyruvate and accumulates within ischemic cells. The development of intracellular acidosis and the accumulation of lactic acid are obligatory consequences of an oxygen lack. However, the extent of acidosis and lactate accumulation and the rate of development of these changes are greater in ischemia than in hypoxic perfusion because ischemia involves not only oxygen lack but also a decreased washout of these potentially deleterious products of metabolism.

When myocardial cells are deprived of oxygen, either by hypoxic perfusion or by ischemia, acidosis and conversion from lactate utilization to lactate production precede by a substantial interval any decline in ATP. This discordance occurs because, despite the cessation of oxidative phosphorylation of ADP to ATP in the absence of oxygen, ATP levels are maintained, at least initially, by transfer of high-energy phosphate from creatine phosphate to ADP and the consequent generation of ATP by a mechanism of limited reserve but operative in the absence of oxygen. Most recent work indicates that changes of myocardial contraction induced by either hypoxia or ischemia are preceded by a decline in ATP and CP content.

Under normal aerobic conditions the heart derives its energy predominantly from the metabolism of fatty acids, lactate, and glucose. Fat is used in preference to glucose because acetyl CoA formed from beta-oxidation of fat exerts a powerful inhibitory influence on pyruvate dehydrogenase. With a reduction in tissue oxygen tension and a depletion of intramitochondrial FAD (because $FADH_2$ accumulates, beta-oxidation of free fatty acids that requires FAD ceases. As a consequence, the formation of acetyl CoA from fat ceases and the brake that acetyl CoA normally exerts on pyruvate dehydrogenase is removed. Glucose utilization thus increases and substrate (glucose) is provided by enhanced breakdown of glycogen. Under conditions of hypoxic perfusion, glycolytic flux increases markedly and glycogen levels become depleted. When substrate for glycolysis is available in excess, the activity of phosphofructokinase (PFK) is rate limiting in the conversion of glucose to pyruvate. Despite the fact that depletion of creatine phosphate enhances PFK activity, enzyme activity is powerfully inhibited by acidosis. Thus, in ischemia, where acidosis is more severe than in perfusion with comparably hypoxic blood, PFK is inhibited and glycolytic flux increases less than would be expected otherwise, or actually diminishes. To the extent that fatty acid uptake and metabolism continue

in ischemic cells, fatty acid is preferentially converted to triglyceride rather than oxidized, and triglyceride accumulates in intracellular droplets, a common histological feature of myocytes that survive in a setting of oxygen lack. In essence, characteristics of ischemic but not yet irreversibly damaged myocardium are (1) lactate production rather than utilization and (2) a marked decrease or cessation of fatty acid uptake and utilization.

These biochemical changes have proved useful in assessing patients with presumed angina pectoris due to coronary artery disease. Investigators have noted that when the coronary sinus or its tributaries are cannulated, and angina is induced by pacing the heart at a rapid rate, lactate is produced by ischemic zones and purine nucleosides and bases are released secondary to catabolism of adenine nucleotides. Even more recently, a regional decrease in the uptake of free fatty acids has been detected by external scanning when carbon-11 isotopes of fatty acids are injected and positron emissions are counted by external coincidence counting. The depletion of purine and pyrimidine nucleotide pools occurs during even brief periods of ischemia and is restored only slowly after reperfusion.

REVERSIBLE AND IRREVERSIBLE CELL INJURY

For many years our understanding of the pathology of myocardial ischemia was limited to studies of infarction in man and was based on macroscopic and standard histological techniques. Using these techniques, little if any change is detectable within the first 12 hours after coronary occlusion. By 18 to 24 hours, areas of infarction appear pale and yellow grossly and by microscopic view myocytes become acidophilic, cross striations are present but obscured, and there is an early but minimal infiltrate of principally polymorphonuclear cells. From 48 to 72 hours there is further loss of muscle striations, cell swelling, interstitial hemorrhage, and pyknotic nuclei. By one week, there is a very prominent inflammatory infiltrate, cell margins are irregular, and the cells appear empty because of resorption of protoplasm and contractile proteins and because of total karyolysis. By day ten the necrotic zone has begun to shrink, the infiltrate consists principally of mononuclear cells and fibroblasts. Fibrosis is clearly evident by two to three weeks, but probably not complete for at least six weeks. At all stages, the infarct has a very irregular contour, the size and extent of transmural damage are highly variable, and within the borders of the infarct there are many islands of viable cells.

Electron micrographs obtained at specific times after experimental coronary artery occlusion and utilizing optimal preservation techniques have revealed changes much earlier. These changes can be correlated with biochemical and physiological alterations and help to define the transition from reversible to irreversible ischemic cell injury. In normal myocytes the nucleus is centrally located in the cell and nuclear chromatin is evenly distributed. Mitochondria are abundant, usually with one per sarcomere, and within each mitochondrion the cristae are tightly packed. Within the cytosol, there are abundant granules of

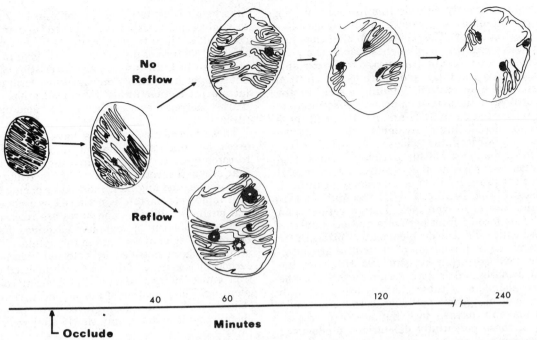

Figure 98. Sequential changes in mitochondrial morphology as a function of ischemia with and without arterial reflow. With permanent ischemia (no reflow), the amorphous matrix densities first are readily detected at 40 minutes. They enlarge and increase in number for the next three to four hours. Also, the mitochondria swell and often show ruptured outer membranes. If arterial reflow is allowed at 40 minutes, granular densities of calcium phosphate appear near the cristae of the involved mitochondria. (With permission from Jennings, R. B.: Relationship of acute ischemia to functional defects and irreversibility. Circulation 53(Supplement I):I-29, 1976.)

glycogen, fat is rare, and with immersion fixation the myofibrils are in a contracted state. The sarcolemmal membrane is scalloped in these contracted cells but is intact and covered with a delicate fuzzy basement membrane. When coronary flow is interrupted for 15 minutes, contractile function ceases and electrical changes are observed, but if flow is restored normal function returns and the cells survive. The ultrastructural changes observed in these reversibly injured cells are confined to a diminished number of glycogen granules and relaxed versus contracted myofibrils.

When ischemia is extended to 20 to 30 minutes there is early evidence of mitochondrial swelling and margination of nuclear chromatin. With 40 to 60 minutes of ischemia, glycogen is virtually absent, the sarcomeres are stretched, the cell volume is increased, and the sarcolemma exhibits defects in its plasma membrane. Mitochondria are also swollen, the cristae are disorganized, and one or more amorphous densities appear within the mitochondrion (Fig. 98). Extreme margination of nuclear chromatin is observed, but there are no detectable changes in the thick or thin filaments other than their relaxed states. Lysosomes, T tubules, and sarcoplasmic reticulum appear normal. From a morphological point of view, the earliest hallmarks of irreversible injury are the appearance of defects in the sarcolemma and the development of amorphous densities without mitochondria. It might be anticipated that these morphological changes would be accompanied by defects in the regulation of cell volume and in the respiratory capacity of mitochondria. The results of in vitro studies of slices of muscle made ischemic for 60 minutes demonstrate clearly that striking defects in cell volume regulation are present.

Similarly, if mitochondria are isolated after 60 minutes of in vivo ischemia, the metabolism of pyruvate is markedly reduced, oxidative phosphorylation is uncoupled, and respiratory rate is reduced. From sequential studies it appears that the earliest feature of irreversibly injured cells is an alteration of the cell membrane and its permeability to ions, particularly calcium.

ACTIVE AND PASSIVE MECHANICS OF ISCHEMIC MUSCLE

The fact that regional myocardial ischemia following coronary artery occlusion leads to localized mechanical dysfunction has been known since the earliest studies of Wiggers and his colleagues. The most illuminating studies of these changes and their temporal course have utilized implanted transducers to monitor left ventricular pressure, coronary blood flow, and the dimensions of segments of the ventricle in normally perfused, marginal, and ischemic zones. Regional function has been assessed early and late after coronary artery occlusion in awake dogs (Fig. 99). Within seconds of interrupting coronary blood flow to a region, shortening of maximally ischemic segments ceases (akinesia). Within a minute, the ischemic segment not only fails to shorten, but actually undergoes holosystolic outward bulging (dyskinesia). The shortening characteristics of ischemic segments are paralleled by essentially mirror image changes of wall thickness. Thus, as the rate and extent of segment shortening diminish, the rate and extent of wall thickening diminish, and with holosystolic bulging of ischemic segments there is a corresponding thinning of the segment during systole. Over a period of hours with permanent occlusion, these dimensional changes in the ischemic zone remain stable. Within the ischemic zone, the end-diastolic segment length does not change significantly from control over a period of days, but beginning at one week and extending until the third and fourth week after occlusion, diastolic segment length tends to shorten by as much as 25 to 30 per cent; the extent of shortening correlates roughly with the extent of replacement fibrosis and represents scar. By contrast, in normally perfused zones, end-diastolic segment length increases and the extent of systolic shortening increases, reflecting compensatory hyperfunction of the noninjured myocardium. To the extent that studies in man have been undertaken at various times after coronary occlusion, and using imaging techniques that are currently less precise than those available to investigators studying animals, comparable results have been reported.

In addition to characterizing systolic contractile events in ischemic, marginal, and normal zones over time, the techniques employed above have been used to study the diastolic properties of ischemic ventricles.

With the onset of the slow phase of ventricular filling after relaxation is complete, the relation between ventricular pressure and the length of any given circumferentially oriented segment is curvilinear and approximates an exponential function. Because of this, the log pressure versus segment length relation is nearly linear and its slope has been used to estimate changes in regional compliance. Within the ischemic zone, but not in normally perfused segments, the slope of this relationship increases within five minutes of occlusion and increases further by 24 hours despite no change in end-diastolic segment length. These changes are compatible with a decreased compliance of the ischemic muscle. By three weeks, end-diastolic segment length has shortened because of scarring and the slope of the log pressure-length relation increases even further, compatible with a further decrease in regional compliance presumably due to fibrous replacement. These observations too are consistent with those in man, suggesting that reduced compliance of the ventricle contributes to the rise of left ventricular end-diastolic pressure observed during angina and early infarctions of significant size. They are also compatible with the

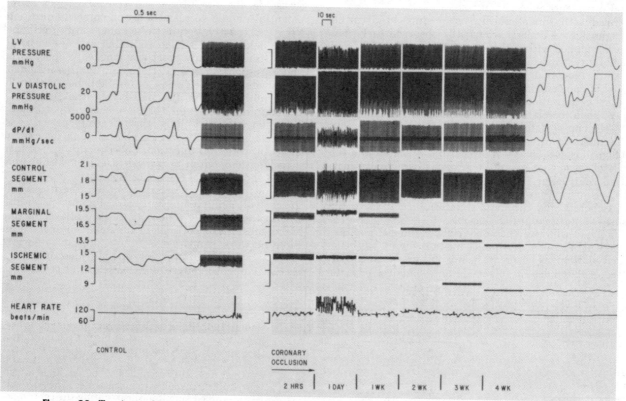

Figure 99. Tracings obtained from an unanesthetized dog in the control state (left panel) and following permanent coronary occlusion for four weeks. The calibrations for the right panels are the same as those shown on the left, the slow tracings are all taken at the same paper speed, and the paper speed during the initial and final tracings is the same. The heart rate (cardiotachometer) is shown in the lower tracings. Normal shortening of all three segments is evident in the left panel. Severe dysfunction is evident after two hours of coronary occlusion in the marginal and ischemic segments, whereas the control segment exhibits increased end-diastolic length, and increased shortening. Severe arrhythmia is present at one day. Subsequently, the control segment exhibits an increasing end-diastolic length and improved shortening. The marginal segment exhibits an increase in dimension at one and two days, and then a progressive shortening. The marginal segment exhibits an increase in dimension at one and two days, and then a progressive reduction in the segment dimension occurs, severe hypokinesis being evident in the tracing at four weeks (shown at rapid paper speed). The ischemic segment exhibits even more severe reduction in the dimension and there is akinesis at four weeks. LV = Left ventricular. (With permission from Theroux, P., Ross, J., Jr., Franklin, D., Covell, J. W., Bloor, C. M., and Sasayama, S.: Regional myocardial function and dimensions early and late after myocardial infarction in the unanesthetized dog. Circ Res 40:162, 1977.)

observed alterations in the diastolic properties of the human ventricle noted at long intervals after infarction with extensive replacement fibrosis. Thus, ischemia affects both the contractile process and the passive diastolic properties of the heart. The regional and global effects of longstanding infarction reflect the consequences of both replacement fibrosis and compensatory hypertrophy of surviving myocardium.

ELECTROPHYSIOLOGY OF ISCHEMIC MUSCLE

Disturbances in the electrical activity of the heart and resulting alterations of cardiac rhythm are an extraordinarily frequent and important consequence of myocardial ischemia. These disturbances noted in patients fall into three broad categories: (1) bradyarrhythmias, which are noted most frequently within the first hour of infarction; (2) single or repetitive ectopic ventricular beats, which increase in the early hours after infarction, persist for one to two days, and then decline; and (3) alterations in atrioventricular and intraventricular conduction.

Bradyarrhythmias due to either sinus bradycardia or transient AV block are usually observed early, are more common with posterior or inferior infarction, and usually respond to atropine, suggesting that they are vagally mediated. In contrast, the alterations of intraventricular conduction and AV block that accompany anterior infarction are unresponsive to atropine and have been correlated with ischemic necrosis interrupting the appropriate specialized pathways of conduction. The major focus of this section will be on electrophysiological consequences of myocardial ischemia and the role of these changes in the genesis of single or repetitive ventricular ectopic activity. These latter disturbances of rhythm are the most frequent consequence of ischemia and the most significant relative to the onset of ventricular fibrillation.

Much of what we know today about the electrophysiological basis of arrhythmias due to ischemia has been derived from experiments using either extracellular needle electrodes or intracellular microelectrodes to study ischemic tissue in animals. Extracellular recordings from epicardial and intramural sites reveal a characteristic temporal sequence of changes following coronary occlusion. These consist of initial elevation of the ST interval between activation and repolarization, a progressive decrease in the amplitude of the local activation potential, delay in local activation, desynchronization of activation, and absent local excitation at many of the sites within the ischemic zone (Fig. 100). It is also of interest that in studies of early ischemia (first 60 to 90 minutes) Purkinje potentials deteriorate in amplitude beneath the ischemic zone, local intramural delays are often very marked (activation occurring within and after the T wave), and these intramural delays are unstable from beat to beat, sometimes producing local 2:1 Wenckebach periods between closely adjacent sites.

At a cellular level, the early effects of ischemia have been studied with microelectrodes in vivo and in tissues removed from ischemic areas and studied in vitro. In vivo recordings from subepicardial muscle cells have shown that within five minutes of coronary occlusion there is a loss of resting membrane potential, a decrease in the amplitude and rate of rise of action potentials, and a decrease of action potential duration. Very early, activation of these subepicardial cells becomes delayed, 2:1 responses are observed, and by 10 to 15 minutes many cells are markedly depolarized and unresponsive (Fig. 101). Generally, these changes are reversible if perfusion is reestablished within 30 to 40 minutes. It is also noteworthy that within an ischemic zone the extent of these changes is spatially nonhomogeneous. Finally, the refractory period of ischemic cells initially shortens, paralleling the change in action potential duration. Subsequently, refractoriness lengthens often to a marked extent despite continued shortening of the action potential.

Following coronary artery occlusion, there is a progressive although nonuniform loss of muscle potentials within the ischemic zone as described above. In contrast, substantial portions of the subendocardial Purkinje network beneath the infarct appear to survive despite transient alterations in their electrical properties. One reason offered for this tendency of Purkinje

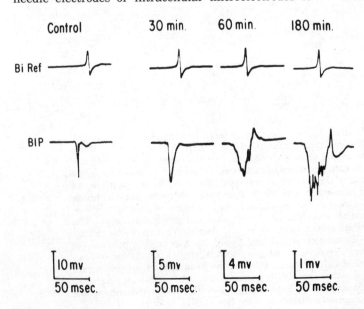

Figure 100. Progressive desynchronization subsequent to coronary occlusion. A bipolar reference electrogram (Bi Ref) recorded from the normal right ventricle is shown here. Below, bipolar intramural electrograms (BIP) recorded from an area of left ventricular ischemia are demonstrated. These signals were recorded simultaneously during the control period and at 30, 60, and 180 min subsequent to coronary artery occlusion. Note the progressive decrease in amplitude of the bipolar potential with increased duration and fragmentation of the complex. Also note that the reference electrogram in the RV remains stable throughout the period of occlusion. (With permission from Boineau, J. P., and Cox, J. L.: Slow ventricular activation in acute myocardial infarction: A source of reentrant premature ventricular contractions. Circulation 48:704, 1973.)

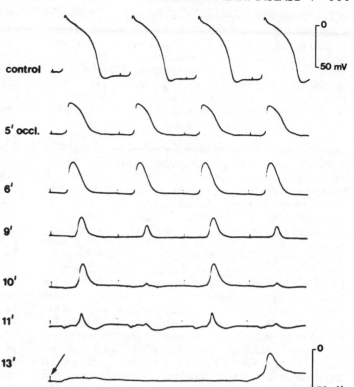

Figure 101. Transmembrane action potentials recorded from the subepicardium of the left ventricle of an in situ pig heart before and after occlusion of the proximal left anterior descending artery. (With permission from Downar, E., Janse, M. J., and Durrer, D.: The effect of acute coronary artery occlusion on subepicardial transmembrane potentials in the intact porcine heart. Circulation 56:219, 1977.)

fibers to survive is their lower oxygen requirements because of a paucity of contractile proteins. A second potential reason is that they may receive some oxygen by diffusion from cavity blood on the basis of proximity even when nutrient coronary flow is interrupted. In vitro recordings from subendocardial Purkinje fibers isolated within 60 minutes after coronary occlusion show that a majority of the cells are viable but depressed with reduced diastolic potential, reduced amplitude and upstroke velocity, and shortened action potential duration. Spontaneous diastolic depolarization is not prominent at this point in time even though arrhythmias in vivo are prevalent. At 24 hours after infarction the number of viable Purkinje cells beneath an infarcted zone is reduced, by perhaps as much as 50 per cent. Viable cells are still evident, however, demonstrating reduced membrane potential and a reduced upstroke velocity and amplitude of the action potential. In contrast to studies of 30 to 60 minutes, however, action potential duration is very markedly prolonged and evidence of spontaneous diastolic depolarization and bursts of repetitive firing are prominent. In chronic infarction (that is, ten days to three weeks) many viable Purkinje fibers are noted on the subendocardial surface of the scar and their action potential characteristics are generally normal.

When otherwise normal ventricular muscle is perfused in vitro with coronary venous blood obtained from ischemic zones, electrophysiological changes ensue in the muscle that are essentially identical to those observed in tissue that is rendered ischemic. The changes induced by the ischemic blood cannot be accounted for by the increase in potassium concentration in blood draining the ischemic area, or by the degree of acidosis or hypoxia, and they are not even reproduced when these changes are simulated in combination. Thus, it appears that the electrophysiological changes of ischemia are attributable to factors that remain to be identified but that are present in the venous effluent of ischemic tissue.

Ischemia induces electrophysiological changes that vary with time after coronary occlusion and with the size of the ischemic zone. When the ischemic area is viewed as a three-dimensional region, the changes and their temporal evolution are nonuniform within the region. The alterations that have been documented appear to form an adequate basis for generating ventricular ectopic events on the basis of either reentry, or repetitive firing, or both. Furthermore, these data support the view that arrhythmias may arise on the basis of different mechanisms, depending upon the time of their occurrence after the initial ischemic insult.

CLINICAL CORRELATIONS

Given the material presented above, it is possible to acquire a reasonably complete pathophysiological understanding of the common and significant manifestations of coronary heart disease. These manifestations have their basis in ischemia and its consequences and in infarction and its consequences. It is important to recall that ischemia is a dynamic process and that ischemia and infarction lead to regional disorders of specialized myocardial function.

The characteristic feature of angina pectoris is chest pain produced by transient myocardial ischemia. We now consider that the most common cause of typical angina is a rise in myocardial demand for perfusion, brought on by exercise, by emotional events, by dreams, and so on. The predisposing anatomic lesion is a flow-limiting stenosis in one or more coronary arteries and inadequately developed collaterals. Under these conditions, coronary vasodilatation, which results from increased myocardial work, is not accompanied by an increased flow. Consequently, distal perfusion pressure drops. A prominent feature of this situation is a marked maldistribution of the available flow with subendocardial underperfusion. The events that precipitate an anginal attack raise either arterial blood pressure, or heart rate, or both, and hence myocardial work. The pain of angina arises because local products of ischemic metabolism (kinins, potassium, acidosis) are capable of exciting receptors at the free ends of unmyelinated sympathetic afferent fibers, which then transmit pain impulses to the spinal cord from the level of C-7 to T-4, hence to the thalamus and to the cerebral cortex. Accompanying the anginal attack are a regional difference in the contractile function and an increased diastolic stiffness of the ischemic zone. The ejection fraction of the ventricle decreases and the heart dilates. Ventricular end-diastolic pressure increases owing to dilatation and to the overall decrease in compliance. Cardiac output is usually maintained by the Starling effect but may drop. Blood pressure may drop because cardiac output is inadequate, because of reflex sympathetic withdrawal induced by stimulation of ventricular stretch receptors, or because of vagally mediated bradycardia and peripheral vasodilatation. The appearance of gallop rhythms reflects reduced ventricular compliance, and an apical murmur of mitral regurgitation may develop resulting from ischemia and reduced contractile function of papillary muscles. The EKG changes reflect predominant subendocardial ischemia and result from discrepancies in membrane potential during the ST-T interval due to marked shortening and loss of the plateau of action potentials in the ischemic zone. Typically, in the patient with angina, chest pain, EKG changes, and hemodynamic alterations are transient; within five to ten minutes of either ceasing the activity that precipitated ischemia or initiating specific therapy with nitroglycerin, these abnormalities revert to normal. However, the depletion of nucleotide pools which develops during even brief periods of ischemia may persist for hours or days.

In 1959, Prinzmetal and his associates described an interesting variant of angina in which pain typically appeared at rest, not with exertion, and the EKG showed ST segment elevation rather than depression. Monitoring of physiological variables in such patients has established that elevations of blood pressure and heart rate do not precede the onset of chest pain as they do in typical angina. Rather, ST elevation is the initial event. It now appears clear from angiographic studies that most, if not all, instances of variant angina arise from focal, or occasionally diffuse, coronary artery spasm. Elevation rather than depression of the ST segment probably reflects transmural ischemia rather than predominantly subendocardial ischemia as seen in typical angina.

Sudden death is a common manifestation of ischemic heart disease. Pathological studies indicate that significant coronary artery disease is usually present. For many years it was felt that sudden death was an early manifestation of infarction. The development of effective community systems for resuscitation of patients with cardiac arrest has shown that a significant proportion of such victims subsequently fail to evolve changes in serum enzymes or in the electrocardiogram, which permit the diagnosis of infarction. We know that paroxysmal, potentially lethal arrhythmias may occur during transient ischemia or repetitively in patients with chronic but otherwise stable coronary heart disease. From these observations, it seems probable that many sudden deaths arise from arrhythmias in acutely ischemic but not infarcted myocardium, from a paroxysmal arrhythmia in chronically scarred but not acutely ischemic myocardium, or from acute electromechanical uncoupling in the ischemic heart, which is an event of uncertain cause in which mechanical function ceases abruptly but the EKG reveals a stable sinus rhythm.

In recent years, much has been written about the subject of acute myocardial infarction. A fundamental question is, what precipitates myocardial infarction? Despite detailed studies of the coronary arteries in a large number of fatal cases, most pathologists have concluded that nothing new appears in these vessels at the time of acute infarction in most patients. Coronary atherosclerosis is present in nearly all cases, but recent reports have emphasized that myocardial infarction sometimes occurs even in the absence of coronary atheroma. Hemorrhage beneath the preexisting plaque has been observed but seldom leads to any further encroachment on the lumen. Perhaps the most relevant recent observation is that patients with acute infarction, studied early during the evolution of infarction, nearly always show a clot in the coronary artery that supplies the ischemic zone. These clots can be dissolved rapidly with streptokinase and, although contractile function of the ischemic segment does not change acutely, most patients demonstrate improvement when studied 7 to 10 days later.

Previous sections of this chapter have presented experimental data regarding the effects of abrupt coronary artery occlusion on blood flow, distribution of blood flow, histological and ultrastructural changes, metabolism, mechanics, and electrophysiology of ischemic muscle. Emphasis has been placed on the regional nature of these changes, nonuniformity within the region, and the evolution of events over time subsequent to coronary occlusion. As clinical data accumulate, there is growing evidence that the insights derived from these experimental models have their clinical counterparts. Infarction and its consequences in man are clearly regional processes. Ischemia that leads to infarction is, at least initially, nonuniform in its extent, and there are increasing data to support the view that the ultimate fate of regions of reduced perfusion but not yet irreversibly damaged cells may be influenced by therapy in the first several hours following the onset of symptoms. Angiographic and radionuclide studies in man have documented the regional nature of perfusion deficits in acute infarction and alterations in the contractile and diastolic properties of the ischemic zone that are comparable to those observed in animals with implanted transducers for monitoring regional flow and function. Hemodynamic studies in man that reflect global cardiac function have demonstrated a continuum from essentially normal data in patients with small uncomplicated infarcts, to profound left ventricular failure in those with massive infarction and shock. In general, the degree of hemodynamic derangement parallels the size of the infarct as reflected by enzymatic, electrocardiographic, and pathological criteria. With infarction of increasing size, cardiac output is reduced progressively, arteriovenous oxygen difference is widened, peripheral resistance increases, and left ventricular end-diastolic pressure measured directly or estimated from pulmonary artery diastolic or wedge pressures is increased. Ventricular function may improve over the weeks that follow infarction; presumably, this reflects restoration of function in initially ischemic but still viable regions, shrinkage and stiffening of the infarcted zone through fibrosis, and compensatory hypertrophy and hyperfunction of residual uninfarcted muscle. From the very onset of ischemia that leads to infarction there is a proclivity for ventricular arrhythmias, which begins within minutes, reaches a maximum from 12 to 36 hours after infarction, and then subsides to a reduced level, but one in which the prevalence of arrhythmias is greater than in the normal heart for months and perhaps years after infarction. Again, in the acute setting a relation has been established between the prevalence of such ectopic activity and estimates of the size of the infarct. Furthermore, in patients with healed infarction there is a similar relation between spontaneous ectopic ventricular activity and the extent of altered ventricular function assessed from angiographic study of left ventricular contractile performance and the number and size of akinetic or dyskinetic scars. A detailed presentation of arrhythmias in infarction is beyond the scope of this chapter, but the picture that has emerged from clinical and experimental studies is one in which ischemia per se contributes to the genesis of early arrhythmias in infarction through its direct effect on the electrophysiology of ischemic cells. Later arrhythmias (weeks or months) probably arise as a consequence of alterations that are unique to zones in which normal cells are intermixed with scar tissue of nonhomogeneous geometry; as a result, intercellular connections are interrupted, conduction is slowed and fractionated, and ectopic rhythms on a reentrant basis predominate. Other lasting alterations of rhythm and conduction, such as AV block and intraventricular conduction disturbances, have been related to involvement of specific sites in the specialized conduction system by ischemia and subsequent scar formation.

When papillary muscles are involved in infarction, either the entire muscle (rarely) or one head of the muscle may rupture. Hence, mitral insufficiency develops in the setting of acute infarction in some patients and may result either from ischemic dysfunction or from rupture. The syndrome of acute mitral regurgitation develops (see chapter on valvular heart disease), which may be sufficiently severe to warrant immediate mitral valve replacement. With transmural infarctions of major proportion, rupture of the heart may occur. This involves the interventricular septum more frequently than the free wall and reflects tears in the necrotic portion of the wall, presumably as a consequence of exaggerated wall stress on the noncontracting necrotic segment during systole. Septal rupture, when it occurs, usually develops within the first six days after infarction—that is, at the peak of the necrotic phase. Ventricular aneurysm is also an infrequent, but important, consequence of myocardial in-

farction. Aneurysms develop as an outpouching of a thin scarred portion of previously infarcted muscle. They may occur anywhere on the left ventricle but are most frequent in the anterior, lateral, and apical regions. In contrast to rupture that occurs early and involves the interplay of wall stress and necrotic tissue, aneurysms develop and expand over a period of weeks or months after infarction, rarely rupture, and thus appear to involve the interplay of wall stress and scar tissue. The hemodynamics of ventricular aneurysm are not unlike those of mitral regurgitation. With left ventricular systole the ventricle transfers some of its end-diastolic volume into expansile aneurysm (rather than the left atrium) and part into the aorta as forward stroke volume. When there is adequate normally functioning left ventricular muscle not involved with the aneurysm, resection of the aneurysm can restore ventricular dynamics and overall cardiac performance to near normal. This situation is also analogous to mitral insufficiency, particularly acute mitral insufficiency with good residual ventricular function, in which mitral valve replacement produces a similar dramatic improvement in cardiac function.

REFERENCES

Ball, R. M., and Bache, R. J.: Distribution of myocardial blood flow in the exercising dog with restricted coronary artery inflow. Circ Res 38:60, 1976.

Downar, E., Janse, M. J., and Durrer, D.: The effect of acute coronary artery occlusion on subepicardial transmembrane potentials in the intact porcine heart. Circulation 56:217, 1977.

Gregg, D. E.: The natural history of coronary collateral development. Circ Res 35:335, 1974.

Hearse, D. J.: Oxygen deprivation and early myocardial contractile failure: A reassessment of the possible role of adenosine triphosphate. Am J Cardiol 44:1115, 1979.

Irvin, R. G., and Cobb, F. R.: Relationship between epicardial ST-segment elevation, regional myocardial blood flow and extent of myocardial infarction in awake dogs. Circulation 55:825, 1977.

Jennings, R. B.: Relationship of acute ischemia to functional defects and irreversibility. Circulation 53(Supp. I):26, 1976.

Kluger, G.: Myocardial release of lactate, inosine and hypoxanthine during atrial pacing and exercise-induced angina. Circulation 59:43, 1979.

Lazzara, R., El-Sherif, N., and Scherlag, B. J.: Early and late effects of coronary artery occlusion on canine Purkinje fibers. Circ Res 35:391, 1974.

Maseri, A., L'Abbate, A., Pesola, A., Michelassi, C., Marzilli, M., and De Nes, M.: Regional myocardial perfusion in patients with atherosclerotic coronary artery disease, at rest and during angina pectoris induced by tachycardia. Circulation 55:423, 1977.

Ramo, B. W., Myers, N., Wallace, A. G., Starmer, F., Clark, D. O., and Whalen, R. E.: Hemodynamic findings in 123 patients with acute myocardial infarction on admission. Circulation 42:567, 1970.

Roberts, W. C., Buja, L. M.: The frequency and significance of coronary arterial thrombi and other observations in fatal acute myocardial infarction. Am J Med 52:425, 1972.

Swain, J. L., Sabina, R. L., McHale, P. A., Greenfield, J. C., Jr., and Holmes, E. W.: Prolonged myocardial nucleotide depletion after brief ischemia in the open-chest dog. Am J Physiol 242:H818, 1982.

Theroux, P., Ross, J., Jr., Franklin, D., Covell, J. W., Bloor, C. M., and Sasayama, S.: Regional myocardial function and dimensions early and late after myocardial infarction in the unanesthetized dog. Circ Res 40:158, 1977.

Pericardial Disease _____

NORMAL ANATOMY

The heart is enclosed within an invaginated sac of serous membrane. The visceral component of this serous sac is a thin mesothelial layer that adheres to the epicardium of the heart and extends a few centimeters onto the great vessels. It is then reflected back as a second layer that adheres to a fibrous sac that also surrounds the heart. The portion of the serous membrane that adheres to the fibrous sac is called the parietal pericardium. The fibrous portion of the parietal pericardium is closed at its neck by fusion with the adventitia of the great vessels and it is attached to the manubrium and xyphoid by pericardiosternal ligaments. The serous membrane is composed of flattened mesothelial cells that transport fluid and electrolytes between the pericardial space and pericardial capillaries. The fibrous sac to which parietal pericardium adheres consists of superficial, middle, and deep layers of collagen interlaced with elastic fibers. The parietal pericardium is distensible and elastic, but its distensibility is limited by its collagen components.

The space between the visceral and parietal serous layers normally holds 15 to 20 ml of an ultrafiltrate of plasma containing 1.5 to 3.5 per cent proteins that serves principally as a lubricant. Pericardial pressure, like pleural pressure, is negative with respect to the atmosphere.

The pericardium receives its vascular supply from branches of the internal mammary arteries, the musculophrenic artery, and the descending thoracic aorta. Venous drainage and lymphatics follow the distribution of the arterial supply. Cardiac lymphatic flow arises in the endocardium and condenses in lymphatic trunks that flow to the epicardium, to the visceral pericardium, to the nodes at the base of the heart, and on to the mediastinal collecting ducts. Vascular and lymphatic channels are located in the adipose tissue beneath visceral pericardium and on the mediastinal surface of the parietal pericardium.

The nerve supply to the pericardium arises from the vagus, the left recurrent laryngeal plexus, and the esophageal plexus. Sympathetic supply is from the first dorsal ganglion, stellate ganglion, and aortic, cardiac, and diaphragmatic plexuses.

NORMAL PHYSIOLOGY

There are widely different views regarding the functional significance of the normal pericardium. The proposed functions should be considered with the perspective that human subjects with genetic or surgical absence of the pericardium function in an entirely normal manner. However, the fact that absence of the pericardium is tolerated well does not mean that the normal pericardium serves no function. Most investigators agree that the fluid-filled pericardial space minimizes friction between the heart and surrounding structures. Most also agree that the fibrous sac and its sternal attachment reduce displacement of the heart and kinking of the great vessels, which might occur during gravitational, accelerating, or decelerating stresses. The pericardial sac can certainly form a barrier protecting the heart from infectious and other inflammatory reactions in the lung and pleural space, and pericardium contains pain receptors and mechanoreceptors capable of eliciting reflex changes in blood pressure and pulse rate. These reflex changes can be prevented by cooling or cutting the vagus nerves.

Considerable controversy exists concerning the mechanical consequences of an intact pericardium versus an open or absent pericardium. At low filling pressures the pericardium appears to exert little or no influence on the diastolic pressure-volume relationship, but at higher filling pressures the pericardium exerts a restrictive influence that limits the change in volume for any given change in pressure (Fig. 102). In acute experiments, regurgitation of the mitral and tricuspid valves develops more easily when filling pressure is

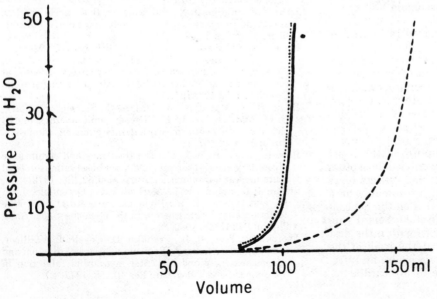

Figure 102. Schematic pressure-volume curves of the isolated dog heart before and after removal of the pericardium. The volume of the pericardiectomized heart, when distended with pressures greater than 5 cm of water, was approximately 50 per cent greater than the volume of the heart with the pericardium present. Solid line, pericardial volume; dotted line, heart within pericardium; dashed line, heart without pericardium. (With permission from Holt, J. P.: The normal pericardium. Am J Cardiol 26:457, 1970.)

raised in the absence of the pericardium. Another consequence of the restrictive influence of the pericardium on ventricular dilatation can be observed when the impedance to left ventricular ejection is abruptly raised while right atrial pressure is maintained constant. With sudden aortic constriction, left ventricular ejection is reduced and left ventricular volume increases. With the pericardium intact, this expansion of the left ventricle within a pericardial space of limited distensibility compromises right ventricular filling and, as a consequence, right ventricular stroke volume falls. Within a few beats, the volume of return to the left heart fails, left ventricular volume and pressure drop, and a new steady state is achieved. Although experiments can and have been designed to demonstrate these mechanical consequences of the pericardium, it should be recalled that pericardial restriction to filling of either ventricle is probably not a very important factor at normal filling pressures.

REACTIONS OF THE PERICARDIUM TO INJURY

Although there are numerous causes of injury, pericardial tissue responds morphologically in a limited number of ways. These responses include acute and chronic inflammation, neoplasia, calcification, and cholesterol effusion.

Acute inflammatory responses are composed of exudates containing fibrin and cells. The type and amount of exudate depend upon the cause of the injury. Acute reactions may resolve or may become chronic with varying amounts of fibrous proliferation. Almost any acute pericardial disease is associated with focal or diffuse fibrin deposits. This type of exudate occurs in acute inflammation associated with increased vascular permeability, allowing plasma proteins, including fibrinogen, to leave vessels and enter the pericardial space. The fibrinogen precipitates as masses of fibrin, which are identified histologically as tangled, eosinophilic networks. There is often an accompanying cellular exudate composed predominantly of neutrophils.

A fibrinous exudate may progress in one of two ways: resolution or organization. Fibrin deposits alone do not provide a chronic process, and most fibrinous reactions resolve through resorption by fibrinolysis. Coupled with effusion, injury, or an infective process, however, a fibrinous reaction may progress to fibrous proliferation. Ingrowth of fibroblasts and capillary buds produces organized, vascularized connective tissue. At this stage, the richly vascular membrane may bleed into the pericardial space, resulting in hemopericardium. Eventually, fibrous adhesions and/or pericardial thickening results.

Accumulation of fluid in the pericardial space is quite common. Fluid exudates are termed serous, bloody, chylous, or lymphous; there is no morphological response to any of these effusions. Blood in the pericardial sac coincidental with pericardial tissue injury may produce fibrous pericardial adhesions.

Serous effusions are common in patients with a low serum albumin and in congestive heart failure. The protein content of these effusions is low, cells are sparse, and the effusion does not imply the presence of pericardial disease. Bloody effusions result from cer-

tain infections (for example, tuberculosis), neoplasms, acute myocardial infarction, trauma, drugs that alter clotting mechanisms, and uremia. Chylous and lymphous effusions are quite rare. Chylopericardium usually occurs with thoracic duct obstruction and seepage of milky substances from pericardial lymphatics into the pericardium. Lymphopericardium, even more rare, results from a pericardial lymphangioma.

The dangers associated with any acute pericardial effusion are those of cardiac tamponade or compression. Pericardial effusion is defined as greater than 50 ml of fluid. The amount of fluid necessary to cause hemodynamically significant effusion varies. It depends upon the time over which the fluid accumulates, the thickness of the pericardium, the weight of the ventricles, and the total blood volume.

An exudation of cells may be of several kinds. Suppurative reactions consist predominantly of polymorphonuclear leukocytes and are caused by pyogenic bacteria such as staphylococci or streptococci. These exudates often progress to fibrous thickening. Mononuclear cell reactions are composed primarily of lymphocytes and macrophages that are localized to interstitial sites. These reactions are classically produced by viruses. The reaction is usually transient and rarely progresses to fibrous proliferation. Acid-fast organisms produce a unique mononuclear exudate, termed a granuloma, consisting of small collections of modified macrophages or histiocytes that are usually surrounded by lymphocytes and giant cells. The granulomatous reaction is characterized by persistence of the etiological agent within the macrophages, probably causing their epithelioid transformation. Fibrous thickening and adhesions are typical after granulomatous reactions.

There are various forms of chronic pericarditis, not all of which produce compression. Chronic adhesive pericarditis refers to the presence of numerous adhesions between visceral and parietal pericardia. The adhesions may be focal with or without effusion. Diffuse adhesions may obliterate the pericardial space without causing constriction. Tuberculosis, viral infections, and pericarditis associated with rheumatic fever sometimes produce a chronic response without constriction. However, in more severe cases, especially those caused by tuberculosis, the pericardial layers become thickened, densely fibrotic, inelastic, and adherent to each other. The pericardial space is obliterated. Calcium deposits are common. The constricting process may result in narrowing at the entrance of the venae cavae or it may involve the atrioventricular groove.

Cholesterol pericarditis is a rare and poorly understood process characterized by a slowly developing effusion that is nonconstricting. The fluid may be clear or turbid, but it has a "gold paint" appearance because of the cholesterol crystals. Both parietal and visceral pericardium become thickened. Cholesterol pericarditis is associated with hypothyroidism, rheumatoid arthritis, and tuberculous pericarditis. The cause of the cholesterol in the pericardial fluid is unknown.

MECHANISMS OF PERICARDIAL DISEASES

Table 4 presents an etiological classification of pericardial disease broadly grouped into those due to

TABLE 4. PERICARDIAL DISEASES

ETIOLOGY	SPECIFIC EXAMPLES	ACCESS TO PERICARDIUM	PATHOGENESIS	HEMODYNAMIC CONSEQUENCES Acute	Chronic
INFLAMMATORY					
A. Infectious					
Bacterial	Staphylococcal Pneumococcal Gram-negative (gonococcal, meningococcal)	direct extension and hematogenous	direct infection with inflammation	tamponade usual	constriction common
	Tuberculosis	lymphatics from breakdown of mediastinal lymph node and hematogenous from primary focus	direct infection with inflammation	slowly progressive effusion; may resolve spontaneously; occasional tamponade	constriction common
Viral	Group B coxsackie	?hematogenous	direct infection with inflammation	variable effusion occasional tamponade	constriction rare
Fungal	Histoplasmosis	direct extension and hematogenous	direct infection with inflammation	variable effusion occasional tamponade	constriction rare
Parasitic	Amebiasis Echinococcosis	direct extension from heart/liver	direct infection with inflammation	tamponade common	constriction common
B. Noninfectious					
Acute "benign" or idiopathic	Similar to viral pericarditis	unknown	?viral infection ?immune response to virus ?autoimmunity	variable effusion tamponade unusual	constriction rare
Traumatic	Post–myocardial infarction (Dressler's syndrome) Post–heart surgery (postperi-cardiotomy syndrome)	?direct innoculation/ trauma	?viral infection ?immune response to virus ?autoimmunity	variable effusion tamponade uncommon (unless cardiac rupture occurs)	constriction rare
	Post-irradiation	direct trauma particularly with doses >4000 rad	direct injury with inflammation acutely; causes of delayed inflammation, effusion unknown	variable effusion with rare tamponade	constriction rare
Associated with chronic renal failure	Particularly in patients on chronic hemodialysis	unknown	unknown	large, progressive effusion, tamponade common with large effusion	constriction uncommon
NEOPLASTIC	Breast Lung	direct extension and via lymphatics	seeding of pericardium with malignant cells; occasionally "sympathetic" and not due to malignancy	tamponade common	survival sufficient to allow constriction is unusual
	Leukemia Melanoma	hematogenous	seeding of pericardium with malignant cells; occasionally "sympathetic" and not due to malignancy	tamponade common	survival sufficient to allow constriction is unusual
CONGENITAL					
Absence of pericardium	Partial or complete		embryologic development defect: when partial, defect most commonly on left	if partial, herniation of left atrial appendage may cause sudden death or strangulation	usually none
Cysts/ diverticula	Cysts most common at right costophrenic angle		abnormal diffusion of mesenchymal lacunae	none	none

inflammatory, neoplastic, and congenital causes and also includes specific examples and a summary of pathogenetic mechanisms and likely hemodynamic consequences. This section will not discuss the pathophysiology of each condition in detail but will touch on both the common and the unique pathogenetic features among the different etiologies, using specific examples to illustrate basic principles. The remaining sections of this chapter will focus on the important hemodynamic consequences of pericardial disease—tamponade and constriction.

Infectious (bacterial, viral, fungal, and parasitic) and neoplastic diseases of the pericardium share the common feature of gaining access to the pericardium by direct extension from contiguous structures, by lymphatic spread, and/or by hematogenous routes. With infectious pericarditis, involvement is most commonly via direct extension from an infected contiguous structure (e.g., pneumococcal pneumonia) or via a hematogenous route (e.g., staphylococcal sepsis). The fluid is purulent with numerous white blood cells. The likelihood of bacterial pericarditis is increased by cardiothoracic surgery or trauma, immunosuppressant therapy, infection of a contiguous structure, and conditions associated with sepsis (e.g., bacterial endocarditis). In bacterial pericarditis, polymorphonuclear leukocytes predominate, and abundant organisms are seen on gram stain and are usually easily cultured. The effusion may increase rapidly, resulting in acute tamponade. With the advent of antibiotic therapy, staphylococcal pericarditis has become the most common etiological agent and is usually caused by a particularly virulent infection with rapid fluid accumulation, marked pericardial thickening and tamponade acutely, and acute/chronic constriction. With tuberculosis, an early pericardial effusion contains predominantly polymorphonuclear leukocytes, but on a more chronic basis monocytes and lymphocytes predominate. The effusion is frequently sanguineous, and acid-fast organisms are rarely seen on stain but in about 30 per cent of cases may be cultured from fluid and cultured or visualized microscopically in pericardial tissue. A tuberculous effusion is typically more indolent than bacterial or fungal/parastic effusions with more gradual progression. Although tamponade may occur, constriction on a chronic basis is particularly common. Viral pericarditis causes a variable degree of serous (and occasionally sanguineous) effusion that infrequently causes tamponade and rarely progresses to chronic constriction. Mononuclear cells predominate and occasionally the virus may be grown from fluid, particularly early in the disease. More commonly, the diagnosis is inferred by a combination of an appropriate clinical syndome and a rise and fall in viral serum antibody titers. Neoplastic disease most commonly involves the pericardium via direct extension from contiguous structures (e.g., lung carcinoma) or via lymphatic spread from the mediastinum (e.g., lung and breast carcinoma) and, more rarely, by hematogenous routes (e.g., melanoma, leukemia). The pericardial effusion is usually sanguineous, and mononuclear cells predominate. Tumor cells may be seen on cell block of a spun sediment of pericardial fluid. The pathophysiology of acute "benign" or idiopathic pericarditis is more controversial, with viral infections, an altered immune response to a virus, and/or autoimmunity the

leading possibilities. The effusion is typically serous and of variable degree, with either acute or chronic hemodynamic compromise rare. The pericarditis syndromes resulting from closed chest trauma, heart surgery (postpericardiotomy syndrome), and postmyocardial infarction (Dressler's syndrome) share a number of features common to acute idiopathic pericarditis, and similar pathogenetic mechanisms have been postulated. Heart reactive antibodies, possibly stimulated by foreign proteins that share cross-antigenicity with heart tissue and/or from heart tissue altered by interaction with a foreign protein (e.g., a virus), have been isolated from patients with these various syndromes. Direct proof of an infectious agent and/or primary role for such antibodies in the disease process, however, is lacking, and they may just be markers of myocardial cell injury. On a more simple level, it may be that a latent viral infection (with finicky growth characteristics) is activated by myocardial infarction, trauma, heart surgery, etc., to produce the syndrome. Another variety of traumatic pericarditis results from irradiation administered to the mediastinum as therapy for a variety of neoplasms. Radiation-induced pericarditis typically develops within the first year after treatment and uncommonly results in acute or chronic hemodynamic complications. In the noninfectious inflammatory pericarditis associated with systemic connective tissue diseases, the mechanism of pericardial involvement remains unproven, but the pericardial fluid is similar to that seen in other serosal cavities such as joints and shows a high protein content (greater than 5.0 grams/dl), low glucose and complement titers, and complement-activating gamma globulin complexes. In rheumatoid arthritis, pericarditis is found in about a third of patients at autopsy, while in systemic lupus erythematosus pericardial involvement occurs at some point in the course of nearly all patients. In both conditions acute and chronic hemodynamic consequences have been reported but are the exception.

CARDIAC TAMPONADE

Cardiac tamponade is defined as compression of the heart due to the accumulation of fluid within the pericardial space. The hemodynamic alterations produced by pericardial effusion reflect the volume and the rate of fluid accumulation. As a point of departure it is useful to consider the pressure-volume relation of the intact pericardium. Pericardial pressure is normally less than atmospheric pressure and closely approximates pleural pressure. With additions of warm saline to the pericardial space, pericardial pressure rises and the relation between volume and pressure describes a curve in which the change in pressure for any given change in volume is small when the volume of pericardial fluid is small, and the change in pressure for any given change in volume is large at higher points on the volume-pressure curve (Fig. 103). The volume-pressure curve demonstrates hysteresis; that is, pressure is higher for any given volume during addition of fluid than during withdrawal. During inspiration pericardial pressure falls, and during expiration it rises. When pericardial pressure and volume are normal, pericardial pressure increases briefly with the onset of ventricular systole but drops during late

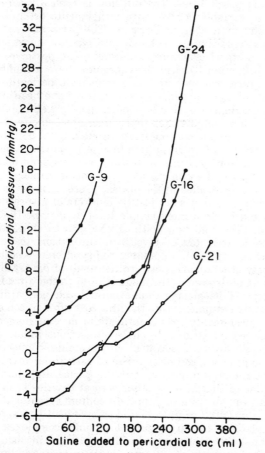

Figure 103. Pressure-volume relationship from four representative experiments, to show effects of infusing warm saline into the pericardial sac. (With permission from Morgan, B. C., Guntheroth, W. G., and Dillard, D. H.: Relationship of pericardial to pleural pressure during quiet respiration and cardiac tamponade. Circ Res 16:496, 1965.)

filling for any given level of venous pressure. The extent of the alterations in cardiac output, blood pressure, heart rate, and ventricular volume correlate with pericardial pressure. Thus the hemodynamic changes that accompany pericardial effusion are influenced by both the volume and rate of accumulation of the effusion.

In addition to these mean changes in hemodynamic parameters, there are certain phasic changes in the venous and arterial pressure pulse that are characteristic of tamponade and helpful in recognizing this condition at the bedside. (For an example of a normal venous wave form see Fig. 30.) Venous pressure is normally only a few millimeters of mercury above atmospheric pressure. Normal venous flow into the right atrium is biphasic. One positive surge in venous return is coincident with the "X" descent of the venous pressure pulse. A second surge of flow into the right atrium coincides with the "Y" descent of the venous pressure pulse. With cardiac tamponade, mean venous pressure is elevated. The "X" descent of the venous pressure pulse is exaggerated and the "Y" descent is abolished or replaced by a gradual positive wave. With tamponade, in contrast to pericardial constriction, inspiration continues to transmit a negative pressure to the right atrium and ventricle, and right atrial pressure drops normally with inspiration (i.e., Kussmaul's sign is absent). In addition, there is usually no early diastolic dip of the right ventricular pressure pulse.

In pericardial tamponade, mean arterial pressure is reduced and the pulse pressure accompanying each heartbeat is reduced because of the smaller stroke volume. Pulsus paradoxus refers to an exaggerated drop in systolic arterial pressure during inspiration (Fig. 104). Normally, the arterial pressure drops during quiet inspiration by more than 5 mm Hg, but almost never more than 10 mm Hg. Studies of aortic blood flow in patients with tamponade show an abnormally great decrease in aortic blood flow velocity and stroke volume during inspiration (Fig. 105). The mechanism responsible for this abnormally great drop in left ventricular stroke volume during inspiration continues to be controversial. One theory proposes that during inspiration the drop in intrapleural pressure is not transmitted equally well to the left ventricle and pulmonary veins, and hence the pressure gradient that favors return to the left heart is diminished, with a resultant fall in stroke volume. This may be the most plausible explanation for the occasional pulsus paradoxus noted in constrictive pericarditis but not for that occurring with tamponade. Another theory is that with inspiration venous return to the right heart is facilitated, which, since it occurs within a closed pericardial space, compromises left ventricular filling and stroke volume. Echocardiographic studies of right and left ventricular dimensions during tamponade provide evidence that this is an important factor. In addition, Shabetai has reported that pulmonary arterial blood flow and velocity increase during inspiration, while aortic flow and velocity decrease in patients with tamponade and a paradoxical systemic arterial pressure pulse. Finally, under both normal and tamponade conditions, inspiration lowers intrathoracic and left ventricular diastolic pressure more than aortic pressure, thereby increasing obligate left ventricular pressure development and contributing to an inspiratory fall in stroke

systole, apparently as a consequence of cardiac ejection and diminution of cardiac volume. When pericardial volume or pressure is increased by additions of fluid, pericardial pressure rises and falls with cardiac activity and essentially parallels the phasic changes in left ventricular pressure. The most important implication of the pericardial pressure-volume relationship is that when tamponade is present, the removal of even relatively small amounts of pericardial fluid will drop pericardial pressure, restore hemodynamics toward normal, and may be life saving.

Cardiac tamponade produces typical changes in cardiac output, blood pressure, and heart rate. Cardiac output and blood pressure are reduced, and heart rate and systemic venous pressure increase. Systemic vascular resistance increases largely as a consequence of reflex activation of the sympathetic nervous system in response to the decreased cardiac output and blood pressure. Angiographic studies have been used to assess ventricular volume during tamponade. These studies have shown that right and left ventricular end-diastolic volume are reduced in tamponade despite the elevated venous pressures. Hence, tamponade compresses the heart and reduces the extent of diastolic

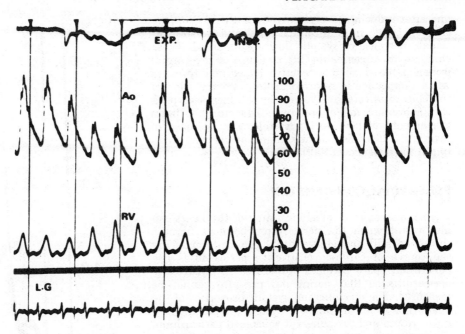

Figure 104. Pressures in a patient with cardiac tamponade and hypovolemia (ruptured dissecting hematoma of the aorta). From top: respiration, aortic (Ao) pressure, right ventricular (RV) pressure, pressure baseline, and electrocardiogram. Note the pulsus paradoxus (25 mm Hg). The right ventricular pressure pulse is abnormal and displays small amplitude and increased diastolic pressure. (With permission from Shabetai, R., Fowler, N. O., and Guntheroth, W. G.: The hemodynamics of cardiac tamponade and constrictive pericarditis. Am J Cardiol 26:481, 1970.)

volume. An old theory that inspiratory traction on the tense pericardium by the diaphragm prevents diastolic filling is refuted by the finding that venous filling is not impaired by tamponade and that respiratory changes in venous return are the important variables in pulsus paradoxus. Despite these and many other potential explanations, the mechanism of pulsus paradoxus remains a topic of investigation and debate.

Inadequate myocardial perfusion may contribute to cardiac depression, since coronary flow is reduced in severe tamponade. When flow probes are used to study phasic left coronary artery blood flow in dogs before

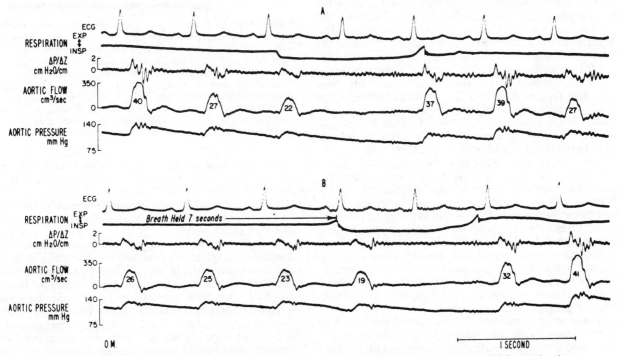

Figure 105. Pressure and flow recordings from patient having pericardial tamponade. ECG, respiration, pressure difference ($\Delta p/\Delta z$), aortic blood flow, and aortic blood pressure are shown from top down in each panel. The stroke volume, cm³, is listed under each flow curve. Data were obtained in Panel *A* during normal respiration and in Panel *B* following a seven-second period in which breathing was suspended in mid-expiration. Note that in both panels the onset of inspiration is followed by the absence of cardiac ejection—that is, complete pulsus paradoxus. (With permission from Ruskin, J., Bache, R. J., Rembert, J. C., and Greenfield, J. C., Jr.: Pressure-flow studies in man: Effect of respiration on left ventricular stroke volume. Circulation 48:79, 1973.)

and after inducing several degrees of cardiac tamponade, a decrease in total coronary flow and a disproportionate decrease of systolic flow are observed. These changes are accompanied by evidence of myocardial ischemia based upon a reactive hyperemia response when tamponade is relieved acutely. Compression of the epicardial coronary vessels by the increased pericardial pressure may therefore be the factor that limits the amount of flow during systole. The decrease in myocardial blood flow during tamponade is most striking in the subendocardial layers.

PERICARDIAL CONSTRICTION

An impairment of diastolic filling of the heart can also result when the pericardium becomes fibrotic, thickened, stiff, and adherent to the epicardium during the course of chronic constrictive pericarditis. The pericardial space becomes obliterated in constrictive pericarditis so that pericardial pressure cannot be measured. The diastolic and systolic properties of the heart thus reflect a "lumped" system composed of the myocardium and the adherent thickened pericardium. Pericardial constriction produces some hemodynamic changes that are indistinguishable from those of tamponade. Hence, cardiac output and blood pressure are reduced and heart rate and venous pressure are elevated. As a consequence of impaired filling, cardiac output can be increased only by an elevation of heart rate, and exercise tolerance is markedly impaired.

In the atrium, mean venous pressure is elevated. The "a" wave is exaggerated because atrial contraction occurs when the ventricle is already filled and the ventricular wall and pericardium are noncompliant. With descent of the tricuspid and mitral valves at the onset of systole, atrial pressures drop precipitously, producing an exaggerated "X" descent. Similarly, when the tricuspid and mitral valves open and ventricular pressure dips to its low point, atrial pressures again drop precipitously, producing an exaggerated "Y" descent. These prominent "X" and "Y" descents may be seen in the jugular venous pulse, providing a bedside clue to the diagnosis of constrictive pericarditis.

Constrictive pericarditis produces a typical and characteristic change in the right and left ventricular pressure recording. At end-systole, ventricular volume is small and atrial and venous pressures are maximal. For a brief period in early diastole ventricular pressure drops to near zero, but then with the onset of rapid ventricular filling the noncompliant ventricular wall is encountered and ventricular pressure rises abruptly to reach a relative plateau that is maintained throughout the remainder of diastole. This pattern produces a characteristic early dip and later plateau in the ventricular pressure pulse (Fig. 106).

It was noted previously that in normal patients flow in the venae cavae and return to the right heart are increased during inspiration. Constriction either limits severely or abolishes the transmission of this negative intrathoracic pressure to the right heart and there is no augmentation of right heart filling by inspiration. In severe cases of constriction, venous pressure may actually rise at the end of inspiration, presumably because the increase in intra-abdominal pressure forces blood toward the heart, but this blood cannot be

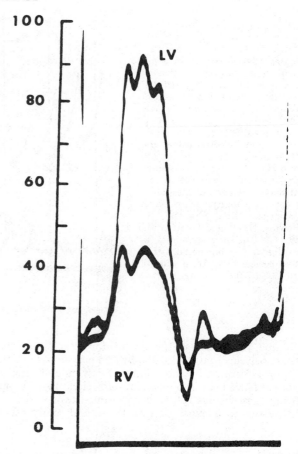

Figure 106. Left and right ventricular pressures from a patient with severe chronic constrictive pericarditis. Note the early diastolic dip and late high plateau recorded from both ventricles and equilibration of the diastolic pressures of the two ventricles. The pulmonary arterial diastolic pressure, the pulmonary arterial wedge pressure, and the right atrial pressure were equal to the right ventricular diastolic pressure. (With permission from Shabetai, R., Fowler, N. O., and Guntheroth, W. G.: The hemodynamics of cardiac tamponade and constrictive pericarditis. Am J Cardiol 26:482, 1970.)

accepted because of the constraint on ventricular filling. In this case venous pressure may rise during inspiration and produce swelling of the neck veins (Kussmaul's sign). Unlike cardiac tamponade, constrictive pericarditis rarely produces a paradoxical arterial pressure pulse.

In both cardiac tamponade and constriction, end-diastolic ventricular pressures are elevated, causing the mean pressures in the left and right atrium to be similarly elevated. Pulmonary artery pressure is also elevated. This sequence produces a situation in which left ventricular end-diastolic, mean left atrial, pulmonary artery diastolic, right ventricular end-diastolic, and mean right atrial pressure are all moderately elevated and nearly equal. This finding is in contrast to most forms of valvular and myocardial disease in which one ventricle is compromised more than the other and pressures are elevated but not to an equal extent.

A brief but special word of comment seems justified concerning the relation between pericardial disease and blood volume. Pericardial effusion and constriction each produce their hemodynamic results primarily as a consequence of limiting severely the extent of diastolic ventricular filling. Elevations of venous pressure are a consequence of this limitation, but they also provide the force that is required to fill either ventricle in the face of external compression or constriction. Thus, in either tamponade or constriction, maintenance of forward cardiac output depends greatly on venous pressure. Therefore, an abrupt decrease of blood volume (for example, with blood loss or after the use of potent diuretics) may drastically reduce cardiac output and arterial blood pressure in the presence of tamponade or constriction. These consequences may develop when venous pressure is lowered only modestly from an elevated but necessarily high level. A second point is that while there are important and distinguishing differences between pericardial disease and myocardial disease, both can lead to reductions of cardiac output below the level that is required to meet the metabolic needs of the body. This situation sets in motion a chain of events that are described in great detail in the chapter on heart failure. At least in a qualitative sense, the mechanisms responsible for salt and water retention, formation of edema, and the consequences of prolonged elevations of venous pressure and augmented neurohumoral activity in heart failure apply when cardiac output is impaired by pericardial disease. One notable exception to this similarity between heart failure and chronic significant pericardial disease is that pulmonary edema is common in the former and rare in the latter. The major reason for this difference is that in pericardial disease the func-

tion of both ventricles is usually compromised to an equal degree, while in valvular, coronary, and myocardial disease the degree of abnormality is often much greater on the left side of the heart than on the right.

REFERENCES

Cortes, F. M.: The Pericardium and Its Disorders. Springfield, Ill., Charles C Thomas Co., 1971.

Engle, M. A., McCabe, J. C., Ebert, P. A., and Zabriskie, J.: The postpericardiotomy syndrome and antiheart antibodies. Circulation 49:401, 1974.

Holt, J. P.: The normal pericardium. Am J Cardiol 26:455, 1970.

Jarmakani, J. M. M., McHale, P. A., and Greenfield, J. C., Jr.: The effect of cardiac tamponade on coronary haemodynamics in the awake dog. Cardiovasc Res 9:112, 1975.

Levine, H. D.: Myocardial fibrosis in constrictive pericarditis. Electrocardiographic and pathologic observations. Circulation 48:1268, 1973.

Robatham, J. L., and Mitzner, W.: A model of the effects of respiration on left ventricular performance. J Appl Physiol 46:411, 1979.

Rubin, R. H., and Moellering, R. C., Jr.: Clinical, microbiologic and therapeutic aspects of purulent pericarditis. Am J Med 59:68, 1975.

Shabetai, R.: The Pericardium. New York, Grune and Stratton, 1981.

Shabetai, R., Fowler, N. O., and Guntheroth, W. G.: The hemodynamics of cardiac tamponade and constrictive pericarditis. Am J Cardiol 26:480, 1970.

Smith, W. G.: Coxsackie B myopericarditis in adults. Am Heart J 80:34, 1970.

Spodick, D. H. (ed.): Pericardial Diseases. Cardiovascular Clinics. Vol. 7. Philadelphia, F. A. Davis Co., 1976.

Mechanisms of Cardiac Dysrhythmias

If the electrocardiogram is used to assess cardiac rhythm, then normal rhythmic activity of the heart can be defined in electrocardiographic terms. The physiological basis of normal activity is developed in detail in the chapter on Excitation of the Heart. Briefly, the sinus node is normally responsible for initiating the electrical impulse that causes cardiac contraction. The frequency of impulse formation within the sinus node determines heart rate and can be related to the metabolic activity of the subject at the time an electrocardiogram is recorded. Under basal conditions this rate varies among individuals but is generally in the range of 60 to 100 beats per minute. This is termed sinus rhythm (Fig. 107). During maximal exercise, however, the sinus node impulse rate speeds with heart rate ranges from 150 to 200 beats per minute (termed sinus tachycardia). During sleep or in conditioned athletes the sinus node rate may drop below 60 beats per minute owing to enhanced vagal tone (this is termed sinus bradycardia). The relation between heart rate and metabolic activity (as reflected by oxygen uptake) is roughly linear in each individual. The origin of the impulse from the sinus node in sinus rhythm leads both to a predictable sequence of atrial activation and to certain typical features of P wave morphology regardless of heart rate. At any given heart rate, impulse formation within the sinus node is more or less regular, except for a modest phasic variation about the mean

heart rate in synchrony with respiration. This phasic variation is mediated by changes in cardiac efferent vaginal nerve activity and is referred to as sinus arrhythmia.

Following excitation of the atria, the electrical impulse is transmitted from the atria to the ventricle through the AV node. Within the AV node, the speed of impulse propagation is extraordinarily slow. As a consequence there is a substantial delay between the P wave and the QRS complex, ranging from 120 to 200 msec in normal subjects. Ventricular excitation is determined by the anatomic distribution of the His-Purkinje system and the speed of impulse propagation within that system and its components. Because the structure and propagation properties of the His-Purkinje system are relatively uniform in normal individuals, there is a more or less uniform morphology to the QRS complex.

Broadly speaking, cardiac dysrhythmias can be defined as any significant deviation from normal rhythm as defined above. More specifically, they represent alterations in the rate, regularity, or site of impulse formation or alterations of impulse propagation that lead to changes in the sequence of atrial or ventricular activation or in the normal coupling of atrial and ventricular activity. The resulting rhythms may be classified as too fast or too slow (tachycardia or bradycardia), ectopic in origin (atrial, junctional, or ventric-

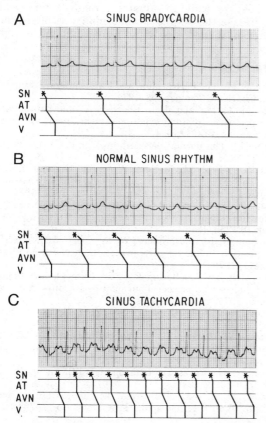

Figure 107. Panels *A, B,* and *C* were taken from the same patient at various times during 24 hours of electrocardiographic monitoring and illustrate responses of the normally dominant sinus node to differing metabolic demands and autonomic balance. (These rhythm strips as well as the others in this section were recorded at a standard paper speed of 25 mm/sec, and each small square therefore equals 0.04 sec and each large square equals 0.2 sec. Heart rate may be obtained by dividing the number of large subdivisions between complexes into 300.) Below each rhythm strip is a ladder diagram that is used to illustrate underlying electrophysiological phenomena. Each horizontal tier corresponds to an anatomical level in the heart beginning with the SA node (SN) and extending through the atria (AT), AV node (AVN), and ventricles (V). An asterisk in a particular level indicates pacemaker activity, and chamber depolarization is indicated by vertical lines. Conduction through various areas is indicated by oblique lines. The more vertical the oblique lines are, the more rapid the conduction. Panel *A* was recorded during sleep and shows sinus bradycardia, with the sinus node remaining dominant at a rate of 50 per minute and with a PR interval of 0.2 sec reflecting the increased vagal tone occurring during sleep. Panel *B* shows normal sinus rhythm and was recorded during work at a desk. Note that the sinus node rate has increased to 75 per minute and that there has been slight shortening in the PR interval (0.18 sec) due to a diminution in vagal tone and the greater metabolic needs of the body. Panel *C*, an example of sinus tachycardia, was recorded during exercise. The sinus node remains dominant but has increased its rate to 163 per minute, while the PR interval has decreased to approximately 0.12 sec. These changes are due to a further decrease in vagal tone, an increase in sympathetic tone, and the metabolic effects of exercise.

ular), or in terms of a site of conduction delay or block (sinoatrial, atrial, junctional, or intraventricular).

Most arrhythmias can be categorized etiologically as (1) disturbances of impulse formation, (2) disturbances of impulse propagation, or (3) combined disturbances of impulse formation and propagation. At a cellular level, the first group includes arrhythmias due to alterations of normal automatic activity, to abnormal automaticity, or to abnormal triggered activity. The second group includes disturbances due to conduction delay, block, and either random or ordered reentry. The third group is typified by parasystolic rhythm and by disturbances of conduction that arise because of delayed propagation or block in regions that have depolarized owing to latent automaticity. Rather than catalogue arrhythmias, this chapter will discuss mechanisms, give electrocardiographic examples, discuss the known features of each from a mechanistic point of view, and briefly highlight the general clinical consequences of arrhythmias. The reader is encouraged to review the chapter on Excitation of the Heart as a preface to this discussion.

DISTURBANCES OF IMPULSE FORMATION

Certain cells or aggregates of cells within the normal heart have the capacity to undergo spontaneous and regular slow diastolic depolarization, which brings the cells to threshold and evokes an action potential that is then propagated away from its site of origin. This phenomenon is referred to as automaticity. It is a normal property of the sinus node, of other specialized atrial fibers, and of parts of the conducting system, including the distal AV node–His bundle junction, bundle of His, proximal portions of bundle branches, and peripheral Purkinje fibers. Nonspecialized fibers that make up the ordinary working muscle of atrium and ventricle and the body of the AV node are not normally automatic.

Of the cells possessing normal automaticity, those in the sinus node initiate impulses at the most rapid rate under most conditions. Assuming normal conduction, impulses that arise in the sinus node are transmitted in an orderly sequence through the atria to the AV node and then over the specialized conducting tissue to the rest of the myocardium and depolarize latent automatic cells in other regions of intrinsically slower rhythmicity. The two major factors that determine the rate of firing, or cycle length, of automatic cells are (1) the slope of diastolic depolarization and (2) the difference between maximal diastolic potential attained at the end of repolarization and threshold potential (Fig. 108). Both factors are capable of influencing automaticity but it is the slope of diastolic depolarization that is the most important determinant of cycle length. Moving from the sinus node to the AV node and the His-Purkinje system, there is gradual diminution in the intrinsic slope of diastolic depolarization. Thus, the sinus node arrives at threshold first and is the dominant pacemaker. Other automatic cells, normally depolarized by the propagated sinus impulse, are latent pacemakers and may, under abnormal circumstances, control the cardiac rhythm. In subsequent parts of this section we will consider in detail factors

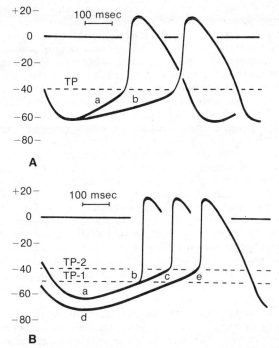

A

B

Figure 108. Transmembrane action potentials typical of those recorded from fibers of the sinoatrial node showing the expected effects of changing the slope of Phase-4 depolarization, the magnitude of the maximum diastolic potential (MDP), and the level of the threshold potential (TP). In *A*, when the slope of Phase-4 is decreased from a to b, more time is required to reach threshold potential and the cycle length is increased. In *B*, under control conditions (TP-1) the fiber depolarizes from a maximum diastolic potential of a and attains threshold at b. If threshold potential shifts to a less negative value (TP-2) the Phase-4 depolarization will not attain threshold until c. If maximum diastolic potential is increased to d, Phase-4 depolarization will not attain threshold until e. Opposite changes in the slope of Phase-4, the value of TP, or the value of MDP would have the opposite effect on cycle length and rate. (With permission from Hoffman, B. F., Rosen, M. R., and Wit, A. L.: Electrophysiology and pharmacology of cardiac arrhythmias. III. The causes and treatment of cardiac arrhythmias. Part A. Am. Heart J 89:119, 1975.)

that modify the frequency or rhythmicity of normally automatic cells. From the point of view of disturbances of rhythm, however, it is apparent that an increase or decrease in the rate of the sinus node can lead to sinus tachycardia or sinus bradycardia respectively. Furthermore, local influences that increase the rhythmicity of latent pacemakers or agents that have a greater capacity to enhance automatic firing of latent pacemakers than that of the sinus node may lead to a situation in which impulses arising from outside the sinus node either interrupt or usurp the normal control of cardiac rhythm by the sinus node. As would be expected from the distribution of these latent pacemakers, such ectopic beats or rhythms may arise from the atrium, AV junction, His bundle, or distal Purkinje cells. Perhaps the most frequent example of isolated beats or sustained rhythms arising from automatic, but normally latent, pacemaker regions are the escape rhythms that develop when impulse formation in the SA node fails, or when AV block prevents sinus impulses from reaching the ventricles.

For many years it has been suspected that electrophysiological characteristics of diseased hearts may differ from normal tissue, and indeed that mechanisms relatively unique to diseased hearts may be responsible for alterations of rhythm. With this possibility in mind, a number of investigators have studied atrial and ventricular muscle and Purkinje fibers, which were partially depolarized by one means or another. In addition, the electrical activity of cardiac fibers removed from diseased hearts of animals and man have been studied. From such studies it has become apparent that certain cells removed from diseased hearts are partially depolarized, and that the electrical activity of partially depolarized cells differs from normally polarized cells obtained from the same specimen. One such difference is that whereas normal atrial and ventricular muscle fibers are quiescent and fail to demonstrate automatic behavior, when these cells are partially depolarized, and especially in the presence of norepinephrine, spontaneous diastolic depolarization may be observed (Fig. 109). Even more recently, atrial

A FAST RESPONSE

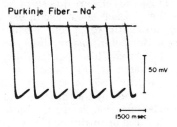

B SLOW RESPONSE

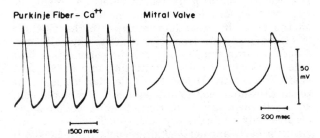

Figure 109. Spontaneous diastolic depolarization and automatic impulse initiation in cardiac fibers with fast and slow response activity. Panel *A* shows action potentials recorded from a canine Purkinje fiber with a maximum diastolic potential of −90 mV and, therefore, fast response activity. This fiber has prominent spontaneous diastolic depolarization and is not being electrically stimulated. Panel *B*, left, shows slow response, calcium-dependent action potentials recorded from a canine Purkinje fiber perfused with a sodium-free medium. Maximum diastolic potential is −65 mV, spontaneous diastolic depolarization is prominent, and the fiber is automatically active. Panel *B*, right, shows slow response action potentials recorded from cardiac fiber in the mitral valve leaflet of a monkey. Maximum diastolic potential is −58 mV. Note the prominent Phase-4 depolarization and automatic activity. The fiber is not being electrically stimulated. (With permission from Wit, A. L., Rosen, M. R., and Hoffman, B. F.: Electrophysiology and pharmacology of cardiac arrhythmias. II. Relationship of normal and abnormal electrical activity of cardiac fibers to the genesis of arrhythmias. Am Heart J 88:518, 1974.)

fibers removed from canine hearts with chronic mitral insufficiency have demonstrated depolarization and automatic activity inducible by norepinephrine. The ionic mechanism responsible for automatic behavior of partially depolarized cells is still uncertain, but indirect evidence indicates that it may differ from the mechanism of spontaneous depolarization in normally automatic cells such as normal Purkinje fibers. The most important point is that abnormal mechanisms of automatic activity may develop in diseased and partially depolarized fibers. Furthermore, in contrast to normal hearts, where automatic activity is confined to the specialized tissues, in diseased hearts rhythms arising from abnormal automatic mechanisms may originate from ordinary atrial and ventricular muscle as well as from specialized tissues. Hence, the number of potential sites of origin of disturbances due to impulse formation outside the sinus node is greatly expanded.

In addition to the normal and abnormal automatic mechanisms noted above, in which a cell or group of cells undergoes repetitive spontaneous diastolic depolarization, there is yet another mechanism of repetitive activity. This mechanism is referred to as triggered activity, because the cells are quiescent for long periods of time in the absence of an excitatory stimulus (in contrast to automatic cells), but when once excited, two or more action potentials or a long run of repetitive responses is observed. This type of activity results from depolarizing afterpotentials, which may be of two types. One type, referred to as early afterdepolarizations, is characterized by the fact that one or repetitive action potentials develop before the membrane potential of the triggered or initial beat has returned to the level it had before the initiating beat. The second type, referred to as a delayed afterdepolarization, is characterized by one or more repetitive action potentials, each of which develops after the membrane potential on the preceding beat has returned to the diastolic level. Delayed afterdepolarizations are typically preceded by a transient period of hyperpolarization that follows recovery from the initiating and subsequent beats (Fig. 110). Delayed afterdepolarizations that reach threshold lead to subsequent firing of the cell, while afterdepolarizations that fail to reach threshold produce only an oscillatory potential. The precise ionic basis for early and delayed afterdepolarizations is still unknown. Triggerable activity of this type has been observed in cells from the floor of the coronary sinus and from cells in the mitral valve obtained from normal

hearts. Ouabain and acetylstrophanthidin have been noted to cause delayed afterdepolarizations and triggerable activity in specialized atrial fibers and in isolated Purkinje fibers. Furthermore, the phenomenon of triggerable repetitive firing observed in isolated preparations is remarkably similar to the response when single stimuli are delivered to the intact heart that has been exposed to digitalis preparations. These physiological studies indicate that afterdepolarizations are a potential basis for either single coupled extrasystoles or bursts of repetitive activity arising from sites outside the sinus node; however, the role of triggered activity in producing clinically significant arrhythmias remains to be proven. Although tachycardias that can be induced and terminated by single, appropriately timed electrical stimuli have generally been attributed to reentry, these same properties appear to characterize triggerable arrhythmias due to afterdepolarization. Thus, the ability to initiate or terminate a tachycardia with a single stimulus is not sufficient to distinguish between these two mechanisms in either the basic laboratory or in clinical situations.

The most important factors that influence rhythmicity of automatic cardiac tissue include (1) autonomic nerve activity, (2) changes in electrolyte concentrations and pO_2, (3) mechanical effects, particularly fiber stretch, and (4) certain cardioactive drugs. Each of these factors affects rhythmicity by changing the slope of diastolic depolarization, the threshold potential, or maximum diastolic potentials. Significant deviations from normal of any or all of these factors may enhance or depress automaticity in the normal pacemaker or enhance automaticity of latent pacemaker cells. If the alteration in automaticity is enough to disturb normal impulse formation, the end result is an arrhythmia, manifested clinically by a change in rate, rhythm, or site of origin of the cardiac impulse (Fig. 111).

Most important among the factors that affect automaticity is the influence of the autonomic nervous system. Alterations of sympathetic and parasympathetic tone are responsible for a number of physiological changes in rhythm. Stimulation of adrenergic nerves and consequent release of norepinephrine increase the slope of diastolic depolarization, resulting in acceleration of the sinus rhythm or sinus tachycardia. In contrast, as predicted from the antagonistic effects of the sympathetic and parasympathetic components of the autonomic nervous system, vagal nerve stimulation and release of acetylcholine decrease the slope of

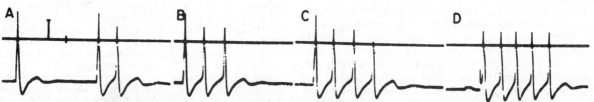

Figure 110. The effects of single driven impulses on a canine Purkinje fiber that was quiescent when exposed to a Na-free solution containing 16 mM Ca and 128 mM TEA Cl. In *A* the first action potential at the far left occurs after electrical stimulation (i.e., is driven) and is followed by an after-hyperpolarization and a delayed after-depolarization. The second action potential in *A* is also driven but is delayed after-depolarization reaches threshold and it is followed by a single nondriven (triggered) action potential. The first action potentials in *B, C,* and *D* are driven and they are followed by several nondriven (triggered) action potentials. The last triggered action potential in each panel is followed by a delayed after-depolarization that fails to reach threshold potential. (With permission from Cranefield, P. F.: The Conduction of the Cardiac Impulse—The Slow Response and Cardiac Arrhythmias. Mt. Kisko, N.Y., Futura Publishing Co., 1975, p. 209.)

SINUS RHYTHM INTERRUPTED BY ACCELERATED VENTRICULAR PACEMAKER

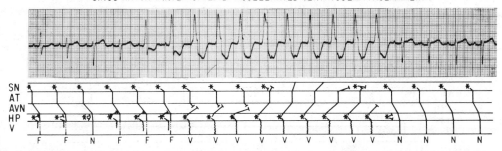

Figure 111. This rhythm strip was recorded from a patient being monitored during the acute phase of myocardial infarction. It is an example of enhanced automaticity in a normally latent pacemaker either in the distal Purkinje system or in working myocardial cells (altered by the effects of ischemia/infarction). In the accompanying ladder diagram, an extra horizontal tier has been added corresponding to His-Purkinje System (HP). Note that the first, second, fourth, fifth, and sixth beats are different from either the normally conducted beats (N) or the beats arising solely from the accelerated pacemaker (V). These intermediate complexes are fusion beats (F) resulting from the ventricle's being activated both by the accelerated pacemaker (indicated by the asterisk in the HP tier) and by the normally conducted impulse. Since the accelerated pacemaker is slightly faster than the sinus node, it gradually usurps control of the ventricles and subsequently even captures the atria via retrograde conduction through the AV node. The accelerated ventricular pacemaker eventually reaches 120 beats per minute and then stops suddenly. The most likely explanation for this sudden cessation of the accelerated pacemaker is exit block from the pacemaker site that allows the subsequent normal antegrade impulses to reset the accelerated pacemaker, making it once again latent.

phase 4 depolarization, resulting in sinus bradycardia (Fig. 107, panel A).

Variations in vagal tone are responsible for other benign alterations of rhythm. Different automatic cells show different sensitivities to autonomic mediators, and in the case of acetylcholine there is a greater depressant effect on the cells of the sinus node than on automatic cells in other regions of the heart. This may result in a shift of the pacemaker from one region to another within the sinus node, to another atrial focus or the distal AV node or His bundle.

In addition to adrenergic and cholinergic enhancement and depression of automaticity in the sinus node, ectopic rhythms may occur if the automaticity of latent pacemaker tissue is increased enough to permit the ectopic site to usurp control from the sinus node. Most commonly, enhanced spontaneous diastolic depolarization of latent pacemakers is the result of an increase in sympathetic activity. Single atrial or ventricular ectopic beats or sustained tachycardia may be induced by this mechanism in the setting of exercise, thyrotoxicosis, caffeine, fatigue, and fever, or in the setting of ischemic heart disease. Spontaneous diastolic depolarization of automatic cells is thought to result from a slow inward Na^+ current at a time when the efflux of K^+ is decreasing because of a decrease in potassium permeability. Changes in extracellular K^+, therefore, influence the rate of diastolic depolarization by altering the gradient for potassium efflux and perhaps membrane permeability to potassium. Hypokalemia increases the rate of diastolic depolarization. When the decreased extracellular K^+ concentration is marked there is also a shift of maximal diastolic potential to a less negative level, contributing to the enhanced automaticity of normal and latent pacemaker tissues.

Hyperkalemia reduces the slope of spontaneous diastolic depolarization, presumably by increasing K^+ permeability. High extracellular K^+ also decreases the maximum diastolic potential (less negative); thus the effect of hyperkalemia on automaticity depends on whether the change in spontaneous diastolic depolarization (reduced rate of firing) or the change in membrane potential (accelerated rate of firing) predominates. Within the physiological range of plasma potassium concentration, these effects of potassium are maximal on latent automatic cells and on digitalis-induced automaticity and minimal on the sinus node and on abnormal automatic mechanisms.

Other electrolytes play a minor role in the genesis of arrhythmias. Hypocalcemia increases automaticity, and hypercalcemia has the opposite effect, probably because of changes in a secondary inward current or a change in potassium conductance and thus the slope of phase 4 depolarization. Disorders of Na^+ metabolism, except when extreme and generally incompatible with life, are not associated with arrhythmias.

DISTURBANCES OF IMPULSE PROPAGATION

Alterations in cardiac rhythm and the form of the electrocardiogram may be caused by abnormalities of impulse propagation (conduction). The resulting disturbances are very often complex, but it appears probable that rhythm disturbances due to abnormal conduction are at least as frequent as, if not more frequent than, those due to abnormal automatic mechanisms. In relation to disturbances of impulse propagation it is useful to consider those factors that lead to slowing of conduction, to block, and to reentry, which is a special circumstance that may arise in the presence of slow conduction and unidirectional block. The potential for abnormal conduction and reentry exists throughout the heart, particularly when normal structures are modified by disease.

The normal impulse, which originates within pacemaker cells of the sinus node, must propagate from those cells across the sinoatrial junction, over the atrial musculature, from atrium over the AV node to bundle

WENCKEBACH SECOND DEGREE AV BLOCK WITH ESCAPE JUNCTIONAL BEATS

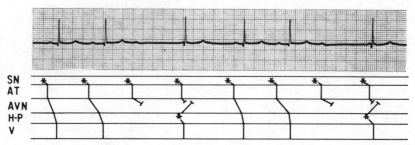

Figure 112. This rhythm strip was obtained from a long-distance runner during sleep. Owing to enhanced vagal tone, the relative refractory period of the AV node is prolonged and sinus node impulses conduct through the AV node at a progressively slower rate (reflected by the increasing PR intervals) until there is complete block of the impulse in the AV node (indicated in the ladder diagram by the line drawn perpendicular to the oblique line in the AV node tier). Following the blocked P wave, the next P wave occurs on time but, before it can conduct, a latent or escape pacemaker from the His bundle (indicated diagrammatically by the asterisk in the H-P tier) emerges and captures the ventricles. The cycle then repeats itself and is an example of Wenckebach second degree AV block. This capability for dramatic variability in conduction time is typical of the AV node and is in contrast to block occurring in the His-Purkinje system, where conduction time is constant both before and after nonconducted beats. That this escape pacemaker is arising above the bifurcation of the bundle branches is indicated by the identical morphology of the escape and normally conducted beats.

of His, down the His-Purkinje system, and to ventricular muscle. As noted previously, propagation from one fiber to another occurs at sites of low-resistance couplings between the cells. In a system of cells the velocity of propagation between any two points in the system will be influenced by the dimensions and geometry of the cells, by the nature and frequency of intercellular connections, by the passive or cable properties of the cells, by the threshold potential, and by the amplitude and velocity of phase 0 of the action potential.

The AV node is a useful basis for discussing mechanisms of delay and block, because here, even in the normal heart, impulse propagation is exceedingly slow and the safety factor for conduction is low. The cells within the AV node are small and loosely arranged with infrequent junctions, and there is a substantial amount of intercellular connective tissue. The cells have a low resting membrane potential by comparison with Purkinje and working myocardial cells, and the upstroke velocity of action potentials is extraordinarily slow. Indeed, within the central portion of the AV node the cells appear to lack the membrane characteristics that allow a fast inward sodium current, and depolarization arises from some other ionic mechanism, possibly similar to the slow response encountered in Purkinje and muscle cells when the rapid sodium-carrying mechanism has been inactivated by partial depolarization. In the AV node the normal delay may become exaggerated by cholinergic influences that depress further the rate of rise of phase 0 of the action potential by early atrial beats that invade the AV node at a time when recovery of the ionic mechanism responsible for phase 0 is incomplete, by hypoxia or by structural consequences of disease that diminish even further the paucity of low-resistance intercellular junctions. First degree AV block (delay), intermittent block of the Wenckebach type, and some cases of complete AV block arise from such mechanisms (Fig. 112).

The sinus node has many structural similarities to the AV node. Furthermore, sinus node cells have a low resting membrane potential, action potentials appear to be of the slow response type, and estimates of the speed of impulse propagation within the sinus are correspondingly very slow. In addition, surrounding the sinus node is a group of perinodal fibers that have a well-developed resting membrane potential and upstroke velocity, but an action potential and refractory period that are longer than those of the sinus node or ordinary atrial muscle. The refractory period of these perinodal fibers may last longer than repolarization. From these characteristics it is not surprising that one may encounter delays of impulse propagation within the sinus node (first and second degree sinoatrial block) and delay or block at the sinoatrial junction when sinus impulses encounter incompletely recovered or refractory perinodal fibers. Disturbances of sinoatrial conduction are recognized less frequently on the EKG than delay or block within the AV node, most probably because the sinus node potential is insufficient to produce a recorded event on the surface EKG, and hence delays of sinoatrial conduction must be inferred. This contrasts with the AV node, in which the P-QRS interval and sequence provide a continuous observable signal of AV node function.

There is now a substantial and growing body of evidence that indicates that insights derived from studies on the AV node have their counterpart in the mechanisms that underlie conduction delay and block in tissues distal to the AV node. Within the node we have seen that impulses that reach the node before the cells have fully recovered excitability from the previous beat can be delayed or blocked. We have seen that within the AV node the structure of cells, their geometry, and the nature and frequency of intercellular connections contribute to slow conduction even under normal circumstances. Finally, we have seen that AV nodal cells normally have a low resting membrane potential and action potentials with a very slow upstroke velocity—that is, slow response. The possibility that one or more of these conditions, observed normally in the AV node, may contribute to delay or block of impulse propagation outside the AV node, has been explored in recent years, and evidence has accrued to support this hypothesis.

Recent studies have demonstrated that action potential duration and recovery of excitability are nonuniform throughout the His-Purkinje system and ventricular myocardium. In general, action potential duration and refractoriness are longer in the Purkinje system than in muscle. Within the Purkinje system, refractoriness may be longer in one bundle branch than in the other, and action potential duration along any given bundle branch and its distal ramifications is not equal. There is also evidence that action potential duration and refractoriness of working ventricular myocardium is not the same in subendocardial and subepicardial zones of the same ventricle. A situation exists therefore in which a supraventricular impulse that successfully traverses the AV node at an early time relative to the last sinus beat may encounter refractoriness or relative refractoriness in specialized tissue or muscle below the AV node. For this reason impulse conduction may be delayed or blocked on premature or early beats even in the absence of pathologic alterations (Fig. 113). One relatively common example of this phenomenon is the fact that in most normal adults the refractoriness of the proximal right bundle branch is longer than that of the left bundle branch. As a consequence, premature atrial beats may reach the right bundle during its relative or absolute refractory period and an intraventricular conduction delay typical of right bundle branch block is observed. In other patients, this same phenomenon may lead to a rate-related bundle branch block, where conduction delay or block is observed at high heart rates but not at normal or slower rates (Fig. 114, panel A). A special case of interest is the so-called Ashman phenomenon. The duration of the cardiac action potential is related to cycle length, so that at slow rates or after a pause action potential duration is long, while at high rates or on early beats action potential duration is reduced. As a consequence, when the heart rate is irregular a functional type of delay or block may be seen when a short cycle follows a long cycle (Fig. 114, panel B). This phenomenon is seen most frequently in the presence of atrial fibrillation, in which intraventricular conduction may be aberrant (usually of right bundle branch morphology) when a short cycle follows a long cycle. Similarly, when a premature ventricular beat is followed by a long compensatory pause, the second sinus beat after the pause may be conducted with intraventricular delay or block. Again, in this situation the interval between the two sinus beats after the pause is shorter than the pause, so that a short cycle follows a long cycle and functional block may be observed owing to propagation into a region that has not fully recovered. Given the nonhomogeneous nature of repolarization throughout the heart, and the nonuniformity of the relation between cycle length and action potential duration, this type of functional and cycle length–dependent delay or block may be encountered anywhere in the specialized tissues or myocardium.

In contrast to the functional types of delay and block within the His-Purkinje system noted above, bundle branch block and AV heart block of a persistent nature occurring in individuals of advanced age or with pathologic conditions involving the heart are nearly always

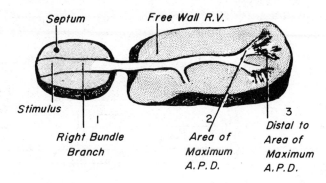

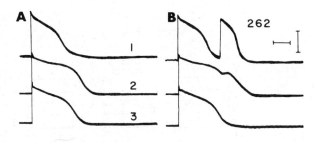

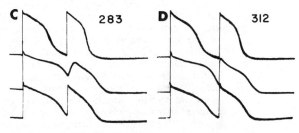

Figure 113. Conduction of test impulses across the area of maximum action potential duration. *A,* Simultaneous driven action potentials recorded from three sites in the right ventricular conducting system: (1) right bundle branch, (2) area of maximum action potential duration (A.P.D.), and (3) Purkinje cell distal to the area of maximum action potential duration. Both the driving impulse (S_1) and the test impulse (S_2) were delivered through small surface electrodes situated on the right bundle branch (drawing). Top, middle, and bottom records in *B, C,* and *D* correspond to 1, 2, and 3. *B,* S_1–S_2 interval was 262 msec. The cell in the top record was almost fully repolarized at this time and responded to S_2 appropriately. The cell in the area of maximum action potential duration was still refractory, however, and showed only a minor graded response. Since the impulse was not conducted, the distal cell showed no response to S_2, *C,* S_1–S_2 interval was 283 msec, the minimum value at which conduction across the area of maximum action potential duration will occur—that is, the functional refractory period of the system. Repolarization was complete in the right bundle branch cell and almost complete in the distal cell, and the R_2 action potentials have appropriate configurations. Repolarization was much less complete in the middle cell, however, and the R_2 action potential configuration has a very slow upstroke. D, S_2–S_1 interval was 312 msec and the R_2 upstroke velocity clearly was much more rapid at site 2. It was still more rapid at sites 1 and 3, although this is not evident in the illustration. (With permission from Myerberg, R. J., Stewart, J. W., and Hoffman, B. F.: Electrophysical properties of the canine peripheral AV conducting system. Circ Res 26:369, 1970.)

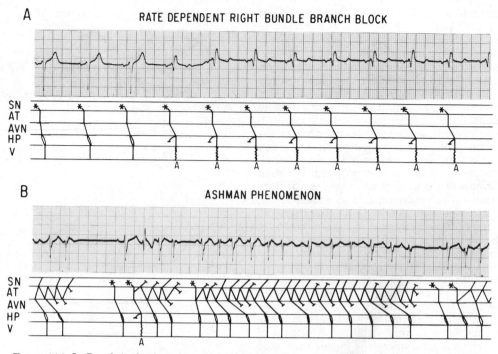

Figure 114. In Panel *A*, the first three beats demonstrate a normal QRS morphology, but as the sinus node rate increases, the impulse encounters refractoriness in the right bundle branch resulting in a rate-related right bundle branch block (note the development of the wide terminal R wave with a QRS duration >0.11 seconds). This variation between normal and right bundle branch block conduction and vice versa occurred repeatedly as the sinus node rate increased to greater than or slowed to less than 65 beats per minute. In the ladder diagram, normal conduction in both bundle branches is indicated diagrammatically by the diverging and converging lines in the HP tier. Block in the right bundle branch is indicated by the perpendicular line interrupting one of these lines. Panel *B*, from a different patient with paroxysmal atrial fibrillation (indicated in the ladder diagram by the recycling, connected lines in the atrial tier), shows four bouts of atrial fibrillation of varying lengths. Sudden terminations of this random atrial re-entry create pauses of varying lengths. The second conducted beat (*A*) following the longest pause has a different morphology because the impulse has encountered a longer refractory period in the right bundle branch that is, in turn, secondary to the long prior cycle. This Ashman phenomenon is seen only once, presumably because the subsequent pauses are of shorter duration, and therefore the functional refractoriness of the right bundle is less.

associated with structural changes in the conducting tissues. There may be a sclerodegenerative process confined to the conducting system in older patients with bilateral bundle branch block and/or fibrosis and calcification of the upper portion of the interventricular septum that appears to arise and spread from the fibrous tissue that makes up the anulus of either the aortic valve, the mitral valve, or both. Scarring of the septum and its conducting fibers may also be observed following myocardial infarction, and interruption of conducting fibers may be observed in diphtheria, in Chagas' disease, in sarcoidosis, and in other infiltrative processes. In these conditions, the His bundle, one or both bundle branches, and fascicles arising from a bundle branch may be involved. The pathological changes may vary from focal degeneration of fibers within a bundle to complete interruption by fibrous tissue. In many instances a conducting fascicle shows cells of reduced size, a breakdown of normal intercellular connections, and extracellular accumulations of fat and fibrous tissue. Physiological studies in man indicate that in the presence of such pathological changes impulse propagation may be delayed or blocked in the altered region, conduction delay or block may be produced at cycle lengths for which conduction

without delay would normally be anticipated, and block may be intermittent. There are no data available concerning the cellular electrophysiology of viable cells within such regions. However, the fact that impulses may propagate successfully and without delay on one beat and fail on the next (for example, in Mobitz Type II AV block) suggests that the viable cells are normal but that the safety factor for conduction is critically low, presumably because of the structural alterations induced by the pathological process. It seems highly probable that conduction delay, intermittent block, and fixed block based upon anatomic discontinuities that interrupt intercellular connections also play a role in other regions—for example, within and around the nonhomogeneous scars resulting from healed myocardial infarction. Indeed, as discussed in the chapter on coronary heart disease, delay and fractionation of impulse propagation within zones of healed infarction have been recorded in both experimental animals and man. In all likelihood, such delay and block account for so-called peri-infarction block and its associated electrocardiographic changes. Intramural delay and block related to cellular discontinuity may also account for certain of the QRS changes on the electrocardiogram in cases of marked hypertrophy and replacement fibrosis related to conditions other than myocardial infarction.

Within the past ten years another group of observations has been made that points to a third potential mechanism of delayed propagation and block within the His-Purkinje system and within ordinary working atrial or ventricular myocardium. Normal Purkinje and myocardial cells have a resting membrane potential of −80 to −90 mV, the upstroke of action potential is rapid (200 to 1000 V/sec), and recovery of excitability is temporally coupled closely to repolarization and is voltage-dependent. The upstroke of these action potentials is the result of a fast inward sodium conductance and can be blocked with tetrodotoxin. Propagation of the action potential is rapid. Even in normally polarized fibers there is now evidence for a second inward current, a current with much slower activation and deactivation kinetics and with a threshold for activation at −30 to −40 mV rather than at −60 to −70 mV, which is the case for the rapid sodium channel. Under normal conditions this is a weak current and is thought to play a role only in determining the absolute membrane potential during the plateau. However, when the membranes of these cells are depolarized to levels of −50 to −60 mV, the rapid sodium channel is inactivated, and when the cells are stimulated an action potential is elicited that has an upstroke velocity of 1 to 10 V/sec and a reduced amplitude (Fig. 115). These action potentials can be augmented by calcium or by norepinephrine and are blocked by manganese and verapamil but not by tetrodotoxin. Propagation of these action potentials is one tenth to one hundredth of the velocity of normal responses. This slow inward current is carried primarily by calcium ions.

The findings described above are of great interest in part because slow response action potentials observed in depolarized Purkinje and muscle fibers are similar in nearly all respects to the normal findings in AV nodal cells. A second observation of interest is that slow response action potentials have been observed in Purkinje and muscle cells removed from hearts of animals subjected to recent myocardial infarction. Furthermore, a common method of inducing slow responses in normal cells is to raise the extracellular potassium concentration, which depolarizes the membrane, and then increase the concentration of norepinephrine, which augments action potentials attributable to the slow current. These conditions—that is, high extracellular [K⁺] and release of norepinephrine—are known to occur within acutely ischemic zones. Finally, depolarized cells from which slow response action potentials can be elicited have been obtained from the atria of patients with chronic atrial dilatation at the time of corrective heart surgery. In these patients, correlations have been established between the degree of depolarization in vitro, the presence or absence of slow responses, and slow atrial conduction and atrial arrhythmias in vivo. These data suggest strongly that slow response action potentials in diseased or dilated tissues may contribute to delay and block in vivo. Again, an analogy between delay and block within the normal AV node and phenomena observed outside the AV node in diseased or depressed regions is suggested. Finally, the possibility that slow response action potentials in the atria, Purkinje system, or ventricle may contribute to certain specific arrhythmias forms the basis of several current therapeutic trials designed to test the antiarrhythmic efficacy of agents that block the slow channel.

Under the category of arrhythmias related to disturbances of impulse propagation are those ectopic beats or repetitive responses that are thought to arise from reentry (Fig. 116). Reentry requires first an initiating beat. The initiating beat may be a normal sinus im-

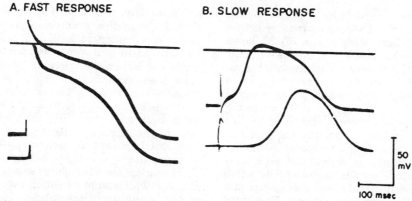

A. FAST RESPONSE **B. SLOW RESPONSE**

50 mV

100 msec

Figure 115. Comparison of the fast and slow response. Panel *A* shows two transmembrane action potentials recorded from different cells in a bundle of canine Purkinje fibers (fast fibers) perfused with normal Tyrode's solution ([K⁺] = 4mM). The reference O line is for the top action potential only. The microelectrodes are located 15 mm apart at either end of an unbranched bundle, and the Purkinje fiber bundle is being stimulated at one end. The action potentials shown in Panel *A* are examples of the fast response. Conduction of the impulse between the two microelectrodes is very rapid; the depolarization phases of both action potentials occur nearly simultaneously. Panel *B* shows transmembrane action potentials recorded from the same two cells, while the Purkinje fiber bundle is being perfused with Tyrode's solution containing a high [K⁺] (16mM) and epinephrine. The high [K⁺] has depolarized the cells to resting membrane potentials of −60 mV, thereby inactivating the fast response. Stimulation of the Purkinje fiber bundle now results in slow response action potentials. Note that the upstrokes of both action potentials are very slow and the action potential amplitudes are low (<80 mV). In addition, conduction between the two microelectrodes is extremely slow; it now takes the impulse 100 msec to propagate the distance of 15 mm between the two microelectrodes. (With permission from Wit, A. L., Rosen, M. R., and Hoffman, B. F.: Electrophysiology and pharmacology of cardiac arrhythmias. II. Relationship of normal and abnormal electrical activity of cardiac fibers to the genesis of arrhythmias. Am Heart J 88:516, 1974.)

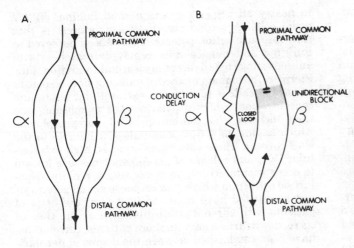

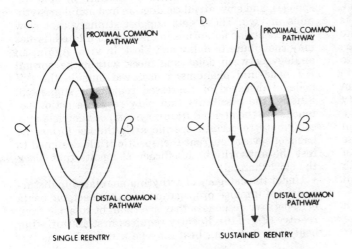

Figure 116. In this diagrammatic representation of re-entry, the re-entry circuit consists of a proximal common pathway, two divergent limbs (the alpha and beta pathways), and a distal common pathway. Normally (Panel *A*), there is uniformity of conduction and refractoriness at each "level" of the heart, resulting in uniform and orderly propagation so that an impulse encountering such divergent limbs conducts synchronously with uniform recovery. In Panel *B* an area of depressed conduction in the beta pathway (resulting from either pathological processes or functional abnormalities) is represented as a stippled zone. The antegrade impulse is blocked in the beta pathway and conducts more slowly through the alpha pathway until it encounters the distal limb of the beta pathway, which it enters in a retrograde direction. If the block in the beta pathway is unidirectional and the impulse traversing the alpha limb and retrograde through the beta limb has traveled slowly enough, the retrograde impulse in the beta pathway may encounter tissue that has recovered sufficiently to be re-excited and the impulse may re-enter this area. This may occur once (Panel *C*), giving rise to a retrograde ectopic impulse or it may occur repetitively (Panel *D*), creating a circulating wave front with surrounding cardiac tissue driven in cadence with the re-entering wavefront in the loop. These panels illustrate diagrammatically the requisite conditions for re-entry—a closed loop, conduction delay, and unidirectional block. (With permission from Gallagher, J. J.: Cardiac arrhythmias. In Wyngaarden, J. B., and Smith, L. H., Jr. (eds.): Cecil Textbook of Medicine. 17th ed. Philadelphia, W. B. Saunders Co., 1985, p. 264.)

pulse or a premature event originating outside the sinus node. The second requirement for reentry is that during the initiating beat some region of the heart must be inexcitable and hence not invaded by the wavefront of the initiating beat. This inexcitable region, however, must either regain excitability at a later time or be excitable if the wavefront approaches it from a direction different from that of the initiating beat. The most important concept embodied in this second requirement is that of one way (or unidirectional) block. Either because of a temporal inequality in recovery of excitability or because of structural alterations that preclude conduction in one direction but not the other, the initiating beat dissociates into two potential pathways for propagation. The third requirement for reentry is that the two pathways that are dissociated by the mechanisms noted above must ultimately be connected, and the conduction time down one path and up the other must be long enough to allow the tissue at the original site of dissociation to recover and be responsive to the returning impulse. Reentry is therefore potentiated by slowed conduction of the reentering wave front. Given this set of requirements reentry then involves continuous propagation over a reentry loop. Single, double, or repetitive responses may occur depending upon the number of times the impulse circulates around the loop.

Perhaps the clearest example of reentry is found in

patients with the Wolff-Parkinson-White syndrome (Fig. 117). In this syndrome, one or more accessory pathways (in addition to the AV node and His bundle) join the atria and ventricles through faults in the anulus of either the tricuspid or mitral valve. Typically, these accessory pathways have a different functional refractory period than the AV node. A premature beat arising within the atrium or ventricle (the initiating beat) may occur at a time when either the AV node or the accessory pathway, but not both, is refractory. The impulse traverses one pathway (for example, from atrium to ventricle), but by the time the wavefront reaches the ventricular end of the other pathway it is excitable and propagation returns to the chamber of the original initiating beat. This cycle may then repeat itself one or more times or repetitively. Because the path is relatively long and because the reentry circuit includes the AV node, where even normal conduction is slow, the likelihood that reentry will occur and will be repetitive is enhanced. It has been established that reentry can occur within the sinus node, within the AV node, and at the junction between Purkinje tissue and ventricular muscle. It seems likely that reentry can also occur within depressed and structurally altered regions of atrial and ventricular muscle. Regardless of the site responsible for reentry, a hallmark of reentry arrhythmias is the ability of single, appropriately timed premature beats to initiate the

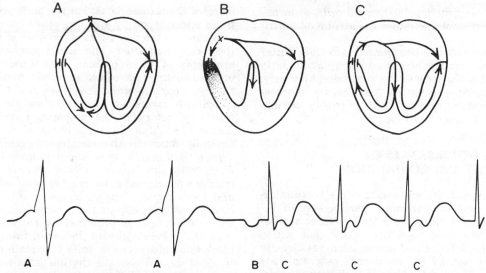

Figure 117. In this diagrammatic example of Wolff-Parkinson-White syndrome, sequence *A* represents sinus rhythm with the impulse conducting through both the AV node and the accessory pathway, resulting in a "fusion" beat with the anomalous activation of the free right ventricular wall represented by the slurred upstroke of the QRS (the Delta wave), with resultant shortening of the PR interval. In sequence *B*, a premature atrial beat (note the different morphology of the P wave) encounters a refractory (stippling) accessory pathway producing a normal appearing QRS. By the time the antegrade impulse from this premature beat reaches the free right ventricular wall, the accessory pathway has recovered sufficiently to allow retrograde conduction and activation of the atria, creating a circuit for continuous recycling (or re-entry) and a paroxysmal tachycardia (sequence *C*). (With permission from Wagner, G. S., and Ramo, B. W.: The physiology of normal and abnormal rhythms. In Wagner, G. S., Waugh, R. A., and Ramo, B. W. (eds.): Cardiac Arrhythmias. New York, Churchill Livingstone, 1983, p. 13.)

arrhythmia and also for single, appropriately timed premature beats to terminate the arrhythmia. These criteria have been satisfied in many clinical instances of atrial, AV nodal, and ventricular tachycardias.

Opponents of the reentry concept have long argued that it was unlikely that conduction could be slow enough in regions outside the AV node for continuous propagation to persist, especially in reasonably focal areas. At the very least, conduction over the reentry loop must persist for 250 to 300 msec to allow surrounding normal tissue to recover after the initiating beat. In this regard, the arguments of opponents have been partially offset by the observation that structural changes and/or slow responses can in fact lead to propagation in reasonably focal areas that is slow enough to permit reentry. In theory and in practice, arrhythmias thought to arise from reentry can be abolished by pharmacological agents that prolong refractoriness of normal tissue, by agents that lead to block within slowly conducting parts of a reentry loop, or most definitively by surgical interruption of a documented reentry circuit.

The exact mechanism of atrial and ventricular fibrillation remains a topic of extensive investigation and debate. The mechanisms that have been proposed for the initiation and maintenance of these arrhythmias are (1) increased automaticity with impulses arising from either a rapidly firing single ectopic focus or multiple foci and (2) repetitive random microreentry. The mechanisms for initiation and maintenance of fibrillation, however, need not be the same, and combinations of abnormal automaticity and conduction may occur to explain the genesis of these arrhythmias.

In both atrial and ventricular fibrillation almost complete electrical disorganization is present. In the presence of a single, rapidly firing ectopic focus, some fibers could fail to respond to every impulse and result in islands of refractory tissue and an irregular spread of excitation. While a single focus with enhanced automaticity might initiate fibrillation, microreentry most probably maintains the disorganized rhythm. Multifocal automatic activity, on the other hand, could explain both the initiation and maintenance of fibrillation without invoking reentry. The major objection to this latter theory is the observation that fibrillation may abruptly terminate; simultaneous cessation of all ectopic automatic behavior would be unlikely. Random reentry, therefore, is the most likely pathophysiological mechanism for fibrillation. A premature impulse, caused either by enhanced automaticity or by a local reentrant mechanism and occurring during the vulnerable period, could lead to multiple wavelets of activity owing to random reentry and hence a totally asynchronous rhythm. This mechanism could explain the propensity for fibrillation to occur in diseases of the atria and ventricles (for example, rheumatic heart disease with atrial fibrosis and dilatation, and ischemic heart disease), which increase the disparity of refractoriness and produce some zones with slow response action potentials. This theory is also compatible with the tendency to develop atrial fibrillation with vagal stimulation and ventricular fibrillation during myocardial infarction complicated by bradycardia, since in both instances inequality of recovery is enhanced. Finally, the multiple wavelet reentry hypothesis is most compatible with the ability of a single electrical shock, simultaneously depolarizing all cells, to terminate fibrillation involving either the atrium or ventricle.

Similar arguments can be mounted to explain flutter (both atrial and ventricular) as an example of orderly reentry in either the atria or the ventricles. Similarly, paroxysmal rapid ventricular tachycardia is most likely explained by orderly reentry within circumscribed areas of either ventricle.

COEXISTING DISTURBANCES OF AUTOMATICITY AND CONDUCTION

Between automaticity and conduction a relation exists that may contribute to understanding certain disturbances not easily accounted for by either mechanism alone. We have seen previously that action potential characteristics and propagation velocity are determined in part by the membrane potential that exists in these fibers at the time of excitation. Normal and abnormal automaticity and afterdepolarizations each represent mechanisms of depolarization. If a fiber or region that is partially depolarized by such mechanisms is invaded by a propagating wavefront, delay or even block may occur depending upon the level to which the membrane has been depolarized. Another possible mechanism of interaction between action potentials in depressed regions is summation and inhibition. In the first, if Purkinje strands are depolarized to a level such that stimulation of either end alone fails to elicit a propagated action potential, excitation of both ends of the strand may give rise to a propagated potential. In the situation of inhibition, an impulse initiated at one end of a strand may excite a depressed central region, while an impulse from the other end of the strand does not. When both ends are stimulated the depressed central region may be rendered inexcitable and propagation fails.

One clinical example of a disturbance related to coexisting alterations of automaticity and conduction is so-called phase 4 block. We have noted before that delay or block may occur when an early impulse invades tissue that has not yet recovered from the previous beat. The impulse is delayed or blocked because refractory tissue is encountered and the block is referred to as a phase 3 block because repolarization is not yet complete. Block or delay on premature beats or at rapid heart rates is thought to reflect such a mechanism. In phase 4 delay or block the disturbance in propagation generally follows a long pause or is observed at very slow heart rates. This disturbance in propagation has been ascribed to phase 4 diastolic depolarization and to delay or block attributable to the loss in membrane potential due to this automatic depolarization. In addition to delays or blocks in the His bundle and bundle branches attributable to a phase 4 mechanism, these changes may also contribute to vulnerability to tachyarrhythmias or fibrillation observed at exceedingly slow heart rates, such as in chronic AV block.

Parasystole is an ectopic rhythm characterized by premature impulses that arise from a focus with its own inherent rate so that each premature impulse occurs at a variable coupling interval after the preceding normal impulse and the cycle length between parasystolic beats is a multiple of the inherent rate of firing of the ectopic focus. For the parasystolic rhythm to be undisturbed by sinus or other ectopic impulses that capture the ventricles, some form of protection of the focus must exist. The actual mechanism for the production of this arrhythmia has not been established, but two theories have been proposed. According to one theory, a high inherent frequency of discharge at the ectopic site keeps the pacemaker and its surrounding tissue refractory to the propagated impulse of the dominant rhythm. Since the observed rate of the parasystolic focus on the electrocardiogram is usually slower than would be required to keep the focus refractory by this theory, certain degrees of exit block from the parasystolic site must be invoked. The second and more popular theory proposes that there is increased automaticity at the parasystolic site and that this ectopic area is protected by entrance block. As with the previous theory, however, intermittent exit block must also occur in order to explain the intermittency of the parasystolic rhythm. This unidirectional, and sometimes bidirectional, failure of conduction may be explained by the concept of slow response fibers at the parasystolic site or by inhibition. Similarly, by the process of summation, sinus beats might facilitate propagation out of a parasystolic site and produce coupling that at first glance appears to arise from reentry but that on closer inspection is more consistent with facilitation of propagation from an otherwise isolated parasystolic focus. The essential point, however, is to recognize that automatic depolarization can influence conduction. Conversely, propagation in and around a parasystolic focus can influence whether or not and when the automatic focus becomes manifest as a basis for beats of ectopic origin.

CLINICAL CONSEQUENCES

The clinical consequences of a given arrhythmia are a function of the clinical setting in which it occurs and the characteristics of the arrhythmia itself, including its mechanism, rate, and the stability of standby or latent pacemakers. Symptomatic manifestations of arrhythmias include palpitations, syncope, chest pain, and congestive heart failure.

The most common clinical manifestation of an arrhythmia is an awareness by the patient of a change in rhythm. The sensations produced by this awareness are called palpitations. Mechanisms responsible for the awareness include being able to detect changes in rate and/or regularity of the heart beat, changes in the inotropic state of the ventricle, and the effects of AV dissociation. In the case of premature beats, some patients may be able to detect the increased stroke volume of the beat terminating the pause after a premature beat. This sensation is commonly characterized by patients as a "thumping" or "hard beat" sensation. Alternatively, the premature beat itself may be detected because AV dissociation produces large a waves that cause sensed distention of the systemic and/or pulmonary venous vasculature. In such instances, patients typically complain of a sharp discomfort, a "flip-flop" sensation, or a sensation of the heart "turning over" in the chest. Increases in the heart rate, regardless of mechanism, may produce a sensation of the heart "racing." Sinus tachycardias resulting from anxiety are commonly sensed in this manner. Reentry atrial and ventricular tachycardias may also produce a sensation of the heart "racing." In such instances, the mode of onset is a helpful differential point, with pacemaker tachycardias characteristically beginning and ending gradually and reentry tachycardias demonstrating a sudden onset and offset. If the tachycardia has a sudden onset and offset and is grossly irregular, then one should suspect random reentry such as atrial fibrillation.

Arrhythmias may also produce symptoms if there is a concomitant fall in cardiac output with inadequate cerebral perfusion, resulting in either presyncope or syncope. Bradycardias (due to AV block, sinus arrest, or long pauses following termination of reentry supraventricular tachycardia—all in the setting of inadequate escape pacemakers) or tachycardias (ventricular tachycardia, ventricular flutter, or extremely rapid atrial tachycardias) may cause inadequate cardiac output. The rate limits at which syncope occurs for each of these arrhythmias may be altered by accompanying cerebral vascular disease *and/or* heart disease. For example, it is unusual for a supraventricular arrhythmia to cause syncope unless the rate is extremely rapid (as may occur with Wolff-Parkinson-White syndrome with very rapid ventricular responses) or unless there is severe underlying heart disease.

Arrhythmias may also cause the symptom of chest pain, most commonly because of the increased oxygen consumption associated with increases in heart rate. Rarely, an extreme bradycardia may produce chest pain because of inadequate coronary perfusion. In both settings, underlying coronary artery disease and/or left ventricular outflow tract obstruction are commonly present.

Finally, arrhythmias may produce symptoms by contributing to congestive heart failure. With mitral stenosis, for example, the development of atrial fibrillation and a rapid ventricular response markedly limits the time available for left atrial emptying and is frequently associated with a sudden increase in symptoms of pulmonary venous congestion. In patients with hypertrophic cardiomyopathy or very poor left ventricular function, the development of atrial fibrillation even with a controlled ventricular response causes a loss of the atrial contribution to left ventricular filling and may result in deterioration of left ventricular function and symptoms of heart failure.

REFERENCES

Cranefield, P. F.: Action potentials, after potentials and arrhythmias. Circ Res 41:415, 1977.

Fisch, C.: Relation of electrolyte disturbances to cardiac arrhythmias. Circulation 47:408, 1973.

Gallagher, J. J., Sealy, W. C., Wallace, A. G., and Kasell, J.: Correlation between catheter electrophysiological studies and findings on mapping of ventricular excitation in the WPW syndrome. In Wellens, H. J. J., Lie, K. I., and Janse, M. J. (eds.): The Conduction System of the Heart: Structure, Function and Clinical Implications. Leiden, The Netherlands, Stenfert Korese B. V., 1976, p. 588.

Hoffman, B. F., and Rosen, M. R.: Cellular mechanisms for cardiac arrhythmias. Circ Res 49:1, 1981.

Hoffman, B. F., Rosen, M. R., and Wit, A. L.: Electrophysiology and pharmacology of cardiac arrhythmias. III. The causes and treatment of cardiac arrhythmias. Part A. Am Heart J 89:115, 1975.

Hordof, A. J., Edie, R., Malm, J. R., Hoffman, B. F., and Rosen, M. R.: Electrophysiologic properties and response to pharmacologic agents of fibers from diseased human atria. Circulation 54:774, 1976.

McDonald, T. F.: The slow inward current in the heart. Annu Rev Physiol 44:425, 1982.

Moe, G. K., and Mendez, C.: The physiologic basis of reciprocal rhythm. Prog Cardiovasc Dis 8:461, 1966.

Vassalle, M.: Automaticity and automatic rhythms. Am J Cardiol 28:245, 1971.

Wit, A. L., and Bigger, J. T., Jr.: The electrophysiology of lethal arrhythmias: Possible electrophysiological mechanisms for lethal arrhythmias accompanying myocardial ischemia and infarction. Circulation 52(Suppl. III):96, 1975.

Heart Failure

Heart failure is a clinical condition or syndrome that may result from a wide spectrum of conditions that affect the heart. Heart failure is not a disease; it is a consequence of diseases that impair the ability of the heart to function as a pump. In this sense, heart failure is analogous to angina pectoris, a clinical condition or syndrome that may result from a spectrum of diseases that compromise coronary blood flow in relation to the metabolic needs of the myocardium. The manifestations of heart failure develop whenever the pumping ability of the heart is inadequate to meet the metabolic needs of the body. It is not surprising, therefore, to find that heart disease may exist with no manifestations of failure. Failure may develop in some patients only under conditions of enhanced metabolic demand; in others, failure may be present even under conditions of basal metabolic demand. Nothing is more important to the successful treatment of patients with heart failure than the recognition that equal attention must be paid to (a) the disease affecting the heart, (b) the level of demand that can be tolerated without producing failure, and (c) the pathophysiological mechanisms that produce failure when pump function is not adequate to meet the demands of the body. Each of these factors is important at all levels of compromised cardiac function. However, at any given level of compromised function one factor may predominate over the others and lead to an appropriate focus for therapy. Hence, in one patient relief of an obstructed valve may correct failure, in another treatment of a hypermetabolic state may relieve failure, and in still another digitalis and diuretics may restore a compensated state in which most normal functions can be carried out without manifestations of failure.

For the most part, conditions that lead to heart failure result from three classes or categories of disease. One category of conditions is that which places a pressure overload on one or the other ventricle, such as aortic or pulmonary valvular stenosis and systemic or pulmonary hypertension. A second category of conditions is that which places a volume overload on one or the other ventricle, such as regurgitation of any cardiac valve and congenital or acquired nonobstructive communications between the systemic and pulmonary circulations (atrial septal defect, ventricular septal defect, patent ductus arteriosus, or AV fistula). The third category of conditions is that which alters the function of normal myocardium or leads to loss or replacement of normal myocardium (myocardial ischemia, scarring, infiltration of the myocardium, toxic insults, and primary or secondary cardiomyopathies). When any condition within the first two categories is allowed to persist for long periods of time, secondary changes may develop in the myocardium that then contribute to reduced pump performance and hence to heart failure. One occasionally sees conditions, particularly acute abnormalities such as aortic or mitral valve regurgitation, in which overt heart failure develops with no evidence of myocardial dysfunction. Much more common, and indeed the usual situation, is one in which myocardial failure, whether primary or secondary, is a component of the problem. Thus, heart failure is rare in the absence of myocardial dysfunction.

In the subsequent sections of this chapter we will deal with the hemodynamic changes that are common to the heart failure state and those uniquely related to specific causes of heart failure. However, because myocardial dysfunction is so common in heart failure regardless of its cause, it is not surprising that investigators have attempted for years to develop an understanding of the structural and biochemical changes within the myocardium that may contribute to or in fact cause myocardial failure.

The heart adapts to a chronic pressure or volume overload or to conditions that cause deletion of some myocardial elements by an increase in mass. This increase in mass, however, occurs in distinctive patterns: with pressure overload end-diastolic volume remains relatively constant and wall thickness increases (concentric hypertrophy); with volume overload, end-diastolic volume increases and the increase in mass is distributed so that wall thickness remains relatively normal (eccentric hypertrophy). There are strong theoretical reasons and practical evidence to suggest that at least within certain limits these adaptive mechanisms are appropriately compensatory and enable the heart to maintain normal pump function despite the overload or condition that led to hypertrophy or dilatation.

Among patients with a chronic volume overload, such as aortic or mitral regurgitation, the increase in end-diastolic volume (dilatation) is proportional to the volume overload. Hence, ejection fraction remains about 60 per cent of diastolic volume, total stroke volume is increased (to equal the sum of forward stroke volume and regurgitant volume), and the size of the ventricular cavity at end-systole is increased only moderately. For many years it has been popular to invoke the Frank-Starling relationship to explain this adaptation of the ventricle to a volume overload. While this "law of the heart" is extremely useful in understanding the response of any given heart to acute hemodynamic changes, it seems singularly inappropriate to our understanding of adaptations to chronic overload, in which the heart becomes different. For example, in acute experiments an increase in ventricular volume is accompanied by lengthening of sarcomeres, yet in chronic volume overloads the average length of sarcomeres is not increased at "normal" operating filling pressures. In chronic volume overload, the diastolic volume-pressure relationship is shifted to the right so that LVEDP is no longer a reliable indicator of end-diastolic volume. Finally, many of the conditions that lead to chronic overload (for example, mitral and aortic regurgitation) reduce the impedance to ventricular emptying, at least during a part of systole, and, as a consequence, wall stress or force is not a simple function of cavity pressure.

More important to our understanding of eccentric hypertrophy are the physical consequences of dilatation and of hypertrophy per se. In the dilated heart, the geometric principles involved in the LaPlace relationship (see p. 886) predict that for a given amount of sarcomere shortening (and hence shortening of any segment of the ventricular wall) a greater stroke volume will be ejected. The LaPlace relation also predicts that a greater force will have to be generated by the sarcomere to eject a larger total stroke volume at normal cavity pressures and it is apparent that this is what occurs. A second important physical principle is that an increase in the number of sarcomeres that bear a given wall stress during systole will decrease the stress on any single sarcomere. Chronic volume overload is accompanied by an increase in muscle mass, and it appears that new contractile elements are laid down both at the periphery of the fiber (to increase fiber diameter) and at the intercalated disks (to increase fiber length). Thus, to the extent that an increase in systolic wall force is needed to eject a larger stroke volume from an enlarged diastolic chamber, hypertrophy provides an important element of this capacity, and in so doing spares the Frank-Starling relation.

With chronic pressure overloads on the ventricle, such as with aortic stenosis or hypertension, end-diastolic volume, stroke volume, and ejection fraction remain nearly normal until very late in the course of the disease. Hypertrophy increases the stiffness of the ventricular wall and tends to shift the volume-pressure relationship to the left, indicating a reduced compliance, and hence an increase in end-diastolic pressure for any given end-diastolic volume. Concentric hypertrophy is due principally to an increase in wall thickness, and this increase in mass is achieved largely by an increase in the intracellular contractile machinery, not by hyperplasia. Again, the increase in muscle mass should be viewed as compensatory, since the effect is to distribute the force that is required to generate higher ventricular pressures over a large number of sarcomeres arranged in parallel; that is, less force is required per sarcomere than would have been the case had hypertrophy not developed.

From the above discussion, several concepts become apparent that are relevant to understanding heart failure. First, any condition that causes an inappropriate pressure or volume overload on the ventricle requires an expenditure of energy by the ventricle that is greater than would be required to maintain forward cardiac output if the overload were not present. Second, to the extent that the Frank-Starling mechanism is involved to maintain forward cardiac output, even under basal conditions, one of the important intrinsic reserves for increasing output is encroached upon. Finally, hypertrophy regardless of cause leads to enhanced stiffness of heart muscle, and to an increase in the metabolic requirements of the heart to achieve any given cardiac output. Thus, without the need to involve a cardiac cellular defect per se, diseases characterized by a chronic pressure or volume overload, and as a consequence hypertrophy or dilatation, may limit the forward cardiac output that can be achieved during physical stress.

There are at least two important corollaries to the observations noted above. First, to the extent that dilatation and hypertrophy enable the heart to maintain a normal cardiac output at acceptable filling pressures, a new steady state can be achieved that is compatible with no symptoms or signs of heart failure during normal activities. Furthermore, if the disease process is not progressive this new steady state is compatible with a normal life expectancy. Thus, it is not surprising that some patients may tolerate mild to moderate hypertension, aortic stenosis, mitral regurgitation, moderate left-to-right shunts, or the consequences of a myocardial infarction without symptoms for many years. A second corollary to these observations is that a normal cardiac output and normal cardiac pressures under basal conditions cannot be used to predict the level of activity that a patient with heart disease can tolerate without developing symptoms and signs of heart failure. Hence, exercise testing with physiological monitoring can play an important role in assessing the cardiac patient beyond its traditional role as a diagnostic test for significant obstructive coronary artery disease.

Heart failure may develop in certain situations in which there is little or no impairment of contractile performance of myocardial muscle. These situations include some cases of isolated mitral stenosis, systemic arteriovenous fistulae, constrictive pericarditis, acute mitral or aortic regurgitation, and large intracardiac communications in infancy, such as ventricular septal defect. Far more frequently, however, dysfunction of myocardial muscle is a component of heart failure whether the primary disease is noncardiac, valvular, or myocardial. Under these conditions, cardiac dilatation develops to an extent that is inappropriate with respect to stroke volume, and as a consequence the effective ejection fraction is reduced below 50 per cent and in some cases to less than 20 per cent. In recent years a number of investigators have attempted to characterize cardiac function in terms of muscle mechanics, using principles adapted from Hill's classic studies of skeletal muscle. Despite the enormous contribution of their efforts to our understanding of myocardial contraction and energetics, the techniques employed to evaluate the intact heart in these terms involve a number of assumptions the validity of which has been questioned. Even under optimal conditions the results are not convincingly more helpful than the simpler assessment of ejection fraction, whether derived from angiographic data or more recently from noninvasive techniques using ultrasound or radionuclide generated images of the left ventricle. The important point is that myocardial contractility, however assessed, is usually diminished in states that had led to heart failure.

In keeping with the clinical observation of a reduced ejection fraction and other indices of contractility in patients with heart failure are the results of several recent studies of cardiac muscle removed from hearts in which hypertrophy and failure were induced by a chronic pressure or volume overload. These studies have shown a decrement in both the velocity and extent of shortening at any given load and a decrease in maximal active tension generated (Fig. 118). Most of the work in this field has suggested that hypertrophy has a deleterious effect on contractility and that muscle removed from failing hypertrophied hearts is quantitatively even more abnormal than muscles removed from hypertrophied nonfailing hearts. These observations, then, are also in keeping with the view that heart failure is not a unique condition, but rather one that develops when a sufficient hemodynamic or metabolic load is placed on compromised myocardium regardless of the cause of the compromised function.

At an ultrastructural level, it is now generally agreed that with hypertrophy there is an increase in the size of myocytes that results from an increase in both radial and longitudinal dimensions of the cell. The increase in cell size is also accompanied by an increase in myofibrillar elements, but by a variable change in the number and size of mitochondria. The most recent data suggest that the concentration of mitochondria decreases relative to myofibrils and that the surface area of mitochondrial membrane (cristae) decreases markedly relative to myofibrillar volume. Studies of this type have raised the important concept that when cells enlarge, all components of the cell do not necessarily participate to a uniform extent in the enlargement, and furthermore that the extent of

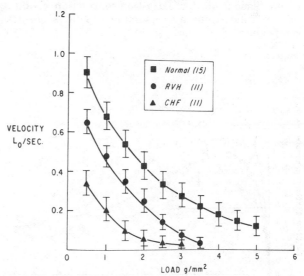

Figure 118. Force-velocity relations of normal, hypertrophied (RVH), and failing (CHF) right ventricular cat papillary muscles. Values given represent averages for each group ± SEM. Velocity has been normalized as lengths per second. (With permission from Spann, J. F., Buccino, R. A., Sonnenblick, E. H., and Braunwald, E.: Contractile state of cardiac muscle obtained from cats with experimentally produced ventricular hypertrophy and heart failure. Circ Res 21:345, 1967.)

change in individual components may vary with the nature of the stimulus that leads to myocyte growth. These studies raise the equally important possibility that the altered function of hypertrophied heart muscle might reflect a structural change in which myofibrillar contractile growth outstrips the ability of even normal mitochondria to provide energy in the form of ATP, or to a change in the spatial or quantitative relation between the contractile elements and membrane components responsible for excitation-contraction coupling. Much remains to be learned in this area of investigation, but it appears clear that the application of ultrastructural techniques and particularly of stereology to the study of hypertrophied and failing hearts will contribute a great deal to our understanding.

At the biochemical level as well, recent work has begun to shed some light on the abnormalities that may cause or at least contribute to myocardial failure. For example, respiratory activity of mitochondria isolated from hypertrophied nonfailing human myocardium is greater than normal, but similar preparations removed from failing human hearts show marked depression of respiratory activity. The capacity for calcium uptake by mitochondria is also depressed in failure. Further studies have indicated that one of the earliest biochemical defects detectable in failing myocardium is a decrease in the ability of isolated fragments of sarcoplasmic reticulum to release and to bind calcium (Fig. 119). Finally, depressed myosin ATPase activity and a decreased affinity of troponin for calcium have been reported in the setting of ischemia, perhaps related to changes in intracellular pH. Again, much remains to be learned before the significance of these observations can be clarified. In the aggregate, however, they seem to point to important differences between normal and failing hearts and to qualitative abnormalities in the function of subcellular components responsible for excitation-contraction coupling and in related energy-consuming functions of these components.

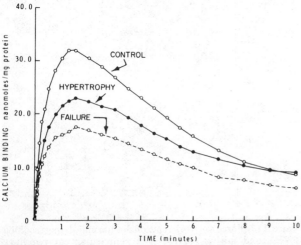

Figure 119. Isolated sarcoplasmic reticulum fragments from control, hypertrophied, and failing rabbit hearts. (With permission from Schwartz, A., Sordahl, L. A., Entman, M. L., Allen, J. C., Reddy, Y. S., Goldstein, M. A., Luchi, R. J., and Wyborny, L. E.: Abnormal biochemistry in myocardial failure. In Mason, D. T.: Congestive Heart Failure. New York, Dun-Donnelley Publishing Corp., 1976, p. 39.)

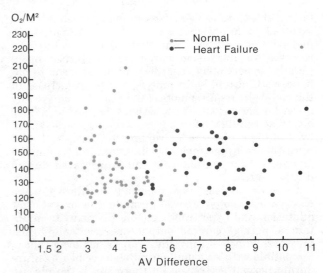

Figure 120. Relation between oxygen consumption and arteriovenous oxygen difference in normal subjects and patients with congestive heart failure. (With permission from Stead, E. A., Jr., Warren, J. V., and Brannon, E. S.: Cardiac output in congestive heart failure. Am Heart J 35:531, 1948.)

In 1944, Warren and Stead published a report on the pathogenesis of heart failure that had a major and lasting impact on the thinking of cardiologists. Prior to that report, it was generally held that venous pressure became elevated in heart failure because blood was dammed up in the venous system behind a ventricle whose ability to pump blood forward was impaired. By making serial observations on patients during the development of heart failure, Warren and Stead pointed out that weight gain, fluid accumulation, and expansion of the blood volume preceded the elevation of venous pressure. From these observations they concluded that the increase in extracellular fluid volume resulted from a decrease in the ability of the kidney to excrete salt and water. Subsequently Stead and his coworkers showed that cardiac output was reduced in most, although not in all, patients with heart failure but that cardiac output was uniformly reduced relative to the metabolic needs of the patients as reflected by their oxygen consumption. Hence, arteriovenous oxygen difference was widened beyond the normal range in nearly all subjects of heart failure (Fig. 120). From the work of a number of investigators it became clear that whenever cardiac output was inadequate to meet the oxygen needs of the body, a redistribution of the cardiac output occurred such that blood flow to areas such as muscle, heart, and brain was preserved at the expense of flow to areas such as the kidney and skin. Furthermore, this distribution abnormality was exaggerated by any condition (such as exercise) that enhanced the metabolic needs of the body above basal levels. The reduction of renal blood flow in heart failure and other mechanisms set in motion by the low cardiac output relative to oxygen needs are fundamental to the mechanism of salt and water retention and its consequences in the patient with heart failure.

It should be apparent from these considerations that hemodynamic measurements in patients with heart failure will reflect (a) the nature of the disease that has led to heart failure, (b) the extent of the disturbance in pump function, (c) the body's metabolic demands at the time of study, and (d) the extent to which extracellular fluid volume has been allowed to expand prior to the time of study. In general, cardiac output is reduced, the arteriovenous oxygen difference is widened and venous pressures in both the systemic and pulmonary circulations are increased.

Early investigations of the mechanism of salt and water retention in heart failure reported that in severe failure glomerular filtration rate (GFR) was reduced to 30 to 50 per cent of normal and that renal plasma flow was reduced to an even greater extent. However, much evidence has been reported subsequently to indicate that in the very early stages of heart failure, although renal blood flow (RBF) is consistently reduced, GFR is within normal limits and hence the filtration fraction is increased. In dogs with experimentally produced valvular lesions, it has been reported that salt retention occurs with reduced RBF and a normal GFR. The infusion of dibenzyline into one renal artery of these dogs caused a marked increase in RBF and in sodium excretion with little or no change in GFR. As a more complete picture of the pathogenesis of salt and water retention in heart failure has evolved, it appears that increased tubular reabsorption of sodium is an early finding in failure, and that this increased sodium reabsorption is accompanied by a decrease in total renal blood flow with or without a concurrent decrease in GFR. The decrease in renal blood flow is related to sympathetically mediated renal vasoconstriction. The most recent evidence suggests that one important consequence of the reduced RBF and the increase in filtration fraction is an increase in the postglomerular capillary colloid osmotic pressure. This increase in capillary colloid osmotic pressure causes an increase in the passive reabsorption of water and sodium by the proximal tubule. To the extent that GFR is also reduced in heart failure, the reduced filtered load of sodium augments the effect of these physical forces acting on the proximal tubule to reduce net sodium excretion in urine, and hence favors sodium retention.

In addition to the effects of a reduced renal blood flow noted above, there is strong evidence to suggest that, by one or more of several possible mechanisms, the decrease in renal blood flow is translated into an increase in renin secretion by the juxtaglomerular (JG) cells of the renal afferent arteriole. One theory is that the JG cells serve a "baroreceptor" function capable of sensing a decreased stretch of the afferent arteriole and responding by renin secretion. It is also clear that enhanced activity of renal sympathetic nerves can liberate renin, a response mediated through activation of beta receptors and that can be blocked by beta-adrenergic receptor antagonists. Whatever the precise mechanism of renin release, the events that follow and lead to enhanced aldosterone secretion are now well known. Increased levels of aldosterone are a common feature of even mild heart failure. The rise in plasma aldosterone level is attributable to increased secretion and to decreased metabolism because heart failure also reduces hepatic blood flow. Aldosterone exerts its principal action on the distal nephron, catalyzing reabsorption of sodium.

A third factor, thought to be hormonal in nature, but still poorly characterized, is felt to play a role in sodium retention in heart failure. In otherwise normal subjects and animals, an infusion of aldosterone leads to initial retention of sodium, but with continued infusion of aldosterone the subject or animal escapes from the sodium-retaining action and edema does not develop. Patients with heart failure fail to demonstrate this escape and continue to retain sodium.

Heart failure also affects pulmonary function and gas exchange. Pulmonary capillaries are incorporated eccentrically into the alveolar septum (Fig. 9 of Section XI) so that the capillary bulges into the alveolus, optimizing the surface area available for gaseous exchange. The smaller remaining portion of the capillary is incorporated into the alveolar septum, hence giving it support. Electron microscopic studies have shown that the portion of a pulmonary capillary that protrudes into an alveolus demonstrates fusion of the basement membranes of alveolar and capillary endothelium, and hence there is no interstitial space. In contrast, within the alveolar septum a substantial interstitial space exists between the basement membranes of alveolar epithelium and capillary endothelium (Fig. 121). This space contains numerous connective tissue elements that give support to the capillary and is also in communication with interstitial spaces throughout the lung and in turn with lymphatic capillaries that converge toward the hilus of the lung. From these anatomic data and supporting physiological studies, a concept has evolved that the component of each capillary incorporated into the alveolar septum is the principal site of pulmonary capillary tissue fluid exchange. Furthermore, to the extent that a net outward movement of fluid and protein occurs from the pulmonary capillary, this will accumulate first in the interstitial space, and the pulmonary lymphatic system will then bear the major responsibility for dispatching any excess back into the intravascular compartment.

Studies from a number of laboratories indicate that in normal animals and in man the volume of extravascular water in the lung (PEV) at any point in time represents approximately 60 per cent of total lung water (extravascular + intravascular). This extravascular volume includes both intracellular and interstitial water. The latter is in a continuous state of exchange resulting from net transcapillary filtration on the one hand and lymphatic drainage on the other. Whenever pulmonary capillary pressure is increased, a new steady state develops in which transcapillary fluid egress is enhanced, pulmonary lymphatic drainage is enhanced, and there is measurable increase in PEV. Several points are noteworthy about this increase in PEV. First, when pulmonary capillary pressure and net fluid egress are enhanced, there is a substantial lag time before lymphatic drainage increases to match the transcapillary leak of fluid. Hence, PEV can increase rapidly. Second, when pulmonary capillary pressure increases, the leak of water exceeds that of protein, tending to dilute the protein concentration of interstitial fluid and hence of pulmonary lymphatic drainage. Third, when a new steady state does develop subsequent to elevation of capillary pressure, the degree of expansion of PEV is correlated closely with the rise in pulmonary capillary and left atrial pressure. Finally, the ability of the lung to minimize the increase in PEV that occurs with any increase in pulmonary

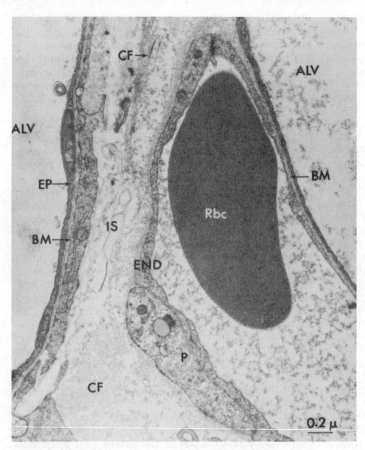

Figure 121. Interstitial pulmonary edema. The interstitial space (IS) of the thick portion of the alveolar septum has been considerably widened by edema fluid during hemodynamic pulmonary edema, whereas the opposite thin part, containing the fused basement membranes (BM), remains unchanged in thickness. In the alveoli, surrounding the red blood cell (RBC) in the capillary is the stroma free hemoglobin that was injected as a tracer. (With permission from Fishman, A. P.: Pulmonary edema: The water exchanging function of the lung. Circulation 46:394, 1972.)

capillary pressure reflects the capacity of the lymphatic drainage system.

The mechanism of fluid accumulation within interstitial spaces of the lung is simple in theory but very complex in practice. One factor that contributes to the complexity is the influence of gravity. All other things being equal, pulmonary capillary pressure will be greater in dependent than in nondependent regions of the lung. A second level of complexity is added by known architectural differences between the peripheral and hilar portions of the lung, which suggests that the rate of fluid egress from capillaries may be greater in hilar zones and that the effectiveness of the lymphatic pump may be less in hilar regions. This situation leads to a bat wing or butterfly chest x-ray appearance in which edema is much more marked centrally than at the peripheral parts of the lung. A third level of complexity is introduced by the fact that local differences in the effectiveness of lymphatic drainage, whether inborn or a consequence of prior diseases, may lead to patchy accumulations of early edema in patterns not predictable from a general knowledge of pulmonary architecture.

Despite these and other complexities that contribute in many cases to difficulty in recognizing pulmonary edema, certain generalities apply. The pulmonary edema that accompanies heart failure is always associated with an increase in pulmonary capillary pressure, and the fluid accumulation is initially interstitial in location. Distention of the interstitial space stimulates pulmonary "J" receptors, which in turn lead to an increase in minute ventilation. Interstitial pulmo-

nary edema decreases lung compliance and vital capacity and increases the work of breathing. When sufficient fluid has accumulated either regionally or throughout the lungs to raise interstitial pressure above atmospheric pressure, the compliance of the interstitial space decreases abruptly, fluid escapes more rapidly from the capillaries into the interstitium, and the alveolar epithelial barrier to fluid movement into the alveoli breaks down leading to alveolar edema. The sequence of radiographic signs of pulmonary edema follows the physiological alterations: venous distention, lymphatic diversion, interstitial edema, and alveolar edema. Blood gas exchange reflects the degree of pulmonary congestion. When edema is principally interstitial, ventilation may be excessive, leading to a reduced arterial pCO_2 and respiratory alkalosis, while pO_2 is relatively well preserved. With more advanced edema ventilation-perfusion inequalities become exaggerated and arterial hypoxia develops. When sufficient alveolar edema develops to obstruct terminal bronchioles, CO_2 elimination is impaired and hypercapnia ensues.

Let us again define heart failure as a condition that develops secondary to diseases that impair the ability of the heart to function as a pump. Furthermore, heart failure develops whenever the output of the impaired heart is for a substantial period of time unable to meet the metabolic demands of the body. The clinical manifestations of heart failure reflect (a) the direct consequences of reduced perfusion, which may be more evident in some organs than in others, (b) the neural and humoral alterations initiated by a cardiac output inadequate to meet metabolic demands, and (c) the consequences of salt and water retention, resulting in expansion of blood volume, elevation of venous pressures, and fluid accumulation in extravascular spaces. Muscular fatigue, particularly during exercise, is a direct consequence of reduced perfusion of skeletal muscles. Increased sweating, tachycardia at rest, and an exaggerated excitational heart rate reflect an increased level of sympathetic nerve activity. Increased sympathetic neural activity is also prominent in causing the redistribution of blood flow characteristic of heart failure, particularly reduced renal blood flow. Reduced renal blood flow and a series of secondary alterations lead to salt and water retention, expansion of blood volume, and an increase in capillary pressure. The rise in capillary pressure is not uniform throughout the body, and in one patient gravity may dominate, leading principally to ankle edema, while in another mitral stenosis may dominate, leading to a relatively early and more marked rise in pulmonary capillary pressure. Whatever the cause, sufficient expansion of blood volume leads to pulmonary vascular congestion, an increase in lung water, and dyspnea. The development of interstitial and alveolar edema represents the extreme consequence of salt and water retention and of elevated pulmonary venous pressure. The combined influences of reduced arterial perfusion and of venous and lymphatic engorgement contribute importantly to hepatic dysfunction in heart failure, to certain cases of protein-losing enteropathy associated with heart failure, and to the extreme condition of cachexia, which sometimes occurs when severe heart failure persists for long periods of time. The general picture, then, is one of inadequate perfusion and its consequences. In any given patient, the primary manifestations of heart failure may reflect the site and nature of the heart disease and the severity or chronicity of heart failure.

REFERENCES

Barger, A. C.: Renal hemodynamic factors in congestive heart failure. Ann NY Acad Sci 139:276, 1966.

Braunwald, E.: The autonomic nervous system in heart failure. In Braunwald, E. (ed.): The Myocardium: Failure and Infarction. New York, H. P. Publishing Co., Inc., 1974, p. 59.

Davis, J. O.: Mechanisms of salt and water retention in cardiac failure. In Braunwald, E. (ed.): The Myocardium: Failure and Infarction. New York, H. P. Publishing Co., Inc., 1974, p. 80.

Dodge, H. T.: Hemodynamic aspects of cardiac failure. In Braunwald, E. (ed.): The Myocardium: Failure and Infarction. New York, H. P. Publishing Co., Inc., 1974, p. 70.

Fishman, A. P.: Pulmonary edema: The water-exchanging function of the lung. Circulation 46:390, 1972.

Paintal, A. S.: Mechanisms of stimulation of J pulmonary receptors. J Physiol 203:511, 1969.

Schwartz, A., Sordahl, L. A., Entman, M. L., Allen, J. C., Reddy, Y. S., Goldstein, M. A., Luchi, R. J., and Wyborny, L. E.: Abnormal biochemistry in myocardial failure. Am J Cardiol 32:407, 1973.

Stead, E. A., Jr., Warren, J. V., and Brannon, E. S.: Cardiac output in congestive heart failure: An analysis of the reasons for lack of close correlation between the symptoms of heart failure and the resting cardiac output. Am Heart J 35:529, 1948.

Warren, J. V., and Stead, E. A., Jr.: Fluid dynamics in chronic congestive heart failure. Arch Intern Med 73:138, 1944.

West, J. B., Dollery, C. T., and Heard, B. E.: Increased pulmonary vascular resistance in the dependent zone of the isolated dog lung caused by perivascular edema. Circ Res 17:191, 1965.

Zelis, R., Flaim, S. F., Liedtke, A. J., and Nellis, S. H.: Cardiocirculatory dynamics in the normal and failing heart. Annu Rev Physiol 43:455, 1981.

Shock

Shock is a state characterized by the inability of the heart and/or the peripheral circulation to maintain an adequate perfusion of vital organs. If left untreated, irreversible damage occurs to organs and tissues throughout the body and death follows. Shock and heart failure have common features: both are syndromes (not diseases), they are defined by a constellation of clinical signs (not by a unique laboratory measurement), and each represents a consequence of profound circulatory alterations that may arise from one or more of many causes. The syndrome is defined by the presence of hypotension, tachycardia, sweating, pallor, cyanosis, hyperventilation, oliguria, and alterations of mental status. Shock is always secondary to some initiating event, such as acute myocardial infarction, trauma, hemorrhage, burns, or infection. At its onset, the physiological alterations that accompany shock reflect the nature of the initiating event. The longer the syndrome persists, however, the more the physiological pictures merge into a common pattern in which consequences of prolonged circulatory failure dominate the picture and initiating mechanisms and features unique to those mechanisms become blurred.

There is a temporal component to the sequence of changes that develop when organ perfusion becomes inadequate. In man, this temporal component to shock is acknowledged by referring to early and late features of the syndrome. In experimental models terms such as compensated, progressive, and irreversible emphasize the timetable to the shock syndrome and phenomena and mechanisms unique to each temporal phase.

The clinical syndrome of shock was first recognized in the middle of the eighteenth century. Nearly one hundred years later patients suffering from shock due to cholera were treated with intravenous fluid. However, at about the same time, experimentalists became interested in shock and the focus of interest shifted to neural control of the circulation and the concept of vasomotor exhaustion as the basis of shock. During World War I, Cannon and Bayliss first studied traumatic shock. They documented that hypotension was a prominent feature of the syndrome and attributed their findings to a postulated decrease in blood volume and cardiac output. It was not until 1943, however, that Cournand and Richards actually measured cardiac output in man and demonstrated that cardiac output was reduced in shock. Their findings also documented a reduction in blood volume and formed the basis of volume replacement therapy. Subsequent to World War II, methods for studying patients with shock improved and were applied extensively. In parallel with these clinical studies numerous animal models of shock have been employed and important physiological mechanisms have been clarified. In animals and man, the ability to prolong life after the onset of shock has led to increasing recognition of alterations in organ function (heart, lungs, liver, kidney, and so on) as a consequence of prolonged circulatory failure. With the development of more sophisticated biochemical methods, function at a cellular level and the role of circulating agents in the pathophysiology of shock have become the focus of recent studies. Despite all of this work, which forms an important and useful basis for treating patients with shock, the puzzle is far from complete. As a consequence, the pathophysiology is still incompletely understood and therapy leaves much to be desired.

HEMODYNAMICS

Several groups have now published the results of hemodynamic measurements in patients with acute myocardial infarction, and in particular results obtained from patients with cardiogenic shock due to myocardial infarction. Mean arterial pressure (by definition) was reduced in all patients. Cardiac output was reduced in all patients by a variable amount but averaged approximately 50 per cent of the output observed in patients with acute infarction without shock. Peripheral arterial resistance was elevated, although the extent of this change was highly variable. The extraction of oxygen from arterial blood was enhanced in the periphery and led to a widening of the arteriovenous oxygen difference. Left ventricular end-diastolic pressure, measured directly or estimated from pulmonary wedge recordings, was elevated and, together with the reduced stroke volume and stroke work of the ventricle, reflected acute left ventricular failure. Right atrial pressure was elevated modestly in many patients as a consequence of venoconstriction. In most studies the correlation betweeen right atrial pressure and left ventricular filling pressure was poor, so that right atrial pressure is a poor guide to assessing left ventricular function.

The first hemodynamic studies in patients suffering from hemorrhage and traumatic shock were reported by Cournand in 1943. Again, mean arterial pressure was decreased (60 to 70 mm Hg), cardiac index was decreased to 50 to 60 per cent of normal, and the peripheral arterial resistance and arteriovenous oxygen difference were increased. Even in Cournand's early studies, right atrial pressure was noted to be decreased in hemorrhagic shock. Subsequent work has confirmed that observation and extended it to include observations of left ventricular filling pressure, which is also reduced with hemorrhage in contrast to cardiogenic shock. In short, the early picture is dominated by depletion of blood volume, reduced cardiac output and peripheral perfusion, and the absence of evidence of myocardial failure.

PERIPHERAL PERFUSION

When cardiac output and arterial blood pressure are reduced, as a consequence of either hemorrhage or acute cardiac failure, blood flow to peripheral organs becomes reduced. The degree to which perfusion of any given organ is reduced reflects the passive pressure-flow relation of that organ, the ability of the vasculature to autoregulate, responsiveness of the vasculature to sympathetic vasoconstrictor influences initiated by hypotension, and the ability of locally produced products of metabolism to promote vasodilatation or to impair the vasoconstrictor effects of catecholamines. Studies of regional blood flow in shock have documented a reduced perfusion to nearly all peripheral organs, but the extent of the reduction is nonuniform. Maximal decreases are observed in skin, in the kidney, and in the intestine. Flow reductions of an intermediate degree are observed in skeletal muscle. At least on a relative basis, the degree of reduced perfusion to the heart and brain is initially small. The preservation of blood flow to the brain reflects the fact that cerebral blood vessels lack sympathetic innervation and do not participate in the intense vasoconstrictor response to hypotension. The heart is densely innervated with sympathetic efferent nerves, but it is apparent from numerous studies that local metabolism dominates in the control of coronary vascular resistance and precludes coronary vasoconstriction even during direct supramaximal stimulation of cardiac sympathetic nerves. In other organs, sympathetic vasoconstriction is a prominent feature of early shock and contributes to a reduction in local flow that exceeds that which would otherwise occur if reduced perfusion pressure were the sole factor determining local flow.

When shock and the accompanying increase in sympathetic activity persist, a significant component of the deleterious effect of enhanced neural activity appears to reflect a transfer of the predominant vasoconstrictor site from precapillary to postcapillary resistance vessels. Vessels on both sides of a capillary bed participate in the early vasoconstrictor response to hypotension. Hence, despite reduced perfusion of the capillary bed, capillary pressure is maintained at normal or reduced levels and there is a tendency for fluid to move from the interstitial space into the capillary. Later, postcapillary vasoconstriction predominates, capillary pressure increases despite arterial hypotension, and a protein-poor ultrafiltrate of plasma leaks from capillaries into the interstitial space, causing a reduction in blood flow and a rise of hematocrit. If cardiac output and arterial pressure can be maintained, either by volume expansion or by assist devices, the deleterious effects of sympathetic peripheral vasoconstriction can be attentuated or blocked by alpha-adrenergic blocking agents. The ability of such agents to increase organ perfusion—for example, to the kidney—is evident in many forms of shock.

DISTURBANCES IN CELLULAR METABOLISM

Whether shock is induced by hemorrhage or by myocardial infarction, the decrease in cardiac output and in regional perfusion has profound effects on cellular metabolism. In part, these changes are a direct consequence of reduced arterial perfusion. An important component of the metabolic change, however, results from activation of neural and hormonal mechanisms in response to hypotension. These latter mechanisms have effects on cellular metabolism that are distinct from those attributable to hypoperfusion per se. The combined effect of hypoperfusion and neural and hormonal influences on cellular metabolism leads to measurable changes in arterial and venous blood that are useful in assessing the degree of shock and its response to treatment.

The reduction in cardiac output that accompanies hemorrhage or myocardial infarction is highly variable. In general, however, the decrease in cardiac output parallels the severity of blood loss in cases of hemorrhage and the extent of myocardial damage in infarction. With modest reductions of cardiac output the metabolic needs of peripheral tissues are met by an increase in oxygen extraction from arterial blood. The arteriovenous oxygen difference is widened, and mixed venous pO_2 drops. However, the product of mixed arteriovenous oxygen difference and cardiac output is normal, and hence oxygen uptake by the patient and by most organs is normal despite hypotension and hypoperfusion.

With more severe reductions of cardiac output, the ability of peripheral organs to extract oxygen is exceeded, oxygen uptake is reduced, and a state of oxygen debt ensues. For example, in patients with acute myocardial infarction, without shock, cardiac index averaged 2.3 ± 0.2 L/min/M²; AVO_2 difference averaged 6.6 ± 0.3 vol %; and systemic oxygen consumption averaged 145 ± 8 ml/min/M². In patients with shock, cardiac index was 1.4 ± 0.09 L/min/M²; AVO_2 difference was 6.8 ± 0.6 vol %; and systemic oxygen consumption was 92 ± 10 ml/min/M².

Shock, therefore, can be viewed as a state of oxygen deficiency. Because the degree of hypoperfusion is nonuniform, the extent of oxygen lack in various organs and tissues is also nonuniform. In those tissues where flow is diminished below the level needed to provide adequate oxygen, cellular metabolism is disturbed. One of the earliest manifestations of this disturbance is a shift to anaerobic metabolism, a state in which glucose is used in preference to fatty acids. Because of oxygen lack, pyruvate formed from the metabolism of glycogen and glucose is converted to lactic acid rather than pursuing its normal course to acetyl CoA and subsequent use in the Krebs cycle. One consequence of this shift to anaerobic metabolism is the rapid development of intracellular acidosis and the release of lactate from these cells into the venous effluent from hypoxic tissues. Lactate released into the plasma is normally cleared by the liver. However, when hepatic blood flow is reduced, uptake and metabolism of lactate are diminished. Studies in animals and man have shown that the clearance of lactate is diminished in shock so that increased production and decreased clearance both contribute to the rise in plasma lactate that is characteristic of shock. Several investigators have established a relation between the blood lactate level and oxygen lack as reflected by oxygen debt. Others have reported that the lactate level in plasma correlates with survival and is a useful guide to therapeutic interventions.

Although acidosis is a prominent and common manifestation of prolonged shock, and even of early shock if it is severe, arterial blood pH is frequently normal in early shock even with modest elevations of lactate. The reason for this is that hyperventilation leads to a compensatory respiratory alkalosis. This feature of shock is discussed in greater detail in the section of this chapter dealing with the lung. As peripheral hypoperfusion persists or worsens, however, the rise in plasma lactate progresses and a state of lactic acidemia ensues. Bicarbonate levels and buffer base fall, and this fall generally parallels the rise in lactate. Approximately 90 per cent of the decrease in buffer base or bicarbonate is attributable to hydrogen ions arising from lactic acid.

With the onset of shock, activation of the sympathetic nervous system leads to important metabolic consequences. One of these effects is hydrolysis of triglycerides in peripheral adipocytes with mobilization of free fatty acids (FFA) and their release into the plasma. Plasma-free fatty acids rise in shock principally because of this peripheral action of catecholamines. A second factor contributing to the rise in FFA is their diminished uptake by oxygen-depleted, anaerobically metabolizing cells throughout the body. Hyperglycemia is a prominent feature of shock even without replacement therapy with glucose-containing fluids. This rise in plasma glucose is also largely attributable to adrenergic mechanisms, principally the effect of catecholamines to stimulate gluconeogenesis and glycogen breakdown by the liver.

In animal studies, a strong case has been made for the release of vasoactive agents other than catecholamines and for their participation in the sequelae of shock. Some of these agents are released directly from ischemic tissues, and others arise from the action of lysosomal and other proteases on circulating precursors. Histamine, serotonin, prostaglandins, and the so-called myocardial depressant factor fall into this group. Much remains to be learned about these substances and their role in shock. At present their role in human shock, and particularly shock arising from hemorrhage or on a cardiac basis, is largely unknown.

THE HEART

A decrease in the pumping capacity of the heart plays a prominent role in shock. In acute myocardial infarction and other cardiogenic causes of shock, depressed myocardial performance is evident early and is the basis of the reduced cardiac output. In hemorrhage and other forms of hypovolemic shock, myocardial performance is normal initially but becomes depressed as shock persists.

Pathological studies in patients who died of shock due to myocardial infarction have shown that ischemic necrosis is extensive and usually involves 40 per cent or more of the left ventricular muscle mass. Angiographic studies in living patients, using either contrast material or radionuclides, have shown large akinetic or dyskinetic regions and a reduction in left ventricular ejection fraction. A detailed discussion of regional changes in myocardial performance, metabolism, and ultrastructure, and the temporal sequence of these changes after the induction of ischemia are presented in the section on coronary heart disease. The major point is that cardiogenic shock develops when these changes involve a large component of the myocardium and when compensatory mechanisms are inadequate to sustain adequate arterial blood pressure and organ perfusion.

In some patients who develop shock as a consequence of hemorrhage, myocardial failure may develop even in the absence of coronary artery disease. Furthermore, in animals subjected to hemorrhage followed by reinfusion of blood hours later, depressed ventricular function has been a uniform finding. Generally, the degree of depressed function has correlated with the duration of shock. Pathological studies in patients and animals have shown focal areas of myocardial necrosis and subendocardial hemorrhage. A second type of myocardial lesion in shock is referred to as a zonal lesion. These lesions consist of apparent zones of hypercontracted sarcomeres, with scalloping of the sarcolemma, fragmentation of Z lines, and displacement of mitochondria. Zonal lesions develop as early as 15 minutes after induction of experimental shock and differ from necrosis and subendocardial hemorrhage in that they are reversible. Both types of lesions can be prevented or markedly reduced in animals by pretreatment with beta-adrenergic blocking agents. The thesis has been developed that these abnormalities develop when enhanced sympathetic drive is imposed on a heart with reduced overall coronary perfusion. In untreated animals the lesions become progressively more extensive and severe as the duration of shock is prolonged.

A third element in myocardial deterioration that develops with prolonged hemorrhagic shock involves the release of agents from ischemic peripheral tissues that have the ability to depress myocardial function. Prominent among these is the myocardial depressant factor (MDF) thought to be a small peptide produced by lysosomal hydrolases in the ischemic pancreas. Increased levels of this factor have been reported in ultrafiltrates of plasma from patients with shock who later demonstrated evidence of cardiac failure. These reports emphasize that depressed cardiac performance can develop as a complication of shock that initially is of a noncardiac cause. The development of a cardiac component in the later stages of noncardiogenic shock leads to a further reduction in cardiac output. Returning to myocardial infarction as an example of cardiogenic shock, we can see that hypoxia, acidosis, sympathetic reflex responses, and the release of potentially depressant factors from peripheral ischemic tissue all serve to perpetuate the primary cause of shock.

THE LUNG

Changes in the function of the lung play a central role in the pathophysiology of the shock syndrome. They highlight a general feature of shock in which initial disturbances of organ function reflect the cause of shock and with which subsequent changes begin to merge regardless of the cause, with the latter changes reflecting organ failure. Hemorrhage that is sufficient to induce systemic hypotension produces immediate changes in lung function that are attributable almost entirely to a decrease in blood volume. The decrease in blood volume decreases venous return and cardiac output. The subject hyperventilates principally because of the stimulation of peripheral chemoreceptors as a consequence of reduced blood flow. The decrease in venous return leads to decreases in right atrial, pulmonary, and left atrial pressures. The volume of blood within the lung is reduced, and at least initially lung compliance is increased and the work of breathing is reduced. Hyperventilation causes the tension of CO_2 to drop in arterial blood, sometimes to levels of 20 to 30 mm Hg. However, the drop in pCO_2 is less than would be predicted from hyperventilation per se. The reason is that when pulmonary pressure and flow are decreased, there is an increase in regions of lung where

pulmonary arterial pressure is less than atmospheric pressure and hence capillary perfusion is diminished or absent. These areas where alveoli are ventilated but not perfused add to the so-called physiologic or alveolar dead space, and ventilation or even hyperventilation of such areas fails to lower pCO_2. Thus, the initial picture is one of decreased pulmonary arterial pressure and flow, decreased pulmonary blood volume, hyperventilation, normal arterial pO_2 because perfused regions of lung are well ventilated, and a decrease in arterial pCO_2 due to hyperventilation of perfused areas. However, the arterial pCO_2 is reduced less than would be predicted from minute ventilation because of ventilation of underperfused areas (that is, an increased alveolar dead space).

If hemorrhagic shock is allowed to persist this initial phase begins to change as a consequence of systemic changes induced by shock per se. Pulmonary vascular resistance increases. In part, this increase in pulmonary vascular resistance is attributable to a rise in circulating vasoconstrictor substances—the most noteworthy with respect to the lung are norepinephrine and serotonin. The rise in plasma norepinephrine levels is prominent in shock and is undoubtedly a part of the neurogenically mediated reflex sympathetic response to hypotension. Serotonin is derived principally from platelet aggregates that are known to form in shock, and aggregation is thought to result from activation of platelet alpha receptors in response to catecholamines. Serotonin is a very potent pulmonary vasoconstrictor, and, at least in dogs, the rise in pulmonary vascular resistance following shock can be markedly attenuated by making the animals thrombocytopenic before hemorrhage. Serotonin is also a potent constrictor of terminal airways. In this phase of shock, the pulmonary picture is determined importantly by circulating substances that influence vascular and airway resistances, by the development of atelectasis in some regions of the lung, and by hypoxic vasoconstriction in atelectatic regions. Total pulmonary vascular resistance is increased, but the resistance changes are nonuniform and the normal mechanisms that closely match ventilation and perfusion on a regional basis are disturbed. Hypoxemia develops, and numerous studies in animals and man have demonstrated that shunting—that is, perfusion of either nonventilated or underventilated alveolar regions—is the dominant basis of the reduced arterial pO_2. Furthermore, whenever shunting is present, the degree of arterial hypoxemia is exaggerated by a low cardiac output. When cardiac output is reduced, the extraction of oxygen by peripheral organs and tissues is increased, and mixed venous pO_2 falls. When significant volumes of mixed venous blood with reduced pO_2 are shunted through the lung without gas exchange, the resulting arterial pO_2 is lower than would occur with a comparable shunt of blood with a higher oxygen tension. In this phase of shock, lung water may increase owing to formation of regional interstitial edema, a factor that contributes to ventilation-perfusion irregularities (see chapter on Heart Failure) and hypoxemia.

When shock has persisted for periods ranging from 12 to 72 hours, a third phase of pulmonary changes may develop that has been referred to as shock lung or adult respiratory distress syndrome (ARDS). Although first recognized in cases of traumatic shock, the pathological alteration of the lung is common to a number of conditions that cause shock. Fortunately, it is a relatively infrequent complication. The clinical picture is dominated by very rapid breathing with a reduced tidal volume due to decreased lung compliance. Rales and wheezes are found on auscultation, and the x-ray shows enlarging zones of interstitial and alveolar edema that tend to coalesce, giving a diffuse haziness to the x-ray. Arterial oxygen tension falls to a marked degree and is not corrected by oxygen administration. Pathologically, there is interstitial and intra-alveolar hemorrhage and the formation of alveolar hyaline membranes. Ultrastructural studies have shown that the junctions between capillary endothelial cells are open so that fluid, protein, blood cells, and platelets lead into the interstitial space. The precise mechanisms responsible for this pathological alteration of the lung are unknown. The histological and ultrastructural picture is one of irreversible tissue injury, and it has been speculated that the process is a consequence of ischemic injury. On the other hand, this lesion can be prevented in one lung when that lung is excluded from the circulation during the period of shock. It follows from this observation that shock lung is not attributable solely to ischemia.

Cardiogenic shock differs from hemorrhagic shock in that cardiac output fails despite a normal or elevated blood volume. Left atrial pressure, pulmonary arterial pressure, and right atrial pressure are elevated, not reduced, during the initial phase. Hyperventilation is prominent as in hemorrhage, but ventilation is stimulated not only by peripheral chemoreceptors but also by receptors in the pulmonary venous system that respond to elevated pulmonary venous pressure. Pulmonary blood volume is increased, lung water increases, compliance is reduced, and the work of breathing is enhanced. The early pulmonary changes are identical to heart failure and pulmonary edema. Hypoxemia develops in proportion to ventilation-perfusion inequalities that largely reflect shunting. The decrease in arterial pO_2 is exaggerated when cardiac output is markedly reduced, leading to a wide AV O_2 difference and a decreased mixed venous pO_2. Until recently, shock lung was an infrequent complication of medical causes of cardiogenic shock, such as myocardial infarction. However, shock lung develops after surgical cardiopulmonary bypass, and with the recent use of assisted circulation and other life support techniques in patients with cardiogenic shock, shock lung has been observed more frequently in patients.

THE KIDNEY

The kidney has been an appropriate target of interest in studies of shock. When cardiac output is reduced, renal blood flow and urine formation are decreased markedly. Because of its uniquely developed capacity to autoregulate, renal flow is reduced less than one might anticipate from a reduction in perfusion pressure per se, but when cardiac output falls and sympathetic vasoconstrictor reflexes are initiated, renal resistance increases and renal blood flow and glomerular filtration rates fall. One reason for the profound interest in the kidney in shock is that urine flow tends to mirror cardiac output; hence the clinician uses urine flow as an index of circulatory function and its response to treatment. A second reason for interest in the kidney is that renal failure due to acute tubular necrosis

develops in many patients who sustain severe shock, even if shock is only brief in duration. Thus, in conditions in which the cause of shock can be corrected and the shock state reversed, a patient's subsequent course is often complicated by acute renal failure.

Nearly 25 years ago, it was demonstrated in humans and animals that the phenomenon of acute tubular necrosis could be prevented in many instances by the administration of hypertonic mannitol. Subsequently, Leaf and coworkers demonstrated that a substantial portion of the energy requirements of the renal tubule and of resting muscle cells is used by the active transport system responsible for extruding sodium from the cell and hence for controlling cell volume. With ischemia, loss in the ability to regulate cell volume is an early (perhaps the earliest) observable derangement in cell function. When flow is restored to cells that have lost this ability there is explosive cell swelling that may or may not be sufficient to contribute to irreversible damage. This phenomenon has now been demonstrated in renal tubular cells, in the retina and brain, in vascular smooth muscle, and in the myocardium. Explosive cell swelling, either by increasing tissue pressure or by leading to obstruction of the microcirculation, can be sufficient to perpetuate ischemia even when perfusion pressure is restored to normal. This line of investigation has contributed an additional important element to the complex role of the microcirculation in shock: it provides a basis for understanding that flow to certain regions is not necessarily restored by restoring perfusion pressure after periods of ischemia sufficient to induce cell injury, and it provides a basis for the therapeutic use of hyperosmolar agents at certain early stages of shock.

REFERENCES

Cournand, A., Riley, R. L., Bradley, S. E., Breed, E. S., Noble, R. P., Lauson, H. D., Gregersen, M. I., and Richards, D. W.: Studies of the circulation in clinical shock. Surgery 13:964, 1943.

de Luz, P. L., Cavanilles, J. M., Michaels, S., Weil, M. H., and Shubin, H.: Oxygen delivery, anoxic metabolism and hemoglobin-oxygen affinity (P50) in patients with acute myocardial infarction and shock. Am J Cardiol 36:148, 1975.

Flores, J., DiBona, D. R., Beck, C. H., and Leaf, A.: The role of cell swelling in ischemic renal damage and the protective effect of hypertonic solute. J Clin Invest 51:118, 1972.

Glenn, T. M., Lefer, A. M., Martin, J. B., Lovett, W. L., Morris, J. N., Jr., and Wangensteen, S. L.: Production of myocardial depressant factor in cardiogenic shock. Am Heart J 82:78, 1971.

Hackel, D. B., Ratliff, N. B., and Mikat, E.: The heart in shock. Circ Res 35:805, 1974.

Jakschik, B. A., Marshall, G. R., Lourik, J. L., and Needleman, P.: Profile of circulating vasoactive substances in hemorrhagic shock and their pharmacological manipulation. J Clin Invest 54:842, 1974.

Moore, F. D.: The effects of hemorrhage on body composition. N Engl J Med 273:567, 1965.

Page, D. L., Caulfield, J. B., Kastor, J. A., DeSanctis, R. W., and Sanders, C. A.: Myocardial changes associated with cardiogenic shock. N Engl J Med 285:133, 1971.

Ramo, B. W., Meyers, N., Wallace, A. G., Starmer, F., Clark, D. O., and Whalen, R. E.: Hemodynamic findings in 123 patients with acute myocardial infarction on admission. Circulation 42:567, 1970.

Swan, H. J. C., Forrester, J. S., Diamond, G., Chatterjee, K., and Parmely, W. W.: Hemodynamic spectrum of myocardial infarction and cardiogenic shock: A conceptual model. Circulation 45:1097, 1972.

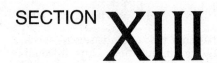

NEUROLOGY

FRED PLUM, M.D., *and* JEROME B. POSNER, M.D.

Pathophysiology as an Approach to Neurologic Diagnosis

A human being can know that he is ill only if his brain tells him so. Thus, all symptoms that signal human bodily dysfunction are ultimately neurologic in origin. However, most physicians use a more restricted definition of nervous system symptoms, i.e., those that reflect physiologic abnormalities *intrinsic* to the nervous system. Even using this definition, one is faced with a potentially bewildering variety of potential complaints (Table 1).

Symptoms of neurologic or muscular disease can arise from any portion of the nervous system from the furthest reaches of the peripheral nerves and the organs they innervate (muscles and skin) to the highest integrative levels of the brain (association cortex). Furthermore, the diseases causing symptoms may af-

fect the nervous system either directly (e.g., toxic destruction of nerve cells) or indirectly (e.g., occlusion of blood vessels to the brain leading to infarction) (Table 2). To relate this entire neurologic section to clinical medicine, this chapter presents first an overview of the pathophysiology of neurologic dysfunction to be detailed in succeeding chapters and then offers a general approach based on using a knowledge of pathophysiology to evaluate symptoms of possible nervous system origin.

PATHOPHYSIOLOGY OF NERVOUS SYSTEM SYMPTOMS

Despite the diversity of symptoms of nervous system disease and their many potential causes, the fundamental pathophysiology of neural dysfunction is simple: Neurons conduct electrical impulses from the dendrites and cell body down the axon and secrete chemical substances (i.e., neurotransmitters, neuroregulators, trophic substances) that carry the signal from one cell to the next. Even neuroendocrine cells, which secrete their chemical substances directly into the bloodstream to affect other cells at a distance, fulfill these fundamental principles. Non-neuronal structures of the nervous system, the glia, blood vessels, and CSF, nourish, metabolically stabilize, and physically support the neurons. Thus, all nervous system disease ultimately arises from a failure of neurons to conduct or transmit impulses appropriately. That failure may be of two types: Impulse conduction may be deficient or absent (hypofunction), or it may be excessive (hyperfunction). Unfortunately, in clinical practice the situation is rarely so simple; most diseases of the nervous system present a mixture of neuronal hypofunction and hyperfunction. In addition, damage to an inhibitory neuron, causing it to cease activity, may result in hyperfunction of the undamaged nerve cell that it previously inhibited. Despite these complexities, one can consider many neurologic disorders as representing neuronal hypofunction, hyperfunction, or a mixture of the two.

NEURONAL HYPOFUNCTION

A particularly clear-cut example of neuronal hypofunction is that which arises from damage to the lower

TABLE 1. SOME SYMPTOMS OF NERVOUS SYSTEM DISEASE

Fatigability	Dizziness and vertigo
Paralysis	Blindness
Incoordination	Loss of bladder and bowel control
Tremor and dyskinesias	Fainting
Seizures	Amnesia
Loss of sensation	Dementia
Numbness and tingling	Inability to speak or comprehend
Pain	speech
Deafness	
Tinnitus	

TABLE 2. SOME PROCESSES CAUSING NERVOUS SYSTEM DISEASE

PROCESS	EXAMPLES
Genetic degenerative disorders	Huntington's chorea, amyotrophic lateral sclerosis (Lou Gehrig's disease)
Infectious disorders	Meningitis, encephalitis, brain abscess
Immune disorders	Myasthenia gravis, multiple sclerosis
Neoplastic disorders	Brain and spinal cord tumors
Vascular disorders	Cerebral hemorrhage, cerebral infarction (stroke), vasculitis
Toxic and metabolic disorders	Drug overdose, hypovitaminosis and hypervitaminosis, narcotic and alcohol addiction
Traumatic disorders	Brain and spinal cord injury

TABLE 3. SOME SYMPTOMS OF NEURONAL HYPOFUNCTION AND HYPERFUNCTION

Hypofunction	Hyperfunction
Paralysis	Paresthesias
Syncope	Trigeminal neuralgia
Muscle atrophy	Seizures
Sensory loss	Scintillating scotomata
Incontinence	Mixed (Release)
Dementia	Spasticity and rigidity
Ataxia	Tremor
Blindness, deafness	Pain (see gate theory)

motor neuron (Table 3). The cell body of the lower motor neuron resides in the ventral horn of the spinal cord. Its axon leaves the spinal cord through the anterior root, enters a peripheral nerve, and terminates on a muscle at the neuromuscular junction. As the Motor System section describes, several pathophysiologic processes can damage the lower motor neuron, leading to complete or incomplete failure of function (hypofunction). Depending on the degree of failure and the number of lower motor neurons involved, a series of characteristic symptoms defines exactly the site of the lesion. For example, if a motor nerve is transected by injury, the distal portion of the nerve deprived of both electrical impulses and nutrition from the cell body first fails to conduct and then dies (wallerian degeneration). Failure of the motor nerve to conduct impulses results in its failure to release acetylcholine at the neuromuscular junction, with the resulting loss of stimulation to the muscle it supplies. There is immediate paralysis of the muscles supplied by that motor nerve, accompanied by a loss of muscle tone. A sharp blow with a rubber hammer to the tendon of the involved muscle elicits no reflex response (absence of deep tendon reflex). After several days the muscles supplied by the motor nerve begin to atrophy noticeably. The distribution of the muscle weakness, along with the combination of paralysis, decreased tone, and muscle atrophy, identifies unequivocally not only the presence of lower motor neuron damage but also which nerve is damaged. Even in this most simple description of lower motor neuron hypofunction, however, complicating *hyperfunction* in the form of muscle fibrillations emerges soon afterward (see p. 1050).

Contrast the findings of lower motor neuron dysfunction with those that occur when it is not the peripheral nerve that is transected but the spinal cord (Table 4). After the initial effects of spinal shock have worn off, the individual with a transected spinal cord remains paralyzed below the level of transection because the corticospinal tracts (upper motor neurons) no longer carry impulses from the brain to the anterior horn cells. Thus, as with a transected nerve, the muscles are paralyzed because the lower motor neuron no longer functions at the brain's command. However, the anterior horn cells are intact, even though deprived of both facilitatory and inhibitory influences from higher centers. The failure of the descending inhibitory fibers leads to increased activity in more caudally located motor-related nerve cells, including the interneurons of the now isolated distal spinal cord. This, in turn, produces increased tone in the paralyzed muscles and increased stretch reflexes. Furthermore, because the lower motor neurons continue to release their normal resting quantities of acetylcholine to the muscles, the muscles do not atrophy to the same degree

that they do in lower motor neuron dysfunction, and fibrillations do not develop. With both peripheral nerve and spinal cord section there is complete failure of the neuron to function normally and the muscle is completely paralyzed for voluntary movement. The clinical findings are entirely different however and provide an immediate diagnosis to the observer with a knowledge of physiology.

At a slightly more complicated level, failure of lower motor neuron function may be either complete or partial and transient or sustained. Section of a motor nerve, as indicated above, is the best example of a complete lesion. Partial lesions can occur in a variety of circumstances, each giving rise to a slightly different set of signs and symptoms characteristic of the type of lesion. For example, in myasthenia gravis (see Neurobiologic Essentials) a lesion of the postsynaptic neuromuscular junction causes increasing but transient weakness with successive effort, related to the temporary saturation of damaged postsynaptic acetylcholine receptors. A different set of clinical findings is found in the so-called myasthenic syndrome, a disorder of unknown cause in which there is decreased release of acetylcholine from otherwise normal nerve endings. In this instance the muscles are weak initially, but as supramaximal stimulus of the nerve increases acetylcholine release, the muscle gains strength as it is exercised.

Turning our attention to the nerve itself, toxic or degenerative diseases tend to cause variable destruction to the lower motor neurons, some dying, some injured but not dead, and some normal. Depending on the degree of failure of function, weakness, but not total paralysis, and atrophy as well as decreased tone and diminished reflexes occur, but, in contrast to nerve

TABLE 4. CLINICAL SIGNS OF UPPER AND LOWER MOTOR NEURON LESIONS

SIGNS	CAUSE
	Lower Motor Neuron
Paralysis	Hypofunction of alpha motor neuron
Atrophy	Failure of neuromuscular transmission
Diminished tone	Hypofunction of gamma motor neuron
Absent tendon reflexes	Hypofunction of both alpha and gamma neurons
Fasciculations	Hyperfunction of damaged alpha motor neurons
Fibrillations	Hyperfunction of denervated muscle fiber
	Upper Motor Neuron
Paralysis	Hypofunction of upper motor neuron
Increased tone (spasticity)	Hypofunction of some upper motor neurons leads to diminished inhibition and resulting hyperfunction of others, including alpha and gamma motor neurons
Increased tendon reflexes	Hyperfunction of alpha and gamma neurons as above
Abnormal nociceptive reflexes (Babinski response)	Release of primitive spinal reflexes by upper motor neuron hypofunction
Late or minor atrophy	Chronic and long-term disuse of muscle

section, the process results in neurons that are damaged but not dead and that often become hyperfunctional (see below).

Many examples of neuronal hypofunction are transient rather than sustained. Simple examples of transient neuronal hypofunction include those produced by injection of local anesthetic agents into nerves (most often sensory nerves for repair of teeth) or compression of nerves against bony structures. If one sits with one's legs crossed, for example, the peroneal nerve on the uppermost leg is compressed between the underlying knee and the head of the fibula behind which it passes. If that posture is maintained for a prolonged period, first large sensory and then motor fibers become blocked. (The pathogenesis is not completely understood but is probably not mere ischemia of the nerve. It is also not a failure of axonal transport of transmitters or nutrients since it develops before even fast transport could play a role.) The foot loses sensation and the muscles supplied by that nerve (dorsiflexors of the foot) become paralyzed. When the compression is released, there is often hyperfunction of the nerve, including paresthesias and sometimes fasciculations. Several metabolic abnormalities may produce either transient or sustained dysfunction of nerves. Such abnormalities often interfere with axonal transport.

More complicated physiologic mechanisms can also have hypofunction as their end result. Hypofunction can be produced in one set of neurons by increased function of another set of inhibitory neurons. One example of this principle occurs when descending serotonergic fibers from the brainstem inhibit incoming nociceptive fibers in the posterior horn, decreasing the sensation of pain (see Sensory Systems). Even so obvious a manifestation of neuronal hypofunction as is produced by section of a sensory nerve may be modified by alterations of excitatory and inhibitory spinal influences on that or adjacent nerves. For example, section of the sensory root of the trigeminal nerve leads to a large area of sensory loss in the face. However, the size of that area can be increased by further lesions of Lissauer's tract and the substantia gelatinosa of the spinal cord and brainstem. Contrarily, facilitation of excitatory fibers by the use of strychnine can considerably decrease the area of sensory loss from section of the fifth nerve, whereas facilitation of inhibitory fibers by the use of L-dopa (a drug metabolized to dopamine in the central nervous system) increases the area of sensory loss. Thus, clinically, even an area of sensory impairment caused by damage to a nerve or root can vary in size, depending on the state of central facilitation or inhibition. Similar increases or decreases in the area of sensory loss can be achieved in experimental animals by selectively sectioning within the spinal cord or brainstem the ventrolateral inhibitory division or the dorsal medial facilitatory division of an entering dorsal root.

NEURONAL HYPERFUNCTION

A simple everyday example of neuronal hyperfunction is the spontaneous discharge of a sensory nerve that results from a direct blow ("bumping one's crazy bone," "seeing stars") or the tingling sensation (paresthesia) that results from spontaneous discharge of a compressed nerve (the foot "going to sleep" when one sits with one's legs crossed). To discharge a normal sensory motor nerve from an external source requires considerable force, such as prolonged compression or a sharp blow. However, if the nerve is already damaged, the threshold falls considerably. Why damage to nerves should lead to hyperexcitability is not entirely clear, but examples abound. Chronic compression of a nerve root such as occurs with a herniated disc (see Sensory Systems) causes pain and often tingling in the dermatomal distribution of that root when it is lightly stretched; normal nerve roots have no such susceptibility. Flexion of the neck stretches the posterior columns; if these structures are scarred or demyelinated, the stretch spontaneously discharges the central area of the axon extending from the dorsal root ganglion and causes paresthesias in the legs (see Lhermitte's sign, p. 1083). A potential mechanism for the above findings is that of ephaptic conduction. The myelin around peripheral nerves normally prevents an action potential in one nerve from discharging its neighbor. Presumably, in demyelinated areas an action potential along a sensory or motor nerve could decrease the membrane potential in its neighbor enough to lead to spontaneous firing. Such ephaptic conduction in a motor nerve actually has been demonstrated in an illness called hemifacial spasm.

Another simple example of neuronal hyperfunction is the fasciculation. In lower motor neuron disease, damaged neurons often fire spontaneously. The pathogenesis of this spontaneous firing is unclear, but it leads to isolated contraction of all of the muscle fibers supplied by that lower motor neuron (motor unit). These contractions are called fasciculations. (Fasciculations also often occur as an isolated phenomenon in normal people, presumably as a result of physiologically rather than pathologically hyperfunctioning lower motor neurons.) When motor units are partly or completely denervated, the terminal axons of the normal remaining neurons then sprout to supply muscle fibers that have lost their neuronal innervation. When there is substantial sprouting the atrophy becomes less, and the individual motor units become larger. These neurons may themselves later become partially damaged by the toxic or metabolic process; the fasciculations they then develop are much larger than the size of a normal motor unit.

Hyperfunction of denervated muscles results in fibrillations. Muscle fibers deprived of an almost continuous supply of acetylcholine across the neuromuscular junction not only atrophy but change their membrane structure. Acetylcholine receptors spread from the site of the neuromuscular junction to involve the entire muscle membrane and become hypersensitive to small amounts of circulating neurotransmitter (denervation hypersensitivity). Spontaneous discharges of the now atrophic muscle fibers (fibrillations) can be recorded with needle electrodes and actually seen beneath the thin surface of the tongue.

A more complicated example of excessive discharge of neurons occurs in the epilepsies. Here a spontaneous hypersynchronous discharge of a group of interrelated central neurons leads to abnormal symptoms (see p. 1147). If the discharge comes from the area of the motor cortex that controls the arm, there may be uncontrollable shaking of the member (focal motor seizure). If it comes from that area of the cortex having to do with the perception of smell, the patient may hallucinate a nonexistent odor. If it comes from the limbic cortex, the patient may suffer feelings of anger, embarrassment, or fear unrelated to any environmental stimulus. When excessively firing neurons generate excessive firing in other neurons, the discharge may spread to involve the entire brain, leading to loss of consciousness and a generalized convulsion.

MIXED HYPOFUNCTION AND HYPERFUNCTION

It is not always easy to define whether a symptom of nervous system dysfunction results from hypofunction or hyperfunction because the disorder may be mixed (for example, see Table 4). As indicated before, even in the simple example of section of a motor nerve, there is resulting hyperexcitability of muscle fibers (fibrillations).

Parkinson's disease similarly reflects a combination of neural hypofunction and hyperfunction. In this condition, destruction of inhibitory nigrostriatal fibers impairs the normally inhibitory striatal output back to the thalamus and cerebral cortex. The result leads to rigidity and tremor, symptoms seemingly of neuronal hyperfunction. Another clinically more subtle "release" finding is that which occurs when failure of one portion of the nervous system leads to hypersensitivity (denervation hypersensitivity) of a connecting area that is no longer receiving appropriate innervation. A clear example occurs with sympathetic denervation of the eye. This generally leads to pupillary constriction because the pupil dilator muscle of the iris no longer receives innervation. However, with time the number of receptors in muscle increases, and they may become supersensitive to circulating norepinephrine. If there is enough circulating norepinephrine, the pupil may paradoxically dilate despite the lack of sympathetic innervation. Denervation hypersensitivity (in this case chemical denervation) probably also underlies the behavioral withdrawal syndrome in patients dependent on narcotic or other sedative drugs.

APPROACH TO PATIENTS WITH SYMPTOMS SUGGESTING NEURAL DYSFUNCTION

The physician encountering a patient complaining of being unwell is faced with a several-fold task. Although the paragraphs above have described the pathophysiology of nervous system disorders, the patient rarely comes complaining that his nervous system is disordered, but rather describes to the physician a symptom or sign that he finds distressing.

CATEGORIES OF SYMPTOMS

The physiology of such symptoms can be viewed as belonging to one of three categories: (1) symptoms caused by an abnormal systemic organ and detected by a normal nervous system, (2) symptoms caused by an abnormal nervous system, (3) symptoms caused by a normal systemic organ but misperceived by an abnormal nervous system. When a person complains of being unwell, it is *always* because the central nervous system has detected a physiologic alteration. In most instances of systemic illness, symptoms reflect a normal nervous system that is receiving and interpreting signals from an abnormal organ. For example, when a patient falls and fractures his hip, the sensory nervous

system carries accurate signals to the brain. Likewise, the patient's tactile sensory system, with its nerve endings in the fingers, can detect on self-examination an otherwise asymptomatic breast cancer. The eyes may see jaundice or a rash, the ears hear an arteriovenous malformation in the head. When symptoms arise from a diseased organ, even if the sensations perceived by the nervous system are nonspecific, e.g., the feeling of malaise that may be the only symptom of liver disease, the physician can usually identify the problem by physical signs such as an enlarged liver or jaundice not noticed by the patient or by laboratory abnormalities such as abnormal liver function tests. However, when the symptoms arise from altered physiology of the nervous system itself, the situation is different in several ways:

(1) The altered nervous system may supply misleading signals such as referred pain; e.g., pain may be restricted to the knee when the L4 nerve root or femoral nerve is disordered without there being any abnormality in the knee itself. If one bumps one's ulnar nerve at the elbow or compresses the peroneal nerve by sitting with crossed legs, the subsequent paresthesias affect, respectively, the fourth and fifth fingers or the foot and do not represent diseases of those organs but rather a misleading signal from the nerves supplying those organs.

(2) Similar symptoms may be produced from nervous system dysfunction at several different levels. Paralysis of a foot may result from a peroneal nerve palsy, an L5 root lesion, a spinal cord lesion, a parasagittal brain lesion, or even from a psychological lesion (conversion reaction). To arrive at a correct localization may be very difficult, although meticulous examination of the nervous system will frequently help the examiner localize the lesion. In the example above, peroneal nerve damage can be distinguished from L5 root damage because the L5 root supplies the hamstring muscles as well as the foot, and the peroneal nerve supplies only the foot. In both of the above lesions, tone is decreased and the muscles become atrophic. On the contrary, in a spinal cord lesion there is no atrophy, tone is increased, and the deep tendon reflexes of the entire leg become hyperactive. In addition, all of the muscles of the leg are somewhat weak, even though muscles supplied by the peroneal nerve may be weaker than other muscles. A parasagittal lesion of the brain usually causes some weakness of the arm as well as the leg, although the changes may be subtle and characterized only by a slight increase in tone and reflex activity. Finally, in a psychological lesion, tone and tendon reflexes are normal, and the distribution of muscle weakness is "nonphysiologic."

(3) Many disorders of the nervous system are transient and disappear by the time the patient sees the physician. Syncopal attacks, seizures, and intermittent vertigo are but a few examples. These disorders leave neither abnormal physical nor laboratory findings at the time of the examination, making the physician entirely dependent on making inferences from the history.

(4) Even when a symptom is present at the time of the examination, it may be unaccompanied by abnormal physical signs or laboratory findings. The nervous system is less amenable than other organs to the time-honored examinations of inspection (the only portion of the central nervous system available to inspection

is the optic nerve) and palpation (one can feel some peripheral nerves but none of the CNS). Percussion and auscultation are likewise rarely useful in examining the nervous system. As a result, the cause of many common neurologic symptoms such as headache, dizziness, and back pain must be inferred from the patient's history rather than confirmed objectively by physical or laboratory findings.

(5) Despite recent advances in diagnostic imaging and in our understanding of the chemistry of the nervous system, many neurologic illnesses cannot be confirmed unequivocally by laboratory examination. In part this occurs because CNS lesions too small to be seen by current imaging techniques nevertheless may produce symptoms, and in part because many disorders of the nervous system result from physiologic rather than structural abnormalities. Dysfunction of the liver or kidneys severe enough to cause symptoms always results in measurable abnormalities of body chemistry, whereas disorders of the nervous system (e.g., migraine) presumably caused by biochemical or physiologic abnormalities frequently are not detectable.

(6) Finally, and most importantly, physiologic changes in the nervous system may so distort peripheral signals or their interpretation that the observer is substantially misled about the nature of the disorder. The higher in the nervous system that the physiologic abnormality is present, the more likely it is that this distortion will occur. This is especially true when the dysfunction exists not in the primary receiving or effector areas of the brain but in the association areas of the cerebral hemisphere, leading to interpretive distortions of perceptions and to changes in mental and cognitive processes. The misleading distortions are more common in those disorders of the CNS we call psychiatric rather than neurologic, but such distortions may exist in both neurologic and psychiatric illness.

Such distortions occur in several forms:

(1) The first are misinterpretations or amplifications of normal bodily sensations. Most normal individuals are subject to frequent, usually brief, foreign sensations that do not portend disease. Examples are twitchings of the eyelid (eyelid myokymia), fasciculations of muscles of the extremity, transient vertigo on changing positions in bed at night, brief ringing in the ears (tinnitus), and a variety of evanescent aches, pains, and paresthesias that come and go with no explanation. Most of us ignore or dismiss these sensations and attend to them only if they become severe, persistent, or disabling. In interpreting these sensations, the brain can err either by amplifying them to the point where the individual is either constantly concerned (hypochondriasis) or by denying them, repressing all evidence of abnormal bodily physiology until it becomes so severe that its associated incapacity becomes crippling.

(2) In "psychophysiologic" illness, brain dysfunction may alter bodily function and produce symptoms that are then reperceived by the brain as abnormalities of the body. An easily understood example is the hyperventilation syndrome: The tense and anxious patient begins to overbreathe, substantially lowering the blood Pco_2. He may be unaware that he is overbreathing, but the ensuing respiratory alkalosis may lead to symptoms of lightheadedness (due to decreased cerebral blood flow engendered by hypocarbia) and paresthesias in the fingers, toes, and around the mouth (engendered by peripheral nerve hyperirritability associated with respiratory alkalosis). Other psychophysiologic abnormalities can lead to other symptoms that, while in themselves a true alteration of the body's physiology, are in fact originally engendered from an ill-functioning brain.

(3) Somatic delusions occur in severe brain abnormalities such as depression, and sometimes early in the development of the dementing illnesses. Patients may complain of pain or dizziness that has no basis in altered peripheral physiology but simply represents a delusional belief about themselves and their bodies. When the symptoms involve afferent systems, these are usually referred to as somatic delusions, and on the efferent side, as conversion reactions. Conversion reactions, sometimes called hysteria, occur in a variety of psychologic illnesses, sometimes representing the lifelong way in which an individual copes with the world, but frequently representing a stress-induced embellishment upon an underlying physical illness. Examples of conversion reactions include blindness, deafness, aphonia, paralysis, and anesthesia.

ANALYSIS OF SYMPTOMS

To deal with the bewildering array of symptoms that can be caused by altered nervous system physiology, physicians must take a systematic approach that has as its purpose the answering of four fundamental questions:

(1) Is a nervous system disorder present? This is essentially a question of physiology that asks if the symptoms of which the patient complains and the signs that the examiner finds are explicable in terms of hypofunction or hyperfunction of the nervous system. If they are, it is likely that the patient is suffering from a disorder of the nervous system. If not, it is likely that the disorder, if the symptoms suggest nervous system disease, is psychological in origin. There is one important caveat: The physician should not place the blame for his own ignorance on the patient. An easy trap for physicians is to make the diagnosis of conversion reaction or psychiatric disease because of their own lack of understanding about altered physiology of the nervous system. One must take great care not to dismiss signs or symptoms simply because they are poorly understood. Equal care must be taken not to overreact to physical symptoms that may prove to be simply a manifestation of psychological stress.

(2) The next question is anatomic. If nervous system disease is present, is it monofocal, multifocal, or diffuse? If monofocal or multifocal, one asks, in succession: Are the lesions peripheral (i.e., at the receptor, muscle effector, synapse, or nerve) or central (i.e., in the spinal cord or brain)? If central, does the disease affect structures above or below the foramen magnum, above or below the tentorium, on the right or the left side? Is the process static, worsening, or improving?

(3) Given the answer or answers to these questions, one can then formulate a pathophysiologic diagnosis

according to whether the evidence suggests a disorder that is genetic, developmental, traumatic, environmental-toxic, infectious, immunologic, degenerative, neoplastic, metabolic, nutritional, physiologic (e.g., epilepsy, migraine), or psychophysiologic (e.g., tension backache, vasodepressor syncope) (Table 2).

(4) Finally, one proceeds to utilize appropriate and specific tests to determine or confirm the exact pathologic cause of the disorder and its etiologic nature. Thus, in evaluation of nervous system disorders, one proceeds from a knowledge of normal physiology and anatomy to pathophysiology to pathology and etiology.

This text attempts to provide the tools to enable the examiner to take the first two of these four steps.

REFERENCES

Barrow, H. S., and Tamblyn, R. M.: Problem-Based Learning. An Approach to Medical Education. Springer Series on Medical Education, Volume 1. New York, Springer Publishing Co., 1980.

Brodal, A.: Neurological Anatomy in Relation to Clinical Medicine. 3rd Ed. New York, Oxford University Press, 1981.

Kandel, E. R., and Schwartz, J. H.: Principles of Neural Science. New York, Elsevier/North-Holland, 1981.

Neurobiologic Essentials

In broad biologic terms the nervous system functions to assure homeostasis. The brainstem controls internal homeostasis by regulating the body's vegetative functions while the forebrain, by generating thought, planning, and motor activities, adjusts the individual to the outer world and to a considerable extent modifies that world to meet the person's inner needs. To accomplish these tasks the human brain and its connections have evolved into an astonishingly complex instrument—many scientists describe it as the most complicated single structure in the universe. Small wonder that efforts to reach a clinical understanding of so complicated an organ system can seem initially intimidating. Fortunately for medical purposes, however, the task becomes easier when one understands some of the principles upon which the nervous system is built and learns to analyze the mechanisms by which disease alters normal physiology and thereby causes symptoms. The purpose of this section is to introduce these principles of pathophysiology.

STRUCTURE OF THE NERVOUS SYSTEM

It is convenient to divide the bewildering number of structures in the central and peripheral nervous system into two functional groups: neural tissues and their supporting structures. *Neural tissues* consist of nerve cell bodies and the processes that connect the neurons to each other, to their receptors, and to their effectors. Neural tissues comprise the executive tissue that performs the unique, message-transmitting functions of the brain and spinal cord. From signals derived from sensory receptors and from the innate knowledge stored in their intracellular genes, nerve cells receive information, code it, transact it through central circuits of varying complexity, and sooner or later incorporate it into an outgoing signal that produces intellectual, motor, or neurosecretory work. Structures supporting the neural tissues include glial cells, myelin sheaths, the blood vessels, and the central meninges and peripheral neural sheaths. These elements variously insulate the nerve cells, nourish them, and maintain their environments within narrow physical and chemical limits. They guarantee the ionic balance of the extracellular fluid, maintain the organ's temperature, remove its waste products, protect it from injury, package it, and deliver to it from the bloodstream the nutrients that the brain requires in large quantity to satisfy its ravenous appetite.

THE NEURON

The term *neuron* includes the entire nerve cell: the nucleus, the perinuclear cytoplasm, known as the *perikaryon*, the dendrites, axons, and their terminal arborizations. The term, *cell body*, refers to the nucleus and perikaryon only. The entire cell, including the terminal arborizations, is enclosed within a phospholipid membrane that separates the cell's intracellular material from the extracellular environment.

The human body contains too many neurons to count accurately—Estimates range from 10 billion to as high as a trillion or more. Within this enormous number, one finds several different anatomic forms and sizes reflecting evolutionary adaptation to specific biologic demands. Despite these gross morphologic dissimilarities, all neurons share certain properties that underlie their principal functions. Once past birth, neuronal cell division does not take place. The perikaryon and the adjacent dendritic cytoplasm contain most of the organelles that manufacture materials that satisfy the nerve cell's intrinsic nutritional requirements (Fig. 1).

As a class, neurons possess a large surface to volume ratio. Indeed, the body of some neurons comprises as little as 1 per cent of the total volume of the cell, with the remainder being occupied by extensive axonal or branching dendritic processes. A common principle in the central nervous system is that, except for small intercellular clefts, the membranes of other cells and their processes tightly abut the entire surface of the nerve cell: Drawings reconstructed from electron micrographs show synaptic boutons and astrocytic processes packed like barnacles all over the surface of the cell body.

The cytoplasm of nerve cells contains a series of structural elements qualitatively similar to those found in other eukaryotic mammalian cells but distributed according to specific need (Fig. 1). Most prominent are clusters of *rough endoplasmic reticulum* (RER) structures whose densely chromophilic cisterns and associated ribosomes give the stained neuron a characteristic floccular appearance, readily observed by light microscopy and termed Nissl substance. *Agranular endoplasmic reticulum* (AER), smooth because of its lack of ribosomes, is grouped most densely about the nucleus, where it also can be detected by light microscopy as the Golgi apparatus. When an axon is injured the chromophilic endoplasmic reticulum disperses, producing a characteristic light microscopic change called chromatolysis.

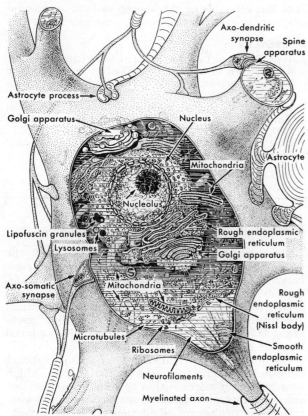

Figure 1. Features of a neuron as seen in electron micrographs. Several dendritic processes are shown with the single myelinated axon appearing at the lower right of the diagram. Astrocytic processes are shown enveloping synapses on the surface of the cell body. Microfilaments and microtubules run down the dendrites and axons. Such subcellular organelles as Nissl bodies (rough endoplasmic reticulum), smooth endoplasmic reticulum, mitochondria, the Golgi apparatus, lysosomes, lipofuscin granules, and ribosomes can be observed. The perforated nature of the nuclear membrane is depicted. (From McGeer, P. L., Eccles, J. C., and McGeer, E. G.: Molecular Biology of the Human Brain. New York, Plenum Press, 1978.)

The endoplasmic reticulum is densest in the perikaryal area from which it extends out into the dendrites for varying distances; the axons contain none. Ribosomes of the RER represent the macromolecular and protein assemblers of the nerve, continuously replenishing cell membranes, and generating the large amounts of transmitter material that stream down the axons to the region of the synapse. Present evidence indicates that the AER participates in the translation of proteins and may be responsible for their further distribution throughout the cell body and the dendrites.

Neurofilaments run throughout the neuron, being most prominent in the perikaryon and the dendrites. These delicate strands are believed to confer structural strength to the cell and may contribute an element of intrinsic mobility to the nerve cell since they contain contractile protein. *Microtubules* are somewhat larger (20 to 40 nM) than neurofilaments. They are distributed in dendrites and, especially, in small-diameter axons. Both microtubules and neurofilaments are believed to contribute to the process of axoplasmic flow.

Neurons also contain *lysosomes,* biologic garbage

disposal units containing specific digestive enzymes. Deficiency of specific lysosomal enzymes occurs in a group of autosomal recessive genetic disorders of children called the *lysosomal storage diseases.* In these conditions the intracytoplasmic accumulation of abnormal amounts of uncatabolized substrates interferes with neuronal action so as to cause symptoms. Nerve cells also contain large numbers of mitochondria, the tiny generators that, by oxidative metabolism, produce stored energy in the form of adenosine triphosphate (ATP). Mitochondria are distributed throughout the neuron but lie especially densely along membrane surfaces and in the synaptic regions, both being areas marked by continuous energy–requiring enzymatic activity.

Axoplasmic Flow

Axoplasmic flow is a bidirectional process by which the neuronal perikaryon sends forth manufactured macromolecules, protein, and mitochondria to supply the far reaches of the cell's dendrites and axons. The peripheral structures, in turn, return metabolic refuse to the central lysosomes and perhaps other messages as well. In both central and peripheral neurons, intracellular material synthesized by the cell body is carried distally, some materials moving at rates as rapid as 400 mm/day, others traveling as slowly as a few millimeters per day. Some neurotransmitters are believed to be shipped in this manner from the perikaryon to the synaptic region, while others are synthesized at the synapse as well. Axonal growth in the developing nervous system as well as the process of sprouting in regenerating axons depends on materials sent distally from the perikaryon by axoplasmic flow. Some macromolecular materials carried to the synapse in this manner may even exert a transsynaptic trophic influence on the next cell. The transport process is energy dependent but not dependent on the particular protein that it carries, since active flow continues at least transiently in the distal segment following section of an axon. As noted earlier, axonal transport is believed to depend in some manner on the activity of microtubules and neurofilaments. Vincristine and some other mitotic inhibitors that disrupt these cytoskeletal structures produce a high incidence of severe and sometimes irreversible peripheral neuropathy. Blockage of axoplasmic flow causes swelling of axons proximal to the site of the block. When pressure on the optic nerve head blocks axoplasmic flow, the resulting swelling (papilledema) can be seen directly with an ophthalmoscope.

The Neural Membrane

An understanding of this remarkable structure illuminates many aspects of neuronal function and disease (Fig. 2). A bimolecular layer of phospholipids makes up the membrane. Its surface is stabilized by structural proteins and studded with a variety of protein *receptors* that respond to specific activating substances. A series of tiny ion-specific channels or pores of varying diameter perforate the membrane and increase or decrease their resistance to the passage of ions under the influence of alterations in adjacent receptor proteins. (The process sometimes is referred to as the receptors opening the gates.) The membrane separates the extracellular fluid, a medium composed of a solution only moderately different from a protein-

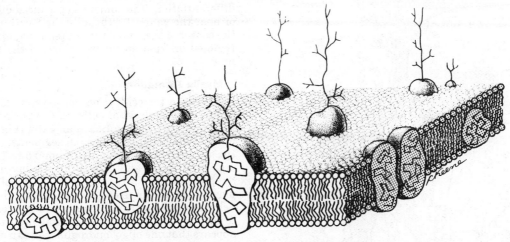

Figure 2. The fluid mosaic model of the plasma membrane, showing polysaccharide chains of glycoproteins protruding into the extracellular space from the surface of the lipid bilayer. (From Fawcett, D. W.: The Cell. 2nd ed. Philadelphia, W. B. Saunders Co., 1981.)

free plasma filtrate, from the intracellular cytoplasm that possesses a very different ionic and protein composition. The transmembrane difference between these two fluids creates an electrical charge of about -70 mV between the inside and the outside of the cell. At rest, the transmembrane potential is maintained by the continuous, energy-requiring pumping of sodium ions outward, coupled with a smaller movement of potassium ions inward, both movements being catalyzed by $Na+$-$K+$–dependent enzyme pumps. A later section will describe the relation among transmembrane voltage, its integration by the cell membrane, and the manner in which such changes control the fundamental firing pattern of the nerve cell.

NEUROGLIAL AND RELATED CELLS

Glial cells include the astroglia, oligodendroglia, and microglia. Microglia probably arise from mesoderm and function mainly as phagocytes. The oligodendroglia form myelin as discussed on the following page.

Astroglia

The astroglia (astrocytes) are numerous, especially in gray matter, where they probably outnumber nerve cells. They possess relatively small bodies but give rise to extensively branching extensions that provide a dense network that fills much of the cortical *neuropil*, that dense background of the gray matter consisting of axons, dendrites, and glial processes in which cell bodies are embedded. Astrocytic processes surround every capillary in the brain, making close contacts with each other and effectively preventing any immediate physical relationship between capillaries and neurons. Their processes also abut extensively on the nerve membrane except in the region of the myelinated

TABLE 5. FUNCTIONS OF THE ASTROCYTES

Guide nerve cell growth during development
Detoxify CO_2, ammonia
Stabilize potassium in extracellular fluid
Maintain water balance in brain
Contribute to metabolic blood-brain barrier
Metabolize neurotransmitters
Repair tissue injury

axon. A number of major functions of the astrocyte are already known, and the future undoubtedly will elucidate many more (Table 5). Thought originally to serve a largely structural function for the brain, astrocytes are now known to make a much more extensive contribution to brain biology. During development they guide the growth of nerve fibers, and later in life they may foster the limited regeneration that occurs following axonal damage in the central nervous system. They provide a crucial role in detoxifying products of brain metabolism, since they contain in exclusive or high concentrations the enzymes glutamine synthetase, carbonic anhydrase, and potassium-dependent ATPase. The result is to assist in maintaining a narrow homeostasis of ammonia, hydrogen ion-CO_2, and potassium in the extracellular fluid of the brain. Furthermore, astrocytes help to buffer the brain against large blood-borne changes in these ions and contribute to the trophic maintenance of the blood-brain barrier (Fig. 3). Astrocytes take up, metabolize, and even may release some neurotransmitters. Moreover, by osmotic pumping they defend the brain's delicate water and osmotic balance. In response to several kinds of injury or metabolic perturbations of the brain, such as hyperammonemia or ischemia, the astrocytes enlarge rapidly and increase their mitochondrial size and number.

Ependyma

Ependymal cells are a specialized form of glia that line the ventricular system of the brain and appear in the center of the spinal cord as isolated "rests." When the embryonic central canal of the spinal cord does not close, a cavitary condition results, known as *hydromyelia*, which is frequently associated with congenital hydrocephalus. Ependymal cells continue to line the hydromyelic structure. Throughout most of the cerebral ventricles, a single layer of cuboidal ependymal cells covers the ventricular surface. The cells are in contact with each other by gap junctions plus occasional desmosomes, forming an architecture that allows full permeability between the ventricular fluid and the extracellular substance of the brain. Thus, cerebrospinal fluid and the brain's extracellular fluid are continuous with each other. Most of the ependymal

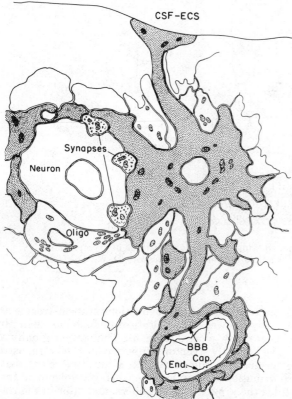

Figure 3. Relationships among the capillary, astrocytes (stippled), neuron, and ventricular ependyma. BBB = blood-brain barrier; Cap. = capillary; CSF = ECS = cerebrospinal fluid–extracellular space; End. = endothelium; Oligo = oligodendroglial cells. (Redrawn from De Robertis, E., and Gerschenfeld, H. M.: Submicroscopic morphology and function of glial cells. Int Rev Neurobiol 3:1–65, 1961.)

cells covering the ventricular surface contain numerous microvilli and cilia. Motility of the cilia is thought to contribute to mixing of the CSF, particularly at the interface between brain and CSF.

In several regions of the nervous system, the structure of the ependymal cells differs from the norm. In the lateral, third, and fourth ventricles, invagination of pial blood vessels into the ventricular system forms the *choroid plexus*, a structure covered by a layer of ependymal cells that do not possess cilia but do possess tight junctions. The tight junctions prevent the free flow of fluid between the blood and ventricular CSF and thereby form the blood-CSF barrier of the plexus. The mechanism prevents the choroidal vessels, which do not have tight junctions, from turning the CSF into a simple ultrafiltrate of plasma.

In the area of the median eminence of the floor of the third ventricle, specialized ependymal cells have lost their cilia but gained a footplate that connects the surface portion of the ependymal cell to choroidal vessels supplying the anterior pituitary glands. These ependymal cells, called tanycytes, take up from the CSF hormones such as thyrotropin releasing hormone and luteinizing hormone releasing factor that have been secreted by the nearby hypothalamus. They then transport them from the ventricles to blood vessels of the pituitary portal circulation whence they reach the anterior portion of the gland itself.

Ependymal cells occasionally undergo neoplastic de-

differentiation. The tumors so produced either arise in or near the ventricles (usually the fourth ventricle), in the center of the spinal cord (often the lumbar or sacral regions) or from ependymal rests in the filum terminale.

Myelin Formation

Myelin in the central nervous system is the product of the oligodendroglial cells; in the peripheral nerves it is produced by the Schwann cells (Fig. 4). Myelin forms coats about the axons in segments, the length of the segment ranging roughly from 0.5 to 1.5 mm. Both oligodendroglial and Schwann cells lay down myelin by progressively wrapping extensions of their cytoplasm around the axon, the single oligodendrocyte or Schwann cell contributing only one segment of myelin to any given axon. In the central nervous system it appears that one oligodendroglial cell can supply single sections of myelin to several different axons. Peripherally, however, each individual myelin segment has its own Schwann cell. Short myelin-free intervals, the nodes of Ranvier, separate the myelin segments in the central and peripheral nervous systems. Myelin, once acquired, is critical to the fiber conduction as is illustrated by the fact that axons lose their capacity to

OLIGODENDROGLIAL CELL

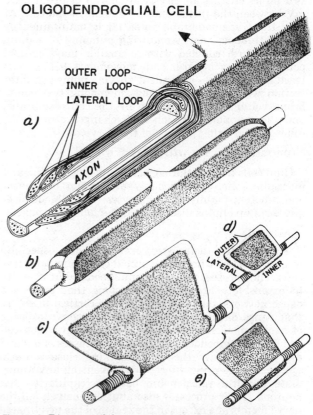

Figure 4. Diagram of the wrapping of myelin around the axon by the oligodendrocyte. In reverse order from *d* to *a* the figure shows the radiation of the inner and outer layers of the sheath as the wrapping is formed. The trapezoid shape of the unrolling sheath prevents the ends of each myelinated segment from thickening as they approach the node of Ranvier. (From Hirano, A., and Dembitzer, H. M.: A structural analysis of the myelin sheath in the central nervous system. Reproduced from *The Journal of Cell Biology*, 1967, Vol. 34, p. 555, by copyright permission of The Rockefeller University Press.)

transmit impulses across demyelinated stretches of three segments or more. This is a critical factor in explaining the dysfunction that occurs in diseases of the central myelin, such as multiple sclerosis, or of the peripheral myelin, such as inflammatory-demyelinative neuropathy, e.g., Guillain-Barre neuropathy.

It is difficult to determine whether myelin contributes anything to nervous system function beyond its influence on nerve conduction and the insulation of one axon from another. There is experimental evidence that demyelinating lesions allow abnormal cross talk (ephaptic transmission) between axons. Some have suggested that certain clinical conditions, such as trigeminal neuralgia and hemifacial spasm, may be a result of such cross talk. In the peripheral nervous system, Schwann cells foster axonal regrowth following axotomy. Centrally, however, oligodendroglial cells appear to perform no similar function. Although central myelin appears capable of regeneration following certain demyelinative processes such as diphtheria, nutritional demyelination, or anoxia, little or no remyelination appears to take place following the inflammatory demyelination of the disease multiple sclerosis. Peripheral Schwann cells, however, generate abundant remyelination following inflammatory-demyelinating disorders of the nerves. Indeed, Schwann cell remyelination sometimes even extends into the central nervous system in cases of severe multiple sclerosis. Little evidence of functional restoration accompanies the latter changes.

NEUROTRANSMISSION

The astonishing quality of the normal mammalian nervous system lies in its capacity to receive, store, process, and transmit an enormous number of independent messages simultaneously without mixing them up. Furthermore, it does all of this rapidly and in a very tiny space. Much of this remarkable accomplishment reflects the evolution of highly efficient and discriminating biologic mechanisms for the several aspects of neurotransmission. These include, among others, (1) a guaranteed unidirectional intracellular and intercellular flow of current, (2) a capacity to vary the conduction speed both within and between cells, (3) a high degree of intercellular membrane insulation preventing false intercellular cross talk, (4) a substantial number of different, yet individually specialized intercellular messengers guaranteeing that only the intended recipients read particular pieces of information, (5) special chemical devices for assuring not only precise and rapid intercellular transmission but an equally rapid decay of the signal, (6) other chemical substances that produce slow-onset, long-lasting changes in postsynaptic reception that modulate the effects of neurotransmitters.

Conduction Within Nerve Cells

In the human nervous system, conduction proceeds electrically within nerve cells and almost entirely chemically between nerve cells or between nerves and their effectors. Normal conduction within the neuron is unidirectional, traveling from dendrite to axon, and has an all-or-none character, i.e., the cell either fires or does not fire. Furthermore, when it fires, the resulting action potential has the same size in all nerves throughout the animal kingdom. Hence the intensity

of neuronal stimulation depends not on the amplitude of its action potential but on the number of potentials traveling down its axon and the frequency at which the cell discharges them.

The nerve action potential consists of the successive depolarization of the nerve membrane triggered initially by the algebraic sum of electrochemical influences acting on its dendrites and cell body. As already noted, an electrical difference separates the inside from the outer surface of the resting neuron. This transmembrane potential, which amounts to approximately −70 mV, the inside of the cell being negative, represents almost the opposite of what one would calculate by simply comparing the ionic composition of the cell's interior with that of the extracellular space. The difference between the passive prediction and the actual potential represents the electrical energy contributed by active metabolic processes within the cell. Normally potassium represents the ion of greatest concentration inside the cell, being about 30 times more concentrated than in the extracellular fluid, while sodium has the greatest concentration in the extracellular fluid, being about 10 times that of the intracellular milieu. The source of the large negative intracellular potential results from the combined effects of constantly greater free diffusion of potassium ions out of the cell than sodium ions in (i.e., a more open potassium channel) and a coupled, energy-requiring $Na+$-$K+$ pump that maintains the biologic concentration of the ions at rest and restores them following their transmembranous movement during the nerve impulse. The importance of this active mechanism can be observed in the promptness by which the extracellular potassium concentration of brain rises in the face of severe anoxia or any other insult that disrupts the nerve cell membrane.

The nerve action potential trips off when, either by neurotransmitter action or some other effect, its membrane permeability to sodium increases, i.e., becomes partially depolarized. Sodium channels open rapidly, and the membrane completely depolarizes and even shifts slightly to the positive side (Fig. 5). The extreme electrical shift progressively slows further sodium movement and creates a strong stimulus for potassium ions to escape the cell. This latter effect, along with membrane pumping, restores the membrane potential and even produces a small overshoot to a more negative (hyperpolarizing) voltage. The process is extraordinarily rapid: The entire depolarizing process generating the nerve impulse requires no more than 1/2000 second. Propagation occurs as the depolarizing current moves into the still unaffected, more distal membrane. A brief postexcitation refractory period prevents the nerve impulse from sending its excitation back into its just depolarized region.

Conduction along nerve fibers depends on the very low resistance afforded by the internal ionic content of the cell together with the high capacitance of the membrane. This same high capacitance also acts to insulate adjacent fibers from each other. In small unmyelinated axons or dendrites the rate of conduction is limited by the diameter of the fiber, providing a relatively inefficient design with which to meet biologic threats that require a prompt reaction in either sensory reception or motor response. The process of myelination, however, greatly accelerates the rate of conduction along axons by providing for the process known

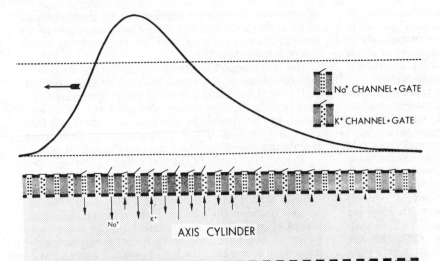

Figure 5. Opening of sodium and potassium gates at an instant during the propagation of a nerve impulse. The *upper part* of the diagram plots the membrane potential along the fiber. In the *lower part,* the opening of the two species of gates is symbolically represented by the angles of the respective gates. The thickness of the membranes on either side is greatly exaggerated with respect to the axis cylinder. (From McGeer, P. L., Eccles, J. C., and McGeer, E. G.: Molecular Neurobiology of the Human Brain. New York, Plenum Press, 1978.)

as saltatory conduction. In saltatory (literally, leaping or dancing) conduction, currents transmitted down the nerve (the action potential) skip that part of the nerve covered with myelin to jump from one node of Ranvier to the next (Fig. 6). The result is that the speed of the action potential becomes equal to the rate at which it transverses the small amounts of axon membrane that lie between the myelin segments; the effective length of the nerve becomes shortened to the sum length of the nerve's individual nodes of Ranvier. The velocity of the action potential can easily be measured in peripheral nerves of man (see p. 1093). A normal conduction velocity of 40 to 60 m/sec may slow to 25 per cent of that value if the nerve partially loses its myelin through disease.

Synapses

Synapses are the discontinuous structures through which nerve cells communicate to each other or to their effector organs. The special case of nerve-muscle synapses is discussed on page 1036.

In the central nervous system, synapses take a variety of forms to adapt to special requirements. Most arise from the processes of terminal axons abutting on either the membranes or spines of the dendrites of adjacent neurons. In addition, one finds axons terminating on perikaryal membranes, coupling in passage with one or more cells while ending on still another.

One even encounters axons that end on the presynaptic structure of another axon. Also, dendrites sometimes contribute presynaptic structures to other dendrites. Finally some axons, such as those arising in the supraoptic nuclei, secrete hormones that directly enter the general circulation to affect distant structures rather than exerting their action immediately on the postsynaptic membrane of another cell.

The direction of the postsynaptic electrical signal that a particular synapse induces on the postsynaptic membrane of the adjacent cell classifies it as excitatory or inhibitory in nature. Excitatory (depolarizing) postsynaptic potentials (EPSPs) increase membrane conductance to sodium while inhibitory (hyperpolarizing) postsynaptic potentials (IPSPs) increase conductance to potassium or chloride. Since thousands of synapses stud the surface of most neurons, the cell membrane is subjected to a constantly changing bombardment. The cell continuously integrates this varying input into the charge on its membrane, thereby at any given instant reaching the decision to fire or not fire to its recipient cells and so on. The end result is human experience composed and translated into behavior.

Neurotransmitters

These are the chemical agents that transmit the signal generated at the terminal axon of one nerve cell to the postsynaptic membrane of its recipient (Table

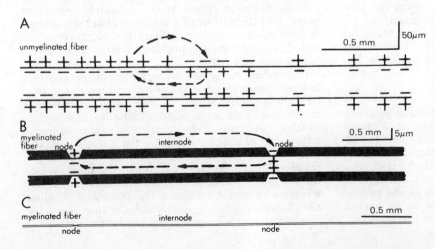

Figure 6. Propagation of impulse along a myelinated fiber with the current flow restricted to the nodes. The dimensions in *B* are transversely exaggerated as shown by the scale, but are correctly shown in *C*. (From McGeer, P. L., Eccles, J. C., and McGeer, E. G.: Molecular Neurobiology of the Human Brain. New York, Plenum Press, 1978.)

TABLE 6. KNOWN AND PUTATIVE NEUROTRANSMITTERS IN MAMMALIAN CNS

NAME	MARKER ENZYME	UPTAKE PROCESS	RECEPTOR TYPES
γ-aminobutyric acid	Glutamate decarboxylase	Yes	$GABA_A$ and $GABA_B$
Glycine	None known	Yes	Strychnine-sensitive
Glutamic acid	None known	Yes	Possibly three
Acetylcholine	Choline acetyl transferase	Yes (for choline)	Muscarinic and nicotinic
Dopamine	Tyrosine hydroxylase	Yes	DA_1 and DA_2
Noradrenaline	Dopamine-β-hydroxylase	Yes	$\alpha_1, \alpha_2, \beta_1,$ and β_2 adrenoceptors
Adrenaline	Phenethanolamine-N-methyl transferase	Yes	As above
5-hydroxytryptamine	Tryptophan hydroxylase	Yes	$5\text{-}HT_1$ and $5\text{-}HT_2$
Histamine	Histidine decarboxylase	No	H_1 and H_2

See also Iverson, L. L.: Neurotransmitter and CNS disease. Lancet 2:914, 1982.

6). Most classic neurotransmitters are synthesized in the perikaryal region of the neuron and sent either in free form or in prepackaged tiny vesicles to the axon's terminal enlargement, called the bouton. There, further vesicular packaging takes place, both of the freshly synthesized material and of transmitter released during previous excitation and reclaimed by the axon. The latter process is known as transmitter reuptake. It is thought that as the depolarization wave of the action potentials spreads to the region of the bouton, it increases the terminal membrane's permeability to calcium, i.e., opens the calcium channel. Calcium ions enter the presynaptic bouton and act on its membrane to stimulate the release of a certain number (quanta) of presynaptic vesicles. These, in turn, act on specialized receptors in the membrane of the receiving neuron to modify its membrane potential.

Chemical neurotransmitters take a number of forms and provide a variety of physiologic functions, many of which are still only partially or incompletely understood despite extensive research effort. Some exert their action with flash-like rapidity, others may modulate subsequent postsynaptic events over periods lasting as long as a minute or more. Most known and putative neurotransmitters are associated with a reuptake process in the parent axon, and all exert their action by coupling to a specific protein receptor on the postsynaptic membrane of the recipient cell. The classic neurotransmitters fall into two general classes, the amino acids and the monoamines.

The known amino acids, namely, gamma-aminobutyric acid (GABA), glycine, and glutamic acid, are believed to serve fast-signaling, point-to-point central nervous system pathways. All three act ionotropically, that is, by affecting specific ion channels in the postsynaptic membrane. GABA inhibits almost all CNS neurons when applied locally, acting to increase the postsynaptic cell membrane's permeability to chloride, thereby hyperpolarizing the membrane. Glycine appears to exert similar functions in the spinal cord. Both L-glutamate and L-aspartate are widely distributed in interneurons of the CNS and have powerful excitant properties mediated by opening sodium channels. Abnormalities of GABA synthesis can lead to epileptic seizures; conversely, some GABA-like substances are effective anticonvulsants.

The monoamines consist of acetylcholine (ACh), the catecholamines, and serotonin. With the exception of the ACh that is synthesized in the craniospinal motoneurons that innervate skeletal muscle, monoami-

nergic neurons in the central nervous system group themselves largely into phylogenetically ancient clumps of cells that lie in the brainstem and basal telencephalic nuclei. From those cell groups they send out projections that are widely distributed, long axoned, and branch extensively along ascending and descending routes to influence the function of multiple specific neuronal structures located at all levels of the nervous system. In the CNS monoaminergic neurons probably provide predominantly a distributed and modulatory influence on biologic functions. Thus these cells create a central autonomic or vegetative nervous system that modifies, but does not primarily initiate, mental activity, emotion, and motor behavior. Partial or extensive degeneration or injury can affect each of the individual monoamine systems, and with some, at least, the resulting neurologic symptoms or disorders can be characteristic, as noted below.

Cholinergic neurons in the CNS, aside from the craniospinal motor neurons, initiate large ascending and descending projections emanating from the brainstem reticular formation, the basal ganglia, and the region of the rostral basal forebrain, including the basal nucleus and adjacent substantia innominata. Muscarinic receptors predominate. Central cholinergic systems play major roles in producing cortical arousal, initiating sleep, controlling the cerebral circulation, and regulating other central autonomic systems. A cholinergic system arising from the basal forebrain plays an important but as yet imprecisely defined role in modulating human memory functions. Alzheimer's disease, the most common form of presenile and senile dementia, for example, is accompanied by a marked reduction in the cholinergic neurons of the basal nucleus of Meynert that project widely to other regions of the cerebral hemispheres.

In the peripheral nervous system, cholinergic neurons innervate all preganglionic fibers of the autonomic system, postganglionic fibers of the parasympathetic system, and a few sympathetic postganglionic fibers. The peripheral cholinergic system illustrates well the difference between nicotinic and muscarinic cholinergic receptor activity. *Nicotinic receptors* are ionotropic and fast acting, responding to stimulation by opening monovalent cation channels in the postsynaptic membrane. *Muscarinic receptors,* on the other hand, exert a slower action, possibly inducing a conformational change in the postsynaptic membrane. This latter alteration, in turn, activates an intracellular second messenger believed to be cAMP for dopamine and cGMP for ACh receptors. A different adenylcyclase-activating receptor responds to norepinephrine. Metabolic activities stimulated by these second messengers induce sustained changes in membrane excitability that modify the cell's response to subsequent stimulation in a relatively prolonged way. In the ACh system the neuromuscular junction and autonomic ganglia have nicotinic receptors and provide fast signaling changes between presynaptic and postsynaptic tissues. Interference of normal ACh transmission across the neuromuscular junction characterizes several diseases of man, including myasthenia gravis, botulism, and the rare myasthenic syndrome that is sometimes associated with systemic cancers. Muscarinic receptors predominate in central cholinergic systems and in postganglionic parasympathetic connections where they regulate the long-action time course of smooth muscle contraction, cardiac rate, and exocrine gland secretion.

The catecholamines in the CNS consist of epinephrine (adrenaline), norepinephrine (noradrenaline), and dopamine. Central epinephrine pathways are limited in number, being found only in small distribution in the pons and medulla where they participate in, among other things, the systems that regulate the blood pressure. Central norepinephrine systems distribute themselves widely throughout both brain and spinal cord, originating largely from small nuclei in the brainstem of which the locus ceruleus is most prominent. The functional effects of these norepinephrine pathways remains largely unelucidated. Physiologic studies suggest that noradrenergic mechanisms play a limited role in regulating vascular resistance in the cerebral circulation. Animal experiments have implicated noradrenergic systems in the physiology of normal reward-seeking behavior. A deficiency in ascending noradrenergic pathways accompanies some forms of genetically determined epilepsy in animals. In man, tricyclic antidepressant agents have the effect of impairing central presynaptic norepinephrine uptake while the antidepressant monoamine oxidase inhibitors slow down norepinephrine synthesis. Norepinephrine excess is thought to participate in the genesis of endogenous and even acquired depressive illnesses while the locus ceruleus degenerates in some cases of senile dementia.

Among the catecholamines, dopamine has received perhaps greatest attention because its known depletion in the striatal-nigral system correlates closely with the development and severity of the human movement disorder called Parkinson's disease. As with other catechol systems, those that project dopamine arise largely in brainstem and basal nuclei, including areas in the ventral tegmentum and substantia nigra from which they send three major projections, the nigrostriatal, mesolimbic, and tuberoinfundibular. Additionally, dopaminergic interneurons appear in a number of other locations, including the olfactory bulb, the retina, the diencephalon, the sympathetic ganglia, and the carotid body.

At the synaptic level, dopamine appears to exert a prolonged modulatory effect influencing the action of other neurotransmitters on the postsynaptic membrane. Functionally, dopamine has several physiologic actions that profoundly but not indispensably influence several biologic activities. The nigrostriatal system

normally acts to facilitate the initiation and balanced control of skeletal muscle movement: Here dopamine deficiency is associated with the known parkinsonism triad of akinesia, rigidity, and alternating tremor. The mesolimbic-mesocortical system is believed to participate in the execution of a number of vegetative-emotional behaviors as well as to influence the general regulation of emotional and thought processes. The clinical effectiveness of several antipsychotic drugs parallels the degree to which they block central dopamine receptors, leading some to speculate that abnormal dopamine metabolism contributes to the symptoms or the course of schizophrenia. In the tuberoinfundibular system, dopamine activity already is known to inhibit prolactin secretion, stimulate growth hormone release, and inhibit ovulation.

Neurons synthesizing serotonin (5-hydroxytryptamine) arise in cell groups within the raphe nuclei of the lower brainstem whence they project to multiple forebrain and diencephalic nuclei, especially in the basal ganglia and hypothalamus. Ascending serotonergic systems have been implicated as contributing to the regulation of sleep-wake cycles, a stable body temperature, and the physiology of aggression. Descending serotonergic pathways modulate pain perception. Lowered serotonin turnover in the forebrain has been an important finding in a number of patients suffering from endogenous depressive illness, but whether the change reflects cause or effect is unknown. Depletion of serotonin from the brainstem is prominent in thiamine deficiency and is believed to contribute to the defects in mental function, pain perception, and other abnormalities that mark the condition.

Neuropeptides

The supraoptic and paraventricular nuclei of the hypothalamus synthesize vasopressin and oxytocin in their cell bodies, package them in macrovesicles, and dispatch the peptide-including vesicle to the posterior pituitary where the hormones are stored for subsequent release into the blood. Neurons widely distributed in the CNS synthesize more than 30 different peptide hormones, and one suspects that many more await future discovery (Table 7). The hypophysiotropic peptides appear to be concerned largely with neural regulation of the pituitary gland. Among the remaining neuropeptides the physiology of even the best understood is only partially discerned presently, and not a clue of explanation exists for the function of many. Certain principles, however, can be established: Many neuropeptides can act as cell-to-cell neurotransmitters, and for several, cell surface–specific protein receptors have been identified on the receptor cell membrane. Also, individual neurons that synthesize one of the classic neurotransmitters also can synthesize and concurrently secrete a neuropeptide. Thus far the local application of neuropeptides on neurons has induced slowly beginning and long-lasting changes in neuroexcitability. The effects of such changes are more consistent with a modulating effect on neurotransmission than a direct cell-cell excitation.

Among the neuropeptides listed in Table 7, the enkephalins and substance P have perhaps the most immediate interest for clinical neurology. Met- and leu-enkephalins bind to endogenous opiate receptors, leading one to speculate that they may modulate the

TABLE 7. PEPTIDES IDENTIFIED IN NEURONS AND NERVE TERMINALS IN MAMMALIAN CNS EXCLUSIVE OF THOSE RELATED DIRECTLY TO ENDOCRINE FUNCTIONS

Pituitary peptides
  Corticotropin (ACTH)
  Growth hormone (GH)
  Lipotropin
  α-melanocyte stimulating
    hormone (α-MSH)
  Oxytocin
  Vasopressin

Circulating hormone
  Angiotensin
  Calcitonin
  Glucagon
  Insulin

Gut hormones
  Avian pancreatic polypeptide
  Cholecystokinin (CCK)
  Gastrin
  Motilin
  Pancreatic polypeptide (PP)
  Secretin
  Substance P
  Vasoactive intestinal
    polypeptide (VIP)

Opioid peptides
  Dynorphin
  β-endorphin
  Met-enkephalin
  Leu-enkephalin
  Kyotorphin

Hypothalamic releasing
    hormones
  Luteinizing hormone
    releasing hormone
    (LHRH)
  Somatostatin
  Thyrotropin releasing
    hormone (TRH)
Miscellaneous peptides
  Bombesin
  Bradykinin
  Carnosine
  Neuropeptide Y
  Neurotensin
  Proctolin

See also Iverson, L. L.: Neurotransmitter and CNS disease. Lancet 2:914, 1982.

activity of multiple points of the pain relay pathway. In addition, they influence breathing functions, modify motor functions through receptor sites in the basal ganglia, and even, in some as yet unexplained manner, influence vision via receptors found in retinal amacrine cells. Their source of synthesis presently is uncertain. *Substance P*, originally identified as a gut hormone, apparently functions as a specific neurotransmitter in certain pathways carrying slow pain sense. Substance P has been identified in cells projecting efferently from the brainstem to the spinal cord, as well as in sensory layers of the spinal dorsal horns of that structure.

The large number of neuropeptides and the many for which cell surface receptors already have been described suggest hitherto unanticipated capacities for nerve cells to vary their chemical transmission to different sets of neurons, thereby establishing continuously changeable central templates of nervous activity, including behavior.

Receptors and Drug Action. As best can be determined, all neurotransmitters and active neuropeptides produce their biologic effects by binding to specific receptors on the membrane of their target cells. Furthermore, most neuroactive drugs appear to exert their effect by acting on specific receptors. These principles have led to much of modern understanding of the pharmacology of neurotransmitters as well as to the discovery of the existence, distribution, and possible functions of the neuropeptide hormones. Studies of receptors also have enhanced the understanding and capacity to synthesize specific neuroactive drugs. In one instance the discovery of a receptor in the brain for the benzodiazepine group of drugs has led to fruitful and testable new theories on the biologic bases of such diverse functions as anxiety, appetite control, and even

the mechanisms whereby receptor-receptor interaction can alter neurotransmission at central synapses.

Ligands. Substances produced by the body that interact with specific membrane receptors are known as ligands. The initial discovery and mapping of the opiate receptors thus led directly to the discoveries of the endogenous endorphins, i.e., their ligands, and established a new era in neuropharmacology. Whether or not discovery of the benzodiazepine receptor will lead to the uncovering of the brain's valium, only time will tell; thus far, at least we have a receptor in search of a ligand.

Denervation Hypersensitivity

Denervation hypersensitivity is a condition in which loss of presynaptic neurotransmitter release induces an increase in receptors for that transmitter either at the specialized postsynaptic membrane site or diffusely along the membrane of the denervated cell. As a result the denervated cell will fire, perhaps excessively, without specific presynaptic stimulation because of small amounts of transmitter that diffuse from nearby sources, from abnormal reinnervation by other axons, or from transmitter-like drugs that diffuse from the bloodstream. The phenomenon appears in several clinical conditions, one example of which is the spontaneous fibrillation that affects denervated skeletal muscle fibers.

FLUID AND ARCHITECTURAL COMPARTMENTS OF THE CENTRAL NERVOUS SYSTEM

Three distinct fluid or semifluid compartments make up the craniospinal central nervous system: The intravascular compartment (blood vessels and blood volume), the extracellular space, and the intracellular space. Dysfunction or damage to any of these can lead to either focal or generalized neurologic dysfunction, depending on the anatomic distribution of the abnormality.

THE CEREBRAL VASCULATURE

Anatomy

Blood vessels and their contents comprise about 10 per cent of the cranial contents. Diseases of the cerebral blood vessels lead to stroke, the most common neurologic disorder of adults and a major cause of death and severe disability in the United States population. Four major extracranial arteries (Fig. 7), namely the paired internal carotids and vertebrals, enter the skull to supply the brain. The internal carotid arteries are particularly susceptible to arteriosclerotic disease at the point where they bifurcate from the common carotid artery in the neck. Occlusion or plaque formation at this point is common and frequently leads to symptoms of stroke in the cerebral hemispheres. The two vertebral arteries are normally somewhat asymmetric, sometimes differing so much in diameter from one another that occlusion of the major side can lead to hindbrain infarction even in childhood. The extracranial arteries are similar in structure to other medium-sized arteries of the body and suffer from similar diseases, i.e., atherosclerosis, fibromuscular dysplasia, and the like.

After the major extracranial arteries enter the skull

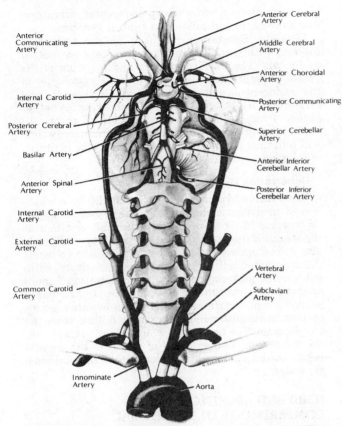

Anterior Cerebral Artery

Middle Cerebral Artery

Anterior Choroidal Artery

Posterior Communicating Artery

Superior Cerebellar Artery

Anterior Inferior Cerebellar Artery

Posterior Inferior Cerebellar Artery

Vertebral Artery

Subclavian Artery

Aorta

Anterior Communicating Artery

Internal Carotid Artery

Posterior Cerebral Artery

Basilar Artery

Anterior Spinal Artery

Internal Carotid Artery

External Carotid Artery

Common Carotid Artery

Innominate Artery

Figure 7. The main arterial supply to the brain, including the major arteries at the base of the brain. The light bands around certain arteries indicate the major areas of susceptibility to atherosclerotic narrowing. (From Barnett, H. J. M.: Cerebrovascular diseases. In Wyngaarden, J. B., and Smith, L. H., Jr. (eds.): Cecil Textbook of Medicine. 17th ed. Philadelphia, W. B. Saunders Co., 1985.)

they interconnect at the base of the brain by communicating arteries that form the circle of Willis. When the circle of Willis is complete, occlusion of one (or sometimes more than one) extracranial artery can be compensated for by increased flow from the other vessels through the circle. When, because of inherent variability or disease, the circle is incomplete (as it is in about 50 per cent of patients), occlusion of a major artery is more likely to cause brain damage. Even then, however, other anastomotic channels from the extracranial arteries can sometimes prevent brain infarction. These include tributaries from the external carotid artery through facial arteries to the ophthalmic artery and thence to the middle cerebral artery, a branch from the anterior spinal artery to the vertebral artery, and a number of usually unimportant dural meningeal arteries. Other factors also play a role in whether or not ischemic necrosis develops in the brain after occlusion of a major extracranial or intracranial artery. These include the level of the systemic blood pressure (when a carotid artery is tied off during the course of head and neck surgery, the likelihood of ischemic infarction of the brain is directly related to the degree of coexistent systemic hypotension), the speed of occlusion (rapid occlusion of extracranial-intracranial arteries is more likely to cause infarction than slow occlusion), and the degree of arteriosclerosis impeding flow in other vessels.

Once beyond the anatomic ring of the circle of Willis, the intracranial arterial bed branches into more or less terminal arteries, i.e., vessels that connect with one another via only delicate and functionally inefficient anastomotic channels. As a result, more than momentary occlusion of the parent trunk or major branches of the anterior, middle, or posterior cerebral arteries or of the major branches of the vertebral or basilar arteries usually leads to ischemic necrosis in at least part of the particular vascular territory. Although a delicate collateral circulation joins the major arterial zones via a diffuse pial arteriolar network, these connections rarely are sufficient to prevent brain damage when a major trunk artery becomes occluded.

Compared to systemic arteries, the intracranial vessels possess thinner walls, have a less well developed muscular coat, and lack elastic tissue. Within the skull the arterial muscularis thins out further at branching points of the major arteries along the base of the brain to create weak points where intracranial aneurysms characteristically develop. Although in such cases the defect in the arterial wall is probably congenital, aneurysms rarely develop in individuals below 10 years of age and characteristically do not rupture until they reach the age of 40 to 60. Also, the presence of hypertension accelerates their formation and rupture. Rupture of a congenital aneurysm is the most common cause of nontraumatic cerebral hemorrhage. The annual incidence of subarachnoid hemorrhage from ruptured aneurysm is about 12 per 100,000 people in the United States.

The small arteries and arterioles of the brain (resistance vessels) are responsible for autoregulation of blood flow (p. 1019). The capillaries of the brain also differ from capillaries elsewhere in the body (except the testis) in that, microscopically, the endothelium lining the intracranial vessels forms a continuous, tightly joined cell-to-cell membrane that extends throughout the brain. This anatomic blood-brain barrier (p. 1020) spares only three small areas: the capillaries of the choroid plexus whose epithelial covering is tightly joined, the infundibular region of the hypothalamus through which hypophysiotropic peptides diffuse, and the area postrema at the caudal end of the fourth ventricle, which is believed to serve as a chemoreceptor zone of the brain to substances diffusing from blood. Prolonged hypertension leads to permanent changes in the arterioles of the brain with areas of medial necrosis, endothelial proliferation, and microaneurysm formation. Proliferative changes may eventually occlude the blood vessel, leading to small areas of infarction, called *lacunes,* that characteristically occur in deep structures of the cerebral hemisphere or the brainstem. The tiny aneurysms, called Charcot-Bouchard aneurysms, may rupture, leading to cerebral hemorrhage.

The venous blood from the brain drains through superficial and deep cerebral and cerebellar veins primarily into an intracranial venous sinus system that is composed of large channels semirigidly encased within the peripheral dural meninges (Fig. 8). Considerable anastomoses interconnect the venous sinuses that lie over the brain's convexity, and form a basal sinus system that extends from the cavernous sinus anteriorly through the peripituitary, sphenopalatine, and superior and inferior petrosal sinuses to the transverse sinuses posteriorly. Additional venous anasto-

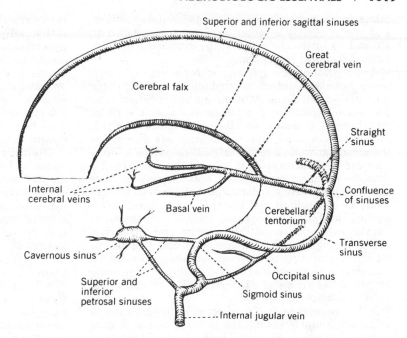

Figure 8. Major cerebral sinuses receiving the cerebral veins. (From Patton, H. D., Sundsten, J. W., Crill W. E., and Swanson P. D.: Introduction to Basic Neurology. Philadelphia, W. B. Saunders Co., 1976.)

moses draining the base of the brain connect with the vertebral venous anastomotic plexus of Batson. Because the system is valveless, this route allows direct communication between the venous system of the brain and that of the thoracic, abdominal, and pelvic organs. The anatomy provides a potential source of metastatic spread of tumor and infection to the nervous system. Smaller, less efficient venous tributaries emerge from the skull via diploic channels to enter the extracranial circulation.

The intracranial dural sinus system also connects directly and without intervening valves via the internal jugular veins to the right side of the heart. The arrangement means that the general intracranial pressure normally responds quickly to changes in the gravitational relationship of the head to the heart as well as to alterations in the level of the systemic venous pressure. Thus, illnesses that increase systemic venous pressure, such as congestive heart failure or, more locally, superior vena caval obstruction, increase the intracranial pressure. The effect can be demonstrated clinically by compressing a jugular vein while performing lumbar puncture and observing the rise that occurs in CSF pressure. This procedure, called the Queckenstedt maneuver, was once used in clinical practice as an aid to diagnosis in spinal tumors. It is potentially dangerous, however, in the presence of either cranial or spinal mass lesions and has been largely abandoned for that reason. Conversely to the above, systemic illnesses, such as dehydration, that reduce systemic venous pressure also reduce intracranial pressure. The superficial cerebral veins possess small constrictions at the point where they enter the venous sinuses, an arrangement that acts to impede flow and prevents the veins from collapsing when we sit or stand.

The intracranial veins are susceptible to several pathologic processes. Normally, anastomotic venous channels are much richer than arterial channels so that occlusion of the venous system less often results in brain infarction than does arterial occlusion. Nevertheless, strategically located obstructions still create a serious risk: Hemorrhagic infarcts can be produced by thrombosis of individual cerebral veins or by sudden occlusion of the posterior portion of the superior sagittal sinus or the dominant lateral sinus. Cavernous sinus occlusion may be asymptomatic or can lead to proptosis of the ipsilateral eye and ocular nerve palsies. Slower occlusion of intracranial sinuses often does not produce infarction but can chronically elevate the intracranial pressure, producing the syndrome of pseudotumor cerebri (p. 1025).

Physiologic Demands

The brain stores no oxygen and virtually no carbohydrate, yet the organ consumes the astonishingly large amount of 156 μ mole of oxygen/100 g/min to manufacture ATP from glucose. Normally this demand is met by a mean organ blood flow of about 50 ml/100 g/min, equaling approximately one-fifth of the total resting cardiac output. Blood flow and tissue metabolism are closely coupled in the nervous system so that regional changes in brain function during activity produce relatively wide and rapid adjustments of local blood flow above and below this mean value. The average blood flow to the metabolically more active gray matter, for example, generally is about 50 per cent above that of the mean for white matter. Furthermore the flow and oxygen consumption of gray matter can double during normal functional activity and even triple or quintuple in zones of epileptic discharge. Conversely if flow slows for any reason, so long as the contents of oxygen and glucose in the blood remain near normal, the tissue can extract more substrate in order to compensate. As a result, little impairment of brain function takes place until local tissue blood flow falls below about 18 ml/dl/min. When flow falls below 15 ml/dl/min, energy failure begins, and, soon afterward, nerve cells begin to die.

Regulation of Blood Flow in the Central Nervous System

The CNS has the capacity to regulate its own blood flow by two important mechanisms. The first is an intrinsic property of arteries termed autoregulation, and the second is a response of the arterial bed to alterations in the chemistry of the extracellular space termed chemical regulation.

Autoregulation is a response wherein arterial resistance vessels maintain a constant rate of capillary pressure-flow in tissue metabolizing at a constant rate. The vessels constrict in response to a rise in arterial intraluminal pressure and dilate in response to a fall. Most of the response appears to originate directly in the muscular wall since the arterial responses to pressure can be demonstrated in vitro in the presence of a constant chemical environment. Some drugs (e.g., halogenated anesthetics, indomethacin) as well as several kinds of generalized and regional brain injuries, including traumatic concussion, seizures, or transient anoxia, can either reset the pressure and blood flow limits through which autoregulation operates or can transiently abolish the mechanism altogether. These considerations imply that neural modulation or some as yet unknown metabolic factors also influence the state of autoregulation.

In the normal brain the effect of autoregulation is to assure a stable circulation to brain tissue despite changes in mean systemic blood pressure that may extend from a low of approximately 60 to 80 torr to a high of approximately 160 to 180 torr (Fig. 9). As one approaches the lower level of the autoregulation range, e.g., a blood pressure of 100/60 torr, mean 80 torr, down to a mean of about 60 torr, CBF begins to decline, at least initially to a somewhat lesser degree than the fall in pressure. Brain homeostasis usually is preserved by an increased extraction of substrate by the capillaries so that no clinical symptoms arise. Below systemic blood pressures of about 60 torr, however, cerebral blood flow falls abruptly. The resulting reduction in capillary perfusion, if abrupt and severe, leads to syncope or, if gradual and less intense, may produce symptoms of generalized cerebral anoxia, including confusion, giddiness, and apprehension. At high systemic mean pressures above about 160 to 180 torr, the

cerebral intravascular pressure tends to "break out" of its normally regulated level and begins to rise. Chronic hypertension or the use of certain drugs can shift the position of the autoregulation curve, as illustrated in Figure 9. Otherwise the resulting high intravascular pressure stimulates pathologic degrees of arterial constriction, or dilatation that can directly damage the arterial vascular wall. Either or both effects can produce focal areas of tissue ischemia and small hemorrhages in the brain.

Clinically, acute damage to autoregulatory mechanisms by hypertension characteristically induces generalized headache. If the process becomes severe the associated multifocal perivascular injury can produce the syndrome of *hypertensive encephalopathy* with clouded consciousness, seizures, or multifocal neurologic changes. Chronic hypertensive disease produces progressive arterial thickening with arteriolar occlusions, resulting in small infarcts scattered through the brain. Chronic hypertension also alters the set point of autoregulation so that any sudden decrease in the blood to a normal level may cause brain ischemia. A more direct and long-lasting impairment of intrinsic autoregulation can accompany major brain damage caused by infarcts, tumors, hemorrhages, or trauma, and results in a pressure-passive vascular system with general vasodilatation, hyperemia, and increased intracranial pressure. As described below, such effects enhance the tendency for pathologic decompensation in brain injury.

Chemical regulation of the cerebral circulation describes the process whereby the CNS resistance arteries locally dilate or constrict in response to areas of regionally increased or decreased metabolism. The result is that with systemic blood pressure within the normal autoregulatory range the rate of local cerebral blood flow is governed largely by the rate of local metabolism. The precise stimuli for normal chemical regulation are unknown. The most powerful known stimulus to cerebral vasodilatation is carbon dioxide, followed in intensity by hypoxemia. Other stimuli also must operate, since blood flow often rises in areas of increased cerebral functional activity without any measurable preceding increase in tissue CO_2 tension or fall in O_2. Probably several metabolic messengers exist, including potassium and adenosine.

Autoregulation to pressure can be temporarily impaired or suspended by intracranial abnormalities and then later return. Abnormal chemical regulation is a more dangerous development that probably occurs only in devitalized nervous tissue.

The Blood-Brain Barrier

The blood-brain barrier (BBB) stands between the intravascular and the extracellular space. It consists of an aggregate of anatomic, physical-chemical, and chemical mechanisms that together maintain the internal milieu of the brain at a different and more stable chemical composition than the blood plasma that constantly circulates through it (Table 8). (Interestingly, peripheral nerve and autonomic ganglia do not possess such a barrier, perhaps making them more susceptible to certain toxins.) The anatomic portion of the BBB consists of the capillary endothelium and the astrocytes. The capillaries of the brain and the nerves have a unique anatomic structure. In contrast to cap-

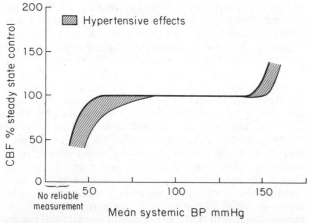

Figure 9. The autoregulatory curve of the cerebral vasculature showing that as long as metabolic demand remains unchanged, cerebral blood flow is normally *(heavy line)* maintained at a constant level in the face of a wide range of systemic blood pressure. With prolonged hypertension the curve shifts to the right *(finer line)*, increasing susceptibility to ischemic symptoms if severe hypertension is too abruptly brought to normal levels.

TABLE 8. CONCENTRATIONS OF MAJOR SOLUTES IN NORMAL PLASMA AND LUMBAR CSF IN HUMANS

	Plasma		CSF
Osmols	295		295
Sodium	140	mEq/l	138
Potassium	4.5	mEq/l	2.8
Chloride	102	mEq/l	119
Bicarbonate	24	mEq/l	22 arterial
pH	7.33		7.41 arterial
Glucose	5	mmol/l	3.5 mmol/l
Lactate	1.0	mEq/l	1.6 mEq/l
Total protein	7.0	g/dl	<50 mg/dl
Leukocytes			1–2 lymphs

Data from Davson, 1967, Fishman, 1980

illary beds elsewhere in the body, except the testis, tight junctions weld the endothelial cells of the brain and spinal cord together in a continuous sheet (Fig. 10). The arrangement provides an equivalent of a double cell membrane (the inner and outer capillary membranes) separating the nervous system's extracellular fluid from the plasma. Surrounding the capillaries on their abluminal side lies the closely spaced layer of metabolically active astrocytic processes.

Penetration of substances across the BBB occurs either by diffusion or active transport. Lipid-soluble substances diffuse across capillary endothelium to a degree proportional to their partition coefficient between oil and water. This principle explains the ready penetration in and out of the brain of carbon dioxide and of anesthetic substances as well as certain drugs. Nonlipid, nonionized substances of small molecular weight (m.w.) (i.e., less than about 20 m.w.) diffuse readily across the membrane, but the diffusion rate falls off rapidly as the molecular weight rises. Urea, for example, with a m.w. about 60, requires approximately four hours to equilibrate between blood and brain. Polarized compounds of all sizes diffuse poorly across the endothelium so that partially ionized substances such as ammonia-ammonium (NH^3–NH^{4+}) diffuse in either direction at a rate proportional to their pK and their partition coefficient as well as the molecular size of the nonionized portion.

Most substrates required for neural metabolism are polarized and are strongly impeded from entering the

brain by simple diffusion. Non-energy-dependent, bidirectional, and stereospecific carrier mechanisms, which behave in a manner somewhat akin to the way that hemoglobin carries oxygen, have evolved to guarantee the selective entry of these substances into the brain by a process called carrier-mediated transport. Independent carrier systems have been identified, for example, for glucose, short-chain monocarboxylic acids, certain neutral amino acids, basic amino acids, certain purines, and certain nucleosides. The cerebral capillaries are rich in mitochondria, and energy-dependent active transport across the capillary endothelium must exist to explain the gradient that separates the lower potassium concentration in brain extracellular fluid from that of plasma. CSF potassium fluctuates little or not at all with changes in serum potassium. Similarly, certain agents known to block organic ion transport systems in the kidney result in an elevation of monoamine metabolites in the CSF, implying that the antimetabolite has closed the normal exit channel for these substances. Astrocytes contribute to the metabolic barrier both by transferring nutrients from blood to the neuron and by limiting the entry of hydrogen ion, ammonia, and potassium to the extracellular fluid. The astrocytes also may contribute a tropic effect on the endothelium, influencing the direction of transport of amino acids across the BBB.

Alterations in the permeability of the BBB can occur with several diseases, and sometimes actually are induced in attempts at therapy. The barrier that normally exists against high molecular weight peptides or proteins can be transiently breached by intense hypertension, either alone or in association with seizures, as well as by producing abrupt plasma hyperosmolarity in the arterial blood going to the brain. Neither effect apparently harms the brain, and the hyperosmotic opening of the barrier has sometimes been exploited to pass otherwise impermeable drugs into the tissue. Increased barrier permeability accompanied by astrocytic swelling (cerebral edema) surrounds many intracranial space-occupying lesions such as tumors, abscesses, and hematomas. When neurologic disability results from brain edema, it appears *not* to be caused by the biochemical alteration of brain extracellular space but because the edema can enhance

Figure 10. Comparison of the ultrastructural features of general (systemic) capillaries and the capillary endothelial cells of the brain. Note the relative absence of pinocytotic vesicles, the greatly increased number of mitochondria, and the presence of tight junctions in brain capillaries, unlike general capillaries, which have clefts, fenestrae, and prominent pinocytotic vesicles. (From Oldendorf, W. H.: The blood brain barrier. In Bito L. Z., Davson, H., and Fenstermacher, J. D. (eds.): The Ocular and Cerebrospinal Fluids. New York, Academic Press, 1977.)

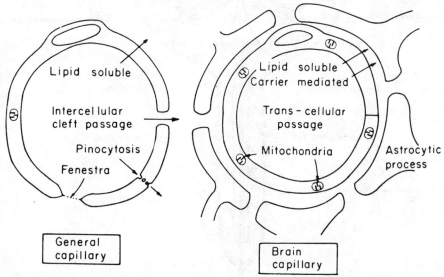

dangerously the initial tissue swelling and the resulting mass effect in the brain (p. 1025). Cerebral infarcts, for example, destroy all tissue in an area of the brain including glial cells and, with time, the capillaries as well. As a result, abnormal BBB permeability progressively increases for a few days after a stroke, accompanied by local failure of the tissue's normal mechanisms for maintaining water balance and, potentially, fatal brain swelling. Clinically, changes in the permeability of the BBB are exploited in radiographic diagnosis. The basis of the approach is that certain radioisotopically labeled or radiopaque molecules to which the barrier normally is impermeable will pass through areas of functional damage so as to outline a radiopaque image of a brain lesion. Glucocorticoid hormones have a salutary effect on edema surrounding brain lesions, such as tumors and abscesses, because they stabilize the injured BBB. This effect is widely used clinically to treat certain types of brain edema.

THE EXTRACELLULAR SPACE

The brain and spinal cord contain two extracellular fluid spaces, one that lies between the cells, termed the extracellular fluid (ECF), and the other consisting of the CSF. The two fluids normally interconnect through the ependymal lining of the ventricular walls as well as through the pial membrane that covers the outer surface of the brain.

The parenchymal ECF normally has a volume of about 200 ml, which is equal to about 15 per cent of the brain and spinal cord. The CSF volume equals another 130 to 150 ml. The cellular, macromolecular, and electrolyte contents of the two fluids differ substantially from that of the blood plasma. Small differences in content also mark different regions of the ECF-CSF. For example, newly formed CSF in the cerebral ventricles has a lower protein (<10 mg/dl) and slightly higher glucose content than does CSF in the cisterna magna (protein 10 to 20 mg/dl) or the lumbar sac (protein 20 to 40 mg/dl). Also, hypophysiotropic peptides can be found in greater concentration in the fluids of the tuberal region of the hypothalamus than elsewhere, while choroid plexus secretions contain slightly higher potassium concentrations than does bulk CSF. Despite these minor changes, however, net concentrations of solute in the ECF of the CNS are maintained within extremely narrow limits even when their counterparts in the blood plasma fluctuate widely (Table 8). Both local and systemic physiologic mechanisms regulate this constancy of cerebral ECF, which is particularly narrowly maintained for hydrogen and potassium ion concentrations. Equal osmolality between plasma and the ECF-CSF normally is achieved by a Donnan equilibrium expressed by a lower protein, a higher chloride, and a slightly higher sodium content in the brain fluids than in the blood.

Formation and Absorption of Cerebrospinal Fluids

About 60 per cent of CSF is formed by the choroid plexus located mainly in the lateral and to a lesser

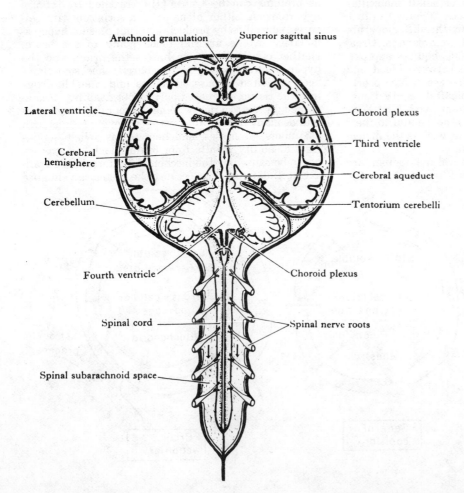

Figure 11. The subarachnoid spaces and circulation of the cerebrospinal fluid. (From Millen, J. W., and Woollam, D. H. M.: The Anatomy of the Cerebrospinal Fluid. London, Oxford University Press, 1962.)

Arachnoid granulation — Superior sagittal sinus
Lateral ventricle — Choroid plexus
Cerebral hemisphere — Third ventricle
— Cerebral aqueduct
Cerebellum — Tentorium cerebelli
Fourth ventricle — Choroid plexus
Spinal cord — Spinal nerve roots
Spinal subarachnoid space

extent in the third and fourth ventricles. Most of the remainder seeps transependymally from the ECF into the ventricular cavities. The combined sources produce approximately 0.3 to 0.4 ml of CSF per minute, a rate that replenishes the bulk of the fluid roughly four times daily (Fig. 11).

CSF production remains constant in the face of wide extremes of intracranial pressures ranging from a low near zero to a high of well over 180 mm of water. Above this upper level, production tends to decline, but not necessarily proportionally. The rate of CSF absorption, however, fluctuates considerably and directly with the height of the intracranial pressure, being less than the formation rate at low pressures and more than formation at abnormally elevated pressures. CSF production in the choroid plexus depends upon several active processes, including chloride transport mediated by the enzyme carbonic anhydrase and potassium transport presumably mediated by a potassium-dependent ATPase. Both the carbonic anhydrase inhibitor acetazolamide and, to a lesser extent, the cardiac glycosides can inhibit CSF secretion, although neither is effective clinically in this capacity.

The CSF normally circulates slowly, trickling downward from the lateral and third ventricles through the aqueduct to exit into the subarachnoid space via foramina located on the roof of the fourth ventricle. The fluid then diffuses rostrally over the surface of the brain, ascending along the basal cisterns to the supratentorial compartment. Most CSF passes over the lateral surfaces of the hemispheres to enter the blood via arachnoid granulations located largely along the longitudinal sinus. Some CSF also appears to be absorbed in the meningeal sheaths covering the spinal dorsal roots. Along its intracranial passage, freshly formed CSF emerging from the ventricles also exchanges, at a slow rate, with the contents of the spinal subarachnoid space. Normally the flow and mixing of CSF are abetted considerably by the vigorous systolic pulsations of the brain. One can observe these pulsations vividly during the radiographic procedure of contrast myelography, in which dye placed at the foramen magnum pulses rhythmically back and forth through the craniospinal junction as the brain expands and contracts with each heart beat. The observation illustrates the shock-absorbing qualities of the spinal canal where, in contrast to the intracranial contents, a relatively large extradural space confers some elasticity to the subarachnoid contents. The CSF can be examined in man by inserting a small needle in the lumbar subarachnoid space (below the level of the first lumbar vertebral body where the spinal cord normally ends) or more rarely into the cisterna magna. Measurement of the fluid's color, red and white blood cells, protein and glucose, and other substances often give clues to nervous system disease.

THE INTRACELLULAR SPACE

The intracellular space makes up the remaining 75 per cent of the normal intracranial contents and is composed mainly of neurons, glial cells, and myelin. (The volume of connective tissue septa and phagocytes in the brain is negligible.) Compared to most other tissues, the brain and spinal cord have a relatively low solute content: Water makes up approximately 79 per cent of the brain's weight, gray matter containing approximately 82 per cent and white matter approximately 70 per cent.

Subsequent sections of this chapter discuss the pathophysiology of how diseases affect the several compartments of the brain and the symptoms that

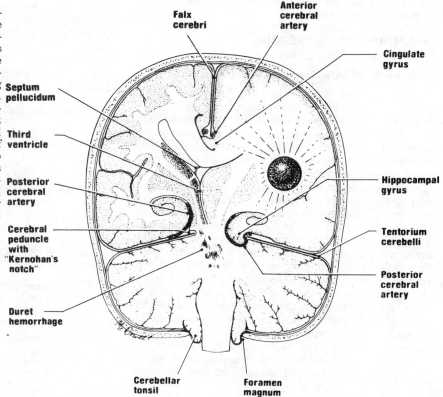

Figure 12. Cerebral herniation patterns evoked by brain metastases. The brain is shown in coronal section, encased in the skull. A brain metastasis and its surrounding edema have caused herniation of the cingulate gyrus under the falx cerebri, compressing the ipsilateral anterior cerebral artery. There is also herniation of the diencephalon across the midline from right to left, compressing the right lateral ventricle and producing obstruction of the left lateral ventricle, leading to hydrocephalus. The third ventricle is likewise compressed. There is herniation of the hippocampal gyrus through the tentorium cerebelli, compressing the posterior cerebral artery and pushing the brainstem from right to left, causing hemorrhage within the brainstem. There is herniation of the cerebellar tonsils through the foramen magnum, and the entire diencephalon and brainstem are shifted downward as a result of the supratentorial mass. (Reproduced by permission from Cairncross, J. G., and Posner, J. B.: Neurological Complications of Systemic Cancer. In Yarbro, J., and Bornstein, R. (eds.): Oncologic Emergencies. New York, Grune and Stratton, 1981.)

result. First, however, it is useful to consider the reactions that disease can induce in these compartments and how some of these reactions potentially threaten the brain even more than the initial disease itself.

GROSS ANATOMIC INTRACRANIAL AND INTRASPINAL COMPARTMENTS

The skull and meninges divide the intracranial contents into the larger supratentorial and smaller subtentorial compartments. The two spaces are separated by the tent-shaped tentorium cerebelli and interconnected through the open incisura of that structure (Fig. 12). The midline falx cerebri further divides the supratentorial cavity into right and left sides, separating and restraining the two hemispheres almost completely above the corpus callosum. These architectural features guarantee to the brain considerable stability within the skull and protect it against the inclemencies of everyday movement and even quite vigorous trauma (e.g., the "sport" of boxing). Conversely, the unyielding nature of the intracranial septa also can contribute importantly to the pathogenesis of the neurologic abnormalities if they resist the brain's effort to adapt to intracranial shifts produced by space-occupying lesions or hydrocephalus. Within the skull, the dura mater, the outer meningeal layer, is plastered tightly against the inner table of the bone except where the dura divides to form the intracranial venous sinuses or extends inward to create the falx and tentorium.

The intracranial contents connect to intraspinal structures through the foramen magnum. Caudal to this point the extradural space contains fat and blood vessels that somewhat separate the spinal meninges from the surrounding bony structures of the spinal column. As noted, the space provides some buffering against the intraspinal arterial pulsations, but also provides a potential reservoir into which infections or metastases may spread.

THE INTRACRANIAL PRESSURE AND ITS ABNORMALITIES

REGULATION OF INTRACRANIAL PRESSURE

The skull and spine enclose the brain and spinal cord in a tightly closed compartment partially vented to ambient conditions by means of direct connections between the dural sinuses and the right side of the heart. At any given moment the intracranial-intraspinal pressure (conveniently expressed as CSF pressure) reflects the dynamically varying algebraic sum of the pressures within the various structures enclosed within the compartment. Mean tissue pressure plus any small added pressure developed to maintain net CSF flow (as determined by the rate of secretion minus the rate of absorption) primarily represents the mean arteriovenous blood pressure in the brain and cord. Except for minor minute-to-minute fluctuations due to postural, respiratory, or other physiologic adjustments, the rate of CSF secretion and absorption as well as blood flow in and out of the brain must remain equal. Otherwise, in the enclosed confines of the skull an unequal ingress and egress would quickly raise the pressure to fatal heights or drop it to near zero.

Normally CSF pressure is approximately equal throughout the skull and spinal cord and averages about 120 to 150 mm of CSF when measured with the subject in the lateral recumbent position. The intracranial pressure changes rapidly if the intracranial blood volume changes. Hyperventilation, by lowering Pa_{CO_2} so as to constrict the arterial bed, drops CSF pressure; CO_2 breathing, by contrast, dilates the cerebral arteries and promptly raises it. The intracranial pressure also is quickly sensitive to changes transmitted from the venous sinuses so that the erect position, which reduces venous sinus pressure, lowers the intracranial pressure (but raises the intraspinal pressure), while the head-down position produces the opposite effect. Maneuvers such as jugular obstruction that elevate the intracranial venous pressure promptly raise both the intracranial and intraspinal pressure.

The intracranial pressure normally possesses a considerable tendency to maintain a steady level even in spite of positional changes or removal of samples of CSF. This damping of pressure fluctuations depends largely on compensatory changes in the volume of the capacitance cerebral veins that reciprocally and rapidly dilate or narrow as the pressure on their walls falls or rises, respectively. Changes in the rate of CSF absorption (i.e., less absorption at low pressures, more at high) abet this capacitance but at a slower time rate.

A variety of conditions, as indicated in Table 9, can raise the intracranial pressure by reducing or impairing the normal elastic properties of the intracranial cavity. In addition to any local destructive effects they may have at the brain, each of these conditions can alter local or generalized intracranial pressure-flow relationships by affecting one or both of the following mechanisms: (1) They interfere with CSF flow and absorption pathways so that increased resistance occurs at one or more points along those channels. (2) If they create an abnormal mass they reduce the compliance of the intracranial spaces by adding nonresilient tissue and vascular volumes that lack normal physiologic regulation. The pathologic reactions of locally impaired autoregulation, inflammation, and spreading edema often accentuate the effects of such masses. Furthermore, most intracranial space-occupying lesions of any size distort or impede the normal pulsatile dynamics of CSF flow within the brain's ventricular

TABLE 9. CAUSES OF INCREASED INTRACRANIAL PRESSURE

Generalized (steady-state forces distributed evenly among all intracranial and architectural compartments)

Acute reversible
Head-down position; Valsalva maneuver; jugular venous compression; acute heart failure; certain anesthetics; intrathecal manometric infusions; generalized seizures

Subacute or chronic
Venous outflow obstruction; pseudotumor cerebri

Localized (forces at least initially distributed unevenly among intracranial fluid and/or architectural compartments). All will be subacute or chronic and, at least immediately, not spontaneously reversible

1. Mass lesions
2. Meningitis
3. Obstructive hydrocephalus

cavities or over its surface. This effect further impairs the elastic properties of the tissue.

ABNORMAL INTRACRANIAL FLOW-PRESSURE CHANGES

Generalized Increased Intracranial Pressure

Several conditions can cause increases in intracranial pressure that are distributed evenly within the skull's anatomic compartments and the brain's fluid compartments (Table 9). When such increases occur briefly, e.g., during coughing or straining, they usually cause no symptoms except for occasional transient headache in a few otherwise normal individuals. Indeed, even prolonged increases in general intracranial pressure usually produce few symptoms except when the pressure rises so high that it interferes with either the venous or arterial circulation of the brain. In the normal brain, the perfusion pressure, i.e., mean intra-arterial minus mean intracranial pressure, must drop below 40 mm Hg before cerebral blood flow declines. Intracranial pressures as high as 800 mm of CSF (60 mm Hg) have been observed in asymptomatic patients with the disorder called pseudotumor cerebri, a relatively benign condition of unknown cause in which the brain becomes diffusely, asymptomatically swollen. Most patients with pseudotumor have generalized headache, however, presumably due to distension or stretching of pain-sensitive cerebral veins at the vertex and base. Most also have swelling of the optic nerve head (papilledema), and some of them experience intermittent obscurations of vision (presumably associated with the appearance of plateau waves (p. 1027). Such obscurations last from seconds to minutes and are believed to reflect transient interference with capillary flow in the optic nerve head. It also is possible that obscurations occasionally can reflect bilateral compression of the posterior cerebral arteries against the tentorium. Even obstruction of the jugular or intracranial sinuses with resulting increased intracranial pressure may produce few or no symptoms except headache and papilledema unless the particular location of the obstruction completely blocks the drainage of specific venous channels so that local brain ischemia occurs.

Mechanisms of Increased Intracranial Pressure with Localized Intracranial Lesions

Focal intracranial abnormalities may cause the intracranial pressure to rise to abnormal levels by either or both of two potential mechanisms: (1) The abnormality may interfere with the normal outflow and absorption of CSF, as discussed in the subsequent section on hydrocephalus. Even small lesions can impede CSF drainage if they lie in or near the ventricular system so as to distort the normal patterns of its fluid movements. Lesions lying more remotely from the ventricles can have a similar effect if they reach sufficient size to compress and distort the intervening brain and thereby alter the ventricular architecture. (2) Intracranial masses may raise the intracranial pressure by introducing a pathologically noncompliant structure that fails to obey the physiologic laws that govern the pressures of the normal brain, CSF, and vascular compartments. Such masses almost always

are abnormally congested and edematous, so that their intrinsic tissue pressure exceeds that of the adjacent normal brain. To maintain equilibrium and retain the elastance of the remaining normal brain and vascular structures, the intracranial pressure must rise to a new equilibrium level.

Localized Lesions Producing Pressure-Flow Abnormalities (Mass Lesions)

Supratentorial Masses or Destructive Lesions. Unless they are small or arise in neurologically silent areas, such as the anterior poles of the frontal or temporal lobes, most focal abnormalities in the brain initially produce functional changes that reflect their site of origin. If they remain untreated, many such lesions enlarge, and their expansion then creates symptoms of more generalized brain dysfunction. Expanding lesions displace previously normal brain tissue and push it contralaterally against the falx cerebri and caudally toward the base of the skull. Because the bones of the skull and the fibrous falx and tentorium resist movement except toward and through the tentorial opening, expanding supratentorial processes ultimately displace the forebrain downward, resulting in the syndromes of either uncal or central transtentorial herniation.

Uncal herniation occurs especially with expanding lesions in the temporal lobe or temporal fossa that force the medially placed temporal uncus and hippocampal gyrus toward the midline so that they herniate over the sharp incisural edge of the tentorium and compress themselves against that structure. As the hernia enlarges, it first compresses the underlying ipsilateral third nerve, then the posterior cerebral artery. Further expansion flattens the adjacent midbrain and shifts it contralaterally against the opposite incisural edge (Fig. 12).

Central transtentorial herniation results when enlargement of one or both of the overlying cerebral hemispheres or their deep basal structures compresses the diencephalon, forcing it downward toward the incisura so that it compresses the midbrain into the subtentorial space (Fig. 12). Sometimes the degree of downward herniation is so great that the brainstem actually buckles.

With both of the above herniation syndromes the intensity of abnormal symptoms and signs depends partly on the causative disease and partly on the rate at which the process develops and advances. The intracranial soft tissues possess considerable capacity to tolerate and adapt to compression and compartmental shifts so long as those displacements develop slowly and without much accompanying inflammation. In accordance with this principle, rapidly enlarging lesions mechanically resulting in acute or subacute supratentorial herniations are likely to produce acutely evolving signs of severe neurologic dysfunction. By contrast, mass lesions of an equal volume that evolve slowly may show their first abnormality in the form of subtle signs of traction or displacement upon remote, more caudally placed intracranial structures. In the latter instance, false localizing signs can occur; examples are sixth nerve palsies resulting from downward traction on the abducens nerve resulting from transtentorial herniation or nystagmus caused by brainstem distortion.

The clinical picture of acutely or subacutely enlarging supratentorial mass lesions has several distinctive features. Localizing symptoms such as frontal headache, focal seizures, or other changes usually appear first and are accompanied by focal hemispheric signs such as sensorimotor defects, aphasia, and visual field abnormalities. Later, as the lesion enlarges, signs of diffuse supratentorial dysfunction develop, indicating that the disease is exerting remote effects on the opposite cerebral hemisphere and the deep-lying diencephalon. Unless the process is far advanced and herniation already has occurred, no evidence of primary brainstem dysfunction will be encountered at this stage: Pupillary and oculovestibular responses remain intact. As the supratentorial lesion and the brain's reaction to it enlarge, the neurologic signs and symptoms evolve in a characteristically orderly rostral-caudal pattern. More rostrally located functions drop out initially, followed by more caudal impairments that successively reflect impairment of the diencephalon and then the brainstem. It is almost as if the structures were being progressively transected from above downward, each plane of function being removed before the next loses its capacities. Once the enlargement produces appreciable diencephalic compression or distorts the deeply located upper brainstem, however, stupor or coma ensues and the prognosis worsens.

Characteristic symptoms accompany the intermediate stages of either uncal or central transtentorial herniation. In *uncal herniation,* as the uncus slides over the tentorial edge and compresses the adjacent third nerve, the ipsilateral pupil begins unilaterally to dilate as a result of partial efferent parasympathetic paralysis. As the process progresses the pupil dilates more widely, and subsequent compression of the posterial cerebral artery against the tentorial edge can produce homonymous hemianopia. With pressure on the midbrain, the patient declines into stupor or deep coma. Shortly thereafter, oculomotor functions of the third nerve become paralyzed, and signs arise of severe unilateral or bilateral corticospinal tract pathway dysfunction. Unless prompt and effective treatment halts the process at this stage, few patients recover without suffering residual brain damage.

The intermediate signs of *central transtentorial herniation* generally reflect the gradual development of diencephalic dysfunction. Forebrain arousal mechanisms are dampened, and patients become lethargic, then drowsy, and eventually stuporous. The pupils shrink to 1 to 2 mm as a result of hypothalamic sympathetic impairment. Distortion and compression of the descending corticospinal tracts produce bilateral abnormalities in skeletal muscle tone as well as abnormal postural responses: Increased resistance to passive stretch, increased tendon reflexes, and decorticate-decerebrate motor posturing (p. 1059) are the result. Concurrently, interruption of descending forebrain oculomotor pathways releases the presence of brisk oculovestibular reflex responses (p. 1118). As the pathologic condition worsens it compresses the midbrain, at which point more severe ophthalmologic signs develop and are followed by evidence of serious and often irreversible vegetative neurologic abnormalities.

Subtentorial Masses. Expanding lesions in the subtentorial compartment produce pathologic reactions in their immediately adjacent tissues that are similar to those outlined above. The effect is to cause dysfunction most immediately in nuclear and internuclear structures adjacent to the lesion and, eventually, to compress and displace either the midbrain upward through the tentorial incisura or the cerebellar tonsils and medulla oblongata downward into or through the foramen magnum. Space is tight in the posterior fossa, and crucial vegetative functions lie packed closely together in the lower brainstem. As a result, life-threatening abnormalities of the respiratory or cardiovascular control systems often precede manifestations of tonsillar or midbrain herniation.

Clinically the close crowding of cranial nerve nuclei, sensorimotor pathways, and vegetative centers in the brainstem means that destructive or compressive subtentorial lesions that affect this area often can be anatomically pinpointed on the basis of their first symptoms and signs. Characteristically with brainstem lesions causing coma one finds cranial nerve palsies and pupils that are pinpoint, unequal, or irregular and fixed. Oculovestibular responses become abnormal or asymmetric, often accompanied by various forms of nystagmus. The breathing pattern frequently becomes ataxic, i.e., irregularly irregular. Large posterior fossa mass lesions or those that destructively affect the midline of the upper brainstem so as to injure the reticular formation often interfere with the normal CSF outflow pathways and produce acute hydrocephalus. Both mechanisms act to reduce the level of arousal. Compression of the cerebellum or brainstem downward against the medulla oblongata with associated cerebellar tonsillar herniation results in stiff neck along with irregularities of respiratory and cardiac rhythm but does not directly impair consciousness. Lesions compressing the vasomotor regions in the floor of the fourth ventricle sometimes produce a characteristic reflex effect of hypertension and bradycardia, although this is uncommon in the adult.

Hydrocephalus. OBSTRUCTIVE HYDROCEPHALUS. The general term *hydrocephalus* refers to dilatation of part or all of the cerebral ventricles due to interference with the normal flow or absorption of CSF anywhere along its course. Except in very chronic examples among the elderly, the condition usually is associated with at least some elevation in the intracranial pressure. *Communicating hydrocephalus* describes the condition in which ventricular fluid passes relatively normally (i.e., communicates) into the cerebrospinal subarachnoid space, but either is delayed in its ascent over the surface of the brain to reach the arachnoid granulations at the vertex or is impeded in traversing the granulations to reach venous sinus blood. Ventricular enlargement from intraventricular obstruction is designated *noncommunicating hydrocephalus* to indicate partial or complete interference with the flow of CSF anywhere between the lateral and fourth ventricles or from the fourth ventricle into the subarachnoid pathways. A now little used term, *hydrocephalus ex vacuo,* describes ventricular dilatation due to primary atrophy of the brain, a condition in which obstruction plays no important role. Brain imaging techniques unequivocally differentiate atrophic hydrocephalus from both forms of obstructive hydrocephalus by demonstrating substantial surface atrophy of the gyral pattern in association with the ventricular enlargement. Overproduction of CSF in the presence of normal intracranial dynamics rarely causes hydrocephalus.

Many conditions can cause hydrocephalus (Table 10), and its development need not require severe or acute obstruction to CSF pathways. Rather the condition tends to occur behind any mechanical distortion or displacement of the normal outflow pathways with its rate of development depending upon the degree of obstruction. This can be very slow when it results from small perturbations of the system, and it occasionally occurs in the absence of an unequivocally elevated CSF pressure. If one produces communicating hydrocephalus in experimental animals, the resulting brain atrophy is maximal in the tissues that lie adjacent to the ventricles, and it lessens radially away from them. A similar distribution of pressure atrophy seems to affect the human brain affected by obstructive hydrocephalus, since at postmortem examination in children with chronic hydrocephalus the cortical mantle remains far better preserved than the underlying white matter. Computerized axial tomography (CT) and magnetic resonance images of obstructive hydrocephalus in adults also show that the greatest reduction of brain tissue solids (i.e., atrophy) lies adjacent to the ventricular system (Fig. 13). These considerations suggest that the impedance to normal CSF flow that occurs in obstructive hydrocephalus gradually damages the periventricular brain parenchyma as it pounds against the unyielding CSF during each cardiac systole.

When hydrocephalus produces symptoms and signs they tend to be of two kinds: (1) evidence of increased intracranial pressure (papilledema, diffuse headache, elevated CSF pressure) and (2) evidence of diffuse brain dysfunction, especially of the cerebral hemispheres (intellectual decline with slowly developing obstructions; drowsiness, delirium, and stupor with rapidly

TABLE 10. CAUSES OF HYDROCEPHALUS

Noncommunicating hydrocephalus
 Mechanism: Obstruction of CSF or distortion of ventricular expansibility anywhere from lateral ventricle to exit foramina of ventricle IV

 Diseases: Mass lesions; inflammation; congenital malformations

 CT: Ventricle(s) large above lesions and often distorted; sulci normal unless obliterated from intracerebral mass-pressure

Communicating hydrocephalus
 Mechanisms: Obstruction to CSF flow or absorption outside the brain anywhere along the intracranial subarachnoid pathway. Most frequent sites: (a) cisterna magna; (b) base of brain in region of the tentorial notch; (c) lateral surfaces and vertex of hemispheres; (d) vertex of hemispheres (pacchionian obstruction)

 Causes: Postinfectious or granulomatous (tbc, sarcoid, etc.); following spontaneous or traumatic subarachnoid hemorrhage; meningeal neoplasm; old-age; idiopathic (remote trauma?)

 CT: All ventricles enlarge symmetrically; sulci obliterated over hemispheres or vertex; increased periventricular lucency

"Ex vacuo": Cerebral atrophy; ventricles diffusely enlarged; sulci diffusely widened; pressure normal or low

developing states). In addition, stretching or pressure atrophy of the motor fibers coursing from the vertex of the cerebral hemispheres around the lateral ventricles may lead to ataxia and signs of corticospinal tract dysfunction in the lower extremities. A similar mechanism involving pathways descending from frontal areas influencing micturition may explain a high incidence of urinary incontinence in patients with chronic hydrocephalus. In all instances these signs of diffuse forebrain dysfunction may be accompanied by additional signs of local neurologic dysfunction caused by the lesion that initiated the hydrocephalus (e.g., a brainstem or cerebellar mass obstructing the fourth ventricle or aqueduct; a case of granulomatous meningitis affecting cranial nerves at the base of the brain). In such complex instances, serial CT scans may reveal increasing ventricular enlargement as well as various forms of ventricular compression and shift. Surgical decompression of the lateral ventricles in many instances can bypass the outflow obstruction and be lifesaving.

Slowly developing hydrocephalus, once the cranial sutures are closed, sometimes can evolve for long periods without producing prominent or even any clinical neurologic changes. CSF dynamics in young persons with pronounced dilatation of the lateral ventricles due to partial aqueductal stenosis, for example, may reach an equilibrium, with the patient remaining asymptomatic until adolescence or even middle adult life. If symptoms attributable to the hydrocephalus finally do arise in such patients, they often reflect perturbation of a previous dynamic equilibrium by a seemingly trivial head injury or intercurrent meningeal infection. At that point, headache, deteriorating intellectual capacity, unexplained lethargy, or unexplained skeletal motor dysfunction may herald the advent of increased supratentorial pressure and the discovery of longstanding substantial ventricular dilatation. Similarly, among older persons many years may pass between a forgotten early episode of head trauma or CNS infection and the discovery in late adult life of a communicating hydrocephalus that has begun insidiously and progressed at an imperceptible rate to produce symptoms of dementia, lethargy, stiff-legged weakness, and occasional urinary incontinence.

Plateau Waves. When disease raises the intracranial pressure to levels above about 20 torr (260 mm CSF), the brain rapidly loses its normal compliance and becomes susceptible to sudden further rises in pressure (plateau waves) that last between 5 and 20 minutes and may be responsible for a variety of transient neurologic symptoms (Table 11). Plateau waves are caused by sudden failure of normal cerebral vascular autoregulation so that an abrupt increase in cerebral blood volume occurs, causing the intracranial pressure to rise (Fig. 14). Plateau waves can be triggered in patients with increased intracranial pressure by normal activity such as coughing or straining, activities that cause only momentary pressure increases in normal individuals. They are also commonly associated with assuming the supine posture and frequently occur spontaneously during periods of rapid eye movement sleep (p. 1143). A plateau wave may increase already high intracranial pressure by as much as 60 to 100 mm Hg.

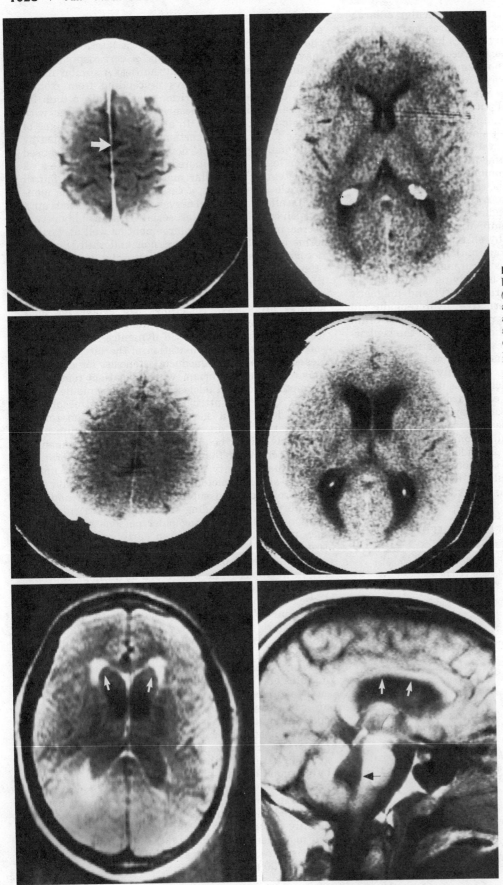

Figure 13. Normal CT scan of brain in a 65-year-old woman *(top)* compared to CT *(middle)* and MR *(bottom)* images of a 68-year-old woman with subacute communicating hydrocephalus caused by carcinomatous meningitis. *Top,* Vertex CT view (left) shows normal subarachnoid sulcal markings along sagittal sinus and falx while horizontal section through the hemispheres (right) illustrates normal ventricular and subarachnoid markings. CT of patient reveals obliterated sulcal markings at vertex (left) with dilated lateral ventricular system (right). MR image similarly discloses ventricular dilatation with periventricular edema (arrows) over frontal horns (left). Midsagittal MR cut shows dilatation of third ventricle with upward bowing of corpus callosum (white arrows) and dilated fourth ventricle (black arrow).

TABLE 11. SOME PAROXYSMAL SYMPTOMS REFLECTING PLATEAU WAVES IN PATIENTS WITH INTRACRANIAL SPACE-OCCUPYING LESIONS

Impairment of consciousness	Flexor or extensor posturing
Confusion, restlessness, agitation	Bilateral extensor plantar responses
Cardiovascular/respiratory disturbances	Generalized weakness
Headache	Clonic movements of arms and legs
Pain in neck and shoulders	Nausea, vomiting, and other autonomic signs
Blurring of vision, amaurosis	Yawning, hiccup
Mydriasis, pupillary areflexia	Urinary and fecal urgency/incontinence
Abducens paresis	
Nuchal rigidity	
Retroflexion of the neck (opisthotonus)	

Modified from Lundberg, N.: Continuous recording and control of ventricular fluid pressure in neurosurgical practice. Acta Psychiatr Scand (suppl) 149:1–193, 1960.

Plateau waves may be asymptomatic or may cause a variety of symptoms ranging from headache to sudden loss of tone in the extremities or even stupor or coma. In patients with generalized intracranial hypertension (as in pseudotumor cerebri), plateau waves, if symptomatic, are usually associated with exacerbation of headache and with visual obscurations (p. 1025). In patients with localized intracranial hypertension (as occurs with brain tumors or obstructive hydrocephalus), in addition to headache, plateau waves may cause a variety of focal symptoms, including hemiparesis,

drop attacks (sudden loss of tone in the lower extremities), or even coma (Table 11).

Intracranial Hypotension

The intracranial pressure is maintained by a constant balance between the formation and absorption of CSF. If the balance is disturbed such that loss of CSF is greater than production, the CSF pressure will decrease. The most common cause of such a decrease in CSF pressure is a leak of fluid out of the CNS such as sometimes occurs following a lumbar puncture (spinal tap). When intracranial hypotension is present, the buoyant effect of the CSF, which normally "floats" a 1500-g brain and decreases its effective mass to about 50 g, disappears. Accordingly, when a patient with intracranial hypotension assumes the upright position, pain-sensitive structures at the vertex and base of the brain are, respectively, pulled upon or compressed by the downward displacement of the brain. Severe headache in the upright position results. Sometimes the abducens nerve is also stretched or compressed by the brain's displacement, resulting in weakness of the lateral rectus muscle and diplopia. When the syndrome of intracranial hypotension follows severe head injury or a lumbar puncture that allows a slowly healing CSF leak, the diagnosis is usually obvious. Much less commonly the syndrome arises from an occult CSF leak secondary to an old basal fracture line or a hitherto unsuspected pituitary adenoma that has penetrated into a nasal sinus. Rarely the syndrome appears spontaneously without explanation in an oth-

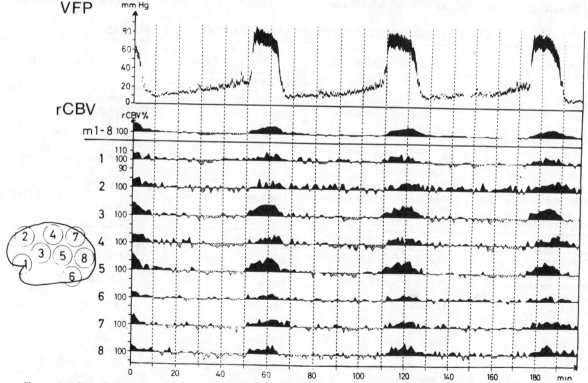

Figure 14. Simultaneous recordings in a patient with pseudotumor cerebri of regional cerebral blood volume (rCBV) and ventricular fluid pressure (VFP) during three consecutive plateau waves. The rCBV was measured in eight regions over the left hemisphere. The mean changes in the eight regions (m 1–8) are shown in the uppermost curve of the rCBV diagram. Note that the rCBV and VFP curves show a very similar course during the three waves. (From Risberg, J., Lundberg, N., and Ingvar, D. H.: Regional cerebral blood volume during acute transient rises of the intracranial pressure (plateau waves). J Neurosurg 31:306, 1969.)

erwise healthy person, lasts a few weeks, and subsides without sequelae, leaving no discoverable trace of its cause.

IMMUNITY AND THE NERVOUS SYSTEM

The immune system and the nervous system relate to each other in three different ways: (1) the two systems are similar both in their major functions and in the mechanisms by which they subserve those functions. For example, both the immune system and the nervous system have the capacity to recognize and respond to novel environmental stimuli. Although the nervous system responds to a much wider variety of stimuli than is represented by the antigens that stimulate the immune system, similar basic mechanisms may apply. Furthermore, both systems are able to recall stimuli previously encountered and to react differently when the stimulus is encountered for a second time. According to Jerne, "both systems thereby learn from experience and build up a memory that is sustained by reinforcement and that is deposited in persistent network modifications which cannot be transmitted to our offspring." (2) The nervous system is a prime target of disorders of the immune system. The first proved autoimmune disease was myasthenia gravis. Perhaps the most well studied experimental allergic immune disorders are experimental allergic encephalitis and neuritis, the former as a model of multiple sclerosis, the latter of postinfectious polyneuritis. Despite the presence of the BBB, which effectively excludes circulating immunoglobulins and, to a lesser degree, lymphocytes or macrophages, the peripheral and the central nervous systems (as well as the muscles) are affected by several immunologically mediated diseases (Table 12). The resulting nervous system damage may be either antibody-mediated or cell-mediated or both. Furthermore, when the immune system fails, the nervous system may become the site of attack of infections and neoplasma formerly prevented by a normally functioning immune system. (3) The nervous system possesses the capacity for modulating the immune system. Such immune modulation by the CNS, whether conducted neurally or humorally, may explain the well-described but poorly defined effects of mood and behavior on the development and natural history of many diseases, including cancer.

The pathophysiology of the immune system is discussed in detail in Section III of this text. In this section we will focus on special immunologic considerations as they affect the relationship between the central and peripheral nervous systems and the immune system.

ANATOMIC CONSIDERATIONS

Two anatomic structures, the BBB by its presence and the lymphatic system by its absence, confer upon the brain a relative degree of immunologic privilege. The BBB effectively excludes all but the smallest quantities of immunoglobulin from the CNS. For example, IgG as measured in the CSF has a concentration between 2 and 4 mg/dl, as opposed to a concentration

TABLE 12. IMMUNOLOGICALLY MEDIATED NEUROLOGICAL DISEASES

DISEASE	TARGET ANTIGENS	CROSS-REACTING ANTIGENS	MEDIATOR
Primarily Antibody-Mediated Immunity			
Myasthenia gravis (and EAMG)	AChR in myoneural junction	Thymocytes; thymic myocytes	Antibody; CMI
Sydenham's chorea	Caudate and subthalamic neurons	Streptococci	Antibody
Paraneoplastic syndromes	Various (myasthenia, polyneuritis, dysautonomia)	Tumors	Antibody; CMI
Systemic lupus erythematosus (SLE in NZB mouse)	Cerebral neurons; choroid plexus	Lymphocytes; other viral and tissue antigens (?)	Antibody; immune complexes
Schizophrenia	Dopaminergic neurons	Unknown	Antibody (?)
Polyarteritis nodosa	Peripheral nerve vessels	Unknown	Immune complexes, CMI (?)
Polyneuritis with myeloma and gammopathy	MAG in myelin	Unknown	Antibody
Primarily Cell-Mediated Immunity			
Multiple sclerosis	Myelin and/or oligodendrocyte antigens (??)	Unknown	Unknown
Post-rabies vaccination encephalomyelitis (and EAE)	PLP, MBP; other myelin proteins, lipids (?)	None	CMI; antibody
Parainfectious encephalomyelitis (EAE with viruses)	Unknown	Viral antigens (?)	Unknown
Long-term relapsing polyneuropathy	Myelin antigens (?)	Unknown	Unknown
(EAN)	P_2 + myelin lipids; other myelin antigens (?)	None	CMI; antibody (?)
Guillain-Barré syndrome	Myelin antigens (?)	Unknown	Unknown
(MD)	Myelin antigens	MD virus antigens (?)	CMI

From Waksman, B. H.: Immunity and the nervous system. Ann Neurol 13:587, 1983.
CMI = T-cell mediated immune reactions; MAG = myelin-associated glycoprotein; MD = Marek's disease; P_2 = characteristic protein of peripheral nervous system myelin; PLP = proteolipid protein; EAN = experimental autoimmune neuritis.
Diseases in parentheses are animal models.

of 1200 mg/dl in the serum. IgG weighs approximately 160,000 daltons; the larger IgM molecule at 900,000 daltons enters the CNS even less well than IgG, with a CSF concentration of 0.005 to 0.025 mg/dl, as compared to 100 mg/dl in the serum. Similarly, complement, a substance often required for antibodies to cause cytotoxicity, is found only at low levels in the CSF when compared with the serum. However, the BBB is not everywhere complete. Immunoglobulins may enter at areas of relative permeability as around the median eminence, the area postrema, posterior root ganglia, and proximal anterior motor root areas. Such incompetence of the barrier may play a role in disease. For example, immunizing injections against myelin galactocerebroside, if continued long enough, will cause demyelination affecting the anterior nerve roots, the region of nerve least well protected by the BBB. The lesion is probably due to the accumulated effects of IgG antibodies, since IgG antibodies are more likely than IgM antibodies to cross even an incompetent BBB. Furthermore, the BBB is not fully developed in the fetus and newborn. When pregnant rats are injected with antiserum against synaptosomal membrane antigens, the offspring behave differently from normal rats, suggesting that maternal antibodies may have crossed the BBB to affect the brain of the developing fetus. In the adult, because the BBB excludes circulating immunoglobulins, injection into the bloodstream of antibodies against nervous system structures does not cause neuropathologic change. However, such passive transfers, accomplished by intraventricular or intraneural injection, successfully produce nervous system abnormalities.

The BBB does not entirely exclude cells of the immune system, but few enter under normal circumstances. The normal CSF white cell count of < 5 cells/cu mm is less than 1/1000 that of peripheral blood, and it is doubtful that even that many lymphocytes enter the brain parenchyma itself. Both lymphocytes and macrophages have the capacity to enter the brain or subarachnoid space by passage through the capillary endothelium. They either pass through the junction between endothelial cells or possibly directly through the cytoplasm of the endothelial cell by a process called *emperipolesis* (literally, "inside, roundabout, wandering"). The entry of such circulating cells through an intact blood-brain and blood-CSF barrier may provide a sanctuary for malignant cells that are eradicated elsewhere in the body by water-soluble chemotherapeutic agents. This principle provides the rationale for employing intrathecal prophylactic chemotherapy for acute leukemia.

There are no CNS lymphatics. The CSF serves one of the functions of the lymphatic system; i.e., it disposes of molecular and cellular debris by bulk flow, but it does not expose the organ to a lymphocyte-rich environment as the lymphatics do for other organs. Furthermore, material leaving the brain is detoxified or immobilized by a tortuous route. CSF contents must drain from the brain first to the subarachnoid space, then through the peripheral circulation, and only then, after recirculation, do they reach the lymphatic system. The pathway guarantees that antigens released by the brain will have later and probably less contact with the lymphatic system than similar antigens released by other organs. There is limited drainage of CSF by

way of olfactory nerves into the nasal submucosa and subsequently into the cervical lymphatic duct and also along exiting spinal roots into paravertebral lymphatics, but these special cases account for only a minority of CSF drainage.

As a result of the presence of the BBB and the absence of lymphatics the brain under normal circumstances is not exposed to immunoglobulins or immunocompetent circulating cells. Likewise, because there are so few immunocompetent cells within the nervous system itself, it does not make its own antibodies. The consequence of these anatomic facts is that the brain is a relatively (but not absolutely) "immunologically privileged" site. Normal organ or tumor tissue implanted in the brain is rejected as it is elsewhere in the body, but more slowly. Viruses introduced directly into the CNS excite a lesser immune response than if they are first introduced into the bloodstream or other organs.

Specifically sensitized immunocompetent cells have the capacity for entering the CNS much more easily than cells that are not specifically sensitized. Thus, transplants of foreign tissues into the nervous system are much more rapidly rejected if the animal has been sensitized against antigens on that organ. Lymphocytes sensitized against antigens shared by CNS and extraneural tissues also enter the CNS more easily. Sensitization to shared antigens may play a role in nervous system reactions such as paraneoplastic syndromes and parainfectious demyelinating disorders, as described later.

Effect of Blood-Brain Barrier Disruption

Injuries to the nervous system as diverse as infections, trauma, and neoplasia increase vascular permeability (decrease BBB function) and alter the protection against an immune response that the nervous system normally enjoys. With infections of the nervous system, lymphocytes and macrophages enter the CNS in large numbers, accumulating in the Virchow-Robin spaces (that potential extracellular space that surrounds the penetrating pial arterioles and venules) and giving rise to the so-called perivascular cuffs that mark the inflammatory response of the brain. Cells may also spread out into the surrounding neuropil and enter the subarachnoid space, leading to an increased number of white cells in the CSF (pleocytosis), a finding that assists the clinician in making a diagnosis of nervous system inflammation. Once ensconced in the nervous system in large numbers, lymphocytes can change to plasma cells, which can then synthesize immunoglobulins. These immunoglobulins likewise find their way into the CSF and inform the clinician of their presence by a rise in the CSF serum immunoglobulin ratio (see below). The sequestration of immunocompetent cells that enter during an acute inflammatory response may continue after the inflammatory response is over, so that the only sign of altered nervous system immunity may be the CNS production of immunoglobulins.

The breakdown of the BBB that accompanies many nervous system diseases also allows protein and other substances that do not normally cross the BBB to enter. A lumbar CSF protein concentration of 20 to 40 mg/dl may rise one or two orders of magnitude, and water-soluble substances such as drugs generally found in the nervous system in only small quantities may now diffuse in. This BBB breakdown with inflammation allows pneumococcal or meningococcal meningitis to be effectively treated with drugs such as penicillin, which usually penetrates the BBB poorly. Likewise, the breakdown of the BBB in tumor tissue allows large, water-soluble, iodinated molecules to mark tumors on a CT scan.

Cerebrospinal Fluid and the Immune System

The CSF in many instances reflects alterations of immunity in the brain. These alterations include the number and nature of white cells, the quantity of protein and immunoglobulin, and the distribution of the immunoglobulins.

Cells. Under normal circumstances, lumbar CSF has fewer than 3 white cells/cu mm, generally all mononuclear, either lymphocytes or macrophages, in a rough ratio of 70 lymphocytes to 1 macrophage. Both T cells and B cells are present and can be identified by appropriate surface markers. Many diseases of the nervous system, particularly immune and inflammatory diseases, cause a rise in the cell count. Acute bacterial infections initially lead to a rise in neutrophils, which are absent from normal CSF. Later in the course of bacterial infections, or with viral infections or other irritative processes of the nervous system, there is a rise in mononuclear cells. Surface markers have to date proved of value only in the diagnosis of lymphoma in the nervous system, where all of the mononuclear cells are from a single clone. Plasma cells, never present in normal CSF, can be found in the fluid when large numbers of lymphocytes have entered the CNS and differentiated into plasma cells.

Protein. Most of the protein in CSF is albumin. Albumin is not synthesized by the CNS, and thus the CSF concentration reflects both its concentration in the serum and its limited access across the BBB. Under normal circumstances the lumbar CSF:serum ratio of albumin varies from 0.0037 in young adults to 0.0052 in the elderly. An increase in that ratio suggests breakdown of the BBB.

Immunoglobulins can reach the CSF either by crossing the BBB or by synthesis within the nervous system. The relative ratio of albumin and IgG in serum and CSF can be compared to give an index of immunoglobulin synthesis: IgG synthesis =

$$\left[\left(IgG_{CSF} - \frac{IgG_S}{369} \right) - \left(Alb_{CSF} - \frac{Alb_S}{230} \right) \times \left(\frac{IgG_S}{Alb_S} \right) \times 0.43 \right] \times 5, \text{ where}$$

369 = number of serum IgG molecules required for one CSF IgG molecule under normal conditions;

230 = number of serum albumin molecules required for one CSF albumin molecule under normal conditions;

$$0.43 = \frac{\text{molecular weight albumin (69,000)}}{\text{molecular weight IgG (150,000)}}$$

Proteins in the CSF, like those in the serum, can be separated by electrophoresis. Under normal circumstances, the CSF immunoglobulins are contained in a diffuse, faintly staining zone in the gamma region. In several inflammatory and immune diseases, the gamma region is not homogeneous but contains one or more sharply defined discrete protein bands (oligoclonal bands). Although these bands are present in a variety of disorders, they are most common in immune diseases, particularly subacute sclerosing panencephalitis, multiple sclerosis, and demyelinating polyneuropathy. The presence of more than two oligoclonal bands in the gamma region is strongly suggestive of an immune disorder of the nervous system.

PATHOPHYSIOLOGY OF IMMUNE DISORDERS OF CNS

Several different immunopathologic mechanisms play a role in neurologic disease (Table 13). It is not certain whether all of these immune mechanisms affect the CNS in human disease, and it is equally uncertain which of the mechanisms plays the major role in those diseases that are believed to be immune mediated. For example, the evidence that immediate-type hypersensitivity reactions such as anaphylactic shock or food allergy affect the nervous system is very weak. Conversely, although there is strong evidence that multiple sclerosis, a relapsing disorder of central myelin, is an immunopathologic disease, the exact mechanism by which the immune system produces the pathologic changes is unclear. The pathophysiology of immune diseases of the nervous system has been worked out best in experimental models, particularly those of experimental allergic encephalomyelitis and experimental allergic neuritis, diseases produced by the injection into an animal of brain and nervous system tissue, respectively, along with Freund's adjuvant, a fatty mixture that intensifies the pathologic effect of the injection on the tissue.

For the immune system to attack the nervous system it must first react to an antigen that directs itself

TABLE 13. PATHOPHYSIOLOGY OF IMMUNE TISSUE DAMAGE

MECHANISM	POSSIBLE HUMAN OR ANIMAL NERVOUS SYSTEM EXAMPLE
Immediate hypersensitivity	No proved clinical examples in the nervous system
Anaphylaxis local or systemic	Brain edema with wasp sting?
Atopic disease	Migraine ???
Antibody mediated	Occur only after blood-brain barrier disruption (except myasthenia)
Complement mediated	Galactocerebrosides—experimental allergic neuritis
Antibody-dependent cell-mediated cytotoxicity	Chronic relapsing experimental allergic encephalomyelitis, ? multiple sclerosis
Blocking antibody	Myasthenia gravis (acetylcholine receptor)
Stimulating antibody	Sydenham's chorea
Basement membrane injury	Goodpasture's syndrome
Immune complex lesions	Role in human CNS disease unclear
Soluble complexes	SLE, polyarteritis nodosa
Arthus reactions	Cerebral vasculitis??
Cell-mediated hypersensitivity	Probably play a role in immune human nervous system diseases
Delayed	Experimental allergic encephalomyelitis and experimental allergic neuritis
Direct	Viral encephalitis

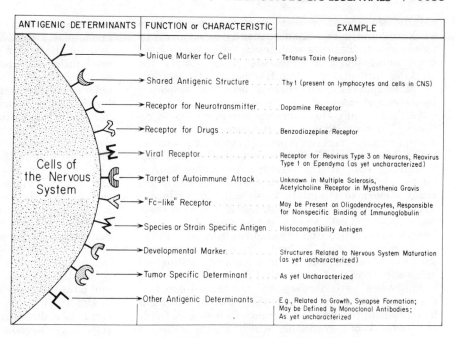

ANTIGENIC DETERMINANTS	FUNCTION or CHARACTERISTIC	EXAMPLE
	Unique Marker for Cell	Tetanus Toxin (neurons)
	Shared Antigenic Structure	Thy 1 (present on lymphocytes and cells in CNS)
	Receptor for Neurotransmitter	Dopamine Receptor
	Receptor for Drugs	Benzodiazepine Receptor
	Viral Receptor	Receptor for Reovirus Type 3 on Neurons, Reovirus Type 1 on Ependyma (as yet uncharacterized)
Cells of the Nervous System	Target of Autoimmune Attack	Unknown in Multiple Sclerosis, Acetylcholine Receptor in Myasthenia Gravis
	"Fc-like" Receptor	May be Present on Oligodendrocytes, Responsible for Nonspecific Binding of Immunoglobulin
	Species or Strain Specific Antigen	Histocompatibility Antigen
	Developmental Marker	Structures Related to Nervous System Maturation (as yet uncharacterized)
	Tumor Specific Determinant	As yet Uncharacterized
	Other Antigenic Determinants	E.g., Related to Growth, Synapse Formation; May be Defined by Monoclonal Antibodies; As yet uncharacterized

Figure 15. Antigenic specificity of the nervous system. Note that a single determinant may serve more than one function. For example, the acetylcholine receptor not only acts as a neurotransmitter receptor but is the target of an autoimmune attack in myasthenia gravis and has been reported to be a viral receptor for rabies virus. Many of the antigenic determinants on nervous system tissue have yet to be characterized. (From Weiner, H. L., and Hauser, S. L.: Neuroimmunology II: Antigenic specificity of the nervous system. Ann Neurol 12:499, 1982.)

against a portion of the nervous system. The surface of nervous system cells contains a bewildering variety of antigenic determinants (Fig. 15). Included are determinants that are unique markers for the cell, determinants that are shared between a cell of the nervous system and a structure outside the nervous system (e.g., viruses, systemic tumor cells), receptors for neurotransmitters, drugs, and many others. The large number of antigenic determinants on cells of the CNS as well as the many determinants that appear to be shared between nervous system cells and other cell types may explain in part why the nervous system is so susceptible to immune attack despite its protection by the BBB.

Immediate-Type Hypersensitivity

In man, immediate-type hypersensitivity is mediated by IgE immunoglobulins and depends on the capacity of immunoglobulin to bind to mast cells and basophils. Various vasoactive substances such as histamine and bradykinin and prostaglandins are released. It is not clear whether the nervous system participates in any reactions of the immediate-type hypersensitivity, but the presence of mast cells in the meninges and in the adventitia of arteries and arterioles of the brain suggests that it may. Isolated case reports describe swelling of the brain after anaphylactic shock, but local anaphylaxis has never been described in the brain. Some postulate that migraine headache may be a disease of immediate-type hypersensitivity, related to the ingestion of food allergens, but convincing evidence for this view is lacking. Systemic mastocytosis is a rare disease of mast cell proliferation in which mast cells release vasoactive substances in excessive amounts. Most of the symptoms are cutaneous or systemic or both, but severe and recurrent headache is a common manifestation of this disorder.

Antibody-Mediated Injury

Antibodies directed against the nervous system can mediate injury in one of several ways: First, the anti-

body may fix complement, causing cell lysis or myelin breakdown. One example is the destruction of myelin that occurs when gangliocerebroside serves as the antigen. As with all antigen-antibody reactions, the circulating immunoglobulin does not cross the normal BBB, but the disease can be produced easily by injecting the antibody intraneurally, i.e., on the nerve side of the blood-nerve barrier (analogous to the blood-brain barrier), or by repeatedly giving intravenous injections of the antigen so as to generate very high circulating levels of antimyelin IgG antibody. In the latter instance the majority of damage occurs at the proximal motor root, a site where the blood-nerve barrier is relatively incompetent.

A second mechanism of antibody damage occurs even in the absence of complement, when antibody-coated cells are lysed by normal lymphoid cells (killer cells). So-called antibody-dependent cell-mediated cytotoxicity is believed to be one mechanism causing chronic relapsing experimental allergic encephalomyelitis, an animal model that closely mimics, clinically and pathologically, human multiple sclerosis.

Because many of the antigenic determinants on the surface of neurons or other cells have functional activity, antibodies binding to these sites can interfere with the function of the cell without necessarily causing inflammation or other pathologic changes. In the nervous system, both stimulating and blocking effects of antibodies have been described. The best example of a blocking effect occurs in the disease myasthenia gravis, where antibodies to the nicotinic acetylcholine receptor bind that structure and prevent the normal effect of ACh on the postsynaptic neuromuscular junction. Because the BBB does not exist in this area, circulating antibodies easily make contact with the postsynaptic receptor. In an example of passive immunization, antireceptor antibody circulating in the blood of pregnant women with myasthenia gravis can cross the placental membrane and produce transient myasthenia gravis in the newborn infant solely due to the presence of blocking antibody. As the antibody is degraded postnatally, the infant recovers from the symptoms of weakness and does not subsequently develop myasthenia gravis. Patients with myasthenia gravis have more immunologic abnormalities than simply the blocking antibody. As a result, removing the antibody by plasmapheresis, although it leads to temporary improvement, does not cure the disease.

Antibodies may also *stimulate* receptors. The injection of brain antibodies into the cerebrum of experimental animals has been reported to produce repetitive trains of electrical discharge that develop into self-sustaining epileptiform activity. Antibodies against neurons in the caudate and subthalamic nuclei of the brain appear to stimulate those cells to produce a hyperactive movement disorder associated with rheumatic fever and called Sydenham's chorea. Likewise it has been postulated that the seizures that occur in the autoimmune disease systemic lupus erythematosus (SLE) may be a result of the circulating antineural antibodies that are found in that disorder.

Antibodies against basement membranes can produce vascular injury, particularly to the basement membrane of the renal glomerulus. One such example is Goodpasture's syndrome, which affects both the glomerulus and the brain's choroid plexus. Despite the morphologic changes of the basement membrane of the choroid plexus, however, there is no evidence that such involvement produces brain dysfunction in this syndrome.

Immune Complex Lesions

Immunologic mechanisms can sometimes damage the nervous system in situations in which there is no clear antigen-antibody reaction directly involving neural structures. In such circumstances, an antigen that operates against extraneural structures and the antibody produced against it may form circulating immune complexes. When these complexes are of appropriate size, they deposit themselves on the endothelial cells of capillaries, often fix complement, and cause vascular damage. A common place for such immune complexes to deposit is in the glomerulus of the kidney, leading to several glomerular disorders. The choroid plexus resembles the structure of the glomerulus of the kidney and also plays host to immune complex deposition. Such deposition has been reported in SLE, in which it has been postulated that choroid plexus depositions may disrupt the BBB function sufficiently to alter the electrolyte composition of the CSF and extracellular space, thus producing physiologic abnormalities. Immune complexes also may deposit themselves in the subendothelial areas of other capillaries in SLE, leading to inflammation and vascular necrosis. The mechanism has been postulated as one cause of the seizures and other neurologic disabilities that often affect patients with SLE. Similar immune complex deposition on the capillaries of peripheral nerves has been postulated to cause the mononeuropathies that occur in the human disease polyarteritis nodosa.

Cell-Mediated Immunity

Cell-mediated immune disorders in the nervous system can occur either through the phenomenon of direct T cell cytotoxicity or by delayed hypersensitivity reactions. In most well-studied clinical and experimental immune disorders of the nervous system, both mechanisms play a role. Much of the damage of viral infections of the nervous system takes place through the mechanism of cell-mediated immunity, and most experimental and clinical demyelinating diseases probably exert their damage via the same mechanism. Furthermore, whatever natural resistance exists against cerebral tumors probably operates through cell-mediated immunity as well. In viral infections of the CNS, the pathologic reaction to the effects of cell-mediated immunity can be much more severe than the brain's reaction to the original viral infection. An example is lymphocytic choriomeningitis of mice. In this disease the virus itself is relatively innocuous, and the acute lesions are entirely due to damage caused by T cells reacting with the viral antigens in the brain. Somewhat similar cell-mediated immune reactions are probably responsible for the demyelination that occurs in multiple sclerosis, postinfectious encephalitis, and polyneuritis, as well as in a variety of other infectious and parainfectious illnesses.

Abnormalities of cell-mediated immunity may also occur as a direct result of abnormalities of immunoregulatory T cells. Decreases in suppressor T cells circulating in the blood have been reported to presage and accompany acute attacks of multiple sclerosis. Increases in suppressor T cells have been reported in a variety of viral infections that affect the nervous system, including Epstein-Barr virus, but their pathogenic role, if any, in these circumstances has not been defined.

Astrocytes may also be important in the development of T cell-mediated immune responses in the CNS. Astrocytes are able to present antigens to T cells "in vitro" and to cause proliferation of those T cells that are able to recognize the antigen. Astrocytes can also synthesize interleukin-1–like factors; such factors promote the secretion of interleukin-2 by T cells to enhance the activity of the natural killer cells. Both properties could result in T cell-mediated CNS damage or in enhanced resistance to CNS tumors.

IMMUNOLOGICALLY MEDIATED NEUROLOGIC DISEASES

Neurologic Diseases and the Immune System

A number of human neurologic diseases are known or thought to be mediated by the immune system (Table 12). These include those that are primarily antibody mediated as well as those that are primarily cell mediated. Each of the disorders is associated with relatively specific pathologic changes in the nervous system. Certain pathologic changes, particularly those of subintimal necrosis of vessel walls, perivascular inflammatory infiltrates, and demyelination, appear common to many immune diseases of the nervous system. A sequence of events leading to nervous system damage that probably occurs in both viral infections and autoimmune disease includes the changes observed in experimental autoimmune encephalomyelitis. As already stated, this disease is produced by injection of brain homogenates or myelin basic protein along with complete Freund's adjuvant. The first pathologic change appears to be an increase in vascular permeability and associated brain edema. Perivascular deposits of fibrin, immunoglobulin, and complement may appear prior to any inflammatory cells. The exact pathogenesis of this BBB disruption is not clear. It may be a result of immune complex damage to endothelial cells or the release of vasoactive substances by sensitized T cells.

Three immunologically mediated human neurologic diseases are of particular importance, both because they are common and because their pathogenesis is better understood than most of the other disorders listed in Table 12. Paraneoplastic syndromes are also discussed here because they are probably immune mediated as well.

Myasthenia Gravis. Myasthenia gravis (see also p. 1047) is a disorder of the neuromuscular junction characterized by weakness of skeletal muscle, particularly of bulbar and respiratory muscles, after exercise. The disorder is caused by production of an antibody against the ACh receptor that damages the postsynaptic neuromuscular junction receptor. ACh receptor dysfunction occurs by several mechanisms. These include complement-dependent damage to the postsynaptic membrane, increased receptor degradation resulting from cross-linking of the receptor by divalent antibody, direct block of receptor function, binding of the antibody to the receptor, and modification of ACh receptor function. Cell-mediated immunity against the ACh receptor has been demonstrated in some myasthenic patients as well. How the autoimmune response gets started is not clear. There must be genetic predispositions, since certain HLA types appear more commonly in patients with myasthenia. In addition, the thymus gland plays a role, both thymoma and thymic hyperplasia being common in patients with this disease. Thymic lymphocytes have a surface antigen that cross reacts with the ACh receptor. Finally, there is a higher incidence of other autoimmune diseases such as hyperthyroidism in patients with myasthenia gravis.

Parainfectious Polyneuropathy. Parainfectious polyneuropathy (Guillain-Barré syndrome discussed subsequently) is an acute inflammatory disorder of peripheral nerve that often follows a viral infection or an immunization. The disorder is characterized by acute or subacute loss of motor function with lesser sensory loss. There is usually complete recovery within a matter of weeks or months. It is believed that the infection or immunization triggers some response of a substance that shares an antigen with peripheral nerve. The resulting immune reaction leads to macrophages attacking peripheral nerve and stripping the myelin from the axon. The component of peripheral nerve involved in the reaction has not been determined. Immune complexes may play a role in the pathogenesis of the disorder as well. Recent studies suggest that plasmapheresis, performed early after onset, can reduce the degree of neurological damage and shorten the course of the illness.

Multiple Sclerosis. A common neurologic disease affecting young and middle-aged people, multiple sclerosis is characterized by relapsing episodes of CNS dysfunction that can involve virtually any region of the brain or spinal cord. Pathologically there are plaques of myelin loss with relative preservation of axons. It is believed that multiple sclerosis is probably an autoimmune disease, but the antigen has not been defined, the mechanism of immune damage is not

entirely clear, and what triggers the autoimmune response is likewise not known.

Paraneoplastic Syndromes. A group of nervous system disorders that occur with greatly increased frequency in patients suffering from cancer, particularly oat cell carcinoma of the lung, paraneoplastic syndromes include a subacute cerebellar degeneration, subacute sensory neuronopathy (see the chapter, Sensory Systems) sensorimotor peripheral neuropathy, neuromuscular disorder (Eaton-Lambert myasthenic syndrome), and a muscular disorder (polymyositis). The disorders are of potentially diagnostic interest because they often occur and produce devastating neurologic disability at a time when the underlying cancer is too small to be detected by standard measures. Paraneoplastic syndromes are believed to be immune mediated in part because inflammatory infiltrates are often found in the affected nervous system tissue and in part because in several of the disorders patients' sera carry circulating antibodies against structures in the CNS. One hypothesis is that the neoplasm shares an antigen with the nervous system, and when the immune system attempts to attack the tumor it attacks the nervous system as well. Proof of this hypothesis is lacking.

Immune Suppression Predisposing to Central Nervous System Dysfunction. Changes in the immune system not only can lead directly to damage of the nervous system, but failure of the system can invite secondary damage of the nervous system. The latter, so-called opportunistic damage, can consist of either infections or malignant neoplasms. Otherwise rare infections of the CNS arise in the setting of damage to either the antibody-mediated immune system or the cell-mediated immune system. Particularly striking has been the high incidence of various nervous system infections in patients with acquired immunodeficiency syndrome (AIDS), where most who succumb have pathologic evidence of either nervous system infection or neoplasia. Examples of opportunistic CNS infections in patients with altered immunity, including AIDS, include parasitic infections such as toxoplasmosis, particularly in the form of brain abscesses, fungal infections such as cryptococcal meningitis, and viral infections, including herpes zoster and probably cytomegalovirus encephalitis. Which organism affects which patient depends in part on exposure to the agent and in part on the exact mechanism of the immune deficiency.

Several congenital diseases of immune suppression are associated with an increased incidence of systemic malignant neoplasms. The nervous system is not specifically singled out in these disorders. However, patients who undergo iatrogenic immune suppression, e.g., after renal or cardiac transplants, suffer a considerably increased incidence of lymphomas, many of which arise primarily in the brain. Whether the relatively immune privileged site of the brain promotes development of the neoplasm there is not clear. Primary lymphoma of the brain is an uncommon tumor in the nonimmune suppressed situation.

Neuroimmunomodulation

The nervous system exerts direct and indirect effects on almost every other system of the body, including the immune system. Neuroendocrine influences on immunity are well established. The increased or decreased output, respectively, of adrenocorticosteroids, decreases or increases the number of circulating lymphocytes. More direct influences are less clear. Certain human diseases of the nervous system such as brain tumors and Huntington's disease appear to result in immunologic abnormalities. Abnormalities of behavior, including psychosis, depression, and stress, lead to impaired lymphocyte reactivity and diminished antibody production. Similar results have been found in experimental animals subjected to stressful situations. Behavioral changes such as depression have been reported to presage the onset of cancer or to lead to a lesser therapeutic response to chemotherapy in patients with established cancer. On the other hand, more optimistic outlooks have been reported to be associated with prolonged survival in established cancer, and some have reported that behavioral treatment of patients with cancer can prolong survival.

Experimentally, destructive lesions of the anterior hypothalamus have been reported to diminish delayed-type hypersensitivity, impair cellular and humoral responsiveness, and decrease anaphylaxis. These responses appear not to be mediated by changes in circulating corticosteroids, but to result from qualitative changes in the function of naturally occurring splenic suppressor macrophages. Electrolytic lesions of the limbic system result in increased lymphocyte blastogenic activity. We presently possess only sketchy knowledge of the effect of the nervous system on the immune system. Future developments may allow therapists to take advantage of such neuroimmunomodulation, both when estimating the prognosis of disease and perhaps in efforts to alter its natural history.

REFERENCES

Beck, D. W., Hart, M. N., Vinters, H. V., and Cancilla, P. A.: Glial cells influence polarity of the blood brain barrier. J Neuropathol Exper Neurol 43:219, 1984.

Bradbury, M.: The Concept of a Blood-Brain Barrier. New York, John Wiley & Sons, 1979.

Cairncross, J. G., and Posner, J. B.: Neurological Complications of Systemic Cancer. In Yarbro, J. W., and Bornstein, R. S. (eds.): Oncologic Emergencies. New York, Grune and Stratton, 1981.

Fishman, R. A.: Cerebrospinal Fluid in Diseases of the Nervous System. Philadelphia, W. B. Saunders Co., 1980.

Goldstein, G. W., and Betz, A. L.: Recent advances in understanding brain capillary function. Ann Neurol 13:389, 1983.

Iverson, L. L., Synder, S. H., Braestrup, C., Nielsen, M., Jessel, T. M., Marsden, C. D., Rossor, M. N., van Pragg, H. M., Sperro, L., and Bloom F. E.: Neurotransmitter and CNS disease. Lancet 2:914–918, 970–974, 1030–1034, 1084–1088, 1141–1147, 1200–1204, 1259–1264, 1319–1322, 1381–1385, 1982.

Kandel, E. R., and Schwartz, J. H.: Principles of Neural Science. New York, Elsevier/North-Holland, 1981.

Kreiger, D. T.: Brain peptides: What, where and why. Science 222:975–985, 1983.

Leibowitz, S., and Hughes, R.A.C.: Immunology of the Nervous System. London, Edward Arnold, 1983.

Ludwin, S. K.: Pathology of demyelination and remyelination of demyelinating disease. In Waxman, S. G., and Ritchie, J. M. (eds.): Basic and Clinical Electrophysiology. New York, Raven Press, 1981, pp. 123–168.

McGeer, P. L., Eccles, J. C., and McGeer, E. G.: Molecular Neurobiology of the Mammalian Brain. New York, Plenum Press, 1978.

Shepherd, G. M.: Neurobiology. New York, Oxford University Press, 1983.

Weiner, H. L., and Hauser S. L.: Neuroimmunology I: Immunoregulation in neurological disease. Ann Neurol 11:437, 1982.

Weiner, H. L., and Hauser, S. L.: Neuroimmunology II: Antigenic specificity of the nervous system. Ann Neurol 12:499, 1982.

Motor System

THE ANATOMY AND PHYSIOLOGY OF NORMAL MOTOR CONTROL

PERIPHERAL NEUROMUSCULAR SYSTEMS

Skeletal Muscle

Skeletal muscle, the largest organ of the body, provides the mechanical instrument by which the brain communicates to the extracorporeal world. From the laborer's shovel of dirt to the soprano's high C, as A. V. Hill, the English physiologist put it, "muscles move the world." The mechanics of our normal body movements reflect the coordinated action of millions of individual striated fibers, grouped functionally into fascicles and individual muscles that insert around bones and joints. One alpha motor neuron, its axon, and the fibers it innervates make up a *motor unit*. The motor units themselves can contain as few as six individual fibers in the muscles controlling the fine movements of the eye or as many as 2000 in the large muscles that produce gross movements of the trunk or limb girdles. In human striated muscle the fibers of any given motor unit distribute themselves widely through many fascicles rather than being grouped into contiguous bundles as they are in some lower mammals. As will be explained, an understanding of this distribution finds practical application when examining human muscle biopsies in attempts to diagnose diseases that cause denervation.

The Myoneural Junction. Each branch of a motor axon joins its muscle fiber at a specialized synapse known as the myoneural junction (Fig. 16). In the presynaptic axon terminal the energy-dependent enzyme, choline acetyltransferase, fueled by a heavy concentration of mitochondria, constantly synthesizes acetylcholine (ACh). Molecules of transmitter are packaged into vesicles, a small discrete number (quanta) of which are discontinuously released at a slow rate from the axon terminals. These few quanta provide repeated, feeble excitation to postsynaptic cholinergic receptors located in subneural clefts of the *motor end-plate*, the specialized membrane that lies on the muscle side of the synapse. The result induces tiny localized depolarizations (miniature end-plate potentials) that are reflected electrically as small spikes whose magnitude of about 1 mV is insufficient to

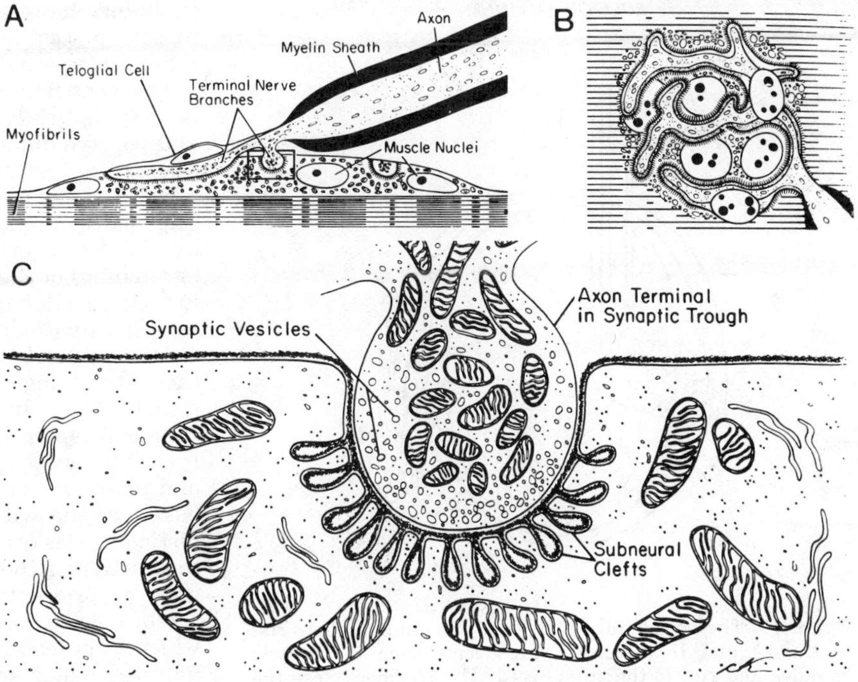

Figure 16. Motor end plate. *A* and *B,* Views from the side and from above, respectively. *C,* Enlarged view (as seen in electron micrographs) of the region outlined by the rectangle in *A.* (From Patton, H. D., Sundsten, J. W., Crill, W. E., and Swanson, P. D.: Introduction to Basic Neurology. Philadelphia, W. B. Saunders Co., 1976.)

depolarize fully the end-plate. When a motor nerve action potential arrives at the axon terminal, the terminal enlargement abruptly and simultaneously releases many quanta of vesicles into the synaptic cleft that excite a proportionately large population of receptors on the motor end-plate. The ensuing depolarization usually exceeds the end-plate threshold by fourfold to fivefold so that sodium ions flood through and into the adjacent muscle fiber, spreading a depolarizing action potential to the ends of the sarcolemmal membrane. As the excitatory impulse spreads it also invades the inside of the muscle fiber, traveling along a series of transverse tubules to the center of the fiber where it mobilizes calcium ions. Calcium, in turn, activates the tiny actin filaments to slide over their myosin filament core. The fiber contracts.

Lower Motor Neurons and the Control of Muscle

Two kinds of motor neurons, larger *alpha* and smaller *gamma,* link the spinal cord and brainstem to striated muscle. The alpha motor neurons represent what Sherrington, the father of modern neurophysiology, called the *final common path.* Clinical parlance sometimes calls the entire structure, including the perikaryon of the motor neuron, its dendrites, axon, and the axon's terminal arborization the *lower motor neuron.* Destruction of the lower motor neuron anywhere along its length produces paralysis and subsequent atrophy of its motor unit. The smaller, gamma, motor neuron also goes to muscle but innervates delicate intrafusal fibers that lie within specialized muscle receptors called *spindles,* described in the following section.

Much of the integration of normal motor activity is carried out directly by alpha motor neurons of the brainstem and spinal cord. These cells respond to signals reaching them from three sources. (1) Five major descending pathways collectively designated the *upper motor neuron* (see also p. 1039) send monosynaptic connections to the lower motor neurons. Among these, the corticospinal, rubrospinal, and midbrainpontine reticulospinal tracts are largely excitatory in action while the vestibulospinal and medullospinal reticular pathways exert mainly inhibitory influences. (2) The above pathways also project to polysynaptic propriospinal neurons and the brainstem-spinal segmental interneuron pools. The net input eventually is integrated by the alpha motor neurons. (3) Monosynaptic and polysynaptic proprioceptive reflex afferents (e.g., stretch reflex afferents) as well as cutaneous and joint afferents convey information from peripheral muscle, tendon organ receptors, skin, and joints to reach the motor neurons of the same and adjacent spinal and brainstem segments. The ultimate connectivity is enormous. It is estimated that the average large spinal motor neuron possesses 40,000 to 80,000 synaptic junction points on its surface.

The Stretch Reflex. The gamma motor neuron and the muscle spindles contribute importantly to motor reflexes as well as to the proprioceptive control of movement.

Muscle spindles are tiny elongated sensors located near the ends of skeletal muscle fibers and distributed in a density that is roughly proportional to the muscle's contribution to fine movement (Fig. 17). Each spindle contains two to twelve tiny intrafusal muscle (fusimotor) fibers cholinergically innervated by the small, gamma (fusimotor) axons of the ventral horn. Each spindle contains at its center a fluid-filled capsule in which lie the receptor endings for two kinds of afferents, called primary and secondary (IA and II fibers). Both afferents discharge when the skeletal muscle is stretched. The primary ending increases or lessens its rate of discharge according to the rate at which stretch occurs, while the secondary ending responds to length alone. Both contribute to the stretch reflex but in different ways.

ROLE OF PALLIDUM

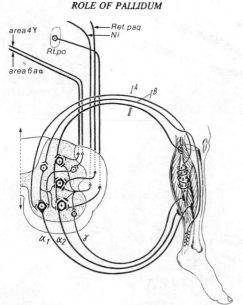

Figure 17. The peripheral reflex loop. The gamma fibers run to the IA and II afferents, which come from the muscle spindles and run to the spinal cord. The IA fibers close the monosynaptic reflex arc for the regulation of muscle length. The II fibers and the IB fibers complete the polysynaptic reflex arc for the regulation of muscle tension and proprioception (pathways not shown). *Rt. po* = pontine reticular formation; *Ret. paq* = periaqueductal reticular formation; *Ni* = substantia nigra. (From Hassler, R. G.: Adv Neurol 40:1–15. Copyright 1984, Raven Press, New York.)

In humans, gamma motor neurons normally activate fusimotor fibers in the spindles of a contracting muscle a few milliseconds after the alpha motor discharge to that muscle begins. The arrangement constantly maintains the sensitivity of the stretch receptor by resetting it to the new shorter length. The spindle is thereby prepared to discharge at any point when contraction (which shortens the muscle) ceases and the muscle begins to relengthen. The sensitivity of the receptor is thus continuously adjusted "in parallel" with the tension imposed on the striated muscle. Concurrently with this spindle adjustment on the shortening muscle, stretch receptors in the relaxed antagonistic muscle fire progressively as length increases. From the receptors, monosynaptic IA afferents increase the excitability of the motor neurons of the stretched muscle and simultaneously provide, by way of group II afferents, polysynaptically mediated proprioceptive information to more rostral centers in the cord and brain.

Tendon organs operate "in series" with striated muscles and are located at the point where the muscle enters its tendon. The organs respond to tension applied by the contracting muscle, discharging a signal via IB afferents that varies directly with the degree of tension applied. They end on a spinal interneuron that, in turn, inhibits the alpha motor neuron of the contracting muscle. An everyday example of the inhibitory function of the tendon organ can be illustrated by its absence in the phenomenon of *muscle cramp*. Cramp arises when a muscle contracts in a fully shortened position, then involuntarily self-sustains the contraction. The shortened muscle places minimal tension on its tendon organ, which accordingly fails to fire its

inhibitory signals. Passively stretching the contracting muscle places tension on its tendon, activates the inhibitory receptor, and stops the cramp.

The connections from stretched spindle receptors monosynaptically reaching synergistic motor neurons and polysynaptically ending on the internuncial pool and more rostral sensory mechanisms provide the afferent limbs of the *phasic* and *tonic stretch reflexes*. The monosynaptic phasic reflex is clinically illustrated by the knee jerk: A briskly delivered lengthening (stretching) of the quadriceps muscle elicited by striking the patellar tendon sends a synchronous volley of excitatory postsynaptic potentials (EPSPs) to converge on the muscle's spinal alpha motor neurons. These then fire a single, synchronous volley to contract the muscle. The polysynaptic, tonic stretch reflex, like its spindle receptor, is both length and velocity dependent. It continuously bombards the spinal internuncial pool and more rostral centers such as the cerebellum and basal ganglia with increasing information as antagonistic muscles are stretched either passively or during contraction of the agonist. The effect provides continuous proprioceptive information to the cerebellum, cerebral cortex, and other higher motor-related areas, which then feed back to the motor neurons to coordinate the motor act. As discussed later on, damage or dysfunction of these long-loop pathways that extend from segmental proprioceptors to higher centers and back underlies many of the abnormalities observed clinically as spasticity, rigidity, tremor, and ataxia.

ORGANIZATION OF DESCENDING MOTOR PATHWAYS

A number of pathways descend from the brain to influence craniospinal alpha and gamma motor control. The complexity of their action as well as the differences between their normal and abnormal influences on movement can easily bewilder even the advanced student. A brief review may help to minimize such confusion.

Development and the Principle of Encephalization

The evolution of the brain has layered increasing complexity on successively advancing but primitive motor systems that arose initially to adapt the organism to simpler tasks. In most instances, new hierarchies of regulation have been added without completely discarding older regulatory mechanisms. Thus the reticular core of the human brain and spinal cord finds its earliest origins in the longitudinal nerve network of the invertebrate nervous system. Segmental reflexes came at a later stage of biologic development as did spatial proprioceptive mechanisms that evolved into the vestibular nuclei, the cerebellum, and their various specialized receptors. By the lizard stage, a primitive forebrain made its appearance, initiating a structure that has been carried forward to primates as the basal ganglia. Further behavioral development has reflected the specificity of action conferred by an evolving cerebral cortex and its accompanying switching-relaying nuclei that make up the complexity of the mammalian thalamus. The progressive enlargement of the forebrain produced the convoluted hemispheres of the higher primates, including humans, and was accompanied by a proportionate enlargement of the motor cortex's guidance control organ, the lateral cerebellum.

Each of these evolved systems participates in motor control, but under normal circumstances the functions of all but the cerebral cortex have become effectively integrated into and somewhat subordinated to the actions of higher levels for the regulation of movement. As a result, one can hardly discern the contributions of more primitive levels of control except by highly sophisticated physiologic analyses of normal persons or by inferences drawn from the effects of neurologic disease. Knowledge of the principle greatly assists the evaluation of neurologic abnormalities and becomes a crucial step in localizing diagnosis.

Damage to the Brain Has Negative and Positive Effects

Because of the ontogenetic development of the human brain, damage to it potentially has two effects. One, the negative effect, *paralyzes* the function initially controlled by the damaged neural structures. The other, the positive effect, by functionally removing the damaged areas of higher control *releases* abnormal motor activities that reflect more primitive levels of neurologic organization. To give an example discussed more thoroughly in later paragraphs: When the corticospinal tract is injured, the hand may lose its skilled movement, a negative effect, but the arm becomes spastic as a result of the release of subcortical mechanisms facilitating the stretch reflex, a positive effect.

Terminology and Physiology of Descending Motor Influences

Neurologists sometimes employ the terms *pyramidal* and *extrapyramidal* motor systems to describe the several descending motor pathways that influence striated muscle movement. (Cerebellar pathways always have been described differently, because while they coordinate movement initiated in other motor centers, they do not independently originate it.) The pyramidal-extrapyramidal concept arose a number of years ago because it was mistakenly believed that voluntary movement in man was controlled by a more or less pure corticospinal tract arising from the large Betz cells in area 4 of the cerebral cortex. This purportedly exclusive pathway decussated in the medullary pyramids (thus the name) and terminated largely monosynaptically on alpha motor neurons of the spinal cord. To accommodate such a view, the extrapyramidal system was interpreted as representing all other descending motor systems. Modern evidence, however, indicates that neither the anatomy, physiology, nor clinical aspects of the pathways underlying motor control make it useful to divide matters in this way. For one thing, the corticospinal tract is not purely precentral motor in its origin, since fibers join it from many areas of the cortex other than area 4. Also, only a fraction of descending axons in the corticospinal tract synapse directly on alpha motor neurons: Many reach other, intermediate, motor centers in the brainstem and spinal cord. This lack of monosynaptic connection means that corticospinal projections differ little from rubrospinal, vestibulospinal, and reticulospinal pathways in terms of their anatomic relationship to the lower motor neuron: Cortical commands become but one component of several major descending brain-

spinal and spinal-spinal systems that eventually converge on the anterior horn cells to synergize voluntary movement with necessary postural responses. Furthermore, although basal ganglia and the brainstem motor control mechanisms have been traditionally grouped together as parts of an extrapyramidal "system," damage to one or the other of these systems produces entirely different neurologic abnormalities, as discussed later in this chapter.

By sharing the common principle of descending from higher levels to regulate coordinated motor activity by way of the segmental internuncial pool, the corticospinal and bulbospinal descending motor tracts actually work *in parallel* with each other. The arrangement can make it difficult or impossible to analyze by clinical means alone the specific contribution of each individual system to normal body movement. Similarly the mechanisms of abnormal movement may be equally difficult to assign to the involvement or release of one particular descending pathway. In evaluating motor disorders that originate in structures above the lower motor neuron one often can be no more specific than to define a level of the nervous system above which motor control no longer works normally; below the level of the lesion motor abnormalities due to damage of the descending pathways often blend together more than they separate into different functional patterns that reflect damage to anatomically identifiable components. As a result, abnormalities of the directly descending motor pathways are best grouped together as *disorders of the upper motor neuron*. The term distinguishes them, as do their signs and symptoms, from diseases of the anterior horn cell or its processes called *disorders of the lower motor neuron* as well as from disorders of the basal ganglia and cerebellum as discussed in the following paragraphs.

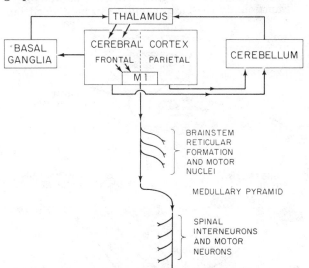

Figure 18. The principal supranuclear influences on motor control, greatly simplified. The cerebral cortex signals both the basal ganglia and the neocerebellum before initiating movement. These latter two structures in turn predominantly feedforward to the cerebral cortex via the thalamus to guarantee the postural supports as well as the rapid, smooth, and coordinated steps necessary for skilled or automatic motor acts. Motor behavior itself is directly controlled by the successive cerebral brainstem and spinal levels of the upper and lower motor neuron systems.

The basal ganglia and cerebellum differ in a major way from the upper motor neuron systems described above in how they influence motor control (Fig. 18). Neither of these structures actually appears to initiate movement. Rather, both systems receive information from the cerebral cortex *before movement starts*, integrate those signals with their own, pre-existing information received from other afferent pathways, and return the processed information back to the cortex where it influences the subsequent corticobulbar spinal signal. In contrast to the descending parallel pathways of the upper motor neuron system, the basal ganglia and neocerebellar outflows both represent cortical-noncortical-cortical feedforward systems that reconverge on the cerebral cortex to influence the coming and continuing pattern of corticobulbar spinal discharge. In the sense that they precede its ultimate messages to lower motor centers and neurons, the basal ganglia and cerebellum can be seen to lie in series rather than in parallel with the upper motor neuron.

BASAL GANGLIA

Functional Anatomy

The structures of the basal ganglia include the caudate, putamen, globus pallidus, and the subthalamic nucleus. The paired nuclei lie deep in the cerebral hemispheres largely anterolateral to the thalamus. They connect closely with each other as well as to the substantia nigra and red nucleus of the midbrain caudally, and to the frontal lobe of the cerebral cortex rostrally. As best can be determined the structures function entirely to regulate motor activity. Recently, however, the observed high incidence of dementia in certain basal ganglia diseases such as Hungtington's chorea, progressive supranuclear ophthalmoplegia, and Wilson's disease has stimulated inquiry into their possible influences on cognitive activity as well.

Functionally the basal ganglia can be divided into

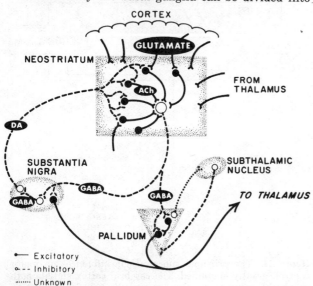

Figure 19. The principal pathways of the basal ganglia, their putative neurotransmitter, and function shown in greatly simplified form. *DA* = dopamine, *ACh* = acetylcholine, *GABA* = gamma-aminobutyric acid. (From Fahn, S.: The extrapyramidal disorders. In Wyngaarden, J. B., and Smith, L. H., Jr. (eds.): Cecil Textbook of Medicine. 17th ed. Philadelphia, W. B. Saunders Co., 1985.)

input and output zones (Fig. 19). The corpus striatum comprises the receiving area, receiving a large projection from the cerebral cortex, the midline thalamic nuclei, and the substantia nigra pars compacta. There is a cascade in the output of the basal ganglia going from the caudate nucleus to the putamen and thence to the globus pallidus. The globus pallidus represents the major output nucleus and divides its projections into three parts. The external segment of the globus pallidus projects to the subthalamic nucleus, which performs an as yet poorly understood function and projects back to the internal segment of the pallidum. The observation that damage to the subthalamic nucleus gives rise to the symptoms of ballism (p. 1053) implies that this loop in some way relates to controlling the postural stability of proximal muscles. Also, the basal ganglia receive important projections from the limbic system and project via the thalamus back to the prefrontal region of the frontal lobe. The functional implications of these connections are not known, although they may relate to some of the behavioral functions alluded to in the preceding paragraph.

The internal section of the globus pallidus sends out three major projections. The smallest and only direct descending pathway goes to the superior colliculus and the midbrain reticular formation where it may contribute to orienting the head, neck, and eyes in space. The second component descends to the reticular portion of the substantia nigra, closing the well-known feedback loop that exists between this structure and the basal ganglia. (Degeneration of the pars reticulata of the substantia nigra underlies the clinical disorder of parkinsonism.) Finally, the major output of globus pallidus projects to the ventral anterior nucleus of the thalamus whence it is relayed back to the premotor and precentral cortex of the frontal lobe.

Neurochemical Anatomy

The neurochemical anatomy of the basal ganglia to the extent that it is known follows the above anatomic lines. The main cortical input to the striatum is glutaminergic while the nigrostriatal input is dopaminergic (Table 14). Dopaminergic synapses probably exist on all neuronal types within the striatum although the functionally most important receptors appear to be localized on the terminals of incoming corticostriate fibers. A small mesencephalostriatal projection appears to be serotonergic. The striatum includes a substantial population of cholinergic interneurons whose principal functions appears to oppose or antagonize dopaminergic activity in the basal ganglia. This action explains the benefit derived from anticholinergic agents in parkinsonism and may also provide insight into the pathophysiology of schizophrenia, since the effectiveness of drugs in relieving symptoms of schizophrenia relates directly to their ability to block the central action of dopamine. The major outputs of the basal ganglia to all of its known projection areas predominantly employ gamma-aminobutyric acid (GABA) as a neurotransmitter and are probably inhibitory in nature.

A number of neuropeptides have been identified in the basal ganglia, including substance P, dynorphin and enkephalin, somatostatin, neurotensin, corticotropin releasing factor, vasoactive intestinal peptide, thyrotropic releasing hormone, cholecystokinin, and oth-

TABLE 14. NEUROTRANSMITTER-RELATED COMPOUNDS ASSOCIATED WITH STRIATAL INPUT—OUTPUT CONNECTIONS

NEUROTRANSMITTER-RELATED COMPOUNDS ASSOCIATED WITH EFFERENT CONNECTIONS		NEUROTRANSMITTER-RELATED COMPOUNDS ASSOCIATED WITH AFFERENT CONNECTIONS	
Compound	Pathway	Compound	Pathway
Certain		*Certain*	
GABA	Striatonigral and striopallidal	Dopamine	Nigrostriatal and tegmentostriatal pathways from cell groups A8,9,10; raphe-striatal from B7; possibly subthalamostriatal
Enkephalin	Striatopallidal to GP$_e$		
Substance P	Striatopallidal to GP$_i$ and strionigral		
Acetylcholine	In the cat, putaminocortical	Serotonin	Fibers from raphe nuclei, principally cell group B7
		Norepinephrine	Afferents from cell groups A1/A2,A5, and A6 (locus ceruleus)
Uncertain			
Angiotensin I/II	Strionigral and striopallidal	Glutamate; Aspartate	Corticostriatal (from neocortex and hippocampal formation); possibly thalamostriatal
Angiotensin converting enzyme			
Homocarnosine	Strionigral	Cholecystokinin	Fibers from the SN and VTA; fibers from the amygdala; fibers from the claustrum or the piriform cortex or both
Cholecystokinin	Strionigral and striopallidal		
Acetylcholinesterase	Strionigral	Acetylcholinesterase	Nigrostriatal
		Histamine	Via medial forebrain bundle
		Vasoactive intestinal polypeptide	Via medial forebrain bundle
		α-MSH; β-Lipotropin/ACTH	Hypothalamostriatal
		Uncertain	
		Acetylcholine	Thalamostriatal
		Monoamine (e.g., phenylethylamine)	Subthalamostriatal
		GABA	Pallidostriatal or nigrostriatal
		Somatostatin	?

From Graybiel, A. M., and Ragsdale, C. W., Jr.: Biochemical anatomy of the striatum. In Emson, P. C.: Chemical Neuroanatomy. Copyright 1983, Raven Press, New York.

ers. The functional significance is not known for any of these agents at the present time.

Functional Considerations

The basal ganglia influence normal motor movement in several complex ways, but the exact mechanisms of these influences have been difficult to unravel during normal motor function. Abnormalities observed with diseases of the basal ganglia, which are discussed later in this chapter, indicate that the structures influence postural control, regulate the speed of initiation and continuity of movement, and facilitate the capacity for simultaneous, mutually independent acts exemplified by movements such as waving goodbye while arising from a chair. They especially influence the proximal muscular control of movement. By feeding forward to the frontal cortex before that region finally signals the muscles to act, they exert a major influence in the planning and execution of movement and in establishing in the axial muscles the platform upon which the corticospinal tract can execute skilled distal activity.

CEREBELLUM

Functional Anatomy

The cerebellum initiates no movement but influences all neurally governed skeletal muscle action, including that which drives the eye movements and even the efferent components of the phasic stretch reflex. Gov-

erning its organization is the principle that each lateral cerebellar hemisphere influences movement on the ipsilateral side of the body while the midline of the cerebellum influences bilateral midline or ipsilateral trunk movements. The cerebellum acts through two major efferent routes to coordinate the movements of skeletal muscle. One pathway influences descending upper motor neuron activity via the latter's projections to the vestibular nuclei, the reticular formation, and craniospinal interneurons. The other consists of a large neocerebellar projection aimed rostrally from the cerebellar output nuclei to the contralateral ventrolateral thalamic nucleus whence the message is relayed to the premotor and motor cortex (Fig. 18). Through these connections the cerebellum imposes feedforward as well as feedback influences on voluntary movement since physiologic analysis shows that some neocerebellar cells related to movement fire a fraction of a second before the motor neurons in the cerebral cortex send their direct commands to the spinal motor neuron pool. Although the cerebellum helps to preprogram and coordinate movement, it does not directly initiate it: Patients with neocerebellar disease may complain of asthenia or inertia, and appropriate testing may even show signs of a mild reduction of muscle strength. The latter effect, however, appears to be mediated entirely through cerebellar influences on the corticospinal system.

The cerebellum directly or indirectly receives signals from every receptor that potentially influences reflex

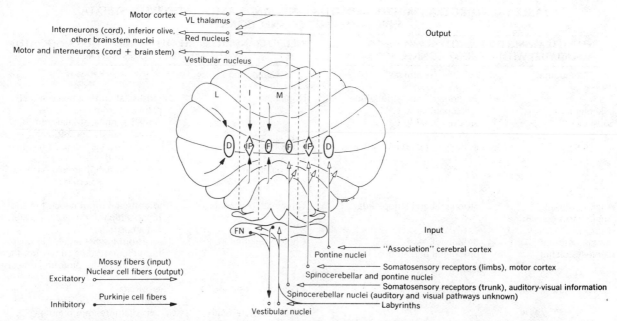

or intended movement, including skin, muscle, semicircular canals, vision, hearing, smell, taste, and programmed thought. Except for crossed projections that reach the cerebellum from the opposite cerebral hemisphere, all cerebellar afferents emanate from the ipsilateral side of the body. Figure 20 diagrams in gross outline the anatomy of these afferent pathways, their major targets in the cerebellum, and the cerebellar outflow nuclei that ultimately project the organ's message to other parts of the nervous system.

A few simple statements may set the stage for physiologic considerations. Afferent pathways destined for the cerebellum reach the structure either directly via *mossy fibers* or after first synapsing in the inferior olivary nucleus, which relays olivocerebellar *climbing fibers* (Fig. 21). Both types of afferents are excitatory in nature, and both send collaterals to the deep cerebellar output nuclei (roof nuclei) as they project toward the cerebellar cortex. Climbing fibers synapse directly on the dendrites of the Purkinje cells whose entire output delivers GABA-mediated inhibitory signals back to the roof nuclei. Mossy fibers synapse with granule cells, which, in turn, disperse their output to millions of cortical parallel fibers, huge numbers of which synapse with each Purkinje cell. The net effect of this circuitry is that the cerebellum's ultimate excitatory output from its roof nuclei consists of initial signals reflecting the immediate influence of incoming stimuli followed within milliseconds by the integrated, graded inhibition of internal cerebellar processing mediated via Purkinje cell circuits. The effect provides prompt damping to the motor action signal. Conversely, when this feedback damping is impaired, os-

cillation in the form of intention tremor results. Although all parts of the cerebellum send some fibers to each roof nucleus, the various anatomic areas of the cortex relate predominantly to particular nuclei, and these then project preferentially to specific areas in the rest of the brain. Thus the dentate nucleus receives its predominant input from the neocerebellar cortex and projects to the contralateral cerebral motor cortex via the ventrolateral nucleus of the thalamus. The fastigial nucleus receives most of its afferents from the cerebellar vermis and projects to the pontine and

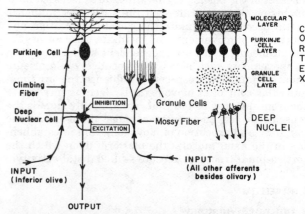

Figure 21. Basic neuronal circuit of the cerebellum. At right are the three major layers of the cerebellar cortex and also the deep nuclei. *E* = excitatory pathway; *I* = inhibitory pathway. (From Guyton, A. C.: Basic Human Neurophysiology. 3rd ed. Philadelphia, W. B. Saunders Co., 1981.)

medullary reticular formation while the nucleus interpositus takes its signals from the intermediate regions of the cerebellum and transmits its messages to the thalamus, the red nucleus, and the reticular formation, thereby bridging and integrating the output of the other deep nuclei.

Although signals from all parts of the body reach all parts of the cerebellum, a general somatotopic relationship still holds, both in terms of body maps and in a manner that reflects the evolutionary development of motor control. Phylogenetically the organ's functions are organized in a medial-to-lateral manner along the sagittal plane. The most primitive controls reside within the basal midline (the vermis) while the control of phylogenetically more recent movements relates to the large exfoliation of the lateral lobes whose development has paralleled the evolution of the human hand. In addition, physiologic studies in animals reveal a series of homotopic body maps lying, respectively, within the roof nuclei, along the paramedian anterior cerebellum, and aside the flocculonodular lobe. Cerebellar body maps drawn from animals give a picture of relatively heavy representation of the trunk and proximal limbs consistent with predominant movement patterns in those species; they reflect the strong association that exists between paramedian structures and the trunk and lower extremities in the human cerebellum.

In the human cerebellum, the nodulus makes up the most posterior portion of the vermis; together with its lateral extension, the flocculus, it interconnects directly with the vestibular nuclei, which serve as its roof nuclei and also provide its principal afferent relay nucleus. The flocculonodular lobe, sometimes called the *vestibulocerebellum,* functions most strongly to regulate by inhibitory modulation the influence of the labyrinthine-vestibular system on eye movements and on erect postural equilibrium. The effects of damage to the structure can be seen in certain degenerative diseases as well as during the early stages of medulloblastoma or other tumors that selectively damage the posterior vermis. Such abnormalities characteristically produce little functional change other than perhaps gaze-evoked nystagmus as long as the patient sits or reclines. Standing or walking, however, induces an immediate gait ataxia, the degree depending on the extent of nodular damage, and often accompanied by falling, especially backward. Damage to the nodulus impairs the normal plasticity of the vestibulo-ocular reflex and, in experimental animals, also abolishes the capacity for motion sickness.

The midline cerebellum extends anteriorly from the nodulus, where it receives information predominantly from spinal-bulbar proprioceptors that reach it via the ascending spinocerebellar tracts and pontine nuclei. The region coordinates these signals with exteroceptive information emanating from visual and auditory pathways. Sometimes called the *spinocerebellum,* the function of the anterior midline region relates primarily to movements during erect activities of the trunk and proximal limbs, especially of the lower extremity. Tumors of this region in children or adults, the effects of alcohol-nutritional disease, paraneoplastic cerebellar degeneration, and, rarely, other toxins can produce relatively selective cortical cell death in this region of the cerebellum. The result causes a distinctive syndrome characterized by broad-based ataxia, a strong extensor thrust of the legs during standing and walking (the positive supportive reaction), and short steppage, en bloc efforts in making turns. Mildly affected patients show neither nystagmus nor ataxia of the individual limbs on point-to-point tests, and few or no abnormalities are usually present in deep tendon reflexes. Patients with more severe cases, perhaps reflecting more extensive degeneration along the vermis and paramedian portions of the anterior cerebellum, also develop hyperactive deep tendon reflexes, lower limb ataxia on heel-to-knee testing, and, rarely, nystagmus.

The lateral portions of the cerebellar hemispheres (the *neocerebellum*) function largely to regulate the speed, skill, and coordination of motor activity in tasks involving learned movement, especially as they relate to the distal upper extremity. Dysarthria occurs with cerebellar damage but has been difficult to localize, correlations having been made with either injuries to the region of the anterior vermis or to the hemispheres, especially the left. In general, disturbances in vocal function are rare with cerebellar disease except when disease involves the roof nuclei and their projections. Despite its large size, much of the physiology of the lateral cerebellar cortex is poorly understood. Even very extensive damage to the structure, for example by surgical removal, induces only a minimum of testable dysfunction so long as the dentate nucleus and its outflow pathway along the superior brachium conjunctivum peduncle are spared. Damage to the latter structures produces immediate and sustained abnormalities in the coordination of appendicular movement as described on page 1068.

THE NORMAL CEREBRAL CONTROL OF MOVEMENT

General Considerations

The cerebral cortex primarily directs voluntary motor acts. Concurrently, it also activates lower, phylogenetically more primitive motor areas that generate the automatic associated activity of skeletal muscles that underpins almost every aspect of normal body movement. To reemphasize a point made earlier, the human cerebral cortex has evolved by a process called *encephalization* to command and guide lower motor centers that at one time in the history of the race operated independently. The reversal of this process by disease, called *dissolution*, provides a key to understanding many disorders of motor function: Damage to higher centers *releases* caudally placed and primitively evolved motor controlling areas to exhibit functions that normally lie hidden within the complexities of evolved higher control. Such pathologic release mechanisms underlie many of the abnormalities in motor control described in the next section of this chapter.

Human motor activity reflects the neural output from several areas of the frontal lobes, continuously integrated with guidance information provided from postcentral cortical perceptual areas (chiefly in the parietal and occipital lobes) as well as from subcortical regions and peripheral receptors. Voluntary movement is a sensorimotor function that requires constant interplay between both effector and receptor areas of the cortex and its subcortical nuclei.

Much of human movement is individually learned and its initiation appears to be preprogrammed in areas of association cortex of the frontal and parietal lobes. Reflecting this preprogramming, electrical recordings from the skull surface show that a burst of unconsciously experienced cerebral activity precedes voluntary acts, even seemingly automatic ones, by several hundred milliseconds. Present thinking is that this *cerebral readiness potential* reflects the activity of programming areas of the brain signaling the cerebellum, basal ganglia, and sensory areas of the cortex to feed forward to the cortex signals that will guarantee the smooth flow of the forthcoming rapidly initiated movement. As discussed in the next section, once the skilled movement begins, peripheral inputs from stretch receptors and other proprioceptors in the body come into play to an amount depending on the rate and amplitude of the movement. The larger and slower the motion the greater is the peripheral influence. At the cortical level, neurons on both the anterior (motor-sensory) and posterior (sensory-motor) side of the central, rolandic fissure fire in accompaniment with every motor act. The findings imply a constant feedback control of the final efferent discharge by local cortical circuits.

Functional Anatomy

The areas of the frontal lobe (Fig. 22) that apply especially to the execution of movement include the primary motor cortex (area 4), lying along the precentral gyrus, the premotor cortex (area 6), lying on the

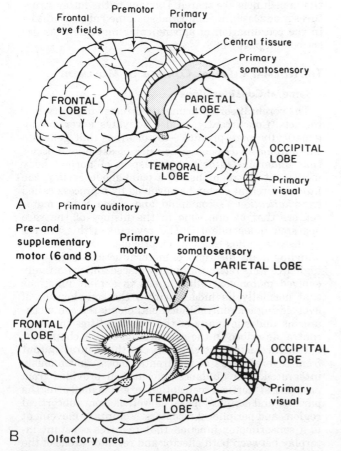

Figure 22. Lateral *(A)* and medial *(B)* views of cerebral cortex areas especially related to the control of movement, as described in text.

lateral surface immediately anterior to area 4, the supplementary motor area (6S), lying on the medial surface immediately anterior to 4, and the lateral and medial prefrontal area, anterior to the premotor cortex. The orbital frontal area of the cortex relates less exclusively to motor behavior.

In addition to these large, well-defined motor regions, specialized areas of the premotor area called the frontal eye fields influence the cortical control of saccadic voluntary eye movement while the occipital lobes send a projection directly to the brainstem to influence reflex visual pursuit movements (p. 1110). Parietal areas 7, influencing visuomotor function, and 5, influencing spatiomotor function, project heavily to the premotor and supplementary motor areas, respectively. These sensory association regions appear to be involved in the cortical preprogramming of stimulus-related movement. The area of the primary sensory cortex, 3,1,2, which lies within the postcentral gyrus, integrates so closely with the precentral gyrus containing area 4 that some authorities consider the two regions to be interdependent and designate them together as the primary sensorimotor cortex.

Experiments studying changes in regional cerebral blood flow in normal man by radiographic tracer techniques demonstrate graphically the complex interrelationships that tie cortical and subcortical areas together in guiding and regulating voluntary movement. In the normal brain, synaptic activity, metabolic requirement, and blood flow are coupled closely and directly together so that when a given structure's blood flow increases or decreases, one can infer that similar changes have occurred in neuronal activity. Studies of changes in cerebral blood flow during movement reveal that widely distributed areas of the cerebrum jointly participate in even highly lateralized, unilateral, programmed skilled movement. For example, during rapid successive finger movement of one hand, blood flow (metabolic activity) increased bilaterally in *both* the supplementary motor areas, in the paracentral and opercular regions of both parietal lobes, and in both premotor areas as well as bilaterally in the putamen, caudate, and thalamus. Only the sensorimotor hand area of the cortex and the globus pallidus that lie contralateral to the moving hand appeared to operate completely or largely unilaterally during the complex skilled movement. In contrast to these widely distributed and largely bilateral flow-metabolic changes during complex activity, simple successive or tonically contracting movements of a single finger appear to require much less extensive cerebral directions: With such simple motions, detectable increases of flow were confined to the contralateral sensorimotor cortex. An additional experiment served to illustrate the cerebral work involved in planning movement; when subjects repeatedly simulated in their minds the preprogrammed successive motor task but did not move the hand itself, cerebral blood flow increased only in the bilateral supplementary motor areas. The changes observed in the paracentral or parietal areas associated with active movement were absent, and no region of the cerebrum unilaterally lit up on the radiation detectors. The findings emphasize the importance of the bilateral supplementary motor cortex in the preplanning of motor acts, the immediate and constant participation of parietal lobe sensory areas in executing those acts, and the fact that only the contralateral sensori-motor cortex is directly involved in giving the final commands to the lower motor neuron pool.

The Corticobulbar-Corticospinal System

Area 4, the region that occupies the precentral gyrus of each hemisphere, contains the primary motor area, sometimes called by physiologists, M1. The area as indicated above closely integrates with the primary sensory cortex, termed S1, as a sensorimotor cortex.

The corticospinal pathway is the executive servant of the forebrain. Ideational (association cortex), pre-motor, proprioceptive, cerebellar, extrapyramidal, and special sensory inputs all feed indirectly or directly into M1 and are integrated there so as to tune, coor-dinate, adjust, and continuously modify the cortical signals that initiate every normal behavioral move-ment we consciously (and most we unconsciously) un-dertake. The primary motor cortex, like the special sensory cortices, is organized into columns, each con-taining six layers of cells; the four upper layers receive information from other cortical and subcortical regions, while layers five and six include the large and small efferent pyramidal neurons that send their axons to the descending corticospinal tract. Studies of single pyramidal neurons in the M1 cortex of monkeys indi-cate that the output of each cortical column relates to movement around a single joint on the opposite side of the body with adjacent neurons innervating related movements rather than adjacent peripheral muscle fibers. Furthermore, each column may participate in more than one movement, depending upon preset in-fluences emanating from other areas of cortex. Al-though each muscle is probably "represented" by many cortical motor neurons, as Hughlings Jackson, the great English neurologist, proposed over a century ago, the cortex "acts in terms of movement not muscles."

Each corticospinal tract contains many more fibers than there are cells in area 4 with areas 6 and 3,1,2 contributing to it. Some axons arise in other more distant cortical areas as well. Among the contributions from area 4, the large pyramidal Betz cells actually contribute but a minority of the fibers; the respective functions of the large versus the many small efferent neurons in area 4 presently are not well understood. At least some of the small cells relate to the control of the gamma, fusimotor muscle spindle system while others project to lower motor centers, e.g., in the red nucleus and the bulbospinal reticular formation. Pre-motor fibers from other areas of the cortex also appear to descend in the corticospinal tract to ipsilaterally located motor neurons so as to influence the bilateral automatic associated trunk and postural responses that underpin skilled voluntary movement. Furthermore, the effects of experiments in animals and of disease in humans indicate that almost every level of the nervous system generates descending motor influences that take routes outside the accepted anatomic boundaries of the corticospinal pathway. As a result, injury or even section of the corticospinal tract anywhere along its length produces only partial motor paralysis, al-ways most affecting acts involving the rapid and skilled activity of the vocal apparatus, the face, or the distal muscles of the extremities.

In human beings only about 20 per cent of the fibers that descend in the corticospinal tract to the bulbar or spinal level appear to end directly on anterior horn motor neurons. The remainder terminate in internun-cial cells adjacent to the motor neurons where they join other descending and segmental pathways con-verging on the final common path. Clinical evaluation of upper motor neuron abnormalities in humans usu-ally can provide an accurate indication of the level of the nervous system where such abnormalities origi-nate. The complexities of the system, however, often make it difficult to identify exactly which among the several components of the upper motor neuron pool is specifically at fault.

THE COMPONENTS OF THE MOTOR ACT

Before considering specific abnormalities in move-ment that result from injury to the motor system, it may be useful to examine the mechanisms that under-lie the peripheral components of learned motor acts. Most motor acts in humans consist of a continuum of a fast start that gradually decelerates into a slower follow-through. The initial fast-off-the-mark muscular events that begin most learned skills or complex motor defense acts follow the onset of a command, an idea, or a sensory stimulus with a latency of only about 200 msec. This interval is too brief to be guided by afferent-efferent proprioceptive reflexes that must travel to the sensory cortex from peripheral joint position and stretch receptors and back. Called *ballistic* (literally "throwing") movements, these fast, cortically gener-ated initial actions are exemplified vividly by the skilled pianist's dancing fingers or the tennis champi-on's quick net play. As a moment's reflection will bear out, however, a fast start initiates almost any sudden change of movement, not only such highly learned activities. Such ballistic activity appears to complete itself independently of peripheral feedback information and in large measure must be preprogrammed by circuits arising locally in the cerebral cortex. Much of it depends upon continued learning and practice. EMG recordings taken during ballistic movements show rapid, bursting muscle discharges alternating between agonists and antagonists at a rate too fast to be regulated by segmental stretch reflexes. The sequence indicates repetitive activation and braking of the mus-cles by automatically generated commands coming from supraspinal centers.

Once anatomically started, learned movement enters a slower, proprioceptively governed targeting phase termed *ramp* or *pursuit movements*. Ramp movements consist of pursuing or tracking acts, such as the smooth follow-through that characterizes the tennis player's baseline stroke or the gradual pursuit activity of the fielder's eyes and head as he follows a baseball as it rises from the bat. Ramp movements of the extremities are influenced heavily in their smoothness and accu-racy by information received from peripheral receptors and relayed polysynaptically to the cerebellum, the basal ganglia, and the cerebral cortex. EMG recordings during such movements show a continuous, necessarily somewhat fluctuating but smoothly contoured, dis-charge so long as the ramp movement persists.

The full physiology of the rapid initiation of move-ment is still incompletely understood. As noted earlier, both the basal ganglia and the cerebellum feed forward to the motor and premotor areas of the cortex rather than sending descending impulses directly to lower motor neurons. The structures contribute in different ways to the rapid-action corticospinal programs that finally govern the initiation of voluntary movement, differences that become evident when disease strikes the basal ganglia or cerebellum. Corticospinal system dysfunction also produces noticeable delays in the initiation of voluntary movement but, again, not in a manner that precisely imitates the effects of either the basal ganglia or cerebellar disease. Even without knowing the precise mechanism, experienced clinical appraisal usually can distinguish readily among these three potentially deranged motor systems when appraising functional difficulties that involve the initiation or follow-through of voluntary motor acts.

PATHOPHYSIOLOGY OF SYMPTOMS AND SIGNS OF MOTOR SYSTEM DYSFUNCTION

Asthenia, Fatigue, and Weakness

Each of these closely related symptoms relates to motor activity in different ways.

Asthenia. Asthenia is a nonspecific feeling of subacute or chronic generalized lassitude. Affected persons describe feeling weak before they start or state that a greater than normal effort is required to initiate tasks of any kind. Such individuals are hesitant to undertake motor activity, fearing that their strength or endurance may be insufficient to the anticipated requirement. The symptom can reflect either physiologic or psychologic abnormalities. Small reductions in motor power or impaired endurance may be difficult for the observer to measure, so that asthenia sometimes reflects the presence of a true but clinically marginal motor weakness such as occurs in mild myasthenia gravis or in the early course of acute polyneuropathy. Similarly, prominent asthenia sometimes accompanies the onset of the myopathy of thyrotoxicosis. The symptom also can accompany acute lateral cerebellar dysfunction, presumably reflecting impairment of that structure's neocortical feedback loop. Asthenia also is expressed as part of the complex difficulty in initiating movement that accompanies parkinsonism. Non-neurogenic asthenia accompanies several systemic non-neuromuscular disorders, including those enumerated below in the paragraph describing fatigue.

Organically based asthenia generally can be identified by its relatively recent onset and the fact that it coincides with other symptoms, signs, or laboratory findings of systemic illness. Subacute or chronic asthenia (neurasthenia, formerly called effort syndrome) contributes prominently to the symptoms of anxiety or depression. Its physiology reflects perturbation originating at the level of the brain rather than of the nerves or muscles; in such instances the symptom may be accompanied by signs of autonomic imbalance, including tachycardia, recurrent sighing, multifocal blushing, and inappropriate sweating of the hands and feet.

Fatigue. An abnormal rate or degree of exhaustion following activity is referred to as fatigue. Abnormal fatigue can be local or generalized in distribution and acute, subacute, or chronic in duration. Many systemic illnesses tend to produce at least a brief sense of generalized lassitude, purposelessness, and easy exhaustion in their wake. Most normal persons have experienced similar sensations following nothing more severe than an intercurrent virus infection. More serious diseases produce even more prominent fatigability. Fatigue is also a notable symptom of certain chronic neurologic disorders such as parkinsonism and, especially, multiple sclerosis, in which its consistency implies a central neurogenic basis. Almost nothing is known of the physiology of either fatigue or asthenia in its chronic state. *Local* acute fatigability with a rapid decline in strength after repeated movement of a particular group of muscles is characteristic of myasthenia gravis (see below). Less easily measurable feelings of muscle tiredness also accompany local peripheral motor neuropathy, radiculopathy, or incipient myopathy. Chronic fatigue that remains unexplained by a careful search for systemic or neuromuscular causes may have a psychogenic basis, but this is less likely than with asthenia.

Acute fatigue states usually have a clearly metabolic or musculoskeletal origin and generally can be referred to the development of acute illness or, more frequently, to episodes of unusual exercise or muscular hyperactivity. Almost all kinds of muscular or neuromuscular weakness lower the threshold for the involved part to tire after vigorous effort, but chronic overwork rarely is a justifiable explanation for persistent somatic fatigue. The timing of fatigue helps in identifying its probable basis: Organically engendered fatigue states are worse in the evening than in the morning. They are accentuated by further activity and typically relieved by sleep. Psychogenic fatigue follows the opposite pattern, victimizing its host maximally in the morning and giving way to a measure of enthusiasm and energy as the day's social pace increases.

Weakness. Weakness is a loss of strength usually complained of as inability to complete a specific and familiar act. Insidiously developing weakness, especially that due to upper motor neuron dysfunction, often goes unrecognized by the sufferer, and patients sometimes ignore even prominent degrees of weakness until it finally becomes apparent to friends ("Your foot drags"; "Why are you limping?") or is brought out by an examiner's tests. Weakness is best appraised or quantified in functional terms: What common acts can the patient not perform? Grading systems of strength such as that published by the British Medical Research Council provide numerical indices, 0 equaling none up to 5 designating normal, but actually say little more about the disability than do classifications that simply quantify weakness as mild, moderate, or severe. A small "Memorandum" published by the Council, however, provides a valuable and inexpensive pictorial guide to testing individual muscles and for judging the specific nerve or root causing specific patterns of lower motor neuron weakness.

The recognition of certain patterns of weakness is a useful diagnostic step, especially when sensory function is appraised concurrently. Loss of strength can reflect disease or dysfunction of muscle, neuromuscular junction, peripheral nerve or root, anterior horn cell, the upper motor neuron, the basal ganglia motor systems, and even hysteria or malingering. Weakness, mainly of muscular origin, also can develop from indirect involvement of the locomotor system as a reflection of generalized metabolic dysfunction such as occurs with hypokalemia, hyperthyroidism or hypothyroidism, certain drug intoxications, and in the setting of the generalized debilitation of starvation or cancer. Painful areas of bone and joint inflammation often induce local, non-neurogenic weakness as part of a psychologic protective response directed at avoiding the further pain that movement would bring. Occasionally, weakness also can be a major complaint with acute disorders of the sensory system, especially certain sensory neuropathies as described on page 1085, even when no direct evidence of interruption of motor control occurs. The following paragraphs describe patterns of weakness that often accompany specific motor disorders and whose recognition can be useful in diagnosis.

Myopathies, diseases intrinsic to muscle, produce weakness because of damage or dysfunction involving the end-organ itself. The category includes three major subgroups, namely, the inherited muscular dystrophies, the inherited and acquired metabolic myopathies, and the inflammatory myopathies. Weakness in myopathy may begin insidiously and progress slowly (all dystrophies and most inherited myopathies), begin recently and progress rapidly (acquired metabolic or inflammatory myopathies), be episodic (periodic paralysis), or remain constant (congenital myopathy). Myotonia (p. 1050) accompanies both a congenital myopathy (Thomsen's congenital myotonia) and a progressive (myotonic) dystrophy. Muscles sometimes are tender in the inflammatory myopathies.

The geography of weakness in myopathy varies depending upon the particular disorder, each of which tends to produce a relatively distinct syndrome. The patterns of weakness in the muscular dystrophies are indicated in Table 15. Pseudohypertrophy (p. 1049) develops in several muscular dystrophies, especially Duchenne's, as well as in congenital myotonia. Except where pseudohypertrophy occurs, however, the involved muscles in most progressive myopathies atrophy late and slowly as their fibers degenerate. Deep tendon reflexes are preserved in most of the myopathies (periodic paralysis and hypokalemia being exceptions), providing a contrast to many neuropathies in which

they are lost early. EMGs (p. 1092) tend to be characteristic: The muscle is silent at rest or may show occasional spontaneous fibrillation potentials, reflecting degenerating fibers. Since individual motor units shrink as their fibers randomly drop out, voluntary activity produces electrical signals of lower amplitude and shorter duration than normal. Sensory changes are absent.

Major junctional disease, i.e., *myasthenia gravis* (MG) and the *Eaton-Lambert Myasthenic Syndrome* (EAMS) are due to autoimmune processes affecting neuromuscular transmission as described in the second chapter of this section. In myasthenia, some postsynaptic receptors degenerate, while the normal amount of ACh released from the nerve terminal by neurotransmission rapidly saturates the remainder. This results in fatigability of repeated effort, the hallmark of the disease. Most often weakness affects the bulbar muscles, particularly the oculomotor groups, and next most frequently those of the neck and proximal limbs. Except for single oculomotor muscles, weakness usually is symmetric. Atrophy occurs late if at all and reflects disuse, since actual denervation does not take place. Fasciculations are absent, and deep tendon reflexes are present or reduced, depending on the degree of initial weakness. The EMG shows successively declining muscle potentials to repetitive motor nerve stimulation. No sensory changes occur.

In EAMS, circulating antibodies, often released from oat cell carcinoma of the lung, interfere with calcium entry into the nerve terminal and reduce the normal probability of the first quantal release of ACh by a nerve impulse. Repeated stimulation improves the defect so that weakness tends to be maximal with first effort and to lessen with repeated tries. Weakness affects mainly the limbs, sparing the extraocular and bulbar muscles. Atrophy does not occur; deep tendon reflexes are reduced; and sensory changes are lacking. The EMG characteristically shows a successive increase in evoked potential size to repeated motor nerve stimulation.

Peripheral nerve weakness can take two major forms. Damage to a single nerve is called *mononeuropathy,*

TABLE 15. CLASSIFICATION OF THE MOST FREQUENT HUMAN MUSCULAR DYSTROPHIES

	DUCHENNE DYSTROPHY	FACIOSCAPULOHUMERAL DYSTROPHY	LIMB-GIRDLE DYSTROPHY	MYOTONIC DYSTROPHY
Genetic pattern	X-linked, recessive	Autosomal, dominant	Autosomal, recessive	Autosomal, dominant
Age at onset	Before age 5	Adolescence	Adolescence	Early or late
First symptoms	Pelvic	Shoulders	Pelvic	Distal; hands or feet
Pseudohypertrophy	+	0	0	0
Predominant weakness, early	Proximal	Proximal	Proximal	Distal
Progression	Relatively rapid; incapacitated in adolescence	Slow	Variable	Slow
Facial weakness	0	+	0	Occasional
Ocular, oropharyngeal weakness	0	0	0	Occasional
Myotonia	0	0	0	+
Cardiomyopathy	0 or late	0	0	Arrhythmia, conduction block
Associated disorders	None (?mental retardation)	None	None	Cataracts; testicular atrophy and baldness in men
Serum enzymes	Very high	Slight or no increase	Slight or no increase	Slight or no increase

Adapted from Rowland, L. P.: Diseases of the muscle and neuromuscular junction. In Wyngaarden, J. B., and Smith, L. H., Jr. (eds.): Cecil Textbook of Medicine. 17th ed. Philadelphia, W. B. Saunders Co., 1985.

while diffuse involvement is termed *polyneuropathy* (p. 1089). An intermediate condition *(multiple mononeuropathy)* occurs when several individual nerves are damaged at various points along their courses. Weakness due to motor mononeuropathy is flaccid, focal, often severe, and follows a functional pattern dictated by the specific muscles that lose their innervation. Pressure or trauma to the nerve is the most common cause. The ensuing reflex or sensory changes depend upon which joint is paralyzed and the anatomy of the particular nerve's sensory distribution, if any. With multiple mononeuropathies, similar principles apply except to produce a multifocal distribution that often takes a patchwork pattern and may blend into the clinical picture of a diffuse polyneuropathy. Weakness due to diffuse polyneuropathy usually affects the two sides of the body symmetrically and involves lower limbs, upper limbs, or cranial nerves, roughly in that order of frequency, sometimes all together. The muscles are flaccid, and weakness most often predominates distally, seldom proximally. With severe weakness, denervation atrophy appears early and can usually be detected within less than two weeks of onset. Deep tendon reflexes are reduced to absent early in the course, and this plus the pronounced early atrophy or the association of sensory changes usually rules out a myopathy. If sensory nerves are affected, paresthesias and sometimes pain affect the paralyzed members. In most acute polyneuropathies weakness predominates over sensory loss.

Electrical changes in the nerves depend on the nature of the neuropathy as described on page 1093. To anticipate briefly, in the inflammatory-demyelinating neuropathies, large fibers are affected preferentially so that conduction velocity slows early. In axonal neuropathies the large most rapidly conducting fibers tend to be spared, and conduction velocities often remain normal. Electrical changes in the muscle following nerve injury depend upon the severity and the time after the onset of denervation that the studies are performed. Immediately following interruption of axonal supply the muscle at rest acts normally and is electrically silent. During efforts to move, it develops a reduction of the number of normal contraction potentials (reduced interference pattern). Sometime after about three weeks, electrical signs of denervation emerge and include fibrillations and fasciculations, described later.

Motor neuron diseases describe a group of axonal neuropathies usually of an infectious, hereditary, or idiopathic nature in which the motor axon and, either immediately or eventually, its anterior horn cell sicken and die. Toxic neuronopathies such as those associated with acute intermittent porphyria may cause a similar but reversible picture but are more commonly classified with the peripheral neuropathies. The development of weakness can be rapid, as with acute poliomyelitis, insidious but moderately rapid, as with amyotrophic lateral sclerosis (ALS), or extremely slow, as occurs with some of the pure motor neuron diseases called progressive muscular atrophy (PMA). Some of the latter can run a course of as long as 30 years or more. The degree of weakness in motor neuron disease depends on the stage of the disease, while the pattern of weakness reflects a bulbospinal motor neuron distribution rather than one of spinal roots or peripheral

nerves. With the acute or subacute forms of motor neuron disease the major damage can affect either lower bulbar or spinal motor nuclei, and upper motor neuron dysfunction characteristically produces spasticity and abnormal reflexes. With the slower PMA, bulbar motor nuclei are involved either very late or, usually, not at all. In either ALS or PMA, oculomotor nuclei are very rarely involved and then only late. If the upper motor neuron is spared as occurs with the hereditary peroneal nerve atrophy (Charcot-Marie-Tooth) group or the various PMAs, flaccid, distally distributed weakness is associated with early muscle atrophy, reduction or absence of regional deep tendon reflexes, the frequent appearance of fasciculations, and either no sensory changes (in progressive muscular atrophy) or minimal loss (in peroneal muscular atrophy). Neurophysiologic studies generally show normal nerve conduction velocities in early stages with slow responses or absence of responses as the disease advances to total paralysis. Affected muscles show EMG evidence of fibrillation, varying sized fasciculations (due to distal sprouting and partial reinnervation as described on p. 1092), and reduced interference patterns during efforts at muscular contraction.

Upper motor neuron (UMN) disease produces changes that contrast in many dimensions with those of the lower motor neuron disorders (Table 4) (although some motor diseases such as ALS attack both the upper and the lower motor neuron system). Weakness in UMN disease can range from minimal to complete and typically affects distal more than proximal parts and movements rather than selective muscles. Deep tendon reflexes are accentuated, and resistance to passive stretch of the weak members is increased (spasticity). Atrophy occurs only after some weeks or months, is moderate in degree, and secondary to disuse, not denervation. Electrical studies of nerve and muscle remain normal except for failure to develop the normal interference pattern during attempted movement.

Akinesia

Akinesia, the absence of or delayed initiation of movement, or *bradykinesia* (slower than normal movement), can be observed in several neurologic and some psychiatric disorders. Bradykinesia is by far the more frequent of the two states. Affected patients, though fully awake and able to understand the need to move, make a paucity of spontaneous body movements compared to normal persons. Few emotional expressions spontaneously cross their faces; their eyelids blink infrequently; they hold head, neck, body, and arms as still as if semiparalyzed; and often they speak slowly, monotonously, and at a low pitch. When they move they are slow to start, commonly labored in their efforts, and may show specific associated abnormalities as indicated in the later discussion of basal ganglia diseases.

Generalized akinesia or hypokinesia can accompany a number of neurologic disorders, especially those of cerebral origin, including many of the metabolic encephalopathies, especially myxedema, starvation, or anoxia-hypercarbia. Generalized akinesia also can be pronounced with disorders causing paramedian damage to the ventromedial diencephalon and to the adjacent medial-inferior surfaces of the frontal lobe. In most instances of the latter condition, both appendicular and vocal muscles are involved (akinetic mutism). Affected persons, although awake, remain apathetically voiceless and appear to possess reduced cognitive awareness as well as severely impaired psychologic motivation. The abnormality has been attributed to interruption of ascending dopaminergic pathways in the hypothalamic region. In most akinetic mutism, however, the administration of either the dopamine precursor, levodopa, or dopamine agonists has little beneficial effect. Bradykinesia also occurs as a symptom of severe psychologic depression, in which it is called *psychomotor retardation*. Whether the motor retardation reflects lack of motivation or relates to the known reduction of 5-hydroxytryptamine and catecholamines found in the brains of severe depressives is not presently known. Reserpine, which depletes the brain of amines, causes bradykinesia as well as depression, while the tricyclic antidepressants, which potentiate central aminergic action, have the opposite effect. The pharmacology is complicated, however, since phenothiazines, which act as dopamine-blocking agents, also cause bradykinesia but do not induce concomitant depression of mood.

As a specific symptom, bradykinesia emerges most often in the syndrome of parkinsonism (p. 1067) in which its appearance relates closely to the known striatal dopaminergic loss in the disease. The initiation of movement is delayed in parkinsonism. In addition, the normal automatic associated skeletal muscle movements, which accompany such physical acts as walking or running, may be reduced or absent. Voluntary movements are both slow to begin and retarded in completion as if the patient were pushing himself through thick mud. Impairment in the initiation of rapid movement also can accompany the motor defects of neocerebellar and UMN disease. In these latter conditions, however, the akinesia is more specifically limited to the very first, ballistic component of the motor act and affects the subsequent components of motor activity less prominently.

Atrophy, Hypertrophy, and Other Physical Changes of Muscle

The size and shape of the bodily musculature varies widely among normal persons. For that reason either symmetrically small or large muscles require cautious evaluation before they can be considered pathologic. Asymmetric or focal changes of either shrinkage (atrophy) or enlargement (hypertrophy) extending beyond the norm for the remainder of the body's size and the person's occupational and recreational habits imply an abnormality that requires medical investigation.

Muscle Atrophy. Aside from the general wasting of starvation, specific atrophy in muscle reflects degeneration, disuse, or denervation. Muscular degeneration occurs gradually in the inherited muscular dystrophies and to a lesser degree and frequency but more rapidly in the acquired myopathies such as polymyositis and thyrotoxicosis. Disuse atrophy can come about by either external immobilization of the muscles or their denervation: When one casts a joint to immobilize it following a fracture, the associated muscles atrophy as rapidly as if their nerves had been cut.

As already noted, muscular atrophy is uncommon in the diseases of the myoneural junction except in occasional patients who suffer prolonged, therapeutically refractory disease so that chronic weakness and immobility gradually give way to disuse atrophy.

Neurogenic atrophy is one of the classic expressions of lower motor neuron disease. Clinically, acute denervation of multiple motor units (e.g., by acute severe polyneuropathy or cutting a nerve) can result in clinically detectable muscle atrophy within as little as 10 days. Subacute or partial denervation as occurs with primary motor neuron disease (e.g., ALS, progressive spinal muscular atrophy) or milder neuropathies produces more slowly developing muscle atrophy whose clinical detection may be delayed by weeks or more after onset. Disease of the upper motor neuron or basal ganglia does not cause focal atrophy, although with profound hemiplegia or prolonged immobility the musculature of an entire limb eventually may waste moderately from disuse. Similarly, damage to parietal somatosensory cortex sometimes is followed by contralateral muscle atrophy in the limbs affected by sensory loss. Electrical studies of the atrophic muscles show no evidence of peripheral denervation, and the effect presumably reflects disuse due to a loss of sensory feedback and associated neglect of the member (p. 1054).

Neurogenic atrophy produces shrinkage of the individual fibers of the denervated motor units. In the absence of severe external immobilization or systemic debilitation, muscular atrophy distributed within patterns consistent with the anatomic supply of peripheral nerve, plexus, root, or anterior horn cells must be considered neurogenic until proved otherwise. Clinical suspicion of neurogenic muscular atrophy can be confirmed by electrical studies of the muscle, which usually begin to show electrical abnormalities about 18 to 21 days following denervation.

Hypertrophy. Muscle hypertrophy most often develops as a physiologic response to exercise and consists of an increase in size of pre-existing muscle fibers without an increase in number. Pathologic hypertrophy marks the course of *congenital myotonia* (Thomsen's disease) presumably because of the prolonged afterexcitation of muscle fibers (myotonia) that is associated with voluntary effort in that condition. Hypertrophy also affects repeatedly used muscles in the movement disorders of dystonia, athetosis, or myokymia, conditions described subsequently. In several muscular dystrophies, especially the Duchenne form (Table 15), many muscle fibers atrophy, while some of the remainder hypertrophy, and still others become overfilled with fat. This latter process gives the impression of an overall enlargement of some muscles. Such *pseudohypertrophy* occasionally can be observed in isolated calf muscles of apparently normal persons as an isolated anomaly of unknown cause.

Tactile Qualities. Skeletal muscle at rest normally is electrically silent, and its palpable qualities represent the non-neurogenic viscoelastic properties of the tissue itself. Normal muscle yields a sense of firm elasticity to touching or squeezing that reflects the trophic state of its fibrillar contents. Quantitative measurements are lacking, but experienced palpation readily discerns that muscles feel softer in comparably aged women than men and firmer in the athletically well conditioned than in the sedentary. Several primary diseases of muscle as well as conditions such as prolonged immobilization due to rheumatic-orthopedic problems, paralysis, sustained neurogenic rigidity, or dystonia can lead to secondary fibrotic and even calcific contractures of muscle that proportionately harden the organ's resistance to palpation. Denervated muscles feel soft unless replaced by connective tissue, while the pseudohypertrophic muscles of dystrophy have a woody, nonresilient feel, reflecting their mesenchymal infiltration.

Percussion of muscle may elicit myotonia or myoedema. *Myotonia* consists of a prolonged involuntary contraction of a group of adjacent muscle fibers following a self-limited voluntary effort or the abrupt percussion of the muscle with a reflex hammer. The condition is due to a hypersensitive postsynaptic muscle membrane that generates self-repetitive depolarizations and muscle afterdischarges following unsustained presynaptic stimulation (percussion can induce myotonia either by precipitating a local stretch reflex or directly depolarizing the fibers themselves). Myotonia may have more than one cause. An increase in sodium conductance of the muscle membrane has been suggested as fundamental to myotonic dystrophy, while an error in chloride permeability has been observed in the muscles of patients and of a strain of goats with congenital myotonia. Myotonia also occurs in some of the periodic paralyses as well as in normal persons taking drugs such as diazocholesterol that affect the lipid composition of muscle membranes.

Myoedema describes the development of a small (0.8 to 1.5 cm diameter) mound of local muscle contraction seen through the skin at the point of percussion with the apex of a reflex hammer. When present, the anomaly is most prominent over the proximal muscles of the upper extremity, but in severe cases can be elicited in almost any muscle. The zone of contraction is electrically silent and reflects direct hyperirritability of the muscle fibers usually associated with weight loss, nutritional insufficiency, or an endocrine disease such as myxedema.

Tenderness or pain results from stimulation of pain-sensitive nerve endings in the muscle. Several conditions can cause muscle pain, including local inflammation or a reduced pain threshold due to disease of the structure's afferent spinal nerve or root. Repeated muscle contraction of an ischemic limb produces severe pain, possibly via the release of potassium from an injured membrane. The pain associated with muscle cramps may have a similar pathogenesis. Pain and muscle stiffness following vigorous unaccustomed exercise may be due to sarcolemmal damage inasmuch as myoglobin can leak from the fiber during very intense muscular activity in unconditioned individuals. The irritating effects of degenerating hemoglobin pigments are believed to cause the pain of muscle hematomas, and the degradation of extracellular myoglobin may have a similar effect.

ADVENTITIOUS MOVEMENTS

Abnormal spontaneous adventitious movements can arise as a result of dysfunction or disease affecting skeletal muscle, motor axon, spinal cord, brainstem, the extrapyramidal motor system, and the cerebral cortex.

Spontaneous Muscle Movements

Myotonia is a stimulus-bound response, as discussed above.

Muscle Fibrillation. The recurrent spontaneous contraction of individual muscle fibers in denervated muscle is called muscle fibrillation. In normally innervated muscle, ACh receptors are concentrated most densely in the motor end-plate, and the general sarcolemmal membrane is resistant to locally applied neurotransmitter. Also, the electrical resistance of the motor end-plate itself is relatively high. Following denervation, acetylcholine receptors increase in number and distribute themselves more diffusely along the sarcolemmal membrane; hypersensitivity sets in within two to three weeks, making the entire membrane anywhere from 100 to 1000 times more sensitive than normal to low concentrations of ACh. Although ACh may no longer be released from the damaged axon terminal, circulating or locally diffusing amounts of transmitter cause the fiber to contract randomly at intervals of 2 to 10 seconds, producing tiny electrical signals of single fiber contractions that can be detected electromyographically. Such fibrillations are so fine as to be invisible to the naked eye except when the muscle is directly exposed.

Fasciculations. Fasciculations in muscle represent recurrent spontaneous depolarizations of the fibers of a single motor unit due to disease, injury, or intrinsic hypersensitivity of the anterior horn cell or its motor axon. Fasciculations can be detected electrically and usually visually. They have a delicate amplitude when they involve only a single motor unit and require close inspection under cross lighting to be seen with the naked eye. Subcutaneous fasciculations appear as quick, randomly, and irregularly occurring linear twitches. Single motor unit fasciculations are more easily observed on the trunk or proximally in the limbs, reflecting the large size of the degenerating motor units in those areas. As disease of the motor cells or their proximal axons progresses, however, individual perikarya die, and degeneration ultimately spreads to the distal axon. Under such circumstances, many of the denervated muscle fibers degenerate, but adjacent axons from still healthy neurons may sprout to reinnervate increasing numbers of fibers that have lost their original axon terminals. The result is that the longer a disease affecting motor neurons lasts, the larger become the motor units. As new neurons or axons then become damaged and hypersensitive, not only their original but all of their adopted motor fibers synchronously twitch together, resulting in increasingly large fasciculations. With chronic conditions such as spinal osteoarthritis of the neck, for example, which can slowly and gradually compress the axons innervating the shoulder girdle and upper extremity, giant fasciculations can incorporate the simultaneous activity of so many motor units that they visibly jerk the arm.

The molecular pathogenesis of fasciculations is not fully understood and may vary from disease to disease. In all instances, however, it involves hypersensitivity of the neuronal membrane to ACh. Although receptors have not been demonstrated on the nerve membrane, drugs such as prostigmine or edrophonium which inhibit acetylcholinesterase enhance fasciculations and, in large enough doses, actually can cause them. Once alpha motor neurons or their proximal axons begin to degenerate in a disease, increasing irritability appears to spread along the entire distal neuronal membrane.

Demonstrating this, anesthetic nerve blocks placed halfway down the axon of a fasciculating motor unit interrupt axoplasmic and electrical transmission from the perikaryon to the distal axon, but the remaining distal axon continues to generate fasciculations (but at a lower frequency) in the motor unit of the muscle.

Fasciculations most often reflect the presence of chronic primary degenerative disease of the anterior horn cell, although they occasionally can accompany any condition, such as disc disease or proximal axonopathies, that gradually damages the ventral horn, ventral root, or proximal motor axon. Diseases of the more distal motor axon, such as polyneuropathy, much less often induce fasciculations. Rarely, *benign fasciculations* occur chronically or recurrently in persons possessing no history or physical or laboratory evidence of neurologic disease. Such benign twitchings affect the calves and feet of many healthy persons, both young and old, especially during times of pressure or anxiety. Less often, such benign twitchings can be a normal occurrence in other parts of the body but should not be so diagnosed without careful evaluation when they are of recent origin.

Myokymia. Myokymia is an uncommon abnormality of muscle producing cascades of continuous, involuntary, fasciculation-like, quivering and rippling fine subcutaneous movements. It is associated with hereditary or acquired disorders of the motor neuron or its axon. The abnormality ceases neither during sleep nor with spinal anesthesia, findings that establish its peripheral origin. Myokymia does stop, however, with curarization, which blocks presynaptic but not postsynaptic excitation of the muscle membrane; the finding proves myokymia's neural origin. As with fasciculations, anesthetic blocks placed at successively more distal points along the axon progressively reduce but do not halt the abnormal movements, indicating that the hypersensitivity to stimulation must extend along the entire axonal membrane. EMG recordings of the resting muscles in myokymia demonstrate cascades of either normal motor units or fractions of motor unit potentials firing continuously and spontaneously at rapid rates ranging from 30 to 300 Hz. Single shocks applied to a peripheral nerve evoke repetitive afterdischarges that appear constantly to reexcite the motor nerve terminals so as to maintain the continuous spontaneous abnormal contractions. Myokymia involving the muscles innervated by the facial nerve can result from neoplasms or demyelinating plaques located in the neighborhood of the output of the facial nerve nucleus in the pons. In the extremities and trunk, myokymia occurs in association with either hereditary or acquired peripheral nerve disorders, or as an idiopathic phenomenon. More intense, presynaptic afterdischarges from the peripheral motor nerve terminals sometimes accompany efforts at voluntary movement in patients with myokymia and give rise to an inability to relax rapidly, a phenomenon called *neuromyotonia*. Myokymic movements often are blocked by benzodiazepines, phenytoin, or carbamazepine.

Tremor

Tremor is an involuntary, rhythmic, or near-rhythmic movement that can emerge under any of three circumstances alone or in combination: during the maintenance of posture, at rest, and while carrying out voluntary motor acts (intention). A mild *physiologic or postural tremor* with a frequency of 8 to 12 Hz can be detected by inspection in most adults during efforts to maintain the steady position of an outstretched extremity or when attempting fine movements such as threading a needle. Such tremor varies widely in degree among normal persons and is made worse by anxiety, fatigue, thyrotoxicosis, the infusion of epinephrine, the post-alcohol withdrawal state, or as the result of an autosomally dominant inherited predisposition. A variety of mechanistic explanations have been proposed to explain physiologic tremor, including that it reflects a central oscillating neural mechanism akin to that which drives the 8-to-12 Hz EEG alpha rhythm of the brain. Other suggestions have been that it is due to an interaction between firing patterns of alpha motor neurons, that it reflects the stimulation of beta-adrenergic receptors in the extremity, or that it involves innate instability of the fusimotor system regulating the feedback loop of the spinal stretch reflex. Physiologic tremor is not troublesome except when it blends into the potentially disabling, more severe forms of inherited "essential" tremor.

Essential Tremor. This disorder, sometimes called *benign familial tremor* because of its usual tendency neither to worsen much nor to incapacitate, can occur at any age of life, beginning most often during young adulthood. When it starts during the late decades of life, it may be called *senile tremor*. The abnormal movements in essential tremor tend to be rhythmic and oscillating and to affect especially the upper limbs, the head, the vocal apparatus, and the breathing muscles in that order of frequency. Absent at rest, the tremor begins with postural maintenance and is accentuated by attempts at voluntary movement. In contrast to acquired neocerebellar intention tremor, however, neither the amplitude of familial tremor nor its regular frequency changes appreciably as the moving body part nears its target. Essential tremor differs from parkinsonian tremor in that EMG recordings show cocontraction of antagonist muscles instead of the alternating contractions described below in parkinsonism. Severe examples of essential tremor may blend into dystonia.

Essential tremor appears to be a variant of physiologic tremor. It has a frequency in young adults of 8 to 10 Hz and is somewhat slower in children and the elderly. Whatever its ultimate origin, the tremor operates through the thalamocortical motor relay and can be blocked by making electrolytic or freeze lesions in the ventrolateral nucleus of the thalamus. Essential tremors diminish considerably after the ingestion of small amounts of alcohol (a well-known cerebellar depressant) and less predictably following anxiolytic agents. About 25 per cent of affected patients are improved symptomatically by the beta blocker, propranolol, acting by as yet undefined mechanisms.

Resting Tremor. The tremor of parkinsonism was identified many years ago as a resting tremor to distinguish it clinically from the prominent action tremor of cerebellar outflow disease. Except in severe cases, however, *parkinsonian tremor* tends to disappear when the body part is completely supported, disappears during sleep, and is most prominent during the tonic muscular activity of maintaining normal posture. Anxiety and fatigue worsen parkinsonian tremor, and while it may increase during the first stages of voluntary movement, intense concentration generally will abolish it while carrying out fine movements, especially during the early stages of its development. Some skilled workers, even surgeons, have been able to continue their craft for a time after the onset of parkinsonian tremor.

Physiologically the tremor of parkinsonism reflects the alternating contractions of agonist and antagonist muscles oscillating at a rate of 4 to 7 Hz. Most affected are the distal joints of the extremities, especially the thumb and index finger ("pill rolling"), and less often the lower facial muscles and the tongue. The tremor is unchanged by blocking muscle spindle receptors, implying that a central oscillator drives it by direct action on the alpha motor neurons. The afferent proprioceptive stimulation of passive movement, however, increases the rate of the underlying tremor. This may explain why cogwheel rigidity in parkinsonism (p. 1067) has a slightly faster frequency (about 9 to 11 Hz) compared to the resting or postural tremor of the disorder.

The pharmacogenesis of parkinsonian tremor is postulated to be based upon cholinergic hyperactivity in the basal ganglia, secondary to a deficiency in striatal dopamine (p. 1067). According to theory, less dopamine leads to more ACh activity, which intensifies GABA output from the putamen to the pallidum. In parkinsonism, rhythmic activity of appropriate frequency has been recorded in the ventrolateral nucleus of the thalamus to which the globus pallidus projects; destruction of this relay nucleus, which stands between the pallidal outflow and the cerebral cortex, abolishes tremor. Just how increased activity of cholinergic striatal neurons might translate into a rhythmic pallidal bombardment of the thalamic relay is unknown.

Intention (Cerebellar) Tremor. Tremor resulting from cerebellar dysfunction takes three forms. One, associated with abnormalities of the archicerebellum, relates primarily to disturbed movements of the trunk and, possibly, eye movements. The most prominent feature is truncal ataxia coupled with an incapacitating oscillation of the body and proximal limbs upon efforts to walk, a condition termed titubation. A second, associated with lesions of the spinocerebellar outflow pathway, affects predominantly the lower extremities and to a lesser degree the trunk. It produces irregular ataxia and tremor on walking that in severe cases blends into the titubation described above. The tremor frequency in both instances is about 5 to 7 Hz and continues as long as the effort of standing or walking is attempted. The third type of cerebellar tremor results from damage to the neocerebellar pathways, including the dentate nucleus and its outflow tract, the superior cerebellar peduncle. This produces the classic cerebellar intention tremor, a coarse 3- to 6-Hz distal oscillation tremor that increases in amplitude and decreases in regularity as the voluntarily moving part approaches its intended object.

Both archicerebellar titubation and the more common neocerebellar intention tremor can be attributed to impairment of the cerebellum's normal feedback control of voluntary body movement in response to changes in tonic stretch receptor afferents. The same physiologic defect produces the characteristic cerebel-

lar defect in rapid successive movements (dysdiadochokinesis). Neocerebellar intention tremor is abolished by ventrolateral lesions of the thalamus. The lesion presumably prevents distorted cerebellar processing from interfering with other preprogrammed influences on movement at the level of the premotor and motor cortex.

Damage to the red nucleus produces in most instances a tremor similar to that which arises from lesions of the dentatothalamic outflow tract. Rubral tremor sometimes appears to have a more proximal distribution in the upper extremities than does dentate tremor and to have a wider amplitude of oscillation. The latter aspect may reflect additional damage to dopaminergic projections from the area to the striatum.

Asterixis. Asterixis is an irregular, flaplike tremor with a frequency interval varying from 2 to 3 Hz to substantially less than 1 Hz. The movement most often accompanies acquired metabolic intoxications of the brain, but arises rarely following acute damage (e.g., infarcts) of the contralateral mesencephalon, thalamus, or even parietal lobe. The abnormality usually is accompanied by an accentuated physiologic postural tremor, seen best with arms outstretched. Asterixis, to develop, requires that an extremity or tongue be tonically, muscularly supported. The first manifestation of the abnormality usually consists of an irregular oscillation of the fingers leading to a sudden dropping deflection of the hands against the wrists followed by a quick recovery to extension. Similar tremors sometimes can affect the tongue and even the proximal extensor muscles of the upper or lower limbs. EMGs recorded during the abnormal movement show a silent period during the sudden drop followed by a rapid contraction of the stretched extensor agonists presumably reflecting synchronous activation of local stretch reflexes.

Chorea

Chorea describes an involuntary movement disorder characterized by nonrhythmic, irregularly distributed, coarse, quick twitching movements affecting groups of muscles in the face, tongue, and proximal and distal extremities. Occasionally, semiathetoid twistings concurrently involve the trunk and chest. Affected patients find it difficult or impossible to maintain a fixed posture or an uninterrupted muscular contraction (e.g., to maintain protrusion of the tongue or fixation of the grip). Muscular effort accentuates the abnormal movements and commonly induces "overflow" activity spreading initially into the ipsilateral then the contralateral limbs, the trunk, or the face. The degree of abnormality varies widely among affected individuals. Less severe afflictions transmit to the observer the impression of being little more than a bad case of the fidgets, while more intense involvements blend into the clinical appearance of ballism or dystonia.

Chorea accompanies two principal illnesses and several less frequent ones (Table 16). *Sydenham's chorea* is a now uncommon, transient CNS sequel to streptococcal disease, akin to rheumatic fever. It affects children and young adults and may recur spontaneously, especially during pregnancy. *Huntington's disease* is a degenerative disorder of the brain characterized by chorea and dementia and inherited in an autosomal dominant pattern that affects adults in their middle

TABLE 16. COMMON CAUSES OF CHOREA

  I. Hereditary
    A. Huntington's disease
    B. Wilson's disease
    C. Ataxia-telangiectasia
 II. Secondary
    A. Infectious
       1. Sydenham's chorea
       2. Encephalitis
    B. Drugs
       1. Levodopa
       2. Estrogen (oral contraceptives)
       3. Phenytoin
       4. Antipsychotic drugs
    C. Metabolic and endocrine
       1. Chorea gravidarum
       2. Thyrotoxicosis
    D. Vascular
       1. Lupus erythematosus
       2. Polycythemia vera
       3. Hemichorea-hemiballism
III. Unknown
    A. Senile chorea

From Fahn, S.: The extrapyramidal disorders. In Wyngaarden, J. B., and Smith, L. H., Jr. (eds.): Cecil Textbook of Medicine. 17th ed. Philadelphia, W. B. Saunders Co., 1985.

years. The disease damages especially the caudate nucleus of the basal ganglia and to a lesser degree the putamen and frontal cerebral cortex. Choreiform movements sometimes blend into dystonic posturings, particularly when Huntington's chorea affects younger adults or nears its final stages. Transient chorea also sporadically complicates the course of postanoxic encephalopathy and several systemic illnesses, including lupus erythematosus and hepatic encephalopathy. Prominent choreiform movements involving the mouth and face accompany a group of rare degenerative oral-facial dyskinesias as well as the now common, permanent *tardive dyskinesia* that complicates the lives of almost one-fifth of patients who have had long exposure to phenothiazine drugs.

Physiologically, chorea mixes features of dysfunction of both the basal ganglia and cerebellum. EMG recordings differ from normal muscle activity only in that they show an abnormal degree of irregularity in the total sum of motor output plus intermittent cocontraction of agonist and antagonist muscles. Phasic stretch reflexes remain normal, but resistance of the muscle to passive stretch is reduced, implying a reduction from normal in the excitability of long-loop tonic stretch reflexes, resulting in lowered stimulation of the gamma motor neuron. As noted, the adventitious movements become worse on action and intensify their frequency and amplitude especially during intended movements as when the hand approaches an aimed-for target.

The pathologic pharmacology of chorea is not well understood, but at least some of its manifestations resemble unbalanced dopamine hyperactivity. Excess levodopa given to patients with parkinsonism induces distal dyskinesias with a choreiform pattern. In addition, levodopa ingested by patients with Huntington's disease, in which GABA is abnormally reduced in the basal ganglia, intensifies the chorea. The phenothiazine drugs have as one of their major actions the blocking of dopamine receptors; in toxic doses they produce parkinsonian-like hypokinesia and rigidity.

The permanently lasting, disfiguring oral-facial-lingual movements of tardive dyskinesia that follow prolonged phenothiazine ingestion have been attributed to the development of denervation hypersensitivity to endogenous dopamine in the long-blocked striatal dopamine receptors.

Ballism

Ballism consists of abruptly beginning, repetitive, wide, flinging movements affecting predominantly the proximal limb and girdle muscles, more often of the upper than the lower extremity. Most examples are unilateral and are then called hemiballismus. The flingings often are accompanied by less prominent and often overlooked distal choreiform activity in the affected limbs or ipsilaterally on the face. Indeed, as ballism subsides with time, all the movements become less intense and take on a choreiform appearance. The disorder is largely confined to elderly persons of either sex.

Ballism results from destructive lesions, usually infarcts but rarely small hemorrhages or neoplasms, that destroy the greater part of the subthalamic nucleus or the proximal part of its projection to the globus pallidus. Neither the physiology nor pharmacology is well understood. Like other dyskinesias the abnormality operates through the extrapyramidal thalamocortical pathway and can be abolished by placing a lesion in the ventrolateral thalamus or by the development of a subsequent hemiplegia. Haloperidol, believed to block dopamine activity, is the most effective antidote. Fortunately most cases subside spontaneously within a matter of a few weeks.

Athetosis

This disorder stands between chorea and dystonia in its pathophysiology and expression. The disorder manifests itself by relatively slow, twisting, writhing, snake-like movements and postures involving the trunk, neck, face, and extremities. The movements can appear at rest but are greatly intensified by efforts to initiate voluntary activity. Coupled with the abnormal movements is an irregular action tremor. Tonic, involuntary (dystonic) contractions of the shoulders, elbows, hands, and feet may involve affected patients at rest. Athetosis occurs mainly in children, the principal sufferers being those who have survived complications of prematurity, perinatal asphyxia, or kernicterus. The fact that classic athetosis almost never accompanies postasphyxial encephalopathy in the adult suggests that its typical pattern reflects abnormal developmental relationships in motor control among the partially damaged striatum, thalamus, and cortex. This inference is strengthened by the pathologic accompaniments of athetosis, which include degeneration of neurons and gliosis in the putamen and to a lesser degree the caudate, accompanied by a unique overgrowth of myelinated astrocytic fibrils. Many affected brains studied at autopsy also show accompanying abnormalities in the cerebral cortex and cerebellum, explaining the high incidence of spasticity and cerebellar dysfunction that involves affected children.

The abnormal physiology and pharmacology of athetosis are poorly understood. Although tonic and often phasic stretch reflexes are increased in most muscles, this appears to be a small component of the disability that gives far more the appearance of a central, non-oscillating, complicated imbalance in the interplay between the basal ganglia and the descending upper motor neuron systems.

Dystonia

Dystonia is a movement disorder consisting of twisting or turning, tonic skeletal muscle contractions, most, but not all, of which are initiated distally. The abnormal movements involve the simultaneous cocontractions of both agonists and antagonists in affected parts, and have a frequency generally more rapid than athetosis. Dystonic movements further differ from athetosis in coming on later in life; indeed, their first appearance may be mistaken for the onset of chorea or even severe familial tremor. Several forms occur only in adulthood.

Dystonia can be inherited or acquired. The inherited forms occur as a primary movement disorder and can follow either autosomal or recessive patterns, with the dominant form being most frequent among persons of Ashkenazi Jewish ancestry. Somewhat similar dystonias arise sporadically or as a component of the signs produced by several pathologic processes that affect the basal ganglia. *Focal dystonias* include writer's cramp and other occupational dystonias, as well as spasmodic torticollis and a restricted flexion dystonia of the foot and ankle. Most focal dystonias appear during the middle years or early senium. The essence of dystonic movement is an abnormal cocontraction of agonist and antagonist muscles arising spontaneously or during attempts at voluntary movement such that the more powerful muscle wins out and moves the joint. The result generates characteristic postures accompanied by twisting semijerking movements that are nonrhythmic in frequency and vary widely in distribution and pattern. Generalized dystonia known as *dystonia musculorum deformans* begins in childhood and usually progresses to involve both sides of the body, eventually giving rise to tragically unattractive postures and almost incomprehensible dysarthria. In the worst cases the development of fixed severe scoliosis and multiple joint and muscle contractures may twist and deform the body into pretzel-like shapes and limit full limb movement. The most common cause of *acute dystonia* occurs as an idiosyncratic hypersensitivity to phenothiazine drugs. The response implies that at some step in its complex pathogenesis dystonia must include a component of cholinergic hyperactivity.

Dystonic movements accompany a variety of specific neurologic diseases that damage the basal ganglia, including Wilson's and Huntington's disease, and several inherited childhood disorders as well as cerebral palsy. Morphologic basal ganglia abnormalities are occasionally found at autopsy in patients with late-onset oral-facial dystonia. The most frequent and prominent dystonias, however, including the inherited or spontaneous dystonia musculorum deformans or the frequently encountered adult spasmodic torticollis, show no recognizable morphologic abnormalities in the brain at autopsy. Specific neuropharmacologic abnormalities have not been reported in any of the idiopathic dystonias.

The abnormality in dystonia must express itself predominantly through the corticospinal outflow on alpha motor neurons since bilateral lesions placed in the ventrolateral and ventromedial nuclei of the thalamus at least transiently can ameliorate even severe cases. Corticospinal hemiplegia has the same effect. As with other disorders of the basal ganglia, anxiety accentuates the abnormal movements while relaxation reduces them. All dystonias disappear during sleep.

Paroxysmal Choreoathetosis and Tonic Spasm. These unusual disorders are related to each other in appearance and probably in pathogenesis. They consist of seizure-like paroxysms of choreodystonic movements that occur in the setting of full consciousness under several circumstances. One variety, called *kinesiogenic* because it is movement induced, can be either familial or spontaneous, affects otherwise healthy persons, lasts less than two minutes per episode, and is precipitated by sudden action or startle. Similar attacks called tonic spasms resemble unilateral, brief spasms of decorticate or decerebrate posturing (p. 1059) except that they occur spontaneously during normal wakefulness. They can occur in advanced multiple sclerosis and following perinatal hypoxia. (Anticonvulsants relieve both these types of short-lasting kinesiogenic spasms, whereas they have no effect on decerebrate posturing.) Presumably the pathophysiology of tonic spasms lies in spontaneous or evoked discharges from collections of damaged, hyperexcitable neurons lying in the basal ganglia or brainstem reticular formation that possess a reduced threshold to reflex stimulation.

Paroxysmal dystonic choreoathetosis, a condition possibly related to the above disorders, consists of choreoathetotic movements, also familial, precipitated by alcohol, tea, coffee, excitement, or fatigue, but not by sudden movement. The episodes can last up to hours at a time, do not occur with structural brain disease, and are not relieved by anticonvulsants.

Tics (Habit Spasms). Tics are sudden, behaviorally related, irregular, stereotyped, repetitive movements of variable complexity that almost always involve similar but not identical groups or fragments of muscles. The abnormalities in mild form are believed to represent a form of learned behavior; more severe, chronic tics, however, often are part of a wider illness of unknown cause called *Tourette's syndrome* or *Gilles de la Tourette's disorder,* in which the various motor tics often are accompanied by random bizarre grunting or barking noises as well as the shouting of scatologic or obscene expletives. Like choreiform movements, which they sometimes resemble, habit spasms are quick, most often involve the muscles about the eyes or mouth, but sometimes affect the distal extremities. Tics disappear with sleep and are aggravated by emotional tension. Most tics, however, can be reduced by voluntary effort, while chorea cannot. This last aspect coupled with a long history of the tic and evidence of either chronic tension-anxiety or other Tourette symptoms usually provides the diagnosis. Confirmatory laboratory tests are lacking.

Myoclonus

The term *myoclonus* describes sudden unexpected abrupt contractions of a single muscle or group of muscles that involve the limbs more than the trunk, and more often than not produce quick flexion in the affected body part. Myoclonus has many causes (Table 17) and can arise from abnormalities at any level of the CNS. Generalized repetitive myoclonus occurs with certain forms of primary epilepsy, can accompany dif-

TABLE 17. FREQUENT CAUSES OF MYOCLONUS

I. Benign myoclonic jerks
  A. Physiologic: sleep jerks, anxiety
  B. Essential myoclonus: familial or sporadic
  C. Nocturnal myoclonus
  D. Associated with petit mal or grand mal seizures
II. Symptomatic myoclonus
  A. Myoclonus epilepsy
  B. Dementias: Creutzfeldt-Jakob, Alzheimer's
  C. Infectious: subacute sclerosing panencephalitis
  D. Lipidoses
  E. Cerebellar degenerations
  F. Hypoxia
  G. Toxins: methyl bromide, strychnine
  H. Drugs: levodopa, tricyclics
  I. Systemic illnesses: uremia, hepatic, dialysis encephalopathy
III. Rhythmic myoclonus
  A. Palatal myoclonus
  B. Ocular myoclonus

From Fahn, S.: The extrapyramidal disorders. In Wyngaarden, J. B., and Smith, L. H., Jr. (eds.): Cecil Textbook of Medicine. 17th ed. Philadelphia, W. B. Saunders Co., 1985.

fuse degenerative diseases of the brain, and, sporadically, appears in normal persons as an accentuated startle response or when drifting off to sleep. Focal or multifocal myoclonus occurs either spontaneously or reflexly, the latter arising in response to either exteroceptive or proprioceptive stimuli. Reflex or action myoclonus is a prominent feature of an inherited degenerative disease of the cerebellum (*Ramsay Hunt's cerebellar dyssynergia*) in which it presumably reflects a loss of normal Purkinje cell inhibition as motor control is initiated. Action myoclonus, with a similar mechanism, also can follow severe hypoxic damage to the brain, and both spontaneous and action myoclonus occur prominently in a slow virus disease of the brain called *Creutzfeldt-Jakob disease.* Spontaneous multifocal myoclonus accompanies several CNS degenerative diseases of childhood as well as the metabolic encephalopathies that result from, among others, uremia, hyperosmolar stupor, penicillin intoxication, and carbon dioxide intoxication. Physiologically, myoclonus represents the spontaneous discharge of clusters of hyperexcitable neurons lacking the usual feedback control from cerebral cortex, cerebellum, or reticular formation. At least some instances have been traced to an apparent central deficiency of the inhibitory neurotransmitter serotonin, and have been treated favorably with serotonin precursors.

Palatal myoclonus is more of a spontaneous tremor than a true myoclonus, at least as the latter term is described above. The abnormality consists of spontaneous, rapid, regular movements with a frequency of 2 to 3 Hz involving the soft palate and less often the adjacent muscles of the pharynx and larynx. Rarely the tremor includes the diaphragm or oculomotor muscles. The abnormal movements persist continuously during wakefulness or sleep in contrast to more rostrally arising tremors. Palatal myoclonus most often follows an infarct that damages structures along the dentatorubro-olivary pathway. The lesion usually lies in the brainstem but sometimes affects the dentate nucleus or the superior peduncle. Palatal myoclonus also can accompany degenerative changes affecting these same pathways in the degenerative disease, olivopontocerebellar atrophy. In most stroke-caused instances a delay of some months separates the initial injury and the appearance of the palatal myoclonus, suggesting the emergence of denervation hypersensitivity in a preolivary pathway. The olive itself may hypertrophy in palatal myoclonus. The serotonin precursor 5-hydroxytryptophan sometimes ameliorates the abnormality.

Hemifacial spasm affects the motor distribution of the facial nerve of either side and is characterized by rapidly recurring painless, nonrhythmic, clonic, fragmentary twitching of any of the facial muscles. The condition persists into sleep and has been associated with longstanding compression of the facial nerve at the base of the brain by a branch of the basilar artery. Ephaptic (fiber to fiber, nonsynaptic) short-circuiting of impulses from one fiber to adjacent ones with denervation hypersensitivity at the site of the compression has been suggested but not proved as the cause of the disorder.

Postdenervation synkinesias consist of the concurrent postdenervation contraction of muscle groups that are innervated by a common axon but lie remote from the site of intended focal muscular activity. The condition results from faulty regeneration or sprouting of peripheral nerve fibers distal to a point of severe compression or transection-resuturing. It is most often seen as a late occurrence following acute facial (Bell's) palsy; in affected persons each automatic blink of the orbicularis oculi, for example, is accompanied by an involuntary twitch of the cheek or corner of the mouth.

ABNORMAL MUSCLE RESISTANCE TO PASSIVE STRETCH

Deep Tendon Reflexes

The deep tendon reflexes provide an index of the level of excitability of the lower motor neuron through its phasic excitation by the monosynaptic stretch reflex (Fig. 17). Elicited by abruptly striking the muscle tendon, the stimulus simultaneously stretches the muscle fibers and discharges IA spindle receptors that synchronously bombard the alpha motor neurons of the stretched muscle: A prompt, visible and palpable contraction normally ensues. The reflex can be *reduced* by damage anywhere along the reflex arc, either centrally or on the afferent or efferent side. On the afferent side, neuropathy, nerve or root trauma, or degenerative nerve or root disease affecting the large proprioceptive afferent fibers can block or disperse the adequate stimulus from synchronously reaching the motor neurons. Centrally, conditions that can reduce alpha motor neuron excitability include such physiologic circumstances as well as psychologic relaxation or athletic conditioning. On the efferent side, pathologic causes of reduced deep tendon reflexes consist of any of the several diseases that affect the alpha motor neurons or their motor axons. Conversely, several conditions can *increase* deep tendon reflexes by enhancing the excitability of the alpha motor neuron either directly or by acting upon its adjacent internuncial pool. These include (1) physiologic excitation caused by psychologic tension states or produced by reticular activation via the Jendrassik maneuver (having the subject either clench the jaws or briskly and isometrically pull his gripped hands against each other while the examiner elicits the reflex), (2) segmental nociceptive stimulation activating facilitatory internuncial pools, (3) anterior midline cerebellar damage or dysfunction that reduces the cerebellar inhibitory influence on the brainstem reticular formation, and (4) spasticity (defined below).

Basal Ganglia (Nonspastic) Rigidity

This form of increased resistance to passive movement accompanies parkinsonism. Pharmacologically, parkinsonian rigidity is closely related in time and mechanism to the degeneration of the dopaminergic nigrostriatal projection that occurs in that disease, and it is usually the first symptom to disappear when treatment is initiated with levodopa. Clinically the resistance is immediately felt with passive movement; in contrast to the tonic stretch reflex, it is velocity independent, tending to maintain steady resistance as long as displacement of the limb avoids the extremes of range of motion. Cessation of motion evokes no counteracting movement, and if the movement is resumed in either direction, immediate resistance of an equal degree is felt. In most instances a sense of regular rachet-like reduced resistance (cogwheeling) with a frequency of 8 to 12 Hz is superimposed on the rigidity, particularly when one applies relatively rapid passive displacement of the wrist, elbow, or knee. Cogwheeling reflects the combined effect of the stretch reflex interacting with the parkinsonian alternating tremor, both superimposed on the continuous motor discharge responsible for the rigidity of the disorder.

Physiologically, parkinsonian rigidity reflects a direct tonic increase in impulses descending from the cerebral cortex upon the spinal alpha motor neuron as a result of abnormal pallidal control of cortical innervation. Both agonist and antagonist innervations are simultaneously coactivated. The rigidity is reduced when the limb is fully supported, and it disappears during sleep. As one moves the joint, involuntary contractions may involve both antagonist and agonist. Although fusimotor activity is enhanced, this component appears insufficient to account for the muscular hyperactivity. Thus the muscular phenomenon resembles most closely that encountered in patients unable voluntarily to relax or performing the Jendrassik maneuver. Although static stretch reflexes are measurably increased with parkinsonian rigidity, deep tendon reflexes usually are not grossly hyperactive nor does one find either abnormal exteroceptive reflexes or evidence of spasticity. Long-latency tonic proprioceptive reflexes are impaired, and it has been postulated that the fundamental fault in rigidity lies with failure of the basal ganglia properly to modulate the cortical feedforward reflex loop that influences forthcoming slow, ramp movements.

Spasticity and Associated Disorders of the Upper Motor Neuron

Spasticity is a condition of abnormal facilitation of the phasic and tonic stretch reflex that can arise as the result of disease or dysfunction affecting the upper motor neuron system at any level lying rostral to the abnormal reflex, from cord to cortex. The least expression of spasticity consists of facilitation of the deep tendon reflexes although, as previously explained, such phasic facilitation need not always be of spastic origin. The major functional abnormality in spasticity consists of a velocity-dependent, pathologic facilitation imposed on the polysynaptic long-loop, tonic component of the stretch reflex. This leads to a progressively increased contraction and resistance of the lengthened muscle against passive or active stretch. This stretch-dependent, tonic muscular hypertonus is what usually is described when one speaks of spastic motor disabilities.

Spastic hyperexcitation of the stretch reflexes affects most markedly the antigravity muscles of the extremities, including in humans the extensor muscles in the lower extremities and the flexor muscles in the upper. The clinical hallmark of spasticity is the *clasp-knife* phenomenon, a two-phased response brought out by tonically and briskly stretching a large muscle around one of its joints such as the knee or elbow. The degree of abnormal counteracting resistance of the lengthening muscle builds slowly, increasing in proportion to the severity of the abnormality in long-loop reflexes as well as to the rate and amplitude at which one applies the stretching force. After a variable arc of movement, the resistance rapidly maximizes, then suddenly collapses in response to afferent inhibitory signals fired from the increasing tension placed upon tendon receptors.

The hyperactive response to passive stretch in spasticity can give rise to *clonus* in which indefinitely repeated rhythmic contractions can be induced in a muscle group by applying an initially rapid then moderately forceful sustained stretch. The flexors of the ankle or wrist are most susceptible to bringing out the phenomenon, but clonus can be induced in almost any muscle in the presence of a severe degree of spasticity. Clonus reflects alpha motor neuron hyperexcitability. Like hyperactive deep tendon reflexes in general, unsustained clonus need not always reflect pathologic changes in the nervous system.

Clonus has a characteristic frequency that varies between 5 and 8 Hz. Views differ whether it reflects an intrinsic hyperexcitation of the stretch reflex or the release of intrinsic oscillatory mechanisms in the spinal cord, perhaps similar to those that operate in physiologic tremor. The mechanism is as follows: The immediate response to the stretch reflex is a contraction of the lengthened muscle that concurrently unloads its spindles, leading to a brief "silent period" in the stretch reflex. As the muscle then begins to restretch under passive force the stretch receptors fire with increasing intensity until the hyperexcitable motor neuron population fires, and the cycle begins over again. Recordings from single muscle afferents in patients with clonus confirm that spindle discharges occur only during the relaxation or lengthening phase of the muscle, which then rhythmically contracts to reinitiate the abnormality.

Several theories have been offered to explain spasticity. One holds that spinal internuncial neurons, relieved of supraspinal descending inhibitory influences, spontaneously enter a state of reverberating reexcitation. The result would be that they constantly bombard the motor neuron with excitatory postsynaptic potentials and chronically lower its resting membrane potential. Such a mechanism cannot always be the cause, however, since ischemic damage to the spinal cord in experimental animals or man selectively kills the small internuncial cells, and is immediately followed by severe spasticity in the affected and distal segments. Another explanation is that the motor neuron, deprived of its normally descending corticospinal and reticulospinal inhibitory influences, intrinsically develops denervation hypersensitivity so that its membrane partially depolarizes in response to low ambient concentrations of neurotransmitter. The time frame for the development of such spasticity contradicts this supposition. A third theory, an anatomic variant of denervation hypersensitivity, postulates that excitatory internuncials below the level of injury send out axonal "sprouts" that converge directly on the motor neurons or on spinal excitatory interneurons. Neither of the latter two theories satisfactorily explains why spasticity generally occurs considerably more rapidly in humans following upper motor neuron lesions located at pontine or higher levels but may be delayed in its appearance for several weeks following severe spinal injuries that produce spinal shock, described subsequently. Since spasticity becomes more intense for months after even partial injuries, it seems possible that more than one mechanism is involved with denervation hypersensitivity or sprouting perhaps accounting for some of the late but not the early changes that one observes.

Spastic Rigidity. This phenomenon occurs rarely as a late complication after bilateral lesions producing classic stretch receptor-dependent spasticity. Affected patients develop a pillar-like tonic rigidity in the muscles of the lower extremity so as to hold the legs constantly in a position of fixed extension. Less frequently the arms are similarly involved, but if so, they may fix in either flexion or extension so that the resulting postures resemble decorticate or decerebrate rigidity as described later. The injury responsible for spastic rigidity usually consists of either ischemic damage to the small neurons in the spinal internuncial pool or lesions of the brainstem reticular formation adjacent to or just rostral to the level of the vestibular nuclei. After the passage of weeks or months, the tonic rigidity continues even after the dorsal roots are anesthetized or cut, implying that its pathophysiology depends entirely on central excitation of anterior horn cells by the upper motor neuron system and not on the stretch reflex. Nevertheless, an element of spasticity always accompanies this form of central rigidity, since stretch stimuli of normal intensity continue to elicit hyperactive deep tendon reflexes and to intensify the rigid posture (unless musculoskeletal fibrosis has occurred). Similar tonic rigidity occurs in mammals with midcollicular decerebrate rigidity in which the addition of either anterior cerebellar ablation or long postlesion survival leads to a state in which deafferentation no longer interrupts the extensor activity.

COMPLEX REFLEX RESPONSES WITH UPPER MOTOR NEURON DYSFUNCTION

Abnormal Somatoceptive Reflexes

The brainstem and spinal cord contain the programmed templates for several coordinated reflex movements that were vital to the activities of our phylogenetic ancestors but have disappeared in humans under the influence of higher levels of motor control regulated by the cerebral cortex. Damage or dysfunction of the origins or pathways of the corticospinal motor system releases these suppressed motor responses, making them clinically useful signs in diagnosis. The released reflexes that contribute most to diagnosis and management in clinical neurology are the Babinski response, the crossed extensor response, flexor spasms, spastic rigidity, spinal shock, and the decorticate and decerebrate postural responses. Absence of the superficial abdominal reflexes and the presence of certain abnormal forebrain reflexes also can signify upper motor neuron dysfunction but are less certain signs of abnormality. Noxious or, less often, tactile stimulation of either cutaneous or visceral receptors provides the adequate stimuli for each of these primitive coordinated responses. The reflexogenous zone varies from reflex to reflex, but all of the responses represent phylogenetically primitive forms of motor organization, incorporated imperceptibly by the central nervous system into more complex motor activity as control of movement in man has evolved.

The Babinski Sign

This, the extensor plantar response, represents a fragment of a phylogenetically ancient spinal triple flexion withdrawal reflex. It comprises the most studied reflex in clinical neurology. The adequate threshold for the reflex consists of a mildly noxious stimulus drawn gradually from the heel toward the small toe along the sole or the lateral inferior surface of the foot. In the presence of severe upper motor neuron disease, mere tactile stimuli are sufficient to elicit the response, and the reflexogenous zone can extend beyond the foot to include the leg and even more proximal parts of the body below the level of the lesion. The foot response consists of extension of the great toe with a lesser degree of extension and lateral fanning of the smaller toes. Concurrently one can palpate and sometimes observe simultaneous cocontraction of the large muscles of the anterior tibial compartment, which extend the ankle on the foot, as well as of the iliopsoas, contracting the thigh on the hip, and the hamstrings, flexing the leg on the thigh.

The extensor plantar response represents the distal component of a short-latency, spinally mediated, flexor withdrawal of the lower limb from noxious stimuli. The reflex mechanism survives in the normal spinal cord, as anyone who has inadvertently stepped on a nail or other sharp object can verify: With toe and foot abruptly extended away from the plantar surface, the leg flexes before any sense of foot pain or even movement reaches awareness. The difference between this one-time, protective flexor response to an unexpected injury and the pathologic Babinski sign lies in the stereotyped nature of the latter, which responds again and again in an identical manner to the same stimulus. Through cerebral inhibition via habituation, normal persons once aware of the noxious stimulus no longer enjoy the protection of the short-latency spinal flexion response. If they did, how could one walk barefoot on the beach on a hot sunny day?

The extensor plantar response provides a cardinal sign of upper motor neuron dysfunction of cerebral, brainstem, or spinal origin. Typically, the closer the upper motor neuron abnormality lies to the spinal level, the shorter becomes the latency between stimulus and response and the more intense is the flexor withdrawal of the foot and leg. The finding implies that multiple rostral levels normally modulate the instinctive response.

The crossed extensor response. This reflex consists of a strong, simultaneous extensor thrust involving the contralateral lower extremity when an adequate stimulus elicits the spinal flexor-Babinski response. It represents a component of the primitive spinal standing and walking reflex and operates normally in all of us during automatic walking or to prevent falling when we reflexly withdraw the contralateral leg after inadvertent plantar injury. It is usually not prominent in clinical conditions except when disease produces chronic, relatively fixed, and severe paraparesis or paraplegia of spinal origin.

Flexor Spasms

Flexor spasms, sometimes called *mass flexion reflexes,* consist of bilateral flexor withdrawal contractions of the lower extremities that arise reflexly from neural structures within the spinal cord and produce bilateral contraction of the flexor muscles of the ankle, knee, hip, and trunk, usually extending as high as the lower abdominal level. Coupled with the reflex, the bowel and bladder sometimes empty automatically. The visceral responses are secondary autonomic reflexes triggered by the sudden increase in intra-abdominal pressure induced by abdominal muscle contraction. Bilateral spinal flexor reflexes can be observed following either partial or complete bilateral lesions of upper motor neuron pathways that affect any level of the CNS extending from the upper lumbar cord forward as far as to the tegmentum of the lower pons. The reflexogenous zone for flexor spasms is maximal on the sole of the foot, but for noxious stimuli often extends as high as the level of the spinal lesion. "Spontaneous" flexor spasms may affect patients with chronic spinal cord lesions. Their presence usually reflects abnormal stimuli arising from decubitus ulcers, urinary tract infections, or bowel distension. In such individuals even intercurrent illness or fever may be sufficient to precipitate the spasms.

Abnormal Forebrain Reflexes

A number of so-called primitive reflexes that reflect normal behavior patterns in developing infants sometimes emerge in adults with frontal lobe or diffuse forebrain dysfunction. These include various abnormalities in gait and posture, persistent avoiding of ophthalmoscopic examinations by diverting the eyes or tightly closing the lids, motor perseveration, reflex sucking and snouting, palmomental reflexes, and other related minor abnormalities. None of them has much diagnostic localizing value.

Reflex grasping of the foot or hand (more often the hand) usually arises in association with large destructive or space-occupying lesions of the opposite frontal lobe. Emergence of the reflex almost always is accompanied by either increased intracranial pressure or dysfunction affecting the ipsilateral frontal lobe as well. The grasp reflex appears to be an exaggerated and distorted flexion reflex that can involve either the upper or lower extremity. Reflex grasping is made up of two components: One is mediated as a short-latency, primitive proprioceptive spinal reflex analogous to the normal finger flexor or flexor plantar response. This phase is elicited by stroking the palmar surfaces of the distal hand or foot and their respective digits; the second phase (the sign of frontal lobe damage) combines the abnormally emergent spinal reflex with motor perseveration. Thus a brisk, brief palmar flexor response without sustained grasping is readily elicited by finger or palmar extension in patients with decerebrate rigidity.

Paratonic rigidity or *gegenhalten* (moving against, motor negativism) is a plastic-like, actively generated increase in muscle resistance that counteracts the examiner's efforts passively to move a patient's extremities, head, or neck. The resistance is felt as constant or nearly so throughout the movement arc and remains of roughly similar intensity regardless of the initial position of the body part. It somewhat resembles the rigidity of parkinsonism but is unaccompanied by cogwheeling resistance and has a behavioral dimension lacking in the rigidity of parkinsonism. In contrast to the latter, paratonia almost disappears if the part is moved very slowly, and it is made worse by rapid passive movement. Paratonic rigidity is greatly enhanced by emotional tension, including brusque urgings to "relax," in which instance the patient may seem to anticipate the examiner and actively move the part in a direction opposite to the passive stretch maneuver. The response has not received detailed physiologic analysis, but appears to reflect a primitive behavioral response signifying limbic system "release" from higher influences.

Spinal Shock

The term describes a state of profound, usually areflexic, inhibitory flaccidity that follows complete mechanical or functional transection of the upper motor neuron pathways in the spinal cord or the lower medullary level of the brainstem. Severe damage to the medulla oblongata rarely provides a clinical cause of spinal shock since such injury usually results in death from associated respiratory and circulatory complications. Similarly, quick death usually follows spinal cord transections above the level of C4 where the phrenic nerves originate. With acute transection or extensive spinal damage below C5, the spinal cord of man almost always temporarily loses all motor activity, including that detectable by electrical testing. At any spinal level, transection abolishes bladder and bowel control, although transient involuntary priapism may remain. Areflexia after the onset of spinal shock lasts for a time inversely proportional to the length of the remaining spinal cord: The higher the transection, the earlier is the return of reflex motor functions. The rate of motor return also is more rapid when patients suffer from no serious complicating neurologic or general medical illness such as urinary, skin, or lung infections.

With transections at the low cervical spinal level or below, most patients develop the extensor plantar response within a few days, and in a few it is immediately elicitable. Usually within a week or so of the injury, the deep tendon reflexes begin to return, and more prominent signs of chronic spasticity follow. Transections affecting the thoracic regions allow the emergence of autonomous sympathetic pressor reflexes; these are supplied by the independently operating spinal intermediolateral sympathetic column and its associated splanchnic outflow.

Flexor reflexes and flexor spasms predominate in the early months following complete spinal transection in man. Extensor activity may develop in the distal segment, but this usually is late and poorly sustained. Among meticulously studied and cared for patients with spinal transection due to injuries received in World War II, the great majority developed predominantly extensor activity, but not on the average until well after six months of recovery. In only a few was the reflex strong enough to permit functional standing.

Brainstem Responses to Noxious Stimuli

These consist of three major patterns: decorticate responses, decerebrate responses, and the mixed response. In contrast to the spinal flexor reflex, which reflects a primitive withdrawal response, the first two and part of the third of these brainstem reflexes represent vestiges of normal postural responses. Their adequate stimulus is nociceptive rather than via the stretch reflex, and their presence represents reflex excitation of the subcortical and brainstem motor pathways upon which the polysynaptic, long-loop stretch reflexes project. Emergence of these abnormal brainstem reflexes reflects the activity of uninhibited vestibulospinal and reticulospinal influences eliciting involuntary reflex movements in distal bulbospinal segments. Their emergence indicates that the portions of the brain from which they emanate remain physiologically intact and imply that the next higher level of motor control, the cerebrum, at least temporarily has been taken out of service.

Abnormal Flexor Responses in the Arm with Extension in the Leg—The Decorticate Response. The adequate stimulus to elicit decorticate posturing consists of applying a moderately noxious stimulus to the skin over the supraorbital nerve, to a fingertip, or to the sternum, as illustrated in Figure 23. "Spontaneous" decorticate responses as well as the decerebrate or mixed decerebrate-spinal responses described below also can arise in response to internal noxious stimuli, including cerebral or subarachnoid bleeding, meningitis, or intracranial pressure waves. Physiologically in the decorticate response, flexor hypertonus predominates in the muscles of the upper extremities and extensor hypertonus in the lower, producing postures reflecting the antigravity functions of the stretch reflex of man. With stimulation the fully developed response consists of a relatively slow tonic flexion of the arm at the elbow, wrist, and fingers with adduction of the upper extremity, coupled with extension, internal rotation, and vigorous plantar flexion of the lower extremity. Less severe lesions of the brain or less vigorous degrees of stimulation can result in a response that is confined to the stimulated member and consists, for example, of no more than stereotyped flexion of the arm.

The decorticate response often appears as a unilateral abnormality, arising on the side of the body opposite to large, deep, contralateral cerebral lesions such as infarcts, hemorrhages, or abscesses. Decorticate responses also appear as a relatively early motor abnormality in the process of downward diencephalic compression during transtentorial herniation.

Abnormal Extensor Response in Arm and Leg—Decerebrate Rigidity. When fully developed in

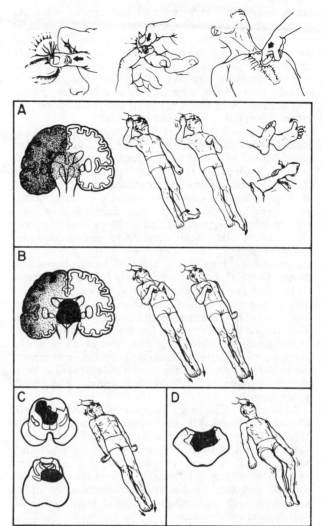

Figure 23. The postures of the decorticate, decerebrate, and mixed brainstem motor responses to noxious stimuli found in patients with acute cerebral-diencephalic dysfunction. *A* shows an incipient decorticate response on the patient's left side secondary to a large deep lesion in the contralateral hemisphere. In *B* the left-sided figure demonstrates bilateral decorticate responses leading in the right-sided figure into a combination of decorticate-decerebrate posturing as the hemispheric abnormality extends downward to affect the diencephalon more severely. *C* depicts bilateral decerebrate posturing reflecting the release of descending reticular-vestibular motor influences emanating from the upper brainstem. In *D* the functional effects of damage lie at the Junction zone where reticulovestibular influences give way to medullospinal ones: With supraorbital pressure the arms extend, but the lower extremities show spinal-type flexion. The cartoons at the top illustrate noxious stimuli commonly employed to elicit the response. (From Plum, F., and Posner, J. B.: The Diagnosis of Stupor and Coma. 3rd ed. revised. Philadelphia, F. A. Davis Co., 1982.)

man, decerebrate rigidity more often than not is bilateral. The response consists of opisthotonus with teeth clenched, the arms stiffly extended, adducted, and hyperpronated, and the legs stiffly extended with feet plantar flexed (Fig. 23). Tonic vestibular and neck reflexes usually can be elicited concurrently. The full response commonly requires the application of an external noxious stimulus. With acute lesions of the brain, waves of shivering and hyperpnea reflecting autonomic hyperactivity may accompany seemingly spontaneous recurrent decerebrate spasms. Individual patients often demonstrate a mixture of decorticate and decerebrate responses on the two sides of the body, and one response may give way to the other over short periods, presumably reflecting relatively minor physiologic changes in the amount of compression or irritation delivered to the upper brainstem.

Physiologically the decerebrate state consists of excessive, synergistic extensor muscle contractions often accompanied by simultaneous cocontraction of flexors as well. Decerebrate rigidity in experimental animals classically results from transections of the midbrain that spare the more caudally placed vestibular nuclei and the adjacent pontine reticular formation. In man, studies employing somatic and auditory evoked potentials indicate that both decorticate and decerebrate reflex responses most often reflect the presence of abnormalities deep in the cerebral hemispheres and diencephalon rather than primarily in the brainstem. Of the two responses the decerebrate posture usually indicates a more caudal (and therefore more dangerous) level of dysfunction, often resulting in the release of excitation by the reticular formation of the midbrain. These postural reflexes do not always require the presence of structural damage. They can accompany the forebrain metabolic depression of several disorders, including hepatic encephalopathy, anoxia, and severe hypoglycemia.

Abnormal Extensor Response in Arms with Flaccid or Weak Flexor Responses in Legs—The Mixed Decerebrate-Spinal Response (Fig. 23). This pattern arises suddenly in patients who have primary hemorrhages, infarcts, or other forms of structural damage involving the pontine tegmentum. The reflex reflects a transition between predominantly upper brainstem and predominantly spinal influences over bulbospinal motor control.

Brainstem Reticular Influences on Movement

The abnormal postural responses described above of decorticate-decerebrate rigidity blending into the mixed response at about the level of the vestibular nuclei and then to spinal shocklike flaccidity below that level are strongly reminiscent of experiments made some years ago by Magoun and Rhines. When the investigators stimulated the rostral reticular formation in midbrain and upper pons, strong facilitatory stimuli converged upon the spinal motor neuron pool. Below about the level of the pontomedullary junction, punctate stimulation of the bulbar reticular formation in the animals abolished movement controlled from more rostral structures as well as all spinal reflexes. The changes imply that in man as in animals the bulbar reticular formation normally supplies inhibitory influences on the alpha motor neurons of the lower brainstem and spinal cord; these influences predominate when abruptly released from more rostral neural control, but gradually lose their dominance with time. By inference, the predominant normal influence of the spinal reticular formation must be similarly inhibitory. Such mechanisms presumably underlie the two-phase transition from flaccidity to spasticity that follows human spinal transections and lower brainstem damage.

SYNDROMES OF MOTOR SYSTEM DISEASE
ABNORMALITIES OF THE CEREBRAL CONTROL OF MOVEMENT

The frontal lobes of man are primarily involved in the planning and expression of behavior. In functional anatomic terms the region can be divided into prefrontal, premotor-supplementary motor, and primary motor areas (Fig. 22). Each of these areas extends along the inner hemispheric surface as well as over its larger lateral convolutional aspect. The prefrontal region also possesses a large orbitofrontal surface that appears to process different information from that integrated by the lateral, dorsal, and frontal polar zones.

The Prefrontal Area

The prefrontal cortex in subhuman primates interconnects with the premotor area, basal ganglia, thalamus, several levels of the limbic system, and the brainstem. The region reaches its largest size relative to the rest of the brain in humans, and this feature plus well known behavioral aberrations associated with frontal lobe damage has attracted considerable effort to unravel its function. Nevertheless it has proved difficult to establish in a precise way how the prefrontal area relates specifically to motor control or even to behavior in general.

Inferences about prefrontal function in humans come from three principal sources: (1) behavioral changes observed with focal epileptic foci and their removal; (2) alterations induced by the now almost discontinued procedure of frontal lobotomy, a procedure in which parts of the frontal lobe were removed in attempts to treat various psychiatric disorders; and (3) preoperative and postoperative changes observed in patients with brain tumors, vascular lesions, or traumatic injuries involving the area. This last approach gives the least exact information, because in such cases both the lesions and their removal tend to be so extensive that by the time they are analyzed they produce dysfunction in adjacent or even geographically remote neurologic structures. As a general rule, unless they produce seizures, few prefrontal lesions produce consistently recognizable abnormal symptoms and signs until they either become very large or extend bilaterally to affect the other frontal lobe as well.

Evidence suggests that different behavioral influences emanate from the dorsolateral-dorsomedial prefrontal cortex and the orbitalfrontal area, respectively. Because small abnormalities seldom produce much damage, any effort at strict localization must be regarded cautiously.

Persons with large frontal lobe lesions may appear unusually bland or apathetic in the face of normally distressing stimuli. As the lesion enlarges patients show a lack of emotional or behavioral spontaneity, possess little initiative, and tend to perseverate in speech or motion. Once started on a task they tend to lock on to environmental stimuli, automatically imitating or anticipating the examiner in their movements. Most lack insight into either their cognitive limitations or their sometimes bizarre behavior. In advanced stages with very large or bilateral prefrontal lesions, hypokinesia blends into a near-motionless, hypovocal (akinetic-mute) state combined with prominent bilateral motor changes consisting of paratonic rigidity. There are usually accompanying signs of mild to moderate contralateral corticospinal tract dysfunction, reflecting extension of dysfunction posteriorly to involve premotor areas.

Disorders of dorsolateral prefrontal function less severe than the above impair motor preprogramming and the capacity to anticipate future requirements. Patients with dorsolateral lesions have difficulty in governing the successive, near-automatic sequence of complicated motor tasks and in adapting overall motor behavior to meet the quick necessity of changing demands. More advanced lesions result in delays or difficulties in carrying out two- or three-stage demands (e.g., "Put your right thumb in your left ear"), produce perseverations of motor movement (the patient may continue to protrude the tongue after the command has changed to "Raise your hand"), or are associated with apathetic failure to respond to motor commands.

Frontal lobe damage restricted to orbitofrontal areas tends to affect personality and emotional behavior more than motor behavior and is discussed in the last chapter of this section.

Lesions injuring the frontal lobe often affect the functions of micturition and, to a lesser degree, defecation. Incontinence with frontal lesions can take either of two forms. Many patients with extensive frontal damage are confused and indifferent to the social conventions that normally surround the management of personal habits. They may evacuate the bowel or bladder randomly, giving little evidence of retaining voluntary sphincter control or even giving attention to the act. More specific sphincter difficulties sometimes result from lesions that damage the posterior extent of the vertex of the dorsolateral and dorsomedial prefrontal region, lowering the threshold for micturition to half or less of the usual bladder volume. The result is repeated episodes of self-aware urgency incontinence accompanied by little or no advance warning but considerable embarrassment for the patient.

Supplementary (Medial) and Premotor (Lateral) Frontal Lobe Cortex

These two regions straddle the vertex of the hemisphere immediately anterior to the primary motor cortex and relate to the regulation of complex voluntary movement (Fig. 22). They preform the templates for complex motor acts and relate learned patterns of movement to spatial (supplementary cortex) and visual (premotor cortex) stimuli coming from the association areas of the parietal lobe. The premotor and supplementary areas also integrate much of the feedforward information coming from the cerebellum and the basal ganglia into their own outflow programs that go to the primary motor cortex and to brainstem motor regions.

Knowledge of the functions of the human supplementary and premotor regions comes from three major sources: (1) stimulating the exposed cortex in awake persons during neurosurgical operations (a painless procedure), (2) correlating the patterns of focal motor epileptic discharges with the anatomic site of abnormal electrical activity, and (3) observing changes in motor behavior that follow destructive lesions or restricted removal of tumors or epileptic scars from the area.

Direct stimulations or epileptic discharges involving the superior-lateral prefrontal region, an area termed the *frontal eye fields,* induce conjugate contraversion of the eyes. With strong stimuli, adversive turning of the head or the head and body can accompany the ocular deviations. Acute destruction of the frontal eye field, area 8, by abnormalities such as large infarcts or surgical removal, results in ipsiversion of the eyes with transient paralysis of conjugate gaze to the opposite side of the body: The eyes "look toward" the lesion. By contrast, as noted above, irritating hemorrhages or seizures affecting a frontal eye field stimulate the eyes to "look away" from the lesion. In such instances the intensity and duration of the oculomotor abnormality are directly proportional to the size and acuteness of the cerebral damage. Unilateral frontal lobe injury rarely affects voluntary eye movement for more than 24 to 36 hours. With pre-existing or concurrent abnormalities in the contralateral frontal eye fields the defect can last substantially longer. Speech arrest is associated with epileptic discharges emanating from the lower end of the premotor region lying adjacent to Broca's area of the dominant hemisphere. *Broca's aphasia* results from destruction of this prefrontal cortical zone (see last chapter of this section). Neglect of motor function on the opposite side of the body as well as forced grasping in the opposite hand accompany many large premotor destructive lesions, especially those extending forward into the prefrontal region.

The supplementary motor region appears to possess motor programming functions even more important than the premotor area. Electrical stimulation of this region or epileptic discharges emanating from it result in complex posturing activity, mainly involving the opposite side of the body and affecting the face and upper limb more than the lower. Nonverbal vocalization or speech arrest may occur concomitantly. Motor changes include raising the contralateral arm, often with the hand elevated above the head, and turning the eyes and head to follow the position of the hand. Often the entire body will rotate away from the stimulated side with the hand leading the retreat. In addition to these postural-type responses, some patients develop repetitive pawing or, rarely, stepping movements. Despite these complex responses to stimulation, abnormalities following destructive damage restricted to the supplementary motor region in man include remarkably subtle clinical changes; most impairments last no more than a few days or weeks unless the lesion extends posteriorly to affect the precentral gyrus. In addition, supplementary motor lesions often interrupt the cerebellocortical motor relay so as to result in moderate ataxia of the contralateral upper extremity accompanying the more usual pattern of corticospinal-type hemiparesis or hemiplegia. Following surgical removal of the supplementary motor area one may detect hypokinesia of the contralateral face and arm as well as forced grasping and reduced vocalization. Most of the alterations subside within weeks, although a few patients are left permanently with a measure of hypokinesia and motor neglect affecting the contralateral arm. Bilateral supplementary motor damage gives rise to profound disturbances in initiating motor control, manifested by paratonia, reflex grasping, and hypokinesia. The impairment of complex movements that follows damage to the supplementary cortex plus the finding that the region generates prominent readiness potentials (p. 1044) reflect the region's role in establishing the programs of movement and coordinating their specific templates.

The Primary Motor Cortex

The primary motor cortex, M1, lies immediately anterior to the central rolandic fissure of the hemisphere. As emphasized in Penfield's cartoon of the upside-down homunculus (Fig. 24), electrical stimulation of the area discloses that the contralateral lower face, tongue, vocal organs, hand, and, to a lesser degree, foot enjoy a greater and more discrete representation than do other parts of the body. Focal seizures arising in this region in humans reflect its organization into simple movements. Beginning in the thumb-hand, the corner of the mouth, or, less often, the foot, these classic attacks described a century ago by the astute English neurologist Hughlings Jackson, and known as *jacksonian seizures,* consist of recurrent rhythmic, focal twitchings. The seizures usually spread gradually from their origin by affecting adjacent muscles or, less often, by jumping from hand to face or vice versa. Almost always their occurrence reflects a structural abnormality in or adjacent to the motor cortex.

An understanding of the pathophysiology of motor abnormalities arising at the level of the cerebral cortex or below relies almost as much on a knowledge of cerebral vascular anatomy and its susceptibilities to disease as it does on the neurophysiology of the system. Accordingly, vascular syndromes and regional syndromes will be discussed together in some of the following sections.

The lateral hemispheric surface of the primary sensorimotor area is served by terminal branches of the middle cerebral artery, while the distal end of the anterior cerebral artery supplies the foot-leg area of the motor cortex on the medial hemispheric surface.

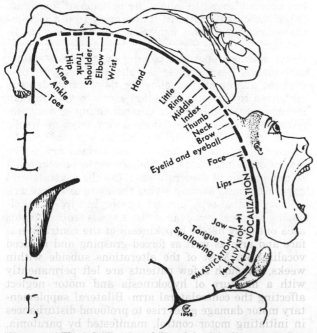

Figure 24. The relative size of the parts of the human primary motor cortex from which movements of different parts of the body can be elicited on electrical stimulation. (From Penfield, W., and Rasmussen, T.: The Cerebral Cortex of Man. New York, Macmillan Co., 1950.)

Focal damage or destruction restricted to the lateral surface of the motor cortex produces weakness largely confined to the lower part of the face or involving the face and the distal hand-arm, all contralaterally. Destruction along the superior-medial surface results in focal impairment of function of the foot and distal area of the leg. Acute vascular occlusion, i.e., cortical branch occlusion of the middle cerebral artery, represents the most common cause of sudden functional loss affecting the face or hand, while sudden isolated foot paralysis (a less frequent occurrence) usually reflects occlusion of the distal portion of the anterior cerebral artery. Because of the artery's distribution to the postcentral gyrus, the latter defect is likely to be accompanied by proprioceptive sensory loss in the foot as well. Focal acute penetrating head wounds can produce acute paralyses that closely resemble the above. Similarly distributed but more gradually developing weaknesses result from enlarging neoplasms or other space-taking or destructive lesions that focally affect the respective regions.

Acute damage confined to the primary motor cortex characteristically produces transient flaccid weakness or paralysis with both the severity of the weakness and hypotonia intensified if damage concurrently involves the postcentral sensory cortex. The latter, hypotonic, influence may reflect the temporary effect of interruption or inhibition of the thalamocortical portion of the long-loop component of the stretch reflex. Rarely, occlusions of small distal cortical arterial branches affecting the hand area produce an acute peripheral sensorimotor loss that is so restricted and glove-like in its distribution that it initially may be mistaken as having been caused by an acute injury to peripheral nerves, especially the radial nerve. The central pathogenesis can be suspected, however, by recalling that acute nontraumatic peripheral neuropathy rarely, if ever, involves simultaneously the ulnar, median, and ulnar nerves at the same distal level. Furthermore, flaccid paralysis with depression of both deep tendon reflexes and muscle tonus never permanently follows damage confined to a unilateral corticospinal pathway. Within hours or days (or sometimes a week or more if the sensory cortex also is involved) deep tendon reflexes increase in the affected limb, and at least some muscle spasticity appears. The larger the frontal lesion, the sooner such manifestations of spasticity arise; spasticity usually emerges immediately when both premotor and motor areas are involved concurrently.

DESCENDING MOTOR PATHWAYS

Functional Anatomy

Axons arising from the precentral motor cortex course through the subcortical hemispheric white matter joined by additional somatotopically congruent fibers from premotor, frontal, and postcentral parietal areas. The combined descending pathways converge via the corona radiata into the *internal capsule* tucked between the globus pallidus and the thalamus (Fig. 25). Within the capsule the corticospinal fibers align themselves in the posterior limb, lying in an anterior-posterior position corresponding to the rostral-caudal distribution of their projection targets: Corticobulbar pathways lie at the genu, adjacent to the anterior

DIENCEPHALON

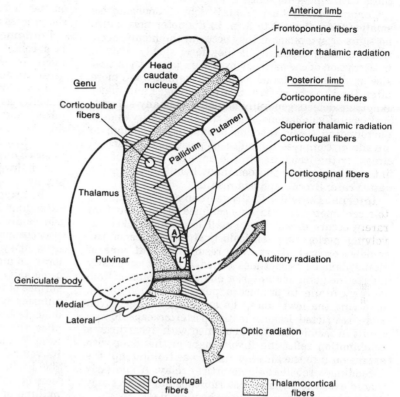

Figure 25. Components of the right internal capsule. (From Carpenter, M. B.: Human Neuroanatomy. 8th ed. Copyright 1983, Williams & Wilkins Co., Baltimore.)

capsular limb, while more caudally directed corticospinal fibers are packed successively behind. The ascending thalamocortical projections, which transmit ascending somatosensory information to the parietal lobe, lie in the capsule in a position somewhat medial but largely posterior to the descending motor pathways. The most posterior portion of the capsule carries the thalamocortical relays for hearing and vision.

Fibers from the posterior limb of the internal capsule descend directly into the cerebral peduncles, twin structures underlying the diencephalon and upper midbrain. Corticobulbar fibers in the peduncle lie medially, with the corticospinal pathways taking a more lateral position. Corticobulbar fibers destined to innervate the oculomotor system depart from the peduncle largely at the level of the diencephalon and midbrain, while axons intended for lower cranial nerves peel off more caudally in the brainstem. A large component of the cerebral peduncles enters the brainstem to influence autonomic functions, the cerebellum, and postural motor control, the last via the rubrospinal and reticulospinal components of the upper motor neuron system. Reflecting the considerable size of these projections to cerebellum and brainstem, the medullary pyramids leaving the brainstem contain less than one-fourth of the number of fibers entering via the cerebral peduncles.

Paralysis of cranial muscles following unilateral peduncular or capsular lesions in humans is seldom severe: Supranuclear (upper motor neuron) weakness in the face is almost confined to the lower half and never complete, while jaw, pharyngeal-laryngeal, and hypoglossal movements characteristically escape almost unscathed. By implication, considerable cortico-

bulbar innervation must come directly or indirectly from both cerebral hemispheres.

Below the cerebral peduncle, descending cerebral motor fibers interweave in a gridlike pattern among the pontine nuclei and the transverse crossing fibers of the afferent cerebellar pathways in the basis pontis. Leaving the brainstem, most corticospinal tract fibers decussate in the medullary pyramids to form the contralateral lateral corticospinal tract; a small proportion extends ipsilaterally into the cord as the ventral corticospinal tract, which descends as far caudally as the midthoracic level. Whichever route they take, however, all evidence indicates that primary motor axons decussate before reaching their final innervation directly or indirectly on the contralateral anterior horn cell. By contrast, the cerebral supplementary motor areas appear to project both ipsilaterally and bilaterally to control midline movements of the head and trunk. The same is to a degree true of pathways extending to spinal cord from brainstem motor centers.

The anatomy of the descending corticospinal pathways and their susceptibility to damage from disease give rise to a number of motor disturbances whose distribution of weakness and accompanying neurologic abnormalities permit accurate localizing diagnosis. Once localized, an evaluation of the natural history (e.g., a sudden onset and appropriate distribution imply vascular disease; a gradual development points to mechanical abnormalities such as neoplasms or bony deformity; a diffuse and symmetric distribution suggests a toxic, metabolic, degenerative, or infectious process; and so on) and the obtaining of appropriate laboratory tests then can lead to precise etiologic diagnosis and guide one to appropriate treatment. The following paragraphs outline the more frequent of these localizing syndromes.

Corona Radiata. Frontal lobe abnormalities smaller than about 2 to 3 cm in diameter may cause no signs or symptoms if they occur in the hemispheric white matter, especially if they form slowly. Partial interruption of the pathway by lesions larger than that size produce a combined paresis of the foot-hand more often than the hand-face. Sensory changes and major language defects generally do not accompany subcortical frontal lobe lesions unless the abnormality and its surrounding tissue reaction become large enough to invade or compress the adjacent parietal or temporal areas, or the lesion lies in the anterior portion of the internal capsule of the dominant hemisphere. In the latter case, Broca's aphasia results.

Internal Capsule. Restricted damage (millimeters to a centimeter or so in size) confined to this structure rarely occurs except with small ischemic strokes involving perforating lenticulostriate branches of the middle cerebral artery. The resulting small zone of tissue damage (sometimes called a *lacune*) typically affects the genu and anterior end of the posterior limb of the capsule to produce a pure motor hemiplegia involving the lower face, the arm, and the leg. Even more restricted lesions in the posterior capsule can result in facial weakness combined with dysarthria, a combination reflecting involvement of the genu with extension into the anterior limb so as to interrupt the ascending cerebellothalamocortical relay. A similarly placed extension from a posterior capsular infarct may add limb ataxia to pure motor hemiplegia.

Deep, larger lesions of the dominant hemisphere involving the posterior limb of the capsule but extending forward into the anterior limb and the adjacent corona radiata produce expressive aphasia sometimes verging on muteness. The motor weakness can predominate in the face or extend to include an entire hemiplegia. Rarely the severe expressive aphasia or muteness appears as an isolated change. Interruption of deep language pathways descending from Broca's area is the presumed mechanism of the language impairment, but satisfactory pathologic examinations are lacking.

Cerebral Peduncles. Fractional damage to these structures occurs with occlusion of arterial branches arising from the apex of the basilar artery or from the adjacent posterior cerebral artery. More gradual injury can result from mechanical lesions such as neoplasms or granulomas arising at the base of the brain. Demyelinating plaques occasionally affect the peduncles. The ensuing signs and symptoms of damage principally reflect the anatomy involved. Complete destruction or interruption of the peduncle results in spastic hemiplegia including the face, arm, and leg. Medially placed lesions interrupt corticobulbar pathways, but spare descending oculomotor fibers. Mild defects appear in the trigeminal motor and vagal somatomotor distribution and are accompanied by severe lower facial weakness, often with the tongue deviating to the side of the facial weakness (hypoglossal paresis ipsilateral to the face). Lesions damaging the lower end of the peduncle at the point where it joins the pons characteristically interrupt the peripheral oculomotor fibers as they emerge from the midbrain. The result produces ipsilateral third nerve paralysis coupled with contra-lateral hemiplegia. A similar combination of signs accompanies damage resulting from external pressure on the midbrain by the medial temporal lobe during the process of transtentorial herniation.

Pontomedullary Pathways. The lower brainstem is a complicated structure containing cranial nerve nuclei interspersed among ascending and descending sensorimotor pathways. The area also contains afferent and efferent cerebellar relays projecting rostrally and caudally as well as a number of nuclear centers that affect more distal bulbospinal motor control. These anatomic considerations provide a substrate for several somewhat differing clinical syndromes whose genesis is based on the contiguous architecture between nuclei and pathways and the geography of the local arterial supply.

The arterial supply of the brainstem and spinal cord extending from the posterior diencephalon caudally can be divided conveniently into paramedian and lateral circumferential branches of the vertebral-basilar arterial system. Starting just above the level of the foramen magnum, the two vertebral arteries each send a medially directed collateral that join on the ventral surface of the medulla to form the cranial origin of the anterior spinal artery (Fig. 26). This vessel plus more delicate branches of the twin vertebral arteries supplies the paramedian medullary structures. At the lower border of the pons the vertebral arteries join on its ventral surface to form the basilar artery (Fig. 7). The basilar, as it courses rostrally, gives off a succession of delicate paramedian branches supplying the midline of the brainstem as well as a series of more stout lateral circumferential arteries termed, in caudal to rostral order, the posterior-inferior (originating from a vertebral artery), anterior-inferior, and superior cerebellar arteries. Finally, at its apex, the basilar splits into two large circumferential arteries, the posterior cerebrals, that supply the posterior lateral thalamus as well as the posterior medial aspect of the hemisphere reaching the occipital pole. The apex of the basilar artery in a delta-like manner divides into many small

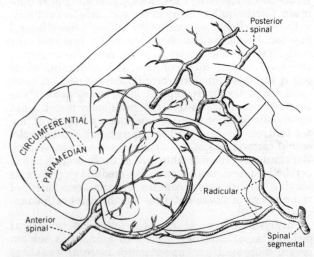

Figure 26. Arterial supply to the spinal cord. (From Patton, H. D., Sundsten, J. W., Crill, W. E., and Swanson, P.D.: Introduction to Basic Neurology. Philadelphia, W. B. Saunders Co., 1976.)

paramedian branches that supply the midline of the posterior diencephalon and the dorsal thalamus.

Corticospinal pathways descend in the basis pontis, lying more medially than laterally with axons destined for upper and lower extremities running in juxtaposition. Corticobulbar fibers projecting to the facial, pharyngeal, and hypoglossal nuclei already have peeled off from the cerebral peduncles. As a result, unilateral paramedian damage of the basis pontis results in contralateral hemiplegia of the arm and leg while bilateral injury produces quadriplegia affecting the same members. If the overlying paramedian tegmentum is affected, appropriate ipsilateral lower motor neuron cranial nerve palsies (V, VI, VII) occur, depending upon the level of the lesion. These may be accompanied by paralysis of conjugate gaze toward the side of the abnormality due to involvement of the ipsilateral parabducens area. Injury to the medial lemniscus impairs contralateral touch, vibratory, and position sensations. Laterally placed lesions interfere more with cerebellar than corticospinal projection pathways, resulting in various patterns of ipsilateral or contralateral ataxia, depending upon which cerebellar brachium is affected.

Severe, acute parenchymal damage to the medullary pyramids is an uncommon clinical problem in humans. The area is well collateralized from the standpoint of its arterial supply. Furthermore, trauma or intramedullary hemorrhages involving the area usually damage the adjacent respiratory and circulatory controlling areas so that death quickly follows unless immediate resuscitation is applied. The few reported patients suffering selective damage to the pyramids have initially suffered a flaccid hemiparesis or quadriparesis presumably reflecting associated involvement of the descending reticulospinal pathways. In those few who have survived, deep tendon reflexes increased within a few days, and muscle spasticity soon followed, following the usual pattern seen with acute spinal lesions. With slow external compression of the medulla such as occurs with local neoplasms or developmental abnormalities of the base of the skull the entire course is that of a progressive spastic motor weakness involving both upper and lower extremities, often on both sides.

A "cruciate hemiplegia" with paralysis of the ipsilateral leg and contralateral arm has been postulated to accompany damage to the lower end of the pyramidal decussation. The envisioned mechanism consists of concurrent interruption of already crossed corticospinal pathways to the leg and as yet nondecussated axons destined for the opposite arm. We are unaware of pathologic verification of such an entity.

Pseudobulbar Palsy

The state of weakness that affects lower cranial nerve functions when disease bilaterally interrupts the descending corticobulbar pathways somewhere between the cerebral cortex and the pons is known as pseudobulbar palsy. Vascular disease is the most common cause, especially that associated with hypertension, which damages the brain's small arterioles and ends up peppering the region of the basal ganglia and internal capsules with tiny infarcts. Appropriately placed bilateral demyelinating lesions, certain degenerative corticospinal tract diseases such as amy-

otrophic lateral sclerosis, and, rarely, infiltrating neoplasms can have similar although usually less prominent effects. Except with degenerative disorders, disease rarely attacks both corticospinal pathways simultaneously. Accordingly, one most often sees pseudobulbar palsy develop following an acute unilateral lesion superimposed on a pre-existing injury to the contralateral corticobulbar system. Acutely, supranuclear bulbar paralysis sometimes may immobilize the tongue, pharynx, face, and jaw so severely as to leave the part almost motionless to voluntary effort, thereby making difficult the distinction from true bulbar palsy of lower motor neuron origin. Pseudobulbar weakness, however, always spares at least some involuntary motor functions so that most patients continue to swallow their own saliva, and all naturally blink the eyes even when unable to do so on command. With milder examples or upon recovery, spastic weakness is the rule, associated with slow awkward movements of jaw, tongue, and larynx. Frequently one observes a slow grinding dysphonia as well as periodic breathing of Cheyne-Stokes type. If the lesions interrupt fibers at the capsular level or above, inappropriately intense, reflexly released laughing or crying occurs, reflecting a disinhibition of descending limbic pathways. The absence of complete facial or sustained pharyngeal paralysis, the lack of muscle atrophy or fasciculations, the presence of the strained unmodulated voice, and the appearance of hyperemotional responses all distinguish chronic pseudobulbar from primary bulbar paralysis.

Spinal Cord

Below the pyramidal decussation corticospinal fibers travel caudally in the dorsal portion of the lateral funiculus of the spinal cord. A variety of abnormalities can affect the corticospinal tract at the spinal level. *Occlusion of the anterior spinal artery* is a rare consequence of arteriosclerotic thromboembolic disease. However, the vessel and its tributaries, which supply the anterior two-thirds of the cord, can be affected by inflammatory or immunologic disorders to cause an acute ischemic anterior myelopathy. The result produces below the lesion an acute bilateral, initially flaccid paraplegia coupled with loss of pain and temperature sensations, reflecting damage to the ventral spinal thalamic pathways. Bowel and bladder control is lost.

Extramedullary mass lesions (e.g., neoplasms, disc lesions, infections) can compress the spinal cord transversely. The result usually impairs both descending motor pathways more or less symmetrically. One finds increased deep tendon reflexes, spasticity, and extensor plantar responses below the lesion. These changes often are accompanied at the level of the lesion by damage to ventral roots, producing reduced tendon reflexes, muscle atrophy, and sometimes fasciculations in the involved spinal segment. The dorsally placed afferent pathways mediating vibratory sensation, proprioception, and touch are affected more than those carrying pain and temperature. Bowel and bladder control is spared until late in the course.

Unilateral spinal cord damage affecting one corticospinal tract and adjacent sensory pathways causes the *Brown-Séquard syndrome*. Distal to the lesion one finds, ipsilaterally, hyperactive deep tendon reflexes, signs of upper motor neuron weakness, spasticity, and the extensor plantar response plus loss of touch, proprioceptive, and spatial sensations. Contralaterally, pain and temperature sensations are impaired. Because of the laminar pattern of the ventral spinothalamic pathway, extramedullary cord compression to this pathway produces analgesia in the distal spinal segments while intramedullary damage results in analgesia beginning one or two segments below the level of the cord dysfunction. All sensory modalities characteristically may be impaired ipsilaterally at the level of the lesion, reflecting injury to the dorsal root sensory entry zone. The effects of functional spinal cord transection are discussed on page 1058.

Disorders of the Lower Motor Neuron

A disorder of the lower motor neuron, as already noted, refers to disease or dysfunction that attacks the perikaryon of the bulbar or spinal motor neuron or any part of its axon along its course from nucleus to nerve terminal. Principal causes of lower motor neuron abnormalities are degenerative diseases such as amyotrophic lateral sclerosis and its congeners (sometimes called motor neuron disease), inherited or acquired peripheral neuropathies, destructive mechanical conditions such as spinal tumors, discs, or infections, trauma, or, less often, vascular occlusions affecting peripheral motor axons.

As described earlier, damage or interruption to the anterior horn cell directly produces trophic changes in skeletal muscle with the rate and severity of the myotrophic and neural abnormalities paralleling each other. Weakness appears immediately following nerve section, and muscle atrophy can be discerned clinically within seven to ten days after severe axonal damage. Lower motor neuron abnormalities reduce the resistance of muscles to passive stretch (hypotonia). The deep tendon reflexes diminish or disappear, and fasciculations and fibrillations develop in the denervated motor units and muscle fibers, respectively. In most instances the anatomic distribution of these changes and the rate of their development provide important leads to their cause.

DISORDERS OF THE BASAL GANGLIA

Pathophysiology of Dysfunction

The functional anatomy and pharmacology of the normal basal ganglia have been described on page 1040, and a preceding section has discussed the patterns and mechanism of most of the individual symptoms and signs that result from basal ganglia disease (Table 18). The following paragraphs recapitulate these clinical changes and describe the pathophysiology of disease in these deep forebrain nuclei.

Basal ganglia dysfunction interferes with normal motor control in one or more of five major ways, depending on the specific anatomic or pharmacologic

TABLE 18. PRINCIPAL SYNDROMES OF BASAL GANGLIA DISEASES

Parkinsonism: Bradykinesia, rigidity, resting and postural tremor, hypophonia, dysarthria, defects in automatic associated movements, resting and reflex postural abnormalities

Chorea
Athetosis
Ballism
Dystonia

errors induced by a particular disease. Defects of basal ganglia origin include (1) dyskinesias, (2) abnormal skeletal muscle resistance to passive stretch, (3) abnormalities in initiating movement and in performing successive or simultaneously independent motor acts, (4) prominent impairment of proximal motor functions that are innervated bilaterally, and (5) defects in automatic postural control.

Dyskinesias. These consist of abnormalities of resting or postural movement that reflect disturbed, feedforward influences on frontal, premotor, and supplementary motor areas of the cerebral cortex. All of the dyskinesias resemble normal body movements, fragments of body movements, or, in the case of dystonia, normal movements "gone wrong" or overdone. Despite their origin in basal ganglia dysfunction, all of the dyskinesias are eventually expressed via the descending corticospinal pathways. Consequently they disappear or largely subside when those pathways are interrupted or severely damaged. Basal ganglia dyskinesias also largely or completely disappear during sleep; they are ameliorated by emotional calmness and accentuated by states of anxiety or emotional tension. Anatomic links that are known to connect the basal ganglia and the limbic system may partly explain this latter effect.

The specific dyskinesias of basal ganglia origin include (1) the alternating tremor of parkinsonism; (2) the slow, twisting, usually action-induced, and mainly proximally located developmental movement disorders of athetosis in which basal ganglia and corticospinal tract dysfunction are combined; (3) the dystonias, individual examples of which may have either a focal or progressive generalized distribution in their pattern; (4) the quick distal irregular movements of chorea; and (5) the proximal flinging movements of ballism.

Abnormal Skeletal Muscular Resistance to Passive Stretch. In basal ganglia disorders, abnormal skeletal muscular resistance to passive stretch can take three forms. One is the continuous agonist-antagonist, steady (lead-pipe) or rhythmic (cogwheel) rigidity of parkinsonism. A second is the irregular, tonic, actively but unpredictably contracting resistance that one encounters when trying to move the body part of a patient affected by athetosis or dystonia. The third is the poorly characterized hypotonia that is occasionally encountered in both Sydenham's and Huntington's chorea.

Abnormalities in the Initiation of Movement or in the Capacity to Perform Successive Motor Acts. These difficulties are grouped together under the general heading of *akinesia* or *hypokinesia*. In parkinsonism they express themselves in delayed initiation and subsequent slowness of onset of movement and in Parkinson's disease as an inability of patients to conduct two independent motor acts successively or concurrently. They also are observed in the inability of patients with chorea to complete smoothly a pursuit voluntary motor act or to maintain a steady contraction or posture. The overflow of automatic movements into posturally inappropriate body parts that characterizes both chorea and dystonia are part of this movement abnormality.

Prominent Impairment of Midline and Other Bilaterally Innervated Movements. While all basal ganglia disorders impair distal motor functions to a more or less severe degree, they differ from primary corticospinal outflow disease in producing in almost every instance equal or greater disturbances in proximal motor control, often bilaterally. Hypovocalism and abnormal speech are prominent in parkinsonism as are a stooped posture, slow and stiff motion of the shoulders and hips, and limitation of the natural appendicular accessory movements that accompany normal walking, climbing, running, and many other activities. A whole category of dopamine-sensitive dyskinesias affect the face and vocal apparatus. Patients with Huntington's disease display a high incidence of bilateral grimacing, jaw opening, tongue working, dysarthria, and twisting of the trunk. Somewhat similar changes in expression and posture affect patients with athetosis and dystonia. The presence of these midline and bilateral disturbances imply that information emanating from the basal ganglia and relayed caudally with the corticospinal system must project bilaterally to vestibulospinal, bulbar reticular, and spinal reticular neuron pools to provide the necessary postural support for skilled movement.

Impaired Postural Control. Abnormalities in automatic postural responses to tilting, falling, skilled movement, and locomotion are observed most prominently in parkinsonism. Labyrinthine-vestibular abnormalities have been described in affected patients, but the most striking feature is an absence of preprogrammed, automatic associated motor responses to sudden postural change. Somewhat similar defects also can affect patients with Huntington's disease, Wilson's disease, and hemiballism.

Major Basal Ganglia Syndromes

The Movement Disorder of Parkinson's Disease

Parkinson's disease and its functional antithesis, Huntington's disease, are the most studied disorders of the basal ganglia. Indeed, much of what we postulate to be the normal physiology of these structures is deduced from abnormalities observed in these two conditions.

Parkinson's disease is largely the functional expression of degeneration of the pigmented dopamine-synthesizing cells that lie in the pars compacta of the substantia nigra (Fig. 27). The cause in most instances is unknown. As a result, the dopamine content and the number of dopamine receptors decline in nigral target cells in the putamen, a structure that also receives the major excitatory input from the cerebral cortex. Dopamine projections also decline in the caudate; the mesolimbic, mesocortical, and hypothalamic dopamine systems degenerate concurrently with those of the nigrostriatal pathway. Lewy bodies, inclusions of uncertain pathogenetic significance but morphologically almost pathognomonic for Parkinson's disease, are found principally in the substantia nigra, locus ceruleus, and the substantia innominata of the basal forebrain as well as being scattered in other areas of the forebrain and brainstem. Noradrenergic neurons degenerate in the locus ceruleus in a proportion of patients.

Behavioral changes are prominent in parkinsonism. Many patients become depressed during the early stages of the illness, and about 25 per cent eventually become demented. Possibly underlying these changes, but not mechanistically easy to explain, is the finding that even nondemented parkinsonian patients show a general reduction of cerebral metabolism below nor-

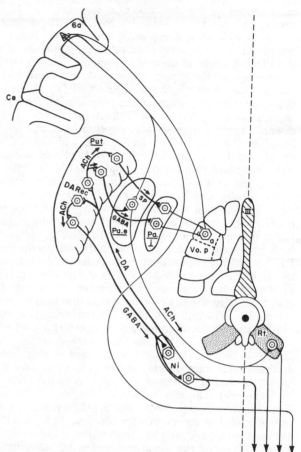

Figure 27. In parkinsonism, the cell loss in the substantia nigra *(Ni)* leads to reduction of the amount of dopamine *(DA)* that is transported to the striatum *(Put)*. Consequently its excitatory action on the DA receptors *(DARec)* is critically weakened. The administration of high doses of L-dopa causes enhanced excitation of the DARec, so that the function of the striatal synaptic mechanism becomes nearly normal. The anticholinergic drugs act on the synaptic mechanism of the cholinergic striatal interneurons. Owing to the DA deficiency in parkinsonism, the excitation of these interneurons is also reduced, so that the pallidal neurons are disinhibited. The action of anticholinergic drugs on the interneurons, however, increases the GABA-ergic inhibition of the pallidum and Ni, and the pallidal neurons are inhibited. Possibly the cholinergic drugs act also on the efferent mechanism of the pallidum, which according to some investigators is cholinergic. *6a* = premotor area 6a; *ce* = central sulcus; *ACh* = acetylcholine; *SP* = substance P; *GABA* = gamma-aminobutyric acid; *Pa.e* and *Pa.i* = pallidum externum and internum; *VoPa* = ventro-oral posterior and anterior thalamic nuclei; *Rt* = formatio reticularis. (From Hassler, R. G.: Adv Neurol 40:1–15. Copyright 1984, Raven Press, New York.

mal; this becomes even more prominent among the demented. Moreover, among those who do become demented, cholinergic neurons disappear from the basal forebrain nuclei in a manner similar to what occurs in Alzheimer's disease (see final chapter of this section).

As is true in many other regulating mechanisms of the human body, the dopamine system of the brain possesses a considerable physiologic reserve. Symptoms of Parkinson's disease usually fail to develop until approximately 80 per cent of nigral neurons have been lost with a commensurate decline in striatal dopamine. Furthermore, the disease is almost specifically caused by the dopaminergic degeneration. As a result, replacement of dopamine by giving the precursor L-dopa nearly completely ameliorates clinical symptoms in early cases. Adding to the evidence of a specific deficiency of dopamine systems is the recent discovery that the piperidine derivative N-methyl-4-phenyl-1-,2,5,6-tetrahydropyridine (NMPTP) produces acute, permanent parkinsonism with clinical features indistinguishable from those of the naturally occurring disease. Typical nigrostriatal degeneration has been found in the brain of an addict who had taken the agent as well as in monkeys given NMPTP experimentally. Levodopa relieves the symptoms of NMPTP poisoning, just as it does those of idiopathic parkinsonism.

The precise way by which the symptoms of tremor, rigidity, akinesia, and loss of postural instability in parkinsonism relate to the loss of striatal dopamine remains poorly understood. Nevertheless, the physiologic abnormalities can be profoundly incapacitating. Patients with parkinsonism have remarkable difficulties in initiating movement. They show an abnormally prolonged motor reaction time whether in response to command or ideation, and some freeze into nearly total immobility. The initiation of movement is delayed, and quick ballistic movements are poorly performed, effects that seriously impair fast-moving, learned skills. The failure to initiate movement is reflected in slow, soft, and relatively unmodulated speech, a molasses-in-January retardation of getting started, and an inability to perform quick acts such as playing the piano or violin. The quickly initiated postural reflexes so necessary to prevent falls or injury are impaired or lost. Finally, patients with parkinsonism suffer from a little-understood failure in the preprogramming of movement. They have major difficulties in carrying out a consecutive or simultaneous series of learned acts such as concurrently patting the head and rubbing the stomach or reaching in the pocket for money while climbing from a bus or taxi. These defects suggest that an intact basal ganglia provides the necessary motor pretemplates upon which the supplementary motor cortex erects the fine control of skilled movements.

Huntington's Disease

The pathophysiology of Huntington's chorea involves the output of the basal ganglia less exclusively than does parkinsonism. Anatomically one finds, in addition to severe atrophy of the striatum, a loss of neurons in layers 3, 5, and 6 of the cerebral cortex, especially in the frontal lobe. Striatal dopamine and epinephrine contents, depending as they do on axons whose perikarya lie in extrastriatal sites, remain normal or actually high. By contrast, the striatal neurons that synthesize GABA and acetylcholine are selectively depleted and they decline markedly in numbers so that the relative concentrations of those transmitters decrease. The overall defect, however, does not resemble a diffuse pharmacologic system degeneration since neurons employing these transmitters in other regions of the brain fail to show consistent reductions. Striatal reductions occur in substance P, angiotensin-converting enzyme, and metenkephalin. These changes are thought to reflect a local loss of the progenitor cells for the substances.

The result of the above anatomic-pharmacologic impairment in Huntington's disease is a major reduction of striatal output, producing a physiologic abnormality that differs substantially from parkinsonism. Furthermore, the effects are less easy to predict because of the diffuseness of the neurochemical lesion. A major feature, however, is that within the striatum the presence of a high concentration of dopamine terminals plus fewer receptor-containing cells implies increased dopamine stimulation of residual receptors. This mechanism may explain at least partially the genesis of the abnormal adventitious movements.

The pathophysiologic contrast between parkinsonism and Huntington's disease is immediately apparent. In the former disorder, extrastriatal dopaminergic neurons die and dopaminergic modulation of striatal output to the cortex fails. The result produces an impoverishment of movements, an increase in muscle resistance to passive stretch, and a failure of rapid movement, but no loss of accuracy of slow movement. There is an oscillating tremor as well as a defect in getting successive acts together, i.e., in sequential motor programming. In Huntington's disease, by contrast, the major striatal output fails with the dopamine modulated pathways being least affected. Quick, inadvertent, unwanted movements appear spontaneously and resemble fragments of normal learned motor activity. When reflex or ideational movements are initiated, reaction time is quick, and the movements start in the correct direction although they often swing wide of the mark as successive, inappropriate motor activity intrudes. Motor programming appears to be intact, but the act becomes repeatedly blocked by the random appearance of subcortical excessive (dopamine) stimulation of the premotor cortex via uninhibited residual striatothalamocortical pathways. In contrast to parkinsonism in which dopamine agonists ameliorate the disorder, they intensify it in Huntington's disease. Finally, muscle resistance to passive stretch is decreased in Huntington's disease, not increased as in parkinsonism. The mechanism of the prominent dementia that accompanies Huntington's disease has not been elucidated. As noted, increasing attention is being given to the connections between the basal ganglia and the limbic system as possibly providing noncortical pathways whose injury could contribute to the abnormal mental functions.

ABNORMALITIES IN THE CEREBELLAR CONTROL OF MOVEMENT

The cerebellum regulates the execution of skilled motor acts and coordinates their smooth postural support. Disease or dysfunction of the cerebellum delays the onset of skilled movement, interferes with its normally smooth trajectory and aim, decomposes the required synergy of its postural supports, and blocks the capacity to perform rhythmic successive movements of the kind required to write, type, speak, or play a musical instrument. The functional anatomy of the cerebellum and its connections is discussed on pages 1041 to 1043, where the regional syndromes that arise in association with damage to the vestibulocerebellar spinocerebellar areas are also described. The following sections describe the defects that arise with damage to the lateral cerebellar areas and the mechanistic abnormalities that produce them.

TABLE 19. THE BASIS OF ABNORMAL CEREBELLAR SIGNS IN HUMANS

SIGN	MECHANISM

Ataxia
  Intention tremor
  Asynergia among muscles
  Decomposition of
    movements around
    separate joints
  Point-to-point error (dysmetria)
    and deviation from the line
    of movement
  Failure of rapid alternating
    movement
    (dysdiadochokinesia)
	All represent errors in preplanning trajectory and impaired proprioceptive feedback loops

Hypotonia
Failure to check voluntary
  movement quickly
Rebound movement after
  release of tonic movement
	Predominantly errors of proprioceptive feedback

Hyperactive deep tendon reflexes	Impaired anterior cerebellar influence on bulbar reticular formation

Clinical Disturbances in Neocerebellar Function

The characteristic abnormalities of impaired neocerebellar control of movement are summarized in Table 19. The changes involve the distal limbs more than the proximal and affect the upper extremities more than the lower. Patients with dentate nucleus or outflow pathway disease have reduced resistance to passive stretch (hypotonia) in the muscles and joints of the affected upper extremity. Ascribed to impaired cerebellar control of the stretch reflex, as described below, the abnormality leads to loose, pendular reflexes and hyperextensibility of joints. Movement is slow to start and difficult to stop, producing overshoot or a failure quickly to check when an arm contracted against resistance is abruptly released. Synergistic movements, those requiring postural supports at several joints, decompose, producing jerky, irregular errors in the range of motion, a phenomenon called dysmetria. As the member nears its target, it oscillates, producing classical intention tremor. Rapid, successive alternating movements are performed awkwardly. If the dyssynergy extends to affect the vocal-lingual apparatus, a scanning, irregular dysarthria appears. Nystagmus sometimes can be detected, but more often this abnormality reflects damage to structures that lie adjacent to the cerebellum rather than arising from injuries within the cerebellum itself.

If cerebellar damage is limited to the hemisphere and fails to involve the roof nuclei, clinical abnormalities may be difficult to detect, especially if the lesion arises slowly and no pressure is exerted on the adjacent brainstem. This principle is especially true with damage to the lateral cerebellum. Mild ipsilateral hypotonia, some awkwardness in rhythmic movements, and subtle defects in point-to-point tests are the most that one can expect. Occasionally even the experienced clinician has difficulty detecting that anything is physiologically wrong. A similar principle applies to cerebellar function after surgical removal of the hemispheres. So long as the roof nuclei are spared,

remarkable degrees of recovery return with time, although finely tuned hand movements such as musicians or machinists require may always remain insufficient for professional use.

The contralateral ventrolateral thalamic nucleus that relays signals from the brachium conjunctivum back to the cerebral cortex modulates and amplifies abnormal cerebellar guidance control signals in as yet incompletely understood ways. Small lesions placed stereotaxically in the posterior portion of this nucleus can greatly reduce or abolish the intention tremor of neocerebellar disease as well as that of parkinsonism and familial tremor. Such lesions have relatively little effect on other aspects of cerebellar dysfunction. Interruption of the thalamofrontal cerebellar-cortical pathway produces uncertain functional abnormalities. Clinical experience indicates that patients with prefrontal cerebral lesions sometimes suffer from a greater degree of ataxia or incoordination in the contralateral limbs than can be explained by the mild corticospinal hemiparesis that is present. These changes have been attributed to interruption of the cerebello-cortical pathway. The older clinical literature, written in days before accurate brain imaging became widely available, described many patients in whom the presence of prominent ataxia secondary to frontal lobe tumors was mistakenly attributed to disease of the cerebellum. Presumably these effects reflected abnormalities in thalamofrontal cerebellar pathways, but the exact pathophysiology is unknown.

The Pathophysiology of Abnormal Cerebellar Motor Control

Two ways by which the cerebellum regulates movement have been studied in relation to neocerebellar ataxia: (1) its influence on ballistic and ramp movements, and (2) its associated influence on the phasic (short-loop) and the tonic (long-loop) components of the stretch reflex.

As described on page 1045, fast-initiating ballistic movements are preprogrammed by the cerebrum, show short reaction times of about 200 msec, and normally are initiated with well-defined timing in which the first agonist and antagonist bursts normally fire alternately for roughly equal periods lasting for 50 to 100 msec each. Subsequent bursts normally may vary somewhat in a manner appropriate to correct the trajectory. Neocerebellar dysfunction disrupts both the timing of these ballistic bursts and the accuracy of the trajectory. In experimental primates, dentate lesions increase the reaction time by which a movement follows an intentional or exteroceptive stimulus by 30 to 50 per cent, and the duration of either the agonist or antagonist bursts or both may lengthen abnormally. The result produces a delay in the onset of movement, a tendency to overshoot or undershoot, and a disruption in rhythmic successive movements.

Ramp movements also are impaired in cerebellar disease, at least partly because of the organ's influence on the fusimotor neuron system and its subsequent effect on the stretch reflex.

Different parts of the cerebellum influence the stretch reflex mechanism in different ways. Stimulation of the anterior vermis in experimental animals raises the threshold of the reflex by reducing descending influences from the cerebellum on the gamma motor neuron. Conversely, ablation or damage to this region of the anterior cerebellum in animals or man increases bulboreticular facilitation of the gamma (fusimotor) motor neuron. Gamma hyperactivity leads to hypersensitivity of the muscle spindle with consequent hyperactivity of the deep tendon reflexes without producing abnormal lengthening and shortening reactions or other manifestations of true spasticity, at least in humans. Stimulation or damage to the lateral cerebellum has an effect opposite to that of the vermis. Stimulation increases tonic descending influences on the gamma motor neuron (not a problem in clinical disorders), whereas damage or dysfunction of neocerebellar outflow reduces the excitability of the fusimotor system. The latter effect raises the threshold for the stretch reflex, thereby reducing or delaying its feedback arc and impairing both phasic and tonic stretch reflexes. Depression of the phasic stretch reflex is responsible for the muscle hypotonia found in cerebellar disease. Delay or abolition of the tonic stretch reflex, on the other hand, interferes with the long afferent arm of the proprioceptive loop that carries postural information from muscles to the sensory cerebral cortex. This, in turn, impairs the short intracortical sensorimotor feedback loop that normally controls the smooth output of area 4 cells projecting back through the cortical-spinal tract. Disease of the neocerebellum must also interrupt the cerebral-cerebellar-cerebral loop that generates normal ramp-pursuit movements.

Abnormalities Inconsistently Associated with Cerebellar Disease

Oculomotor Paralysis. Internal and external oculomotor palsies arise as a result of dysfunction produced outside the cerebellum rather than within the structure itself. Space-occupying lesions of the cerebellum, however, sometimes cause secondary oculomotor palsies because of compression of the brainstem. Deep cerebellar hemorrhages may dissect into the ipsilateral brachium pontis to compress or damage the underlying abducens-para-abducens nuclei of the pons. The usual result is partial conjugate gaze paralysis toward the side of the lesion, less often that of a selective weakness of the ipsilateral external rectus muscle. Saccadic undershoots or overshoots (ocular dysmetria) occur commonly with degenerative diseases that affect the region of the fastigial nucleus and dorsal vermis.

TABLE 20. OCULAR MOTOR ABNORMALITIES IN "PURE" CEREBELLAR DEGENERATIONS

---

1. Inaccurate (dysmetric) saccades; normal velocities and latencies
2. Fixation abnormalities: square wave jerks (saccadic intrusions) and increased slow drift
3. Impaired smooth pursuit with head still or moving (VOR cancellation); impaired OKN; impaired fixation suppression of caloric-induced nystagmus
4. Post-saccadic drift (glissades)
5. Gaze-evoked nystagmus (occasionally centripetal nystagmus)
6. Rebound nystagmus
7. Downbeat nystagmus
8. Positional nystagmus
9. Increased VOR gain
10. Alternating hyperdeviation on lateral gaze (skew)

From Leigh, R. J., and Zee, D. S.: The Neurology of Eye Movements. Philadelphia, F. A. Davis Co., 1983. VOR = Vestibular-ocular reflex; OKN = optokinetic nystagmus.

Nystagmus. The association of nystagmus as a specific sign of cerebellar disease or dysfunction remains an uncertain matter. Nystagmus of a variety of kinds can result when cerebellar mass lesions compress the underlying brainstem or dissect into it in the region of the vestibular nuclei and adjacent reticular formation. Table 20 lists a variety of oculomotor abnormalities attributed to pure cerebellar degenerations, i.e., conditions that appear not to affect simultaneously other, extracerebellar, neural systems. Downbeat nystagmus (perpendicular nystagmus with a slow upward and fast downward component often seen with the eyes at rest) occurs commonly in association with congenital malformations or neoplasms involving the region of the vestibulocerebellum, but all such disorders affect the lower brainstem as well, so that their pure cerebellar origin is questionable.

Brainstem and More Remote Dysfunction Accompanying Cerebellar Mass Lesions. The posterior fossa provides a confined cavity occupied tightly by structures that often lie close to their peripheral receptors or effectors. As a result, when abnormalities compress or distort the brainstem, tug on its associated peripheral nerves, or impede its CSF outflow pathways, blatant signals of neurologic dysfunction often quickly follow. Such is the case with cerebellar mass lesions that reach a sufficient size to expand the organ. Several pathophysiologic principles tend to apply: (1) The cerebellar hemispheres possess considerable plasticity in their function. Accordingly, small hemispheric lesions commonly produce no abnormal symptoms or signs. (2) Rapidly expanding lesions, such as hemorrhages or metastatic tumors, cause abnormal symptoms and signs at a smaller size than do slowly involving ones. (3) Cerebellar mass lesions that enlarge sufficiently to cause detectable clinical signs usually produce signs of both ipsilateral and midline cerebellar dysfunction. (4) Prominent nystagmus, particularly with a vertical or asymmetric quality, implies brainstem dysfunction and should be respected accordingly. (5) Nausea, vomiting, hiccup, or oculomotor paralyses always imply lower brainstem dysfunction and with expanding cerebellar lesions also imply either compression or invasion of the lower brainstem in the region of vital autonomic centers. (6) Papilledema associated with posterior fossa lesions, with or without ventricular dilatation by CT, signals potential decompensation of the secretion-absorption balance of the CSF. The sign warns of the possibility of herniation of the brain through the apertures of the tentorium or foramen magnum. Diagnostic lumbar puncture can induce such a complication as can a hesitatingly slow approach to surgically decompressing the lateral ventricles in conditions such as cerebellar hemorrhage or other rapidly expanding posterior fossa abnormalities. (7) Dementia, delirium, or confusional states accompanying cerebellar mass or destructive lesions are never caused by cerebellar destruction itself. Rather such mental changes imply the presence of either longstanding obstructive hydrocephalus or the codevelopment of lesions of the cerebral hemispheres such as degenerative changes or additional metastases.

THE PATHOPHYSIOLOGY OF ATAXIA AND GAIT DISTURBANCES

At this point it may be helpful to synthesize material presented in previous sections on this subject. The nonspecific term, *ataxia,* describes incoordination of intentional movement applied most often to disturbances affecting the lower extremities, less often the upper, and sometimes to abnormal oculomotor movements. Ataxia affecting the vocal apparatus is termed *dysarthria.* Such terms as *dysmetria* (defective motor judgment of distance), *dyssynergia* (incoordination of compound movements about two or more joints), *intention tremor* (increasing oscillatory tremor involving a member as it approaches its goal), and *dysdiadochokinesia* (decomposition of the act of attempted rhythmic alternating movement) represent specific examples of ataxic movement.

Ataxia in the literal sense can result from any abnormality in motor function whether induced by faulty peripheral sensory mechanisms or by disturbances of descending corticospinal, basal ganglia, or cerebellar control. When weakness is present, it may become difficult or impossible to ascertain how much additional incoordination can be attributed specifically to other mechanisms. Accordingly, the analysis of ataxia as a diagnostic problem most often lies in distinguishing between sensory ataxia and cerebellar ataxia.

Proprioceptive (Sensory) Ataxia

Potentially incapacitating ataxia can result from damage to the proprioceptive afferents anywhere along their route from the peripheral nerve via dorsal root, and dorsal spinal funiculus to thalamus and postcentral cortex. The functional defect results from a variable loss of knowledge of the location of the body part combined with relatively preserved strength in the member. Information carried by long loop reflexes is blocked so that ramp movements are interfered with. Furthermore, a lack of accurate spatial information reaching the sensory cortex impairs the programming necessary at that level to initiate subsequent accurate ballistic activity.

The distribution of ataxia often provides clues to its mechanism. Most spinal nerve or nerve root lesions as well as spinocerebellar tract degenerations cause a bilateral defect that characteristically (1) affects the lower more than the upper extremities; (2) impairs position as much as or more than vibratory sensation but may sometimes be difficult to quantify by bedside testing; (3) results in absence of or greatly reduced deep tendon reflexes; and (4) induces a broad-based, weaving gait that with severe sensory loss becomes high stepping, lurching, sometimes leg flinging, or pounding, and is worse in the dark (rombergism). Spinal dorsal column lesions produce similar symptoms except that the loss of position sense may be more selective in the involved leg or legs, the signs may be less equally symmetric, the tendon reflexes can be preserved, and pathologic reflexes may be present if the abnormality also involves the descending corticospinal pathways. Brainstem lemniscal involvement resembles spinal impairment, but is seldom bilateral and rarely severe. Patients with peripheral or spinal sensory ataxia are subjectively well aware of their deficits. They are also aware that their lack of coordination is not due to "dizziness," which distinguishes them from patients with vestibular disorders. Parietal or thalamoparietal proprioceptive impairment produces an ataxia that is usually unilateral and (1) affects the contralateral upper extremity as much as

or more severely than the lower, (2) disproportionately or selectively impairs position sense rather than vibration, and (3) may go partially unrecognized or be denied by the patient (anosognosia).

Cerebellar Ataxia

As already noted, the motor abnormality associated with cerebellar lesions depends on the localization of the abnormality in the cerebellum and whether adjacent or related neural structures are involved.

Drunkenness

Drunkenness, whether due to alcohol or depressant drug intoxication, results mainly from bilateral labyrinthine-vestibular dysfunction and is accompanied by sensations of both vertigo and dizziness. Few patients with cerebellar disease walk the streets with as much incapacity as a severe alcoholic. Severely intoxicated patients reel, lurch, twist, and fall. Lesser degrees of intoxication produce unsteadiness, a tottering, cautious gait with the feet placed moderately widely apart coupled with clumsiness, dysarthria, and nystagmus in all directions.

Vestibular Ataxia

Chronic unilateral impairment of the vestibulosensory system can occur with lesions anywhere along the peripheral pathway, including labyrinthine destruction by disease or drugs, eighth nerve damage from cerebellopontine angle tumors, or compression, injury, inflammation, or neoplasms damaging the vestibular complex in the brainstem. Patients with such abnormalities tend to drift toward the side of impairment and then quickly correct the deviation in the opposite direction. Turning accentuates their unsteadiness and induces missteps. Bilateral damage to the vestibular nuclei in the brainstem results in a narrow-based ataxia with poor compensating movements in the limbs, drifting or falling to either side, and a tendency to retropulsion and falling backward. Patients with vestibular dysfunction depend heavily on visual proprioception so that closing the eyes accentuates the gait disorder.

Spastic Ataxia

Combined abnormalities of the spinal dorsal columns and cortical spinal tracts produce a characteristic broad-based, tottering, and sometimes pounding gait with the knees sometimes held high but the legs always moving stiffly. The condition occurs with demyelinating diseases and other intrinsic spinal disorders such as vascular malformations, cyanocobalamin deficiency, arachnoiditis, and, occasionally, neoplasms.

Patients with frontal lobe disease can suffer any of several gait disorders depending upon the anatomic distribution of the lesions. Unilateral injury to the foot-leg area of the somatosensory cortex produces a focal monoparesis, while bilateral motor-premotor damage results in a relatively narrow based, stiff-legged impairment, sometimes accompanied by scissoring of the legs. More anteriorly placed premotor and prefrontal abnormalities resulting from deep bilateral tumors, multiple cerebral infarctions, or communicating "low pressure" hydrocephalus sometimes produce an ataxia that has been called *gait apraxia.* The disorder consists of severe difficulty in walking or otherwise initiating movement of the lower extremities so long as the feet are placed firmly on the floor. The feet appear glued in place, and attempts to walk often induce short shuffles or even hops before the legs get moving. Walking, once (or if) it begins, proceeds as a halting and broad-based movement made easier by guidance or support. Patients with advanced cases may be unable to get under way at all and, unless they are supported, they tend to retropulse or to fall backward, even from a sitting position. A degree of clinically obvious dementia consistently accompanies the gait disorder.

Patients with frontal ataxia of this type consistently show a greater ability to move their legs on command when lying supine than when standing. Examination of the lower extremities discloses increased paratonic resistance to passive movements coupled with bilateral plantar grasp responses, extensor thrust responses, and usually accentuated tendon reflexes. These reflex abnormalities and physiologic dysfunctions, rather than the elusive mechanisms of an ill-defined apraxia, best explain the difficulty in movement.

Gait Disturbances in the Elderly

Any of several specific visual, somatosensory, or motor diseases may impair walking in elderly persons. Less easily classified but fairly typical walking difficulties include a tendency to walk with slow, short, mincing, and unsteady steps. Fairly common is a stooped position coupled with a moderately broad-based, unsteady gait sometimes associated with CT evidence of a chronic communicating hydrocephalus. Among the very elderly a gait disturbance arises that closely resembles the bilateral vestibular ataxia, described above. At present no satisfactory pathologic or physiologic studies illuminate the mechanism.

Retropulsion

A tendency to step or fall backward from the standing position or to fall back while sitting can be a symptom of several serious, acquired midline abnormalities of the brain. The physiology of the symptom is poorly understood. It accompanies midline tumors of the posterior cerebellum as well as degenerative disorders affecting the central vestibular mechanism bilaterally, and can be observed in association with bilateral lesions affecting the walls of the third ventricle, the basal ganglia, and the medial orbital region of the frontal lobes. Occasionally the abnormality is associated with large, unilateral frontal lobe neoplasms that produce an increase in the intracranial pressure and a shift of the hemispheres toward the opposite side. Retropulsion of posterior fossa origin is especially dangerous, as it often comes on suddenly and is accompanied by a loss of the normal postural protective mechanisms that guard against injury during falling.

Hysterical Gait

Hysteria can mimic a variety of hemiparetic, steppage, or ataxic gait disorders. With a hemiparetic type, the pattern usually gives itself away by atypical dragging behind of the affected leg during a series of hops or supported steps. The most obviously factitious hysterical disorder is a lurching, irregularly based, sometimes bent-forward walk in which the patient grasps any object in an effort to reach for support and reels from side to side inconsistently. Such patients may sink to the floor, but they almost never endure an unsupported, self-injuring fall. Accompanying signs of altered muscular tonus or abnormal reflexes remain absent, and the bizarre movements not only differ from the expected pattern of sensory or cerebellar dysfunction but often change from examination to examination.

REFERENCES

Auger, R. G., Daube, J. R., Gomez, M. R., and Lambert, E. H.: Hereditary form of sustained muscle activity of peripheral nerve origin causing generalized myokymia and muscle stiffness. Ann Neurol 15:13, 1983.

Brookhart, J. M., and Mountcastle, V. B. (eds.): Handbook of Physiology. Section I, The Nervous System. Volume II, Motor Control, Parts 1 and 2. Edited by Brooks, V. B. Bethesda, Md., American Physiological Society, 1981.

Cooper, J. R., Bloom, F. E., and Roth, R. H.: The Biochemical Basis of Neuropharmacology. New York, Oxford University Press, 1982.

Denny-Brown, D.: The Basal Ganglia and Their Relations to Disorders of Movement. London, Oxford University Press, 1962.

Desmedt, J. E., and Godauz, E.: Voluntary motor commands in human ballistic movements. Ann Neurol 5:415, 1979.

Freund, H.-J.: The pathophysiology of the premotor syndrome in man. Brain, 1984. In press.

Gilman, S., Bloedel, J. R., and Lechtenberg, R.: Disorders of the Cerebellum. Philadelphia, F. A. Davis Co., 1981.

Kremer, M.: Sitting, standing, and walking. Br Med J 2:63, 1958.

Lance, J. W., and McLeod, J. G.: A Physiological Approach to Clinical Neurology. 3rd ed. London, Butterworths, 1981.

Magoun, H. W.: Caudal and cephalic influences of the brainstem reticular function. Physiol Rev 30:459, 1950.

Marsden, C. D.: The mysterious motor function of the basal ganglia. The Robert Wartenberg Lecture. Neurology 32:514–539, 1982.

Medical Research Council, War Memorandum No. 7. Aids to the Investigation of Peripheral Nerve Injuries. London, Her Majesty's Stationery Office, 1952.

Mountcastle, V. B. (ed.): Textbook of Physiology. 14th ed. St. Louis, C. V. Mosby, 1980.

Plum, F., and Posner, J. B.: The Diagnosis of Stupor and Coma. 3rd ed. 3rd revised printing. Philadelphia, F. A. Davis Co., 1982.

Roland, P. E., Larsen, B., Lassen, N. A., and Skinhøj, E.: Supplementary motor area and other cortical areas in organization of voluntary movements in man. J Neurophysiol 43:118, 1980.

Walton, J. (ed.): Disorders of Voluntary Muscle. 4th ed. Edinburgh, Churchill Livingstone, 1981.

Young, R. R., and Delwaide, P. J.: Spasticity. N Engl J Med 304:28, 1981.

Sensory Systems _____

ORGANIZATION OF THE NORMAL SENSORY SYSTEM

An organism perceives its internal milieu and environment only through its sensory systems. Although philosophers may disagree whether a tree falling unobserved in the forest actually falls, there is no disagreement that a human being can be aware of the existence of that tree only if he sees it, hears it, touches it, smells it, reads about it, or is told about it by another individual. Furthermore, when portions of the senory system are diseased, the organism can no longer accurately perceive its internal needs or external stimuli and cannot interact with them to full effect. So important are the sensory systems to the activity of the person that an acutely deafferented limb becomes almost as useless as if it were paralyzed. In most instances, partial sensory loss is more disabling to a patient than partial motor loss.

For purposes of convenience the sensory systems are usually divided into three physiologic entities. The *somatosensory system* is designed to perceive environmental stimuli that contact the organism directly. The sensory modalities of touch, pressure, pain, temperature, and proprioception are components of the somatosensory system. The *special sensory system* is designed in general to perceive stimuli arising at a distance from the organism. The highly specialized receptors of vision, hearing, and olfaction are examples. Taste and vestibular sensation are also part of the special sensory system, even though they perceive internal as well as external stimuli. The *visceral sensory system* perceives changes in the internal environment and possesses detectors for both the general functions of pressure and pain and the more specialized functions of osmolality, blood pressure, oxygenation, and the like.

The following sections discuss the anatomy, physiology, and pathophysiology of first the somatosensory and then each of the special sensory systems. In some instances the sensory arm of coordinated activity of the organism is so inextricably linked with integration and motor output (e.g., the stretch reflex) that they cannot be easily separated. Thus the sensory arc of the stretch reflex is discussed on page 1037 with the motor system, and some aspects of visceral sensation are discussed in the section on the autonomic nervous system. Some aspects shared by all sensory systems, such as receptors, are discussed in the paragraphs below.

RECEPTORS

All sensory systems interact with the environment through receptors. Receptors transduce the energy of the incoming stimulus into an electrical potential usable by the nervous system. Different receptors are specialized to detect and transduce a variety of environmental stimuli (Table 21). Highly specialized receptors detect photons (vision), molecular structure (taste and smell), temperature, or mechanical deformation (e.g., touch and pressure). In some instances the environmental stimulus is detected only after it is altered from its original form to mechanical energy. For example, sound waves cause mechanical deformation of the hair cells of the cochlea, which leads to their firing. Angular and linear acceleration distorts the hair cells of the semicircular canals and stimulates them to discharge. Receptors also vary in relationship to the sensory nerve ending. In its simplest form the receptor is a free nerve ending of a small unmyelinated nerve fiber (C fiber, p. 1075). Small myelinated fiber nerve endings remain sheathed in Schwann cells (p. 1012) and myelin. With many larger fibers the nerve ending is specialized, for example, the pacinian corpuscle (p. 1079). In other instances the sensory receptor is independent from the nerve ending, for example, hair cells of the hearing and vestibular system. A synaptic potential must be generated from the receptor to the nerve ending before an environmental stimulus can be perceived.

Whether simple or complicated, all receptors share certain properties. When they are stimulated by an appropriate environmental agent, they produce a graded receptor potential that, if sufficient in magnitude, discharges the sensory nerve to generate an all-or-none action potential that travels toward the central

TABLE 21. SENSORY SYSTEMS

SYSTEM	FORM OF ENERGY	RECEPTOR ORGAN	RECEPTOR CELL
Somatosensory			
Temperature	Temperature	Skin, hypothalamus	Nerve terminals and central neurons
Pain	Various	Skin and various organs	Nerve terminals
Touch	Mechanical	Skin	Nerve terminals
Pressure	Mechanical	Skin and deep tissue	Encapsulated nerve endings
Muscle stretch	Mechanical	Muscle spindle	Nerve terminals
Muscle tension	Mechanical	Tendon organs	Nerve terminals
Joint position	Mechanical	Joint capsule and ligaments	Nerve terminals
Special sensory			
Taste	Ions and molecules	Tongue and pharynx	Taste bud cells
Smell	Molecules	Nose	Olfactory receptors
Balance			
Linear acceleration (gravity)	Mechanical	Vestibular organ	Hair cells
Angular acceleration	Mechanical	Vestibular organ	Hair cells
Hearing	Mechanical	Inner ear (cochlea)	Hair cells
Vision	Electromagnetic (photons)	Eye (retina)	Photoreceptors
Visceral sensory			
Common chemical	Molecules	Various	Free nerve endings
Arterial oxygen	O_2 tension	Carotid body	Cells and nerve endings
Toxins (vomiting)	Molecular	Medulla	Chemoreceptor cells
Osmotic pressure	Osmotic pressure	Hypothalamus	Osmoreceptors
Glucose	Glucose	Hypothalamus	Glucoreceptors
pH (cerebrospinal fluid)	Ions	Medulla	Ventricle cells
Vascular pressure	Mechanical	Blood vessels	Nerve terminals

Modified from Shepherd, G. M.: Neurobiology. New York, Oxford University Press, 1983.

nervous system. Receptors differ not only in the nature of the stimulus they are capable of detecting but also in the necessary intensity of the stimulus that can produce a response. A few photons of light are sufficient to trigger a response in a visual receptor. Movement of the tympanic membrane a distance of 10^{-8} cm (about the diameter of a hydrogen ion) can stimulate a hair cell, although neither of these mild stimuli may be perceived in the central nervous system. On the other hand, certain free nerve endings require intense stimulation, often of a degree sufficient to damage surrounding tissue, before they respond. These high threshold receptors carry information perceived in the central nervous system as pain. Another important characteristic of some receptors is their tendency to cease firing when a stimulus persists unchanged (adaptation). The phenomenon of adaptation is well developed in many touch-pressure receptors and its opposite, lack of adaptation, in most pain receptors. Accordingly, although one is usually unaware of the pressure and touch of wearing shoes and socks within a few minutes after they are put on, one remains acutely aware of a stone or nail in the shoe compressing the foot until the offending object is removed.

Receptors play a role in the "doctrine of specific nerve energies," which states that each afferent nerve has its own specific physiologic "energy" and can transmit only one kind of sensory modality, no matter how stimulated. Thus, electrical stimulation of a cold receptor produces a sensation of cold and not of electricity. A blow to the eye that discharges the optic nerve causes one to "see stars," i.e., produces a sensation of light rather than pressure. A blow to the head discharges many sensory systems and may cause seeing stars, ringing in the ears, and dizziness, all properties of the sensory units stimulated by the mechanical trauma. Some free nerve ending receptors are polymodal, responding to more than one stimulus, and high-intensity stimulation of receptors, including bright light and loud sound, often produce pain as well as the primary sensation. The doctrine of specific nerve energy applies not only to receptors but also to the sensory units, i.e., the several ascending neural systems, to which they are attached. Electrical stimulation of specific nerves, i.e., auditory or optic, produces a sensation of sound and light even when the receptors themselves are not stimulated.

A useful physiologic subdivision of receptors is into exteroceptors, teleceptors, and enteroceptors. Exteroceptors receive stimuli from the environment coming in direct contact with the body (e.g., pressure or touch); teleceptors perceive stimuli at a distance from the body (e.g., light, sound, heat, and cold); and enteroceptors perceive the internal environment (e.g., osmolality, blood pressure). The term *proprioceptor* includes all of those receptors that identify for the organism its position in space, including receptors in muscles and tendons and the hair cells in the semicircular canals and otolith. Pain receptors or nociceptors are exteroceptive, teleceptive, and enteroceptive.

THE SOMATOSENSORY SYSTEM

ANATOMY AND CLINICAL PHYSIOLOGY OF SOMATIC SENSATION

Two major sensory pathways subserve both exteroception and conscious proprioception. Together these make up the somatosensory nervous system. The first pathway, often called the spinothalamic system (Fig. 28), subserves the sensations of pain, temperature, and crude touch and consists largely of free receptor nerve endings and small myelinated and unmyelinated fibers. Most of the fibers ascend to the brain in the spinothalamic tract of the spinal cord and brainstem. The second pathway subserves the functions of light touch, position sense, and tactile localization and consists predominantly of specialized receptors connected to larger myelinated fibers. The second system can be subdivided further into those fibers that perceive the external environment (cutaneous and subcutaneous receptors) and those that perceive the position of the organism in space (proprioception—muscle and joint position sense). Those fibers that carry messages that reach consciousness travel through the medial lemniscus in the brainstem and thus are often called the lemniscal system. Although these systems are considered separately below, they interact at several levels, particularly in the dorsal horn of the spinal cord (p. 1075). Failure of normal interaction between these systems is believed to be responsible for some painful nervous system disorders (see gate theory, p. 1076).

Spinothalamic System

Figure 28 schematically outlines our current understanding of pain and temperature pathways. The receptor for pain and temperature is the free or sheathed nerve ending of small myelinated or unmyelinated nerves. There is not complete agreement on the adequate stimulus for discharging all of these receptors. Some receptors respond only to heating, cooling, or high intensity mechanical stimuli. Others respond to more than one modality (polymodal receptors). Itch and tickle are believed to be detected by free nerve endings.

Pain receptors (nociceptors) are probably stimulated either by strong mechanical deformation or by extremes of hot or cold. It is believed that tissue damage from mechanical or thermal injury liberates chemical substances that lower the firing threshold of the mechanonociceptors and thermonociceptors so that previously innocuous mechanical or thermal stimuli pro-

TABLE 22. CLASSIFICATION OF NERVE FIBERS ACCORDING TO THICKNESS OF MYELIN SHEATHS AND VELOCITY OF CONDUCTION

TYPE OF FIBER	DIAMETER (μ)	VELOCITY (m/sec)
Ia fibers (A, α) From anulospiral endings	Approx. 17	70–120
Ib fibers (A, α) From tendon organs of Golgi	Approx. 16	70–100
II fibers (A, β, and γ) From flower-spray endings and Merkel's touch menisci	Approx. 8	15–40
III fibers (A, δ) Pain, temperature, pressure	Approx. 3	5–15
IV or C fibers Pain, temperature, heavy touch	Approx. 0.2–1	0.2–2

From Duus, P.: Topical Diagnosis in Neurology. Stuttgart, Georg Thiem Verlag, 1983, p. 6.

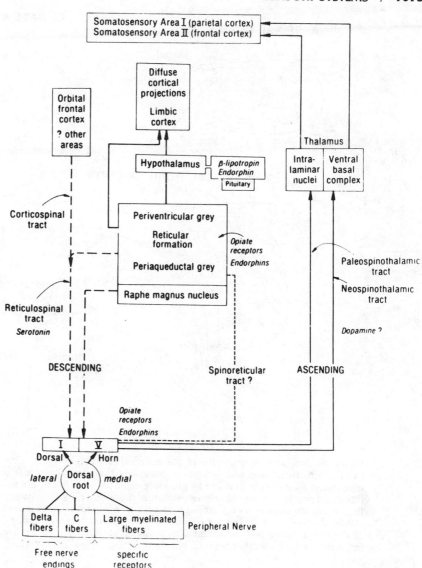

Figure 28. Pain pathways. (From Posner, J. B.: Pain. In Wyngaarden, J. B., and Smith, L. H., Jr. (eds.): Cecil Textbook of Medicine, 16th ed. W. B. Saunders Co., Philadelphia, 1982, p. 1941.)

duce pain, and noxious stimuli produce exaggerated, more prolonged discharges. Substances liberated by tissue damage that lower the threshold of pain receptors include potassium, acetylcholine, histamine, serotonin, prostaglandins, and bradykinin. There is some evidence that the lowering of nociceptor threshold is mediated by prostaglandins. Aspirin analgesia may result from that drug's ability to inhibit prostaglandin synthesis.

Free nerve endings occur on two sets of peripheral fibers: small (6 μ), thinly myelinated, A delta fibers, which conduct at about 35 msec, and unmyelinated C fibers (1 to 2 μ), which conduct at about 0.5 msec (Table 22). This dual set of fibers explains the phenomenon of "double pain." A noxious stimulus elicits first a sharp, pricking, well-localized pain mediated by the more rapidly conducting fibers, and the C fibers mediate a burning, poorly localized, exceedingly unpleasant "second pain." The rate of discharge is determined by the intensity of the stimulus. Recording from a single C fiber in man after applying heat stimuli to the skin, one can relate the rate of discharge in C fibers to the intensity of the stimulus. Thus at a

discharge rate of 0.3/sec there is no pain, but at 0.4/sec the subject perceives pain; at 1.5/sec the pain becomes severe. Stimulation of a C fiber at 3/sec causes unbearable pain. Warmth and itch are conducted by C fibers, cool and tickle by A delta fibers.

All primary sensory afferents have their cell bodies in the dorsal root ganglion. Pain fibers enter the spinal cord via the dorsal root, lateral to the large myelinated (touch and proprioception) fibers. Experimental section of the lateral portion of the dorsal root decreases the perception of pain but leaves large fiber modalities intact. Nociceptive and thermoceptive fibers enter the cord, ascend or descend for one or two segments in the medial portion of Lissauer's tract, then enter the more ventrally placed dorsal horn. Lesions of the medial portion of Lissauer's tract contract the dermatomal field of a single root, indicating that it carries excitatory fibers from adjacent roots, and lesions in the lateral portion expand the dorsal root dermatome, indicating that it carries inhibitory fibers.

The dorsal horn consists of six laminae, with lamina 1 being the most dorsal. Laminae 2 and 3 taken together are often referred to as the substantia gela-

A. SPINAL CORD

C. GATE CONTROL THEORY

B. DORSAL HORN CIRCUITS

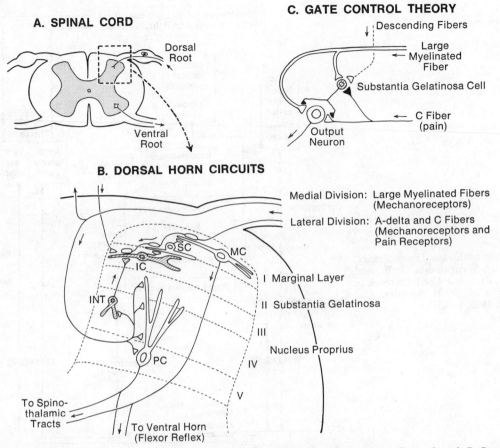

Medial Division: Large Myelinated Fibers (Mechanoreceptors)

Lateral Division: A-delta and C Fibers (Mechanoreceptors and Pain Receptors)

I Marginal Layer

II Substantia Gelatinosa

III

Nucleus Proprius

IV

V

Figure 29. Somatosensory circuits in the mammalian spinal cord. *A,* Cross section of spinal cord. *B,* Some of the main neuron types and synaptic connections that have been identified in the dorsal horn. The large myelinated fibers are believed to be glutaminergic; pain fibers contain substance P, somatostatin, vasoactive intestinal peptide, or possibly cholecystokinin; descending fibers contain norepinephrine or serotonin. (Based in part on discussions with Carole La Motte). *C,* Simplification of gate-control theory of Melzack and Wall (1965). Postulated excitatory terminals shown by open profiles; inhibitory, by shaded profiles. *I–V* = laminae of the dorsal horn; *MC* = marginal cell; *SC* = stalked cell; *IC* = islet cell; *INT* = interneuron; *PC* = projection cell. (From Shepherd, G. M.: Neurobiology. New York, Oxford University Press, 1983.)

tinosa, but the functional boundaries of this area are not clearly defined. Fibers subserving pain probably end in all six laminae, with laminae 1 and 5 being most important (Fig. 29). The site of the interaction between neurons in the dorsal horn is an important one for modulating sensory input. The *gate theory* proposes that impulses from the more rapidly conducting large myelinated fibers (lemniscal) inhibit conduction centrally of the late-arriving smaller spinothalamic fibers ("close the gate") and that when there is an abnormality of that interaction, previously innocuous stimuli cause pain (p. 1084). In human experiments the pain produced by C fiber stimulation can be diminished by simultaneous stimulation of larger fibers. Descending fibers from the cerebral cortex and from brainstem structures also modulate this system. These descending pathways also inhibit incoming pain fibers. Most thermosensitive fibers terminate in lamina 1.

The ascending pain pathways in the spinal cord are characteristically divided into two groups: the neospinothalamic tract, which is believed to subserve the perception of intensity and localization of pain, and the phylogenetically older paleospinothalamic tract, which is believed to subserve the arousal and emo-

tional components of pain. The axons of the neospinothalamic tract arise from the dorsal horn, cross the anterior commissure, and ascend in the anterolateral quadrant of the spinal cord. The axons terminate in the ventral basal complex of the thalamus, principally within the posterolateral ventral nucleus ipsilateral to the side of their ascent. The thalamic terminations of these fibers coincide to a large extent with those of the dorsal column, and the pathway shows somatotopic localization at the thalamic level, the face and upper body being represented most medially. Third-order neurons from the thalamus project to somatosensory area I (sensorimotor cortex), with the same somatotopic localization as other sensory modalities. Lesions made in the neospinothalamic pathway at either the thalamus or the cortex rarely relieve pain, and in fact lesions in this pathway at the thalamic level often lead to chronic so-called thalamic pain. The paleospinothalamic tract, whose cells of origin in the dorsal horn receive C fiber input, also crosses in the anterior commissure and ascends in the spinal cord, closely applied to, but more ventral than, the neospinothalamic tract. Fibers ascending in the spinothalamic tract have a somatotopic localization, with fibers from the sacrum and lower extremity moving more laterally as incoming fibers from trunk and upper extremities assume a medial placement. As a result, dysfunction of the spinothalamic tract, if medially placed, may produce the phenomenon of "sacral sparing," i.e., loss of pain and temperature in trunk and lower extremities with normal sensation in the sacral areas. The phenomenon of sacral sparing, however, does not always indicate that the lesion is intrinsic to the cord, since external spinal cord compression sometimes can yield sacral sparing, presumably by interfering with the vasculature to the more medially but not laterally placed fibers.

Lesions of the spinothalamic tract usually lead to loss of pain and temperature sensation, but occasionally may cause a spontaneous burning pain similar to that noted with peripheral nerve (causalgia) or thalamic lesions (thalamic pain). These painful phenomena are probably a result of spontaneous discharge of damaged fibers, but why they discharge spontaneously is not known. Many of the fibers of the paleospinothalamic tract give collaterals to the reticular formation of the brainstem, but some reach the thalamus, terminating in several nuclei, particularly the nucleus centralis lateralis and the intralaminar nuclei. None of these fibers projects to the centromedian nucleus despite the fact that lesions in this nucleus have been reported to relieve pain. The intralaminar nuclei of the thalamus project to somatosensory area II both ipsilaterally and contralaterally with some degree of somatotopic localization. The intralaminar nuclei also project diffusely, affecting large regions of both the frontal and parietal lobes. There is no somatotopic localization in these latter projections. A third spinal ascending pathway that may play a role in nociception is the spinoreticular pathway, also referred to as the archispinal-lemniscal pathway. Phylogenetically the oldest of the nociceptive pathways, it consists of projections from small myelinated and unmyelinated fibers. It originates in the dorsal horn and ascends via multiple synapses in the dorsal horn, mostly ipsilaterally but to a lesser degree contralaterally, to terminate in the brainstem reticular formation, particularly that of the pons and medulla. The role the spinoreticular pathway plays in the conscious perception of pain in man is unclear, but it is unlikely to be major because spinal cord hemisection in humans usually eliminates contralateral pain perception, thus ruling out a significant contribution by ipsilateral pathways. Possibly the existence of such a multisynaptic ipsilateral pathway may explain why some anterolateral cordotomies (surgical sections of spinothalamic pathways) fail. Temperature fibers ascend in the spinothalamic tract (and to a lesser extent in the spinocervical tract) intermixed with pain fibers. Anterolateral cordotomy almost always diminishes temperature as well as pain sensation.

Pain and temperature fibers from the face enter the brainstem and the mid pons and then descend ipsilaterally as far as the upper cervical segments of the spinal cord (descending trigeminal tract). There is somatotopic localization in the descending tract. The fibers of the ophthalmic branch of the trigeminal supplying the forehead and cornea are placed more ventrally and descend more caudally than the fibers of the maxillary division, which in turn are more ventral and caudal than the fibers of the mandibular division.

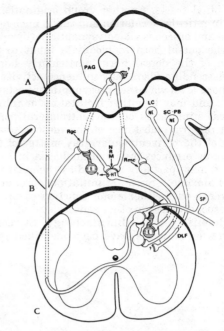

Figure 30. The endogenous pain control system: *A,* midbrain level; *B,* medullary level; *C,* spinal level.

The periaqueductal gray *(PAG),* an important locus for stimulation-produced analgesia, is rich in enkephalins *(E)* and opiate receptor, though the anatomic details of the enkephalinergic connections are not known. Microinjection of small amounts of opiates into PAG also produces analgesia.

Serotonin *(5-HT)*-containing cells of the nucleus raphe magnus *(NRM)* and the adjacent nucleus reticularis magnocellularis *(Rmc)* receive excitatory input from PAG and, in turn, send efferent fibers to the spinal cord.

Efferent fibers from the NRM and Rmc travel in the dorsolateral funiculus *(DLF)* to terminate among pain-transmission cells concentrated in lamina I and V of the dorsal horn. The NRM and Rmc exert an inhibitory effect specifically on pain-transmission neurons. The pain transmission neurons, which are activated by substance P *(SP)* containing small-diameter primary afferents, project to supraspinal sites, and indirectly, via the nucleus reticularis gigantocellularis *(Rgc),* contact the cells of the descending analgesia system in the PAG and NRM, thus establishing a negative feedback loop.

Catecholamine-containing neurons of the locus ceruleus *(LC)* in rats and subceruleus-parabrachialis *(SC-PB)* in cat may also contribute to pain-modulating systems in the DLF. *(NE*-norepinephrine.) (From Basbaum, A. I., and Fields, H. L.: Endogenous pain control mechanisms: Review and hypothesis. Ann Neurol 4:455, 1978.)

Fibers originating in the brainstem reticular formation receive input from several sources, including almost certainly the paleospinothalamic and spinoreticular pathways, and ascend in a polysynaptic projection to wide areas of the thalamus. The anatomy and physiology of the reticular formation are becoming increasingly important in our understanding of pain perception. Electrical stimulation of this area produces analgesia, and the area may serve as the site of action for narcotic drugs.

Spinal sensory mechanisms are influenced by descending as well as afferent impulses called the endogenous pain control system (Fig. 30) and consisting of several sets of descending fibers. One set originates in the orbital-frontal cortex and probably travels via corticospinal tracts. Another group originates in the midbrain reticular formation and raphe nucleus of the medulla and descends via polysynaptic pathways. Both reach the dorsal horn to modulate input to all the laminae of the dorsal horn, particularly lamina 5. These descending fibers may influence activity at the dorsal horn level via either presynaptic or postsynaptic contacts and may be either facilitatory or inhibitory. Electrical stimulation of the ventrolateral portion of the central gray substance of the mesencephalon as well as of the periventricular gray matter of the hypothalamus produces profound analgesia in both animals and man, partially reversed by the opiate antagonist naloxone. Such stimulation produces no interference with either motor function or the organism's responsiveness to other sensory stimuli.

Biochemistry and Pharmacology. Stereospecific receptors for narcotics have been identified in brain and spinal cord. These opiate receptors exist in highest concentrations in the brainstem reticular formation, thalamus, and limbic system, the areas where narcotic analgesics are believed to act. The receptors bind both narcotic agonists and antagonists. Several subpopulations of receptors occupy different cerebral and spinal regions and probably mediate different pharmacologic effects. In addition, several peptides called collectively the endorphins, which have morphine-like properties, have been isolated from brain. These analgesic peptides, enkephalin and beta-endorphin, are localized to discrete but different areas of the central nervous system, and are believed to be neuromodulators of specific pain pathways. Both bind to the opiate receptor and can be displaced by opiate antagonists.

Neurotransmitters, including dopamine, serotonin, substance P, gamma-aminobutyric acid, and norepinephrine, also appear to be important in pain modu-

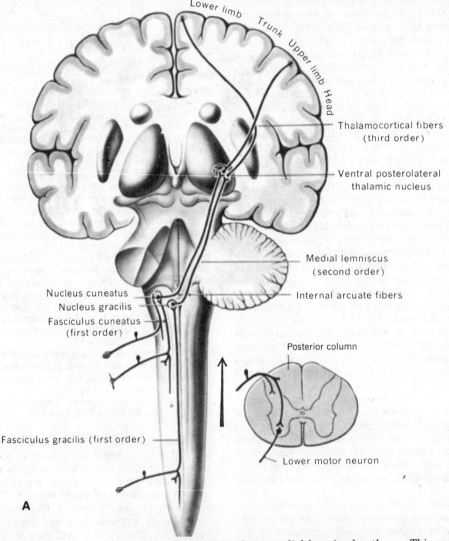

Figure 31. Large fiber sensory pathways. *A,* Posterior column-medial lemniscal pathway. This pathway is composed of (1) neurons of the first order with cell bodies in the spinal ganglia and with axons that ascend in the posterior column to the nuclei gracilis and cuneatus; (2) neurons of the second order with cell bodies in the nuclei gracilis and cuneatus and with axons that decussate as the internal arcuate fibers in the lower medulla and ascend in the medial lemniscus to the thalamus; and (3) neurons of the third order with cell bodies in the thalamus and with axons that project to the cerebral cortex (postcentral gyrus). Collateral branches of the neuron of the first order pass to the posterior horn, the anterior horn, and the posterior column; the last are descending association fibers.

Illustration continued on opposite page.

lation. Dopamine enhances the effect of both morphine analgesia and brainstem stimulation and may be the transmitter that subserves ascending inhibitory pathways to the brainstem reticular formation. Serotonin also has an inhibiting effect on pain perception and is probably the transmitter of descending inhibitory pathways that arise in the raphe nucleus of the medulla. GABA may be an inhibitory transmitter modulating pain and the level of the dorsal horn of the spinal cord. Substance P is found mainly in dorsal horns of the spinal cord. Its activity is inhibited by morphine. Norepinephrine, localized primarily in brainstem structures, can likewise either enhance or inhibit pain, depending on the dose.

Lemniscal System

The lemniscal system consists primarily of larger myelinated fibers, subserving the functions of light touch, position sense, tactile localization, and unconscious proprioception. Those fibers come from muscle and, possibly, joints and ascend in the spinocerebellar tract to reach the cerebellum and assist in maintaining the organism's position in space. They must include relays to the postcentral gyrus, where the organism has a map of the external world and its position in that world (see discussion of parietal lobe in the following chapter). These pathways are diagrammed in Figure 31. The pathway begins with receptors that are specialized sensory nerve endings. An example is the pacinian corpuscle, a low threshold mechanoreceptor widely distributed in the dermis, both glabrous and hairy skin, the connective tissue of muscles, the periosteum of bone, and the mesentery of the abdomen. The corpuscle consists of a nerve ending surrounded by multiple concentric layers of cellular membranes, with fluid between each two layers. The structure itself

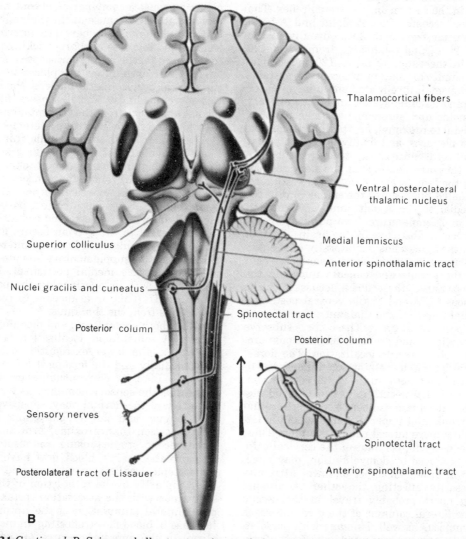

Figure 31 *Continued. B,* Spinocerebellar tracts, spinovestibular tract, and spinoreticular tract. The spinocerebellar tracts include (1) the uncrossed posterior spinocerebellar tract that passes through the inferior cerebellar peduncle and terminates in the paleocerebellum, and (2) the crossed anterior spinocerebellar tract that passes through the superior cerebellar peduncle and terminates in the paleocerebellum. The spinovestibular tract includes fibers that terminate in the vestibular nuclei. The spinoreticular tract is composed of crossed and uncrossed fibers that terminate in some brainstem reticular nuclei. (From Noback, C. R., and Demarast, R. I.: The Human Nervous System: Basic Principles of Neurobiology. 3rd ed. New York, McGraw-Hill Book Co., 1981, pp. 181, 186.)

may be as large as 1 mm in diameter. When the capsule of the corpuscle is deformed, there is a brief receptor potential that ceases if deformation is maintained, thus leading to rapid adaptation of the nerve potential. The release of deformation produces another receptor potential, also brief. If the membranous surrounding of the sensory nerve ending is removed, the receptor potential persists for a much longer time. Thus the corpuscle is ideally suited to detect rapidly changing stimuli. Its threshold is lowest for a vibratory stimulus of about 200 Hz. Other receptors such as Merkel's discs, Meissner's corpuscles, and free nerve endings around hair follicles also detect mechanical deformation but adapt much less rapidly. Sensory nerves ending in touch and pressure receptors are mostly of the A-beta size (Table 22), myelinated fibers ranging from 6 to 12 μ in diameter and conducting at a rate of about 30 to 70 m/sec. Receptors from extrafusal muscle fibers and from Golgi tendon organs have been described in the section on the stretch reflex. The fibers from these receptors are A-alpha and A-beta, ranging in diameter from 5 to 20 μ, usually in the range of 15 to 20 μ, and conducting from 30 to 120 m/sec, mostly in the range of 90 to 120 m/sec. The fibers of the lemniscal and proprioceptive systems combine with the small myelinated and unmyelinated fibers of the spinothalamic system and with efferent fibers of the motor and autonomic systems to form, moving from distal to proximal, first peripheral nerves, and then nerve plexuses, and finally nerve roots that enter the spinal cord. Since these structures subserve all modalities they are detailed in the next section, after we follow the lemniscal system to the brain.

Large myelinated fibers enter the spinal cord in the dorsal root medial to the A-delta and C fibers that subserve pain and temperature. Two pathways carry the entering mechanofibers toward the brain. The first or lemniscal pathway ascends ipsilaterally in the dorsal column, carrying incoming fibers, usually without synapsing, to the gracile and cuneate nuclei in the medulla. After synapse, these fibers decussate as the medial lemniscus to ascend to the ventral posterolateral and medial nuclei of the thalamus, thence to be relayed to the postcentral gyrus. These fibers subserve functions of conscious (and probably unconscious) proprioception as well as tactile localization. The dorsal column—medial lemniscus retains somatotopic localization throughout its length. In the spinal cord, incoming fibers from the lower extremities are moved medially in the dorsal column as fibers from more cranial levels of the trunk and upper extremities enter laterally to form the more lateral cuneate column. Thus, small lesions of posterior columns of the cervical cord, such as those produced by demyelination, may affect proprioception in either an upper or lower extremity without necessarily affecting the other. Additional touch-carrying fibers probably travel in the second pathway in the lateral columns of the cord and reach the medial lemniscus as well. Humans with dorsolateral lesions of the cervical cord often experience vibratory sense loss in the lower extremities. Furthermore, one can identify in the cat a well-developed pathway, the spinocervical column, that carries large-fiber proprioception and is intermixed with the corticospinal tract in the lateral portion of the cord.

Fibers of the lemniscal system join those of the neospinothalamic tract at the mesencephalic-diencephalic junction to reach the thalamus. Fibers of the paleospinothalamic tract have, by this time, left the spinothalamic system to synapse in the reticular formation of the midbrain. The thalamus organizes the incoming information somatotopically, placing the lower extremities more laterally in the ventral posterolateral nucleus, the upper extremities more medially in that nucleus, and the face even more medially in a separate nucleus called the ventral posteromedial nucleus. There also appears to be a modality–specific somatotopic localization with cutaneous afferent nerves being represented more posteriorly than those from joint and muscle. These two nuclei of the thalamus, ventral posterolateral and ventral posteromedial, lie just ventral to the lateral posterior nucleus of the thalamus, the structure that carries ascending fibers from the dentate nucleus of the contralateral cerebellar hemisphere. Thus, lesions affecting this thalamic complex may cause a combination of contralateral sensory loss and ataxia. Because at the thalamic level neocerebellar and lemniscal fibers are intermixed, discrete lesions lead to a loss of sharp pricking pain as well as to impaired tactile and proprioceptive sensation.

The lower extremities are placed more laterally in the ventral posterolateral nucleus, the upper extremities more medially. Facial sensory fibers enter the medial lemniscus from the trigeminal nerve in the mid pons and end in the ventral posteromedial nucleus.

After synapsing in the thalamus, third-order sensory fibers (1: dorsal root ganglion, 2: gracile or cuneate nucleus, 3: thalamus) then project to the somatosensory cortex. The entire output of sensory fibers from the thalamus appears to reach either S1, the primary somatosensory cortex located just posterior to the rolandic fissure, or S2, the second somatosensory cortex, located rostral to the sylvian fissure and posterior to S1 but overlapping with it in its anterior extent. The third area, the supplementary somatosensory cortex, is located in the medial portion of the hemisphere coterminus with or overlapping the posterior medial extent of S1. This area appears to receive no direct projections from the thalamus.

S1 has both somatotopic and modality-specific localization. A somatotopic localization is maintained in the cortex, the lower extremities being represented most medially and the face most laterally, the arm in between. Like its corresponding primary motor homunculus, the sensory homunculus represents a gross distortion of the normal body, sensitive areas such as lips, tongue, and fingers possessing a much larger representation than proximal arm and leg (Fig. 32). More recent studies using radioisotopic tracers to measure the brain's blood flow have confirmed this somatotopic localization in man and have indicated the complexity of the interaction of the primary sensory areas with the association cortex. Not only does contralateral stimulation of the lip or face cause an increase in blood flow (reflecting an increase in metabolism) in the appropriate area of the sensory motor cortex (SM), but asking the subject to focus attention on an area of the body without actually stimulating it causes a similar increase in flow. There is, in addition, focal activation in the superior frontal region, mid frontal region, and parietal region on the border between the superior and inferior parietal regions. Blood

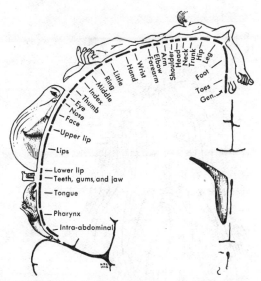

Figure 32. The somatosensory homunculus, representing the body surface as projected onto the postcentral gyrus of the human cerebral cortex. (From Penfield, W., and Rasmussen, T.: The Cerebral Cortex of Man. New York, Macmillan Co., 1950.)

flow changes in these association areas are similar whether attention is directed toward the hand or the lip.

A second form of localization in the cortex is by sensory modality. Several physiologic studies on monkeys' somatosensory cortex indicate a differential representation of modalities in separate areas, touch and pressure being represented close to the monkey analogue of the rolandic fissure and deep somatic sensation being represented both more anteriorly and more posteriorly. "SM2" receives only modest direct thalamic input and has no fine somatotopic localization, but the region receives fibers from somatosensory cortex 1 and probably has an integrative function.

The third form of structure of the somatosensory cortex is that of cortical columns. The column is the basic functional unit of the somatosensory cortex. It consists of a column 1 to 300 μ in diameter running perpendicular to the cortex, all units of which receive fibers from the same receptive field of the body.

The connections of the somatosensory cortex are quite complex. In the monkey SM1 has important reciprocal connections with SM2 and SM3 as well as both primary and supplementary motor cortex. The reciprocal connections of the somatosensory and motor cortices are so intimately linked physiologically that the banks surrounding the rolandic fissure often are called collectively the sensory motor cortex.

The primary sensory cortex makes major interconnections with association areas located more posteriorly in the parietal lobe. These areas also receive visual and auditory input. The combination of somatosensory, visual, and auditory messages allows the parietal lobe to progressively abstract information to create an internal map from which the subject attends to the spatial world of his body and the outer world that surrounds it. The integrative actions of the parietal lobe, including those having to do with visual-spatial orientation and praxis, are described in the chapter on Regional Abnormalities of Cerebral Function.

The Peripheral Sensory System

The *sensory unit* is analogous to the lower motor neuron in the motor system (p. 1037) and can be defined as a single primary afferent nerve fiber with all its terminal branches, including, where applicable, the non-neural transducer receptors. Unlike the motor system, where the cell body of the lower motor neuron lies within the spinal cord, the cell bodies of the peripheral somatosensory system lie in the dorsal root ganglion or in their cranial analogue, the trigeminal ganglion. From these extramedullary ganglia, each somatosensory unit bifurcates into a long peripheral axon that terminates in a cutaneous or subcutaneous receptor and a long or short central axon, which enters the spinal cord to synapse along one or more of the pathways described above. The dorsal columns can be considered a part of the peripheral sensory system in that they respond to injury in the dorsal root ganglion. Moreover, the dorsal root ganglia contain the cell bodies of both the spinothalamic and lemniscal somatosensory systems. Unlike nuclei of the central nervous system, dorsal root ganglia do not possess a blood-brain barrier and thus are susceptible to attack by circulating toxins that would not normally cross the blood-brain barrier. The predilection of some toxins for sensory neurons reflects the lack of a blood-nerve barrier in the dorsal root ganglion.

Peripheral Nerves. The peripheral nerves that subserve cutaneous sensations are indicated in Figure 33. Most of these nerves are mixed and carry motor as well as sensory fibers. A few, such as the lateral cutaneous nerve of the thigh and the sural nerve of the leg, carry only sensory fibers. Although the architecture illustrated in Figure 33 applies to most persons, there is considerable individual variability. Thus, damage to the ulnar nerve usually results from sensory abnormalities involving the fifth and the medial half of the fourth finger, sparing the lateral half of the fourth finger, which is usually supplied by the median nerve. (The C8 root generally supplies the entire fourth and fifth fingers.) In a few individuals, however, only a small portion of the medial fourth finger is supplied by the ulnar nerve, whereas in others the entire fourth finger may suffer sensory loss. The exclusive field of each peripheral nerve also varies individually and even within each individual by modality. If a peripheral sensory nerve is cut, there is a small central area of anesthesia, i.e., loss of all sensation, which represents the area exclusively innervated by the parent nerve. Surrounding the area of anesthesia is an intermediate zone where sensation to touch and tactile localization is lost, but noxious stimuli and extremes of temperature are perceived, although poorly localized. This wider area represents the receptive field for pain and temperature of neighboring nerves. Finally, surrounding the intermediate zone and fading into the normally innervated areas, there is an area where touch, cold, or pinprick elicits hyperesthesia. The zones of altered but not absent sensation result from a wider cutaneous distribution of nerve endings that supply the spinothalamic system than those supplying the lemniscal system, leading to the altered perception.

Nerve Plexuses. Peripheral nerves from the arm and leg rearrange themselves in the brachial and lumbosacral plexus (Fig. 34). Differences in sensory and motor distribution of the plexuses as opposed to

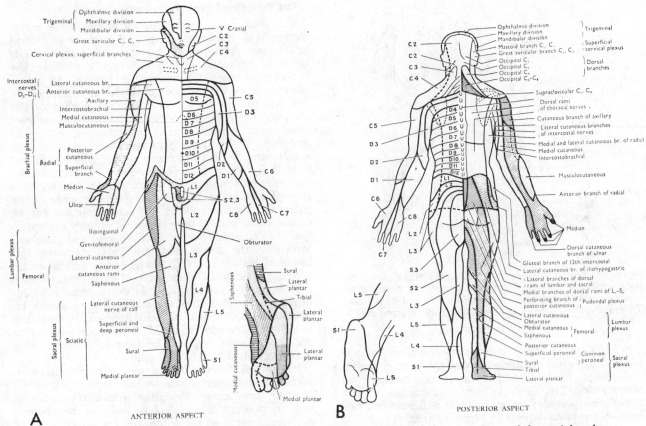

Figure 33. Cutaneous areas of distribution of spinal segments and of the sensory fibers of the peripheral nerves. *A*, Anterior aspect; *B*, Posterior aspect. (From Walton, J. N.: Brain's Diseases of the Nervous System. 8th ed. Oxford, Oxford University Press, 1977.)

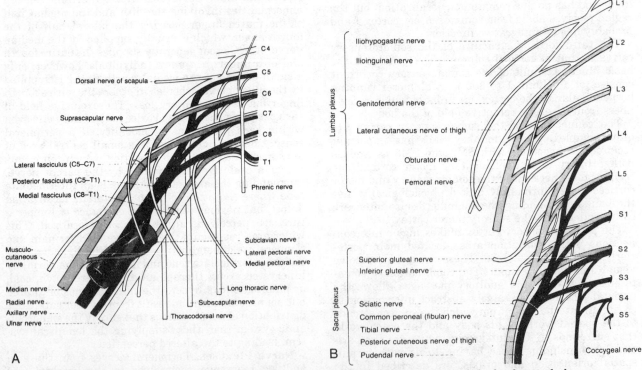

Figure 34. Peripheral nerves of the arm rearranged in the brachial plexus *(A)* and the lumbosacral plexus *(B)*. (From Duus, P.: Topical Diagnosis in Neurology. Stuttgart, Georg Thiem Verlag, 1983, pp. 33, 34.)

peripheral nerves and roots (see below) allow one to make a localizing diagnosis of a lesion on the basis of the neurologic examination. Like the peripheral nerve, the distribution of the plexus may vary somewhat among individuals. Thus the brachial plexus may be *prefixed*, containing a larger contribution from the C4 and C5 roots and a smaller representation from T1, or *postfixed* with a lesser representation from C4 but a greater contribution from T1 and T2. Such minor variations usually do not reduce the reliability of the clinical examination. Nerves of the trunk and abdominal wall do not form plexuses but instead move proximally from the skin and muscles toward the intervertebral foramen to become the spinal root.

Spinal Roots. Mixed spinal nerves converge onto the anterior spinal roots that carry motor fibers and the posterior roots that carry sensory fibers (Fig. 33). The dorsal root ganglion sits along the posterior spinal root. Several properties of spinal roots and dorsal root ganglia make them of clinical interest. As with peripheral nerves and plexuses, myelinated root fibers are covered by Schwann cells. Proximal to the dorsal root ganglion but before entry into the spinal cord, myelinated fibers lose their Schwann cell covering to be succeeded by glial cell myelin. A small, relatively denuded area called the zone of Obersteiner-Redlich lies between Schwann cell and glial cell myelin. Some pathologists believe that this zone is particularly susceptible to attack by disease. It appears to be the site, for example, where syphilis attacks the sensory nervous system. As alluded to above, the lack of a blood-brain barrier in the dorsal root ganglion makes that structure also sensitive to attack by circulating toxins. For example, when the human anticancer drug doxorubicin is given to animals, it selectively damages dorsal root ganglia cells, presumably because of the lack of a blood-nerve barrier at that area. Fortunately neurotoxicity is not observed in humans treated with this drug, illustrating the importance of considering possible species specificity when evaluating the results of studies on the nervous system.

PATHOPHYSIOLOGY OF SOMATOSENSORY DISORDERS

DEFINITION AND MECHANISMS OF SYMPTOMS

Somatosensory disorders may diminish, increase, or distort sensation, depending on the pattern and intensity of their damage: *Diminution* or absence of function in the exteroceptive system is called *hypoesthesia* or *anesthesia*, respectively. Diminution or loss of pain sensation is called *hypalgesia* or *analgesia;* loss of temperature sensation, *thermanesthesia* or *thermhypesthesia*; and so on. Diminution or absence of sensation is easily explicable in pathophysiologic terms as a result of damage to sensory nerve fibers anywhere along their course from the receptor to the brain. More difficult to explain in pathophysiologic terms are hyperfunction and distortion.

Hyperfunction of the exteroceptive sensory system is characterized either by a lowered threshold to stimulation or by spontaneous discharges of sensory fibers. There are several common examples of a lowered threshold to sensory stimuli: *Hyperesthesia* of cutaneous receptors is a phenomenon that occurs in some instances of physical (e.g., sunburn) or chemical abnormalities of cutaneous receptors, or sometimes is associated with systemic viral infections, leading to increased appreciation of light touch and perception of previously non-noxious stimuli as painful. In illness, hyperesthesias probably result from an abnormality of the receptors of unknown cause, lowering their threshold. In some instances it may result from closer contact of the sensory receptor with the environment, as when a safecracker rubs his fingers with sandpaper to increase their cutaneous perception. Spontaneous discharges of the sensory system usually cause either pins and needles sensations (paresthesias from discharges in large peripheral A-delta fibers in the lemniscal system) or a burning sensation that may or may not be painful (small myelinated or unmyelinated peripheral fibers in the spinothalamic system). In the peripheral nervous system a lowered threshold to discharge is often encountered when a previously damaged nerve is regenerating. If a peripheral nerve is sectioned and begins to regenerate, the newly regenerated fibers are not fully myelinated and have a lower threshold to discharge. A light tap over the area of regeneration will produce paresthesias in the distal distribution of the nerve (Tinel's sign). Tinel's sign can be used to trace the time course of a regenerating nerve as it grows at the usual rate of 1 to 3 mm/day. Similar paresthesias in response to a light tap can be found at sites of nerve compression where the nerve is partially demyelinated. Paresthesias in the distribution of the median nerve when the wrist is lightly tapped suggest compression of the nerve at that site (carpal tunnel syndrome). This finding is a quantitative rather than a qualitative one, since a firm enough tap will discharge any nerve, as anyone can attest who has ever bumped his elbow ("crazy bone") and noted the resulting ulnar nerve paresthesias. In the central nervous system a similar phenomenon occurs when the posterior columns are partially demyelinated in their cervical portion. In this situation, if the neck is flexed, mild stretch is undergone by the posterior columns sufficient to cause them to discharge. The patient perceives an electric shock-like sensation down the back and lower extremities. This phenomenon (Lhermitte's sign) commonly occurs in multiple sclerosis, a disease that causes demyelination of nervous system structures, but can accompany other forms or dorsal column damage as well. Because there are no pain fibers in the posterior columns, Lhermitte's sign, although unpleasant, is not painful. On the contrary, when a sensory nerve root is compressed and its fibers demyelinated, a light tap or pull on the nerve root, as may occur with sudden movement of the back, will produce painful paresthesias in the distribution of the nerve root, since at this site lemniscal and spinothalamic fibers are intermixed.

The pathophysiology of the lowered threshold that accompanies damage to nerve fibers is not fully understood. One factor is failure of normal interaction between lemniscal and spinothalamic systems. In most instances of painful peripheral nerve disease there is selective loss of small nerve fibers, whereas when large fibers are selectively lost there is usually sensory loss without pain. A second condition that explains some threshold abnormalities is *ephaptic conduction*. A nerve impulse passing through a damaged or demyelinated area can evoke a discharge in nearby nerve fibers without making a synaptic connection (ephaptic conduction). Thus a light touch may fire not only the nerve fibers attached to the receptor stimulated but also other fibers that subserve touch, pain, or even motor functions. There is good evidence in humans suffering from spontaneous abnormal discharges of the facial nerve (hemifacial spasm) that ephaptic conduction causes the abnormal facial movement. Ephaptic conduction has been used to explain why in the syndrome of trigeminal neuralgia (p. 1096) a light touch in the distribution of the trigeminal nerve often leads to a painful discharge. A third factor relates to physiologic changes that occur centrally after peripheral nerve section or crush. Among the changes that have been recorded after such lesions are spontaneous firing of cells of the dorsal root ganglion, changes in neuropeptide and drug receptor density in the posterior horn, and alterations of the receptive field of peripheral nerves in the posterior horn and the tract of Lissauer. All such alterations could lower the threshold for nerve discharge and lead to spontaneous pain.

Spontaneous discharges of the sensory system can occur from any site where the system is damaged. In the peripheral nerves, spontaneous discharge leads to unpleasant and sometimes painful paresthesias in the distribution of that nerve. A good everyday example of the spontaneous discharge of a nerve that accompanies release of compression comes from sitting with the legs crossed for an extended period: At first the foot loses sensation; then, when the legs are uncrossed to relieve compression on the external peroneal nerve, a spontaneous discharge of an unpleasant pins and needles sensation occupies the previously insensate area. In the central nervous system, focal epileptic seizures are the best example of spontaneous discharges (p. 1148). When seizures originate from the somatosensory cortex they are characterized by paresthesias, usually not painful, in a contralateral portion of the body. Because the area around the lips and thumb have such a wide representation in somatosensory cortex, they are a common site for the seizures to begin. The paresthesias then generally march from that site along the homunculus to involve much of the rest of the body as well, in a pattern resembling that of the jacksonian seizures that arise from the motor cortex (p. 1062).

Distortion of sensory input leads to *dysesthesia*, usually an unpleasant or painful sensation produced by a stimulus that is ordinarily painless, or to hyperpathia. *Hyperpathia* follows damage to the small-fiber spinothalamic system that elevates the threshold to noxious stimuli but, once that threshold is exceeded, amplifies the stimulus into a severely painful or unpleasant sensation. (Hyperalgesia and hyperpathia together are usually now referred to as allodynia.) *Causalgia*, a condition that follows traumatic peripheral nerve injury, causes both painful paresthesias and hyperpathia and is characterized by spontaneous burning pain that is exacerbated by touch or pressure.

We can observe the full gamut of abnormalities of sensation in ourselves when we put pressure on a peripheral nerve, causing the area to "go to sleep." Because peripheral nerve compression leads to dysfunction first of large myelinated fibers and only sub-

sequently of small myelinated and unmyelinated fibers, sensations of touch and light pressure disappear first, accompanied by preserved sensation to noxious stimuli, including extremes of temperature, pinprick, and pressure. With continued compression, all sensation may disappear, although usually firm pressure will lead to an unpleasant, vaguely localized burning sensation. When the compression is released, spontaneous discharges of the large peripheral fibers lead to pins and needles paresthesias associated with an unpleasant hyperesthetic sensation in response to light touch or pressure. Most persons are also familiar with local anesthetic injections that, in contradistinction to compression, preferentially diffuse to and affect unmyelinated and small myelinated fibers. Following such an injection, discomfort from noxious stimuli and temperature stimuli rapidly disappears. Light touch and pressure sensations are initially distorted so that the lightest touches are not felt and more firm touch or pressure may be perceived as a poorly localized paresthetic or pins and needles sensation. Finally anesthesia ensues.

Strictly speaking, humans suffer from very few "pure" sensory disorders. Because the sensory pathways are so intimately intermixed with motor pathways throughout most of their peripheral and central course, structural diseases, such as tumors, infarcts, or hemorrhages, rarely cause purely sensory disorders. Instead the sensory loss is usually mixed with motor, autonomic, or movement abnormalities as a result of damage to nearby nonsensory pathways. Only in those areas where sensory fibers are isolated will structural lesions cause purely sensory loss. Examples are entrapment neuropathies of pure sensory nerves (such as the syndrome of meralgia paresthetica—sensory loss in the distribution of the lateral cutaneous nerve of the thigh), compression of the sensory portion of the nerve root in a herniated disc, a small syrinx (p. 1091) damaging only spinothalamic fibers crossing in the anterior commissure of the spinal cord, or small infarcts or tumors restricted to the sensory thalamus or somatosensory cortex. Furthermore, there are few diseases of the nervous system that affect sensory fibers as a system, and those that do are rare, in contradistinction to the fairly common degenerative diseases of the motor system (such as motor neuron disease) or of the cerebellar system (spinocerebellar degenerations). The best example of widespread sensory system disease is so-called subacute sensory neuronopathies, in which actual or presumed toxins cause degeneration of dorsal root ganglion cells (p. 1088). The second possible example is a very rare disorder called congenital universal indifference to pain, which is characterized by normal sensation except for the absence of appreciation of pain anywhere in the body. The pathophysiologic basis of the condition is not known.

Because of the paucity of pure sensory loss in disease, the disorders described below usually encompass both sensory and motor changes, although the emphasis in this chapter is on the sensory loss.

Contrary to the paucity of pure syndromes of sensory loss, pain as an isolated symptom is common. Headache, back pain, and neck pain are the most common reasons for referral of a patient to a neurologist. The pathophysiology of these conditions is considered separately, beginning on page 1094.

DISORDERS OF PERIPHERAL NERVES

General Considerations

Disorders of the peripheral nerves (neuropathies) are common and may appear as manifestations of a wide variety of disease processes, including genetic, traumatic, metabolic, immune, and vascular disorders. Table 23 classifies some common neuropathies, and the following paragraphs describe the pathophysiology of the symptoms and signs caused by these disorders. To understand the pathophysiology of the signs and symptoms of a patient with a peripheral nerve disorder, one must first consider the gross anatomy of the lesion(s), i.e., single nerve, multiple nerves, nerve plexus, nerve root, or dorsal root ganglion. Second, one must assess the impact of the pathologic process on nerve fibers of various size; i.e., does the process involve predominantly large fibers (lemniscal system) or small fibers (spinothalamic system)? Third, one must consider which cellular component of the nerve is damaged by the pathologic process; i.e., does the damage most affect the axon, the myelin sheath, the cell body, or all components more or less equally? Consideration of these three pathophysiologic factors often will allow a strong inference as to the etiologic agent underlying the neuropathic disorder.

Anatomically, peripheral nerve lesions can be divided into those that are symmetric and generalized, the so-called polyneuropathies, and those that are focal or multifocal (mononeuropathy or mononeuropathy multiplex). Included among the mononeuropathies are disorders not only of the peripheral nerve but the nerve plexuses or nerve roots as well. As their name implies, mononeuropathies usually produce symptoms within the distribution of one or several discrete nerves (only a portion of the nerve distribution may be involved, depending on the site and extent of the lesion), whereas the polyneuropathies generally produce symptoms that affect the most distal extremity of all nerves, leading to the so-called stocking-glove loss of sensation. Thus a polyneuropathy such as that caused by the neurotoxic anticancer drug vincristine begins with tingling in the tips of all ten fingers and all ten toes, whereas bilateral ulnar palsies caused by compression begin with tingling only in the tips of the fifth and ulnar halves of the fourth fingers. The distinction may become difficult when mononeuritis multiplex involves so many individual nerves as to give the appearance of a polyneuropathy, a problem that sometimes arises with widespread vascular disorders of nerve (e.g., polyarteritis nodosa). Complicated rearrangement of peripheral nerve fibers in the large brachial and lumbosacral plexuses also sometimes makes localizing diagnosis difficult. Careful sensory and motor testing, along with electrical recording of denervated muscle, often clarifies the situation. The anatomic classification has important etiologic implications. Most mononeuropathies or mononeuropathy multiplex are caused either by local trauma, compression, tumors or by vascular disorders, whereas most polyneuropathies are caused by toxic, metabolic, or immune disorders.

Peripheral nerve injuries can also be classified by the *cell* or *fiber size* most involved, i.e., large-fiber neuropathy, small-fiber neuropathy, pan-neuropathy. This classification has both etiologic and clinical implications. Large-diameter fibers and their cell bodies subserving the lemniscal system and small-diameter fibers and their small cell bodies subserving the spinothalamic system have differing susceptibilies to various insults. In the mononeuropathies, for example, compression of a nerve is more likely to produce large-fiber damage, leaving the small fibers relatively intact, whereas local anesthetic injection into a nerve does just the opposite. Certain hereditary and metabolic

TABLE 23. ANATOMIC CLASSIFICATION OF PERIPHERAL NEUROPATHY

TWO OVERALL TYPES—	1. SYMMETRICAL GENERALIZED 2. FOCAL AND MULTIFOCAL
1. Symmetrical Generalized Distal Axonopathies	Neuropathies (Polyneuropathies) Toxic—many drugs, industrial and environmental chemicals Metabolic—uremia, diabetes, porphyria, endocrine Deficiency—thiamine, pyridoxine Genetic—HMSN II Malignancy associated—oat-cell carcinoma, multiple myeloma
Myelinopathies	Toxic—diphtheria, buckthorn Immunologic—acute inflammatory polyneuropathy (Guillain-Barré) chronic inflammatory polyneuropathy Genetic—Refsum disease, metachromatic leukodystrophy
Neuronopathies somatic motor	Undetermined—amyotrophic lateral sclerosis Genetic—hereditary motor neuronopathies
somatic sensory	Infectious—herpes zoster neuronitis Malignancy-associated—sensory neuronopathy syndrome Toxic—pyridoxine sensory neuronopathy Undetermined—subacute sensory neuronopathy syndrome
autonomic	Genetic—hereditary dysautonomia (HSN IV)

2. Focal (Mononeuropathy) and Multifocal (Multiple Mononeuropathy) Neuropathies
   Ischemia—polyarteritis, diabetes, rheumatoid arthritis
   Infiltration—leukemia, lymphoma, granuloma, Schwannoma, amyloid
   Physical injuries—severance, focal crush, compression, stretch and traction, entrapment
   Immunologic—brachial and lumbar plexopathy

From Schaumburg, H., Spencer, P., and Thomas, P. K.: Disorders of Peripheral Nerves. Philadelphia, F. A. Davis Co., 1983.

neuropathies have a predilection for involving small fibers, whereas immune and certain deficiency disorders often affect large fibers. In addition to the etiologic implications there are important clinical implications.

Those diseases of peripheral nerves that affect both large and small fibers diminish all sensory modalities to approximately equal degree. If small or large fibers are involved preferentially there is a "dissociated sensory loss." When small fibers are predominantly affected, pain and temperature sensation are involved out of proportion to light touch, vibration, and position sense. Because autonomic fibers are also small, trophic changes in skin and joints may accompany such small-fiber peripheral neuropathies, but because motor fibers and the afferent portion of the stretch reflex are subserved by large fibers, these functions are relatively preserved despite sometimes profound loss of pain and temperature sensation. Such selective small-fiber damage is sometimes encountered in diabetes and is common in some of the hereditary neuropathies as well as in toxic-nutritional neuropathies. Large-fiber loss is more common in demyelinating neuropathies and may lead to profound loss of localizing touch and proprioception with relative preservation of crude touch, pinprick, and temperature sensations. Such disorders are commonly accompanied by paresthesias and less often by spontaneous pain. The deep tendon reflexes disappear because damage to large afferent fibers interferes with the afferent volley of the stretch reflex, and weakness usually develops.

Neuropathies can also be classified on the basis of the *cellular component* most affected (Fig. 35). Pathologic attack on a peripheral nerve may affect primarily the myelin sheath (demyelinating neuropathies), the axon, in which case the myelin sheaths degenerate secondarily (axonal neuropathy), or the cell body itself, a situation that usually leads to loss of axon and myelin sheath as well (neuronopathy). Some disorders may be mixed. By considering the cellular component most affected, one can often not only predict the underlying etiologic factor but also determine prognosis for recovery. The clinical differentiation of neuropathies by cellular component (Table 23) is described below.

Demyelinating Neuropathy

Myelinated axons are embedded in Schwann cells along their entire length. Each Schwann cell supplies 1 to 2 mm of myelin to the axon. Between contiguous Schwann cells along an axon there is a ring-shaped constriction called the node of Ranvier. At the node of Ranvier the axon is denuded of both myelin and Schwann cell sheaths. Nerve conduction is much more rapid in myelinated than unmyelinated fibers and is generally proportional to the size of the axon. Rapid conduction along myelinated fibers is saltatory, i.e., rather than the impulse being conducted along the entire length of the fiber, it jumps from node of Ranvier to node of Ranvier. The distance between the nodes of Ranvier determines the speed of conduction. Clinical examples of damage to the myelin sheath or Schwann cell (myelinopathy, demyelinating neuropathy) are inflammatory polyneuropathy (e.g., Guillain-Barré syndrome) and direct compression of nerve (e.g., carpal tunnel syndrome). Loss of nerve function is characterized either by slowing of nerve conduction across partially myelinated or demyelinated segments or by complete failure of conduction (conduction block) if several contiguous segments lose their myelin. Because the axon remains intact and if, as is usually the case, the Schwann cells remain undamaged so that they can replace the damaged myelin, recovery is often rapid and complete. Pathologically, loss of myelin usually begins at the node of Ranvier and works back toward the center of the myelinated segment. In most clinical conditions, single myelin segments are lost randomly along the length of the nerve, with preserved myelin segments in between. Frequently the spinal roots are more heavily involved than the more distal nerve. When remyelination occurs it usually produces a thinner sheath than previously, and internodal segments may be shortened.

Clinically, demyelinating neuropathy is characterized by failure of large myelinated fiber function, leading to decreased light touch, position, and vibration sense as well as reduction or absence of deep tendon reflexes. A relative sparing of lightly myelinated or unmyelinated fibers leads to partial preservation of temperature and pain sensation, although these modalities may become involved if the disorder is severe. Electrical studies of demyelinated nerves (p. 1093) reveal that the conduction velocity is slowed, often to 20 to 25 per cent of normal values, and the action potential is small because of dispersion.

Axonal Neuropathy

Damage to the axon (axonal neuropathy, dying-back neuropathy) results either from direct injury to the nerve, with degeneration of axons distal to the injury (wallerian degeneration), or, more commonly, from metabolic or toxic injury, leading to diffuse axonal degeneration. When such injury occurs the axon no longer can transport vital nutrients to its most distal portions. The result is axonal degeneration, beginning distally and slowly dying back toward the cell body. If the axonal injury is sufficiently distal the cell body escapes damage. More proximal injuries may result in dispersion of the rough endoplasmic reticulum in the nucleus (central chromatolysis). Severe injury to the entire axon may result in death of the cell body. In demyelinating neuropathies the loss of myelin does not damage axons, but when the axon is damaged the myelin sheath also undergoes degeneration. Furthermore, the central extension of the sensory axon also undergoes degeneration and secondary demyelination along with adjacent astrocytic proliferation, leading to easily identifiable pathologic changes in the posterior columns of the spinal cord. If the damage is severe enough there may even be trans-synaptic degeneration in specific sensory systems, for example, the neurons of the gracile nucleus. Clinically, axonal neuropathy is usually characterized by an equal loss of all modalities, although in certain instances smaller cells carrying sensations of pain and temperature are lost out of proportion to larger cells carrying those of vibration and position. Because most axonal failure begins distally the first symptoms are usually sensory, involving paresthesias or sensory loss in the tips of the fingers and toes. Only later, when sensory loss spreads more proximally, does motor involvement occur as well. Remember that sensory axons carrying sensation from fingers and toes begin there, whereas the motor axons

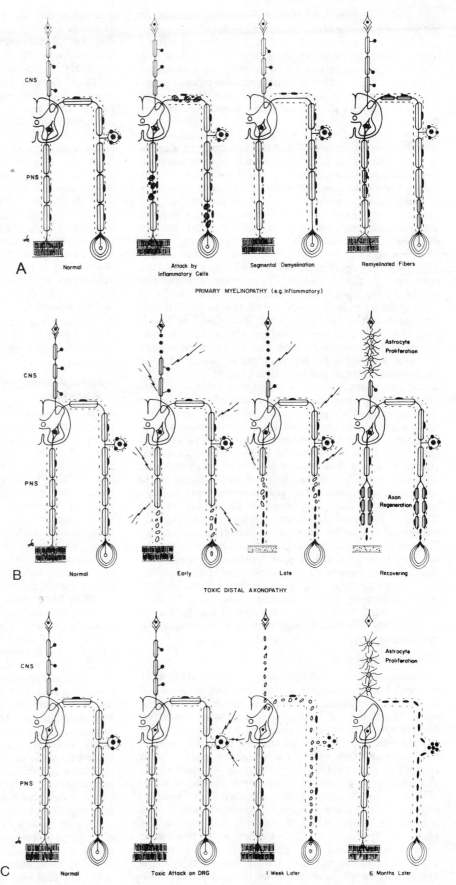

Figure 35. Neuropathies according to affected cellular component. *A,* The cardinal pathologic features of an inflammatory PNS myelinopathy. Axons are spared as is CNS myelin. Following the attack, the remaining Schwann cells divide. The denuded segments of axons are remyelinated, leaving them with shortened internodes. *B,* The cardinal pathologic features of a toxic distal axonopathy. The jagged lines (lightning bolts) indicate that the toxin is acting at multiple sites along motor and sensory axons in the PNS and CNS. Axon degeneration has moved proximally (dying-back) by the late stage. Recovery in the CNS is impeded by astroglial proliferation. *C,* The cardinal features of a rapidly involving toxic sensory neuronopathy. The *jagged lines* (lightning bolts) indicate that the toxin is directed at neurons in the dorsal root ganglion *(DRG).* Degeneration of these cells is accompanied by fragmentation and phagocytosis of their peripheral-central processes. The Schwann cells remain; there is no axonal regeneration. (From Schaumburg, H., Spencer, P., and Thomas, P. K.: Disorders of Peripheral Nerves. Philadelphia, F. A. Davis Co., 1983, p. 8.)

that move fingers and toes are shorter, ending in muscles in the forearm, proximal area of the hand, calf, and proximal part of the foot. Unlike demyelinating neuropathy, recovery is usually slow, proceeding at a regeneration rate of 1 to 3 mm/day for a damaged axon. Electrically, axonal neuropathies are characterized by normal or only 10 to 15 per cent slower conduction velocities and by small sensory action potentials.

In both demyelinating and axonal neuropathies the sensory loss is maximal distally, leading in diffuse polyneuropathy to the typical stocking-glove distribution and sometimes in severe neuropathy to sensory loss in the medial anterior trunk, the most distal extent of thoracic and lumbar nerves. A recently described *central distal axonopathy* can be caused by several toxic substances and may underlie several human degenerative diseases. This disorder is characterized by selective vulnerability in that portion of the sensory axon between the dorsal root ganglion and the spinal cord, sparing that portion of the axon directed peripherally. As with peripheral axonopathies there is dying back of the axon in the posterior column (or with motor disorders, in the lateral column) from distal to proximal, with loss of the surrounding myelin sheath from gliosis of the posterior column. Central motor pathways are also affected with degeneration of distal portions of the corticospinal tracts. Clinically the sensory loss is usually characterized by the subacute onset of paresthesias and lemniscal system sensory loss similar to that in large-fiber peripheral neuropathy. However, unlike the situation in the peripheral neuropathies, deep tendon reflexes are usually hyperactive because the fibers of the monosynaptic stretch reflex are spared (the afferents not reaching the posterior columns), and the reflex inhibitors descending the corticospinal tracts are involved. Because of the corticospinal tract damage there may be spastic paraparesis accompanying the disorder. However, there may be loss of ankle jerks, reflecting the mild peripheral axonal involvement. Electrical studies of the peripheral nerves may be normal, but there are gross disorders in sensory conduction. The reason the distal portion of the sensory axon is relatively spared is not known, but differences in the microenvironment (axons surrounded by glial rather than Schwann cell myelin) and functional capacity (less efficient axonal transport in sensory-directed fibers) have been proposed as causes.

Neuronopathy

Damage to the cell body itself (neuronopathy) may be focal, as when herpes zoster infection attacks the dorsal root ganglion, or more generalized, as in some toxic disorders and in the paraneoplastic syndrome termed subacute sensory neuronopathy. Neuronopathy is characterized by death of the cell body with secondary degeneration of the axon and its myelin, both centrally and peripherally, leading to pathologic changes in the periphery of the nerve similar to those of axonal neuropathy. Toxic neuronopathies tend to affect sensory rather than motor neurons because the sensory cell body in the dorsal root ganglion is not protected by the blood-CNS barrier as is the motor neuron in the spinal cord. Clinically there is usually a rapid onset of sensory loss, with complete or relative sparing of motor function. Like the peripheral neuropathies, the disorder usually begins distally and proceeds proximally, but sometimes may affect proximal and distal segments at onset, and more often affects the trunk than axonal neuropathies. Because cell bodies in the gasserian ganglion are as vulnerable as those in the dorsal root ganglion, loss of facial sensation is rare except in the most severe demyelinating and axonal neuropathies but is common in neuronopathies. Large cells may be more affected than small cells, leading to proprioceptive and deep tendon reflex loss greater than pain and temperature loss. Electrical studies of sensory nerves usually reveal absence of or small potentials, with variable slowing. If the neurons are not irreversibly damaged, recovery may occur, but it is frequently slow and incomplete.

The motor analogue of the sensory neuronopathies is anterior horn cell disease. Poliomyelitis is an inflammatory disease restricted to anterior horn cells that once occurred in epidemic proportions in the United States, but is now fortunately rare—the result of development of antipolio vaccine. Several degenerative diseases, the most common of which is amyotrophic lateral sclerosis, affect anterior horn cells, leading to a motor neuronopathy, sparing sensory fibers. The clinical characteristics of such a lower motor neuron dysfunction are described in the first chapter of this section.

Pathophysiology of Neuropathic Syndromes

The diagnosis of a peripheral neuropathy involving sensory fibers is established by the distribution of the sensory loss. *Mononeuritis* by definition is an illness in which there is damage to a single peripheral nerve. Because it is a local disease, local factors are usually responsible for its pathogenesis. Most mononeuritides result from nerve compression, either by extrinsic or intrinsic factors; for example, Saturday night palsy, a mononeuritis of the radial nerve, is caused by extrinsic compression of that nerve between an external object such as the arm of a chair and the unyielding humeral bone around which the radial nerve winds. Compression usually occurs when an intoxicated person sleeps soundly with the outstretched arm resting over a chair or other hard object. Distal radial nerve palsy caused by compressing a cutaneous branch of the radial nerve leads to sensory loss restricted to the dorsum of the thumb. The most common examples of intrinsic compression are the so-called entrapment neuropathies (e.g., carpal tunnel syndrome—in which the median nerve is compressed by the flexor retinaculum of the wrist—or meralgia paresthetica—in which the lateral femoral cutaneous nerve of the thigh is entrapped as it passes through the inguinal ligament). These two entrapment neuropathies are the most common; many other nerves may be trapped at one or more sites along their course. Less common than the entrapment neuropathies are mononeuropathies caused by infiltrating or compressing tumor, ischemia, infarction of the nerve by focal vascular disease (e.g., vasculitis, diabetic mononeuropathy), or direct trauma.

Because most single mononeuropathies are compressive, large fibers suffer disproportionately. If a motor nerve is involved, weakness is an early symptom. When predominantly sensory nerves are involved, paresthesias and loss of the sensation of light touch and proprioception are early symptoms. Pain may occur at the site of compression. The diagnosis is made by the distribution of sensory and motor loss, and the exact site can be localized by electrical studies (p. 1092).

Multiple mononeuritis (mononeuritis multiplex) is a condition in which multiple single nerves are damaged. The most common cause of mononeuritis multiplex is vasculitis leading to ischemia or infarction of multiple nerves. The vasculitis may be the result of immunologic disorders such as polyarteritis nodosa and rheumatoid arthritis as well as, sometimes, diabetes. Arteriosclerotic vascular disease is a much rarer cause of mononeuritis multiplex. Even more rarely, there are patients who have a genetic predisposition to a compression neuropathy, the biology of which is unknown. Such patients may develop a mononeuritis multiplex picture without suffering an underlying systemic disease such as vasculitis.

Vasculopathies of peripheral nerves occlude vessels, with resulting ischemia or infarction of that portion of the peripheral nerve supplied by that vessel. If the vascular disorder is limited, only one nerve may be involved, and the development of collateral circulation may eventually allow for reversal of the neuropathy so produced. Diabetic mononeuropathy, particularly affecting the oculomotor nerve, represents such an instance: The disorder is characterized by acute failure of oculomotor function, often associated with pain, but within two or three months the symptoms resolve. Clinically, ischemia affects both large and small fibers, leading to both motor and sensory loss of all modalities. Pure sensory loss occurs only when sensory nerves are involved.

Polyneuropathies are caused by a large variety of disorders. Among these are toxic axonopathies caused by drugs, industrial and environmental chemicals, metabolic disorders such as uremia and diabetes, and some genetic disorders (Table 23). The exact clinical picture depends on which fibers have borne the brunt of the pathogenetic attack. In most instances there is distal and symmetric sensory and motor loss. In the demyelinating neuropathies, motor loss is usually out of proportion to the sensory change, and, of course, in the sensory neuronopathies the motor fibers are spared.

NERVE PLEXUSES AND ROOTS

The large nerve plexuses and the roots that supply them are extensions of the peripheral nerves, and they are susceptible to the same disorders that affect peripheral nerves. However, some disorders of nerve plexuses and roots are more or less unique to those structures and deserve special consideration. For example, the posterior cord of the brachial plexus is particularly susceptible to compression by tumors arising in the apex of the lung (Pancoast tumor), and portions of the lumbosacral plexus are particularly susceptible to invasion by genitourinary tumors. The inferior portion of the brachial plexus may be compressed between normal tissues as it leaves the neck to enter the arm (thoracic outlet syndrome), and, because of its relatively exposed position, the brachial plexus and its attached cervical nerve roots are particularly susceptible to direct trauma. Stretch injury to the brachial plexus or its nerve roots is another disorder almost unique to that anatomic area. Stretching

of a peripheral nerve or nerve plexus may cause damage ranging from temporary disruption of the myelin sheath to total transection of the nerve. Such stretch injuries are seen with increasing frequency in motorcycle accidents, because motorcycle drivers now wear helmets and often survive the associated head injury. The stretch injury may be sufficiently mild to produce only demyelination in all or part of the brachial plexus, leading to transient paralysis, or it may be sufficiently severe to avulse the brachial plexus from the attached roots. Clinically there are both motor paralysis and sensory loss. Mild injuries may be relatively painless, but with avulsion injuries there is often severe pain of a causalgic nature (p. 1097) at the onset of the injury, which persists unchanged for life. Avulsion injuries are accompanied by a characteristic myelographic change in which the iodinated dye injected into the spinal canal can be seen to exit through the torn root sleeves of the involved cervical roots.

Either the brachial or, less commonly, the lumbosacral plexus may be the site of an acute demyelinating disorder called acute brachial or acute lumbosacral neuropathy and probably caused by immune attack upon the myelin sheath. Why the disorder localizes to one brachial or lumbosacral plexus is unknown.

The disorder is characterized by the acute painful onset of motor and, to a lesser extent, sensory dysfunction in a patchy distribution suggesting a plexus rather than single or multiple peripheral nerves. It often occurs in otherwise healthy individuals and is usually followed by full recovery. The disorder is thought to be related to other acute demyelinating neuropathies such as the Guillain-Barré syndrome, but the reason for its localization to a single area is unclear.

In the *nerve root* the most common and characteristic disorder is compression by a herniated intervertebral disc. With the degeneration of aging or following trauma to the disc, disc material herniates through a weakened anulus fibrosus to compress the nerve root as it exits through the intervertebral foramen. Compression of the nerve root leads to edema and demyelination, which, in turn, cause dysfunction, more often sensory than motor, in the distribution of that root. A swollen and demyelinated nerve root is particularly sensitive to stretch, and thus the patient finds that movement such as bending or raising the legs, which stretch on the nerve roots but are normally painless, cause severe pain, again in the distribution of the involved root. Herniated discs are probably the most common cause of peripheral nerve dysfunction in civilized man. In the dorsal root ganglion, the most common and characteristic disorder is herpes zoster. The body is usually invaded by the varicella-zoster virus in childhood, with a resulting varicella infection. The virus reaches one or more dorsal root ganglia and lies dormant for years, until an unknown trigger (sometimes trauma or immune suppression) reactivates the virus, leading to a varicella rash restricted to the dermatomal distribution of the involved dorsal root ganglion. In some individuals the herpetic infection after healing may cause chronic pain in the dermatome (postherpetic neuralgia [p. 1097]).

Although nerve plexuses and nerve roots are often affected by different pathophysiologic processes, as indicated above, it is sometimes very difficult to differentiate between the two sites on clinical grounds alone.

This is particularly true when nerve roots are involved in the paravertebral space just before they conjoin to form the plexuses. In general, single nerve root lesions are more likely to cause pain and paresthesias in an easily localizable and discrete dermatomal distribution, whereas the pain of plexus lesions is more diffuse and less clearly localized. Furthermore, single root lesions do not usually cause severe muscular weakness, since most major muscles are innervated by more than one root. When there is muscle weakness and sensory change the distribution differs between root and plexus, as indicated in Table 23. The distribution of motor weakness can be confirmed by electrical studies showing denervation in muscles innervated by either roots or plexus. Sensory and motor conduction velocities can sometimes identify the site of conduction block, further assisting in the differentiation.

SPINAL CORD

Just proximal to the dorsal root ganglion, myelinated fibers lose their Schwann cells, which are replaced by oligodendroglial cells, making the incoming dorsal root fibers part of the central nervous system. The dorsal root entry zone and the spinal cord as part of the central nervous system are susceptible to all of the pathophysiologic processes that affect neurons and pathways of the brain. Anatomic peculiarities of the spinal cord determine some of the differences between lesions that affect it and those that affect the brain. For example, in the spinal cord the gray matter is located centrally, surrounded by white matter, whereas in the cerebral hemispheres, gray matter, except for the basal ganglia, is located peripheral to white matter. An enlarging central canal of the spinal cord (hydromyelia), analogous in some respects to hydrocephalus in the brain, compresses surrounding gray matter in the spinal cord, whereas hydrocephalus first compresses subcortical white matter. Furthermore, the greatest distance between lemniscal and spinothalamic pathways is in the spinal cord, making lesions of the spinal cord much more likely to produce dissociated sensory loss than lesions elsewhere in the nervous system. The nature of the sensory loss with spinal cord disorders depends on the anatomy of the lesion and, to some degree, its rate of development. Slowly growing

compressive (e.g., meningiomas) or invasive tumors can produce truly astounding destruction or distortion of the spinal cord with minimal symptoms, whereas acutely developing compressive or invasive lesions (e.g., metastatic tumors to extradural space or spinal cord) can produce major signs and symptoms while they are quite small. The small size of the spinal cord usually guarantees that large and rapidly developing lesions of a segment of the cord affect all motor, sensory, and autonomic function of the body (Fig. 36B) below that segment. Smaller lesions are more selective: At the root entry zones or in the posterior horn, spinal lesions affect all modalities ipsilaterally, but only in the involved segments. There is usually demyelination of the continuing posterior column (Fig. 36A).

Lesions of the posterolateral columns (Fig. 36E) produce profound loss of position and vibration sense accompanied by normal crude touch, pain, and temperature sensation. Paresthesias are common, but pain is rare, probably because most of the large-fiber–small-fiber interaction occurs at the dorsal root entry zone, before fibers enter the posterior columns. Strictly speaking, lemniscal fibers, unlike other pathways in the spinal cord, are part of the peripheral nervous system in that their cell body originates in the dorsal root ganglion, just like the cell body of the sensory peripheral nerve, rather than in the central nervous system. Thus in sensory neuronopathies there is loss of axons both centrally and peripherally despite the fact that they have the same origin. Several toxic, metabolic, and deficiency disorders can involve the posterior columns. In some instances the posterior column degeneration is secondary to that of peripheral nerve. Less commonly, as in central distal axonopathies, the posterior column is primary, and then corticospinal tracts are usually involved as well as the sensory pathways, so that most such patients have hyperactive reflexes and extensor plantar responses in addition to the sensory changes. The reason for the "metabolic sensitivity" of these large axons is not known.

Lesions that damage the spinothalamic tract or the fibers that cross to it from the contralateral posterior horn cause loss of pain and temperature sense but spare the sensations of vibration, position, and localizing touch. Such *dissociated sensory loss* is common

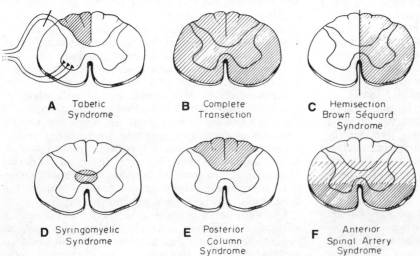

A Tabetic Syndrome **B** Complete Transection **C** Hemisection Brown Séquard Syndrome

D Syringomyelic Syndrome **E** Posterior Column Syndrome **F** Anterior Spinal Artery Syndrome

Figure 36. Some of the sites of lesions that produce characteristic spinal cord syndromes (*shaded areas* indicate lesions). (From Adams, R. D., and Victor, M.: Principles of Neurology, 2nd ed. New York, McGraw-Hill Book Co., 1981, p. 113.)

in syringomyelia (Fig. 36D), where an enlarging central canal impinges on fibers crossing in the anterior commissure from the posterior horn to the spinothalamic tract of the opposite side. The sensory loss is bilateral and affects only the areas supplied by the damaged fibers. Motor function may be normal. Dissociated sensory loss also occurs with infarction of the anterior portion of the spinal cord from occlusion of the anterior spinal artery (Fig. 36F). With anterior spinal artery occlusion, corticospinal tracts are involved as well, although the dorsal columns are spared. When only one side of the spinal cord is damaged (Fig. 36A), proprioceptive loss is ipsilateral, and loss of pain and temperature is contralateral. The entire body below the level of the lesion is usually affected, although pain and temperature sensation may be spared in the sacrum because the sacral fibers of the spinothalamic tract are in the most peripheral portion of the spinal cord and may escape damage from an intrinsic lesion. There is usually a small band of decreased sensation to all modalities, resulting from damage to the posterior horn at the level of the lesion. This so-called Brown-Séquard syndrome sometimes results from tumors either compressing or invading the spinal cord and is a common presenting syndrome in radiation myelopathy or multiple sclerosis.

Lesions of the spinal cord are rarely confused with those of peripheral nerves even when the latter show dissociated sensory loss, because the sensory loss in spinal cord lesions usually affects both the proximal and distal parts of the trunk and extremities and is restricted to segments below the level of the spinal cord that is damaged. Thus by the time a polyneuropathy causes substantial sensory loss above the knees, nerve fibers supplying the fingertips are usually involved as well, whereas a thoracic spinal cord lesion below T2 always spares the arms. Furthermore, motor signs of upper motor neuron disease, particularly extensor plantar responses, usually correctly identify the central nature of a spinal cord disorder rather than pointing to a peripheral disturbance.

BRAINSTEM

Lesions of the brainstem are characterized by the combination of lower motor neuron–cranial nerve dysfunction and upper motor neuron–trunk and extremity dysfunction. This combination occurs only with brainstem lesions and, when combined with the characteristic ocular findings and abnormal breathing patterns characteristic of brainstem disorders, makes localization relatively easy.

Sensory changes occurring with abnormalities of the brainstem are also characteristic. In the lower brainstem or in the spinal cord, the spinothalamic and proprioceptive pathways remain separated. Lateral lesions of the medulla cause loss of pain and temperature sensation on the same side of the face (a result of damage to the descending root of the ipsilateral trigeminal nerve) and the opposite side of the body. This sensory abnormality is usually accompanied by other signs of lateral medullary damage (Wallenberg syndrome), but spares proprioceptive pathways because of their more dorsomedial position. Higher in the brainstem, as the two pathways converge in their route toward the thalamus, damage causes contralateral loss of all modalities, usually accompanied by cranial nerve

palsies, ataxia (from the cerebellar outflow), and motor weakness.

The pathologic processes that affect the brainstem are similar to those that affect brain and spinal cord. Because of the dense packing of cranial nerve and long tract fibers in the brainstem, small vascular or demyelinating lesions are likely to produce characteristic complexes of symptoms, most of which are designated by eponyms. Small midbrain infarcts provide an example of how proximate but discrete lesions can produce widely different clinical symptoms. A ventrally placed infarct involving the cerebral peduncle and the exiting third nerve produces Weber's syndrome (ipsilateral third nerve palsy and contralateral hemiparesis without sensory changes), whereas a slightly more dorsally placed lesion produces Benedikt's syndrome (ipsilateral third nerve palsy and contralateral tremor and hemiataxia).

CEREBRUM

In the *thalamus*, damage to the ventral posterolateral nucleus causes contralateral decrease in all modalities on the body and face. Sensory loss is often accompanied by dysesthesias. A *thalamic syndrome* often appears four to six weeks after acute thalamic damage and has been attributed to the development of denervation hypersensitivity of sensory neurons in the midbrain reticular formation that previously interconnected with the now-damaged thalamus. Affected patients develop spontaneous pain in the distribution of the contralateral sensory loss, usually associated with a dysesthetic response to touch and hyperresponsiveness to pinprick once threshold is exceeded. The thalamic syndrome is rare but causes a particularly unpleasant pain intractable to most therapeutic endeavors. Conversely, surgical lesions of the intralaminar nuclei, which receive fibers from the paleospinothalamic tract, often decrease pain without affecting sensory thresholds.

Damage to the *cerebral cortex* causes sensory loss in which the synthetic qualities of sensation are involved out of proportion to crude sensation. Pain sensation is usually preserved, although the patient may describe a pinprick as feeling less sharp on the involved side. The distribution of sensory impairment follows that of the sensory homunculus. Depending on the cortical location of the lesion within that distribution, touch and vibration sensibilities are usually relatively preserved as well. Position sense loss is often profound; in addition, affected patients are unable to distinguish between one and two points touching the finger or foot, and cutaneous sensations, even though identified, may not be localized. Patients may be unable to identify the nature of objects placed in their hand, even though they can describe certain of the object's physical qualities (astereognosis). Patients with large cortical sensory lesions are often relatively inattentive to sensation arising from the opposite side of the body. The impairment is intensified if there is a distracting stimulus to the same side. Thus the patient presented with two symmetric cutaneous sensory stimuli may fail to identify the one contralateral to the cortical lesion even though the strength of the stimulus exceeds threshold (extinction). With less severe damage, if two nonhomologous stimuli are presented (for example, to the left hand and to the right side of the face), the patient may perceive the stimulus on the involved side as occurring homologous to the stimulus on the uninvolved side ("You touched both sides of my face"). Such sensory extinction phenomena are characteristic of parietal lobe lesions, particularly those affecting the nondominant hemisphere. Smaller or more restricted lesions of the parietal lobe may lead to subtle changes in sensory function, with only synthetic modalities such as stereognosis, two-point discrimination, and graphesthesia (ability to identify numbers or letters traced on the palm or fingertip) involved.

The sensory cortex, when damaged, is relatively susceptible to the development of spontaneous discharges or to prolonged discharges after stimulation. Small lesions of the sensory cortex, even those too small to cause discernible sensory loss, may present themselves as sensory seizures. The seizure is perceived by the patient as a paresthetic sensation, sometimes but not usually painful, that affects the contralateral part of the body supplied by the discharging area of the cortex. Because the cortical representation of the thumb and lip are so large, seizures characteristically begin in this area and, as the discharge spreads over the cortex, the patient may perceive the paresthesias moving up the arm and subsequently over the face and leg. Because the sensory and motor cortices are so inextricably linked, a motor seizure may accompany the sensory changes. Seizures usually last only a few minutes, and in some instances may be followed by a period of sensory loss in the distribution of the seizure analogous to the motor loss that sometimes follows motor seizures (Todd's paralysis). The pathophysiology of the sensory loss following sensory seizures is not certain. It appears not to be due to metabolic exhaustion of the neuron. At times, sensory seizures can be precipitated by cutaneous stimulation, and at other times they can be aborted by cutaneous stimulation.

ELECTRICAL DIAGNOSIS OF SENSORY AND MOTOR DISORDERS

Electrical measurement of nerve and muscle potentials in human beings with neurologic disease often yields important information in four areas: (1) the distinction between muscle and neural disease causing weakness, (2) the identification and diagnosis of disorders of the neuromuscular junction causing weakness and fatigability, (3) the site and distribution in the peripheral or central nervous system of abnormalities causing sensory or motor disturbances, (4) the pathology of peripheral nerve disease causing sensory or motor loss (i.e., axonal versus demyelinating neuropathies). The common electrical tests that assist in defining the above physiology include electromyography, neuromuscular transmission studies, measurement of conduction velocity in peripheral nerves, and measurement of velocity and wave form in the central nervous system by means of evoked potentials.

Electromyography

Electrical potentials from muscle fibers can be recorded by means of a surface electrode or by placement of a small concentric needle electrode into the muscle itself (Fig. 37). Normal muscles are electrically silent at rest. With mild voluntary contraction, individual motor unit discharges can be identified; these units vary in amplitude and width but are generally under 3 µv and less than 5 msec long. With maximal contraction the baseline on the oscilloscope is no longer visible, being obscured by the contraction of many motor units (called a complete interference pattern). As noted in the previous chapter, the Motor System, primary disease of muscle is characterized by motor unit potentials of small amplitude and short duration, with a normal interference pattern. These findings represent the dropout of individual muscle fibers within the motor unit, leading to the small size and duration of the motor unit potential. A normal interference pattern represents normal numbers of smaller motor units. When the muscle membrane is unstable, as in myotonic dystrophy, or when there is inflammation of the muscle leading to irritability of nerve endings, as in inflammatory myopathies, the muscle membrane may discharge when the needle is inserted or moved. Disease of the lower motor neuron is characterized by abnormal spontaneous activity of two types: (1) *Fibrillation potentials* are discharges of single muscle fibers, a result of a fiber's loss of innervation so that the membrane is supersensitive to circulating acetylcholine. (2) *Fasciculation potentials* are spontaneous discharges of entire motor units that occur when disease of the anterior horn cell or peripheral nerve make the motor unit irritable.

In lower motor neuron disease of long standing, sprouting of distal axons supplies muscle fibers that have lost their motor units and leads to motor unit potentials of increased amplitude and increased duration, often with bizarre polyphasic forms. Furthermore, because there are fewer motor units, even though larger, the interference pattern on voluntary contraction becomes incomplete. With upper motor neuron disease the electromyogram is usually normal except that motor units are decreased or absent when the patient attempts to contract the muscle.

When the electromyogram shows evidence of peripheral nerve disease, the distribution of the muscles involved can often be measured better by electrical testing than by physical examination, since subtle changes in electrical activity may not be reflected in diminished strength and that distribution may help the clinician distinguish peripheral nerve, nerve plexus, or nerve root disease.

Tests of Neuromuscular Transmission

Surface-stimulating electrodes can be placed over a peripheral nerve and the muscular activity resulting from stimulation of that nerve recorded by either surface or needle electrode in the muscle (Fig. 38). As described on page 1047, abnormalities of neuromuscular transmission include myasthenia gravis, in which repetitive stimulation of the nerve leads to rapid decrement in the size of the evoked muscle potential, and the myasthenic syndrome, characterized by an incrementing response to repetitive nerve stimulation. The electrical activity is reflected clinically in the fatigability of the muscle to repetitive voluntary contraction at the bedside. Other disorders of neuromuscular transmission that can be detected by such studies include botulism, spider bite and snakebite poisoning, and magnesium intoxication.

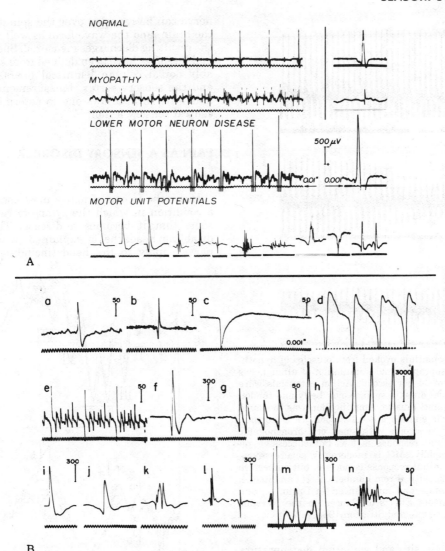

Figure 37. Potentials recorded in electromyography. *A,* Motor unit potentials during voluntary contraction in a normal person, in muscular dystrophy *(myopathy),* and in amyotrophic lateral sclerosis *(lower motor neuron).* Potentials on left are displayed with a slow time base; on right, with a fast time base. *B,* Isolated potentials: *(a)* end-plate noise (small negative deflections) and an associated muscle fiber spike from normal muscle; *(b)* fibrillation potential; and *(c)* positive wave from denervated muscle; *(d)* high-frequency discharge in myotonia; *(e)* bizarre repetitive discharge; *(f)* fasciculation potential, single discharge; *(g)* fasciculation potential, repetitive or grouped discharged; *(h)* synchronized repetitive discharge in muscle cramp; *(i)* diphasic, *(j)* triphasic, and *(k)* polyphasic motor unit action potentials from normal muscle; *(l)* short-duration motor unit action potentials in progressive muscular atrophy; *(m)* large motor unit action potentials in progressive muscular atrophy; *(n)* highly polyphasic motor unit action potential and short-duration motor unit action potential during reinnervation. Calibration scales are in microvolts. (From Department of Neurology and Department of Physiology and Biophysics, Mayo Clinic and Mayo Foundation: Clinical Examinations in Neurology. 3rd ed. Philadelphia, W. B. Saunders Co., 1971, pp. 276 and 285.)

Nerve Conduction Velocities

One can measure the rate of both sensory and motor conduction in appropriate peripheral nerves. Motor conduction is measured by placing stimulating electrodes at several sites along the nerve and recording the resulting action potential by means of a surface electrode over the innervated muscle. The delay from time of stimulation to muscle contraction divided by the distance of the stimulus from the recording electrode is called the conduction velocity and is generally measured in meters per second. Representative con-

duction velocities from various fibers are given in Table 22. Sensory conduction can be measured by stimulating a cutaneous nerve in the finger or toe and recording proximally from that nerve. Furthermore, since the stimulation of the peripheral nerve conducts both orthodromically and antidromically, one can often record the conduction in motor roots by noting the length of time from peripheral stimulation to discharge of the anterior horn cell and return of the impulse to the original stimulating electrode. In some badly damaged nerves no conduction takes place at all. If the nerve is

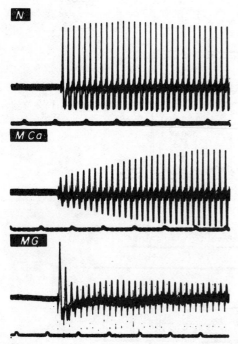

Figure 38. Action potentials evoked from muscles of hypothenar eminence by supramaximal stimulation of ulnar nerve at wrist at a rate of 54 per second. Action potentials were recorded by electrodes on skin surface over belly and tendon of abductor digiti quinti muscle. Amplification was the same in each record. Time signals are 0.1 second. *N* is normal. *MCa* is myasthenic syndrome with small cell bronchogenic carcinoma. The initial response is low, but successive responses increase rapidly. *MG* is moderately severe myasthenia gravis. The initial response is normal, but successive responses decrease rapidly. (From Lambert, E. H., and Rooke, E. D.: Myasthenic state and lung cancer. In Brain, L., and Norris, F.: The Remote Effects of Cancer on the Nervous System. New York, Grune and Stratton 1965, p. 73.)

damaged at a single site and wallerian degeneration has not taken place distally, it may be possible to identify the site of the conduction block by stimulating both proximally and distally to the block. For example, with the ulnar nerve compressed at the elbow, one may get a normal velocity and action potential if the electrode is placed distal to the elbow but no muscle potential at all if the stimulation is proximal to the elbow. The conduction velocity is determined in part by the nature of the pathologic process in the nerve: Demyelinating neuropathies lead to very slow conduction, whereas axonal neuropathies lead to relatively normal rates of conduction. Conduction velocities measure the velocity in only the most rapidly conducting fibers so that it may be normal despite the loss of large numbers of smaller, more slowly conducting fibers.

Evoked Potentials

Evoked potentials, the electrical activity that occurs in central pathways in response to stimulation of a peripheral nerve, can be measured by means of a recently developed and powerful technique. Evoked potentials may be measured in the visual, auditory, or somatosensory system (Fig. 39). In the sensory system the central response to stimulation of a peripheral

nerve can be recorded over the spinal cord as well as the brain, and the wave form as well as the latency of the resulting discharges measured. Specific wave forms and latencies have been defined from spinal cord (probably dorsal column lemniscal fibers), the thalamus, and the sensory cortex. Measurement of the velocity and wave form allows one to determine the site of a central sensory lesion.

PAIN AS A SENSORY DISORDER

HEADACHE

Headache is one of man's most common afflictions, a condition in which the symptom can be so troublesome that it becomes a disease. The frequency of disabling headache is explained in part by the rich nerve supply to the head (including afferent nerve

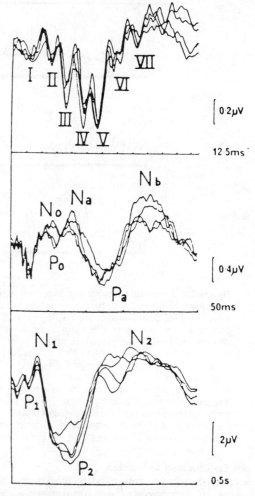

Figure 39. The three epochs of the auditory evoked response are illustrated as elicited by a 60 dB Hl click delivered once per second. Positivity to the vertex is represented as an upward deflection. The earliest (0 to 10 msec) period is called the brainstem auditory evoked response, while later epochs are labeled middle (0 to 50 msec) and long latency (100 to 500 msec) responses. (From Hecox, K., and Hogan, K.: Neuro-otologic disorders. In Rosenberg, R., and Grossman, R.: The Clinical Neurosciences: Neurology/Neurosurgery. New York, Churchill Livingstone, 1983, p. I:182.)

fibers from trigeminal, glossopharyngeal, vagus, and the upper three cervical nerves) and in part by the psychologic implications of head pain, causing anxiety about even modest headache, whereas pain of equal severity elsewhere in the body might be ignored. Head pain can result from distortion, stretching, inflammation, or destruction of pain-sensitive nerve endings as a result of intracranial or extracranial disease in the distribution of any of the aforementioned nerves. However, most head pain arises from extracerebral structures, in particular blood vessels and muscles, and has a benign prognosis.

Vascular Headaches

The term *vascular headache* applies to a group of clinical syndromes of unknown etiology in which the final step in pathogenesis of the pain appears to be dilatation of one or more branches of the carotid artery, leading to stimulation of pain-sensitive nerve endings supplying that artery (Table 24). There may be a release of noxious substances by either the arterial wall or the nerve ending, causing a substantially lowered pain threshold. Such substances as serotonin, substance P, bradykinin, histamine, and prostaglandins alone or in combination have all been implicated in the pathogenesis of vascular headache. Most vascular headaches are unilateral in distribution, often but not always throbbing in quality, and recur over months or years. Individual headaches are frequently precipitated by identifiable environmental (e.g., hangover headache) or psychologic factors. During the course of a vascular headache the involved arteries may be tender to the touch, and compression of the carotid artery may temporarily relieve the pain, but it returns with increased severity when compression is released. Most vascular headaches can be relieved by

TABLE 24. PATHOPHYSIOLOGIC CLASSIFICATION OF HEADACHE

Vascular Headache
  Migraine headache
    Classic migraine
    Common migraine
    Complicated migraine
    Variant migraine
  Cluster headache
    Episodic cluster
    "Chronic" cluster
    Chronic paroxysmal hemicrania
  Miscellaneous vascular headaches
    Carotidynia
    Hypertension
    Hangover
    Toxins or drugs
    Occlusive vascular disease
Muscle Contraction (Tension) Headache
  Common tension headache
  Depressive equivalent
  Conversion reaction
  Temporomandibular joint dysfunction
  Atypical facial pain
  Cervical osteoarthritis
Traction-Inflammation Headache
  Cranial arteritis
  Increased or decreased intracranial pressure
  Extracranial structural lesions
  Pituitary tumors
Cranial Neuralgias

prompt administration of vasoconstrictive agents, and many recurrent headaches can be prevented by one of several vasoactive drugs.

Classic migraine is unique among vascular headaches in that well-defined symptoms of neurologic dysfunction (see below) precede or, less often, accompany the headache. The neurologic symptoms are usually visual, consisting of bright flashing lights (scintillation or fortification scotomas) beginning in the center of a homonymous visual half-field and radiating, over 10 to 30 minutes, outward toward the periphery. Less commonly the visual abnormalities are monocular (retinal) or consist of hemianopic loss of vision in place of or following the scintillating scotomas. Other neurologic disturbances include unilateral paresthesias, usually involving the hand and perioral area, aphasia, hemiparesis, or hemisensory defects.

It was originally believed that the pathophysiology of the neurologic symptoms consisted of cerebral vasoconstriction with ischemia and that the headache represented compensatory vasodilatation. Indeed, there is decreased cerebral blood in the involved hemisphere during the aura of classic migraine (the neurologic symptoms). The decrease in blood flow appears to always start in the posterior portion of the hemisphere and march anteriorly at the rate of 1 to 5 mm/min, the blood failing to cross major interhemispheric sulci. The decrease in cerebral blood flow, however, is not sufficient to cause cerebral ischemia. The slow march across the hemisphere, which may not be accompanied by neurologic symptoms, is reminiscent of spreading depression produced by focal trauma in experimental animals. The trigger for this spreading depression in migraine has not been established.

Muscle Contraction (Tension) Headache

Muscle contraction or tension headaches are characterized by a steady, nonpulsatile, unilateral or bilateral aching pain, usually beginning in the occipital regions but also often involving frontal or temporal regions as well. The headaches are so called because they are frequently accompanied by tight and tender muscles at the site of the most severe pain, particularly in the posterior cervical, temporal, and masseter areas. They are probably the most common cause of headache in the adult.

The pathogenesis of tension headaches is unclear, but continuously contracting muscles or the nerves supplying them may release vasoactive substances such as lactate, serotonin, bradykinin, and prostaglandins, which lower pain threshold. Thus some of the same substances implicated in migraine may also play a role in tension headache and explain why the two syndromes frequently overlap. Tension headaches are commonly accompanied by skeletal muscle contraction about the neck, face, and jaw, and palpation of those muscles may reveal sharply localized painful areas or nodules, injection of which with local anesthetics transiently relieves the headache. Sometimes massage has a similar effect. Patients are frequently aware that sustained contraction of muscles leads to headache. Tension headache may also be a result of sustained contraction of muscles to prevent head movement that may increase the pain of structural disease of the eye, ear, nose, paranasal sinuses, teeth, scalp, or intracranial contents.

Tension headaches are recurrent, often present every day, usually beginning in early afternoon or evening, with a dull occipital or frontal pain that may spread to grip the entire head "in a vise." These headaches are more frequent in women, in individuals who are tense and anxious, and in those whose work or posture requires sustained contraction of posterior cervical, frontal, or temporal muscles.

Atypical Facial Pain

A syndrome characterized by steady aching face pain, usually unilateral, localized to the lower part of the orbit, maxillary area, and sometimes the jaw is known as atypical facial pain or atypical facial neuralgia. The pain begins without a known precipitating episode and may last for hours to days. It may spread to involve the head or neck, and muscles of the jaw and neck are often tender. Autonomic symptoms may include sweating, flushing, and pallor. The disorder usually affects women, often in early middle age. Patients affected with the disorder are tense, anxious, and often chronically depressed. The pathogenesis of the illness is unknown. The autonomic changes have led some to suggest that the syndrome is a migraine variant, and the muscle tenderness and depression have led others to suggest that it be classified with musculoskeletal tension pain. Still others suspect it may be a conversion symptom.

Traction/Inflammation Headache

Most intracranial as well as many extracranial headaches result from structural lesions that either inflame or distort pain-sensitive structures in and around the head. Examples of inflammatory extracranial lesions causing headache include cranial arteritis (a granulomatous angiitis characteristically involving the superficial temporal artery); acute infections or inflammatory lesions of the leptomeninges (meningitis); acute sinus and dental infections; and some acute or chronic ear infections. Distortion of pain-sensitive structures also can cause pain. Tumors of the eye, sinus, or ear occasionally cause headache. Within the intracranial cavity, the brain itself is pain insensitive. Those intracranial structures that are pain sensitive include the pial arterial vessels at the base of the brain, the large venous sinuses, portions of the dura near the venous sinuses, and the branches of the fifth, ninth, and tenth cranial nerves at the base of the brain. Compression, distortion, or especially traction of these structures causes headache. Brain tumors and other mass lesions within the brain distort these pain-sensitive structures, making headache a common symptom of brain tumor even though brain tumor is not a common cause of headache. Alterations of intracranial pressure from causes other than tumor, whether that pressure is elevated or decreased, can also cause headache if they shift the brain against its tethering structures. The headache that sometimes follows a lumbar puncture is an example of distortion of pain-sensitive structures from decreased intracranial pressure.

Neuralgia

Spontaneous discharges of cranial nerves are an uncommon but distinctive cause of head pain. Called cranial neuralgias, the most common is trigeminal neuralgia. Similar abnormalities occur in the glosso-pharyngeal, vagus, and intermediate nerves. Neuralgia is characterized by sudden lightning-like paroxysms of pain in the distribution of the involved nerve. In trigeminal neuralgia it usually affects the second or third division or both. The pain is often triggered by a light touch to the face, talking, or brushing teeth (trigeminal neuralgia) or by swallowing (glossopharyngeal neuralgia). Many observers believe that neuralgic pain results from discharge of pain fibers within the nerve, triggered ephaptically at a site of nerve damage (p. 1083) by an incoming touch or proprioceptive impulse.

Symptomatic trigeminal neuralgia occurs with tumors in the gasserian ganglion, in multiple sclerosis at the root entry zone of the trigeminal nerve, and with brainstem infarcts involving the descending root of the trigeminal nerve. Tumors in the tonsil and pharynx sometimes cause symptomatic glossopharyngeal neuralgia, but such large structural lesions are the exception. Some think that most neuralgias are caused by compression of the nerve by arteries or veins in the posterior fossa (the compression leading to demyelination, which, in turn, allows for ephaptic transmission).

NECK AND BACK PAIN

Neck or back pain, whether localized or radiating into the extremities, is one of man's most common afflictions. Fortunately, despite its frequency, most neck or back pain is transient and neither life threatening nor associated with obvious pathologic abnormalities.

Anatomy and Physiology of the Spine

The functional unit of the spine is composed of two segments. The anterior segment contains two adjacent vertebral bodies separated by an intervertebral disc. The function of the anterior segment is to bear weight and support the shock to the spine of such activity as walking and running. The posterior segment is composed of the vertebral arches, the transverse processes, the posterior spinous processes, and the paired articulations known as facets with the facet joint between them. The posterior segment is a non-weight-bearing structure that has the function of protecting the contained spinal cord and nerves as well as allowing the spine to be mobile in both extension and rotation.

Not all of the structures of this unit are pain sensitive. The vertebral body, at least its periosteum, is pain sensitive (therefore, compression fractures are, at least initially, painful), whereas the intervertebral disc is not in itself pain sensitive. However, if the intervertebral disc bulges and compresses the posterior longitudinal ligament, pain may result even if the nerve root itself is not involved. Posteriorly the synovial-lined facet joints are pain sensitive, although the intraspinal ligaments holding the posterior elements together are not. The paravertebral muscles surrounding and supporting the spine are pain sensitive, particularly when they are overstretched or when they go into spasm. In the neutral position, the nerve root occupies only a small portion of the intervertebral foramen from which it exits the spinal canal. However, when the spine is extended, i.e., in hyperlordotic posture, the intervertebral foramen becomes smaller, potentially causing impingement on a nerve root and also leading to overlap of the facet joints, the latter allowing for irritation of the pain-sensitive synovial membranes. This is the reason that on examination of patients with intervertebral disc disease or with pain originating from the facet joints, the pain may be relieved somewhat by flexion of the spine and exacerbated by extension or lordosis. It is also the reason that hyperlordosis, a common postural abnormality, sometimes leads to chronic low back pain and why most back exercises have as their goal the production of a flat or slightly flexed but certainly not hyperlordotic lumbar spine.

Another anatomic finding of clinical importance in evaluating low back pain is that lumbar roots exit through that portion of the intervertebral foramen that is above the intervertebral disc. Thus, even though the L4 root exits between L4 and L5, herniation of a disc between these vertebral bodies occurs just below the exit of the L4 root and thus the herniated disc will usually compress the L5 and not the L4 root. A herniated disc between the L5 and S1 vertebral body will usually compress the S1 root and not the L5 root. If, however, the disc protrudes more medially, much less common than a laterally protruding disc, an L4-5 disc may involve the caudally directed sacral roots rather than the L5 lumbar root. Only if the disc completely extrudes into the vertebral canal will an L4-5 disc compress the L4 root. In the cervical spine the roots exit above a vertebral body with the same number (i.e., C4 root exits between C3 and C4). Thus a herniated C4-5 disc may compress the C6 or C5 root but not the C4.

Neck or back pain may be severe and disabling and can originate from any of the pain-sensitive structures in the spine or surrounding muscles, the description giving no sure clue as to its etiology. Only if pain radiates in a clear dermatomal distribution can the physician infer that a nerve root has been damaged or compressed by the process. Most acute neck and back pain occurs after unaccustomed exercise and probably results from muscle strain, the pain originating pathophysiologically in a manner similar to muscle contraction headaches (p. 1095). More chronic neck or back pain is usually associated with vertebral arthritis or intervertebral disc disease, the former causing pain by compression of small nerve twigs supplying the facet joints and the periosteum of the vertebral bodies, the latter causing pain by compression of the nerve root.

OTHER PAIN SYNDROMES

In pain syndromes, lightning pains resulting from tabes dorsalis and reflex sympathetic dystrophies resulting from nerve or extremity injuries are believed to result from nerve damage allowing for ephaptic transmission similar to the pathogenesis of trigeminal neuralgia and hemifacial spasm. The lightning pains of tabes are acute, stabbing pains in the trunk or lower extremities that occur with structural lesions of the dorsal roots. Unlike trigeminal neuralgia, they appear not to be triggered by touch but instead occur spontaneously. The term *reflex sympathetic dystrophy* applies to pain, hyperalgesia, hyperesthesia, and autonomic changes, including hyperhidrosis or hypohidrosis, as well as localized osteoporosis and trophic changes in skin, subcutaneous tissue, and muscle.

If the injury has involved a peripheral nerve, particularly the sciatic or median nerve, the syndrome is called *causalgia* (hot pain). If the injury has not involved a peripheral nerve, the condition is known as post-traumatic painful osteoporosis, Sudeck's atrophy, post-traumatic spreading neuralgia, minor causalgia, shoulder-hand syndrome, or reflex dystrophy, the particular term depending on the outstanding symptom. The pain of causalgia is believed to be caused by ephaptic transmission from major or minor nerve injury. Because sympathetic nerve fibers travel with major nerve trunks, they may also be inappropriately stimulated ephaptically, explaining the autonomic and trophic changes. When there has been no clear nerve injury, the pathogenesis of the pain may be similar to that of thalamic pain, resulting from minor injury making pain receptors hypersensitive to otherwise non-noxious stimuli or lowering the threshold sufficiently to lead to spontaneous pain.

Postherpetic Neuralgia

Postherpetic neuralgia refers to severe and prolonged burning pain with occasional lightning-like stabs in the involved dermatome after an attack of herpes zoster. Severe postherpetic neuralgia is usually a disease of elderly patients and, like most chronic pain, is exacerbated by emotional upset and relieved to some degree by distraction. The pathophysiology of postherpetic neuralgia is not fully understood. Some observers believe that there is selective destruction of large fibers after herpes zoster and that the resulting unmodulated input from small fibers causes the pain and discomfort. An alternate possibility is that the injury itself may lower nociceptor threshold.

Phantom Limb Pain

Phantom limb pain is a chronic and severe pain appearing to be localized in an amputated or totally denervated limb. All patients experience phantom sensations after amputation, but in only about 10 per cent is it painful, usually when there has been severe pain prior to operation. The pain is frequently similar to that suffered before amputation, or at times it may resemble muscle pain with the phantom seeming to be in a cramped or uncomfortable position. In most instances the pain lessens and disappears with time, but in occasional patients it is a chronic and severe problem. The pathophysiology of phantom limb pain is not understood. In some instances a neuroma (a tangle of partially regenerated nerve fibers without covering myelin sheaths) develops in the severed nerve in the amputation stump. The neuroma, when stimulated, may be a source of intense pain. Anesthesia or extirpation of the neuroma generally does not relieve phantom limb pain.

Myofascial Pain Syndromes

Pain arising from skeletal muscle is common. Unaccustomed exercise causes soreness and tenderness in the involved muscles, but is rarely a source of patient complaint. Prolonged tonic contraction of skeletal muscles, however, has an underlying pathogenesis of psychologic tension, resentment, and anxiety and may produce pain in which the cause is not immediately apparent to the patient. Examples are tension headache arising from chronic contraction of paraspinous muscles at the base of the skull; pain anteriorly in the chest from contraction of the pectoralis major; posterior thoracic or lumbar pain from paraspinous muscle contraction; and abdominal pain from rectus muscle contraction. The pain is initially localized over the area of muscle contraction but may spread widely into a distribution characteristic for the muscles involved. The muscles are usually tender to palpation, and there is often a particularly tender area somewhere in the muscle, called a trigger area, that, when palpated, reproduces the entire distribution of the spontaneous pain. The pathophysiology of myofascial pain is not well understood. Some observers have reported microscopic changes at trigger points (so-called fibrous nodules), suggesting that a tonic contraction may lead to structural changes in the muscle. Others have suggested that release of noxious substances such as lactic acid from chronic contracting muscles might be responsible for the pain and tenderness associated with this syndrome.

SPECIAL SENSORY SYSTEMS

VISUAL SYSTEM

Information from detailed and color-coded visual perception provides our best sense of the nature of the surrounding world. The size of the system reflects its importance: Each optic nerve contains a million fibers, outnumbering the input of the cochlear system by a ratio of 15:1 and exceeding in number the ganglion cells found in the total number of somatosensory dorsal ganglia of the spinal cord. One estimate indicates that as many as 60 per cent of forebrain axons are linked to the visual system.

Anatomy and Physiology of the Visual Pathways

The Globe and Retina

Light waves must traverse the normally clear structures of the aqueous humor, lens, and vitreous humor to reach the photoreceptive rods and cones of the retina. Abnormalities of form or transparency of these anterior structures (e.g., myopia [see below], corneal scar, cataracts) account for most visual abnormalities. Normally the incoming light path is shielded by pigmentation that lies in the choroid and outermost retinal layer. Dynamically this natural shielding is greatly strengthened by the pigmented iris under the control of the pupilloconstrictor muscle and the light-sensitive pupillary reflex.

The smooth muscles of the ciliary bodies serve to shorten or relax the suspensory ligaments of the lens to focus light images more precisely on the retina. Many human eyes are either too long (myopia) or too short (presbyopia) for the lens to thicken or flatten sufficiently to focus the incoming image sharply. In children, with their more elastic lenses and attachments, the lens often can adjust to compensate for such congenital nearsightedness or farsightedness, but the refractory disturbance progresses with age as the lens loses its natural elasticity—thus, the increasing need for refractive lenses as life progresses.

The retina derives directly from neural ectoderm

and developmentally is part of the brain rather than peripheral nerve ganglion. It is an inside-out structure with the receptors placed nearest to the outer ocular choroid and the ganglion cells, whose axons form the optic nerve, lie on the innermost surface (Fig. 40). The structure contains five kinds of nerve cells: rods, cones, horizontal cells, amacrine cells, and ganglion cells, as well as a special glial cell, the Müller cell. Light-sensitive rods outnumber the color- and pattern-sensitive cones by a ratio of nearly 20:1. The rods distribute themselves over the more peripheral retina, declining in number toward the periphery, so that retinal photosensitivity decreases centripetally away from the central macular area. The macula contains densely packed cones, especially in the tiny fovea, where cones comprise the exclusive receptor population. Also, in the fovea the innermost retinal layers that overlap the receptors in other areas are absent, an anatomic advantage that further enhances the sensitivity of the cones. The number and proportion of cones decline rapidly as one moves outward across the adjacent macula so that almost all sensitivity for color vision is lost outside an area comprising the macula's six to eight degrees of total arc.

Cone cells are individually sensitive to blue, green, or red light and, like the rods, depend upon specialized intracellular photosensitive pigments for these speci-

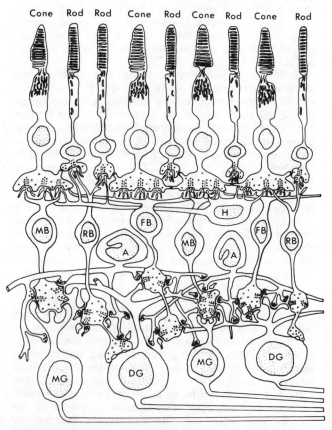

Figure 40. The organization of the primate retina. *MB*, midget bipolar; *RB*, rod bipolar; *FB*, flat bipolar; *H*, horizontal cell; *A*, amacrine cell; *MG*, midget ganglion cell; *DG*, diffuse ganglion cell. (From Gardner: Fundamentals of Neurology, 6th ed., and previously published by Dowling, J. E., and Boycott, B. B.: Proc R Soc Lond B 166:80–111, 1966.)

fications. Rhodopsin, a conjugated chromoprotein that depends upon vitamin A for its synthesis, comprises the pigment in the rod cells. Accordingly, vitamin A deficiency results in night blindness. Similar but individually distinct conjugated pigments provide the separate cover sensitivities of the three populations of cones. Genetic failure to synthesize one of these pigments accounts for selective color blindness. With either rods or cones, isomerization of the photosensitive pigment by light comprises the first step in visual excitation.

In the retina, information about incoming light stimuli is either relayed directly to the brain via a three-neuron afferent pathway (receptor to bipolar cell to ganglion cell) or, more frequently, is distributed from receptors to several surrounding ganglion cells by way of local circuit neurons. Direct relays occur mainly in the central foveal area where most of the color-sensitive cones are packed, while distributed circuits are located more peripherally. Complex excitatory-inhibitory circuits within the retina assure that adjacent ganglion cells either respond maximally or are inhibited by opposite kinds of light stimuli, thereby enhancing the responses to contrasts and the detection of movement.

In the neural map of the retina, the receptor fields of contiguous ganglion cells are excited by stimuli that arise in contiguous parts of visual space. The cone-containing macular fovea detects the center of the visualized world and forms the center of the *visual field*, i.e., what the eye sees. The two eyes normally possess identical visual fields except for small crescents of sight in the nasal edge of each retina that perceive stimuli arising from an extreme lateral (temporal) position in relation to either globe (Fig. 41). (The nasal protuberance blocks such stimuli from reaching the contralateral eye.)

The geometry of the globe is such that the right half of space is detected by the left half of each retina and vice versa, while the vertical morphology of objects is inverted. Receptor fields in each retina normally develop so that homologous points of the right or left visual fields project to homologous left or right areas respectively of the nasal receptor fields of one eye and of the temporal receptors of the other. Ganglion cells from these homologous fields seeing the right or left half of visual space send their axons, in turn, to the lateral geniculate body of either side. The geniculates then transmit the signals to adjacent cell columns in the occipital cortex. The result is that each successive unilateral level of visual processing from retina to cortex reconstructs vertically an accurate topologic map of the opposite half of the surrounding world.

The macula lies on the temporal side of the optic nerve. The large number of macular ganglion cells project axons to the lateral (temporal) portion of the optic nerve (Fig. 41) to form the *maculopapillary bundle,* which carries central vision and provides the majority of input from the retina to the lateral geniculate body and visual cortex. The bundle is susceptible to damage by several immunologic, toxic, nutritional, and genetic disorders.

Because of the substantial bulk of the retinal maculopapillary fibers, axons from the retinal areas that lie laterally, superiorly, or inferiorly to the macula must arch over or under the bundle to reach the optic nerve. Damage to these *arcuate fibers* leads to crescent-

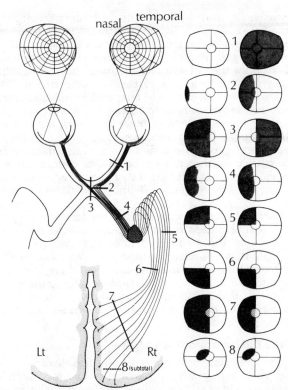

Figure 41. Visual fields that accompany damage to the visual pathways. *1,* Optic nerve: unilateral amaurosis. *2,* Lateral optic chiasm: grossly incongruous, incomplete (contralateral) homonymous hemianopia. *3,* Central optic chiasm: bitemporal hemianopia. *4,* Optic tract: incongruous, incomplete homonymous hemianopia. *5,* Temporal (Meyer's) loop of optic radiation: congruous partial or complete (contralateral) homonymous superior quadrantanopia. *6,* Parietal (superior) projection of the optic radiation: congruous partial or complete homonymous inferior quadrantanopia. *7,* Complete parieto-occipital interruption of optic radiation: complete congruous homonymous hemianopia with psychophysical shift of foveal point often sparing central vision, giving "macular sparing." *8,* Incomplete damage to visual cortex: congruous homonymous scotomas, usually encroaching at least acutely on central vision. (From Plum, F.: Visual and ocular abnormalities. In Wyngaarden, J. B., and Smith, L. H., Jr. (eds.): Cecil Textbook of Medicine. 16th ed. Philadelphia, W. B. Saunders Co., 1982, p. 1953.)

shaped blind spots, as discussed later. Ganglion cells lying immediately superior, inferior, or nasal to the disc project their axons in straighter, topographically oriented lines.

Optic Nerve Chiasm and Tract

Behind the eye the optic nerve proceeds in a somewhat redundant course across the orbit for a distance of approximately 20 mm, passes through the orbital foramen, and traverses the sphenoid bone to reach the *optic chiasm.* In the chiasm, nerves from the nasal half of each retina decussate and join the fibers from the temporal half of the contralateral retina. The resulting intermingled bundles independently serve the respective left and right homonymous visual fields (Fig. 41).

Within the chiasm, fibers from the inferior halves of the nasal fields decussate before the superior nasal fibers cross. The decussating fibers from each nasal retina commonly loop forward somewhat into the extreme posterior portion of the contralateral optic nerve.

As a result, unilateral optic nerve tumors sometimes produce small, arcuate, contralateral visual field defects without necessarily invading the chiasm itself.

At the posterior end of the chiasm the temporal fibers from the one eye and the nasal fibers from the other join to form the respective *optic tracts*. The crossed nasal and uncrossed temporal fibers emanating from homonymous receptor fields in the two eyes remain at first separated in the optic tracts, but gradually comingle to converge upon neighboring layers of the lateral geniculate bodies. As a result, damage to the optic tract posterior to the chiasm usually causes homonymous but unequal (i.e., noncongruent) defects in the ipsilateral temporal and contralateral nasal field.

Each optic tract passes around the ipsilateral cerebral peduncle deep to the temporal lobe to reach on either side the six-layered lateral geniculate relay nucleus that lies adjacent to the posterior end of the posterior limb of the internal capsule. Fibers from the ipsilateral (temporal) retina terminate on geniculate layers 2, 3, and 5, while contralateral fibers from homonymous retinal points end on adjacent cells in layers 1, 4, and 6.

The Geniculocalcarine Radiation

The geniculate body projects to the striate cortex via the optic (or geniculocalcarine) radiation, another structure whose anatomic susceptibility contributes an important component to clinical diagnosis. As the radiation first leaves the geniculate body, it sends its axons for a short distance anterolaterally around the lateral ventricle, then fans out into a continuously joined inferior, medial, and superior distribution of fibers that ultimately turn occipitally to reach the calcarine cortex (Fig. 41). The inferior fibers first pass forward over the lateral surface of the temporal horn, in most brains reaching almost as far anteriorly as the temporal horn's anterior tip. They then loop inferiorly (Meyer's loop) and head for the occipital pole. The temporal loop serves the receptor fields of the inferior portion of the ipsilateral temporal and contralateral nasal retinas, the ipsilateral fibers usually lying somewhat nearer to the surface of the temporal lobe than the contralateral. The medially placed fibers of the optic radiation, after their initial forward passage, turn occipitally and pursue a nearly horizontal course to the striate cortex. The superior fibers of the radiation, serving principally the superior quadrants of the ipsilateral temporal and contralateral nasal retinas, turn

somewhat dorsally from the geniculate body to enter the inferior portion of the parietal lobe before heading for the superior bank of the calcarine cortex.

Area 17 of the occipital lobe comprises the primary visual or striate cortex (called striate because of the grossly visible line of Gennari, which contains the abundant geniculocalcarine myelinated axons converging onto layer 4 of the cortex). The striate cortex begins on the hemisphere's external surface at the occipital pole and extends along the medial surface, straddling the calcarine fissure forward for a distance of about 8 cm. The small external surface of the occipital pole and the adjacent one-third of the medially placed calcarine cortex represent the macula. Representation of successively more peripheral retinal areas extends continuously forward, with the upper bank of the fissure receiving fibers from the superior and the lower bank from the inferior retina.

Visual Cortex

The striate cortex, like other sensory areas of the brain, is organized into columns perpendicular to the cortex (Fig. 42). In area 17, individual *orientation columns* are maximally sensitive to small straight lines of light flashed upon the retina, each column possessing a specific angular orientation. Adjacent columns show maximal responsiveness to stimulus lines of slightly changing axes. Groups of adjacent orientation columns are clustered together into larger columns that predominantly respond to one eye or the other. These adjacent *ocular dominance columns,* in turn, alternate from eye to eye, with contiguous ocular discrimination and dominance columns serving contiguous areas in the visual fields.

Neurons within the visual cortex respond to fairly elemental but increasingly complex visual stimuli, depending upon the cortical layer in which they reside as well as upon their distribution between the primary (area 17) and association (18 and 19) areas. *Simple cells* lie in area 17 and receive afferents from geniculate neurons representing one or the other eye. *Complex* and *hypercomplex cells* lie above and below simple cells in the same column, as well as in adjacent and more remote columns, extending into the peristriate cortex where they abstract signals of an increasingly elaborate nature. Extensive feedback loops interconnect the striate cortex and the geniculate body, as well as the visual cortex and the tectum, each providing further discriminations to visual function. In comparison to somatic sensory systems in which the receptors

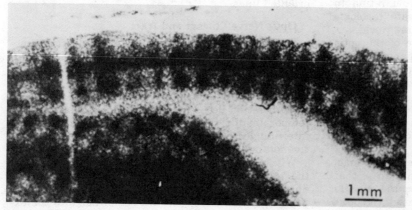

Figure 42. Deoxyglucose autoradiograph showing orientation columns of the monkey visual cortex following binocular exposure to vertical stripes only. All layers are labeled; layer *IVc,* where the cells are normally not orientation selective, is labeled as a continuous band. (From Hubel, D. H., Wiesel, T. N., and Stryker, M.: Anatomical demonstration of orientation columns in macaque monkey. J Comp Neurol 177:361, 1978.)

1 mm

provide most of the discrimination that differentiates among stimuli, the visual system depends on the brain itself for an enormous amount of processing.

Areas 18 and 19 of the occipital lobes receive their sensory afferent projections predominantly from the striate cortex, with area 18 containing mostly complex neurons and area 19 several orders of hypercomplex cells. Area 19 in turn connects richly with more forward areas of the cerebral hemispheres. A ventral visual pathway, known to be critical for object vision, extends forward into the temporal lobe, while a dorsal pathway, believed to relate to spatial visual perception, extends into the inferior parietal lobule. Both the primary and association visual cortex also have strong reciprocal connections with the brainstem via the superior colliculi.

Visual Influence on the Brainstem

The superior colliculi as well as the underlying tectal area and midbrain receive connections from the retina and receive and transmit strong interconnections to the striate and peristriate cortex of the occipital lobes. The retinal pathways provide the afferent stimulus to the pupillary light reflex, while the occipital pathways influence visual pursuit movements as well as the accommodation and fixation reflexes. Both systems synapse directly or indirectly on midbrain nuclei that project to the lower brainstem and spinal cord to influence ocular and skeletal motor responses to visual stimuli.

Vascular Supply

The eye receives its blood from the ophthalmic artery (a branch of the internal carotid), long and short ciliary arteries, and the retinal artery branch from the ophthalmic in the orbit. The short and long ciliary arteries travel along the surface of the optic nerve, supplying its outer surface; at the globe they pierce the outer sclera and branch out to irrigate the outer layer of the retina. The *central retinal artery* approaches the eye along each optic nerve in the skull and orbit, piercing the inferior aspect of the nerve's dural sheath at about 6 to 10 mm behind the globe. At that point it enters the center of the nerve and travels forward into the eye to emerge at the center of the nerve head and branch into superior, medial, inferior, and lateral branches. Anastomotic branches derived from the choroidal and posterior ciliary arteries supply the retinal nerve head as well as the macular region. Venous drainage from the retina and nerve head flows primarily via the central retinal vein, which lies alongside the incoming retinal artery and leaves the body of the nerve in the orbit where the artery enters it.

The region of the optic chiasm is supplied by small filamentous arterial branches arising directly from the carotid artery on either side as the vessel loops past the chiasmatic areas. Posterior to the chiasm, the anterior choroidal artery provides most of the blood supply to the optic tract as well as the lateral geniculate body. The latter also is irrigated by the posterior choroidal artery emanating from the posterior cerebral artery. Primary ischemic damage to the optic chiasm, tract, and lateral geniculate body from primary arterial occlusive disease is uncommon, since each structure receives anastomotic supply from several adjacent arteries.

The middle and superior portions of the geniculocalcarine radiation receive their blood supply from branches of the middle cerebral artery, while branches of the posterior cerebral artery largely supply the inferior temporal loop. In most human brains the middle cerebral artery irrigates areas 18 and 19 on the external surface of the cerebral hemisphere, with the posterior cerebral artery supplying areas 17, 18, and 19 on the medial surface, including the receptors for central vision. Sometimes the two circulations anastomose at the occipital pole so that macular sparing occasionally follows occlusion of the posterior cerebral artery.

Pathophysiology and Regional Diagnosis of Visual Impairment

Definitions

Amblyopia refers to partial loss of vision; *amaurosis*, to blindness. *Scotomas* are areas of relative or complete visual loss leaving comparatively better vision in the remaining field of the particular eye. The blind spot, the area of retina occupied by the optic nerve, is an example of such a scotoma. Abnormalities in vision due to lesions affecting structures lying anywhere from the retina to the occipital pole produce distinctive changes in the visual field. Visual defects impairing half or nearly half of a field are termed *hemianopic*. Those affecting less than this, if they extend to the periphery, are termed *partial field defects,* often with the additional designation of *quadrantic* (superior or inferior), *sector* (less than the full quadrant), or *altitudinal* (superior or inferior), according to the distribution. A visual defect that involves similar parts of the right or left half-field in the two eyes is called homonymous; identical errors of homonymous involvement are termed *congruent*. Unilateral scotomas have a retinal origin. Bilateral scotomas can reflect abnormalities anywhere from retina to occipital pole: The more symmetric the scotomas, the more posterior is their causative lesion likely to lie; bilaterally homonymous and congruent scotomas usually reflect occipital lobe damage. Abnormalities of the macular area or its projections produce central *scotomas*. Scotomas that lie near the macular area are sometimes called *paracentral*, whereas those that extend from the periphery into the macular field of vision are designated *cecocentral*. Involvement of the arching axons in the retina characteristically produces *arcuate scotomas*. Central scotomas always interfere with visual acuity.

Examination Techniques

The disordered visual system lends itself to accurate diagnosis by both bedside examination and laboratory investigation. Loss of visual acuity, if correctable by lenses or by looking through a pinhole to collimate incoming light, is non-neurogenic. Uncorrectable acuity to 20/50 or less implies involvement of macular fibers. The retina and optic nerve are the only portion of the brain that can be visualized by the examiner (using the ophthalmoscope). Visual field abnormalities can be detected either by bedside or laboratory examination (tangent screen on perimeter).

Electroretinography is a specialized electrophysiologic test that uses a corneally placed electrode to record the potential that a visual flash stimulator evokes in the light-sensitive structures of the retina. The technique has clinical application in the early diagnosis of retinal degenerations where it shows abnormalities before gross changes become visible with the ophthalmoscope.

Visual evoked responses (VERs) consist of computer-averaged electrical signals recorded over the occipital region of the scalp following the repetitive delivery of a standard visual stimulus to one or the other eye. The recorded signal largely reflects activity transmitted from the cones in the foveal area to the visual cortex. Most VER units in clinical use employ for the stimulus a rapidly alternating pattern of light and dark squares, total luminance being held constant. Latency between stimulus and scalp response is measured for each eye, as is the respective amplitude of the response. The results are compared to each other and to standardized norms. In clinical use the test has been most valuable for identifying clinically inapparent defects in the macular conducting system such as occur in demyelinating disease. VERs also have been applied to the testing of postoptic nerve visual field responses, but thus far other diagnostic measures have been found to give more information about these functions. Computed tomography and magnetic resonance imaging can identify small lesions of the visual system.

Regional Abnormalities of Vision

The Globe

Glaucoma produced by impaired absorption of the aqueous humor results in high intraocular pressure that gradually compresses the retinal circulation and may damage ganglion cells by a similar mechanism. The result is gradual loss of vision with reduced nighttime vision, halos around illuminated lamps, and often pain in the affected eye. Uncommonly, rapid visual loss can occur with few or no premonitory symptoms. Since perimacular fibers suffer first, vertical extension of the blind spot and paracentral ring scotomas are characteristic. The diagnosis comes from tonometric measurement of high intraocular pressure.

Retinal tears and detachments give rise to unilateral distortions of the visual image, seen as sudden inappropriate angulations or curves of unusually straight-edged objects (metamorphopsia). Small retinal tears create areas where contiguous receptor areas angulate against one another to produce a strong suggestion of duplicate images, providing a rare organic cause of monocular diplopia. Hemorrhages into the vitreous humor or unilateral infections or inflammatory lesions of the retina can produce scotomas that resemble those resulting from primary disease of the central visual pathway. Ophthalmoscopy gives the answer.

Vitreous atrophy, a common problem of aging, pulls on the peripheral retina, causing the sufferer to see lightning-like flashes in the peripheral visual field. They are distressing to the patient and often to the unaware physician but are of no pathologic consequence. At all levels of the visual pathway, abnormalities affecting the central portions of either one or both visual fields attract the patient's attention far earlier and more prominently than do peripherally distributed impairments. This rule applies to both pregeniculate and postgeniculate visual defects so that with loss of peripheral vision due to retinal degeneration or compression of the optic chiasm some patients may go for months or years without being aware of their abnormality.

Disorders affecting the visual structures of the eye can be divided conveniently into those that grossly damage the retinal structures and those that primarily affect the axons of the optic nerve.

Retina

Both acquired and inherited diseases commonly affect the retina. Acquired disorders characteristically affect a single eye or the two visual fields asymmetrically, while inherited diseases characteristically produce bilateral and fairly symmetric retinal abnormalities.

Acquired Retinal Damage. Most retinal changes resulting from acute trauma or neoplasms are obvious upon gross or ophthalmoscopic inspection. The inflammatory lesions of chorioretinitis affect initially the outer retinal layer. Causes include, among others, herpes simplex, syphilis, tuberculosis, cytomegalic infection, toxoplasmosis, cryptococcus, histoplasmosis, and sarcoidosis. The ensuing visual defect depends upon the site of the inflammatory lesion. Some of these chorioretinal inflammations have a characteristic appearance, but etiologic diagnosis usually depends upon the findings of serologic testing or the presence of associated lesions elsewhere in the body. Usually scotomas secondary to unilateral chorioretinitis do not impair functional vision unless they intrude upon the macula.

Retinal vascular disease primarily damages the inner retinal layers and includes hypertensive retinopathy, diabetic and other proliferative microangiopathies, and obstruction of either the central retinal artery or one of its branches. Among these conditions, hemorrhage from diabetic microangiopathy and arterial or, less often, venous occlusions are the most frequent and the most likely to produce severe visual impairment.

Most retinal artery occlusion results from systemic emboli arising either from plaques along the course of the internal carotid artery system or, less often, directly from the heart. Many patients with recurrent brief unilateral amaurosis fail to show any source of emboli by arteriography, however, and it may be that platelet emboli also can arise spontaneously in the intravascular compartment. Occlusion of the ophthalmic artery produces either transient (amaurosis fugax) or permanent monocular visual loss, depending on whether or not the offending embolus rapidly disintegrates and passes on through the retinal circulation. If it disintegrates, one often can observe embolic particles passing through the peripheral portion of the retinal arteries as vision returns. Such emboli, if white, are composed of platelets and fibrin products and rapidly dissolve. Yellow, refractile emboli, however, contain insoluble cholesterol and tend to lodge permanently at arterial bifurcations, producing permanent distal ischemic damage and a sector field defect but seldom fully occluding vision. Permanent occlusion to the retinal artery system anywhere from its origin to the fundus usually produces a characteristic ophthalmoscopic appearance of a narrow, bloodless artery, areas of ischemic spasm, or hemorrhages accompanied by unilateral amaurosis or scotomas.

Pathologic studies indicate that most permanent occlusions of the central and peripheral retinal arteries result from acute thrombosis superimposed on a previously narrowed lumen. Inflammatory occlusions of the retinal artery are discussed subsequently.

Central retinal vein occlusion occurs in younger adults as well as in those who have reached the arteriosclerotic years. The condition most often results from thrombophlebitis, some relating to atherosclerotic lesions in the adjacent retinal artery. In contrast to central artery occlusion, vision seldom is severely impaired, especially when the condition occurs in younger patients. An exception occurs when back-pressure hemorrhage leaks into the overlying vitreous.

Hereditary Retinal Degeneration (Dystrophies). Primary neurologic disorders affecting the eye include conditions involving either the outer pigmentary epithelium and receptor cells or the inner retinal layers consisting of the ganglion cells and their axons. The initiating neuropathologic changes often are understood poorly because of a lack of early specimens for study.

Peripheral or outer layer retinal dystrophies affect the pigmentary epithelial layer of the retina and its adjacent overlying receptor cells. Nearly all are characterized by initially normal development followed by later deterioration of selected retinal elements.

Retinitis pigmentosa is an outer retinal dystrophy that begins insidiously in early adult life, first affecting the peripheral portions of the retina. Damage to the visual pigment of the rod receptors results in early defects in night vision. Concurrent degeneration of the pigmented epithelial cells leads to ophthalmoscopically visible precipitation of spidery black pigment along the retinal blood vessels. Some sufferers lose functional vision by midlife, while others retain indefinitely at least a vestige of central visual acuity. The mode of genetic transmission varies. Most examples follow an autosomal dominant pattern with incomplete penetrance, but families showing autosomal recessive or X-linked patterns have been described.

Patterns of outer retinal degeneration resembling retinitis pigmentosa also accompany general neurologic and systemic defects in several less common genetically transmitted disorders. These include some of the mucopolysaccharidoses, abetalipoproteinemia, hereditary phytanic acidemia (Refsum's disease), and the various syndromes named for Laurence-Moon-Biedl, Sjögren-Larsson, Hallgren, Alstrom, Usher, Cockayne, Hallervorden-Spatz, Pelizaeus-Merzbacher, and Alport. The retinal degeneration that accompanies certain examples of olivopontocerebellar degeneration also arises in the outer pigmented receptor layer.

Macular retinal degeneration occurs in three principal forms:

(1) *Incidental macular degeneration* can complicate almost any structural lesion affecting the retina, including tumors, inflammation, trauma, and vascular abnormalities. Visual impairment usually begins abruptly or subacutely, commonly is asymmetric or unilateral, and involves scotomas that appropriately reflect damage to localized central receptor fields in the retina.

(2) *Hereditary macular degeneration* occurs most often in the macular degenerations characterized by widespread and progressive lipid accumulation and degeneration in both retinal and central nervous system ganglion cells. Severe visual impairment is an early manifestation and characteristically progresses to functional blindness; there are usually associated generalized neurologic abnormalities. Closely akin to hereditary macular degeneration is *hereditary optic atrophy* (Leber). The disorder, which may have several modes of genetic transmission, including X-linked recessive, originates in the retinal ganglion cell. It predominates in males, the male:female ratio ranging from 3:2 to 9:1 in different study groups. Macular axons are first affected, with unilateral or bilateral central visual loss beginning abruptly or subacutely, most often in young men in their early 20s, and unaccompanied by other symptoms. In most patients there is eventual progression to complete blindness. The optic fundi show the typical appearance of primary optic atrophy. Neurologic dysfunction outside the visual system is rare.

(3) *Senile macular degeneration* describes a variety of degenerative changes affecting the retinal pigmentary epithelium, Bruch's membrane, and the choriocapillaries of the elderly eye. The initial abnormality may represent gradual failure in the metabolic process by which the normal rods and cones constantly phagocytose and resynthesize their photosensitive pigment. Whatever the precise first step, the process affects central visual acuity of as many as 30 per cent of persons who reach the age of 80 years. Ophthalmoscopy often discloses ill-defined pigmentary changes in the macular area coupled with tiny excrescences of phagocytic debris (drusen) scattered over the retina.

Optic Nerve

The position of the optic nerves in the skull makes them vulnerable to mechanical damage from abnormalities lying anywhere from the optic globe to the chiasm. Whether trauma, neoplasm, aneurysm, or infection causes the injury, such paraneural disturbances usually begin unilaterally, first affect the outside of the nerve (and therefore the periphery of the visual field), and produce early peripheral optic atrophy but late visual disturbances. Lesions inside the nerve include tumors, vascular occlusions, toxic and nutritional disturbances, and a limited number of inflammations, of which demyelinating disease is the most common. Most such parenchymal lesions directly injure the maculopapillary bundle, making loss of vision a prominent early symptom.

Papilledema describes elevation of the optic nerve head in the optic fundi and results from one of two general causes: (1) when an ischemic, inflammatory or demyelinative lesion affects the nerve head itself or (2) when increased back pressure occurs in the central retinal veins as a result of local venous obstruction or an increase in intracranial or cavernous sinus pressure. Severe disc swelling is easily identified with the ophthalmoscope and is a result of interference with axoplasmic flow, leading to accumulation of axoplasm in the nerve head.

The distinction between *retrobulbar neuritis* and *optic neuritis* producing papilledema (papillitis) deserves a brief pathogenetic explanation. Inflammatory or demyelinating lesions that affect the optic nerve behind the point in the orbit where its artery and vein enter and leave it (retrobulbar neuritis) produce axonal damage and central visual defect without any accompanying swelling of the retinal nerve head. When, however, similar lesions affect the nerve immediately at or behind the nerve head, they produce vascular engorgement: The structure inside its tight dural sheath swells forward into the eye to produce ophthalmoscopically typical papilledema. Both these forms of optic neuritis, since they damage the parenchyma of the nerve, impair the central or paracentral visual pathways, and both usually produce complaints of pain as well as blindness or shadows in front of the eye.

In contrast to the disc swelling associated with optic neuritis, the papilledema caused by increased intracranial pressure seldom causes visual impairment and then under one of three circumstances: (1) Acute seconds-long episodes of amaurosis may occur that can be attributed to intermittent acute rises in intracranial pressure (plateau waves) that interfere with the retinal circulation (p. 1027). (2) Acute bilateral sustained visual loss may sometimes follow abrupt surgical relief of longstanding severely increased intracranial pressure. The pathogenesis of this rare event is incompletely understood, but it may result from sudden lowering of previously high pericapillary and perivenular pressure, leaving those vessels in the optic nerves vulnerable to a sudden surge of blood under high arterial pressure that stretches and ruptures their endothelia, damaging the surrounding nerve. (3) Progressive loss of peripheral vision accompanies longstanding severe papilledema and is attributed to pressure atrophy of the most peripherally lying fibers in the tightly sheathed optic nerve.

Additional points that differentiate the papilledema of optic neuritis from that due to increased intracranial pressure are that the former is usually unilateral, is often accompanied by a reddened disc due to associated inflammation, and is associated with abnormal VERs, with normal CT scans of the orbit and intracranial structures, and with a normal lumbar puncture pressure.

Primary degeneration of retinal ganglion cells or retrobulbar compression or demyelination of the fibers of the optic nerve eventually produces *primary optic atrophy* in which the axons and blood vessels shrink, leaving a pale white optic disc sharply demarcated at its edge from the relatively normal appearing surrounding retina (full moon in a midnight sky). The usual appearance of *optic atrophy* following longstanding papilledema differs from the above. Even though there is reduction of the optic nerve fibers in such circumstances, the chronic edema at the disc margin induces extensive glial scarring of the disc and the adjacent retina. The result is a grayish pallor of the disc plus adjacent retinal scarring that obliterates the normally sharp demarcation between the disc and the surrounding retina.

Pregeniculate Visual Pathways

Almost all lesions impairing the visual pathways between the optic nerves and the lateral geniculate bodies compress, distort, or invade from the surface inward. Exceptions include gliomas, in children espe-cially, that arise in the chiasm or extend into it from the hypothalamus, as well as rare examples of small arterial occlusions that affect branches of the internal carotid arteries to produce asymmetric central scotomas. The latter most often accompany large intracranial neoplasms or aneurysms arising adjacent to the chiasm. Lesions involving or compressing the optic chiasm produce nonhomonymous visual abnormalities such as bitemporal hemianopia that affect the unilateral fields incongruously and frequently asymmetrically. Intrinsic or extrinsic neoplasms and parachiasmal arterial aneurysms are the common causes. Lesions compressing the chiasm can arise from its superior, lateral, or inferior aspect and include craniopharyngiomas, pituitary adenomas, dermoid cysts, meningiomas arising from the sphenoid bone, and large aneurysms of the carotid artery. The patient often is unaware of visual impairment until the deficit encroaches on central vision in one or both eyes.

The anatomic position of the *optic tracts* makes isolated visual abnormalities arising from these structures comparatively rare. Since fibers serving identical points in the homonymous half-fields do not fully comingle in the tracts, lesions of these structures characteristically produce incongruous and usually incomplete homonymous hemianopias. Mild and sometimes subtle optic hemiatrophy can accompany longstanding tract lesions. Pupillary reactions usually appear normal by clinical testing.

Geniculate Ganglion, Visual Radiation, and Occipital Cortex

Damage to these structures results from infarcts or hemorrhages, trauma, neoplasms, or, rarely, inflammatory or degenerative disorders involving the cerebral white matter. The site of the lesion usually can be deduced from the resulting visual field defects (Fig. 41), especially if an accompanying CT scan is available. Lesions affecting the visual radiations in the temporal lobe or at the inferior bank of the calcarine cortex produce homonymous partial or complete superior quadrantic field defects. Most of these are fully congruent, occasional exceptions being observed in the horizontal outer margins of field defects occurring with temporal lobe lesions. Lesions damaging the parietal radiation or, more often, the superior bank of the calcarine cortex produce congruent, homonymous partial or complete inferior quadrantanopia. As elsewhere in the system, postgeniculate damage to the visual radiations can go long unrecognized unless hemianopia intrudes on macular vision. Even then, psychophysical adjustments shift the foveal point so that the visual image is permanently split in a few patients with occipital lesions unless the adjacent parastriate cortex is involved and produces defects in visual association function.

Postgeniculate amaurosis can be differentiated from pregeniculate causes by the presence of (1) a normal funduscopic appearance, (2) intact direct and consensual pupillary light reflexes, and (3) anatomically appropriate lesions on CT. When the injury to the visual radiation concurrently involves the right parietal lobe, patients may be unaware of or even deny the existence of visual loss (p. 1162). VER studies will distinguish cortical visual loss from hysteria or malingering if any doubt exists following CT.

Bilateral damage to the optic visual radiation or occipital cortex produces *cortical blindness,* partial or complete. Partial damage involving adjacent areas of the superior and inferior banks of the calcarine cortex is rare, but can follow, occasionally, traumatic (e.g., shrapnel) or, less often, ischemic injuries. Damage to structures at or near the occipital pole results in homonymous congruent central or paracentral scotomas that are usually but not always hemianopic. Aside from the history and CT findings, differentiation of such scotomas from bilateral optic nerve defects depends on finding their congruity by visual fields, the absence of pupillary reflex abnormalities, and, if necessary, the finding of normal VERs.

Visual Hallucinations

Owing to its complex organization and extensive anatomic connections, the visual system is prone to develop spontaneous interiorly generated images. The slow time-constant of metabolic changes in the retinal visual pigments explains the low-intensity afterimages that normally occur when one shifts central vision from a bright to a dark surface or that follow an inadvertent bright flash before the open eyes. Compressing the normal eyeball under the closed lid or even moving the eyes against the closed lids evokes *phosphenes,* largely unsteady images with a bright center, a dark surround, and a wide flickering margin. The entirety somewhat resembles Kuffler's diagram of the on-off circular fields of retinal receptor activity. Electrical stimulation of the striate cortex produces flickering white lights, reminiscent in their description of the scintillating scotomas of migraine or of elaborations of the diagrams produced by Hubel and Wiesel to illustrate the light bars that constitute the ideal stimulus for simple striate receptor cells. Epileptogenic lesions in this area produce similar hallucinations. Electrical stimulation of the surgically exposed parastriate or lateral temporal lobe produces more complex and often animate visual images.

Endogenously arising visual hallucinations most commonly occur in toxic-delirious states, especially accompanying the use of or withdrawal from intoxicating drugs. Such hallucinations characteristically appear as animate, moving forms exhibiting disconnected and often frightening fragments of complex activity. Structural damage to several loci along the visual pathways can generate hallucinations. Complex inanimate or animate visual illusions or hallucinations can occupy either the blind or seeing fields in association with damage arising anywhere from the retina to the cerebral cortex. *Peduncular hallucinations,* for example, consisting of multicolored, geometric, kaleidoscopically changing images, have been described in association with lesions of the cerebral peduncles at the base of the diencephalon and also in association with injuries that lie almost anywhere along the rostral territorial distribution of the basilar artery. Nevertheless, most evidence associates formed, animate or inanimate, repetitive visual hallucinations with destructive irritative lesions involving area 19 of the visual cortex or its projections anteriorly in the parietal or temporal lobes. Hallucinations evoked by lesions affecting the occipital or occipital-parietal part of this system tend to possess a stereotyped pattern and to have a still-frame rather than cinematic quality.

Temporal lobe hallucinations by contrast can be either still-frame or consist of fragments of memory juxtaposed in chaotic sequence and associated with other features of psychomotor seizures. Like *palinopsia,* the phenomenon of perseveration of full visual images, cerebrally initiated visual hallucinations commonly arise in or adjacent to areas of impaired or blind visual fields.

PUPILLARY FUNCTIONS

Neural mechanisms controlling the pupil travel widely through the nervous system so that changes in pupillary activity often provide a clue in neurologic diagnosis.

The Anatomy of Pupillary Pathways

Retinal influences on the pupil take origin in ganglion cells receiving maximal stimulation from receptors located in and adjacent to the macular area. The centrally traveling axons largely traverse the maculopapillary bundle and follow the crossed and uncrossed pregeniculate visual pathways into the optic tracts. From the tracts they diverge to synapse in pretectal interneurons whence they project to both parasympathetic Edinger-Westphal nuclei atop the midbrain third nerve complex. As a result, afferent stimuli from either retina affect parasympathetic outflow bilaterally. From Edinger-Westphal nuclei, paired parasympathetic efferent fibers leave the midbrain accompanying each emergent third nerve to travel in the interpeduncular space across the petroclinoid ligament and the edge of the tentorium. After traversing the cavernous sinus, they approach the globe via the superior orbital fissure and synapse in the ciliary ganglion of the orbit, which sends short ciliary nerves into the eye to reach the pupillary muscles.

The principal *sympathetic control of the pupil* originates in the ventrolateral hypothalamus (first-order neuron), from whence fibers descend ipsilaterally to the lower brainstem tegmentum and then to the cervical cord where they lie superficially and synapse with preganglionic neurons in the intermediolateral cell column of the upper three thoracic segments. Preganglionic fibers (second-order neurons) emerge with the ventral roots of C8, T1, and T2 and ascend in the neck, passing through the inferior and middle cervical ganglion to synapse in the superior cervical ganglion adjacent to the base of the skull. Postganglionic (third-order neurons) pupillary fibers accompany the internal carotid artery through the skull and diverge from it to follow the ophthalmic branch of the trigeminal nerve, passing via the nasociliary branch to reach pupillodilator muscles of the eye.

Diagnosis of Pupillomotor Abnormalities

Topologic diagnosis of pupillary abnormalities follows the above principles (Fig. 43). Lesions of one retina or prechiasmatic nerve produce little or no pupillary change at rest, since pupillomotor efferents bilaterally remain under the control of the afferent stimuli emanating from the other intact eye. Direct stimulation by flashlight of the visually impaired eye either does not evoke a response or evokes a reduced direct and consensual constrictor response (afferent

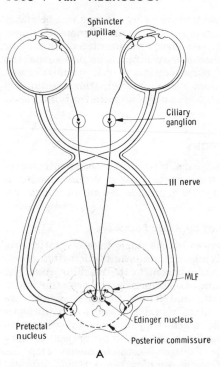

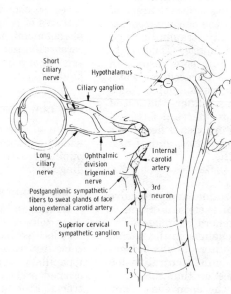

Figure 43. *A*, The parasympathetic pupilloconstrictor pathway; *B*, The sympathetic pupillodilator pathway. (From Plum, F., and Posner, J. B.: The Diagnosis of Stupor and Coma. 3rd ed. rev. Philadelphia, F. A. Davis Co., 1982.)

A

B

pupil), while swinging the light to shine on the normal receptors of the other eye elicits brisk constriction of both pupils (the swinging flashlight test). Chiasmal or tract lesions produce pupillary defects proportional to the degree that the lesions encroach on fibers of the maculopapillary bundle; in any event, pupillary changes tend to be a late sign. Lesions compressing or damaging the tectal region interrupt the light reflex bilaterally to produce mid-position or moderately wide (greater than 5 mm) and light-fixed pupils. Pupillary constriction on accommodation is preserved until late stages. Damage to the midbrain tegmentum and third nerve nuclei destroys the preganglionic parasympathetic pupillary control, but in the brainstem such injuries also interrupt sympathetic pupillary pathways descending from the hypothalamus. The result is pupils 3 to 5 mm in diameter that are irregular, often unequal, and in fixed mid position. Interruption of the emerging third nerve in the ventral midbrain or along the proximal part of its course produces a mid-dilated pupil 6 to 7 mm in diameter. For not fully understood reasons, injury to the third nerve in the cavernous sinus or anterior to it sometimes misleadingly spares the pupil. Sympathetic paralysis of the eye with ptosis and miosis (Horner's syndrome) can result from lesions anywhere along the course of the first-, second-, or third-order sympathetic neuron. Topical diagnosis of pupillary defects is reached by identifying associated signs of dysfunction in the brainstem or neck or along the carotid artery but can be assisted by pharmacologic testing. Failure of the affected eye to dilate after instilling 1 per cent hydroxyamphetamine indicates a postganglionic (third-order neuron) lesion.

Central pupillary problems may occur in relative isolation. These include *essential anisocoria*, a lifelong, idiopathic difference in the size of the two pupils. Reflex reactions are normal. The disparity remains constant during constriction and dilatation. *Adie's tonic pupil*, which is characteristically medium to large (3 to 6

mm), shrinks little or not at all in response to light and reacts slowly to accommodation, but constricts with the instillation of dilute pilocarpine (0.02 per cent) or mecholyl 2.5 per cent. The abnormal pupil is associated with absence of or diminished deep tendon reflexes. The condition usually affects one eye or occasionally both, is more frequent in women 25 to 45 years of age, and carries no serious implications. Its cause is unknown. *Argyll Robertson pupils* are small, 1 to 2 mm, unequal, irregular, and fixed to light; they constrict to accommodation. Their principal cause at one time was tertiary neurosyphilis; now Argyll Robertson changes are encountered most often with diabetes and certain autonomic neuropathies. Unexplained unilaterally or bilaterally dilated pupils as an isolated finding can result from accidental or intentional instillation of mydriatics (e.g., with malingering). Failure of the pupil to constrict promptly with instillation of pilocarpine 1 per cent provides the diagnosis if the history is withheld.

OCULOMOTOR SYSTEM

Anatomy and Physiology

Each eye, encased in the protective bones of the skull and face, can move in six primary directions: medially, laterally, superiorly, inferiorly, and rotationally in a clockwise or counterclockwise direction. The eye movements are controlled by six muscles that, in turn, are innervated by three cranial nerves. The lateral rectus, supplied by the abducens nerve, is a pure lateral deviator of the globe. The medial rectus, supplied by the oculomotor nerve, is a pure medial rotator of the eye. The other muscles depend for their function on the position of the eye. In the externally rotated position the superior rectus is a pure elevator and the inferior rectus a pure depressor of the eye. They are both innervated by the oculomotor nerve. In this externally rotated position, the superior oblique muscle, supplied by the trochlear nerve, is an intorter, and the inferior oblique, supplied by the oculomotor nerve, is an extorter. As the eyes move medially, well beyond the primary position, the superior oblique muscle becomes a depressor and the inferior oblique an elevator, the superior and inferior recti, respectively, intort and extort. The functions of the muscles are easily understood when one inspects a figure depicting the angle and position of their insertion in the globe (Fig. 44). The eyelid is maintained in its open position by actions of the levator muscle, a voluntary muscle supplied by the oculomotor nerve, and Müller's muscles, sympathetically innervated smooth muscle in the upper and lower lid that serve to maintain elevation and depression of the lid, respectively. The voluntary levator muscle is innervated by the oculomotor nerve and the sympathetic muscles by the cervical sympathetic chain (see the following chapter).

The oculomotor nerves (third cranial nerves) originate in paired nuclei and the periaqueductal gray of the mesencephalon. Within the nucleus there is somatotopic localization for each of the muscles. All of the muscles except the superior rectus are innervated by ipsilateral neurons. Superior rectus axons cross in the brainstem to join the oculomotor nerve of the opposite side. The pupilloconstrictor fibers are the most medially located. The oculomotor nucleus is small and located near other important structures, so it is rarely selectively involved in brainstem lesions such as infarcts. When it is, the ipsilateral eye closes because of paralysis of the levator muscle, the pupil becomes unreactive to light, and the globe deviates laterally because of paralysis of the medial rectus muscle. The inferior rectus and inferior oblique muscles are also paralyzed, but the ipsilateral superior rectus remains intact, the superior rectus of the opposite side being paralyzed. Axons from the cell bodies of the oculomotor nerve exit from the ventral aspect of the midbrain, passing through the red nucleus and substantia nigra and just medial to the cerebral peduncle. Small infarcts in these areas of emergence cause loss of oculomotor function and, depending on the site, either contralateral tremor (cerebellar pathways passing through the red nucleus) or contralateral hemiparesis (involvement of cerebral peduncles).

The two oculomotor nerves lie close together in the interpeduncular fossa of the midbrain, making them simultaneously susceptible to compression by basilar aneurysms. They then pass between the superior cer-

Figure 44. *Above,* The actions of the extraocular muscles and, *below,* the medial and lateral recti (lateral gaze to right side). (From Patten, J.: Neurological Differential Diagnosis. London, Harold Starke, Ltd., 1977, p. 31.)

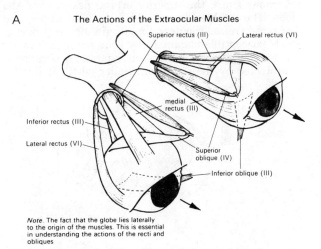

A The Actions of the Extraocular Muscles

Superior rectus (III)

Lateral rectus (VI)

medial rectus (III)

Inferior rectus (III)

Lateral rectus (VI)

Superior oblique (IV)

Inferior oblique (III)

Note. The fact that the globe lies laterally to the origin of the muscles. This is essential in understanding the actions of the recti and obliques

The Actions of the Medial and Lateral Recti (lateral gaze to R side)

Adducting eye (action of III nerve)

Medial rectus (III)

These muscles usually act as a pair in conjugate gaze to either side. The medial recti act together in convergence. The central pathways for these movements are discussed in Chapter 7

Lateral rectus (VI)

Abducting eye (action of VI nerve)

B

ebellar and posterior cerebral arteries on their respective sides, making them susceptible to compression between the arteries (cerebral herniation syndrome, p. 1025). The oculomotor nerve is also susceptible to compression by aneurysms of the posterior communicating artery, a particularly common cause of third nerve palsy. The oculomotor nerves then enter the cavernous sinus, where they lie in the lateral wall along with fibers of the trochlear and abducens nerves and the first and second divisions of the trigeminal nerve as well as sympathetic fibers surrounding the carotid artery. Within the cavernous sinus, aneurysms of the carotid artery can also compress the oculomotor nerve, but generally other ocular nerves are involved as well. Along with the other ocular nerves, the oculomotor nerve then enters the globe through the superior orbital foramen and bifurcates into a superior and inferior branch. The superior branch innervates the superior rectus and the levator, and the inferior branch innervates the other muscles.

The trochlear nerve (fourth cranial) arises from the midbrain, just below the oculomotor nerve, and, in fact, is actually a caudal extension of that nerve. Axons of the trochlear nucleus exit from the dorsal midbrain (the only cranial nerve to exit dorsally) where they cross just caudal to the inferior colliculus, cross along the under surface of the tentorium, and enter the cavernous sinus, the superior orbital fissure, and the globe. The trochlear nerve is a long, thin nerve, and its course around the dorsal midbrain makes it particularly susceptible to damage by head trauma. It is not involved in cerebral herniation syndromes because it is protected by the tentorium under which it lies for much of its course. It can, however, be damaged by acute concussion injuries to the head that transiently jolt the edge of the tentorium against the dorsum of the midbrain. The superior oblique muscle, which it innervates, passes through a bony eye in the medial wall of the orbit (the trochlea), which may at times interfere with the smooth contraction of that muscle, leading to brief episodic diplopia. Eye injuries may fracture the trochlea, also leading to diplopia.

The abducens nerve (sixth cranial) originates in the tegmentum of the caudal pons, just below the floor of the fourth ventricle. Fibers course through the pons to exit from its ventral surface, then ascend along the clivus to enter the cavernous sinus, superior orbital fissure, and orbit. The abducens nerve is the longest of the cranial nerves. Its length and long upward course make it susceptible to trauma and particularly to compression by increased intracranial pressure and herniation syndromes. Lateral rectus weakness from sixth nerve dysfunction may be the only sign of increased intracranial pressure, and bilateral lateral rectus weakness is a common remote sign of several kinds of brain tumors in children.

Because the visual system plays such an important role in relating the organism to its environment, movement of the eyes must be very finely controlled and linked to visual and vestibular pathways. The ocular nuclei are interconnected by a large myelinated fiber bundle, the median longitudinal fasciculus, which carries fibers from vestibular and other systems and serves to yoke the eye muscles. Thus contraction of one lateral rectus is associated with cocontraction of the opposite medial rectus and inhibition of the con-

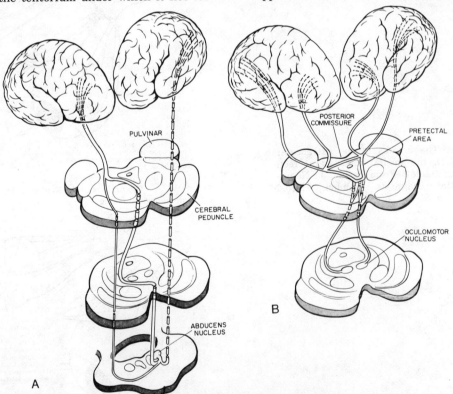

Figure 45. *See legend on opposite page.*

tralateral lateral rectus and ipsilateral medial rectus. Eye movements are controlled voluntarily from the frontal eye fields (Brodman's area 8). These centers regulate rapid (saccadic) voluntary eye movements in all directions. Saccades are ballistic movements that change fixation at rates up to 700 per second. Fibers from the frontal eye fields destined to control lateral

eye movements descend through the brain and brainstem, cross in the upper pons, and synapse at the pontine reticular formation near the abducens nucleus. Second-order neurons can control the abducens nucleus and, through the medial longitudinal fasciculus, the opposite oculomotor nucleus. Fibers controlling voluntary and vertical gaze travel through the regions of

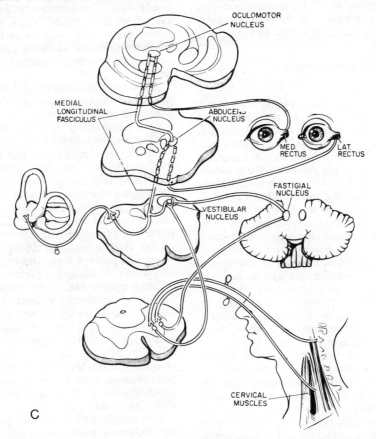

C

Figure 45. The supranuclear pathways and internuclear connections subserving conjugate gaze and eye movement, respectively.

A, Lateral conjugate gaze. The pathways from the "frontal eye fields" are shown descending in two bundles through the midbrain, crossing to the contralateral midbrain and upper pons to synapse in the contralateral midpons close to or within the abducens nucleus. The pathway from the parieto-occipital eye fields, which probably has both ipsilateral and contralateral components, is shown descending ipsilaterally to synapse in or near the abducens nucleus in the pons.

B, Vertical conjugate gaze. These pathways are shown originating from the "frontal and occipital eye fields" of both hemispheres and descending through the ipsilateral hemisphere to the pretectal area of the upper midbrain. Some of the fibers cross in the posterior commissure, and others cross in the midbrain tegmentum ventral to the sylvian aqueduct. The fibers then descend, probably through the midbrain tegmentum, to reach both contralateral and ipsilateral oculomotor nuclei. The anatomy of these pathways is less well worked out than that of the pathways subserving lateral conjugate gaze.

C, The internuclear connections between the nuclei subserving eye movement and how they are influenced by proprioceptive, cerebellar, and labyrinthine fibers. At the *lower right,* proprioceptive fibers from posterior cervical muscles and ligaments are shown entering the spinal cord to reach the vestibular nuclei, either directly or via a relay through the fastigial nucleus of the cerebellum. In the *left middle* of the drawing, vestibular fibers from the labyrinth are shown reaching the ipsilateral and contralateral vestibular nuclei of the medulla. In the *middle right* of the drawing, fibers from the cerebellum are shown leaving the fastigial nucleus to reach ipsilateral and contralateral vestibular nuclei. Fibers from the vestibular nuclei then ascend in the medial longitudinal bundle to reach the abducens nucleus. Fibers from the abducens area cross in the midpons and ascend in the medial longitudinal fasciculus to reach the contralateral oculomotor nuclei. As shown in the drawing, the left abducens nucleus, which moves the left eye laterally, is linked to the right oculomotor nucleus, which moves the right eye medially via the medial longitudinal fasciculus, which also links incoming fibers from cervical muscles, cerebellum, and labyrinth, allowing these structures to influence conjugate movement of the eyes by oculovestibular and oculocephalic reflexes.

(From Plum, F., and Posner, J. B.: The Diagnosis of Stupor and Coma. 3rd ed. rev. Philadelphia, F. A. Davis Co., 1982.)

the pretectal and posterior commissural nuclei to reach the oculomotor nuclei bilaterally. Fibers from the posterior parietal area serving slow, tracking, or pursuit eye movements probably descend ipsilaterally to supply the same oculomotor nuclei. Fibers from cervical muscles and the vestibular system as well as from the cerebellum also impinge on the oculomotor nuclei to assure that the eyes move so that the organism can maintain fixation during head and body movement. These pathways are schematically shown in Figure 45.

Disturbance of Ocular Movements

Definitions

Abnormal, *disjunctive* eye movements can result from abnormalities in the action of the individual ocular muscles, the oculomotor myoneural junctions, the oculomotor nerves or nuclei, and the medial longitudinal fasciculus. The term *strabismus* describes malalignment of one eye with respect to the other. Nonparalytic strabismus is due to an intrinsic imbalance of ocular muscle tone and is usually congenital. Paralytic strabismus results from defects in ocular muscle innervation. In *comitant strabismus* the relationship between the two ocular axes remains constant in all directions of gaze; in *noncomitant strabismus* they change; and in *latent strabismus* the imbalance is brought out only by covering one eye to prevent fixation. Latent strabismus can appear in otherwise normal individuals who are fatigued, intoxicated, or develop acute febrile illness. In congenital comitant strabismus, present at birth or soon thereafter, there is a strong risk that, if it is uncorrected, the subject will suppress vision in the nondominant eye during early development when it normally forms connections to the visual cortex. The result is unilateral, permanent reduction of vision in the nondominant eye *(amblyopia ex anopia)*. Strabismus beginning later in life after binocular fusion develops produces sudden diplopia that gradually disappears as the subject automatically suppresses the image from the misaligned eye (much as physicians do when using a monocular microscope or the ophthalmoscope). Postinfancy visual suppression does not lead to permanent visual loss.

Defects in ocular movements resulting from faulty action of the eye muscles or their peripheral innervation from the third, fourth, or sixth cranial nerves or their nuclei in the brainstem are called *ocular paralyses* or palsies. This contrasts with disorders in eye movement or conjugate gaze due to abnormalities of the medial longitudinal fasciculus or supranuclear structures, which are called *gaze paralyses*.

Ocular Paralyses

Ocular paralyses are identified at the bedside by examining the full range of eye movements and estimating the distribution of muscle weakness. With severe ocular paresis the involved eye is often deviated in the direction of the functional muscles, a result of loss of tone in the paralyzed muscle. With mild to moderate paresis, the patient may be able to align the eyes in forward gaze but fails to move the eye fully in the direction of the paretic muscle. In addition, as the eyes move conjugately in the direction of the paretic muscle, the weak eye lags noticeably. Even though the eye may be aligned in forward gaze, it may drift in the direction of stronger muscles when the eye is covered, only to snap back into alignment when it is uncovered. With the mildest ocular paresis the defect may be detected only by covering one eye with a transparent red glass and asking the patient who complains of diplopia to describe the position of the two images. The distance between the images is greatest when the patient looks in the direction of the paralyzed muscle and perceives the image seen in the paralyzed eye as being projected further from the vertical or horizontal midline than the image from the normal eye.

Although the cardinal sign of ocular paresis is diplopia, other manifestations of imbalance may occur. Thus a patient with paralysis affecting the dominant eye may inadvertently stumble over objects or miss intended targets when he reaches for them. Particularly when the paralyzed eye is the dominant one, a patient who continues to use the paretic eye for visual fixation may bump into things when he walks or reach wrongly for objects when he attempts to pick them up, because the image is displaced. Most ocular pareses remain stable over a long period. The exception is ocular paralysis accompanying myasthenia gravis, in which ocular fatigue leads to diplopia that rapidly resolves when the patient rests the muscle by closing the eye or looking in another direction.

Some compensation for ocular paresis may be produced by involuntary head turning. Patients with lateral rectus palsy turn the head away from the paralyzed eye to prevent looking in that direction, while patients with superior oblique palsy characteristically tilt the head in the opposite direction to compensate for the lack of intorsion. In children this phenomenon can be so prominent that it leads to misdiagnosis of abnormalities of the cervical rather than the ocular muscles.

The simplest of the ocular pareses is that produced by abducens paralysis. The lateral rectus alone is involved except when the lesion affects the nucleus of the abducens nerve, in which case there is a gaze palsy (see below) as well. Most isolated abducens lesions result from either increased intracranial pressure or diabetic mononeuropathy. Trochlear lesions are relatively common and may arise as isolated lesions after head trauma or associated with diabetic neuropathy; often they are of unknown cause. Isolated oculomotor palsies are particularly common with compression of the third nerve by aneurysms or herniation syndromes or by damage to that nerve in diabetes. Mixed ocular pareses occur with lesions in the cavernous sinus or at the superior orbital fissure. These lesions may be vascular, inflammatory, or neoplastic. A particularly acute and often puzzling problem arises with the advent of sudden ocular paralysis and visual loss that accompanies sudden hemorrhage or infarction of a previously silent pituitary tumor. The abrupt expansion of the tumor compresses the overlying optic chiasm and the laterally placed cavernous sinus to compress both the optic and oculomotor nerves.

Abnormalities of Conjugate Gaze

Acute damage to a frontal eye field (e.g., by hemorrhage or infarct) results in 24 to 72 hours of inability to direct the eyes contralaterally. Bilateral damage to the gaze areas of both frontal lobes or their descending pathways may produce inability to move the eyes voluntarily despite preserved visual reflex tracking movements (sometimes called oculomotor apraxia, but actually a pseudobulbar defect). Vertical eye movements are particularly susceptible to damage by midbrain lesions. Parinaud's syndrome, consisting of wide light-fixed pupils and loss of upward gaze, which is at first voluntary and later reflex as well, results from compression of the dorsal midbrain. The lesion interrupts incoming pathways from the light reflex and the cerebral eye fields destined for the pretectal area and midbrain tegmentum. Pineal tumors and posterior transtentorial herniations are the most frequent causes. Damage to either para-abducens area paralyzes lateral conjugate gaze to the side of the lesion. Thus with conjugate gaze paralysis of forebrain origin, the eyes "look" toward the lesion, whereas with conjugate gaze paralysis of brainstem origin the eyes look away from the lesion.

Lesions of the median longitudinal fasciculus (MLF) characteristically produce *internuclear ophthalmoplegia* (INO) with which the eyes in the primary position at rest either may be parallel or show a mild skew deviation, but move disjunctively in lateral gaze. (Skew results from any of a number of lesions involving the brainstem and has little localizing value.) Characteristic of fully developed INO is that during lateral gaze toward the side of the interrupting lesion the ipsilateral eye abducts and shows nystagmus, whereas the contralateral, adducting eye completely or partially fails to move nasally because of failure of ascending impulses to reach the opposite third nerve nucleus. Classically, adduction for near-vision convergence is relatively well preserved. INO may be unilateral or bilateral, partial or complete, depending upon the location of the lesion and the degree of damage to the paired MLF structures. Demyelinating and small vascular (e.g., systemic lupus erythematosus, hypertension) lesions are the most common cause of unilateral INO isolated from other ocular palsies or brainstem

signs. Larger brainstem lesions damage one or more oculomotor nuclei plus the MLF, often producing bizarre combinations of disjunctive eye movements coupled with nuclear oculomotor paralyses. Partial ophthalmoplegia from myasthenia gravis can sometimes resemble inconstant INO and should be tested for in doubtful cases.

In addition to ocular and gaze pareses, a variety of repeated abnormal eye movements affect some persons. The most common is nystagmus resulting from vestibular dysfunction. Nystagmus and some other abnormal eye movements are discussed on page 1147.

SMELL AND TASTE

Olfaction

The capacity to detect odor provides humans with both strong limbic signals and potential safety warnings. Smell contributes importantly to the anticipation and ingestion of food since much of what we "taste" derives from olfactory stimulation during the ingestion and chewing of food. In lower animals, olfactory detection of pheromones plays an important role in many kinds of behavior, especially sexual. That particular system is extraordinarily sensitive, with a single molecule of a sex pheromone eliciting a detectable response.

The nose is to olfaction as the external ear is to hearing. Odoriferous molecules in the air enter the nasal passage to reach olfactory receptors that lie in a roughly dime-sized area of specialized pigment epithelium that arches along the superior aspect of each side of the nasal mucosa (Fig. 46). The receptor cell is a bipolar cell with a long, thin dendrite reaching the surface of the nasal mucosa to detect aromatic molecules as they dissolve. The centrally directed axons traverse the cribriform plate to reach the olfactory bulb on the ventral surface of the frontal lobe. Unique to neurons, these olfactory cells degenerate and regenerate with a life span of about 60 days. Just as taste buds (see below) detect 4 primary tastes, olfactory

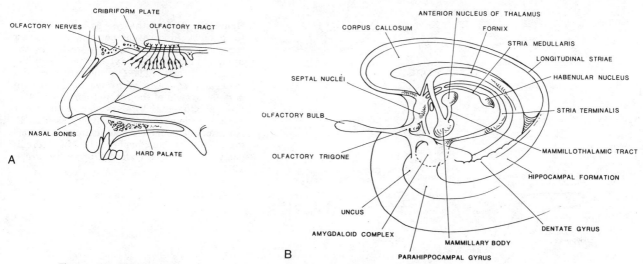

Figure 46. Olfactory structures. *A*, Lateral view of olfactory nerves penetrating the skull through the cribriform plate. *B*, Medial aspect of the temporal lobe and interconnections with the limbic lobe and diencephalic structures in the limbic system. The cortex of the temporal lobe has been removed to expose the deep fiber pathways. (From Daube, J. R., and Sandok, B. A.: Medical Neurosciences. Boston, Little, Brown and Co., 1978.)

receptors are believed to detect as many as 32 *primary* odors, allowing humans to identify more than 1000 distinct odors. Second- and third-order neurons project directly and indirectly from the olfactory bulb to the prepiriform cortex and parts of the amygdaloid complex of the same and opposite side of the brain, representing the primary olfactory cortex.

Olfactory sense can be reduced (hyposmia), absent (anosmia), or distorted (dysosmia). Dysosmia may result from local disease, but occasionally is a psychiatric symptom. Anosmia can be partial or complete, inherited or acquired. Thus, anosmia or hyposmia for specific selective odors occurs rarely as an autosomal or recessive inherited trait. Congenital anosmia accompanies certain autonomic and endocrinopathic disorders, notably hypogonadotropic hypogonadism.

Most acquired disturbances of smell result from transient or sustained diseases of the nasal mucous membranes that deaden or dry out the receptor area. Such disorders seldom are complete and commonly respond to local treatment. More severe and often permanent anosmia results from basal skull fractures avulsing the olfactory nerves, frontal fossa brain tumors affecting the central pathways, and, much less often, herpes zoster, vitamin B_{12} deficiency, and multiple sclerosis. Sudden idiopathic anosmia usually associated with loss of taste has been reported, probably a result of a local neurotropic viral infection. No satisfactory treatment has been found for such neurogenic anosmias. Affected patients must be warned explicitly to avoid gas heating and to install smoke

alarms to compensate for the life-threatening hazards of the defect. *Parosmia* is a distortion of olfactory perception (normal odors perceived as foul smells) that may occur without prior anosmia or during the recovery phase from anosmia.

Hallucinations of smell, usually of a foul quality, occur with epileptogenic lesions affecting the region of the amygdala and are termed uncinate fits (p. 1156).

Gustatory Function

Taste, like smell, has both vegetative and survival values, the latter more crucial to our primitive ancestors than it is today. The impairment or loss of taste is a serious complaint with a variety of illnesses in some of which a concurrent olfactory loss is actually at fault.

The brain abstracts its specific sense of taste from signals fed from taste buds and associated receptors that lie on the dorsal surface of the tongue and in the adjacent faucial areas (Fig. 47). Unlike olfactory receptors but similar to hair cells of the auditory system, the taste buds are not neurons but make synaptic connections with centrally directed taste neurons. The individual taste receptors live about 10 days. Fungiform papillary buds on the anterior region of the tongue respond mainly to sweet, sour, and salt stimuli, while foliate and circumvallate papillae located along the base of the tongue and adjacent areas detect predominantly bitter qualities. The distribution of selective taste receptors may vary from time to time within the individual to help guide food selection according to

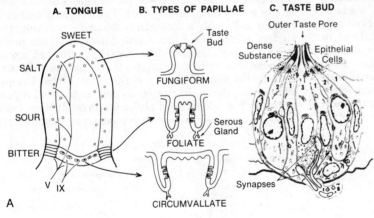

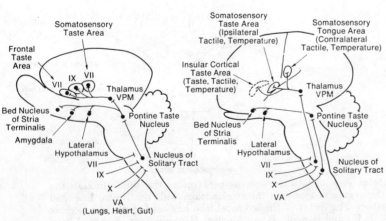

Figure 47. Taste pathways. *A,* Distribution of taste buds, innervation pattern, and lowest threshold regions for different tastes in the human tongue. *B,* Main types of taste papillae, containing taste buds. *C,* Fine structure of a taste bud. *D,* Taste pathways in the central nervous system of the rat and monkey. *VA* = visceral afferents; *VPM* = ventral posterior medial nucleus of the thalamus. Based on R. Norgren (personal communication) and Norgren, 1978. (From Shepherd, G. M.: Neurobiology. New York, Oxford University Press, 1979.)

nutritional need. Taste receptors on the anterior two-thirds of the tongue are innervated by branches of the chorda tympani division of the intermediate and facial nerves, and the chorda tympani is especially susceptible to injuries or infections that affect the facial nerve on its route through the middle ear and petrous bone. Glossopharyngeal nerve fibers supply the taste receptors of the posterior two-thirds of the tongue and fauces. Both innervations project to the nucleus tractus solitarius of the medulla and then ascend in the brain via a series of relays to reach the postcentral somatosensory cerebral cortex. Taste receptors on the tongue have an innately relatively high threshold, which increases further with age, often making specific testing difficult for diagnostic purposes.

Loss and reduction of the sense of taste are termed *ageusia* and *hypogeusia*, respectively; distortion is called *dysgeusia*. Disorders that cause taste abnormalities include Bell's palsy, an acute unilateral loss of facial nerve function that usually reduces taste perception on the involved side of the tongue. On the contrary, loss of trigeminal function causing somatosensory loss on the tongue usually does not affect taste. Epileptic discharges occasionally cause gustatory hallucinations. Depressive or paranoid delusions also can affect the sense of taste, more often distorting taste or smell than destroying them. Among systemic problems, aging, hepatitis, cancer, and various forms of drugs are the main causes of taste reduction or distortion. Investigation of the symptom of taste loss or abnormal taste involves first a clinical search for local mucous membrane or neurologic disease, followed by a systematic review of medications being taken, inquiry into possible exposure to toxic fumes and, if necessary, a more exacting inquiry into possibly hidden systemic illness.

HEARING AND EQUILIBRIUM

The neural pathways subserving hearing and those most important for equilibrium and spatial orientation are anatomically proximate through much of their course, from their end-organs in the inner ear (Fig. 48) to their termination in the cortex. Because of the close anatomic linkage, disorders that affect hearing often affect equilibrium as well, and vice versa. For this reason they are considered together here. Despite their major anatomic similarities, there are substantial pathophysiologic differences that make clinical examination of the two systems quite different: (1) The auditory system is physiologically relatively isolated, so that its function and dysfunction can be tested independently of other neural systems. The vestibular system, on the other hand, has many close physiologic linkages with the motor system (particularly the cerebellum, oculomotor system, and the autonomic nervous system) and can be tested only indirectly by noting secondary effects on oculomotor and cerebellar functions. Abnormalities of the auditory system lead only to loss or distortion of hearing, tinnitus, or both. Abnormalities of the vestibular system may cause symptoms that mimic disorders of other neural structures. Such symptoms include dizziness or vertigo, ocular abnormalities (nystagmus), motor abnormalities (including ataxia or sudden falls), and autonomic abnormalities (including nausea and vomiting and even syncope).

Anatomy and Physiology of Hearing

In normal hearing, sound waves are transmitted from the tympanic membrane via the three ossicles of the air-filled middle ear (air conduction) to the oval

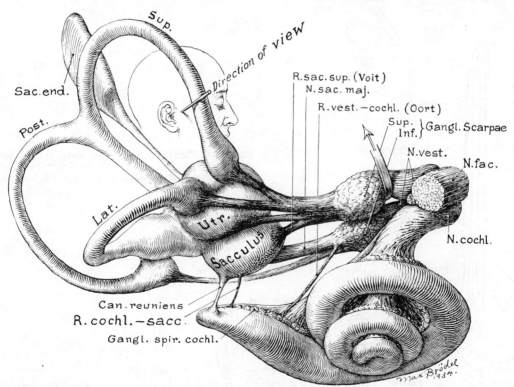

Figure 48. Semidiagrammatic drawing of the innervation of the labyrinth. The orientation of the afferent vestibular and cochlear nerve trunks can be seen to the right. (Drawing by M. Brödel in Hardy, M.: Observations on the innervation of the macula sacculi in man. Anat Rec 59:403–418, 1934.)

window, to which is attached the basilar membrane of the fluid-filled cochlea. The ossicles serve to increase the gain from tympanum to oval window about 18-fold, compensating for the loss that sound waves moving from air to fluid would otherwise suffer. In the absence of this system, sound may reach the cochlea by vibration of the temporal bone (bone conduction) but with much less efficiency (approximately 60 dB loss). Hair cells lying along the cochlear basilar membrane detect the vibratory movement of that membrane and transduce vibration into nerve impulses. The nerve impulses are then relayed via nerve cells that synapse at the base of hair cells and have their bodies in the spiral ganglion to reach the cochlear nucleus of the ipsilateral pontine tegmentum (Fig. 49). Auditory frequency receptors are distributed unevenly along the basilar membrane. Hair cells sensitive to higher frequencies (above 2000 to 4000 Hz) are localized along the basilar turn of the cochlea, while receptors sensitive to lower frequencies are distributed along the full length of the structure. The sensitivity of the basilar turn to noise trauma somewhat explains why partial deafness characteristically affects the perception of higher more than lower frequencies. Within the brainstem, auditory signals ascend from the ventral and dorsal cochlear nuclei to reach the superior olivary nuclei of both sides. Thus, nervous system lesions central to the cochlear nucleus do not cause monaural hearing loss, nor, conversely, do unilateral lesions

cause any deafness. From these structures the pathway projects by way of the lateral lemnisci to the inferior colliculi. Each inferior colliculus transmits to both its ipsilateral and contralateral medial geniculate bodies, which, in turn, send the final projection to the transverse auditory gyrus lying in the superior portion of their ipsilateral temporal lobe.

The normal ear can detect sound frequencies ranging between about 20 and 20,000 Hz, with the upper range dropping off rapidly with advancing age. The ear is most sensitive between 500 and 4000 Hz, in part because the middle ear has a resonant frequency about 3000 Hz. Normal speech resonates at frequencies of 2000 Hz and below. Standard clinical audiograms record hearing frequencies only below 8000 Hz. The intensity of sound is quantified by decibels, a logarithmic abstraction calculated from the smallest perceptible difference in intensity that the normal ear can discriminate. Loss of 30 to 40 dB (about 100-fold decrease) impairs normal conversation; an 80 dB loss indicates deafness.

Symptoms of Auditory Dysfunction

As noted, only two symptoms result from disease of the auditory system: The first is hearing impairment, sometimes associated with distortion as well as decrease in the intensity of sound, and the second is

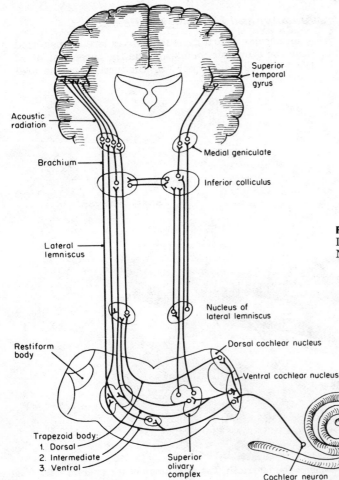

Figure 49. Central auditory pathways. (From Baloh, R. W.: Dizziness, Hearing Loss and Tinnitus: The Essentials of Neurotology. Philadelphia, F. A. Davis Co., 1984.)

tinnitus, a sound heard in the ear or head not arising from the external environment. Hearing loss is termed conductive (external and middle ear), sensorineural (cochlea and auditory nerve), or central (brainstem and cerebral hemispheres), according to the anatomic location of the abnormality. Most deafness is conductive or sensorineural.

Conductive hearing loss is characterized by equal loss of hearing at all frequencies and by well-preserved speech discrimination once the threshold for hearing is exceeded. With sensorineural hearing loss, low-frequency tones are typically heard better than those of high frequency, and it may be difficult to hear speech that is mixed with background noise. Furthermore, because of recruitment (see below), small increases in the intensity of sound may cause discomfort. With hearing loss resulting from cochlear disease (usually due to selective destruction of hair cells), diplacusis and recruitment are common problems. With diplacusis, an individual hears a pure tone as if it were a complex mixture of tones, or the pitch of a pure tone sounds different in the ear with the involved cochlea than it does in the normal ear. Recruitment is the abnormally rapid growth in the sensation of loudness as the intensity of the sound is increased, leading to greater ability, once threshold is exceeded, to detect small increments in intensity in the damaged ear than in the normal ear. The exact pathophysiology of these symptoms is unknown, but both occur when there is selective damage to hair cells in the cochlea.

Tone decay, a symptom of acoustic nerve dysfunction, is the inability to continue to hear a tone at the same intensity over a sustained period. Adaptation and fatigue in damaged acoustic nerve fibers appear to be the pathophysiology of this symptom.

Central hearing loss is uncommon, but when present is characterized by loss of more speech perception than pure tone perception. If cortical, hearing loss requires bilateral temporal lobe damage with the primary receiving areas (Heschl's gyrus) being destroyed; hearing is diminished or absent even for pure tone. If association areas in the superior temporal gyrus are damaged, a patient may hear the sounds but be unable to comprehend their meaning.

Hearing Tests

Hearing may be tested either at the bedside or in the laboratory. Bedside tests, e.g., of perception of whispered sounds, hearing a watch ticking, and listening to a tuning fork at various frequencies, can often define the nature of hearing loss and frequently distinguish between conductive and sensorineural loss. More sophisticated laboratory tests include pure tone and speech audiometry and evoked potential responses with repeated clicks (similar in all principles to visual evoked potentials [p. 1094]).

Causes of Hearing Loss

Conductive Hearing Loss

Conductive hearing loss arises from abnormalities of the external or middle ear and can raise hearing threshold no more than 60 dB, since bone conduction persists intact. Obstruction in the external auditory meatus (the most common cause of conductive hearing loss) impairs air transmission to the tympanum. This benign condition is most often caused by *impacted cerumen,* but occasionally results from canal infection or similar causes. A *fluid-filled middle ear,* a result of middle ear infection (otitis media), reduces movement of the ossicles against the oval window.

Otosclerosis is a process in which the annular ligament that attaches the stapes to the oval window overgrows and calcifies. It reduces ossicular transmission via the window to the cochlear basement membrane.

Sensorineural Hearing Loss

Genetically determined deafness, usually from hair cell aplasia or deterioration, may be present at birth or develop in adulthood. The diagnosis of *hereditary deafness* rests on the finding of a positive family history. In many instances, inheritance is through a recessive gene or a dominant gene with low penetrance, making it difficult to determine the genetic nature of the disorder. *Intrauterine factors* resulting in congenital hearing loss include infection (especially rubella); toxic, metabolic, and endocrine disorders; and anoxia associated with Rh incompatibility and difficult delivery.

Acute unilateral deafness usually has a cochlear basis. Bacterial or viral infections of the labyrinth, head trauma with fracture or hemorrhage into the cochlea, or vascular occlusion of a terminal branch of the anterior-inferior cerebellar artery all can damage extensively the cochlea and its hair cells. An acute, idiopathic, often reversible, unilateral hearing loss strikes young adults and is presumed to reflect either a viral infection or a vascular disorder of the cochlea. Sudden unilateral hearing loss, often associated with vertigo and tinnitus, can result from a perilymphatic fistula. Such fistulas may be congenital or follow stapes surgery or severe or mild trauma to the inner ear.

Drugs fairly often cause sudden bilateral hearing impairment. Salicylates, furosemide, and ethacrynic acid can potentially produce transient deafness when taken in high doses. More toxic to the cochlea are the aminoglycoside antibiotics (gentamicin, tobramycin, amikacin, kanamycin, streptomycin, and neomycin). These agents can destroy cochlear hair cells in direct relation to the height of their serum concentrations and the cumulative duration of drug exposure, causing permanent hearing loss. Some anticancer chemotherapeutic agents, particularly cisplatin, cause severe ototoxicity by a similar mechanism.

Subacute relapsing cochlear deafness occurs with *Meniere's syndrome,* a condition associated with fluctuating hearing loss and tinnitus, recurrent episodes of abrupt and often severe vertigo, and a sensation of fullness or pressure in the ear. Recurrent endolymphatic hypertension (hydrops) is believed to cause the episodes. Pathologically the endolymphatic sac is dilated and the hair cells become atrophic. The resulting deafness is subtle and reversible in the early stages, but subsequently becomes permanent and characterized by diplacusis and loudness recruitment. The disorder is usually unilateral. When bilateral (<20 per cent of cases) it begins in one ear before the other.

Gradually progressive hearing loss with age, *presbycusis,* reflects deterioration in the cochlear receptor system with degeneration of the hair cells, especially at the base. As a result, higher tones are lost early, with audiograms showing a characteristically sharp decline at each successive frequency above 2000 Hz. The recurrent trauma of noise-induced hearing loss affects approximately the same cochlear region and is almost as frequent, particularly among those with exposure to loud military or industrial noises. Loud blaring modern music has become an offender recently. The increasing tone loss starts initially above a slightly higher threshold of about 4000 Hz, but moves down toward speech frequencies with repeated exposure.

Hearing loss from direct damage to the acoustic nerve in the petrous canal occasionally results from abscess within or trauma to the surrounding bone; severe, abruptly beginning, deafness marks the event and is usually associated with acute vertigo due to concurrent vestibular nerve injury. Progressive unilateral hearing loss that arises insidiously and worsens by almost imperceptible degrees is characteristic of benign neoplasms of the cerebellopontine angle such as acoustic neurinomas. Bilateral gradual eighth nerve deafness is uncommon, but when it occurs it suggests the angle tumors of neurofibromatosis.

Central Hearing Loss

Central hearing loss is unilateral only if it results from damage to the pontine cochlear nuclei on one side of the brainstem. Such can occur with ischemic infarction of the lateral brainstem, e.g., due to occlusion of the anterior-inferior cerebellar artery, a plaque of multiple sclerosis, or, rarely, invasion or compression of the dorsal lateral pons by a neoplasm or hematoma. Bilateral degeneration of the cochlear nuclei accompanies some of the rare recessively inherited disorders of childhood.

Because of the extensive cross innervation of the supranuclear auditory pathways, clinically important unilateral hearing loss never results from neurologic disease arising rostral to the cochlear nucleus. Bilateral hearing loss could in theory result from bilateral destruction of central hearing pathways anywhere along their course. In practice, involvement of neighboring structures in brainstem or hemisphere usually leads to such severe neurologic disability that the hearing loss becomes an unimportant additional sign. Two exceptions occur: In rare instances, bilateral hearing loss has been reported as an early sign of pineal region tumors, presumably from compression of the inferior colliculi. Most affected patients also have other signs of brainstem tectal dysfunction, including loss of upward gaze. Bilateral infarctions of the anterior transverse gyrus of the temporal lobe may also cause central deafness, but usually it is accompanied by aphasia as well because of involvement of the nearby Wernicke's area in the dominant hemisphere. *Spatial orientation* for sound depends upon the integrity of several of the neural structures and pathways carrying auditory information in the brainstem to as well as in the auditory cortex itself. Lesions lying anywhere along this path can impair function.

Tinnitus

Tinnitus generally refers to noises that arise spontaneously in one or both ears. Tinnitus may be classified as *objective*, i.e., the patient is hearing a sound arising externally to the auditory system, a sound that can usually be heard by the examiner with a stethoscope, or *subjective*, i.e., the sound arises from an abnormal discharge of the auditory system and cannot be heard by the observer. Objective tinnitus usually has benign causes such as noise from temporomandibular joints, opening of eustachian tubes, or repetitive contraction of the stapedius muscle. Sometimes in a quiet room individuals can hear the pulsatile flow in the carotid artery or a continuous hum of normal venous outflow through the jugular bulb. The latter can easily be obliterated by gentle compression of the jugular vein. Pathologic objective tinnitus occurs when patients hear turbulent flow in arteriovenous anomalies or tumors (e.g., glomus jugulare tumor). Objective tinnitus may also be an early sign of increased intracranial pressure. Such tinnitus, which can be obliterated by pressure over the jugular vein, probably arises from turbulent flow of compressed venous structures at the base of the brain. The symptom is also transiently relieved by decreasing intracranial pressure, for example, by lumbar puncture.

Subjective tinnitus can arise from anywhere in the auditory system. The sounds most frequently complained of are metallic ringing, buzzing, blowing, roaring, or, less often, bizarre clangings, poppings, or nonrhythmic beatings. A degree of tinnitus, heard as a faint moderately high-pitched metallic ring, can be observed by almost everyone who concentrates their attention on auditory events in a quiet room. Sustained, louder tinnitus accompanied by audiometric evidence of deafness occurs in association with either conductive or sensorineural disease. The phenomenon can be a manifestation of salicylate, quinine, or quinidine toxicity. Tinnitus observed with otosclerosis tends to have a roaring or hissing quality, while that associated with Meniere's syndrome often produces sound that varies widely in intensity with time and quality, sometimes including roarings or clangings. Tinnitus with other cochlear or auditory nerve lesions tends to be higher pitched and ringing.

Anatomy and Physiology of the Vestibular System

The paired vestibular end organs lie within the temporal bones proximate to the cochlea. Each end-organ consists of three semicircular canals that detect angular acceleration and two otolithic structures, the utricle and saccule, that detect linear (gravitational) acceleration. Like the cochlea, these organs possess hair cells projecting into a fluid-filled (endolymph) membrane. The hair cells of the three semicircular canals, each of which is oriented at right angles to the others, are concentrated in the ampulla, where they are embedded in a gelatinous mass called the cupula. Movement of the head causes the endolymph to flow either toward or away from the cupula, distorting the hair cells and, depending on the direction of endolymphatic movement, either stimulating or inhibiting their firing. Since the hair cells of the semicircular canal are tonically active, both excitation and inhibition change the rate of discharge. Furthermore, the two sets of semicircular canals are approximately mirror images of each other, so that rotational movement of the head that excites one canal will inhibit the analogous canal on the opposite side. The hair cells of the otolithic apparatus, the utricle and saccule, are concentrated in an area called the macula. The macula of the utricle lies approximately in the plane of the horizontal canal, and the macula of the saccule is essentially vertical. The hair cells are embedded in a membrane that also contains calcite masses or otoliths; the density of otoliths is considerably greater than that of the endolymph. As the head is moved the force of gravity on the otoliths distorts the hair cells, producing firing of these organs.

A discharge of hair cells from either semicircular canals or otoliths is detected by nerve fibers at the base of the hair cells. These fibers have their cells of origin in Scarpa's ganglion. The nerve fibers travel in the vestibular portion of the eighth nerve contiguous with the acoustic nerve. The vestibular portion of the eighth nerve is divided into superior and inferior vestibular nerves. The fibers of the horizontal and vestibular canals as well as the utricle and anterior saccule comprise the superior vestibular nerve, while those of the posterior canals comprise the inferior vestibular nerve. Nerve fibers from various portions of the semicircular canal terminate in different vestibular nuclei at the pontomedullary junction. There are also direct connections between the semicircular canals and many portions of the cerebellum, with the greatest representation in the flocculonodular lobe, the so-called vestibulocerebellum. Efferent fibers from the brainstem travel through the vestibular nucleus to reach the hair cells of the semicircular canal and utricles. Efferent fibers are inhibitory in nature and may, like the efferent fibers of the cochlea, have as their function selecting inputs to which the brain will attend. From the vestibular nuclei, second-order neurons make important connections to the vestibular nuclei of the other side, to the cerebellum, to motor neurons of the spinal cord, to autonomic nuclei in the brainstem, and, most importantly for the examining clinician, to the nuclei of the oculomotor system. Fibers from the vestibular nuclei also ascend through the brainstem and thalamus to reach the cerebral cortex, where the vestibular system is bilaterally represented. The exact site of cortical representation is unclear. Clinical evidence points to both superior temporal and inferior parietal lobes being possible sites (Fig. 50).

Symptoms and Signs of Vestibular Dysfunction

The vestibular system is a finely tuned, tonically discharging system. Any imbalance in discharge between the paired peripheral vestibular end-organs or their primary receiving areas in the vestibular nuclei, if not caused by a true movement of the head or body, produces a mismatch between vestibular input and other sense organs (especially the eyes and proprioceptive apparatus) and leads to an illusory sensation of movement in space called vertigo. Vertigo is the only direct symptom of a vestibular abnormality, but because the vestibular system influences other neural systems, vertigo may be accompanied by autonomic symptoms (nausea, vomiting, diaphoresis), motor symptoms (ataxia, past pointing, falling) or ocular symptoms (oscillopsia—a visual sensation that the environment is moving). Also because of the close

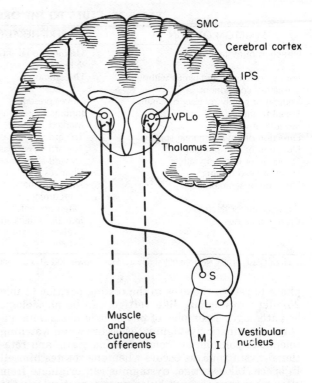

Figure 50. Vestibulothalamocortical projections. S = superior nucleus; L = lateral nucleus; M = medial nucleus; I = inferior nucleus; $VPLo$ = nucleus ventralis posterior lateralis pars oralis; IPS = intraparietal sulcus; SMC = sensorimotor cortex. (From Baloh, R. W.: Dizziness, Hearing Loss and Tinnitus: The Essentials of Neurotology. Philadelphia, F. A. Davis Co., 1984.)

interconnection among neural systems, the sensation of vertigo can be produced by abnormalities of the visual or somatosensory system as well as, much more commonly, the vestibular system.

Vertigo may be mild or severe, physiologic or pathologic. *Physiologic vertigo* occurs when there is a mismatch among the vestibular, visual, and somatosensory systems induced by an external stimulus. Common examples of physiologic vertigo include motion sickness, height vertigo (the sensation that occurs when one looks down from a great height), and visual vertigo (the sensation sometimes felt when one watches a motion picture of a roller coaster or other violent movement). *Pathologic vertigo* usually arises from an abnormality of the vestibular system, but less commonly can be produced by visual or somatosensory disorders. *Severe vertigo* is a sensation usually well described by the patient and easily recognized by the physician. *Milder vertigo*, however, may easily be confused with the light-headedness of syncope, the unsteadiness of ataxia, and the psychogenic symptoms of anxiety or dissociation.

The major clinical *sign* of a disordered vestibular system is *nystagmus*, a rhythmic to-and-fro movement of the eyes. There are two types of nystagmus: In pendular nystagmus the eyes oscillate at equal rates. Pendular nystagmus is usually congenital, a result of poor vision or, rarely, brainstem disease. Jerk nystagmus has two components, a slow phase resulting from vestibular or visual input and a compensatory fast

TABLE 25. CLUES TO THE ORIGIN OF VESTIBULAR NYSTAGMUS

SYMPTOM OR SIGN	PERIPHERAL (END-ORGAN)	CENTRAL (NUCLEAR)
Direction of nystagmus	Unidirectional, fast phase opposite lesion	Bidirectional or unidirectional
Purely horizontal nystagmus without rotatory component	Uncommon	Common
Vertical or purely rotatory nystagmus	Never present	May be present
Visual fixation	Inhibits nystagmus and vertigo	No inhibition
Severity of vertigo	Marked	Mild
Direction of environmental spin	Toward slow phase	Variable
Direction of past-pointing	Toward slow phase	Variable
Direction of Romberg fall	Toward slow phase	Variable
Effect of head turning	Changes Romberg fall	No effect
Duration of symptoms	Finite (minutes, days, weeks) but recurrent	May be chronic
Tinnitus and/or deafness	Often present	Usually absent
Common causes	Infectious (labyrinthitis), Meniere's disease, neuronitis, vascular, trauma, toxic	Vascular, demyelinating, neoplastic

From Glaser, J. S.: Neuro-ophthalmology. Hagerstown, Md., Harper and Row, 1977.

phase to return the eyes to the resting position (Table 25). Jerk nystagmus, like vertigo, can be physiologic or pathologic. Examples of physiologic nystagmus include optokinetic nystagmus, as occurs when watching telephone poles go by from a moving train, and rotational nystagmus, as occurs when one rotates himself in space. Like vertigo, nystagmus can originate from sites other than the vestibular system, particularly the visual or cerebellar systems, and may occur either with or without vertigo. Vestibular nystagmus arises when there is unbalanced input from the two vestibular systems. For example, stimulation of the horizontal canal on the left side increases the output from the left horizontal canal relative to the right and causes a reflex movement of the eyes toward the right. There is a rapid compensatory (nonvestibular) movement of the eyes back to the midline, so that in the awake patient the net movement of the eyes is only a few degrees. In the comatose patient, vestibular stimulation may produce full conjugate lateral deviation of the eyes with only slow return to the midline. Nystagmus is named for the direction of the rapid component. Thus, stimulation of the left horizontal canal that drives the eye slowly to the right with a compensatory movement to the left is called left beating nystagmus.

Purely horizontal fine nystagmus at the extremes of gaze is a common finding without pathologic significance. It is more common with fatigue or poor lighting. When bidirectional gaze-evoked nystagmus is prominent or involves vertical as well as horizontal movements to an equal degree, excessive sedative or anticonvulsant drug ingestion is probably the cause.

Several unusual forms of nystagmus have neurologic localizing qualities: *Dissociated nystagmus*, i.e., unequal in the two eyes, implies a brainstem lesion. *Seesaw nystagmus* involves the eyes reciprocally rising and falling, then reversing the reciprocal directions. The phenomenon accompanies parasellar tumors or, less often, upper brainstem damage. *Convergence* or *retractory nystagmus* consists of horizontal jerk nystagmus that changes its direction periodically. A typical sequence would be jerk nystagmus 90 seconds to the left, followed by a 10-second inert pause, followed by jerk nystagmus 90 seconds to the right, with the sequence then repeating itself. The finding has been associated with a variety of posterior fossa abnormalities, especially those involving the region of the craniocervical junction. *Down-beat* nystagmus produces downward jerks with the eyes in the primary gaze position; it often reflects a craniocervical abnormality, such as the Arnold-Chiari malformation, but can occur with parenchymal lesions such as multiple sclerosis. Some subjects have the capacity to induce *voluntary nystagmus*, which is extremely rapid, occurs in short bursts of 10 to 15 seconds or so, is present on the extremes of gaze, and may be unequal in the two eyes. It is doubtful whether cervical disease produces clinically significant nystagmus.

Other abnormalities of conjugate eye movements include *ocular bobbing*, consisting of fast conjugate downward eye jerks followed by slow return to the primary gaze position. The phenomenon accompanies severe displacement or destruction of the pons or, much less often, metabolic central nervous system depression. *Ocular myoclonus* consists of continuous rhythmic, pendular oscillations, most often vertical with a rate of two to five beats per second. Often it accompanies palatal myoclonus and has a similar pathogenesis. *Ocular flutter* consists of brief, intermittent, horizontal oscillations arising from the primary gaze position. It blends into *opsoclonus*, a pattern of rapid, chaotic, conjugate, repetitive, saccadic eye movements ("dancing eyes"). Both of these disorders usually reflect cerebellar dysfunction, but can emerge as a remote effect of systemic neoplasms, especially neuroblastoma in children. *Ocular dysmetria* consists of saccadic overshoots or undershoots of conjugate eye movement during rapid following of a visual object. It reflects cerebellar dysfunction.

Vestibular Tests

The vestibular system cannot be examined directly in the human being, but, because of its intimate connections with the oculomotor nuclei, it can be tested by observing the effect upon eye movements of vestibular stimulation (*vestibulo-ocular reflexes*). The *caloric test* can be performed at the bedside:

With the patient lying supine and the head elevated approximately 30 degrees, water either 7°F above or below body temperature is douched against the tympanic membrane. In the normal situation, cold water produces nystagmus away from the side of stimulation (because of inhibition of the horizontal semicircular canal), and warm water produces nystagmus to the side of stimulation (because of stimulation of the semicircular canal). In the comatose patient whose oculomotor system is intact, caloric stimulation produces tonic deviation toward the side receiving the cold water infusion. Similarly, the vestibular nuclei can be stimulated by rapid turning of the head (*oculocephalic reflex*). In the comatose patient, turning the chin toward the left causes deviation of the eyes toward the right and vice versa, sudden flexion of the neck produces upward deviation of the eyes, and extension of the neck downward deviation of the eyes. In the awake patient, visual fixation may inhibit these movements. In the unconscious patient, caloric and oculocephalic stimulation may help identify oculomotor paralyses as well as vestibular dysfunction. Because nystagmus is often inhibited by the visual fixation of the open eyes, accurate quantitative evaluation requires electrical recording of the eye movement with the eyes closed. *Electronystagmography* can be performed in the resting position, with the head rotated into various positions to provoke nystagmus, and before, during, and after caloric stimulation. Electronystagmography is often helpful in identifying the pathology of the vestibular system and localizing it when identified.

Causes of Vertigo

Examples of physiologic vertigo have already been given.

Pathologic Vertigo

Vertigo can be caused by disease of either the peripheral or central vestibular apparatus (Table 26). In general, peripheral vertigo is more severe, more likely to be associated with hearing loss and tinnitus, and often leads to nausea and vomiting. Nystagmus associated with peripheral vertigo is frequently inhibited by visual fixation. Central vertigo is generally less severe than peripheral vertigo and is often associated with other signs of central nervous system disease. The nystagmus of central vertigo is not inhibited by visual fixation and frequently is prominent when vertigo is mild or absent.

TABLE 26. CAUSES OF VESTIBULAR VERTIGO

PERIPHERAL CAUSES	CENTRAL CAUSES
Peripheral vestibulopathy	Brainstem ischemia
Labyrinthitis and/or	Cerebellopontine angle tumors
vestibular neuronitis	Demyelinating disease
Acute and recurrent	Cranial neuropathy
peripheral vestibulopathy	Seizure disorders (rare)
"Benign" positional vertigo	Heredofamilial disorders
Meniere's syndrome	Spinocerebellar degenerations
Vestibulotoxic drugs	Friedreich's ataxia
Post-traumatic vertigo,	Olivopontocerebellar atrophy,
metastatic tumor, etc.	etc.
Other focal peripheral disease	Other central causes
Infection	Brainstem tumors
Ischemia	Cerebellar degenerations
Otosclerosis	Paraneoplastic syndromes
Perilymph fistula	
Cervical arthritis	

Peripheral Vertigo

Benign positional vertigo is an extremely common disorder of middle age. Typically the patient first experiences severe whirling vertigo when turning over or first lying down in bed at night. Less commonly he may experience similar symptoms when he sits up from a lying position or when he turns suddenly while standing or walking. Usually the symptoms are greatest when the patient lies on his side with the affected ear undermost. The vertigo is sudden in onset, very severe, and may be accompanied by nausea and vomiting. The pathophysiology of the disorder is not established, but some investigators have postulated that debris from otoliths may enter the posterior canal and artificially stimulate that canal or impede the movement by its endolymph when it is in the dependent position (Fig. 51).

Peripheral Vestibulopathy. This disorder, also called acute labyrinthitis or vestibular neuronitis, may occur as a single bout or may recur repeatedly over months or years. Characteristically the patient has acute onset of severe vertigo, often associated with nausea and vomiting. This may follow a respiratory infection, but often there is no preceding illness. The vertigo may be so severe that the patient is unable to sit or stand without vomiting or ataxia, preferring to lie absolutely still in bed with the involved ear uppermost and often refusing to move. Nystagmus is invariably present, usually horizontal or rotatory, and directed away from the involved labyrinth. The severe symptoms usually improve substantially within 48 to 72 hours, allowing the patient to be up and about. However, for weeks or months following the episode affected subjects often note that sudden movements of the head produce mild vertigo or nausea. The pathogenesis of the illness is not entirely known. Although

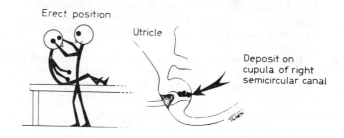

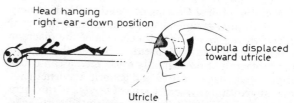

Figure 51. When the patient is in the erect position the ampulla of the semicircular canal is located inferior to the other structures of the vestibular labyrinth. With the patient in the head-hanging right-ear-down position the ampulla of the posterior semicircular canal assumes a superior position, thus reversing the direction of gravitational force on deposits located upon the cupula. (From Schuknecht, H. F., and Ruby, R. R. F.: Cupulolithiasis. Adv Otorhinolaryngol 20:435, 1973.)

the disorder is called *acute labyrinthitis*, suggesting a viral infection of the labyrinth, recent EEG and evoked potential studies suggest that in many patients there are accompanying eighth nerve or brainstem abnormalities, leading some to refer to the disorder as *vestibular neuronitis*.

In some patients, attacks (usually less severe) of acute vestibulopathy recur over many months or years. There is no way of predicting whether an individual with a first attack will have repetitive attacks. In the patient suffering from repetitive attacks, the differential diagnosis includes Meniere's syndrome and otosclerosis. At least 25 per cent of patients with otosclerosis suffer from vertigo. In both of these disorders, hearing tests will be abnormal as well. Labyrinthine fistulas have been reported to produce episodic vertigo. Fistula testing by a skilled otolaryngologist should establish that diagnosis.

Meniere's Syndrome. Meniere's syndrome is also described on page 1115. The disorder accounts for about 10 per cent of all patients with vertigo. The diagnosis is established primarily on the basis of the hearing tests.

Vestibulotoxic Drug-Induced Vertigo. Several drugs that damage the auditory system (p. 1115), such as the aminoglycosides, also may damage the labyrinth. The patient may suffer acute vertigo, either along with or independently of hearing loss and tinnitus. Unfortunately many patients being treated with the drug are bedridden and are unaware of labyrinthine failure until they recover from their acute illness and attempt to ambulate. Then they discover that they are unsteady on their feet, the environment tends to jiggle in front of their eyes (oscillopsia), and they feel vertiginous. Younger patients adapt after some weeks to the labyrinthine failure; older patients may be permanently disabled. Usually there is no nystagmus, but the patient is ataxic. Caloric tests may demonstrate absence or hypoactivity of the labyrinth, and the Bárány rotation test may fail to elicit either vertigo or nystagmus.

Post-Traumatic Vertigo. Head injury may lead to benign positional vertigo or may produce a more vaguely described, rather constant feeling of dizziness or vertigo, usually associated with anxiety, difficulty in concentrating, headache, and phonophobia. Vertigo in this complex of symptoms called the *post-traumatic syndrome* is probably peripheral in origin, but its exact pathogenesis is unknown. The post-traumatic syndrome often follows a mild head injury, and the vague vertiginous feelings may persist for weeks or months.

Other Peripheral Causes of Vertigo. Vertigo may be an additional symptom in patients suffering from *sudden hearing loss*. The pathogenesis of the disorder is unknown, but may be vascular. Bacterial infection of the labyrinth or occasionally otitis media can cause vertigo, as can degenerative and genetic abnormalities of the labyrinthine system. *Cervical vertigo* is the term given to the vertiginous feelings associated with head movement in patients with cervical osteoarthritis or spondylosis. The disorder probably is caused by unbalanced input from cervical muscles to the vestibular apparatus. Acute neck strain may be occasionally associated with vertigo. Local anesthetics injected into one side of the neck can produce vertigo and ataxia by

a similar lack of balanced input. There is no nystagmus in these disorders.

Central Vertigo

Central causes of vertigo, less common than peripheral causes, are usually characterized by less severe vertigo than that resulting from peripheral lesions, absence of hearing loss and tinnitus, and concomitant neurologic signs of brainstem or cerebellar dysfunction. When central vertigo is usually accompanied by other neurologic signs or symptoms, the localization is strongly suggested by history and physical examination.

Cerebrovascular Disease. Vertigo accompanied by nausea and vomiting commonly accompanies ischemia, infarction, or hemorrhage affecting the brainstem or cerebellum. Occipital headache usually accompanies the symptoms, as do other neurologic signs suggesting brainstem or cerebellar dysfunction. Rarely, vertigo is the sole symptom of *transient ischemic attacks* of the brainstem, but most patients suffering such attacks will, if carefully questioned, report headache, diplopia, facial or body numbness, and ataxia as well. Even in the absence of other symptoms, however, in elderly patients with risk factors for cerebrovascular disease, such as hypertension, diabetes, heart disease, or hyperlipidemia, the possibility of posterior fossa vascular disease should be investigated.

Cerebellopontine Angle Tumors. Most tumors growing in the cerebellopontine angle (e.g., acoustic neuroma, meningioma) grow slowly, allowing the vestibular system to accommodate and thus usually producing a vague sensation of dysequilibrium rather than acute vertigo. Affected patients frequently complain of tinnitus, hearing loss, and a sensation of being pulled or pushed to one side when walking. Occasionally, episodic vertigo or positional vertigo heralds the presence of a cerebellopontine angle tumor. Virtually all such patients also have retrocochlear hearing loss.

Demyelinating Disease. Acute vertigo may be the first symptom of *multiple sclerosis*, although only a small percentage of young patients with acute vertigo eventually develop multiple sclerosis. Such central vertigo is often accompanied by nystagmus and other signs of brainstem dysfunction. A history of transient neurologic deficits suggests multiple sclerosis, and CT or, if available, magnetic resonance imaging may reveal demyelinating plaques. The presence of oligoclonal bands in the cerebrospinal fluid supports the diagnosis. Vertigo in multiple sclerosis is usually transient and often associated with other neurologic signs of brainstem disease, in particular internuclear ophthalmoplegia or cerebellar dysfunction. Vertigo may also be a symptom of *parainfectious encephalomyelitis* or, rarely, *parainfectious cranial polyneuritis*. In these instances, accompanying neurologic signs establish the diagnosis.

Cranial Neuropathy. A variety of acute or subacute illnesses affecting the eighth cranial nerve may produce vertigo as an early or sole symptom. The most common is *herpes zoster*. The *Ramsay Hunt syndrome (geniculate ganglion herpes)* is characterized by vertigo and hearing loss associated with facial paralysis and sometimes pain in the ear. The typical zoster lesions, which may follow the appearance of neurologic signs, are found in the external auditory canal and sometimes over the palate. Whether herpes zoster is ever responsible for vertigo in the absence of the full-blown syndrome is not certain. *Granulomatous meningitis* or *leptomeningeal metastases* and cerebral or systemic *vasculitis* may involve the eighth nerve, producing vertigo as an early symptom. In these disorders, cerebrospinal fluid analysis usually suggests the diagnosis.

Seizure Disorders. Patients suffering from temporal lobe epilepsy occasionally suffer vertigo as the aura. Vertigo in the absence of other neurologic signs or symptoms is never caused by epilepsy or other diseases of the cerebral hemispheres.

Other Central Causes. Many structural lesions of the brainstem or cerebellum, particularly if rapid in onset, may cause vertigo. In a few instances, *paraneoplastic brainstem* or *cerebellar degeneration* may be associated with vertigo. As with *brainstem tumors,* cerebellar degenerative diseases, and other structural disease of the brainstem and posterior fossa, there are usually other neurologic symptoms, and there are almost always signs of brainstem or cerebellar dysfunction in addition to the vertigo and nystagmus.

REFERENCES

Baloh, R. W.: Dizziness, Hearing Loss, and Tinnitus: The Essentials of Neurotology. Philadelphia, F. A. Davis Co., 1984.

Chiappa, K. H.: Evoked potentials in clinical medicine. New York, Raven Press, 1983.

Dyck, P. J., Thomas, P. K., Lambert, E. H., and Bunge, R. (eds.): Peripheral Neuropathy, Vols. I and II. Philadelphia, W. B. Saunders Co., 1984.

Glaser, J. S.: Neuro-ophthalmology. Hagerstown, Md., Harper & Row, 1978.

Johnson, E. W.: Practical electromyography. Baltimore, Williams and Wilkins, 1983.

Leigh, R. J., and Zee, D. S.: The Neurology of Eye Movements. Philadelphia, F. A. Davis Co., 1983.

Schaumberg, H., Spencer, P., and Thomas, P. K.: Disorders of Peripheral Nerves. Philadelphia, F. A. Davis Co., 1983.

Wall, P. D., and Melzack, R. (eds.): Textbook of Pain. New York, Churchill Livingstone, 1984.

The Autonomic Nervous System

The previous chapters have been concerned primarily with the methods by which the organism relates to and functions in its external environment. Most of these "somatic systems" are under voluntary control. The autonomic nervous system is primarily concerned with the task of maintaining a stable internal environment (called homeostasis by Cannon). It does this by controlling such vital functions as blood pressure, body temperature, ingestion of food and water, sexual function, and elimination of products of metabolism. As the name *autonomic* implies, the system is largely autonomous or independent of voluntary control. However, the division between autonomic and somatic nervous systems is neither anatomically nor functionally absolute. For example, both the somatic and autonomic nervous systems supply the urinary bladder, and although the bladder can function autonomously, the mature nervous system converts it into an organ essentially under voluntary control. The same is true of bowel and sexual function. Even those target organs that receive a pure autonomic nervous supply such as heart or blood vessels can be influenced by the cerebral cortex. Experiments in man have shown that individuals can exert some degree of control over blood pressure, utilizing biofeedback and conditioning techniques. However, despite these overlaps between the autonomic and somatic systems, and their close functional relationship, the two systems are in large measure anatomically and physiologically independent and are susceptible to different pathologic insults.

ANATOMY AND PHYSIOLOGY

GENERAL PRINCIPLES

The autonomic nervous system consists of the hypothalamus, the brainstem parasympathetic and spinal sympathetic and parasympathetic nuclei and their connections (Fig. 52). The hypothalamus can roughly be divided into endocrine and nonendocrine portions. The endocrine portions produce and secrete releasing factors that affect the pituitary gland and thus exert control over the entire endocrine system. The endocrine hypothalamus is discussed in detail in Section VIII of this book and will not be considered here except to indicate that there are close interconnections between it and the nonendocrine hypothalamus. At times the division is arbitrary. For example, water balance controlled by the hypothalamus through the release of antidiuretic hormone from the posterior pituitary is considered here as part of the autonomic or nonendocrine hypothalamus. The nonendocrine hypothalamus is part of the limbic system (see the following chapter) and has extensive connections with those portions of the temporal and frontal lobe that play an important role in emotion and behavior (Fig. 53). Descending influences from cerebral cortex (see below) impinge on the hypothalamus and other portions of the autonomic nervous system, but are not considered anatomically part of the system. Thus the hypothalamus stands between these biologically comprehensive, internally and externally directed regulatory mechanisms, serving as a kind of command post that receives afferent signals of visceral, somatic, and emotional need or sufficiency, then integrates the sum and translates the message to coordinate internal homeostasis with outward behavior.

Historically the autonomic system has been divided into two major efferent pathways—sympathetic and parasympathetic (Fig. 52). As indicated below, the sympathetic pathways have their final central nervous system cells of origin in the intermediolateral cell columns of the thoracolumbar spinal cord; and those of the parasympathetic pathways, in several cranial nerve nuclei and in the gray matter of the sacral spinal cord. Unlike the somatic motor system, the spinal cord autonomic neuron is not the final common path. There

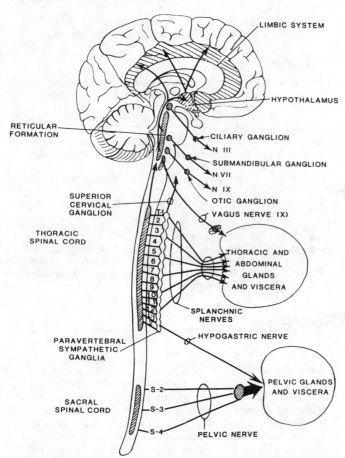

Figure 52. The major components of the autonomic nervous system. (From Daube, J. R., and Sandok, B. A.: Medical Neurosciences. Boston, Little, Brown and Co., 1978.)

is always a synapse and a peripheral ganglion before autonomic fibers reach their target organ.

The major target of postganglionic sympathetic and parasympathetic neurons is the smooth muscle of the viscera. Unlike skeletal muscle supplied by somatic nerves, there are no discrete neuromuscular junctions, the transmitter being released from varicosities at

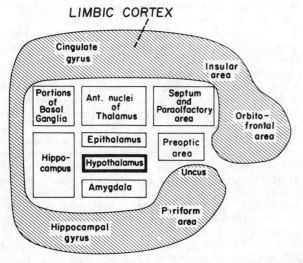

Figure 53. The limbic system.

various points along the axon. Some of these release sites lie very close to the muscle cell membrane while others are located at some distance. The result is that some smooth muscles are activated directly and others by a generalized diffusion of the transmitter. Thus, discharge of the autonomic nervous system cannot yield the fine point-to-point relationship possible in the somatic nervous system, but instead functions to produce a kind of mass action-like response.

Smooth muscle innervated by the autonomic nervous system is of two types: unitary and multiunit. Unitary muscles are characterized by spontaneous activity initiated in pacemakers within the tissue that spread throughout the whole muscle as if the muscle were a single unit. Such activity characterizes the smooth muscle of the gastrointestinal tract and uterus. Unitary smooth muscle is sensitive to stretch, responding with a contraction even when deprived of its nervous system innervation. The function of the autonomic nervous system is to coordinate and regulate spontaneous contractions of these organs. Multiunit smooth muscles are not spontaneously active, and each unit requires nervous innervation for contraction. Muscles supplying the iris, ciliary muscle, and some blood vessels are of the multiunit variety. Some smooth muscles do not fall clearly into one group or the other, but combine properties of both, and thus the division is not absolute.

Chemical Transmitters (Table 27)

Both sympathetic and parasympathetic systems synapse in peripheral ganglia with acetylcholine as the chemical transmitter. The systems differ, however, in that chemical transmission at the target organ from the sympathetic fibers is generally by norepinephrine and from the parasympathetic fibers by acetylcholine (Table 27). However, some sympathetic fibers, e.g., sweat glands, uterus, blood vessels of skeletal muscles and pilomotor muscles, are cholinergic rather than adrenergic. The adrenal gland (a modified sympathetic ganglion) secretes epinephrine as well as norepinephrine.

The action of chemical transmitters is determined not only by the structure of the chemical transmitter but also by the nature of the receptor it contacts. Acetylcholine receptors in autonomic ganglia have nicotinic properties, whereas acetylcholine receptors at the target organ are generally muscarinic (so classified by Dale because of the differing effects of the alkaloids nicotine and muscarine on the receptor). Most acetylcholine receptors of the central nervous system are muscarinic as well. The differences in muscarinic and nicotinic receptors have important clinical implications. Anticholinergic drugs such as atropine and scopolamine block muscarinic but not nicotinic receptors. As a result they produce parasympathetic paralysis (dilated pupils, tachycardia, absence of sweating) and, if they cross the blood-brain barrier as scopolamine does, abnormalities of memory and behavior. They do not, however, produce muscle weakness. Anticholinesterase drugs (e.g., prostigmine) enhance the action of acetylcholine at both muscarinic and nicotinic sites. Thus one of the side effects of the treatment of myasthenia gravis (see the chapter, Neurobiologic Essentials) is hyperactivity of the parasympathetic system leading to abdominal cramps, diarrhea, increased salivation, and visual blurring. Such side effects can often be ameliorated by the use of atropine-like drugs without any decrease in the salutary effects of increased muscle strength.

Adrenergic receptors are also of at least two types: alpha receptors stimulated mainly by norepinephrine are largely excitatory and lead to vasoconstriction, pupillary dilatation, and pilomotor contraction in the skin. Beta receptors stimulated by both epinephrine and norepinephrine are either excitatory or inhibitory and lead to vasodilatation of intramuscular blood vessels; relaxation of the duodenum, bronchi, and intestinal walls; and tachycardia. Alpha and beta receptors can each be subdivided into two or more different receptors having different properties. Alpha$_1$-receptors are postsynaptic, and alpha$_2$-receptors are presynaptic on the nerve terminal, probably inhibiting the release of neurotransmitter as a feedback mechanism. Beta$_1$-receptors are responsible for increased heart rate and contractility, whereas beta$_2$-receptors mediate relaxation of the smooth muscle of the bronchi and blood vessels. Pharmacologists have taken advantage of the difference in receptors to develop agents that act either as agonists or antagonists at specific receptors. One example is propranolol, an antagonist of beta-adrenergic receptors. The drug decreases heart rate and relaxes peripheral blood vessels, making it useful for the treatment of systemic hypertension. Other pharmacologic effects are summarized in Table 27.

Peptides

Small peptides seem also to act as neurotransmitters or, more likely, neuromodulators in the autonomic nervous system as they appear to do in the brain (see the chapter, Neurobiologic Essentials). Peptides such as vasoactive intestinal polypeptide, bombesin, substance P, and enkephalin are found in the gut as well as the brain and appear to modulate the effects of the autonomic nervous system on their target organs. Such peptide modulators may coexist in the same pair of terminals with the more classic neurotransmitter norepinephrine. Their exact function and relationship to the classic transmitters is not fully established.

Sympathetic and Parasympathetic Convergence

The sympathetic and parasympathetic nervous systems are separate in the central nervous system, but they converge at the end-organ, where they confer different properties. Historically it was believed that the two systems had opposite effects on the target organ, one being inhibitory and the other excitatory. In many instances this observation was true. Sympathetic nervous innervation dilates the pupil; the parasympathetic nervous system constricts it. Sympathetic fibers produce tachycardia; parasympathetic fibers (vagal) produce bradycardia. However, the system is more complicated than that. Some organs are supplied solely by the sympathetic or parasympathetic nervous system (e.g., sweat glands are sympathetic); in other organs the two systems may both be excitatory (increased release of saliva after either parasympathetic or sympathetic stimulation). Table 28 summarizes the differing effects of parasympathetic and sympathetic stimulation on the target organs that have both types of innervation.

CENTRAL PATHWAYS

Cerebral Cortex

Although the autonomic nervous system is generally accepted to begin in the hypothalamus, important pathways descend from the cortex that converge on the hypothalamus and on lower structures to exert control over the entire autonomic nervous system. The two major sites of cortical control of autonomic function are in the frontal lobe and in the limbic portions of the temporal lobe. Best understood are the frontal lobe pathways that originate anterior to the motor strip and exert inhibitory control over the detrusor muscle and probably over bowel function as well. Perurethral striated muscle appears to be represented more posteriorly, in the medial portion of the sensorimotor cortex. From the detrusor motor area there are reciprocal connections with the locus ceruleus of the autonomic nervous system via fibers that pass through the basal ganglia. These fibers have as their major function the inhibition of the micturition reflex (contraction of the detrusor muscle of the bladder and retraction of the internal sphincter); they probably also play a somewhat lesser role in control of both bowel and sexual function. Bilateral lesions of the premotor frontal lobes, such as sometimes occur with occlusion of the anterior cerebral arteries or rupture of an anterior communicating artery aneurysm, result in "urgency incontinence." This is characterized by a brief warning of bladder fullness followed by involuntary emptying of the bladder without ability to inhibit the detrusor reflex for more than a few seconds. Lesions in this area sometimes produce bowel incontinence and have also been reported occasionally to produce urinary retention. Stimulation of the medial sensorimotor cortex, such as occurs in epileptic attacks, may be associated with genital sensations (usually not erotic).

Less well defined pathways, also from the frontal lobe, occasionally affect the autonomic nervous system as well. Abnormalities of the frontal lobe may affect control of temperature, sweating, and blood flow contralaterally in the body, leading to hyperhidrosis, excess warmth or coolness, changes in color (redness or pallor), and even focal or generalized areas of edema. Ipsilateral and contralateral pupillary dilatation have been described with epileptic discharges from the frontal lobe. The effects of prefrontal cortex on behavior are described in the following chapter.

Fibers from the limbic portion of the temporal cortex also impinge on the autonomic nervous system. Stimulation of medial temporal cortex, especially around the amygdala, evokes changes in blood pressure, respiratory patterns, and behavioral patterns associated with fear or anger. Although the pathways are not clearly worked out, most of these effects are mediated through the autonomic nervous system.

Hypothalamus

The origin of the autonomic nervous system is in the hypothalamus (Fig. 54). The hypothalamus integrates input from the internal milieu both by receiving fibers from the visceral autonomic nervous system and by containing receptors that measure osmolality, body temperature, serum glucose concentration, and circulating hormone levels. The hypothalamus also has reciprocal connections with the limbic and frontal

TABLE 27. SOME PHARMACOLOGIC AGENTS OF RELEVANCE TO THE AUTONOMIC NERVOUS SYSTEM

SUBSTANCE	ACTIONS	SOME CLINICAL USES
Adrenergic Agents		
Noradrenaline: postganglionic adrenergic neurotransmitter (Levophed bitartrate)	Increased cardiac rate and excitability with little change in output. Constriction of blood vessels of muscle, skin, and viscera with increased total peripheral resistance. Increase in systolic and diastolic blood pressure. Stimulation of smooth muscle of pregnant uterus and sphincters, relaxation of smooth muscle of intestine and bladder with little effect on bronchi	In hypotension, by continuous infusion. An undue rise in blood pressure suggests denervation (and hence oversensitivity) of peripheral blood vessels
Adrenalin	Increase in heart rate, cardiac output, and cardiac excitability. Dilatation of vessels of skeletal muscle and heart. Constriction of vessels of skin and viscera. Total peripheral resistance decreased. Increase in systolic and decrease in diastolic blood pressure. CNS stimulation with tremor, anxiety, and increased respiration. General relaxation of smooth muscle with sphincter contraction	In cardiac arrest to increase excitability; also to reduce bleeding, and as a bronchodilator
Isoproterenol hydrochloride (Isuprel hydrochloride)	Increases cardiac output, relaxes smooth muscle, especially bronchial and gastrointestinal	As a bronchodilator; as a cardiac stimulant in heart block
Ephedrine	Similar to adrenalin but relatively greater effect on CNS causing tremor, anxiety, and insomnia	As a bronchodilator; also used in Stokes-Adams syndrome and narcolepsy
Dextroamphetamine (Dexedrine)	CNS stimulation; decreases appetite and may increase blood pressure	In depression, obesity, and narcolepsy
Metaraminol (Aramine)	Blood pressure elevation	For hypotension
Nylidrin hydrochloride (Arlidin)	Dilates skeletal muscle arteries, increases cardiac output and pulse rate	In peripheral vascular disease
Adrenergic Inhibiting Agents		
A. Alpha adrenergic blocking agents*		
Phenoxybenzamine, dibenzyline	Inhibition of vasoconstriction with increase in peripheral blood flow; tachycardia	Raynaud's syndrome, causalgia, and phlebitis; also has been used in acute hemorrhagic shock to limit deleterious vasoconstriction
Tolazoline (Priscoline)	Vasodilatation and cardiac stimulation; usually increased blood pressure	In Raynaud's syndrome, causalgia, phlebitis, and other peripheral vascular syndromes
Phentolamine	Vasodilatation usually with decreased blood pressure	In diagnosis of pheochromocytoma; also used in Raynaud's syndrome, causalgia, phlebitis, and other peripheral vascular syndromes
B. Beta adrenergic blocking agents		
Propranolol hydrochloride (Inderal)	Reduces rate and metabolism of heart	For angina, cardiac arrhythmias, circulatory disorders in tetanus, and benign essential tremor
C. Antiadrenergic agents		
Reserpine	Decrease in noradrenaline stores, blood pressure, and heart rate; sedative and tranquilizing effects	For hypertension
Methyldopa (Aldomet)	Decarboxylase inhibitor; decrease in blood pressure and heart rate	For hypertension
Cholinergic Agents		
Acetylcholine	The neurotransmitter for skeletal muscle, parasympathetic and sympathetic ganglia, postganglionic parasympathetic effector sites, adrenal medulla and certain postganglionic sympathetic effector sites; can cause either excitation or inhibition	As a test for integrity of postganglionic sympathetic fibers
Methylcholine	Similar to acetylcholine but less rapidly destroyed by cholinesterases	As a test for integrity of parasympathetic supply to the pupil
Carbachol	Similar to acetylcholine but unaffected by cholinesterases	For stimulation of bowel and bladder
Bethanechol chloride (Urecholine chloride)	Similar to carbachol	For stimulation of bowel and bladder
Pilocarpine	Similar to acetylcholine by direct action on autonomic effector cells and by ganglionic stimulation	In glaucoma

TABLE 27. SOME PHARMACOLOGIC AGENTS OF RELEVANCE TO THE AUTONOMIC NERVOUS SYSTEM (*Continued*)

SUBSTANCE	ACTIONS	SOME CLINICAL USES
Neostigmine methylsulfate (Prostigmine methylsulfate)	Inhibits acetylcholinesterase allowing acetylcholine to accumulate at cholinergic sites; may also have direct cholinomimetic action	In myasthenia gravis and myasthenic syndrome; for paralytic ileus, atonic bladder, and glaucoma
Ambenonium chloride (Mytelase)	Similar to neostigmine	In myasthenia gravis and the myasthenic syndrome
Edrophonium chloride (Tensilon chloride)	Similar to neostigmine	Diagnosis of myasthenia gravis and the myasthenic syndrome
Atropine sulfate (and other belladonna alkaloids and their synthetic substitutes)	Selective inhibition of muscarinic action† of acetylcholine, both excitatory (as in the heart) and inhibitory (as in the gut)	In hyperactive carotid sinus reflex, heart block, peptic ulcer, and acetylcholinesterase poisoning; also in parkinsonism and for motion sickness, gustatory sweating, and asthma; also for mydriasis
Hexamethonium chloride (Methium chloride)	Selective inhibition of neurotransmission in autonomic ganglia	In hypertension
Trimethaphan camphorsulfonate (Arfonad)	Similar to hexamethonium	To produce control of hypertension for brief period

Baker, A. B., and Baker, L. H. (eds.): Clinical Neurology, vol. 4. Philadelphia, Harper and Row, 1984.
*Most alpha blocking agents act selectively against *excitatory* effects of adrenergic nerves or agents. Beta blocking agents selectively block the *inhibitory* effect on most organs but block the excitatory effect on the heart.
†Muscarinic actions of acetylcholine are on structures innervated by postganglionic cholinergic nerves at parasympathetic effector sites plus the cholinergic sympathetic nerves.

lobes, as described above, as well as with the brainstem reticular formation. In general, anterior nuclei are concerned with parasympathetic activity and posterior nuclei with sympathetic activity. However, the tightly packed, interwoven contents of the hypothalamus make it difficult or impossible to assign specific signs and symptoms to any but a few local areas. Ventromedial and posteriorly located lesions tend to produce greater functional abnormalities than those located elsewhere, because their position inevitably interrupts fibers leading to the endocrine and descending autonomic nervous systems. Except when they affect unilateral descending sympathetic projections, clinically detectable changes in autonomic function due to hypothalamic disorders always imply the presence of bilateral lesions.

Brainstem and Spinal Cord

Descending pathways from the hypothalamus to the autonomic nervous system are largely ipsilateral and serve to influence both the sympathetic and parasympathetic nervous systems. The course taken by descending fibers from the hypothalamus through the brainstem and spinal cord is not entirely known. Most appear to descend in the lateral tegmentum of the midbrain, pons, and medulla, and then occupy the lateral aspect of the lateral columns of the spinal cord to synapse finally in the intermediolateral cell columns. Lesions in the lateral hypothalamus or lateral medulla produce sympathetic dysfunction characterized by Horner's syndrome (miosis from uninhibited parasympathetic constriction of the pupil, ptosis from the paralysis of the sympathetic elevator of the upper eyelid and depressor of the lower eyelid, and anhidrosis). Because these lesions are central and supply the entire sympathetic outflow, the anhidrosis involves the entire ipsilateral body. Bladder, bowel, and blood pressure functions, however, are rarely affected by unilateral lesions of the brainstem or cord.

PERIPHERAL PATHWAYS

The spinal and peripheral pathways of the sympathetic and parasympathetic nervous systems are illus-

trated in Figures 52 and 55. For both systems the efferent autonomic pathway consists of two neurons, a preganglionic myelinated neuron originating in the brainstem or spinal cord and exiting with cranial nerves or spinal roots to synapse with a cell in an autonomic ganglion. The postganglionic fibers are unmyelinated and synapse directly on the target organ. The systems differ in that the preganglionic sympathetic axons are short, synapsing near the site of exit from the spine (Figure 55). The postganglionic neurons travel long distances to reach the target organ. Conversely, parasympathetic preganglionic axons are long, the autonomic ganglia residing near the cell body, and the postganglionic axons are short.

Sympathetic System

The final central neurons of the sympathetic nervous system originate in the intermediolateral cell column of the thoracic and lumbar spinal cord, beginning at the first thoracic segment and ending at the first or second lumbar segment. These neurons have received suprasegmental projection from the cell bodies of the posterior and lateral hypothalamic areas and from brainstem catecholinergic neurons via reticulospinal projections. The axons of the sympathetic cell bodies in the intermediolateral cell column leave the spinal cord through the anterior root to enter a sympathetic ganglion that resides in the paravertebral space of each spinal segment. The entire chain of sympathetic ganglia is interconnected by the sympathetic trunk, carrying a mixture of preganglionic and postganglionic fibers, since some of the preganglionic fibers do not synapse in the sympathetic ganglion at the level of their spinal segment but instead traverse it to a ganglion closer to the target organ where they make their final synapse. For example, the pupillodilator fibers depart the spinal cord from the first and second thoracic segments but do not synapse until they reach the superior cervical ganglion close to the base of the skull (Fig. 52).

After synapsing, most ganglionic fibers generally travel with spinal nerves or sometimes with major

TABLE 28. SUMMARY OF THE INNERVATION AND FUNCTION OF MAJOR AUTONOMIC EFFECTORS

	PREGANGLIONIC NEURON	POSTGANGLIONIC NEURON	FUNCTION
Head Structures			
Eye: pupillary and ciliary muscles			
Sympathetic	Cord segments T1 to T2	Superior cervical ganglion	Pupillary dilation (mydriasis); accommodation for far vision
Parasympathetic	Edinger-Westphal nucleus (oculomotor nerve—III)	Ciliary ganglion	Pupillary constriction (miosis); accommodation for near vision
Lacrimal gland			
Sympathetic	Cord segments T1 to T2	Superior cervical ganglion	Vasoconstriction
Parasympathetic	Lacrimal part of superior salivatory nucleus (facial nerve—VII)	Sphenopalatine ganglion	Tear secretion and vasodilation
Parotid, submandibular, and sublingual salivary glands			
Sympathetic	Upper thoracic cord segments	Superior cervical ganglion	Salivary secretion (mucous, low enzyme, vasoconstriction)
Parasympathetic			
Parotid gland	Inferior salivatory nucleus (glossopharyngeal nerve—IX)	Otic ganglion	Salivary secretion (water, high enzyme, vasodilation)
Submandibular and sublingual glands	Superior salivatory nucleus (facial nerve—VII)	Submandibular ganglion	Same as above
Thoracic Viscera			
Heart			
Sympathetic	Cord segments T1 to T4	Upper thoracic to superior cervical chain ganglia	Acceleration of heart rate and force of contraction; coronary vasodilation
Parasympathetic	Dorsal motor nucleus (vagus nerve—X)	Cardiac plexus	Deceleration of heart rate and force of contraction; coronary vasoconstriction
Esophagus			
Sympathetic	Thoracic cord segments	Thoracic and cervical chain ganglia	Vasoconstriction
Parasympathetic	Dorsal motor nucleus (vagus nerve—X)	Intramural plexuses	Peristalsis and secretion
Lungs			
Sympathetic	Cord segments T2 to T6	Thoracic chain ganglia	Bronchial dilation
Parasympathetic	Dorsal motor nucleus (vagus nerve—X)	Pulmonary plexus	Bronchial constriction
Abdominal Viscera			
Stomach and intestine			
Sympathetic	Cord segments T5 to T12 (thoracic splanchnic nerves)	Celiac and superior mesenteric ganglia	Inhibition of peristalsis and secretion; sphincter contraction
Parasympathetic	Dorsal motor nucleus (vagus nerve—X)	Intramural plexuses	Peristalsis and secretion
Adrenal medulla			
Sympathetic	Cord segments T8 to T11 (thoracic splanchnic nerves)	The adrenomedullary cells are derived from neural crests but have no dendrites or axons. They are endocrine cells	Secretion of epinephrine and norepinephrine directly into the blood
Parasympathetic (none)			
Descending colon			
Sympathetic	Cord segments T12 to L2 (lumbar splanchnic nerves)	Inferior mesenteric ganglion	Inhibition of peristalsis and secretion; vasoconstriction
Parasympathetic	Cord segments S2 to S4 (pelvic splanchnic nerves)	Intramural plexuses	Peristalsis and secretion
Pelvic Viscera			
Sigmoid colon, rectum and anus, bladder, gonads and associated ducts and organs, and erectile tissue			
Sympathetic	Cord segments T12 to L2 (lumbar splanchnic nerves)	Inferior mesenteric ganglion (hypogastric nerves)	Inhibition of peristalsis and secretion; anal and bladder sphincter contraction; vasoconstriction; ejaculation
Parasympathetic	Cord segments S2 to S4 (pelvic splanchnic nerves)	Intramural or specific organ plexuses	Peristalsis and secretion; bladder detrusor muscle contraction; penile and clitoral erection

From Patton, H. D., Sundsten, J. W., Crill, W. E.,. and Swanson, P. D.: Introduction to Basic Neurology. Philadelphia, W. B. Saunders Co., 1976.

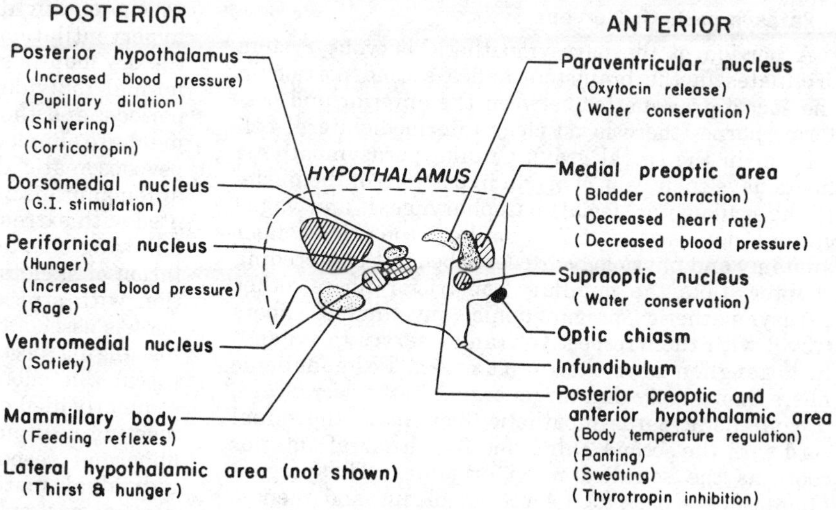

POSTERIOR

ANTERIOR

Posterior hypothalamus
(Increased blood pressure)
(Pupillary dilation)
(Shivering)
(Corticotropin)

Paraventricular nucleus
(Oxytocin release)
(Water conservation)

HYPOTHALAMUS

Medial preoptic area
(Bladder contraction)
(Decreased heart rate)
(Decreased blood pressure)

Dorsomedial nucleus
(G.I. stimulation)

Perifornical nucleus
(Hunger)
(Increased blood pressure)
(Rage)

Supraoptic nucleus
(Water conservation)

Optic chiasm

Ventromedial nucleus
(Satiety)

Infundibulum

Posterior preoptic and
anterior hypothalamic area
(Body temperature regulation)
(Panting)
(Sweating)
(Thyrotropin inhibition)

Mammillary body
(Feeding reflexes)

Lateral hypothalamic area (not shown)
(Thirst & hunger)

Figure 54. Autonomic control centers of the hypothalamus. (From Guyton, A. C.: Textbook of Medical Physiology, 5th ed. Philadelphia, W. B. Saunders Co., 1976.)

blood vessels to reach their respective target organs. Since there is no direct sympathetic outflow from the cervical, lower lumbar, or sacral spinal cord, the head and neck and abdominal and pelvic viscera that receive a sympathetic supply must do so through outflow from the thoracic ganglia. Abdominal and pelvic viscera are supplied by splanchnic nerves and the celiac, mesenteric, and hypogastric plexuses. Sympathetic fibers destined for the face and eye exit through the upper thoracic segments and travel through the sympathetic trunk to reach the superior cervical ganglia. There they synapse. The postganglionic fibers destined for the pupil follow the internal carotid artery and subsequently the ophthalmic nerve into the orbit. Postganglionic pseudomotor (sweat) fibers to the face follow the external carotid artery. The long course of sympathetic fibers to the head and neck from the thoracic vertebral bodies makes them susceptible to compression and damage by a variety of diseases (see Horner's syndrome in the preceding chapter).

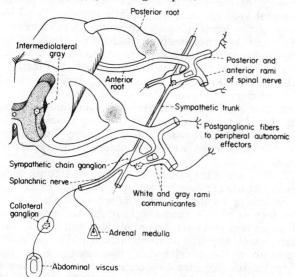

Posterior root

Intermediolateral gray

Posterior and anterior rami of spinal nerve

Anterior root

Sympathetic trunk

Postganglionic fibers to peripheral autonomic effectors

Sympathetic chain ganglion

Splanchnic nerve

White and gray rami communicantes

Collateral ganglion

Adrenal medulla

Abdominal viscus

Figure 55. The origin of the routes taken by the sympathetic preganglionic and postganglionic fibers. (From Patton, H. D., Sundsten, J. W., Crill, W. E., and Swanson, P. D.: Introduction to Basic Neurology. Philadelphia, W. B. Saunders Co., 1976.)

Afferent fibers concerned with the transmission of visceral sensation travel along either splanchnic or somatic nerves to reach the dorsal root ganglion, then follow the classic sensory pathways described in the preceding chapter. The functions of various portions of the sympathetic nervous system are outlined in Table 28. Local failure of autonomic function usually results from trauma interrupting sympathetic fibers or from tumors compressing them. As a result the sympathetic fibers are unable to carry out their normal functions. More rarely, when tumors compress the sympathetic trunk, there may be initial hyperactivity followed by failure of function. An example is the Horner's syndrome caused by tumors originating in the apex of the lung. Compression of the sympathetic trunk by the tumor usually leads to ptosis, miosis, and anhidrosis of the ipsilateral face and neck. There is also often slight reddening and increased temperature ipsilaterally on the face, a result of vasodilatation due to sympathetic failure. On occasion the development of the Horner's syndrome is preceded by a period of mydriasis and excessive sweating, the result of irritation of the sympathetic trunk or perhaps ephaptic conduction from partial demyelination (see the preceding chapter). Similarly, focal areas of increased sweating and piloerection on the trunk have been described with tumors compressing paravertebral sympathetic ganglia. A generalized loss of sympathetic function is usually characterized by severe problems of blood pressure control (p. 1133).

When postganglionic sympathetic fibers are disrupted, target organ receptors become supersensitive to their appropriate neurotransmitter. Thus with postganglionic sympathetic denervation, circulating or injected catecholamines may cause hyperactivity of the sympathetic nervous system. In fact, denervation hypersensitivity was first described by Cannon, based on his experiments with the sympathetic nervous system. Two clinical examples of such denervation hypersensitivity are the excessive mydriasis that occurs after instillation of dilute solutions of norepinephrine into the eye after postganglionic sympathetic denervation and the excessive rise in blood pressure that follows infusion of norepinephrine-like substances in some patients with Shy-Drager's syndrome (see below).

Parasympathetic Nervous System

A portion of the parasympathetic nervous system originates in the brainstem and a second portion in the sacral gray matter between the anterior and posterior horns (there is no clear intermediolateral cell column in the sacral gray). Cranial parasympathetic fibers have their cells of origin in portions of the nuclei of the oculomotor, facial, nasopharyngeal, and vagus cranial nerves (Fig. 52). Pupillary constrictor fiber anatomy and physiology are described in the preceding chapter. Like the pupillary constrictor fibers, other parasympathetic preganglionic myelinated fibers travel with their respective cranial nerves to synapse in a ganglion near the target organ. Postganglionic fibers then supply that target organ. In the sacral cord, preganglionic parasympathetic fibers leave the spinal cord with the second, third, and fourth sacral anterior roots as the so-called nervi erigentes. The preganglionic fibers pass to the vesical plexus and then to numerous ganglia in the walls of the bladder, rectum, and other pelvic organs to subserve the specific functions outlined in Table 28. More specific anatomy relating to abnormalities of bladder, bowel, and sexual function as affected by the parasympathetic nervous system is described below.

Parasympathetic afferents include those that carry baroreceptors, chemoreceptors, and stretch receptors from the lungs and the walls of the carotid artery, heart, and aorta to the CNS. These fibers are extremely important for the reflex control of circulation and respiration.

Like the sympathetic nervous system, denervation hypersensitivity also occurs in the parasympathetic nervous system. *Adie's or tonic pupil* is a disorder of unknown cause that affects postganglionic parasympathetic fibers to the pupil. The pupil dilates, and there is only a delayed or slow response to light stimulation or attempts at near vision. Distillation of dilute solutions of the parasympathomimetic agent, carbachol, produces prompt constriction of the parasympathetically denervated pupil, which does not occur in a normal pupil (such a response will also not occur if the pupil has been dilated by instillation of the parasympathetic blocking agent atropine, and this forms the basis for distinguishing a structural parasympathetic lesion causing pupillary dilatation from a chemical one). A therapeutic example occurs when parasympathetic denervation of the bladder leads to urinary retention. In some instances, injection of parasympathomimetic agents may restore partial bladder function. Because these agents are primarily muscarinic, they do not have an effect on receptors at the somatic neuromuscular junction.

PATHOPHYSIOLOGY OF AUTONOMIC DISORDERS

The autonomic nervous system may be affected by the wide range of pathophysiologic processes that affect other portions of the nervous system. Because of the close interconnections between the autonomic system and the emotional brain (limbic system), and the important functions of the autonomic system in controlling involuntary organs, emotional upset is often manifested through autonomic abnormalities (so-called psychosomatic disorders). The sweating, tachycardia, hyperventilation, and mydriasis that accompany fear; the dry mouth, sweaty palms, and diarrhea that many normal individuals suffer during school examination periods; and the blushing associated with embarrassment are simple, everyday examples of mild autonomic psychosomatic disorders. More severe, stress-related autonomic disorders include the incontinence associated with extreme fear, vasodepressor syncope (see the following chapter) associated with inappropriate dilatation of skeletal muscle blood vessels, gastric ulceration with stress, and constriction of coronary artery vessels associated with anger. As John Hunter said of his angina pectoris, "My life is in the hands of any rascal who chooses to annoy and tease me." (He subsequently died during an argument at a hospital board meeting.) Autonomic influences act in subtle ways, and abnormal responses to life stress are often highly individual matters, not easy to separate from the nervous system's routine adjustments to living. Clinical sensitivity to the possibility that the brain rather than the target organ sometimes causes the symptoms represents perhaps the most important first step in detecting pathologic autonomic adjustments to life stress.

Like the physiologic processes that lead to psychosomatic disorders, structural pathologic processes affecting the autonomic nervous system may be either focal or generalized. If the disease process is a focal one affecting only a part of the autonomic nervous system, autonomic signs and symptoms are usually accompanied by other abnormalities resulting from involvement of nearby neural or non-neural structures. Thus a focal lesion of the first thoracic root may cause Horner's syndrome, but Horner's syndrome is likely to be accompanied by motor and sensory loss in the hand and by pain in an upper thoracic distribution. Compression of the cauda equina leading to autonomic bladder and bowel dysfunction is likely to result in absence of ankle jerks and weakness in the small muscles of the feet as well as involvement of the external anal sphincter (a somatic muscle). Focal lesions of the hypothalamus often affect the endocrine as well as the nonendocrine hypothalamus; in addition, they commonly interrupt fibers passing from the cerebral cortex to the brainstem that mediate functions other than autonomic. Occasionally, focal lesions of the autonomic nervous system occur in isolation. Perhaps the best example is Horner's syndrome (see the chapter, Motor System), since the long course of preganglionic fibers through the neck places these fibers at a distance from other nonautonomic neural structures.

Except when they occur in the hypothalamus, focal lesions of the autonomic nervous system are rarely life threatening. Failure of sweating or vasoconstriction of the face or of one limb does not substantially affect homeostasis, and even loss of bladder and bowel function (which requires bilateral lesions of the parasympathetic system), although distressing, does not threaten life. An exception occurs with local lesions of the hypothalamus in which, as indicated below, abnormalities of salt and water balance as well as those of temperature control may be life threatening. Even here it is usually the neighborhood symptoms of endocrine failure and loss of consciousness that are more likely to threaten life than the autonomic symptoms themselves.

Generalized loss of autonomic function occurs in certain system degenerations (e.g., see autonomic insufficiency below) and can interfere with homeostasis to the point of being life threatening. Such disorders are uncommon but important to recognize because of their potential severity. In addition, diffuse, moderate sympathetic-parasympathetic dysfunction can accompany occasional cases of otherwise typical parkinsonism and is seen as a component of several of the late-life cerebellar or olivopontocerebellar degenerative disorders. Similarly, many elderly patients gradually lose the briskness of their autonomic reflexes and suffer an insidious decline in orthostatic circulatory control, sexual function, heat regulation, urinary and rectal sphincter continence, and bowel motility.

HYPOTHALAMIC DISORDERS

Most clinical disorders of the hypothalamus are focal and result from either mass lesions, such as tumors or abscesses, or vascular lesions, including hemorrhages and infarcts. Because most functions of the hypothalamus are bilaterally represented, a lesion of the hypothalamus has to be large and affect many structures other than the nonendocrine hypothalamus to produce autonomic dysfunction. The endocrine system and the fibers of passage controlling behavior and consciousness are examples of such structures. Rarely a mass lesion or a system disorder may predominantly affect a specific nucleus of the hypothalamus, leading to prominent loss of one or more autonomic functions.

Hunger and Satiety

The forebrain, especially the limbic system, provides a major influence on feeding behavior in man; hypothalamic disorders account for no more than a tiny fraction of human obesity or emaciation, making it all the more important to recognize when it occurs.

In experimental animals, stimulation of the ventromedian region of the hypothalamus inhibits feeding, whereas lesions destroying this region produce hyperphagia and weight gain that later stabilizes at a new elevated set point. The changes may be mediated by autonomic influences on the digestive tract and on insulin secretion to enhance appetite. Conversely, stimulation of the lateral hypothalamus induces feeding in excess of caloric requirement, whereas damage to the region results in a temporarily severe aphagia that slowly recovers to maintain chronically lowered body weight. Both hyperphagia and hypophagia due to hypothalamic dysfunction can occasionally be observed in man.

Hypothalamic Obesity. Most patients with hypothalamic obesity have shown at autopsy diffuse or large lesions of the structure. A few, however, have suffered from precisely placed abnormalities of the ventromedian hypothalamus. Examples include leukemic infiltration, with the most severe damage localized in the ventromedian region; others have consisted of discrete tumors in this area. Affected patients have experienced remarkable combinations of food-seeking behavior, including ravenous hyperphagia, decreased motor activity, and sometimes enormous obesity.

The hypothalamus integrates a set point that roughly regulates the individual's body weight. In patients who develop hypothalamic obesity, the continuation or remission of hyperphagia depends on whether (1) the neurologic abnormality is fixed and (2) the new disease-related set point for weight has been reached. Patients with obesity following brain surgery or severe closed head trauma that affects the hypothalamus illustrate this principle. Characteristically, such persons eat ravenously and gain weight quickly following the injury until they reach their new set point, at which time they become normophagic, and weight is stabilized at a new, higher set point.

Emaciation. Sometimes emaciation accompanies hypothalamic disease in man, but the associated lesions usually have been large and their specificity uncertain. Efforts to link hypothalamic disease and anorexia nervosa have been unsuccessful.

Temperature Regulation

The preoptic anterior hypothalamus contains separate receptors for warmth and cold as well as for pyrogens. Diurnal changes in central excitability and in the level of circulating ovarian hormones provide additional nonspecific stimuli. In turn, the hypothalamus activates varying combinations of behavioral autonomic and endocrine responses that conserve or dissipate body heat. Diseases in the region can be responsible for hypothermia or, rarely, hyperthermia.

Hypothermia (Relative Poikilothermia). Poikilothermia, defined as a fluctuation in body temperature of greater than 2° C with changes in ambient temperature, is the most common central abnormality of heat regulation in man. Most such cases are detected by a lowered body temperature. Poikilothermia results from damage to the posterior hypothalamus and rostral mesencephalon. Damage to this area impairs not only autonomic heat-regulating pathways but also those that control the sense of thermal discomfort and the behavioral regulation of body temperature as well. As a result, many patients with poikilothermia are unaware of this condition and do little to avoid it. At ordinary ambient temperatures of 20° to 25° C, the degree of hypothermia tends to be proportional to the degree of functional hypothalamic impairment. Relative poikilothermia resulting from impaired hypothalamic-autonomic function frequently affects elderly persons (senile hypothermia), making them dangerously susceptible to lowered environmental temperatures. Chronic poikilothermia also accompanies several degenerative disorders that affect the hypothalamus in children and adults. Poikilothermia regularly follows extensive damage to the posterior hypothalamus or midbrain by stroke, trauma, neoplasm, encephalitis, or thiamine deficiency. Such central hypothermia must be differentiated from that caused by metabolic disorders such as acute or chronic sedative drug ingestion, hypoglycemia, and myxedema.

Paroxysmal Hypothermia. Sustained hypothermia (as opposed to relative poikilothermia) is rare in humans. Less uncommon is paroxysmal hypothermia, consisting of attacks of lowered body temperature that vary widely in frequency from daily to more than a decade apart. Such attacks usually begin abruptly, last from minutes to days, and are characterized by sweating, flushing of the skin, and a fall in body temperature, usually to 32° C or lower. Fatigue, decreased mental responsiveness, hypoventilation, hypotension, cardiac arrhythmias, ataxia, lacrimation, and asterixis may accompany the temperature drop. The attacks subside either slowly (hours to days) or rapidly with shivering and peripheral vasoconstriction. During hypothermia, mechanisms for both heat production and heat dissipation respond normally, but around a lower temperature set point. Most affected patients have had direct evidence for hypothalamic disease; several have suffered from congenital agenesis of the corpus callosum. In some instances, anticonvulsant therapy stops the attacks.

Hyperthermia. Chronic fever never results fromn hypothalamic disease, and even acute neurogenic fever is rare. The most frequent causes of acute neurogenic hyperthermia include gross head injury, surgical trauma, or spontaneous bleeding into the region of the anterior hypothalamus, and hemorrhage in the adjacent meninges or the third ventricle. With neurogenic hyperthermia the body temperature can rise to potentially fatal levels of 42° C or higher as a result of active heat production unbalanced by heat dissipation. The cardiovascular changes that normally accompany fever are disproportionately lacking. If standard cooling measures fail, small (2 mg) doses of morphine can ameliorate neurogenic fevers in which the temperature is dangerously high.

Salt and Water Balance (see also Section X)

The hypothalamus controls body water content and osmolality via coordinated mechanisms regulating affective thirst, drinking behavior, and the release of antidiuretic hormone (ADH) via the paraventricular and supraoptic nuclei. Hypothalamic or limbic system disease can produce four principal disorders of water balance, including ADH deficiency (diabetes insipidus), inappropriate ADH secretion, neurogenic (essential) hypernatremia, and episodic hyperdipsia. Osmoreceptors and volume receptors appear to reside in different areas of the hypothalamus. Osmoreceptors and central thirst receptors have been identified within the preoptic region. These respond to afferent stimulation from peripheral thirst receptors as well as to local sodium concentrations and circulating levels of the peptide angiotensin. Volume receptors appear to lie more laterally in the hypothalamus and project to the PV and SO nuclei by pathways different from those that carry osmoreceptor signals. Peripherally, thirst is stimulated or quenched by signals arising from receptors lying within the mouth and interstitial fluids, while different receptors arising from heart, large-capacitance systemic veins, and carotid baroreceptors signal volume control needs. Differential peripheral stimulation of the two systems or selective damage to the central osmoreceptor-thirst area explains some examples of inappropriate ADH secretion and most if not all cases of neurogenic (essential) hypernatremia.

Neurogenic (Essential) Hypernatremia. This disorder is marked by four features: (1) elevated plasma sodium level unaccompanied by circulating volume deficiency, (2) preserved renal tubular responsiveness to ADH, (3) inadequate secretion of ADH in response to osmotic stimuli, and (4) the absence or deficiency of appropriate thirst (hypodipsia) despite otherwise rela-

tively normal conscious behavior. True essential hypernatremia is rare; most cases of serum hyperosmolarity accompanying intracranial disease result from a nonspecific combination of dehydration and stupor-impaired drinking behavior.

Essential hypernatremia in its milder and more chronic forms often elevates the plasma sodium only modestly, and such patients characteristically lack symptoms except for a remarkable absence of thirst. Close attention often discloses considerable fluctuation in daily sodium values above the 150 mEq/l mark. When sodium levels climb to the range of 160 to 170 mEq/l, affected patients develop weakness and sometimes fever as well as muscle tenderness and cramping that may progress to fatigue, ataxia, and even myoglobinuria. Mental symptoms include lethargy, anorexia, depression, and irritability. With elevations of serum sodium above 180 mEq/l, most patients become confused or stuporous, and some will die. Patients with essential hypernatremia fail to experience thirst, but many retain persistent habitual drinking, although at a volume insufficient to maintain normal serum osmolality. They commonly lack clinical evidence of dehydration; only mild hypovolemia or even normovolemia can accompany serum sodium levels as high as 200 mEq/l or more. Associated hypokalemia usually contributes to the muscular symptoms. Urine volumes may be low or normal, but are always more dilute than appropriate for the serum hyperosmolality. The administration of exogenous ADH induces a more concentrated urine. Either an acute water load or a hypertonic saline load, however, can produce an increase in free water clearance, reflecting the failure of central osmoreceptors to respond to the latter stimulus.

The hypothalamic defect that produces essential hypernatremia is inexactly localized. Almost all affected patients have had associated neurologic or endocrine abnormalities, but many lack radiographic evidence of central nervous system abnormalities. Some give a history of diffuse head trauma, while in others space-occupying lesions destroy the entire hypothalamic region by the time of death. In a few patients, restricted tumors have involved the preoptic and tuberal region. The mechanisms of essential hypernatremia remain unsettled. The absence of thirst is critical, and this, along with direct measurements showing that serum vasopressin levels fail to increase when sodium levels rise but fall when blood volume increases, indicate either that osmoreceptor function is selectively uncoupled from the behavioral and hormonal control of water balance or that mechanisms that regulate natriuresis are distinct from ADH control.

Hyperdipsia and Self-Induced Water Intoxication. Excessive water drinking in the absence of either hypovolemia or serum hyperosmolality is termed primary hyperdipsia and must be differentiated from the compensatory hyperdipsias of conditions such as diabetes insipidus, diabetes mellitus, or polyuric renal failure. In the absence of inappropriate ADH secretion, symptoms of severe hyperdipsia, i.e., hypervolemia, hyponatremia, and clinical water intoxication accompanied by stupor, delirium, and convulsions, are infrequent. The problem never arises, to our knowledge, as the result of primary central nervous system disease. Most severe hyperdipsia occurs in persons with acute psychiatric disorders who drink excessively to overcome delusional fears. Occasionally, acute water intoxication occurs in alcoholics with gastritis or in youngsters drinking huge amounts of fluids on a dare, e.g., during ritual hazing or tea-party games.

BRAINSTEM, SPINAL, AND PERIPHERAL AUTONOMIC DISORDERS

Abnormalities of the autonomic nervous system can have their effects on many organs of the body. The abnormalities commonly encountered in clinical practice are those of bladder and bowel dysfunction, sexual dysfunction, abnormalities of cardiovascular regulation (cardiac rhythm and blood pressure), and abnormalities of sweating. Autonomic respiratory abnormalities are less common than the above. Pupillary disorders, although common, rarely cause major symptoms.

Bladder and Bowel Dysfunction

The bladder is a hollow pelvic structure composed of the interlacing smooth muscle fibers of the detrusor covered by its internal mucous membrane and outer serosa. The smooth muscle and its resistance to stretch are determined predominantly by the viscoelastic properties of its wall rather than by direct neurogenic mechanisms. With progressive filling of the bladder, the normal intravesical pressure rises slowly, remaining below about 15 cm of water until average capacities, between 400 and 600 ml, are reached, at which point the intravesical pressure rises either abruptly, owing to the onset of the micturition reflex, or more gradually, owing to reaching the elastic limits of the wall itself. Normal adult micturition volumes average between 200 and 400 ml, but with acute urinary retention the structure can stretch abnormally to accommodate 1 liter or more, while chronic infection and hypertrophy may contract it to a capacity of no more than 60 to 100 ml.

Urine enters the bladder from the paired ureters and normally leaves via the membranous urethra. In both sexes the lower detrusor musculature joins with elastic tissue to form an involuntary internal sphincter that normally can resist passively induced intra-abdominal–intravesical pressures as high as 150 mm Hg. The more distal urethra is encircled by voluntarily controlled striated muscle innervated by the somatomotor pudendal nerve. More competent in men than in women, this external sphincter can withstand briefly the intraurethral detrusor-induced pressure of normal micturition, but is unnecessary to normal urinary continence.

The act of voiding represents a stretch-induced parasympathetic reflex of smooth muscle facilitated by brainstem and spinal mechanisms, normally inhibited or released by forebrain regulatory influences. The actual neuromuscular sequence consists of initial voluntary relaxation of the skeletal muscle of the pelvic floor followed by the disinhibited reflex discharge, which contracts the detrusor, assimilates and relaxes the musculoelastic tissue of the internal sphincter, and empties the organ by a fusion of successive detrusor contractions.

The complete reflex mechanism for micturition exists within the spinal cord (Fig. 56). The afferent route of the arc depends upon fibers that originate in stretch receptors in the bladder wall and travel centrally via

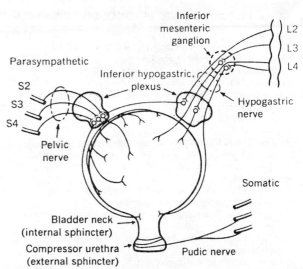

Figure 56. Somatic and autonomic motor innervation of urinary bladder showing possible interconnections permitting sympathetic-parasympathetic neuron interactions in hypogastric ganglia and plexuses. (From Koizumi, K., and Brooks, C. M.: The autonomic system and its role in controlling body functions. In Mountcastle, V. B. (ed.): Medical Physiology, 14th ed. St. Louis, C. V. Mosby Co., 1980, p. 912.)

sacral roots 2 to 4. Efferent preganglionic fibers arise in the lateral columns of the sacral segments of the conus medullaris, whence they travel in the cauda equina to and through the lower sacral foramina to synapse with their final ganglia over the outer surface of the bladder and the region of the proximal urethra. Centrally, afferent proprioceptive signals travel rostrally via the lemniscal system, while descending inhibitory influences originate in the paramedian prefrontal cerebral cortex. These latter pathways are joined in the brainstem and upper spinal cord by reflex-facilitating fibers that enhance complete reflex bladder emptying. The pathway descends in the spinal cord within the lateral funiculus to synapse upon the sacral preganglionic neurons. Sympathetic fibers to the bladder originate in the lower thoracic and upper lumbar intermediolateral cell column and reach the bladder via the hypogastric nerves and inferior hypogastric ganglia. Sympathetic fibers innervate the proximal urethra and the bladder, but their primary effects are on blood vessels in the bladder wall. The hypogastric nerves also carry some afferent pain fibers from the bladder wall.

Cerebral Disturbances in Micturition (Table 29). Damage to the bilateral prefrontal area lowers the micturition reflex threshold, resulting in a proportionately smaller bladder capacity. The chief symptoms are sudden, sometimes uncontrollable urgency with moderately large volumes, usually of less than 250 ml, but complete bladder emptying. The cystometrogram shows a normal bladder pressure–volume filling curve but a reduced micturition reflex threshold, with a comparably reduced threshold to filling sensation. Clinical evaluation or computed tomography of the head readily discloses evidence of structural frontal lobe disease.

Dementia leads to incontinence of indifference (a loss of bladder training) in which visceral physiology remains intact but social restraints depart. Patients

TABLE 29. NEUROGENIC BLADDER DISTURBANCES

Incontinence
Stress: Small volumes, brief urgency, women more than men
  Normal in 50 per cent of giggling girls
  Multiparas with cystocele, other outflow damage
  Increases with normal aging
Retention-overflow: Dribbling or small volumes, pain in pelvis
  or flanks, palpable bladder
  Causes as listed with retention
  Severe cystitis (small bladder volume)
Confusional: Small or large volumes, usually shameless
"Spastic": Large volumes, sporadic occurrence, prominent
  urgency, emptying complete
  Prefrontal lesions
  Extramedullary advanced spinal compression
  Occasionally partial outlet obstruction
  Circumstance: Bedridden or crippled elderly with facilities
    remote
Spinal: Moderate volumes, brief urgency, frequent occurrence,
  high residual urine
  Intramedullary cervical-thoracic-lumbar lesions (multiple
    sclerosis, neoplasms, etc.)
  Occasionally with partial peripheral denervation

Retention
Acute or chronic outflow obstruction
Acute neurologic disease
  Peripheral: Autonomic polyneuropathy, pelvic trauma, cauda
    equina compression, conus lesions
  Central: Poliomyelitis, spinal transection
Drugs (usually plus local structural problems)
  Anticholinergics, antidepressants, opiates
Psychogenic
Postanesthetic

with severe physical disabilities such as hemiplegia and advanced arthritis may develop pseudoincontinence because of difficulty in reaching the toilet or, occasionally, as a depressed, angry and frustrated response to the limitations of their condition.

Spinal Disturbances of Micturition. Gradual extramedullary spinal cord compression produces few changes in bladder function until late in the course when the reflex is facilitated along with somatic motor reflex pathways. Urgency with moderately reduced voiding volumes results. Incontinence occurs only with advanced or sudden cord compression. Intramedullary spinal lesions can directly affect the descending parasympathetic pathways, releasing the reflex from higher inhibition and impairing brainstem-originating pathways that facilitate complete detrusor emptying. The reflex threshold drops and urgency frequency with moderate volumes results, often leaving a high post-voiding residual volume. Sporadic reflex incontinence is common.

Acute spinal transection produces reflex inhibition in the distal segment (spinal shock), with loss of voiding reflexes as well as of somatomotor ones. Acute retention develops, stretching the smooth muscle wall and producing a flat pressure-volume curve with no reflex. Overflow dribbling incontinence ensues. Reflex recovery is marked by increasingly large, randomly spaced, reflex partial bladder emptyings that in many instances can be trained by skill and patience into complete self-stimulated reflex voidings.

Peripheral (Preganglionic or Somatic Afferent) Defects in Voiding. These can result from disease of either efferent or afferent peripheral nerves (e.g., oc-

casional inflammatory neuropathy, diabetic neuropathy, tabes dorsalis, pelvic carcinoma), of the cauda equina, or of the conus medullaris. Depending upon the rate of neuritic progression, the bladder gradually dilates, with sensations of fullness disappearing commensurately with the degree of mechanical stretching, or vice versa. Normal sensations of urgency disappear, and the reflex progressively loses its effectiveness. Residual urine volumes increase. Ultimately, moderate to severe retention occurs, with or without spontaneous dribbling or occasionally with spurting, small-volume, overflow incontinence. In the absence of cystitis, the cystometrogram shows a flat filling curve on which, in time, autonomous ganglion-induced local detrusor contractions increasingly become superimposed. Spontaneous parasympathetic activity eventually leads to nearly continuous autonomous local detrusor activity, producing a hypertrophied bladder wall with decreased bladder capacity and a steep pressure-volume curve.

Disturbances of Bowel Function. Bowel innervation is similar in many respects to that of the bladder. Parasympathetic stimulation contracts the rectal musculature but relaxes the internal sphincter. The voluntarily controlled external sphincter of the anus, which is supplied by the pudendal nerve, enables reflex evacuation to be resisted voluntarily. Similar to the bladder, when the rectum is distended with feces, there is reflex contraction of the rectum leading to a defecation reflex. Disorders of bowel function are similar to those of bladder function, and since the central and peripheral pathways are proximate, an affected patient often suffers from both disorders. The most common symptom of bowel dysfunction is constipation, although incontinence can occur in the same disorders that result in incontinence of urine.

Sexual Dysfunction

Disorders of sexual function are common in both male and female. Relatively little is known of the pathophysiology of sexual dysfunction in the female. Organic disturbances of *male* sexual function are limited almost entirely to loss of libido, failure to attain an erection of sufficient strength to carry out sexual intercourse (impotence), and failure to attain normal ejaculation-emission. Masters and Johnson define impotence somewhat generously as greater than a 25 per cent failure during attempted intercourse. Failure to reach orgasm or the presence of premature or delayed ejaculation with normal libido and erectile capacity almost always reflects a psychogenic rather than an organic problem.

Neural control over male sexual activities arises within forebrain limbic areas, generating sexual drives that, in turn, are chronically stimulated by the effects of circulating androgens (Fig. 57). Descending pathways travel with the parasympathetic outflow. Parasympathetic sacral efferents control penile tumescence by inducing vascular engorgement and also stimulate a large proportion of the severally originating pelvic contractions that initiate ejaculation and lead to the sensation of orgasm. Concurrently, sympathetic stimulation contracts the seminal vesicles and closes the bladder neck to prevent retrograde emission, thereby guaranteeing anterograde ejaculation. Genital sensory fibers reach the spinal cord via the S2 to S4 dorsal roots and thenceforth ascend in the lemniscal system.

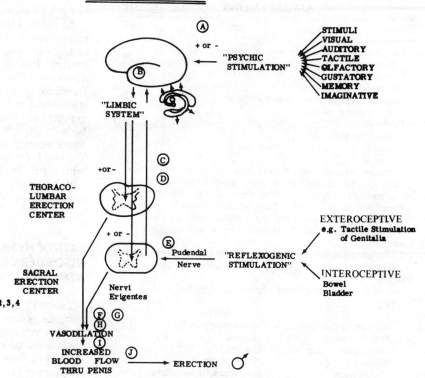

HUMAN PENILE ERECTION

Figure 57. The pathways involved in human penile erection. A to J = potential sites of lesions that could cause erectile dysfunction. (From Weiss, H. D.: The physiology of human penile erection. Ann Intern Med 76:793–799, 1972.)

Considerable evidence gained from the study of sexual function in paraplegics with an isolated, distal thoracic and lumbosacral spinal cord indicates that the cord contains all the necessary reflexes to complete sensory-induced erection and ejaculation.

Male impotence is common and increases with age to affect at some time almost half the population over 55 years; at that age psychogenic causes appear to be primary in only about 25 per cent. Therapeutic drugs and alcohol excess represent the most frequent causes of male impotence. Aging itself, however, eventually becomes a cause, and about 25 per cent of males of 70 years or more have erection failure attributable to aging alone.

Impotence has several possible causes, as indicated in Table 30, and more than one can operate in a given patient. In perhaps 10 per cent of cases no satisfactory explanation can be found. Psychologic factors are always important. They account for as many as half of the overall cases and must be inquired into carefully even when adequate organic reasons appear to exist.

Sweating Abnormalities

Anhidrosis, a relatively uncommon complaint, occurs as part of a rare, probably autosomal recessive, disorder in which it is associated with congenital insensitivity to pain. Anhidrosis due to congenital absence of the sweat glands is similarly rare. Anhidrosis also follows preganglionic or postganglionic sympathetic denervation produced by disease or surgical procedures and can occur in the appropriate territorial distribution of any diseased or damaged peripheral nerve.

Hyperhidrosis, defined as sweating in excess of apparent thermal requirements, is a common response to anxiety, especially among persons less than 30 years old. Longstanding severe hyperhidrosis causing constantly dripping hands and feet is an uncommon but socially troublesome disorder of unknown cause. Emotional factors seem to contribute little. Severe cases can be relieved by sympathectomy directed at the most affected areas, usually the upper extremities. The procedure is best limited to either the upper or lower extremities, since compensatory accentuation of preexisting sweating tends to affect nondenervated parts. Total sympathectomy produces too many undesirable side effects to be recommended. Hyperhidrosis localized to a particular body part occasionally occurs in association with irritation of the related preganglionic fibers or ganglia by an infection or neoplasm and deserves careful attention from that standpoint.

Cardiovascular Dysfunction

The autonomic system exerts profound effects on the cardiovascular system via both sympathetic and parasympathetic connections to heart and blood vessels. The afferent portion of the autonomic nervous system plays a major role in regulating blood pressure through baroreceptors in the great vessels and heart. Thus the autonomic nervous system plays a role in the pathogenesis of hypertension, tachyarrhythmias (sympathetic system), and bradyarrhythmias (vagal nerve) and probably in coronary artery disease. Markedly increased sympathetic outflow from the brain sometimes occurs with seizures or subarachnoid hemorrhage and produces enough vasoconstriction of coronary vessels to lead to ECG changes suggestive of ischemia as well as small areas of ischemic infarction in the myocardium. Among the diseases classically considered neurologic, the most common cardiovascular manifestation of autonomic dysfunction (except for syncope, see the following chapter) is the postural hypotension that accompanies autonomic insufficiency. This disorder is described in detail subsequently. Fail-

TABLE 30. PRINCIPAL ORGANIC CAUSES OF MALE SEXUAL FAILURE

Drugs
Endocrine
  Secondary: pituitary adenoma; idiopathic or acquired
    hypogonadotropic hypogonadism; hyperprolactinemia
  Primary gonadal failure
  Advanced diabetes mellitus
  Hypothyroidism, hyperthyroidism (rare)
Chronic systemic illnesses
  Cirrhosis
  Chronic renal failure
  Disseminated malignant disease, etc.
Neurogenic
  Temporal lobe disorder, trauma, epilepsy, neoplasm, stroke
  Intramedullary spinal lesions, paraplegia; demyelinating
    disorders; neoplasms; syrinx; Shy-Drager dysautonomia
  Peripheral nerve disorders. Somatic or autonomic
    neuropathies; pelvic neoplasms; granulomas, trauma,
    structural lesions of cauda equina or conus medullaris
Urologic
  Complete prostatectomy; priapism; local trauma or neoplasms;
    Peyronie's disease; rectosigmoid "cleanouts"
Vascular
  Severe aortic atherosclerosis; lower aortic bypass
  Drugs:

Alcohol	Guanethidine
Anticancer chemotherapy	Immunosuppressives
Anticholinergics	Lithium
Antiparkinson agents	Opiates
Barbiturates and	Phenothiazine
congeners	Several antihypertensive
Benzodiazepines	ganglionic blockers
Bethanidine	Several diuretics
Cannabis	Tricyclic and MAO-inhibitor
Cimetidine	antidepressants

ure of blood pressure regulation leading to postural hypotension similar to that of idiopathic autonomic insufficiency also accompanies some of the peripheral neuropathies, particularly those that accompany diabetes and amyloidosis, and sometimes an acute probably autoimmune polyneuropathy called acute pandysautonomia.

TESTS OF AUTONOMIC FUNCTION

As with other aspects of neurologic disease, the physician learns most about a given patient's disease of the autonomic nervous system by taking a careful history. Psychosomatic disorders as well as structural disorders affecting bladder and bowel function, sexual function, or blood pressure control can often be exquisitely localized by a detailed history of the patient's symptoms. When that history is combined with a bedside examination, most of the information relevant to autonomic nervous system disease can be obtained. Table 31 details tests of autonomic function, most of which can be performed at the bedside but a few of which require the assistance of a radiologic or clinical chemistry laboratory.

PATHOPHYSIOLOGY OF SPECIFIC DISORDERS OF THE AUTONOMIC NERVOUS SYSTEM

Table 32 lists some specific syndromes of autonomic nervous system diseases. In many of the disorders the pathophysiology and even the pathologic locus of the disease is unknown. Some of the disorders are described in detail elsewhere in this chapter or in other chapters of this section.

HYPOTHALAMIC SYNDROMES

Diabetes insipidus resulting from destruction of the supraoptic paraventricular neurons or their axons generally is caused by tumors involving the pituitary or hypothalamus or trauma to that area. Although rare, idiopathic diabetes insipidus as a result of specific failure of these nuclei has been reported. The converse of diabetes insipidus is *inappropriate ADH secretion* resulting in excessive retention of water despite continued renal secretion of sodium (see Section X). This results in hypo-osmolality of the serum, which if severe

TABLE 31. TESTS OF AUTONOMIC FUNCTION

I. *Parasympathetic*
  A. *Pupil.* Reflex arc: CN II → Edinger-Westphal nucleus → CN III → ciliary ganglion. Dysfunction: absence of responses to light and accommodation. Test for denervation hypersensitivity using 2.5% Mecholyl eye drops: Normally there is no pupillary change but with postganglionic denervation the pupil constricts (Adie's pupil).
  B. *Lacrimation.* Reflex arc: CN V → superior salivatory nucleus → CN VII → sphenopalatine ganglion → lacrimal n. Produce reflex tearing by repeatedly touching the cornea with a cotton wisp or have the patient sniff an irritating substance such as ammonia. Tearing is present in postgeniculate lesions, but may be absent in pregeniculate lesions of the peripheral facial nerve. Tearing can be quantified by inserting one end of an absorbent paper strip into each conjunctival sac (Schirmer tear test).
  C. *Salivation.* Reflex arc: CN VII → superior salivatory nucleus → CN VII → chorda tympani → lingual nerve → submaxillary ganglion. Inspect the submaxillary duct for salivary production after having the patient suck or chew a lemon. Reflex salivation may be absent in pregeniculate or postgeniculate salivary lesions, or in CN VII lesions, but may be preserved if the lesion is distal to the branching of the chorda tympani.
  D. *Heart rate.* Reflex arc: CN IX → dorsal motor nucleus of CN X → vagus nerve → cardiac ganglia → SA and AV nodes.
    1. *Carotid sinus massage.* Gently massage unilaterally the area of the carotid bifurcation and simultaneously monitor the heart rate. Up to 30% of young people will have no change in heart rate. Older persons and hypertensives often have marked slowing. The vagal type of carotid sinus hypersensitivity is marked by asystole.
    2. *Standing.* Have the patient stand; note the heart rate change. Normal response is a 10 to 20 beats per minute increase. Young persons generally have a more marked response than the elderly. The increase in standing heart rate may be absent in autonomic insufficiency.

TABLE 31. TESTS OF AUTONOMIC FUNCTION (*Continued*)

      3. *Atropine.* 1.0 mg atropine IV normally increases the heart rate from 30 to 40 beats per minute. In autonomic insufficiency the response may be less.

  E. *Gastrointestinal tract.* Parasympathetic lesions (e.g., diabetic neuropathy) may result in abnormal motility. Barium study is useful in documenting abnormal retention and motility patterns, particularly in small bowel. Insulin hypoglycemia results in an increase in gastric acidity. This response is absent in autonomic insufficiency.

  F. *Bulbocavernous reflex.* Reflex arc: squeezing of the glans penis elicits reflex contraction of the bulbocavernous muscle.

  G. *Anal sphincter reflex.* Evaluate anal sphincter on rectal examination.

II. *Sympathetic*

  A. *Pupil* (see preceding chapter). Cocaine Test: Failure of one pupil to dilate after instillation of 4% cocaine into the conjunctival sac indicates sympathetic denervation (cocaine prevents reuptake of normally released transmitter).

  B. *Blood pressure regulation.* Blood pressure is a balance between vasoconstrictor and vasodilator action on the arterioles.

    1. *Carotid sinus massage.* Normal: Systolic drop of less than 10 mm Hg in young persons, increased response in hypertensives and the elderly. Marked drop in the vasodepressor form of carotid sinus sensitivity (increased baroreceptor sensitivity due to arteriosclerosis).

    2. *Postural response.* Take the blood pressure with patient supine and after standing. Erect posture normally gives a mean pressure rise of 5 mm Hg. With advancing age the diastolic rise is abolished, and the systolic fall is more pronounced. Sitting has less effect and cannot be substituted for standing or tilting. Prior hyperventilation may accentuate postural hypotension.

    3. *Mechanical phlebotomy.* Inflate thigh cuffs to subdiastolic pressure for 10 minutes. Normal persons show a mean pressure reduction of less than 10 mm Hg. In autonomic insufficiency there is a gradual but steady pressure fall.

    4. *Valsalva maneuver.* Have the patient expire against a closed glottis for 20 to 30 seconds. Monitor the blood pressure to assess the fall in pulse pressure. Within 30 seconds after release of forced expiration there should be a reactive overshoot of diastolic blood pressure that is roughly proportional to the pulse pressure reduction during forced expiration. The overshoot may be absent with autonomic insufficiency, heart failure, or reduced blood volume.

    5. *Cold pressor reflex.* Reflex arc: Spinothalamic tract → suprapontine but infrathalamic central relay → descending sympathetic pathways. Place the patient's hand to the wrist in ice water (4° C) for 1 minute. Take blood pressure every 30 seconds. The average normal response is a blood pressure increase of 16–20/12–15 mm Hg. Response is minimal, absent, or inverted in autonomic insufficiency. With spinothalamic lesions below the midbrain, the response will be minimal or absent.

    6. *Denervation hypersensitivity.* NOREPINEPHRINE: Infuse a concentration of 1 μg/cc IV for 5 minutes at the rate of 0.05 μg/kg/min. The normal pressor response is 0–23/0–19 mm Hg. (Average 8/9 mm Hg) Marked pressor responses occur in peripheral autonomic insufficiency. NEO-SYNEPHRINE: Inject 2.5 mg IM. The average normal pressor response is 4/6 mm Hg with a range up to 15/10 mm Hg. Marked pressor responses are present in autonomic insufficiency.
Denervation hypersensitivity is due to failure of the denervated blood vessels to store norepinephrine. Direct-acting pressor amines (norepinephrine or Neo-Synephrine) are not inactivated by the vessel wall. Ephedrine and similar amines act by releasing norepinephrine and will be inactive in peripheral autonomic denervation.

    7. *Nitroglycerin.* Give 0.4 mg sublingually. Normally, blood pressure falls less than 15/5 mm Hg. A pronounced fall may occur in autonomic insufficiency because of inadequate compensatory vasoconstriction.

    8. *Rapid saline or blood infusion.* Infuse 3000 cc of normal saline in 1 hour. Take blood pressure every 5 minutes during the infusion and calculate the average blood pressure during the infusion. Normal persons have little change in blood pressure (less than 5-mm Hg increase in mean pressure). Patients with autonomic insufficiency may show a mean pressure rise of 20–35 mm Hg and blocking of postural hypotension. Rapidly infusing blood will give similar results.
In autonomic insufficiency there will also be an increase in urine flow and sodium excretion during rapid saline infusion. The mechanism is not understood.

	Normal	Auto. Insufficiency
Average urine flow	6 cc/min	23 cc/min
Sodium excretion	15 mEq/hr	80 mEq/hr

The urine should be collected through an indwelling catheter.

III. *Regional Vascular Reactions*

  A. *Axon reflex.* Inject 0.1 cc of 1:1000 histamine intradermally. In complete peripheral denervation the flare is absent; even in severe peripheral neuropathy the flare may remain because of overlapping neurons. This reflex is independent of central connections.

  B. *Evaluation of reflex dystrophy.* Pain is prominent, commonly burning in quality, and accompanied by vasospasm, sweating with skin atrophy, hair loss, and osteoporosis as manifestations of chronicity. Common causes are injury to a limb (Sudeck's atrophy), injury to a nerve (causalgia), referred pain with immobilization (shoulder-hand syndrome). To evaluate sympathetic component, use either systemic (400 mg Etamon IV) or local ganglionic blockade. Note change in skin color, temperature, sweating, and alteration of pain after blockade.

  C. *Plethysmography:* Requires special equipment, but useful in studying reflex thresholds and response and changes in regional flow with ganglionic blockade.

IV. *Sweating*

May be judged clinically. Axillary sweating remains even in autonomic insufficiency. Inspect for areas of spontaneous sweating. Rub the fingers lightly across the skin; even minor amounts of sweat can be detected in this manner.

  A. *Colorimetric Testing.* Paint the patient with one of the following solutions, allow it to dry, then dust the painted area with the appropriate powder. Water discolors the area and indicates preserved sweating.

    1. Tincture ferric chloride, USP diluted with 3 parts alcohol. Tannic acid powder.

    2. Minors solution (15 g iodine, 100 cc castor oil, and 900 cc dilute alcohol). Starch.

  B. *Thermoregulatory sweating.* To accentuate sweating, place the patient in heat chamber (respirator with lights on, bed with heat lamps and foot bridge, etc.). The rectal temperature must increase 0.5–1.0° C for the test to be valid, and there may be a 30-minute latent period. Sweat response depends on intact sympathetic efferents from hypothalamus to skin. Excess local heat (43–46° C) to skin can cause local sweating.

  C. *Axon reflex sweating.* Inject 0.1 cc of either 1:10,000 acetylcholine or 1:100,000 nicotine sulfate intradermally or use faradic stimulation. Sweating takes place 1 to 2 min after injection, covers an area 5 cm in diameter from point of injection. Response tests the integrity of local nerve supply to the sweat glands.

  D. *Integrity of sweat glands.* Inject 1:1000 pilocarpine intradermally. Sweating occurs over the wheal. This demonstrates that the sweat glands are intact and capable of reacting to stimuli.

TABLE 32. DISORDERS OF THE AUTONOMIC NERVOUS SYSTEM

I. Hypothalamic syndromes
  A. Abnormalities of temperature regulation
    1. Poikilothermia (hypothermia)
    2. Hyperthermia (central fever)
  B. Abnormalities of appetite
    1. Hypothalamic obesity
    2. Hypothalamic emaciation (diencephalic syndrome)
    3. Hypodipsia with absence of thirst
  C. Abnormalities of fluid and electrolyte balance
    1. Diabetes insipidus
    2. Inappropriate ADH secretion
    3. Essential hypernatremia
  D. Abnormalities of memory and emotion
    1. Wernicke-Korsakoff syndrome
    2. Rage reaction
  E. Abnormalities of sleep and consciousness
    1. Hypersomnia
    2. ? Kleine-Levin syndrome
    3. ? Narcolepsy
II. Generalized dysautonomia
  A. Primary involvement of the autonomic nervous system
    1. Familial dysautonomia (Riley-Day syndrome)
    2. Idiopathic orthostatic hypotension
    3. Autonomic failure as a remote effect of cancer
    4. Acute or subacute pandysautonomic neuropathy
    5. Autonomic failure with multiple system atrophy (MSA-Shy Drager)
    6. Autonomic failure with Parkinson's disease
  B. Autonomic dysfunction with other disease of the nervous system
    1. Myelopathy
      a. Spinal trauma
      b. Spinal tumor
      c. Syringomyelia
    2. Diabetic autonomic neuropathy
    3. Guillain-Barré syndrome
    4. Porphyric neuropathy
    5. Amyloid neuropathy
    6. Botulism
    7. Tabes dorsalis
    8. Wernicke's encephalopathy
  C. Dysautonomia secondary to drugs
    1. Neurotoxic drugs
    2. Tranquilizers
    3. Ganglionic blocking agents
    4. Miscellaneous drugs
III. Restricted autonomic dysfunction
  A. Cardiovascular
    1. Cardiac arrhythmias
    2. Essential hypertension
    3. Syncope
  B. Gastrointestinal tract
    1. Irritable bowel syndrome
    2. Achalasia of the esophagus
    3. Gastric atony (often due to diabetes)
    4. Colonic ileus (Ogilvie's syndrome)
    5. Megacolon (Hirschsprung's disease)
  C. Skin
    1. Generalized or focal anhidrosis
    2. Generalized or focal hyperhidrosis
    3. ? Congenital insensitivity to pain
  D. Bladder (Table 29)
  E. Sexual function (Table 30)
  F. Pupil
    1. Horner's syndrome
    2. Holmes-Adie syndrome (tonic pupil)
  G. Miscellaneous forms of restricted autonomic dysfunction
    1. Peripheral nerve injury
    2. Causalgia
    3. Reflex sympathetic dystrophy
    4. Aberrant regeneration (crocodile tears)
    5. Raynaud's syndrome

enough can lead to encephalopathy and seizures. The disorder also has been reported with head injury or with involvement of the hypothalamus by tumor or inflammation. It can occur as an early manifestation of generalized polyneuropathy (Guillain-Barré syndrome [see the preceding chapter]), probably the result of afferent autonomic failure.

Sexual abnormalities have also been reported with hypothalamic dysfunction. Adrenogenital dystrophy resulting from abnormalities of tuberal nuclei, the tuberoinfundibular tracts, or both combines obesity with delayed sexual development. Tumor involving the hypothalamus can cause this disorder, but at other times the cause is unknown. *Sexual precocity* has also been reported with hypothalamic abnormalities, including pineal tumors. Disturbances of sleep, including narcolepsy and the Kleine-Levin syndrome (see the following chapter), may result from abnormalities of the hypothalamus or lower brainstem. The exact pathophysiology is unknown. Trauma involving the hypothalamus, particularly the tuberal nuclei, can lead to erosion, ulceration and hemorrhage of the gastric mucosa (Cushing's ulcers). The disorder usually occurs after massive trauma to the brain, and the exact site of the lesion is unknown.

AUTONOMIC INSUFFICIENCY

Diffuse loss of autonomic function may accompany severe peripheral neuropathy or be a part of so-called acute pandysautonomia, an acute, probably autoimmune, peripheral neuropathy restricted to autonomic nerves. Other disorders that are associated with autonomic insufficiency are Wernicke's disease, the congenital Riley-Day syndrome, and autonomic ganglion dysfunction from ingestion of ganglioplegic agents. Tabes dorsalis is commonly accompanied by autonomic insufficiency. Destruction of the spinal cord as occurs with syringomyelia, trauma, or spinal tumors may also be accompanied by autonomic insufficiency. Pontine hemorrhage may disrupt descending sympathetic pathways in the brainstem, thereby causing sympathetic dysfunction but not more widespread insufficiency.

Idiopathic autonomic insufficiency or the *Shy-Drager syndrome* is a rare degenerative disorder of unknown cause that strikes during middle age, causing progressive autonomic dysfunction; severe disability or death may occur within 5 to 15 years of onset. Associated extrapyramidal abnormalities and lesions of pigmented brain nuclei may play a prominent role in the pathogenesis of symptoms. Histologic examination at autopsy has disclosed various changes, ranging from the severe to the barely detectable. Degenerative abnormalities may affect autonomic ganglia in the periphery, the preganglionic intermediolateral cell column in the spinal cord, or autonomic centers in the hypothalamus, nigrostriatal system, pontine nuclei, and globus pallidus. Postmortem biochemical studies have revealed marked depression of dopamine β-hydroxylase, which converts dopamine to norepinephrine, in sympathetic ganglia, whereas tyrosine hydroxylase, the rate-limiting enzyme in catecholamine biosynthesis, is decreased in locus ceruleus.

At least two entities may constitute idiopathic autonomic insufficiency. The first may consist of autonomic insufficiency alone, whereas the second may be characterized by autonomic insufficiency in association with a variety of neurologic signs, including movement disorders resembling Parkinson's disease. The degree of clinical overlap between these groups, however, is consistent with the existence of a broad continuum rather than distinct entities.

Symptoms of autonomic dysfunction predominate early in the course. Characteristically, initial difficulties consist of sexual impotence; urinary hesitancy, urgency, or incontinence; anhidrosis; or a combination of these. These early symptoms are frequently unrecognized and undiagnosed. Within months to years, the hallmark of the disorder, postural hypotension, appears. This may be manifested as dizziness, giddiness, or frank syncope upon standing. Less frequently, patients complain of generalized weakness, cervico-occipital discomfort, or leg weakness upon standing. Attendant autonomic symptoms include intermittent diplopia, dysphagia and diarrhea, fecal incontinence or constipation. A parkinsonian disorder, consisting of bradykinesia, coarse tremor and rigidity, is common and tends to progress inexorably. Myoclonus, gait disturbance, and signs of olivopontocerebellar dysfunction may also occur.

Physical signs of autonomic dysfunction parallel the aforementioned symptoms. Orthostatic hypotension, a greater than 30/20 mm Hg fall in blood pressure upon assumption of the erect position, constitutes the fundamental sign. Other signs include absence of sinus arrhythmia and absence of the normal overshoot in diastolic pressure during phase IV of the Valsalva maneuver. Autonomic dysfunction may express itself in Horner's syndrome, in parasympathetic pupillary changes, or as anhidrosis even with elevated ambient temperature. Muscle wasting, fasciculation, and extensor plantar responses occasionally have been observed.

MISCELLANEOUS DISORDERS

A few other disorders of the autonomic nervous system deserve mention. After recovery from a facial palsy (Bell's palsy), misdirection of regenerating parasympathetic fibers can result in fibers originally innervating salivary glands now reaching the lacrimal gland, so that lacrimation occurs when the patient eats (crocodile tears). Gustatory sweating, i.e., sweating on the face during eating, is another such reflex phenomenon that occasionally is seen in normal individuals.

Raynaud's phenomenon is characterized by painful blanching of the fingers on exposure to cold. This disorder commonly accompanies connective tissue diseases. It has been reported as a side effect of cancer chemotherapy. Its pathophysiology is unknown, although it probably results from hyperactivity of the sympathetic vasoconstrictor response, possibly following partial postganglionic denervation.

Reflex sympathetic dystrophy and causalgia resulting from minor injury to the peripheral nerves or extremities is described in the preceding chapter.

Congenital megacolon is a rare disease affecting infants and children, usually male, resulting from absence of ganglionic cells in Auerbach's plexus. The parasympathetic denervated segment of the colon is constricted. Proximal to that area the colon becomes massively dilated.

REFERENCES

Appenzeller, O.: The Autonomic Nervous System. 2nd ed. New York, American Elsevier, 1976. *The only available comprehensive monograph of recent origin.*

Bannister, R.: Autonomic Failure: A Textbook of Clinical Disorders of the Autonomic Nervous System. Oxford, Oxford University Press, 1983.

Boller, F., and Frank, E.: Sexual Dysfunctions in Neurological Disorders. New York, Raven Press, 1982.

Hald, T., and Bradley, W. E.: The Urinary Bladder: Neurology and Dynamics. Baltimore, Williams and Wilkins, 1982.

Plum, F., and Van Uitert, R.: Non-endocrine diseases and disorders of the hypothalamus. Res Publ Assoc Res New Ment Dis 56:415–473, 1977.

Alterations of Consciousness: The Cerebral Hemispheres and Higher Brain Function

SUSTAINED DISORDERS OF CONSCIOUSNESS

Definitions

Consciousness describes a state of forebrain neural activity producing behavioral awareness of the self and the environment. Both the degree and perceptual-conceptual content of normal consciousness can vary widely, depending upon elements of arousal, attention, emotion, intellectual capacity, learning, and memory. Among these ingredients, arousal, learning, and memory are critical. Without them, mental capacities could neither awaken, nor when awake could they recognize their own identity or incorporate new or familiar sensations into perceptions. From the more immediate medical standpoint, *consciousness* reduces itself into two major dimensions: wakefulness and psychologically recognizable mental activity. Its antithesis, *coma,* is a state of complete, eyes-closed mental unresponsiveness in which neither behavioral nor electrophysiologic evidence of normal psychologic responses to stimulation can be observed. Anatomically the content of consciousness reflects primarily the functions of the association cortex regions of the cerebral hemispheres and their closely related subcortical nuclei, while the level of arousal represents primarily the functional expression of structures located in the ventral diencephalon and upper brainstem.

Between the antipodes of full consciousness and coma lie gradations of mental content and arousal that reflect the effects of different degrees, anatomic locations, and acuteness of brain damage or dysfunction.

The terms *obtundation* and *drowsiness* describe states of impaired alertness or wakefulness in which patients continue to respond to verbal stimuli. *Stupor* is a state in which subjects arouse when subjected to vigorous and sustained stimulation, but sink back to unresponsiveness as soon as external stimuli are withdrawn. *Amnesia, aphasia,* and *dementia* are conditions that reduce specific components of the content of consciousness, but leave normal arousal and sleep-wake cycles relatively or completely intact. The *vegetative state* describes a degree of dementia so profound that no recognizable mental activity exists: Affected patients preserve their autonomic-vegetative functions, including normal circadian patterns of sleeping and waking. Put another way, in the vegetative state arousal is preserved, but the content of consciousness is lost. The terms *akinetic mutism* and *coma vigil* describe variations on the vegetative state in which severely brain-damaged individuals give the appearance of being especially alert and attentive, but fail to reveal evidence for any consistently recognizable cognitive functions. The *locked-in state* describes the condition of patients who are awake and retain mental content, but, because of paralysis of descending or efferent motor pathways, cannot express themselves by speech, regulation of facial expression, or movement of the limbs. The site of the lesion in such cases usually interrupts motor pathways in the base of the pons or, less often, the midbrain. Sparing of the brainstem tegmentum in these areas explains why consciousness is retained. Rarely, generalized polyneuropathy can cause such severe paralysis that it produces a locked-in state.

MECHANISMS OF CONSCIOUSNESS AND UNCONSCIOUSNESS

The Physiology of Arousal

Normal consciousness depends upon a close physiologic interaction between the cerebral cortex and both specific and nonspecific afferent systems that project to it via ascending pathways in the diencephalon and brainstem. Specific systems are exemplified by the lemniscal or spinothalamic pathways that carry fast-acting, somatotopically organized, modality-specific information from appropriate peripheral receptors and connect in a point-to-point pattern to specific thalamic relay nuclei. The latter, in turn, project the incoming specific sensory information to topographically organized somatosensory areas of the cortex. Nonspecific systems, by contrast, are self-exciting in function, diffusely organized in their anatomy and projections, and exert predominantly a modulatory, tonic influence on more rostrally placed brain structures. Within the functions of consciousness, specific ascending systems and their targets act largely to define the perceptual content of the conscious state, while the nonspecific systems largely govern the level of arousal and degree of attention.

Normal and Abnormal Arousal. A number of nonspecific ascending systems have been identified in the brainstem or basal forebrain, several being neurotransmitter specific (Table 33). Among these, the pathways crucial to arousal lie within the general area of the brainstem-diencephalic paramedian reticular formation. The portions of this structure that particularly relate to arousal extend forward in the brainstem tegmentum from approximately the level of the midpons to the region of the anterior hypothalamus (Fig. 58). Evidence is still incomplete as to exactly which set of neurons and connections within the reticular formation is critical for generating and maintaining arousal. It does not appear that a single neurotransmitter system is responsible.

At the level where the midbrain joins the posterior diencephalon, the ascending reticular activating system (RAS) divides into two branches: One projects more dorsally, forward to the intralaminar and midline thalamic nuclei, while the other more ventrally enters the lateral hypothalamus. Both of these receiving areas, in turn, project diffusely to the cerebral cortex with clinical studies suggesting that the ventral hypothalamic relay plays an especially important role in influencing wakefulness.

Both sensory and emotional stimulation influence normal arousal. Anatomically the RAS receives collateral fibers from all modality-specific afferent pathways as well as a rich feedback influence from limbic and

TABLE 33.   SOURCES OF ASCENDING AFFERENTS TO CEREBRAL CORTEX

	PATHWAY	TRANSMITTER
I. Specific System		
Thalamus-specific nuclei	Internal capsule	Not known
II. Nonspecific systems		
A. Thalamus-intralaminar and midline nuclei	Internal capsule	Not known
B. Monoamine systems		
1. Locus ceruleus and ventrolateral medulla	Lateral hypothalamus	Norepinephrine
2. Dorsal and superior central raphe nuclei	Lateral hypothalamus	Serotonin
3. Paranigral area	Lateral hypothalamus (Nigrostriatal bundle)	Dopamine
C. Basal-hypothalamopontine system		
1. Nucleus basalis and associated cell groups	Basal forebrain	Acetylcholine
2. Lateral hypothalamus	Basal forebrain	α-MSH, ? others
3. Tuberomammillary hypothalamus	?	GABA
4. Pedunculopontine and laterodorsal tegmental nuclei	Lateral hypothalamus	Acetylcholine
5. Periventricular gray matter of IV ventricle	?	Substance P Others unknown
6. Parabrachial nucleus of pons	Lateral hypothalamus	Not known

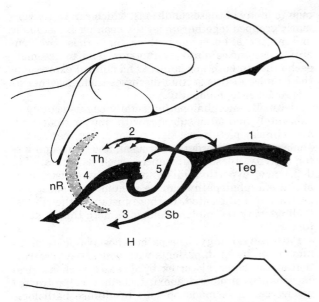

Figure 58. Some main features in the fiber projections assumed to be related to the ascending activating system. Fibers from the reticular formation of the brainstem *(1)* ascend through the tegmentum *(Teg)*. Caudal to the thalamus they bifurcate into a dorsal leaf *(2)*, which is lost in the intralaminar *(Th)* and dorsomedial thalamic fields, and a ventral leaf *(3)*. This runs ventrally and laterally through the subthalamus *(Sb)* and hypothalamus *(H)* and thereby swings ventrally to the thalamic reticular nucleus *(nR)*. Axons of cells in the "nonspecific" thalamic projections have a rostral component *(4)* that perforates the reticular nucleus and continues rostrally in the inferior thalamic peduncle. Another component *(5)* turns caudally and runs back to the tegmental level. (From Scheibel, M. A., and Scheibel, A. B.: Structural substrates for integrative patterns in the brainstem reticular core. In Jasper, H. H., et al. (eds.): Reticular Formation of the Brain. Boston, Little, Brown and Co., 1958.)

neocortical portions of the forebrain. The thalamic projections of the RAS appear to modulate or "gate" a normally inhibitory effect that the nonspecific intralaminar thalamic nuclei otherwise exert on the specific thalamic relay nuclei. In this manner the RAS enhances arousal by inhibiting tonic intrathalamic inhibition.

How the hypothalamic branch of the RAS mediates its effects on arousal is less well understood than the above, although the behavioral effects are well established, especially in clinical work. Anterior hypothalamic stimulation in the cat induces a sleeplike state, while posterior hypothalamic stimulation generates arousal. Anterior hypothalamic destruction in animals results in hyposomnia or insomnia, while posterior lesions induce in either animals or human beings a state of prolonged hypersomnolence or even sleeplike unarousable coma. These effects of ventral hypothalamic lesions on arousal are both more profound and more durable than comparable damage to the more dorsal RAS pathway. Thus acute damage to the midbrain or upper pontine RAS in man produces a brief stage of unarousable unresponsiveness, lasting for several days or more. If well cared for, however, patients with injury to this area always reawaken within days or weeks. Furthermore, gradual or staged destruction to the midbrain reticulum in experimental animals may never produce coma at all. Similarly, damage

received bilaterally by the posterior dorsal medial thalamus in man is followed by 24 hours or so of unresponsiveness, following which a relatively apathetic and amnesic but wakeful condition ensues.

The loss of arousal classically associated with acute damage to the brainstem RAS probably reflects acute reticular "shock," i.e., a stage of transient, damage-associated, rostral inhibition, perhaps akin to the state of physiologic depression that temporarily affects the distal portion of the acutely transected spinal cord. By contrast to these relatively evanescent effects on awakening, bilateral severe damage to the posterior hypothalamus appears to affect more specific arousal-inducing areas and can be followed by prolonged hypersomnolence or coma.

Mechanisms of Impaired Arousal with Intracranial Structural Lesions. Most examples of acutely arising stupor and coma can be explained as representing the effects of (1) damage or dysfunction of the nonspecific RAS, (2) widespread impairment of cerebral cortical receiving areas, or (3) a combination of these two pathologic processes.

Compression and blocking of conduction within the RAS can accompany expanding intracranial masses when, as described in the second chapter, such masses either originate supratentorially and produce secondary downward compression-herniation of the diencephalon or when they arise in the subtentorial fossa so as directly to squeeze the brainstem (Fig. 12). Destruction of the same areas by infarcts, abscesses, or trauma produces similar clinical effects. With supratentorial masses the expanding brain initially presses upon the diencephalon and displaces it in a rostral-caudal manner to produce signs and symptoms of *central herniation* (p. 1025). Initially, at least, RAS impairment is reflected by generalized obtundation, stupor, or coma unaccompanied by evidence of focal cranial nerve abnormalities. *Lateral transtentorial herniation-compression,* by contrast, tends to herniate the uncus at the same time that the mass lesion compresses the diencephalon. The result is that as the uncus squeezes upon the third nerve, oculomotor weakness accompanies or may even precede the state of reduced arousal. Compressive lesions in the posterior fossa, most of which arise in the cerebellum, tend to produce ipsilateral cranial nerve paralyses at the same time that they blunt arousal. Clinically it is critical to distinguish between destructive and compressive lesions of the RAS. Neural tissue can fully recover from considerable compressive force, but once the tissue actually begins to herniate downward or upward through the sharp-edged tentorium, reticular destruction and other tissue damage soon follow. At this point, irreversible neural injury begins.

Metabolic depression of the RAS, usually accompanied by at least some measure of cerebral depression, underlies the reduced arousal that results from most anesthetic agents, sedative drugs, and coma-producing systemic metabolic encephalopathies. Barbiturate anesthetics, for example, especially block synaptic transmission in the reticular formation more than they do in the cortex. Similarly, acute depression of the RAS has been noted experimentally during acute concussion. During recovery from acute occurring metabolic coma, improvement in general mental alertness usually lags considerably behind functional return of specific motor systems. Thus the diffusely organized RAS appears to be both more susceptible to metabolic depression and slower to recover than the large, ascending oligosynaptic systems.

THE METABOLIC AND DIFFUSE ENCEPHALOPATHIES

Once arousal occurs the content of consciousness depends on cerebrally mediated functions. Forebrain abnormalities, depending on their size, location, and acuteness, can produce focal, multifocal, or diffuse changes in conscious behavior. At their most severe, acute diffuse forebrain abnormalities result in unresponsive coma with a clinical picture indistinguishable from that resulting from damage or depression of the RAS at the midbrain-hypothalamic level. An example of this principle can be seen in the form of severe hypoxia that occurs with carbon monoxide poisoning. Such injuries can severely attack the cerebral white matter. The process interrupts a large proportion of the normal corticocortical and corticodiencephalic connections, but spares the cell bodies of the cortical mantle as well as those in the subcortical projection nuclei. The result disconnects the cerebral cortex from the subcortex and thereby causes an acute stage of deep coma followed by a prolonged vegetative state, despite the absence of direct injury to the nerve cells of either the cortex or the RAS. The effect emphasizes that any alteration of consciousness ultimately expresses itself as a failure of forebrain information processing.

Causes and Manifestations

Many disorders can produce diffuse or multifocal disturbances of forebrain function. Table 34 lists the main ones, all of which can result in generalized abnormalities in conscious behavior ranging in severity from delirium or confusion through to stupor or coma. Certain clinical and pathogenic factors are com-

TABLE 34. PRINCIPAL CAUSES OF METABOLIC OR MULTIFOCAL ENCEPHALOPATHY

Deprivation of oxygen, substrate, or metabolic cofactors
  Hypoxia-hypoxemia
  Ischemia
  Hypoglycemia
  Deficiency states: thiamine, niacin, pyridoxine,
    cyanocobalamin, folate
Diseases of extracerebral organs
  Nonendocrine: liver, kidney, lung, pancreas
  Endocrine: pituitary, thyroid, parathyroid, adrenal, pancreas
  Systemic disease: sepsis, porphyria, cancer, endocarditis
Exogenous poisons
  Sedatives
  Acid poisons
  Psychotropics
  Miscellaneous
  Chronic polydrug ingestion
Fluid, electrolyte, and acid-base disorders
  Water and sodium
  Lithium, magnesium, calcium, phosphorus derangements
  Systemic acidoses-alkaloses
  Hypothermia or hyperthermia
Infectious-inflammatory disorders
  Meningitis-encephalitis, infectious and immunogenic
Cerebral vasculitis
Seizures or postictal states
Post-traumatic coma (concussion)
Withdrawal or isolation deliria
Subarachnoid hemorrhage

mon to many of these conditions, which can be conveniently grouped together under the heading of metabolic and multifocal encephalopathies. Since these two general causes of cerebral dysfunction tend to resemble each other in both mechanical and clinical expression, the balance of this section discusses them together as metabolic encephalopathy.

Metabolic encephalopathy usually begins acutely or subacutely and often subsides with time or treatment. The clinical picture consists of confusion, behavioral abnormalities, disorders of arousal, and abnormal motor activity. In some instances, such as vitamin B_{12} deficiency, hyperthyroidism, or hypothyroidism, metabolic encephalopathy can be insidious in onset and protracted if untreated. In those instances the clinical findings may resemble a dementia more than a delirium.

Pathophysiology. The pathogenesis of acute delirium or confusion in patients with widespread destruction of the cerebral cortex by diseases such as viral encephalitis, profound anoxia-ischemia, or protracted hypoglycemia is made obvious by diffuse pathologic changes affecting the cerebral cortex. With anoxia-ischemia, for example, the mildest visible abnormalities observed microscopically consists of microvacuoles in neuronal cytoplasm of the neocortex and hippocampus. The microvacuoles represent swollen mitochondria, and this change is probably reversible. With more severe insults one observes dissolution of rough endoplasmic reticulum and generalized pallor of neuronal staining. Finally the nuclei shrink and become hyperchromatic and irregular. Basophilic rings and granules appear in the swollen cytoplasm. These changes are not reversible. After severe, prolonged and irreversible insults, all neurons in the cerebral cortex may die, or the third, fifth, and sixth layer of the cortex may degenerate selectively so that the naked dye detects a thin line of spongy necrosis. Anoxic changes also affect the basal ganglia to cause grossly visible focal necrosis of the globus pallidus. Occasionally such processes produce diffuse demyelination of the cortical white matter. Characteristically the brainstem and spinal cord are spared unless anoxia-ischemia has been overwhelmingly severe and rapidly fatal.

Changes that are similarly diffuse but biochemical rather than morphologic are believed to affect brain cells in the reversible metabolic encephalopathies. In hepatic coma, for example, unusual glial cells with ballooned and lobulated nuclei appear in wide areas of the cerebral cortex and basal ganglia, presumably reflecting the astrocytic response to the need for detoxification of ammonia that takes place in this disorder. In inflammatory illnesses caused by viruses or bacteria, local neuronal lesions may result, but perivascular cuffs of lymphocytes also can be observed in widely distributed portions of the cerebrum and brainstem.

So far, we understand in only a few instances how systemic illnesses specifically interfere with cerebral metabolism, but examples of these serve as models to suggest possible mechanisms for others. The following paragraphs outline some of our knowledge of normal and abnormal cerebral metabolism.

Glucose

Glucose is the brain's only substrate under physiologic conditions. Other substances, such as ketone bodies generated from fat stores during starvation, can serve as partial substrates for brain metabolism, but they never fully replace glucose requirements. Glucose is transferred across the blood-brain-barrier by a process termed facilitated transport. Under normal circumstances, each 100 g of brain utilizes about 31 μM (5.5 mg) of glucose per minute, an amount that represents almost the body's entire basal consumption. Under aerobic conditions 85 per cent of brain glucose uptake is oxidized to form CO_2, water, and energy. The remainder is accounted for by production of lactate, pyruvate, and other intermediates and by the synthesis of structural chemicals. Under anaerobic conditions, lactic acid is the end-product of glucose metabolism, but the energy produced during such glycolysis is insufficient to maintain neuronal function. The brain contains about 2 g of reserve glucose and glycogen. That reserve plus the continued reduced supply from the blood allows the brain of a severely hypoglycemic patient to survive for about 90 minutes without suffering irreversible injury. The blood glucose concentration at which cerebral metabolism fails and clinical symptoms develop varies from patient to patient and to a certain extent depends upon the rate at which the blood glucose declines. In general, however, levels in the adult below 1.5 mM/l (27 mg/dl) cause confusion and below 0.5 to 1 mM/l produce coma.

Oxygen

Oxygen, the other substance vital for normal cerebral function, is not stored by the brain, and a few seconds of asystole or very low inspired oxygen concentrations promptly induce coma. After a variable period, usually only a few minutes, either profound hypoxia or ischemia causes irreversible neuronal damage. The normal brain consumes about 156 μM (3.5 ml) of oxygen per 100 g per minute and produces an almost equal amount of carbon dioxide. Oxygen consumption by the brain represents about 20 per cent of that of the entire body at rest. This net high cerebral consumption rate remains remarkably constant in normal man whether awake or asleep, although regional consumption varies widely according to local functional changes. Significant deviations in oxygen consumption accompany brain dysfunction. Seizures, for example, can increase the brain's demand for oxygen by as much as fourfold and usually are associated with a greatly increased blood flow. Conversely, sedative drugs may decrease the brain's metabolic demand so that sedative drug overdose or anesthesia is usually associated with decreased cerebral blood flow and oxygen uptake. Metabolic encephalopathy or hypothermia has a similar effect. Clinically, delirium usually accompanies cerebral oxygen uptakes below 2.5 ml 100 g/min, and when the uptake falls below 2.0 ml, most patients become unconscious. The degree of hypoxia necessary to cause clinical symptoms depends not only on the blood oxygen tension but also on hemoglobin concentration, cerebral blood flow, serum pH, and the rate of acclimatization.

Acclimatization markedly changes the cerebral tolerance to anoxia by a combination of raising hemoglobin concentrations, increasing cerebral blood flow, and, possibly, by altering tissue metabolism. Estimates based on alveolar gas measurements indicate that healthy climbers breathing air at the peak of Mt. Everest had an arterial Po_2 of 28 torr, a Pco_2 of 7.5 torr, and a pH of 7.7. The degree of compensatory hyperventilation is extraordinary and suggests that cerebral blood flow almost certainly responded to the vasodilatory stimulus of hypoxemia rather than to the vasoconstrictor stimulus of hypocapnia. Even so, the climbers suffered sustained impairment of tasks requiring repetitive fast movements as well as transient declines in verbal learning and short-term memory. In general, Pao_2 values that fall acutely below 50 torr in a previously healthy person at sea level cause mental changes, while declines below 25 torr result in coma.

Blood

As noted earlier, the total brain blood flow of 800 ml/min amounts to about 15 per cent of the cardiac output. Initially, at least, when the blood flow declines, the brain compensates by extracting more oxygen and glucose to maintain its normal metabolism. If, however, the capillary partial pressure of oxygen becomes too low, clinically reflected in a cerebral venous blood Po_2 below about 20 mm of mercury (or hemoglobin saturation of 35 per cent), it fails to sustain normal metabolism, and consciousness usually becomes impaired or lost. Increases in blood flow similarly can compensate for loss of oxygen-carrying capacity due to anemia. With hemoglobin concentrations below about 8 g/dl, cerebral blood flow must almost double to assure an adequate oxygen supply. Any limitation of this response makes severe anemia a potential contributor to cerebral hypoxia.

Other Substances

In addition to glucose or oxygen, the brain requires other substances such as enzymes, vitamins, amino acids, and electrolytes to maintain metabolism, synthesize transmitters, preserve cellular structure, and maintain membrane potentials. Abnormalities of any of these essentials can lead to metabolic brain dysfunction. The unique function of nervous tissue is to transmit electrical impulses both within cells and, by synaptic transmission, between them. The integrity of intracellular transmission depends not only on energy derived from oxidative metabolism to maintain the sodium pump but also on the presence of finely controlled intracellular and extracellular electrolyte balances. Thus, for example, either severe increases or decreases of extracellular sodium produce behavioral changes and delirium. Lithium, a cation with thermodynamic properties similar to both sodium and potassium, changes behavior in manic patients and in overdose similarly can lead to severe delirium or coma. As remarked earlier, altered neurotransmitters likewise can affect the state of consciousness: The phenothiazine neuroleptics act against the hallucinations and disordered thought processes of schizophrenia in direct proportion to their effectiveness in blocking central dopamine receptors. Also, drugs that enhance the central activity of serotonin and norepinephrine activity counteract the mood and behavioral expressions of depressive illness. Most psychotropic drugs in overdose produce delirium and sometimes coma. Severe alterations in amino acid or amine metabolism may have the same effect. A striking example of the latter is observed in the severe toxic delirium that large doses of scopolamine and other anticholinergic agents induce. Interference with transmitter function may occur when the synthesis, breakdown, or release of the agent is inhibited or when a foreign substance having a structure similar to a transmitter competes for sites on the postsynaptic receptor. It has been postulated that the generation of such "false transmitters" may explain how hallucinogenic drugs act or may contribute to the mechanism of hepatic coma. At present no biochemical common denominator has been found among the many metabolic encephalopathies.

Pathogenesis of Symptoms and Signs

Disturbances in arousal, mental content, motor function, pulmonary ventilation, and cerebral electrical activity are the clinical hallmarks of the metabolic-multifocal encephalopathies.

Arousal and Cognitive Changes

With acute encephalopathy the combination of reticular and diffuse cerebral dysfunction almost always first produces impaired attention and arousal, i.e., a clouding of consciousness, often mixed with an abnormal mental content. In the early stages, patients may appear quietly perplexed; even when hypervigilant and distractible, they tend to lapse off into intermittent sleep. Restlessness, lethargy, emotional lability, and vivid nightmares may ensue, randomly reflecting loss of cortical control on limbic and hypothalamic systems. The normal hypothalamically engendered diurnal sleep-wake cycle may reverse itself. As the illness progresses or with severe encephalopathies almost from the start, progressive stupor and sometimes coma develop, reflecting increasing dysfunction of the RAS.

Patients with slowly developing, mild metabolic-multifocal encephalopathy show their most prominent abnormalities in the cognitive sphere. Memory for recent events declines, and accurate orientation slips away, at first for time, then for place. Perceptual errors creep in, intensifying the confusional state while, with more advanced delirium, visual and sometimes auditory hallucinations intrude. Severely delirious patients can lose contact completely, behaving in a dreamlike manner, showing no recognizable awareness of the environment.

Motor and Oculomotor Changes

Tremor, asterixis, and multifocal myoclonus, abnormalities defined in the chapter on Motor System, are characteristic of metabolic-diffuse encephalopathies. Physiologic studies of these changes suggest that they reflect abnormalities in motor coordination arising at subcortical or even spinal levels. Most patients with severe metabolic encephalopathy develop paratonic resistance to passive movement of the extremities or trunk. Many of those with severe cases of anoxia, hypoglycemia, hepatic coma, or multifocal vascular coma also show signs of bilateral corticospinal tract dysfunction with increased deep tendon reflexes, extensor plantar responses, and even decorticate or decerebrate postural responses. By contrast, except during the initial moment of poisoning, severe sedative drug overdose or grave postanoxic coma can depress the brainstem reticular motor areas to cause diffuse motor flaccidity. The key to the metabolic origin of all of these motor abnormalities consists more in recognizing their characteristic distribution than in searching for disease-specific patterns. Motor dysfunction in meta-

bolic brain disease reflects diffuse cerebral and brainstem involvement. Except for unusual cases of hypoglycemic or hepatic encephalopathy, the changes are almost always bilateral and usually fairly symmetric in their distribution. By contrast, motor dysfunction secondary to localized disease of either the forebrain or brainstem usually begins by producing focal or unilateral signs and seldom becomes completely symmetric except when devastating bilateral brainstem damage evolves.

Central autonomic pathways are resistant to metabolic depression so that pupillary reactions as well as circulatory and ventilatory control mechanisms escape the early depressive effects of all but a few metabolic encephalopathies. Except with severe asphyxia or a limited number of drugs that produce anticholinergic effects (e.g., hyoscine, scopolamine, or the sedative glutethimide) pupillary light reactions are almost always preserved in metabolic coma. Accordingly the absence of the pupillary light reaction, especially if unilateral or asymmetric, strongly suggests a structural lesion. Also, most metabolic encephalopathies depress forebrain functions more than they do those of the brainstem. As a result, intact or unusually brisk oculocephalic responses characterize the early stages of many of the metabolic encephalopathies, while unilateral neuro-ophthalmologic abnormalities always mean a focal lesion. The combination of preserved pupillary reactions (signifying intact midbrain autonomic function) and absence of oculovestibular reflexes (reflecting absence of brainstem oculomotor responses) in an acutely ill patient always means metabolic encephalopathy, usually due to drug poisoning.

Ventilatory Changes

Many disorders producing metabolic encephalopathy affect the pattern of breathing. *Hyperventilation* can be caused by metabolic acidosis (i.e., diabetic ketoacidosis, uremia, systemic lactic acidosis, organic acid poisoning) or can reflect abnormal chemical or reflex stimulation of the central respiratory drive producing respiratory alkalosis (e.g., hepatic coma, salicylism, sepsis, pulmonary infarction, pulmonary congestion). *Hypoventilation* in a patient with altered consciousness usually reflects either acute respiratory depression from drugs (opiates, barbiturates, glutethimide) or the late stages of chronic respiratory insufficiency (primary pulmonary insufficiency or neuromuscular ventilatory failure).

Electrophysiologic Changes

The electroencephalogram in metabolic encephalopathy differs from the individual's normal EEG. The changes are symmetric, in keeping with the diffuse nature of the process. Drug withdrawal deliria produce low-voltage rapid, 12- to 20-Hz changes in the EEG. Most other encephalopathies slow the record from its normal 8.5- to 13-Hz activity, retarding the frequencies roughly in proportion to the severity of the depressed cerebral state. EEGs with focal or unilateral slow activity suggest a structural rather than a metabolic or multifocal disorder of the brain.

ALTERED CONSCIOUSNESS IN PSYCHIATRIC DISORDERS

Nonphysiologic disturbances of behavior sometimes resembling the delirium, stupor, or coma caused by organic diseases or drugs are encountered frequently among patients presenting to hospital emergency rooms. Malingering, conversion reactions, or the manic phase of bipolar affective disease all can cause agitated and sometimes uncontrollable or violent behavior. Conversely, deception, conversion, severe psychologic depression, and schizophrenic catatonia all can imitate depressed levels of arousal. Among awake persons the main differential features are mainly psychologic: Psychiatric patients, unless schooled malingerers, give bizarre and inconsistent answers to the mental status examination or often fail to respond at all. If the patient is disoriented, the condition often extends to the self: "Who am I?" always reflects psychiatric illness. The episode of agitated or depressed behavior may coincide with a threatening life experience or arise conveniently in an effort to avoid disciplinary action. The EEG in such cases will not be slow unless the person has taken depressive drugs. By contrast, organically confused or delirious persons usually are at least intermittently lethargic, are always oriented to self unless completely out of contact with the environment, usually have slow EEGs, often show signs of systemic illness, and frequently have abnormalities in the motor system.

Psychogenic stupor or pseudocoma can be recognized by its lack of physiologic abnormalities. Affected persons may fail to respond by word or movement to voice or noxious stimuli, but analyses of their somatic functions reveal no abnormality. Efforts to open the closed eyelids commonly meet resistance and, if successful, are followed by brisk closure rather than the slow reshutting of the palpebral fissure that accompanies natural sleep or true coma. If turned on their sides, patients with psychogenic pseudocoma often turn the eyes conjugately toward the surface of the bed if the lids are forcefully opened. Pupillary reactions remain normal unless mydriatics have been self-instilled; oculovestibular tests elicit only the normal, quick-phase nystagmus unless the effort induces the subject to make brisk avoiding eye movements. Muscle tonus is normal or inconsistently directed against the examiner's manipulations of the patient's limbs. No pathologic motor reflexes are found. The EEG contains a normal awake record, usually with fast activity or muscle artifact reflecting an underlying state of emotional tension rather than organic brain depression.

SLEEP

Sleep is a recurrent state of behavioral unconsciousness from which the person can be awakened by appropriate external or internal stimulation. Sleep rhythmically affects all members of the animal kingdom, yet its biologic causes or physiologic advantages remain almost entirely unknown. Sleeping and waking are linked strongly to environmental influences: Reptiles sleep when cold and arouse progressively with heat, and several mammals hibernate in winter. During warmer weather most mammals, if left to their natural state, link their waking hours to natural or simulated daylight. Curiously the true circadian cycle of human beings kept in the dark for long periods settles in at about 25 rather than 24 hours.

The Stages of Sleep

Normal adult human sleep consists of alternating cycles of what appears to be a progressive deactivation of central nervous system function followed every 90 minutes or so by roughly 20-minute periods of excessive activation of certain autonomic and limbic functions (*activated sleep*). During the deactivated stages often called *slow-wave sleep* (SWS), the EEG slows progressively from theta into delta activity with patterns that resemble the slow tracings associated with certain forms of pathologic coma. Muscle tone decreases, body temperature declines, pulse rates and respiratory volumes go down, and blood pressure falls. Four successive stages characterize SWS based on the subject's behavioral resistance to arousal and the degree of EEG slowing. In SWS stage four some persons become almost unarousable, and extensor plantar responses can be obtained at least briefly. It is widely believed that the hypotension and bradycardia of deep SWS predispose to concurrent myocardial or cerebral ischemia.

Activated or *REM sleep* is marked by several dissociations between the behavioral state of unconsciousness and aspects of neurophysiologic hyperactivity. The EEG quickens and assumes an awake-like desynchronized pattern. Rapid eye movements (REM) jerk conjugately from side to side, pulse and respiratory rates accelerate, body temperature rises, and penile or clitoral engorgement takes place. Dreams, while they also accompany SWS, possess a more vivid and memorable dimension during REM. Paradoxically, skeletal muscle tonus declines, a change that reflects hyperactivity of the bulbar inhibitory reticular formation just as some of the previous components represent hyperactivity of more rostrally placed facilitatory neural centers.

The Pattern of Sleep

SWS usually initiates the night, with normal young adults descending into stage four within about 45 minutes and then experiencing their first brief REM episodes roughly 45 minutes after that. As the night wears on, SWS and REM periods alternate, with stages three and four disappearing about halfway through the night and REM episodes lengthening toward morning. Sleep changes its pattern through life. Normal newborns sleep about two-thirds of the day, filling about half that time with REM. By age 10 years and thereafter, REM occupies about one-fourth total sleep time, while the amount of stage four SWS gradually declines to 5 per cent or less by age 60 years.

Physiology and Pharmacology of Sleep

Neither is well understood. Sleep is influenced strongly by structures located at both hypothalamic and brainstem levels. The hypothalamus and adjacent pontine-midbrain reticular formation set the circadian regulation of the sleep-wake cycle. Stimulation of the anterior basal hypothalamic region induces SWS in animals, while damage to this area induces prolonged insomnia. Conversely, high frequency stimulation of the midbrain reticular formation or especially the lateral posterior hypothalamus induces EEG desynchronization and arousal in animals, whereas inflammation or destruction of these areas in animals and man results in profound hypersomnia (sleeping sickness) or coma. A second "clock" appears also to reside in the pontine tegmentum since humans with extensive midbrain hypothalamic damage or animals with transections at the midbrain level regain rhythmic sleeping and waking changes that correlate (in animals) with recordings of autonomous electrophysiologic cycling in pontine nuclei.

Early theories on the pharmacology of sleep focused on the postulate that sleeplike coma reflected merely the deafferentation of the forebrain from the reticular formation. The theory became untenable when it was realized that malformed newborns without cerebral hemispheres as well as adults with severely damaged ones can show normal sleep-wake cycles. Subsequent speculations have postulated that both the raphe nucleus and the nucleus tractus solitarius of the brainstem possess important sleep-stimulating functions making sleep an active rather than a passive function of brain. Based on several kinds of experiments, aminergic theories have emerged suggesting that either serotonergic or cholinergic excitation originating in the low brainstem may induce sleep, while noradrenergic activation engenders wakefulness. Alternatively, several investigators have isolated from the CSF of fatigued animals chemical agents that appear to promote sleep. Up to the present none of these pharmacologic hints explains satisfactorily the full cycling pattern of normal sleep, much less its self-evident but physiologically elusive restorative values to the brain.

Pathophysiology of Abnormal Sleep States

Although most normal adults average seven to nine hours of sleep per day, equally healthy persons can be satisfied with as little as four or may feel the need for as much as ten or more. As with other autonomic functions, medical concern usually arises only when there is a distinct change in sleep patterns. Everyday conditions or circumstances that produce limbic reticular excitation are likely to be associated with insomnia-hyposomnia while those that depress or damage the basal hypothalamic or related brainstem sleep-influencing areas are likely to cause hypersomnia. A limited number of disorders also affect the sleep state secondarily or occur as primary abnormalities of the sleep-regulating mechanism.

Hyposomnia-Insomnia. Most hyposomnia has a nonorganic cause. Furthermore, except during fairly severe sleep deprivation little beyond feelings of drowsiness and fatigue beset the insomniac. Reaction times and, sometimes, judgment declines after 24 hours or so of continuous working wakefulness. Briefer periods of non-sleep or merely reducing total sleep times gives no consistent abnormalities. Prolonged insomnia, over 72 hours or so, often precipitates intermittent confusion, perceptual delusions, and occasional hallucinations. No evidence indicates that chronic functional hyposomnia harms either the human mind or body. Most self-reported hyposomniacs actually sleep much more they believe; what they recall is their awakenings, not the often abundant sleep that lies between.

Diseases associated with insomnia include any that produce anxiety, severe pain, or other somatic discomfort such as dyspnea. CNS causes of insomnia include

occasional cases of encephalitis, syphilitic general paresis, and an idiopathic restless myoclonus that affects the extremities during the late middle and elderly years. Patients with diseases affecting the respiratory controlling areas of the pontomedullary reticular formation often are afraid to sleep lest they stop breathing (see sleep apnea, below).

Hypersomnia. Excessive sleepiness occurs in one of four settings: (1) as a symptom of anxiety or depression, (2) in association with lesions that distort, compress, inflame, or damage the posterior hypothalamic-midbrain reticular formation, (3) in association with several metabolic encephalopathies, especially those producing sedation or caused by hypoventilation of any cause resulting in pronounced hypoxemia and hypercarbia, (4) as the most prominent symptom of a group of conditions called sleep disorders. Of the above four causes only 2 and 3 produce radiographic or systemic laboratory abnormalities, and only those two are consistently associated with abnormal EEG tracings not explained by mere drowsiness or sleep.

Sleep Disorders. The sleep disorders include chronic *narcolepsy-cataplexy,* a syndrome in which relatively normal symptoms become intensified to the point of threatening incapacity. Narcoleptics suffer from an excess of socially inappropriate, uncontrollable drowsiness with a tendency to drop immediately into brief periods of REM sleep. Many also experience episodes of cataplexy, brief states of muscular atonia precipitated by sudden emotional changes such as fear or laughter. The condition also includes the presence of vivid dreamlike reveries called *hypnagogic hallucinations,* and so-called *sleep paralysis,* the feeling upon awakening that one cannot move. The sleep disorders also include the rare *Kleine-Levin syndrome,* an episodic disorder of older boys and young men who spontaneously and without explanation undergo recurrent, weeks-long bouts of overeating and SWS. The condition gradually disappears with increasing maturity.

Parasomnias. Parasomnias consist of the appearance during sleep of several annoying or frightening experiences, including enuresis, recurrent nightmares, night terrors, sleep walking, sleep talking and bruxism (grinding of the teeth). None of these conditions has a satisfactory physiologic explanation.

Sleep Apnea. This condition occurs as a brief and inconsequential symptom in many adults, most often as a momentary enhancement of the kind of palatal-glottic partial obstruction that leads to snoring. More serious respiratory arrest occurs under three circumstances. (1) *Glottic obstruction,* sometimes termed secondary sleep apnea, occurs mostly in moderately obese, middle-aged, and frequently semialcoholic males. The pathogenesis lies more in the collapse of a fat-compromised airway plus an excess of sedation than in any neurologic deficit. More severe secondary sleep apnea can occur in the overly obese, in whom several factors coincide to produce a combination of frequent nocturnal obstruction combined with apparent central hyposensitivity to carbon dioxide retention and hypoxemia as respiratory stimulants. The result can be narcoleptic-like daytime drowsiness and, sometimes, confusion coupled with evidence of reversible cardiopulmonary insufficiency. (2) *Central or primary sleep apnea* is an uncommon phenomenon that can follow primary pontine-medullary disease such as occurs with poliomyelitis, multiple sclerosis, syringomyelia, or local neoplasms. The condition also can follow surgical attempts to section the spinothalamic tract in the cervical cord that inadvertently interrupt descending respiratory pathways. In some cases no cause can be found. In this condition the reticular depression of SWS further dampens an already hypofunctioning respiratory control mechanism. As a result, breathing becomes first irregularly irregular (ataxic), then develops longer and longer pauses, and finally stops. Fortunately, rising blood CO_2 levels usually stimulate the affected person into gasping wakefulness. Less favorable outcomes are well known, however, and a similar condition in infants is believed to underlie unexplained crib deaths. (3) *Self-induced drug overdose.* Accidental drug overdose causing apnea has become less of a problem since the benzodiazepines supplanted barbiturates for routine sedative use. Most semiaccidental drug-induced apnea results from a combination of heavy alcohol ingestion plus the impulsive ingestion of a larger-than-usual dose of sedative. Vigorous external stimulation usually overcomes the potentially alarming situation.

BRIEF AND EPISODIC LOSS OF CONSCIOUSNESS

This heading includes a group of disorders that interfere with arousal or self-awareness for short periods (Table 35). The duration may last as briefly as a few seconds to as much as a few hours but rarely longer. In some of the conditions, such as circulatory syncope, the state of impaired consciousness is immediately apparent to both patient and observers. In others, such as nonconvulsive seizures or some of the self-limited amnesias, only the patient may be aware that an unremembered lapse of time has passed. All represent potential diagnostic problems, especially since their brief nature often precludes direct observation, and objective physical or laboratory abnormalities often are lacking by the time the patient reaches the doctor.

SYNCOPE AND OTHER NONCONVULSIVE STATES

Syncope describes a state of brief unconsciousness usually accompanied by sudden generalized loss of motor strength due to reduction or interruption of blood flow to the brain. All but a small percentage of syncopal attacks result from a reduction of cardiac output due to impaired cardiac filling, asystole, or severe arrhythmia. The remainder arise as a consequence of fluctuating cerebral blood flow in association with severe stenosis affecting more than one large parent artery in the neck.

TABLE 35. PRINCIPAL CAUSES AND APPROXIMATE FREQUENCIES (%) OF BRIEF LOSS OF CONSCIOUSNESS

Syncope	
Vasovagal/psychophysiologic	55
Cardiovascular	10
Central nervous system	
First seizure	10
Other	5
Drug-metabolic	5
Undiagnosed, including hysteria	15

Mechanisms of Syncope and Allied States

Abrupt global loss of consciousness usually reflects diffuse failure of the brain's circulation rather than the presence of focal ischemia to the nonspecific arousal systems or any other focal areas of the cerebrum. Given a normal oxygen and glucose content of the arterial blood, it requires a reduction of approximately 60 per cent in local blood flow for neuronal failure to occur. So long as cerebral arterial perfusion pressure remains above about 70 torr, the process of cerebral autoregulation, described in the chapter Neurobiologic Essentials, guarantees near-normal blood flow to the tissue unless either local arterial obstruction or an overwhelming reduction in arterial blood volume takes place. In the absence of severe hypoxemia or hypoglycemia the development of syncope always implies an acute reduction in cerebral perfusion pressure, usually secondary to a drop in systemic blood pressure. The process of neuronal failure develops rapidly: It takes only about 10 seconds of complete ischemia for integrated neuronal function to stop in the brain, and the EEG disappears after about 12 seconds. Lesser reductions of perfusion pressure, especially when accompanied by anoxemia, globally reduce cerebral blood flow and oxygen delivery and may account for some of the symptoms of cerebral insufficiency that occur in patients with very severe heart failure such as occurs following myocardial infarction.

Cardiac mechanisms leading to syncope can be grouped into two large categories: those that primarily affect cardiac filling (Table 36) and those that primarily affect cardiac emptying. The former are more common, especially in young persons, and less dangerous than the latter in their implications. As inspection of the table indicates, abnormalities of cardiac filling result either from disorders of autonomic cardiovascular reflex control or from systemic diseases. Primary disturbances of cardiac output, on the other hand, are more often caused by heart disease itself. Either filling or emptying defects reduce the cardiac output, which, if it falls by more than about half, results in severely lowered systemic blood pressure and produces a critical drop in cerebral blood flow. *Cerebral vascular disease* requires unusual conditions to cause brief or intermittent unconsciousness. Most episodic neurologic dysfunction resulting from cerebral vascular disease reflects transient ischemic attacks (TIAs) most often arising in the territorial distribution of one of the internal carotid arteries or of the basilar artery. In either distribution the vascular anatomy of the affected artery means that the ischemic episode most often impairs neural structures regulating focal motor or sensory function. Even TIAs that affect the brainstem usually spare the RAS because the core of the pons and midbrain enjoys a rich collateral vascular supply. The one condition in which syncopal-like episodes accompany cerebral vascular disease occurs when atherosclerosis gradually but severely narrows or occludes two or more of the major internal carotid or vertebral arteries in the neck. Under such circumstances a single or only two parent cervical arteries may gradually be forced to provide the necessary blood supply to large areas of the brain, e.g., a single carotid may irrigate both cerebral hemispheres. When this happens, the further development of intrinsic stenosis, the passage

TABLE 36. PRINCIPAL MECHANISMS OF SYNCOPE

I. Impaired right heart filling, cardiac rate slow and abnormal (mainly reflex)
  A. Vasodepressor syncope (vasovagal)
    1. Psychophysiologic (including hyperventilation)
    2. Visceral reflex (micturition, pain, gastrointestinal dilatation, acute vertigo)
    3. Carotid sinus, type 2 (reflex, severe hypotension)
  B. Orthostatic hypotension
    1. Reduced blood volume (hemorrhage, acute salt and water loss, protein loss, enteropathy, burns)
    2. Hypotensive drugs
    3. Neurogenic and idiopathic
  C. Mechanically impaired right heart venous return (cough, syncope, acute pulmonary infarction, fainting lark, near-term pregnancy, pericardial tamponade)
II. Impaired cardiac output
  A. Vasovagal attacks (transient sinus arrest)
    1. Psychophysiologic (uncommon)
    2. Visceral trauma (glossopharyngeal neuralgia, swallow syncope, tracheal stimulation, dilatation of hollow viscus)
    3. Carotid sinus, type 1 (transient asystole)
  B. Cardiac arrhythmia or asystole
    1. Extreme tachycardia > 160–180 minute
    2. Severe bradycardia < 30–40 minute
    3. Heart block: Morgagni-Adams-Stokes syndrome
    4. Ventricular fibrillation
III. Cerebral ischemia (rare)
  A. Severe cervical arterial obstructive disease plus transient ischemic attack (TIA) in remaining single carotid or vertebral artery
  B. Transient acutely increased intracranial pressure (plateau waves)
  C. Basilar migraine

---

of an embolus from the heart or a vascular plaque through the remaining vessel, or even the small drop in systemic arterial pressure that accompanies sudden standing can intermittently reduce flow to large areas of the brain. A global reduction in cerebral function results, producing episodic confusion or syncope.

Transient global amnesia, a condition described more fully with the amnesias on page 1164, represents an episodic and selective abnormality of cerebral memory mechanisms in which affected individuals lose recent memory suddenly and for periods of up to several hours. No abnormality in arousal function accompanies the severe memory loss. The disorder is believed to result from transient vascular insufficiency affecting the posterior diencephalon or adjacent hippocampal structures.

Distinction of Syncope from Seizures

Only a few types of seizures can cause brief episodic unconsciousness in a form that might be confused with syncope.

Convulsive syncope describes a circumstance that occurs more often in children than adults in which the sudden cessation of blood flow to the brain precipitates a brief tonic convulsion or a series of symmetric clonic twitches in the extremities. Not an expression of epilepsy, the motor abnormality almost immediately follows the loss of consciousness and represents a diffuse depolarization of cerebral neurons as a result of abruptly developing anoxia. No postsyncopal EEG abnormalities accompany the condition, nor do other manifestations of generalized epilepsy develop.

Akinetic seizures affect children with certain forms of severe generalized epilepsy and are characterized by sudden inhibition of motor control producing limpness with falling or pitching to the ground. No change in blood pressure is involved, nor do systemic circulatory changes such as pallor or sweating develop. The neurogenic pathogenesis is reflected in the frequency of the spells, their characteristic appearance, and an abnormal EEG. The brief absences of *petit mal epilepsy* are characterized by 3-Hz blinking or bodily movements. The transient loss of consciousness is not associated with falling, loss of color, or other autonomic changes. The EEG is almost always abnormal and diagnostic.

Partial complex (psychomotor) seizures of temporal lobe origin sometimes generate episodic periods of confusion or delirium called dreamy states. The episodes are unlike syncope in many ways. The attacks usually last for a period of 0.5 to 3 minutes or more; falling does not occur unless the seizure discharge spreads to produce a generalized convulsion. Rarely, bradyarrhythmia can occur. The EEG usually shows paroxysmal abnormalities that reflect the temporal lobe genesis of the disorder.

Hypoglycemia

Episodic hypoglycemia of whatever origin can cause brief, recurrent episodes of altered or reduced consciousness. The pathogenesis lies in the failure of glucose supply to the brain. Hypoglycemia has an unexplained propensity to affect different areas of the brain in a sometimes unpredictable manner. As a result, hypoglycemic attacks can vary in their expression from person to person and from attack to attack in the same person. Most attacks depress functions of the forebrain more than the brainstem so as to produce episodic confusion, hypersomnolence, or a slow dysarthric ataxic state resembling alcohol intoxication. Convulsions can occur, especially in children. In other instances stroke-like episodes, psychomotor attacks, transient amnesia, or diffuse flaccid coma may accompany degrees of hypoglycemia no more severe than sometimes are observed to accompany only mild confusion. Abrupt changes in blood sugar or depletion of glycogen reserves in the brain or liver may partially explain the more severe neurologic responses.

Concussion

Concussion describes a state of brief, total unresponsiveness due to head trauma, invariably associated with periods of retrograde and anterograde amnesia. The total duration of such concussive episodes usually is less than 8 to 12 hours and nearly always less than 24. Concussive injuries in humans are rarely witnessed medically, except, perhaps, during boxing bouts. Monitoring of experimentally induced concussion injury in primates, however, reveals a consistent set of physiologic abnormalities. The response typically follows intense blows that produce sudden acceleration or deceleration of the head in the sagittal plane, a physical circumstance particularly designed to perturb paramedian structures, including the RAS. Coma characteristically accompanies the moment of impact and is associated with a depression of corneal and, often, pupillary and oculovestibular reflexes that lasts for several seconds to minutes. For 15 to 20 seconds animals become apneic and diffusely flaccid, changes readily observed at a distance in knocked-out fighters. First breathing, then muscle tonus, and finally pupillary and corneal reflexes return, followed by reawakening in a manner of minutes to hours. Anterograde amnesia lasts for several hours more, with a duration that correlates directly with the severity of the brain injury.

The behavioral changes in animals suggest diffuse depression in the brainstem reticular formation. Electrophysiologic recordings support this inference, showing temporary post-traumatic abolition of electrical activity in brainstem reticular neurons. Neuropathologically, animals killed shortly following experimental concussion show petechial hemorrhages and neuronal loss in the lower brainstem. Neither experimental observations nor those on humans provide a satisfactory explanation for the periods of antegrade amnesia.

Acute Intracranial Hypertension

Sudden rises in the intracranial pressure that approach the mean systolic blood pressure create an unusual cause of brief loss of consciousness that is potentially fatal. The rise abruptly impedes cerebral perfusion so that widespread loss of function and syncope, sometimes accompanied by convulsive movements, takes place. Such increases in pressure can result from severe plateau waves (see the chapter, Neurobiologic Essentials) or from abrupt rupture of blood under arterial pressure into the subarachnoid space or a cerebral ventricle, as occurs with ruptured cerebral aneurysms or acute cerebral hemorrhage. If the plateau wave subsides or the intracranial bleeding stops, consciousness quickly returns so long as brain parenchyma is not directly damaged in critical areas.

Seizures

A *seizure,* or epileptic attack, is the clinical event caused by an intense, uncontrollable, paroxysmal discharge of abnormally hyperactive and hypersynchronous CNS neurons. The cerebral eruption itself is called a *seizure discharge* and usually is recognized by its appearance on a surface EEG or other electrical recording from the brain. In almost any illness producing epileptic attacks, such new electric seizure discharges are far more frequent than clinical attacks and appear on the EEG as brief, self-limited phenomena that spread so little to adjacent or remote brain structures that they produce no detectable alteration in either overall brain function or the person's physical or mental behavior. In the absence of clinical seizures, the finding of paroxysmal discharges on an EEG may support a suggestive history of epilepsy or identify a focal origin for past seizures, but by itself the EEG neither defines the epileptic condition nor gives more than a guideline for treatment.

Seizures and seizure discharges can occur in anyone given a sufficient stimulus. Either singly or recurrently, seizures arise under three major circumstances: (1) sporadically from acute injuries, inflammations, electric shocks, or the effects of drugs, chemical, or anoxic insults on the brain, (2) recurrently and sometimes increasingly, as part of any of several fixed or progressive intrinsic diseases of the brain, and (3) as part of a chronic, genetically influenced illness called epilepsy, whose cause is either unknown or reflects a long-sustained complication of a minor degree of brain scarring most often but not always received during the early years of life.

Recurrent seizures are conventionally considered to arise largely spontaneously as a result of intrinsically abnormal brain mechanisms. This principle applies even to some of the epilepsies that can be induced by stimulation, such as petit mal or photosensitive epilepsy, since spontaneous attacks also characterize those conditions. Accordingly, although reflexly induced patterned motor responses such as flexor spasms, decorticate and decerebrate posturing, and tonic spasms may involve somewhat similar physiologic abnormalities at the neuronal level, they are traditionally dealt with separately and discussed in the chapter, Motor System. An additional, practical reason for this distinction is that these purely reflex hyperactivities only seldom respond to the anticonvulsant drugs that control most seizures.

Almost all seizures, with the exception of a limited group of myoclonic disorders, which can affect the lower brainstem and spinal cord, arise within the forebrain. Accordingly the recording of the surface electrical activity of the brain becomes an important part in understanding the pathophysiology of seizures just as it adds insight into normal and abnormal sleep and other states of altered consciousness.

The Electroencephalogram

For over 50 years it has been recognized that high-gain amplifiers connected to electrodes applied to the scalp would record more or less rhythmic and symmetric electrical activity emanating from the surface of the brain. The resulting EEG contains potentials ranging in frequency from 1 to 50 Hz and with amplitudes ranging from about 20 to as much as 200 mV or more (Fig. 59). The typical EEG frequencies recorded in healthy adults are 8.5 to 13 Hz called alpha, 13 to 30 Hz called beta, 4 to 7 Hz called theta, and 0.5 to 4 Hz called delta. Wakeful persons at rest typically show a dominant alpha rhythm that accelerates into less rhythmic, faster frequencies (i.e., desynchronizes) during concentrated thought, attention, states of emotional tension, and after ingesting certain drugs. Some otherwise normal persons have these higher frequencies at rest. Frequencies of 8 Hz and slower occur normally during drowsiness or sleep. When such slower waves appear during wakefulness, however, they com-

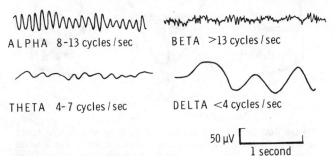

Figure 59. Basic EEG rhythms. (From Solomon, G. E., Kutt, H., and Plum, F.: Clinical Management of Seizures. 2nd ed. Philadelphia, W. B. Saunders Co., 1983.)

monly reflect an abnormality of brain function. Localized areas of slowing, sharp waves, or spike-like waves characteristically reflect focal structural disturbances in brain function, while paroxysmal slow, sharp, or sharp-slow activity is typical of epilepsy. Diffuse EEG slowing accompanies many of the metabolic encephalopathies as well as the pathologic decortication that can follow severe anoxia or major closed head trauma.

The Basis of the EEG. The neurons of the cerebral cortex project a huge number of dendrites toward the cortical surface. At rest a state of constantly changing, partial depolarization affects this intertwined dendritic mesh and generates the undulating, symmetric potentials that make up the EEG. The wakeful alpha rhythm of the EEG reflects the pacemaking influence of the activated nonspecific thalamic reticular formation on the cortical neuropil. As noted, when the cortex goes into greater action, its surface activity desynchronizes, but the sum of the massive dendritic activity remains so great that it still hides the tiny axonal potentials that accompany normal degrees of specific afferent, efferent, or transcortical neural signaling. Seizure discharges, however, because of the intensity and relatively large cortical areas captured by their paroxysmal, accelerated, hypersynchronous bursting activity, break through the background and produce intermittent abnormalities that can be visualized on the EEG.

Slower theta and delta rhythms also can be synchronous between the hemispheres, and in such instances reflect the rhythmic pacemaking of thalamic mechanisms that are deactivated by either normal sleep or pathologic influences such as metabolic encephalopathy. Focal EEG slowing also represents a change in massed surface dendritic activity in the region of the focus, but in this case the altered rhythm is believed to reflect the intrinsic frequency of a cortical area whose connections to the normal thalamic pacemaker have become partially or completely interrupted.

Seizure Mechanisms

Clinical seizures are of two types, focal or generalized (Fig. 60). Focal seizures most often arise from specific, anatomically restricted lesions of gray matter such as

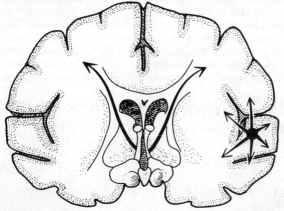

Figure 60. Generalized seizures arise deep within the brain and may have a metabolic, genetic, or unknown origin. Partial seizures arise from a specific focal cerebral region and are caused by scars, tumors, or malformations. (From Solomon, G. E., Kutt, H., and Plum, F.: Clinical Management of Seizures. 2nd ed. Philadelphia, W. B. Saunders Co., 1983.)

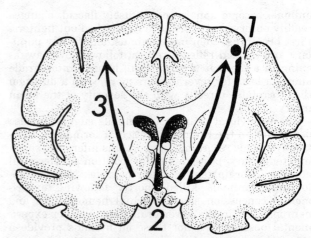

Figure 61. Spread of the epileptic discharge. If a focal seizure discharge (1) activates the centrally placed activating system (2) or diencephalon, the ensuing massive discharge (3) stimulates the hemispheres diffusely and synchronously, and consciousness is lost. (From Solomon, G. E., Kutt, H., and Plum, F.: Clinical Management of Seizures. 2nd ed. Philadelphia, W. B. Saunders Co., 1983.)

scars, tumors, arteriovenous malformations, or focal areas of inflammation. (An exception to this rule of structural abnormality sometimes occurs in children with a benign form of focal motor epilepsy called rolandic epilepsy.) Generalized seizures, by contrast, represent either a diffuse epileptogenic propensity of brain cells or the presence of a deep, cryptic epileptogenic abnormality involving centrally located subcortical activating mechanisms. Overlap occurs between focal and generalized seizures in that focally originating ictal discharges can become generalized in their expression if they happen to arise in a cortical brain area that possesses a strong anatomic projection back into the diencephalic gray matter. In this instance the remote focus quickly transmits its hyperactive hypersynchrony to the central pacemaker, which, in turn, captures both sides of the forebrain in the succeeding generalized attack (Fig. 61).

As already noted, EEGs in patients having illnesses potentially causing clinical seizures record many brief self-contained paroxysmal discharges that have no measurable effect on the person's mental function or physical activity. The following principles influence the genesis of these paroxysmal brief discharges and whether or not they evolve into clinical seizures.

All seizures start in gray matter, arising preferentially in certain anatomic areas but rarely or never in others. The frontal lobes, the limbic system of the medial temporal lobes, the diencephalic reticular formation and, to a lesser degree, the occipital lobe are preferential epileptogenic sites. By contrast, discharging foci almost never are found in the parietal lobe, and they seldom exist on the lateral surface of the temporal lobe or, except for myoclonus, in gray matter that lies caudal to the diencephalon.

Genetic factors influence susceptibility to both generalized epilepsy and at least some forms of focal epilepsy. Intrinsic epilepsies, such as petit mal absences, express themselves along readily identified genetic lines, usually as an autosomal dominant trait with limited penetration. Inherited factors also may influence susceptibility to seizures that occur as a consequence of brain injury. Patients with chronic focal seizures originating in the temporal lobe, for example, show an above-normal incidence of seizure disorders of all kinds in their blood relatives. Furthermore, the incidence of seizures varies widely among persons suffering similar brain injuries from trauma or neoplasms, implying that endogenous factors may influence the epileptic threshold.

In focal epilepsy local brain mechanisms causing seizure discharges to start, spread, or stop are only partially understood. Electrical studies in animals of epileptogenic hippocampal tissue show repeated sudden depolarizing shifts of the affected region occurring at somewhat unpredictable intervals. Whether some neurons in the area intrinsically possesses the capacity to discharge bursts of impulses to the dendrites of adjacent cells or whether the trigger lies in the failure of some naturally inhibiting or metabolic factor coming from other neurons or even adjacent glial cells is debated. In any event, the initial depolarizing burst appears to originate in a relatively small number of neurons that discharge to adjacent excitatory circuits much like the spreading ripples of a pond. The surrounding excitation in turn becomes self-reinforcing and spreads via anatomically preferential pathways to involve more and more of the brain. An implicit step in the postulated mechanism is that the epileptogenic area fails to possess the normal inhibitory feedback mechanisms that ordinarily limit such self-reverberating activity. Reflecting such a failure, the EEG in humans with focal seizures commonly shows spike foci or sharp and slow waves overriding the normal brain waves in the region of the epileptic focus.

Mechanisms that explain focal seizures may not similarly apply to the pathogenesis of generalized seizures, especially those with a strong genetic tendency or having their basis in intrinsic metabolic diseases of the brain. Several hypothetical abnormalities are possible to explain generalized seizures: (1) Intrinsic neuronal membrane changes could lead to a generalized abnormality in ionic conduction, increasing neuronal excitability. (2) Deficiencies in inhibitory or excesses in excitatory neurotransmitters might upset the normal balance between facilitation and inhibition in the brain. (3) Deficiencies in genetically regulated intracellular enzymes could alter the capacity of the cell to carry out the ion pumping that is necessary constantly to repolarize the membrane in the face of naturally occurring dendritic bombardment.

Some seizure discharges may alter brain function even without producing clinical attacks. This appears particularly to be a problem with foci involving the limbic system along the medial temporal lobe where, as discussed in a later section, certain behavioral disorders appear to be particularly associated with right- or left-sided epileptogenic discharges. Quantitative radionuclide scanning in such patients characteristically shows reduced brain metabolism surrounding the seizure focus even when clinical epilepsy no longer occurs. Furthermore, the associated behavioral changes somewhat resemble the effects of amputating the particular temporal lobe. In this instance abnormally discharging foci in the brain appear capable of chronically altering everyday behavior even though clinically recognizable epileptic attacks rarely or never occur. Some investigators believe that a similar mechanism may predispose to behavioral abnormalities in the major psychoses.

Classification and Pathogenesis of Seizure Types

Both focal and generalized seizures include several subtypes depending on the site of the focus and the age when the attacks begin. Table 37 lists the major varieties according to two widely used classifications. Figure 62 diagrams the typical EEG recordings of the most common subtypes.

In both focal and generalized seizures the discharge is believed to begin in a relatively restricted area of the brain representing either a focal hyperexcitable

TABLE 37. CLASSIFICATION OF SEIZURES

INTERNATIONAL CLASSIFICATION OF EPILEPTIC SEIZURES	OLDER CLINICAL CLASSIFICATION
I. Partial seizures (seizures beginning locally)	Focal cerebral
A. Partial simple seizures without impairment of consciousness	
1. With motor symptoms	Focal motor
2. With special sensory or somatosensory symptoms	Focal sensory
3. With autonomic symptoms	
B. Partial complex seizures with impairment of consciousness	Focal cerebral—psychomotor, temporal lobe seizures
1. With impairment of consciousness only	
2. With cognitive symptoms	
3. With affective symptoms	
4. With psychic symptoms	
5. With automatisms	
6. Compound forms	
C. Partial seizures secondarily generalized	Focal cerebral—that become generalized
II. Generalized seizures (bilaterally symmetric from the start)	
A. Absences (petit mal)	Petit mal
B. Bilateral massive epileptic myoclonus	Myoclonic
C. Infantile spasms	Myoclonic-infantile spasms
D. Clonic seizures	Generalized
E. Tonic seizures	Generalized
F. Tonic-clonic seizures	Generalized-grand mal
G. Atonic seizures	Minor motor
H. Akinetic seizures	
III. Unclassified epileptic seizures (due to incomplete data)	Unusual seizure variants

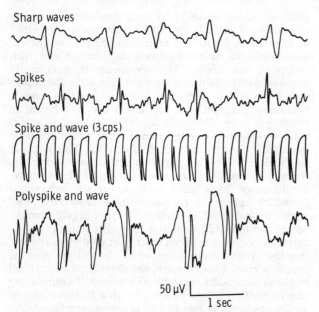

Sharp waves

Spikes

Spike and wave (3 cps)

Polyspike and wave

50 µV
1 sec

Figure 62. Paroxysmal EEG patterns seen in patients with epilepsy. (From Solomon, G. E., Kutt, H., and Plum, F.: Clinical Management of Seizures. 2nd ed. Philadelphia, W. B. Saunders Co., 1983.)

abnormality or an area of low epileptogenic threshold and to spread along preferential pathways whose anatomy explains the clinical attack. Thus the onset of a focal seizure often has diagnostic value, since it may reveal where an abnormality lies. Seizures emanating from the frontal lobe cortex adjacent to or in the primary motor strip, for example, both capture the activity of motor neurons originating in M1 and concurrently spread horizontally across the cortex. The result produces focal seizures as described in the chapter, Motor System.

Generalized seizures are believed to start in the reticular formation or, possibly, basal ganglia of the diencephalon whence the hypersynchronous hyperexcitability captures the thalamocortical relay to cause diffuse cerebral effects whose pattern somewhat depends upon the patient's age when the disorder begins. In children, some generalized seizures take the form of brief "absences" lasting 10 to 20 seconds, during which the child blankly loses contact with his surroundings and may blink or nod in synchrony with a 3-Hz EEG abnormality. The child abruptly recovers when the seizure passes and usually matures normally. Other youngsters suffer more serious atonic or myoclonic attacks from such presumably thalamoreticular epileptic disorders. In adults, generalized seizures occur with patterns that may be tonic, tonic-clonic, or purely clonic (Table 37).

Clinical seizures may interrupt normal consciousness either not at all, partially, or completely, depending on the area of the brain from which they arise and to which they spread. Some focal seizures producing motor, somatosensory, and visual sensory changes fail to spread beyond their cortical areas of origin, and fully alert self-awareness continues unabated while the attack runs its course. By contrast, complex seizures of temporal lobe origin can produce self-limited confused states that partially interfere with awareness of the surroundings and often impair subsequent mem-

ory of the ictal period. The person's overall behavior may not be detectably impaired, even his capacity to respond appropriately during the attack. More extensive temporal lobe attacks that spread their discharges bilaterally to occupy limbic systems in both temporal lobes and beyond characteristically produce complex, vacant behavior, often filled with semipurposeful and autonomic automatisms in which the victim loses contact with the environment as well as any memory of the events. No matter where their initial focus, seizures that spread to central diencephalic pacemaker mechanisms and then project diffusely to the cerebrum block consciousness altogether. Usually such seizures either massively stimulate or inhibit bilateral cerebral-spinal motor systems for the duration of the attack and the several minutes or so of the postictal period.

The duration of seizure discharges varies widely according to their cause. Brief, seconds-long attacks occur in petit mal or akinetic epilepsy of children and may, as noted, somewhat resemble syncope. Partial complex seizures of temporal lobe origin generally last up to about three minutes or so and may be followed by two or three minutes more of postictal confusion. Similar periods frame most tonic and tonic-clonic generalized ictal events. Repetitive attacks with crises succeeding each other without respite can occur in almost any of the acquired or intrinsic seizure disorders. Called *status epilepticus,* this condition can produce either prolonged behavioral abnormalities, as occurs with petit mal or psychomotor status, or can consist of repeated multifocal seizures or life-threatening grand mal convulsions that continue for hours or days, depending upon the underlying illness and its treatment. A rare form of focal motor epilepsy termed *partial continuous epilepsy* can even persist for weeks or months, defying all therapeutic efforts.

ABNORMALITIES OF THE CEREBRAL CORTEX

ORGANIZATION OF THE CORTEX

The Primary and Association Areas

The human cerebral cortex contains densely packed layers and columns of cells lying in a convoluted sheet on top of millions of intracortical and subcortical axons and dendrites that link together different areas of each hemisphere as well as homotypic regions of the two hemispheres. Despite these potentially intimidating complexities, certain guiding principles govern the way the cortex operates, especially when it comes to understanding the structure as it relates to neurologic and organic behavioral disease. This section attempts to outline these principles.

A longstanding and convenient anatomic classification divides the cortex into primary motor, primary sensory, and association areas. Among these the association cortex occupies by far the greatest fraction, more, in fact, than in any other animal species. The regions considered as association cortex transact most of the higher integrative functions of the brain (Fig. 63).

In the frontal lobe, as the reader will recall, only the precentral gyrus represents the primary motor area. The entire remainder of that massive anterior

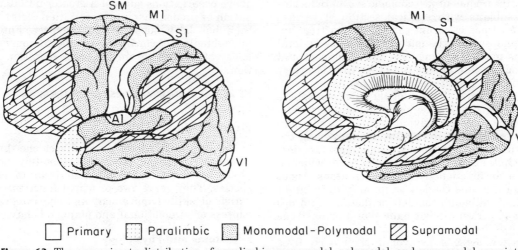

Primary ☐ Paralimbic ▦ Monomodal-Polymodal ▨ Supramodal ▧

Figure 63. The approximate distribution of paralimbic, monomodal, polymodal, and supramodal association cortex as seen on the surface of the cerebral hemispheres. Note the relatively small amount of cortex devoted to specific receptor and final executive motor *(M1)* activity. M1 = Primary motor cortex; S1 = primary sensory cortex; A1 = primary auditory cortex; V1 = primary visual cortex; SM = Supplementary motor cortex.

structure consists of association cortex devoted to organizing the planning, purposefulness, coordination, and emotional content of all forms of expression and motor action. Similarly in the parietal lobe, only the postcentral gyrus appears to be devoted exclusively to somesthetic responses. The remaining parietal cortex integrates spatial, visual, and auditory information to form perceptual presets that influence reflex coordinated motor responses and, at more advanced stages of processing, are integrated into complex memories and the learning of motor acts. Vision appears to be the exclusive province of the occipital lobe, an area that encompasses a large specific visual association cortex as well as the primary visual cortex. The temporal lobe contains the primary receptor cortical areas for audition and olfaction while its extensive association areas relate vision and spatial perception to movement. The posterior temporal areas also serve as zones where pathways carrying perceptual information converge into areas processing memory and become linked to instinctual emotions and autonomic responses. These latter integrations both influence one's immediate reaction to stimuli and modulate autobiographic learning.

An important principle of organization in the association cortex is that of distribution and convergence. Individual incoming specific sensory signals received from both internal and external receptor systems converge upon primary receiving areas of the occipital, parietal, and temporal lobe cortices. There they are processed into second-order signals and distributed immediately to sensory-specific, monomodal association areas in the parietotemporal lobes, as well as to adjacent polymodal association regions in the parieto-temporal and frontal areas (Fig. 63). These latter similarly receive second-order signals from other sensory areas. Each monomodal and polymodal sensory region interconnects with each other and also distributes its received signals more widely, repeating at each successively wider step the frontal-parietal interconnection. Ultimately the multistaged, ever more widely distributed process includes interconnections

with the limbic system. Finally the process converges back upon supramodal areas of parietotemporal and frontal lobe cortex. At this final stage the information conveyed by perception, motor associations, and emotions becomes linked to specific memories and programs that relate to particular learned perceptual and motor integrations. Damage to such supramodal areas or interruption of their projections into the hippocampus or frontal lobe executive cortex can directly disrupt or destroy the cortical templates for either learned, organized perceptions or well-learned motor acts. The result produces abstract behavioral abnormalities as well as the various linguistic (aphasia), perceptual (agnosia), and complex motor (apraxia) disorders discussed later in this chapter. Since homotypic regions of the cerebral hemispheres are closely wired together across the corpus callosum, only functions such as language that are lateralized strongly to one hemisphere or the other are likely to suffer major permanent disruptions from focal unilateral lesions of association cortex. Conversely, small or slowly developing lesions that arise in association areas but do not damage strongly lateralized polymodal functions may cause few or no recognizable behavioral changes in their early stages.

Functional Lateralization in the Hemispheres

The primary motor, somatosensory, and visual cortices of each hemisphere exclusively serve contralateral motor-sensory functions, while the auditory and olfactory primary areas appear to relate predominantly to signals arising from contralateral origins. Cognitive and emotional processing regulated by the association cortex is less consistently assigned to one hemisphere or the other, and controversy surrounds several aspects of the lateralization of these functions. Information concerning such lateralization comes from four general sources. One consists of anatomic examination of the two halves of the normal cerebrum; a second derives from CT, surgical, and postmortem estimations of the abnormal anatomy of clinically well studied cases; the third emanates from neuropsychologic evaluations performed on subjects with surgical section of various parts of the corpus callosum carried out to treat intractable epilepsy; and the fourth includes behavioral observations made following injection of amobarbital (Amytal) sodium into one or the other carotid artery to anesthetize the ipsilateral cerebral hemisphere.

Anatomically, several areas of the left hemisphere differ from the right. The region of the auditory association cortex in the left sylvian fissure (the planum) is larger than the right in most brains, providing the anatomic substrate for syntactic language function. The left occipital and right frontal lobes are wider in most persons for functionally unknown reasons. About two-thirds of the time the left occipital horn is larger than the right, although this left predominance drops to less than 40 per cent in left-handed or ambidextrous persons.

All but a few persons discover in their early lives that one hand, usually the right, automatically shows a preference for performing simple skilled tasks and, eventually, writing. Similar automatic preferences govern the use of a dominant, usually ipsilateral, foot in kicking and hopping. Eye preference is less consistently evident. The anatomic basis of manual dominance relates in some way to hemispheric language dominance: Left handers show less or no anatomic preponderance of the size of the left temporal planum as well as less or reversed asymmetry in ventricular size, as noted.

Among cognitive functions, language is strongly lateralized to one hemisphere, usually the left, in 90 per cent of adults. The right hemisphere, by contrast, appears to transact the major processing involved in recognizing and expressing music and to show substantial advantage over the left in recognizing harmonic pitch.

In most persons the right hemisphere proves to possess superior capacities for discriminating visuospatial functions, although not to the degree by which language is dominantly distributed in the left hemisphere. Patients with right inferior parietal lobe damage suffer greater visual spatial difficulties than do those with comparably sized lesions on the left. Similarly, analyses following unilateral temporal lobectomy indicate greater impairment of visuospatial memories after right- than left-sided ablations. Studies on patients with callosally sectioned brains also indicate superior capacities in the right hemisphere over the left for making visuospatial integrations.

Several efforts have been made to identify lateralized differences between the hemispheres in regulating emotional and nonverbal perceptual functions. Temporofrontal regions on the right seem predominantly to serve the capacity to recognize or impart emotional tone (prosody) to speech. Right-sided lateralization of several other affective responses seems to exist. Patients with large lesions of the right hemisphere commonly show little despair, i.e., remain relatively euphoric, in the face of severe contralateral losses of function, whereas depression of mood is commonly associated with comparably placed lesions of the left hemisphere. Oppositely, uncontrollable laughing as a manifestation of epilepsy occurs primarily with seizures arising from left-sided foci.

Although still fragmentary in many instances, the above observations suggest a greater unilateral distribution or predominance of association cortex functions than has been suspected in the past. Future work undoubtedly will clarify the specific anatomy and physiology of how the brain transacts cognition and emotion.

REGIONAL ABNORMALITIES OF CEREBRAL FUNCTION

Frontal Lobes

The frontal lobes comprise almost one-third of the cerebral cortex and are proportionately larger and phylogenetically newer in man than in any lower species. They serve two principal functions—the execution of skilled movement and the integration and expression of emotional and planned behavior.

Anatomy and Physiology

The frontal lobe couples emotional, intellectual, and perceptual stimuli to motor behavior in still incompletely understood ways. The connections of the region include, among others, prominent reciprocal pathways from the medial dorsal nucleus of the thalamus and the mesencephalic reticular formation (the two serving memory and arousal) as well as from the hypothalamus and amygdala. Frontal cortical areas interconnect with every other lobe of the cerebral hemispheres, including limbic areas in the cingulate gyrus, the septal area, and the temporal lobe, as well as with temporoparietal language areas and parietal lobe sensory association areas. Because of the redundancy of their connections, damage to frontal association areas usually must be large in area, bilateral in distribution, or injure a strongly lateralized function to produce clinically detectable signs and symptoms.

The somatotopically organized rolandic motor cortex (Fig. 24) relates closely to the postcentral, similarly topographically organized, sensory cortex. As noted in the chapter, Motor System, studies show that the primary sensorimotor regions of the cerebral cortex are linked closely together in tight feedback loops so that prerolandic and postrolandic cortical areas discharge concurrently in the process of executing the smoothly governed control of contralateral voluntary movement. Within the frontal lobe, only the rolandic cortex relates in a specific relatively point-to-point manner to motor function. The remainder of the large frontal lobe structure is given over to association cortex. Immediately anterior to the primary motor area (area 4) lie the premotor and supplementary motor regions 6 and 8 that integrate the organization of skilled voluntary movement (Fig. 64). More anteriorly are found the behaviorally related supramodal prefrontal zones. The orbitofrontal and inferomedial regions relate predominantly to the autonomic and emotional components of behavior, while the lateral cortex appears to exert its major influence on attention, planning, and intellectual function.

Both the premotor and prefrontal regions increase their activity during tasks involving directing the person's attention to the choosing and planning of future acts. Considerable lateralization of certain functions exists in these regions. The inferior premotor region on the dominant, usually left, hemisphere includes Broca's area, which relates to the expression of

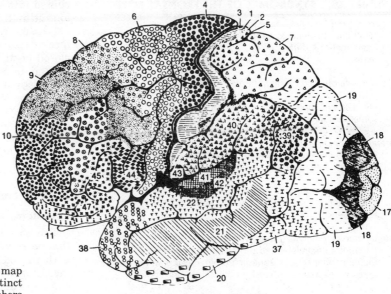

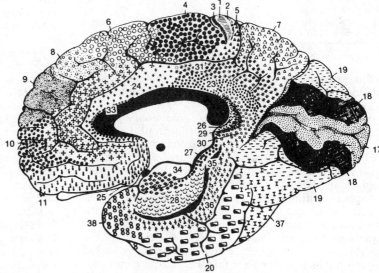

Figure 64. Brodmann's (1909) cytoarchitectural map of the human cerebral cortex. Anatomically distinct areas are designated by symbols, and their numbers are indicated.

language. The same region in the right hemisphere appears to influence the emotional tone or prosody of spoken language. (Prosody is the quality that modulates the tone and melody of speech to convey shades of meaning.) More superiorly lie the frontal eye fields (area 8), which, when stimulated, induce adversive eye movement. Functionally these latter regions appear to be involved in the coordinated direction of visual attention and interconnect closely to visually related area 7 in the parietal lobe, just as the supplementary motor cortex interconnects to the somatosensory related parietal area 5.

Studies in man and monkey indicate that the frontal lobe premotor regions exercise their functional activity bilaterally during both the advanced planning and immediate modification of voluntary movement. The more anterior, prefrontal, parts of the superolateral and superomedial frontal cortex appear to function especially strongly in tasks requiring that the individual give selective attention to one of many stimuli. In addition, the premotor regions appear to participate in tasks involving choosing and synthesizing an imme-

diate succession of behavioral motor acts as well as in planning for future ones.

Clinical Pathophysiology

Table 38 summarizes the principal regional syndromes of the frontal lobes. The nature of *motor dysfunction* following injury to the primary or association motor areas of the frontal lobe has already been described in the chapter on the motor system and will be briefly summarized here. Abnormalities of the primary motor strip produce paralysis or seizures that predominantly affect distal, fine focal movements of the contralateral face, hand, and foot. By contrast, seizure abnormalities affecting the premotor and supplementary areas produce more complex contralateral movements, often including adversion of the eyes, limbs, or body. Lesions that depress or damage the prefrontal regions, if they impair motor function at all, produce hypokinesia accompanied by increased muscular resistance to passive movement. Patients may be unable to relax on command and find it difficult to carry out complex instructions. They may show contralateral

TABLE 38. SYNDROMES OF THE FRONTAL LOBE

Posterior orbitofrontal damage (bilateral and extensive)
Apathetic; inattentive; hypovocal; delayed responsiveness; hypokinetic; indifference-incontinence. Blends into akinetic mute

Anterior orbitofrontal or medial frontal-frontal polar (usually bilateral)
Distractible; short attention span; facetious; logorrhea; sometimes aggressive; "pseudopsychopathic"

Lateral prefrontal unilateral
Either no detectable change or subtle disturbances in planning, anticipation, and attention span

Large or bilateral prefrontal-lateral surface
Hypokinetic; apathetic; much like posterior orbitofrontal but less severe

Lateral supplementary or premotor
Paratonia; contralateral grasp reflexes; urgency incontinence; Broca's aphasia (dominant); ideomotor apraxia. If seizures: adversive oculomotor and motor; speech arrest

Primary motor
Focal distal paralysis (often sensorimotor) or seizures; hand > face > foot. Dysarthria or anarthria

reflex grasping or groping as well as motor·neglect. Bladder and sometimes bowel urgency-incontinence may occur.

Knowledge of the *autonomic and emotional effects* of damage to the inferomedial and orbitofrontal regions comes from physiologic studies in monkey and man as well as from evaluations in humans with various restricted lesions, including those resulting from now seldom used surgical efforts to control psychiatric symptoms. Stimulation or ablation of a number of frontal polar and inferior frontomedial points can induce minor changes in cardiovascular and respiratory functions. Similarly, small lesions in the region of the anterior cingulate gyrus, corpus callosum, or septal region produce few or no symptoms. Large abnormalities in these areas, however, encroach on the underlying diencephalon, producing effects that resemble the alterations associated with large prefrontal lesions described below, plus a somewhat greater degree of reduced arousal than with pure frontal lesions.

Unilateral fixed prefrontal injury often is accompanied by few or no detectable neurologic symptoms. Bilateral damage, however, cutting across or penetrating both prefrontal areas, especially on the inferior and medial surfaces, is followed by a fairly characteristic behavioral pattern, including a flat or inappropriate affect, a disregard for the future consequences of unsocial behavior or of pain, and inability to maintain concentration or take initiative. Sustained attention declines, childishness and vulgarity are common, and abstract intellectual problems present impossible hurdles. Although a few patients may become chronically hyperdistractible and overactive, much more common, especially with large lesions, is a condition of apathetic, relatively mindless, inattentive, underspoken, and hypokinetic behavior that in its extreme form blends into emotionless, motionless, wakeful mutism. Even this apathetic state, however, can be interrupted into an aggressive overreaction by mildly noxious stimuli such as venipuncture.

Damage restricted to the anterior orbitofrontal surface or its connections to the limbic system can follow closed head injury or accompany large tumors. Uninhibited impulsiveness is characteristic, often accompanied by a lack of insight that reduces the subject's awareness of the future implications of external or internal events. Some physicians have capitalized on this effect in neurosurgical procedures that divide the connections between the cingulum and orbitofrontal surface in an effort to improve incapacitating obsessive behavior or relieve the anxieties of severe cancer pain.

Parietal Lobes

Anatomy and Physiology

The parietal lobes provide the cortical mechanisms that perceive somatosensory events and integrate them with the memory of past experiences and with other incoming sensory perceptions to provide awareness of ongoing somatic and extracorporeal events. The parietal lobe contributes to the function of attention and generates the mental "map" that provides internal awareness of the body and the world that surrounds it.

The primary somatosensory cortex, lying immediately posterior to the rolandic fissure, receives its information from the opposite side of the body distributed in a pattern that closely resembles the adjacent, prerolandic motor homunculus (Fig. 32). As with the motor cortex, face, hand, and foot are spatially "overrepresented." Studies in humans following small surgical procedures for removal of tumors or other lesions indicate that the primary sensory cortex provides the critical properties for recognizing the position of body parts in space, identifying the position of stimuli in or on the body, discriminating differences in the weights of lifted objects, discriminating multiple simultaneous somatic stimuli (e.g., smooth from rough, two points from one point), and abstracting the nature of objects from their tactile form (i.e., providing somesthetic recognition or stereognosis). Lesions confined to the primary sensory area do not affect threshold for the sense of vibration, pain, temperature, or simple touch. In the natural course of disease, however, damage to the postcentral gyrus often accompanies lesions that extend considerably deeper and more widely in the hemisphere. When that occurs, other sensations normally mediated by thalamic or polymodal mechanisms may suffer proportionately.

Knowledge about the topographic and functional organization of the posterior parietal association cortex is in a more primitive state. Small lesions of the parietal lobe in humans often produce few or no clinically detectable changes, possibly because the extensive connectivity of the area provides functional redundancy with other regions of association cortex. Accordingly when one finds evidence suggesting parietal lobe dysfunction, it implies either that the abnormality affects the postcentral gyrus, that it is very large, or both.

Large posterior parietal lobe lesions, at least acutely, can produce devastating neurologic difficulties (Table 39). The findings in such cases, plus examinations of patients with cortical excisions and the results of

TABLE 39. LATERALIZING COGNITIVE ABNORMALITIES OF THE POSTERIOR PARIETAL LOBE LISTED IN DESCENDING ORDER OF THEIR APPROXIMATE FREQUENCY*

Right-Sided	Left-Sided
Constructional apraxia	Constructional apraxia
Contralateral spatial neglect	Right-left confusion
Contralateral sensory extinction	Calculation defects
Apathetic indifference	Impaired recognition of distal body parts
Dressing apraxia	Agraphia or conduction aphasia‡
Motor impersistence	
Denial of abnormality (anosognosia)	Ideomotor or ideational‡ apraxia
Nonverbal spatial amnesia† (faces, other specific objects)	

*The more frequent signs can accompany relatively small lesions while those at the bottom of the lists reflect the presence of extensive damage, often extending beyond parietal lobe boundaries.
†Usually implies bilateral lesions.
‡Implies extension into posterior temporal lobe.

experiments in laboratory primates, indicate that the posterior parietal area integrates visual and, to a lesser degree, auditory stimuli with somesthetic perceptions to provide progressive abstractions of spatial orientation and attention. As noted, the postcentral area projects information to both the prefrontal and premotor areas of the frontal lobes as well as to temporal regions related to memory and limbic functions. In monkeys the posterior parietal area also reciprocally interconnects with the pulvinar and reticular formation of the brainstem. These connections provide the anatomic substrate for some of the parietal influences that direct the monkey's attention to incoming spatial stimuli received peripherally in the visual field. It seems likely that such pathways for guiding attention must also exist in man. Evidence in humans subjected to small posterior parietal cortical resections for the removal of epileptogenic lesions suggests that the superior portion of the parietal association cortex concerns itself predominantly with the further integration of somesthetic spatial perception, while the inferior area, encroaching on the marginal gyrus of the temporal lobe, serves a more multimodal function where somatosensory spatial, visual, and auditory perceptions converge upon areas dealing with memory and emotion. In the dominant hemisphere this area appears to participate in verbal memory as well.

Pathophysiology

Restricted parietal lobe damage in man is relatively uncommon and most often accompanies benign or small metastatic brain tumors or their surgical removal. Occasionally, vascular lesions, such as small branch occlusions of the distal middle cerebral artery, can injure both the prerolandic and postrolandic areas to the exclusion of other regions of the brain. The resulting distal local sensory loss coupled with weakness involving the hand, or less often, the foot may initially resemble the changes of a unilateral peripheral neuropathy.

Parietal lobe damage limited to the postcentral gyrus produces the restricted "cortical" somatosensory defects described in a preceding paragraph. Larger cortical lesions extending deep to the cortex of either hemisphere can additionally encroach upon frontal

motor pathways to produce monoparesis or hemiparesis. Similarly, they can extend deep toward the thalamus to impair primary sensory modalities, or extend posteriorly to cause signs and symptoms of posterior parietal lobe dysfunction.

The symptoms resulting from posterior parietal lobe injury depend upon the size of the lesion and the rate of its development (Table 39). Small lesions commonly cause no symptoms or produce changes lasting only a few days. Large lesions involving the posterior parietal lobe produce several well-defined syndromes. Such damage tends especially to follow vascular occlusions of the internal carotid or middle cerebral artery, particularly of the latter's postsylvian branches. Cerebral hemorrhages, malignant brain tumors, or brain abscesses also can produce rapid progression with similarly severe neurologic dysfunction. The resulting disabilities, particularly when the lesion affects the nondominant hemisphere, can produce striking symptoms. Even when somesthetic or visual thresholds are not detectably elevated, one finds defects in attention such that when both sides of the body or visual field are tested simultaneously the subject fails to perceive the one arising contralateral to the lesion. In more advanced cases, disturbances in the recognition of contralateral spatial relationships emerge. With worsening of the defect, spatial disorientation may develop along with constructional or dressing apraxia (p. 1161), as well as inattention or neglect of the opposite side of the body and the extracorporeal space subtended by the contralateral visual field. Very large lesions in the nondominant hemisphere can produce additional devastating incapacities. Affected victims not only ignore the contralateral extracorporeal world but lose their awareness of internal spatial relationships (maps) as well. Thus some patients affected with severe right parietal-frontal damage act and speak as if only the functionally intact, right half of the body ever existed. They behave as if all memory of the previously healthy left side had departed their awareness and, as a result, may deny its ailments (anosognosia) even when confronted directly with the crippled example. For instance, patients with such severe perceptual disorders when presented with their own functionless and usually insensate hand may disclaim its possession saying, "It can't be mine, it doesn't work." Sometimes such severe disturbances in the recognition of external and internal space extend to include the spatial realm served by the still intact hemisphere so that affected individuals show bilateral defects in attention or even develop a global confusional state or delirium. Apathetic inattention and emotional flatness commonly accompany extensive damage to the nondominant side.

Lesions associated with severe abnormalities in spatial orientation and contralateral neglect rarely are confined entirely to the parietal lobe cortex. Rather the structural changes usually involve much of the underlying white matter and extend deeply into the thalamus or forward to interfere with frontal lobe motor or premotor systems. Visual pathways as well as those connecting the parietal lobe to the reticular and limbic systems are similarly impaired. Most patients with acute parietal lobe lesions large enough to impair attention and spatial perception will be lethargic, slow, and mentally confused. Reflecting the interruption of occipital-tectal pathways, the head and eyes may deviate toward the side of the cerebral damage; contralateral visual fields usually show a homonymous lower quadrant or hemianopic field defect.

Some authorities have attributed the right-sided predominance of lesions causing hemispatial neglect, denial of disability, and disregard for half of one's body to the fact that the effects of similarly large lesions on the left hemisphere cannot accurately be tested because of associated aphasia. This seems unlikely to be the only factor, however, since the right hemisphere functions preferentially in relation to spatial tasks in either hand, as noted following section of the corpus callosum. Furthermore, only right-sided damage appears capable of inducing bilateral spatial disorientation.

Injuries restricted to the posterior parietal lobe of the left hemisphere result in less profound contralateral inattention than outlined above. Patients with left parietal lesions sometimes have difficulty selecting right from left as well as in identifying distal body parts (finger agnosia). They often show considerable difficulty in making arithmetic calculations, even of a simple nature. The close relationship between the left parietal lobe and language function is described below in the section on aphasia.

Temporal Lobes

Anatomy and Physiology

The temporal lobes serve as major convergent areas for signals arising from all parts of the cortex. The structures have three major surfaces. The superior surface forms the inferior bank of the sylvian fissure, the medial inferior aspect faces on the tentorium and sphenoid bone, and the lateral convolutions face outward against the temporal bone. The superior surface, including the transverse (auditory) gyrus and the region immediately posterior to it, contains the primary auditory cortex and its association area. In the dominant hemisphere this region is indispensable for language processing, and damage to it results in Wernicke's aphasia, as described below. The comparable nondominant zone may provide the necessary processing for musical recognition and melody composition. On the medial inferior surface lies the parahippocampal gyrus that connects with the cingulate gyrus posteriorly and with the subcallosal gyrus of the septal area anteriorly. The resulting ring of gray matter surrounding the diencephalon is termed the *limbic cortex*. Located posteriorly within the parahippocampus is the hippocampus proper, a structure that relates in a major way to the storage and retrieval of autobiographic memory. Although both hippocampal regions usually must be damaged to produce severe memory loss, in most persons injury to the left side impairs at least some measure of verbal memories, while damage to the right may interfere more with visual-spatial recall. Anteromedially the uncal region and the anterior end of the hippocampal gyrus contain the primary olfactory cortex. Neoplasms or scars in this region give rise to *uncinate seizures,* brief paroxysms of intense, unpleasant, and unfamiliar smell. The underlying amygdaloid complex provides stout interconnections between the rest of the cerebrum and the olfactory system lying immediately anterior to it, as well as with the hypothalamus and other nuclei that comprise the subcortical components of the limbic system. Interconnections between brainstem and cortex relayed via this region provide emotional and autonomic modulations that affect the encoding, storage, and retrieval of acquired memory and link instinctive and learned emotional and visceral responses to immediate sensory stimuli.

The functions of the part of the superior temporal cortex that lies anterior to the auditory cortex, as well as that which occupies the lateral and inferior surfaces, are less well understood in man. Various patterns of intensely perceived memories or even dreamlike sequences have been elicited by electrical stimulation of these regions in epileptic patients. In monkeys the middle and inferior temporal gyri have been found to make up a major polymodal integrating way station interposed between the posteroinferior parietal area and the inferolateral premotor frontal region. Studies of cerebral blood flow changes in humans during attentional tasks indicate that the lateral inferior temporal areas participate in processing responses to visual spatial stimuli involving saccadic eye movements. Undoubtedly this represents but one of several complex functions integrated by the area.

Pathophysiology

In monkeys, bilateral removal of the temporal lobes produces a remarkable disorder called the Klüver-Bucy syndrome. The condition is characterized by an indiscriminate tendency to examine objects manually, visually, and orally without regard to their meaning (psychic blindness). In addition, the animals show anterograde memory loss, endless distractibility, emotional placidity, and a marked increase in sexual activity. Much of the disorder can be traced to (a) a visual spatial agnosia due to bilateral interruption of the connections between the lateral inferior temporal cortex and the frontal lobe, (b) memory loss secondary to bilateral hippocampal removal, and (c) placidity and loss of sexual restraint associated with removal of the amygdala. Somewhat similar but more complex behavior changes have appeared in humans with extensive bilateral temporal lobe damage due to encephalitis, severe head trauma, or the degenerative dementias of Pick's and Alzheimer's diseases.

Some of the best inferences about temporal lobe function and dysfunction come from the study of patients with seizures that originate in this region of the brain. Such attacks, if well localized, characteristically mimic or make a caricature of the normal function of the area. The association of olfactory hallucinations with the region of the uncus already has been mentioned. Seizures arising from mesial basal temporal lobe structures, including the hippocampal and amygdaloid region and their adjacent cortex, characteristically produce memory disturbances in which the subject feels as if he is reliving a previous experience (déjà vu = already seen) or that the environment suddenly seems entirely unfamiliar (jamais vu = never seen). Both déjà vu, and less often, jamais vu episodes can occur in mild forms among about half the normal population; only when particularly abrupt in onset or intense in nature should they be considered as possible epileptic phenomena. In the form of seizures, déjà vu and jamais vu attacks especially relate to the right temporal lobe ictal foci. Patients affected by such limbic system discharges also may experience fragments of forced thinking, brief hallucinations of verbal memory, or undergo a more sustained sense of being caught for a minute or so in an irresistible, vivid dream, complete with voices addressing them. The attacks illuminate the way that temporal lobe mechanisms integrate emotional and perceptual experiences into cohesive patterns of recall rather than simply chaotic fragments of past sensory stimuli. Seizures arising in more superior or lateral aspects of the temporal lobe may block language formation, produce hallucinations of hissing, roaring, or clicking, or create a brief illusion of intense floating vertigo, changes reflecting a focal origin in or near the auditory or vestibular cortex. Visual distortions of size and shape also occur, presumably reflecting involvement of the association areas of the lateral temporal lobe cortex.

Many persons with temporal lobe epilepsy possess interictal personality features that distinguish them from the normal population. These traits also may reflect damage to the emotional-anatomic functions of this part of the brain. Such individuals tend to be humorless, self-absorbed, circumstantial, and given to excessive detail as well as intellectual preoccupations. As a group they appear prone to religiosity and philosophic ruminations, and many are given to quick, intensive emotional responses, whether of anger or sadness. Some studies have detected differences in behavioral traits, depending on the side of the temporal lobe lesion. In these analyses, patients with left temporal lobe seizure foci tended toward hypergraphia, kept extensive notes or diaries, and showed a preoccupation with verbally related complex or cosmic ideas. By contrast, nonverbal excesses of mood or emotional responses were associated more often with right temporal lobe foci (Table 40). As noted earlier, the personality changes suggest that the epileptic tissue in the temporal-limbic system must interfere with or reduce function in the affected area, especially since metabolic studies employing positron emission demonstrate abnormally low interictal brain metabolism in temporal lobe areas that contain epileptogenic foci.

Some believe that temporal lobe seizures arising from the amygdaloid region can result in unprovoked assault, but this conclusion lacks strong supporting evidence. Unprovoked aggression is extremely rare as

TABLE 40. ABNORMALITIES ASSOCIATED WITH UNILATERAL TEMPORAL LOBE DAMAGE OR CHRONIC SEIZURE FOCI

Right	Left
Often Lost After Damage or Removal	
Memory for harmonies, musical constructions, nonverbal visual and spatial patterns	Posterior: Wernicke's and related noncomprehension aphasias
Recognition for emotional tonality of speech	Anterior: Reduced verbal memory and learning
Sometimes Associated with Temporal Lobe Epilepsy	
Emotional deepening, easy anger, aggression, sadness	Reduce self-esteem
	Increased absorption and sobriety
	Circumstantiality
	Hypergraphia
	Religiosity, philosophic preoccupations

a specific manifestation of epileptic attacks except when unsuspecting observers attempt to restrain affected individuals during the course of an attack. Somewhat stronger evidence, however, does suggest that the poorly inhibited emotional responses of some temporal lobe epileptics leads them to severe rage responses and sometimes violence in response to relatively minor stimuli. Another remarkable dimension of temporal lobe epilepsy is that most affected males have a subnormal libido not accompanied by abnormalities in circulating testosterone levels.

Whether or not abnormal temporal lobe mechanisms can result in severe emotional symptoms or even psychosis is a controversial and unsettled issue. An unexpectedly high incidence of limbic system tumors has been reported from autopsies in patients chronically hospitalized with a diagnosis of schizophrenia. Furthermore, patients with temporal lobe epilepsy demonstrate an abnormally high incidence of schizophrenia-like psychosis. Even if this association truly exists, however, available information tells one little about precise mechanisms. Some authorities believe that schizophreniform illnesses are associated with left temporal lobe epilepsy while bipolar or affective psychoses are associated with right temporal lobe abnormalities. When prominent behavior abnormalities do occur, they usually follow the onset of epilepsy and sometimes begin only after successful medical or surgical treatment halts the usual manifestations of the seizure disorder.

FOCAL DISTURBANCES OF HIGHER BRAIN FUNCTION

Language and Speech

Verbal language comprises the process by which the forebrain applies symbolic terms and grammar to objects and concepts to formalize its knowledge of sensory perceptions, memories, emotional responses, and the stream of preverbal inner thoughts. The neuroanatomy of the mechanisms that accomplish language is known from three sources. One comes from the postmortem study of patients in whom language impairment has been carefully evaluated. The second consists of the change produced in language by stimulating various regions of the cerebral cortex during neurosurgical procedures. The third derives from tomographic brain imaging, including CT, nuclear magnetic resonance, and positron emission tomographic (PET) scans, which disclose much of the structure and, with PET, the metabolism of language in the intact patient.

Anatomic Considerations

Although wide areas of both hemispheres contribute to language function, the critical regions are concentrated in two principal cortical zones, a posterior predominantly receptor-integrative area and an anterior region devoted predominantly to language expression (Fig. 65). The principal posterior portion of the language cortex occupies the posterior aspect of the superior temporal gyrus, extending from approximately the transverse auditory (Heschl's) gyrus back to the end of the sylvian fissure. This, the *Wernicke area*, represents the region where auditory sensory perceptions appear to be integrated with inner thought and memory to generate the fundamental abstractions and grammar of language. The region of the adjacent

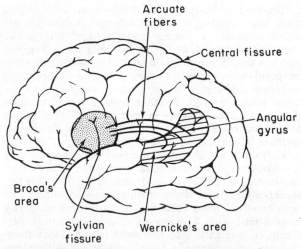

Figure 65. The language areas of the dominant hemisphere.

angular and supramarginal gyri as well as of the superiorly adjacent parietal operculum and the ventro-lateral nuclear complex of the thalamus contribute importantly but in a clinically less predictable manner to the fundamental synthesis of language. The angular gyrus region appears to integrate visual percepts into the language mechanism, while the region of the parietal operculum contains the arcuate fasciculus, which interconnects the posterior and anterior zones. More anteriorly, *Broca's area,* lying in the inferolateral frontal lobe just anterior to the primary motor cortex and extending under the surface into the frontal operculum and insula, is critical to the normal verbal or written semantic expression of speech. Lesions surrounding the Wernicke area that interrupt pathways projecting into it but not the speech cortex itself, disrupt selective aspects of posterior language function while peri-Brocal lesions produce partial impairments in the expression of language. Some evidence indicates that verbal and written expression may return following damage to small areas or even removal of this anterior region. As a rule, however, severe injury to the primary language zones of the adult results in at least some permanent functional impairment.

Language function is strongly lateralized in most human brains. Anatomically the left hemisphere usually contains a longer sylvian fissure than the right. Furthermore, the planum of the left temporal lobe (the superior temporal area lying in the sylvian fissure in back of the posterior edge of the transverse gyrus) is larger than the right in two-thirds of brains, the anatomic difference already being evident in the brains of infants. Clinically, language laterality in patients can be estimated in two major ways, one by correlating the side of temporofrontal brain lesions with the presence or absence of aphasia, the other, used in persons with normal speech, by observing the effect of injecting the short-acting anesthetic amobarbital sodium into an internal carotid artery. The injection briefly anesthetizes the ipsilateral cerebral hemisphere, including whatever language activities it possesses, giving preoperative knowledge of the risks of surgery to the particular side of brain. Both analyses indicate that in almost all right-handed persons the left hemisphere is heavily dominant for speech and that aphasia resulting from damage to the left posterior language areas sel-

dom fully recovers. Among left-handers and the strongly ambidextrous, about 70 per cent show a left hemisphere language dominance or predominance. Of the remaining 30 per cent, about half show strong language representation in each hemisphere, while the remainder are right dominant. A feature of many left-handers or ambidextrous persons is that damage to the major language area on either side may produce acute symptoms of aphasia, but a higher percentage recover than do right-handers with comparable dominant hemispheric lesions.

Language function in children represents a special case. Most youngsters who suffer a severe hemispheric brain injury when less than six years of age recover normal or near-normal capabilities whether or not aphasia accompanies the early postinjury period. Even among such children, however, transient aphasia follows damage to the left temporal frontal area nine times more often than to the right.

The Physiology of Language

Studies of cerebral blood flow or metabolism in humans during language and speech reveal extensive participation by areas outside the classic dominant Wernicke and Broca regions. Although left hemispheric activity predominates in most persons, the comparable regions of the right hemisphere participate to a lesser degree. During reading the visual cortex and premotor frontal eye fields increase their activity, while the supplementary motor cortex participates in both silent and articulated speech. Increased activity in the prefrontal region regularly and predictably accompanies all aspects of programmed, serial language. Subcortical structures of the dominant hemisphere also play a role: The thalamus appears to relate to word retrieval, while increased caudate activity can be observed during tasks involving both the planning and articulation of speech. During tests involving the recognition or formation of musical sounds, right-hemispheric temporofrontal areas increase their activity more than comparable areas on the left.

Considerable sublocalization seems to exist in the association cortex devoted to language. Perisylvian and inferior frontal areas, for example, are closely linked to orofacial motor functions. The temporal lobe and adjacent cortex appear to function largely in the storage of language, while the inferior frontal area provides verbal retrieval. Grammatic functions and nominal memories appeared to depend upon different areas of the superior temporal cortex, the latter being situated more posteriorly.

Aphasia

Aphasia or dysphasia describes an impairment or loss of language function as a result of damage to the specific language areas of the cerebrum. The condition must be distinguished from *dysarthria,* a disturbance in the articulation of speech, as well as from defects in sensory systems that prevent perceptions from reaching the language cortex. Persons deaf and blind from peripheral causes can learn a language as long as the brain is intact, while disease of the motor system, cerebellum, or the vocal apparatus can cripple or halt the outflow of words but does not produce aphasia.

The pattern of aphasia depends on the part or parts of the speech brain that are irreversibly damaged so that the ultimate nature of a language impairment may not become clear until several days after an acute lesion produces more global dysfunction. Language represents the integration and expression of many aspects of brain function, and injuries to its mechanism can result in several somewhat varying symptom complexes. Among its properties are (1) the comprehension of symbols, (2) the ability to transform perceptions or inner thoughts into words, (3) the ability to express symbols. Most aphasic disorders can be classified by testing comprehension of language, fluency of output, and ability to repeat phrases (Table 41).

Lesions damaging the dominant posterior superior temporal gyrus and its adjacent area characteristically destroy the capacity to recognize the sensory symbols of language or to transform inner thoughts into meaningful words. The result is *Wernicke's aphasia.* Affected patients cannot recognize spoken, written, or symbolic instructions except, perhaps intermittently, to obey the simplest verbal commands, e.g., "Stop!" Despite the severe injury to comprehension, the brain preserves its memory storehouse of individual words so that they characteristically are expressed correctly. Patients with Wernicke's aphasia speak fluently with a natural rhythm, although the result provides an incomprehensible flow of neologisms, agrammaticisms, and pressured speech that risks being mistaken for psychotic behavior. Insight is lost, and prognosis for total recovery is poor. Lesions to the parietal operculum adjacent to the Wernicke area give rise to *conduction aphasia,* a condition in which arcuate fibers connecting the posterior with the anterior language area are interrupted, but the auditory association cortex remains intact. Anatomic lesions have been described by CT in the supramarginal gyrus and auditory or insular cortices. In conduction aphasia patients speak fluently, but make many errors similar to what occurs in Wernicke's aphasia. Comprehension of language heard or read remains relatively normal, but the ability to repeat phrases is severely impaired.

Focal lesions of the dominant hemisphere lying posterior to the Wernicke area can destroy selectively one or another dimension of language perception. *Alexia* (inability to comprehend written language while re-

taining relatively good general vision, especially in the left visual field) without *agraphia* (inability to write language despite the preservation of related motor function) results when a lesion destroys the left visual radiation or cortex and, in addition, extends to involve the splenium of the corpus callosum. The splenial placement interrupts the projection that otherwise would connect the unaffected right visual cortex to the language areas of the left hemisphere. Such patients, despite their inability to comprehend the written word, can speak and write normally, in contrast to those with a combination of *alexia with agraphia* in which normal auditory comprehension, thought, and speech remain, but the comprehension of both visual and written language symbols is lost. The abnormality is rare and has been stated to follow lesions of the left angular gyrus. *Pure word deafness* describes the condition in which auditory language perception is lost selectively despite intact hearing for noises and the preservation of other language capabilities. This rare phenomenon folows bilateral focal damage to the auditory cortex of the superior temporal gyrus. Reportedly it also can accompany subcortical white matter damage in the left temporal lobe that injures the adjacent left auditory cortex and disconnects the transcallosal fibers from the right temporal lobe destined for Wernicke's area.

Broca's aphasia is characterized by severe disturbances in the output of speech and writing, either spontaneous or in response to command. Comprehension of simple language constructions is relatively well preserved, although complex syntactic relations are misunderstood and things heard usually are better comprehended than things read. Patients with Broca's aphasia often are depressed. Largely because of vascular distributions, many also have an associated right hemiparesis or hemiplegia, but this is the result of an extension of the lesion to involve the nearly internal capsule. Enlargement of the lesion into the adjacent premotor cortex may explain an associated motor apraxia observed in some patients. More restricted inferior frontal cortical lesions may result in slow, effortful, dysarthric speech with good comprehension,

TABLE 41. CLASSIFICATION OF APHASIAS

	Expression	Comprehension	Repetition	Other Signs	Localization
Broca's (expressive)	Nonfluent	+	−	Right hemiparesis worse in arm; mood depressed	Lower posterior frontal
Wernicke's (receptive)	Fluent	−	−	Often none; may be euphoric and/or paranoid	Posterior superior temporal area
Conduction	Fluent	+	−	Often none; cortical sensory loss in right arm; depressed	Usually parietal operculum
Global	Nonfluent	−	−	Right hemiparesis worse in arm; flat affect	Massive peri-sylvian lesion
Transcortical motor	Nonfluent	+	+		Anterior to Broca's area or supplementary speech area
Transcortical sensory	Fluent	−	+		Surrounding Wernicke's area posteriorly
Transcortical mixed (isolation syndrome)	Nonfluent	−	+		Both of the above
Anomic	Fluent	+	+		Lesion of angular gryus or second temporal gryus

After Geschwind, N.: The organization of language and the brain. Science 170:940–944, 1970.
+ = relatively or fully intact.
− = definitely impaired.

normal syntax, and preserved ability to write normally.

Global aphasia describes the severe loss of all major aspects of language function. Acutely affected patients are often mute and have an accompanying right hemiplegia. Shortly thereafter it becomes apparent that they neither can comprehend language nor correctly express it except, perhaps, in the form of brief expletives or phrases. Insight, as judged from other behavior, is poor, as is prognosis for full recovery.

A group of aphasic disorders are characterized by the ability of the patient to repeat phrases or even long sentences after the examiner. Such an ability to repeat implies that Wernicke's and Broca's areas as well as the primary connections between them must be intact so that the responsible lesions must lie near to but not within the primary speech areas. These aphasias with good repetition have been classified as: (1) transcortical motor (similar to Broca's), (2) transcortical sensory (similar to Wernicke's) and (3) the isolation syndrome (caused by a large lesion producing a global type of aphasia except for normal repetition). Included in this group of disorders is *anomic aphasia,* associated with a lesion of the angular gyrus and characterized by rambling, lengthy, empty, and poorly focused speech, with transparent circumlocutions— talking around forgotten words. However, the diagnosis of anomic aphasia deserves words of caution: Nonspecific difficulties in word finding are common in many persons, especially the elderly and can accompany damage of several kinds affecting either hemisphere. Such word-finding problems commonly appear in nonspecific confusional states accompanying general medical problems in older persons and often disappear largely or entirely when the general illness subsides.

Epileptic *speech arrest* has been reported in association with focal abnormalities or electrical stimulation of several areas of the dominant cerebral cortex. The susceptible regions, all in the dominant hemisphere, include the temporoparietal-occipital confluence, the region of the angular gyrus, the inferior premotor area, the prerolandic and postrolandic facial-oral representation, and the superior premotor (Fig. 66).

Nonaphasic Speaking Defects

Any process that interferes with the nuclear or supranuclear innervation of the larynx, pharynx, tongue, mouth, or lips can interfere with the capacity for clear articulation. Disturbances of speaking associated with cerebellar dysfunction, basal ganglia disease, and most cortical spinal tract dysfunction parallel the motor defects seen in other skeletal muscles with those disorders.

Mutism. The inability to speak, mutism, has several causes. Acutely it appears in association with vascular lesions of the left frontal lobe involving either a part of Broca's area or its conducting pathways. Under such circumstances, mutism coupled with right hemiplegia, as indicated above, reflects the presence of a relatively large brain lesion and gives way to a less complete language disturbance within a few days. Acute mutism also can arise as an isolated symptom of a restricted frontal vascular lesion, in which case the disability usually disappears within a few days to a week or so without leaving residual expressive symptoms. More sustained mutism develops as a symptom of extensive bilateral basal forebrain damage where it is accompanied by apathy, inattention, and hypokinesia. Sustained mutism and behavioral withdrawal also can accompany severe psychiatric disorders. The latter illnesses usually occur in younger patients and are unaccompanied by signs, symptoms, or laboratory findings that would indicate structural frontal lobe disease. *Anarthria,* the inability to speak because of abnormal innervation or mechanical disease of the vocal apparatus, differs from mutism in that affected patients make sounds and usually express vividly their frustration over being unable to speak. Occasionally, anarthria will reflect a hysterical disorder, in which case the alert, attentive patient usually displays an insouciant indifference to his or her lack of vocal capacity. Neurogenic causes of anarthria include either severe

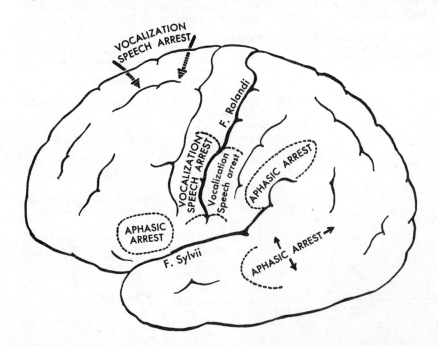

Figure 66. Areas where epileptic discharges have been found to interfere with speech. (From Penfield, W., and Rasmussen, T.: The Cerebral Cortex of Man. New York, Macmillan Co., 1950.)

bulbar or pseudobulbar palsy, conditions readily diagnosed by the presence of other signs and symptoms of nuclear or supranuclear paralysis.

Spasmodic Dysphonia. Spasmopdic dysphonia is a bizarre and rare form of dysarthria that produces a spastic, hoarse difficulty in speaking, but fails to affect the capacity to laugh, cough, or even sing articulately. The disorder once was considered to represent a hysterical symptom, but affected patients tend to lack other psychopathologic symptoms. Furthermore, many of these patients show other signs of dystonia, such as torticollis or blepharospasm, or neurologic abnormalities affecting brainstem-evoked responses or functions of the vagus nerve. The condition is most often regarded as being a monosymptomatic dystonia.

Prosody. The melodic intonations of normal speech, prosody, appear to depend predominantly upon right hemispheric functions. Loss of the modulation of speech as well as of associated gestures and facial expressions accompanies damage or dysfunction of the right inferior perisylvian area.

The Etiology of Aphasia. Although brief disturbances in language function can result from seizures or transient attacks of vascular insufficiency, the development of a true aphasia, i.e., a selective disturbance in language function not part of a global decline in the intellect and lasting for more than a few hours, reflects a focal structural lesion of the brain. The most common cause is vascular damage, either from infarction or hemorrhage, in the distribution of the middle cerebral artery or, less often, the posterior or anterior cerebral arteries. Occlusions of the last-mentioned may damage the pulvinar or disconnect right hemispheric sensory signals from the language areas in the left hemisphere. The second most frequent cause of aphasia is severe head trauma. Neoplasms and other space-occupying lesions engender most of the remaining cases. None of these causes of aphasia typically produces very discrete brain lesions, and several, such as vascular disease, tend to generate either multifocal brain damage or large lesions whose effects extend considerably beyond the classic language zones. Verbal language represents an exclusively human function, so that aphasia can be studied only in the damaged human brain. The anatomic variability of the lesions that cause aphasia necessarily leads to an equally inconsistent patterning of its major symptoms. The examiner must constantly recall these principles when trying to localize the anatomy and diagnose the cause of a language defect.

Apraxia

Apraxia refers to a disturbance of ability or an inability to perform learned motor acts even though the person can attend to instructions and retains sufficient perceptual, memory, and language functions to understand the command and possesses the motor capacity to carry it out. As a symptom isolated from more widespread deterioration of psychologic powers, apraxia is uncommon, even rare. It has been considered to occur in four principal forms: (1) *Ideational apraxia* is a rare phenomenon implying that the brain has lost the learned memory for a specific act. While they may be able to imitate, affected patients are unable to conceive of the commanded behavior and to carry it out in proper sequence. The disorder affects both sides of the body and includes all motor parts that would normally be involved in the desired action. The defect characteristically varies in intensity, being worsened by fatigue or tension. An additional factor that makes evaluation difficult is that most ideational apraxia is associated with extensive defects in language or spatial functions. When focal or unilateral lesions exist, they most often consist of large strokes involving the posterior temporoparietal area of the dominant hemisphere. (2) *Ideomotor apraxia* consists of the inability to carry out relatively simple gestures (wave goodbye; salute the flag; light a match) either in response to a verbal command or, less often, by imitation. Affected patients usually have little difficulty in including similar gestures in their naturally occurring behavior. Nevertheless, suitable testing indicates that they comprehend the command and recall the nature of the simple act that is required. Patients with ideomotor apraxia tend to have insight into their motor capacity and may shrug or smile helplessly as tentative efforts fail to carry out the command accurately. Specific lesions most often associated with ideomotor apraxia lie in the region of the temporoparietal or parietal areas of the dominant hemisphere, and most affected patients have an associated conduction aphasia. This finding as well as studies of commissourotomy patients imply that most motor apraxia represent failure to be able to transmit to the motor system commands received by visual verbal areas of either hemisphere. (3) *Kinetic or motor apraxia.* Some patients with partial Broca's aphasia may have great difficulty carrying out motor commands involving the face or hand of either side of the body despite their apparent ability to understand what is said. The defect is considered to reflect damage to a premotor area in the dominant hemisphere that regulates the serial action for certain learned motor functions. Affected patients appear to understand instructions and may even haltingly repeat them verbally, but are unable to imitate with either hand the simple acts as indicated under ideomotor apraxia above. By contrast, some of these functions, e.g., combing the hair, using a toothbrush, may be carried out in automatic settings such as when performing the morning toilet. It is difficult to separate the manual motor difficulties from the wider disruption of language function that occurs in most affected patients. (4) *Callosal (anterior disconnection) apraxia.* Lesions that damage the transcallosal motor pathway between the left and right frontal lobes can produce apraxia affecting the left hand in response to verbal but not visually mediated commands. The disorder has been attributed to interruption of signals that transmit verbally related motor engrams from the left, dominant premotor area to the premotor areas of the right hemisphere. The condition must be differentiated from transient motor arrest due to seizures emanating from the right frontal area as well as from the general hypokinesia that accompanies parkinsonism or pseudobulbar palsy.

Constructional apraxia and dressing apraxia are more specifically reproducible abnormalities than the above. They consist of disorders of skilled movements that relate more to damaged perceptual mechanisms than to motor impairments. Constructional apraxia describes difficulty in arranging or copying objects in accordance with their normal spatial relationships.

Dressing apraxia refers to the inability properly to relate the shape and parts of garments to the appropriate part and form of the body so as to clothe oneself. In isolation, both constructional and dressing apraxia relate to large lesions that destroy or damage the spatial integrating functions of the posterior right parietal lobe and its transcortical-subcortical connections. Alternatively they tend to be prominent features of the bilateral temporoparietal abnormalities that accompany Alzheimer's disease or certain other vascular-degenerative dementias. Constructional apraxia is the more common of the two defects, follows damage to either parietal lobe, and affects interpretations of material presented to either visual field or carried out by either side of the body. Dressing apraxia is less common and when associated with severe left somatosensory defects or denial tends more selectively to affect that side of the body. Both abnormalities tend to clear as acute damage to the parietal lobe subsides, suggesting that their development reflects polymodal dysfunction emanating from areas outside the immediate area of tissue destruction. Sustained bilateral dressing apraxia sometimes accompanies neoplasms involving the junctional area between the occipital and parietal lobe cortex on the right side.

Several motor abnormalities sometimes have been called apraxia that are probably better considered to be combinations of pseudobulbar palsy and the effect of abnormal supranuclear reflexes. *Gait apraxia,* described on page 1071, is due to a combination of bilateral pyramidal and extrapyramidal weakness of the lower extremities plus paratonic rigidity and the presence of plantar grasping reflexes. Similarly, *oculomotor apraxia,* a term applied to complete or partial inability to look conjugately in a particular direction on command, is best understood as a bilateral interruption of the descending supranuclear oculomotor pathways from the frontal eye fields. The effects of the voluntary paresis or paralysis are accentuated by the sparing of an uninhibited, occipitally originating, visual fixation reflex. Characteristically, patients affected with the disorder must blink to block fixation before they can voluntarily redirect gaze toward a new point. They easily follow visually fixated objects.

Agnosia

Agnosia describes a rare psychologic defect in which the individual fails to recognize a complex stimulus despite preserved sensory processing and intact naming. The abnormality reflects, as Tueber put it, "a normal percept . . . stripped of its meaning." Careful analysis indicates that most if not all instances of agnosia relate to damaged central perceptual mechanisms, their integrations into polymodal memory mechanisms, or a combination of the two.

Visual Agnosia

Visual agnosia is the most frequently encountered disturbance of this group, but often is difficult to evaluate because of associated aphasia or dementia. The disorder consists of failure to recognize and name individual members of familiar classes of objects such as pictures, faces, or colors despite retaining sufficient visual discrimination to copy them. The abnormality arises in association with bilateral inferior occipital-temporal lobe lesions. It appears to reflect a combination of impaired visual processing and either disconnection from or direct damage to memory areas that delineate and name singular characteristics among overall groups (e.g., a particular face among faces in general).

Auditory Agnosia

Although extremely rare, auditory agnosia has been observed in two forms. *Pure word deafness* describes an inability to understand spoken language despite relatively intact audiometric functions and the ability to read, write, and speak in a close to normal manner. Affected patients tend to lose their capacity to perceive various qualities of musical sound as well. Closely linked to word deafness is *emotional deafness,* observed occasionally with right temporal lobe damage, in which the subject loses the normal capacity to distinguish prosodic intonations that convey phonemic or emphatic modulations of spoken language.

Spatial Agnosia and Neglect

The perceptual contributions of the nondominant posterior and posterior-inferior parietal lobe in forming and recognizing spatial relationships for the person's outer world and inner body map already have been described. Disturbances in such spatial functions can include not only failure to recognize the form and nature of sensory stimuli reaching the right hemisphere but can extend into loss of recognition and denial that the left side of the body or the world that surrounds it exists at all. This is the uncommon condition termed *anosognosia.* Less severe forms of contralateral spatial inattention called *neglect* occur more frequently and can accompany damage restricted to the right posterior parietal area, the frontal premotor association areas, the striatum, or the right thalamus. Severe denial seldom lasts indefinitely except following large frontoparietal abnormalities of the right hemisphere, but minor degrees of contralateral inattention may persist indefinitely following major damage to either the parietal or frontal association cortex of the right hemisphere.

Memory, Learning, and Their Impairments

Memory has two major sources. Instinctual memory represents information coded in the genes and passed from generation to generation in ways that are still poorly understood. Acquired or autobiographic memory depends upon percepts that fall on the senses and the process by which the brain encodes, stores, and retrieves them. Acquired memory is identical to learning and is the property with which this chapter deals. Disturbances of memory-learning include two dimensions: defects in past memory, called *retrograde amnesia,* and the inability to form new memories from ongoing events, called *anterograde amnesia.*

Patterns of Memory Acquisition

The components of memory can be grouped into three major epochs, immediate, intermediate, and remote. (Psychologists sometimes identify only two categories, immediate and remote.) *Immediate memory or recall* consists of holding in the mind material just heard or read with no necessary intervening process of memory storage. The capacity to register and then repeat the received stimuli lasts until the subject's mind is interrupted by some other stimulus; it is tested by such simple measures as repeating after the examiner a series of numbers. Except for grossly confused or delirious subjects, patients with organic brain disease usually show little or no defect in immediate memory.

Intermediate memory covers the time span beginning within a few seconds past and extending backward for 24 to 48 hours or more. It is tested by inquiring into knowledge of current events, the content of recent meals, or asking the subject to repeat three unrelated words 2 to 5 minutes after having been given them. As with immediate memory, inattention may impair the answers. *Long-term memory* begins beyond that epoch, but this too has its gradations, for childhood memories tend to be singularly well recalled even as more recent ones begin to fade. As a result, standard I.Q. tests that examine primarily words and functions learned before the age of 14 years often give normal or near-normal scores even in adults who have suffered from diseases that severely damage or destroy intermediate and anterograde memory.

The Anatomy of Memory

Memory has both a distributed and focal anatomy. Many regions of the cerebral hemispheres nonspecifically process the initial sensory stimuli that go into learning about the outer and inner world. As previous sections indicate, several polymodal convergent areas of the association cortex not only encode higher abstractions for sensory signals and learned movement, but both store and retrieve the memories for certain dimensions of those functions. Subcortical regions involved in intensifying or blocking the translation of perceptions or skilled movements into memory are only partly known, but relate closely to the limbic system. Structures located in the medial thalamic and probably hypothalamic regions as well as in the ascending brainstem reticular formation and basal forebrain activating systems are known to play an important role in the encoding and, probably, retrieval of memory. Reflecting their widespread processings, loss of at least some learned function can accompany large lesions affecting any lobe of the brain.

In addition to the above distributed contributions, certain structures make especially important contributions to the integration of adult memory, especially verbal-symbolic memory. In experimental primates, both the hippocampus and amygdala have been implicated in this regard. In humans, evidence suggests that at the cortical level the hippocampus appears to play the most important role in the retrieval of recent memories and the laying down of new ones. Unilateral damage to the human hippocampus results in relatively subtle defects, left hippocampal damage being followed by modest impairments in verbal memory, while right hippocampal injury may produce difficulties in visual spatial memories and the recognition of musical tones. Occasional patients with acute inferomedial left temporal lobe damage develop fairly severe but transient amnesia for places, events, and verbal memories. If the opposite hemisphere is spared, this almost always subsides in three to four days, leaving no clinically detectable residuals.

In contrast to the above-mentioned mild or evanescent effects of unilateral injury, bilateral damage or surgical removal of the hippocampus and adjacent structures in the adult produces devastating effects. What ensues are profound and usually permanent deficits in intermediate memory, affecting especially the verbal-visual and spatial spheres. The degree of associated retrograde amnesia is proportional to the extent of hippocampal damage, but rarely extends back beyond late adolescence. Severe defects in forming anterograde learning accompany the retrograde loss. At the subcortical level, bilateral damage to the dorsal-medial nuclei of the thalamus and, less consistently, to the ventral-medial hypothalamus, including the region of the mammillary bodies, results in a profound multidimensional disturbance of retrograde and anterograde memory. The prominent memory loss that accompanies Huntington's disease, which affects the striatum, suggests that the basal ganglia also may contribute to the normal memory process.

The Physiology of Memory

An understanding of the steps that the brain takes to encode perception into stored memory and, subsequently, to retrieve the percept and insert it into the larger whole of acquired information or skill has hardly passed beyond informed guesswork. The receptive column of each cortical sensory processing area receives incoming information and then progressively abstracts it in adjacent association areas to compare the constructed signals with past experience. This stage, at least for several modalities, provides at least some level of recognition. Such local processing is fairly advanced, for example, in the postcentral cortex, which appears to contain the necessary machinery both to synthesize the three-dimensional pattern of objects and to compare their form with past perceptions in the process called stereognosis. The left temporal auditory association cortex appears to provide a similar function for language. Nevertheless, at least in adult life both these and other semicomplete percepts must be processed further by hippocampal mechanisms before comprehensive learning can proceed and be retrieved.

An increase in cellular connections develops during normal learning and, conversely, a reduction in dendritic synapses accompanies the memory failure of Alzheimer's disease. In ways that remain little understood, cerebral memory mechanisms appear to be related to the integrity of cholinergic projections that arise from the basal nucleus, innominate substance, and diagonal band region of the basal forebrain and project diffusely to the cerebral cortex, amygdala, and other regions. Ascending catecholaminergic pathways also appear to play a role. Blocking of the cholinergic transmitter projections affects the learning capacities of lower animals, and the degeneration of these pathways is a prominent accompaniment to the dementia of Alzheimer's disease.

How learning takes place at the cellular level remains largely unknown. In some species at least the process appears to depend upon sensitization of synaptic channels by genetically governed cyclic $3',5'$-adenosine monophosphate (cAMP) release. Kandel and his associates, working with sea molluscs (Aplysia), have found that during conditioned learning serotonin release stimulates the synthesis of cAMP. The cAMP, in a genetically regulated process, then dissociates subunits from a protein kinase in neuron terminals.

Several subsequent steps ensue, eventually facilitating the release of an increased amount of transmitter, which intensifies activity at the learning synapse. Whether or not such elementary building blocks for cellular learning in one primitive species are specific only to the particular invertebrate strain or underlie the broader biologic process of learning throughout the animal kingdom remains to be seen.

Clinical Memory Disorders

Many middle-aged or elderly persons report a progressive but relatively isolated difficulty in recalling proper names and recent events of minor importance. Whether or not this "benign forgetfulness" foretells the later development of a more malignant, progressive dementia cannot be discerned from presently available evidence.

Korsakoff's Syndrome. Korsakoff's syndrome is a severe disturbance of recent memory that occurs most often as a sequel to acute and frequently repeated attacks of severe thiamine deficiency. The fully developed disorder includes profound recent and intermediate memory loss, lack of insight, disorientation to time and place, and confabulation. In Western countries, nutritional Korsakoff's syndrome most frequently affects alcoholics and often accompanies or follows the florid signs and symptoms of the confused or delirious states called Wernicke's encephalopathy or delirium tremens. Korsakoff's syndrome, however, can follow any circumstance in which thiamine-free calories provide the major or only sustained source of nutrition. The memory failure in thiamine deficiency is accompanied consistently by bilateral damage of the dorsal medial nucleus of the thalamus. Other structural abnormalities affect the mammillary bodies and pulvinar as well as various areas of the cortex, including the hippocampus.

Severe retrograde and anterograde memory loss producing a Korsakoff syndrome also can follow global cerebral anoxia-ischemia, severe status epilepticus and subarachnoid hemorrhage. All of these conditions can selectively damage vulnerable neurons in the hippocampus that normally relate to the functions of learning and memory. Even modest head trauma temporarily interrupts memory-mediating neural connections in the hippocampus and diencephalon: Concussive injuries frequently produce an initially severe degree of retrograde and lesser anterograde amnesia. In most instances of concussion, the retrograde memory loss almost fully disappears with time. Concurrently, anterograde learning increasingly improves. A less fortunate prognosis accompanies prolonged post traumatic coma. When this lasts more than 2-3 weeks, most patients, particularly those over 25 years old, never fully recover their memory faculties.

Permanent or prolonged amnesia occasionally can follow bilateral cerebral infarction, large brain tumors, or surgical operations. Such cases also have shown bilateral damage either of the hippocampus, the medial diencephalon, or both structures. The encephalitis caused by H. simplex virus characteristically leaves severe and often permanent amnesia in its wake. The disease has a predilection to produce necrotic and inflammatory lesions that destroy the limbic system lying along the medial surfaces of the temporal lobes.

Transient Global Amnesia (TGA) is a condition marked by an abnormal period of acute confusion, lasting from several minutes to as much as 12 hours or so, during which the affected person remains fully awake and can identify himself but suffers a severe deficit in recent and intermediate memory. The memory loss is maximal at the beginning, usually with total disorientation to time and place, then gradually disappears as the attack wears off. Most TGA attacks come on in middle-aged or elderly persons and appear to reflect temporary vascular insufficiency, either to bilateral hippocampal or paramedian thalamic regions that take their blood supply from the apex of the basilar artery. Patients with TGA usually remain bright, attentive, and distressed by their acute confusion. They tend repeatedly to ask where they are and what is going on until, within a few hours, the disorientation gradually disappears. Most TGA attacks neither leave residual limitations nor carry a strong risk of recurrence. Status epilepticus with partial complex or nonconvulsive generalized (petit mal) seizures can produce an amnesic state somewhat similar to TGA. In these instances the seizure discharges temporarily occlude synaptic pathways involved in normal memory. Attacks of such "minor status" are distinguished by dull, slow-witted, and inattentive behavior, a history of previous seizures, and characteristic EEG abnormalities.

Psychogenic Memory Impairment. This can involve either recent or remote recall, usually in clinically recognizable patterns. Among patients with severe systemic illnesses, preoccupation, forced inattention, or reduced arousal can result in inconsistent responses to testing, with patients able to give accurate answers to some questions about current events but not to others. Severe depressive illnesses sometimes reduce patients to near muteness or incomprehensible monosyllables. In general, organic disturbances in memory are marked by variability in what is remembered, emotionally reinforced material being recalled better than neutral events. With organic memory loss, disorientation is worst for time, less for place and persons, and never for self. In most instances, events of the recent past are unevenly forgotten more than are remote memories. Furthermore, the providing of cues often improves recall. By contrast, hysterical or factitious amnesia tends to be greatest for emotionally important events, removes from the patient's memory well-defined blocks of past events while leaving intact the recall of preceding or following experiences, affects remote memories equally with recent ones, resists improvement with cues, and sometimes even includes disorientation to self. Asking "Who am I?" or "What's my name?", unless spoken during a severe delirium or a proved epileptic seizure, provides a confident sign of malingering.

GENERALIZED DISTURBANCES OF HIGHER BRAIN FUNCTION—THE DEMENTIAS

Definition and Classification

The term *dementia* describes a sustained or permanent, multidimensional decline in intellectual powers so as partially or completely to incapacitate the individual's normal behavioral, social, or economic adjustments. Different aspects of the mind deteriorate, depending upon the causative diseases, but all dementias involve a reduction or loss of recent memory coupled with impaired learning, reduced attention, loss of capacity for abstract thinking, a decline in intellectual quickness, and difficulties in planning and completing future action. Language functions, level of arousal, insight, and attention to social amenities are affected in some but spared in others, depending mainly on the anatomic distribution of the causative disease. Common to all dementias, however, is the diffuse or multifunctional aspect of the mental decay, an aspect that contrasts to the focal losses that characterize selective perceptual abnormalities such as isolated amnesia or aphasia. Table 42 lists the most frequently encountered causes of dementia.

Dementia differs by definition from *amentia*, i.e., mental retardation, in which intellectual function fails to develop normally from the start. It also must be differentiated from the transient or reversible states of mental disruption or decline, which are termed delirium or confusion. *Pseudodementia* is a state in which abnormal psychiatric conditions of catatonia, depression, or hysteria so severely preclude a subject's capacity to respond that satisfactory testing of the mental status is not possible, giving the false impression of a primary intellectual loss.

A few long-lasting yet potentially reversible conditions that diffusely impair mental function stand midway between the reversible acute deliria and the chronic irreversible organic dementias (Table 43). As their categorization implies, these disorders all have a specific known cause of endogenous or exogenous origin, and all are uncommon. They deserve attention beyond their incidence, because proper treatment often may be followed by considerable or, occasionally, complete clinical improvement.

Among the prolonged but reversible encephalopathies, *chronic toxic confusion* in the elderly has become increasingly a problem as a by-product of both indiscriminate drug use and the sometimes necessary taking of prescription drugs. By the time the normal brain reaches the age of 70 years or so it undergoes a substantial loss of neurons, some estimates being that as many as 10,000 or more nerve cells die each day after the age of 30 years. As a result, as age proceeds, neurotropic drugs affect an ever decreasing number of sensitive cells and synapses and exert a commensurately increasing pathophysiologic effect. Furthermore, many drugs or their active metabolites have prolonged

TABLE 42. THE PRINCIPAL CAUSES AND APPROXIMATE FREQUENCIES (%) OF PROGRESSIVE DEMENTIA

1. Senile dementia, Alzheimer type	50
2. Multi-infarct (arteriosclerotic)	
3. Combination of 1 and 2	25
4. Alcoholic-post-traumatic	5
5. Communicating hydrocephalus	
6. Huntington's	15
7. Intracranial mass lesions	
8. Uncommon or mixed with above: Chronic drug use; Creutzfeldt-Jakob; metabolic (thyroid, liver, nutritional); degenerative (spinocerebellar, amyotrophic lateral sclerosis, Parkinsonism, multiple sclerosis, Pick's, Wilson's, epilepsy); static dementia	10

TABLE 43. POTENTIALLY REVERSIBLE CHRONIC ENCEPHALOPATHIES RESEMBLING DEMENTIA

Infections
  Neurosyphilis
  Chronic fungal meningitis
Whipple's disease

Endogenous metabolic disorders
  Chronic portal-systemic encephalopathy (ammonia intoxication)
  Uremia
  Recurrent hypoglycemia
  Porphyria
  Wilson's disease
  Hypocalcemia or hypercalcemia; hypoadrenalism or hyperadrenalism
  Panhypopituitarism
  Niacin deficiency: pellagra
  Cyanocobalamin deficiency (B_{12})

Drugs and toxins

Alcohol	Antineoplastic agents
Psychotropic agents	Cardiac glycosides
Anticonvulsants	Steroids
Anticholinergics	Mixed therapeutic programs in elderly

Brain disorders
  Chronic subdural hematomas
  Low-pressure communicating hydrocephalus

serum half-lives so that repeated doses lead to progressive systemic accumulation of the drug or its toxic products. What follows is that small amounts of medication can produce an insidiously beginning and gradually increasing deterioration in mental function. The complexity of the interactions between drugs and the aging brain and the varying capacities of today's medications to involve different brain systems make the ensuing symptoms somewhat unpredictable. Chief offenders are any of the barbiturates, the benzodiazepines, phenothiazines, butyrophenones, tricyclic antidepressants, MAO inhibitors, anticholinergics, adrenal cortical steroids, methyldopa (Aldomet), and digitalis. Combinations of drugs represent especially frequent culprits.

Pathophysiology

Dementia, being multidimensional and predominantly psychologic in the components of its specific losses, always reflects damage or dysfunction in the association cortex of the cerebral hemispheres or in the subcortical nuclei that interrelate with the association cortex. Structural changes in the brain almost always accompany and underlie the psychologic deficits of dementia (Table 44). Depending upon its cause, dementia can begin acutely, subacutely, or insidiously. Thereafter the process, again depending upon its cause, can either remain static, as occurs following an episode of severe cerebral anoxia or head trauma, or become progressive, as is the case with most of the other disorders listed in Table 44.

Physiologic studies of dementia usually reflect the diffuse and bilateral nature of the cerebral deficit. In almost all instances the EEG is slow. Patterns of cerebral metabolism measured by metabolic tomography or as reflected in cerebral blood flow studies show differences that vary from disease to disease. In parkinsonism, for example, even before dementia appears

TABLE 44. PATHOLOGIC DISTRIBUTION IN THE MAJOR DEMENTIAS

Condition	Cortical Changes	Subcortical	Course
Predominantly cortical			
Alzheimer's disease	Association cortex; plaques, tangles, loss of large pyramidal cells	Loss of large cells basal nucleus complex; neuronal loss locus ceruleus, amygdala	Progressive
Postanoxic, postictal, posthypoglycemic	Diffuse laminar necrosis; hippocampal vulnerability; occasionally diffuse demyelination	Occasionally striatal or thalamic necrosis	Fixed
Pick's disease	Focal frontotemporal cortical atrophy		Progressive
Obstructive hydrocephalus	White matter atrophy; gray matter compression?	Basal ganglia—thalamic compression?	Reversible
General paresis (syphilis)	Inflammation and cell loss frontal → other cortex	Striatum; occasionally hypothalamus, thalamus	Arrestable
Mixed cortical-subcortical			
Trauma	Diffuse or multifocal	Basal ganglia or diencephalon	Fixed or improving
Vascular	Multiple infarcts	Multiple infarcts	Stair step
Parkinson's with dementia	Alzheimer-like changes	Same plus substantia nigra degeneration	Progressive
Huntington's	Mild to moderate frontal atrophy	Caudate and putamen degeneration	Progressive
Predominantly subcortical			
Vascular		Bilateral paramedian thalamic infarction; paramedian midbrain, pontine reticular formation	Fixed
Progressive supranuclear ophthalmoplegia		Neuronal loss and gliosis, basal ganglia, red nucleus, periaqueductal gray	Progressive
Wilson's disease	Variable cell loss and gliosis	Gliosis, cell loss, sometimes cavitation in striatum	Progressive or arrestable
Creutzfeldt-Jakob disease	Neuronal loss and gliosis	Neuronal loss and gliosis basal ganglia; thalamus, brainstem	Progressive

glucose uptake by the brain may decline diffusely below normal with no visible focal accentuations. Alzheimer's disease (AD) also produces a general decline in metabolic activity, but the functional abnormalities tend to be accentuated in the region of the temporo-parietal-occipital association cortex. In Huntington's disease (HD), functional activity declines significantly in the caudate and putamen, while cortical metabolism remains relatively intact even in patients with easily detectable clinical dementia. The mechanisms of these functional differences remain poorly understood, but the diffuse changes in parkinsonism do correlate with the overall hypokinesia of that disorder, while the more focal changes in AD and HD generally reflect the

expected anatomic substrate of many of the most severe symptoms.

The precise molecular cause has not been found in any of the degenerative dementias. Several, however, have an at least partially genetic etiology and must be regarded as examples of inherent programming for premature neuronal death. Thus a dominant gene with apparently complete penetrance governs the expression of HD. AD may have almost as strong a genetic predisposition, but the late age of onset and perhaps other variables make it more difficult to map the true pattern of its inheritance. Many other inherited degenerative disorders, including the spinocerebellar ataxias and the muscular dystrophies, also produce an associated mental decline. The specific gene-enzyme failure has not been found for any of these conditions. Considerable progress, however, recently has been made toward identifying the abnormal Huntington gene.

Pharmacologic efforts have been made to identify the mechanism of some of the dementias, although in no instance has a cause-effect relationship been established. Nigral dopamine content is reduced in parkinsonism, but the alteration correlates primarily with the movement disorder rather than with the intellectual loss, which affects only about 25 per cent of cases. When the latter occurs, it correlates best with the superposition of Alzheimer-like anatomic changes upon the Parkinson brain. In AD, cholinergic neurons in the basal forebrain degenerate, and the acetylcholine-synthesizing enzyme, choline acetyltransferase (CAT), concurrently declines in the amygdala, the hippocampus, and throughout the cerebral cortex. Whether the cholinergic decay directly causes the cortical dysfunction and degeneration in AD or is only an associated finding is not known, although anticholinergic drugs greatly accentuate the behavioral impairments in affected patients. Furthermore, the relative decline in CAT in different regions of the brain correlates both with the local extent of the silver-staining plaques that serve as the anatomic hallmarks of AD and the observed maximal declines in cerebral metabolism. Concentrations in the brain of the neuropeptide somatostatin also go down in AD but with unknown functional effects. Noradrenergic pathways arising from locus ceruleus decay in some patients.

Neurotransmitter changes in other dementias are either not established or more difficult to interpret. In HD, both gamma aminobutyric acid (GABA) and its synthesizing enzyme, glutamic acid decarboxylase, are reduced disproportionally to other neurotransmitters in the striatum, pallidum, and substantia nigra. The number of small Golgi-type neurons that utilize GABA as a neurotransmitter decline greatly in the striatum. This may explain the decrease of GABA, but leaves unanswered the mechanism of the also reduced levels of CAT, dopamine, cholecystokinin, angiotensin-converting enzyme, and substance P in the basal ganglia. While the loss of striatal inhibitory neurons provides a reasonable explanation for the development of chorea in HD, it gives little hint as to what causes the mental deterioration. Inasmuch as the cerebral cortical changes in HD are both variable and sometimes modest, it seems possible as noted earlier that in HD the severe degeneration in the striatum, a structure that enjoys extensive connections with both the frontal lobe and the limbic system, may be directly involved in producing the impaired mental and emotional function of the disease. Similar functional mechanisms may explain the pathophysiology of some of the other disorders listed in Table 44 in which severe subcortical abnormalities are unaccompanied by consistent neuropathological alterations in the cerebral cortex.

REFERENCES

Baer, D. M., and Fedio, P.: Quantitative analysis of interictal behavior in temporal lobe epilepsy. Arch Neurol 34:454–467, 1977.

Blackwood, W., and Corsellis, J. A. N.: Greenfield's Neuropathology. Chicago, Arnold-Yearbook, 1976.

Brodal, A.: Neurological Anatomy in Relation to Clinical Medicine. 3rd ed. New York, Oxford University Press, 1981.

Brookhart, J. M., and Mountcastle, V. B. (eds.): Handbook of Physiology. Section I, The Nervous System. Volume VI, Higher Functions of the Nervous System, Parts 1 and 2. Edited by Plum, F. Bethesda, Md., American Physiological Society, 1986.

Coyle, J. T., Price, D. L., and DeLong, M. R.: Alzheimer's disease: A disorder of cortical cholinergic innervation. Science 219:1184–1190, 1983.

Cummings, J. L., and Benson, D. F.: Dementia, A Clinical Approach. Boston, Butterworths, 1983.

Delgado-Escueta, A. V., Ferrendelli, J. A., and Prince, D. A.: Basic mechanisms of the epilepsies. Ann Neurol 16:S1–158, 1984.

Delgado-Escueta, A. V., Mattson, R. H., King, L., et al.: The nature of aggression during epileptic seizures. N Engl J Med 305:711, 1981.

Geschwind, N.: Disconnexion syndromes in animals and man. Brain 88:237–294, 585–644, 1965.

Hécaen, H.: Apraxia. In Filskov, S. B., and Boll, T. J. (eds.): Handbook of Clinical Neuropsychology. New York, John Wiley & Sons, 1981.

Heilman, K., and Valenstein, E. (eds.): Clinical Neuropsychology. Oxford, Oxford University Press, 1979.

Hier, D. B., Mondlock, J., and Caplan, L. R.: Behavioral abnormalities after right hemisphere stroke. Neurology 33:337–344, 1983.

Ingvar, D. H.: Serial aspects of language and speech related to prefrontal cortical activity. Human Neurobiol 2:177, 1983.

Jones, E. G., and Powell, T. P. S.: An anatomical study of converging sensory pathways within the cerebral cortex of the monkey. Brain 93:793–820, 1970.

Kandel, E. R., and Schwartz, J. H.: Molecular biology of learning: Modulation of transmitter release. Science 218:433–443, 1982.

Kapoor, W. N., Karpf, M., Wieand, S., Peterson, P. A., and Levey, G. S.: A prospective evaluation and follow-up of patients with syncope. N Engl J Med 309:197, 1983.

Mesulam, M.-M. (ed.): Principles of Behavioral Neurology. Philadelphia, F. A. Davis Co., 1985.

Milner, B.: Hemispheric specialization: Scope and limits. In Schmitt, F. O., and Worden, F. G. (eds.): The Neurosciences. Third Study Program. Cambridge, Mass., MIT Press, 1974, pp. 77–89.

Ojemann, G. A.: Brain organization for language from the perspective of electrical stimulation mapping. Behav Brain Sci 6:189, 1983.

Penfield, W., and Jasper, H.: Epilepsy and the Functional Anatomy of the Human Brain. Boston, Little, Brown and Co., 1954.

Plum, F., and Posner, J. B.: The Diagnosis of Stupor and Coma. 3rd ed. 3rd revised printing. Philadelphia, F. A. Davis Co., 1982.

Roland, P. E.: Astereognosis. Arch Neurol 33:543–550, 1976.

Roland, P. E.: Cortical regulation of selective attention in man. A regional cerebral blood flow study. J Neurophysiol 48:1059, 1982.

Terry, R. D., and Katzman, R.: Senile dementia of the Alzheimer type. Ann Neurol 14:497, 1983.

Teuber, H. L.: Alterations of perception and memory in man. In Weiskrantz, L. (ed.): Analysis of Behavioral Change. New York, Harper and Row, 1968.

Victor, M., Adams, R. D., and Collins, G. H.: The Wernicke-Korsakoff Syndrome. Philadelphia, F. A. Davis Co., 1971.

West, J. B.: Human physiology at extreme altitudes on Mt. Everest. Science 223:784, 1984.

Woods, B. T., and Teuber, H.-L.: Changing patterns of childhood aphasia. Ann Neurol 3:273–280, 1978.

PATHOPHYSIOLOGY OF THE GASTROINTESTINAL TRACT

Introduction _____
MARVIN H. SLEISENGER, M.D.

Pathophysiology of the gut is not only the accurate description of signs, symptoms, laboratory findings, and disorders of that organ system based upon altered physiology. It is also, in part, the explanation of their evolution. Thus, pathophysiology is linked to normal physiology as well as to the pathogenesis of disease and disorder.

With this definition as a guide the short discussions that follow will deal primarily with the pathophysiologic basis of important clinical information about diseases of the gastrointestinal system—that is, the symptoms, the physical signs, and the important laboratory data. The discussions will be centered chiefly on the various component organs of the gastrointestinal tract (with the exception of liver and gallbladder, which are dealt with in a separate section). The pathophysiology of malnutrition and of dietary intolerances is described in part in the discussion of the small intestine but more extensively in the part of this book on nutrition.

Many symptoms and physiologic abnormalities in the gastrointestinal tract, with or without associated systemic aberrations, are not readily confined to a single part of this extensive organ system as defined in the chapter headings. In this case to serve brevity the appropriate discussion has been assigned, sometimes somewhat arbitrarily, to a single part that deals with the organ most prominently affected, such as diarrhea in the part on the small intestine and constipation in the part on the colon. Some pathogenetic factors such as psychological stress are impossible to confine to a single discussion, so will be considered both in relation to the peptic ulcer disease in the part on the stomach and to irritable bowel disease in the part on the colon.

The discussions that follow are designed to present an up-to-date summary of the scientific basis for an understanding of the pathogenesis and pathophysiology of a remarkably diverse and important group of diseases, which collectively account for approximately 10 to 15 per cent of the illness sufficient to cause hospital admission in the United States. A more extensive discussion of these diseases can be found in the *Cecil Textbook of Medicine,* of which this is a companion volume.

Pathophysiology of the Esophagus _____
IRA S. GOLDMAN, M.D.

ANATOMY AND EMBRYOLOGY

The esophagus, a tubular organ extending from the mouth to the stomach, is approximately 35 cm long in adults. It begins at the level of the pharyngeal constrictors—where the cricopharyngeous muscle constitutes the upper esophageal sphincter. The esophagus passes through the posterior mediastinum to the diaphragm. The proximal third of the esophagus is composed of striated skeletal muscle, whereas the distal two thirds consists of smooth muscle in both longitudinal and circular layers. The esophagus has a mucosa composed of a nonkeratinized stratified squamous epithelium, a submucosa, but no serosa.

The pathophysiology of a variety of esophageal diseases is directly related to the anatomy of the diaphragmatic hiatus through which the esophagus passes. The opening is relatively large and is surrounded with loose areolar tissue. Since it is a soft, mobile organ lying adjacent to many structures, the esophagus is subject to compression. Thus, difficulty in swallowing may be experienced by a patient who has any of a number of anatomic abnormalities involving the chest—a large goiter, an aneurysm of the aorta, a dilated left atrium, or enlarged hilar lymph nodes.

The esophagus receives the majority of its blood supply from small branches of the thoracic descending aorta. The upper third of the esophagus is supplied by branches of the inferior thyroid artery, while the lower third is supplied from the left gastric artery. The venous drainage of the esophagus is likewise split into three portions. The upper third drains into the superior vena cava, the middle third into the azygos system, and the lower third into the portal vein via the gastric veins. All three drainage systems have anastomotic connections.

The parasympathetic autonomic innervation of the esophagus consists of fibers from the spinal accessory nerve that supply the high cervical portion of the esophagus and fibers from the vagus nerve that innervate the remainder. Fibers from the vagus synapse with nerve cells of ganglia in the muscle layers, sending out postganglionic fibers to the individual muscle cells. The sympathetic innervation is from cervical sympathetic ganglia and from ganglia in the thoracic sympathetic chain.

In embryologic development, the gut and respiratory tract start out as a single tube, with division by the second month of development. It can be readily seen that failure of separation in normal development can be associated with various connections between the two systems. The most common such abnormality is a *tracheoesophageal fistula*, which often results in aspiration in newborns. Similarly, abnormalities in the development of the esophageal vascular supply or neurologic innervation may cause clinical problems.

PHYSIOLOGY

The esophagus functions as an integrated motor unit consisting of muscular action by the pharynx, hypopharynx, and the esophagus, which serves to transfer food and fluids from the mouth into the stomach. The components of the esophagus that integrate the swallowing mechanism are the upper esophageal sphincter (UES), the body of the esophagus, and the lower esophageal sphincter (LES).

PHARYNX AND UPPER ESOPHAGEAL SPHINCTER

The pharyngeal muscles and tongue play a major part in the propulsion of fluid and food into the upper esophagus. Following a signal from the brainstem swallowing center, swallowing initiates a series of pressure rises in the pharynx. Immediately distal to this area is a zone of high resting pressure in the esophagus called the upper esophageal sphincter (UES). Relaxation of the UES coincides, and is coordinated with, the appearance of the retropharyngeal pulsion wave. Relaxation of the UES allows the tongue and pharyngeal muscles to thrust food or fluid into the esophagus.

BODY OF THE ESOPHAGUS

The primary muscular process in the body of the esophagus is a moving contraction wave that moves down to, but not through, the lower esophageal sphincter and is known as *primary peristalsis*. Immediately following a swallow, this wave causes an increase in the baseline pressure of the esophagus, reaching a high level and being propagated as a wave distally at the rate of 2 to 3 cm per second (Fig. 1). Several factors influence the amplitude and the occurrence of this peristaltic wave. The amplitude varies from one end of the esophagus to the other, is higher when liquids are swallowed than when dry solids are swallowed, and also varies according to intragastric or intra-abdominal pressure by heightened peristaltic contrac-

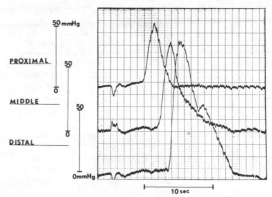

Figure 1. Normal peristalsis in the body of the esophagus. A Honeywell probe with recording tips 5 cm apart is in the body of the esophagus. A small jog in the baseline of all three tracings is a movement artifact signaling the onset of swallowing. A high monophasic wave is recorded sequentially by the three tips. (From Sleisenger, M. H., and Fordtran, J. S. (eds.): Gastrointestinal Disease. 3rd ed. Philadelphia, W. B. Saunders Co., 1983.)

tions. The velocity of peristalsis increases with warm substances and decreases with cold ones.

A peristaltic wave can also be initiated by material that has remained in the esophagus or that has been refluxed into the esophagus from the stomach. This peristaltic contraction is caused by esophageal distention and is termed *secondary peristalsis*.

Physiologic control over the body of the esophagus appears to be primarily cholinergic under normal circumstances and is not subject to the wide variety of hormonal influences that are seen to influence the lower esophageal sphincter. Recent evidence, however, does indicate a role of enkephalins and other peptides in esophageal motility.

LOWER ESOPHAGEAL SPHINCTER

The lower esophageal sphincter is a segment of circular smooth muscle in the wall of the esophagus, 2 to 4 cm in length, just proximal to the gastroesophageal junction. Its resting pressure is generally 10 to 30 mm Hg above intragastric pressure, and it is thus a barrier to gastric reflux. The LES pressure rises together with increases in intra-abdominal and intragastric pressures, maintaining the gastroesophageal pressure gradient. The second principal function of the LES is relaxation in response to the peristaltic wave of the body of the esophagus. With relaxation of the LES, the bolus of food or liquid is propelled into the stomach.

Several factors have been identified that influence LES pressure. As previously mentioned, intragastric pressure affects LES pressure and parasympathetic innervation seems to play a role, although vagotomy seems to have little effect on resting pressure or the relaxation of the LES. Investigation of the extensive LES response to hormones and to pharmacologic agents has been very active in recent years. Some of these hormonal and pharmacologic influences are listed in Table 1.

SYMPTOMS OF ABNORMAL FUNCTION

Normally, most people are totally unaware of esophageal function. Symptoms are produced by dis-

TABLE 1. SOME AGENTS INFLUENCING HUMAN LES PRESSURE

	RAISE	LOWER

Hormones	Gastrin
	Motilin
	Prostaglandin
	PGE$_{2\alpha}$
		Estrogen and
		  progesterone
		Glucagon
		Secretin
		Cholecystokinin
		Prostaglandin
		  PGE$_2$

Pharmacologic Agents	Metoclopramide Bethanechol Histamine Pentobarbital Indomethacin Antacids	Atropine Theophylline Meperidine
Other	Protein in diet Coffee	Smoking Fat in diet Alcohol

Modified from Sleisenger, M. H., and Fordtran, J. S. (eds.): Gastrointestinal Disease. 3rd ed. Philadelphia, W. B. Saunders Co., 1983, p. 419.

turbances of the normal swallowing mechanism, ulceration of the esophagus, and obstruction of the esophageal lumen. The pathophysiologic consequences of these disorders most frequently result in one or more of 3 symptoms: (1) *dysphagia* (difficulty in swallowing), interference with the normal rate of progress of food or liquid from the mouth to the stomach; (2) *odynophagia* (painful swallowing); and (3) *heartburn* (pyrosis), pain unassociated with swallowing caused by the action of acid gastric juice on the lower esophagus. It often is associated with reflux esophagitis. All of these symptoms are perceived with varying degrees of awareness and intensity by the patient and may exist alone or in combination.

DYSPHAGIA

Patients describe dysphagia as the "hanging up" or "sticking" of food and, in extreme instances, of liquids as well. Dysphagia is not usually associated with pain (odynophagia); however, dysphagia and odynophagia may coexist. Patients with dysphagia are aware that a bolus is not progressing normally or has completely halted and can usually indicate on the surface of their bodies the approximate site of delay. However, the reference points for accompanying odynophagia may not exactly correspond to the levels of delay or obstruction. Dysphagia may be of variable intensity, frequency, and duration, depending upon the underlying problem. For example, it may induce a patient to throw his head back, raise his shoulders, swallow repeatedly, engage in a Valsalva maneuver—with success—or wash the bolus down with liquid. In such an instance, it is likely that the patient has a motor disorder. In more extreme instances (progressive occlusion caused by stricture or tumor of the esophagus) neither food nor liquid can pass—everything swallowed is regurgitated. Oropharyngeal dysphagia is a particular kind of awareness of difficulty in swallowing that is felt in the pharynx. This is distinct from *globus hystericus*, a feeling of a persistent "lump" in the throat not primarily related to swallowing. Oropharyngeal dysphagia is most commonly associated with central nervous system disease or generalized muscle diseases. Proximal dysphagia, high in the esophagus or in the pharynx, indicates a disorder of pharyngeal striated muscle or of a diffuse muscular weakness such as *scleroderma, dermatomyositis,* or *amyotrophic lateral sclerosis.* When such a motor disorder is high and severe, affecting the pharynx and cervical esophagus, the patient may choke even while attempting to swallow liquids, which then pass up the hypopharynx and out of the nose. Intermittency of dysphagia—affecting both solids and liquids—suggests a motor disorder such as achalasia, either cricopharyngeal or of the LES (see below).

ESOPHAGEAL PAIN

Esophageal pain may or may not be associated with swallowing. Indeed, the esophagus is thought to be the cause of a large proportion of noncardiac chest pain syndromes. Both odynophagia and pain unrelated to swallowing may be associated with inflammation of the esophagus and mucosal disruption as seen most commonly in the *distal esophagitis* caused by reflux of acid peptic juice and less commonly in such infections as *Candida* or *herpes esophagitis.* Esophageal motility disorders are also common causes of pain, both at rest and with swallowing. In either case, it is due to simultaneous prolonged contraction of the esophageal body; the underlying failure of neuromuscular control of the esophagus is poorly understood. It is particularly noted in so-called *diffuse spasm of the esophagus* in which the esophagus contracts incoordinately and with increased pressure. The pain is caused by esophageal muscle spasm and because of its substernal location is often confused with cardiac pain. The similarity of this pain to angina pectoris includes radiation at times to the jaw, neck, or arm. The differential diagnosis of these two types of pain is often difficult.

At times, if the pain is due to esophageal irritation or inflammation associated with reflux, this can be ascertained by the Bernstein test. In this test dilute hydrochloric acid and saline are slowly perfused alternately into the esophagus of the patient, who is unaware which solution is being perfused. Frequently, those who have reflux or symptoms suggesting angina pectoris will complain of their usual type of discomfort only when HCl is the test perfusate. Similarly, other patients with unexplained chest pain have manometric evidence of esophageal spasm. Relief of the chest pain and manometric evidence of relief of spasm may be demonstrated with the use of some of the newer calcium-blocking agents, such as nifedipine.

DISEASE STATES

GASTROESOPHAGEAL REFLUX

Etiology

Reflux of gastric contents (including pepsin and hydrochloric acid) follows diminution of lower esophageal resting pressure below a critical level. This is generally caused by a transient complete relaxation of the LES, rather than low resting pressure. The lower esophageal sphincter is normally the primary barrier protecting the esophagus from the damaging effects of acid gastric juice from the intact stomach. However, other important factors may contribute to the pathogenesis of reflux esophagitis. Among these are (1) diminished efficiency of esophageal clearing, (2) impaired esophageal mucosal resistance, and (3) decreased efficiency of gastric emptying.

Patients with reflux tend to have lower resting LES pressures than normal persons, but the overlap is great (Fig. 2).

Diminution of the resting lower esophageal sphincter pressure may or may not be associated with a discernible disorder or disease. The disorder is common—in one study 7 per cent of normal individuals experienced daily reflux, and 36 per cent of the population had at least one episode of reflux a month. Neither the presence or absence of reflux nor LES pressures correlate with fasting plasma gastric levels. Deficiency of gastrin, a known stimulator of the LES (Table 1), is therefore an unlikely explanation for reflux.

In some patients a hypotensive LES and reflux are associated with a sliding hiatus hernia. The essential pathophysiologic event is LES incompetence, however,

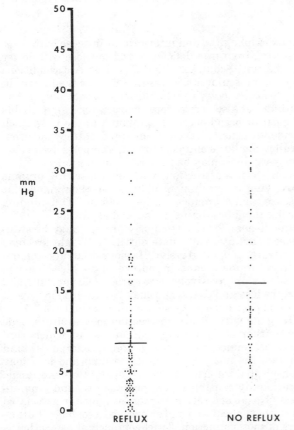

Figure 2. Sphincter pressures and esophageal reflux. Each dot represents the mean sphincter pressure in millimeters of mercury above gastric pressure of one individual. Separation into groups was made by demonstrating the presence or absence of reflux with an intraesophageal electrode after loading the stomach with 300 ml of 0.1 N HCl. Although the means of the two groups are statistically significant, p <0.001, there is a fair amount of overlap. (From Sleisenger, M. H., and Fordtran, J. S. (eds.): Gastrointestinal Disease. 3rd ed. Philadelphia, W. B. Saunders Co., 1983.)

not the anatomic abnormality of a pouch of stomach of varying size that is located above the diaphragm. Effective therapy depends upon restoration of a functional sphincter, usually occurring when the terminal 4 cm of esophagus and the gastric pouch are restored to their normal subdiaphragmatic location.

Patients with nasogastric intubation may experience reflux of gastric contents into the esophagus, because the nasogastric tube prevents closure of the sphincter. In other patients a disease in which the smooth muscle of the LES atrophies, such as scleroderma, may impair function of the sphincter. Low LES pressure is also common in normal pregnancy and in women using oral contraceptives, pointing to the role of hormones in lowering resting LES pressure and causing gastroesophageal reflux.

Another mechanism may be operating in those with reflux who develop symptoms of inflammation—namely, an abnormal "clearing" of the esophagus of refluxed gastric juice. Such individuals require a larger than normal number of peristaltic waves to clear acid juice from the esophagus. As noted, certain foods such as fat, alcohol, and chocolate, as well as smoking, lower LES pressure (Table 1) and thereby may play roles in the pathophysiology of reflux and the pathogenesis of esophagitis. Delayed gastric emptying also increases the potential for postprandial reflux.

Clinical Manifestations

Regardless of the cause, reflux is associated with *heartburn*. This is a sharp burning distress, often wavelike, felt for a variable distance from the tip of the sternum up to the suprasternal notch. Sour gastric juice may often be tasted ("water brash"). The discomfort occasionally is caused by mucosal inflammation; however, in most cases the mucosa is normal both grossly and histologically. In some way the refluxed material stimulates mucosal sensory nerve fibers. Factors that promote or exaggerate reflux will heighten the frequency and intensity of symptoms. These include lying flat after meals, bending over, lifting heavy objects, performing other actions of straining with Valsalva maneuvers, and wearing binders or corsets that create abdominal compression.

Consequences of Long-Term Reflux

Continued reflux of acid gastric juice often leads to chronic inflammation of the lower esophagus—in some instances the involvement reaches as high as the aortic arch. In some of the latter cases, squamous epithelium is transformed to a columnar form (Barrett's epithelium) and the mucosa at the junction is easily ulcerated. Strictures often result from such ulceration and, in turn, a chronic ulcer may become sufficiently fibrosed to become a stricture (Barrett's ulcer and stricture). Stricture may also complicate esophagitis and peptic ulcer of the lower third of the esophagus that is not associated with such epithelial cell transformation. In either event, progressive gradual narrowing of the lumen of the esophagus is associated with dysphagia and often, if active inflammation continues, odynophagia. Persistent substernal pain is present in addition to heartburn, particularly if the inflammation is severe or if a peptic ulcer is active. Chronic, persistent bleeding from these ulcers as well as from chronic esophagitis is common, causing iron deficiency anemia. Long-continuing irritation and inflammation of the esophagus caused by reflux and associated with metaplasia may predispose to carcinoma of the esophagus.

Diagnostic Testing

Reflux of ingested barium can be demonstrated fluoroscopically in up to 20 per cent of the patients with reflux, almost always those with symptoms and marked reflux. It may be demonstrated in many of the remaining 80 per cent by giving a large drink of barium, placing the patient head down, and giving water to sip. Swallowing relaxes the LES; if the sphincter is incompetent, barium will be seen to reflux.

Manometry. The resting pressure of the LES is 20 ± 10 mm Hg. The usual technique for measuring it is with open tipped catheters that are slowly perfused with water and subsequently "pulled through" the gastroesophageal junction. As noted, pressures in patients with symptomatic reflux are lower than in asymptomatic normal subjects, but the overlap between the groups is wide (Fig. 2).

Measuring pH (with Manometry). Reflux of acid can be documented by a pH sensor—a special probe attached to a pressure-measuring catheter—placed 5 cm above the LES. The sphincter is identified by the change in pressure from stomach to lower esophagus on gradual withdrawal. The pH at this point in the esophagus normally is about 6.0; however, when patients with a hypotensive LES and reflux perform a Valsalva maneuver or have abdominal compression applied, the pH may drop to 2.0 or below. In some patients reflux may be shown only by instilling 300 ml of 0.1 N HCl into the stomach via the catheter, withdrawing it and the pH probe to the desired location, and repeating the maneuvers designed to stress the sphincter.

Radionuclide Scanning. This technique involves drinking 300 ml saline containing 100 microcuries ^{99m}TC sulfur colloid followed by scanning with a gamma camera. If no reflux into the esophagus is noted, the upper abdomen is compressed with a tight binder and the stomach and lower esophagus are rescanned. About 90 per cent of patients with reflux symptoms can be shown to have the radioisotope in the lower esophagus.

Esophagoscopy. Endoscopy is useful in discovering whether symptoms of reflux are associated with visible changes in the esophageal mucosa. Diagnoses such as Barrett's esophagus or dysplasia can be made only with esophageal biopsy.

Treatment of Reflux. Therapy is not the major consideration in this textbook on pathophysiology. It is notable, however, that current medical management of gastroesophageal reflux is based on a reversal insofar as possible of those factors described in its pathogenesis, as summarized in Table 2.

ESOPHAGEAL OBSTRUCTION

Organic diseases frequently obstruct the esophageal lumen in varying degrees and with markedly different rates of progression. Regardless of the nature of the disease, luminal narrowing causes dysphagia. It is relentlessly progressive in malignancy of the esophagus, variably so in strictures caused by unremitting

TABLE 2. MEDICAL TREATMENT OF GASTROESOPHAGEAL REFLUX

1. *Combat reflux*
   Elevate head of bed
   Reduce fluid intake after evening meal

2. *Increase sphincter competence*
   Avoid fats, chocolate, and caffeine in diet
   Avoid tobacco and alcohol
   Avoid anticholinergic Drugs
   Decrease intra-abdominal pressure
     Lose weight
     Avoid tight clothing, braces
     Avoid straining maneuvers
   Use drugs: Urecholine, metoclopramide

3. *Reduce intraluminal acid content*
   Use antacids
   Use histamine-2 antagonists (cimetidine, ranitidine)
   Radiate parietal mass

4. *Increase esophageal acid-clearing*
   Urecholine
   Metoclopramide

Modified from Hurwitz, A. L., Duranceau, A., and Haddad, J. K. (eds.): Disorders of Esophageal Motility. Philadelphia, W. B. Saunders Co.,1979, p. 131.

reflux esophagitis, and intermittent in those with webs resulting from iron deficiency and in those with lower esophageal (Schatzki) rings. The last two conditions are fibromuscular strictures that narrow the lumen. In the *Schatzki ring,* dysphagia may be not only intermittent but also very severe; characteristically, a bolus of meat or bread obstructs proximal to the ring. Such incidents usually result from rapid eating and from swallowing large chunks of meat. Temporarily ineffective peristalsis may be in part at fault.

Long-term obstruction, whether caused by organic narrowing of the lumen or by severe neuromuscular disease, may produce serious effects. Outstanding among them are malnutrition and aspiration.

Insufficient food, particularly protein, may be swallowed to maintain adequate nutrition. Weight loss may be severe and progressive. Lesions that are inflammatory or malignant in nature often bleed slowly, causing a progressively severe iron deficiency anemia. Weight loss and dysphagia may be present for several months before patients seek medical attention.

Patients with severe obstruction may aspirate. This may either occur during swallowing, in which case there is immediate choking and discharge of fluid through the nose; or accumulated fluid and food may be aspirated into the tracheobronchial tree and lungs, occasionally causing severe pneumonitis and lung abscess. Nasal aspiration is more commonly associated with pharyngeal and upper cervical esophageal disorders of motor function. Tracheobronchial aspiration is characteristically associated with either progressive organic obstruction of the esophagus or severe motor disorder of the body and LES, particularly achalasia (see below). Pulmonary aspiration is often a nocturnal event and is usually heralded by a period of weeks or months of coughing during the night or early in the morning. Ultimately, a large amount of material may be aspirated with serious consequences to the lungs.

DISEASES OF STRIATED MUSCLE

Disease that affects the striated muscle will involve the pharyngeal, hypopharyngeal, and cervical esophageal muscles, the tongue, and the upper esophageal sphincter. These muscles may be affected by primary muscle disease or by lesions in the central nervous system or peripheral nerves.

Primary Muscle Disease

Primary muscle disease will usually affect all the muscles just listed. Difficulties in the upper esophageal sphincter will be compounded by loss of propulsive force in the pharyngeal muscle above it. Table 3 lists some of the processes that involve these muscles.

These motor disorders often have remarkable and characteristic abnormalities, which may be studied by two principal techniques—radiographic and manometric. For diseases of the striated musculature, the radiographic approach is the superior one, particularly cineradiography. This method directly visualizes the defective component of swallowing or of esophageal transit. Since the striated musculature is located quite proximally, manometric study is more difficult than for diseases and disorders of the body of the esophagus or those affecting the lower esophageal sphincter. Indeed, accurate pressure measurements of pharyngeal and hypopharyngeal contractions are nearly impossible to obtain. Several of these disorders have other characteristic diagnostic tests and therapies such as the edrophonium (Tensilon) test for myasthenia gravis.

Primary Nerve Diseases

The diseases of the nervous system that alter the function of the striated muscle of the esophagus are listed in Table 4. These range from lesions of the brainstem to peripheral nerve degeneration. Lesions of the brainstem interfere with coordination of the tongue and pharynx; these are most common following cerebrovascular accidents. Involvement of peripheral nerves by toxins may be rarely encountered in diphtheria and tetanus. Both poliomyelitis and amyotrophic lateral sclerosis may involve the lower motor neurons of the brainstem and thereby lead to loss of peripheral nerve function and, in turn, to striated muscle paresis and atrophy. Indeed, the serious consequences of failure of the pharyngeal musculature are well known in these diseases, particularly aspiration pneumonia. Striated muscle function may also be impaired in multiple sclerosis and in Huntington's chorea.

TABLE 3. PRIMARY MUSCLE DISEASES AFFECTING STRIATED MUSCLE

Myasthenia gravis
Myotonia dystrophica
Dermatomyositis-polymyositis
Amyloidosis
Oculopharyngeal muscular dystrophy
Thyrotoxicosis
Myxedema

From Sleisenger, M. H., and Fordtran, J. S. (eds.): Gastrointestinal Disease. 3rd ed. Philadelphia, W. B. Saunders Co., 1983, p. 427.

TABLE 4. PRIMARY NERVE DISEASES THAT IMPAIR OROPHARYNGEAL FUNCTION

Poliomyelitis
Brainstem lesions
Amyotrophic lateral sclerosis
Huntington's chorea
Multiple sclerosis
Parkinson's disease
Diphtheria
Tetanus

From Sleisenger, M. H., and Fordtran, J. S. (eds.): Gastrointestinal Disease. 3rd ed. Philadelphia, W. B. Saunders Co., 1983, p. 428.

Dysfunction of the Cricopharyngeus Muscle

Some patients who have a prominent cricopharyngeal muscle noted on cineesophagrams may also have difficulty in swallowing, presumably because of failure of this muscle to relax normally. It is thought that the upper esophageal sphincter (UES) is disordered. Despite dysphagia in some of these patients, however, manometric measurements do not usually substantiate dysfunction of the cricopharyngeus muscle. Indeed, pressure within this so-called "cricopharyngeal bar" is usually normal, and elevated pressures in the UES correlate neither with dysphagia nor with radiographic prominence of the cricopharyngeus muscle (Fig. 3). Furthermore, the cricopharyngeus muscle appears to relax normally in patients with this syndrome. Lack of such correlations notwithstanding, dysphagia in some patients has been relieved either by careful bougienage or by cutting the cricopharyngeus muscle. Often sphincterotomy is necessary, in addition to resection, for successful treatment of a pulsion diverticulum of the cervical esophagus that is often associated with this condition.

DISEASES OF SMOOTH MUSCLE

This category primarily includes achalasia (cardiospasm) and diffuse esophageal spasm as the prototype conditions. There is often overlap between these two categories; achalasia and diffuse esophageal spasm may be really just part of a spectrum of related motor disorders.

Achalasia

Strictly defined, achalasia is failure of the LES to relax and permit a bolus to enter the stomach. Failure of normal relaxation, in these instances, is traceable to absence or disease of the ganglion cells of the myenteric plexuses of the smooth muscle. This damage to the ganglion cells may be idiopathic, so-called achalasia or "cardiospasm" of the esophagus. It may be due to a toxin, as in Chagas' disease, or it may be due to the invasive effects of malignancy, particularly carcinoma of the distal esophagus or cardia of the stomach. The concentration of vasoactive intestinal peptide (a potent smooth muscle relaxant) containing nerve fibers is greatly reduced in patients with achalasia; the significance of this observation is still unclear.

Idiopathic achalasia is a prime example of a disorder

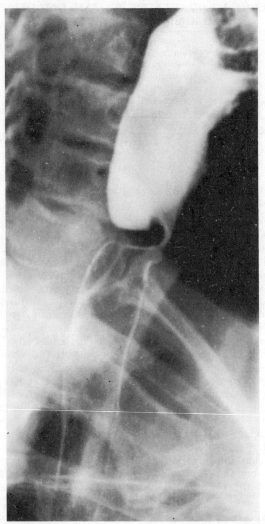

Figure 3. Cricopharyngeal "spasm." A prominent indentation is seen in the column of barium at the level of the cricopharyngeus muscle. The pharynx is somewhat dilated above this point. Such x-rays are obtained because of a history of dysphagia. (From Sleisenger, M. H., and Fordtran, J. S. (eds.): Gastrointestinal Disease. 3rd ed. Philadelphia, W. B. Saunders Co., 1983.)

of smooth muscle function of the esophagus. It is characterized pathologically by the diminution or absence of ganglion cells of the myenteric plexuses in the lower third of the esophagus. Since receptive relaxation of the LES and peristalsis of the body with which it is coordinated are both under intrinsic parasympathetic control, both functions are impaired in this disease. Thus, in achalasia, peristalsis in the body is either severely impaired or is absent and the LES does not relax with swallowing. Dysphagia, therefore, has two causes—lack of normal propulsion through the body and failure of relaxation of the LES.

Manometry. The motor abnormalities are best shown by manometry in which open-tipped catheters are spaced at adequate intervals to register changes in intraesophageal pressure. A classic example of the findings may be seen in Figure 4 (please compare with Figure 1). Manometry reveals normal function of the upper esophageal sphincter in achalasia and, indeed, some peristalsis may be demonstrated in the upper esophagus. In contrast to the normal situation, resting

pressure in the body of the esophagus is usually elevated. Uncoordinated, low-amplitude, simultaneous nonperistaltic contractions unrelated to swallowing may also be noted. The important finding is that swallowing does not result in normal peristaltic activity in the body of the esophagus. Equally striking is the elevated resting pressure in the LES and, characteristically, failure of the lower esophagus to relax with swallowing. In some patients the pressure will fall somewhat, but the LES pressure always remains above the gastric baseline, thus creating a persistent barrier.

Pharmacologic Responses

In achalasia the response of the esophagus to parasympathomimetic agents is extremely interesting, informative of the pathophysiology, and considered by some to be diagnostic. Essentially, the organ behaves as though parasympathetically denervated and follows Cannon's law of autonomic denervation—that is, denervation produces hypersensitivity to the humoral neurotransmitters of the particular system. Thus, an injection of a parasympathomimetic agent such as methacholine (Mecholyl) in very small amounts (0.1 to 0.2 mg subcutaneously) will cause an immediate, sharp, and sustained rise in pressure throughout the body of the esophagus when the parasympathetic system has been denervated, as in achalasia. This hypersensitivity of the body of the esophagus to parasympathomimetic medications is best shown if balloons are used instead of open-tipped, perfused catheters (Fig. 5).

Radiologic Phenomena

The failure of normal propulsion of a radiopaque substance or object (barium-coated marshmallow) may be readily demonstrated by fluoroscopy in most patients with achalasia, and the defect in peristalsis and

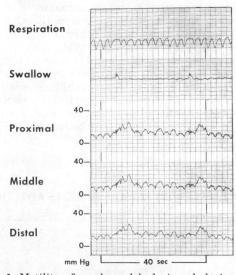

Figure 4. Motility of esophageal body in achalasia. In this tracing, three tips located 5 cm apart are in the body of the esophagus of a patient with achalasia. Note the elevated resting pressure of 10 mm Hg. Swallowing causes a broad, low amplitude simultaneous pressure wave to be seen in all three leads. No peristalsis is seen. (From Sleisenger, M. H., and Fordtran, J. S. (eds.): Gastrointestinal Disease. 3rd ed. Philadelphia, W. B. Saunders Co., 1983.)

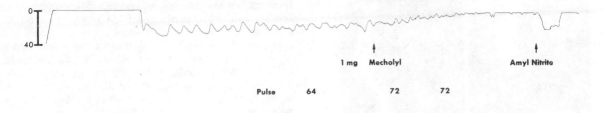

| Pulse | 64 | | 72 | 72 |

1 mg Mecholyl   Amyl Nitrite

Figure 5. Positive Mecholyl test. The balloon was positioned in the lower two-thirds of the esophagus. When air is released into the balloon, it expands to a volume of 30 ml. The normal esophagus only allows a 10-ml volume to exist before contraction empties the balloon. Spontaneous rhythmic activity is observed. After subcutaneous injection of 1 mg of Mecholyl, pulse rises slightly and air is excluded from the balloon until the recording pen shows zero balloon volume. Temporary relaxation of the tightly contracted esophagus is caused by inhalation of amyl nitrite. Time is shown at the bottom of the tracing. Each small mark is 10 seconds; the larger marks are minutes. (From Sleisenger, M. H., and Fordtran, J. S. (eds.): Gastrointestinal Disease. 3rd ed. Philadelphia, W. B. Saunders Co., 1983.)

failure of sphincter relaxation can be more clearly documented by cineradiography. In patients with achalasia, often a barium-covered marshmallow will not be propelled normally down the esophagus; it will "hang up" at the LES. Either fluoroscopy with barium or cineradiography will show the smooth conical narrowing at the distal end of the esophagus with intermittent spurting of material into the stomach, representing intermittent relaxation of the sphincter sufficient to allow material to pass into the stomach (Fig. 6). Numerous uncoordinated nonperistaltic contractions—so-called tertiary contractions—may be noted by either method.

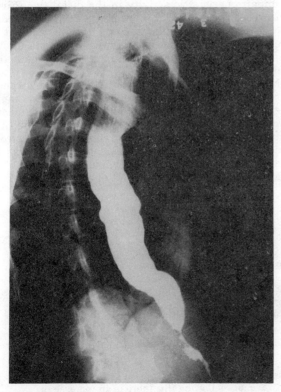

Figure 6. Achalasia of the esophagus. This is the classic appearance of the dilated esophagus terminating in a narrowed segment. Fluid and mucus float on top of the more dense barium. (Courtesy of Dr. F. E. Templeton.)

Sequelae of Achalasia

In effect the patient with unremitting chronic achalasia has an obstruction of the esophagus, and since it is at the lower end of the organ, several pathologic complications may result. The muscle wall proximal to the LES may become weakened to the point of forming an epiphrenic diverticulum. Presumably, the wall becomes weaker because of repeated effort to overcome the obstruction offered by an abnormally behaving sphincter. Chronic obstruction also results in stasis of food and liquid in the lower segment of the esophagus, leading to irritation and esophagitis. Further, the incidence of carcinoma of the lower third of the esophagus is increased above normal for age and sex in patients with achalasia, probably secondary to chronic stasis and irritation.

Clinically, the patient with unremitting and untreated achalasia will develop progressive dilation of the esophagus. In advanced stages food and fluid collect and regurgitation becomes more frequent and extensive, the serious consequence of which is aspiration. Frequent bouts of bronchopneumonia are not uncommon, and an occasional patient may suffer from a lung abscess. Progressive weight loss and nutritional deficiences of many kinds secondary to diminished food intake—particularly of protein and the water-soluble vitamins—are inevitable in the untreated patient.

Diffuse Spasm

Disordered esophageal motility may result in diffuse spasm, characterized by pain, either at rest or more particularly following the ingestion of either very hot or cold liquid (odynophagia). In some patients substernal pain radiates directly to the back, is unrelated to food, and may awaken patients from sleep. Dysphagia with or without odynophagia may be the particularly notable symptom associated with swallowing hot or cold substances.

Motility. The cardinal pathophysiologic feature of motility disorders is a distinct motor abnormality, noted by both radiologic and manometric examinations. Following a swallow, peristalsis is noted to traverse only the upper third of the esophagus. Thereafter, the motor movement is uncoordinated and irregular, characterized by the aforementioned "tertiary contractions." Radiographically, there is a corkscrew

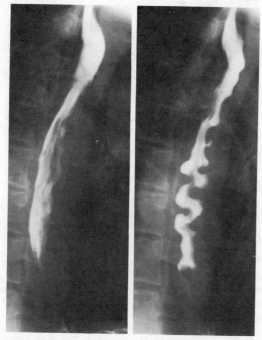

Figure 7. Diffuse spasm. Two spot films were taken within seconds of one another. A fairly normal appearance on the left is replaced by numerous contractions which form pseudodiverticula. (Courtesy of Dr. C. A. Rohrmann.)

pattern—an exaggerated sacculation shown in Figure 7. On occasion, the lower half or more of the body of the esophagus may seem to contract as a unit, and barium is propelled cephalad, rising into the hypopharynx and pharynx.

Manometric examinations corroborate the abnormal radiologic findings of swallowing seen in the upper third of the esophagus. The simultaneous contractions of high amplitude, seen by cineradiography in the lower two thirds, are also recorded manometrically. Pressures as high as 80 mm Hg may be reached. These contractions are prolonged, and frequently patients complain of pain. In most patients the LES relaxes normally; however, in some the resting pressure is high (Fig. 8).

The pathophysiologic changes in motor activity on

manometry also include exaggerated responses to both methacholine and pentagastrin. Although resting pressure in the body of the esophagus as recorded by intraluminal balloons is normal, it rises significantly after the injection of methacholine in most patients.

The major pathologic finding in the esophagus in most, but not all, patients with diffuse spasm is thickening of the smooth muscle. However, it is not known whether this precedes or follows the appearance of the abnormal motor behavior.

MOTOR DISORDERS OF THE ESOPHAGUS IN SYSTEMIC ILLNESS

Collagen Vascular Diseases

Of the diseases in this group, *scleroderma* most frequently affects the esophagus. It is a diffuse systemic disease involving the skin, joints, kidneys, lungs, spleen, heart, and gastrointestinal tract. Of the organs of the gut, the esophagus usually is the first and most severely affected. The disease slows motor activity throughout the gut, but particularly in the esophagus. The basic pathologic lesion is progressive atrophy of smooth muscle and replacement by fibrous tissue. The importance of vasculitis in the pathogenesis and pathophysiology of the gut dysfunction is demonstrated by the early appearance of Raynaud's phenomenon in most patients, often correlated with manometric evidence of impaired motor activity of the esophagus, long in advance of dysphagia and other clinical evidence of esophageal disease.

Scleroderma affects the esophagus in two ways: (1) it impairs peristaltic activity in the distal two thirds of the esophagus, and (2) it lowers the resting pressure in the LES. The net effect is to reduce the gradient of pressure between stomach and lower esophagus, allowing reflux of acid peptic juice, and to impair the clearance of this fluid.

Motility. Radiologically, the findings may range from inability of an asymptomatic patient to empty the esophagus of a column of barium while recumbent to complete esophageal atony. Involvement of the LES may be inferred from the free reflux of barium from the stomach into the lower esophagus. Peristalsis in the body of the esophagus is diminished or absent.

Manometry demonstrates diminished to absent per-

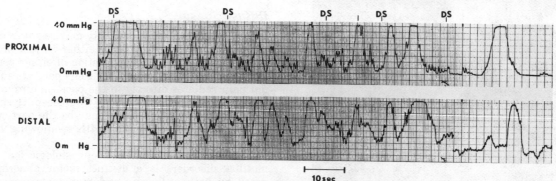

Figure 8. Manometric evidence for diffuse spasm. This record is obtained from two infused catheters whose tips are 5 cm apart. A dry swallow (DS) causes a peristaltic wave, but following this there is an increase in the baseline pressure lasting over 80 seconds. There are also spontaneous simultaneous contractions unrelated to swallowing. At the end of the period of spasm, a final dry swallow sets off another peristaltic wave. (From Pope, C. E., II: Postgrad Med 61:118, 1977. Reprinted by permission.)

istalsis in the distal two thirds of the esophagus. Resting pressure in the LES is diminished to a point that a zone of high resting pressure cannot be demonstrated between stomach and esophagus. Thus, the two organs form a common cavity. This finding explains the presence of air in the esophagus and also the continuous column of barium constituted by the lower esophagus and the stomach during conventional fluoroscopy. The abolition of the normal resting pressure renders the lower esophagus vulnerable to reflux of acid gastric juice. The damage to the LES is not entirely the result of muscle atrophy and fibrosis. There is an impaired response to edrophonium, an anticholinesterase agent, suggesting malfunction of the nervous control of the LES. The sphincter is not entirely unresponsive, however, and may show a rise in pressure following the administration of methacholine or metaclopramide.

Other diseases characterized by vasculitis also may affect the esophagus, particularly systemic lupus erythematosus, dermatomyositis-polymyositis, and other mixed disorders. The common denominator seems to be Raynaud's phenomenon. As indicated earlier, impaired motor activity may be detected manometrically in a high percentage of patients with Raynaud's phenomenon before esophageal symptoms develop. However, there is good correlation between the degree of Raynaud's phenomenon and the eventual clinical severity of esophageal involvement. Both lupus and dermatomyositis-polymyositis are characterized by impaired peristalsis in the body of the esophagus and a hypotensive lower esophageal sphincter.

Diabetes Mellitus

Patients with diabetic neuropathy may have impaired motor function of the esophagus; presumably, the disorder is caused by impaired innervation of the smooth muscle by involvement of the intrinsic autonomic nervous system by the underlying disease. Manometrically, the pathophysiologic defects are impaired peristalsis, decreased amplitude of peristaltic waves, and a high incidence of purposeless "tertiary contractions." Most individuals with these abnormalities are not symptomatic.

Alcoholic Neuropathy

Ingestion of ethanol may be associated with both impairment of primary peristalsis and diminution of the resting pressure in the lower esophageal sphincter. Perhaps these changes explain the heartburn often found in persons who are drinking alcohol. Chronic alcoholics do not have problems with motor power of the esophagus unless they develop neuropathy. In such instances the primary peristaltic activity of the lower half of the esophagus is impaired, often severely, and sphincter function also may be abnormal.

Presbyesophagus

With advancing age, disordered peristaltic activity, detected manometrically, may be manifested by decreased amplitude of peristaltic contractions together with reduced peristaltic activity following swallowing and by a decrease in LES pressure. However, no clearcut symptomatology can be attributed to these changes, and no elderly patient should be assumed to have "presbyesophagus" unless a complete work-up (including esophagoscopy) fails to detect other diseases.

The Esophagus and Intestinal Pseudo-obstruction

A rare condition known as intestinal pseudo-obstruction is characterized by intermittent ileus and dilation of the small and large intestine presenting clinically with distention and obstruction. These patients also have difficulty with swallowing. Dysphagia is associated with diminished peristalsis and inability of the lower esophageal sphincter to relax properly.

REFERENCES

Benjamin, S. B., and Castell, D. O.: Chest pain of esophageal origin: Where are we, and where should we go? Arch Intern Med 143:772, 1983.

Castell, D. O.: The lower esophageal sphincter. Ann Intern Med 83:390, 1975.

Castell, D. O., Knuff, T. E., Brown, F. C., et al.: Dysphagia. Gastroenterology 76:1015, 1979.

Christensen, J.: Effects of drugs on esophageal motility. Arch Intern Med 136:532, 1976.

Clouse, R. E., Staiano, A., Landau, D. W., et al.: Manometric findings during spontaneous chest pain in patients with presumed esophageal "spasms". Gastroenterology 85:395, 1983.

Cohen, S.: Motor disorders of the esophagus. N Engl J Med 301:184, 1979.

Dodds, W. J., Dent, J., Hogan, W. J., et al.: Mechanisms of gastroesophageal reflux in patients with reflux esophagitis. N Engl J Med 307:1547, 1982.

Helm, J. F., Dodds, W. J., Riedel, D. R., et al.: Determinants of esophageal acid clearance in normal subjects. Gastroenterology 85:607, 1983.

Liöbermann-Meffert, D., Allgewer, M., Schmid, P., et al.: Muscular equivalent of the lower esophageal sphincter. Gastroenterology 76:31, 1979.

Pope, C. E., II: The esophagus. Physiology. In Sleisenger, M. H., and Fordtran, J. S., (eds.): Gastrointestinal Disease. 3rd ed. Philadelphia, W. B. Saunders Co., 1983, p. 414.

Pope, C. E., II: The esophagus. Motor disorders. In Sleisenger, M. H., and Fordtran, J. S. (eds.): Gastrointestinal Disease. 3rd ed. Philadelphia, W. B. Saunders Co., 1983, p. 424.

Pope, C. E., II: The esophagus. Gastroesophageal reflux disease (reflux esophagitis). In Sleisenger, M. H., and Fordtran, J. S. (eds.): Gastrointestinal Disease. 3rd ed. Philadelphia, W. B. Saunders Co., 1983, p. 449.

Pope, C. E., II: The esophagus. Rings and webs. In Sleisenger, M. H., and Fordtran, J. S. (eds.): Gastrointestinal Disease. 3rd ed. Philadelphia, W. B. Saunders Co., 1983, p. 476.

Richter, J. E., and Castell, D. O.: Gastroesophageal reflux: Pathogenesis, diagnosis, and therapy. Ann Intern Med 97:93, 1982.

Vantrappen, G., Janssens, J., Hellemans, J., et al.: Achalasia, diffuse esophageal spasm, and related motility disorders. Gastroenterology 76:450, 1979.

The Stomach

CLIFFORD W. DEVENEY, M.D.

The stomach connects the esophagus with the duodenum. It is the most dilated portion of the gastrointestinal tract, measuring about 10 to 12 cm in maximal transverse diameter and 25 to 30 cm in length.

The stomach is divided into five segments (Fig. 9): the cardia, fundus, body, antrum, and pylorus. The gastric cardia is limited to the small segment of proximal stomach that surrounds the gastroesophageal junction and the fundus is a pouch or dome-like structure extending from the cardia along the greater curvature to the body. The body is the middle third of the stomach, extending from the cardia and fundus caudally to the incisura angularis. The body and fundus contain parietal cells and constitute the acid-secreting portion of the stomach. The antrum extends distally from the incisura angularis to the pyloric sphincter. Each area of the stomach has a distinctive type of mucosal gland. The boundaries between different segments are indistinct; there is usually an overlap, with mixed glands where two areas meet. The stomach is composed of four tissue layers: the mucosa, submucosa, muscularis propria, and serosa.

Mucosa

The surface of the mucosa is studded with the openings of gastric pits that extend deeply into it. These are lined by the gastric glands that contain secretory cells (see Fig. 10). The difference in the cells making up these glands characterizes the different anatomic portions of the stomach. The cardiac glands contain clear-staining mucous type cells and resemble antral glands; the fundus and body contain the oxyntic glands with a high proportion of oxyntic (parietal) and chief cells; in the antrum, glands containing clear-staining mucous cells predominate. The gastric mucosal cells are columnar and secrete mucus. These mucus-secreting cells actively divide at the necks of the glands and migrate upward to replace cells lost by desquamation. Surface epithelial cells are renewed about every 24 to 72 hours. The *oxyntic glands* in the body and fundus contain parietal cells, chief cells, and also mucous neck cells and endocrine cells.

The *parietal cells,* which secrete hydrochloric acid and intrinsic factor, are large and pyramidal cells that are most prominent in the midportion of the gland and

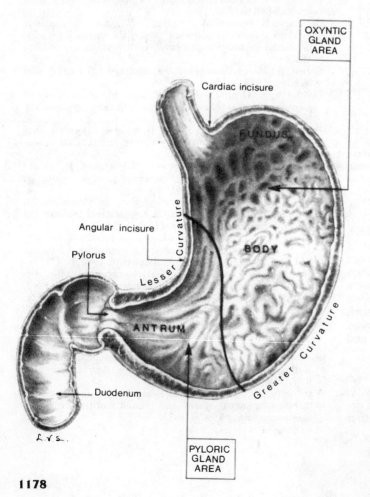

Figure 9. Names of the parts of the stomach. The line drawn from the lesser to the greater curvature depicts the approximate boundary between the oxyntic gland area and the pyloric gland area. No prominent landmark exists to distinguish between antrum and body (corpus). The fundus is the portion craniad to the esophagogastric junction. (Reproduced with permission from Way, L. W. (ed.): Current Surgical Diagnosis and Treatment. 6th ed. Los Altos, CA, Lange Medical Publications, 1983.)

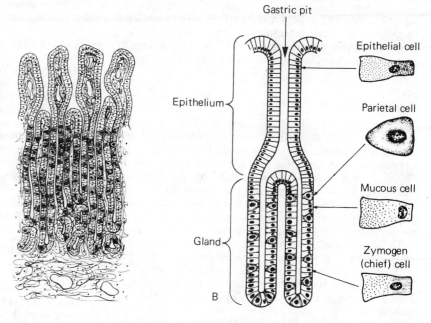

Figure 10. *A*, Histologic features of the mucosa in the oxyntic gland area. Each gastric pit drains 3–7 tubular gastric glands. The neck of the gland contains many mucous cells. Oxyntic (parietal) cells are most numerous in the mid portion of the glands; peptic (chief) cells predominate in the basal portion. *B*, Drawing from photomicrograph of the gastric mucosa. (Both figures reproduced with permission from Way, L. W. (ed.): Current Surgical Diagnosis and Treatment. 6th ed. Los Altos, CA, Lange Medical Publications, 1983.)

are packed with mitochondria. These cells have a complicated canalicular network that opens into the lumen of the gastric gland. They contain cytoplasmic vesicles that are reduced in number when stimulated, at which time the canalicular network becomes more prominent and the number of mitochondria diminishes.

The *chief (zymogen) cells,* which secrete pepsinogen, are most prominent in the deepest portion of the gland and are characterized by the presence of large, highly refractile zymogen granules. These granules, which are secreted during stimulation, contain pepsinogen, the precursor of pepsin.

The *mucus neck cells* also contain granules that take a PAS stain, indicating the presence of glycoprotein. Their secretion, however, is different from that of the surface mucous cells, as indicated by some differences in the staining of the mucous granules of each cell type.

Endocrine and paracrine cells, scattered throughout the glands of the proximal and distal stomach, have prominent secretory granules that contain peptide hormones identifiable by immunohistochemical techniques. Each cell usually contains only one peptide hormone. Most of the endocrine cells have a brush border that abuts on the lumen. It is believed that the luminal border of the cell acts as a chemoreceptor that senses intraluminal contents and releases hormones in response. Gastrin, somatostatin, glucagon, and bombesin-like immunoreactivities have been localized to these cells. In addition, serotonin is found in some of the endocrine cells and histamine is found in mast cells. These hormones or messengers presumably control gastric acid and pepsin secretion. The peptides are either released into the blood and reach their target through the circulation (endocrine function) or they are released and act locally (paracrine function). For example, bombesin causes gastrin release and gastric acid secretion. Somatostatin inhibits both gastric acid secretion and gastrin release; gastrin and histamine are potent stimuli for acid and pepsinogen secretion. It is speculated that gastrin acts through the blood-

stream and histamine, bombesin, and somatostatin act locally.

The antrum contains *pyloric glands,* which open into gastric pits that are deeper than those in the body and fundus. Most of the cells appear similar to mucous neck cells and to cells in the Brunner's glands of the duodenum. The most prominent endocrine cells in the antrum contain gastrin (G cells) and release it into the circulation.

Gastric mucosa, like mucosa elsewhere in the gastrointestinal tract, also contains a lamina propria and a muscularis mucosae. Deep to the mucosa is the submucosa containing connective tissue and small arteries and veins, some lymphoid elements, and submucosal neuroplexuses.

Smooth Muscle

The gastric wall has three muscle layers—longitudinal (outer), circular (middle), and oblique (inner). The longitudinal muscle layer covers the lesser and greater curvatures, and the circular inner layer surrounds the entire organ except for a short distance near the esophagogastric junction. In contrast to the longitudinal layer, the innermost or oblique coat of muscle extends over the anterior and posterior surfaces and is not prominent along the curvatures. At the distal end of the stomach the pyloric portion of the organ is thicker; its musculature consists principally of circular muscle that surrounds the gastroduodenal junction. In terms of motor function, the stomach may be divided into proximal and distal portions. The proximal stomach including the fundus and the proximal corpus expands to accommodate food or drink. It maintains a constant intragastric pressure over large volume changes, and it determines in large part the rate at which liquids leave the stomach. The distal stomach—including the antrum—generates forceful peristaltic contractions that grind or disperse solid food into small particles and control the emptying of solid food.

The gastric musculature enables the stomach to stretch or expand to hold a recently ingested meal and to grind solid food mechanically into small particles. It subsequently empties this meal into the duodenum in a uniform, predictable fashion for about three hours postprandially.

Nervous System

The nervous system of the stomach, like that of the rest of the gastrointestinal tract, is intrinsic and can function independently of extrinsic innervation; this nervous system is called the *enteric nervous system* (ENS). The ENS consists principally of two plexuses, the myenteric (Auerbach's) and the submucous (Meissner's) plexus. The myenteric plexus lies between the circular and longitudinal smooth muscles and the submucous plexus lies in the submucosa.

These plexuses receive input from the central nervous system via the vagi (parasympathetic) and the splanchnic nerves via the celiac ganglia (sympathetic). These nerves integrate the CNS with the enteric nervous system and modify actions of the enteric nervous system.

Some reflexes are primarily mediated through the sympathetic or parasympathetic nerves, but many reflexes represent an interaction of these nerves with the ENS. In general, the direct actions of sympathetic nerves are inhibitory. For example, decreasing duodenal pH or intestinal distention inhibits gastric motility. The efferent arm of this reflex is adrenergic or sympathetic.

The vagus (cholinergic) nerve mediates relaxation of the gastric fundus; it coordinates peristalsis in the body and antrum and relaxation of the pylorus. The vagus also enhances acid and pepsin secretion to all stimuli.

The sympathetic nerves are mainly adrenergic, and the presynaptic vagi are cholinergic. Many of the postsynaptic vagal fibers as well as many of the enteric nerves are neither cholinergic nor adrenergic. Several gastrin (ENS) nerves contain peptides and probably use these peptides as transmitters. Vasoactive intestinal peptide (VIP), substance P, somatostatin, enkephalins, bombesin, and cholecystokinin (CCK) have been identified in these nerves and are probable neurotransmitters. Serotonin is a transmitter for some nerves, and ATP may also serve as a neurotransmitter.

Nerves are seen in close proximity to smooth muscle, blood vessels, and mucosal cells. It is believed that afferent nerves of the ENS sense chemical stimuli from the lumen—such as proteins, amino acids, and fats—and distention from the wall of the stomach. Impulses are sent to the ganglia in the myenteric and mesenteric plexuses, which also receive impulses from the CNS. These reflexes from CNS and ENS afferent fibers are integrated in the myenteric and mesenteric plexuses and efferent nerves originating from these ganglia control motility, secretion, absorption and blood flow—that is, the process of digestion. As noted, the neurotransmitters for this system are not only adrenergic and cholinergic but also peptidergic (peptides). Table 5 lists the pharmacologic effects of several peptides found in gastric nerves. Although their physiologic actions are not known, these peptides have pronounced effects on smooth muscle and mucosal cells and may well be neurotransmitters.

GASTRIC ACID SECRETION

Gastric secretion consists principally of hydrochloric acid, pepsinogen, and mucus. Hydrochloric acid is actively secreted by the parietal cells and can be concentrated as high as 150 mEq/l, a concentration of hydrogen ion one million times that in the blood. Gastrin, histamine, and acetylcholine stimulate the parietal cell to secrete acid. All of these substances probably play a physiologic role in acid secretion since all are present in gastric mucosa.

CELLULAR MECHANISMS OF ACID SECRETION

The enzyme responsible for acid secretion is a potassium-primed ATPase that is located uniquely in the apical cell membranes of the parietal cell. The enzyme "pumps" hydrogen ion into the lumen in exchange for potassium in a process requiring ATP. Histamine, gastrin, and acetylcholine are all potent secretagogues in vivo, but the secretory effect of all is significantly reduced by histamine H-2 receptor antagonists—cimetidine, ranitidine, and famotidine. This initially led to the belief that gastrin and acetylcholine did not act directly on the parietal cell but rather through histamine as the final mediator for acid secretion. However, in vivo studies using gastric glands or parietal cells have demonstrated characteristic differences in the modes of action of histamine, gastrin, and acetylcholine and therefore imply that there are separate receptors on the parietal cell for these three secretagogues (Fig. 11).

TABLE 5. ACTIONS OF SEVERAL PEPTIDES FOUND IN THE GASTRIC NERVES*

PEPTIDE	ACTION
(1) Bombesin	(1) Release of gastrin contraction of smooth muscle.
(2) Enkephalins	(2) Diffuse action on smooth muscle.
(3) Cholecystokinin	(3) Affects antral smooth muscle and pylorus; overall effect delays gastric emptying.
(4) Substance P	(4) Contracts smooth muscle.
(5) Somatostatin	(5) Numerous inhibitory actions; inhibits gastric acid and pepsinogen secretion, delays gastric emptying.
(6) Vasoactive intestinal polypeptide (VIP)	(6) Causes smooth muscle relaxation and increases blood flow.

*These actions pertain only to possible actions on the stomach. The exact role of these transmitters is unknown.

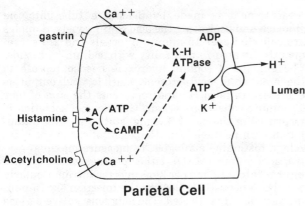

*A
C = Adenylcyclase

Figure 11. The parietal cell with three receptors, histamine, gastrin, and cholinergic. Histamine, gastrin, and acetylcholine all act to stimulate a potassium hydrogen ATPase (the hydrogen pump at the luminal side of the cell). However, the characteristics of each compound differ enough to suggest that each compound acts at a different receptor. Histamine causes increases in intracellular adenylcyclase and cyclic AMP, which in turn activate or increase the amount of the sodium potassium ATPase. Cholinergic drugs and gastrin cause influx of Ca^{++}, which in turn activates the potassium hydrogen ATPase.

Histamine produces dose-dependent acid secretion. The action of histamine correlates with cyclic AMP and adenylcyclase levels in the cells and is potentiated by phosphodiesterase inhibitors. Thus it appears that histamine works by increasing cyclic AMP. The action of histamine is completely blocked by H-2 receptor antagonists. In vitro, the reaction of parietal cells to *acetylcholine* is transient, peaking at 15 minutes, and is blocked by atropine but not by H-2 blockers. Extracellular calcium is necessary for the acid secretory response to acetylcholine but not to that of histamine. If the cells are exposed to acetylcholine and small amounts of histamine, the response is no longer transient. Acetylcholine and histamine together strongly potentiate each other. In vivo, either H-2 receptor antagonists or anticholinergics significantly reduce acid secretion because either can block the potentiation that occurs between histamine and acetylcholine.

Gastrin produces a small but significant increase in acid secretion in parietal cells. When gastrin is given with a phosphodiesterase inhibitor, it becomes a potent secretagogue. This response is blocked by histamine blockers (H-2 antagonists). Gastrin does not activate adenylcyclase or increase cAMP as histamine does. The augmentation of the gastrin response by a phosphodiesterase inhibitor suggests that the action of gastrin, at least in part, is modulated through endogenous release of histamine. However, for gastrin to evoke any acid secretion, calcium must be present in the medium, whereas histamine alone does not require calcium. Thus, although the action of gastrin on the parietal cell requires small amounts of histamine within the cell, the mechanism of action is different from that of histamine alone. This implies a separate gastrin receptor on the parietal cell membrane.

The reason H-2 blockers substantially reduce acetylcholine-stimulated acid secretion in vivo is that acetylcholine and histamine strongly potentiate one another; the blocking of the histamine receptor removes that potentiation. The response to gastrin is reduced by H-2 blockers presumably because gastrin evokes acid secretion by releasing endogenous histamine. Even though the actions of gastrin and acetylcholine are substantially reduced by H-2 blocking agents, these two secretagogues probably act directly on the parietal cell.

PHYSIOLOGY OF ACID SECRETION

Normally, basal acid secretion ranges from 2 to 10 mEq H^+ per hr. After a meal, acid secretion increases and peaks within two hours (Fig. 12). In vivo, gastric acid secretion has been traditionally divided into three phases:

1. *Cephalic phase.* The thought of food, prompted by appetizing sights or smells, will cause acid secretion. This effect, which can be abolished by vagotomy, can be demonstrated by sham feeding in animals. The animals are allowed to eat but the food is diverted through a cervical esophagostomy and does not reach the stomach. These classical studies in animals can be simulated by studies in humans (Fig. 13).

2. *Gastric phase.* The presence of a meal in the stomach causes gastric acid secretion by several mechanisms. The protein content of the meal causes release of the potent gastric secretagogue gastrin from the antral G cells. The bulk of the meal stretches the

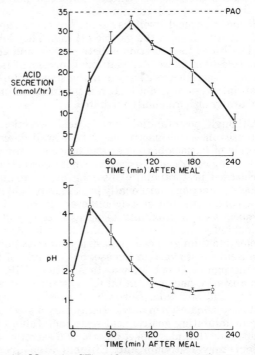

Figure 12. Mean ($\pm$ SE) acid secretion (top) and intragastric pH (bottom) following a sirloin steak meal in healthy subjects. On day 1 (top) after the meal was eaten, acid secretion was measured by in vivo intragastric titration to pH 5.5 in 6 subjects. On day 2 (bottom), intragastric pH in 10 subjects was allowed to seek its natural level after the meal was eaten. The mean basal acid secretion rate (top) and basal pH (bottom) before the meal are shown at 0 minute. Peak acid output (PAO) is also indicated. (From Sleisenger, M. H. and Fordtran, J. S. (eds.): Gastrointestinal Disease. 3rd ed. Philadelphia, W. B. Saunders Co., 1983.)

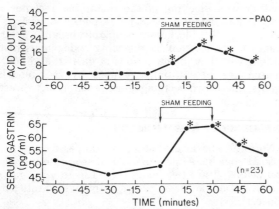

Figure 13. Effect of sham feeding for 30 minutes on mean acid output (top) and serum gastrin concentration (bottom) in 23 healthy subjects. During sham feeding, mean acid output and serum gastrin concentration increased significantly (p<0.05). After sham feeding ended, acid output and serum gastrin concentration decreased toward basal levels. Mean peak acid output (PAO) to 6 μg per kg of pentagastrin in these subjects is also shown. Acid output during sham feeding increased to approximately 50 per cent of PAO to pentagastrin. (From Sleisenger, M. H., and Fordtran, J. S. (eds.): Gastrointestinal Disease. 3rd ed. Philadelphia, W. B. Saunders Co., 1983.)

stomach and activates cholinergic stretch receptors in the wall of the stomach. These cholinergic nerves act on the parietal cell to stimulate acid secretion. In addition, the meal itself has some buffering capacity and usually elevates the gastric pH to 5. The elevated pH facilitates the secretion of both gastrin and acid.

3. *Intestinal phase.* An additional increment in gastric acid secretion occurs when the meal enters the small intestine. It is not known if the intestinal phase is neurally or hormonally mediated.

Although postprandial gastric acid secretion and increases in serum gastrin have been well described, the role of various hormones and other substances in controlling gastric acid secretion is not known. Gastrin is released postprandially into the bloodstream and probably functions hormonally to stimulate acid secretion. Histamine and acetylcholine are present in the stomach wall in proximity to parietal cells and they undoubtedly act locally to stimulate acid secretion. Cholecystokinin also causes gastric acid secretion and bombesin causes gastrin release, but the role of these two hormones is not known. In addition, VIP, GIP, somatostatin, and secretin inhibit gastrin release and gastric acid secretion. However, it presently appears that only somatostatin may actually play a physiologic role in inhibiting gastric acid secretion. Table 6 lists compounds that may affect gastric acid secretion.

Secretory Patterns and Clinical Measurement of Acid. Most patients with duodenal ulcer secrete acid at a normal rate; therefore, measurement of acid has little value in the diagnosis of peptic ulcer disease except in the case of gastrinoma (Zollinger-Ellison syndrome), in which acid secretion is extremely high, and in recurrent peptic ulcer disease after surgery to determine if vagotomy is complete. Nonetheless, the role of acid secretion is important in the treatment of peptic ulcer disease, since all successful therapy for peptic ulcer reduces acid concentration.

Measurement of Gastric Acid Secretion. The measurement is made by placing a tube into the stomach and aspirating the acid continuously. Samples are collected over 15-minute intervals and are subsequently titrated to neutrality with sodium hydroxide. The amount of sodium hydroxide needed represents the amount of acid present. Gastric acid output is expressed in mEq H^+ and represents the sum of four 15-minute collection periods. Gastric acid secretion is measured in the basal (fasting) state and after stimulation with pentagastrin (the agent of choice) or betazole, a histamine analogue. To measure maximal gastric acid output (MAO), either pentagastrin 6 μg per kg or betazole 1.5 mg per kg is injected intramuscularly or subcutaneously. Following the injection six 15-minute samples are collected. The four consecutive periods with the highest acid secretion are called the MAO and the two consecutive periods with the highest secretion are called peak acid output (PAO). Both MAO and PAO are expressed in mEq H^+ per hr. The peak response will be seen within 30 to 90 minutes of injection and tends to be earlier when pentagastrin is used.

Other substances that have been used to test acid secretory response in humans include insulin, tolbutamide, and 2-deoxyglucose. These agents act by producing hypoglycemia or by blocking CNS glucose, utilization that causes the vagus nerves to stimulate acid secretion. Thus these agents have been used primarily to test the integrity of the vagus nerve. Since acid response to lowering of blood sugar is not entirely dependent on the vagus, however, and since tests are not without danger, they should be used rarely or never.

Patterns of Secretion. Table 7 presents a summary of acid secretion measured basally and following various stimuli in normal subjects and in patients with duodenal ulcer disease. There is overlap between the upper limit of normal and the mean value for the patients with duodenal ulcer, both for basal secretion and in response to histamine, betazole, or pentagastrin stimulation. Thus, a significant number of normal people secrete acid comparable in amount to those with duodenal ulcer; a large number of patients with duodenal ulcer secrete amounts of acid that may be considered in the high normal range.

TABLE 6. HORMONES AND SUBSTANCES THAT MAY AFFECT GASTRIC ACID SECRETION OR DUODENAL pH

ACTION	STIMULATION	INHIBITION
Acid secretion	Gastrin	VIP
	CCK	GIP
	Histamine	Somatostatin
	Acetylcholine	Secretin
Gastrin release	Bombesin	Secretin
		Somatostatin
		VIP
		GIP
		Glucagon
Pancreatic bicarbonate secretion	CCK	PP
	Secretin	
	VIP	
Delay of gastric emptying of acid into duodenum	CCK	

CCK, cholecystokinin; VIP, vasoactive intestinal peptide; GIP, gastric inhibitory peptide; PP, pancreatic polypeptide.

TABLE 7. BASAL AND MAXIMAL STIMULATED GASTRIC ACID SECRETION IN NORMAL SUBJECTS AND IN PATIENTS WITH DUODENAL ULCER

	SEX	N	ACID OUTPUT (mEq/hr)			
			Normal		Duodenal Ulcer	
			Mean	ULN	Mean	LV-DU
Basal	M	615	2.4	?6.6	5.3	0.1
	F	634	1.3	?4.1	2.9	0.1
Histamine	M	25	23.1	42.0	45.9	# 0
	F	20	12.3	30.2	32.0	18.8
Betazole	M	75	34.4	59.8	42.4	6.2
	F	45	16.8	40.0	30.8	13.4
Pentagastrin	M	18	25.0	45.0	43.0	15.0

N = number; ULN = upper limit of normal (mean + 2SD); LV-DV = lowest value in duodenal ulcer.
Modified from Sleisenger, M. H., and Fordtran, J. S. (eds.): Gastrointestinal Disease. 2nd ed., Philadelphia, W. B. Saunders Co., 1978.

Clinically, gastric analysis has limited application. It is not used in routine cases of duodenal or gastric ulcer. It is helpful, however, if gastrin levels are high and gastrinoma is suspected. Patients with gastrinoma usually secrete 15 to 100 mEq H+ per hour compared to 2 to 10 mEq H+ per hour in patients without gastrinoma. Gastric analysis is also helpful in determining if a previous vagotomy was complete. Complete vagotomy reduces acid secretion by 60 to 70 per cent; thus basal acid secretion should be less than 5 mEq H+ per hour after vagotomy and stimulated acid secretion should be less than 20 mEq H+ per hour.

Response to a Test Meal. The best physiologic stimulus for gastric acid secretion is the ingestion of food. The mean secretory response of patients with duodenal ulcer to a protein meal is significantly higher than that of normal subjects (Fig. 14). The measurement of gastric acid secretion following a meal involves either frequent aspiration and neutralization of the gastric acidity with sodium bicarbonate—the total amount of acid secreted over a period of time being equal to the mEq of sodium bicarbonate added to maintain a pH of 5.5—or by calculations from data derived from measurements of acid in aspirates from separate tubes in the stomach and duodenum.

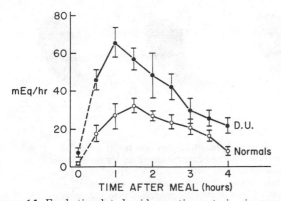

Figure 14. Food-stimulated acid secretion rate in six normal subjects and seven patients with duodenal ulcer. Mean ± SE. Basal acid secretion is shown for comparison at 0 time. (From Fordtran, J. S., and Walsh, J. H.: Reproduced from *The Journal of Clinical Investigation*, 1973, vol. 52, p. 645, by copyright permission of The American Society for Clinical Investigation.)

PEPSINOGEN SECRETION

Pepsinogens are secreted from the chief cells in response to the same stimuli as for gastric acid secretion. Pepsinogens are also contained in mucous cells of cardiac, oxyntic, and pyloric glands and are activated to pepsins when the pH is less than 5. Pepsins are enzymes that cleave peptide bonds, particularly those containing phenylalanine, tyrosine, or leucine. Pepsin works optimally at a pH of 2 and is inactivated when the pH is greater than 5.

Mucous and Bicarbonate Secretion

Gastric mucus, a gel of glycoprotein and water secreted by mucosal cells throughout the stomach, coats and lubricates the mucosa and affords protection against abrasion. Whether it acts as a buffer against gastric acid is not clear. The secretion of mucus has not been as well studied as that of acid or pepsin because of difficulty in measuring mucus. It does appear that vagal stimulation (as well as topical application of acetylcholine), secretin, and prostaglandin E_2 analogues all increase gastric secretion of mucus.

Gastric mucosal cells also secrete bicarbonate, which is postulated to layer out over the mucosal cells and remain relatively undiffused because it is covered by mucus. If this is true the bicarbonate would act locally to neutralize acid and protect the mucosal cell from acid digestion (Fig. 15).

Intrinsic Factor Secretion

Intrinsic factor, a mucoprotein of about 60,000 daltons, is essential for the absorption of cobalamin (vitamin B_{12}) with which it forms a complex that is bound to specific receptor sites in the ileum. It is secreted along with acid by the parietal cell. The common stimulants of acid secretion also increase intrinsic factor secretion; these include vagal stimuli, cholinergic agents, histamine, and gastrin.

When acid secretion is subnormal, secretion of intrinsic factor is usually depressed as well. Since only a small amount of intrinsic factor is required for normal B_{12} absorption, most patients with diseases that reduce the number of parietal cells still secrete suffi-

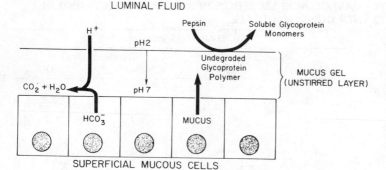

Figure 15. Model for surface neutralization of H^+ by HCO_3^- within unstirred layer of gastric mucous gel. HCO_3^- secretion into gel by superficial mucous cells would keep pH near mucosal surface alkaline. Undegraded mucous glycoprotein polymer is continuously secreted into mucous gel by superficial mucous cells, and gel is continuously solubilized by luminal pepsin. (Modified from Allen, A., and Garner, A.: Gut 21:249, 1980.)

cient intrinsic factor so that they do not become B_{12} deficient. Intrinsic factor and B_{12} absorption are discussed further under Nutrition and Hematology.

GASTRIC MOTILITY AND EMPTYING

The accommodation of a food bolus and the emptying of the meal into the duodenum are functions of gastric motility. The proximal stomach (the fundus and proximal corpus) relaxes to accommodate the meal bolus and maintains a tonic pressure of 10 to 30 cm H_2O to control the emptying of liquids. The distal corpus and antrum, including the pylorus, grind solid food into small particles and essentially determine the emptying rate of these particles.

Postprandial or Digestive Cycle

When food is swallowed, the muscles in the proximal corpus and fundus relax, reducing the intragastic pressure. This phenomenon is called *receptive relaxation* and is mediated at least partially through the vagus. In addition, the proximal stomach does not increase intragastric pressure as the volume of food increases. This characteristic is called *accommodation* and can be demonstrated by placing a balloon in the stomach and infusing increasing volumes into the balloon. As the volume goes from 0 to 300 ml the intragastric

pressure increases from 0 to 10 cm of water. When volume is increased from 300 to 600 or 800 ml there is virtually no change in pressure. This ability to accommodate a meal is a function of the proximal stomach only and is mediated at least in part through the vagus nerve. Thus, resection of the proximal stomach—that is, fundectomy—or section of the vagi will reduce the storage capacity of the proximal stomach. The antrum does not participate in the relaxation and accommodation of food.

The distal stomach (antrum and distal corpus) has characteristic peristaltic contractions. These contractions begin from a point in the middle of the greater curvature, called the gastric pacemaker, and proceed distally, becoming stronger as they reach the pylorus. As the contractions near the pylorus, the pylorus also closes. Solid food particles are moved along by these contractions. However, when they reach the closed pylorus, the solids are consequently squeezed between the peristaltic waves and the pylorus and then repulsed more proximally. This process is called *propulsion* and *retropulsion* and results in reducing particles to a size of 0.5 mm to 1.0 mm before they are passed into the duodenum (Fig. 16). Particles that cannot be broken down to such sizes are not emptied during the normal digestive cycle but instead are emptied during phase III contractions of the fasting cycle.

The emptying of liquids is determined by the pressure gradient across the pylorus. The proximal stomach

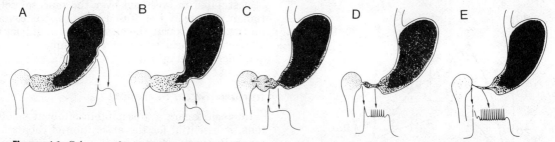

Figure 16. Schema of gastric processing and emptying of solid food. Intracellular electrical potentials, gastric contractions, and the effects of contraction on gastric contents are diagrammed. In Panel A, solid food fills the proximal stomach and corpus. Gastric peristalsis begins with gentle contractions of the corpus. Paced by the electrical slow wave, the wave of contraction travels distally, compressing and kneading the solid food and breaking off small pieces (Panel B). These pieces are propelled into the antrum by progressively stronger waves, and small particles of food are accelerated through the still open pylorus by the force of contraction (Panel C). Antral contraction proceeds, and food is squirted through the narrowing pylorus and through the central orifice of the contraction wave (Panel D). The pylorus closes during the terminal antral contraction (Panel E), and all material is forced back to the corpus. Another wave then starts in the corpus, and the cycle is repeated. This pattern of activity results in the mixing and grinding of solid food and in the selective passage of small food particles into the duodenum. (From Sleisenger, M. H., and Fordtran, J. S. (eds.): Gastrointestinal Disease. 3rd ed. Philadelphia, W. B. Saunders Co., 1983.)

determines the intragastric pressure and therefore the emptying rate of liquids. In contrast, the antrum and pylorus primarily determine the emptying rate of solids. Liquids empty more rapidly than solids. Ninety per cent of liquids will have left the stomach within one hour while three hours are required to empty 80 per cent of solids.

Several factors influence the rate of gastric emptying. Increased volume and gastric distention increase the emptying rate. Meals of high osmolarity and high nutrient content decrease the rate of gastric emptying, as does acid in the duodenum. Nutrients and osmolarity probably act on receptor cells in the duodenum and jejunum. These receptor cells in turn either liberate hormones or initiate a neural reflex that slows gastric emptying. Several peptide hormones such as gastrin, CCK, secretin, VIP, and gastric inhibitory peptide (GIP) affect gastric emptying when infused intravenously. These hormones could be released by cells in the duodenum and jejunum; however, it is not known if their action is physiologically important.

Fasting Cycle

During fasting there is a cyclical pattern of contractions that occurs every 100 minutes. Each cycle is divided into four phases (I, II, III, and IV). Phase I is a 60-minute period with virtually no peristalsis followed by phase II, lasting 15 minutes and with sporadic contractions. Phase III has forceful, coordinated contractions that begin in the stomach and move to the ileum. The pylorus is open during phase III contractions and undigested solids are cleared from the stomach. Phase IV is similar to phase II. The primary event occurring in the fasting cycle is the clearance of large undigested particles from the stomach.

Gastric emptying normally occurs in an orderly, predictable fashion. The meal enters the stomach already mixed with salivary amylase and is mixed with pepsin and acid. Protein and carbohydrate digestion begins. The solid food is "ground" into particles in the antrum. The meal is then emptied into the duodenum in an orderly fashion over several hours with most particulate matter no larger than 5 mm. Any indigestible large particulate matter will be emptied during phase III of the interdigestive complex.

The pathophysiology of the stomach can be divided into motility and secretory disorders.

MOTILITY DISORDERS

In patients who have not had previous gastric surgery, most motility disorders result in delayed gastric emptying. The abnormality may be mild and produce only vague symptoms of postprandial bloating or fullness, or more severe and cause nausea, vomiting, and weight loss. Delayed gastric emptying without a mechanical cause is called *gastroparesis* and may have several causes that involve the ENS or smooth muscle (Table 8). Opiate analgesics such as morphine, codeine, and meperidine cause gastric stasis, nausea, and vomiting by acting both through the CNS and peripherally. Several disorders of the muscular system, including myotonic dystrophy and muscular dystrophy, can also produce gastric stasis. Gastroparesis is probably most commonly seen in the patients with diabetic neurop-

TABLE 8. CONDITIONS ASSOCIATED WITH GASTROPARESIS

1. **METABOLIC**
   Hyperglycemia, hypokalemia, hypocalcemia, ketoacidosis, myxedema
2. **NEUROLOGIC**
   Brain tumors, diabetic neuropathy, tabes dorsalis
3. **DRUGS**
   Opiates, anticholinergics, ganglionic blockers
4. **DISEASES OF THE STOMACH**
   Atrophic gastritis, peptic ulcer, outlet obstruction

athy and familial autonomic nervous dysfunction. The emptying of solids is usually affected to a greater degree than liquids, and it is often necessary to perform gastric emptying studies of solid meals to confirm the diagnosis of gastroparesis.

Patients with diabetic gastroparesis have a marked reduction in gastric motor activity with absence of interdigestive motor complexes. The decrease in postprandial motor activity causes incomplete "grinding" or "sieving" of solids to the size required for passage through the pylorus and the absence of interdigestive motor complexes means that any indigestible debris or large particles will not be emptied between meals. This combination results in slow emptying of solids and in the accumulation of food debris in the stomach (*bezoars*). Diabetic gastroparesis is probably caused by neural dysfunction. Dopamine antagonists (metoclopramide, domperidone) and cholinergic agents (bethanechol) can restore gastric muscular contractility and alleviate the symptoms somewhat. However, if gastroparesis is caused by a muscular disorder—for example, scleroderma or aganglionosis—dopamine antagonists or cholinergic agents are of little benefit. In severe cases of gastroparesis unresponsive to medications, surgical removal of the antrum may be effective. Idiopathic gastroparesis may rarely develop in otherwise healthy individuals.

DELAYED GASTRIC EMPTYING SECONDARY TO MECHANICAL OBSTRUCTION

Congenital Abnormalities Causing Obstruction

Congenital hypertrophic pyloric stenosis, caused by hypertrophy of the pyloric sphincter that produces an obstruction at the gastric outlet, can be used as a prototype of this group of disorders. Onset of symptoms usually occurs three to four weeks after birth, but on rare occasions symptoms may be minimal initially and clinically manifested only later, in early or even middle adulthood. The disorder is four times more common in males than females. Although the cause is unknown, it may be the result of excessive pyloric contractions prenatally, resulting in muscle hypertrophy and narrowing of the outlet. The main symptom—severe, projectile vomiting—may be initially sporadic but soon becomes continuous. Since the gastric outlet is obstructed, the emesis is free of bile. Because very little or no food passes into the intestine, the infant fails to gain weight and to thrive. The metabolic effects are those of prolonged vomiting, dehydration, sodium and chloride loss, and metabolic alkalosis. The consequences of vomiting are discussed later in this section.

Patients with *congenital volvulus of the stomach* may also have intractable vomiting, particularly after meals. In this instance the obstruction is usually due to a rotation along the longitudinal axis of the stomach. Food cannot enter the stomach because of obstruction at the esophagogastric junction; consequently the patients vomit ingested food that cannot enter the stomach.

Other congenital disorders that may cause delayed gastric emptying secondary to obstruction include:

(1) *congenital duodenal obstruction,* which may be caused by duodenal atresia, stenosis, the presence of a membranous ring in the duodenum, extrinsic compression by congenital peritoneal bands, or a duplication of the duodenum. Both atresia and stenosis commonly occur distal to the duodenal papilla, so that the vomitus, as opposed to that from pyloric obstruction or volvulus of the stomach, is bilious in most instances.

(2) *Annular pancreas* represents the anomalous presence of a ring of pancreatic tissue in the second portion of the duodenum. This results from failure of one of the buds of the embryonic ventral pancreas to degenerate, such that it continues to grow around the right side of the duodenum to join the other two parts of the pancreas, constituting a ring or an extrinsic obstructive band.

(3) *Malrotation of the intestine* may be associated with external compression by bands of mesentery crossing over the duodenum or with a hypertrophied hepatoduodenal ligament (Fig. 17). In these cases vomiting usually begins one or two days after birth, but

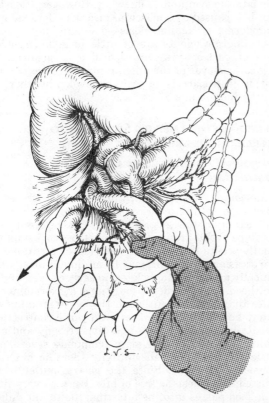

Figure 17. Malrotation of the intestine and a hypertrophied hepatoduodenal ligament causing duodenal obstruction. (Reproduced with permission from Way, L. W. (ed.): Current Surgical Diagnosis and Treatment. 6th ed. Los Altos, CA, Lange Medical Publications, 1983.)

rarely after several months of age. If obstruction is unrelieved, duodenal dilatation, perforation, and peritonitis will follow.

Acquired Gastric Outlet Obstruction

In adults without previous gastric surgery, gastric obstruction is usually caused by ulcer or tumor. These patients present with early satiety, nausea, vomiting of food without bile, and weight loss. Their symptoms may develop acutely or over several weeks to months. The diagnosis is usually made by a roentgenographic barium contrast study of the stomach that demonstrates the obstruction. The treatment is surgical resection of the obstruction (antrectomy) or bypass (gastrojejunostomy). If the obstruction is secondary to peptic ulcer, an operation that reduces gastric acid secretion (vagotomy or antrectomy and vagotomy) should also be performed.

Consequences of Delayed Gastric Emptying and Vomiting

In mild forms patients will complain of early satiety, postprandial bloating, belching, and occasional nausea. They may consume less to avoid these symptoms and may lose weight. They may also modify the diet to avoid high-residue foods that do not empty well.

In more severe cases the same symptoms will be present but nausea and vomiting will be frequent. If gastric outlet obstruction is nearly complete, patients will regurgitate more than they consume and consequently will become dehydrated. Gastric juice contains about 50 mM H^+, 50 to 70 mM Na^+ and 90 to 120 mM Cl. Thus with repeated vomiting the patient will become alkalotic, hyponatremic, and hypochloremic. The kidneys will retain Na^+ and water and will consequently secrete K^+ and H^+ in the urine to neutralize excess HCO_3^-. This augments the alkalosis and also produces hypokalemia. The consequences of severe dehydration and hypokalemia are discussed in detail in Section X.

When correcting dehydration, metabolic alkalosis and hypokalemia secondary to gastric outlet obstruction, one must replace the sodium or the kidneys will continue to secrete K^+ and H^+ to neutralize HCO_3^- and the alkalosis and hypokalemia will be difficult if not impossible to correct.

If gastric dilatation occurs suddenly it can cause cardiac arrhythmias, mainly bradycardia. If the stomach becomes chronically dilated it can reach volumes as large as 10 liters, and therefore distend the abdomen sufficiently to interfere with breathing.

MOTILITY AFTER GASTRIC SURGERY

Most operations for peptic ulcer involve section of the vagus nerve and a bypass or division of the pyloric sphincter (pyloroplasty). Severing of the vagus nerve has two adverse physiologic consequences: (1) It destroys the phenomenon of receptive accommodation so that the stomach cannot relax and stretch to accommodate food as effectively. (2) It also results in a relative paralysis and discoordination of the antral muscles that delays the emptying of solids. On reception of a meal, intragastric pressure increases more rapidly than normal, and as a result liquids empty much more rapidly than normal. The disruption of the pylorus reduces pyloric sphincter pressure and increases the emptying rate of both solids and liquids. Therefore, following vagotomy and bypass or pyloroplasty, liquids empty more rapidly. Solids may empty rapidly, normally, or more slowly depending on the balance among the antral dysmotility, absent pyloric pressure, and increased intragastric pressure. Proximal gastric vagotomy denervates only the fundus and body of the stomach and leaves the pylorus intact and the antrum innervated. After this operation, emptying of liquids is more rapid presumably because of loss of receptive accommodation; however, emptying of solids is normal because the antrum and pylorus function normally (Fig. 18).

If the gastric emptying of solids and liquids is extremely rapid, a condition called the *dumping syndrome* may result. The symptoms of the syndrome are flushing, diaphoresis, lightheadedness, cramping abdominal pain, and diarrhea, which occur about 30 minutes postprandially. The symptoms may be mild or so severe that the patient does not want to eat for fear of provoking them. Symptoms are most easily produced by liquid meals with a high carbohydrate content. The cause of the dumping syndrome is the rapid emptying of a large volume of hyperosmolar solution into the small intestine. This solution releases several vasoactive substances (serotonin, bradykinin) from the intestine that may be the cause of flushing and hypotension. The hyperosmolar solution also produces the cramping and diarrhea. Dumping is most often successfully treated by altering patients' eating habits so that they consume smaller, low carbohydrate and low osmolality meals with minimal liquids. Occasionally, dumping is unresponsive to dietary manipulations and requires an operative procedure to delay gastric emptying.

Delayed gastric emptying after surgery is usually mild and does not produce symptoms. If delayed emptying is severe, an obstruction to the gastric outlet

should be excluded. These patients are usually not responsive to bethanechol or metoclopramide.

NAUSEA AND VOMITING

Definition

Vomiting is the rapid evacuation of gastric contents in retrograde fashion from stomach through the mouth. The feeling of nausea, which usually precedes vomiting, is a most unpleasant sensation that is associated with diminished gastric motor activity, increased pressure in the duodenum, and reflux of duodenal contents into the stomach. *Retching* accompanies vomiting and consists of spasmodic respiratory movements opposed by expiratory contractions of the abdominal muscles. The glottis and distal end of the stomach are closed and the proximal end of the stomach is open. Retching increases with abdominal pressure and pushes the cardia into the mediastinum. Because the pressure surrounding the cardia is less in the mediastinum than in the abdomen the cardia becomes patent to reflux of gastric contents. Vomiting itself is the forceful and sustained contraction of the abdominal muscles with the cardia of the stomach open and the pylorus contracted. The cardia of the stomach is raised into the mediastinum, overcoming the possible resistance of the gastroesophageal sphincter to retropulsion of material from stomach through esophagus, pharynx, and mouth.

Mechanism of Vomiting

Vomiting is under central nervous system control. Bilateral vomiting centers exist in the dorsal portions of the lateral reticular formation of the medulla. These centers are activated by so-called chemoreceptor trigger zones (CTZ) (Fig. 19). Vagal afferents also may stimulate the vomiting centers, bypassing the chemoreceptor trigger zones.

The principal pathway for nausea and vomiting caused by drugs is via stimulation of the chemoreceptor trigger zones; this pathway also mediates the nausea and vomiting of motion sickness, uremia, diabetic ketoacidosis, and general anesthetics.

Additional stimuli of the vagal afferents that pass directly to the vomiting center include (1) distention of the smooth muscle of the gut, particularly when vomiting is sudden; (2) substances noxious to the mucosa of the stomach, such as copper sulfate, mustard, and ethanol in large volumes; and (3) irritation and inflammation of the peritoneum. Thus a large number of diseases and disorders that affect the intestine, bile ducts, ureters, and peritoneum are associated with nausea and vomiting. Hence, the symptom complex often is nonspecific and not helpful in differential diagnosis of intra-abdominal disorders. Also, there are obvious pathways to the vomiting center that are stimulated by noxious smells and tastes; however, the location of the supramedullary receptors that are involved is not known.

Types of Vomiting

Important features of vomiting are its amount, duration, content, and timing in relationship to meals.

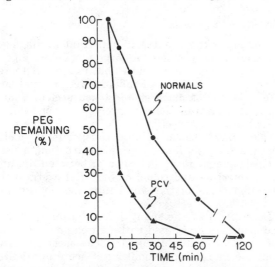

Figure 18. Polyethylene glycol (PEG) meal marker remaining in the stomach after infusion of a 700 ml amino acid meal in ten normal subjects and in eight patients after parietal cell vagotomy (PCV). Early gastric emptying is extremely rapid in patients after vagotomy because of loss of gastric accommodation. (From Sleisenger, M. H., and Fordtran, J. S. (eds.): Gastrointestinal Disease. 3rd ed. Philadelphia, W. B. Saunders Co., 1983.)

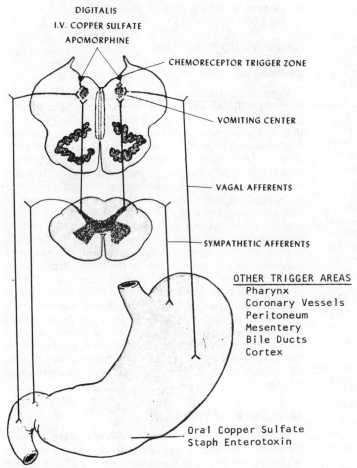

MOTION SICKNESS
DIGITALIS
I.V. COPPER SULFATE
APOMORPHINE

CHEMORECEPTOR TRIGGER ZONE

VOMITING CENTER

VAGAL AFFERENTS

SYMPATHETIC AFFERENTS

OTHER TRIGGER AREAS
Pharynx
Coronary Vessels
Peritoneum
Mesentery
Bile Ducts
Cortex

Oral Copper Sulfate
Staph Enterotoxin

Figure 19. The interrelation of the vomiting center, the chemoreceptor trigger zone, and peripheral trigger areas. (Modified from Wang, S. C., and Borison, H. L.: Gastroenterology 2:1 1952.)

These factors often characterize a particular category of underlying disease. The following general statements regarding them may be made.

Timing in Relationship to Meals

When a patient vomits during or immediately after a meal, it is more likely to be psychogenic, although such vomiting, particularly after a heavy meal, may be caused by edema and spasm of the pylorus associated with a pyloric canal ulcer. Persistent vomiting an hour or more after a meal is more compatible with gastric outlet obstruction, acute pancreatitis, or a motility disorder of the stomach (diabetic neuropathy, postvagotomy). Vomiting of material eaten many hours previously also fits in the category of organic obstruction. Often patients with chronic outlet obstruction will have large, dilated stomachs and on examination will be noted to have a *succussion splash*. This sign is important in distinguishing psychogenic from organic obstruction in patients with chronic vomiting. Alcoholics, pregnant women, and uremics have nausea and vomiting early in the morning on arising. Some patients with increased intracranial pressure may have vomiting unassociated with meals or nausea. The majority of patients who present with an initial episode of vomiting usually have a viral gastroenteritis or bacterial food poisoning and their illness is self limiting.

Quality of Vomitus

Content of the vomitus is important in diagnosing the underlying problem. A large amount of ingested food suggests a gastric outlet obstruction; if there is blood in the vomitus, an inflammatory or malignant disease of the stomach should be suspected. Vomitus with bile indicates that the problem is not pyloric or gastric outlet obstruction.

Odor may also be helpful; thus, a fecal smell to vomitus suggests low intestinal obstruction, a fistula between the stomach and colon or between the upper small intestine and colon, or bacterial overgrowth of the stomach or of the small intestine (longstanding obstruction).

Description of the many intra-abdominal diseases and disorders associated with nausea and vomiting is not possible in this discussion. The spectrum ranges from the nausea and vomiting of acute appendicitis, which follows the onset of epigastric pain, to the feculent vomiting of far-advanced colonic obstruction in an elderly individual. Nausea and vomiting that follow recent onset of persisting abdominal pain indicate an abdominal illness that often requires hospitalization, and, in some cases, surgery.

TABLE 9. CAUSES OF NAUSEA AND VOMITING

1. Direct gastric or intestinal irritation
   Gastroenteritis, gastritis

2. Intestinal obstruction
   Gastric outlet obstruction, small bowel obstruction

3. Inflammation within the abdominal cavity
   Appendicitis, cholecystitis, intra-abdominal abscess

4. Motility disturbances
   Gastroparesis

5. Drugs
   Opiate analgesics, anticancer drugs

6. Hormonal changes
   Pregnancy

7. Neurologic
   Psychogenic, increased intracranial pressure

The different causes of nausea and vomiting are summarized in Table 9.

Drug Therapy of Nausea and Vomiting

Nausea and vomiting result from a stimulus to the vomiting center by impulses from afferent pathways of the gut, from the chemoreceptor trigger zones that have been activated by circulating substances, or from neural pathways in other parts of the brain, in particular the vestibular apparatus. Hence drugs are used that affect or interrupt these pathways, or depress either the chemoreceptor zone or the vomiting center itself. Chlorpromazine (a phenothiazine), dimenhydrinate, cyclizine, and meclizine all depress the vomiting center; trimethobenzamide acts on the chemoreceptor trigger zone. Antihistamines depress the vestibular mechanism and therefore may be effective for nausea and vomiting of motion sickness and of pregnancy. Phenothiazines are used effectively for nausea caused by drugs, radiation, and surgery. For the control of the nausea and vomiting of radiation and chemotherapy for cancer, delta-9 tetrahydrocannabinol, a component of marijuana, is said to be effective when taken by mouth. However, early positive reports are unconfirmed. Metoclopramide suppresses the chemoreceptor trigger zone and peripheral receptors of the gastrointestinal tract and may be effective in treatment of nausea and vomiting in many different clinical states.

MUCOSAL DISEASE

The most common diseases involving gastric mucosa are peptic ulcers (gastric and duodenal), gastritis, and gastric cancer. Abnormalities in gastric acid and pepsin secretion or mucus secretion accompany these diseases in most instances. When considering the pathophysiology of the gastric mucosa, one should understand the concept of the gastric mucosal barrier and the meaning of gastritis. The principal abnormalities seen in gastroduodenal mucosa that produce symptoms are peptic ulcers and tumors, and both of these entities are related to gastritis or defects in the gastric mucosal barrier.

GASTRIC MUCOSAL BARRIER

Although the stomach secretes acid and pepsin in high concentrations, it does not usually undergo autodigestion. The ability of the gastric mucosa to withstand gastric juice is attributed to the impermeability of the apices of the mucosal cells and the tight junctions between the cells. This phenomenon is called the *gastric mucosal barrier*. If hydrogen ion diffuses back across the mucosa, it is said that the gastric mucosal barrier is damaged or broken. When the barrier is damaged, the mucosal potential difference decreases. Normally the mucosal cell is negatively charged with respect to the lumen. Several drugs or chemicals such as topical aspirin, alcohol, bile salts, and several types of detergents damage the mucosal barrier. Disorders that reduce mucosal blood flow, such as hemorrhage and shock, will also damage the mucosal barrier. The concept of the mucosal barrier is pertinent because it allows assessment of the integrity of the mucosa. If back diffusion of H^+ is occurring, the gastric mucosal barrier is damaged and the mucosa is damaged and susceptible to autodigestion and ulcer formation.

Clinically, the gastric mucosal barrier is thought to be acutely damaged in patients who are severely stressed by such conditions as shock, sepsis, burns, CNS injury, and chronically damaged in patients with gastritis and in those taking aspirin and other nonsteroidal antiinflammatory agents. All of these patients are prone to develop gastric ulcers.

Gastritis

Gastritis encompasses many entities and can be divided into several categories. *Specific gastritis* has distinctive histologic features and is associated with a specific disease process—that is, sarcoidosis, eosinophilic gastritis, and hypertrophic gastropathies—and will be discussed at the end of this section. The vast majority of gastritis is nonspecific—that is, neither the gross nor microscopic appearance is specific for the etiology.

Nonspecific Gastritis. This group of disorders may be either erosive or nonerosive. In *erosive gastritis* there are mucosal defects that do not extend beyond the muscularis mucosa. The defects are most often small (0.5 to 2.0 mm) and multiple, and they often bleed. This type of gastritis is most often seen in patients under severe physical stress—for example, after severe trauma, in sepsis, and after burns. The gross appearance is that of numerous punctate or linear areas of denuded epithelium and hemorrhage. Light microscopy may show only trivial inflammation. The most striking histologic finding is mucosal cell loss seen with the scanning election microscope.

Nonspecific nonerosive gastritis, which may occur anywhere in the stomach, is the most common type of gastritis. It may be divided into three histologic patterns: superficial gastritis, atrophic gastritis, and gastric atrophy. *Superficial gastritis* connotes inflammation that is limited to the area of the pits only but without involving the glands (Fig. 20A). The pit cells may become anaplastic, becoming more cuboidal and with mitotic figures more prominent. There is also evidence that these cells secrete less mucus. *Atrophic gastritis* occurs when the inflammatory cells extend

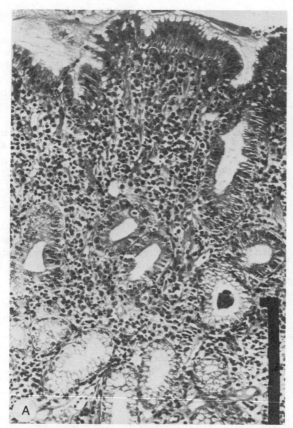

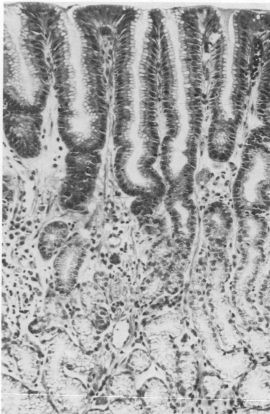

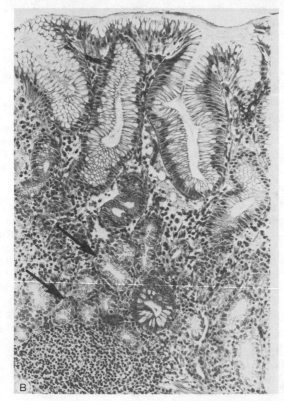

Figure 20. *A,* Superficial antral gland gastritis. The lamina propria inflammatory cells are concentrated in the upper half of the mucosa. The antral glands (bracketed zone) are intact. Compare with adjacent section which shows normal antral gland mucosa. Hematoxylin and eosin stain, ×120. *B,* Atrophy of the fundic gland mucosa. Biopsy from the midbody greater curvature in an achlorhydric patient. The surface epithelium and the pits are normal. There is only a minimal increase in the number of lamina propria inflammatory cells. The normal fundic gland elements (parietal and chief cells) are absent. There is pseudopyloric metaplasia as evidenced by the clear-staining mucous type glands (arrows). A lymphoid aggregate lies deep in the mucosa (lower left). Hematoxylin and eosin stain, ×120. (From Sleisenger, M. H., and Fordtran, J. S. (eds.): Gastrointestinal Disease. 3rd ed. Philadelphia, W. B. Saunders Co., 1983.)

more deeply to involve and destroy glands, leading to relative hyposecretion of gastric acid. In *gastric atrophy,* parietal and chief cells are significantly reduced in the fundic and body glands but no inflammation is seen (Fig. 20*B*).

Two other histologic features may be seen in all forms of nonspecific nonerosive gastritis: (1) *Intestinal metaplasia* occurs when the mucosal cells assume the appearance of intestinal goblet cells. The process is usually patchy, but when it is extensive with loss of gastric glands, the resultant mucosa can be indistinguishable from that of the small intestine (Fig. 21). (2) *Antralization* of the proximal stomach occurs when normal fundal and body glands are replaced by the clear-staining mucous glands that look like antral glands.

Nonspecific nonerosive gastritis occurs in up to 50 per cent of people over 40 years of age, especially in the antrum. This disease is more prevalent and severe in areas where gastric cancer and gastric ulcer are also more common. Patients with nonspecific nonerosive gastritis are most often asymptomatic. Gastritis is seen with virtually all gastric ulcers and usually persists after the ulcer heals. This suggests that the gastritis either predisposes to gastric ulcer formation or is caused by the same process that causes the gastric ulcer. Gastritis often develops after surgery for peptic ulcer, presumably because bile acids reflux into the stomach and the gastric pH is elevated.

Severe gastric atrophy will produce *pernicious anemia* when insufficient parietal cells are left to secrete enough intrinsic factor for adequate vitamin B_{12} absorption. Pernicious anemia, a megaloblastic anemia that is secondary to vitamin B_{12} absorption, appears to be an autoimmune disease with 90 per cent of the patients having antibodies to gastric parietal cells and 60 per cent having antibodies to intrinsic factor. People with pernicious anemia have an increased incidence of gastric cancer, about three times that of a comparable population without pernicious anemia.

Specific Gastritis. Characteristic lesions may form in the stomach in certain systemic illnesses such as sarcoidosis or may be part of an illness localized in the gastrointestinal tract as in eosinophilic gastroenteritis or Menetrier's disease. In sarcoidosis involvement of the gastrointestinal tract is rare, but when it occurs the stomach is often involved. Essentially the findings are microscopic noncaseating granulomas in a normal-appearing gastric mucosa. When granulomas are seen, it is important to rule out other causes such as tuberculosis.

In *eosinophilic gastritis* all layers of the stomach may be infiltrated by eosinophils. Extensive mucosal infiltration can cause ulceration and involvement of the muscle layers and can cause delayed gastric emptying or even gastric outlet obstruction in severe cases. The etiology is unknown.

Menetrier's disease is characterized by enlargement of the mucosal folds, particularly in the fundic area. When this rare disease is extensive, there is a reduction in the number of parietal and chief cells with replacement by mucus glands. Gastric acid output is decreased and plasma proteins are lost from the mucosa. The diagnosis is made by a barium contrast upper gastrointestinal roentgenographic study that demonstrates large rugal folds. Most patients require no

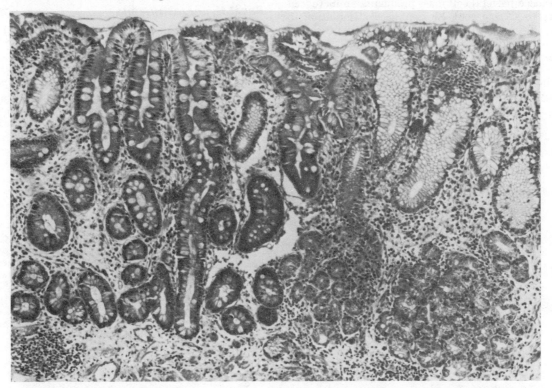

Figure 21. Intestinal metaplasia of the fundic gland zone. The left half of the biopsy shows full-thickness mucosal intestinal metaplasia with rudimentary villi and numerous goblet cells. Hematoxylin and eosin stain, ×75. (From Sleisenger, M. H., and Fordtran, J. S. (eds.): Gastrointestinal Disease. 3rd ed. Philadelphia, W. B. Saunders Co., 1983.)

treatment. Partial gastric resection is sometimes required when protein loss is severe. The risk of gastric cancer may be increased in patients with Menetrier's disease, but this is unclear.

PEPTIC ULCER

Definition. Peptic ulcers are lesions in the mucosa of the duodenum or stomach that have been caused by and become vulnerable to digestion by acid and pepsin. This leaves an area denuded of mucosa and further susceptible to digestion. Ulcers most often occur at the junction between the body and antrum of the stomach on the antral or nonacid-secreting side, and 1 cm proximal or distal to the pylorus. Ulcers within 1 cm proximal to the pylorus are called prepyloric ulcers. Ulcers occurring more proximally in the stomach are called gastric ulcers.

Pathogenesis. Chronic nonspecific nonerosive gastritis and hyposecretion of acid are commonly found with gastric ulcers. Acid and pepsin are major causative agents for ulcers; any surgical procedure that reduces acid secretion (vagotomy, antrectomy) or drugs that reduce or neutralize acid (antacids, H-2 receptor antagonists) promote ulcer healing.

Patients with duodenal and prepyloric ulcers tend to secrete more acid and pepsin than do normal subjects, basally and in response to any stimulus (Table 7, Fig. 22). However, there is an overlap between normal individuals and patients with duodenal ulcer, so that some patients will have normal acid secretion. Four factors might cause these patients to be hypersecretors: (1) increased parietal cell mass producing an increased capacity to secrete acid, (2) increased stimulation to secrete, (3) increased sensitivity of the parietal cell to a normal stimulus, and (4) decreased inhibition of acid secretion and gastrin release.

Increased Parietal Cell Mass. Patients with duodenal ulcers have on the average about 1.5 to 2.0 times as many parietal cells as do normal subjects. These figures are deduced from estimates of the number of parietal cells histologically and from maximal acid secretory capacity (pentagastrin or betazole stimulation), which is a reflection of parietal cell mass.

Increased Stimulation of Secretion. Patients with duodenal ulcer have a higher basal acid secretion than normal and a higher basal in relation to maximal acid secretion. This suggests that there is excessive stimulation of acid secretion. There is ample evidence that excitation of the vagus nerve produces acid secretion and that section of this nerve reduces acid secretion. There is, however, no evidence that patients with duodenal ulcer have excessive "vagal tone." The cause of this increased "basal tone" of gastric stimulation in patients with duodenal ulcer is unknown.

Increased Sensitivity of the Parietal Cell. The parietal cell in patients with duodenal ulcer is more sensitive to pentagastrin. That is, less pentagastrin is required to produce half maximal stimulation of acid secretion (Fig. 23). This increased sensitivity to gastrin may reflect increased vagal tone or relative deficiencies in inhibitory factors.

Decreased Inhibition of Acid Secretion and Gastrin Release. Gastrin is a major stimulant of gastric acid secretion. Basal gastrin is normal in patients with duodenal ulcer, and the antrum contains normal amounts of gastrin. However, in patients with duodenal ulcer, gastrin release following a meal is more pronounced and the serum gastrin stays elevated for a longer period of time even though these patients are secreting excessive amounts of acid. This suggests that these patients may have a defect in the inhibition of gastrin release by antral acidification (Fig. 24).

Basal Hypergastrinemia

There are seven uncommon causes of basal hypergastrinemia associated with duodenal ulcer: *gastrinoma, hypercalcemia, massive small bowel resection, renal failure, gastric outlet obstruction, antral G cell hyperplasia, and antral exclusion.* In the evaluation of a patient with severe, intractable, or recurrent duodenal ulcer, gastrin levels should be measured. If

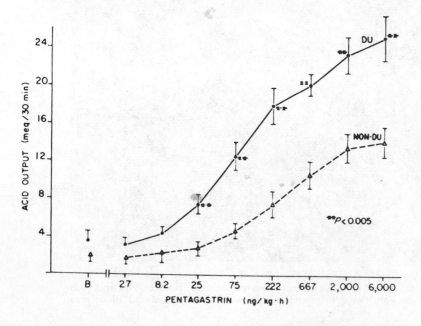

Figure 22. Mean acid output in 20 duodenal ulcer patients and 20 nonulcer subjects during infusion of graded doses of pentagastrin. The data represent the mean ± SE. (From Isenberg, J. I., et al.: J Clin Invest 55:330, 1975.)

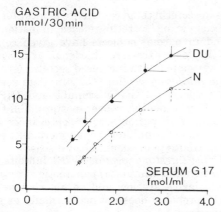

GASTRIC ACID
mmol/30 min

SERUM G 17
fmol/ml

Figure 23. Comparison of the relationship between mean serum heptadecapeptide gastrin (G17) and mean gastric acid output after graded peptone meals in duodenal ulcer (DU) and normal (N) subjects. The horizontal and vertical bars represent 1 SE. For each incremental change in serum gastrin, gastric acid secretion was greater in DU patients than in normal subjects. (From Lam, S. K., Isenberg, J. I., and Grossman, M. I.: J Clin Invest 65:555, 1980.)

hypergastrinemia is present, these conditions should be considered.

Gastrinoma is a tumor that releases large amounts of gastrin resulting in excessive acid secretion and severe ulcer disease. Reduction of acid secretion can often be accomplished with H-2 receptor antagonists (cimetidine, ranitidine) and with selective anticholinergics (pirenzepine). The tumor should be resected if feasible, but this is possible in only 10 per cent of

patients. When tumor resection and pharmacologic agents fail to control hyperacidity, total gastrectomy will abolish acid secretion and is reasonably well tolerated by these patients.

Hypercalcemia stimulates increased secretion of gastrin and gastric acid. In patients with hyperparathyroidism, removal of a parathyroid adenoma with return of the serum calcium level to normal usually also allows the serum gastrin and gastric acid secretion to become normal. However, the relationship between hypercalcemia and duodenal ulcer disease is by no means constant. In general, if severe duodenal ulcer disease is present in a patient with hyperparathyroidism, the cause is more likely to be gastrinoma (as part of so-called multiple endocrine neoplasia [MEA] type I) than it is to be a direct effect of hypercalcemia. This syndrome is described in Section VIII.

Extensive small bowel resection is often associated with hypergastrinemia and increased gastric acidity, most likely from loss of an enterogastrone—a hormone from the intestine that inhibits gastrin release and gastric acid secretion. This increased acid secretion usually subsides within a few months, so that treatment with H-2 receptor antagonists is usually sufficient.

Renal failure may be accompanied by hypergastrinemia and gastric hyperacidity, probably because of decreased catabolism of the large molecular forms of gastrin by the diseased kidneys. Treatment consists of antacids and H-2 blocking agents.

Gastric outlet obstruction results in antral distention with presumed secondary increase of gastrin secretion. Decompression of the stomach with a nasogastric tube

Figure 24. Acid secretory rates and serum gastrin in response to an amino acid-cornstarch meal in patients with duodenal ulcer. Acid secretion was measured using intragastric titration at a pH of 5.5 (left) and 2.5 (right). *Top panels:* Acid secretory rates have been normalized as the percentage of the maximal secretion in response to histamine for duodenal ulcer patients (DU) and normal subjects. * = p<0.05. *Bottom panels:* Serum gastrin concentrations in the same normal and DU subjects in the fasting state and at 30-minute intervals after the meal. (From Walsh, J. H., Richardson, C. T., and Fordtran, J. S.: J Clin Invest 55:462, 1975.)

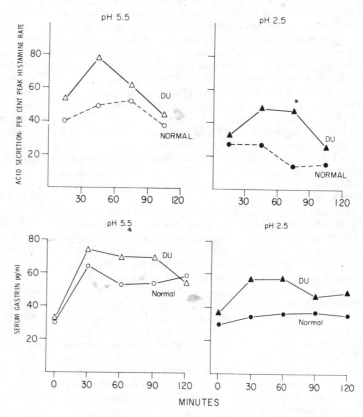

usually results in a return of the gastrin levels to normal.

Antral G cell hyperplasia, a condition of unknown etiology, results in functional hyperactivity of the antral G cells. This condition is even rarer than hypergastrinemia from gastrinoma. Treatment consists of H-2 blocking agents or antrectomy.

The *excluded antrum syndrome* describes the condition after distal gastrectomy when some antrum is left attached to the duodenal stump. This remnant will now be excluded from the acid produced by the stomach because intestinal continuity is reestablished with a gastrojejunostomy. This excluded antrum will occasionally produce excessive amounts of gastrin, probably because of the absence of acid inhibition. The excess amount of gastrin can produce a syndrome similar to that seen with gastrinoma. It is extremely rare to see the retained antrum syndrome now because removal of all the antrum at surgery is relatively simple.

Effects of Other Hormones and Agents on Acid Secretion

Several substances other than gastrin either stimulate or inhibit acid secretion. Their possible roles in duodenal ulcer and acid hypersecretion will be reviewed here.

Histamine, a potent gastric secretagogue, is present in gastric mucosa and almost certainly acts locally to stimulate acid secretion. Parietal cells respond to histamine in a dose-related manner. However, there is no evidence that patients with duodenal ulcer have excessive amounts of gastric histamine in the gastric mucosa.

Acetylcholine potentiates the effect of gastrin and of histamine on acid secretion. The vagus is primarily a cholinergic nerve and secretion of the vagus reduces acid secretion. This reduction can be partially reversed by giving intravenous cholinergic agents. It may be that patients with duodenal ulcer hypersecrete acid because of excessive vagal tone but this is not proved.

Bombesin releases gastrin probably by acting directly on the G cell. Bombesin-like immunoreactivity (BLI) is present in the antral mucosa and may serve as a physiologic stimulus for gastrin release. Bombesin release is not inhibited by antral acidification. Theoretically, excess bombesin could produce the exaggerated gastrin response to a meal and the diminished inhibition of gastrin release by acid that characterize duodenal ulcer disease.

Cholecystokinin (CCK) is a weak agonist of acid secretion and probably does not act to stimulate acid secretion. It potentiates secretin-stimulated pancreatic bicarbonate secretion and delays gastric emptying. Pancreatic bicarbonate neutralizes acid in the duodenum and the rate of gastric emptying governs delivery of acid to the duodenum. Low CCK levels could therefore theoretically contribute to ulcer formation by allowing more rapid emptying of acid into the duodenum and by decreasing bicarbonate secretion.

Secretin inhibits meal-stimulated gastrin release and gastric acid secretion, but secretin is liberated in such small quantities that it would have little effect on the stomach. Secretin does, however, stimulate pancreatic bicarbonate secretion, and duodenal acidification stimulates secretin release. Although abnor-

malities in secretin could contribute to ulcer formation, studies comparing secretin release in patients with ulcer and in normal subjects have given conflicting results. In fact, excessive duodenal acidification is usually associated with increased secretin levels.

Gastric inhibitory peptide (GIP) inhibits acid secretion in response to many stimuli, and GIP levels increase after a meal. However, postprandial GIP levels are higher in patients with peptic ulcer than in controls. Thus, it is unlikely that abnormalities in GIP levels contribute to duodenal ulcer disease.

Vasoactive intestinal peptide (VIP) inhibits gastric acid secretion and stimulates pancreatic secretion, but the serum levels are low and do not change after a meal. VIP probably does not act normally as a circulating hormone.

Somatostatin inhibits gastrin release and gastric acid secretion in response to virtually all stimuli. The location of somatostatin in cells near the antral G cells suggests that it may serve as a paracrine inhibitor of gastric acid secretion. That is, somatostatin secreted locally may act to inhibit gastrin release and therefore gastric acid secretion. It is possible that decreased somatostatin activity contributes to duodenal ulcer formation, but experiments testing this possibility are preliminary and contradictory.

Patients with duodenal ulcers have on the average lower *duodenal pH's* than do normals, presumably because of a tendency for more rapid acid secretion and gastric emptying. Bicarbonate from pancreatic juice is the principal neutralizer of duodenal acid. Bicarbonate responses to graded doses of acid instilled intraduodenally are reported to be normal in patients with duodenal ulcer. There is no evidence that the duodenal mucosa is abnormal or more susceptible to acid digestion.

Mucosal Defense. One must also consider deficiencies in mucosal defenses as a possible cause of duodenal ulcers. Since many patients with duodenal ulcers do not secrete increased amounts of acid it is logical to assume that there may be some defect in mucosal defenses in the duodenum. Decreases of cellular turnover, mucus production, mucosal bicarbonate secretion, or blood flow, or of the synthesis of prostaglandins may occur in these patients and could contribute to ulcer formation, but these potential factors have not been quantified.

GASTRIC ULCER

Patients with gastric ulcer usually secrete less acid than normal both in the basal and stimulated states. As noted above, diffuse gastritis is usually present, which may contribute to formation of the ulcer. It tends to remain after the ulcer has healed. Histologically, there is extensive round cell infiltration of the lamina propria, the gastric mucosa is reduced in height, and intestinal metaplasia is often seen.

Most patients with gastric ulcer reflux duodenal contents including bile salts into the stomach. Bile salts have been demonstrated experimentally to damage the mucosal barrier, produce mucosal damage, and lead to back diffusion of H+ ions. Thus, duodenal-gastric reflux of bile salts may well produce mucosal damage and cause the mucosa to become more sensitive to acid and pepsin. The injured mucosa secretes less acid but in turn is less resistant to acid and pepsin.

Peptic Ulcer Symptoms and Complications

The symptoms and complications of duodenal and gastric ulcers (peptic ulcers) are the same. The most common symptom is burning *epigastric pain*. The pain is constant, may radiate into the back, and may or may not be relieved by food, antacids, or H-2 receptor antagonists.

When an ulcer erodes into an artery, gastrointestinal *hemorrhage* occurs. This most common complication of peptic ulcer disease occurs in about 20 per cent of patients with duodenal ulcer. The hemorrhage is often precipitous and the patient may present with vomiting blood (hematemesis) or passing bloody stools (melena). If the patient secretes acid, the blood usually turns black and has the appearance of coffee grounds. Although bleeding often stops spontaneously, surgery is indicated when the hemorrhage is brisk and the patient requires five or more units of blood transfusions.

If the ulcer erodes completely through the bowel wall, *perforation* occurs and gastric contents spill in the abdominal cavity with a resultant peritonitis. These patients present with sudden onset of acute abdominal pain that is severe and unrelenting. The diagnosis is usually made from the patient's history and the presence of free air in the abdominal cavity as seen on an upright abdominal radiograph. Surgery is indicated for this condition to close the perforation and cleanse the peritoneal cavity of gastric acid and bile.

Gastric *outlet obstruction* occurs when there is substantial edema and pyloric spasm acutely or cicatrix formation and pyloric stenosis chronically. These patients usually present with a history of early satiety, intermittent nausea, and vomiting of food without bile. These patients have usually had a long history of ulcer disease and may have weight loss related to diminished nutrition secondary to nausea and vomiting. They may also present with dehydration and metabolic alkalosis. The diagnosis is made with upper gastrointestinal contrast radiographs. It is often not apparent if the obstruction is secondary to ulcer or to malignancy. Patients are initially treated with a nasogastric tube for decompression and with intravenous fluids. The obstruction will sometimes resolve but surgery is often required.

GASTRIC CARCINOMA

Gastric carcinoma is an adenocarcinoma arising from the gastric epithelium. The incidence of this disease varies widely in different parts of the world. For example, in the United States the incidence is 10 per 100,000 per year while in Japan the incidence is 70 per 100,000. Gastric adenocarcinomas may be grouped by their gross characteristics of growth. The extremes are polypoid and exophytic or ulcerative and invasive.

The development of gastric cancers is probably associated with the oral intake of some type of carcinogen. Epidemiologic studies suggest that gastric carcinoma is associated with a high intake of starches and barbecued or smoked meats and a low intake of vegetables and fresh fruits.

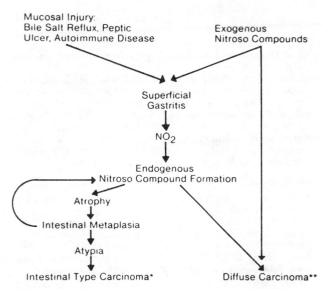

Figure 25. Possible mechanisms for the pathogenesis of gastric cancer. Note that exogenous nitroso compounds may produce gastritis and subsequently induce carcinoma. Gastritis and hyposecretion of acid predispose to the formation of endogenous nitroso compounds which are carcinogenic. * Population in high risk area. ** Persons receiving high dose of carcinogen, or genetically sensitive to low dose. (From Stemmermann, G. N., and Mower, H. F.: J Clin Gastroenterol 3(Suppl 2):23, 1981.

Severe atrophic gastritis with gastric intestinalization is almost always present in patients with gastric cancer. These patients usually secrete less acid than normal; about 20 per cent will be achlorhydric. It is not known if gastritis is a precancerous lesion per se, if the gastritis is the result of exposure to carcinogens, or if the relatively high pH and hypoacidity of acid that accompany gastritis lead to the formation of carcinogens within the stomach. Nitrosamines are known experimental gastric carcinogens. In animals these compounds initially produce superficial gastritis, gastric ulcer, and intestinal metaplasia. If exposure is continued, cancer eventually develops. Thus, nonspecific nonerosive gastritis may represent repeated exposure to carcinogens. It is also known that a relatively high gastric pH favors the intragastric conversion of nitrates (NO_3) to nitrites (NO_2) and subsequent formation of nitrosated amines, which are carcinogens. The possible mechanisms of gastric cancer formation are outlined in Figure 25.

REFERENCES

Enteric Nervous System and Endocrinology

Bloom, S. R., and Polak, J. M.: Alimentary endocrine system. In Sircus, W., and Smith, A. N. (eds.): Scientific Foundations of Gastroenterology. Philadelphia, W. B. Saunders Co., 1980, p. 101.

Gershon, M. D., and Erde, S. M.: The nervous system of the gut. Gastroenterology 80:1571, 1981.

Gastric Acid Secretion

Fordtran, J. S., and Walsh, J. H.: Gastric acid secretion rate and buffer content of the stomach after eating. Results in normal subjects and in patients with duodenal ulcer. J Clin Invest 52:645, 1973.

Koelz, H. R., Muller-Lissner, S. A., Malinowska, D. H., et al.: The stomach and duodenum in gastroenterology. Annual 1:33–78, 1983.

Schiller, L. R., Walsh, J. H., and Feldman, M.: Distention-induced gastrin release: Effects of luminal acidification and intravenous atropine. Gastroenterology 78:912, 1980.

Soll, A. H., and Grossman, M. I.: Cellular mechanisms in acid secretion. Annu Rev Med 29:495, 1978.

Walsh, J. H., Richardson, C. T., and Fordtran, J. S.: pH dependence of acid secretion and gastrin release in normal and ulcer subjects. J Clin Invest 55:462, 1975.

Gastric Motility

Hunt, J. N.: Mechanisms and disorders of gastric emptying. Annu Rev Med 34:219, 1983.

Kelly, K. A.: Motility of the stomach and gastroduodenal junction. In Johnson, L. R. (ed.): Physiology of the Gastrointestinal Tract, Vol. 1. New York, Raven Press, 1981, p. 393.

Kroop, H. S., Long, W. B., Alavi, A., et al.: Effect of water and fat on gastric emptying of solid meals. Gastroenterology 77:997, 1979.

Malagelada, J. R.: Regulation of gastric emptying in health and disease. Viewpoints on Digestive Diseases 13:17, 1981.

Meyer, J. H.: Gastric emptying of ordinary food: Effect of antrum on particle size. Am J Physiol 239:G133, 1980.

Pellegrini, C. A., and Ryan, T.: Management of gastric motility disorders. Contemp Surg 22:15, 1983.

Schiller, L. R.: Motor function of the stomach. In Sleisenger, M. H., and Fordtran, J. S. (eds.): Gastrointestinal Disease. 3rd ed. Philadelphia, W. B. Saunders Co., 1983, p. 521.

Gastritis

Correa, P.: The epidemiology and pathogenesis of chronic gastritis: Three etiologic entities. In van der Reis, L. (ed.): Frontiers of Gastrointestinal Research. Vol. 6, The Stomach. New York, S. Karger, 1980, p. 98.

Guth, P. H.: Pathogenesis of gastric mucosal injury. Annu Rev Med 33:183, 1982.

Stemmermann, G. N., and Mower, H.: Gastritis, nitrosamines, and gastric cancer. J Clin Gastroenterol 3(Suppl. 2):23, 1981.

Strickland, R. G., and Mackay, I. R.: A reappraisal of the nature and significance of chronic atrophic gastritis. Am J Dig Dis 18:426, 1973.

Weinstein, W. M.: Gastritis. In Sleisenger, M. H., and Fordtran, J. S. (eds.): Gastrointestinal Disease. 3rd ed. Philadelphia, W. B. Saunders Co., 1983, p. 559.

Ulcer

Baron, J. H.: Current views on pathogenesis of peptic ulcer. Scand J Gastroenterol (Suppl)80:1, 1982.

Gibiński, K.: Step by step towards the natural history of peptic ulcer disease. J Clin Gastroenterol 5:299, 1983.

Grossman, M. I., Kurata, J. H., Rotter, J. I., et al.: Peptic ulcer: New therapies, new diseases. Ann Intern Med 95:609, 1981.

Isenberg, J. I.: Peptic ulcer. DM 28:1, December, 1981.

Soll, A. H., and Isenberg, J. I.: Duodenal ulcer diseases. In Sleisenger, M. H., and Fordtran, J. S. (eds.): Gastrointestinal Disease. 3rd ed. Philadelphia, W. B. Saunders Co., 1983, p. 625.

General References

Grossman, M. I. (ed.): Peptic Ulcer: A Guide for the Practicing Physician. Chicago, Year Book Medical Publishers, Inc., 1981.

Johnson, L. R. (ed.): Physiology of the Gastrointestinal Tract. New York, Raven Press, 1981.

Sircus, W., and Smith, A. N. (eds.): Scientific Foundations of Gastroenterology. Philadelphia, W. B. Saunders Co., 1980.

Sleisenger, M. H., and Fordtran, J. S. (eds.): Gastrointestinal Disease. 3rd ed. Philadelphia, W. B. Saunders Co., 1983.

van der Reis, L. (ed.): Frontiers of Gastrointestinal Research. Vol. 6, The Stomach. New York, S. Karger, 1980.

Pathophysiology of the Small Intestine

MARTIN F. HEYWORTH, M.D.

The major functions of the small intestine are (1) digestion and absorption of food components, (2) transport of nonabsorbed luminal material to the colon, and (3) "immunologic surveillance" of luminal contents, with the development of an immune response against microorganisms and other antigenic materials.

Abnormalities in each of these areas will be considered. Other aspects of small intestinal pathophysiology will also be discussed—namely, protein loss, abnormal water and electrolyte secretion, endocrine abnormalities, and small intestinal ischemia.

SMALL INTESTINAL MOTILITY

NORMAL MOTILITY

Movement of small intestinal contents occurs as a result of organized contractions of the intestinal wall. Smooth muscle contraction in this site occurs in re-sponse to depolarization of muscle cell membranes. Two major types of depolarization are recognized: slow waves, which are repetitive depolarizations of the muscle membrane, and spike potentials, which are rapid bursts of depolarization intermittently superimposed on slow waves. The frequency of slow waves in the small intestine ranges from approximately 12 per minute in the duodenum to 8 per minute in the ileum. Spike potentials are necessary for muscle contraction to occur in the intestine, and the strength of this contraction depends on the intensity of spike potentials.

Intestinal motility is strongly influenced by neurologic and hormonal factors. Local parasympathetic and sympathetic nerves have opposite effects on small intestinal motility; it is increased by parasympathetic activity and decreased by sympathetic stimulation. The actual mechanisms by which autonomic nervous stimuli influence intestinal motility are not well understood. Autonomic nerves probably act both on smooth muscle cells of the intestinal wall and also on intra-mural neurons belonging to the enteric nervous system. Intestinal smooth muscle cells have adrenergic receptors. Stimulation of these receptors inhibits smooth muscle contraction. Besides catecholamines and acetylcholine, other neurotransmitters and local hormones may influence small intestinal contraction. These substances include serotonin, enkephalins, and possibly also ATP and vasoactive intestinal peptide (VIP).

Between meals, the small intestine shows periods of quiescence alternating with vigorous electrical and motor activity. During these phases of activity, a wave of spike potentials spreads down the small intestine from the stomach or duodenum. This electrical activity is accompanied by a wave of muscle contraction that also spreads distally along the small intestine. This motor activity is termed the interdigestive migrating motor complex and, in human subjects, it occurs at intervals of approximately 90 minutes. The migrating motor complex prevents stasis of intestinal contents and helps to minimize bacterial growth in the small intestinal lumen. The migrating motor complex may be triggered by *motilin,* which is a gastrointestinal peptide hormone. In addition, there is evidence that the enteric nerve plexuses play a part in generating the motor complex. Food ingestion leads to alteration of the electrical and motor activity of the small intestine. Instead of the organized migrating motor complex, random spike and motor activity occurs immediately after meals. The type of food influences the extent to which the migrating motor complex pattern is disrupted; this disruption is particularly marked after ingestion of triglycerides.

ABNORMAL MOTILITY

Small intestinal motility can be abnormally increased or decreased. In circumstances that cause reduced motility, bacterial colonization of the small intestine can occur, leading to malabsorption and diarrhea. These particular topics will be dealt with more fully later in this chapter. Meanwhile, some of the disorders associated with abnormal small intestinal motility will be discussed briefly.

Intestinal motility is reduced in *systemic sclerosis* and *idiopathic intestinal pseudo-obstruction.* In these conditions, the small intestine is able to generate electrical slow waves, but spike potentials and contraction in response to intestinal distention do not occur. In advanced systemic sclerosis, abnormalities are present in both the innervation and smooth muscle of the small intestine. Patients with idiopathic intestinal pseudo-obstruction have episodes of "functional" intestinal obstruction, with abdominal pain and vomiting. The cause of this disorder is not known. Bacterial colonization of the small intestine commonly occurs in patients with systemic sclerosis involving this organ. These patients develop malabsorption and steatorrhea (visible fat in the stools).

Several endocrine disorders can lead to abnormal motility of the small intestine. *Thyrotoxicosis* can lead to diarrhea, and *myxedema* to constipation. Although the frequency of small intestinal slow waves can be increased in thyrotoxicosis and decreased in myxe-dema, it is not clear whether these electrical abnormalities are responsible for the intestinal symptoms occurring in thyroid disease. Loss of intestinal muscle tone may be severe in myxedema, leading to ileus and pseudo-obstruction. Patients with *diabetes* can develop symptoms of small intestinal dysfunction, particularly diarrhea. The mechanism of the diarrhea is frequently obscure, although autonomic neuropathy and, rarely, bacterial colonization of the small intestine may both play a part in its development. *Irritable bowel syndrome* appears to be mainly associated with abnormal motility of the colon. However, increased motility of the small intestine may contribute to abdominal pain and diarrhea in a number of patients with irritable bowel syndrome.

ELECTROLYTE AND WATER SECRETION

Although absorption is a major function of small intestinal epithelial cells, there is evidence that these cells also secrete electrolytes and water under normal circumstances. When this secretory activity is increased, so-called secretory diarrhea results. Electrolytes and water are mainly secreted by small intestinal epithelial cells located in the crypts rather than on the villi. The pathophysiology of secretory diarrhea has been studied in some detail, but there is relatively little information about normal intestinal secretion. Active chloride secretion is known to occur in the normal human jejunum, and sodium secretion has been demonstrated in the guinea pig ileum. The mechanisms by which normal intestinal epithelial cells secrete electrolytes are not understood. Cyclic AMP may play a part in normal chloride secretion, but this remains speculative at present.

NORMAL DIGESTION AND ABSORPTION

Digestion and absorption of food components are major functions of the small intestine. In this discussion, normal digestion and absorption will be considered, and abnormalities in each of these areas will be discussed.

STRUCTURE OF THE SMALL INTESTINAL EPITHELIUM

A number of anatomic specializations ensure that the epithelial cell area available for absorption in the small intestine is very large. These specializations include *valvulae conniventes,* which are circumferential folds of mucosa and submucosa, particularly prominent in the distal duodenum and upper jejunum. *Villi* are numerous smaller mucosal projections (Fig. 26), and *microvilli* are regular finger-like projections of the apical membranes of epithelial cells (Fig. 27). Epithelial cells arise by mitosis from progenitor cells in the crypts, and migrate toward the apices of villi. It requires between four and seven days for small intestinal epithelial cells to migrate from crypts to the tips of villi, where they are then shed into the intestinal lumen. Absorptive cells of the small intestinal epithelium are columnar in form. Microvilli on the apical surfaces of these cells form a "brush border," which lines the intestinal lumen. Microvillus membranes are

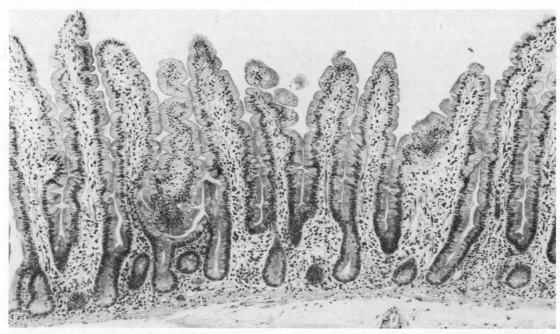

Figure 26. Light micrograph of a section of mucosa obtained by peroral biopsy from the jejunum of a healthy human subject. Normal villi are present. Hematoxylin and eosin stain. (From Sleisenger, M. H., and Fordtran, J. S. (eds.): Gastrointestinal Disease. 3rd ed. Philadelphia, W. B. Saunders Co., 1983.)

covered with a closely adherent glycoprotein coat known as the *glycocalyx*. This coat and the underlying membrane contain enzymes that are important in digestion, and receptors for binding and transport of important substances. For example, disaccharidases and peptidases are part of the microvillus surface of intestinal absorptive cells. In addition, the microvillus surface of ileal absorptive cells bears a receptor for intrinsic factor-bound vitamin B_{12}. Absorptive cells in the jejunum lack this receptor. It has been suggested that receptors for bile salts, iron, and calcium are also located on microvillus membranes, and it is known that these membranes can transport sodium, glucose, and amino acids.

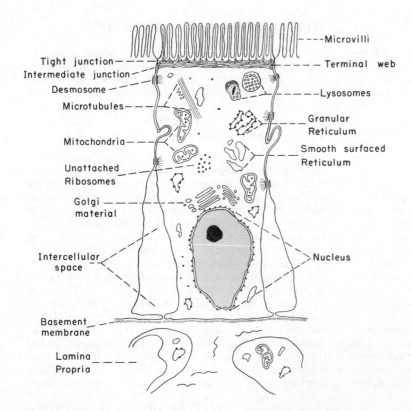

Figure 27. Schematic diagram of an intestinal absorptive cell. (Redrawn from Trier, J. S., and Rubin, C. E.: Gastroenterology 49:575, 1965. © 1965 The Williams & Wilkins Co., Baltimore.)

Adjacent epithelial cells achieve intimate contact at tight junctions, which are located in the apical region of lateral cell membranes (Fig. 27). These junctions appear to prevent luminal macromolecules from entering between epithelial cells, although water and small ions may be able to cross the junctions. Spaces between adjacent epithelial cells do not remain constant in size but enlarge during active absorption. Apart from low molecular weight substances that may cross tight junctions between epithelial cells, other materials pass through the cells during the process of absorption. These materials then leave absorptive cells either across the lateral plasma membrane or the basal membrane of the cells. Finally, absorbed substances cross the continuous basement membrane located just below the bases of absorptive cells (Fig. 27), and enter capillaries or lymphatics in the lamina propria.

WATER AND ELECTROLYTE ABSORPTION

As discussed previously, the small intestinal epithelium is able to secrete electrolytes and water. Under normal circumstances, however, absorption of these materials exceeds secretion, leading to net movement of electrolytes and water from the lumen to the intestinal mucosa. The total amount of fluid presented to the adult human small intestine is normally 7 to 9 liters per day, and comprises fluid secreted into the gastrointestinal lumen in addition to ingested fluid. Absorption of electrolytes by the small intestinal epithelium is the result of several different mechanisms. These include passive and active processes. There is no evidence that water is actively absorbed. Movement of water across the epithelium follows that of electrolytes and other low molecular weight solutes.

Sodium absorption occurs by various processes. The simplest of these is *electrogenic absorption* in which sodium enters epithelial cells passively, moving down an electrochemical gradient. This gradient is generated by active pumping of sodium ions out of the cells across their basolateral membranes, through the action of a sodium-potassium ATPase. Sodium uptake by epithelial cells is also linked to glucose and amino acid absorption. In the case of *glucose-linked sodium absorption,* glucose and sodium appear to enter cells through the action of a carrier molecule located on the brush border. Because glucose and amino acid uptake is linked to sodium absorption, sodium is necessary for the absorption of these organic compounds. Sodium is also absorbed across the intestinal epithelium as a result of *solvent drag.* In this process, passive absorption of water occurs in response to glucose uptake, and sodium is also absorbed passively along with the water. *Exchange of sodium with hydrogen ions,* across the epithelial cell brush border, constitutes another mechanism of sodium absorption in the human small intestine. In addition, bicarbonate/chloride exchange can occur across the apical membranes of ileal and colonic epithelial cells (Fig. 28).

Absorption of chloride in the small intestine takes place by more than one mechanism, including bicarbonate/chloride exchange. Chloride is also absorbed passively, either across epithelial cells or via tight junctions, in response to the electrical gradient created by absorbed sodium. In *congenital chloridorrhea,* chloride-bicarbonate exchange in the ileum and colon is impaired. Exchange of sodium for hydrogen in the

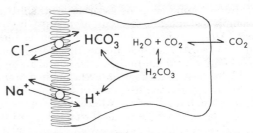

Figure 28. Ion exchanges across the apical membrane (brush border) of an ileal absorptive cell. Sodium is exchanged for hydrogen, and chloride for bicarbonate. The H_2CO_3 shown in this diagram is generated by the action of carbonic anhydrase. (From Sleisenger, M. H., and Fordtran, J. S. (eds.): Gastrointestinal Disease. 3rd ed. Philadelphia, W. B. Saunders Co., 1983.)

small intestine of patients with this condition is normal. More hydrogen than bicarbonate is lost via the feces, leading to metabolic alkalosis. Because passive chloride absorption is normal, patients with this disorder can be treated with oral sodium chloride or potassium chloride. Although diarrhea persists, this treatment can prevent excessive chloride depletion.

Potassium is absorbed passively in the small intestine, in response to electrochemical concentration gradients.

IRON ABSORPTION

There are two main forms of dietary iron: heme iron, which is present in meat, and non-heme iron, which is largely present in vegetables—including fruits and nuts. Heme iron is much more readily absorbed than non-heme iron. In an average Western diet, most of the iron is in the non-heme form (15 to 20 mg per day), with only a small amount of heme iron (1.5 to 3.0 mg per day). Important factors that influence iron absorption include the valency of the iron and whether it is bound in the form of insoluble complexes in the food. Ferrous iron (Fe^{++}) is absorbed more readily than the trivalent ferric form.

Iron absorption mainly occurs in the duodenum and upper jejunum. Iron-containing heme is absorbed intact by mucosal cells. Absorption of heme iron is not influenced by luminal substances that affect non-heme iron absorption. Following absorption, iron is released from heme in mucosal cells, by the action of heme oxygenase. This iron is in the divalent ferrous form and mainly enters the portal venous blood. Non-heme iron, largely contained in vegetable foods and eggs, is relatively unavailable for absorption. Gastric hydrochloric acid releases some non-heme iron from these foods and tends to maintain the iron in a soluble form. Other luminal substances also influence the solubility of non-heme iron, and thus affect its absorption. Agents that increase iron solubility include ascorbic acid and amino acids released during protein digestion. Solubility of non-heme iron is reduced by various anions, such as phosphate, phytate, and oxalate, and by phosphoproteins. These substances bind iron in the gastric and intestinal lumen, and reduce its availability for absorption. It is uncertain whether dietary fiber can also bind iron and reduce its uptake by intestinal epithelial cells.

There is evidence that an active transport process is responsible for iron absorption by epithelial cells. When iron is presented to these cells as soluble complexes with amino acids or ascorbic acid, splitting of the complexes appears to occur at microvillus membranes. After epithelial cell uptake, iron is incorporated into ferritin located inside the cells. The iron may remain within epithelial cells, bound in ferritin, and will be lost if these cells are sloughed from the villi. Alternatively, the iron may be transported to the bases of epithelial cells, from where it enters the portal venous blood. The mechanisms of iron transport across epithelial cells, and iron release from the serosal aspect of these cells, are not yet clear.

The absorption of iron is regulated by the amount of iron in the body and by the activity of erythropoiesis. Iron absorption increases during depletion of body iron stores and vice versa. Similarly, absorption of iron is directly proportional to erythropoietic activity. It is not known how body iron content and erythropoiesis actually influence iron absorption. Ferritin may play a part in the regulation of iron absorption, but this remains uncertain. Increased absorption of iron appears to be the underlying abnormality in "idiopathic" hemochromatosis.

CALCIUM ABSORPTION

Calcium is absorbed in the ionized form. Much of the calcium in milk and other dairy products becomes ionized after contact with gastric acid. Calcium in vegetables is bound to organic anions such as oxalate and phytate, and is not readily available for absorption. The absorption of calcium is a complex process that is influenced by a number of factors, including vitamin D and parathormone. Calcium tends to remain in solution at a low pH, and to precipitate under alkaline conditions. Substances that form soluble complexes with calcium—including bile acids, amino acids, and low molecular weight sugars—can increase its absorption. Conversely, substances that form insoluble compounds with calcium, such as oxalate and phosphate anions, and long-chain fatty acids, decrease calcium absorption.

Calcium uptake by small intestinal epithelial cells requires energy and is dependent on vitamin D. This vitamin occurs in several different forms. 25-Hydroxy-vitamin D is a weak stimulator of calcium absorption, and is normally converted into 1,25-dihydroxy-vitamin D in the kidneys. The dihydroxy vitamin is a potent stimulator of intestinal calcium absorption. It promotes the synthesis of a microvillus membrane carrier protein, which transports calcium into epithelial cells. The 1,25-dihydroxy-vitamin D appears to act by stimulating DNA transcription; the resulting RNA is then translated into carrier protein. Patients with vitamin D deficiency have impaired absorption of calcium.

Various hormones influence calcium transport across the intestinal mucosa. Parathormone stimulates intestinal uptake of calcium in parathyroidectomized rats. The effect of parathormone on calcium absorption requires vitamin D. Parathormone increases the conversion of 25-hydroxy-vitamin D to 1,25-dihydroxy-vitamin D in the kidneys, by increasing the activity of a 1-alpha hydroxylase enzyme. There is little evidence that parathormone has any direct effect on calcium absorption. Intestinal uptake of calcium can be stimulated by growth hormone and may be decreased by glucocorticoids, estrogens, thyroxine, phenytoin, and thiazides. Of the low molecular weight sugars that increase calcium uptake, lactose is the most active in this respect. Calcium absorption and its relationship to parathyroid hormone and vitamin D metabolism are discussed more fully in Section VIII.

FOLATE ABSORPTION

Folic acid (pteroylmonoglutamic acid) has a three-part molecular structure, consisting of a pteridine derivative, a para-aminobenzoic acid residue, and a residue of L-glutamic acid. Folic acid derivatives are important in many biochemical processes. These include purine and pyrimidine synthesis and amino acid metabolism. Because folic acid plays an important part in the synthesis of nucleic acids, its deficiency adversely affects rapidly dividing cells. These include erythrocyte precursors and intestinal epithelial cells.

In the diet, folates mainly occur as polyglutamates. These substances need to be hydrolyzed before they can be absorbed. Approximately 60 per cent of dietary folate is present in vegetables, cereals, and fruit, with about 40 per cent in meat, fish, and dairy products. Cooking of food destroys a large proportion of its folate. The liver is able to store folate in the form of 5-methyl-tetrahydrofolate, and normally contains enough folate to keep the body supplied for approximately four months. The daily folate requirement is about 100 to 200 μg. The pentaglutamate appears to be the most common dietary form of folate, although folates with four and six glutamate residues are also common in food. Folate is mainly absorbed in the upper jejunum with some absorption occurring in the lower jejunum.

Polyglutamate forms of folate are hydrolyzed in the small intestine. The site of hydrolysis has not been clearly identified, but may be the brush border or the lysosomes of absorptive epithelial cells. The hydrolytic enzyme pteroylpolyglutamate hydrolase removes glutamate residues from polyglutamates. The resulting monoglutamate form of folate is then reduced and methylated within epithelial cells to form 5-methyl-tetrahydrofolate. This compound and a relatively small proportion of unchanged pteroylmonoglutamate then leave epithelial cells and pass into the mesenteric venous circulation (Fig. 29). Two mechanisms by which

INTESTINAL LUMEN	INTESTINAL EPITHELIUM	MESENTERIC CIRCULATION

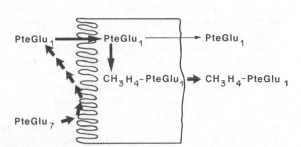

Figure 29. Digestion and absorption of pteroylpolyglutamates (shown here as PteGlu$_7$). Folate (PteGlu$_1$) and 5-methyl-tetrahydrofolate (CH$_3$H$_4$-PteGlu$_1$) enter the blood. (Modified from Rosenberg, I. H.: N Engl J Med 293:1303, 1975.)

folate enters absorptive cells from the intestinal lumen have been suggested: (1) a carrier-mediated, saturable system operating at a low luminal concentration of folate, and (2) a passive transport process occurring at higher folate concentrations. Under normal circumstances, there is an enterohepatic circulation of folate. Most of the folate in bile appears to be in the form of methyl-tetrahydrofolate.

Absorption of folate is impaired in a number of circumstances. These include diseases of the intestine leading to generalized malabsorption and the rare condition of congenital folate malabsorption. In this disorder, pteroylmonoglutamate absorption is impaired, without malabsorption of other substances. The anticonvulsant phenytoin can induce folate deficiency, possibly through interference with its intestinal absorption. Sulfasalazine is known to diminish folate absorption. Alcoholism may be associated with folate deficiency, partly because of inadequate dietary folate.

VITAMIN B$_{12}$ ABSORPTION

Vitamin B$_{12}$ occurs in a number of chemically related forms. Of these, methylcobalamin and deoxyadenosyl-cobalamin are biologically active. Vitamin B$_{12}$ plays an important but indirect role in DNA synthesis through its interactions with folate. Deficiency of this vitamin leads to impaired production of erythrocytes as well as disease of the central nervous system. Most of the dietary vitamin B$_{12}$ occurs in animal products—including meat, eggs, cheese, and milk. Liver is a particularly rich source of the vitamin. Vitamin B$_{12}$ in animal products is actually of bacterial origin, and includes B$_{12}$ produced in the rumen of ungulates and absorbed into their tissues. Although bacteria in the human colon synthesize vitamin B$_{12}$, it cannot be absorbed from this site.

Vitamin B$_{12}$ is bound to proteins in food and appears to be liberated from these by acid and pepsin in the human stomach. The vitamin B$_{12}$ then binds to carrier proteins called R proteins, at an acid pH in the gastric lumen. The role of R proteins is not well defined. These proteins reach the gastric lumen in saliva and are glycoproteins with a molecular weight of around 60,000 daltons. Vitamin B$_{12}$-R protein complexes pass from the stomach into the upper small intestinal lumen, where the R proteins are degraded by pancreatic protease enzymes. Free vitamin B$_{12}$ is liberated and then binds to intrinsic factor, which is a glycoprotein secreted by gastric parietal cells. Human intrinsic factor has a molecular weight of 44,000 daltons. Complexes of intrinsic factor and vitamin B$_{12}$ become attached to receptors on the microvillus membranes of epithelial cells in the ileum. The binding process requires calcium and a neutral pH. The receptor protein has a molecular weight of around 200,000 daltons and does not bind vitamin B$_{12}$ in the absence of intrinsic factor. In human subjects, intrinsic factor receptors are present from the mid-small intestine to the lower end of the terminal ileum. After attachment of vitamin B$_{12}$-intrinsic factor complexes to ileal cell surfaces, the complexes are split by an unknown mechanism. Liberated vitamin B$_{12}$ enters absorptive cells and appears to pass into the mitochondria of these cells. After a period of about 6 hours, the B$_{12}$ leaves epithelial cells and enters the portal venous blood. The fate of intrinsic factor after it binds to ileal absorptive cell surfaces is unknown. Absorption of intrinsic factor has not been convincingly demonstrated.

In the blood, vitamin B$_{12}$ is transported attached to binding proteins known as transcobalamins. Two of these (transcobalamins I and III) transport vitamin B$_{12}$ to the liver. These particular transport proteins appear to be identical with two of the R proteins that bind vitamin B$_{12}$ in the gastric lumen. Another serum transport protein, transcobalamin II, transports vitamin B$_{12}$ to tissues other than the liver.

A small proportion of dietary vitamin B$_{12}$ is absorbed without becoming bound to intrinsic factor. Absorption by this mechanism appears to involve diffusion across intestinal epithelial cells. Under normal circumstances, there is an enterohepatic circulation of vitamin B$_{12}$. The vitamin is bound to R proteins in bile, and these complexes are split in the small intestinal lumen. The liberated vitamin B$_{12}$ is then absorbed by the mechanisms described previously. The human liver normally stores about 5,000 µg of vitamin B$_{12}$. Approximately 1 µg of the vitamin is required daily for metabolic activities.

ABSORPTION OF OTHER WATER-SOLUBLE VITAMINS

Little is known about the mechanisms by which other water-soluble vitamins are absorbed by the human small intestine. There is some evidence that thiamine (vitamin B$_1$) and riboflavin (vitamin B$_2$) are absorbed by active transport. Nicotinic acid and pantothenic acid appear to be absorbed by passive diffusion. Ascorbic acid (vitamin C) is readily absorbed by the human small intestine, although the mechanism of absorption is unknown. Clinical deficiency of the vitamins considered in this paragraph is usually the result of inadequate dietary intake. Whether malabsorption can lead to significant deficiency of these substances is not clear. Thiamine deficiency can occur in chronic alcoholism, largely because of poor dietary intake of the vitamin. In addition, there is some evidence that alcoholism leads to impaired thiamine absorption.

FAT DIGESTION AND ABSORPTION

The normal daily intake of fat in a Western diet is approximately 60 to 100 grams. This fat consists mainly of triglycerides, formed between glycerol and long-chain fatty acids (Fig. 30). Triglycerides are hydrolyzed by lipase in the lumen of the gastrointestinal tract. A small amount of triglyceride is hydrolyzed in the stomach, through the action of a lingual lipase. However, the bulk of triglyceride hydrolysis occurs in the duodenum, as a result of the action of pancreatic lipase. This enzyme splits the outer (α) ester linkages of triglycerides, releasing the fatty acids and leaving β-monoglycerides and some diglycerides. For maximal activity of lipase, an additional pancreatic protein is necessary. This is a small enzyme known as *colipase,* which binds to triglycerides in the presence of bile salts. Lipase then forms a complex with colipase, leading to hydrolysis of the triglycerides.

The products of triglyceride hydrolysis are solubilized by the action of bile salts. Monoglycerides and

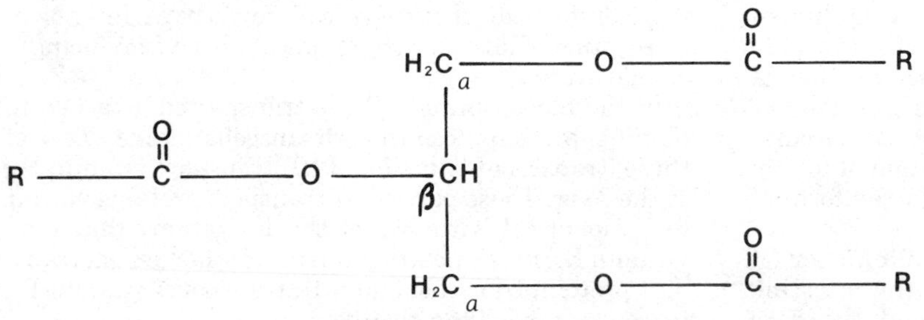

Figure 30. Diagram of a triglyceride molecule. Fatty acid residues are shown as R-CO, and the alpha and beta carbon atoms of the glycerol "backbone" are labeled. In most dietary triglycerides, long-chain fatty acid residues are present, each containing 16–18 carbon atoms.

long-chain fatty acids are relatively hydrophobic, but aggregate with bile salts to form micelles. These consist of an outer hydrophilic region, facing the aqueous environment of the intestinal lumen, and an inner hydrophobic core. Micelles, which form when the bile salt concentration exceeds a level of 2 to 5 mM (the critical micellar concentration of bile salts), are disk-shaped structures with a diameter of approximately 400Å. The hydrophilic side chains of bile salts cover the surface of micelles, while the hydrophobic steroid nuclei of these molecules interdigitate with long-chain fatty acids, monoglycerides, cholesterol, and phospholipids, in the core of micelles.

Monoglycerides and long-chain fatty acids are transported in micelles to the absorptive surfaces of small intestinal epithelial cells. There are two significant barriers to the absorption of hydrophobic substances such as long-chain fatty acids and monoglycerides. The first of these is the unstirred water layer over the surface of epithelial cells. The other principal barrier is the mucous layer that covers the apical membranes of epithelial cells. It is not clear where micellar disaggregation occurs during the process of fat absorption. Micelles may penetrate the unstirred water layer and then release monoglycerides and fatty acids that penetrate the mucous coat, or the micelles may actually pass through this mucous layer to disaggregate at the outer surface of the cell membrane. Monoglycerides and fatty acids pass through the apical membrane of epithelial cells, and reach the endoplasmic reticulum of these cells. It appears that a low molecular weight cytoplasmic protein—known as *fatty acid binding protein*—is partly responsible for transporting long-chain fatty acids from the apical membrane to the endoplasmic reticulum.

Within the endoplasmic reticulum, fatty acids become conjugated to coenzyme A (CoA), through the action of fatty acid CoA ligase. These activated fatty acids are then conjugated to monoglycerides, leading to the formation of diglycerides. This step is catalyzed by monoglyceride acyltransferase. Triglyceride formation then occurs, following the interaction of diglycerides and fatty acid-CoA. The enzyme that catalyzes triglyceride formation is known as diglyceride acyltransferase. Triglycerides accumulate in the Golgi apparatus of epithelial cells, and are then transported in vesicles to the basolateral membranes of the cells. Microtubules may be partly responsible for this vesicular transport. Before leaving epithelial cells, triglycerides are incorporated into chylomicrons. Figure 31 outlines the steps involved in fat digestion and absorption.

Chylomicrons (Fig. 32) vary in size from 75 to 600 nm. The core of a chylomicron consists mainly of triglyceride, and the outer coat region contains phospholipid and apoproteins. Chylomicrons leave intestinal epithelial cells by crossing the basolateral cell membranes, and then enter lacteal vessels from where they reach the thoracic duct lymph and venous blood. Although apoproteins constitute only about 1 per cent of the total mass of a chylomicron, they play a crucial role in the formation of chylomicrons and their exit from epithelial cells. Apoprotein B is absent in patients with *abetalipoproteinemia*. This is a rare genetic disorder, in which chylomicrons cannot be formed and fat accumulates within intestinal epithelial cells. Because chylomicrons do not form in this disease, transport of fat across basolateral membranes of epithelial cells is impaired. In addition to fat malabsorption, patients with this disease have abnormal erythrocyte membranes, central nervous system demyelination, and retinal abnormalities.

ABSORPTION OF BILE SALTS

Bile salts are glycine or taurine conjugates of bile acids. In human subjects, the primary bile acids known as *cholic acid* and *chenodeoxycholic acid* are synthesized from cholesterol in the liver. These bile acids are then conjugated to glycine or taurine in hepatocytes, and pass into the duodenal lumen via the bile. Approximately 25 per cent of the primary bile salts are deconjugated by bacteria in the ileum, liberating free bile acids. Most of these bile acid molecules are reabsorbed and subsequently reconjugated with glycine or taurine in the liver. Bacterial dehydroxylation of primary bile acids also occurs in the small intestinal lumen. This reaction converts cholic acid into *deoxycholic acid* and chenodeoxycholic acid to *lithocholic acid*. Approximately 50 per cent of the deoxycholic acid is then absorbed, conjugated to glycine or taurine in the liver, and secreted in the bile. Most of the lithocholic acid appears to become adsorbed to colonic bacteria, and to be excreted by this mechanism. Deoxycholic acid and lithocholic acid are classified as secondary bile acids. The tertiary bile acid *ursodeoxycholic acid* appears to be mainly formed by the action of bacteria on chenodeoxycholic acid in the small intestinal lumen. The chemical structures of some important human bile acids are shown in Figure 20 in Section XV.

Bile salts are recycled via an enterohepatic circulation. They are absorbed intact in the distal ileum by an active process that requires sodium. After entering portal venous blood, they pass into liver parenchymal cells and are then secreted into the bile, still in the form of glycine or taurine conjugates. Unconjugated bile acids are more hydrophobic than bile salts. Absorption of bile acids occurs by passive diffusion in all regions of the small intestine.

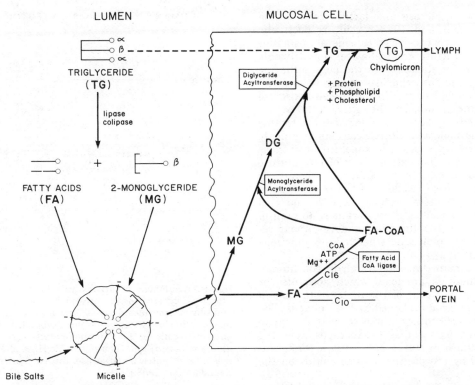

LUMEN   MUCOSAL CELL

Figure 31. Diagrammatic summary of fat digestion and absorption. In this diagram, 2-monoglyceride is synonymous with β-monoglyceride, and DG indicates diglyceride. Carbon chain lengths of fatty acids are shown as C_{10} and C_{16}. (From Sleisenger, M. H., and Fordtran, J. S. (eds.): Gastrointestinal Disease. 3rd ed. Philadelphia, W. B. Saunders Co., 1983.)

ABSORPTION OF MEDIUM-CHAIN TRIGLYCERIDES

As mentioned previously, most of the fatty acid residues in dietary fat have long chains of 16 to 18 carbon atoms (see Fig. 30). Triglycerides with fatty acid residues 6 to 10 carbon atoms in length—known as medium-chain triglycerides (MCT)—are absorbed more readily than long-chain triglycerides. MCT are able to pass directly from the intestinal lumen into the absorptive epithelial cells without requiring hydroly-sis. After oral administration of MCT to human subjects, approximately 30 per cent of the intake is absorbed by this direct mechanism. While pancreatic lipase hydrolyzes long-chain triglycerides to β-monoglycerides and fatty acids, it readily splits beta and alpha ester linkages of MCT, liberating fatty acids. These acids are more water soluble than long-chain fatty acids, and are able to pass directly across absorptive cells into the portal venous blood. Within absorptive cells, intact MCT and medium-chain monoglycerides are hydrolyzed to fatty acids that also pass into the portal vein. Because MCT are assimilated more readily than long-chain triglycerides, they are a useful dietary supplement for patients with malabsorption.

ABSORPTION OF CHOLESTEROL AND FAT-SOLUBLE VITAMINS

Cholesterol becomes incorporated into micelles in the intestinal lumen, and subsequently diffuses across the apical membranes of absorptive cells. It is then transported in chylomicrons, from epithelial cells to intestinal lymph. Vitamins A, D, K, and E are fat-soluble. They become incorporated into micelles in the intestinal lumen, together with long-chain fatty acids, monoglycerides, and cholesterol. The absorption of these vitamins is discussed in the section on nutrition.

CARBOHYDRATE DIGESTION AND ABSORPTION

The principal dietary carbohydrates are starch, sucrose, and lactose. In a normal Western diet, starch accounts for approximately 60 per cent of the dietary

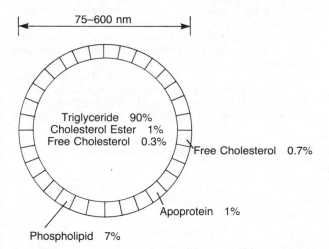

75–600 nm

Triglyceride 90%
Cholesterol Ester 1%
Free Cholesterol 0.3%

Free Cholesterol 0.7%

Apoprotein 1%

Phospholipid 7%

Figure 32. Schematic diagram of a chylomicron. This is shown as a cross-section of a sphere that consists of an outer coat region and a core. Percentages indicate the proportion of total chylomicron mass contributed by each component. (From Sleisenger, M. H., and Fordtran, J. S. (eds.): Gastrointestinal Disease. 3rd ed. Philadelphia, W. B. Saunders Co., 1983.)

carbohydrate, with sucrose and lactose constituting around 30 per cent and 10 per cent, respectively. Dietary carbohydrates present in considerably smaller amounts include fructose and trehalose. Nonutilizable carbohydrates in the diet include the polysaccharide cellulose, and the oligosaccharides stachyose and raffinose. In ruminants, bacteria in the rumen hydrolyze cellulose. In human subjects, however, cellulose remains undigested, as mammalian enzymes are unable to hydrolyze the molecule. Starch consists of glucose residues joined by two types of linkage. In one of these linkages, the first carbon atom (C–1) of one glucose residue is joined via oxygen to the fourth carbon (C–4) of the adjacent glucose residue. In the other type of linkage, an oxygen atom bridges the C–1 and C–6 positions of two adjacent glucose residues. Joining of glucose residues by 1–4 linkages produces linear regions of the starch molecule, whereas 1–6 junctions are branching points.

There are two main types of starch in the human diet. One of these is amylose, which accounts for approximately 20 per cent of the dietary starch and consists of glucose residues joined by 1–4 linkages. The other 80 per cent of dietary starch consists of amylopectin, in which 1–6 as well as 1–4 linkages occur. All the glucose residues in starch are in the α configuration, as defined by the position of side chains on the C–1 atom.

Three major processes are involved in carbohydrate digestion and absorption: (1) the digestion of starch to form oligosaccharides, (2) the breakdown of oligosaccharides at the surface of epithelial absorptive cells, and (3) the absorption of monosaccharides by these cells. Starch is hydrolyzed by amylase, which breaks 1–4 α linkages between glucose residues in the interior of the starch molecule. The enzyme does not break 1–4 linkages that are adjacent to a 1–6 link. In addition, 1–6 linkages resist cleavage by amylase. By the action of amylase, starch is hydrolyzed to maltose, maltotriose (a trisaccharide), and oligosaccharides which contain approximately 8 glucose residues. These are known as α-limit dextrins. They are formed by the hydrolysis of amylopectin and contain glucose residues joined by 1–4 and 1–6 linkages. A limited amount of starch digestion occurs through the action of salivary amylase, but this is terminated by gastric acid. Pancreatic amylase digests starch in the duodenum.

Oligosaccharides are hydrolyzed by enzymes located on the apical surface of small intestinal epithelial cells. Table 10 summarizes the names and functions of human intestinal oligosaccharidases. Sucrase and α-dextrinase are linked noncovalently to form a double

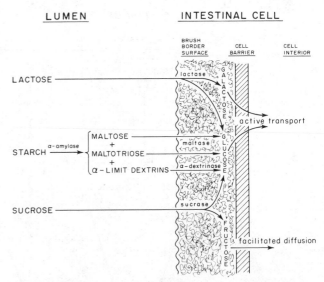

LUMEN   INTESTINAL CELL

Figure 33. Summary of carbohydrate digestion and absorption. Starch is digested in the intestinal lumen. Lactose, sucrose, and oligosaccharides derived from starch are hydrolyzed to monosaccharides by enzymes on the brush border surface of absorptive cells. In this diagram, maltase is synonymous with glucoamylase. (From Sleisenger, M. H., and Fordtran, J. S. (eds.): Gastrointestinal Disease. 3rd ed. Philadelphia, W. B. Saunders Co., 1983.)

molecule. This dual enzyme is sometimes called *sucrase/isomaltase*. Oligosaccharide hydrolysis mainly occurs in the jejunum. The steps involved in carbohydrate digestion and absorption are summarized in Figure 33.

Glucose, galactose, and fructose are released by the action of oligosaccharidases. Glucose and galactose are absorbed across the apical membrane of epithelial cells by an active process that requires sodium. There is evidence that these sugars bind to a carrier protein that also binds sodium, and the sugar and sodium are then transported across the apical membrane of the absorptive cell. After crossing the membrane, sugar molecules and sodium ions are released from the carrier protein, inside the cell. Sodium ions are actively pumped out of the cells, across their basal and lateral membranes, providing the energy needed for sugar and sodium uptake via the apical membrane. Glucose and galactose pass through epithelial cells, cross the basolateral cell membranes by the action of a carrier that does not require sodium, and then reach the portal venous blood. Fructose is absorbed by a different process from that which mediates the uptake of glucose

TABLE 10. BRUSH BORDER OLIGOSACCHARIDASES OF THE HUMAN SMALL INTESTINE

ENZYME	SUBSTRATES	PRODUCTS
Glucoamylase (Maltase)	Glucooligosaccharides, including maltose, maltotriose, and α-limit dextrins (splits α 1–4 links)	Glucose; residual oligosaccharides with α 1–6 link
Sucrase/α-dextrinase (Sucrase/isomaltase)	Sucrose; glucooligosaccharides, including maltose, maltotriose, and α-limit dextrins (splits α 1–4 and α 1–6 links)	Glucose, fructose
Lactase	Lactose	Glucose, galactose
Trehalase	Trehalose	Glucose

Modified from Sleisenger, M. H., and Fordtran, J. S. (eds.): Gastrointestinal Disease. 3rd ed. Philadelphia, W. B. Saunders Co., 1983, p. 852.

and galactose. There is evidence that fructose absorption is energy-independent, although a carrier protein appears to be involved. The mechanism of fructose absorption is sometimes called *facilitated diffusion.*

The slowest event—that is, rate-limiting step—in the digestion and absorption of most carbohydrates is the transport of hexose sugars across intestinal epithelial cells. In the case of lactose, however, hydrolysis by lactase proceeds more slowly than uptake of the hydrolysis products glucose and galactose.

PROTEIN DIGESTION AND ABSORPTION

Protein digestion starts in the stomach, as a result of the action of gastric pepsin. Maximum activity of pepsin occurs at low pH. Pepsin-mediated digestion is a relatively unimportant process, and the bulk of protein digestion occurs in the small intestine.

Pancreatic protease enzymes are secreted into the duodenal lumen. These enzymes are released from the pancreas as inactive precursor molecules from which peptides are cleaved in the duodenum to yield active proteases. Pancreatic trypsinogen is converted into the active protease enzyme trypsin, through the action of duodenal enterokinase. Trypsin itself converts additional trypsinogen molecules to trypsin, besides generating active forms of other pancreatic proteases—including chymotrypsin and carboxypeptidases A and B. Pancreatic proteases can be divided into two functional types: (1) *endopeptidases* (trypsin, chymotrypsin, and elastase), which hydrolyze peptide bonds in the interior of whole protein molecules to yield peptide fragments, and (2) *exopeptidases* (carboxypeptidases A and B), which split peptide linkages at the C terminal end of peptide fragments, releasing free amino acids. Within protein molecules, peptide linkages (CO-NH) are responsible for joining amino acid residues, and these bonds are broken by peptidase enzymes. As a result of the action of pancreatic proteases, dietary proteins are converted into small peptides containing 2–6 amino acid residues, free neutral amino acids, and free basic amino acids (arginine and lysine).

Oligopeptides containing 2–6 amino acid residues are hydrolyzed by oligopeptidase enzymes of intestinal epithelial cells. These enzymes are located on apical membranes of the cells (approximately 10 per cent of total cellular peptidase enzymes) and also within the epithelial cell cytoplasm (90 per cent of cellular peptidases). Several epithelial cell peptidase enzymes have been recognized in human subjects and experimental animals. *Aminopeptidase,* which occurs on the apical cell membrane and in the cytoplasm of epithelial cells, removes individual amino acids from the N terminal end of oligopeptides. There may be more than one type of aminopeptidase in the intestinal epithelium. Peptides containing 4–6 amino acid residues are broken down to dipeptides, tripeptides, and free amino acids by aminopeptidase located on apical membranes of epithelial cells. Limited hydrolysis of di- and tripeptides also occurs through the action of this brush border enzyme. However, proline-containing dipeptides are resistant to hydrolysis by this mechanism. Furthermore, the aminopeptidase is unable to remove N terminal amino acids from larger oligopeptides when these particular amino acids are adjacent to a proline residue.

Dipeptidyl peptidase, which is a brush border enzyme, removes N terminal dipeptide units from oligopeptides. The peptide linkages that are most susceptible to breakage by this enzyme are those adjacent to a proline residue.

Dipeptides and tripeptides that have not been hydrolyzed at the apical membranes of epithelial cells are transported into these cells. Uptake of the peptides across the brush border membrane appears to be an energy-dependent process that may require sodium. Within the cytoplasm of epithelial absorptive cells, splitting of di- and tripeptides can occur through the action of several different enzymes. These include (1) glycyl-L-leucine dipeptidase, which hydrolyzes dipeptides containing neutral amino acids, (2) aminotripeptidase, which hydrolyzes various tripeptides, and (3) proline dipeptidase, which cleaves proline-containing dipeptides. Amino acids liberated within epithelial cells subsequently enter the portal venous blood.

Amino acids within the intestinal lumen are absorbed by at least four different mechanisms, depending on the type of amino acid, that are responsible for the uptake of:

1. Neutral aromatic and aliphatic amino acids
2. Dibasic amino acids, such as lysine and arginine
3. Dicarboxylic amino acids (glutamic and aspartic acids)
4. Imino acids (proline and hydroxyproline) and glycine.

These processes require the presence of sodium and do not occur at equal rates. The first two mechanisms appear to be examples of active transport. There is evidence that uptake of free amino acids by intestinal epithelial cells proceeds more slowly than peptide hydrolysis by brush border enzymes or epithelial cell uptake of intact di- and tripeptides.

A number of rare genetic abnormalities of amino acid transport have been described. In *cystinuria* there is impaired intestinal and renal tubular absorption of cystine, arginine, and lysine. In *Hartnup disease* intestinal absorption of free neutral amino acids is impaired. Unlike the transport of free amino acids, uptake of di- and tripeptides by intestinal epithelial cells is normal in cystinuria and Hartnup disease. Patients with these disorders therefore absorb adequate quantities of dietary peptides and do not develop protein malnutrition.

ABNORMAL DIGESTION AND ABSORPTION

A number of diseases cause abnormalities of digestion and absorption. Detailed consideration of the clinical and pathologic features of these diseases would not be appropriate for the present chapter. Instead, an attempt will be made to survey the different mechanisms that underlie malabsorption, while briefly pointing out the disease entities that can be responsible for these various pathophysiological mechanisms.

PATHOPHYSIOLOGICAL MECHANISMS

Table 11 outlines the pathophysiologic mechanisms of abnormal digestion and absorption. Although much of this table is self-explanatory, it may be helpful to

TABLE 11. PATHOPHYSIOLOGIC CLASSIFICATION OF ABNORMAL DIGESTION AND ABSORPTION

AFFECTED MECHANISM	PATHOPHYSIOLOGIC REASONS	CAUSES	MAIN DIETARY COMPONENTS SHOWING IMPAIRED ASSIMILATION
I. Luminal digestion (fat, protein)	Deficiency of pancreatic enzymes	Chronic pancreatitis, pancreatic carcinoma, cystic fibrosis, resected pancreas	Fat, protein, vitamin B_{12} (rarely)
	Inactivated pancreatic enzymes	Zollinger-Ellison syndrome	
II. Luminal solubilization (fat)	Bile salt deficiency	Biliary tract obstruction, absent or diseased terminal ileum, small intestinal bacteria	Fat Fat-soluble vitamins Calcium
III. Availability of ingested nutrients	Uptake of nutrient by luminal organisms	Small intestinal bacteria, fish tapeworm	Vitamin B_{12}
	Absence of binding agent that promotes absorption	Intrinsic factor deficiency	Vitamin B_{12}
	Binding agents reducing absorption	Organic anions (phytate, oxalate)	Iron, calcium
		Cholestyramine	Fat, fat-soluble vitamins, calcium
IV. Epithelial cell digestion or transport	Disaccharidase deficiencies	Genetic; epithelial damage	Carbohydrate
	Absent transport mechanism for glucose and galactose	Genetic	Carbohydrate
	Nonformation of chylomicrons	Abetalipoproteinemia	Fat
	Impaired amino acid transport	Cystinuria, Hartnup disease	Free amino acids
	Impaired vitamin B_{12} transport	Genetic	Vitamin B_{12}
	Loss of normal epithelial cells	Partially resected small intestine, celiac disease, Crohn's disease, tropical sprue, radiation enteritis, eosinophilic gastroenteritis, intestinal ischemia, colchicine	Multiple
V. Lymphatic transport	Lymphatic obstruction	Whipple's disease, lymphoma, tuberculosis, Crohn's disease, lymphangiectasia	Multiple

The term "assimilation" in the right column embraces both digestion and absorption.

clarify a number of points. Considered in the order of their appearance in the table, these are:

I. *Abnormalities of luminal digestion.* Deficiency of pancreatic proteases can lead to vitamin B_{12} malabsorption. It will be recalled that vitamin B_{12} normally reaches the duodenum bound to R proteins, which are then degraded by pancreatic proteases so that the B_{12} can be released for binding to intrinsic factor. When pancreatic protease levels are deficient, B_{12} remains bound to R proteins in the small intestinal lumen and is unable to bind to intrinsic factor. B_{12} absorption is therefore impaired.

In the Zollinger-Ellison syndrome, hypergastrinemia occurs as a result of a gastrin-secreting tumor of the pancreas. Stimulated by the gastrin, excessive acid secretion occurs in the stomach, and the pH of the duodenal contents is lower than normal. Because of the low pH pancreatic enzymes are inactivated, leading to impaired digestion of fat and protein.

II. *Abnormalities of luminal solubilization.* Absorp-

tion of bile salts normally occurs in the terminal ileum; absence or disease of this intestinal segment can therefore lead to bile salt deficiency. Significant bile salt malabsorption often follows surgical resection of the terminal ileum. Crohn's disease involving the terminal ileum can also lead to bile salt malabsorption.

Abnormal bacterial colonization of the small intestine can occur because of several underlying conditions. These include diseases associated with reduced motility, small intestinal diverticula, and loops of small intestine that have been bypassed, either surgically or as a result of disease—for example, Crohn's disease. Bacteria in the small intestine can deconjugate bile salts. This leads to impaired formation of micelles, with resulting fat malabsorption.

III. *Reduced availability of ingested nutrients.* Besides causing fat malabsorption, abnormal bacterial colonization of the small intestine can lead to malabsorption of vitamin B_{12}. The bacteria are able to bind vitamin B_{12}, which therefore becomes unavailable for absorption by the ileum. Small intestinal infestation with the fish tapeworm *Diphyllobothrium latum* can lead to vitamin B_{12} deficiency, because the worm utilizes the host's dietary B_{12}.

Intrinsic factor deficiency occurs in pernicious anemia and following gastrectomy. In pernicious anemia, there is loss of gastric parietal cells. Because these cells secrete hydrochloric acid and intrinsic factor, individuals with pernicious anemia have achlorhydria in addition to vitamin B_{12} deficiency.

The anion-exchange resin cholestyramine is able to bind bile acids in the intestinal lumen. These bile acids are therefore unavailable for micelle formation, and this leads to malabsorption of fat and fat-soluble vitamins.

IV. *Abnormalities of epithelial cell digestion or transport.* A number of types of disaccharidase deficiency have been described. The commonest of these is *lactase deficiency,* which occurs in a high proportion of individuals in certain African and Asian ethnic groups. It also occurs, but with a lower prevalence, in other individuals. This type of lactase deficiency appears to be recessively inherited. *Sucrase/α-dextrinase deficiency* is a rare genetic abnormality that also shows recessive inheritance. Genetic deficiency of the brush border enzyme *trehalase* has been documented in a small number of individuals. The disaccharide substrate for this enzyme, trehalose, is found in mushrooms. Besides these genetic abnormalities, disaccharidase deficiencies occur as a result of epithelial cell damage—for example, in *celiac disease, Crohn's disease, tropical sprue, viral enteritis,* and *radiation enteritis.* Lactase deficiency is the best known disaccharidase deficiency occurring in association with these diseases. Genetic impairment of glucose and galactose transport by epithelial cells is a rare disorder. It appears to be recessively inherited and presents clinically during infancy.

Nonabsorbed oligosaccharides and monosaccharides are metabolized by colonic bacteria, to produce short-chain fatty acids, carbon dioxide, and hydrogen. Individuals with carbohydrate malabsorption develop abdominal distention, flatulence, and diarrhea after ingesting relevant sugars.

Genetic impairment of vitamin B_{12} transport by ileal absorptive cells ("familial selective vitamin B_{12} malabsorption") is a rare disorder. In this condition, B_{12}/intrinsic factor complexes bind normally to ileal absorptive cells, but transport of B_{12} through these cells appears to be impaired.

As listed in Table 11, a number of diseases can cause loss of normal epithelial cells. In most of these diseases, atrophy of small intestinal villi is a prominent feature. As a result of villus atrophy, the absorptive surface area of the small intestine is greatly reduced. In addition, intestinal epithelial cells are frequently abnormal in these diseases. For example, epithelial cells in *celiac disease* are often cuboidal or relatively flat, in contrast to their normal columnar appearance. Furthermore, the microvilli of these cells are commonly shortened and fused in celiac disease, and cytoplasmic abnormalities can be seen in the cells by electron microscopy. It is likely that all these abnormalities contribute to malabsorption.

Radiation and colchicine affect dividing cells, including those of the intestinal epithelium. In addition, the antibiotic neomycin can produce shortening of small intestinal villi, for reasons that are not clear. Steatorrhea may occur in patients taking neomycin.

V. *Abnormalities of lymphatic transport.* Transport of absorbed nutrients via intestinal lymphatic vessels may be impaired in a number of diseases. *Whipple's disease* is a rare condition in which the small intestinal lamina propria is densely infiltrated with macrophages. These macrophages contain bacilli and may compress lymphatic vessels in the lamina propria. In *small intestinal lymphoma, tuberculosis,* and *Crohn's disease,* lamina propria lymphatic vessels may also be obstructed by mononuclear leukocytes. Furthermore, small intestinal lymphatics can be obstructed by lymphoma in the mesentery or in mesenteric lymph nodes. *Primary intestinal lymphangiectasia* is a rare condition in which intestinal mucosal lymphatic vessels are greatly dilated. Flow of lymph within these vessels appears to be abnormally slow, and lymphatic transport of chylomicrons away from the small intestine is impaired.

A number of disorders that can cause malabsorption are not mentioned in Table 11. Impaired digestion of fat and protein can follow total or partial gastrectomy, probably because food passes abnormally rapidly through the duodenum, allowing insufficient time for adequate mixing with pancreatic enzymes and bile. Patients with *amyloidosis* involving the small intestine may develop malabsorption for reasons that are not clear. Possible mechanisms include small intestinal ischemia resulting from amyloid infiltration of mesenteric arterial branches, reduced small intestinal motility with bacterial colonization of the lumen, and amyloid in the lamina propria acting as a "barrier" to the transport of absorbed nutrients. Malabsorption can occur in various parasitic infestations of the small intestine, including *giardiasis* and *strongyloidiasis.* The mechanisms responsible for this malabsorption are uncertain, although epithelial cell damage by parasites may play a part. Finally, a number of laxatives can cause mild steatorrhea, possibly by increasing the rate at which small intestinal contents are transported through the lumen. An increased transit rate would decrease the time available for assimilation of nutrients.

CLINICAL MANIFESTATIONS

The clinical, hematologic, and biochemical results of malabsorption will be considered only briefly. Patients with malabsorption may develop steatorrhea, weight loss, and muscle wasting, or may present with various specific nutritional deficiencies. These deficiencies may be single or multiple. Important nutrients that may be deficient in patients with malabsorption include vitamin D, calcium, vitamin K, iron, folate, and vitamin B_{12}, in addition to protein. Deficiency of these particular nutrients can, respectively, lead to osteomalacia, muscle weakness and tetany (vitamin D and calcium), impaired blood clotting (vitamin K), microcytic hypochromic anemia (iron), megaloblastic anemia (folate and B_{12}), and muscle wasting and hypoalbuminemia (protein). Several mechanisms can underlie the calcium deficiency associated with steatorrhea. These include vitamin D deficiency and binding of calcium to nonabsorbed long-chain fatty acids in the intestinal lumen. Magnesium is an essential nutrient, although relatively little is known about its mechanism of absorption in human subjects. Deficiency of magnesium can result from malabsorption and produces clinical features similar to those of calcium deficiency, including tetany and muscle weakness. All of these deficiency syndromes have been described in greater detail in the section on nutrition.

Patients with malabsorption can lose excessive amounts of water, sodium, potassium, and bicarbonate via the gastrointestinal tract. The mechanisms of this increased water and electrolyte loss include (1) an osmotic effect of luminal oligosaccharides and monosaccharides, (2) a cathartic effect of long-chain hydroxy fatty acids and nonabsorbed bile acids, which appear to stimulate colonic water and electrolyte secretion, and (3) a possible increase in the secretion of water and electrolytes by the small intestinal epithelium in celiac disease. Hydroxy fatty acids are produced by the action of intestinal bacteria on nonabsorbed long-chain fatty acids.

TESTS FOR MALABSORPTION

The investigation of patients with impaired digestion or absorption has three main objectives: (1) the identification of specific nutritional deficiencies, (2) the documentation of impaired digestion or absorption, and (3) identification of the disease causing these various abnormalities. Table 12 summarizes a number of important diagnostic tests. It will be noted that tests for nutritional deficiency are not mentioned in Table 12. These tests include the measurement of hemoglobin concentration, prothrombin time, and serum calcium, albumin, iron, folate, and vitamin B_{12} levels.

Brief discussion of several tests mentioned in Table 12 may be helpful. The tests will be considered in the order of their presentation in the table.

Fecal Fat. Measurement of the amount of fat in stools collected over a period of three days provides information about the efficiency of fat digestion and absorption. In healthy individuals consuming 80 to 100 grams of fat per day, the 24-hour fecal fat content is approximately 3 to 5 grams. The fecal fat level is greater than this in patients with impaired fat digestion or absorption. Fecal fat measurement does not identify the cause of impaired fat digestion or absorption.

¹⁴C-Triolein Test. Triolein is a triglyceride (trioleoyl glycerol) that can be prepared from radioactive precursor molecules so that each of the three oleic acid residues is labeled with ¹⁴C. In the small intestine, this ¹⁴C-labeled triolein is digested and absorbed by mechanisms identical to those for normal dietary triglycerides. Following digestion and absorption of ¹⁴C-triolein, ¹⁴CO₂ is produced by tissue metabolism and is then exhaled via the lungs. This ¹⁴CO₂ can be quantified in a liquid scintillation counter. Individuals taking part in the triolein test are given ¹⁴C-triolein orally, and subsequently exhale through a tube into hyamine-containing scintillation fluid. ¹⁴CO₂ trapped by the hyamine is then quantified. In the ¹⁴C-triolein test, patients who have impaired fat digestion or absorption show reduced levels of ¹⁴CO₂ in exhaled air, when compared with healthy subjects. Like the fecal fat test mentioned earlier, the ¹⁴C-triolein test can provide information about the efficiency of fat digestion or absorption, without identifying reasons why these processes may be abnormal. A variant of the triolein test has been developed, using triolein labeled with the nonradioactive isotope ¹³C. In this version of the test, exhaled ¹³CO₂ is quantified with a mass spectrometer.

¹⁴C-Bile Salt Breath Test. When given orally to healthy individuals, the bile salt cholyl-¹⁴C-glycine passes along the small intestinal lumen and is largely absorbed in the terminal ileum. This absorbed material then participates in the bile salt enterohepatic circulation. Under normal circumstances, only a small proportion of orally administered cholyl-¹⁴C-glycine remains unabsorbed after passing along the small intestinal lumen. The unabsorbed cholyl-¹⁴C-glycine enters the colon, where bacteria deconjugate it to cholic acid and ¹⁴C-glycine. This glycine is metabolized by colonic bacteria, with the production of ¹⁴CO₂, which is absorbed in the colon and ultimately exhaled via the lungs.

In patients with impaired bile salt absorption, resulting from absence or disease of the terminal ileum, an excessive proportion of orally administered cholyl-¹⁴C-glycine reaches the colon. This leads to an increased rate of ¹⁴CO₂ excretion in exhaled air. Decon-

TABLE 12. INVESTIGATION OF PATIENTS WITH IMPAIRED DIGESTION OR ABSORPTION

TEST	INFORMATION PROVIDED BY TEST
Fecal fat ⎱ ¹⁴C-triolein test ⎰	Fat digestion and absorption
¹⁴C-bile salt breath test	Fate of intraluminal bile salts
Pancreatic function tests	Secretion of pancreatic enzymes and bicarbonate
Schilling test	Vitamin B_{12} absorption
Breath hydrogen ⎱ D-xylose absorption ⎰	Carbohydrate digestion and absorption
Small intestinal x-rays	Anatomic abnormalities of small intestine
Mucosal biopsy of small intestine	⎰ Mucosal histology ⎱ Epithelial cell disaccharidase activities
Stool microscopy	Presence of intestinal parasites

jugation of cholyl-^{14}C-glycine can also occur in the small intestine if this is colonized by bacteria. The resulting $^{14}CO_2$ is absorbed by the intestine, and is subsequently exhaled. After oral administration of cholyl-^{14}C-glycine, the rate of $^{14}CO_2$ exhalation is greater in patients with bacterial colonization of the small intestine than in healthy individuals.

Pancreatic Function Tests. These tests assess the ability of pancreatic exocrine cells to secrete enzymes and bicarbonate in response to different stimuli. In two of these tests, pancreatic secretion is stimulated by intravenous secretin or cholecystokinin, and duodenal fluid is then aspirated through a tube. The activities of pancreatic enzymes and the bicarbonate concentration in this duodenal fluid are determined. Another pancreatic function test (Lundh test) involves giving a liquid test meal by mouth and collecting duodenal fluid at intervals over a period of several hours. In this procedure, the test meal contains fat, protein, and carbohydrate. Trypsin activity is measured in duodenal fluid obtained during this test; it normally increases after the test meal has been given. In patients with pancreatic disease causing impaired digestion or absorption, pancreatic function tests may reveal subnormal output of pancreatic enzymes or bicarbonate.

The Schilling Test. In this test of vitamin B_{12} absorption, 0.5 to 1.0 μg of radioactive vitamin B_{12} is given by mouth. The radioactive isotope used to label the B_{12} molecule is usually ^{57}Co or ^{58}Co. When the radioactive vitamin B_{12} is given orally, a "loading" dose of 1000 μg of nonradioactive B_{12} is also given, by intramuscular injection. The purpose of this loading dose is to saturate hepatic binding sites for B_{12}, thus reducing the chance that any radioactive B_{12} that has been absorbed by the intestine might be retained in the liver. After giving the radioactive and the nonradioactive B_{12}, urine is collected for 24 hours. The amount of radioactivity appearing in the urine indicates the amount of radioactive B_{12} that was absorbed in the small intestine and then excreted via the kidneys. In comparison to healthy individuals, patients with impaired B_{12} absorption show diminished urinary excretion of an oral dose of radioactive B_{12}. This form of the Schilling test does not identify the mechanism of impaired B_{12} absorption. Intrinsic factor deficiency and ileal disease can be distinguished by comparing the urinary excretion of radioactive B_{12} given orally with and without added intrinsic factor. If vitamin B_{12} deficiency is the result of bacterial colonization of the small intestine, an oral dose of radioactive B_{12} will be poorly absorbed. In this condition, vitamin B_{12} absorption may become normal after the intestinal bacteria have been destroyed by antibiotic treatment. Whole body counting, after giving radioactive vitamin B_{12} by mouth, is an alternative method to the Schilling test for assessing B_{12} absorption.

Breath Hydrogen. In patients with impaired digestion or absorption of carbohydrates, oligosaccharides and monosaccharides can enter the colon. Here they are metabolized by luminal bacteria to yield various products, including hydrogen gas. Some of this hydrogen is absorbed by the colon and ultimately exhaled via the lungs. After oral intake of relevant sugars, patients with disaccharidase deficiency or impaired monosaccharide absorption show increased levels of breath hydrogen. In addition, patients with bacterial colonization of the small intestine may exhale more hydrogen than normal subjects because of carbohydrate metabolism by small intestinal bacteria. Hydrogen levels in exhaled air can be measured by gas chromatography.

D-Xylose Absorption. This pentose (5-carbon) sugar is absorbed in the small intestine both by passive diffusion and by active transport via the same pathway utilized by glucose and galactose. In comparison with the other two monosaccharides, D-xylose has a low affinity for this active transport process. After D-xylose absorption, a limited amount of it is metabolized, and the rest is excreted in the urine. In the xylose absorption test, D-xylose is given by mouth in a dose of either 5 g or, more commonly, 25 g. Urine is then collected for a five-hour period, and the amount of D-xylose in this urine sample is determined. Under normal circumstances, at least 4 g of xylose will be excreted in a 5-hour urine sample collected from an individual given 25 g of xylose by mouth. Lower levels of urinary xylose are seen in various conditions. These include impaired absorption of monosaccharides in patients with small intestinal diseases such as celiac disease, renal disease causing impaired xylose excretion, and ascites, because some of the xylose may be retained in the ascitic fluid. In addition, bacteria in the small intestinal lumen can metabolize D-xylose. Therefore, urinary excretion of oral xylose may be subnormal in patients with bacterial colonization of the small intestine. If the bacteria are destroyed by antibiotic treatment, the xylose absorption test may then be normal.

Measurement of plasma xylose levels can be helpful in assessing xylose absorption. One hour after xylose is given by mouth, the plasma xylose level will be lower in patients with impaired absorption than in healthy subjects. By contrast, plasma xylose levels at this point in time are likely to be similar in healthy individuals and patients with renal impairment or ascites. As mentioned previously, measurement of urinary xylose often fails to distinguish reduced absorption from ascitic retention or impaired urinary excretion of xylose, when xylose has been given orally. Xylose absorption does not require prior digestion, so it is sometimes used to distinguish malabsorption due to pancreatic exocrine deficiency (in which it should be normal) from that caused by intestinal disease (in which it tends to be abnormal).

Radiographs of the Small Intestine. In patients with impaired digestion or absorption, barium sulfate radiographs of the small intestine may be helpful by revealing anatomic abnormalities. These include small intestinal diverticula, which may be colonized by bacteria, and areas of luminal narrowing or fistulas between loops of small intestine—features of *Crohn's disease.*

Mucosal Biopsy of the Small Intestine. Several diseases that are responsible for impaired digestion or absorption have a characteristic histologic appearance (Table 13). In patients with parasitic diseases such as *giardiasis,* mucosal biopsy of the small intestine may be diagnostic by revealing parasites and allowing them to be identified. Mucosal biopsy may also be valuable in patients with suspected disaccharidase deficiency,

TABLE 13. HISTOLOGIC APPEARANCES OF SMALL INTESTINE IN DISEASES CAUSING IMPAIRED DIGESTION OR ABSORPTION

DISEASE	MAJOR HISTOLOGIC ABNORMALITIES
Celiac disease	Villus flattening, crypt hyperplasia, increased lymphocytes and plasma cells in lamina propria
Whipple's disease	Numerous macrophages in lamina propria, bacilli in macrophages, broad villi, dilated lymphatics in lamina propria
Lymphoma	Malignant lymphocytes or histiocytes in wall of intestine, villus flattening
Tropical sprue	Villi short and broad, increased lymphocytes and plasma cells in lamina propria
Crohn's disease	Granulomas, increased lymphocytes and plasma cells in wall of intestine, villus flattening, ulceration
Eosinophilic gastroenteritis	Numerous eosinophils in wall of intestine
Amyloidosis	Amyloid in muscle layers, blood vessels, and lamina propria
Lymphangiectasia	Dilated lymphatics in lamina propria
Abetalipoproteinemia	Epithelial absorptive cells distended by lipid

by providing tissue for direct measurement of epithelial cell disaccharidase activities.

SMALL INTESTINAL PROTEIN LOSS

Several diseases can cause excessive loss of plasma protein from the gastrointestinal tract ("protein-losing gastroenteropathy"). In patients with impaired digestion or absorption of dietary proteins, excessive loss of endogenous protein via the intestine can occur. This may contribute to protein malnutrition. Patients with excessive loss of protein can develop hypoalbuminemia with resulting edema or ascites. Under normal circumstances, small amounts of plasma proteins enter the lumen of the gastrointestinal tract. Studies with marker proteins such as ^{51}Cr-albumin have suggested that up to 1 per cent of plasma protein is normally lost into the lumen of the gastrointestinal tract per day. The rate of plasma protein loss is greater than this in patients with protein-losing gastroenteropathy.

It is not known how plasma proteins normally reach the lumen of the gastrointestinal tract. Some leakage of plasma protein into the lumen may occur at the tips of small intestinal villi, in association with normal sloughing of epithelial cells. However, this is conjectural. Several mechanisms may account for disease-associated leakage of protein into the gastrointestinal lumen. These include mucosal ulceration in which plasma proteins reach the lumen by leaking from the ulcerated area. Excessive gastrointestinal loss of plasma protein can also be seen in mucosal diseases without ulceration. The underlying mechanisms of plasma protein leakage in these diseases are not known. Damage to epithelial cells, with or without loss of these cells, may be partly responsible, but precisely how this might cause plasma protein leakage is unclear. Protein loss into the lumen of the gastrointestinal tract also occurs in patients with impaired flow of lymph within intestinal lymphatic vessels. This can occur in *primary intestinal lymphangiectasia* and in other diseases that cause increased hydrostatic pressure inside lymphatics. In diseases of this general type, protein loss into the gastrointestinal lumen appears to be the result of leakage from within lymphatic vessels.

In addition to protein, lymphocytes may also leak out of dilated intestinal lymphatics and be lost from the body via the gastrointestinal lumen. The blood lymphocyte count in patients with primary intestinal lymphangiectasia can be abnormally low because of this process. Some diseases that cause excessive protein loss from the gastrointestinal tract are listed in Table 14. By contrast with the nephrotic syndrome, in which low molecular weight plasma proteins are frequently lost selectively, plasma protein loss via the gastrointestinal tract appears to be nonselective.

Investigation of patients with suspected protein-losing gastroenteropathy has two principal aims: (1) to show that excessive protein loss is actually occurring via the gastrointestinal tract and (2) to identify the disease process responsible for this loss. Radiolabeled proteins can be used to quantify gastrointestinal protein loss; an intravenous injection of the protein is given and stools are collected over a period of several

TABLE 14. CAUSES OF EXCESSIVE LOSS OF PLASMA PROTEINS FROM THE GASTROINTESTINAL TRACT

TYPE OF LESION	DISEASE
Mucosal ulceration	Erosive gastritis, Crohn's disease, ulcerative colitis, pseudomembranous enterocolitis
Mucosal disease without ulceration	Giant hypertrophic gastritis (Menetrier's disease), celiac disease, tropical sprue, blind loop syndrome, *Capillaria philippinensis* infestation*
Impaired lymphatic flow, with leakage of lymph into lumen of intestine	Primary intestinal lymphangiectasia, lymphoma of small intestine, Whipple's disease, constrictive pericarditis, tricuspid valve regurgitation

Modified from Sleisenger, M. H., and Fordtran, J. S. (eds.): Gastrointestinal Disease. 3rd ed. Philadelphia, W. B. Saunders Co., 1983, p. 283.

Capillaria philippinensis is a nematode worm that colonizes the small intestinal mucosa. It occurs in the Philippines and elsewhere in Southeast Asia.

days. The amount of radioisotope excreted in the stools is compared with the total dose of the isotope that was given intravenously, in order to determine the rate at which protein is entering the gastrointestinal lumen. One of the most useful proteins for studying the rate of gastrointestinal protein loss is ^{51}Cr-labeled albumin. The radioisotope ^{51}Cr has the advantage that it is not secreted into the gastrointestinal lumen in significant quantities if it becomes detached from the carrier protein. A further advantage is that ^{51}Cr is poorly absorbed from the lumen of the gastrointestinal tract. Other macromolecules that may be useful for quantifying gastrointestinal protein loss include ^{67}Cu-labeled ceruloplasmin and ^{59}Fe-labeled iron–dextran. Radioactive iodine–labeled macromolecules are unsuitable for this purpose, because any iodine that becomes detached from the carrier molecule can then be secreted into the gastrointestinal lumen or absorbed from this site. Plasma alpha$_1$-antitrypsin can act as a "natural" marker of gastrointestinal protein loss. It normally enters the intestinal lumen in small amounts; however, unlike other plasma proteins, it resists destruction by pancreatic proteases. The fecal concentration of alpha$_1$-antitrypsin can be measured immunologically and compared with the level in plasma to provide information about the rate of gastrointestinal protein leakage. The advantage of this particular marker protein is its nonradioactivity.

Diagnostic techniques for identifying diseases causing protein loss overlap with techniques used to identify causes of malabsorption (see above).

DIARRHEA

Diarrhea can be defined as an abnormal increase in the amount of fluid excreted via rectum. When the fecal water content exceeds 200 ml per 24 hours, diarrhea can arbitrarily be said to occur. Increased stool frequency is a common feature of diarrhea.

Four general types of diarrhea are recognized: (1) *osmotic* diarrhea, (2) *secretory* diarrhea, (3) diarrhea resulting from *defective ion absorption*, and (4) *motor* diarrhea.

OSMOTIC DIARRHEA

Osmotic diarrhea results from the effect of poorly absorbed solutes in the lumen of the gastrointestinal tract. Solutes that can cause osmotic diarrhea include oligosaccharides, monosaccharides, and poorly absorbed ions such as magnesium, sulfate, and phosphate. Oligosaccharides and monosaccharides in the intestinal lumen do not cause diarrhea under normal circumstances, but can do so in patients with disaccharidase deficiencies or with impaired absorption of monosaccharides. Under these circumstances, the low molecular weight sugars remain in the intestinal lumen instead of being absorbed, and exert an osmotic pressure in the ileum and colon. Colonic bacteria metabolize low molecular weight sugars to produce short-chain fatty acids—including butyric and propionic acids—which appear to be readily absorbed and utilized as energy sources by colonic epithelial cells. Therefore, colonic bacteria may limit the osmotic diar-

rhea resulting from poorly absorbed low molecular weight sugars.

When poorly absorbed solutes are present in the lumen of the small intestine, the intraluminal osmotic pressure is greater than normal. Because of this, water enters the intestinal lumen bringing sodium and chloride passively in the same direction (solvent drag). Although sodium, chloride, and water are then absorbed to some extent in the distal small intestine and colon, the poorly absorbed solute remains in the lumen of the intestine and continues to exert an osmotic effect. Therefore, the fecal water content is greater than normal. Since osmotic diarrhea is dependent on ingested sources of osmotically active substances, it characteristically ceases when the patient fasts. Furthermore, there is a fecal solute gap in that the normal fecal electrolytes account for less of the fecal fluid osmolality than normal.

SECRETORY DIARRHEA

As discussed earlier in this chapter, electrolytes and water are absorbed and also secreted by the small intestinal epithelium. If secretion exceeds absorption, secretory diarrhea can result. Abnormally increased secretion of electrolytes and water by the colon—for example, in response to hydroxy fatty acids and nonabsorbed bile acids—can also lead to secretory diarrhea.

Some causes of secretory diarrhea are indicated in Table 15. The profuse secretory diarrhea that occurs in cholera can be considered as a prototype of the pathogenesis of this group of disorders. The clinical and pathophysiologic features of this disease are caused by a potent exotoxin released by the causative organism, *Vibrio cholerae*, in the small intestinal lumen. In cholera, the intestinal mucosa is histologically normal and is not invaded by the causative bacterium. Cholera toxin is a protein molecule with a molecular weight of 84,000 daltons. The molecule consists of two different types of subunit—designated A and B—with five B subunits surrounding a single A subunit. The toxin molecule becomes attached to epithelial cell membranes through binding of the B subunit to a receptor on the membrane—ganglioside G_{M_1}—and the A subunit binds to adenylate cyclase on the inner surface of the cell membrane, activating this enzyme. Following enzyme activation, the concentration of cyclic AMP inside epithelial cells increases. The cyclic

TABLE 15. CAUSES OF SECRETORY DIARRHEA

Bacterial exotoxins	*Vibrio cholerae, Escherichia coli, Shigella* species, *Yersinia enterocolitica*
Hormones and neurotransmitters	Vasoactive intestinal peptide, prostaglandins, calcitonin, serotonin (5-hydroxytryptamine)
Bile acids (in colon)	
Laxatives	Ricinoleic acid, phenolphthalein, dioctyl sodium sulfosuccinate, bisacodyl, anthraquinones
Intestinal distention (partial intestinal obstruction)	

AMP stimulates secretion of chloride and bicarbonate by epithelial cells. Because of the electrochemical gradient established by anion secretion, sodium also leaves the cells. In cholera, electrolyte and water secretion by epithelial cells exceeds absorption of these substances. The colon is unable to absorb the large volume of fluid presented to it by the small intestine, and this leads to profuse watery diarrhea. Cholera toxin does not interfere with glucose-linked sodium absorption by epithelial cells. Because of this, cholera can be treated by giving patients an oral solution of glucose and sodium chloride. However, these patients also usually need a large amount of intravenous fluid replacement.

A number of other bacterial exotoxins cause secretory diarrhea. Toxigenic *Escherichia coli* produce a heat-labile and a heat-stable toxin, both of which cause secretory diarrhea. The heat-labile toxin acts like cholera toxin, by stimulating epithelial cell adenylate cyclase. The heat-stable toxin appears to activate guanylate cyclase, increasing the level of cyclic GMP inside epithelial cells. There is some evidence that cyclic GMP increases ion secretion by the cells, leading to secretory diarrhea. Other bacteria, including *Shigella* species and *Yersinia enterocolitica,* produce exotoxins that appear to stimulate electrolyte and water secretion by epithelial cells. However, the precise mechanisms responsible for this increased secretion are not yet clear.

Various other substances—including hormones, laxatives, and other drugs—are able to promote electrolyte and water secretion by the small intestinal epithelium. Some of these materials act by increasing the cyclic AMP level in epithelial cells. Vasoactive intestinal peptide (VIP) and prostaglandin E1 stimulate adenylate cyclase, whereas xanthine derivatives such as theophylline inhibit the enzyme phosphodiesterase that hydrolyzes cyclic AMP. Serotonin, calcitonin, and glucagon stimulate ion secretion by intestinal epithelial cells. The mechanisms responsible for this effect are not known, although serotonin may act by increasing the intracellular concentration of calcium. Laxatives may induce secretion of electrolytes and water in both the small intestine and colon. Laxatives with this property include ricinoleic acid, phenolphthalein, and anthraquinone derivatives. It is not clear whether this increased secretion is mediated by cyclic AMP.

Secretory diarrhea associated with intestinal distention may be the result of increased permeability of the intestinal epithelium, with leakage of electrolytes and water into the intestinal lumen. Endocrine tumors that cause secretory diarrhea will be discussed later.

Diarrhea from Defective Ion Absorption

In congenital chloridorrhea, diarrhea is associated with defective chloride absorption. As discussed previously, ileal and colonic absorption of chloride, in exchange for bicarbonate, is impaired in this disease. As a consequence of losing excessive amounts of chloride, patients with this condition develop metabolic alkalosis.

Diarrhea from Motor Abnormalities

Abnormally increased motility of the small intestine or colon can lead to diarrhea through mechanisms that are not clear. However, intestinal contents pass along the lumen more rapidly than normal when the intestinal motility is increased, and the time available for water and electrolyte absorption is therefore reduced. Consequently, the amount of stool water may be abnormally increased. Irritable bowel syndrome and thyrotoxicosis are examples of disorders in which diarrhea is associated with increased intestinal motility.

Diarrhea is a feature of diseases that cause mucosal ulceration of the colon, such as bacillary dysentery and ulcerative colitis. In these conditions, plasma, blood, and pus gain entry to the colonic lumen via areas of ulceration and are present in diarrheal stools. However, other factors also appear to contribute to the diarrhea that occurs in these diseases. In bacillary dysentery, increased fecal loss of water and electrolytes can occur as a result of intestinal secretion induced by *Shigella* exotoxins. In active ulcerative colitis, secretion of electrolytes and water by the colonic mucosa may be increased, possibly in response to locally synthesized prostaglandins. The reasons why diarrhea occurs in patients with carcinoma of the colon, or intestinal parasitic diseases such as giardiasis, are largely unknown.

RESULTS OF DIARRHEA

Patients with diarrhea can lose substantial amounts of water, sodium, chloride, and potassium in their fecal fluid. Such losses are particularly large in patients with secretory diarrhea caused by *Vibrio cholerae* toxin or a vasoactive intestinal peptide (VIP)-secreting pancreatic tumor. These patients may excrete several liters of fecal fluid per day, and can rapidly become dehydrated and electrolyte-depleted. If water and electrolytes are not replaced, death may soon follow. Metabolic acidosis is common in patients with severe diarrhea, because of excessive bicarbonate loss in the stools. In contrast, bicarbonate retention is a feature of congenital chloridorrhea, and leads to metabolic alkalosis.

IMMUNOLOGY OF THE SMALL INTESTINE

Like the respiratory tract, the gastrointestinal tract has a large epithelial surface area that is exposed to environmental antigenic materials. In the case of the gastrointestinal tract, these include dietary antigens, normal microbial flora, and pathogenic organisms. Much of the gastrointestinal mucosa of healthy individuals consists of "immunologically active" cells. These include antigen-presenting cells (macrophages and dendritic cells), lymphocytes, and plasma cells. In addition, mast cells, eosinophils, and neutrophil polymorphonuclear leukocytes are present within the gastrointestinal mucosa.

The small intestinal mucosa is able to mount immunologic responses against luminal pathogenic organisms and bacterial toxins. On the other hand, food antigens and normal microbial flora in the intestinal lumen do not usually elicit significant immune responses. It is not known how the gastrointestinal tract is able to classify luminal antigenic materials as either "harmful" or "harmless"—that is, to determine whether or not an immune response should be mounted against a particular antigenic stimulus. In this discussion, different aspects of the normal immunologic behavior of the small intestine will be summarized first. Intestinal features of immunodeficiency states will then be considered. Finally, immunologic aspects of a number of gastrointestinal diseases will be discussed, with particular reference to the pathogenesis of these diseases.

DISTRIBUTION AND PROPERTIES OF IMMUNOLOGICALLY ACTIVE CELLS IN NORMAL SMALL INTESTINE

Most of the immunologically active cells within the small intestine are found in the mucosa. These cells are distributed in three principal compartments: (1) Peyer's patches, (2) diffusely in the lamina propria, and (3) the epithelium of intestinal villi.

Peyer's patches, part of the so-called "organized lymphoid tissue" of the gastrointestinal tract (along with the tonsils, lymphoid tissue of the appendix, and solitary lymphoid follicles in the small intestine and colon), consist of groups of lymphoid follicles located in the mucosa and submucosa of the small intestine.

There is considerable evidence that immunologic responses against luminal antigens are initiated in Peyer's patches. The epithelium over Peyer's patch lymphoid follicles contains cells termed *M cells,* which appear to be specialized for "sampling" luminal antigens. The cytoplasm of M cells extends down from the epithelial surface in a shell-like configuration, enclosing lymphocytes and macrophages (Fig. 34). Intact protein molecules and virus particles can be transported from the intestinal lumen, through the cytoplasm of M cells, to the subjacent macrophages and lymphocytes. It is reasonable to infer that transport of luminal antigenic materials through M cells may be the first step in the local immunologic response to these materials.

Lymphoid follicles within Peyer's patches each contain a germinal center filled predominantly with dividing B lymphocytes. The follicles are separated from each other by interfollicular zones that contain mainly T lymphocytes. The patches enlarge after birth, in response to antigenic materials within the intestinal lumen, are largest in adolescence, and then decrease in size in later life. Germ-free mice challenged with oral bacteria and viruses show growth of Peyer's patches, and the development of germinal centers in their lymphoid follicles. Lymphocytes appear in Peyer's patches by different mechanisms; T cells and some B cells enter directly from the blood, whereas other B cells arise by mitosis in germinal centers.

Peyer's patches are important for intestinal immunologic responses. For example, if *Shigella* organisms or cholera toxoid are introduced into small intestinal loops of rabbits or rats, vigorous local production of specific IgA occurs if the loops contain Peyer's patches, but the response is subnormal in their absence. IgA is not actually released from the patches, but they initiate immunologic responses—whether antibody-mediated or cell-mediated—that take place elsewhere in the gut.

Inside Peyer's patches, presentation of antigen to lymphocytes may occur by the action of local antigen-presenting cells. Introduction of antigens into the small

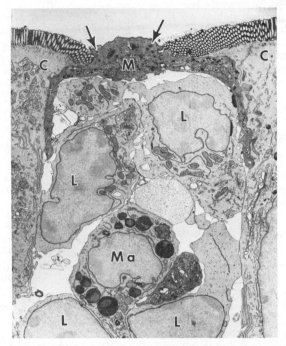

Figure 34. Electron micrograph of mouse Peyer's patch epithelium. An M cell is shown (M), with adjacent columnar epithelial cells (C). Below the M cell, there are four lymphocytes (L) and a macrophage (Ma). Horseradish peroxidase was introduced into the intestinal lumen and has been taken up by the M cell (vesicles containing peroxidase are indicated by arrows). (Modified from Owen, R. L.: In Nieuwenhuis, P., van den Broek, A. A., and Hanna, M. G., Jr. (eds.): In Vivo Immunology; Adv Exp Med Biol, 149:509, 1982. New York, Plenum Publishing Corporation. Used by permission.)

intestinal lumen can lead to the appearance, in Peyer's patch germinal centers, of B lymphocytes bearing surface immunoglobulin (Ig) directed against those antigens and destined to become Ig-secreting plasma cells. During this maturation process, the B cells migrate out of Peyer's patches, enter mesenteric lymph nodes, and then pass into thoracic duct lymph. From here, the cells enter the blood and circulate to the lamina propria of the gastrointestinal tract (and to mucosae of the respiratory tract, female genital tract, and mammary glands) to secrete immunoglobulins, particularly IgA. B lymphocytes within germinal centers of Peyer's patches initially bear IgM on their surfaces, but can "switch" from IgM to IgA expression under the influence of a population of Peyer's patch T cells. Terminal differentiation of IgA-expressing B cells into IgA-secreting plasma cells appears to be driven by a separate and distinct population of helper T lymphocytes, probably located in mesenteric lymph nodes.

The lamina propria normally contains numerous lymphocytes and plasma cells, arranged in an apparently random fashion, as well as macrophages, eosinophils, and mast cells. Under normal circumstances in the human intestinal lamina propria approximately 70 to 80 per cent of the plasma cells contain IgA, 15 to 20 per cent contain IgM, and the rest contain IgE or IgG. Most of the lymphocytes within the lamina propria and within the epithelium of intestinal villi are T cells, the functions of which are largely unknown. Most of the T cells in the lamina propria of the human small intestine belong to the helper/inducer subset while those within the intestinal epithelium appear to be cytotoxic/suppressor T cells, some of which cytologically resemble natural killer (NK) cells, or even mast cells. Indeed, populations of intestinal lymphocytes have been shown to exert spontaneous, antibody-dependent (K-cell), and lectin-induced (putative T-cell) cytotoxicity.

IMMUNOLOGIC EFFECTOR MECHANISMS IN THE SMALL INTESTINE

Immunologic effector mechanisms can be classified as either humoral (antibody-mediated) or cell-mediated (see discussion in section on immunology).

Humoral Mechanisms

In healthy human subjects, IgA accounts for most of the immunoglobulin produced by the small intestine. IgA is released from plasma cells in the lamina propria, as double molecules (dimers) of the immunoglobulin. These consist of two molecules of monomeric IgA joined by a polypeptide called the J chain. Much of the dimeric IgA is exported from the lamina propria into the intestinal lumen, which is the main site where the IgA exerts its biologic effects. To reach the intestinal lumen, dimeric IgA in the lamina propria binds to a glycoprotein on the basal and lateral surfaces of intestinal columnar epithelial cells, known as secretory component. Dimeric IgA bound to secretory component (secretory IgA) is transported through intestinal epithelial cells, crosses the apical membranes of these cells, and enters the intestinal lumen. In addition, it can leave the lamina propria via intestinal lymphatic vessels, enter thoracic duct lymph, and hence reach the blood (Fig. 35).

Experimentally, specific IgA in the intestinal lumen prevents cholera toxin and pathogenic bacteria from binding to the apical surfaces of epithelial cells. IgA may be important in the elimination of protozoan parasites from the intestine as well. For example, *Giardia lamblia* trophozoites obtained from the human small intestinal lumen have been found to be coated with IgA.

Secretory IgA also reaches the intestinal lumen via bile, which it presumably enters from the plasma by crossing bile ductule epithelial cells and possibly hepatic parenchymal cells. Biliary IgA is largely dimeric, and its secretory component seems to be added to the IgA molecules while these are being transported from plasma to bile across bile ductule epithelium or hepatocytes. The significance of IgA transport from plasma to bile is not yet entirely clear. There is some evidence that this transport process may help to rid the plasma of immune complexes consisting of antigens bound to IgA. The physiologic functions of intestinal IgM, IgE, and IgG are obscure.

Cell-Mediated Mechanisms

At present, very little is known about the role of cell-mediated immunologic effector mechanisms in the normal small intestine. Mice fed with tumor cells from allogeneic donor animals will develop precursors of tumor-directed cytotoxic T cells in their Peyer's patches. Similarly, intraperitoneal injection of allogeneic tumor cells into mice is followed by the appearance of anti-tumor cytotoxic T lymphocytes in the small intestinal lamina propria. T cells are probably involved in the immunologic response of the intestine to protozoan and helminth parasites, but whether they kill parasites directly or act as helper cells for production of anti-parasite immunoglobulin is not known.

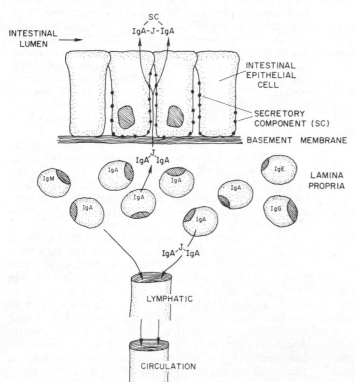

Figure 35. Transport of IgA into the intestinal lumen. Dimeric IgA containing J chain is secreted by plasma cells in the lamina propria. After coupling to secretory component (SC) on the basal and lateral surfaces of epithelial cells, dimeric IgA is transported (as secretory IgA) through the cells into the lumen. Dimeric IgA produced in the lamina propria can also enter lymphatic vessels and then reach the blood. (Modified from Kagnoff, M. F.: In Johnson, L. R. (ed.): Physiology of the Gastrointestinal Tract. New York, Raven Press, 1981. Used by permission.)

INTESTINAL FEATURES OF IMMUNODEFICIENCY SYNDROMES

A number of immunodeficiency syndromes predispose to gastrointestinal infection. Traditionally, immunodeficiency states have usually been classified as abnormalities of either B cell or T cell function, in addition to "combined" T and B cell abnormalities in some cases of childhood immunodeficiency. While this classification still provides a useful framework for discussion, it is now known that abnormally low immunoglobulin production may be the result of abnormal T cell behavior rather than a sign of intrinsic B cell malfunction. Thus, reduced activity of helper T cells or increased activity of suppressor T cells may lead to depressed production of immunoglobulin by B cells and plasma cells.

B Cell Disorders. *Selective IgA deficiency* occurs in approximately 1 in 700 adults. This does not appear to be a single disorder; most of the affected individuals have reduced IgA levels in serum and intestinal secretions, while a small proportion have deficient IgA levels in only one of these sites. There is evidence that selective IgA deficiency is the result of intrinsic failure of B cells to produce IgA in some patients, and the result of excessive suppressor T cell activity in others. Selective IgA deficiency is frequently associated with diarrhea, although the mechanism of this association is not always clear. Chronic intestinal *Candida albicans* infection has been described in association with secretory component deficiency and absence of IgA in the intestinal fluid.

"Common variable immunoglobulin deficiency" (CVID) refers to a heterogeneous group of abnormalities, in which affected individuals have reduced serum immunoglobulin levels. Most of these individuals have a subnormal level of serum IgG, frequently in association with low serum IgM and IgA levels. As in the case of selective IgA deficiency, there is evidence that CVID can reflect intrinsic failure of B cell development in some patients or elevated activity of suppressor T cells in others. CVID usually presents clinically in childhood, adolescence, or early adult life. Approximately 60 per cent of patients with CVID have been found to have diarrhea, which is commonly associated with steatorrhea and intestinal *Giardia lamblia* infection. *"Nodular lymphoid hyperplasia"* (NLH) refers to the presence of abnormally large nodules of lymphoid tissue in the small intestinal lamina propria. It usually occurs in association with CVID or selective IgA deficiency; probably because of immunoglobulin deficiency, patients with NLH often have giardiasis. Nearly all of the cells in the hyperplastic lymphoid nodules are IgM-expressing B cells. IgA-bearing B cells are absent from these nodules, suggesting that NLH may represent failure of intestinal B-cell switching from IgM to IgA expression.

X-linked immunoglobulin deficiency is a severe inherited immunodeficiency syndrome in which plasma cells and B lymphocytes are lacking in the intestine and elsewhere. These patients can develop giardiasis and steatorrhea, but gastrointestinal problems are less frequent than in common variable immunoglobulin deficiency.

T Cell Disorders. In *thymic hypoplasia* (DiGeorge syndrome) embryonic development of the third and fourth pharyngeal pouches is defective, leading to impaired formation of the parathyroids and the thymus. Infants with this disorder can develop chronic diarrhea and malabsorption. The pathogenesis of these gastrointestinal problems is not clear, but they are sometimes associated with oral *Candida albicans* infection. Infants with *"severe combined immunodeficiency"* have genetic impairment of T and B cell function, related in some instances to deficiency of the enzyme adenosine deaminase. Chronic oral *Candida albicans* infection, diarrhea, and malabsorption are prominent features of severe combined immunodeficiency. It is not known whether intestinal virus infections are partly responsible for the diarrhea which occurs in infants with T cell deficiency syndromes.

Since 1980, *acquired immune deficiency syndrome* (AIDS) has been increasingly recognized in certain groups of individuals. These include homosexual males, intravenous drug abusers, Haitians, and hemophiliacs who have received intravenous infusions of blood clotting factors. There is strong evidence that AIDS is caused by a retrovirus designated HTLV-3, which infects human helper T cells. Patients with AIDS have reduced numbers of helper T lymphocytes in the blood. The ratio of helper:suppressor T lymphocytes in the blood of healthy individuals is normally around 2:1 but can fall to less than 1:1 in AIDS. Opportunistic infections are common in patients with AIDS, including a number of infections involving the intestine. A variety of organisms are responsible for these infections, including *Cryptosporidium* species. This protozoan parasite colonizes the luminal surfaces of epithelial cells in the small intestine (Fig. 36) and, for unknown reasons, causes profuse watery diarrhea. Another protozoan parasite, *Isospora belli,* and *Mycobacterium avium–intracellulare* also cause opportunistic infection of the small intestine in AIDS. Macrophages within the intestinal lamina propria of some patients with AIDS have been shown to contain large numbers of *M. avium-intracellulare* organisms in their cytoplasm. It is not known whether intestinal helper T lymphocytes are depleted in patients with AIDS or whether such depletion might predispose to the intestinal infections that occur in these patients.

GRAFT VERSUS HOST DISEASE

In human subjects, graft versus host disease (GVHD) is usually seen as a complication of bone marrow transplantation. GVHD occurs when an immunodeficient host receives immunocompetent lymphocytes from a donor whose histocompatibility antigens differ from those of the recipient. The donor lymphocytes perceive their new antigenic environment as foreign and consequently mount an attack against the recipient's tissues. Although the precise mechanisms of this attack are still unclear, there is evidence that donor T lymphocytes are responsible for graft versus host reactions. The skin, gastrointestinal tract, and liver are the principal sites affected in human GVHD. Necrosis of the small intestinal mucosa and of colonic epithelial cells has been observed in this disorder. Patients with GVHD affecting the gastrointestinal tract can develop profuse watery diarrhea, abdominal pain, and ileus. In addition, they may have impaired absorption of nu-

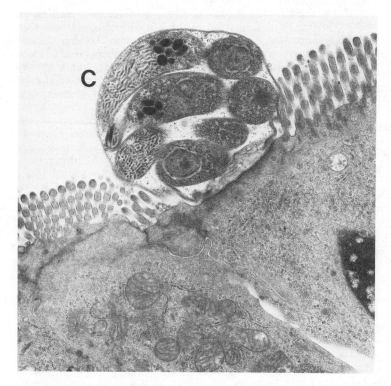

Figure 36. Electron micrograph of a *Cryptosporidium* organism (C) on the surface of a jejunal biopsy specimen from a patient with acquired immune deficiency syndrome. The organism is attached to an epithelial cell. (Modified from Owen, R. L., and Brandborg, L. L.: Clin Gastroenterol 12:575, 1983.)

trients, and loss of plasma albumin into the lumen of the intestine.

ALPHA CHAIN DISEASE

In this condition, the small intestinal mucosa becomes infiltrated with a clone of plasma cells that produce an abnormal form of IgA. The protein consists of incomplete heavy chains of IgA and lacks κ or λ light chains. In patients with alpha chain disease, this abnormal protein can be demonstrated in the serum, and in fluid obtained from the lumen of the small intestine. Fully developed alpha chain disease has the histologic and clinical features of a malignant lymphoma. In this phase of the disease, the small intestinal wall is heavily infiltrated with malignant lymphoid cells. The lymphoma can also spread to mesenteric lymph nodes and other extraintestinal sites. At an earlier stage in the development of alpha chain disease, however, the clonal expansion of intestinal plasma cells may be benign. At this stage of the disease, treatment with broad-spectrum antibiotics may lead to remission. The main clinical features of alpha chain disease are diarrhea, steatorrhea, weight loss, and signs of hypoproteinemia. Pathophysiologically, the disease causes malabsorption and protein loss into the small intestinal lumen. When there is overt lymphoma of the small intestine, local hemorrhage and obstruction can occur. Although the pathogenesis of alpha chain disease is not understood, it is possible that it represents an abnormal response to an unidentified infectious organism. The disease is mainly found in the Mediterranean area and the Middle East, and is largely seen in individuals exposed to an unhygienic environment.

CELIAC DISEASE

Some of the histologic features of celiac disease have already been mentioned, namely atrophy of small intestinal villi and morphologic abnormalities of absorptive epithelial cells (Fig. 37). Patients with celiac disease also have an increased number of lymphocytes and plasma cells per unit volume of small intestinal lamina propria. IgA-, IgM-, and IgG-containing plasma cell populations are expanded in the small intestine of most patients with this disorder.

Gluten—a complex mixture of proteins found in wheat, barley, and rye flour—is responsible for the mucosal damage in celiac disease, but the actual mechanism by which the damage occurs is not yet clear. Gluten is an almost universal component of North American and European diets, but only a small proportion of individuals eating these diets actually have celiac disease. Therefore, unknown host factors are important in the genesis of the disorder. The results of HLA typing suggest that genetic factors play a part in the development of celiac disease. Thus, approximately 80 per cent of patients with this condition are HLA-DR3–positive. By contrast, approximately 20 per cent of individuals in a healthy control population bear this HLA antigen. Around 80 per cent of individuals with celiac disease are also HLA-B8–positive, but this may simply reflect the fact that HLA-DR3 and HLA-B8 frequently occur in the same individual—an example of so-called linkage disequilibrium. Genes coding for HLA-DR antigens may be associated with genes that determine the intensity of immunologic responses (see immunology section). Therefore, patients with celiac disease who are HLA-DR3–positive may have an immune response gene that "encodes" an abnormally vigorous immunologic response to gluten. At present, this is a hypothesis and not an established fact.

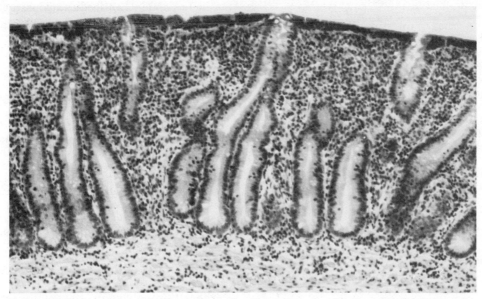

Figure 37. Light micrograph of a section of mucosa from the duodenojejunal junction of a patient with active celiac disease. The mucosal surface is flat, villi are absent, and crypts are hyperplastic. There is increased cellularity of the lamina propria. Crypt hyperplasia in active celiac disease is associated with increased mitotic activity of crypt epithelial cells. (From Sleisenger, M. H., and Fordtran, J. S. (eds.): Gastrointestinal Disease. 3rd ed. Philadelphia, W. B. Saunders Co., 1983.)

Immunologic events seem likely to be important in the pathogenesis of celiac disease. Continued exposure of the intestinal mucosa to gluten is necessary for maintenance of a severely abnormal histologic picture in celiac disease. Several attempts have been made to identify the components of gluten that are necessary for histologic damage in this disorder. *Gliadin* (a mixture of alcohol-soluble proteins) and polypeptides obtained by pepsin-trypsin digestion of gluten will activate celiac disease in asymptomatic patients with this condition. In the presence of gluten, jejunal biopsy specimens from patients with celiac disease synthesize larger quantities of IgA and IgM than corresponding specimens from healthy individuals, and a substantial proportion of that total immunoglobulin is directed against gluten. There is no direct evidence, however, that antigluten antibodies are responsible for the intestinal mucosal damage that occurs in celiac disease. It is not yet known whether cytotoxic T lymphocytes are involved in the pathogenesis of celiac disease.

CHRONIC INFLAMMATORY BOWEL DISEASE

The term "chronic inflammatory bowel disease" embraces Crohn's disease and ulcerative colitis. Of these diseases, ulcerative colitis mainly affects the colon. Nonetheless, it is convenient to consider both diseases together in the present discussion, under the general heading of inflammatory bowel disease (IBD). The various immunologic phenomena described in these disorders show considerable overlap between the two conditions. Furthermore, the significance of most of these phenomena is equally uncertain in the case of both diseases.

The causes of Crohn's disease and ulcerative colitis are unknown. It has frequently been suggested that these diseases may have an infectious origin, although there is no conclusive evidence in favor of this possibility. Both diseases are characterized by episodes of activity alternating with remission. During active phases, the intestinal wall contains abnormally large numbers of lymphocytes and plasma cells. In ulcerative colitis, these cells are mainly present in the lamina propria, whereas in Crohn's disease they are frequently distributed in all layers of the intestinal wall. IgG-containing plasma cells are markedly increased within the intestinal lamina propria of patients with IBD, in comparison with normal intestine, possibly as an immunologic response to antigens that have penetrated the damaged intestinal wall from the lumen. As with other immunologic features of IBD, the increased number of intestinal plasma cells is likely to be the result of more fundamental abnormalities and may provide no direct clues to the pathogenesis of IBD. Increased numbers of T lymphocytes have been demonstrated in the lamina propria, submucosa, and muscle layers of intestine obtained from patients with active Crohn's disease. The functional significance of these T cells is unknown. In comparison with healthy individuals, patients with Crohn's disease can have reduced numbers of T lymphocytes in the blood, possibly because of increased sequestration of these cells in the intestinal wall.

Antibodies against colonic epithelial cells are often demonstrable in the sera of patients with IBD, but of unknown significance. No convincing evidence has ever been obtained that they are responsible for damaging colon cells in vivo. Blood lymphocytes, especially those with Fc receptors, obtained from patients with IBD can exert a cytotoxic effect on colon epithelial cells in vitro. Antibody-dependent cell-mediated (K-cell) cytotoxicity may be involved in this reaction, but the significance of these observations remains unclear.

Intestinal Lymphangiectasia

Patients with primary intestinal lymphangiectasia often lose excess proteins and lymphocytes into the intestinal lumen from the abnormal dilated lymphatic vessels. The serum levels of IgG, IgA, and IgM can be greatly reduced in such patients, in comparison with the levels seen in healthy individuals. Patients with intestinal lymphangiectasia can also have markedly subnormal numbers of lymphocytes in the blood. Because of lymphocyte depletion, these patients may show impaired delayed hypersensitivity as judged by skin testing. Furthermore, lymphocyte depletion in patients with intestinal lymphangiectasia can allow prolonged acceptance of skin allografts by these individuals.

Eosinophilic Gastroenteritis

In this uncommon disorder, excessive numbers of eosinophils infiltrate the mucosa, submucosa, muscle layers, or serosa of the gastric antrum or small intestine. Patients with this condition also have eosinophilia, and can develop malabsorption and loss of plasma proteins into the gastrointestinal lumen.

The pathogenesis of eosinophilic gastroenteritis is not known. It has been suggested with little evidence that this condition represents an allergic response to dietary antigens. In a small number of patients with the disorder, jejunal biopsy specimens have been examined before and after introduction of particular types of food into the lumen of the intestine, but with no convincing evidence that jejunal mucosal eosinophils increase after food challenge. Association of eosinophilic gastroenteritis with asthma, urticaria, and atopic eczema has been described. A possibly distinct form of eosinophilic gastroenteritis has been described in infants in whom the number of eosinophils in the blood and small intestinal mucosa is increased. Ingestion of cow's milk by these infants was shown to induce vomiting, diarrhea, increased loss of plasma albumin in the feces, and an increased eosinophil count in the blood. Several of the infants with this condition have had asthma and eczema. Whether this infantile disorder represents an allergic reaction to cow's milk proteins is not yet clear.

Food Allergy

In human subjects, allergic reactions to a number of types of food have been demonstrated. The best-documented mechanism of food allergy involves IgE antibodies against dietary antigens. Patients with this type of allergy can develop asthma, eczema, urticaria, or rhinorrhea after eating foods to which they are allergic. Types of food associated with this form of allergy include milk, eggs, fish, and nuts. In some affected individuals, serum IgE can be shown to be directed against dietary antigens. The clinical features of IgE-mediated allergic reactions occur because histamine and other "vasoactive" substances are released from mast cells. This release is triggered by the binding of antigen to IgE molecules attached, via their Fc portions, to mast cell surface membranes. Additional mechanisms of food allergy have been proposed, but have not yet been well documented in human subjects.

Serum IgA and IgG antibodies against dietary antigens have been demonstrated in a number of individuals. The significance of these antibodies is unclear, and there is little evidence that they lead to clinical problems.

BACTERIOLOGY OF THE SMALL INTESTINE

Although bacteria are present in the small intestinal lumen of healthy human subjects, the total number of these microorganisms is much smaller than the number of bacteria in the normal colon. Several factors limit the growth of bacteria in the small intestinal lumen of healthy individuals: (1) Gastric acid limits bacterial colonization of the jejunum. (2) Small intestinal peristalsis propels bacteria and other intestinal contents into the colon. (3) Trapping of bacteria in small intestinal mucus may facilitate their peristaltic transport into the colonic lumen. (4) Unconjugated bile acids may inhibit the growth of anaerobic organisms of the genus *Bacteroides*.

In healthy individuals, the jejunum contains up to 10^4 bacteria/g of total contents. By contrast, larger numbers of bacteria are normally present in the lumen of the ileum (10^5 to 10^8/g). Within the human colonic lumen, the total number of bacteria is normally around 10^9 to 10^{12}/g of contents. Bacteria in the normal human jejunum comprise aerobes and facultative anaerobes. Identical organisms and some strict anaerobes are found in the normal human ileum. Anaerobic bacteria that occur in the normal ileum include bacteroides and clostridia. Most of the bacteria in the lumen of the normal human colon are strict anaerobes.

Blind Loop Syndrome

The term "blind loop syndrome" refers to the combination of excessive bacterial colonization of the small intestine and malabsorption of one or more nutrients. Several features of this syndrome have already been discussed—the syndrome will be considered here only briefly.

A variety of anatomic and functional abnormalities can be responsible for the blind loop syndrome; the existence of an actual blind loop of small intestine is not necessary for the development of the syndrome. Various anatomic abnormalities of the small intestine can lead to excessive local bacterial colonization. These include diverticula, strictures, fistulas joining loops of small intestine, and blind-ended afferent loops of duodenum constructed during Billroth II gastrectomy. In addition, a gastrocolic fistula can lead to colonization of the small intestine by colonic bacteria. Excessive growth of bacteria in the small intestinal lumen can also be caused by impaired peristalsis—for example, in patients with scleroderma or idiopathic intestinal pseudo-obstruction. Absence of gastric acid (achlorhydria) is another factor that can promote excessive bacterial colonization of the small intestine. In patients with blind loop syndrome, the bacterial flora of the small intestine resembles that of the normal colon. Strict anaerobes (including bacteroides, anaerobic lactobacilli, and clostridia), and some aerobic bacteria colonize the small intestine of such patients.

As mentioned previously, vitamin B_{12} deficiency is an important consequence of the blind loop syndrome since intraluminal bacteria bind the vitamin, thus reducing its absorption by the patient's intestine. Both free and intrinsic factor-conjugated vitamin B_{12} can be bound to intestinal bacteria. Aerobic organisms such as *Escherichia coli* bind the vitamin much more avidly when it is free than when it is in the conjugated form. By contrast, anaerobic organisms of the genus *Bacteroides* can bind unconjugated and conjugated B_{12} almost equally well. Fat absorption is impaired in the blind loop syndrome, largely because micelle formation in the small intestinal lumen is defective. Bacterial deconjugation of bile salts is thought to be the underlying abnormality that impairs micelle formation. As an additional factor, there is some evidence that unconjugated bile acids can damage absorptive cells of the small intestinal epithelium.

Structural changes have been noted in the small intestinal mucosa of patients with the blind loop syndrome. In such patients, intestinal villi are sometimes shorter than normal, and the microvilli of epithelial cells can also be abnormal. As a result, disaccharidase and peptidase levels in the apical membranes of epithelial cells can be reduced in this syndrome.

TROPICAL SPRUE

Caucasians and members of indigenous population groups can develop tropical sprue, a disorder of unknown cause characterized by malabsorption and usually chronic diarrhea. Associated histologic abnormalities of the small intestinal mucosa range from moderate shortening and thickening of intestinal villi to actual flattening of the intestinal mucosa with loss of villi. Malabsorption of various nutrients can occur in tropical sprue, including folate, vitamin B_{12}, fat, and vitamin D, comparable to gluten-sensitive enteropathy.

There is evidence that intestinal bacteria are involved in the pathogenesis of tropical sprue, but their actual role is not clear. Exotoxin-producing bacteria—including *Escherichia coli* and organisms of the genus *Klebsiella*—have been cultured from the small intestinal contents of patients with tropical sprue. Toxins produced by these bacteria may contribute to the chronic diarrhea of tropical sprue by promoting intestinal secretion of electrolytes and water. Oral antibiotics are often effective therapeutically, leading to improvement in the histologic appearance and absorptive capacity of the intestinal mucosa.

ENDOCRINE TUMORS AND THE SMALL INTESTINE

The normal gastrointestinal mucosa contains a variety of types of hormone-producing cells. Neurons within the intestinal wall also contain a number of peptides, which may function as neurotransmitters. Peptides that have been demonstrated in small intestinal endocrine cells and/or neurons include somatostatin, secretin, cholecystokinin, gastric inhibitory peptide, substance P, motilin, and vasoactive intestinal peptide. In addition, neurons containing peptides identical or similar to enkephalins and bombesin are found in the gastrointestinal tract. Relatively little is known about the physiologic function of most peptide hormones produced in the human small intestine. Furthermore, the roles—if any—of most of these substances in human disease have not been defined. Apart from carcinoid tumors (p. 1220), important endocrine tumors that have an effect on the small intestine are located in extraintestinal sites.

GASTRINOMA

Most gastrin-secreting tumors arise in the pancreas. In addition, a small percentage of gastrin-secreting tumors can originate in nonpancreatic sites, particularly the wall of the duodenum. In more than two thirds of patients with gastrinoma, the tumor is malignant.

The Zollinger-Ellison syndrome, which occurs in patients with pancreatic gastrinoma, is characterized by intractable peptic ulceration, usually of the duodenum or jejunum. This ulceration is the result of markedly increased gastric acid secretion, which, in turn, is a consequence of elevated plasma gastrin levels. Peptic ulcer disease is described more fully on pp. 1192–1194. Gastrin-secreting tumors can also lead to diarrhea. Several mechanisms may contribute to the pathogenesis of diarrhea in this syndrome: (1) Hydrochloric acid may cause diarrhea by damaging epithelial cells in the proximal small intestine. (2) Gastrin may directly contribute to diarrhea by inhibiting sodium and water absorption in the jejunum. (3) Gastrin-secreting tumors can lead to steatorrhea, as a result of the inactivation of pancreatic lipase by acid in the small intestinal lumen. When lipase is inactive, triglyceride hydrolysis is impaired. (4) Micelle formation can also be impaired in patients with Zollinger-Ellison syndrome, because the solubility of bile acids in the intestinal lumen is reduced at low pH. Impaired formation of micelles contributes to fat malabsorption in this syndrome. (5) Malabsorption of vitamin B_{12} is also associated with the Zollinger-Ellison syndrome. The reason for impaired vitamin B_{12} absorption is not entirely clear, but the absorptive defect is not corrected by giving intrinsic factor orally. It is reasonable to speculate that vitamin B_{12} remains bound to R proteins in the small intestinal lumen of patients with Zollinger-Ellison syndrome, because pancreatic proteases (which normally liberate B_{12} from R proteins) are inactivated by the low pH. According to this hypothesis, vitamin B_{12} would not become available for binding to intrinsic factor.

VIPOMA

The term VIPoma indicates a tumor that secretes vasoactive intestinal peptide (VIP). Most VIP-secreting tumors arise in the pancreas; the cells of these pancreatic tumors are commonly thought to be of neural crest origin. Pancreatic VIPomas can be benign or malignant.

VIP-secreting tumors of the pancreas produce a characteristic clinical picture: profuse watery diarrhea, hypokalemia resulting from fecal loss of potassium, and subnormal or absent secretion of gastric acid. These effects are usually attributed to circulating VIP, which is known to promote electrolyte and water secretion by small intestinal epithelial cells (as discussed earlier). Some investigators have suggested that other hormonal substances besides VIP might be responsible for the clinical features observed in patients with pancreatic VIPoma. However, the present consensus is that VIP is responsible for the clinical picture in most—if not all—of these patients.

In a number of individuals with watery diarrhea, hypokalemia, and gastric hypochlorhydria or achlorhydria, the responsible tumor is a ganglioneuroma or ganglioneuroblastoma of the adrenal medulla rather than a pancreatic neoplasm. There is evidence that these patients' gastrointestinal problems are the result of VIP secreted by the adrenal tumor.

SOMATOSTATINOMA

A small number of patients with a somatostatin-producing tumor of the pancreas have been described. Such patients have diarrhea and steatorrhea associated with increased intestinal motility, reduced pancreatic enzyme secretion, and impaired contraction of the gallbladder. These abnormalities can be attributed to increased plasma levels of somatostatin.

MEDULLARY CARCINOMA OF THE THYROID

This tumor arises from calcitonin-producing C cells of the thyroid gland that are derived embryologically from the neural crest. Patients with medullary carcinoma of the thyroid can develop secretory diarrhea. This is caused by calcitonin and/or prostaglandins that are secreted by the tumor cells. It is not known how calcitonin induces electrolyte and water secretion by intestinal epithelial cells. Evidence exists that secretory diarrhea occurring in response to prostaglandins is the result of increased cyclic AMP levels within the intestinal epithelium.

CARCINOID TUMORS

These tumors consist of cells that are able to convert the amino acid L-tryptophan to 5-hydroxytryptophan and usually also to 5-hydroxytryptamine (serotonin)

L-TRYPTOPHAN

    | Tryptophan hydroxylase
    ↓

5-HYDROXYTRYPTOPHAN

    | Aromatic L-amino acid
    | Decarboxylase
    ↓

5-HYDROXYTRYPTAMINE (SEROTONIN)

    | Monoamine oxidase
    ↓

5-HYDROXYINDOLE ACETALDEHYDE

    | Aldehyde dehydrogenase
    ↓

5-HYDROXYINDOLE ACETIC ACID (5-HIAA)

Figure 38. Metabolism of L-tryptophan and its derivatives, in patients with carcinoid syndrome. 5-HIAA is excreted in the urine. (Modified from Sleisenger, M. H., and Fordtran, J. S. (eds.): Gastrointestinal Disease. 3rd ed. Philadelphia, W. B. Saunders Co., 1983.)

(Fig. 38). Like other endocrine cells of the gastrointestinal tract, the normal precursor cells of carcinoid tumors are believed to arise embryologically in the neural crest. More than 90 per cent of carcinoid tumors occur in the gastrointestinal tract—particularly in the appendix, terminal ileum, and rectum. Carcinoid tumors can also arise in the stomach and in the bronchial mucosa.

Metastasis of gastrointestinal carcinoid tumors to the liver leads to the carcinoid syndrome. This is characterized by episodes of flushing of the face and chest and increased motility of the gastrointestinal tract, with vomiting, abdominal pain, and diarrhea, and also bronchoconstriction. Patients with the carcinoid syndrome also frequently develop endocardial fibrosis of the right side of the heart, with tricuspid regurgitation and pulmonary valve stenosis. Carcinoid tumors in the intestinal wall and mesenteric lymph nodes may elicit extensive local fibrosis. This leads to kinking and distortion of the small intestine.

Carcinoid tumors produce a variety of pharmacologically active substances. Serotonin is one of the important products of these tumors and may be responsible for the associated increased gastrointestinal motility. In addition, serotonin may provoke the endocardial and peritoneal fibrosis that accompanies the carcinoid syndrome. In contrast to carcinoid tumors occurring in other sites, primary carcinoid tumors of the stomach frequently lack the decarboxylase enzyme responsible for converting 5-hydroxytryptophan into serotonin (Fig. 38). Consequently, these tumors generally release 5-hydroxytryptophan into the blood rather than serotonin. Besides metabolic products of L-tryptophan, carcinoid tumors can secrete histamine and prostaglandins and can cause the production of various peptides. These peptides include bradykinin, lysyl-bradykinin, and calcitonin. All of these biologically active substances are likely to contribute to the systemic features of the carcinoid syndrome.

SMALL INTESTINAL ISCHEMIA

The blood supply of the stomach, small intestine, and colon is largely provided by three major arteries. These are the celiac axis, superior mesenteric artery, and inferior mesenteric artery. Anastomotic vessels link the proximal branches of these three major arteries. The anastomoses connect branches of each individual major artery and also link the territories of the three major vessels. Because of these anastomoses, occlusion of a single proximal branch of one of the major arteries rarely leads to infarction in the wall of the gastrointestinal tract. By contrast, occlusion of the superior mesenteric artery close to its origin from the aorta is a relatively frequent cause of small intestinal infarction. This occlusion can occur for a variety of reasons—including local atheroma, dissecting aortic aneurysm, or an embolus that becomes lodged.

The small intestine receives most of its blood supply via branches of the superior mesenteric artery. The distal branches of this vessel appear to be end arteries—that is, vessels without local anastomotic connections. Therefore, occlusion of these distal branches within a circumscribed area—for example, in patients with vasculitis—can lead to local infarction of the intestinal wall. Small intestinal infarction can also occur because of mesenteric venous thrombosis and in patients with no evidence of occlusion in the mesenteric arteries or veins ("nonocclusive intestinal infarction"). In patients without vascular occlusion, small intestinal infarction can occur because of reduced blood flow in the mesenteric circulation. This clinical picture is seen in patients with severe cardiac failure. When mesenteric blood flow is reduced, the small intestinal mucosa is more susceptible to ischemic damage than the muscle layers.

Chronically reduced mesenteric blood flow, usually the result of atherosclerosis, can lead to intestinal ischemia without overt infarction. Clinically, chronic ischemia of the small intestine may be associated with abdominal angina or steatorrhea. Patients with abdominal angina develop pain in the abdomen after meals. This pain reflects the increased oxygen requirement of the small intestine during digestion and absorption of food, occurring in the face of an impaired arterial blood supply. Small intestinal blood flow normally increases after meals through mechanisms that are not well understood, although local peptide hormones may be involved.

REFERENCES

Bienenstock, J., and Befus, A. D.: Some thoughts on the biologic role of immunoglobulin A. Gastroenterology 84:178, 1983.
Creutzfeldt, W. (ed.): Gastrointestinal hormones. Clin Gastroenterol Vol. 9, No. 3, 1980.
Dobbins, J. W., and Binder, H. J.: Pathophysiology of diarrhoea: Alterations in fluid and electrolyte transport. Clin Gastroenterol 10:605, 1981.
Doe, W. F.: Immunological aspects of the gut. In Lachmann, P. J., and Peters, D. K. (eds.): Clinical Aspects of Immunology, Vol. 2. 4th ed. Oxford, Blackwell Scientific Publications, 1982, p. 985.
Doe, W. F.: Immunodeficiency and the gastrointestinal tract. Clin Gastroenterol 12:839, 1983.
Johnson, L. R. (ed.): Physiology of the Gastrointestinal Tract. New York, Raven Press, 1981.
King, C. E., and Toskes, P. P.: Small intestine bacterial overgrowth. Gastroenterology 76:1035, 1979.
Sleisenger, M. H. (ed.): Malabsorption and Nutritional Support. Clin Gastroenterol Vol. 12, No. 2, 1983.
Sleisenger, M. H., and Fordtran, J. S. (eds.): Gastrointestinal Disease. 3rd ed. Philadelphia, W. B. Saunders Co., 1983.
Snape, W. J., Jr.: Pseudo-obstruction and other obstructive disorders. Clin Gastroenterol 11:593, 1982.

The Pancreas
JAMES H. GRENDELL, M.D.

The pancreas is a small organ (approximately 100 grams) that serves several important functions. It is the master exocrine digestive gland of the alimentary tract, secreting approximately two liters of protein- and bicarbonate-rich fluid into the duodenum each day. In addition the pancreas is vitally important as an endocrine organ—the source of insulin, glucagon, and other peptides produced by the islets of Langerhans. Inflammation of this gland or a significant loss of its function can have a variety of serious consequences. This chapter will be concerned only with the exocrine pancreas. Its endocrine function is discussed elsewhere.

ANATOMY

The head of the pancreas lies within the curvature of the duodenum with the body and tail retroperitoneal, transverse, and directed cephalad toward the hilum of the spleen (Fig. 39A). The exocrine pancreas is composed of clusters of secretory acini containing the acinar cells that are primarily responsible for digestive enzyme secretion. Myriads of ductules drain these acini and are formed from specific ductular epithelial cells, which are mainly responsible for water and electrolyte secretion. The ductules drain into intralobular ducts that join to form interlobular ducts, ultimately entering the central duct of Wirsung (Fig. 39B), which runs the length of the organ. This duct enters the duodenum at the duodenal papilla, usually alongside the common bile duct. In most individuals the sphincter of Oddi surrounds both ducts. In about one third of individuals,

the duct of Wirsung and the common bile duct form a common channel before terminating at the ampulla of Vater. In about 70 per cent of persons the minor duct (of Santorini) runs from the body of the gland in a separate course to enter the duodenum just proximal to the duodenal papilla. In about 10 per cent, the main duct drains into the accessory papilla. The islets of Langerhans, containing the cells of the endocrine pancreas, lie between the lobules.

The pancreas is strategically situated close to a number of important structures in the posterior abdomen. The common bile duct passes through the head of the pancreas before entering the duodenum. A variety of major abdominal vessels including the aorta, inferior vena cava, splenic artery and vein, and superior mesenteric artery and vein are all in close proximity to the gland. In addition, the distal stomach, pylorus, loops of jejunum, and transverse colon are adjacent structures.

PHYSIOLOGY

COMPOSITION AND FORMATION OF PANCREATIC JUICE

Water and Electrolyte Secretion

Pancreatic juice is isotonic with extracellular fluid at all rates of secretion. Water enters the ductules passively along osmotic gradients, whereas the secretion of electrolytes and other solutes is active. The principal cations, Na^+ and K^+, are secreted at fixed

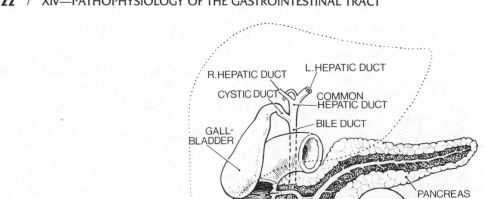

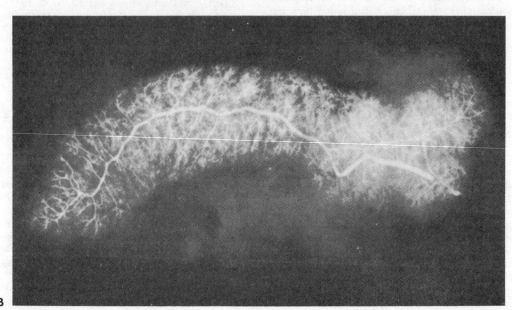

Figure 39. *A,* Connections of the ducts of the gallbladder, liver, and pancreas. (From Bell, G. H., Emslie-Smith, D., and Paterson, C. R.: Textbook of Physiology and Biochemistry. 9th ed. Churchill Livingstone, New York, 1976.) *B,* Roentgenogram of human pancreas after removal from the body and filling of the ducts with a solution of barium injected through the sphincter of Oddi. Note gradual tapering in the size of the ducts and filling of the terminal ducts and acini. (From Kreel, L., Sandin, B., and Slavin, G.: Clin Radiol 24:154, 1973.)

concentrations. The concentrations of the two principal anions, HCO_3^- and Cl^-, vary reciprocally and together total about 150 mEq/l. At high flow rates, HCO_3^- concentrations are high and Cl^- concentrations are low. At low flow rates, this ratio is reversed (Fig. 40). The HCO_3^- secreted by the pancreas neutralizes HCl delivered to the small intestine from the stomach, raising the pH to levels at which the pancreatic enzymes are catalytically active (pH > 3.5 to 4.0). In addition, neutralization of stomach acid by pancreatic bicarbonate probably has a protective effect on small intestinal mucosa.

Enzyme Proteins: Content and Function

At least 90 per cent of the protein content of pancreatic juice consists of digestive enzymes that are responsible for much of the intraluminal digestion of complex nutrients in the small intestine. The most important of these in humans are *amylase,* which splits starches into maltose, maltotriose, and limit dextrins; *lipase,* which splits triglycerides into fatty acids and monoglycerides; and the *proteolytic enzymes* (trypsin, chymotrypsin, elastase, and the carboxypeptidases), which cleave proteins and polypeptides into oligopep-

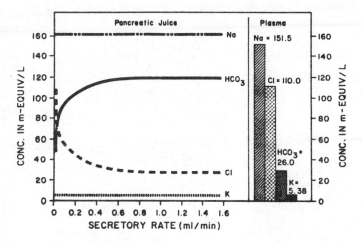

Figure 40. Relationship of pancreatic secretion and concentration of electrolytes. (Adapted from Bro-Rasmussen, F., Kilman, S. A., and Thaysen, J. H.: Acta Physiol Scand 37:97, 1956.)

tides and free amino acids. Pancreatic juice also contains a small peptide cofactor called *colipase,* which combines stoichiometrically with lipase. Colipase prevents inhibition of lipase activity by bile salts and lowers the pH optimum of lipase from 8.5 to 6.5, the normal luminal pH in the proximal intestine.

Amylase and lipase are secreted by the acinar cell in active form, but the proteases are secreted into the duct lumen as inactive proenzymes (zymogens). The small intestinal peptidase enterokinase converts the proenzyme trypsinogen to trypsin, which then activates all of the other proenzymes.

CONTROL OF PANCREATIC SECRETION

Pancreatic secretion is controlled by both hormonal and neural mechanisms (Fig. 41). The major hormonal stimuli are the gut hormones secretin and cholecystokinin (CCK), which are released following a meal. *Secretin* mainly augments water and bicarbonate se-

cretion through a mechanism involving an increase in intracellular cyclic AMP. *Cholecystokinin* substantially increases enzyme secretion through a mechanism increasing intracellular ionized calcium. CCK also potentiates the effect of secretin in stimulating water and bicarbonate secretion. Other gut hormones or potentially hormonally active peptides—for example, gastrin, vasoactive intestinal polypeptide, somatostatin, glucagon, and pancreatic polypeptide—at pharmacologic doses or in experimental systems can act as either stimulants or inhibitors of pancreatic secretion. However, a physiologic role has yet to be established for any of these substances. A diagrammatic summary of pancreatic secretion is shown in Figure 42.

PROTECTIVE MECHANISMS AGAINST AUTODIGESTION

The range of pancreatic enzymes necessary for adequate digestion of a meal poses a risk to the organ

Figure 41. Interaction of acetylcholine and gastrointestinal peptides with pancreatic acinar cells. (Courtesy of Dr. J. D. Gardner, National Institute of Arthritis, Metabolism and Digestive Diseases, Bethesda, Maryland, 1979.)

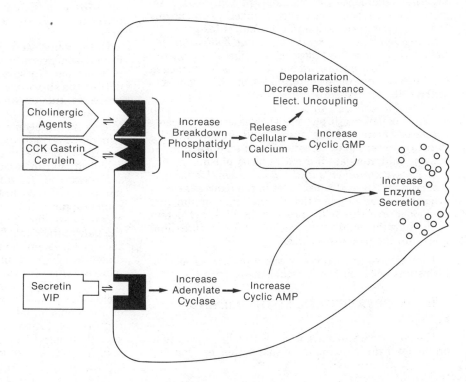

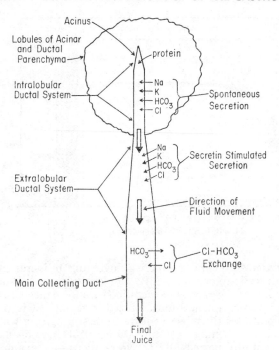

Figure 42. Diagram of pancreatic acinus and duct system ("pancreon"). Sodium bicarbonate is probably also secreted in the acinus. The effects of inhibitors of sodium transport suggest that active transport of sodium occurs proximally. Secretin stimulates a bicarbonate "pump" to add a solution of bicarbonate in the extralobular ducts. (From Swanson, C. H., and Solomon, A. K.: J Gen Physiol 62:426, 1973.)

itself of autodigestion. A variety of protective mechanisms appear to have evolved to deal with this potential problem:

1. *Secretion in inactive proenzyme (zymogen) form.* As described above, the enzymes most capable of causing tissue damage—for example, proteases—are secreted into the pancreatic duct in inactive proenzyme form, requiring activation in the small intestine.

2. *Sequestration in membrane-bound compartments.* Before their secretion, most of the digestive enzymes in acinar cells are stored in membrane-bound zymogen granules and are separated from the other components of the cell.

3. *Presence of enzyme inhibitors.* Should small amounts of pancreatic enzyme, such as trypsin, become activated before arriving in the small intestine, inhibitors are present in pancreatic tissue and juice. Similar enzyme inhibitors are present in blood plasma.

4. *Pressure gradients in the duct system.* Under normal circumstances the pressures in the pancreatic duct are substantially higher than in the common bile duct or duodenum. This helps prevent the reflux of potentially harmful substances such as bile or intestinal juice into the pancreatic duct.

The relative importance of these protective mechanisms has not been firmly established.

STUDIES OF PANCREATIC STRUCTURE AND FUNCTION

The exocrine pancreas is a relatively inaccessible organ for examination, for visualization by imaging

techniques, or for biopsy. Fortunately, there are a number of new approaches now available that supplement the traditional studies, which were largely confined to evaluating the secretory capacity of the organ. Since the emphasis in this book is on pathophysiology, the reader is referred to other sources for a more extended discussion of these methods and their usefulness in diagnosis.

Pancreatic Enzymes in Body Fluids. Amylase activity is used almost exclusively for this purpose. Serum lipase was used in the past to reflect the presence of pancreatitis, but it is more difficult to measure and offers no real advantage over the measurement of amylase. About one third of normal serum amylase activity is derived from the pancreas (as determined by isoenzyme patterns); the rest comes largely from the salivary glands. An increase in the pancreatic amylase activity in serum usually but not always indicates injury to acinar cells. With acute injury amylase activity increases within the first few hours (2 to 12) and then usually returns to baseline in 3 to 5 days. In acute pancreatitis (see below) the renal clearance of amylase is sometimes determined as well, since it is enhanced in this condition (clearance > 4 per cent of that of creatinine) because of diminished renal tubular reabsorption of the enzyme. Some believe that this determination is of value in differentiating the hyperamylasemia of pancreatitis from that associated with other disorders. With the recent development of radioimmunoassays for trypsin, determination of serum trypsin immunoreactivity in various pancreatic diseases is being evaluated to determine if it is more sensitive or specific than determination of serum amylase activity.

Imaging Techniques. In the past the study of the pancreas was limited to use of a plain film of the abdomen and an upper gastrointestinal series, which might reveal pancreatic calcification or an alteration in the duodenal loop, respectively, but which were insensitive to the early appearance of pancreatic disease. Some of the newer methods will be described briefly.

ULTRASONOGRAPHY. Sound waves that are reflected from tissue interfaces are recorded and displayed. With no radiation exposure, this noninvasive technique can outline the size of the pancreas and detect pseudocysts, abscesses, tumors, and calcification (Fig. 43).

COMPUTED TOMOGRAPHY (CT SCAN). The computed tomogram has been remarkably successful in outlining pancreatic structure (Fig. 43). It has allowed the demonstration of mass lesions, dilated pancreatic ducts, calcifications, abscesses, and pseudocysts.

ENDOSCOPIC RETROGRADE CHOLANGIOPANCREATOGRAPHY (ERCP). With the aid of the fiberoptic endoscope, radiographic contrast material can be injected through a small catheter directly into the biliary tree and/or the pancreatic duct. This allows direct visualization of the duct system and may help in the differential diagnosis of chronic pancreatitis from carcinoma of the pancreas (Fig. 44).

MAGNETIC RESONANCE IMAGING (MRI). This new technology is just now being applied to the diagnosis of intra-abdominal diseases. It may allow a better contrast resolution between normal and abnormal tissues than does CT.

SELECTIVE ANGIOGRAPHY. The ability to inject con-

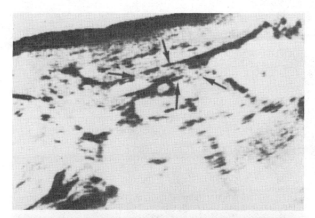

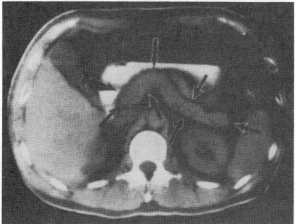

Figure 43. Normal pancreas demonstrated by ultrasound (above) and computed tomography (below). (Courtesy of Dr. Eugene P. DiMagno, Mayo Medical School, Rochester, Minnesota.)

trast material in a highly selective manner into the arterial supply of the pancreas or of one of its lesions together with excellent means of image amplification may be helpful in diagnosis, especially of pancreatic neoplasms.

Biopsy. With ultrasound or CT guidance the pancreas can usually be safely biopsied percutaneously using the "fine needle" technique. This avoids the necessity for a laparotomy.

Studies of Pancreatic Exocrine Function. These tests are difficult to perform and to interpret for at least two reasons: (1) a wide range exists of normal pancreatic secretion both basally and in response to stimulation, and (2) these tests depend on the necessarily incomplete aspiration by a tube of duodenal fluid that is a variable mixture of pancreatic fluid, bile, gastric juice, and succus entericus. In the *secretin* and the *secretin-cholecystokinin tests,* duodenal aspirate is evaluated for volume, bicarbonate, and amylase after these pancreatic secretagogues are given intravenously to fasting patients. In the *Lundh test* the mean tryptic activity of duodenal aspirate is measured after a test meal. Table 16 summarizes the range of normal responses to these tests.

Because of the need for duodenal intubation and the problems involved in ensuring complete aspiration of duodenal contents in these direct tests of pancreatic function, several indirect "tubeless" tests—the *benti-*

romide and *fluorescein dilaurate tests*—have been developed. In these tests, marker substances attached to carriers are administered orally. These markers are cleaved from their carriers by pancreatic enzymes, absorbed from the intestine, and excreted in urine. Thus the amount of the marker excreted reflects pancreatic function. Although the sensitivity of these "tubeless" tests is fairly high in moderate-to-severe pancreatic insufficiency, it is not very good in milder disease. In addition, conditions that interfere with either intestinal absorption or urinary excretion may result in false-positive studies.

PANCREATIC DISEASE

ACUTE PANCREATITIS

The distinction between "acute" and "chronic" pancreatitis has been a difficult one. Clinically defined, acute pancreatitis produces a discrete episode of symptoms resulting from inflammation of that organ without subsequent residual pain or exocrine insufficiency. This definition has been extended by some to require that the pancreas return to its normal morphologic and functional state following the episode of disease. However, in clinical practice this latter criterion is quite difficult to apply because pancreatic tissue is not ordinarily available for biopsy and precise tests of pancreatic function are infrequently performed. Therefore, in this discussion, the terms acute and chronic pancreatitis will be used in the clinical sense.

Clinical Picture

The patient with acute pancreatitis most commonly presents with epigastric pain, nausea, vomiting, abdominal distention, and ileus. Other signs may include low-grade fever, mental confusion, shock, and rarely jaundice and/or ascites. Basilar rales, atelectasis, and left-sided pleural effusion may be found. Rarely, scattered areas of subcutaneous fat necrosis may lead to tender red nodules in the skin, or necrotizing hemorrhagic pancreatitis may result in discoloration in the flanks caused by hemoglobin catabolism (Grey-Turner's sign) or discoloration around the umbilicus (Cullen's sign).

Most frequently, these clinical findings of acute pancreatitis must be differentiated from other acute intra-abdominal catastrophes such as a perforated viscus, mesenteric ischemia, acute cholecystitis, or intra-abdominal sepsis. The most useful laboratory study for this purpose is the serum amylase level, as noted above. The pancreas may be diffusely enlarged by ultrasonography or CT scan. ERCP is contraindicated unless an impacted common duct stone is suspected, since this study may exacerbate the disorder. Pancreatic biopsy is similarly not indicated.

Pathogenesis

The central event in the development of acute pancreatitis appears to be "autodigestion" of the organ caused by premature activation of the digestive enzymes normally contained in the gland—by this process the protective mechanisms described previously

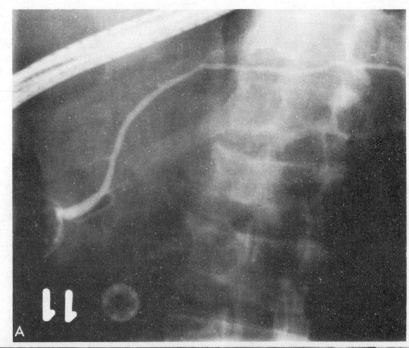

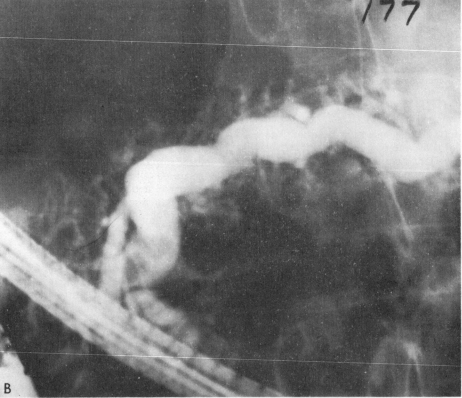

Figure 44. *A,* Normal pancreatic ductogram as demonstrated by ERCP, contrasted with *B,* dilatation of ductal system in chronic pancreatitis. (Courtesy of Dr. Stephen E. Silvis, Chief, Specialized Diagnostic and Treatment Unit, Medical Service, Veterans Administration Medical Center, Minneapolis, Minnesota.)

TABLE 16. RANGE OF NORMAL RESPONSES TO SECRETORY TESTS OF THE PANCREAS

1. *Secretin test*
   Volume (ml/80 min): 117–392
   HCO_3^- concentration (mEq/liter): 88–137
   HCO_3^- output (mEq/80 min): 16–33
   Amylase output (units/80 min): 439–1921
2. *Secretin + CCK*
   Volume (ml/80 min): 111–503
   HCO_3^- concentration (mEq/liter): 88–144
   HCO_3^- output (mEq/80 min): 10–86
   Amylase output (units/80 min): 441–4038
3. *Lundh test*
   Mean tryptic activity (IU/liter): 61

From Meyer, J. H.: Pancreatic physiology. In Sleisenger, M. H., and Fordtran, J. S. (eds.): Gastrointestinal Disease. 3rd ed. Philadelphia, W. B. Saunders Co., 1983, p. 1434.

are overcome. Trypsin is capable of activating the other proenzymes (zymogens). Therefore, only the activation (by some means) of trypsinogen would be necessary to initiate autodigestion (Figs. 45 and 46). How this occurs is unknown. A role for intracellular lysosomal enzymes as a trypsinogen activator has been proposed to explain how autodigestion occurs under certain circumstances. Table 17 lists some of the clinical etiologies that have been associated with acute pancreatitis.

Ethanol. There are several lines of evidence suggesting mechanisms by which chronic excessive ethanol intake may lead to pancreatitis. Alcoholic patients (and animals chronically fed ethanol) have been observed to develop duct obstruction by proteinaceous plugs that originally precipitate in the smaller ducts and later may calcify to form calculi. It has been proposed that alcohol abuse may result in a deficiency of an inhibitor protein whose normal function is to prevent the formation of calculi in the ducts. Trypsin activity—absent in pancreatic juice of normal individuals—has been reported to be measurable in pancreatic juice of patients with alcoholic pancreatitis and of some alcoholic individuals without clinically apparent pancreatitis. The presence of activated trypsin appears to be a consequence of an increase in the ratio of trypsinogen to trypsin inhibitor in pancreatic juice. How important these alcohol-related abnormalities are in the evolution of alcoholic pancreatitis remains to be determined.

Gallstones. Gallstones have been recovered in the stools of a high percentage of patients with acute pancreatitis and no history of excessive alcohol use.

This suggests that some alteration in pancreatic duct pressure, or the reflux of infected bile into the duct system associated with passage of a gallstone, may lead to the initiation of autodigestion. There is other evidence that obstruction and an increase in pancreatic duct pressure may play a role in the pathogenesis of pancreatitis. Some cases of pancreatitis appear to be related to dysfunction of the sphincter of Oddi or to pancreas divisum and other congenital abnormalities of the duct system. However, obstruction alone is probably not the primary cause of pancreatitis because generalized dilatation of the pancreatic duct system is not commonly found in pancreatitis and obstruction of the pancreatic duct by tumors does not usually produce pancreatitis.

Hyperlipoproteinemia. An increased incidence of acute pancreatitis has been observed in patients with certain forms of hyperlipoproteinemia characterized by very high serum triglyceride concentrations, and recurrences in these patients can be reduced by treatment to control the lipoprotein abnormality. In the presence of extremely high serum triglyceride concentrations, small amounts of pancreatic lipase entering the pancreatic circulation via secretion across the basolateral surface may liberate free fatty acids that are toxic to pancreatic tissue.

Miscellaneous. Acute pancreatitis following the sting of a particular West Indian scorpion (*Tityus trinitatis*) and that reported after organophosphate poisoning may have a similar pathogenesis—excessive cholinergic stimulus of pancreatic secretion. In some animals, hyperstimulation with CCK or homologous peptides or hyperstimulation due to cholinesterase inhibition has been shown to produce pancreatitis. The pancreatitis seen in some patients with kwashiorkor may relate to an inadequate supply of the amino acid substrate necessary for the high rate of protein secretion by the pancreas. However, toxic factors in the diet may also play a role in that the incidence of this type of pancreatitis varies greatly among regions with similar levels of protein–calorie intake. Acute pancreatitis following abdominal trauma or retrograde injection of contrast material during pancreatography is probably related to disruption of the pancreatic duct system.

Apart from these rather sketchy concepts of pathogenesis, little is understood about the mechanisms of injury for the numerous other clinical conditions associated with acute pancreatitis (Table 17).

Pathophysiology

Involvement of the Pancreas. Activation of trypsinogen to trypsin can lead to the subsequent activation of a variety of potentially destructive enzymes (Figs. 45 and 46). For example, phospholipase A can cause severe damage to pancreatic parenchymal and adipose tissue, and its effects are accentuated by bile acids. Elastase attacks the elastic fibers of blood vessels, resulting in hemorrhage. In addition to these and other digestive enzymes capable of participating in autodigestion, there is evidence that trypsin can trigger in both pancreatic tissue and blood the production of bradykinin and kallidin, two vasoactive peptides that produce vasodilation and increased vascular permeability and that are chemotactic for neutrophils. This generation of bradykinin and kallidin from kini-

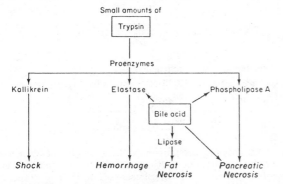

Figure 45. Hypothesis for pathogenesis of acute pancreatitis.

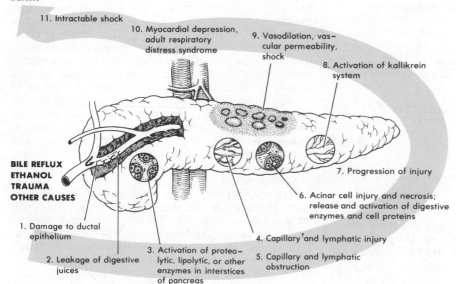

Figure 46. The pathophysiology of acute pancreatitis is not fully understood, but, as the model implies, a series of events seems probable, beginning with the release of toxic substances into the parenchyma and ending with shock and death. Damage to the ductal epithelium or acinar cell injury may result from bile reflux, increased intraductal pressure, ethanol ingestion, or trauma. (Modified from Webster, P. D., III, and Spainhour, J. B.: Hospital Practice 9:59, 1974. Original drawing by Nancy Lou Gahan Makris.)

nogens may be a direct result of trypsin or an indirect effect caused by tryptic activation of kallikreininogen to kallikrein (Fig. 47).

All of the major signs, symptoms, and complications of acute pancreatitis are explicable on the basis of the consequences of extensive damage to the ductules, acini, and islets of the pancreas. The degree of damage may be highly variable, and so are the clinical consequences.

The *pain* of acute pancreatitis is caused by edema, extravasation of plasma and red cells, release of digested protein and lipids, and distention of ductules. The principal cause appears to be the stretching of the capsule caused by swelling, collections of exudate, diapedesis of red cells, and accumulation of products of cellular digestion. These materials also seep out of the gland, surround it, and dissect into the retroperitoneal space, into the lesser sac, and down into the gutters. The spread of this material in such a manner stimulates the sensory nerves of the peritoneum and retroperitoneal space and accounts for intense pain in the back and flanks when the gland is extensively damaged. During an acute attack the pain will gradually become generalized over the abdomen as the peritoneum becomes irritated chemically and, in rare instances, bacterially. The stretching of the gland likewise will cause *nausea* and in many instances *vomiting*. As pain increases and persists, a paralytic ileus with marked abdominal distention may ensue, particularly if the intraperitoneal and retroperitoneal inflammation is widespread. Gastric motility ceases, the gastroesophageal sphincter relaxes, and the result is nausea and emesis.

The extensive injury to tissue and the inflammatory reaction, necrosis, and inflammation are responsible for the *fever* that is seen in almost two thirds of patients with acute pancreatitis. In the majority of patients with pancreatitis, fever is not caused by infection; it is caused by the absorption into the general circulation of pyrogens—probably proteins—derived principally from polymorphonuclear leukocytes, which play an important part in inflammatory reaction and necrosis.

The fever of acute pancreatitis is present usually for a few days and tends to be sustained, with minor fluctuations between 38° and 39°C; higher spikes of temperature indicate marked necrosis and severe inflammation. Persistence of fever beyond four or five days, or higher spikes to 40°C or more, may indicate either septic complications such as *pancreatic abscess*

TABLE 17. RISK FACTORS IN ACUTE PANCREATITIS

1. Alcohol abuse
2. Gallstones
3. Abdominal trauma
4. Infections: mumps, coxsackievirus, hepatitis, other viruses
5. Ischemic vascular disease
6. Hyperlipoproteinemias
7. Hypercalcemia
8. Drugs: steroids, diuretics, isoniazid, immunosuppressives
9. Duodenal disease: periampullary diverticula, Crohn's disease
10. Postoperative state, especially after gastrectomy
11. Immunologic disorders: polyarteritis, SLE
12. Cancer of the pancreas
13. Pancreatitis of pregnancy
14. Pancreas divisum
15. Hereditary: several forms

Modified from Brooks, F. P.: Diseases of the Exocrine Pancreas. Vol 20. In Smith, L. H., Jr. (ed.): Major Problems in Internal Medicine. Philadelphia, W. B. Saunders Co., 1980, p. 8.

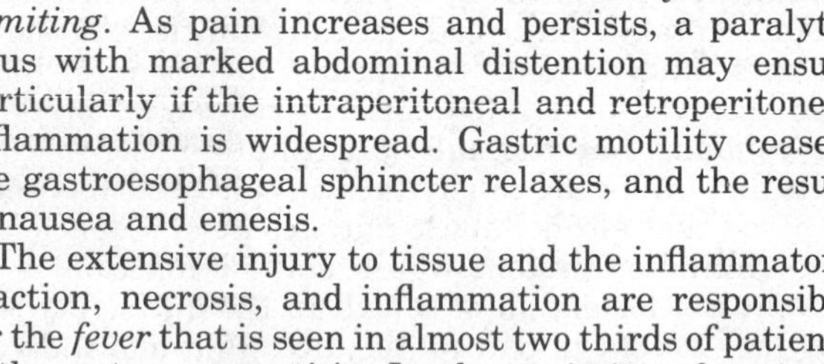

Kininogens (α_2 -globulins in plasma, lymph)

Inhibited by:	Stimulated by:
α_1-antitrypsin	Kallikrein—Kallikreininogen (pancreas)
Aprotinin	Trypsin—?

Bradykinin
Kallidin → vasodilatation, edema, pain

Figure 47. Possible mechanism for the activation of vasoactive polypeptides and their participation in the pathophysiology of acute pancreatitis. (From Sleisenger, M. H., and Fordtran, J. S. (eds.): Gastrointestinal Disease. 3rd ed. Philadelphia, W. B. Saunders Company, 1983.)

or *infected pseudocyst* or an associated *cholangitis* in patients with underlying biliary tract disease.

Complications of Acute Pancreatitis. ILEUS. As the inflammatory process in moderate-to-severe pancreatitis extends out from the retroperitoneum along the leaves of the mesentery, extensively dilated loops of intestine may fill with substantial amounts of fluid ("third space"). The pathophysiologic mechanism responsible for this process—which is a general response to peritoneal inflammation of any cause—has not been elucidated. Visceral reflexes probably play an important role. In less severe cases, the ileus may be confined to localized areas of bowel adjacent to the pancreas. On abdominal radiography this can result in a *sentinel loop* (dilated segment of jejunum overlying the pancreas) or *colon cut-off sign* (dilated segment of transverse colon).

CARDIOVASCULAR. The combination of both marked peripheral vasodilation caused by release of vasoactive substances such as bradykinin and kallidin and of profound volume loss caused by exudation of plasma and hemorrhage into the retroperitoneal space and fluid loss into dilated bowel may result in hypotension and—if severe—shock. This may result in myocardial or cerebral ischemia and contributes to the impairment in renal function often seen in severe pancreatitis.

PULMONARY. A variety of abnormalities found in chest radiographs in acute pancreatitis are the direct result of the inflammation present just below the diaphragm. These include elevation of the diaphragm, basilar atelectasis, and the presence of pleural fluid with a high concentration of amylase. In addition, moderate hypoxemia (Pa_{O_2} 50 to 70 mm Hg) may occur without any radiographic abnormalities. This appears to be the result of intrapulmonary right-to-left shunting that is caused by either the effects of vasoactive substances released in pancreatitis or pulmonary vascular microthrombi, formed as a result of subclinical disseminated intravascular coagulation (DIC).

ADULT RESPIRATORY DISTRESS SYNDROME (ARDS). This may occur in 5 to 10 per cent of patients with severe acute pancreatitis—it is one of the most serious complications. These patients have diffuse bilateral pulmonary infiltrates and severe hypoxemia. These findings result from a reversible disruption of the alveolar-capillary membrane with transudation of edema fluid despite normal pulmonary capillary hydrostatic forces. Several theories have been proposed to explain this. One suggests that circulating phospholipase A or free fatty acids damage pulmonary surfactant and thus produce pulmonary edema. Another theory proposes that disruption of the alveolar-capillary membrane by activated complement is the precipitating event. Adult respiratory distress syndrome is discussed more fully in the section on respiration.

IMPAIRED RENAL FUNCTION. Impairment in renal function ranging from mild renal tubular dysfunction to acute renal failure can be observed in acute pancreatitis. In milder cases, this may be manifested mainly as impaired reclamation of low molecular weight proteins by the proximal tubule, the basis for the elevated amylase-to-creatinine clearance ratio described in acute pancreatitis. At the other end of the spectrum, anuric renal failure may be seen, even in the absence of severe hypovolemia and shock. In some of these patients, increased renal vascular resistance and reduced renal blood flow and oxygen uptake have been described.

ENDOCRINE ABNORMALITIES. Transient *hypocalcemia* develops in about 30 to 40 per cent of patients with acute pancreatitis. Although rarely is the degree of hypocalcemia a clinical problem, its development is associated with a worse prognosis as a manifestation of the severity of the inflammatory process. In part the fall in serum calcium concentration reflects the loss of albumin from the vascular space. However, a true fall in the concentration of ionized calcium may be present. In part this is due to sequestration of calcium in saponified fat in the retroperitoneum and mesentery. There also appears to be a defect in the normal homeostatic mechanisms, which fail to compensate for this loss of circulating calcium. Studies of parathormone (PTH) levels in acute pancreatitis have yielded conflicting results, and the reason for impaired calcium homeostasis remains obscure.

The effects of pancreatic inflammation on the function of the islets of Langerhans may lead to mild, transient *hyperglycemia*. This appears to be the result of an increase in glucagon secretion relative to that of insulin.

CHRONIC PANCREATITIS

Clinical Picture

The usual incidence of the signs and symptoms of chronic pancreatitis is listed in Table 18. The three cardinal features of chronic pancreatitis are *pain, pancreatic exocrine insufficiency,* and *diabetes mellitus* (endocrine insufficiency). These manifestations will be discussed further under the heading of pathophysiology below. In general, severe, intractable abdominal pain tends to dominate the clinical picture. When this occurs in the setting of a risk factor for chronic pancreatitis (see below), especially in the presence of the classical triad of *pancreatic calcification, steatorrhea,* and *diabetes mellitus,* the diagnosis is evident and requires no further studies. Unfortunately, only a minority of patients (< one third) exhibit all these features; therefore, further studies may be indicated.

Measurement of serum amylase or lipase is of no help in the diagnosis of chronic pancreatitis because these enzyme levels are usually normal. Scattered calcifications in the pancreas may be seen by a plain abdominal radiograph or with greater sensitivity by CT. Ultrasonography may demonstrate pseudocysts or

TABLE 18. SYMPTOMS AND SIGNS IN CHRONIC PANCREATITIS

	PERCENTAGE OF PATIENTS
1. Abdominal pain	90
2. Weight loss	100
3. Jaundice	20–30
4. Steatorrhea	5–30
5. Diabetes	30–65
6. Gastrointestinal bleeding	9–15
7. Pancreatic ascites	2
8. Palpable abdominal mass (pseudocyst)	5

From Brooks, F. P.: Diseases of the Exocrine Pancreas. Vol 20. In Smith, L. H., Jr. (ed.): Major Problems in Internal Medicine. Philadelphia, W. B. Saunders Co., 1980, p. 41.

dilated pancreatic ducts. ERCP can be extremely useful in visualizing the characteristic beading in the ducts, the "chain of lakes" sign.

Malabsorption is best demonstrated by direct analysis of fecal fat. In the malabsorption of pancreatic insufficiency, presumably caused by enzyme and colipase deficiency, the intestinal mucosa is normal. The absorption of xylose is therefore normal, since it does not require digestion in contrast to the impaired absorption of fat and protein. These studies for malabsorption are indirect indices of pancreatic exocrine deficiency. The direct measurements using the secretin or secretin-CCK tests described above usually show a marked reduction in volume, bicarbonate concentration and output, and amylase output from the normal levels shown in Table 16. Similar abnormalities have been noted for the tryptic activity in the Lundh test and in the absorption and urinary excretion of the marker substances in the newer "tubeless" tests of pancreatic function (bentiromide and fluorescein dilaurate tests).

Pathogenesis

The primary etiology of chronic pancreatitis in adults in developed countries is chronic excessive ethanol use. The potential pathogenetic mechanisms already discussed under acute pancreatitis appear to be active on a subclinical basis long before the first symptom or sign of acute or chronic pancreatitis is seen (Table 17). The result is chronic progressive atrophy and fibrosis of the gland, calculi in the ducts, and distortion of the ductal system with—in some patients—occasional episodes of acute pancreatitis. Other etiologies associated with the development of chronic pancreatitis include hypercalcemic states, hyperlipoproteinemia, trauma, and longstanding protein-calorie malnutrition. There are also rare groups of patients who appear to develop chronic pancreatitis on a hereditary basis. In childhood the most common cause of chronic pancreatitis is cystic fibrosis. Notably, biliary tract disease (gallstones) rarely if ever causes chronic pancreatitis, in contrast to its frequent association with acute pancreatitis.

Pathophysiology

The current understanding of the pathophysiology of some of the most frequent clinical features of chronic pancreatitis will be discussed briefly.

Pain. The great majority of patients with chronic pancreatitis have pain ranging from mild and intermittent to disabling and unremitting. Classically the pain is deep and boring, beginning in the epigastrium and penetrating to the back, but it may assume many patterns. The pathophysiologic basis for this is usually uncertain. Increased pressure in the pancreatic ductal system caused by the presence of calculi or areas of stenosis and entrapment of neural structures in advancing chronic inflammation and fibrosis have both been suggested as explanations. In only a relatively small number of patients can a more definite source of pain such as a rapidly enlarging pseudocyst be identified.

The traditional approach to the treatment of intractable pain has been surgical: either drainage of the ductal system if it appears to be obstructed or removal of a large part (or even all) of the gland. These approaches have been only moderately successful, at best, in providing long-term relief of pain. A significant reduction in pain in patients with chronic pancreatitis given oral pancreatic digestive enzyme supplements has been reported recently. These enzyme supplements may suppress pancreatic secretion by a "negative feedback" mechanism involving the proximal small intestine, thus "putting the pancreas at rest."

Exocrine Insufficiency. Loss of functional acinar tissue may ultimately result in pancreatic exocrine insufficiency. Because of the gland's great secretory reserve, this is observed only as the result of near total loss of secretory function. Lipase output, for example, must be reduced by more than 90 per cent before an increase in stool fat excretion (steatorrhea) is seen (Fig. 48). For amylase an even greater degree of reduction must be present to result in clinically significant starch malabsorption. However, once enzyme secretion falls below a critical level, further small decrements in enzyme output result in major increases in malabsorption. Malabsorption is discussed more extensively under Pathophysiology of the Small Intestine.

Attempts to treat pancreatic insufficiency by replacement with exogenous digestive enzymes are limited by the following:

AMOUNT. Commercially available pancreatic enzyme preparations are not very potent compared with the meal-stimulated secretory output of a normal pancreas.

TIMING. Gastrointestinal motility and secretion are superbly coordinated so that food, pancreatic enzymes, and bicarbonate, along with bile, all arrive in the proximal small intestine at the same time.

DISPERSION. Pancreatic enzymes are secreted as a liquid suspension that readily mixes with intestinal chyme. Exogenous replacement enzyme preparations

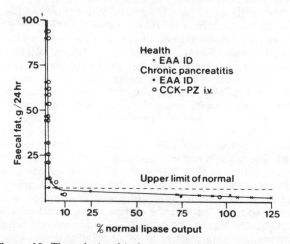

Figure 48. The relationship between 24-hour fecal fat excretion and pancreatic lipase output in healthy individuals following intraduodenal perfusion with essential amino acids (× EAA ID) and in patients with chronic pancreatitis following intraduodenal perfusion with essential amino acids (● EAA ID) or intravenous injection of cholecystokinin-pancreozymin (○ CCK-PZ i.v.). Note that fecal fat excretion remains normal (below broken line) until lipase output falls to less than 10 per cent of normal. (From DiMagno, E. P., Go, V. L., and Summerskill, W. H.: N Engl J Med 288:813, 1973.)

are ingested in solid form and do not disperse as rapidly or uniformly in the small intestine.

ACID INACTIVATION. Pancreatic digestive enzymes have pH optimums near pH 7.0. At pH 3.5 to 4.0, these enzymes are rapidly inactivated. In patients capable of secreting HCl, a substantial loss of enzyme potency occurs as the enzyme supplement passes through the stomach.

These problems can usually, at least in part, be overcome by using large quantities of high potency enzyme preparations (amount), taking the supplements throughout the course of meals and with snacks (timing and dispersion), and reducing gastric acidity—if necessary—by use of H_2-antagonists or some antacids. An enteric-coated pancreatic enzyme supplement designed to release its contents in the duodenum and jejunum has also been developed and may be useful when acid inactivation makes conventional preparations ineffective.

Diabetes Mellitus. Loss of about 90 per cent or more of functioning islet cells may result in diabetes mellitus caused by a reduction in insulin secretion. Although blood glucose concentrations may be very labile and difficult to control in this setting, diabetic ketoacidosis and renal or vascular complications are rare.

Other Manifestations of Chronic Pancreatitis. A variety of other abnormalities can result from chronic pancreatitis.

1. *Pseudocysts* (Fig. 49) are encapsulated collections of fluid that can occur in the setting of clinically acute pancreatitis as exudate and inflammatory debris walled off by a barrier formed by adjacent serosal, mesenteric, and peritoneal surfaces. In the setting of chronic pancreatitis, pseudocysts may also develop as retention cysts resulting from atrophy of acinar tissue. Pseudocysts may result in pain, obstruction of the biliary tree or gastric outlet by mass effect, hemorrhage due to erosion into a major vessel, and free rupture into the peritoneal cavity. In addition, cyst contents are subject to infection.

2. *Pancreatic ascites* characterized by fluid high in digestive enzyme concentration can be observed. This is caused by leakage of pancreatic juice from a pseudocyst or from the ductal system.

3. *Common bile duct obstruction* may develop from constriction of the common bile duct as a result of fibrosis in the head of the pancreas or compression by a pseudocyst. Longstanding high-grade obstruction may result in the development of secondary biliary cirrhosis.

4. *Splenic and portal vein thrombosis* may occur secondary to involvement of these vessels by acute pancreatic inflammation or to compression by a pseudocyst.

HEREDITARY OR CONGENITAL DISEASES OF THE PANCREAS

A variety of hereditary or congenital disorders of the pancreas, usually presenting in childhood, may produce malabsorption. Inadequate pancreatic enzyme activity in the intestinal lumen results from these disorders. They include diseases in which overall pancreatic enzyme secretion is reduced (cystic fibrosis, Schwachman's syndrome), isolated enzyme deficiencies—for example, of lipase, colipase, trypsin, or amylase—and failure of activation of pancreatic enzymes in the small intestine (enterokinase deficiency). These will not be discussed here as separate entities.

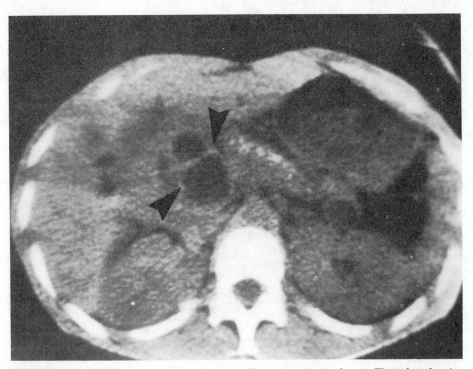

Figure 49. Computed tomography in patient with pancreatic pseudocyst. Three low-density fluid collections are visible in the head of the pancreas (arrowheads), while an additional cyst is seen in the tail of the gland. (From Sleisenger, M. H., and Fordtran, J. S. (eds.): Gastrointestinal Disease. 3rd ed. Philadelphia, W. B. Saunders Co., 1983.)

CARCINOMA OF THE PANCREAS

Carcinoma of the pancreas, the fourth most common cause of death from cancer in the United States (after malignant tumors of the lung, colon, and breast), almost always originates in ductal rather than acinar cells. Islet cell tumors, which occur very rarely, will not be considered here. The incidence of carcinoma of the pancreas seems to be steadily increasing in developed countries, in sharp contrast to carcinoma of the stomach, which is steadily decreasing in incidence. Since very little is known about the etiology, the pathogenesis, or the pathophysiology of carcinoma of the pancreas, this discussion will be comparatively brief despite the medical importance of this tumor.

Clinical Picture

Some of the most frequent symptoms and laboratory abnormalities associated with carcinoma of the pancreas are summarized in Table 19. The most frequent symptom is that of dull epigastric pain, often penetrating to the back, associated with insidious weight loss. The pain has no characteristic features. Associated with this pain the patient may have anorexia, nausea, and vomiting and sometimes a strange aversion to meat. Emotional disturbances have been described as occurring more frequently than in association with other malignant tumors, especially anxiety and depression. Obstructive jaundice is frequent, especially with carcinoma of the head of the pancreas, and may be associated with an enlarged, palpable gallbladder (Courvoisier's sign). Other abnormalities that may occur include the rapid onset of diabetes mellitus, thrombophlebitis (Trousseau's syndrome), acute pancreatitis, endocrine paraneoplastic syndromes (especially ACTH secretion and pseudohyperparathyroidism with hypercalcemia), an abdominal bruit resulting from involvement of the splenic artery and upper gastrointestinal bleeding. An epigastric mass may be felt, especially with carcinoma of the body and tail of the pancreas.

The most useful laboratory studies are those for imaging the pancreas, especially ultrasonography, CT scan, and ERCP. The use of the fine needle for percutaneous biopsy, as described earlier, has been of great diagnostic help. Serum tumor markers—carcinoembryonic antigen, α-fetoprotein, and the galactosyl-transferase isoenzyme II—have not been proven to be of assistance in making an early diagnosis. The secretin and secretin-CCK tests generally show pancreatic exocrine secretion that is diminished but of normal composition. These tests are rarely indicated in these patients, however.

Pathogenesis

As is the case for most malignant tumors, the cause of carcinoma of the pancreas is unknown. Nor is it known why these tumors are almost always (> 90 per cent) of ductal rather than acinar cell origin. Epidemiologic associations have been reported with advancing age, smoking, diabetes mellitus, some but not all forms of chronic pancreatitis, and dietary habits (increased consumption of animal fat and protein). An association with excessive consumption of coffee has been reported, but this has not yet been confirmed.

Pathophysiology

The pathophysiology of most of the clinical manifestations of carcinoma of the pancreas is usually very clear or very obscure. Many features result from direct invasion or compression of normal tissues by the neoplasm or by the dense, fibrotic, desmoplastic reaction that it produces in its immediate vicinity. This is the presumed cause of the pain, obstructive jaundice, upper gastrointestinal bleeding, gastric outlet obstruction (nausea, vomiting), and other localized abnormalities. The pathogenesis of the more generalized paraneoplastic syndromes, such as ectopic production of hormones or thrombophlebitis, is still obscure. The explanation awaits our obtaining a better understanding of the biology of neoplasia per se.

REFERENCES

Acosta, J. M., Rossi, R., and Ledesma, C. L.: The usefulness of stool screening for diagnosing cholelithiasis in acute pancreatitis: A description of the technique. Am J Dig Dis 22:168, 1977.

Brooks, F. P.: Diseases of the Exocrine Pancreas. Philadelphia, W. B. Saunders Co., 1980.

Grendell, J. H.: Nutrition and absorption in diseases of the pancreas. Clin Gastroenterol 12:551, 1983.

Grendell, J. H., and Cello, J. P.: Chronic pancreatitis. In

TABLE 19. SYMPTOMS AND ROUTINE LABORATORY TESTS IN CARCINOMA OF THE PANCREAS

SYMPTOM*	PERCENTAGE	LABORATORY TEST†	PERCENTAGE ABNORMAL
Abdominal pain	74	Alkaline phosphatase	82
Jaundice	65	5′-Nucleotidase	71
Weight loss	60	LDH	69
Diarrhea	27	SGOT	64
Weakness	21	Albumin	60
Constipation	8	CEA (> 5.0 ng/ml)	57
Hematemesis/melena	7	Bilirubin	55
Vomiting	6	Amylase	17
Abdominal mass	1	α-Fetoprotein	6

*Modified from Anderson, A., and Bergdahl, L.: Am Surg 42:173, 1976.
†Modified from Fitzgerald, P. J., Fortner, J. G., Watson, R. C., et al.: Cancer 41:868, 1978.
Reprinted from Cello, J. P.: Carcinoma of the pancreas. In Wyngaarden, J. B., and Smith, L. H., Jr.: Cecil Textbook of Medicine. 17th ed. Philadelphia, W. B. Saunders Co., 1985, p. 778.

Sleisenger, M. H, and Fordtran, J. S. (eds.): Gastrointestinal Disease. 3rd ed. Philadelphia, W. B. Saunders Co., 1983, p. 1485.

Moossa, A. R.: Diagnostic tests and procedures in acute pancreatitis. N Engl J Med 311:639, 1984.

Soergel, K. H.: Acute pancreatitis. In Sleisenger, M. H., and Fordtran, J. S. (eds.): Gastrointestinal Disease. 3rd ed. Philadelphia, W. B. Saunders Co., 1983, p. 1462.

Stafford, R. J., and Grand, R. J.: Hereditary disease of the exocrine pancreas. Clin Gastroenterol 11:141, 1982.

Wilson, J. S., and Pirola, R. C.: Pathogenesis of alcoholic pancreatitis. Aust NZ J Med 13:307, 1983.

The Colon

C. RICHARD BOLAND, M.D.

STRUCTURE AND FUNCTION IN THE NORMAL COLON

ANATOMICAL AND STRUCTURAL CHARACTERISTICS

General Considerations

The colon and rectum measure approximately 1.5 m in length, including a small cul-de-sac, the cecum, and the appendix, which are located at the extreme proximal end of the organ. There are substantial differences in structure and function between the proximal (cecum, ascending and transverse colon) and distal (descending and sigmoid colon, rectum) portions of the colon. The proximal colon, which receives its blood supply from the superior mesenteric artery, is larger in diameter than the distal colon. Blood group antigens are expressed on cell surface membrane glycoconjugates and in colonic mucins. The motility patterns in the proximal colon are primarily antiperistaltic; they favor the absorption of water, sodium, and chloride (which also continues in the distal colon) in addition to the specific absorption of conjugated and unconjugated bile acids. The distal colon, which receives its blood supply from the inferior mesenteric artery, slowly propels the intestinal contents toward the rectum and continues to absorb fluid from, and segment, the feces. Blood group–active glycoconjugates are absent from cell membranes in the distal colon, and the mucin also lacks these carbohydrate moieties.

The wall of the colon contains essentially the same muscular coats as in the small bowel except that the longitudinal muscle forms three separate bands—the taeniae coli—which are about 0.6 to 1.0 cm in width and run from the tip of the cecum to the rectum, converging at the base of the appendix. Between the taeniae are outpouchings called *haustrae,* separated by folds. The size and shape of the haustrae are determined by the state of contraction of the smooth and longitudinal muscle layers. Covering the serosal surface of the colon are the *appendices epiploicae,* which are fatty structures attached to the peritoneum. In contrast to the small bowel, the colon does not have a mesentery for its entire length, containing such a structure only for a short distance along the transverse and sigmoid colon.

The muscle coat found immediately beneath the serosa is composed of an inner circular muscular layer forming a tight spiral circumferentially along the course of the colon, and an outer longitudinal muscle layer that is distinctive because it is composed of three separate longitudinal strips (the taeniae coli). The ganglion cells of the myenteric plexus of Auerbach may be found between the circular and longitudinal muscle layers, with the majority being located along the external surface of the circular muscle coat. Unmyelinated postganglionic fibers are also found in the circular muscle layer and communicate with the submucosal plexus of the nerves.

Cellular Proliferation

The crypt is the basic epithelial unit of the colon. Cells in the lower half of the crypt are progenitor cells capable of proliferating and replacing the mature cells shed from the luminal aspect of the crypt. Once committed to terminal differentiation, the epithelial cell migrates up the crypt in contact with a basally paired fibroblast. It appears that once the goblet cell discharges its mucin, it continues to function as an absorptive cell; thus goblet cells and absorptive cells have a common origin.

The epithelial cell has a turnover time of 32 to 96 hours in the human colon and 96 to 192 hours in the rectum. In the basal state, between 15 to 25 per cent of the cells in the crypt are actively synthesizing DNA, and the proliferative index is generally higher in the rectum than in the colon. The majority of DNA synthesis occurs in the lower crypt, and cells near the mucosal surface normally cease proliferating. Endocrine cells are also present in the crypt, but less is known about their patterns of migration and turnover.

Ileocecal Valve

The ileocecal valve behaves like a sphincter. Anatomically, it is composed of an upper and lower lip; at their corners of fusion they taper to form transverse folds that are part of the cecal wall. Functionally, the sphincter prevents reflux of material from the cecal lumen back into the distal ileum; however, if sufficient pressure is exerted—as, for example, during a barium enema radiographic examination—the material will reflux into the terminal ileum. As a sphincter, the ileocecal valve permits the delivery of ileal content into the cecum in an intermittent, discontinuous, but orderly fashion.

Anatomy, Physiology, and Innervation of the Anorectal Sphincters

The anus has an internal and external sphincter. The internal anal sphincter is circular smooth muscle

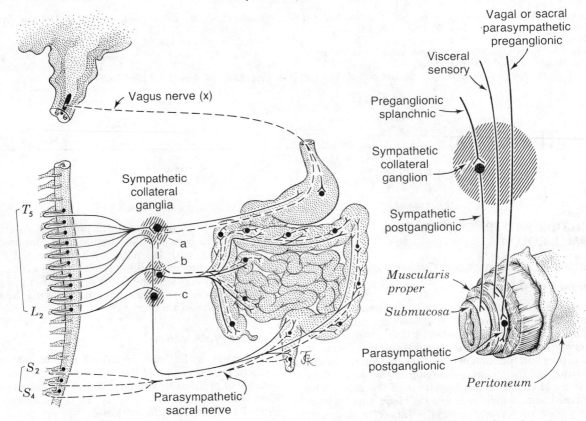

Figure 50. Autonomic innervation of the colon and rectum. (Courtesy of Dr. Albert L. Jones.)

and the external sphincter is striated muscle located in various layers of the anorectum. Other striated muscle groups besides the external sphincter are involved in the act of defecation. These include the levator ani, some fibers of which move the rectum forward and upward toward the pubis on contraction while others elevate the pelvic floor and provide support for abdominal viscera.

The innervation of the anorectum is diagrammed in Figure 50. The autonomic motor innervation of the internal sphincter is most important in defecation. The sympathetic supply is via the hypogastric nerves in the fifth lumbar segments, and the parasympathetic supply is via the nervi erigentes in the first, second, and third sacral segments. The sympathetics induce contraction of this sphincter and the parasympathetics inhibit it. In contrast, the parasympathetic nerve supply to the rectum is motor, not inhibitory as it is for the internal sphincter. The sympathetic system is inhibitory for the rectum but stimulates the internal sphincter. The external sphincter has only somatic pudendal innervation, and its relaxation is caused by reduction in frequency of the existing motor impulses.

Rectal Continence and Defecation

The maintenance of continence of the internal and external anal sphincters is important and complicated. Small amounts of material in the rectum are not sufficiently stimulating to overcome the tonically contracted internal sphincter; also, the anal canal remains closed when intra-abdominal pressure increases. With increasing distention of the rectum, the internal anal sphincter relaxes. The external anal sphincter is under voluntary control, and increasing distention of the rectum is brought to the subject's awareness. Voluntary relaxation of the external sphincter is accompanied by increasing abdominal pressure (generated by contracting abdominal muscles and diaphragmatic contraction against a closed glottis), allowing for expulsion of the rectal contents.

During transient distention of the rectum the internal sphincter relaxes and the external sphincter contracts (Fig. 51). The normal resting pressure of the internal sphincter, 3 to 7 cm proximal to the external anal margin, is 25 to 85 cm of water. This can be ascertained by the insertion of small balloons constructed in tandem so that simultaneous recordings may be made in both sphincters. Basically both sphincters are in a tonic state of contraction and the internal sphincter will maintain its heightened pressure despite transection of the spinal cord.

Afferents from the rectum and efferents to the descending colon are linked so that rectal distention leads to contraction of the left colon, serving to evacuate the remaining contents of the descending colon into the ampulla. Impulses are also carried to the cortex, which may then initiate the mechanism for voluntary defecation. The act increases intra-abdominal pressure and relaxes both the pelvic floor and the external anal sphincter.

Pressure in both sphincters increases with increased intra-abdominal pressure, except when such an increase is associated with defecation, at which time activity in both sphincters markedly diminishes. Pressure in them rises again following defecation, the so-

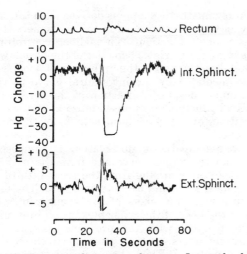

Figure 51. Transient distention of rectum. Internal sphincter relaxes and external sphincter contracts. Distention of the rectal balloon is indicated by an up-going arrow above the time scale, and deflation by a down-going arrow. Resting pressure recorded from each balloon is assigned a zero value. Increase in pressure above this level is termed positive and decrease below this level negative. (From Schuster, M. M., et al.: Bull Johns Hopkins Hosp 116:70, 1965.)

called *closing reflex*. In the intact person conscious behavior dominates defecation; however, it can be largely controlled by reflex, as after transection of the spinal cord above the lumbosacral area. In this situation the chief mediators of the efferent arc are the parasympathetic nerves from the sacral cord, stimulated by receptors for tension in the rectal musculature. In this way paraplegics remain continent. However, defecation is inefficient because striated muscle contraction is not normal.

The Anal Canal

The terminal 3 cm of rectum is the anus or anal canal. The separation between rectum and anal canal is marked by longitudinal folds called the *columns of Morgagni*, which terminate in the anal papillae. The anal canal terminates at the mucocutaneous junction, at which point the lining of the canal changes from columnar epithelium to stratified squamous epithelium

identical with skin. The transition is not sudden but is rather gradual, with an intermediary cuboidal type of epithelium. Several plexuses of veins may be found in the anus—the internal hemorrhoidal plexus in the submucosal space at the level of the columns of Morgagni and the anal papillae, and the external hemorrhoidal plexus in the subcutaneous tissue near the anal verge.

The muscular pelvic diaphragm is important in the defecation reflex and in the function of the sphincters. Components of the levator ani muscles—puborectalis, pubococcygeus, and ileococcygeus—make up this pelvic diaphragm, which is joined in its most posterior portion by the small coccygeus muscle. The fibers of the levator ani form a puborectal sling within which the lower rectum turns posteriorly. Contraction of the levator ani raises the pelvic diaphragm, the rectum, and the anus, and narrows the anal-rectal angle, contributing to anal continence, which is maintained principally by the contraction of the external sphincter.

The internal sphincter of the anal canal is part of the smooth muscle of the rectum. It extends from the distal tip of the rectum to within 1 cm of the anal orifice. The external sphincter circumscribes the anal canal and is separated from the internal sphincter by a thin layer of elastic fibers and longitudinal muscle that represents an extension of the outer longitudinal muscle coat of the rectum. Superiorly, its fibers blend with those of the levator ani muscle; it is attached posteriorly to the coccyx and anteriorly to the peritoneal body. Distally, the external sphincter ends subcutaneously at the anal margin.

Colonic Bacteria

Large numbers of bacteria reside in the colon, mainly gram-negative anaerobes, numbering 10^9 to 10^{12} organisms per gram feces. The principal anaerobes are bacteroides, lactobacilli, and clostridia (Table 20). They carry out some important functions, among which are the deconjugation and dehydroxylation of bile acids, and the hydration of unsaturated fatty acids. Bacterial metabolites of bile acids and sterols have been postulated to be of importance in the pathogenesis of colon cancer.

The anaerobic bacteria vastly outnumber the aerobic

TABLE 20. GASTROINTESTINAL FLORA IN THE HUMAN

	STOMACH	JEJUNUM	ILEUM	FECES
Total bacterial count	$0-10^3$	$0-10^5$	10^3-10^7	$10^{10}-10^{12}$
Aerobic or facultative				
Anaerobic bacteria				
Enterobacteria	$0-10^2$	$0-10^3$	10^2-10^6	10^4-10^{10}
Streptococci	$0-10^3$	$0-10^4$	10^2-10^6	10^5-10^{10}
Staphylococci	$0-10^2$	$0-10^3$	10^2-10^5	10^4-10^7
Lactobacilli	$0-10^3$	$0-10^4$	10^2-10^5	10^6-10^{10}
Fungi	$0-10^2$	$0-10^2$	10^2-10^3	10^2-10^6
Anaerobic bacteria				
Bacteroides	Rare	$0-10^2$	10^3-10^7	$10^{10}-10^{12}$
Bifidobacteria	Rare	$0-10^3$	10^3-10^5	10^8-10^{12}
Gram-positive cocci*	Rare	$0-10^3$	10^2-10^5	10^8-10^{11}
Clostridia	Rare	Rare	10^2-10^4	10^6-10^{11}
Eubacteria	Rare	Rare	Rare	10^9-10^{12}

*Includes *Peptostreptococcus* and *Peptococcus*.

enteric flora such as *E. coli,* Proteus, and Klebsiella. These anaerobic organisms may be found in large numbers in abscesses and in peritonitis following gut perforations; however, their significance in the production of human disease is still debatable. It appears that the anaerobes are less clinically significant in the development of acute abdominal pathologic processes. The enteric flora are largely confined to the colon by means of effective small bowel clearing mechanisms and an intact functioning ileocecal valve.

Physiological Considerations

The main functions of the colon are the movement and storage of feces prior to discharge, the absorption of fluid and electrolytes, and the secretion of fluid, mucus, bicarbonate, and potassium. These functions are intimately interrelated but shall be considered first individually.

Neural Control of the Colon

The innervation of the colon takes on special significance in understanding abnormalities of colonic motility. The nerve supply of the colon is entirely autonomic and consists of an extracolonic network of ganglia, plexuses, and fibers and another network composed of myelinated and nonmyelinated fibers, along with the ganglion cells of nerve plexuses in the submucosa and between the two layers of smooth muscle.

The parasympathetic system is composed of the vagus nerve and the sacral nerves, or nervi erigentes, from the sacral spinal cord. The latter consists of long, preganglionic fibers that terminate at synapses within the myenteric and submucosal plexuses. The sympathetic division, on the other hand, has preganglionic fibers that emerge as splanchnic nerves from the thoracic spinal cord and synapse in the preaortic ganglia. Postganglionic fibers then follow the blood vessels to the colon wall.

The splanchnic nerves, which are the efferent nerves of the sympathetic system, pass through the chain of paravertebral sympathetic ganglia. They usually synapse in the preaortic sympathetic ganglion chains. In their course from the spinal cord to these chains they pass through the white ramus, where they join with the nerve fibers from the dorsal root ganglion cells, which are the afferents providing the sensory innervation of the colon. Fibers of these sympathetic sensory afferents terminate in the plexus of the submucosa and intermuscular layers.

In view of their importance in transit time and defecation, special emphasis on innervation of the cecum and rectum is warranted. The extrinsic nerve supply to the cecum and part of the transverse colon is via the superior mesenteric plexus, which sends out both vagal and sympathetic nerve fibers to the colon. From a point in the distal transverse colon down to the rectum, the innervation is derived from the thoracolumbar outflow via the inferior mesenteric plexus. Some vagal fibers, however, are also derived from the celiac and aortic plexuses.

The sympathetic supply of the rectum is from the upper and lower divisions of the hypogastric nerves.

The parasympathetic supply is derived from the sacral outflow of the cord contained in the pelvic nerves. The extrinsic supply functions as a modifier, controlling to some extent the intrinsic behavior of the bowel, which is more directly under the influence of local reflex activity mediated by the intramural nerve plexuses. For example, despite transection of the cord, colonic and rectal function continue because of the intrinsic innervation, and greater local activity of the rectum supervenes.

The parasympathetic innervation is composed of fibers from the vagus nerve and from the nervi erigentes, the latter arising from the second, third, and fourth sacral segments of the spinal cord. The myelinated preganglionic fibers of the vagus ramify profusely at the level of the celiac plexus and intermingle indistinguishably with the pre- and postganglionic sympathetic fibers as they pass down through the preaortic plexuses. They then proceed to the colon, coursing through the mesentery in company with the colonic branches of the superior mesenteric artery. The nervi erigentes are a bundle of myelinated nerves intermingled with sympathetic nerves of the hypogastric plexuses. The parasympathetic fibers of the sacral outflow enter the colon in its distal portion and may be found as far proximally as a point in the distal transverse colon. These fibers from the vagus and nervi erigentes are preganglionic myelinated fibers that synapse in the ganglia of the submucosal plexuses of Meissner. This network of myenteric plexuses is the intrinsic innervation of the intestine and may function independent of external stimulation and connections. The levator ani, coccygeus, and external anal sphincter muscles are supplied by motor fibers from the fourth sacral segment of the spinal cord, which emerges with the root of the pudendal nerve.

The afferent impulses that respond to stretch and spasm of the colonic musculature are mediated by autonomic afferent fibers. They pass from the bowel wall through the sympathetic ganglia (preaortic and prevertebral) to the white ramus and into the posterior root ganglion and thence to the posterior columns of the spinal cord, where they synapse. The anal epithelium, composed of skin as well as mucous membrane, has extremely sensitive receptors that are responsive to stimuli that produce itch as well as pain. These impulses, in contrast to those of the colonic wall, are carried by somatic afferent pathways. These anatomic considerations account for some of the functional differences between the proximal and distal colon, and the specialized activity of the rectum and anus. A more general description of the autonomic nervous system is contained in the section on neurology.

ABSORPTION AND SECRETION

Water and Electrolytes

The colon is extremely important in reducing the amount of water that is excreted per rectum daily. Depending on whether the observations are made from ileostomy effluent or from ileal intubation, from 500 to 1500 ml of water enters the colon each day. Approximately 150 ml is excreted in the stool. Water absorption is therefore very efficient and can be expanded if necessary. The colon actively absorbs sodium and chlo-

TABLE 21. COLON ABSORPTION AND SECRETION OF H_2O AND ELECTROLYTES (PER DAY)

	H_2O (ml)	NA$^+$ (mEq)	K$^+$ (mEq)	CL' (mEq)	HCO$_3$' (mEq)
Terminal ileum	1500–1800	180–220	5	117–157	63
Stool	100–150	5	9–13	2	3
Net absorption or secretion	1350–1700	175–215	4–8	115–155	60*

*Represents the difference between ileal fluid and stool, *not* net absorption. In fact, HCO_3 is secreted into colon but is converted to CO_2 (see text).
From Sleisenger, M. H., and Fordtran, J. S. (eds.): Gastrointestinal Disease. 2nd ed. Philadelphia, W. B. Saunders Co., 1978, p. 1524.

ride while it secretes potassium and bicarbonate (Table 21). The primary glycoprotein secretion of the colon is *mucin,* which serves both protective and lubricating functions. Potassium concentration in stools is approximately 90 mEq per liter of stool water, while sodium is only 40 mEq per liter. This difference is due in part to some exchange between sodium and potassium in the colon. Chloride concentration is low, about 15 mEq per liter, because of an active exchange with bicarbonate in the ileum and colon. Bicarbonate is about 30 mEq per liter, its concentration being reduced by reaction with organic acids present in the colon. Colonic bacteria produce a variety of short-chain, volatile fatty acids (VFA), including acetate, proprionate, and butyrate, which increase the osmolality of stool water over plasma.

Ammonia is also produced in the colon. Most of it is in the form of the ammonium ion, NH_4+, and will pass out in the stool. The more acidic the pH of the colonic contents, the less ammonia will diffuse back into the blood.

Considering the volume and electrolyte concentration of stool water, it is estimated that about 5 mEq of sodium, 5 to 15 mEq of potassium, and 2 mEq of chloride are excreted each day by the colon. The colon normally absorbs about 1350 ml water, 200 mEq sodium, and 150 mEq chloride, and secretes 4 to 8 mEq potassium per day. The colon will continue to absorb sodium, chloride, and water until the luminal concentration of sodium is below 20 mEq/l. A coupled transport of chloride and bicarbonate seems apparent. More chloride than sodium is absorbed from equimolar solutions, and bicarbonate secretion accounts for the difference. Most bicarbonate in colon is converted to CO_2 by organic acids such as butyrate and acetate. Thus, stool bicarbonate is very low.

Studies of the colon by a perfusion technique in which isotonic sodium chloride solution without glucose is perfused indicate that the colon can absorb approximately 2.5 liters of water, 400 mEq of sodium, and 550 mEq of chloride in the 24-hour period during which it would also secrete 45 mEq of potassium and 250 mEq of bicarbonate into the perfusion solution. The human colon has the capacity to absorb over 5 liters per 24 hours and double its electrolyte absorption when presented with larger ileal outputs, demonstrating the reserve function that may be called upon to maintain homeostasis during small intestinal disease. Absorption in the right colon is greater than that in the transverse colon, which in turn is greater than that in the descending colon. The absorptive capacity of the rectum is relatively slight. Thus, fecal water and electrolytes may be normal in clinical states in which an increased ileal effluent enters the colon—for example, adult celiac disease and after ileal resection.

Fluid and electrolyte transport may be influenced by several factors. Sodium absorption is enhanced during periods of decreased intake or increased losses. The colon behaves in some ways like the renal tubule in that sodium and chloride are absorbed throughout the colon, but sodium is exchanged for potassium only in the distal colon, and both processes are responsive to aldosterone. During periods of active salt conservation—that is, increased aldosterone states—the ratio of sodium to potassium in stool falls below 0.3.

Rat colon will absorb calcium, dependent upon vitamin D. Whether the human colon absorbs calcium is unknown, but magnesium appears to be absorbed by human colon. Glucose is absorbed insignificantly and unabsorbed carbohydrate in colon is converted by bacterial action to short-chain VFA. The major fraction of VFA is converted to carbon dioxide and water, or absorbed.

Bile Acids

Bile acids are absorbed from the colon by nonionic (passive) diffusion. This mechanism is important in the absence of the distal small intestine, helping to maintain the total bile salt pool of the body, since 5 to 20 per cent of this pool enters the colon per day. The process is quantitatively important because only 300 to 600 mg of bile acids are excreted in the stool daily. The mucosa is more permeable to bile acids after their deconjugation and dehydroxylation. Dehydroxylation in the colon may also be important because there is some evidence that the resulting compounds may affect bile acid synthesis and cholesterol metabolism. On the basis of conversion of cholic acid to deoxycholic acid, the amount of bile acid absorbed from rat colon is estimated to be about 10 mg per day, or half the cholic acid pool. The corresponding figure in humans would be about 600 to 650 mg per day.

Effect of Bile Acids on Transport. Unconjugated bile acids affect the transport of water and electrolytes in the colon. When conjugated bile acids are not normally absorbed in the distal small intestine—as, for example, following ileal resection or because of extensive ileal disease—these substances are hydrolyzed and metabolized by colonic bacteria. Diarrhea caused by bile acids has been termed *cholerrheic enteropathy.* This condition is due in part to the inhibition of electrolyte and water absorption from the colon by unconjugated dihydroxy bile acids, particularly the metabolite of cholic acid, deoxycholic acid.

The effect of these substances on absorption by normal colon in humans and in the dog, although completely reversible, is clinically important with regard to water, sodium, chloride, and bicarbonate absorption. Potassium secretion increases, but not in proportion to the failure of normal water and sodium absorption. Inhibition is not the exclusive property of unconjugated bile acids, as conjugated dihydroxy bile acids will also block water and electrolyte absorption.

Thus the human colon will secrete water, sodium, potassium, and bicarbonate when perfused with conjugated bile acids. The primary effect in humans may be stimulation of secretion of sodium, which promotes secretion of water, which in turn will bring other electrolytes into the lumen. Investigators are divided in their opinions on whether bile acids and hydroxy fatty acids stimulate adenyl cyclase activity, raising cyclic AMP levels and producing active secretion, or whether net secretion is a result of a change in membrane permeability.

Bacterial enzymes in high concentrations in the colon produce a large number of secondary fecal bile acids, particularly deoxycholic acid, via 7-alpha dehydroxylation. Deoxycholic acid, derived from the primary bile acid cholic acid, is present in significant concentrations in normal stool and will inhibit colonic water and electrolyte transport at lower concentrations than will the primary bile acids.

Volatile Fatty Acids (VFA)

A major component (perhaps half) of stool anion solutes is the short-chain acids. They are composed mainly of acetate, proprionate, and butyrate, with acetate being 60 per cent of the total amount. Normal feces contain about 80 to 90 mEq/l VFA, but only 1.0 to 3.0 mEq/l is in ileal fluid. VFA may rise markedly in some instances of diarrhea due to decreased absorption. Some VFA is absorbed by the colon; this is likely to be the fate of a large but undetermined part of colonic VFA. The rate of nonionic diffusion of VFA through the mucosa is slow and favored by low pH; uptake of the ionic form may account for 40 per cent of absorption. What effects these substances have on colonic function are not clear. Volatile fatty acids in high concentration may cause an osmotic diarrhea; however, their concentration may also fall in diarrhea, when more rapid colonic transit diminishes their production. Nonvolatile fatty acids have been shown to cause water and electrolytes to be secreted by the colon. Hydroxy fatty acids, converted by colonic bacteria from unabsorbed long-chain fatty acids, are present in the colon, and are potent secretogogues.

Other Solutes

A number of other substances may be absorbed by the human colon, including amino acids, oxalate, medium-chain triglycerides, and some drugs, notably corticosteroids and aminophylline.

MOTILITY OF THE COLON

The reservoir and excretory functions of the colon depend upon a sequence of closely coordinated motor activities, some of which are clearly reflex responses. Generally, these components of colonic motility are due to smooth muscle contraction, either segmentally restricted or involving large portions of muscle, and they only infrequently produce a significant forward motion of colonic contents. Transit time is slow, about 24 hours for passage from cecum to anus.

PATTERNS OF COLONIC MOTILITY

The myoelectric activity of the colon may be divided into two types: slow waves and spike bursts (Fig. 52). The *slow waves* represent phasic changes in the electrical potential across the membranes of colonic smooth muscle. The activity arises in the circular muscle layer, spreads rapidly circumferentially, and moves slowly in both proximal and distal directions. Electrical slow waves are generated from a source near the mid-transverse colon and migrate in opposite directions. This *pacemaker* region accounts for the antiperistaltic nature of motility in the proximal colon and the slow propulsive activity distally. Slow waves determine the frequency of colonic contractions.

Spike bursts are transient electrical responses activated by the slow waves within the muscle that signal the initiation of muscular contractions. The dominant slow wave frequency in the human colon is 6 to 10 cycles per minute. The distal colon has infrequent *migrating spike bursts* associated with prolonged contraction, which may be responsible for the mass propulsion of feces.

The three taeniae are distributed along the mesentery equidistantly around the serosal aspect of the colon. Contraction of these longitudinal muscle bundles results in shortening and sacculation of the colon. Circular muscular bands are found intermittently that form the haustrae, and may produce segmentation of the colonic contents.

The myoelectrical activity of the colon may be modulated by feeding, serum electrolytes—including so-

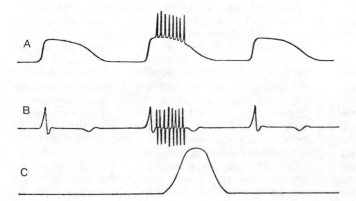

Figure 52. Diagram of the relationships between electrical slow waves, spike bursts, and muscle contraction. *A,* Transmembrane potentials recorded by an intracellular electrode in a single smooth muscle cell, demonstrating three cycles of slow waves with a spike burst in the middle cycle. *B,* Extracellular electrode signal from a group of intestinal smooth muscle cells. *C,* Tension in smooth muscle cells measured by a pressure transducer. Note that the onset of a contraction occurs with a spike burst. (From Christensen, J.: N Engl J Med 285:85, 1971.)

dium, chloride, and calcium—hormones—including gastrin, glucagon, and cholecystokinin—neurotransmitters, and a wide variety of drugs. A number of *reflex* motor patterns have also been described in the colon, demonstrating the complex neural control and interrelationships between different segments of the gastrointestinal tract.

Reflex Activity in the Colon

Entry of food into the upper small bowel initiates a reflex response at the ileocecal sphincter, perhaps hormonally mediated, leading to passage of material from the distal small intestine into the cecum. Associated with this passage of small bowel contents is an increase in colonic segmenting activity, and later mass movements appear. This response to food is probably not dependent upon the release of either gastrin or any other peptide from the stomach, since individuals who have undergone total gastrectomy continue to have mass movements after meals. Other hormones besides gastrin and secretin—particularly cholecystokinin-pancreozymin—may play a role in this integrated scheme; however, experimental evidence to support such a role for this hormone is not yet at hand. The response does not depend upon the vagus nerve, because it is present after either truncal or selective vagotomy. Whether it is dependent in some way on the rate of entry of food into the upper small intestine or upon the action of 5-hydroxytryptamine or prostaglandins remains to be determined.

Mass movement does not correlate with increased segmenting activity. On the contrary, segmenting activity of the left colon decreases or disappears as it shortens to receive material propelled into it from the proximal colon. After the material has arrived, segmenting activity resumes, initiating the "to-and-fro" motion that mixes contents and moves them slowly over very short distances. Finally, a bolus will be moved into the rectum, which responds to distention by initiation of the defecation reflex (see below). Also, the rectum may rapidly become distended as a result of the mass movement of material into it from a more proximal location.

Role of the Autonomic Nervous System

What is the role of the autonomic nervous system in colonic motor function? The answer is far from clear, and although both excitatory and inhibitory autonomic nerves are present, the main effect seems to be inhibitory, with some of this effect being mediated by adrenergic nerves. It is assumed that slow waves may be the pacemaker that the autonomic system, and possibly hormones, modulate. The parasympathetic system is thought to be excitatory; however, methacholine may inhibit muscular contraction and ganglionic blocking agents depress activity, an observation that supports the notion that the principal role of these nerves is inhibitory, particularly in the distal colon.

Pharmacology of the Colon

Autonomic drugs have been shown to alter slow wave activity and the frequency of accompanying spike bursts, consistent with an important modifying and integrating role for the autonomic nervous system. Cholinergic agents such as carbachol prolong slow wave activity and increase the frequency of spike bursts. Acetylcholine is the parasympathetic transmitter for excitation of colon muscle, being released by postganglionic nerve terminals. Its role in maintaining gut motor function and transit is vividly demonstrated by the atony that follows its inhibition by anticholinergic agents such as atropine. Its action can be simulated by methacholine (Mecholyl) or bethanechol (Fig. 53).

In vitro, acetylcholine causes contraction of muscle strips. Noncholinergic excitatory nerves are also present in the wall, but the transmitter of these impulses is not known. The action of acetylcholine can be potentiated by the cholinesterase inhibitor neostigmine. The effect of parenteral acetylcholine or methacholine on colon motor activity is to increase the pressure segmentally on the right side and, apparently, to reduce or abolish phasic activity on the left. This effect has been interpreted to be a simulation of "mass movement" of material from right to left associated with the temporary disappearance of segmental contraction and haustrae in the left colon. Apparently, normal myenteric innervation is required for this effect on the left colon, because it is absent in approximately 50 per cent of patients with congenital megacolon (Hirschsprung's disease).

Adrenergic agents such as norepinephrine relax isolated colonic muscle strips; however, when both alpha and beta receptors are blocked, epinephrine causes contraction. Norepinephrine released in tissue may also cause relaxation because it inhibits acetylcholine release. Agents that block alpha receptors, such as guanethidine and phentolamine, may be employed to combat intestinal ileus, which is often caused in part by sympathetic (inhibitory) overactivity.

Other pharmacologic agents produce changes that appear more complex. Alpha-adrenergic drugs such as epinephrine increase spike activity in low concentrations and decrease it in high concentrations, the excitatory action being increased by the beta-adrenergic antagonist propranolol, and inhibited by the alpha-receptor antagonist phenoxybenzamine. Beta-adrenergic stimulation with isoproterenol shortens slow wave duration and suppresses spike activity.

In addition to the autonomic drugs, other agents produce significant but poorly understood changes in myoelectric activity. Serotonin, morphine, and ouabain all prolong slow wave duration and increase spike activity. In the case of morphine, this remains to be correlated with the marked constipating effect that is observed clinically. Pentagastrin in humans has been shown to increase the frequency of slow wave activity in the rectosigmoid.

Effects of Eating, Emotion, and Exercise on Colonic Motility

The effect of eating upon the movement of material from the ileum into the colon and then its sudden transit by "mass movement" from right to left colon has been described. It appears to be independent of the extrinsic innervation of the large bowel, as well as of

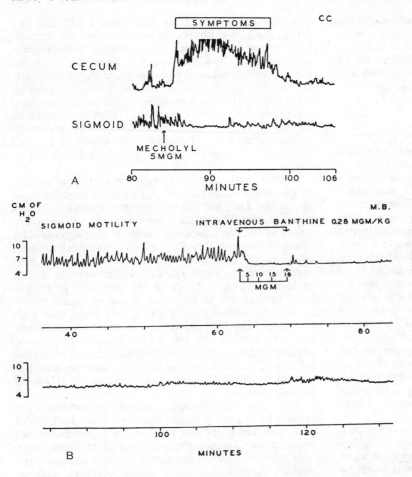

Figure 53. *A*, Balloon-kymographic recordings of motility of the cecum and sigmoid colon, showing coordinated action of methacholine on these regions of the bowel. (From Kern, F., Jr., and Almy, T. P.: J Clin Invest 31:555, 1952.) *B*, Intravenously administered Banthine promptly abolishes contractions of the sigmoid. This occurred after only 5 mg had been administered. (From Kern, F., Jr., et al.: Am J Med 11:67, 1951.)

longitudinal conduction of impulses in the spinal cord, because it is noted after transection of the cord. As noted, although gastrin may be involved (because eating is associated with the release of this hormone), mass movements are not abolished by total gastrectomy. Movement of contents into the cecum and diminution of pressure in the ileocecal valve, facilitated by reflex activity, somehow is associated with both segmentation and mass movements. Within three minutes of eating, the number of segmental contractions of the colon markedly increases, particularly in the sigmoid. The increase is about 25 per cent above the basal level in terms of numbers of contractions; however, the amplitude may also be greater.

However, the effect of eating on the colon is normal in patients with complete achlorhydria (pernicious anemia). Since these patients probably do not stimulate normal release of secretin or cholecystokinin-pancreozymin, the role of these hormones in mass movement is presently unclear. No correlation of colonic response to food with gastric acid output (and hence stimulation of upper intestinal hormone release) is found in patients with duodenal ulcer disease and acid hypersecretion. Perhaps the most important effects of small bowel activity upon colonic motor functions are mediated through release of 5-hydroxy-tryptamine, kinins, or prostaglandins.

Emotion appears to play an important role in colon motility, although reports of this association have been conflicting. In some experiments in which stress interviews were employed in patients with abnormal bowel habits, the evocation of certain emotional responses was associated with characteristic changes in motility patterns (Fig. 54). For example, anger and hostility aroused in individuals might be associated with increased phasic activity and an increase in the amplitude of the waves; contrariwise, depression with weeping or feelings of resignation has been associated with an abolition of all phasic activity in the left colon. Other investigators have not found a relationship between the emotional state of the patient and the motor activity of the left colon; in any event, it is difficult to interpret these experiments. Clinically, emotion is thought to play an important role in the function of the colon during certain periods in the course of both ulcerative colitis and irritable colon.

Exercise has long been noted to affect bowel habit, being a recognized antidote in some people for intermittent constipation. Motility studies have been done in which telemetering capsules were used to indicate that physical activity increases colon motor activity, particularly propulsive movements after meals.

ABNORMALITIES OF COLONIC FUNCTION

The preceding section has reviewed normal colonic physiology and suggested some of the principles of colonic dysfunction. The primary activities of the colon are the transport of fluid and solute—that is, absorp-

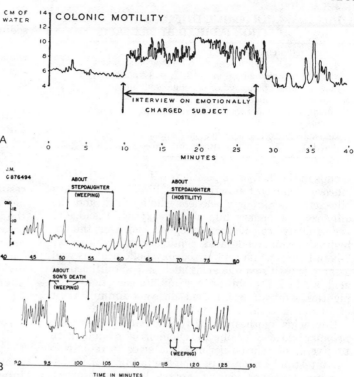

Figure 54. Changes in colonic motility associated with emotionally charged events. *A,* Increases in colonic motility during a stressful interview. (Reprinted by permission of the publisher from Alterations in colonic function in man under stress; experimental production of sigmoid spasm in healthy persons by Almy, T. P., Kern, F., Jr., and Tulin, M., Gastroenterology, vol. 12, p. 436. Copyright 1949 by The American Gastroenterological Association.) *B,* Changes in motility patterns in a patient with a history of both diarrhea and constipation. Note the changes in motility with the changes in emotional status. (From Almy, T. P., et al.: Am J Med 10:60, 1951.)

tion—and motility; disorders of these functions will be the main focus of this discussion. However, the effects of many disease states or drugs involve perturbations of *both* absorptive and motor functions, and the relative contribution of each cannot always be determined. The basis of disease and disability caused by colonic *gas, ischemia,* and *neoplasia* will also be given consideration.

ABNORMALITIES OF TRANSPORT OF WATER AND ELECTROLYTES

The Absent Colon (Table 22)

It is appropriate to begin by considering the effect of removing the colon. In general, there are no major pathophysiologic consequences of total colectomy. Normally the colon absorbs 1 to 1.5 liters of water and 100 to 200 mEq of sodium chloride daily and is capable of increasing the recovery of fluid and electrolytes lost from the small intestine during periods of reduced absorption or *net* secretion. The colon, unlike the small intestine, responds to aldosterone to maintain salt and water balance during deprivation or excessive losses. In the absence of a functional colon, this adaptive mechanism is lost, and the patient with an ileostomy or a functionally compromised colon is at greater risk for complications of increased ileal output.

The colon participates in the enterohepatic circula-

TABLE 22. CONSEQUENCES OF COLECTOMY

More vulnerable to increases in ileal fluid output.
Disappearance of secondary bile salts.
At increased risk for urinary calcium and urate stones.
At no risk for urinary oxalate stones secondary to steatorrhea.

tion of bile acids, and in the absence of an active fecal flora, secondary bile acids are no longer produced. The colon is also responsible for the absorption of excess oxalate caused by fat malabsorption. Therefore, patients with sufficient ileal disease to produce malabsorption of bile acids are spared the consequences of hyperoxaluria and urinary oxalate stones. However, as the kidney increases its reabsorption of water and electrolytes to compensate for enteric losses, as many as 5 per cent of patients with ileostomies may develop urinary tract stones composed of calcium salts or sodium urate.

Resection or dysfunction of a sufficient quantity of terminal ileum will result in depletion of the bile acid pool, causing steatorrhea. Malabsorbed bile acids and the byproducts of fat malabsorption, hydroxy-fatty acids, are cathartic substances. Whereas the amount of steatorrhea is related to the length of the ileal resection, the severity of diarrhea, the fecal weight, transit time, and electrolyte composition are related to the amount of *colon* resected. Therefore, the consequences of ileal dysfunction can be assessed accurately only with knowledge of the reserve capacity of the colon.

Diarrhea Associated with Malabsorption of Fat and Bile Acids: Steatorrhea and Cholerrheic Enteropathy (Table 23)

Dietary triglycerides and bile acids may produce diarrhea; it may be difficult to determine which of these two is responsible for the diarrhea in certain clinical situations. The presence of excess bile acids in the colon may produce colonic secretion and stimulate motility, but not all bile acids affect the colon equally. Dihydroxy bile acids with alpha-linked hydroxyl

TABLE 23. CHOLERRHEIC ENTEROPATHY: COLONIC SECRETION INDUCED BY BILE SALTS

Structural requirements of the bile salts:
  dihydroxy bile acids (chenic acid, deoxycholic acid)
  α-linked hydroxyl groups in the 3, 7, or 12 positions
  may be either conjugated or unconjugated salts
Secretion not produced by:
  trihydroxy or monohydroxy bile acids (cholic acid or
    lithocholic acid)
  keto-substituted bile acids (ketolithocholic acid)
  dihydroxy bile acids with β-linked-OH (ursodeoxycholic acid)

groups in the 3, 7, or 12 positions will specifically alter mucosal transport function. The dihydroxy primary bile acid, chenic (or chenodeoxycholic) acid, and the dihydroxy secondary bile acid, deoxycholic acid, are very effective colonic secretagogues. However, the trihydroxy primary bile acid, cholic acid, the dihydroxy 7-beta-hydroxy bile acid, ursodeoxycholic acid, as well as keto-substituted bile acids such as 7-ketolithocholic acid, all lack the ability to stimulate secretion. Conjugation of dihydroxy bile acids does not diminish their effects on mucosal secretion.

Bile acids synthesized by the human liver are the *primary* bile acids (cholic and chenic); their conjugation to glycine or taurine permits bile acids to remain in the intestinal lumen to participate in micellar formation until 95 per cent of dietary lipid is absorbed, whereupon the conjugated bile acids are reabsorbed in the terminal ileum. However, during their sojourn in the intestine, approximately one quarter to one third of the primary bile salt pool is converted to *secondary* bile salts by anaerobic bacteria. Any residual chenic acid that escapes reabsorption, and the deoxycholic acid produced by bacterial 7-dehydroxylation, may produce cholerrheic enteropathy. To treat this disorder, a substance that binds bile acids such as an anion-exchange resin (cholestyramine or colestipol), or an aluminum-based antacid, may be given.

Steatorrhea classically produces a bulky and greasy, but not watery, stool. However, the escape of triglycerides from the small intestine exposes them to colonic flora that may hydrate the fatty acid chains at sites of unsaturation. Hydroxy-fatty acids with chain lengths of 12 or more carbon atoms ("long chain") are clinically important secretagogues. It is of interest that castor oil contains a long chain unsaturated hydroxy fatty acid—ricinoleic acid—which is a potent secretagogue. Ricinoleate also alters motor function in the colon, underscoring the difficulty in separating the relative roles of secretion and motility in the pathophysiology of diarrhea. Although some controversy remains about the relative importance of hydroxylation at sites of unsaturation in the carbon chain to the ability of fatty acids to induce colonic secretion, it is clear that fatty acids must be hydrolyzed from the parent triglycerides to alter intestinal electrolyte movement. Therefore, the fecal flora and the failure to absorb *hydrolyzed* fat are the central key issues in the production of secretagogues from malabsorbed lipid.

Anaerobic colonic flora also metabolize nonabsorbed carbohydrate substrates into large quantities of volatile short-chain fatty acids (VFA) such as acetic acid, proprionic acid, and butyric acid. VFAs provide an important source of metabolic fuel for colonic epithelium. The presence of butyric acid in the experimental colon produces dramatic increases in the absorption of sodium. Although little data exist on the subject, it is tempting to suggest that a perturbation in colonic flora that produces a fall in colonic butyrate production—such as during antibiotic therapy—may reduce the capacity of the colon to absorb salt and water.

Diarrhea Associated with Malabsorbed Carbohydrate

Carbohydrates that escape intestinal absorption may per se produce an increase in fecal osmolality. However, metabolism of this substrate by colonic bacteria results in the production of VFAs and gas (carbon dioxide, hydrogen, and methane). By overwhelming the colon with a hyperosmolar load, these substances produce cramping abdominal pain, borborygmi, flatulence, and watery diarrhea. Different responses to carbohydrate malabsorption are accounted for by individual variations in colonic flora, which may be altered by antibiotics. Furthermore, modest acidification of the fecal content to pH 5 to 6 significantly inhibits the formation of hydrogen gas from malabsorbed carbohydrate sources.

This phenomenon may be manipulated for therapeutic purposes by the use of *lactulose*. Lactulose is a synthetic disaccharide that is not absorbed from the intestine by virtue of the nonhydrolyzable beta (1,4) linkage between galactose and fructose. Lactulose is not metabolized until it reaches the colon, where it undergoes degradation by bacteria into organic acids, producing a drop in the pH of colonic contents from 7.0 to approximately 5.0, which favors the trapping of ammonia as NH_4^+ in the colon. The metabolism of lactulose results in the liberation of an increased number of osmotically active particles, producing diarrhea. The concerted action of fecal acidification and shortened fecal transit time reduces the absorption of substances that produce hepatic encephalopathy. The administration of an appropriate dose of *lactose* to a lactase-deficient individual may accomplish a similar beneficial result in hepatic failure.

Inflammatory Bowel Disease (IBD)

Perhaps no gastrointestinal disease is surrounded with more controversial issues than IBD. Numerous mechanisms have been suggested for the pathogenesis of both *ulcerative colitis* and *Crohn's disease* of the colon, without any promise of a prompt resolution. Although distinctions between these two diseases can usually be made clinically, overlap exists between both the clinical picture and the pathophysiologic principles.

Ulcerative colitis is a disease of the colonic epithelium, characterized by recurrent episodes of inflammation associated with hypermotility, excess losses of fluid, electrolytes, mucus and serum proteins, and the appearance of frank bleeding in the stool. Some evidence indicates that the inflammatory process and epithelial secretion are mediated by mucosal prostaglandins. Sulfasalazine, the mainstay of therapy against colonic IBD, inhibits the production of metabolites of arachidonic acid, prostaglandins and leukotrienes as does 5-aminosalicylate, strongly suggesting that this moiety (rather than the sulfapyridine portion of the molecule) is the active therapeutic agent. Nonsteroidal antiinflammatory drugs such as salicylates inhibit the prostaglandin synthetase system, but are ineffective therapeutically. The principal drug for treating severe IBD—corticosteroids—inhibits lipoxygenase and cyclooxygenase, preventing breakdown of arachidonic acid into leukotrienes and prostaglandins.

Extreme degrees of inflammation in ulcerative colitis may occasionally (<5 per cent of cases) involve the smooth muscle layer and proceed to a total cessation of motor activity and catastrophic dilatation of the colon. This complication, toxic megacolon, may result in perforation or may heal, possibly leaving a fixed stenotic segment of colon.

Crohn's disease of the colon is an infiltrative, transmural disease that may be clinically indistinguishable from ulcerative colitis, and may be associated with extensive disease of the small intestine and upper gastrointestinal tract. Because of the prominent transmural nature of Crohn's disease, it may produce deep mucosal fissures, fistulous connections between segments of bowel or between bowel and skin (particularly in the perianal region), and obstructive symptoms caused by exuberant cellular infiltration and narrowing of the bowel lumen. Gross rectal bleeding is less common in Crohn's colitis than in ulcerative colitis.

The pathogenesis of IBD remains a major problem confronting investigators. All forms of infectious agents have been implicated: several viruses, slow-growing mycobacteria, cell wall–deficient bacteria, *Clostridium difficile* toxin, and combinations of these. Abnormalities of lymphocyte function have been reported, including defective suppressor T cell activity, suggesting that perhaps trivial acute inflammation may progress to chronic disease because of a deficiency in the arm of the inflammatory process that limits the activity. IBD may cluster in families, in regions, or in time, supporting the concept of a transmissible infectious agent in this disease. However, a recently described structural deficiency in the mucin of patients with ulcerative colitis (present in active and inactive disease) raises the possibility of an inherited, biochemical basis for susceptibility. Finally, cigarette smoking correlates negatively with the incidence of ulcerative colitis; relapses in activity may follow the discontinuation of tobacco. This suggests that additional pharmacologic factors may influence the activity of the disease. Much work remains to define the roles of factors involved in the causation and modulation of IBD.

ABNORMALITIES OF COLONIC FLORA

The pathophysiology of diarrhea caused by infectious agents is described in greater detail in the section on the small intestine. Topics specific to the colon will be addressed here.

Cell-free lysates of the parasite *Entameba histolytica* stimulate the secretion of salt and water in the experimental colon and ileum. The secretion appears to be mediated by serotonin produced by the protozoa, as it may be blocked by an antibody to, or known antagonists of, serotonin. Hormone-like substances and neurotransmitters have been detected in other bacteria and protozoa, but their role in producing colonic secretion during infection is as yet unexplored.

The shigella bacterium, an invasive agent that produces colonic secretion, elaborates an enterotoxin that stimulates mucosal secretion similar to that seen with *Vibrio cholerae*, a noninvasive organism. However, unlike the cholera enterotoxin, shigella toxin produces a delayed response (100 minutes vs 15 to 30 minutes) and cytotoxic changes in columnar epithelium. Still other shigella toxins are secretogogues and neurotoxins, explaining some of the variable manifestations of this infection.

Diarrhea is not uncommon during or following the administration of a variety of antibiotics, particularly by the enteral route. As mentioned above, the production of VFA, which are products of the bacterial degradation of nonabsorbed carbohydrates, facilitates the capacity of the colon to absorb fluid and electrolytes. Although not yet proved, a reduction in VFA may reduce net absorption in the colon and increase stool water. In addition, perfusion of the intestine with the antibiotic clindamycin acutely reduces the transport of fluid and electrolytes, and induces net secretion in the rat ileum.

A more serious complication of antibiotic use is the emergence of the anaerobe *Clostridium difficile,* which causes pseudomembranous colitis. This is recognized as a relatively common and potentially serious form of diarrhea. This entity should be distinguished from the historically more prominent entities pseudomembranous *entero*colitis (which may be a problem in newborns and may complicate the course of some seriously ill adults, but is not related to antibiotics) and *pseudomembranous colitis* caused by enterotoxin-producing *Staphylococcus aureus* (which does not necessarily follow antibiotic use).

C. difficile may be a normal bowel inhabitant in small numbers, which emerges when its bacterial competition has been eliminated by broad-spectrum antibiotics. Alternatively, this anaerobe may colonize the susceptible individual in a nosocomial setting and produce disease without antecedent antibiotic use. The organism is noninvasive, but its lysis releases a potent toxin that produces nonselective cytopathic effects to colonic epithelium, causing the disease. This property also affects cultured human amniotic cells and is the basis of the bioassay for the toxin. The resulting colitis and its attendant diarrhea may persist long after the offending antibiotic is withdrawn, demonstrating that although antibiotics may alter colonic transport function by a direct mechanism, the basis of this disease lies in the cytopathic toxin.

The antibiotics most often implicated in producing pseudomembranous colitis are broad-spectrum antibiotics with prominent activity against anaerobic bacteria (exclusive of *C. difficile*). These include clindamycin and lincomycin (the most important offenders), all of the members of the penicillin and cephalosporin families, and less often virtually every other antibiotic with the notable exceptions of vancomycin (to which *C. difficile* is usually sensitive) and the aminoglycosides. Tetracyclines and erythromycin are relatively uncommon offenders, in spite of their activity against anaerobic bacteria and their frequent usage.

Unresolved issues regarding *C. difficile* include the frequent presence of the organism and toxin in the stools of 25 to 50 per cent of asymptomatic neonates and 3 per cent of healthy adults, the role of *C. difficile* toxin in chronic inflammatory bowel disease, and the role of the toxin in patients with antibiotic-associated diarrhea without pseudomembrane formation. An additional clinical conundrum is an explanation for *focal* pseudomembranous disease produced by *C. difficile*—that is, disease in the proximal colon that spares the rectum.

HORMONES AND COLONIC SECRETION

Hormones must be taken into account in describing the pathophysiology of the colon, but their role in producing dysfunction appears to be less important than in the small intestine. Since many "hormones" may function primarily as paracrine or neurotransmitter substances, one cannot rely upon peripheral blood levels to indicate their role in normal or abnormal states.

Vasoactive intestinal polypeptide (VIP) produces prominent effects in the colon in several experimental settings. In the human colon, VIP virtually abolishes net water absorption and inhibits the transport of sodium and chloride. VIP stimulates active chloride secretion in the rat colon by increasing the activity of adenyl cyclase, augmenting mucosal levels of cyclic AMP. Thus, the diarrhea that is associated with either infusions of VIP or VIP-secreting tumors is partially caused by its effects on colonic as well as upon small intestinal function.

Enteroglucagon is richly represented in colonic mucosa, but little is known about its role in salt and water homeostasis. Other peptide hormones have variable effects upon secretion and absorption in different species, but little is known about their roles in the pathophysiology of any discrete disorder. Basal levels of pancreatic polypeptide, and both basal and postprandial responses of motilin, enteroglucagon, and VIP are significantly greater in hospitalized patients with acute diarrhea (of a variety of causes) than among controls, whereas plasma levels of gastrin, gastric inhibitory polypeptide (GIP), and pancreatic glucagon are normal. However, the role of these hormones in the genesis of acute and chronic diarrheal states is purely speculative at this time.

The gut hormone with perhaps the greatest impact upon colonic function is cholecystokinin (CCK), the effects of which exemplify overlapping of secretory and motor functions in colonic disorders. (The effects of CCK and thyroid hormone on the colon will be discussed later in this chapter.)

EFFECTS OF LAXATIVES AND OTHER DRUGS ON COLONIC SECRETION

Formerly most laxatives were considered to act either as osmotic cathartics or as stimulants of intestinal motility. It is now generally appreciated that most agents used to relieve constipation or diarrhea affect absorptive *and* motor function in the colon.

Exogenously administered agents such as the detergent laxative dioctylsulfosuccinate (DOSS, initially thought to be a "bulk agent"), ricinoleic acid (the dihydroxy fatty acid present in castor oil), magnesium sulfate (sometimes referred to as a "saline cathartic,"

thought to produce passive movement of solvent down an osmotic gradient), and all of the so-called "stimulant cathartics" that have been studied (phenolphthalein, bisacodyl, oxyphenisatin, cascara, and senna) produce net secretion of fluid into the colon. These agents also result in the stimulation of motor activity in the colon, and it is not clear whether this action can be isolated from the secretory effects of the agents. The two effects will certainly be synergistic in opposing the absorptive function of the colon, but enhanced motility per se appears to be an inadequate explanation for the increase in fecal water produced by these agents.

On the reverse side of the coin, antidiarrheal agents such as opiates (morphine, codeine) and their congeners (synthetic enkephalins, diphenoxylate, loperamide) stimulate net absorption of sodium, chloride, and water from the ileum and colon. Some of these agents have been shown specifically to inhibit colonic secretion mediated by cyclic AMP or cyclic GMP. Changes in absorptive function take place in concert with alterations in motility to enhance the recovery of fluid from the colonic contents.

Two naturally occurring constituents of the feces may stimulate net secretion of fluid and electrolytes into the colon, namely certain bile acids and fatty acids. Dihydroxy bile acids and long chain hydroxy fatty acids alter membrane permeability, produce net intestinal secretion, appear to stimulate active secretion of chloride ion, and produce changes in mucosal morphology and motor function. Chloride secretion produced by ricinoleate appears to be mediated by cyclic AMP. The fecal effluent induced by the above agents is essentially isotonic NaCl and HCO_3^-.

ABNORMALITIES OF MOTOR FUNCTION

As discussed, the colon is richly innervated from within (the myenteric nervous system) and by the autonomic nervous system. A functional ileocecal valve prevents reflux of colonic contents (and its specialized flora) back into the small intestine. The anus and rectum regulate the passage of feces. Colonic contents are churned in the proximal colon to facilitate the completion of absorption, and the distal colon regulates the aboral flow of feces and their segmentation. The circular and longitudinal smooth musculature are coordinated by mechanisms mentioned previously to facilitate the role of the colon as a reservoir and excretory organ.

FUNCTIONAL DISORDERS OF COLONIC MOTILITY: CONSTIPATION, IRRITABLE BOWEL SYNDROME (IBS), AND DIVERTICULOSIS

The clinical symptoms and complications of disorders of colonic motility range from the minor to severe discomfiture of irritable bowel syndrome (IBS) to death from perforated diverticula.

Stress, anxiety, emotionally charged events, travel, and other external stimuli affect bowel function. Studies of motility during stressful interviews or discussions of disturbing personal experiences have demonstrated colonic spasm in association with feelings of hostility and an inhibition of motor activity during periods of weeping (Fig. 54). Changes in colonic motor function occurring with emotional stress are not specific for IBS and may be seen in persons who do not usually suffer gastrointestinal symptoms with distress. These patterns of abnormal motility are not uniformly seen among patients with IBS, nor are such changes consistently present with serial testing of affected individuals. Furthermore, little insight has been gained into the factors that determine which patients will suffer disabling gastrointestinal symptoms after minor stress, nor the factors that modulate the frequency of such symptoms.

In spite of these limitations, some general pathophysiologic principles have been established. First, a wide range of normal is recorded for colorectal transit time and frequency of bowel evacuation. Therefore, the perception of constipation will depend upon the patient's cultural and personal expectations, since no standards exist to define normality. Numerous disease states that produce an "atonic" colon will produce unquestionable, objective fecal inertia. However, so-called "functional" constipation has been associated with a heightening of motility in circular smooth muscle—that is, nonpropulsive motor activity—whereas "functional" diarrhea has been associated with relaxation of circular smooth muscle and a relative paucity of motor activity. Patients with longstanding chronic idiopathic constipation requiring daily laxatives have responded to the opiate antagonist naloxone within 24 hours with an increase in fecal water and passage of feces, suggesting that the constipation in that setting was caused by an excessive effect of endogenous opiates.

Irritable Bowel Syndrome. IBS encompasses patients whose complaints of abdominal pain, diarrhea or constipation, or both lead them to believe they are ill. No morphologic or biochemical indices have been found to define the disorder, and the term "irritable" in no way implies inflammation nor any insight into pathogenesis. Symptoms of IBS are best explained by perturbations in motility. Motility studies in the rectosigmoid colon on IBS patients reveal a higher than normal incidence of 2 to 3 cycle per minute slow wave activity, which leads to increased colonic motor activity during periods of stimulation. Slow wave activity comprises approximately 40 per cent of the motility tracing in IBS patients, as opposed to 10 per cent in normals. Powerful, prolonged 2 to 3 cycle per minute contractions ("spasms") have been associated with episodes of abdominal pain in these patients. It has been suggested that this motor activity is associated with nonpropulsive haustration of the colon. Stimuli such as meals and drugs that are normally well tolerated may trigger this dysmotility in the IBS patient. Intravenous injections of cholecystokinin can reproduce abdominal pain in these patients. Administration of this hormone increases colonic spike activity without altering slow wave rhythms, and the level of this hormone normally rises in response to a meal. Abdominal pain in this setting may be a reflection of hyperresponsiveness of colonic smooth muscle to ordinary stimuli, which results in heightened but *nonpropulsive* motor activity. An abnormally prolonged postprandial increase in colonic spike and motor activity has been observed in IBS patients (Fig. 55). Administration of the anticholinergic agent clidinium bromide does not affect the frequency of slow colonic waves or resting spike and

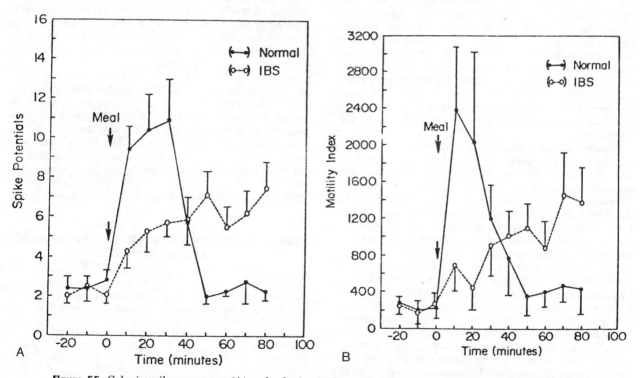

Figure 55. Colonic spike responses *(A)* and colonic motility index *(B)* are compared between IBS patients and normal controls. The IBS patients have a delayed and prolonged increase in postprandial spike and motor activities compared to controls. (From Sullivan M. A., Cohen, S., and Snape, W. J., Jr.: Colonic myoelectrical activity in irritable-bowel syndrome. Effect of eating and anticholinergics. N Engl J Med 298:880, 1978.)

motor activity but does reduce the intensity and duration of the prolonged postprandial colonic motor responses.

Studies utilizing a rectal balloon to distend the colon and record myoelectric activity there demonstrate an increase in 3 to 4 cycle per minute slow waves and an increase in the motility index in IBS patients over normal subjects. Contrary to what had been previously reported, IBS patients with prominent diarrhea had 6 to 9 cycle per minute phasic activity, which correlated with the symptoms elicited by this technique. Patients who complained of constipation were least likely to have 6 to 9 cycle per minute activity, demonstrating some of the discrepancies that unfortunately characterize attempts to understand this disorder. Inflation of the rectal balloons reproduced the painful symptoms experienced by these patients, who appeared to be more sensitive to distention than were controls. Specific foods have been shown to provoke specific symptoms in some IBS patients. It is not clear whether the provocative foods elicit a direct pharmacologic response, an allergic response, or simply produce modest amounts of gas in unusually sensitive individuals.

Some investigating groups have attempted to divide IBS patients into diarrhea-predominant and constipation-predominant groups. The diarrhea predominant group has historically been characterized by painless dilatation of the colon coupled with a passive, dependent personality. Diminished motor activity has been reported in this latter group, which was abolished when the patients wept, but subsequent studies have demonstrated increased colonic motility in this clinical setting. It is difficult to understand how diarrhea could result from hypomotility unless the circular, segmenting activity selectively ceased while the longitudinal motor activity continued unabated. The constipation-predominant group of IBS patients has historically been characterized as having prominent abdominal pain, a tense, hostile personality, and increased myoelectric activity in the resting and stimulated colon. Again, this concept has been challenged, and much remains to be understood concerning specific motor patterns associated with the clinical poles of the IBS spectrum.

Colonic Diverticulosis. This disorder is much more clearly related to abnormalities of colonic motor function. Epidemiologically, diverticulosis is linked with populations ingesting a low residue diet and increases in frequency with advancing age, suggesting that this disorder is a maladaptive response to inadequate fecal bulk. The circular smooth muscle is hypertrophied in the colons of such individuals, and this phenomenon precedes the development of the diverticula. An increase in phasic activity and intracolonic pressures of 50 to 90 mm Hg may be recorded in these patients. Segments of colon containing diverticula contract excessively in response to cholinergic stimulation (prostigmine), opiates (morphine), and meals. Intracolonic pressure within these segments eventually forces mucosa through points of weakness in the circular colonic musculature, usually at the site of entry of the penetrating arterial branch of the mesenteric vessel on the mesenteric site of the taenia coli. Although most diverticula remain silent, weakness in the bowel wall and the continued presence of high intracolonic pres-

sure may lead to perforation, spilling of colonic contents into the peritoneum, and peritonitis. Although this inflammatory process is usually self limited, it accounts for the episodes of pain, fever, and leukocytosis seen in diverticulitis. This may heal without complication, or the inflammatory process may surround the colon, producing colonic obstruction, necessitating surgical intervention. Less often, the diverticulum may impinge upon and erode into the mesenteric arterial branch and produce brisk hemorrhage. Although diverticula are far more numerous in the sigmoid and descending colon than in the proximal colon, diverticular hemorrhage has been reported equally from the right and left colon. It is not clear whether diverticula in the right colon are unique or whether bleeding from undiagnosed angiodysplasia has been mistakenly attributed to otherwise innocuous diverticula in this region.

Patients with diverticulosis but no diverticulitis may complain of cramping left lower quadrant pain, often in response to certain foods or stress. The pain is probably secondary to spasm in the region of the diverticula. Therefore, it appears that excessive motor function, primarily nonpropulsive contraction of hypertrophied circular smooth muscle, is responsible for the chronic symptoms of this disease, in addition to its pathogenetic role. As such, diverticulosis appears to be closely related to the pole of the IBS spectrum associated with pain and constipation.

AGANGLIONOSIS, PSEUDO-OBSTRUCTION, AND MEGACOLON

A wide group of chronic colonic dysmotility syndromes characterized by inadequate propulsion of feces may be grouped together, from which a growing list of discrete entities has emerged (Table 24). These syndromes all share a clinical picture of bowel obstruction without an occluding lesion.

Hirschsprung's disease, or *congenital megacolon,* is the best characterized of these hypomotility diseases. In this condition, the intramural ganglionic plexus is congenitally absent from the distal colorectum. The segment of involved bowel is variable, usually involves the rectum and distal sigmoid, but has occasionally involved the entire colon. The aganglionic segment is tonically contracted, and the bowel is dilated proximally. The anal sphincters fail to relax in response to parasympathomimetic drugs but denervation hyper-

TABLE 24. SYSTEMIC DISORDERS CAUSING REDUCED COLONIC MOTILITY

Scleroderma	Parkinson's disease
Polymyositis	Familial visceral myopathy
Dermatomyositis	Pheochromocytoma
Systemic lupus erythematosus	Familial autonomic
Hollow visceral myopathy	dysfunction
Acute intermittent porphyria	Hypoparathyroidism
Amyloidosis	Chagas' disease
Ceroidosis	Uremia
Myxedema	Hypokalemia
Diabetes mellitus	Hypercalcemia
Myotonic dystrophy	Hirschsprung's disease
	Drugs

sensitivity to muscarinic stimulation is not seen. The extent of the aganglionic segment (documented morphologically using full-thickness biopsy and barium enema) must be established, since complete surgical removal of this segment is usually the most reasonable remedy.

A dilated, hypomotile colon is more often an *acquired* abnormality; however, the pathogenesis of this clinical syndrome is recognized in only a minority of cases. The pathophysiologic basis has recently come to light for some of the patients grouped under the rubric "chronic intestinal pseudo-obstruction." One inherited disorder, called *hollow visceral myopathy,* is characterized by atrophy and vacuolization of the longitudinal and circular smooth muscle and its replacement by collagen. Additional ultrastructural changes in smooth muscle are evident at electron microscopy. At least one family has been reported in which the longitudinal smooth muscle layer was affected with relative sparing of the circular layer. These diseases are inherited as autosomal dominant characteristics, and afflicted patients may also have abnormalities in the upper gastrointestinal tract and urinary tract smooth muscle.

In a second familial syndrome with a similar clinical picture, the smooth muscle is morphologically intact, but the neurons of the myenteric plexuses are reduced in number and are morphologically abnormal. This has been termed *familial visceral neuropathy,* and cases that have similar involvement in the spinal and celiac ganglia and central nervous system have been given the more general name *familial autonomic dysfunction.*

Other generalized disorders of neural control or function may affect the gastrointestinal tract and produce a hypomotile colon. Included among these are rare syndromes such as acute intermittent porphyria and gastrointestinal ganglioneuromatosis. Multiple sclerosis and Parkinson's disease are more common neurologic syndromes in which simple constipation or megacolon may develop. Perhaps the most frequent cause of altered motility is disordered autonomic control secondary to *diabetes mellitus.* In general, this complication is seen in association with peripheral neuropathy and other manifestations of autonomic neuropathy. Slow wave activity and the response to exogenously administered cholinergic stimulation remain intact in these patients; however, the normal colonic response to a meal is deficient. Although the most prominent gastrointestinal symptom of diabetic neuropathy is constipation, diarrhea may be a more disabling complication. Since no specific treatment is available for autonomic neuropathy, one should be careful to exclude bacterial overgrowth caused by hypomotility or in association with small intestinal diverticulosis.

Hypomotility may result from smooth muscle disease in the colon. Gastrointestinal smooth muscle atrophy affects about 40 per cent of patients with *scleroderma.* These patients also have normal colonic slow wave activity but have absent responses to meals and a diminished response to cholinergic stimulation, caused by atrophy and fibrosis of the smooth muscle layer. The defect early in scleroderma is best explained on the basis of a neurologic disorder; however, the disease is characterized by a striking morphologic and functional failure of smooth muscle later in its course.

Constipation, colonic dilatation, and hypomotility may be seen in *dermatomyositis, polymyositis,* and *systemic lupus erythematosus.* The pathophysiology in these situations is presumably similar to that of scleroderma, but none has been studied intensively and all are complicated by the potential for coexisting vasculitis. Infiltration of the muscle layer or neural elements or both in *amyloidosis, ceroidosis,* or *myxedema* may produce a similar picture.

Acute massive dilatation of the colon may be seen in the postoperative state or in acutely ill patients requiring ventilatory support. These profound hypomotility states can produce very large cecal diameters (in which the risk of cecal perforation becomes extreme), necessitating colonoscopic decompression or surgical cecostomy. Postoperative ileus has been traditionally attributed to a combination of factors including the perioperative medications and manipulation of the bowel at laparotomy, presumably mediated by hyperactivity of the sympathetic nervous system. Neither general anesthesia per se nor the extent of handling and exposure of the gut during laparotomy appear to be primary factors in determining the duration of postoperative ileus. It is more likely that medications with prominent anticholinergic effects and narcotics play a major role in prolonging ileus in the postoperative period. One should expect depression of contractible activity for 40 to 48 hours postoperatively in the right colon (location of the pacemaker); however, recovery of the left colon, which determines the clinical recovery from ileus, may take several more days in some cases.

Even less is known about the acquired megacolon observed in the acutely ill patient on ventilatory support. The hypomotility may be caused by a combination of drug therapy and excessive activity of the sympathetic nervous system, and the condition may be complicated by excessive amounts of air ingested by the awake patient attempting to gasp while intubated. Some patients respond to cholinergic drugs (neostigmine), others do not; thus the pathophysiologic basis, presumed to involve autonomic imbalance, remains obscure. The problem is most commonly associated with respiratory failure, and is usually ameliorated by extubation. More aggressive intervention, however, may be necessary when the cecum dilates over 12 cm in diameter. The cecum is used as the weathervane for intervention, since its larger circumference results in the greatest wall tension (assuming that intraluminal pressure is evenly distributed throughout the colon), and its thin wall is therefore most susceptible to perforation.

DISORDERS OF THE ANAL SPHINCTER

Normal function of the anus has previously been discussed in detail, and a relatively short list of disorders is attributed to this sphincter. The most serious of these problems is a loss of coordination during defecation. Distention of the rectum results in reflex and voluntary relaxation of the smooth and striated muscle and sphincters, respectively. Some investigators have suggested that abnormal tone and motor mechanics—that is, failure of relaxation—are a cause of chronic constipation and recommend anorectal myotomy for patients with abnormal manometric tracings. The prevalence of this disorder is a matter of some debate. Hyperactivity of the anal sphincter has been implicated in the pathogenesis of anal fissures and hemorrhoids. This, too, is a disputed question, and it is not clear whether the hypermotility is the cause or is simply a secondary reflex effect. Nonetheless, anal myotomy has been employed for both conditions.

At the opposite end of the spectrum, incontinence may result from relaxation of the anal sphincter. Anal incompetence may be related to trauma to the sphincter (obstetric, surgical, or other), but many cases appear to be related to idiopathic denervation. Diabetes mellitus may result in abnormal internal anal sphincter function and episodes of fecal incontinence. Lesions of the sacral roots must be extensive to reduce tone seriously in the external anal sphincter. Spinal cord lesions above the level of the sacrum leave an active anal sphincter, and normal defecation may usually be accomplished by rectal distention in paraplegic individuals.

HORMONAL EFFECTS ON COLONIC MOTILITY

The past decade has witnessed great progress in gathering information on gastrointestinal hormones and regulatory peptides; however, the roles of these agents in colonic function and malfunction remain relatively unexplored. Cholecystokinin stimulates colonic motility, and an exaggeration of the colonic response may underlie symptoms in some patients with IBS. Endorphins and enkephalins—the endogenous opiates—are present in the gut and may play a role in functional diarrhea. In contrast to the small intestine, where motility is inhibited by enkephalins, tonic nonpropulsive contractions are stimulated by these agents in the colon, and this response is blocked by naloxone. The control of colonic motility is complex, and the factors that modulate the relative activation of circular as opposed to longitudinal musculature, and the factors producing coordinated, propulsive activity as opposed to simultaneous, nonpropulsive motility remain to be elucidated. The role played by the central nervous system in the control of motility is uncertain. Injection of very small amounts of somatostatin or of cholecystokinin octapeptide into the lateral ventricles of the rat brain modulates the frequency of migrating motor complexes of the intestine in a dose related manner, suggesting key central nervous system involvement in the control of motility.

Sex hormones may also modulate motility. Gastrointestinal transit time is significantly prolonged in the luteal phase of the menstrual cycle, when progesterone levels are highest. This may account for cyclic variations in bowel function in women. Transit times are also significantly prolonged during the third trimester of pregnancy, supporting the observation that progesterone inhibits colonic motor function.

EFFECTS OF DRUGS AND FIBER ON COLONIC FUNCTION

Drugs play an important and often overlooked role in colonic function (Table 25). Cholinergic stimulation

TABLE 25. DRUGS INDUCING CONSTIPATION

Analgesics
Anesthetic agents
Antacids (calcium and aluminum compounds)
Anticholinergics
Anticonvulsants
Antidepressive agents
Barium sulfate
Bismuth
Diuretics
Drugs for parkinsonism
Ganglionic blockers
Hematinics (iron especially)
Hypotensives
MAO inhibitors
Metallic intoxication (arsenic, lead, mercury, phosphorus)
Muscle paralyzers
Opiates
Psychotherapeutic drugs
Laxative addiction???

From Sleisenger, M. H., and Fordtran, J. S. (eds.): Gastrointestinal Disease. 3rd ed. Philadelphia, W. B. Saunders Co., 1983.

of colonic smooth muscle increases motor activity; the synaptic junctions at the ganglion are nicotinic but the receptors on the smooth muscle itself are muscarinic. Therefore, methacholine, bethanechol, and neostigmine all cause stimulation of colonic motor function. Muscarinic antagonists such as atropine, propantheline, and pirenzapine inhibit colonic motility, increase colonic transit time, and in so doing, may relieve pain due to spasm. Other drugs appear to cause the direct relaxation of colonic smooth muscle (nonmuscarinic), such as the so-called "antispasmodic" agents such as dicyclomine and tridihexyl chloride.

Adrenergic nerves from the sympathetic nervous system generally counteract and modulate parasympathetic activity. Alpha-adrenergic agonists (such as phenylephrine and clonidine) stimulate colonic motility, whereas beta agonists (such as isoproterenol) are inhibitory. The side effects of beta-adrenergic blockade are of primary interest, since these drugs are used widely in clinical practice. Propranolol (a nonselective beta blocker) and metoprolol (a selective beta$_1$ antagonist) produce significant increases in sigmoid colonic pressures, perhaps by inhibiting beta-adrenergic input and unmasking tonic alpha-adrenergic activity. Propranolol also prevents the stimulation of adenyl cyclase by secretogogues through a mechanism that may be independent of simple adrenergic antagonism. The clinical manifestations of the "beta blockers" are not consistent, however, reflecting the complex interplay among the various factors controlling motility. Propranolol has been reported to decrease the number of bowel movements and the degree of fat excretion in two hyperthyroid patients. However, propanolol produces *greater* increases in sigmoid pressure in patients with IBS than in normal people, and symptoms of IBS will be unmasked in some patients treated with this drug.

Most opiates (morphine, codeine) cause an increase in nonpropulsive motility in the colon, and stimulate absorptive function. Anal sphincter tone is augmented, and attention to the rectal defecatory reflex may be diminished, which can produce severe constipation. Atropine may relieve the spasms induced by opiates but does not restore propulsive motility. Meperidine

(Demerol) does not cause the sigmoid colon to generate pressures as high as those seen with morphine, does not increase segmental pressure, and actually diminishes phasic activity. Diphenoxylate and loperamide—congeners of meperidine—inhibit mass movement and decrease longitudinal and circular muscle activity in the colon. As such, these drugs are used empirically in diarrhea for their constipating effects. Pentazocine (Talwin), a synthetic opiate with weak antagonist activity, decreases intraluminal colonic pressure and may be a preferable agent for patients who require an opiate but also have a dysmotility syndrome such as IBS or diverticulosis.

Psychoactive drugs should be mentioned because of their widespread use and potential to alter colonic motility substantially. Sedative drugs (benzodiazepines, barbiturates) may reduce both segmental and propulsive activity in the colon. The tricyclic antidepressants and phenothiazines may produce severe constipation on the basis of their anticholinergic activity. They may be a particular problem in the inactive institutionalized patient who requires large doses of these drugs. The development of atonic megacolon is not rare in this circumstance.

DIETARY FIBER

Dietary fiber is nondigestible complex carbohydrate that adds bulk to stool. However, dietary fiber is far from inert; it provides a nutritional source for colonic bacteria and is a substrate for the production of VFAs. Fiber stimulates the net secretion of fluid into stool. Transit time of stool is reduced. By increasing the colonic diameter without increasing intrinsic wall tension, dietary fiber reduces intraluminal pressures (LaPlace's law). This observation has led to the use of bran for IBS and diverticulosis. Other beneficial effects are postulated regarding colonic carcinogenesis (see below). Dietary bran does not appear to affect plasma lipids or iron significantly, but its effects on the absorption of calcium, zinc, other trace elements and drugs are still uncertain and deserve more study.

INTESTINAL GAS

ORIGINS

Excessive belching, passage of flatus, distention, and active borborygmi are common gastrointestinal complaints. The production of intestinal gas is a combined function of the host (including the adequacy of brush border enzymes, pancreatic function, mucosal absorptive function, and intestinal flora) and the diet. The fasting gut may contain approximately 200 ml of gas, but this rises rapidly following a meal. It was once thought that swallowed air was the major source of gas in the intestinal lumen. Chemical analysis has revealed that aerophagia usually makes an insignificant contribution and that most colonic gas is generated from the metabolism of dietary substrates. Carbon dioxide is generated from the neutralization of gastric acid by pancreatic bicarbonate, and although 500 to 600 ml may be produced with each meal, it is rapidly absorbed into the blood. Hydrogen gas is generated from the bacterial degradation of *undigested* carbohydrate sources. The amount of expired hydrogen can be used to estimate the completeness of absorption of a carbohydrate substrate or to detect bacterial contamination of the upper gastrointestinal tract. As a result, the hydrogen breath test has proved clinically valuable in the diagnosis of disaccharidase deficiency and the blind loop syndrome.

The bacterial flora will determine the composition of colonic gas. Therefore, certain individuals will produce larger amounts of hydrogen and methane, depending upon the dietary intake and colonic flora. The final composition of rectal gas is a function not only of production but also of the relative rates of absorption from the lumen. Thus, rapidly diffusible gases such as carbon dioxide and hydrogen will be lower in the final "product," whereas nitrogen (which may actually diffuse down its concentration gradient from blood to lumen) will be relatively higher.

ERUCTATION

Among individuals who belch frequently, the air that is eructated can be shown to have been recently swallowed into the esophagus. Such patients state that the belching results from thoracic or epigastric discomfort. It is likely that the discomfort is caused by swallowed air that has not been quickly regurgitated, and that an enlarging gastric bubble causes the distress that necessitates the belching. Repeated belching may be also associated with gastric outlet obstruction. However, the vast majority of individuals who belch frequently in order to relieve distress are anxious (constantly swallowing air, thus the word "aerophagia"). The pathophysiology of the symptom complex of aerophagic belching is usually explicable on this basis, although the exact mechanism for the establishment of the habit is not clear.

DISTENTION AND BORBORYGMI

These symptoms, often associated with "gas pains," have classically and erroneously been thought to be caused by excessive gas. Actually individuals with "gas pains" generally have the same amount of gas in the gut as normal subjects, both fasting and postprandially. In addition, the percentages of oxygen, nitrogen, carbon dioxide, hydrogen, and methane were identical for the two groups.

The origin of these gastrointestinal complaints is related to a disturbance in motility rather than excessive amounts of gas. Patients with prominent pain have slower transit times for gas and have more severe symptoms associated with similar degrees of distention compared to normals. In fact, gas infused into the jejunum of patients complaining of chronic abdominal pain has a tendency to reflux back into the stomach rather than to pass directly into the colon. Patients who complain of painful distention from intestinal gas overlap with the larger group of IBS patients who also seem to have disordered motility, and appear to have lower thresholds for pain in the gut than normal controls.

EXCESSIVE FLATUS

This is a complaint that is obviously subjective; documentation of excessive amount of gas per rectum per day is extremely difficult. Flatus is passed on the average 10 to 15 times per day; the amounts vary. It is reasonable to suppose, however, that it is abnormal for individuals to exceed 20 or more passages per day.

The pathophysiology of this complaint is that the patient has been ingesting foods that are substrates for gas formation. This would indicate either the ingestion of carbohydrates not normally digestible by humans (such as raffinose and stachyose in beans), or the ingestion of ordinary carbohydrates by intolerant individuals. Examples of the latter are patients who are lactase-deficient or who have bacterial overgrowth of the small gut, or malabsorption caused by small intestinal or pancreatic disease. These patients have excessive gas owing to bacterial action on unabsorbed carbohydrate, which is hydrolyzed in the colon (or in the small gut if there is bacterial overgrowth), at which time the hexoses are acted upon further with release of hydrogen and carbon dioxide. Some patients have increased frequency of flatus following any meal, and this is most likely caused by a hyperactive gastroileocolic reflex that characterizes many patients with irritable colon syndrome.

If analysis of flatus demonstrates high concentration of hydrogen and carbon dioxide, malabsorbed carbohydrate is the probable culprit. If on the other hand most of the gas that is analyzed has a high concentration of nitrogen, swallowed air is more likely to be the cause. As discussed, most of these patients have emotional problems, and the psychodynamics are not well understood. Anxiety plays a major part, particularly as manifested in phobias related to the possibility of harboring a serious or incurable illness.

ISCHEMIC COLITIS

As with the small intestine, the response of the colon to vascular insufficiency depends on several factors, including the location and extent of occlusive disease, and possible associated systemic disorders. Thus ischemia of the colon may accompany nonthrombotic infarction of the small intestine in patients with cardiac failure, or may result from interruption of the colonic blood supply during an abdominal aortic aneurysmectomy or abdominoperineal resection. It may follow aortoileac reconstruction. Ischemic colitis attributed to loss of the inferior mesenteric artery or important collaterals appears to occur less commonly after abdominoperineal resection of the rectum.

Colonic ischemia may result from localized occlusive disease in the inferior mesenteric artery or in its critical collateral channels. Less commonly, the syndrome is associated with hypercoagulable states, amyloidosis, vasculitis, obstructing colorectal cancer, or the use of oral contraceptive agents. Oral contraceptive-associated ischemic colitis is typically segmental in its distribution. A cause and effect relationship has not been conclusively established for this association; similar colonic lesions of uncertain cause have been observed in young persons not using these agents. These same reservations apply to small bowel infarction and mesenteric venous thrombosis associated with oral contraceptives.

The syndrome of ischemic colitis may be quite variable in its extent, severity, and prognosis. Extensive infarction, gangrene, or perforation may result from

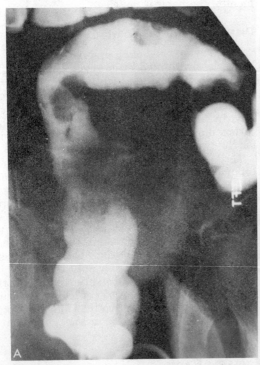 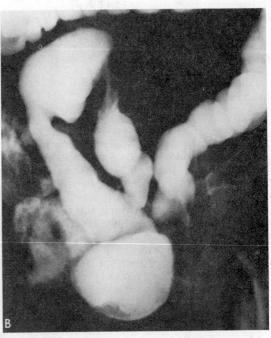

Figure 56. Ischemic colitis secondary to amyloid disease. *A,* Large impressions in the sigmoid colon reflect intramural hemorrhage. Sigmoidoscopy showed blue nodular masses. *B,* Follow-up study, three weeks later, shows healing with two strictures present in sigmoid colon. (Courtesy of Dr. Henry I. Goldberg.)

occlusive disease, nonocclusive ischemia, or surgical interruption of the blood supply affecting all or a portion of the colon. There are less catastrophic variants of ischemic disease of the colon, which seem to be associated with more localized or segmental ischemia. Particularly vulnerable are those areas of the colon that lie on the "watershed" between two adjacent arterial supplies—that is, the splenic flexure (superior and inferior mesenteric arteries) and the rectosigmoid area (inferior mesenteric and internal iliac arteries)—but in small vessel disease any portion of the colon may be affected.

Most patients with ischemic colitis are over 50 years of age and have evidence of vascular disease, usually atherosclerotic. They characteristically present with abrupt onset of lower abdominal cramping pain, rectal bleeding, and variable vomiting and fever. Barium enema examination will often show the characteristic picture of intramural hemorrhage and edema, including "thumbprinting," tubular narrowing, "sawtooth" irregularity, and sacculation. In some patients, the clinical process may subside completely, with disappearance of symptoms and return of radiographs to normal. In many, however, a residual stricture will remain, particularly in patients who have had significant ischemia of the muscular layers of the bowel (Fig. 56).

COLONIC NEOPLASIA

Pathophysiology includes the explanation of problems that stem from disorders of cellular proliferation and differentiation—neoplasia. The transformation of a normally proliferating colonic epithelial cell into a malignant one involves a critical genetic event (*initiation*) that may be modulated by other important genetic or epigenetic events referred to as *tumor promotion*.

CARCINOGENESIS

Colonic neoplasia is generally assumed to be caused by an as yet unidentified group of dietary carcinogens. Fecal mutagens have been reported to be more frequent in the stools of people from certain regions that have higher incidences of colonic cancer. The wide range of incidences for colonic cancer observed internationally may be caused by differences in exposure to these carcinogens, but also may be caused by the effects of *promotional agents*. Bile acids have been identified as potent tumor promoters in animal models of neoplasia. Diversion of the biliary flow reduces tumor formation; amplification of the delivery of bile to the colon augments tumorigenesis. The chronic use of bile acid–binding resins in humans, which would increase

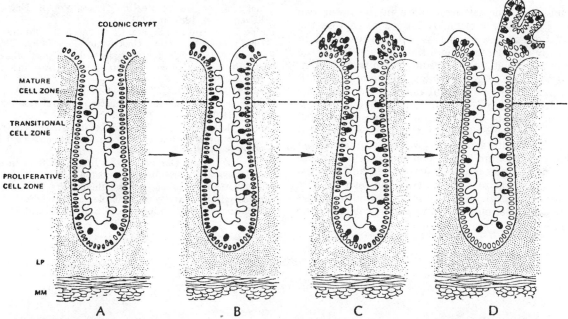

Figure 57. Epithelial proliferation in colonic polyps: a sequence of events to account for the location of abnormally proliferating colonic epithelial cells before and during the formation of polypoid neoplasms in man. *A* shows the location of proliferating and differentiating epithelial cells in the normal colonic crypt. Dark cells illustrate thymidine labeling in cells that are synthesizing DNA and preparing to undergo cell division. As cells pass from the proliferative zone through the transitional zone, DNA synthesis and mitosis are repressed, and migrating epithelial cells leave the proliferative cell cycle to undergo normal maturation before they reach the surface of the mucosa. *B* shows the development of a phase I proliferative lesion in colonic epithelial cells as they fail to repress the incorporation of ^{3}H-thymidine into DNA and begin to develop an enhanced ability to proliferate. The mucosa is flat and the number of new cells born equals the number extruded, without an excess cell accumulation in the mucosa. *C* shows the development of a phase II proliferative lesion in colonic epithelial cells. The cells incorporate ^{3}H-thymidine into DNA and also have developed additional properties that enable them to accumulate in the mucosa in increasing numbers. *D* shows further development of abnormally retained proliferating epithelial cells into pathologically defined neoplastic lesions including tubular and villous adenomas. (From Lipkin, M.: Cancer 34:878, 1974.)

the colonic delivery of bile, has been reported to be associated with colon cancer. It has been suggested that cholecystectomy, which would result in a constant flow of bile into the gut, increases the risk of cancers in the proximal colon; however, this observation has failed corroboration in a recent, larger study.

The fecal flora may play a role in colonic carcinogenesis. Experimental carcinogens undergo metabolic "activation" by intestinal bacteria, and differences in cancer incidence may be related to the flora supported by a given host. Secondary bile acids have been specifically implicated as carcinogenic. Their concentration depends in part upon bacterial 7-alpha-dehydroxylase, which is induced by a high fat diet. Other bacterial enzymes including nitroreductase, beta-glucuronidase, and azoreductase are capable of "activating" procarcinogens to proximate carcinogens in rodents, and all three enzymes are induced by a high-beef diet. Contrariwise, dietary fiber will *dilute* fecal carcinogens and tumor promoters by its sheer bulk and ability to induce colonic secretion, and may also *bind* carcinogens and bile acids, further reducing their contact with the epithelium. Thus, a complex relationship exists among the dietary factors, fecal flora, and the modification of potential carcinogens and promoters within the colonic lumen.

PROLIFERATION AND DIFFERENTIATION

Normal cell renewal takes place in the lower two thirds of the colonic crypt. A failure to repress the proliferation process normally, which goes hand in hand with disordered differentiation, is seen in the crypts of adenomatous epithelium, which is the benign form of neoplasia (Fig. 57). An expansion of the proliferative zone is seen in rectal biopsies from patients with ulcerative colitis. Normal-appearing colonic crypts in patients with *familial polyposis coli* and *Gardner's syndrome* also show this failure of normal epithelial cell maturation. The process by which *benign* neoplastic epithelium (which demonstrates disordered cellular maturation but does not invade adjacent tissues nor metastasize to distant organs) evolves into *malignant* neoplastic epithelium is not known, but it appears that most malignant neoplastic colonic tissue

has evolved from benign neoplastic tissue. It is not yet known whether this process is inexorable, or whether it may be controlled by factors in the colonic environment.

The epithelial-mesenchymal interaction may be important in influencing differentiation and the potential for transformation of the colonocyte. Fibroblasts cultured from biopsies of normal skin from asymptomatic persons carrying the gene for *familial polyposis coli* have several characteristics that are more similar to the malignant than the normal phenotype. Other perturbations of the behavior of epithelial cells in vitro—that is, excess tetraploidy in dividing cells—have been observed in cells cultured from biopsies of normal-appearing skin from persons carrying the gene for Gardner's syndrome and familial colon cancer without polyposis. Thus, when considering the normal maturational process and its relationship to carcinogenesis, one is required to consider the epithelial cell in the context not only of the fecal environment but also of the epithelial-mesenchymal relationship.

REFERENCES

Binder, H. J.: Colonic secretion. In Johnson, L. R. (ed.): Physiology of the Gastrointestinal Tract, Vol. 2. New York, Raven Press, 1981, p. 1003.

Connell, A. M. (ed.): Motility and its disturbances. Clin Gastroenterol Vol. 11, No. 3, 1982.

Connell, A. M.: Dietary fiber. In Johnson, L. R. (ed.): Physiology of the Gastrointestinal Tract, Vol. 2. New York, Raven Press, 1981, p. 1291.

Faulk, D. L., Anuras, S., and Christensen, J.: Chronic intestinal pseudoobstruction. Gastroenterology 74:922, 1978.

Feldman, M., and Schiller, L. R.: Disorders of gastrointestinal motility associated with diabetes mellitus. Ann Intern Med 98:378, 1983.

Jacob, H., Brandt, L. J., Farkas, P., and Frishman, W.: Beta-adrenergic blockade and the gastrointestinal system. Am J Med 74:1042, 1983.

Lasser, R. B., Bond, J. H., and Levitt, M. D.: The role of intestinal gas in functional abdominal pain. N Engl J Med 293:524, 1975.

Simon, G. L., and Gorbach, S. L.: Intestinal flora in health and disease. Gastroenterology 86:174, 1984.

Sullivan, M. A., Cohen, S., and Snape, W. J., Jr.: Colonic myoelectrical activity in irritable-bowel syndrome: Effect of eating and anticholinergics. N Engl J Med 298:878, 1978.

PATHOPHYSIOLOGY OF LIVER DISEASE

DAVID ZAKIM, M.D.

The practice of medicine traditionally has been based on clinical experience, and medical education traditionally has emphasized the acquisition of an enormous amount of factual material, which represented primarily the sum total of this clinical experience. The need to learn facts has expanded rapidly in the recent past because of burgeoning knowledge of the chemical and physical principles underlying life processes themselves and the physiology of the interdependency of organ function in complex animals. At the same time, however, this expansion of understanding of the chemistry, physics, and physiology of health and disease provides principles for organizing concepts about the basic causes of disease. This leads in turn to the realization that decisions on the management of disease processes must depend on an understanding of their mechanisms. Decisions about treatment made in the absence of logical thinking about the principles that govern the normal behavior of cells and organs do not provide patients with the maximal benefits to be gained from modern medicine. This idea is illustrated easily in the context of liver disease simply by considering what is meant by the term "cirrhosis." This term is used to describe irreversible changes in the morphology of the liver. Often, but not always, affected patients manifest a characteristic set of symptoms and signs, as for example, ascites, esophageal varices, encephalopathy, and functional renal failure. Identical morphological abnormalities and the clinical disorder that we associate with the diagnosis "cirrhosis" tell us little about the cause of the cirrhosis in a given patient because there are several distinct, identifiable causes of cirrhosis. Certainly, we will delineate more of these in the future. Doing so is not an idle intellectual activity, for in those instances in which the etiology of cirrhosis is understood we are able to alter its natural course and even to prevent cirrhosis from developing in some genetically predisposed patients.

Most classic diseases should be viewed as the "final common pathway" for expression of a myriad of distinct functional defects, because the number of ways in which disturbances of function at the subcellular level can manifest clinically and pathologically are limited as compared with the possible causes of each "common final pathway." Identification of the organ that is malfunctioning and causing an obvious clinical manifestation also depends on understanding the physiology of health and the pathophysiology of disease. Ascites, for example, is a common manifestation of liver disease, but not all patients with ascites have liver disease. Diagnosis and treatment of disease depend, therefore, on developing rational solutions to two interrelated problems. First, the manifestations of illness—i.e., the symptoms, signs, and laboratory abnormalities—must be elucidated and integrated into a scheme that allows the physician to identify the organ causing them. Second, the specific etiology for the dysfunction must be identified so that treatment can be directed to interrupting the natural course of illness and not structured to provide only relief of obvious symptoms. Thus, the goal of treatment is to alter the course of the disease process causing dysfunction.

The regulatory processes maintaining stability of function usually are multiple. This is true at the subcellular level and in the context of the interdependency of organ function in intact animals. We often overlook this important biological principle as we try to define "the cause" of specific dysfunctions, when in reality there are several causes. Different causes may be the ultimate problem in different patients. Failure to appreciate this point leads to a search for a panacea.

A CONCEPTUAL APPROACH FOR UNDERSTANDING HEPATIC FUNCTION

In the pathophysiology of liver disease one must consider the function of the liver per se, the factors responsible for the functional integrity of liver cells, and the agents in the environment that alter the function of these factors. The role of the liver in supporting the overall function of the organism is reasonably well understood, as are the mechanisms for some but not all aspects of that function. For example, the detailed steps and the enzymology for each step in the pathways for hepatic synthesis of glucose are known. The critical factors by which the integrity of liver cells is maintained are largely unknown except for the obvious need to generate ATP. Environmental agents capable of inducing liver disease are known (e.g., ethanol abuse, infection with viruses), but the biochemical pathways involved in the genesis of liver disease by these agents are obscure. The exception to this generalization is liver disease secondary to hepatic metabolism of a selected number of organic xenobiotic molecules, such as acetaminophen. The purpose of the following discussion is to outline what is known now, although in an incomplete fashion, about liver function and the causes of dysfunction.

The liver carries out approximately 1500 identifiable chemical functions important for viability of the host. Conceptually, however, the important hepatic functions can be grouped in broad categories (as summarized in Table 1), and these will form the basis for further discussions.

TABLE 1. MAJOR HEPATIC FUNCTIONS

Integration of energy metabolism in intact animals
   a. Storage of glycogen that can be used as a source of plasma glucose
   b. Surveillance of intake of glucose
   c. Synthesis of fatty acids as storage form for excess calories
   d. Metabolism of fatty acids to ketones
Storage and metabolism of vitamins
Synthesis of plasma proteins
Chemical detoxification of endogenously produced and exogenously administered chemical toxins and mechanical filtration of bacteria
Maintenance of normal salt and water balance
Secretion of bile

MORPHOLOGY

Cellular Composition. Ninety-four per cent of the liver cells are parenchymal (hepatocytes). The remaining 6 per cent of cells are of three major types: (1) The *Kupffer* and *endothelial cells* that line the luminal side of the hepatic sinusoids. The Kupffer cells are fixed macrophages, the largest group of such cells in animals. The endothelial cells of liver differ from those in other tissues in that they lack a basement membrane and their cytoplasmic extensions have clusters of openings, which are referred to as sieve plates. (2) The *perisinusoidal cells,* which are the lipid-storing cells separated from the sinusoids by overlying endothelial cells. The lipid-storing cells of unknown function normally contain numerous droplets of fat and large amounts of vitamin A. (3) *Fibroblasts* within the space of Disse, i.e., between the parenchymal cells and the sinusoids. The plates of liver cells are encircled by bundles of collagen fibers that are probably synthesized by these fibroblasts.

Anatomical Arrangement of Cells. Hepatic parenchymal cells are arranged in cords. The cells are bound to each other via specialized structures on their lateral sides, called "tight junctions." These represent a fusion of the plasma membranes of the two adjacent cells such that adjacent cells have a common portion of membrane that serves to cement them together in tight junctions and in the process to form bile canaliculi (Fig. 1). Two adjacent cells each contribute one side of

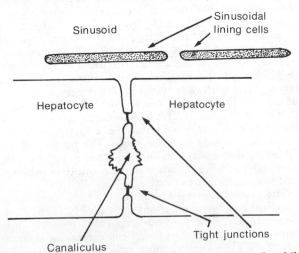

Figure 1. Schematized view of the morphology of a bile canaliculus and its relation to tight junctions.

a bile canaliculus. The tight junctions appear to hold together the parenchymal cells along a hepatic cord, and to seal off bile canaliculi from communication with other regions within the liver. The scanning electron micrograph in Figure 2 shows the cordlike structure of parenchymal cells, the course of bile canaliculi through the areas between adjacent cells, and the relationship between the cells and the sinusoids. The bile canaliculi seen in this figure have been split lengthwise. The viewer hence is looking at one half of each canaliculus, the other half having been removed. The bile canaliculi empty into bile ducts in the portal area. The connection between a bile canaliculus in the liver parenchyma and a bile duct in the portal tract is called the canal of Herring.

The plasma membrane of the liver cell is covered with microvilli over the portions that border the sinusoidal surface and the region forming the bile canaliculus. Microvilli are not usually present on the lateral sides of the cell.

Normally, the cords of liver cells are one cell thick, so the cell has extensive contacts with the sinusoidal space. The sinusoids are lined by endothelial cells that have large discontinuities. These allow free passage of all but the formed elements in blood. As shown in Figure 3, microvilli of the plasma membrane of parenchymal cells extend through these holes directly into the sinusoidal space. Large protein molecules and aggregates, such as lipoproteins, hence can pass freely from the vascular spaces to the space of Disse, which is the area between liver cells and the sinusoidal membrane. The sizes of discontinuities in the sinusoidal membranes have a selective effect on what elements pass into the space of Disse. Small, but not large, chylomicrons, for example, are taken up by the liver because of the size of the "holes" in the membranes. The dimensions of the openings, which may have significance for normal function, can change in pathological states. Figure 4 illustrates another type of cell present in the sinusoid (Kupffer cells), as well as the relationship between liver cell cords, sinusoids, and the space of Disse.

Heterogeneity of Parenchymal Cells. Although liver parenchymal cells appear identical they are functionally different because of their organization with respect to the hepatic blood supply. Blood from the portal veins and hepatic artery is distributed through the liver in large branches coursing through the portal tracts. Blood enters the sinusoids via branches of these major vessels, and flows from the portal areas to central collecting vessels called central veins. Each such vein is surrounded by a number of radiating cords of hepatic cells and their sinusoids. The functional lobular element in the liver is centered on a central vein. The lobule is a hexagonal array of cords with a portal area at each of the six corners of the hexagon. A single central vein drains the blood from one lobule (Fig. 5). Across the lobule, from portal area to central vein, there is an oxygen gradient. Cells nearest the corner of the hexagon have the most abundant supply of oxygen, whereas those at the center probably have a barely adequate oxygen supply. The declining oxygen tension across the lobule probably accounts for the preferential susceptibility of cells in the central vein region of the lobule to the effects of many toxins. In addition to the oxygen differential, the concentration of some key enzymes is different within cells adjacent

Figure 2

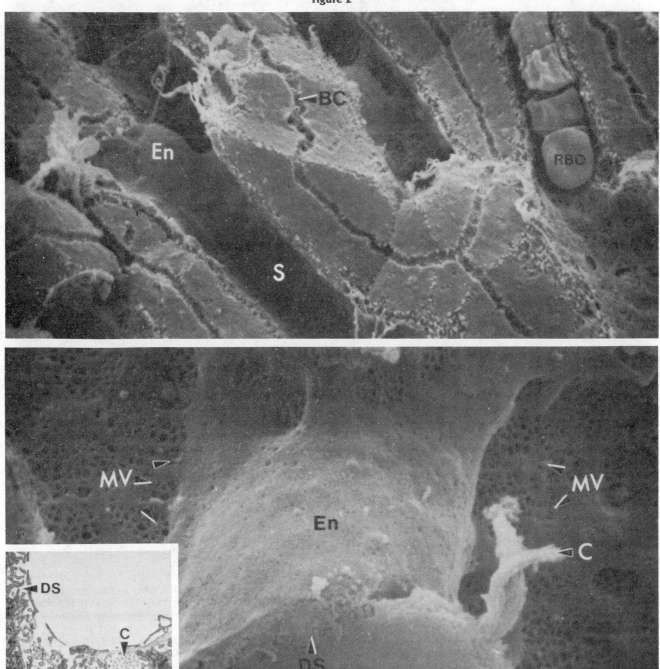

Figure 3

Figure 2. A scanning electron micrograph of rat liver. The liver cells appear as one-cell-thick plates dispersed between the blood vascular spaces of sinusoids *(S)*. The bile canaliculi *(BC)* are clearly seen centrally located between adjacent liver cells. *En,* endothelial cell; RBC, red blood cell (approximate magnification × 2000). (From Jones, A. L., and Schmucker, D. L.: Gastroenterology 73:833, 1977. Reprinted with permission.)

Figure 3. A scanning electron micrograph *(SEM)* of rat liver endothelium. Note the thickened area of the endothelial cell that overlies the nucleus *(En)*. The endothelium is fenestrated, and numerous microvilli *(MV)* can be observed protruding into the lumina through the fenestrae. Bundles of collagen *(C)* can be seen extending out of the perisinusoidal space or space of Disse *(DS)*. Compare with transmission electron micrograph (TEM, inset). (SEM approximate magnification × 14,000; TEM × 5000). (From Jones, A. L., and Schmucker, D. L.: Gastroenterology 73:833, 1977. Reprinted with permission.)

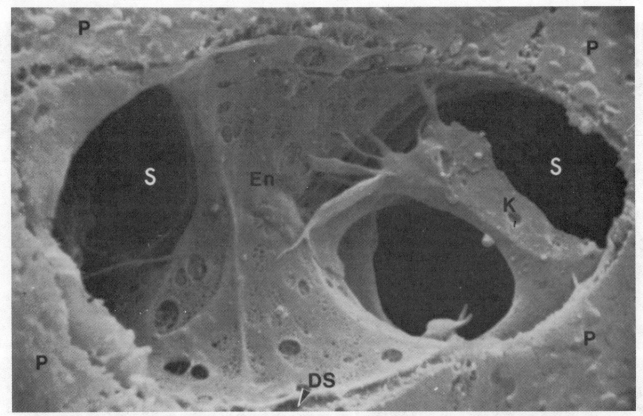

Figure 4. A bifurcation of a liver sinusoid *(S)* demonstrating the relationship of Kupffer cell *(K)* to the endothelium *(En)* and surrounding parenchymna *(P)*. The surface pits noted in the Kupffer cell may represent areas of endo- or exocytotic activity. *DS*, space of Disse. (Approximate magnification ×7500). (From Jones, A. L., and Schmucker, D. L.: Gastroenterology 73:833, 1977. Reprinted with permission.)

to the portal tracts as compared with those near the central vein. The amounts of glucose-6-phosphatase and phosphoenolpyruvate carboxykinase, enzymes crucial for hepatic synthesis of glucose, are three times greater in periportal hepatocytes than in those near the central vein. The hepatic lobule can be divided into three sections, called zones, depending on their relative distances from the hepatic veins and portal tracts (Fig. 6).

THE HEPATIC BLOOD SUPPLY

Hepatic blood flow is approximately 1500 ml per minute, or about 25 per cent of cardiac output, but varies with posture, exercise, and alimentation. Blood reaches liver parenchymal cells by two routes—the portal vein (70 per cent) and the hepatic artery. Blood pressure in the portal vein is quite low—about 10 mm Hg. This is sufficient to perfuse the liver, because resistance within the branches of the portal vein and sinusoid is low. A high sinusoidal pressure, as in occlusion of the hepatic veins or in diffuse parenchymal disease, has serious consequences for function, as will be delineated below. Blood from the hepatic artery (approximately 30 per cent of total flow) eventually enters the sinusoids. However, the high pressure in the arterial circulation does not enhance perfusion in the sinusoids, because the high arterial pressure is dissipated prior to this point.

Oxygen tension in the portal vein is relatively low compared with that in the arterial circulation. Admixture of arterial and venous blood in the sinusoids undoubtedly increases the oxygen available to cells from portal blood alone. Nevertheless, liver cells can survive the low oxygen tension in portal vein blood alone; the arterial blood supply to liver can be occluded acutely and completely without producing infarction.

Liver disease may alter the normal relationship between hepatocytes and their blood supply. Sudden acute collapse of the reticular fibers in the liver secondary to massive necrosis or chronic death of liver cells, followed by regeneration, leads frequently to increasing resistance to flow of blood within the sinusoids. As the resistance to flow in the sinusoids increases, portal vein pressure increases passively, and perfusion of hepatocytes with portal vein blood diminishes. At the same time, the fraction of blood flow contributed by the hepatic artery increases, which indicates a dynamic regulation of pressure in the hepatic arteries proximal to the sinusoids. In experimental animals acute occlusion of the portal system leads to a reciprocal increase in hepatic arterial blood flow.

In patients with increased resistance to sinusoidal flow, the arterial pressure is transmitted to the sinusoids, whereas in normal liver, as mentioned above, arterial pressure dissipates before the sinusoid. The adaptive changes in the regulation of pressure within the arterial system of the liver maintain blood flow in

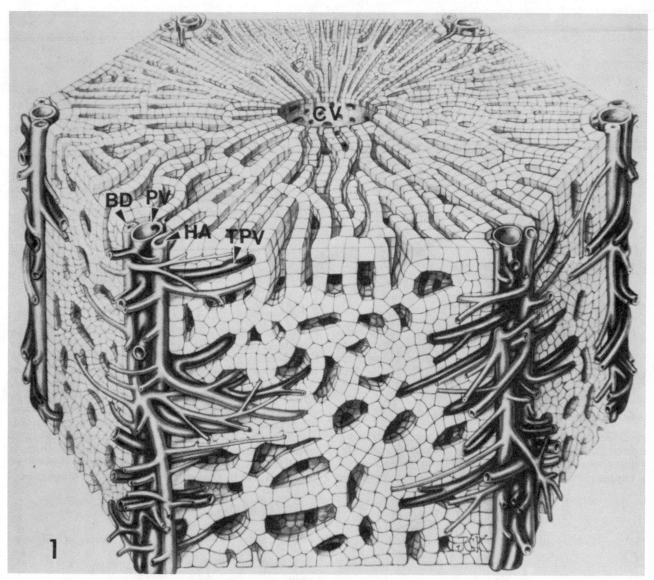

Figure 5. A diagrammatic representation of the current concepts of the liver lobule. *BD*, bile duct; PV, portal vein; HA, hepatic artery; *TPV,* terminal portal venule; *CV*, central vein. (From Jones, A. L., and Schmucker, D. L.: Gastroenterology 73:833, 1977. Reprinted with permission.)

a setting of increased sinusoidal resistance. It is unlikely, however, that transmission of hepatic arterial pressure to the sinusoids exacerbates pressure increases that are due to the basic disease process itself, since ligation of the hepatic artery of cirrhotic livers in experimental animals does not lower the pressure in the portal vein.

As pressure in the portal vein rises, blood seeks a pathway of flow with lower resistance, producing collateral channels where tributaries of the portal system are in close proximity to those of the systemic venous system. The major anastomosis of the high pressure portal blood to blood under low pressure in the vena cava is between the coronary veins (portal side) and azygos veins (caval side) in the submucosa of the esophagus. Hence, veins in the esophagus dilate as pressure and flow are transmitted to them from the portal vein in instances of heightened resistance to flow along portal channels. A significant amount of portal blood that normally bathes hepatocytes can be diverted in patients with liver disease.

Continual necrosis and regeneration of liver cells in the face of toxic stimuli can lead to derangement in the normal interaction between cells and portal blood without affecting the measurable functions of surviving cells. The biochemical function of individual liver cells may be normal in this instance, yet the function of the liver as an integrated organ may be abnormal. Disorders of cell function and abnormalities in blood flow sometimes have separate roles in determining the clinical and laboratory manifestations of liver disease. It is important to understand and differentiate abnormal liver function that rests on derangement of blood flow from that secondary to failure in the function of individual cells.

INTEGRATION OF ENERGY METABOLISM BY THE LIVER

Individual cells cannot store all the materials needed to sustain energy generation. Energy metabolism in

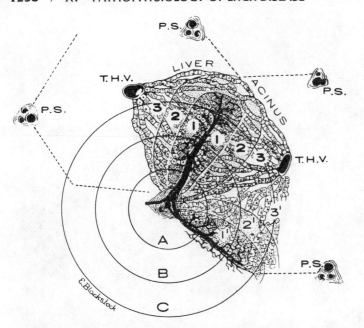

Figure 6. Schematic view of blood flow to hepatocytes. Blood flows from the portal area to enter sinusoids, and then centrally to the terminal hepatic vein (T. H.V.). Numbers indicate the lack of equality between hepatocytes in different portions of the functional unit of liver cells. Thus, Zones 1, 2, and 3, respectively, represent areas supplied with blood of first, second, and third quality with regard to oxygen and nutrients. (Adapted with permission from A. M. Rappaport. In Schiff, L. (ed.): Diseases of the Liver, 4th ed. Philadelphia, J. B. Lippincott, 1975.)

intact animals is therefore interrelated and interdependent in various organ systems. These interactions can be appreciated by considering what happens as patterns of metabolism shift from the fed to the postabsorptive to the fasting state (Figs. 7 to 9).

GENERAL PROPERTIES OF THE FED STATE (Fig. 7)

When a mixed diet is ingested, glucose is distributed from the gut to all tissues, where it can be stored for later use or oxidized immediately to produce high-energy bonds. The latter sustains energy-requiring

vital functions such as maintenance of the ion gradients in excitable tissue, secretory functions of liver and kidney, and synthesis of structural elements. The disposition of ingested glucose depends on the characteristics of specific tissues. The brain and the red cells, which rely on glucose but cannot synthesize its storage forms, oxidize glucose immediately for energy production. In muscle, on the other hand, most of the glucose taken up at rest is stored as glycogen to be used later when the muscle is working. The livers of fed animals oxidize very little of the glucose taken up, converting most instead to glycogen to a maximum storage capac-

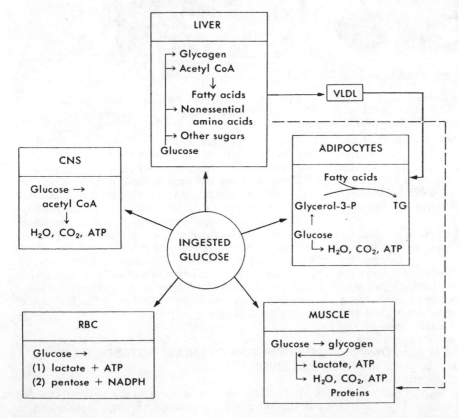

Figure 7. Pattern of supply and utilization of glucose in the fed state. Ingested glucose is shown in the lumen of the intestine. Of the sugar absorbed, 50 per cent is removed by the liver. The figure does not show that all absorbed sugar passes into the portal vein and thus into or through the liver. (From Zakim, D., and Boyer, T. D. (eds.): Hepatology: A Textbook of Liver Disease. Philadelphia, W. B. Saunders Co., 1982.)

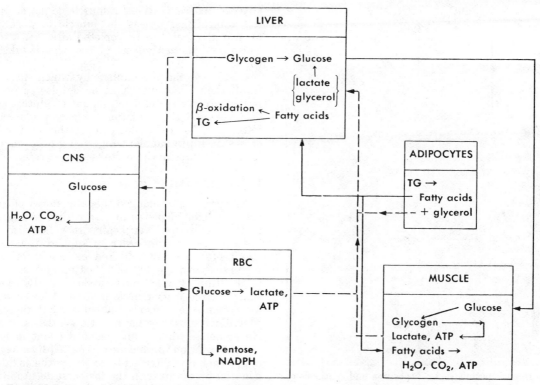

Figure 8. Pattern of supply and utilization of glucose in the postabsorptive state. Notice the reversal in the direction of supply of carbon atoms (as glucose and fatty acids) between liver and adipose tissue compared with Figure 7. Also, compared with the fed state, the liver is the sole source of plasma glucose in the postabsorptive state. (From Zakim, D., and Boyer, T. D. (eds.): Hepatology: A Textbook of Liver Disease. Philadelphia, W. B. Saunders Co., 1982.)

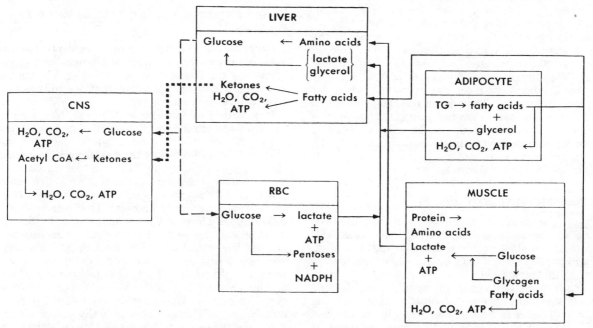

Figure 9. Pattern of supply and utilization of glucose in the fasted state. Compared with Figure 8, (1) liver glycogen is depleted, (2) amino acids derived from muscle protein are delivered to the liver to support synthesis of glucose, and (3) the liver supplies the central nervous system with two oxidizable substrates, glucose and ketone bodies. Not shown in the figure is that ketones are also good substrates for skeletal and cardiac muscle. (From Zakim, D., and Boyer, T. D. (eds.): Hepatology: A Textbook of Liver Disease. Philadelphia, W. B. Saunders Co., 1982.)

SINUSOIDAL GLUCOSE

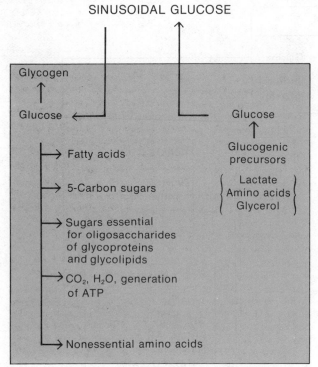

Figure 10. Hepatic pathways for disposition and synthesis of glucose.

ity of 65 grams of glycogen per kilogram of liver tissue. Glucose above that needed to saturate hepatic stores of glycogen can be metabolized in a variety of ways (Fig. 10). In an especially important pathway excess glucose is converted to fatty acids, which are esterified and secreted in the form of very low density lipoproteins for transport to storage depots in adipocytes.

Fat absorbed during a meal reaches tissues in the form of the triglycerides of chylomicrons. The amount in excess of caloric needs will be stored in adipose tissue. The amino acids of ingested protein are also distributed widely to meet the needs of tissues for synthesis of proteins. The critical metabolic events in liver in the fed state, therefore, are (1) conversion of glucose to glycogen, which can be used as a rapid source for plasma glucose in the postabsorptive state, and (2) the conversion of excess glucose to fatty acids for storage in adipose tissue.

THE POSTABSORPTIVE STATE (Fig. 8)

Two major metabolic events occur in the shift from eating to the postprandial state: (1) the liver adds glucose to the blood rather than removing it, and (2) adipose tissue releases fatty acids rather than storing them, as during a meal.

The synthesis of hepatic glycogen during feeding ensures survival in the postabsorptive state or during a fast. Glycogen is broken down readily to glucose, which supplies the specific and unique requirements of the central nervous system and red cells for this oxidizable substrate and which is also available to muscle during fasting. Unlike liver glycogen, muscle glycogen is not stored for use during fasting, nor is it available to other tissues. The purpose of muscle glycogen in fed and fasted animals is to support work.

Glycogen concentrations in muscle do not decline during a brief fast unless the muscle is working, and muscle glycogen can be repleted after work ends because the liver can release glucose that is taken up by the muscle.

A shift in the mechanism by which most tissues fulfill their basal metabolic needs also occurs in the postabsorptive state. The amount of glucose oxidized declines, and the oxidation of fatty acids increases. Fatty acids, stored in fat cells in the form of triglycerides, begin to supplant ingested glucose as the fuel for most tissues in the postabsorptive state.

THE FASTED STATE (Fig. 9)

As fasting is prolonged, hepatic stores of glycogen are completely depleted in man within 48 hours. Prior to this time the liver begins to synthesize glucose (gluconeogenesis) in order to support the metabolic needs of the brain and red cells. Gluconeogenesis increases progressively with fasting and become maximal within 24 to 48 hours, predominantly from amino acids derived from muscle protein. Adipose triglycerides release fatty acids into blood, but these do not contribute substrate for hepatic synthesis of glucose. Nevertheless, this is an essential event in the shift from utilization of glucose by the fed liver (synthesis of glycogen and fatty acids) to its synthesis (gluconeogenesis) by the liver in the fasted state. Additionally, enhanced fatty acid oxidation by the fasted liver produces ketones that supplant glucose as a fuel for 75 per cent of the metabolic needs of the central nervous system during a prolonged fast, therefore sparing this amount of breakdown of muscle protein, which would otherwise be the limiting fuel in a complete fast.

UNIQUE METABOLIC EVENTS IN LIVER DURING THE FED STATE

Other sections of this text cover in depth the metabolic pathways for synthesis of glycogen and glucose, glycolysis, the Krebs cycle, etc. (Section VI). Only the key events in these pathways that are unique to the liver will be discussed here.

Regulation of Uptake of Glucose. The liver metabolizes approximately 50 per cent of glucose entering the portal vein during a meal, but it does not remove glucose from the blood in the postabsorptive or fasted states. Hepatic glucose uptake is carrier-mediated, but it is not insulin-dependent, nor is it an active process. The liver cell does not concentrate glucose, but depends on its rapid metabolic disposal. This means that the mechanisms for metabolism of glucose in the liver must be able per se to "measure" the concentration of glucose in portal blood. The most reasonable way to accomplish this goal is to monitor the glucose concentration at its point of entry into metabolic pathways, for this ensures that intermediates of metabolism will not accumulate. The reaction on which all further metabolism of glucose depends is the phosphorylation of glucose to glucose-6-P, catalyzed by a specific hepatic type of hexokinase that is called "glucokinase."

[1] $glucose + ATP \rightarrow glucose-6-P + ADP$

The activity of this enzyme, in contrast to that of other hexokinases, is sensitive to concentrations of glucose

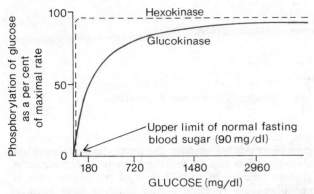

Figure 11. Rate of phosphorylation of glucose by glucokinase and hexokinase as a function of glucose concentration.

that are in the physiological range (Fig. 11). The affinity of glucokinase for glucose is relatively poor as compared with hexokinase isoenzymes from other tissues, which are saturated by a glucose concentration of about 5 mg/dl. The activity of hepatic glucokinase is half its maximal rate at a glucose concentration of 180 mg/dl, an affinity that allows the liver to "measure" the amount of glucose in blood. That is, the rate of phosphorylation of glucose catalyzed by glucokinase depends directly on the concentration of glucose in portal blood. Hence the liver detects when glucose is ingested and adjusts hepatic uptake in an appropriate way.

Glucokinase is an adaptive enzyme. Its hepatic content depends on the presence of insulin and glucose and can change markedly within 24 to 48 hours. Fasting normal rats reduce their hepatic glucokinase, which returns to normal when glucose is fed. Repletion

of diabetic animals with insulin restores the level of glucokinase to normal.

The Synthesis of Fatty Acids. Any substance metabolized to acetyl CoA can serve as a precursor of fatty acids, but synthesis occurs only when there is an excess of calories in the diet. Fatty acid synthesis, primarily an hepatic function in man, is shut off quickly during fasting or in the absence of insulin. In addition, there are adaptive changes in the amounts of enzymes unique to the fatty acid synthesizing pathway. Activities are high when experimental animals are fed excess carbohydrate calories, and low in those whose diet contains no sugar or in fasted or diabetic animals. This regulation ensures that synthesis of fatty acids for storage occurs only during intake of excess calories.

UNIQUE METABOLIC EVENTS IN LIVER DURING THE POSTABSORPTIVE STATE

The critical metabolic event in the postabsorptive state is a switch from the synthesis of glycogen to its breakdown. An associated change is increasing oxidation of fatty acids as a source of energy for the liver.

Breakdown of Glycogen. The synthesis and the breakdown of glycogen proceed via different pathways (Fig. 12). Separation of anabolism and catabolism, as opposed to synthesis and degradation along a single, reversible pathway, is a general property of metabolic systems. Its purpose is to allow independent control of each process, precise modulation of rates, and rapid activation/deactivation of the separate limbs of a pathway. The rate of the synthetic pathway of glycogen metabolism is regulated by the activity of glycogen synthetase. Catabolism of glycogen is regulated by the activity of phosphorylase. Glycogen synthetase and

Figure 12. The enzymes that regulate synthesis and catabolism of glycogen in liver.

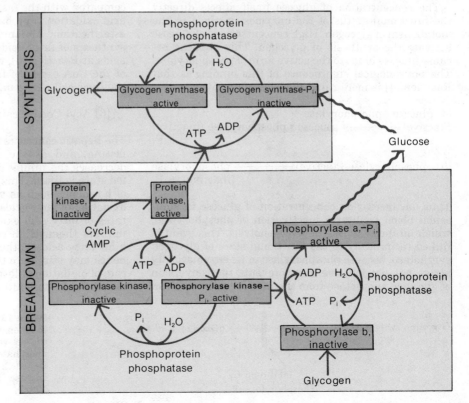

$$[2] \text{ (phosphorylase-P)}_a \text{(active)} \underset{\text{kinase}}{\overset{\text{phosphatase} \nearrow P_i}{\rightleftarrows}} \text{phosphorylase}_b \text{(inactive)}$$

$$\begin{array}{cc} \text{ADP} & \text{ATP} \\ \text{ATP} & \text{ADP} \end{array}$$

$$[3] \text{ glycogen synthetase}_a \text{(active)} \underset{\text{phosphatase} \searrow P_i}{\overset{\text{kinase} \nearrow}{\rightleftarrows}} \text{glycogen synthetase-P (inactive)}$$

phosphorylase occur in liver as active forms (designated by the subscript "a") and inactive forms (designated by the subscript "b"). For example, phosphorylase$_b$ has low activity when compared with phosphorylase$_a$ and hence it is referred to as the "inactive" form of phosphorylase.

Phosphorylase$_a$ (active) is a phosphorylated form of phosphorylase$_b$ (inactive) (Reaction [2]). Glycogen synthetase$_a$ (active) is a dephosphorylated form of glycogen synthetase$_b$ (inactive) (Reaction [3]). The most salient point illustrated by Reactions [2] and [3] is the reciprocal relationship in the control of glycogen synthetase and phosphorylase. The activities of the kinases catalyzing Reactions [2] and [3], which have specificities for phosphorylase and for glycogen synthetase, are linked to each other functionally such that either glycogen synthetase or phosphorylase, but not both, is predominantly in the enzymatically active form. Which of these enzymes is active can depend on the hepatic concentrations of cAMP and glucose. The concentration in liver of cAMP obviously will be under the control of the effects of various hormones (Section VIII), but hormonal changes probably are not necessary for regulating the changes in glycogen metabolism during a meal and in the postabsorptive state. Variations in the concentration of glucose alone can modulate these processes.

The concentration of glucose itself affects directly the functional status of the enzymes involved in the metabolism of glycogen. High concentrations of glucose activate the synthesis of glycogen. This happens because glucose binds to the active form of phosphorylase. The physiological significance of this binding is that Reaction [4] is more rapid than Reaction [5].

$$[4] \text{ glucose} \cdot \text{phosphorylase-P(active)} \longrightarrow \text{glucose} \cdot \text{phosphorylase (inactive)} + P_i$$

$$[5] \text{ phosphorylase-P(active)} \longrightarrow \text{phosphorylase (inactive)} + P_i$$

Thus, an increasing concentration of glucose in sinusoidal blood facilitates inactivation of phosphorylase, which inhibits the rate of glycogenolysis. This event is linked reciprocally to the functional state of glycogen synthetase, because phosphorylase in its enzymatically active but not inactive form prevents the conversion of glycogen synthetase from the inactive to active form

(Fig. 13). The sequence of events in the transition of glycogen metabolism from the fed to the postabsorptive state therefore is a decreasing hepatic concentration of glucose leading to stabilization of the active form of phosphorylase relative to the inactive form because Reaction [5] as compared with [4] becomes the predominant pathway for inactivation of phosphorylase. This leads in turn to a decrease in the concentration of the active form of glycogen synthetase because, as shown in Figure 12, increasing concentrations of the active form of phosphorylase prevent conversion of glycogen synthetase from the inactive to the active form.

The normal liver stores limited amounts of glycogen. Restrictions on the storage appear to be set by interactions between glycogen and the enzymes of its synthesis and catabolism. High concentrations of glycogen inhibit phosphorylase phosphatase (Reaction [3]) and glycogen synthetase phosphatase. Therefore, the hepatic concentration of glycogen indirectly turns off its own synthesis.

Oxidation of Fatty Acids. There are two metabolic pathways for fatty acids in the liver: oxidation and esterification to triglycerides that are then secreted in the form of lipoproteins.

The relative importance of esterification and oxidative pathways for fatty acids depend on the nutritional state. Oxidation of fatty acids is limited in the fed as compared with the fasted liver. The regulation of fatty acid oxidation is probably modulated independently of esterification. Malonyl CoA, an intermediate in the synthesis of fatty acids, inhibits the oxidation of fatty acids at Reaction [6], which is the step for the transfer of the CoA esters of fatty acid from the cytoplasm of the liver cell to the mitochondrial compartment.

$$[6] \text{ Acyl-CoA} + \text{carnitine} \rightarrow \text{acyl-carnitine} + \text{CoA}$$

The hepatic concentration of malonyl CoA falls during fasting, and as the concentration of malonyl CoA decreases the inhibition of fatty acid oxidation in the fed state is lifted. This formulation explains the effects of hormones such as glucagon and insulin on hepatic oxidation of fatty acids. Glucagon markedly stimulates rates of fatty acid oxidation in liver, whereas insulin inhibits them. High concentrations of fatty acids inhibit fatty acid synthesis via a direct mechanism and hence may stimulate their own oxidation directly. The rate of oxidation of fatty acids in liver increases within about eight hours after the onset of fasting.

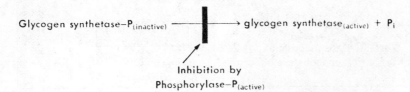

Figure 13. Conversion of glycogen synthetase to its enzymatically active form is blocked by the active form phosphorylase. P_i, inorganic phosphate. (From Zakim, D., and Boyer, T. D. (eds.): Hepatology: A Textbook of Liver Disease. Philadelphia, W. B. Saunders Co., 1982.)

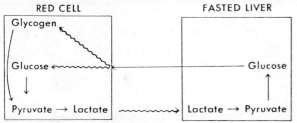

MUSCLE FUNCTIONING
ANAEROBICALLY OR
RED CELL

FASTED LIVER

Figure 14. Recycling of carbon between muscle and liver and red cells and liver during a prolonged fast. The red cell does not store glycogen. (From Zakim, D., and Boyer, T. D. (eds.): Hepatology: A Textbook of Liver Disease. Philadelphia, W. B. Saunders Co., 1982.)

Unique Metabolic Events in the Liver During the Fasted State

As fasting persists and liver glycogen is depleted, the liver begins to synthesize glucose from amino acids and lactate. The amino acids are derived largely from muscle protein. The source of the lactate is anaerobic metabolism of glucose by red cells and by muscle (Fig. 14). Production of glucose from lactate and the recirculation of glucose from liver to red cells and muscle do not deplete protein stores, but the continuing requirement of the central nervous system for glucose comes at the expense of the carbon stored in structural proteins of muscle. It is important in order to spare these proteins that the utilization of glucose by the brain decrease as fasting is prolonged. This is achieved during a long fast via a switchover by some but not all parts of the brain to the use of ketones as a fuel in place of sugar. These ketones are produced in the liver.

Hepatic Production of Glucose. The liver in fasting man continually produces glucose from glycogen, amino acids, lactate, and glycerol. This process is stimulated by glucagon, glucocorticoids, and growth hormone but inhibited by insulin. The characteristic of liver that allows for this synthesis is the presence of enzymes catalyzing reversal of the three irreversible reactions in the glycolytic pathway, which are Reactions [7] to [9].

[7] glucose + ATP $\xrightarrow{\text{(glucokinase)}}$ glucose-6-P + ADP

[8] fructose-6-P + ATP $\xrightarrow{\text{(phosphofructokinase)}}$ fructose-1,6-P + ADP

[9] phosphoenolpyruvate + ADP $\xrightarrow{\text{(pyruvate kinase)}}$ pyruvate + ATP

Glucose-6-phosphatase catalyzes the hydrolysis of glucose-6-phosphate, which overcomes the irreversibility

of Reaction 7. Synthesis of fructose-6-P from fructose-1,6-P, is catalyzed by fructose diphosphatase:

[10] fructose-1,6-P + $H_2O \longrightarrow$ fructose-6-P + P_i

Pyruvate is converted to phosphoenolpyruvate in a sequence of two reactions catalyzed by pyruvate carboxylase (Reaction 11) and phosphoenolpyruvate carboxykinase (Reaction 12):

[11] pyruvate + CO_2 + ATP $\xrightarrow{\hspace{2cm}}$ oxaloacetate + ADP

[12] oxaloacetate + GTP $\xrightarrow{\hspace{2cm}}$ phosphoenolpyruvate + GDP

Starvation and/or an absence of insulin increase the amounts of the enzymes catalyzing Reactions [10] to [12]. These adaptive changes, complete after about 48 hours of fasting, maximize the liver's capacity to synthesize glucose. At the same time that adaptive changes enhance the rate of hepatic gluconeogenesis, there is a reciprocal decline in the rate of glycolysis, owing to the low levels of insulin associated with fasting.

Fatty acids are a storage form for energy, but they do not contribute to the synthesis of glucose. Lactate produced in nonhepatic tissues (see later) contributes about 15 per cent of the glucose carbon, and a small amount comes from glycerol. The remainder is supplied by amino acids, of which alanine is the major precursor of glucose. Leucine is the only amino acid that is not glucogenic. Protein is the limiting factor during starvation: when protein is depleted, muscle function fails, including respiration.

Glucose production by the liver is maximal after about four days of fasting but declines if fasting continues. The fall in glucose production after four days of fasting is unrelated to changes in the levels of gluconeogenic enzymes, hormones, or hepatic extraction of gluconeogenic substrates. There is, however, diminished availability of the most important gluconeogenic precursors, owing to decreased catabolism of protein in muscle. Urinary loss of nitrogen, for example, is maximal after four days of complete fasting, but then begins to taper off. The signal for these changes seems to be a rising concentration of ketones in the blood, which interferes with release of alanine from skeletal muscle.

Production of Ketones. The *oxidation of fatty acids* can be viewed as proceeding in two separate, sequential pathways. The first is the β-oxidation cycle in which the length of fatty acids is shortened progressively by two carbons. Since the major fatty acids in mammals contain an even number of carbon atoms, a 4-carbon tail, acetoacetyl CoA, remains after shortening is completed (Reaction 13):

[13] $\underset{\textit{Palmitoyl CoA}}{CH_3-(CH_2)_{14}-\overset{\overset{O}{\|}}{C}-S-CoA}$ + (6) FAD + (6) NAD^+ $\xrightarrow[\text{in mitochondria}]{\beta \text{ oxidation}}$ (6) $\underset{\textit{Acetyl CoA}}{CH_3-\overset{\overset{O}{\|}}{C}-S-CoA}$ +

$\underset{\textit{Acetoacetyl CoA}}{CH_3-\overset{\overset{O}{\|}}{C}-CH_2-\overset{\overset{O}{\|}}{C}-S-CoA}$ + (6) $FADH_2$ + (6) NADH + (6) H^+

Reduced flavin nucleotide

Reduced pyridine nucleotide

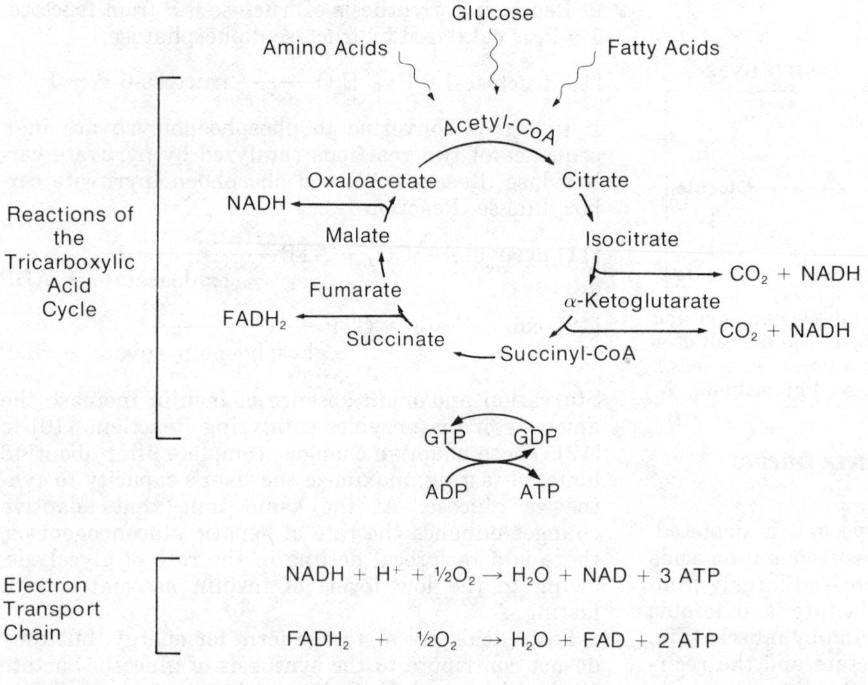

Figure 15. The pathways of the tricarboxylic acid cycle.

Reactions of the Tricarboxylic Acid Cycle

Glucose
Amino Acids
Fatty Acids
Acetyl-CoA
Oxaloacetate
Citrate
NADH
Isocitrate
Malate
CO_2 + NADH
Fumarate
α-Ketoglutarate
$FADH_2$
CO_2 + NADH
Succinate
Succinyl-CoA

GTP GDP
ADP ATP

Electron Transport Chain

$$NADH + H^+ + \tfrac{1}{2}O_2 \rightarrow H_2O + NAD + 3\ ATP$$

$$FADH_2 + \tfrac{1}{2}O_2 \rightarrow H_2O + FAD + 2\ ATP$$

$FADH_2$ and NADH formed during shortening are reoxidized in the electron transport system of mitochondria in reactions coupled to the synthesis, respectively, of two and three molecules of ATP. Removal of each 2-carbon unit from a long-chain fatty acid generates five molecules of ATP. The second sequence in the complete combustion of fatty acids is the oxidation of acetyl CoA and acetoacetyl CoA in the tricarboxylic acid cycle, yielding CO_2, H_2O, and additional ATP (Fig. 15). The complete metabolism of fatty acids in these two sequences occurs only when small amounts of fatty acids are metabolized in the β-oxidation cycle. Acetyl CoA and acetoacetyl CoA accumulate when fatty acids are oxidized rapidly. Acetoacetyl CoA is reduced to β-hydroxybutyryl CoA in this setting, and both compounds are hydrolyzed within the liver to the ketone bodies β-hydroxybutyrate and acetoacetate. Accumulated acetyl CoA also is converted to ketone bodies (Fig. 16). Ketosis, therefore, is a consequence of high rates of fatty acid oxidation.

Most tissues contain the β-oxidation pathway for fatty acids, but only the liver produces ketone bodies. The brain does not use fatty acids as a fuel but will oxidize ketones via the tricarboxylic acid pathway. For this reason, complete oxidation of fatty acids does not occur in the liver of fasted animals.

DISORDERS OF ENERGY METABOLISM IN LIVER DISEASE

Abnormal Glucose Metabolism

A general problem in any patient with liver disease is to separate the manifestations due to liver dysfunction directly from those secondary to involvement of other organs. Specifically, how does one determine whether abnormalities of glucose metabolism reflect intrinsic disease of the liver or involvement of the pancreas, or both? It is clear that abnormalities of glucose metabolism are common in patients with liver disease and take one of only two forms, i.e., defective removal of glucose by the liver, or a failure to make it.

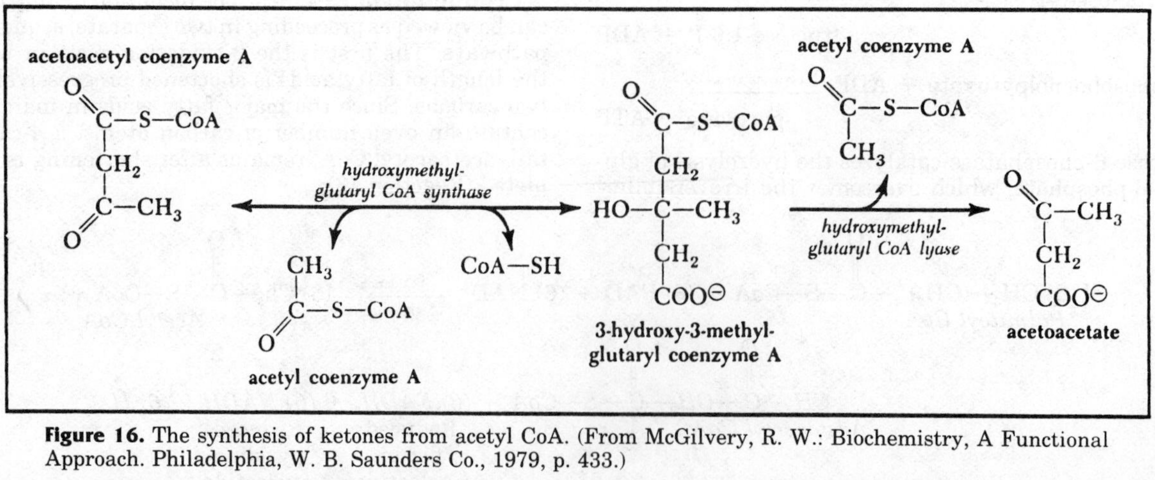

Figure 16. The synthesis of ketones from acetyl CoA. (From McGilvery, R. W.: Biochemistry, A Functional Approach. Philadelphia, W. B. Saunders Co., 1979, p. 433.)

Hyperglycemia

Interposition of the liver between the splanchnic and systemic circulations has important consequences for the metabolism of glucose for two reasons. First, uptake of glucose by the liver depends on the presence of high concentrations of glucose in the blood. Second, liver removes one half the absorbed glucose. Patients with significant shunting of portal blood can have diabetic-like glucose tolerance tests in the absence of derangements of pancreatic and hepatocyte function simply because splanchnic glucose bypasses the hepatocyte and spills into the peripheral blood. This results in an increase in the maximal concentration of glucose in systemic blood after oral glucose and an apparently decreased fractional rate of removal of glucose from blood. As a result, glucose tolerance is abnormal significantly more often after oral than after intravenous glucose challenge. In a study of unselected cirrhotics, oral glucose tolerance was abnormal in 76 per cent of patients, whereas intravenous glucose tolerance was abnormal in only 8 per cent. Liver disease usually does not interfere with the metabolism of glucose in nonhepatic tissue.

The postglucose concentration of immunoreactive insulin in peripheral blood is greater in cirrhotics than in normals. Diversion of blood away from the liver can explain this, since 50 per cent of the insulin secreted by the pancreas is inactivated in a single pass through the liver.

In addition to abnormal blood flow, failing hepatic cell function may alter glucose tolerance. Shunting of blood deprives hepatocytes of insulin needed for maintaining normal amounts of glycolytic enzymes and suppressing gluconeogenesis.

Abnormalities of hepatic blood flow or dysfunction of hepatocytes do not account for fasting hyperglycemia in patients with chronic forms of liver disease. Fasting hyperglycemia in cirrhosis reflects an intrinsic abnormality in the regulation of hepatic gluconeogenesis. Cirrhotics with fasting hyperglycemia probably have a form of diabetes secondary to insulin deficiency. A reasonable differentiation between diabetes and glucose intolerance due only to liver disease can be made sometimes on the basis of a subnormal insulin response to oral glucose. Less than normal concentrations of insulin in peripheral blood after glucose loading cannot be explained by liver disease.

No treatment is indicated in patients who have abnormal oral glucose tolerance tests associated with chronic liver disease but no insulin deficiency. This type of hyperglycemia has not been shown to increase the risk of accelerated atherosclerosis, retinal vessel disease, and renal failure. On the other hand, cirrhotic patients who also are insulin-deficient may benefit from therapy for their glucose intolerance.

Hypoglycemia

Hypoglycemia is uncommon in cirrhotics, except when cirrhosis and hypoglycemia are manifestations of glycogen storage diseases, suggesting that, even in terminal forms of chronic liver disease, the capacity of individual hepatocytes to synthesize glucose is quite large. It is possible, however, that hypoglycemia is uncommon in liver disease because of gluconeogenesis in the renal cortex (a normal function of this tissue).

Patients with acute fulminant hepatitis often will be hypoglycemic, especially in the terminal stages of the illness. All hepatic functions fail in these instances, and the hypoglycemia can be explained by an absence of gluconeogenesis.

The most common cause of hypoglycemia in patients with liver disease is the combination of ethanol abuse and fasting. In this setting, ethanol inhibits the synthesis of glucose from amino acids, lactate, and glycerol. Oxidation of ethanol, catalyzed by alcohol dehydrogenase, increases the hepatic concentration of reduced pyridine nucleotides (NADH). High levels of NADH inhibit gluconeogenesis by limiting the entry of precursors (lactate, amino acids, and glycerol) into the gluconeogenic pathway. This inhibition is reversed as soon as ethanol is oxidized completely, and the hepatic level of NADH returns to normal. Ethanol, on the other hand, does not interfere with production of glucose from glycogen. Thus, hypoglycemia secondary to ethanol ingestion does not occur unless glycogen stores are depleted completely, by fasting. Since it takes approximately 48 hours of fasting to deplete hepatic glycogen, ethanol-induced hypoglycemia occurs under carefully controlled conditions only in patients fasted for this length of time. Alcoholics who have fasted for a shorter period of time may present with this syndrome, since their dietary habits are notoriously poor and they probably begin a period of fasting with less than a normal amount of hepatic glycogen, and hence are more susceptible to hypoglycemia during alcoholic binges. Patients with established alcoholic cirrhosis are not at greater risk for alcohol-induced hypoglycemia than those with normal hepatic morphology. The unknown degree of depleted hepatic glycogen in the former (as well as in other different liver diseases) becomes the determining factor of the risk.

Hypoglycemia secondary to reduced hepatic production of glucose occurs in many inborn errors of metabolism in which there is a defective enzyme for the breakdown of glycogen. Deficiency of glucose-6-phosphatase is the most difficult of these to deal with clinically, and the one that leads to the most troublesome hypoglycemia, because glucose-6-P is the final common intermediate in the production of glucose from glycogen, amino acids, and lactate.

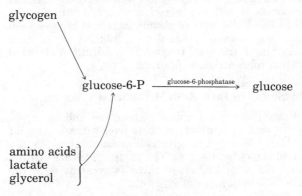

Absence or deficiency of glucose-6-phosphatase blocks release of glucose from glycogen as well as synthesis of glucose from amino acids and lactate. Other enzyme deficiencies associated with *glycogen storage disease* do not affect the synthesis of glucose from other carbon sources. Many inborn errors of metabolism interfere with the production of glucose indirectly. For example, ingestion of fructose leads to severe hypoglycemia in patients lacking hepatic fructose-1-P aldolase, an enzyme not involved in the pathways of glycogenolysis or gluconeogenesis. It seems that accumulation of fructose-1-P inhibits both gluconeogenesis and the release of glucose from glycogen. Inhibition of hepatic gluconeogenesis also occurs in children who are unable to oxidize branched-chain amino acids (leucine, isoleucine, and valine)—so-called maple syrup urine disease. Accumulation of leucine in blood is the most likely cause of hypoglycemia in these patients in that leucine inhibits gluconeogenesis in normal people. Hypoglycemia also occurs in methylmalonic aciduria and (rarely) in children with galactose intolerance.

An important cause of hypoglycemia in some parts of the world is ingestion of "hypoglycin," a chemical present in the seeds of unripe akee fruit. Hypoglycin inhibits hepatic gluconeogenesis and produces "Jamaican vomiting sickness." Interestingly, it is not toxic when ingested by well-nourished people.

Lactate Metabolism in Patients with Liver Disease

Lactate release from muscle, brain, and red cells is metabolized in the liver. The amount of lactate formed by tissues is increased under anaerobic conditions because of the block in mitochondrial oxidation. Lactic acidosis hence is a complication of anoxia. In addition, inhibition of hepatic metabolism of lactate may be a primary factor in the accumulation of lactate in blood, even in the absence of anoxia, since extensive injury to the liver interferes with the metabolism of lactate formed in other tissues. Ingestion of ethanol also blocks clearance of lactate by liver, irrespective of the liver morphology. NADH produced during the oxidation of ethanol shifts the equilibrium between pyruvate and lactate in favor of lactate for as long as the concentration of NADH is high (Fig. 17). This shift interferes with hepatic uptake of lactate because the latter depends on the further metabolism of lactate to pyruvate. Ethanol ingestion alone usually does not produce a severe enough accumulation of lactate to embarrass acid-base balance. Lactic acidosis in alcoholics is associated almost always with other serious medical problems, or with the ingestion of other toxins. On the other hand, the level of plasma lactate is high enough after ingestion of ethanol to inhibit renal tubular secretion of uric acid, frequently resulting in elevated plasma concentrations of urate.

DISORDERS OF FATTY ACID METABOLISM

Fatty liver is a common histological finding in patients with or without intrinsic liver disease. The fat in "fatty liver" is triglyceride accumulating in the cytoplasm of hepatocytes. The triglycerides are synthesized via esterification of three fatty acids with the three alcohol groups of glycerol.

When the release of fatty acids from adipose tissue is stimulated, their uptake by liver increases as the concentration of free fatty acids rises in the blood. The fatty acids taken up by the liver usually exceed what can be utilized for energy needs or structural purposes. The excess is re-esterified to triglyceride and excreted as lipoproteins, completing a circulation of fatty acids between liver and fat depots. This circulation (Fig. 18) appears to be the only mechanism for returning fatty acids to storage depots. The liver, therefore, reclaims fatty acids that are released from adipose tissue but not metabolized. The process and control of lipolysis are described in detail in Section VI.

The frequency of fatty liver reflects the number of normal and pathological states that stimulate release of fatty acids from adipose cells and/or limit the capacity of the liver to secrete VLDL. This is so because the liver responds passively to increased concentrations of fatty acids in the blood. Liver clears a fixed fraction of these over a wide range of concentrations. Stimulation of lipolysis alone thus has the potential for creating a fatty liver because it increases the amounts of fatty acids delivered to, and taken up by, the liver. The enhanced lipolysis of triglycerides in fat depots of obese patients, as compared with lean controls, accounts for the frequent association of obesity and fatty liver. Even when functioning normally, the liver will not secrete all the fatty acids delivered to it in obesity. A small amount is stored in esterified form (triglyceride). Liver biopsy reveals mild accumulations of triglyceride in liver cells in as many as 50 per cent of obese patients. This finding is a physiological consequence of the obese state and does not signify an abnormality of liver function. Similarly, fatty liver is common in patients with a variety of endocrine disorders. Diabetes leads to enhanced rates of lipolysis in fat tissue, a reaction that is normally suppressed by insulin. The diabetic, especially when poorly controlled, accumulates fatty acids in blood secondary to increasing mobilization of fat and will store variable amounts of these as triglycerides in the liver. Starvation similarly leads to mobilization of fatty acids, and accounts in this manner for much of the fatty liver of fasted patients who are not yet malnourished. Administration of corticosteroids, or excessive endogenous production, produces fatty liver for the same reason. Fatty liver can be produced too in experimental animals simply by feeding them excessive amounts of carbohydrates. Fat accumulation in this instance results from excessively high rates of synthesis of fatty acids stimulated by the ingested carbohydrate. This mechanism may explain the fatty liver in patients hyperalimented parenterally. Thus, the rate of synthesis of fatty acids in liver is stimulated by the large amounts of glucose given to these patients and probably exceeds the capacity of the liver to secrete them as triglyceride.

The genesis of fatty liver is more complex in patients who are fasted for prolonged times, or who suffer from protein-calorie malnutrition. Deficiencies of lipotropic

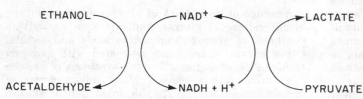

Figure 17. Coupling of the oxidation of ethanol to the reduction of pyruvate.

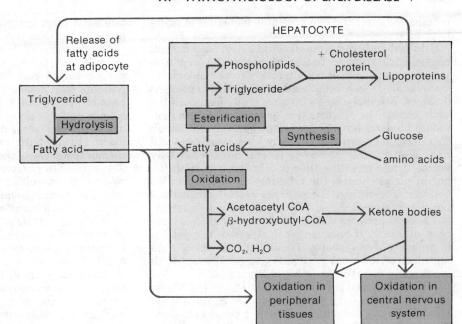

Figure 18. Central role of the liver in the metabolism of fatty acids.

substances interfere with secretion of very low density lipoproteins (VLDL) (see Section VI) and lead, in this way, to excess hepatic triglycerides. Fatty liver in the severely malnourished hence can be due not only to increased mobilization of fat from adipose tissue but also to diet-induced defects in the capacity of the liver to resecrete it. The severe fatty liver in kwashiorkor is associated with low levels of VLDL in serum, suggesting that the liver is secreting an inappropriately small amount of VLDL. Accumulation of hepatic fat is an almost constant finding in *obese patients* with a *jejunoileal bypass* and probably reflects protein-calorie imbalance. There is no clear causal relationship in these patients, however, between the fatty liver and development of a rapidly fatal form of liver disease. The fatty liver of *pregnancy* and of *Reye's syndrome* seems to be only one aspect of a more serious and far-reaching derangement of hepatocyte function. Toxic hepatitis may cause fat accumulation in the liver. The mechanisms of fat accumulation after poisoning with carbon tetrachloride, yellow phosphorus, and similar agents most likely reflect impaired capacity to synthesize and secrete VLDL.

Fatty liver is the most frequent abnormality in liver biopsies from patients who abuse *ethanol*. Accumulation of fat secondary to ethanol ingestion is mutifactorial. Ethanol stimulates synthesis of fatty acids in the liver by supplying large amounts of acetyl CoA. It interferes, too, with normal regulation of fatty acid synthesis. The oxidation of ethanol inhibits the entry of long-chain fatty acids into the β-oxidation cycle, diverting them instead to triglyceride. Ethanol may stimulate release of fatty acids from adipose tissue as well, but this point is controversial. Ethanol clearly does not interfere acutely with the synthesis and secretion of VLDL. Ethanol, in fact, increases the output of VLDL by liver, leading frequently to hyperlipidemia, that remits with abstention. Synthesis of VLDL may be inhibited, on the other hand, in the chronic alcoholic who is malnourished and/or has chronic irreversible liver disease. Ethanol can produce a fatty liver in the absence of liver disease.

The finding of fatty liver on biopsy poses two questions: (1) Is the accumulation of triglyceride an appropriate response of the liver to derangements in other systems, or is there a primary defect in hepatic secretion of triglycerides? (2) Does the excess triglyceride in liver have pathogenetic significance? The first question can be answered by careful consideration of the patient's overall status and an understanding of the potential mechanisms for producing fatty liver. The second question is difficult to answer with certainty. Fatty liver per se probably has no deleterious effects on hepatic function. Many alcoholic patients may have fatty liver for years without evidence of progressive liver disese. The fatty liver associated with severe malnutrition also seems to have no negative effect on hepatic function. Although patients receiving parenteral hyperalimentation may have elevated levels of SGOT and alkaline phosphatase in association with fatty liver, the relationship between these abnormalities is uncertain.

There are no specific treatments for mobilizing triglyceride from human liver. Reversal of fatty liver occurs in response to correction of the primary abnormality, whether hepatic or nonhepatic. Treatment in any individual with significant fatty liver thus is directed at the primary abnormality associated with the accumulation of fatty acids rather than the manifestation per se.

Abnormalities of Ketogenesis. The production of ketones by the liver during a long fast protects the mass and contractile strength of muscle protein. We know little about the control of these processes in patients with liver disease. Simple questions such as nitrogen balance in fasted patients with cirrhosis as compared with normal controls have not been studied. This specific problem may have clinical relevance in that one frequently observes rapid, extensive wasting of muscle not due to myopathy in patients with alcohol-induced cirrhosis. Theoretically a quantitatively small defect in rates of production of ketones in fasted patients with liver disease could have a profound effect on nitrogen metabolism. Ketone production by rat liver is impaired after the experimental induction of acute liver injury.

Ethanol-Induced Ketosis. Mild ketosis is a normal physiological response to fasting. Accumulation of acetoacetate and β-hydroxybutyrate severe enough to cause acidosis is a complication of insulin-dependent diabetes. Ethanol abuse also may rarely be associated with ketosis. In all instances, patients with ethanol-induced ketosis have been chronic abusers of ethanol; they have been drinking steadily for several days and have been fasting for one to several days. They may not be drinking at the time of admission to hospital, but in such instances the drinking has been curtailed because of vomiting. The patients are dehydrated but not hypoglycemic. Blood pH may be reduced slightly, but several patients with alcohol-induced ketosis have been alkalotic. If blood sugar is elevated, the patient is probably also diabetic. Treatment consists of fluid and electrolyte replacement plus glucose. Therapy with insulin and bicarbonate is not indicated.

Ethanol-induced ketosis probably reflects the effects of starvation on fatty acid metabolism. Ethanol itself tends to have an antiketogenic effect because it stimulates the esterification of fatty acids, thereby diverting them from β-oxidation. Why this fails to happen in ketotic patients is open to speculation.

SYNTHESIS OF LIPOPROTEINS

Hepatic Synthesis. The synthesis of lipoproteins is an important hepatic function. The essential features of metabolism in the liver consist of the synthesis of the components and assembly of high density lipoproteins (HDL) and very low density lipoproteins (VLDL). The detailed metabolism of lipoproteins is discussed in Section VI, to which the reader is referred.

Abnormalities of Lipoprotein Metabolism. Patients with mechanical obstruction of the bile ducts or intrahepatic cholestasis have elevated levels of cholesterol in their blood. Concentrations of plasma phospholipid are increased, too, but these usually are not measured in the clinical laboratory. The plasma cholesterol in patients with cholestasis is carried principally in an abnormal particle referred to as lipoprotein X, which has the density of an LDL but differs from it in terms of lipid and protein components. As compared with LDL, lipoprotein X contains less protein and more phospholipid and cholesterol. In addition, more than 90 per cent of the cholesterol of lipoprotein X is unesterified, whereas 55 per cent of LDL cholesterol is unesterified. This difference has important implications for the life span of red cells in patients with liver disease, as will be discussed later. Finally, the major protein in lipoprotein X is albumin, which is not a constituent of LDL. Particles of lipoprotein X look like red cells stacked in arrays when visualized with the electron microscope. The lipids of lipoprotein X are probably arranged as a vesicle of bilayered membranes. LDL, in contrast, consists of a globular core surrounded by phospholipid, protein, and cholesterol. Current thinking is that lipoprotein X forms as a consequence of excessive synthesis of cholesterol, an event known to follow complete obstruction of the bile duct or selective occlusion of the biliary system in a single lobe of the liver. Excess cholesterol, albumin (the major protein of lipoprotein X), phospholipids, and perhaps bile salts form the membranes of the abnormal lipoprotein that then is secreted into the sinusoid.

The presence of lipoprotein X in blood is not innocuous. It leads to xanthomatous deposits in skin. It may play a causal role in accelerated atherosclerosis in patients with *primary biliary cirrhosis*. Also, the presence of lipoprotein X is related to the frequent hemolytic anemia in patients with cholestasis of any etiology. Unesterified (or free) cholesterol, when present in plasma lipoproteins, exchanges with lecithin of red cell membranes. Thus, the free cholesterol in lipoprotein X can be incorporated into the red cell, accompanied by transfer of lecithin from the red cell to the lipoprotein. This exchange increases the amount of cholesterol in the red cell membrane, which expands its surface area. Excess surface area gives red cells the appearance of target cells. Further increases of cholesterol in the membrane cause formation of spurs. Red cells with excess membrane are subject to early destruction as they circulate through the spleen. All conditions that increase the amount of unesterified cholesterol in lipoproteins produce a similar effect on red cell morphology and longevity. On the other hand, hyperlipemic states in which the ratio of esterified to unesterified cholesterol is normal do not lead to hemolytic anemia or to excess cholesterol in the red cell membranes. (Patients with the hereditary forms of hypercholesterolemia do not have red cell abnormalities.) Liver has an essential role in the normal catabolism of VLDL, and defects in this process occur in patients with liver disease. Abnormal lipoproteins in liver disease hence are not restricted to the occurrence of lipoprotein X.

Triglycerides are released from VLDL through the activity of lipoprotein lipase, which catalyzes their hydrolysis to fatty acids and glycerol. This reaction takes place in close proximity to adipocytes, so that the fatty acids of triglycerides are transported directly from VLDL to storage depots in fat cells. The triglyceride-rich core of VLDL particle becomes progressively smaller as lipids are removed in this manner. There is an associated requirement to reduce the amount of surface elements per particle. This is achieved by transfer of free cholesterol, phospholipid, and protein from the surface of VLDL to HDL in exchange for cholesterol esters, which enter the residual core region of VLDL. When released from the liver, however, cholesterol in HDL is almost completely unesterified. The synthesis of cholesterol esters in HDL must precede exchange, a step that is vital for the metabolism of VLDL. Esterification proceeds within circulating HDL and is catalyzed by lecithin cholesterol acyl transferase (LCAT), as shown in Figure 19. LCAT is made in the liver, and its synthesis is defective in many patients with liver disease. Additionally, the activity of this enzyme is inhibited by bile salts in the plasma. In the absence of sufficient LCAT, the levels of free cholesterol in all types of lipoproteins are elevated and cholesterol esters depressed. LCAT deficiency thus explains the well-known abnormality in the ratio of free to esterified plasma cholesterol in patients with liver disease. LCAT deficiency also is a primary mechanism for shortened red cell survival (hemolytic anemia) in patients with liver disease who do not have cholestasis. For example, abnormal amounts of free cholesterol are present in HDL, VLDL,

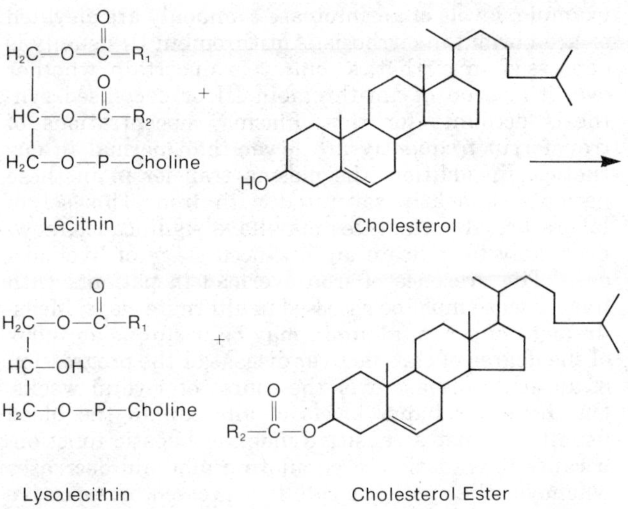

Figure 19. The reaction catalyzed by lecithin-cholesterol acyl transferase (LCAT).

and LDL from patients with less than normal amounts of LCAT. Free cholesterol in these lipoproteins exchanges with red cell lipids, leading to abnormalities identical to those in patients with lipoprotein X. Reduced activity of LCAT does not account, however, for the appearance of lipoprotein X in cholestatic patients. Lipoprotein X is present prior to deficiency of LCAT. Finally, LCAT deficiency leads to hypertriglyceridemia as nonmetabolized VLDL accumulate.

METABOLISM OF CHOLESTEROL AND BILE ACIDS AND THEIR DISORDERS IN LIVER DISEASE

CHOLESTEROL

Cholesterol is essential for normal function of all cell membranes. It is synthesized by all cells in a pathway consisting of three major steps: (1) synthesis of mevalonic acid from acetyl coenzyme A; (2) the polymerization of five molecules of mevalonic acid to produce squalene; and (3) the conversion of squalene to cholesterol. Regulation of the synthesis of cholesterol is effected by modulating the amount of β-hydroxyglutaryl-coenzyme A reductase, the enzyme catalyzing the synthesis of mevalonic acid. Its biosynthesis, transport, and metabolism are described in detail in Section VI. Hepatocytes synthesize cholesterol in excess of their own structural needs. A teleological explanation for this is utilization of the excess for synthesis and secretion of triglyceride-rich lipoproteins. Cholesterol, however, is a potential toxic compound because of its effects on blood vessels. At the same time, mammals have a limited capacity for metabolizing cholesterol to compounds that are excreted. The problem of limiting the toxic potential of excess cholesterol made in the liver is solved, in large part, by using it as a source of cholesterol in nonhepatic tissues. Cholesterol synthesized in the liver and secreted by it in the form of VLDL is transported to nonhepatic tissues. LDL remaining after the release of triglycerides from VLDL are the transport particles. They bind to receptors on the surface of nonhepatic cells, and are internalized by

endocytosis. The esterified cholesterol contained previously in the LDL is released to the interior of the cell, where it is hydrolyzed by cholesterol esterase. The free cholesterol then is incorporated into the membranes of nonhepatic cells. Uptake of cholesterol by nonhepatic tissues suppresses their endogenous synthesis. Thus, cholesterol synthesized in liver becomes the major source of cholesterol for other cells.

BILE ACIDS

Mammals lack the enzymatic machinery for breaking down the ring system of cholesterol. It is converted to bile acids and steroid hormones in man, but only the former pathway is significant quantitatively for disposal. Synthesis of bile acids from cholesterol, which occurs only in the liver, involves hydroxylation of the steroid nucleus (Fig. 20) followed by oxidation and shortening of the hydrocarbon chain attached at position 17. Cholic acid and chenodeoxycholic acid (lacking the hydroxyl at position 12) are the principal bile acids made by liver. These are secreted into bile as salts, conjugated with glycine or taurine. Conjugation is not essential for secretion, but enhances its rate and is significant physiologically in the gut.

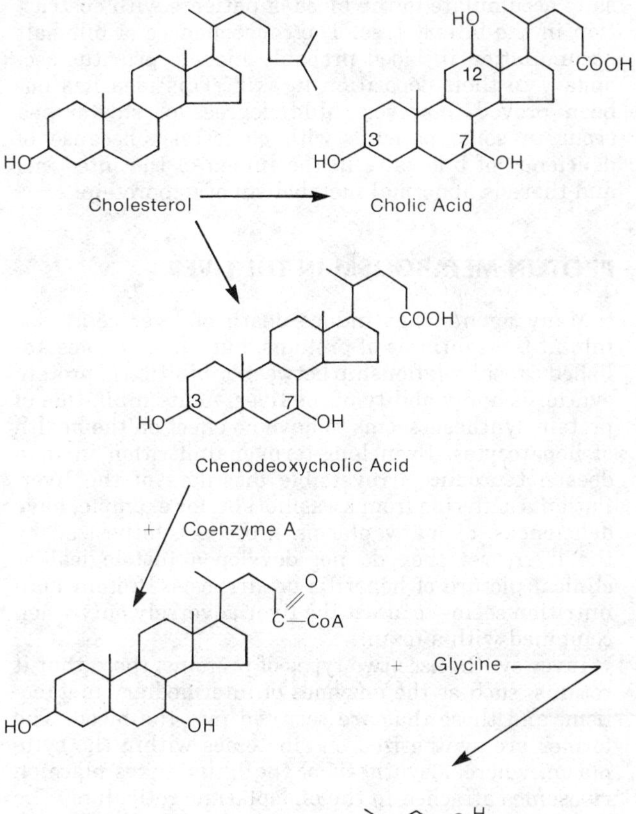

Figure 20. The conversion of cholesterol to bile acids and bile salts.

Bile salts are important determinants of the amount and composition of bile, because they enhance the excretion of biliary water, cholesterol, and phospholipid. They appear to be absolutely essential for absorption of fat-soluble vitamins. Unconjugated bile acids are not as efficient as the conjugated forms for intestinal absorption of fat. Unconjugated bile acids also inhibit intestinal absorption of salt and water. The adult human liver normally synthesizes about 400 to 600 mg of cholic acid per day, and 200 to 300 mg of chenodeoxycholic acid. Creation of a bile fistula, as occurs after inserting a T tube or administering resins (e.g., cholestyramine) that bind bile acids increases the conversion of cholesterol to bile acids. This technique can effect long-term lowering of cholesterol levels in plasma. The enterohepatic circulation of bile acids and their salts, as well as the pathophysiology of cholelithiasis, is considered later, in the section on the gallbladder, pages 1293–1294.

Obstructive jaundice obviously is associated with diminished transfer of bile salts from liver cells to bile. However, unconjugated cholic acid is removed from blood at a normal rate in jaundiced patients unless hepatocellular function is poor. The rates of bile acid conjugation also are normal in this setting. Hence, bile salts accumulate in the blood of patients with obstruction in the biliary tree. The consequences of bile salt accumulation in blood probably include pruritus secondary to their deposition in skin. This idea has not been proved, however. Mild degrees of steatorrhea occur in some patients with cholestasis because of deficiency of bile salts in the lumen of the intestine, and there is abnormal metabolism of lipoproteins.

PROTEIN METABOLISM IN THE LIVER

Many agents that induce death of liver cells also inhibit the synthesis of proteins, but there is no established causal relationship between inhibition of protein synthesis and viability of the liver. Acute inhibition of protein synthesis seems to have no effect on the health of hepatocytes. Even long-term malnutrition in man does not produce irreversible disorders of the liver. Patients suffering from kwashiorkor, for example, have deficiencies of many plasma proteins synthesized by the liver, yet they do not develop a histological or clinical picture of hepatitis or cirrhosis. Protein malnutrition seems to affect the liver adversely only when combined with a toxin.

Liver synthesizes two types of proteins: those that it retains, such as the enzymes of intermediary metabolism, and those that are secreted into the blood. The former are synthesized on ribosomes within the cytoplasm, whereas synthesis of the latter takes place on ribosomes attached to the endoplasmic reticulum. The cell biology of protein secretion is described in Section I.

Plasma proteins synthesized by the liver include albumin, transferrin, ceruloplasmin, haptoglobin, α_1 acid glycoprotein, clotting factors, several types of antiproteases, some of the complement factors, and C-reactive protein. The levels of these proteins are quite variable in patients with liver disease, so that their concentrations in plasma may not reflect the extent of liver disease, except in end-stage liver failure. For example, levels of antiprotease commonly are elevated or are normal in cirrhosis. Antithrombin III usually is depressed in cirrhotics, but it is uncertain whether overutilization of antithrombin III or decreased synthesis accounts for this. Plasma concentrations of transferrin frequently are lower than normal in cirrhotics. In addition, the plasma transferrin in these patients is nearly saturated with iron. This set of laboratory abnormalities may have significance, however, only to indicate an advanced stage of liver disease. The presence of iron overload in patients with liver disease must be assessed in alternate ways. Measurement of serum albumin may be useful as an index of the degree of chronic liver disease or the progression of an acute disease over the course of several weeks. On the other hand, levels of albumin in the blood usually are not a sensitive index of hepatic function, because degradation of circulating albumin decreases whenever the synthetic rate is depressed, irrespective of the mechanism of the former effect. Levels of albumin in sera usually are low in patients with chronic liver disease. The changes in its rate of degradation may allow for normal concentration of albumin in blood despite impaired synthesis.

Deficiencies of albumin, transferrin, ceruloplasmin, lipoproteins, and several other plasma proteins, as occur in patients with acquired forms of liver disease, have relatively little importance for the continued health or longevity of the patient. They reflect only the severity of liver disease. Clinically important abnormalities of protein synthesis in patients with acquired forms of liver disease are restricted to disorders of synthesis of clotting factors. Liver synthesizes clotting factors I (fibrinogen), II (prothrombin), V (proaccelerin), VII (proconvertin), IX (Christmas factor), X (Stuart factor), XI (plasma thromboplastin antecedent), and XIII (fibrin stabilizing factor). Deficiencies of factors I, XI, and XIII are unusual, except in end-stage liver disease. Deficiencies of the other factors are common. Synthesis of clotting factors is assessed most often with the one-stage prothrombin time, which is sensitive to the levels of factors II, V, VII, and X. In most cases of acute hepatic failure with an overall deficiency of protein synthesis, the prothrombin time will be prolonged secondary to deficiency of factor VII. The basis for this is the short half-life in blood of factor VII (4–6 hours) as compared with those for factors II (3–5 days), V (20–30 hours), and X (2–3 days). The short half-life of factor VII accounts for the laboratory constellation of markedly prolonged prothrombin times and normal levels of serum albumin in patients with fulminant hepatic necrosis. The long half-life of albumin masks an abrupt decline in its synthesis.

The mixture of normal and abnormal levels of serum proteins in a given cirrhotic patient is unpredictable. Some patients have prolonged prothrombin times and normal levels of albumin, whereas others have abnormal levels of albumin and normal prothrombin times. In addition, a cirrhotic patient may have a normal prothrombin time but a prolonged partial thromboplastin time secondary to deficient factor IX, which has a plasma half-life of about 24 hours. The pattern of deficient proteins also is of no use as a prognostic indicator, because we do not yet understand the chemical and pathophysiological basis for such findings. Measurements of albumin and prothrombin time hence are both essential in assessing the status of protein synthesis by liver. Levels in the blood are indices of the balance between rates of synthesis and degradation. A normal level of a plasma protein is not firm evidence for normal rates of synthesis by liver.

The syntheses of effective clotting factors II, VII, IX, and X depend on vitamin K. Precursors of the vitamin K-dependent clotting factors accumulate in the liver after administration of vitamin K antagonists, indicating that the vitamin-dependent steps occur after assembly of their primary structures. Thus, if the prothrombin time is prolonged secondary to deficiency of protein synthesis, administration of vitamin K will not correct it. Rather, vitamin K is involved in the addition of a carboxyl residue to glutamic acid in the protein precursors of clotting factors. When administration of vitamin K corrects abnormalities in the clotting factors in patients with liver disease, it does so by mechanisms distinct from the synthesis of protein. Some patients with relatively mild forms of acute hepatitis have prolonged prothrombin times that respond promptly to vitamin K. The cause of the apparent vitamin K deficiency in these patients is unclear, and has no prognostic significance.

ABNORMALITIES OF PROTEIN METABOLISM IN PATIENTS WITH LIVER DISEASE

In addition to quantitative abnormalities of protein synthesis, qualitative abnormalities in the plasma proteins occur in some patients with liver disease. The latter include protein abnormalities associated with hepatoma, abnormalities of lipoproteins associated with cholestatic states, a dysfibrinogenic state in some patients with acute and chronic forms of liver disease, and poorly defined abnormalities of proteins that seem to be associated with acquired defects in the function of platelets.

Defective Catabolism of Proteins. The liver is an important site for the degradation of plasma proteins. An abnormality in the degradative process has clinical significance for at least one plasma protein: plasminogen activator. Clotted blood from patients with cirrhosis tends to lyse on standing, an abnormality due to stimulation of fibrinolysis by elevated amounts of plasminogen activator. There is a marked decrease in the rate of degradation of this protein in liver disease, which serves to promote thrombolytic activity even when antiplasmin levels are normal. Manipulations that enhance the synthesis of plasminogen activator, such as surgical procedures, trauma, and certain drugs, induce marked elevations of plasminogen activation in cirrhotics and can precipitate acute fibrinolysis. The products of fibrinolysis are themselves cleared by the liver, a process that also is defective in cirrhosis. Fibrinolytic products hence accumulate in patients with liver disease, leading to further abnormalities of hemostasis.

Protein Abnormalities in Patients with Hepatoma. All cells within a given animal contain identical genetic material and are capable, in theory, of producing the same proteins. The heterogeneity of cell function is based on selective transcription of some regions of DNA and repression of others by mechanisms not yet identified in eukaryotic cells. The regulation of DNA transcription is disordered in tumor cells, and

carcinogenesis is characterized by a dedifferentiation of cells. Hepatoma cells thus are dedifferentiated liver cells and produce in many instances proteins not found in adults. The most frequent abnormality of this sort in patients with hepatoma is production of α-fetoprotein, which is synthesized by normal fetal liver but disappears from the blood within a few days of birth. Alpha-fetoprotein crosses the placenta and so is present normally in maternal blood. It may be present in the plasma of patients with acute hepatitis and rarely in patients with alcoholic liver disease. Levels of α-fetoprotein do not increase when adult liver regenerates rapidly, as for example after partial resections. The significance of α-fetoprotein in blood remains obscure, except in patients with hepatoma, in whom it may be used as a clinical marker.

Dysfibrinogenemia in Liver Disease. Fibrinogen is a glycoprotein. The fibrin monomer in some patients with liver disease as compared with normals has an increased content of sialic acid, which is the terminal sugar of branched-chain oligosaccharides. This excess of sialic acid residues, which carry a negative charge, interferes with normal polymerization of fibrin monomers. There are other abnormalities of the oligosaccharide chains of fibrin monomer in affected patients, but the excess of sialic acid seems to account completely for the dysfunction of fibrin. Thus, selective removal of the excess sialic acid from abnormal fibrin monomers restores normal capacity for polymerization. It is uncertain, however, whether the presence of this abnormal type of fibrinogen is significant for clotting in patients with liver disease. Fibrin monomer is not the only glycoprotein with abnormal oligosaccharide composition in patients with liver disease. The activities of several glycosyl transferases, including sialytransferase, are increased in blood from patients with hepatocellular disease.

MECHANISMS FOR DETOXIFYING ENDOGENOUS AND EXOGENOUS TOXINS

One of the critical functions of the liver is to detoxify a variety of potentially lethal materials. The liver is equipped for this purpose with a broad array of different enzymes. In addition, there appear to be within each family of enzymes for detoxification a number of enzymes with broad, overlapping specificity for substrates. This allows us to cope with an ever-increasing number of toxic, man-made chemicals.

DETOXIFICATION OF AMMONIA

Large amounts of ammonia are produced in the course of metabolism of amino acids, and from bacterial action in the large bowel. Ammonia is poorly tolerated by the body possibly because of its effects on energy metabolism in the brain. Ammonia is detoxified by the liver.

FORMS OF AMMONIA IN THE BLOOD

The principal chemical forms of ammonia in blood are ammonium ion [NH_4^+] and ammonium hydroxide:

$$[14] \quad NH_4^+ + OH^- \rightleftharpoons NH_4OH.$$

Alkaline Side (High OH⁻)   Acidic Side (High H⁺)

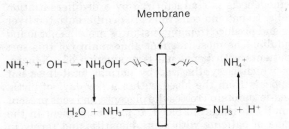

Figure 21. The effect of a pH gradient on the transfer of NH_4^+ across cell membranes.

A small amount exists as ammonia gas (NH_3), which is in equilibrium with ammonium hydroxide. (The partial pressure of ammonia at given values of blood pH and total nitrogen as ammonium can be determined from nomograms.) The quantity, or partial pressure, of ammonia is important because this is the only form that penetrates cell membranes. Membranes do not allow passage of ammonium ion and ammonium hydroxide. The pK for the equilibrium between ammonium ion and ammonium hydroxide is approximately 9.0. The equilibrium is shifted in favor of ammonium ion as the pH is lowered. Ammonium ion thus is the principal form of ammonia at physiological pH. Differences between intracellular and extracellular pH generate gradients that concentrate NH_4^+ on the side of the membrane with the lower pH, which is the intracellular side. The chemical pathway for producing such gradients is outlined in Figure 21. Hypokalemia, which produces extracellular alkalosis and intracellular acidosis, augments the normal tendency to transfer ammonia to the inside of cells. Shifts in ammonia from the extracellular to intracellular space can be significant within the range of pH changes encountered clinically, even though these are distant from the pK of the ammonium hydroxide–ammonium ion equilibrium.

PRODUCTION OF AMMONIA

Ammonia is produced by deamination of amino acids. The most important of these is oxidative deamination of glutamic acid, catalyzed by glutamate dehydrogenase. This reaction has a central position in the metabolism of amino acids and nitrogen, since it represents a common pathway for the nitrogen involved in transaminase reactions. Thus,

[15] α-ketoglutarate + amino acids ⇌ glutamic
acid + α-ketoacids

[16] glutamic acid + NAD $\xrightarrow{\text{glutamate dehydrogenase}}$
α-ketoglutarate + NADH + NH_3

Gluconeogenesis in the liver increases deamination via the above pathway. Additionally, renal production of ammonia is enhanced by acidosis, hypokalemia, and high rates of gluconeogenesis. Exercising muscle also forms significant amounts of ammonia. Production of ammonia in the large bowel is due to the metabolism of enteric bacteria that oxidatively deaminate amino acids, thereby releasing nitrogen in the form of ammonia. In addition, urea in the lumen of the bowel is split by urease, yielding ammonia.

METABOLISM OF AMMONIA IN THE LIVER

Liver normally removes 80 per cent of the ammonia in portal blood in a single passage. Ammonia is metabolized by conversion to glutamine (Reaction [21]) and urea (Fig. 22).

[17] glutamic acid + NH_3 + ATP $\longrightarrow$
glutamine + ADP + P_i

The former is not quantitatively important for detoxification, but nitrogen incorporated into glutamine is utilized for the synthesis of several essential compounds, for example, purines, pyrimidines, and amino sugars. Glutaminase catalyzes the release of ammonia from glutamine in an important reaction for maintenance of acid-base balance in the kidney.

Conversion to urea is the more significant pathway for detoxifying ammonia. Half the nitrogen for urea synthesis comes from ammonia directly. Note that this ammonia is trapped as carbamyl phosphate, in a re-

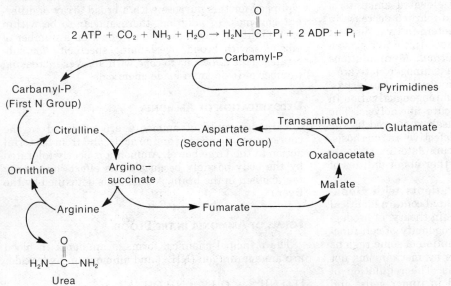

Figure 22. The synthesis of urea from ammonia.

action consuming 2 moles of ATP per mole of product formed (Fig. 22). Synthesis of urea thus is an energy-dependent pathway. Aspartate contributes the second molecule of ammonia. The nitrogen of aspartate is derived from transamination reactions. It may come from glutamate or from other amino acids.

Normal liver has a large capacity for synthesis of urea and hence for detoxification of ammonia. The excretion of urea varies with protein metabolism but averages about 13 grams per 24 hours. This is considerably less than the maximum capacity, since the synthesis of urea is adaptive. There are no specific data on levels of urea cycle enzymes in patients with liver disease in whom there is faulty detoxification of ammonia.

Hepatic Coma

A number of mechanisms have been proposed as explanations for the stupor that occurs in patients with liver disease: excess ammonia, production of false neurotransmitters and short-chain fatty acids, abnormalities in the transport of amino acids into the brain, excess serotonin, and a liver-dependent defect in the utilization of glucose by the brain. There is a factual base to support each idea. A number of amines that could act as neurotransmitters are synthesized by bacteria-catalyzed decarboxylation of amino acids in the intestine. Short-chain fatty acids, such as butyrate, valerate, and isovalerate, also are produced in the gut. Normally, these substances are taken up and metabolized by the liver. In cirrhosis, however, shunting of portal blood allows them to bypass metabolism in the liver and thus to enter the central nervous system where they can interfere with transmission of impulses and metabolism. At this point, it is not worthwhile to try any longer to find *the* cause of hepatic coma. The syndrome is a nonspecific manifestation of disordered cerebral function. Several factors acting in concert could produce it, and the significance of any single etiology varies. Of the factors implicated in the genesis of hepatic coma, the level of ammonia in the blood correlates best with the clinical status of patients in "hepatic coma": blood ammonia levels are elevated in about 75 per cent of patients with this syndrome. Moreover, since the tissue level of ammonia, rather than the plasma level per se, is toxic, measurement of amounts in tissue—if they could be done—might in-

crease the diagnostic accuracy of determining ammonia in patients with hepatic coma. Most importantly, therapies that decrease ammonia levels often ameliorate the signs and symptoms of stupor. Finally, the key role of ammonia in hepatic coma is underscored by the presence of stupor in children with inborn defects in the function of urea cycle enzymes. These children have otherwise normal liver function, morphology, and blood flow, yet display the clinical characteristics of patients with coma secondary to liver failure. The histological abnormalities in brains from children with genetically determined deficiencies of urea cycle enzymes also are identical to abnormalities in patients with chronic liver disease and hepatic encephalopathy. Thus, although it is unproved that ammonia is the only active toxin in hepatic coma, certainly ammonia is a significant factor.

The best biochemical explanation for the toxicity of ammonia is interference with metabolism in the brain. By reacting with α-ketoglutaric acid to produce glutamic acid and glutamine, ammonia steals oxidizable substrates from the energy-metabolizing pathways of the brain (Fig. 23). Precursors of α-ketoglutarate or substrates beyond the block caused by ammonia theoretically should replace the metabolites stolen from the Krebs cycle by the scheme depicted in Figure 23. It is not possible to increase the rate of metabolism of glucose and ketone bodies in brain, however, nor will added fuels such as citrate and succinate penetrate into the mitochondria of brain cells. Diminished entry of glucose or ketone bodies into the brain would amplify any depletion of α-ketoglutarate related to excess ammonia in brain cells. Since ammonia interferes in a general way with energy generation in the brain, its apparent clinical effect on central nervous system function could amplify—or be amplified by—other etiological factors implicated in the syndrome of hepatic coma, e.g., abnormal transport across the blood-brain barrier, deficiency of branched-chain amino acids, receptor dysfunction, false neurotransmitters, or short-chain fatty acids.

Treatment of ammonia intoxication rests on decreasing the ammonia load entering the circulation and minimizing the tendency of ammonia to pass from the plasma into cells of the central nervous system. Reduction of protein in the diet decreases the amount of ammonia produced by bacteria in the gut as well as that synthesized by liver in the absorptive period. In

Figure 23. Ammonia-induced "steal" of substrates from energy-yielding pathways produces a functional blockade of the Krebs cycle.

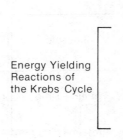

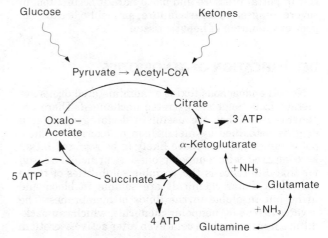

Glucose   Ketones

Pyruvate → Acetyl-CoA

Citrate → 3 ATP

Oxalo-Acetate

α-Ketoglutarate

+NH₃ Glutamate

5 ATP   Succinate

4 ATP   +NH₃

Glutamine

Energy Yielding Reactions of the Krebs Cycle

patients with intestinal bleeding, the protein in the gut must be removed by purgatives and enemas. In addition, antibiotics are useful in decreasing the population of enteric bacteria and thereby lessening ammonia production within the bowel. Finally, the amount of ammonia absorbed from the gut can be reduced by acidifying the luminal contents. This is achieved currently by feeding lactulose, a nonabsorbed sugar that is metabolized by enteric bacteria, to acidic products. Acidification of the gut lumen has the net effect of converting ammonia (NH_3) to ammonium ion (NH_4^+), which is not absorbed.

Endogenous production of ammonia during the metabolism of amino acids can be reduced by feeding glucose, since this obviates the need to synthesize glucose from the carbon skeletons of amino acids. Maintenance of normal acid-base balance and normokalemia decrease ammonia production by the kidney and help to trap NH_4^+ in the plasma compartment. Renal excretion of urea is an important factor in hepatic coma as well. Urea not excreted by the kidney enters the intestinal fluid, where it is split into ammonia and carbon dioxide by bacterial urease. Good renal function and/or sterilization of the gut can decrease this source of ammonia. Administration of α-keto acids, such as α-ketoglutarate, has been employed as a means for detoxifying ammonia. The rationale for this approach is to trap nitrogen as amines. Unfortunately, it has no proved therapeutic efficacy.

Although ammonia accumulates in the blood of patients with cirrhosis, it is not established whether shunting of blood past the liver and/or failure to detoxify ammonia delivered to hepatocytes is the principal cause for hyperammonemia. Many patients with cirrhosis and significant portal hypertension, *including demonstrable esophageal varices,* do not suffer from hepatic coma or hyperammonemia. Moreover, some patients with bleeding esophageal varices tolerate the potential toxicity of blood in the intestinal lumen quite well. The extra load of ammonia is detoxified in these patients despite significant diversion of portal blood. The weight of evidence, therefore, is that the major reason for accumulation of ammonia in the blood of patients with liver disease is diminished capacity of individual hepatocytes to metabolize it, not simply the shunting of blood away from the liver. We may expect to see hepatic coma, therefore, in conditions in which hepatocyte function fails in the absence of abnormalities in portal pressure and blood flow. It occurs, too, in severe congestive heart failure, probably because of poor oxygenation of hepatic tissue.

DETOXIFICATION OF XENOBIOTICS

Not all endogenous toxins or administered drugs are metabolized. Some are excreted unchanged. There are general rules that are useful in deciding whether a drug is detoxified by metabolism or excretion. Thus, polar compounds are more likely to be secreted intact as compared with nonpolar ones. A principal reason for this difference is the variable solubilities of these materials. Polar chemicals are soluble in blood and urine but insoluble in the lipids of membranes. The reverse is true for nonpolar chemicals, which can back-diffuse from urine into cells even after active secretion.

Removal of most nonpolar compounds from the body depends, therefore, on their prior conversion to water-soluble derivatives. The liver contains elaborate systems for increasing the solubility of water-insoluble compounds. The strategies displayed by these systems are introduction of polar groups via an oxidative reaction, hydrolysis, and/or conjugation with polar groups. Biological activity usually is destroyed by such derivatization. Liver is the primary and sometimes exclusive site for these reactions. Normal liver function hence is essential for limiting the pharmacological effects of a diversity of substances and for removing endogenously produced toxins. A detailed knowledge of the pathways for drug metabolism is not essential; a general understanding, however, is required to anticipate interactions between drugs and their potential toxicity. In addition, detailed knowledge of the metabolism of ethanol, bilirubin, and ammonia is important because of the frequency with which the physician encounters clinical and laboratory disorders related to these substances.

HEPATIC UPTAKE OF NONPOLAR COMPOUNDS

Since they are insoluble in water, nonpolar chemicals in blood are bound to plasma proteins, especially albumin. Protein-bound drug is in equilibrium with a small amount in true solution. The relative amounts of bound and free drug depend, in each instance, on the avidity of protein binding and solubility in water. Only the unbound fraction penetrates the plasma membrane of the hepatocyte (Fig. 24). There is no evidence that drugs are concentrated within the liver by an active process; but, because of their solubility in lipids, nonpolar compounds can move passively through the external or plasma membrane into the cell. Continuous uptake requires constant removal by binding to intracellular proteins, metabolism, and secretion of metabolites into bile and blood. Clearance rates are determined, therefore, by several factors, and different compounds are cleared by the liver at widely varying rates. Unfortunately, we do not know the rate-limiting step in the disposal of most drugs.

Drugs can rebind to intracellular proteins once inside the hepatocyte (Fig. 24). This binding traps the drug and thus prevents back-diffusion. In addition, by providing a storage capacity for intracellular drug, the liver cell pulls the equilibrium in the direction of free drug (Fig. 24). Two proteins have been identified in the liver cell that may be involved in the uptake of drugs and endogenous nonpolar compounds. These have been designated Y and Z. The former is also

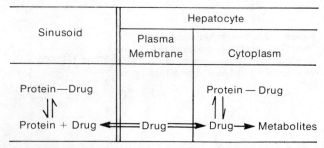

Figure 24. Schematic view of uptake of nonpolar drugs by hepatocytes.

TABLE 2. DRUG-METABOLIZING REACTIONS CATALYZED BY CYTOCHROME P$_{450}$ IN LIVER

TYPE OF REACTION	REPRESENTATIVE COMPOUND
Aliphatic Hydroxylation $R—CH_2—CH_2—CH_3 \longrightarrow R—CH_2—CHOH—CH_3$	*Pentobarbital*
Aromatic Hydroxylation 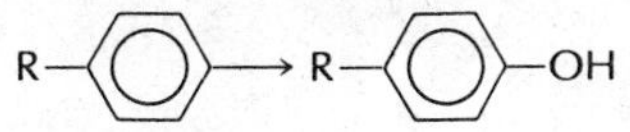 $R—\bigcirc \longrightarrow R—\bigcirc—OH$	*Acetanilid*
N-Deacylation $R—N\begin{smallmatrix}CH_3\\CH_3\end{smallmatrix} \longrightarrow R—N\begin{smallmatrix}H\\H\end{smallmatrix} + 2HCHO$	*Aminopyrine*
Oxidative Deamination	*Amphetamine*
N-Oxidation $(CH_3)_3—N \longrightarrow (CH_3)_3—N{=}O$	*Trimethylamine*
N-Hydroxylation $R_1—N—H \longrightarrow R_1—N—OH$ (with R_2)	*Aniline*
O-Dealkylation $R—O—CH_3 \longrightarrow R—OH + HCHO$	*Codeine*
S-Demethylation $R—S—CH_3 \longrightarrow R—SH + HCHO$	*Methylthiopurine*
Desulfuration $R—SH \longrightarrow R—OH$	*Parathione*
Sulfoxide Formation 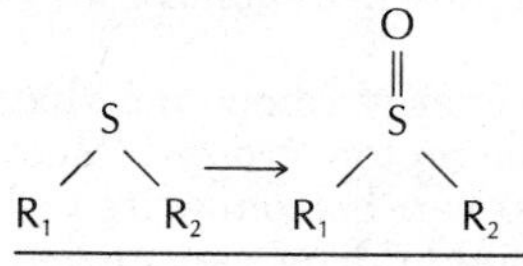 $\begin{smallmatrix}S\\R_1 \quad R_2\end{smallmatrix} \longrightarrow \begin{smallmatrix}O\\\|\\S\\R_1 \quad R_2\end{smallmatrix}$	*Chlorpromazine*

known as "ligandin," and comprises about 5 per cent of the soluble protein (the nonmembranous components) of the liver cell. Binding to Y is nonspecific. The property required is a significant proportion of hydrophobic residues. Thus, ligandin binds a large number of organic compounds, including bilirubin, BSP, and indocyanine green. Since there is only a single type of binding site, different compounds compete for the same site. Administration of one substance that binds to ligandin interferes with hepatic clearance of others.

CHEMICAL MECHANISMS FOR DETOXIFICATION

The latitude between therapeutic efficacy and intolerable toxicity for most drugs is related to the presence of many nonspecific mechanisms for metabolizing drugs (Table 2). Basically, however, there are two general types of chemical modifications, referred to as Phase I and Phase II reactions. Phase I reactions involve the modification of a functional group (oxidation of an alcohol to an aldehyde) or introduction of a polar group. Phase II reactions are characterized by the addition of a conjugating group. Either general type of reaction can destroy pharmacological activity.

In addition, each enhances the polarity, and hence the solubility in water, of the compounds metabolized. Some compounds, as illustrated below, are metabolized by both types of reactions.

The Cytochrome P$_{450}$ System

The largest variety of drugs is metabolized by a system of enzymes referred to as the cytochrome P$_{450}$ system, which consists of two proteins—an NADPH cytochrome P$_{450}$ reductase and cytochrome P$_{450}$. Both are located in the endoplasmic reticulum of the liver cell. The cytochrome P$_{450}$ is so named because of its typical absorption of light at 450 nm when combined with carbon monoxide, which inhibits its function. The combined activities of NADPH cytochrome P$_{450}$ reductase and cytochrome P$_{450}$ catalyze the hydroxylation of aliphatic chains and aromatic rings, removal of alkyl groups from oxygen, nitrogen, and sulfur, oxidative deamination, formation of sulfoxides, and the removal of sulfhydryl groups. Each of these reactions is oxidative and proceeds according to the following general scheme:

$$[18] \quad \text{reduced drug} + NADPH + H^+ + O_2 \xrightarrow[\text{and Cytochrome P}_{450}]{\text{NADPH Cytochrome P}_{450}\text{ reductase}} \text{oxidized drug} + NADP + H_2O$$

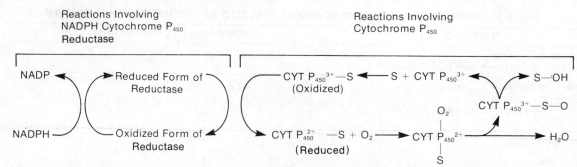

Figure 25. The flow of electrons in the cytochrome P_{450} system. S is any substrate.

The general mechanism is outlined in Figure 25. The substance metabolized (S) binds to cytochrome P_{450}. NADPH binds to the NADPH cytochrome P_{450} reductase and is oxidized to NADP. The reductase enzyme is reduced as it accepts an electron from NADPH, and then passes the electron to the cytochrome P_{450}-drug complex, which becomes reduced. Oxygen, the final electron acceptor, attaches to the latter, leading to oxidation of the substrate, production of water, and reoxidation of the cytochrome P_{450}. The cytochrome P_{450} system is called a "mixed function oxidase" because one atom of the O_2 molecule goes to the substance oxidized and the other to water. It is likely that several specific forms of cytochrome P_{450} account for the variety of drugs metabolized by this system. Examples are listed in Table 2.

Induction of Cytochrome P_{450}

Most of the compounds metabolized by the cytochrome P_{450} system induce synthesis of the two enzymes composing it. This response is nonspecific in that a single compound can induce synthesis of enzymes that metabolize it and nonrelated drugs. There hence is a broad potential for interaction among drugs. For example, phenobarbital, which is oxidized via cytochrome P_{450}, is an inducer. When administered with other agents that are metabolized by cytochrome P_{450}, it will alter their therapeutic dose. In addition, it enhances the rate of its own inactivation in liver. Therapeutic agents thus can modify both their own metabolism and that of other drugs. Induction is caused, too, by chemicals not considered to be therapeutic compounds. Cigarette smoke is an effective inducer of the cytochrome P_{450} system. Ethanol also is an inducer. While some drugs are detoxified by cytochrome P_{450}, the toxicity of a wide range of agents is enhanced by metabolism according to the scheme in Figure 25. Nonspecific induction of drug-metabolizing enzymes can be critical for the hepatotoxicity of some therapeutic agents.

PHASE I REACTIONS NOT CATALYZED BY CYTOCHROME P_{450}

Endoplasmic reticulum of liver contains amine oxidases that catalyze the oxidation of secondary and tertiary amines. In addition, mitochondrial enzymes deaminate naturally occurring amines such as catecholamines, tryptophan derivatives, serotonin, and drugs. Many drugs hence are oxidized in liver by enzymes that are not a part of the P_{450} system. Other Phase I reactions are the hydrolysis of esters (procaine), amides (nicotinamide), and reduction of the azo group ($-N-N-$), and the nitro group ($-NO_2$). Liver also catalyzes the oxidation of purines to uric acid through the action of xanthine oxidase. Several alcohols and aldehydes are oxidized by nonspecific alcohol and aldehyde dehydrogenases. Ethanol is metabolized by this system. The details of ethanol oxidation are presented later, in a separate section.

Phase II Reactions (Table 3)

Phase II reactions, characterized by the addition of a functional group to the parent compound, are detoxifying. None leads to the activation of a drug or to the production of a toxin. Conjugation reactions have the following general scheme:

[19] acceptor + donor X → acceptor X + donor

The donor X usually is a high-energy compound that can react with a variety of acceptor groups. Most organic compounds, as a result, can be conjugated in several different reactions; a single drug can appear in the urine as several different types of conjugates. The potential multiplicity of conjugated products has physiological significance because the activities of conjugating enzymes are low. That a single compound can be metabolized in a variety of pathways protects against its accumulation. Phase I and Phase II reactions can have concerted effects in the detoxification of compounds. For example, hydroxylation of aromatic compounds is a common type of reaction catalyzed by cytochrome P_{450}. Addition, in this way, of an —OH group provides a substrate for conjugation with glucuronic acid or sulfate. Similarly, removal of alkyl groups from nitrogen or oxygen provides substrates for conjugation reactions.

CLINICAL CONSIDERATIONS IN PRESCRIBING DRUGS FOR PATIENTS WITH LIVER DISEASE

We can expect defects in (1) the uptake of drugs by the liver, secondary to abnormalities of blood flow; (2) the transfer of drug from blood to hepatocyte; (3) deficiencies of enzymes that metabolize drugs; and (4) abnormal secretory mechanisms. Yet it is possible to assess clinically only the overall rate of drug disappearance, which includes all the mechanisms just cited. We know little about the exact defects that account for faulty metabolism of drugs generally present in patients with liver disease. Half-times ($t_{1/2}$) for the rate of disappearance of many drugs are increased in this group of patients, but there are no chemical tests of

TABLE 3.   VARIETIES OF PHASE II REACTIONS

TYPE OF CONJUGATING REACTION	DONOR SUBSTRATE	ACCEPTOR SUBSTRATE
Glucuronidation	UDP-glucuronic acid	Aromatic—OH (Steroids) Aromatic—COOH (Bilirubin) Aromatic—NH$_2$ Aromatic—SH (Thiophenol)
Acetylation	Acetyl-CoA	Aromatic—NH$_2$ Aromatic—SO$_2$—NH$_2$ R—CH$_2$—NH—NH$_2$ R—NH$_2$
Methylation	S-Adenosyl-methionine	R—NH$_2$ (Norepinephrine) R—SH R—OH (Norepinephrine)
Sulfation	Phosphoadenosine-phosphosulfate	R—NH$_2$ R—OH (Tyrosine)
Mercapturic acid	Glutathione	Polycyclic
Detoxification of CN$^-$	S$_2$O$_3^=$	CN$^-$

liver function or signs and symptoms of liver disease that correlate with alterations of $t_{1/2}$ for disposal of drugs. In addition to alterations in the intrinsic capacity of the liver to remove drugs from the body, liver disease may affect the efficacy of a given dose of drug because of deficiencies in the synthesis of albumin, which increases the concentration of free drug (unbound). Since the concentration of free drug determines therapeutic and toxic effects, a changing ratio of free to bound drug will alter its toxic potential irrespective of abnormalities in the rate of detoxification by the liver. Moreover, the extent of protein binding is related inversely to the volume of distribution of drug in body water. As the fraction bound decreases in response to deficient binding protein, the volume of distribution rises. Half time for removal of drug can be prolonged on this basis alone.

It is essential to proceed cautiously when prescribing medication for patients with liver disease, especially for agents that are detoxified by the liver. Many patients with serious forms of liver disease are alcoholics. Their levels of drug-metabolizing enzymes may appear normal, in terms of clinical response to a given dose, while they are taking ethanol but may be significantly lower than normal when they are abstinent and off all medications. Finally, the central nervous system of patients with liver disease is more sensitive than normal to the effects of sedatives and analgesics. This occurs in the absence of demonstrable abnormalities of drug detoxification.

DETOXIFICATION OF ETHANOL

Liver is the primary site for the metabolism of ethanol. Two pathways are available. The predominant one, which accounts for 90 per cent of ethanol metabolism, is catalyzed by nonspecific alcohol and aldehyde dehydrogenases in the soluble portion of the cell:

[20] CH_3—CH_2OH + NAD $\xleftarrow{\text{alcohol dehydrogenase}}$
Ethanol

$$CH_3\text{—CHO} + NADH + H^+$$
Acetaldehyde

[21] CH_3—CHO + NAD $\xleftarrow{\text{aldehyde dehydrogenase}}$
$$CH_3\text{—COOH} + NADH + H^+$$
Acetic acid

Alcohol dehydrogenase is saturated at the relatively low ethanol concentration of 46 mg per dl of plasma. The rate of oxidation of ethanol is constant (zero order) as long as the ethanol concentration is at this level or greater. It equals 10 grams of ethanol per hour in a 70-kg man. Although we think generally that metabolic rates are limited by enzyme activities, this is not true for the oxidation of ethanol, which depends instead on the rate of conversion of NADH to NAD, i.e., the reoxidation of NADH formed during oxidation of ethanol. A variety of metabolic intermediates can accept the H from NADH, thereby regenerating NAD:

$$\left.\begin{array}{l}\text{Pyruvate}\\\text{Dihydroxyacetone-P}\\\text{Glyceraldehyde}\\\text{Oxaloacetate}\end{array}\right\} + NADH + H^+ \longleftrightarrow \left\{\begin{array}{l}\text{Lactate}\\\text{Glycerol-1-P + NAD}\\\text{Glycerol}\\\text{Malate}\end{array}\right.$$

If levels of hydrogen acceptors such as pyruvate are low, they can limit the rate of ethanol oxidation. Thus, ethanol oxidation proceeds more slowly in the fasted, as compared with the fed, state. This, plus more rapid absorption from the gut, may account for the feeling of a heightened euphoric effect of ethanol when taken on an "empty stomach." There is some adaptation to chronic ingestion of ethanol in that the rate of oxidation increases. Adaptation occurs in this setting because of an enhanced rate of reoxidation of the reduced pyridine nucleotide (NADH) produced as ethanol is oxidized. The amount of alcohol dehydrogenase in liver does not increase in the chronic alcoholic.

Acetaldehyde produced from ethanol is oxidized rapidly in the liver to acetyl CoA, with the additional release of NADH. Nevertheless, a small amount accumulates in the blood (50 μg per dl) after ingestion of ethanol. Since acetaldehyde, like all aldehydes, is highly reactive, its production may lead to some of the observed but as yet unexplained effects of ethanol ingestion on the central nervous system, liver, heart, and other organs.

A number of the metabolic consequences follow from the oxidation of ethanol (Table 4) because of changes in the ratio of reduced pyridine nucleotide to oxidized pyridine nucleotide (NADH/NAD). Abnormalities such as hyperlipidemia, hypoglycemia, or hyperuricemia may be transient manifestations of drinking and not reflections of permanent disturbances of lipid, carbohydrate, and purine metabolism. Acute elevation of plasma uric acid as a consequence of ethanol intake, nevertheless, may precipitate an acute attack of gout.

In contrast with all other drugs, the oxidation of ethanol releases energy that can be conserved in the form of ATP. The NADH generated by the oxidation of ethanol to acetic acid is reoxidized in mitochondria. Acetic acid can be oxidized further to carbon dioxide and water, releasing additional energy. Ethanol hence is a fuel with a caloric value of 7 calories per gram. This accounts, in part, for its capacity to suppress appetite.

Alcohol dehydrogenase from human liver can also oxidize methanol to formaldehyde. The latter is then oxidized to formic acid, which is toxic. Since ethanol and methanol are metabolized by the same enzyme, administration of ethanol can minimize the toxicity of methanol by blocking its oxidation and allowing it to be excreted unchanged.

Microsomal cytochrome P_{450} and catalase can also catalyze conversion of ethanol to acetaldehyde, but the amounts of ethanol metabolized by pathways other than alcohol dehydrogenase are small under all circumstances.

The apparent resistance of alcoholics to many therapeutic agents now can be explained biochemically: chronic ethanol intake speeds the rate of metabolism of certain drugs through inducing increased P_{450}. There

are, however, many types of cytochrome P_{450}. Which ones are induced by ethanol remains to be elucidated.

Ethanol inhibits drug oxidation by cytochrome P_{450}. Irrespective of the amount of cytochrome P_{450} in liver, ethanol, when present, inhibits the metabolism of drugs by this enzyme. The rate of metabolism of barbiturates in a chronic user of ethanol will be low as compared with a nondrinker if the barbiturate and ethanol are present simultaneously. By contrast, the rate of metabolism of barbiturate will be greater in the former patient, as compared with the latter, after the ethanol is metabolized. We see an apparent paradoxic situation in drinkers: heightened susceptibility to the effects of drugs while they are drinking, but resistance to the same drug as soon as ethanol is metabolized completely. After admission to hospital and cessation of drinking, the inductive effects of ethanol disappear, and the rate of drug metabolism may then be slow even in the absence of ethanol.

DETOXIFICATION OF BILIRUBIN

Bilirubin is the catabolic product of heme pigment. The largest precursor pool is hemoglobin of red cells, the breakdown of which accounts for 80 per cent of the 250 to 300 mg of bilirubin excreted per day. In addition to catabolism of senescent red cells, a small amount of bilirubin is formed from heme pigment of red cell precursors in the bone marrow, i.e., immature forms of red cells that are destroyed prior to leaving the marrow. The extent of this ineffective erythropoiesis in some disorders is large enough to add significantly to the total amount of bilirubin produced from hemoglobin. Bilirubin is formed too by breakdown of heme-containing proteins other than hemoglobin, as for example, cytochrome P_{450}, catalase, and several other oxidizing enzymes. Catabolism of these enzymes in liver is the source of 20 per cent of bilirubin in the normal state.

The first step in the formation of bilirubin is removal of the heme prosthetic group from hemoglobin and other heme-containing proteins. Heme then is oxidized by a microsomal enzyme designated heme oxygenase (Fig. 26), releasing iron, carbon monoxide, and biliverdin. The latter is reduced to bilirubin in a reaction catalyzed by biliverdin reductase. The sequence of reactions that lead from heme-protein to bilirubin is effected within the reticuloendothelial system of spleen and bone marrow, and within liver cells and probably tissue macrophages. The capacity to make bilirubin from heme is quite large and seldom is unable to keep pace with the rate of catabolism of red cells. In addition, the activity of heme oxygenase increases in hemolytic states. Enhanced destruction of red cells and turnover of heme-proteins other than hemoglobin always increase the load of bilirubin delivered to the liver for detoxification.

The natural conformation of bilirubin is folded to yield a surface containing an array of hydrophobic residues. The hydrophilic regions of the molecule are buried within the fold. Bilirubin hence is insoluble in aqueous media but soluble in the lipid regions of membranes. This gives rise to several interrelated difficulties. For example, the major portion of bilirubin is formed both normally and in pathological states in

TABLE 4. SOME EFFECTS OF ETHANOL OXIDATION ON METABOLISM IN LIVER

METABOLIC EFFECT	CLINICAL CONSEQUENCE
Inhibition of gluconeogenesis	Hypoglycemia in fasted patients
Inhibition of fatty acid oxidation	Fatty liver
Provision of excess carbon for synthesis of fatty acids	Hyperlipidemia
Inhibition of lactate uptake by liver	Lactic acidemia; hyperuricemia secondary to diminished renal secretion of lactate
Increased production of ketone bodies	Mild ketosis
Increased oxygen utilization	Increased susceptibility of liver to anoxia

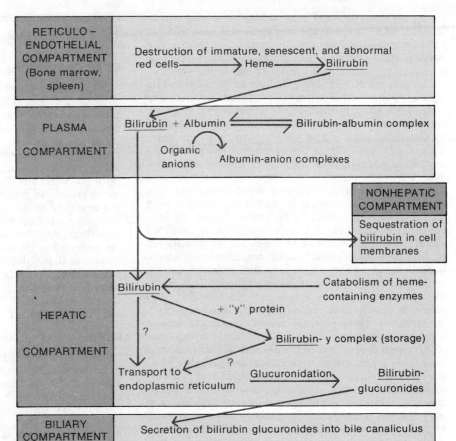

Figure 26. Physiology of bilirubin metabolism in man.

spleen and bone marrow, whereas detoxification and excretion take place only in the liver. It is necessary, therefore, to transport bilirubin from its sites of synthesis to the liver. Unconjugated bilirubin is toxic, however, because of its great avidity for cellular membranes. The problems of transport and modulation of toxicity of bilirubin while in transit to the liver are solved by its binding with high affinity to albumin, in a ratio of 2 moles per mole of albumin. The plasma-binding capacity in adults is large enough that more than 60 mg of bilirubin can be bound to albumin per dl of plasma. The fraction of bilirubin not bound is the only portion that enters cells. Unbound bilirubin in plasma is taken up preferentially by liver as compared with other organs. There are three reasons for this: (1) hepatocytes may have a unique, selective, carrier-mediated transport system for unconjugated bilirubin; (2) the liver contains nonspecific mechanisms for trapping bilirubin; (3) hepatocytes are the only cells that effectively detoxify and excrete bilirubin.

No transport system for bilirubin in plasma membranes of hepatocytes has been identified.

Two intracellular proteins that bind bilirubin have been purified from liver. Of these, Y-protein has the greater affinity for bilirubin. The physiological significance of Y and Z proteins for the metabolism of bilirubin is uncertain, and recent evidence suggests that they are not important in this regard. Storage of bilirubin as complexes with Y and Z proteins is limited by their amounts, and the most important process for continuously removing bilirubin from blood is its secretion into the bile. This requires prior addition of

glucuronic acid residues to one or both the propionic acid groups of bilirubin, catalyzed by glucuronyltransferase, an enzyme localized in the endoplasmic reticulum.

Addition of bulky acidic groups to bilirubin forces the folded structure to open, thus allowing hydrophilic residues, especially the carboxyl of glucuronic acid, to interact with water. The glucuronides of bilirubin (mono- and di-) are water-soluble. They are secreted actively into the bile.

The maximal rate of glucuronidation is greater than the maximal rate of excretion of bilirubin glucuronides into the bile: bilirubin glucuronide not secreted into bile re-enters the blood via a pathway not yet identified. Its solubility in blood allows for excretion via glomerular filtration. This excretion into urine limits the increase in levels of plasma-conjugated bilirubin to about 30 mg per dl of plasma even in complete obstruction of the biliary tract. Obviously, levels may be higher in patients who also have renal failure.

Bilirubin glucuronides entering the intestinal lumen by way of the bile are not reabsorbed. About half the daily load is degraded by intestinal bacteria to urobilinogens, which are colorless. The metabolic fate of the remainder of enteric bilirubin glucuronides is unknown. A small portion (10 to 15 per cent) of urobilinogens are absorbed and undergo enterohepatic circulation. In addition, urobilinogens are excreted in the urine.

Many components in the pathway of bilirubin metabolism are inducible. Administration of phenobarbital, for example, increases the levels of Y protein and glucuronyltransferase. Phenobarbital also can stimulate output of bile, but the mechanism of this effect is not understood. Phenobarbital, in some instances, can lower plasma levels of bilirubin in jaundiced patients. It is rarely a useful agent in this regard, however.

The amount of bilirubin glucuronide excreted in bile equals the amount of bilirubin produced in the steady state. Increasing production, as in hemolytic diseases, leads to increased uptake, conjugation, and secretion by the liver until a new steady state is established. This occurs, however, at the expense of increasing the amount of unconjugated bilirubin in the plasma. Moreover, although secretion of bilirubin glucuronide into bile keeps pace with synthesis under conditions of a normal load of bilirubin, it is limited as compared with conjugation when abnormally large amounts of bilirubin are taken up by the liver. Bilirubin in the blood hence accumulates in any of the following situations: increasing rates of heme breakdown, interference with hepatic uptake of bilirubin, defective glucuronidation, or an impaired capacity to secrete bilirubin glucuronide. Abnormal plasma levels of both bilirubin and bilirubin glucuronide occur when bilirubin production is increased. Thus, elevated plasma concentrations of bilirubin during hemolysis are a natural consequence of increased production, in the absence of abnormalities of uptake, conjugation, or secretion; and jaundice, during a hemolytic episode, is not an indication of intrinsic disease of the liver. Similarly, conditions in which there is ineffective erythropoiesis (pernicious anemia) may lead to jaundice in the absence of liver disease. Usually plasma contains a greater proportion of bilirubin glucuronide than of unconjugated bilirubin during hemolysis; occasionally the reverse may occur. No certain conclusions can be drawn at this time as to hepatic defects on the basis of levels of conjugated and unconjugated bilirubin.

Defects in hepatic uptake of bilirubin have been implicated in the production of jaundice. Deficiencies in Y or Z protein are not documented in human liver, but there is circumstantial evidence that interference with the function of these proteins is associated with elevation of bilirubin in the blood in that administration of organic anions that compete with bilirubin for binding to Y and Z proteins produces jaundice that is reversed quickly when the offending drug is discontinued. Although unproved in newborn humans, levels of Y proteins are quite low in newborn rats and other experimental animals. Normal levels are attained in the first few weeks of life. Such deficiency may contribute to physiological and pathological forms of jaundice in newborns. As noted, however, the significance of intracellular binding proteins for the metabolism of bilirubin remains to be established.

The capacity to glucuronidate bilirubin is low in newborns because of the absence of the appropriate glucuronyltransferase and relative deficiency of the donor substrate, UDP-glucuronic acid. Levels of both enzyme and substrate reach adult levels in the first few days of life. Immaturity of the glucuronidating mechanism is probably the most significant factor in causing physiological jaundice in the newborn, as well as dangerous accumulations of plasma bilirubin in prematures and infants suffering from hemolytic disease. It is unknown whether defects of glucuronidation contribute to jaundice in adult life, since levels of glucuronyltransferase have not been measured accurately in patients with acquired forms of liver disease. There are, however, instances of congenitally determined defects in glucuronyltransferase.

GILBERT'S SYNDROME

Mild degrees of congenital deficiencies in bilirubin conjugation are common, and a surprisingly large number of otherwise healthy individuals have moderate elevations of plasma unconjugated bilirubin. This condition is called *Gilbert's syndrome*. Since fasting augments the bilirubin concentrations in blood from all types of individuals (normals as well as cirrhotics), patients with the Gilbert's syndrome frequently become jaundiced during intercurrent illnesses, and the abnormality in bilirubin metabolism often is discovered at such times. It is important to recognize this condition in order to avoid unneeded diagnostic procedures and to reassure the patient. The best evidence indicates that Gilbert's syndrome is due to a deficiency of glucuronyltransferase. Severe congenitally determined deficiencies of this enzyme occur rarely. They are associated with high levels of unconjugated bilirubin in plasma.

OTHER CAUSES OF JAUNDICE

Large amounts of bilirubin glucuronide accumulate in patients with mechanical obstruction of the biliary system, and in those suffering from some type of chemical defect in the production of bile (intrahepatic cholestasis). Unconjugated bilirubin also accumulates in these situations, for reasons that are not clearly established. A large number of therapeutic agents, viral hepatitis, alcoholic liver disease, and congenital disorders of metabolism interfere with bile secretion. None of these mechanisms can be defined in terms of their abnormal chemistry, including the anatomic pathway by which bilirubin glucuronide leaves the liver cell to enter the plasma (see also section on formation of bile). The amounts of bilirubin and bilirubin glucuronide in the blood of jaundiced patients are variable, unpredictable, and have never been correlated carefully with the rates of production, uptake, and conjugation of bilirubin.

TOXICITY OF BILIRUBIN

Several clinical studies suggest greater than expected rates of postoperative renal failure in patients operated on for relief of bile duct obstruction. Bilirubin glucuronide has been implicated as a toxic agent in these patients, but there are no demonstrated toxic effects of bilirubin glucuronide in vitro. On the other hand, unconjugated bilirubin is an uncoupler of oxidative phosphorylation in isolated mitochondria. It has serious toxic effects on central nervous function where it produces the syndrome of kernicterus. Binding of bilirubin to albumin prevents this toxin from entering the central nervous system in most patients with high levels of unconjugated bilirubin in the blood. The major exception is infants, in whom the level of albumin is less than that in adults. Since many organic anions—sulfonamides, salicylates, fatty acids, hematin—compete with bilirubin for binding to albumin, and since acidosis limits the binding of bilirubin to albumin, administration of organic anions together with acidosis decreases the capacity of a given amount of albumin to sequester bilirubin, allowing the unbound toxic fraction to increase. Low plasma proteins, medical complications requiring administration of drugs, overproduction of bilirubin, and an immature glucuronidating system all enhance the susceptibility of infants to the toxic effects of bilirubin by allowing it to escape from the circulation into the cells. Some children and young adults with complete absence of glucuronyltransferase (Crigler-Najjar syndrome) and extreme levels of unconjugated bilirubin in the blood do not suffer from its central nervous system toxicity. Possibly the binding capacity of plasma proteins is large enough to prevent passage of bilirubin across the blood-brain barrier during infancy in these patients. Unfortunately, however, kernicterus has developed in such patients in adult life.

SECRETION OF BILE

Bile formation is the pathway for excretion of a large number of detoxified chemicals. It also allows entry of bile salts into the lumen of the small intestine, where they facilitate nearly complete absorption of fat. Elaboration of bile involves two processes: secretion of the fluid component, and separate but related secretion of the dissolved or suspended solid components. The latter comprise sodium salts, bile salts, cholesterol, phospholipid, bilirubin glucuronides, and the detoxification products discussed in the chapters on drug metabolism. Unfortunately, we have little knowledge of the detailed chemical mechanisms that account for the formation of bile. The smallest biliary vesicles, the canaliculi, are formed by specialized regions of the plasma membranes of two adjoining hepatocytes. Adjacent cells form a channel between them that is sealed off from the intracellular space by fusion of their membranous structure (see Figs. 1 and 2). The portion of membrane within the lumen of the bile canaliculus contains numerous microvilli, which have an abundance of the enzyme ATPase. The apparatus for bile formation consists of active transport systems for bile salts, organic anions other than bile salts, and organic cations, and of ATPase. The hydrostatic pressure within biliary vesicles is greater than that in the sinusoid, indicating that bile flow cannot be driven by the pressure within the hepatic vascular system. Formation of bile must be an active process. Bile flow probably depends on active secretion of bile salts and sodium from the hepatocyte into the canaliculus. Water then flows passively in the same direction because of the osmotic gradient created by concentrating solutes in the lumen of the bile canaliculus. Evidence that active secretion of bile salts generates passive flow of water is found in the well-established observation that bile salts are choleretic when given to man. Critical aspects of this phenomenon, however, remain obscure. Thus, bile salts are not in true solution in bile, but are dispersed as micellar aggregates containing other lipophilic components such as cholesterol and phospholipids. The osmotic force of a given amount of bile salt in bile is less, therefore, than for an equal amount (mole per mole) of solute in true solution. For a compound in true solution, there will be a linear relationship between volume of water secreted per mole of solute. Linearity of this relationship should not be observed for a compound not in solution. Nevertheless, dependence of volume of bile flow on amount of bile

salt secreted is a linear one. The reason for this is unknown. We also do not understand why the volume of water secreted per mole of bile salt is dependent on the species studied. It may be that active secretion of Na as compared with bile salts is more important for solvent flow into bile, and the choleretic effect of bile salts reflects the effect of the latter on active secretion of Na^+. There is precedent for this idea in that bile acids stimulate salt and water secretion by the large bowel. Resolution of these uncertainties will shed new light on the role and mechanism of water flow into the bile.

Extrapolation of the rate of flow as a function of bile salt to zero bile salt suggests that biliary water is formed even in the absence of bile salts. That portion of biliary volume formed in the absence of bile salts, called the bile acid–independent fraction, is believed to be generated by the activity of ATPase in the canalicular membrane, which presumably pumps sodium from the hepatocyte to the bile canaliculus, thereby creating an osmotic gradient. Water flows passively along this gradient from liver cells to bile. There is no direct proof for this mechanism, but drugs that inhibit ATPase in vitro reduce bile flow when administered to intact animals. In addition to actively transporting bile salts and sodium across the canalicular membrane, the hepatocyte concentrates organic anions (such as BSP and bilirubin glucuronides) in the bile. Many of these organic anions are choleretic, suggesting that they are secreted actively, that is, against a concentration gradient. On the other hand, most biliary anions are amphipathic; they contain hydrophobic and hydrophilic regions. These properties facilitate incorporation of bile salts into micelles, which reduces their effective chemical concentrations and augments secretion. The significance of solutes other than bile salts and sodium as osmotic determinants of bile flow is unknown. We also do not know how the solutes that appear eventually in the bile traverse the interior of the hepatocyte to reach the area of the canalicular membrane.

There is evidence, in fact, that solutes in sinusoidal blood equilibrate with bile faster than they do with the cytosol of hepatocytes. Moreover, substances that do not enter hepatocytes can be excreted in bile. Observations like these suggest that compounds can enter bile via direct transport from the sinusoids or via a paracellular route. This process, if it occurs, is not well understood.

How many transport systems are there in the canaliculus for organic ions? Studies of patients with the *Dubin-Johnson* and *Rotor's* syndromes indicate that there are at least two and perhaps more. These patients fail to excrete conjugated bilirubin into bile and so are jaundiced. In addition, there is defective transport of BSP and a variety of organic anions. Secretion of taurocholate (a bile salt) is normal, however. Moreover, the secretory defects are not identical in patients with each of these disorders. The biliary tree of Dubin-Johnson patients is not visualized by oral or intravenous cholecystographic dyes, indicating abnormal hepatic transport of these substances. The gallbladders of patients with Rotor's syndrome are visualized after administration of oral, but not intravenous, contrast materials. It is reasonable to conclude, therefore, that there are several separate transport mechanisms for organic anions.

In addition to stimulating the flow of water into bile, active transport of bile salts is important for biliary secretion of cholesterol and phospholipids. Administration of bile salts increases the amounts of cholesterol and phospholipid in bile. Decreasing the amount of bile salts circulating within the liver diminishes the output of these substances via biliary radicles. A pathogenetically significant feature in the relationship between biliary excretion of cholesterol and phospholipids, on the one hand, and bile salts, on the other, is the lack of a one-to-one relationship in the outputs of cholesterol and phospholipid. Thus, the secretion of phospholipid falls to a greater extent when the availability of bile salt declines. The tendency of cholesterol to precipitate in bile and form stones is enhanced in this setting. In contrast, the excretion of phospholipid is increased by bile salt administration to a greater extent than is that of cholesterol, thereby enhancing the solubility of cholesterol in the bile ducts. These physiological findings have been put to good use. Oral administration of bile salts can lead to dissolution of cholesterol gallstones.

CLINICAL STATE OF DEFECTIVE BILE SECRETION

Defective secretion of bile (cholestasis) is perhaps the most common abnormality of hepatic function and is encountered clinically in three distinct clinical settings: biliary tract obstruction, hepatic cell injury, and selective damage to the bile secretory mechanism (Table 5).

Bile secretion fails when there is *mechanical obstruction to the flow of bile*. If obstruction is at the level of the common bile ducts, as in patients with carcinoma of the head of the pancreas, jaundice ensues. The substances secreted normally into the bile appear instead in the blood. Obstruction of only a segment of the biliary tree is associated with functional hypertrophy of the unobstructed portions of the liver, and jaundice is not seen in such patients.

A second cause of failure to secrete bile is *generalized toxic injury to liver cells*. A third setting in which cholestasis is evident is *selective injury to the bile secretory apparatus*, referred to as intrahepatic or functional cholestasis. There is, in these situations, no other evidence of hepatocyte dysfunction, and the bile ducts are patent. The first and third causes of cholestasis cannot be differentiated by chemical tests. Chemical changes in the blood are identical, initially, irrespective of the etiology of the cholestatic state. It also is not possible to make a specific diagnosis on the basis of liver biopsy. Mechanical obstruction can be excluded only by visual demonstration of the patency of the bile duct system. Despite the absence of chemical differences among patients with mechanical and functional cholestasis, these disorders have significantly different clinical histories. Complete mechanical obstruction of the biliary tree ends in cirrhosis. Additionally, there is a high risk of infection within the bile ducts, with spread to the liver in some patients who have persisting, more malignant obstruction. Neither of these outcomes supervenes in patients with a functional form of cholestasis (defective secretory mechanism). Usually, the latter disorder is short-lived, which may account for the different effects of mechanical and functional cholestasis on liver morphology. Occasionally, however, cholestasis secondary to drug toxicity (functional failure of the secretory mechanism) persists for more than a year without progression to cirrhosis or complication by infection. There is, of course, an important difference between mechanical obstruction of the biliary tree and intrahepatic cholestasis. In mechanical failure bile secretion fails because of a block in its exit into the duodenum. As hydrostatic pressure in the bile duct rises, the capacity of the hepatocyte to pump against this pressure will fail. In contrast, functional cholestasis reflects a primary failure in the mechanism of bile secretion. The latter event seems to be less toxic to the liver as compared with a mechanical block to the flow of bile.

Intrahepatic cholestasis in the absence of widespread abnormalities of hepatocyte function is frequently generated by a diversity of agents, has a variable course, and is poorly understood. Outstanding examples are *drug-induced liver injury* secondary to phenothiazines, esters of erythromycin, and testosterone; cholestasis during the *third trimester* of otherwise normal *pregnancies*; and during ingestion of *oral contraceptives*. It may be the dominant feature in patients with *viral hepatitis*, and sometimes even in patients with *alcoholic hepatitis*. An especially interesting form presents as intermittent episodes of cholestasis in the absence of inciting causes. Affected patients may have as many as 20 or more such attacks of varying duration between which there are no detectable chemical or morphological abnormalities in the liver. This entity of *relapsing cholestasis* has a benign course.

The most serious form of intrahepatic cholestasis is referred to as *primary biliary cirrhosis*. Its cause also is unknown. Liver biopsy of affected patients reveals abnormalities in small bile ducts. There is an inflammatory reaction, together with necrosis of the wall of the biliary ducts within portal tracts. These channels eventually become occluded. Whether primary biliary cirrhosis represents a unique illness or a nonspecific reaction to selective injury along the course of the biliary tree is unknown.

THE CAUSE OF BILE SECRETORY FAILURE

Failure of the bile secretory mechanism occurs in patients with severe generalized injury to hepatocytes, as seen, for example, in viral- and alcohol-induced hepatitis. It also can fail selectively, in that failure to form bile is the only or predominant manifestation of hepatocellular injury. We do not know, for either of the above two settings, why liver cells stop secreting

TABLE 5. CLASSIFICATION OF CHOLESTASIS

TYPE	CAUSE
Mechanical obstruction	Gallstones; tumor; chronic fibrosis anywhere along the course of biliary tree; enlarged lymph nodes; inflammation of intraportal bile ductules
Liver cell failure	Massive acute necrosis of liver cells; chronic loss of liver cell parenchyma
Functional failure of bile secretion	Drugs; sepsis; viral hepatitis; alcoholic hepatitis

bile at normal rates. The most reasonable explanation for intrahepatic cholestasis is defective transport of bile salts and/or sodium into the bile canaliculi. An alternative hypothesis is that the permeability of the canalicular membrane is altered in functional cholestasis, allowing actively secreted ions to diffuse back into the hepatocyte. The result is the same in either case, i.e., a diminished osmotic gradient for movement of water from hepatocyte to bile when the ion gradient is impaired. There is no way to decide, on the basis of current data, which of these two mechanisms describes what happens in cholestasis. It may be, in fact, that different agents produce cholestasis by separate mechanisms. Another major unanswered question in cholestasis is which ion pump fails—that for bile salts or that for sodium, or both. Currently defects of the ATPase–sodium-pumping mechanism are thought most likely to be at the root of functional cholestasis. A few drugs known to induce cholestasis poison the canalicular ATPase in in vitro studies, but it would be premature to conclude that failure of the sodium pump underlies all cholestatic illnesses.

EFFECTS OF THE LIVER ON THE ENDOCRINE SYSTEM

A single circulation through the liver destroys the activity of 50 per cent of insulin secreted into the pancreatic vein. Metabolism in the liver also can inactivate other peptide hormones, such as glucagon. It is unlikely, however, that derangements of any of these functions produce significant clinical abnormalities.

Hypogonadism and feminization are common findings in patients with ethanol-induced cirrhosis. Most likely, however, hypogonadism is due not to hepatocellular disease but to ethanol abuse per se. Thus, hypogonadism is observed more often in alcoholic patients, but not in patients with viral-induced forms of chronic liver disease. Feminization of males, on the other hand, appears to be caused by liver dysfunction and does not depend on the etiology of the liver disease.

Alcoholic men have decreased levels of testosterone in plasma associated with atrophy of germ cells and Leydig cells. Although levels of gonadotropins are normal in alcoholic patients, they are inappropriate for the decreased levels of testosterone. Alcoholic patients, therefore, appear to have a primary abnormality of the hypothalamic-pituitary axis, but ethanol also has direct effects on the testes that can account for hypogonadism, as for example inhibition of the synthesis of steroid hormones.

Alcoholic women also have hypogonadism that probably occurs independently of the effects of ethanol on the liver. Whatever underlies the hypogonadism of alcoholic men is likely to be the cause of this problem in women as well.

The liver modifies the structure and function of steroid hormones. It has been suggested, therefore, that abnormal metabolism of androgens and estrogens underlies the feminization in men with cirrhosis. Elevated levels of estrogens have not been a constant finding in cirrhosis, however. It has been proposed that the distribution of estrogen between liver and peripheral tissues may be modified by liver disease, allowing for greater effect on peripheral tissues of a given amount of estrogen. This could result from disruption of the enterohepatic circulation of steroids and/or a decreased hepatic binding capacity for estrogenic steroids.

Estrogens and weakly androgenic steroids are excreted by the liver into the bile, from which they enter the gut. They then are reabsorbed and enter the portal blood. Normally they will be removed from portal blood by the liver, but in patients with liver disease and portal hypertension they will bypass the liver. This abnormality of blood flow allows for possible greater utilization of steroids in peripheral tissues and for the conversion in these sites of weak androgens to estrogens. Since the concentration of estrogen-binding proteins in liver is decreased in patients with chronic or acute fulminant liver disease, the capacity of the liver to remove estrogen presented to it is diminished by liver disease. This mechanism also facilitates expression of estrogenic steroids in nonhepatic tissues.

The liver metabolizes a variety of steroids by adding hydrogen to unsaturated bonds in the ring system and by conjugation with glucuronic acid. Both reactions destroy physiological activity and facilitate excretion. The metabolism of steroids is decreased in patients with hepatocellular disease; and, as a result, the halftimes of steroids in the blood may be prolonged abnormally. Since the secretion of hormonally active steroids is under feedback inhibition, decreased rates of catabolism in patients with liver disease may not lead to increases in their concentration in plasma. For example, plasma levels of cortisol are normal in patients with liver disease despite its increased biological halflife in serum. On the other hand, the rate of secretion of cortisol by the adrenal cortex is low in patients who have significant liver disease and thus an impaired capacity to metabolize cortisol. Tests of adrenal cortical function that are based on secretion of cortisol, e.g., secretory rate or 24-hour urinary excretion of 17-hydroxysteroids, suggest diminished function in such patients because of abnormally low rates of catabolism. The results of tests that reflect secretion hence may be difficult to interpret in patients with liver disease. It thus is better to rely on direct measurements of plasma cortisol.

ROLE OF THE LIVER IN THE METABOLISM OF VITAMINS (See also Section VII)

There seem to be few clinically significant effects of liver disease on the metabolism of vitamins, despite the frequent occurrence of vitamin deficiency in patients with cirrhosis. Although vitamins undergo important transformations within the liver and are stored there in large amounts, acute and chronic liver diseases do not affect vitamin metabolism in a manner that has been clinically identified. There are two exceptions to this generalization—the metabolism of vitamins A and D. In addition, the distribution of folate to tissues other than the liver depends on an intact enterohepatic circulation.

VITAMIN A METABOLISM

Vitamin A is adsorbed as the free alcohol (Fig. 27) but is esterified within the small intestine. Vitamin A

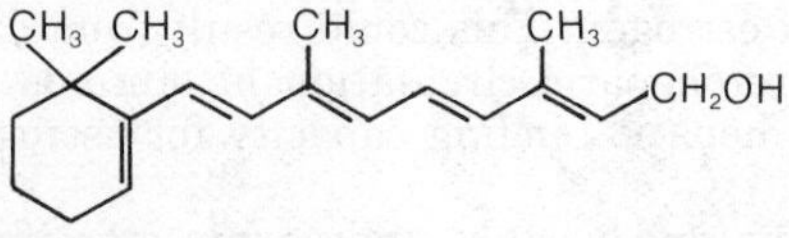

Figure 27. Chemical structure of vitamin A.

esters, transported to the liver in chylomicrons, are not available to other tissues until they are processed in the liver. In the liver, the esters are hydrolyzed, re-esterified, and stored in the cytoplasm within droplets of lipid, some in the Ito cells, but the majority in hepatic parenchymal cells. The release of vitamin A alcohol from hepatic stores of the ester is dependent on its being bound to two proteins synthesized in the liver: (1) a specific retinol binding protein and (2) prealbumin, which serves also as a carrier protein for compounds other than retinol. Synthesis of binding proteins is depressed in chronic liver disease, thereby limiting mobilization of vitamin A stored within the liver. Levels of retinol in plasma fall in this setting and symptoms of deficiency develop, most notably night blindness. Surveys of patients with cirrhosis demonstrate a high incidence of reduced vitamin A levels in blood and faulty dark adaptation. Most often, however, these findings reflect nutritional deficiency rather than intrinsic liver disease, since oral supplementation with vitamin A restores plasma levels to normal. There are some cirrhotic patients with a permanent deficit in their capacity to synthesize the binding proteins and hence to mobilize vitamin A from stored esters. Night blindness in these individuals does not respond to supplementation with vitamin A.

Synthesis of vitamin A–binding protein is diminished in vitamin A–deficient animals but returns to normal after administration of vitamin A. Zinc deficiency, which occurs in alcoholic patients, also depresses the synthesis of retinol-binding proteins. Affected patients can manifest night blindness that is unresponsive to administration of vitamin A but is cured by administration of zinc.

Excess vitamin A is hepatotoxic. Vitamin A partitions into membranes, altering their stability. Lysosomes are one organelle affected in this manner in that vitamin A excess facilitates the breakdown of lysosomes, which leads to release of proteolytic and lipolytic enzymes. This mechanism may be the cause of the toxicity of vitamin A.

VITAMIN D METABOLISM

Irradiation of precursors in the skin produces cholecalciferol (vitamin D_3), which is hydroxylated sequentially at the 25 position in the liver and then at the 1 position in the kidney to produce 1,25-dihydroxyvitamin D_3, the most active form of vitamin D (see Section VIII). Hydroxylation in the liver must precede that in the kidney. The rate of 25-hydroxylation, which is separate from the cytochrome P_{450} system, seems to be abnormally slow in patients with cirrhosis, especially those with so-called primary biliary cirrhosis. These patients frequently have osteomalacia and less than normal levels of 1,25-dihydroxy vitamin D_3 in plasma. Depressed levels return to normal when patients are treated with large amounts of oral vitamin D_3, suggesting that the functional effect of enzyme deficiency can be overcome by excess substrate. Treatment with vitamin D should be undertaken cautiously, however, because it is toxic when present in excess.

HEPATIC METABOLISM OF FOLATE

Folic acid is stored in the liver as polyglutamates. Release of folate from stores in liver cells to peripheral tissues occurs indirectly, however, in that folate is excreted actively into the bile in concentrations three- to four-fold greater than plasma. An intact enterohepatic circulation appears essential in rat and presumably by analogy in man for the distribution of hepatic folate to tissues. The folate antagonism of ethanol appears to be mediated via interference with the enterohepatic cycle for folate metabolism. Ethanol prevents the secretion of folate into bile through unknown mechanisms. There are no current data relating to the metabolism of folate and its enterohepatic circulation in patients with cholestasis.

PATTERNS OF CLINICAL ABNORMALITIES IN PATIENTS WITH LIVER DISEASE

So far the major functions of the liver have been discussed in order to develop rational schemes that facilitate understanding the principal manifestations of liver diseases. The symptoms, signs, and chemical abnormalities in patients with liver disease are nonspecific, and therefore an etiological diagnosis rarely can be made on these grounds alone. The pathophysiology of all degrees of liver cell failure is the same whether it is induced by *alcohol, viral hepatitis, carbon tetrachloride,* or *excess iron.* Patients with liver disease present with variable types of dysfunction. Moreover, derangements at the clinical and laboratory levels differ from patient to patient even for those suffering the effects of identical etiological agents. Finally, different types of liver functions may deteriorate selectively. For example, albumin levels may be normal despite inability to synthesize clotting factors, and, conversely, levels of albumin may be abnormal despite normal levels for clotting factors. Similarly, a patient with cirrhosis may have ascites and/or esophageal varices, yet have well-preserved hepatocyte function as reflected by levels of albumin, clotting factors, bilirubin, ammonia, utilization of fuels, and tolerance of drugs. How, then, can the physician evaluate the status of liver disease in a given patient in order to determine the chronicity and extent of dysfunction? Recognizing general patterns of abnormalities associated with disorders of liver function, therefore, is valuable.

PATTERNS OF LIVER DYSFUNCTION

It is possible to identify patterns of liver dysfunction (Table 6). Thus, a patient with mechanical obstruction to bile flow presents a set of signs, symptoms, and laboratory abnormalities that can be explained completely by the obstruction. The patient with mechanical obstruction will have no evidence, initially, of liver cell failure or of vascular changes such as esophageal varices and ascites. Long-standing, unrelieved mechanical obstruction, however, causes eventual hepatocellular failure. Toxic reactions to a large number of

TABLE 6. CLINICAL PATTERNS OF LIVER DYSFUNCTION AS REFLECTED BY CLINICAL FINDINGS AND LABORATORY ABNORMALITIES

TYPE OF LIVER DYSFUNCTION	MANIFESTATION OF LIVER DYSFUNCTION
Cholestatic	Failure to form bile
Vascular	Portal hypertension; esophageal varices; ascites
Mild to moderate hepatocellular	Evidence of cell necrosis such as elevated transaminase levels; mild functional abnormalities such as transient decreases in protein synthesis
Severe hepatocellular	Evidence of failure of protein synthesis; detoxification of ammonia, bilirubin, and drugs

drugs, especially phenothiazines and certain estrogens and androgens, also are often purely cholestatic, and there have been epidemics of acute viral hepatitis in which the picture of cholestasis dominated the clinical and laboratory abnormalities without evidence of hepatocellular dysfunction or death of individual cells.

In some patients with cirrhosis, the clinical and laboratory findings reflect a predominant derangement of a vascular nature, that is, esophageal varices or ascites (or both). These patients may have no significant hepatocellular or cholestatic defects. The synthetic, detoxifying, and excretory functions of individual hepatocytes are well preserved, despite destruction of the normal lobular structure of the liver. Although pure patterns of cholestasis and/or vascular derangements are not typical for patients with parenchymal disease of the liver, they may be present in an occasional patient.

Mild hepatocellular disease is typical in a patient with *acute viral* hepatitis. The patient complains of nausea and vomiting, is jaundiced, and has a high level of transaminase enzymes in plasma. The latter reflects death or serious injury to liver cells, but the function of remaining hepatocytes is adequate for maintaining synthetic and detoxifying activities. The number of dead cells on biopsy is relatively small, and does not explain adequately the failure to excrete bilirubin. It is likely, therefore, that intrahepatic cholestasis accompanies typical, mild, viral hepatitis. Whether the cholestasis is due to the effect of infection on the bile canaliculi specifically or to a more generalized toxic effect on hepatocytes is unknown. Nevertheless, patients with acute viral hepatitis have combined patterns of cholestasis and hepatocellular dysfunction.

Moderate to severe hepatocellular dysfunction implies a generalized toxicity to all liver cells and/or extensive destruction. The end result is the same. The cellular functions of the liver fail. There is an inability to synthesize proteins or to detoxify endogenous compounds and drugs. Moderate to severe hepatocellular dysfunction characterizes both acute and chronic forms of liver disease. The prototype of the acute, severe hepatotocellular pattern is seen most often as a manifestation of *drug toxicity* (halothane), *poisoning* (carbon tetrachloride), and severe *viral hepatitis*. The constellation of signs, symptoms, and chemical abnor-

malities we have called patterns in Table 6 can be present in both acute and chronic types of liver disease. Most often, patients with acute and chronic disease present mixed patterns, i.e., overlapping of the pure patterns. For example, a typical patient with so-called acute alcoholic hepatitis has cholestasis (increased amounts of conjugated bilirubin and bile acids in the plasma), hepatocellular dysfunction (low levels of albumin and clotting factors, incipient hepatic coma, undue sensitivity to the effects of drugs), and vascular abnormalities (esophageal varices, sodium retention, ascites). The severity of each of these depends on the extent of disease and obviously varies in different patients. In addition, it is common to see evidence of acute and chronic disease in the same patient; an example is *alcoholic hepatitis,* which is a reversible lesion, superimposed on *cirrhosis,* which is a permanent, irreversible change in the liver. Moreover, hepatocellular failure in chronic forms of liver disease is accompanied almost always by vascular changes, i.e., esophageal varices and ascites. On the other hand, the severe hepatocellular pattern occurs in a pure form in the early stages of acute liver disease. It is followed quickly by evidence of vascular changes. We need to ask, therefore, how acute and chronic forms of liver disease can be differentiated. Careful history of the patient's exposure to toxic agents and previous illnesses is more reliable in this regard than are current signs and chemical abnormalities. It is often necessary to assess the presence of chronic liver disease by biopsy.

THE PATHOPHYSIOLOGY OF HEPATIC INJURY

The pathophysiology of liver disease is independent, in most instances, of the etiologic agent. The judgment that liver dysfunction is the basis for a clinical problem must be followed by determining its cause.

The major causes of liver disease in developed countries are *alcohol ingestion, viral hepatitis,* and administration of *pharmacological agents. Parasitic infestations* are important vectors for liver disease in undeveloped regions where drug-induced liver injuries are less significant as compared with their incidence in the West. There is a large miscellaneous group of liver disorders secondary to *inherited defects* in *enzyme function.* Some of the latter, such as glycogen storage disease, fructose intolerance, Wilson's disease, and hemochromatosis, lead eventually to cirrhosis. Why this is so is unclear in almost all instances. Clearly accumulation of Cu is toxic to the livers of patients with Wilson's disease, but the biochemical connection between cause (Cu) and effect (hepatic dysfunction) is unknown. The same is true in most other diseases of the liver, whether acquired or genetically determined, which is why the treatment of liver disease is limited primarily to management of complications rather than treatment of cause. We want to consider here what is known about the pathogenesis of the most common types of liver disease.

TOXICITY OF ETHANOL

There is a positive epidemiologic correlation between deaths due to cirrhosis and the per capita consumption of ethanol. Moreover, cirrhosis is a leading cause of death or an associated finding at autopsy in about 20 to 30 per cent of those classified as alcoholics. Alcohol abuse is an associated finding in about half the cases of cirrhosis in the Western world. On the other hand, alcohol abuse does not produce cirrhosis in all abusers, nor is there an identifiable amount of alcohol, or duration of intake, the leads to cirrhosis in all those who drink. Approximately 10 to 20 per cent of alcoholic patients without overt clinical signs of liver disease have cirrhosis on liver biopsy. A similar number of asymptomatic alcoholic patients have the histological lesion of alcoholic hepatitis. Clearly, therefore, chronic ingestion of ethanol often leads to serious forms of liver disease. The unresolved problem is the mechanism of ethanol-induced liver disease. The caloric value of ethanol suppresses appetite and ethanol interferes with gastrointestinal function so that ingested nutrients may not be absorbed. Many alcoholics are therefore malnourished. Malnutrition associated with alcoholism, as opposed to direct toxic effects of ethanol, has been viewed in the past as the inciting factor for cirrhosis in the alcoholic. Malnutrition, however, does not produce irreversible liver disease. As an alternative theory, alcohol has been postulated to cause cirrhosis per se.

Although ethanol produces liver disease to a variable extent in different people, it does have toxic manifestations in all those who drink it—even in those who consume only moderate amounts. Some of these were discussed in the chapters on energy metabolism and hepatic detoxification of ethanol (pp. 1277–1278). In addition, ethanol has acute effects that are not explained in terms of current knowledge of its metabolism (Table 7). Most of the toxic effects due to ingestion of ethanol have been demonstrated in volunteers consuming a normal hospital diet. Ethanol also has toxic effects on liver in experimental animals ingesting apparently adequate diets. It is proposed, therefore, that ethanol is uniformly toxic to human liver, and that the identified toxic reactions (see Tables 3 and 7, and discussions of fatty liver, glucose metabolism, and energy metabolism, pp. 415, 889, 891) are precursors of alcoholic hepatitis and eventually cirrhosis. This idea may seem reasonable, but the demonstrable toxic effects of ethanol have not been shown to have a causal relation to alcoholic hepatitis and/or cirrhosis. There are data, in fact, to suggest that ethanol per se is not the cause of liver disease in abusers of alcohol. A question, which at first seems absurd, is what is the

TABLE 7. TOXIC EFFECTS OF ETHANOL

Disruption of mitochondrial membranes

Interference with oxidative phosphorylation

Hypofunctioning endoplasmic reticulum

Leakage into plasma of intracellular enzymes (SGOT) and enzymes of the plasma membrane

Inhibition of protein synthesis

Minimal areas of necrosis of liver cells

Inhibition of microtubular function of "tubulin" transport of proteins out of hepatocytes

effect of continued ingestion of ethanol on the course of liver disease in patients admitted to the hospital with decompensated alcoholic hepatitis? If this disease can be explained by direct toxicity of ethanol, continued administration of ethanol should lead to a worsening of the patient's condition. Two well-controlled studies examined this aspect of the alcohol problem. In each, administration of large amounts of ethanol did not impede clinical and laboratory recovery from decompensated, alcohol-induced liver disease in patients eating a normal hospital diet. The conclusion to be drawn from these results is that ethanol and some other as-yet-unidentified environmental factor combine to produce liver disease in the susceptible host. It is reasonable to suggest that the environmental factor is dietary. We are confronted, therefore, with an apparent paradox. Neither malnutrition nor ethanol ingestion causes serious liver disease, yet abuse of ethanol plus malnutrition produces liver disease in some patients. The cirrhogenic potential of ethanol is due to interactions with environmental factors, presumably with serious forms of liver disease requiring, in addition, a susceptible host. In a study of monkeys fed a nutritionally adequate diet, only about half developed hepatitis and cirrhosis after ingestion of large amounts of ethanol. Moreover, hepatitis may heal in this setting despite continued ingestion of ethanol. The best evidence available indicates that ethanol alone does not produce liver disease. Thus, ethanol-induced liver disease in primates is prevented by supplementing the diet with choline. Moreover, administration of ethanol to rats leads to liver disease only in combination with a protein- and choline-deficient diet. Liver disease does not occur, except for benign fatty infiltration, if the deficient diet alone is fed, or if ethanol is administered with a nutritionally adequate diet. Further, the inflammation and progression of fibrosis, and cirrhosis due to the combined effects of ethanol and dietary deficiency, remit when a nutritionally adequate diet is fed with ethanol. The liver of rats, like that in monkeys and humans, thus is affected by the *combination* of ethanol and dietary factors.

Clinical Patterns in Patients with Alcohol-Induced Liver Disease

Liver disease in alcoholics presents a variety of distinct patterns of evolution (Fig. 28). Patients admitted to the hospital because of decompensated liver disease have alcoholic hepatitis, alcoholic hepatitis superimposed on cirrhosis, or cirrhosis complicated by liver cell failure and/or the pattern of vascular disorders. It is reasonable to assume that patients with alcoholic hepatitis only are in an early course of their disease. Those with cirrhosis are in a later phase.

Alcoholic hepatitis often has an apparently abrupt onset in a patient who has been drinking for months to years. Quite frequently, the disease is precipitated by an increase in alcohol intake in response to emotional trauma, accompanied by decreased appetite and food intake. Biopsy of the liver shows acute changes but no evidence of cirrhosis. Nevertheless, many patients with acute alcoholic hepatitis will develop cirrhosis in a matter of weeks to months even while abstaining from ethanol. Whether or not this occurs

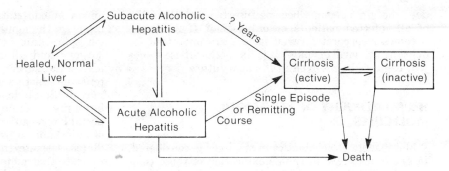

Figure 28. The course of alcohol-induced liver disease as determined by liver biopsy. The entities in the boxes can be identified on clinical grounds. Activity refers to evidence on biopsy of continued inflammation.

after the first episode of acute hepatitis, those patients who continue to drink will have a relapsing course, i.e., repeated admissions for acute alcoholic hepatitis. Eventually, many—if not all—will develop cirrhosis and experience the permanent, irreversible complications of this abnormality. Abstention from ethanol is the only effective therapeutic device altering the natural course of liver disease in such patients, that is, those who have had an episode of alcoholic hepatitis. Irrespective of the importance of dietary factors in the genesis of alcohol-induced liver disease, the patient with clinically overt alcoholic hepatitis has a demonstrated susceptibility to the toxic effect of ethanol, alone or in combination with dietary deficiencies.

Obviously, some patients with the clinical syndrome of alcoholic hepatitis have this lesion superimposed on cirrhosis. A large number of alcoholics with a history of heavy drinking for 20 to 30 years have this constellation of abnormalities the first time they experience overt decompensation of liver function. The course of disease in these patients is not clear in that we do not know for certain the events that caused the underlying cirrhosis. Presumably, they have had a long-standing, subclinical alcoholic hepatitis that destroyed liver cells at a rate slow enough to avoid acute episodes of clinical disease. Approximately 15 to 20 per cent of alcoholics who are well clinically and have normal or minimally abnormal chemical function are found to have alcoholic hepatitis on biopsy of their livers. Destruction of liver cells seems to proceed at a slow, constant rate in these patients until they experience the hepatocellular and vascular complications of cirrhosis. Onset of jaundice, ammonia intoxication, functional impairment of the kidneys, ascites, or bleeding esophageal varices (i.e., end-stage disease) may be the first signs of serious liver disease. Biopsy reveals long-standing, already irreversible changes, plus hepatitis. The factors that determine which type of clinical course the disease takes in different individuals are unknown.

VIRAL HEPATITIS

It has been traditional to think of viral hepatitis as two distinct diseases caused by related viruses. One was transmitted orally or parenterally, had a short incubation period, acute onset, and almost universally excellent prognosis. This form was called viral hepatitis. Now it is called type A hepatitis. The other was transmitted by administration of blood, had a long incubation period, and clinical disease often was of insidious onset. This form, previously referred to as serum hepatitis, now is known as type B hepatitis. The prognosis of type B hepatitis is usually good, but

in a significant number of patients this disease causes death, either from an acute episode or after a chronic course. Discovery that the Australia antigen was a marker for infection by type B, plus laboratory techniques for identifying infection due to type A virus, has changed our concepts of the "disease" viral hepatitis. There are cases of hepatitis that are not due to infection with either type A or type B virus. Obviously, viral hepatitides are not limited to these entities.

Type A viral hepatitis most likely reflects the cytopathic effects of the virus. The disease typically presents with a combined picture of mild hepatocellular and cholestatic abnormalities. Onset is acute and resolution usually rapid. In a few instances, necrosis has been extensive enough to cause death. Chronic disease does not develop, however. A small number of patients die of acute disease; all the rest recover completely. *Type B hepatitis* differs in many significant respects from type A disease. Most importantly, it is not clear that infection of liver cells with type B virus has cytopathic effects. Thus, virus can be demonstrated in almost all liver cells for days to weeks prior to clinically apparent injury. Virus, in some cases, can disappear without injury. In other instances, virus may persist indefinitely, yet cause no chemical or clinical decompensation of hepatocytic function. It has been suggested, for these reasons, that acute injury in type B hepatitis is mediated via immune reactions to virus-altered hepatocytes, although proof of this concept is lacking. Chronic, slowly progressing hepatic disease is frequent after acute type B infection, and substantial clinical and laboratory evidence is compatible with an immune mechanism in the chronic phase of the illness. On the other hand, patients with chronic disease are infected persistently with the virus, and immunosuppressive therapy of chronic active hepatitis in patients with type B antigen in their sera is not useful.

The pathophysiological consequences of type B hepatitis and the course of the illness are similar to what is depicted in Figure 28 for alcoholic liver disease. Patients may present with acute disease that subsequently either heals or becomes chronically active. They may be seen first during the chronic stages. They may not become sufficiently ill to seek medical attention until cirrhosis has developed. A variety of clinical constellations is likely, therefore, in this group of patients, depending on the phase of illness.

Obviously, patients infected with hepatitis B virus display variable patterns of illness. What we need to determine are the factors in the patients that account for chronicity. This level of understanding depends on developing answers to several crucial questions about the events of the viral infection itself. For example, does the viral genome become inserted into the DNA of all infected patients or only some? If it always becomes incorporated, what factors are important for deleting the viral genome? It is likely that these issues will begin to be resolved in the near future.

HEPATOTOXICITY OF XENOBIOTIC MOLECULES

Metabolism of xenobiotics in the liver is considered, in general, to lead to the detoxification of these compounds. Metabolism of xenobiotics in the liver can lead, however, to the formation of toxic intermediates that cause disease ranging from acute hepatitis to hepatocellular carcinoma. The enzyme system primarily responsible for converting nonreactive xenobiotics to highly reactive species is the microsomal cytochrome P_{450}. The extent of hepatic necrosis due to carbon tetrachloride (CCl_4) is diminished, for example, by prior administration of agents that block its metabolism. It seems, therefore, that CCl_4 itself does not injure the liver but is converted to a toxin via the cytochrome P_{450} system. The reaction responsible for converting CCl_4 to a toxic intermediate appears to be the generation of free radicals, $\cdot CCl_3$, during removal of a chloride ion. Free radicals are highly reactive intermediates that peroxidize unsaturated fatty acids in a self-sustaining chain reaction. A small amount of free radical can damage cells severely, since peroxidation of lipids disrupts the structure and function of intracellular and plasma membranes. The metabolism of CCl_4 by the P_{450} system is prototypic of reactions involved in the metabolism of halogenated hydrocarbons that are useful general anesthetics, and production of free radicals during dehalogenation of hydrocarbons is an important clinical problem today because of the wide use of these drugs as anesthetic agents.

Halothane, the first of these agents to be used widely, causes liver disease in some patients sporadically and in experimental animals. By contrast, CCl_4 causes hepatic injury in all exposed animals. It is unclear why the toxicity of carbon tetrachloride is more uniform than that of halothane. Unfortunately, this discrepancy in toxic potential obscured possible similarities in the mechanisms of tissue damage secondary to halothane- and CCl_4-induced toxicity and led temporarily to the view that halothane toxicity reflected a hypersensitivity to this agent. The presence of eosinophilia in some affected patients was taken as support for the involvement of the immune system as a primary agent in halothane hepatitis. An immune reaction in the course of tissue damage after halothane more likely follows from the modification of proteins by metabolites of halothane, and any hypersensitivity reaction would be against these modified, endogenous proteins.

Halothane is a volatile anesthetic and is excreted rapidly via the lungs. Nevertheless, as much as 25 per cent of administered halothane is metabolized, normally to trifluoroacetic acid by the hepatic P_{450} system. In the presence of anoxia, however, halothane is reduced by P_{450} to $F_3C - \overset{\text{H}}{\underset{\text{Cl}}{C}} \cdot$, a toxic, free radical intermediate, plus Br^-. Since the oxygenation of liver depends primarily on venous flow, liver normally borders

on an anoxic state, especially in the central venous region of the lobule. A multitude of factors can diminish splanchnic flow and thereby portal flow during surgery and after; so in most patients undergoing abdominal surgery there is ample opportunity for extensive reductive metabolism of halothane. Portal flow may decline independently of changes in the systemic blood pressure; furthermore, small decreases in Po_2 in portal blood can augment significantly the metabolism of halothane to free radicals and other toxic intermediates. Despite the considerable body of evidence to indicate that metabolism to toxic intermediates is the mechanism of halothane-induced hepatitis, we do not understand why halothane hepatitis occurs sporadically, or more importantly why the second exposure to this agent, but not the first, usually is associated with severe hepatitis.

Generation of free radicals is not the only chemical pathway by which liver produces toxins. Unsaturated ring systems can be oxidized to epoxides by cytochrome P_{450} (Reaction [22]):

[22]

Naphthalene   *Naphthalene-1,2-epoxide*

These are highly reactive alkylating agents that add to macromolecules, thereby destroying function. The hepatic toxicity of epoxide formation is related to interference with the function of the proteins of the cell. In view of the large number of pharmacologically active compounds containing an unsaturated ring system, the potential for drug toxicity secondary to epoxide formation is quite large. They add rapidly to proteins and are converted to other, less toxic intermediates.

Hepatotoxicity is an increasingly important problem after overdoses of acetaminophen (shown below) and in patients receiving isoniazid.

$$H-N-COCH_3$$

OH

Untoward reactions to each of these drugs follow their metabolic activation in the liver. In the case of acetaminophen, the parent compound is oxidized to the reactive, toxic intermediate by cytochrome P_{450}. The toxic intermediate arises from hydroxylation of the nitrogen, which produces a reactive, alkylating agent. The pathway for production of toxic metabolites after administration of isoniazid is somewhat more complicated and depends on prior acetylation of the parent drug (Fig. 29). Hydrolysis of acetylisoniazid releases acetylhydrazine. Hydrazines are potent hepatotoxins because they are metabolized by the cytochrome P_{450} system to reactive compounds that bind covalently to macromolecules. The toxicity of isoniazid in animals is enhanced, therefore, by prior administration of in-

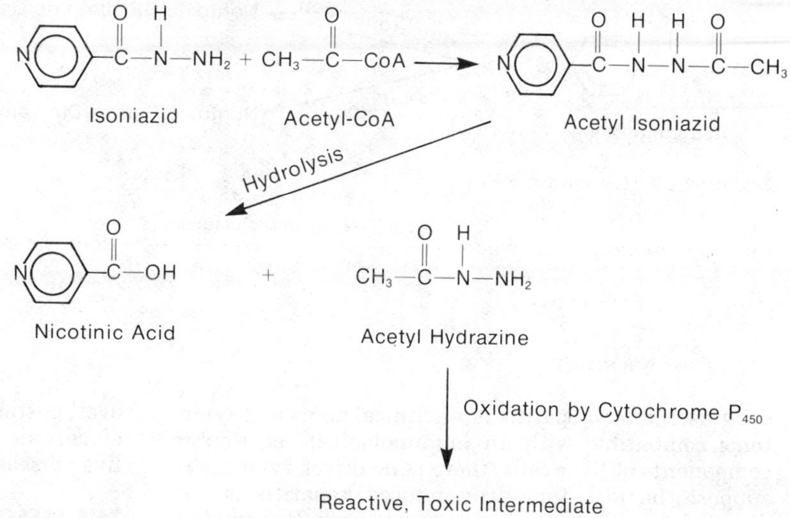

Figure 29. Pathway for conversion of isoniazid to a hepatotoxin.

ducers of cytochrome P_{450}. Since acetylated isoniazid, but not the parent drug, is hydrolyzed to release the hydrazine derivative ($-NH-NH_2$) as the essential step in the toxicity of isoniazid, we might expect that the rate of acetylation of isoniazid could influence its clinical toxicity. Acetylation of drugs, including isoniazid, is under genetic control, and two classes of acetylators—rapid and slow—can be described on the basis of pharmacological studies. Isoniazid-induced liver injury occurs more often in rapid acetylators as compared with slow acetylators. Eighty per cent of Orientals are "rapid acetylators." The frequency is far below this level in other groups studied. Unexplained as yet is why the risk of serious forms of isoniazid-induced hepatitis is much higher in older patients than in young ones. Perhaps this is related to the "activation" of acetylhydrazine to toxic compounds.

Drugs containing acetyl- or isopropyl-substituted hydrazines can produce the same type of toxic hepatitis seen during treatment of some patients with isoniazid. For example, the structure of iproniazid

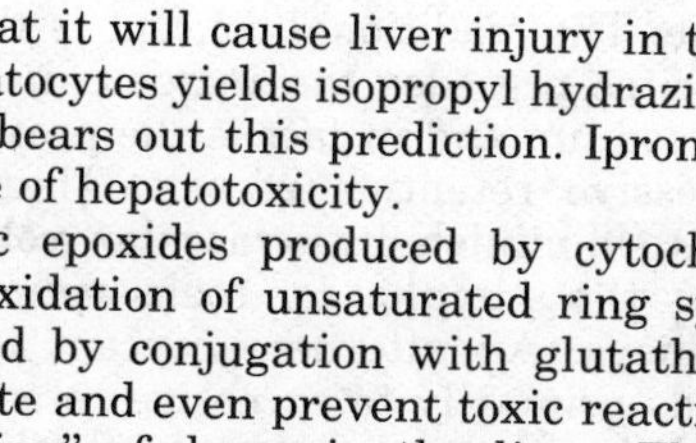

HYDRAZINE
GROUP

Iproniazid

suggests that it will cause liver injury in that hydrolysis in hepatocytes yields isopropyl hydrazine. Clinical experience bears out this prediction. Iproniazid has a high degree of hepatotoxicity.

The toxic epoxides produced by cytochrome P_{450}-catalyzed oxidation of unsaturated ring systems can be detoxified by conjugation with glutathione which can modulate and even prevent toxic reactions caused by "activation" of drugs in the liver. The potential interactions among Phase I and Phase II drug-modifying reactions are exemplified best by considering the chemical basis for hepatic necrosis secondary to ingestion of acetaminophen.

The phenolic group of acetaminophen can be conjugated with glucuronic acid or sulfate. Acetaminophen, on the other hand, can be oxidized by cytochrome P_{450} to toxic intermediates (Fig. 30). Prior conjugation prevents this oxidation. Finally, the toxic intermediates, when formed, can be detoxified by reaction with glutathione. Therapeutic doses of acetaminophen are metabolized largely to the glucuronide and sulfate conjugates, which are nontoxic. A small amount must be oxidized normally to toxic derivatives, however, because about 4 per cent of a *therapeutic* dose is excreted as a conjugate of glutathione. As the dose of acetaminophen is increased, conjugations with glucuronic acid or sulfate become saturated. Acetaminophen becomes available in this setting for oxidation by cytochrome P_{450}. Alternatively, more of the toxic oxidation products may be generated from a given dose of acetaminophen if the amount of cytochrome P_{450} is increased, as occurs when there is previous administration of an inducer. Serious toxicity, i.e., massive hepatic necrosis, is avoided so long as the toxins formed react with glutathione. Thus, reduction of the amount of glutathione in liver, induction of cytochrome P_{450}, or very large intakes of drug enhance the toxicity of acetaminophen. Retrospective studies of patients with acetaminophen-induced hepatic necrosis indicate that drug toxicity was potentiated by chronic ingestion of inducers of cytochrome P_{450}.

DRUG TOXICITY VERSUS HYPERSENSITIVITY

A large number of foreign compounds injure the liver. For some, such as carbon tetrachloride, the incidence of injury is high and is related to dose. Other agents, such as the phenothiazines, produce hepatic injury less often, and in a manner not predicated on dose or duration of intake. The difference between the incidence of injury after administration of carbon tetrachloride and after that of phenothiazines has led to a distinction in terminology. Unless a drug produces a uniformly severe hepatitis in all patients ingesting some given amount, there is a tendency to think of the drug-induced reaction as idiosyncratic, a hypersensitivity reaction, or even an allergic phenomenon. Whereas chemicals like carbon tetrachloride are considered true hepatotoxins, phenothiazines are thought to be sensitizing agents. Although some patients with

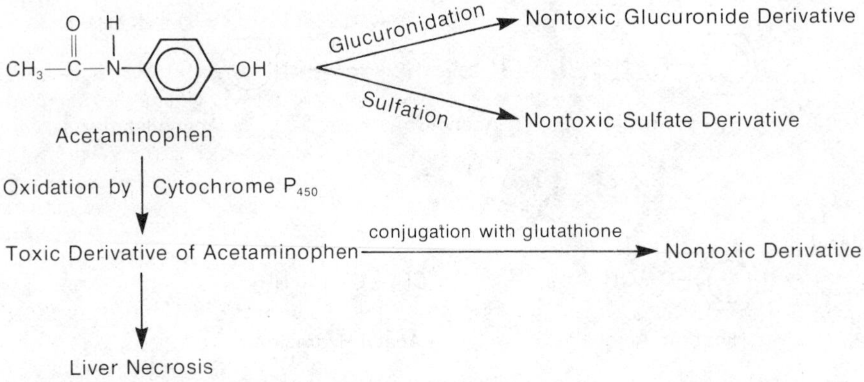

Figure 30. Multiple pathways for the metabolism of acetaminophen in liver.

drug-associated hepatitis have clinical signs and symptoms compatible with an immunological reaction to components of liver cells, there is no direct evidence to support the idea that drug-induced hepatitis is mediated primarily by immune mechanisms. Immunological or allergic phenomena, like rash and eosinophilia when they occur, may indicate sensitization to complexes of proteins and toxins or other components released by dying hepatocytes. In contrast, recent studies with halothane, acetaminophen, and isoniazid, as outlined above, indicate that the hepatic toxicity due to these drugs, which seemed unpredictable until now, reflects conversion to toxic chemicals. Therefore, it is unrealistic to distinguish arbitrarily between "true hepatotoxins" and sensitizing agents on the basis of the uniformity of toxicity in a given population. As illustrated above with acetaminophen, the toxic potential of a drug depends on several identifiable factors that vary from patient to patient and that are different at different times in the same patient. These include the amounts of enzyme(s) that produce nontoxic derivatives or activate the parent compound to a toxic agent, and the availability of cofactors for detoxifying metabolites.

Another important factor, especially in patients taking many different drugs, is competition for detoxification pathways. At present, we have little specific data on individual differences in the capacity to metabolize drugs via Phase I and Phase II reactions. Nevertheless, limited studies indicate that such differences exist in the absence of induction of cytochrome P_{450} or of competition between different drugs. Another significant variable in drug toxicity is binding in plasma. Large amounts of free, or unbound, drug can enter hepatocytes and be metabolized to reactive intermediates because detoxifying pathways are overloaded at relatively low concentrations. This may occur simply in response to administration of an inappropriate amount of drug. Alternatively, defects in plasma binding may allow excessively large amounts of a given agent to gain access to the liver. For example, hepatotoxicity due to furosemide appears when the amount given exceeds plasma-binding capacity.

An attempt should always be made to interpret toxic hepatitis in terms of the factors elucidated above rather than to invoke hypersensitivity reactions as an all-encompassing mechanism. At the same time, attention to the principles of drug metabolism in the liver will reduce the incidence of serious drug hepatotoxicity, which accounts for about 25 per cent of hepatic necrosis in the U.S. Mortality in this condition is high. Moreover, postnecrotic cirrhosis and/or a histological picture of chronic active hepatitis may follow drug-induced liver diseases.

THE EFFECT OF LIVER FUNCTION ON SALT AND WATER BALANCE

There are three major changes in kidney function in patients with liver disease: sodium retention, inability to excrete a water load, and an unstable, abnormal pattern of blood flow in the kidneys. These defects in renal function are functional in that they are reversible. Each can occur independently of the others, but typically abnormally avid retention of sodium precedes the defect in excretion of water. The instability of blood flow can lead eventually to functional renal failure, the so-called hepatorenal syndrome, and hence presents clinically as a late manifestation of functional renal disease in patients with various forms of hepatic disease. Nevertheless, abnormal patterns of intrarenal blood flow can be demonstrated in patients with well-compensated liver disease, who have no clinical evidence of renal retention of salt and water. It has not been possible, as yet, to identify the feature of liver disease that leads to the above three functional disorders of kidney function. It appears, however, that some aspect of sinusoidal outflow block, as opposed to splanchnic venous hypertension, leads to the abnormalities of kidney function, at least in experimental animals. Obviously, several intrahepatic defects might lead independently to the abnormalities to be described.

SODIUM RETENTION

There are two theories as to the cause of excessive reabsorption of sodium by kidneys of patients with liver disease. The traditional concept is that development of ascites precedes the increase in renal reabsorption of sodium and in fact is the proximate cause of the excessive retention of salt. Thus, ascites is considered to diminish intravascular volume, which then acts as the stimulus for reabsorption of sodium by the kidneys. An alternate concept is that liver disease leads primarily to excessive retention of salt, which coupled with local factors in the liver leads to ascites. Evidence available today indicates that (1) the intravascular volume of patients with liver disease and ascites is normal to expanded; (2) excessive retention of sodium occurs in some patients with liver disease in the presence of normal GFR; and (3) these patients reabsorb excess sodium even in the absence of ascites. In addition, in experimentally induced cirrhosis retention of salt occurs prior to development of ascites. Some feature(s) of liver disease seems, therefore, to signal the kidney to conserve sodium beyond the amount needed to maintain normal intravascular volume. Local factors within the liver (see Development of Ascites) lead to the accumulation of fluid within the peritoneal cavity.

Patients with liver disease and ascites undergo a diuresis during head-out immersion in water (Fig. 31), an observation interpreted as reflecting a diminished "effective" intravascular volume in these patients because head-out immersion increases vascular volume centrally. The exact meaning of the effects on renal handling of sodium during head-out immersion in water of patients with liver disease must remain uncertain, however, until the specific agents acting to cause reabsorption of excess salt by the kidney are identified more carefully. Thus, head-out immersion does more than induce a sodium diuresis in patients with ascites and a normal GFR. It also can correct creatinine clearance in patients with liver disease and abnormally low clearance. The mechanism by which this happens is unknown, but obviously these data raise the possibility that head-out immersion has effects on intrarenal blood flow in patients with advanced forms of liver disease.

The extracellular fluid volume and absorption of sodium in the proximal tubule are normally inversely related. The amount of sodium reaching the distal tubule increases as extracellular fluid volume expands. Finally, a level of distal tubular sodium is reached that exceeds absorptive capacity, even in the presence of excess mineralocorticoid. Sodium diuresis then ensues. This volume-dependent mechanism overrides the stimulus of mineralocorticoids and allows normal subjects to "escape" from the sodium retention due to excess mineralocorticoid. There seems to be a disturbance in the normal relationships between proximal retention of sodium and extracellular fluid volume in edematous states. Reabsorption of sodium in proximal tubules is excessive in patients with ascites, despite increasing retention of sodium and water. Sodium reaching the distal tubule will be retained avidly because levels are insufficient to overload the absorptive capacity, especially when there is excess aldosterone. The sodium retention in cirrhotics could reflect a failure of the normal escape mechanism in addition to primary retention of salt, but there is insufficient evidence to allow for a final conclusion.

The scheme discussed above provides a reasonable explanation for retention of salt in patients with liver disease, but there remain two unanswered questions: (1) What factor promotes proximal reabsorption of sodium in patients with liver disease? (2) What is the signal for increased production of renin, which leads ultimately to the excessive aldosterone? There is, unfortunately, no completely satisfactory explanation for the Na^+ retention in cirrhotic patients. Infusion of isotonic saline into the portal vein produces a greater urine flow than infusion into the vena cava, under conditions that do not alter the rate of glomerular filtration. There are suggestions, too, that liver contains nerve roots sensitive to plasma osmotic pressure and/or the concentration of sodium. The conclusions to be drawn from these experiments are that normal liver senses changes in sodium balance and releases an unknown humoral substance that promotes renal excretion of sodium. But no such "hormone" has been isolated, despite efforts to find it. The idea that liver secretes a substance that acts on the proximal renal tubules, although attractive, remains an unsubstantiated hypothesis.

It is easy to understand why the plasma level of aldosterone is high in patients with liver disease; however, we do not know what stimulates hypersecretion of renin. In the absence of detailed answers to either of questions (1) or (2) above, treatment of sodium retention in liver disease can be symptomatic only.

FAILURE TO EXCRETE A WATER LOAD

Failure of the ascitic patient to secrete a water load reflects a diminishing rate of glomerular filtration and

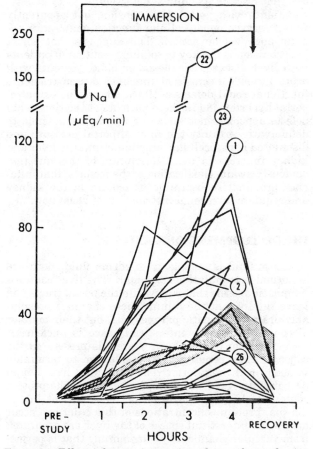

Figure 31. Effects of water immersion after an hour of quiet sitting (prestudy) on rate of sodium excretion ($U_{Na}V$) in 26 patients with alcoholic liver disease. The circled numbers represent individual patients. The shaded area represents the mean ±SE for 14 normal subjects undergoing an identical study while receiving an identical 10 mEq sodium/100 mEq potassium diet. Eleven of the patients manifested an absent or sluggish natriuretic response. In contrast, the remaining 15 patients manifested an appropriate or "exaggerated" natriuretic response compared with normal controls. In general, the increase in $U_{Na}V$ was associated with a concomitant increase in potassium excretion. (From Zakim, D., and Boyer, T. D. (eds.): Hepatology: A Textbook of Liver Disease. Philadelphia, W. B. Saunders Co., 1982.)

probably increased plasma levels of ADH. The former mechanism leads, in the extreme case, to frank renal failure with azotemia, the so-called hepatorenal syndrome. The kidney defect in hepatorenal syndrome is functional and potentially reversible. Kidneys from patients dying with the hepatorenal syndrome function normally when transplanted to patients with normal liver function. Renal failure in patients with end-stage liver disease is associated with a reduction of blood flow to the kidney plus a shunting of intrarenal blood from cortical to medullary regions. The most reasonable explanation for these findings is increased vascular resistance in the kidney in the face of a falling peripheral vascular resistance, which diverts blood away from the kidney. Within the kidney, there is a maldistribution of blood. An intense constriction of cortical blood vessels directs renal blood flow to medullary areas. Glomerular filtration decreases, and azotemia supervenes. Radiographic studies of the renal vasculature confirm the presence of cortical constriction and diversion of blood away from the glomeruli. These changes are reversed quickly post mortem in that kidneys from deceased patients do not demonstrate the abnormalities that were present during life.

Renal vascular resistance depends on many factors. The most important of these appear to be the renin-angiotensin system, the bradykinin-kallikrein system, and sympathetic amines. Angiotensin II is a potent vasoconstrictor; as mentioned earlier, it is present in excess amounts in patients with liver disease. It is possible, therefore, that renal vasoconstriction reflects increased levels of angiotensin II. On the other hand, peripheral vascular resistance is diminished in patients with the hepatorenal syndrome. Invoking angiotensin-induced vasoconstriction in the kidney as a cause of its increased vascular resistance perforce then poses the idea of differential effects of angiotensin II on the systemic and renal vascular systems. There are no data on this point. In contrast to angiotensin II, bradykinin has a vasodilating effect on the kidney. Plasma bradykinin levels are diminished in patients with cirrhosis and functional renal failure, resulting in diminished effector for vasodilatation in the presence of excessive constrictor activity. These abnormalities could have a concerted effect on vascular resistance in the kidney, producing the severe vasoconstriction of cortical vessels seen on x-ray. In addition, false neurotransmitters, produced by bacterial action in the gut and not detoxified by the diseased liver, can contribute to this effect. By interfering with the normal action of sympathetic amines, false transmitters may lower peripheral vascular resistance, thereby shunting blood away from the kidney, or contribute to the maldistribution of blood flow within the kidneys.

We have considered so far that abnormalities of salt and water balance in patients with liver disease are separate entities. Obviously, this is not so. Thus, as glomerular filtration rate decreases secondary to functional vascular changes within the kidney, the sodium load to the proximal and distal tubules decreases. This augments any tendency to retain sodium. Indeed, small changes in intrarenal blood flow could account for sodium retention in the absence of other mechanisms. In any case, the amount of sodium reaching the distal tubules can become exceedingly small in patients with liver disease. Some patients with ascites are resistant to the diuretic effect of spironolactone, because their distal tubules receive almost no sodium. Additionally, it is possible to explain renal tubular acidosis in cirrhotic patients who retain sodium with great avidity. Nearly complete absorption of sodium proximally leaves no ions to exchange with H^+ distally. Renal excretion of acid falls, and the patient becomes acidotic. Osmotically induced natriuresis in such patients increases the load of sodium delivered to the distal tubules, and acidification of the urine is enhanced.

At what point in the progress of liver disease does functional renal impairment occur? There is no certain answer to this question. Abnormalities in renal blood flow and hemodynamics and abnormal retention of sodium can be demonstrable in well-compensated, non-ascitic patients with cirrhosis. The defect in renal sodium excretion in cirrhosis is not based on a contracted intravascular volume secondary to formation of ascitic fluid. Patients with ascites have abnormalities that predate its clinical detection.

Patients with portal hypertension, but apparently well-preserved hepatocellular function, may retain sodium and develop ascites. This suggests that portal hypertension is the key to sodium retention in patients with liver disease. On the other hand, patients with acute massive necrosis of the liver demonstrate the functional renal defects outlined above. The extent of portal hypertension in these patients at the time renal defects appear is not known. So, it is not possible to define with certainty the roles of portal pressure and disordered hepatocellular function in linking liver and kidney function in man. Resolution of this question obviously awaits clarification of the factor(s) that influence proximal reabsorption of sodium in the kidney and regulate intrarenal distribution of blood flow.

THE DEVELOPMENT OF ASCITES

Ascitic fluid is analogous to edema fluid. Both are abnormal accumulations of lymph. The liver contains lymphatic vessels that run within the portal tracts and leave the liver at the hilum. These channels presumably drain the hepatic parenchyma, but their manner of connection to the interstitial space is unclear. A second system of lymphatic vessels is present in the capsule. They penetrate the diaphragm to terminate in nodes near the inferior vena cava. Most liver lymph probably derives from the space of Disse. The protein content of liver lymph is 90 per cent of that in the plasma. Protein concentrations of this order can occur only if the interstitial spaces of the liver are separated from vascular channels by a membrane that is permeable to large molecules. The membrane separating sinusoids from the space of Disse is the only one in the liver that fulfills this criterion.

Loss of fluid from capillaries depends on the balance between oncotic and mechanical pressures in the capillary and interstitial tissue. Plasma oncotic pressure in capillaries is due primarily to albumin and equals 30 cm of water when levels of albumin are normal. The tissue oncotic pressure is about 15 cm of water. A mechanical pressure of 15 cm of H_2O on the inside of the capillary hence will lead to a net transudation of fluid from capillary lumen to interstitial space. This is not true in the liver. The space of Disse (the interstitial space in the liver) is separated from hepatic sinusoids by a membranous structure that is permeable to everything but the formed elements of the blood. There hence are no effective oncotic forces between these two regions. The direction of flow of plasma components into the space of Disse depends only on the gradient of mechanical pressure between it and the sinusoid. Formation of hepatic lymph is thus sensitive to small pressure changes within the sinusoid. Whereas an increase of mechanical pressure of 15 cm of water is required to form an excess of lymph in interstitial spaces, a 1- to 2-cm elevation of pressure increases the amount of hepatic lymph in the space of Disse.

Fluid and protein within the space of Disse flow in a direction opposite to the flow of blood in the sinusoids. It is reasonable to infer that they reach lymphatic channels within the portal spaces, which drain ultimately into the thoracic duct. To a certain extent, excess hepatic lymph production is accommodated by flow into the thoracic duct, but this is a limiting factor for direct re-entry of hepatic lymph into the circulation. Experimental occlusion of the hepatic vein is associated with increased formation of hepatic lymph that weeps from the surface of the liver into the peritoneal cavity. Similarly, exudation of hepatic lymph from the liver's surface can be seen in patients with increased resistance to flow of blood in the hepatic sinusoid secondary to destruction of the normal hepatic acinar unit (cirrhosis). In addition to differences in the pressures required to form excess hepatic versus tissue lymph, ascitic fluid in patients with cirrhosis contains a relatively high concentration of albumin as compared with lymph coming from mesenteric vessels. Many ascitic fluids in patients with cirrhosis cannot be classified as transudates because the protein concentration of the hepatic lymph is high as compared with that in plasma. The presence of hepatic lymph in the peritoneal cavity reduces the fluid-retaining capacity of the osmotic forces within mesenteric capillaries and hence may promote transudation of additional ascitic fluid across the mesentery.

It has been taught for many years that hypoalbuminemia is a critical factor in the formation of ascites in patients with cirrhosis. This formulation is incompatible with the present concept of factors regulating lymph flow. The amount of hepatic lymph formed by the flow of plasma into the space of Disse has no relationship to the plasma concentration of albumin. *Resistance to sinusoidal blood flow is the important determinant in the generation of ascites.* Low concentrations of albumin can contribute to the production of ascites, but only for that portion formed by ultrafiltration across mesenteric capillaries. Small amounts of ascitic fluid are generated by this mechanism. It is unusual to find ascites in patients with portal hypertension secondary to occlusion of the portal vein. Ascites becomes a problem when the cause of portal hypertension is resistance to outflow of blood from the liver, i.e., at the level of the sinusoid and beyond. This is the circumstance for excessive formation of hepatic lymph.

Ascitic fluid is reabsorbed quite readily. As much as 900 ml can be mobilized per day during diuresis (natriuresis) of ascitic patients. Ascitic fluid can be formed continuously in patients with cirrhosis but can be absorbed rapidly enough to prevent its accumulation, that is, up to a volume of about 900 ml per day. Clinically apparent collections of ascites mean that the rate of formation exceeds the rate of removal. *Retention of salt* is the key factor, since ascites accumulates with positive sodium balance and recedes during negative sodium balance. Refractory ascites is failure to achieve adequate sodium excretion. The connection between positive salt balance and formation of ascites in cirrhotic patients must be an expanding plasma volume, especially on the venous side of the circulation.

Expansion of the plasma volume increases the amount of blood in the venous, as opposed to the arterial, circulation. The former normally contains most of the blood volume. High resistance to blood flow in the sinusoids creates an access route for portal blood to reach a low pressure sump: the hepatic lymph in the peritoneal cavity. Simply stated, excess salt and water, which are retained by the cirrhotic for the reasons outlined above, will follow the pathway of least resistance and accumulate in the compartment with minimal pressure. The pathway of least resistance for exit of fluid from the circulation of the cirrhotic is via hepatic sinusoids into the space of Disse, from which excess volume can escape, via lymphatic channels, to the peritoneal cavity. The best available evidence suggests that ascitic fluid does not collect at the expense of normal vascular volume. Depletion of intravascular volume in cirrhotics is seen almost exclusively after inappropriately vigorous diuresis. Since 900 ml is the maximum amount of ascitic fluid reabsorbed per day, water losses in excess of this volume can decrease the intravascular volume of an ascitic patient.

THE ENTEROHEPATIC CIRCULATION OF THE BILE SALTS AND DISORDERS OF THE BILIARY TREE

Current concepts of how bile is elaborated at the level of the individual hepatic cell have been discussed above. Total biliary volume is not dependent solely on canalicular secretion, however. Secretin, cholecystokinin, and gastrin stimulate ductular secretion of water, bicarbonate, and chloride ion to a lesser extent. Of these, secretin is the most potent choleretic and gastrin the least. Vagal stimulation also is choleretic. Whether the bile ducts modify canalicular bile in ways other than adding water and alkali is uncertain, because the exact composition of bile secreted by canaliculi is not known. Secretion of bicarbonate by the bile ducts neutralizes bile salts and most likely contributes to neutralizing acid when the gastric, pancreatic and biliary secretions mix in the small intestine. The pH of bile is slightly acidic, however, since the pK_a's of bile salts are quite low.

About one half the bile secreted at any moment reaches the duodenum in the fasting state. The remainder enters the gallbladder, which serves two functions. The first is concentration of the bile. The second is delivery of bile to the intestine during digestion. These are interrelated.

The role of the gallbladder in sequestering bile salts and the enterohepatic circulation of bile acids: The daily rate of synthesis of bile acids from cholesterol is approximately 500 to 700 mg. The total amount of bile salts in man is 2.5 to 4 grams. These are distributed, at any given time, almost exclusively in the gallbladder bile and in the juices of the small intestine. It is known, however, that the liver secretes between 15 and 35 grams of bile salt per day. Clearly, there is (1) a rapid recirculation of bile salts, and (2) considerable conservation of those that reach the intestine. The total loss of bile salts in the stool in a normal steady state does not exceed their rate of synthesis.

The enterohepatic circulation of bile salts is outlined in Figure 32, using glycyl cholate as an example. Once secreted into the intestine, there are three alternative fates for glycyl cholate: (1) The bile salt can be absorbed intact. This is thought to occur to a small extent along the length of the small intestine. Most bile salt is absorbed actively, however, in the terminal ileum. (2) A portion of the bile salt can be deconjugated through the action of bacterial enzymes. Bile acid, cholate in the example given, is released. The cholate is absorbed passively in the upper small intestine and actively in the terminal ileum. (3) Bacterial enzymes can dehydroxylate cholate to produce deoxycholate, a so-called secondary bile acid, that is, one not produced in the liver. Deoxycholate is absorbed in the same manner as cholate. Conjugated bile salts are not substrates for the dehydroxylating enzyme. Prior deconjugation is required for the synthesis of secondary bile acids.

Reabsorbed bile acids and salts are removed by the liver with great efficiency, about 70 per cent in a single passage through the liver. The unchanged glycyl cholate is resecreted intact. Cholate and deoxycholate are converted to glycyl and tauryl salts, and then resecreted into canalicular bile. Only relatively small amounts of the bile salts and acids are lost in the stool during recycling between liver and intestine.

The enterohepatic circulation of chenodeoxycholate is similar in pattern to that for cholate. There is a major difference, however, in that dehydroxylation of chenodeoxycholate at the 7 position produces lithocholate, which is converted to a sulfate derivative on recirculation to the liver. The glycyl and tauryl "salts" of lithocholate are poorly soluble in water, but addition of sulfate at the 3 position increases their solubility. In addition, chenodeoxycholate is absorbed more efficiently in duodenum and jejunum as compared with the other bile acids.

The rate of bile secretion by canaliculi is not constant but varies with feeding. Let us consider, first, the events during fasting. Bile that enters the gallbladder is concentrated, because up to 90 per cent of the water is absorbed by the gallbladder. Inorganic ions also are absorbed so that the osmotic pressure in gallbladder bile does not increase. Since bile contains little protein, its salt concentration is greater as compared with plasma in order to maintain a physiological osmolality. Bile salts, in contrast to inorganic ions, remain in the lumen of the gallbladder and hence are concentrated. The biological reason for concentrating bile salts in this manner is not clear. On the other hand, the capacity of the gallbladder is limited to about 50 ml. By removing water and inorganic salts, the gallbladder can continue to accept bile secreted by the liver during fasting. For example, the bile salts that pass directly from bile duct to intestinal mucosa are conserved by the terminal ileum. We can expect that one half of these will enter the gallbladder after resecretion into canalicular bile. Eventually, the processes of enterohepatic recirculation and reabsorption of water sequesters nearly the entire pool of bile salts in the gallbladder. If a meal is eaten at this time, all of the bile salt pool is delivered promptly to the small intestine, where it has an important function in ensuring complete absorption of fat and fat-soluble vitamins.

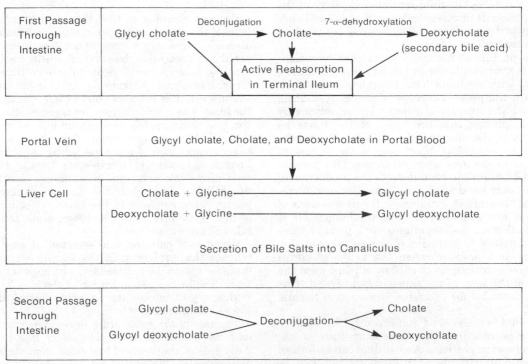

Figure 32. Enterohepatic circulation of glycyl cholate.

The rate (volume) of secretion of bile depends on the amount of bile salts available to be secreted. Bile secretory rates are low in the fasted state because the bulk of the bile salt pool is stored in the gallbladder. Upon eating, however, these enter the intestine, to be reabsorbed eventually into portal blood. Since bile acids circulate rapidly between liver and intestine during periods of active absorption, the amount of bile salt entering liver cells increases during a meal, as compared with fasting, and the rate of bile formation increases. Recirculation of bile salts works to keep a maximal amount of bile salt in the upper portion of the small intestine during meals. The gallbladder does not store bile salts during the day in people eating meals during this time.

The enterohepatic circulation of bile salts is an elaborate, elegant biological system for maximizing intestinal absorption of foods requiring emulsification prior to absorption. Man can function well without a major component of this system—the gallbladder, which seems only to introduce the maximal possible amount of bile salts into the duodenum at the start of a meal. In addition, some species lack a gallbladder. What, then, is the importance of the gallbladder? Possibly, by maximizing absorptive capacity, it had survival value in situations in which food was scarce, and meals unpredictable and spread far apart.

DEFECTS IN THE ENTEROHEPATIC CIRCULATION OF BILE ACIDS

The capacity of the terminal ileum to actively conserve (absorb) bile acids and salts may be destroyed by disease, as in regional enteritis of this segment of the small intestine. Extensive loss of bile acids into the stool results. Hepatic synthesis of cholate and chenodeoxycholate increases in response to excessive loss of bile salts via any route (stool, or T-tube drainage of the biliary tree), and patients with absent or defective reabsorption of bile acids reach a steady state in which daily synthesis equals losses. If losses are large, however, the total pool of bile acids will be reduced in the new steady state because synthetic rates cannot compensate completely. Fat absorption will be less than complete in this setting, and mild to moderate steatorrhea will ensue. A reduced bile salt pool does not produce severe malabsorption, however. In addition to altering absorption, intestinal losses of bile acids secondary to ileal disease interfere with colonic function: bile salts escaping absorption in the terminal ileum enter the colon, where they are deconjugated rapidly by colonic bacteria. The free bile acids stimulate secretion of salt and water by colonic mucosa, producing diarrhea. Disease of the terminal ileum also enhances the likelihood of gallstone formation. The basis for the relationship between ileal function and gallstones is discussed later.

Hepatic disease affects enterohepatic circulation of bile acids by interfering with their removal from portal blood. This may be due to shunting of portal blood away from liver cells in patients with portal hypertension. In addition, uptake of bile acids by hepatocytes seems to be an extremely sensitive index of their function, especially when bile acids are measured in blood two hours after a meal. Increases above normal in plasma concentrations of bile acids are considered

to reflect the portion escaping uptake by the liver. Elevated levels of bile acids are observed in patients with acute and chronic forms of liver disease that appear mild on the basis of other types of liver "function" tests, i.e., transaminase, bilirubin, clotting factors, etc. Abnormal levels of bile acids after a meal have no value, nevertheless, in establishing the cause of liver disease.

Mild degrees of malabsorption are not uncommon in patients with cirrhosis, but it is not known whether defects in the hepatic-uptake limb of the enterohepatic circulation of bile acids contribute to this abnormality.

THE ROLE OF BILE ACIDS IN THE GENESIS OF GALLSTONES

Two types of stones form within the biliary tree—pigment stones and cholesterol stones. The former are combinations of bile pigments and calcium which are insoluble and precipitate in the gallbladder. Bile salts have no significance in the pathogenesis of these, but they do have an important function in the genesis and treatment of cholesterol stones.

Cholesterol is insoluble in water. It is dispersed in bile as a complex with lecithin (phosphatidylcholine) and bile salts, which combine to form a mixed micelle. In brief, the essential characteristic of micelles is that they contain molecules with amphipathic properties; i.e., they have both hydrophobic and hydrophilic portions. When arrayed in micelles, the hydrophobic segments of different molecules are on the interior of the structure, where they interact with each other. Water is excluded from this region. The hydrophilic residues are on the surface, in contact with water. The phenolic hydroxyl group of cholesterol is its hydrophilic residue. It interacts with oxygen atoms of the polar head groups of phospholipids. The hydroxyl groups of the bile acid and the carboxyl of the conjugated amino acid interact with water. Since these all are located on the same side of the planar ring system of the bile acid, the bile salts have a hydrophobic surface and a hydrophilic one. Cholesterol within a micelle will not precipitate out of the bile. Precipitation of cholesterol in bile depends on how much can be incorporated into micelles and how much is free in solution. Micelle formation is determined by the amounts of lecithin and bile salts secreted by the canaliculi. Cholesterol precipitates from bile when there is insufficient lecithin and/or bile salt to keep it "solubilized," that is, dispersed as part of a micelle.

The relative amounts of cholesterol, phospholipid (lecithin), and bile salts secreted by the canaliculi are not independent of each other. At low rates of bile formation, which occur when there is limited bile salt available to hepatocytes, the secretion of cholesterol is excessive in relation to phospholipid. This type of bile tends to be saturated with cholesterol and is likely to allow formation of cholesterol stones because secreted cholesterol is not incorporated completely into stable micelles. This reflects relative deficiency of both phospholipid and bile salts. Bile is supersaturated with cholesterol in 25 per cent of fasted individuals who do not have cholesterol stones. This group is especially at risk for the eventual development of stones. In contrast, high rates of bile secretion by hepatocytes, which are produced by infusing bile salts (or during a meal), are accompanied by a relatively large secretion of phospholipid as compared with cholesterol. Bile, in this setting, is not saturated with cholesterol. The saturation of bile with cholesterol varies with the time of day, even in the normal individual without evidence of stones.

Defining samples of bile as being supersaturated with cholesterol or containing an amount of cholesterol that is solubilized adequately by the bile salts and phospholipid present in the bile does not completely delineate patients with and without gallstones. There appear to be other factors involved, and these are referred to as nucleation factors. Nevertheless, on the basis of the above physiological description, we can conclude that the size of the bile salt pool is important for production of gallstones. Small pools will lead to secretion of bile that contains inadequate phospholipid and bile salt to "solubilize" all the cholesterol secreted. This is why the incidence of gallstones is high in patients with ileal disease. The size of the bile salt pool is not the only factor in the production of cholesterol stones. Thus, there are patients who seem to add an inappropriately large amount of cholesterol to the normal amounts of bile salts and lecithin secreted. This seems to be true of patients who are grossly obese; such patients can be considered to have a primary abnormality in production of bile, whereas those with ileal disease have a secondary abnormality. Interestingly, patients with primary derangements in bile production, from the point of view of saturation of bile with cholesterol, respond to exogenously administered bile acids. Thus, oral ingestion of chenodeoxycholate increases the amount of this bile salt in the bile of patients with cholesterol stores. At the same time, the bile of these patients becomes unsaturated with respect to cholesterol; and stones already present dissolve. Cholate is much less useful as a therapeutic agent for the treatment of bile supersaturated with cholesterol as compared with chenodeoxycholate. A possible reason for this difference is that chenodeoxycholate, as compared with cholate, forms micelles at a significantly lower concentration (the critical micelle concentration).

The synthesis of cholate and chenodeoxycholate is regulated in some manner by their levels in portal blood; i.e., there is feedback inhibition. Loss of bile acids via the stool removes inhibition and allows synthesis to accelerate. It is proposed that feedback inhibition is oversensitive (that is, inhibited by relatively low concentrations of bile acid) in some patients with cholesterol stones. This would lead to a reduced pool of bile salts on a primary basis and cause supersaturation of bile followed by cholesterol stones. This concept is undocumented.

MOTOR FUNCTION OF THE GALLBLADDER

The biliary tree in man is separated from the duodenum by the sphincter of Oddi. There also may be a sphincteric mechanism in the cystic duct. Contraction of the gallbadder during a meal must occur concomitantly with relaxation of these sphincters if bile is to flow into the small intestine. Integration of motor functions within the biliary tract is effected by chole-cystokinin and pancreozymin, which are released from duodenal mucosa in response to influx of gastric contents. These hormones stimulate contraction of the gallbladder and relaxation of the sphincter of Oddi.

REFERENCES

Alpern, R. J.: Renal sodium retention in liver disease—Medical Staff Conference, University of California, San Francisco. West J Med 138:852, 1983.

Beker, S. (ed.): Diagnostic Procedures in the Evaluation of Hepatic Diseases. New York, Alan R. Liss, Inc., 1983.

Blanckaert, N., and Schmid, R.: Physiology and pathophysiology of bilirubin metabolism. In Zakim, D., and Boyer, T. D. (eds.): Hepatology: A Textbook of Liver Disease. Philadelphia, W. B. Saunders Co., 1982, p. 246.

Cohen, S.: A review of hypoglycemia and alcoholism with or without liver disease. Ann NY Acad Sci 273:338, 1976.

Conney, A. H., Pantuck, E. J., Hsiao, K.-C., et al.: Regulation of drug metabolism in man by environmental chemicals and diet. Fed Proc 36:1647, 1977.

Epstein, M. (ed.): The Kidney in Liver Disease, 2nd ed. New York, Elsevier, 1983.

Glomset, J. A., Norum, K. R., and Gjone, E.: Familial lecithin: Cholesterol acyltransferase deficiency. In Stanbury, J. B., Wyngaarden, J. B., Fredrickson, D. S., et al. (eds.): The Metabolic Basis of Inherited Disease. 5th ed. New York, McGraw-Hill Book Co., 1983, p. 643.

Green, J. R. B.: Mechanism of hypogonadism in cirrhotic males. Gut 18:843, 1977.

Hofmann, A. F.: The enterohepatic circulation of bile acids in man. Clin Gastroenterol 6:3, 1977.

Howell, R. R., and Williams, J. C.: The glycogen storage diseases. In Stanbury, J. B., Wyngaarden, J. B., Fredrickson, D. S., et al. (eds.): The Metabolic Basis of Inherited Disease. 5th ed. New York, McGraw-Hill Book Co., 1983, p. 141.

Jones, A. L., and Schmucker, D. L.: Current concepts of liver structure as related to function. Gastroenterology 73:833, 1977.

Lickley, H. L. A., Chisholm, D. J., Rabinovitch, A., et al.: Effects of portacaval anastomosis on glucose tolerance in the dog: Evidence of an interaction between the gut and the liver in oral glucose disposal. Metabolism 24:1157, 1975.

Mitchell, J. R., and Jollows, D. J.: Metabolic activation of drugs to toxic substances. Gastroenterology 68:392, 1975.

Newsholme, E. A.: Role of the liver in integration of fat and carbohydrate metabolism and clinical implications in patients with liver disease. Prog Liver Dis 5:125, 1976.

Popper, H., and Schaffner, F. (eds.): Progress in Liver Diseases 7. New York, Grune and Stratton, 1982.

Scharschmidt, B. F.: Cholestasis—Medical Staff Conference, University of California, San Francisco. West J Med 138:233, 1983.

Small, D. M.: The etiology and pathogenesis of gallstones. Adv Surg 10:63, 1976.

Smith, L. C., Pownall, H. J., and Gotto, A. M., Jr.: The plasma lipoproteins: Structure and metabolism. Annu Rev Biochem 47:751, 1978.

Unikowsky, B., Wexler, M. J., and Levy, M.: Dogs with experimental cirrhosis of the liver but without intrahepatic hypertension do not retain sodium or form ascites. J Clin Invest 72:1594, 1983.

Walser, M.: Urea cycle disorders and other hereditary hyperammonemic syndromes. In Stanbury, J. B., Wyngaarden, J. B., Fredrickson, D. S., et al. (eds.): The Metabolic Basis of Inherited Disease. 5th ed. New York, McGraw-Hill Book Co., 1983, p. 402.

Wilkinson, S. P.: Hepatorenal Disorders. New York, Marcel Dekker, Inc., 1982.

Zakim, D., and Boyer, T. D. (eds.): Hepatology: A Textbook of Liver Disease. Philadelphia, W. B. Saunders Co., 1982.

PATHOPHYSIOLOGY OF SKIN

THOMAS B. FITZPATRICK, M.D.,
and NICHOLAS A. SOTER, M.D.

The skin (and its tissue paper–thin epidermis) envelops the body and contains the internal fluid milieu, and therefore plays a major role in the human's ability to maintain homeostasis. Inasmuch as it is composed of epithelial, mesenchymal, glandular, and neurovascular elements, the skin is much more than an inert body sheathing. It can prevent damage to underlying tissues from many external physical stimuli, such as ultraviolet radiation, by virtue of its melanin pigment, and also from mechanical forces by the adipose and connective tissue that acts as a pad over muscles and bones. With its capacity for self-regeneration following injury, the skin continuously provides a barrier that impedes the entrance of noxious chemicals and of harmful microbiologic agents. With its vast, complex, and readily adaptable vascular network, the skin plays a vital role in thermoregulation and in the inflammatory response.

What is unique about skin in the perspective of general medicine? For the clinician, the skin is a mirror of internal disease. It is a microcosm of the major epithelial and mesenchymal elements present in all organs, and it is directly visible to the eye of the clinician. Thus, the lesions of multisystem disease are often displayed for the physician in the detection of diseases of other organs. Furthermore, dynamic pathologic processes, such as inflammation and neoplastic growths, and alterations in hemodynamics or in fluid balance, or in cell kinetics, are reflected clinically as erythema, desquamation, nodules, ulcers, and the like. Such changes are readily studied, by easily obtainable biopsy specimens, with light and electron microscopy and with immunofluorescence techniques. The "gross" pathology and the microscopic histology can therefore be investigated in disorders arising in the skin, or in disorders associated with diseases of other organs that also involve the skin.

The integrity of the integument is vital for motion. A breakdown of the skin surface can be likened to corrosion of the metal surface of a delicate instrument. It is obvious that an intact, healthy skin of the hands is essential for the performance of intricate tasks, and that a fissured, thickened, dry skin can temporarily or permanently disable a skilled craftsman, whether a surgeon, a dentist, or a machine tool operator.

The integument, a multifunctional interface, mediating influences of the environment on the organism, is a major determinant in the life and behavior of all species. Behavioral patterns of the individual and of the group are also affected by the integument—for example, reactions of avoidance to individuals with various scars and disfigurements. Sometimes the disfigured are neglected and isolated. The relegation, in the past, of the dermatologic ward to some sequestered part of the hospital is only one expression of the general aversion, even by physicians, to the unaesthetic nature of skin disease.

The skin is a unique organ for the study of experimental pathology and for exploring fundamental mechanisms of disease, inasmuch as it is the most accessible solid tissue. The one-gene–one-enzyme concept was initiated by Sir Archibald Garrod's study of albinism. Transplantation immunity was evolved by a series of studies using mouse skin, conducted by Sir Peter Medawar and his collaborators. These experiments, done to develop methods for treating severely burned patients with homografts, proved that the rejection phenomenon results from delayed hypersensitivity reactions. This was the beginning of transplantation immunity, but it did not solve the problem of the severely burned patient. Now some 40 years later with the advances in cell biology of the principal epidermal cell (the keratinocyte), there are some new approaches to the treatment of the extensively burned patient. Large sheets of a patient's own keratinocytes can be grown in tissue culture for grafting after burns, thus avoiding the rejection phenomenon.

STRUCTURE AND FUNCTION

GENERAL VIEW OF SKIN

Human skin is a tough but flexible and self-repairing membrane that invests the contents of the body; a "live clothing" that covers, contains, and protects because "nature abhors exposed mesenchyme." It is layered, not homogeneous. There are three principal layers (Table 1): (1) the outermost, and only visible layer, the *epidermis*; (2) the *dermis*, which is what one feels when the skin is palpated, since the epidermis is paperthin; (3) the *panniculus adiposus* (subcutaneous tissue), which acts as a cushion between the bone and the epidermis and dermis. Each layer is structurally and functionally unique, but the epidermis and dermis are interdependent throughout prenatal and postnatal life.

The epidermis is a mixture of cells of different embryonic origin and function; the dermis is a melange, composed of a dense fibrous connective tissue stroma, a complex network of blood and lymphatic vessels and nerves, specialized glands and appendages derived from the epidermis, and a population of various types of cells: histiocytes, macrophages, mast cells, and mononuclear cells. The panniculus adiposus is a specialized layer of connective tissue containing, predominantly, fat cells. Because of its special function as a

TABLE 1. INTEGRATION OF STRUCTURE, FUNCTION, AND PATHOLOGY OF HUMAN SKIN

ANATOMIC COMPARTMENT	PRINCIPAL FUNCTIONS	
EPIDERMIS—STRATUM CORNEUM	Protective Layer	
Dried, flattened keratinocytes; a multicellular membrane	Permeability Barrier	The barrier layer of the skin that impedes the entrance of microorganisms and toxic substances and retains water and electrolytes
EPIDERMIS—MALPIGHIAN LAYERS	Body's Sheath	Contains and encloses milieu intérieur
Highly cellular; no blood vessels or nerves:		
Keratinocytes 80%	Synthesis of Keratin Precursors	Synthesis of tonofilaments and keratohyalin, and transformation into stratum corneum cell
Melanocytes 5–10%	Synthesis of Melanin	Protection against damaging ultraviolet radiation by melanin in the malpighian layer and stratum corneum
Langerhans' cells 5–10%	Immunologic Function	Involved in cell-mediated immune reactions
BASEMENT MEMBRANE	Support and Attachment for Epidermis	During development, provides substratum for developing epidermis, and may play some part in epidermal differentiation; postnatally, provides point of limitation and attachment for basal keratinocytes
Light microscopy: PAS-positive zone at epidermal-dermal interface	Epidermal-Dermal Adherence	
Electron microscopy: Basal lamina of ectodermal origin; a fibrilloamorphous layer beneath basal keratinocytes; subbasal lamina fibrous elements of papillary dermis; anchoring fibrils and microfibrils		? Permeability barrier
		Attach basal lamina firmly to dermis
DERMIS		
Loose connective tissue consisting of:		
Fibrous protein:	Mechanical Protection	Passively protects against trauma, and maintains the body's integrity by virtue of the envelopment of the body with a strong and flexible composite material—i.e., collagen and ground substance
collagen		
reticulin		
elastin		
Ground substance	Main Support Structure of Skin; Water Binding	Actively determines wound repair, provides both a reservoir and a diffusion medium for regulating the distribution of water, salts, hormones, and other substances; contains essential elements (cells, mediators) of inflammatory and immunologic reactions
cells		
fibroblasts		
macrophages		
mast cells		
lymphocytes		
VASCULATURE		
A three-dimensional meshwork with two predominant planes that comprise plexuses oriented parallel to the surface and located in the papillary dermis and deep in the reticular dermis	Thermoregulation	Carries oxygen and nutrients to skin
	Skin Color	A major factor in thermoregulation through a series of AV shunts
LYMPHATICS		
Composed of lymph capillaries, postcapillary lymph vessels, and deep lymph vessels	Drainage System	Removal of cells, solutes, and proteins
NERVES		
Schwann cells, neurites, and connective tissue sheaths:		
Somatic sensory	Sensory Perception	Mediation of touch, pain, temperature, and itch
Autonomic	Secretomotor	Control of vessels, glands, and piloreaction
APPENDAGES		
Eccrine sweat glands	Thermoregulation	Eccrine sweat glands secrete water and salts
Apocrine sweat glands		Apocrine sweat glands secrete lipids and proteins
Sebaceous glands	Lubrication	Sebaceous glands secrete lipids
Hair follicles	Protection	Hair protects from sun, wind, and physical trauma; hair has a social function
	Heat Insulation	Presence of thick, fatty tissue helps conserve body's heat
PANNICULUS ADIPOSUS		
Connective tissue specialized in the formation of fat		Serves as a mechanical shock absorber, reducing trauma to underlying tissue
Contains large blood vessels, lymphatics, and nerves		Provides a reserve depot of calories; during starvation this metabolic reservoir is rapidly drained
		Larger blood vessels through countercurrent flow help conserve heat

TABLE 1. INTEGRATION OF STRUCTURE, FUNCTION, AND PATHOLOGY OF HUMAN SKIN (*Continued*)

BIOLOGIC PROCESS	PATHOLOGY	REPRESENTATIVE DISEASE
Desquamation	Altered rate of desquamation Malformation of stratum corneum (often more porous)	Psoriasis, exfoliative dermatitis Ichthyosis vulgaris Ichthyosiform dermatoses
	Acantholysis by autoantibodies	Pemphigus
Keratinogenesis and keratinization	Disturbances in keratinogenesis	Ichthyosiform dermatoses
Melanogenesis and transfer of melanosomes	Increased melanization Decreased melanization	Addison's disease Albinism
Antigen recognition and processing	Proliferation of Langerhans' cells	Contact eczematous dermatitis
Morphogenesis and epidermal-dermal interaction	Thickening of basement membrane Lysis of basement membrane	Lupus erythematosus
	Lysis of basement membrane by autoantibodies	Pemphigoid
Synthesis or maturation of collagen, etc.	Solar degeneration of collagen Elastic tissue degeneration	Solar elastosis Pseudoxanthoma elasticum
Inflammatory reactivity Wound healing	*Papillary dermis:* most strictly cutaneous disorders involve the papillary dermis; superficial venules are usually involved in inflammatory reactions (erythema, edema, and extravasation) *Reticular dermis:* systemic diseases usually involve the lower-lying reticular dermis	Urticaria Scleroderma
Inflammatory reactivity Wound healing	Dilatation/constriction Occlusion (intravascular thrombosis) Acute, subacute, and chronic inflammation of venules	Raynaud's phenomenon Purpura fulminans Necrotizing vasculitis
Draining of exudate, especially proteins and cells from sites of inflammation	Dilatation of lymphatics	Lymphangitis, streptococcal
Afferent impulse transmission	Inflammation of peripheral nerves	Herpes zoster (hypesthesia, anesthesia, or hyperesthesia)
Efferent impulse transmission		Pruritus
Eccrine sweat secretion	Profuse sweating (salt loss) Cessation of sweating Congenital absence of sweat gland Resorption malfunction Mechanical occlusion of duct	Heat cramps, heat exhaustion Anhidrosis or heat hyperpyrexia, heat stroke Anhidrotic ectodermal dysplasia Cystic fibrosis Anhidrosis, miliaria
Apocrine sweat secretion Secretion of lipids Formation of hair	Inflammation of apocrine glands Comedo formation Altered production and malformation	Hidradenitis suppurativa Acne Alopecia, hirsutism
Fat synthesis	Fat necrosis Septal inflammation (acute and chronic) Loss of fat cells	Panniculitis associated with pancreatitis Erythema nodosum Lipodystrophy

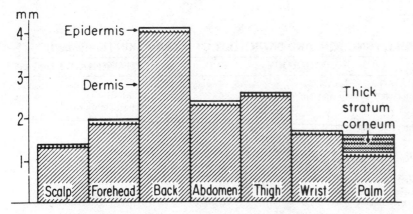

Figure 1. Diagrammatic representation of regional variations in thickness of skin. (From Fitzpatrick, T. B., Arndt, K. A., Clark, W. H., Jr., Eisen, A. Z., Van Scott, E. J., and Vaughan, J. H. (eds.): Dermatology in General Medicine. New York, McGraw-Hill Book Co., 1971.)

mechanical cushion, the panniculus is quite thick in certain regions (buttocks and abdomen) and virtually absent in other areas (face, dorsum of the hands).

The skin is the largest organ in the body, weighing 3 to 4 kg, two to three times the weight of the liver, and it constitutes approximately 6 per cent of the body weight. The average thickness (mm) of each of the three layers is as follows:

	Epidermis	Dermis	Subcutaneous
AVG (mm)	0.07–0.17	1.7–2.0	4.0–9.0
MAX	1.56	3.0	30
MIN	0.042	0.6	0.6

The skin varies in thickness in different regions of the body: thickest on the back and thinnest on the scalp and palm, thicker on the dorsal and extensor than on the ventral and flexor surfaces, thicker in men than in women (Fig. 1).

THE FUNCTIONAL HISTOLOGY OF THE SKIN

This section is an elaboration of the material presented in Table 1. This table should be followed for integration of *structure, principal functions, biologic processes, pathology,* and *clinical disease.*

Epidermis: Stratum Corneum. Scraping the skin with a sharp instrument results in the appearance of barely visible flakes of skin. This is the *stratum corneum,* or horny layer, which is the outermost layer of the epidermis. The anucleate, cornified epidermal cells of the stratum corneum have a thick cell membrane that is chemically resistant. The horny layer is 10 μm thick, but on specialized regions, such as the palms, it is 500 μm thick.

The horny layer is the principal barrier against the transfer of water and various ions, molecules, and microorganisms. The stratum corneum, however, is supple and elastic and withstands shearing and compression. A thickened stratum corneum—two to three times normal, as in certain genetic keratinization disorders—is much more impervious, but it is also inelastic, and makes grasping motions of the hand impossible. Because the skin is in equilibrium with dry air, the water content of the stratum corneum is comparatively low. Water loss through the stratum corneum is apparently a passive diffusion process, and the rate of water loss is a function of the difference in the concentration gradient on the two sides of the stratum corneum.

Epidermis: Malpighian Layer. The epidermis is composed of four cell types: (1) keratinocytes, arranged as an organized, stratified epithelium with epithelial appendages that project into the lower dermis (sweat glands, sebaceous glands, and hair follicles); (2) melanocytes; (3) Langerhans' cells, and (4) Merkel cells. Of these cell types, by far the most numerous is the keratinocyte, which comprises 80 per cent of the cells of the epidermis and is therefore the main structural element of the epidermis. Without keratinocytes there is no epidermis; melanocytes can be completely absent, as in vitiligo, and yet the epidermis functions normally except as a density filter for ultraviolet radiation.

The malpighian layer can be subdivided on the basis of the three stages of differentiation of the keratinocyte (Fig. 2): (1) the almost cuboidal germinal *basal cells,* which lie on the basal lamina; (2) the *stratum spinosum,* which is several layers of polyhedral cells above

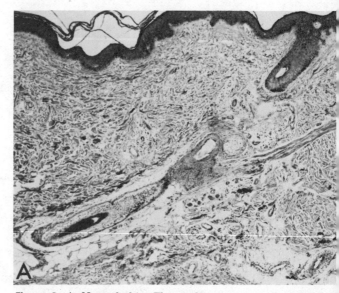

Figure 2. *A,* Normal skin. The epidermis crosses the upper portion of the micrograph. The narrow zone of dermis immediately deep to the epidermis is the papillary dermis, while most of the micrograph shows the collagen bundles of the reticular dermis. Traversing the picture from lower left to upper right there is a pilar unit with its associated arrector pili muscle. ×40. (Micrograph by Wallace H. Clark, Jr., M.D.)

Illustration continued on opposite page

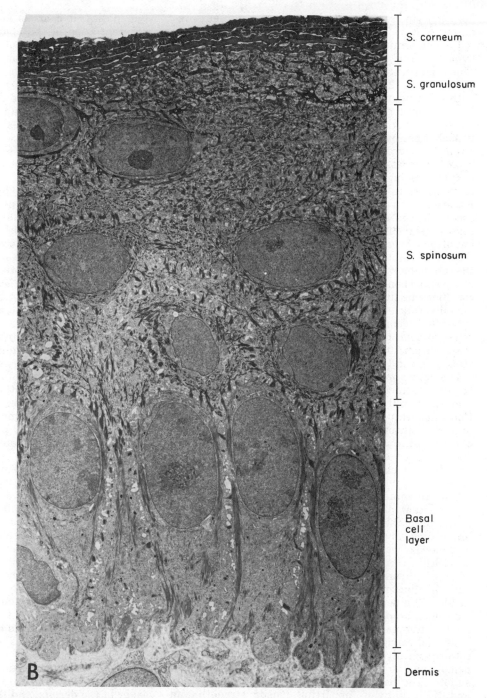

S. corneum

S. granulosum

S. spinosum

Basal
cell
layer

Dermis

B

Figure 2. *Continued. B*, Electron micrograph shows epidermis with four or five of the lowermost layers of the stratum corneum. × 2900. (From Fitzpatrick, T. B., Arndt, K. A., Clark, W. H., Jr., Eisen, A. Z., Van Scott, E. J., and Vaughan, J. H. (eds.): Dermatology in General Medicine. New York, McGraw-Hill Book Co., 1971.)

the basal cells; and (3) the *stratum granulosum*, composed of darkly staining, flattened, nucleated cells that contain distinctive keratohyaline granules.

As the surface layers of the epidermis are lost, the maintenance of a constant thickness of the epidermis depends on a replacement of lost keratinocytes by mitotic proliferation in the germinal basal cell layer. There are structurally and functionally distinct populations of basal cells. Some of the basal cells may represent the epidermal stem cell population; others may have an anchoring function. Above the basal layer, the epidermal cells are organized into units, in which a number of germinative and differentiated cells are surmounted by a single flat stratum corneum cell. These vertical columns of stacked cells may influence

ordered cell movement during differentiation and desquamation.

The major structural protein of the epidermis is keratin, which has a helical configuration and is organized into intracellular intermediate filaments. Keratins consist of a family of polypeptides of molecular weights ranging from 40 to 70 kilodaltons (kd). As yet no specific keratin markers for diseases have been described, but one can relate specific keratins to morphological and functional events. For example, the characteristic keratins of hyperproliferative epidermis are somewhat different from those in normal keratinizing epidermis. Keratins are not unique to the skin; they occur in other epithelia, such as esophagus and cornea. This differentiation and maturation of the keratinocyte from basal cell to stratum corneum requires 26 days.

The epidermis as a tightly knit membrane is secured by a "locking" mechanism between epidermal cells. This complex structure between keratinocytes is called a *desmosome*. The cytoplasm of keratinocytes is filled with prominent intercellular filaments that attach to the internal face of the desmosome, thereby providing a rigid but flexible network of keratinocytes connected to each other by desmosomes, and ensuring the tensile strength by this kind of "wiring" system of intracellular filaments.

Synthesis of fibrous and nonfibrous epidermal proteins occurs in the cytoplasm of the living epidermis. Keratinization begins in the basal cell layer. As cells ascend in the epidermis, synthesis of new filaments ceases and a change in orientation of fibers occurs; the bundles of fibers become aligned to the surface of the skin. The viable cells are then dramatically changed: the cell membrane becomes thickened and a thick layer is deposited beneath the cell membrane. Keratinization concludes in the stratum corneum, when the cell organelles (nuclei, mitochondria, ribosomes) disappear, the cells become dehydrated, the cell membranes become further thickened, and the water content decreases from 70 per cent in the viable keratinocytes to 10 per cent in the stratum corneum.

The active protein synthetic processes that are present in keratinocytes are evident in the ultrastructure: there is a well-developed endoplasmic reticulum and Golgi apparatus and a well-developed ribosomal system. Keratinocytes also possess the capacity for phagocytosis, which permits degradation of ingested materials. A good example of phagocytosis is the active transfer of melanosomes to keratinocytes by melanocytes.

The Basement Membrane Zone. The anatomic region situated between the epidermis and the dermis is the dermal-epidermal junction or basement membrane zone. The basement membrane, although a homogeneous band when examined with periodic acid–Schiff (PAS) stain and light microscopy, consists of four components: (1) basal cell plasma membrane with hemidesmosomes; (2) a clear zone or lamina lucida; (3) a dense basal lamina, consisting of a basement membrane of epidermal origin; and (4) subbasal lamina fibrous elements—anchoring fibrils, microfibrils, and collagen. The lucent zone contains the noncollagenous glycoproteins laminin, fibronectin, bullous pemphigoid antigen, and the proteoglycan heparan sulfate. The basal lamina contains type IV collagen and KF-1 antigen, imparting tensile strength and elasticity.

The basement membrane has three roles: it anchors the epidermis to the dermis, provides mechanical support for the epidermis, and acts as a barrier to cells and molecules, larger than 40 Kd. The basement membrane is the central tissue element in several dermatologic diseases: systemic lupus erythematosus, bullous pemphigoid, and dermatitis herpetiformis.

Dermis. The mechanical strength of the skin is in the dermis. This is the part that "sculptures" the skin with flexure lines, furrows, and folds; fingerprints are simply alternating patterns of dermal ridges and sulci. The richly vascular dermis is the "mother" tissue to the epidermis, which possesses no blood vessels or lymphatics. It controls and specifies the growth and differentiation of the epidermis and plays the major role in the development of the various specialized patterns of the epidermis. This control is by inductive interactions between the dermis and the epidermis. Dermal inductive agents may act selectively on a series of "epithelial genes" and direct the type of differentiation—the thick epidermis of palms and soles, or the thin epidermis of the flexural skin. The dermis, which is 1 to 4 mm in thickness, is made up of tough fibroelastic tissue that comprises 20 per cent of wet weight and serves to protect against mechanical injury. Because it binds water, the dermis is a reservoir for body water and electrolytes; and because it contains a complex, rich, vascular network, it has a major role in temperature regulation. Its network of nerves provides the sensory contact of the body with the environment.

Most of the fibrous protein of the dermis is collagen, which has a high tensile strength. Only a small portion of the dermis is elastic tissue. The amorphous ground substance of the dermis is a viscoelastic gel that serves as the matrix for the fibrous proteins and consists mainly of mucopolysaccharides, hyaluronates, and chondroitin sulfates. The function of the ground substance in the dermis is not fully understood, but it is thought to provide mechanical strength and to contribute resistance when the skin is compressed.

A mixed population of cells is found in the dermis: fibroblasts (which synthesize collagen), mast cells (which play an important role in inflammation), lymphocytes in small numbers, and monocyte-macrophages, termed "dermal phagocytes." The structure of the dermal phagocyte changes, depending on the level of phagocytic activity.

Vasculature. The skin color is largely due to the melanin content in the epidermis but it also reflects the content of blood in a complex and rich system of arteries, arterioles, capillaries, venules, and veins. The function of the vascular system in the dermis is largely one of temperature regulation, although this system also supplies the nutrient and metabolic needs of the dermis and the epidermis. It also serves to store large quantities of blood in the skin, which can be directed to other parts of the body. This occurs via a specialized vascular architecture that includes a large subcutaneous venous plexus and arteriovenous anastomoses between the arteries and the venous plexus, located in areas frequently exposed to cold (feet, hands, lips, nose, and ears).

The extensive three-dimensional vascular network contains two predominant planes: one in the papillary layer of the dermis, and the other deep in the dermis. The vertical communicating vessels connect the superficial and deep large-vessel networks. (Fig. 3*A* and *B*.) The cutaneous microvasculature is described in greater detail later in this chapter.

Lymphatics. The lymphatics remove cells, water, protein, and other products from the extracellular environment of the dermis in a centripetal, one-way path. The lymphatics are disposed as large sinuses in the papillary dermis, draining into collecting trunks that follow the course of the communicating vascular channels to the subcutaneous lymphatic trunks. The large trunks of lymphatics in the subcutaneous layer have thick walls containing muscles and valves to ensure a one-way direction, while in the papillary

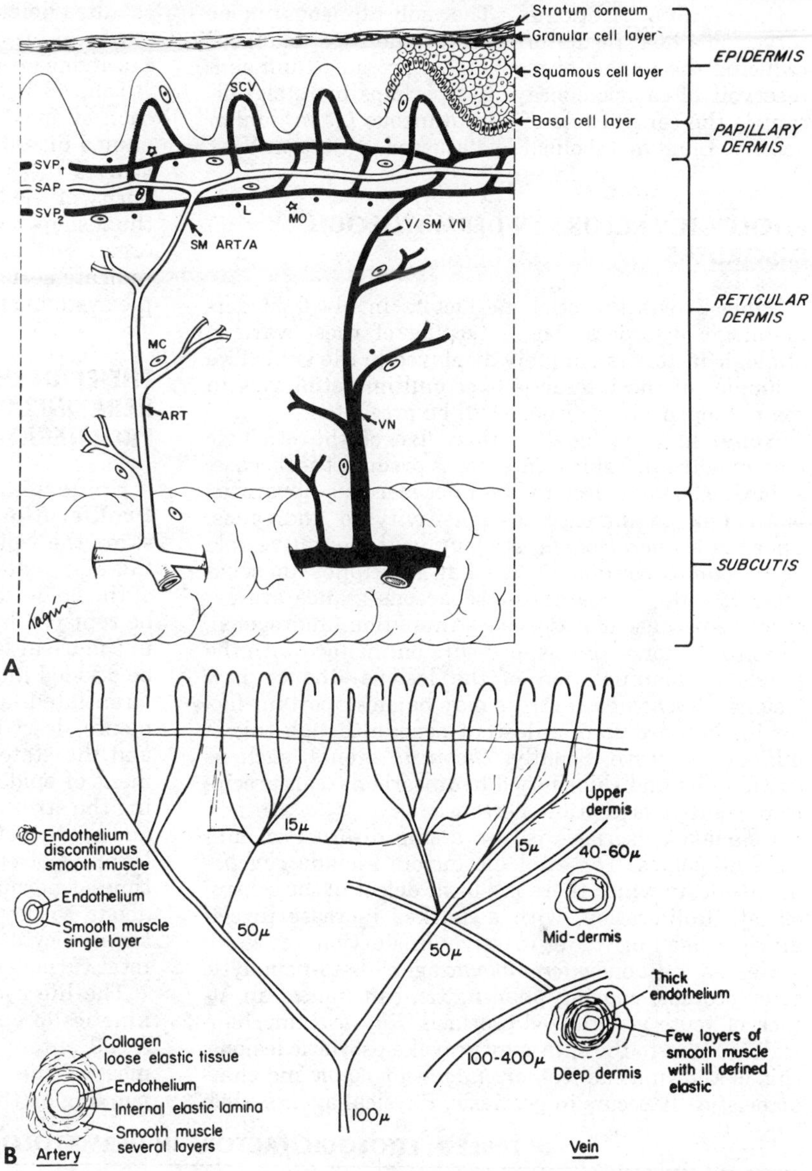

Figure 3. *A*, Vascular network in adult skin. (From Soter, N. A., and Mihm, M. C., Jr.: Cutaneous necrotizing venulitis. In Moschella, S. L. (ed.): Dermatology Update: Reviews for Physicians. New York, Elsevier-North-Holland, 1979.) *B*, Diagram of vascular pattern and structure in adult skin with relative sizes of the vessels. (From Jarratt, A. (ed.): The Physiology and Pathophysiology of the Skin. Vol. 2. London and New York, Academic Press, 1973.)

dermis they have thin walls lined by only a single layer of endothelial cells.

Nerves. The skin is the antenna of the body, the sensing organ, composed of a vast network of free and encapsulated nerve endings that convey impulses to the central nervous system for integration. A series of mosaics of various sensitivities are spread on the skin surface. Some receptors are free nerve terminals that sense temperature (heat and cold); other free nerve terminals mediate pain and itch. Mechanoreceptors include specialized, encapsulated corpuscles (Meissner's and pacinian) and unencapsulated nerve terminals, forming nets around hairs. The autonomic nerve supply of the skin appears to be entirely sympathetic. The autonomic terminals are adrenergic, cholinergic, and pruinergic. Blood vessels and the errector pili muscles are supplied with both adrenergic and cholinergic fibers; eccrine sweat glands are exclusively supplied with cholinergic fibers, while sebaceous and apocrine glands have no detectable nerve supply.

There are no demonstrable free nerve endings in the nonhairy epidermis. In the superficial dermis, unmyelinated fibers predominate, but it is impossible to designate from the morphology whether they are somatic, sensory, or autonomic. In the subepidermal region, the perineural sheath is lost and the Schwann cell–axonal processes are in direct contact with the collagen.

The subcutaneous and mid-dermis contain nerves with an epineural sheath of layers of collagen fibers, blood vessels, mast cells, and fibroblasts, within which there is a perineural sheath of endothelium-like cells and collagen that encloses a compartment occupied by myelinated and unmyelinated fibers and endoneural collagen.

Appendages. The structure and function of the appendages are so intimately connected that the functional histology will be discussed elsewhere in this chapter, in the sections dealing with sebaceous glands, sweat glands, and hair.

Panniculus Adiposus. The subcutaneous layer serves as a heat insulator, as a "cushion" or "bumper" reducing the impact of mechanical pressure, and as a reservoir of caloric energy. But perhaps more significant is the central role of subcutaneous fat in human obesity. Lipid metabolism is discussed in Section VI.

ETIOLOGIC FACTORS IN DERMATOLOGIC DISORDERS

Table 2 lists the etiologic factors involved in dermatologic disorders. The interplay of these various etiologic factors is uniquely displayed in the skin. Two examples of the interactions of multiple etiologies in the pathogenesis of disease will be presented.

Acne. In acne, no less than five of the etiologic factors listed in Table 3 interact to produce the disease. A basic *genetic* defect in the pilosebaceous apparatus is thought to increase its sensitivity to androgens. There is a *microbiologic* etiology in the putative role of *Propionibacterium acnes* that multiplies in sebaceous glands. Furthermore, sebaceous glands are overactive because of *endocrine* stimulation (androgens). *Physical* factors—that is, pressure on the face with the hands or manipulation of the lesions—induce new lesions. *Psychological* stress may be an important factor in the flare-up of quiescent acne, although this is difficult to prove. Finally, *chemical* agents, such as cutting oils and chlorinated hydrocarbons, can precipitate acne in susceptible persons.

Psoriasis. Psoriasis is also a skin disorder of multiple etiologies. The etiologic factors include *genetic-metabolic*, in which there is a basic defect in the control of cell proliferation, with a marked increase in cell division leading to a massive production of white scales. At least one *microbiologic* agent, beta-hemolytic streptococcus, causing pharyngitis, can induce an attack of acute generalized psoriasis. *Physical* (mechanical) trauma to the skin may provoke psoriatic lesions: this is known as an *isomorphic phenomenon* and characteristically occurs in psoriasis. Physical agents, such

as ultraviolet light, can also bring about a marked flare of psoriasis. *Chemical* agents, such as practalone, can induce psoriasis.

Table 3 lists a few examples of diseases caused by each of the 12 etiologic factors. There are over 3000 named disorders of the skin—the majority arising *sui generis* in the skin. Although comprising only a minority of the total number of dermatologic alterations, the lesions that are manifestations of disease in other organ systems are more important because they may indicate serious general medical problems—for example systemic scleroderma.

THE EPIDERMIS: DISORDERS OF KERATINIZATION AND OF EPIDERMAL PROLIFERATION

Epidermal Differentiation, Morphogenesis, and Proliferation. The stratified squamous epithelium of skin, the epidermis, is a renewing cell population. Cellular material in the superficial stratum corneum of the epidermis is shed into the outer environment, to be replaced by new cells constantly formed by mitosis in the basal layer (Fig. 4). The epidermis (Fig. 2B) can be divided into three compartments—germinative, differentiated, and cornified. The size of these compartments, described previously, varies with body location and the state of tissue normalcy. The third compartment of epidermal cells, the stratum corneum overlying the stratum granulosum, is considered a nonviable end product of epidermal cell differentiation. By isotope labeling of epidermal proteins, the average turnover time of normal stratum corneum was estimated to be about 15 days. By means of desquamation rates and keratinocyte counts in normal human epidermis, a total turnover time of 30 days was calculated.

The life cycle of cells can be analyzed to study the kinetics of epidermal cell proliferation. After mitosis, a cell enters the G_1 interphase period and carries on most of the metabolic activities of the cell line. Depending on the cell type, G_1 may vary in duration from

TABLE 2. ETIOLOGIC FACTORS IN DERMATOLOGIC DISORDERS

Immunologic and Inflammatory	Physical Biologic Chemical Genetic Metabolic Endocrine Developmental Degenerative Psychologic Nutritional	Proliferative and Neoplastic

Skin Disease and Skin Manifestations of Multisystem Disease

TABLE 3. EXAMPLES OF DISEASE PROCESSES ILLUSTRATING ETIOLOGIC FACTORS IN DERMATOLOGY

ETIOLOGIC FACTOR	DISORDER	CLINICAL FINDINGS	MECHANISM
Physical: cold	Cryoglobulinemia	Urticaria; arthritis; purpura	Thrombosis of small vessels by immune globulin complexes
Chemical	Arsenical intoxication	Palmar hyperkeratoses; squamous cell carcinoma of skin, bladder, and lung	?Somatic mutation
Microbiologic	Herpes zoster	Pain; unilateral vesicles in the distribution of a sensory nerve	Viral replication in a peripheral ganglion and retrograde spread to the skin
Genetic	Xeroderma pigmentosum (autosomal recessive)	Severe actinic damage, including sun-induced malignancies (melanoma, carcinoma, sarcoma)	Defective repair replication of DNA
Endocrine	Addison's disease	Diffuse generalized brown hyperpigmentation	Increased secretion of pituitary hormones (ACTH and α-MSH), which stimulate melanogenesis
Developmental	Congenital melanocytic "garment" nevus	Extensive, raised, hairy pigmented plaques that cover the "bathing trunk" area, or the shoulders	Spontaneous mutation leading to increased numbers of altered melanocytes
Metabolic	Gout	Salmon-pink nodules on the helix of the ear and the digits of the hands and feet	Deposits of crystals of monosodium urate that provoke an acute inflammation
Nutritional	Scurvy	Perifollicular hemorrhagic lesions on the shins Delayed wound healing	Increased capillary fragility Failure to form normal collagen
Psychological	Hyperhidrosis	Marked increase in sweating on palms, soles, and axillae	
Degenerative	Lipodystrophy	Progressive loss of subcutaneous fat leading to a bizarre cachectic appearance	?Insulin-antagonizing polypeptide
Immunologic	Serum sickness (penicillin)	Hypersensitivity reaction with generalized urticaria, angioedema, arthralgia, and lymphadenopathy	Chain of events beginning with antibody production and formation of antigen-antibody complexes, and complement activation
Neoplastic	Dematomyositis with carcinoma of ovary, breast, and other organs	Periorbital edema, diffuse red telangiectatic macular and papular eruption of face and upper trunk, muscle weakness of shoulder girdle, neck, and arms	Possibly hypersensitivity to tumor antigens

a few hours to months. After appropriate stimulation, the cell begins the DNA synthesis (S) period during which DNA is doubled in preparation for mitosis. A relatively short postsynthetic G_2 phase then occurs prior to mitosis. The mitotic period (M), usually the shortest of the four periods, follows. The G_1 period repeats, during which the two daughter cells will separate, one to remain in the proliferative cycle and the other to differentiate, moving outward to the stratum corneum.

The cell cycle in skin can be studied using the intradermal injection of ^{3}H-thymidine as a pulse DNA label. A difference in cell kinetic behavior has been noted between normal and psoriatic cells. The rapid turnover of psoriatic epidermis is accounted for not only by the larger germinative cell population per unit area but also by the rapid rate of individual cell reproduction as compared with normal skin.

Epithelial tissues lining portions of the body, such as the mouth and vagina, are described as squamous mucosae. Buccal mucosa has features that resemble the epidermis of psoriasis. The transient time is shortened, and there are certain similar histopathologic features. Vaginal mucosa, in which cell reproduction and maturation are influenced by specific hormones, provides a unique epithelium for investigation of cell proliferation kinetics. Atrophic postmenopausal vaginal cells have a low-label index similar to normal epidermis, while under estrogen stimulation the labeling index is similar to that of oral mucosa or psoriatic epidermis.

Internal and external factors influence epidermal cell proliferation. Diurnal variations in mitotic activity occur in human skin. A tissue-specific epidermal mitotic inhibiting substance called *chalone* has been described but never isolated or characterized. An epidermal growth factor, cyclic nucleotides, and prostaglandins have also been suggested as regulators of epidermal proliferation, especially as shown by studies in psoriatic epidermis. External factors that affect epidermal proliferation are those that injure the skin, such as ultraviolet radiation.

Epidermal Lipids. The lipid content of epidermis has been estimated to be in the range of 10 per cent of the dry weight. Dermal lipid content is only 4 per cent of dry weight but varies with the number of sebaceous glands and hair follicles. Sebum has abundant squalene and wax esters, along with triglycerides and free fatty acids. The epidermis also contains triglycerides, free fatty acids, cholesterol, and cholesterol esters but no squalene or wax esters. In addition, 7-dehydrocholesterol has been demonstrated, thus establishing the epidermis as a site for the synthesis of the precursor for vitamin D.

Biosynthesis of epidermal lipids appears to be regulated to some extent by total body metabolism. The skin can use fatty acids as well as glucose for oxidative metabolism, so that cutaneous lipogenesis is partially determined by the availability of exogenous fuels.

The composition of lipids of whole epidermis reflects the lipid content of epidermal cells at successive stages of maturation. Stratum corneum lipids differ from those of living epidermis in their higher content of sterol esters and lack of phospholipids. Polar and nonpolar neutral lipids accumulate during the terminal stages of keratinization in the epidermis and may serve a functional role in the barrier and be involved in cell cohesion.

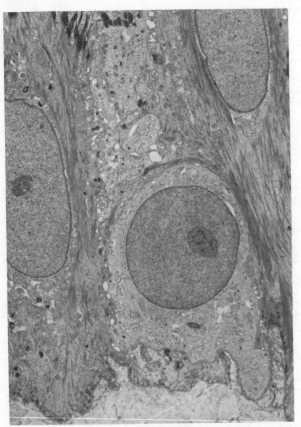

Figure 4. Parts of two basal epidermal cells and the basal lamina of epidermis enclosing a melanocyte. Note filaments in epidermal cell cytoplasm and premelanosomes in melanocyte and its processes. Desmosomes between basal cells and suprabasal cells are apparent at top of figure to left of center. × 10,560. (From Fitzpatrick, T. B., Arndt, K. A., Clark, W. H., Jr., Eisen, A. Z., Van Scott, E. J., and Vaughan, J. H. (eds.): Dermatology in General Medicine. New York, McGraw-Hill Book Co., 1971.)

Abnormalities of epidermal lipid metabolism have been noted in disorders characterized by hyperproliferative and hyperkeratotic states with resultant abnormalities of keratinization and the integrity of the barrier function, such as essential fatty acid deficiency, Refsum's disease, and psoriasis.

Epidermal Proteins. The proteins of the epidermis may be divided into two groups: the fibrous structural proteins, which are a major constituent of keratin, and the nonfibrous proteins, especially epidermal enzymes. These include the oxidative enzymes of the citric acid cycle, the enzymes involved in glycogen synthesis, the enzymes of the Embden-Meyerhof pathway, those of the hexose monophosphate shunt, and enzymes of nucleic acid metabolism. Certain proteolytic enzymes, esterases, hydrolytic enzymes, phosphatases, and enzymes involved in lipid synthesis are also present in epidermis.

Epidermal protein synthesis starts in the basal cell layer and continues throughout the malpighian layers, but different polypeptides appear to be made in the various layers of the epidermis. The keratin of the living layers contains cysteine, whereas that of the stratum corneum has cystine, which results in intrachain and interchain disulfide crosslinks. As the physiochemical properties of keratin change, it becomes more insoluble.

In the superficial portion of the epidermis, keratohyaline granules are composed of two classes of proteins. One is rich in histidine and arginine and acts as a matrix material surrounding filaments in the stratum corneum. The other protein is rich in cystine and appears to give rise to the cornified envelope of the cell. The lamellar bodies known as membrane-coating granules, which also contain hydrolytic enzymes, release their contents into the intercellular space and give rise to sheets composed of lipid and protein. These sheets are probably the principal diffusion barrier in the stratum corneum. The final events in keratinization occur in the stratum corneum. The filaments become aligned parallel to the surface of the skin, and cellular organelles are lost. The water content of the epidermis decreases from 70 per cent in the living cells to 10 per cent in the stratum corneum.

Disorders of the epidermis and of keratinization may be genetic or acquired. Abnormalities of increased epidermal proliferation occur in such entities as psoriasis and lamellar ichthyosis. An increase in the saturated hydrocarbons n-alkanes was noted in scales from some patients with lamellar ichthyosis. This finding suggests that n-alkanes may be involved in the abnormal desquamation in this disorder. Decreased shedding of the stratum corneum occurs in ichthyosis vulgaris.

THE EPIDERMAL-DERMAL INTERFACE: DISORDERS AFFECTING THE BASEMENT MEMBRANE AND THE COHESION OF KERATINOCYTES

The epidermal-dermal interface has an organized system of fibrillar and laminar structures as previously described. Disturbances of the epidermal-dermal interface can result in cavities containing fluid that are known as *vesicles* or *blisters* when small, and *bullae* when large. The site of cleavage may be within the lamina lucida or at the basal lamina and its sublaminar connective tissue. For example, in bullous pemphigoid the damage is associated with the deposition of complement proteins and frequently of immunoglobulins in the lamina lucida. In the recessive form of dystrophic epidermolysis bullosa, a genetic disorder with bullae over areas of pressure, there is absence or rarefaction of the anchoring fibrils.

Dermoepidermal separation can occur within the epidermis by loss of adhesion of cells (acantholysis), by edema within the intercellular spaces (spongiosis), or by cytolysis. Spongiosis occurs in inflammation and may be the most common cause of epidermal vesiculation and separation. Abnormalities of adhesion occur primarily in the pemphigus group of disorders. During cytolysis, separation of epidermis is related to epidermal cell rupture and death. Separation may occur as the result of damage to the papillary dermis and arises by destruction of the dermal connective tissue, such as in porphyria cutanea tarda.

THE MELANIN PIGMENTARY SYSTEM: DISORDERS LEADING TO CHANGES IN SKIN COLOR

Variation in skin color depends solely on the *epidermal melanin unit*, a functional and structural unit composed of specialized dendrite-shaped, pigment-producing glands, the *melanocytes* (Table 4), associated with a cluster of keratinocytes that are supplied with pigment particles by one single melanocyte (Fig. 5). These pigment particles, which are called *melanosomes*, are secreted into the keratinocytes in a process apparently unique in all of biology, in which a cell secretes into another cell and is therefore called *cytocrine*.

In the hair and skin of humans, characteristic coloration is determined not by variations in the number of melanocytes, but by the number of melanosomes and their melanin content present in the keratinocytes. However, melanin is formed from tyrosine by the action of the enzyme *tyrosinase*, and is deposited on melanosomes within the melanocyte. The color of the skin, as viewed clinically, is related to the number of these melanized melanosomes *present in the keratinocytes*. In certain human disorders with a defect in melanosome transfer, melanocytes may contain many heavily melanized melanosomes, but the skin looks white (hypomelanosis) because of the reduction in the number of melanosomes in keratinocytes.

Three factors determine the level of melanin pigmentation in humans: genes, exposure to sunlight, and pituitary hormones (melanocyte-stimulating hormones, MSH, and ACTH). In normal pigmentation, only genes and sunlight are major determinants. Genetic factors fix the basic level of skin color present in the habitually sun-shielded areas; this is called *constitutive* skin color and it is the major factor in racial pigmentation. When the skin is exposed to sunlight, or when high levels of MSH or ACTH are present (as in Addison's disease), the basic level of skin color increases and the familiar "tan" is observed, several days after exposure to sunlight or following the injection of ACTH or MSH. This is called *facultative* skin color and is also under genetic control, as there is considerable variability in the depth of tanning inducible in different white persons.

The additive interaction of three or four gene pairs is believed to be adequate to account for the variation in skin color in the various races. These few interacting loci probably explain the wide variation in constitutive skin color over the globe. In addition to the polygenic series responsible for constitutive skin color, there are other genes, as in human albinism, that act "individually" to partly or completely dilute melanin pigmentation. The genetic influences in humans may be as complex as in mice, in which more than 70 genes at 40 loci influence skin and hair color.

TABLE 4. TERMINOLOGY OF VERTEBRATE MELANIN-CONTAINING CELLS

Melanoblast: a cell that serves at all stages of the life cycle as a precursor of the melanocyte (and melanophore).

Melanocyte: a cell that synthesizes a specialized organelle, the melanosome.

Melanophore: a type of melanocyte that participates with other chromatophores in the rapid color changes of animals by intracellular aggregation and dispersion of melanosomes. (Among vertebrates, melanophores have been clearly demonstrated in fish, amphibians, and reptiles.)

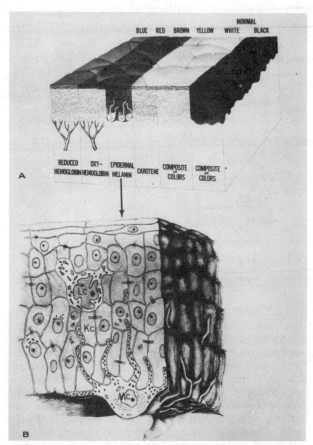

Figure 5. *A,* Schematic representation of the components of normal skin color. *B,* Epidermal melanin unit consisting of a melanocyte and associated pool of keratinocytes. Langerhans' cell is located among the suprabasal keratinocytes. Mc, melanocyte; Kc, keratinocyte; Lc, Langerhans' cell. (From Stanbury, J. B., Wyngaarden, J. B., and Fredrickson, D. S.: The Metabolic Basis of Inherited Disease. 4th ed. New York, McGraw-Hill Book Co., 1978.)

MELANIN BIOSYNTHESIS

The interrelationship of melanocyte, melanosome, tyrosinase, and tyrosine is shown in Figure 6, which presents the components of the cellular and biochemical elements based on levels of organization. For purposes of a discussion of the pathophysiology of melanin disorders, it is possible to consider clinical pigmentation at the tissue (epidermal melanin unit), cell (melanocyte), organelle (melanosome), macromolecule (tyrosinase), and molecule (tyrosine) levels.

In the light microscope, melanin occurs as a brown particle, but not all black or brown pigments are melanin. In humans, brown or black cytoplasmic particles are present in a variety of cells: in the neurons of the central nervous system (for example, substantia nigra), in the cells of the chromaffin system (adrenal medulla, sympathetic ganglia, and so on), and in the cells composing the melanin system. The pigment (called "neuromelanin") in the pigmented nuclei of the brain stem (substantia nigra) and in the chromaffin system is derived from tyrosine by the action of an enzyme called tyrosine hydroxylase. In the melanin system, the brown pigment is formed from tyrosine by

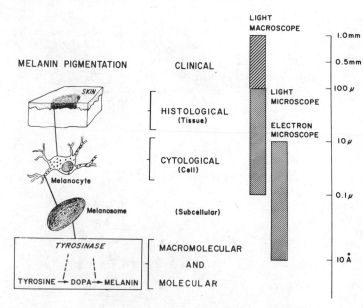

Figure 6. Levels of organization of the melanin pigmentary system. (From Fitzpatrick, T. B., Arndt, K. A., Clark, W. H., Jr., Eisen, A. Z., Van Scott, E. J., and Vaughan, J. H. (eds.): Dermatology in General Medicine. New York, McGraw-Hill Book Co., 1971.)

the action of a copper-containing aerobic oxidase, *tyrosinase*. Brown-black melanin, called *eumelanin*, is produced in the melanocytes as a high molecular weight, random polymer of many different indoles. Reddish brown macromolecular pigments are also produced in melanocytes and are called *pheomelanin*; pheomelanin contains nitrogen, as does eumelanin, but it also contains sulfur and is formed by the tyrosinase oxidation of tyrosine and subsequent reaction with cysteine. Both eumelanin and pheomelanin are produced in the melanocyte, but the biosynthesis of pheomelanins is a deviation from the pathway leading to eumelanins, the key step being the reaction of cysteine with dopaquinone.

In the conversion of tyrosine to melanin, tyrosine is oxidized to dopa and then to dopaquinone, which then cyclizes to leukodopachrome. The first two steps in the reaction are probably catalyzed by the aerobic oxidase tyrosinase. The balance of the metabolic pathway of tyrosine to melanin is nonenzymatic: leukodopachrome is oxidized to dopachrome, which rearranges with loss of carbon dioxide to 5,6-dihydroxyindole, followed by an oxidative polymerization by way of indole-5,6-quinone or its semiquinone.

Melanosomes are assembled from at least four elementary components: structural proteins, tyrosinase, "membranes," and, possibly, certain auxiliary enzymes. The structural and enzymic proteins segregate within the membrane-limited vacuoles to form a matrix consisting of several concentrically arranged protein sheets. Four steps of melanosome development are currently recognized (Fig. 7). The various melanosomal components are under genetic control, the key regulatory steps being associated with the transcription and translation of information coded within appropriate "pigmentary" genes. The qualitative attributes of melanosomal components are specified by nucleotide sequences within DNA; transcriptional and translational control mechanisms may interplay to affect not only the number of melanosomes synthesized but also certain qualitative attributes of individual melanosomes.

Some genetically programmed faults in the organization of the matrix are known in human pigment disorders; these result from either abnormalities in the primary structures of the melanosomal proteins or imbalances in the quantities in which they are presented for melanosome assembly—for example, the formation of macromelanosomes in neurofibromatosis, which will be discussed below.

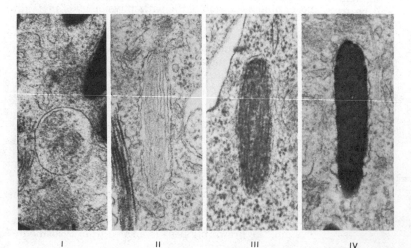

Figure 7. Stages in the development of the melanosome. **Stage 1:** A spherical, membrane-delineated vesicle may be called a melanosome if it (1) is shown to contain tyrosinase by electron microscopy combined with histochemistry, or (2) contains filaments that have a distinctive periodicity. **Stage II:** The organelle is ellipsoid and shows numerous membranous filaments, with or without cross-linking, having a distinctive periodicity. **Stage III:** The internal structure, characteristic of Stage II, has become partially obscured by electron-dense melanin. **Stage IV:** The oval organelle is electron-opaque without discernible internal structure. (From Fitzpatrick, T. B., Arndt, K. A., Clark, W. H., Jr., Eisen, A. Z., Van Scott, E. J., and Vaughan, J. H. (eds.): Dermatology in General Medicine. New York, McGraw-Hill Book Co., 1971.)

Melanocytes among all cells in the body are uniquely capable of synthesizing tyrosinase, which, when incorporated within melanosomes, initiates events leading to the synthesis of melanin. Melanocytes derive from the neural crest, and the *melanocyte system* comprises melanocytes not only of the skin and mucous membrane but also of the eye (the uveal tract and retinal pigment cells), the ear (in the stria vascularis), and of the central nervous system (leptomeninges). For the most part, all melanocytes other than the epidermal and hair melanocytes form measurable amounts of melanin only in embryonic life. Hair bulb melanocytes are active during the anagen stage of the hair growth cycle, and epidermal melanocytes form melanin only in response to appropriate stimuli—exposure to ultraviolet light or to pituitary hormones.

Melanocytes have dendritic processes that permit them to secrete melanosomes into keratinocytes. Keratinocytes may play an active role in the phagocytizing of portions of the melanosome-laden dendrites of melanocytes. The process consists of two steps: a cytophagic process and melanosome dispersion. The transferred melanosomes exist in keratinocytes as discrete particles (nonaggregated) or as two or more particles within membrane-limited vesicles (aggregated). Whether melanosomes become aggregated or remain discrete depends on the size of the organelle; small ellipsoidal melanosomes aggregate within the phagosomes in the keratinocytes and undergo degradation; larger melanosomes appear to do neither. The skin of African and American blacks and of Australian aborigines contains melanosomes in the keratinocytes that are large and discrete (nonaggregated); those in the keratinocytes of unexposed skin of Asiatics, whites of European ancestry, and American Indians are small and predominantly aggregated and in membrane-limited organelles within phagolysosomes (secondary lysosomes). In the phagolysosomes the melanosomes undergo degradation by the action of acid phosphatase and probably other lytic enzymes.

In Figure 8, the ten steps in the morphologic and metabolic pathway of melanin pigmentation are depicted. As an example, cyclic AMP may serve as a second messenger in melanocytes (step 4, Fig. 8); MSH activates tyrosinase by eliciting the conversion of an inactive form of the enzyme to active tyrosinase; also cyclic AMP appears to stimulate mitotic activity of melanocytes. There are specific receptor sites for MSH on the cell surface of the melanocyte; MSH leads to a stimulation of adenylate cyclase and a subsequent increase in the intracellular concentration of cyclic AMP and activation of tyrosinase. The binding of MSH occurs on the surface of melanocytes at sites related to the Golgi complex; MSH appears to be internalized in vesicles within the melanocytes. Thus, the "instructions" resulting from the attachment of MSH to the melanocyte cell receptors are carried out in a "compartmentalized manner" in the Golgi complex.

Pathophysiology of Pigmentary Disturbances

Disturbances of melanin pigmentation can be divided on the basis of color change into three types: (1) leukoderma (white or lighter than the individual's normal color); (2) melanoderma (brown hypermelanosis); and (3) ceruloderma (blue hypermelanosis).

The various disorders and their etiologic factors are set forth in Table 5.

At least eight etiologic factors can lead to alterations in pigmentation in humans (Table 5). To this list could be added an immunologic basis for pigmentation change, illustrated by the decreased pigmentation that occurs in patients with malignant melanoma (around the primary or metastatic lesion), or in a vitiligo-like hypomelanosis that infrequently appears at a site distant from the primary or the metastatic skin lesions. Selected disorders will be discussed in which the mechanism of the pigment alteration is reasonably well understood.

Migration and Differentiation of Melanoblasts into Melanocytes—Steps 1 and 2 (Fig. 8). In the disorder called *piebaldism*, melanoblasts either fail to

Figure 8. Morphological and metabolic pathway of melanin pigmentation. (From Fitzpatrick, T. B., Eisen, A. Z., Wolff, K., Freedberg, I. M., and Austen, K. A.: Dermatology in General Medicine. 2nd ed. New York, McGraw-Hill Book Co., 1979.)

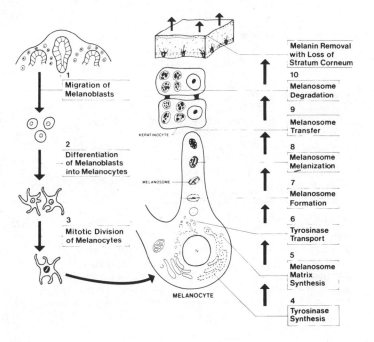

TABLE 5. DISTURBANCES OF HUMAN MELANIN PIGMENTATION

CAUSATIVE FACTORS	HYPOMELANOSIS[a]	HYPERMELANOSIS[a]	
	White	Brown	Gray, Slate, or Blue[b]

Genetic	Piebaldism[b]
	 Woolf's syndrome[b]
	 Waardenburg's syndrome[b]
	 Vitiligo[b, c]
	 Hypomelanotic macules in tuberous sclerosis[b, d]
	 Nevus depigmentosus[b, d]
	 Ziprkowski-Margolis syndrome[b]
	 Incontinentia pigmenti achromians[b]
	 Incontinentia pigmenti[b]
	 Albinism, oculocutaneous:[e, f, g]
	   Tyrosinase-negative
	   Tyrosinase-positive
	   Yellow mutant
	   Hermansky-Pudlak syndrome
	   Chediak-Higashi syndrome
	   Cross-McKusick-Breen syndrome
	 Albinism, ocular[b, f, g]
	 Albinoidism, oculocutaneous[e, f, g]
	 Phenylketonuria[e, f, g]
	 Fanconi's syndrome[f]
	 Homocystinuria[e, g]
	 Histidinemia[e]
	 Menkes' kinky hair syndrome[g]
	 Canities, premature[g]
		Café-au-lait and freckle-like macules in neurofibromatosis[b]
		 Melanotic macules in polyostotic fibrous dysplasia (Albright's syndrome)[b]
		 Ephelides (freckles)[b]
		 Lentigines[b]
		 Lentigines with cardiac arrhythmias[b]
		 Seborrheic keratosis[b]
		 Melanocytic nevus[b]
		 Neurocutaneous melanosis[b]
		 Xeroderma pigmentosum[b]
		 Acanthosis nigricans[b]
		 Dyskeratosis congenita[b]
		 Fanconi's syndrome[b]
			Oculodermal melanocytosis (nevus of Ota and nevus of Ito)[b, n, o]
			 Dermal melanocytosis (Mongolian spot)[b, n, o]
			 Blue melanocytic nevus[b, n, o]
			 Incontinentia pigmenti[b, n, o]
			 Franceschetti-Jadassohn syndrome[b, n, o]

Metabolic factors		Hemochromatosis[e] Hepatolenticular disease (Wilson's disease)[e] Porphyria (congenital erythropoietic, variegata, and cutanea tarda)[e] Gaucher's disease[k] Niemann-Pick disease[k]	Hemochromatosis[e, o] Amyloidosis, cutaneous macular[b, n, o]
Endocrine factors	Hypopituitarism[e] Addison's disease[b] Hyperthyroidism[b]	ACTH-producing and MSH-producing pituitary and other tumors[e] ACTH therapy[e] Pregnancy[k] Addison's disease[e] Estrogen therapy[l] Melasma[b, m]	
Nutritional factors	Chronic protein deficiency or loss,[g, h] kwashiorkor, nephrosis, ulcerative colitis, malabsorption Vitamin B$_{12}$ deficiency[g]	Kwashiorkor[b] Pellagra[k] Sprue[k] Vitamin B$_{12}$ deficiency[k]	Chronic nutritional insufficiency[b, o]
Chemical and pharmacologic agents	Hydroquinone monobenzylether[b] Hydroquinone[b, d] Miscellaneous catechol and phenol components[b] Chloroquine and hydroxychloroquine[g] Arsenical ingestion[b] Mercaptoethyl amines[b] Corticosteroids, topical and intradermal[b, d] Retinoic acid, topical[b, d]	Arsenical intoxication[e] Busulfan administration[e] Photochemical agents (topical or systemic drugs, tar)[b] Berlock dermatosis[a] 5-Fluorouracil, systemic[e] Cyclophosphamide[e] Nitrogen mustard, topical[b] Bleomycin[b]	Fixed drug eruption[b, o]

migrate or fail to thrive once they have migrated to the skin. This is an autosomal dominant trait that produces the familiar white forelock as well as white vitiligo-like spots (Fig. 9) in a striking pattern on the forehead, anterior trunk, and legs. In piebaldism there are few or no melanocytes in the skin. There are, however, melanocytes present in the few pigmented "islands" scattered through the large white macules; these contain spherical and granular melanosomes rather than the normal ellipsoidal melanosomes.

Mitotic Division of Melanocytes—Step 3 (Fig. 8). Reduction of melanocyte replication occurs in *graying* or *whitening of hair*. During the gray hair phase there is a gradual diminution of tyrosinase activity of the hair bulb, and in the final phase when the hair becomes white there is a total loss of melanocytes. The number

TABLE 5. DISTURBANCES OF HUMAN MELANIN PIGMENTATION (*Continued*)

CAUSATIVE FACTORS	HYPOMELANOSIS[a] White	HYPERMELANOSIS[a] Brown	HYPERMELANOSIS[a] Gray, Slate, or Blue[b]
Physical agents	Burns (thermal, ultraviolet, ionizing radiation)[b, i] Trauma[b, i]	Ultraviolet light (suntanning)[b] Thermal radiation[b] Alpha, beta, and gamma ionizing radiation[b] Trauma (e.g., chronic pruritus)[b]	
Neoplasms	Leukoderma acquisitum centrifugum (including halo nevus)[b] Malignant melanoma: Around primary neoplasms[b] Vitiligo-like hypomelanosis[b, d] Around nevi and metastatic melanoma[b]	Malignant melanoma[b, n] Mastocytosis (urticaria pigmentosa)[b] Acanthosis nigricans, with adenocarcinoma and lymphoma[b]	Slate-gray dermal pigmentation with metastatic melanoma and melanogenuria[e, o]
Inflammation and infection	Sarcoidosis[b, d] Pinta[b] Yaws[b] Syphilis, secondary[b] Syphilis, endemic, nonvenereal[b] Onchocerciasis[b] Leprosy[b, d] Tinea versicolor[b, d] Post-kala-azar[b] Pityriasis alba[b, d] Eczematous dermatitis[b, d] Discoid lupus erythematosus[b] Psoriasis[b] Vagabond's leukoderma[b] Miscellaneous postinflammatory hypomelanoses[b, d]	Postinflammation melanosis (exanthems, drug eruptions)[b] Lichen planus[b] Lupus erythematosus, discoid[b] Lichen simplex chronicus[b] Atopic dermatitis[k] Psoriasis[b] Tinea versicolor[b]	Pinta in exposed areas[b, o] Erythema dyschromicum perstans[b, n, o] Riehl's melanosis[b, n, o]
Miscellaneous factors	Alezzandrini's syndrome[b] Vogt-Koyanagi-Harada syndrome[b] Scleroderma, circumscribed or systemic[b] Canities[a] Alopecia areata[i] Horner's syndrome, congenital and acquired[f] Idiopathic guttate hypomelanosis[b]	Scleroderma, systemic[e] Chronic hepatic insufficiency[e] Whipple's syndrome[e] Encephalitis, chronic[b] Lentigo, senile ("liver spots")[b] Cronkhite-Canada syndrome[b] Catatonic schizophrenia	

[a]Listing includes the pigmentation disorder itself or the condition with which it is associated.
[b]Pigment change is circumscribed.
[c]Total loss of pigment in the skin and hair may occur.
[d]Loss of pigmentation is usually partial (hypomelanosis); viewed with Wood's lamp, the lesions are not completely devoid of pigment (amelanosis), as in vitiligo.
[e]Pigment change is diffuse, not circumscribed, and there are no identifiable borders.
[f]Pigment is decreased in the iris.
[g]Pigment is decreased in the hair.
[h]Hair is gray or reddish.
[i]There is a loss of melanocytes.
[j]Regrown hair is white.
[k]Pigment change may be diffuse or circumscribed.
[l]Nipples are affected.
[m]Idiopathic or due to progestational agents.
[n]Areas of brown may be admixed with the slate-gray and blue discoloration.
[o]Gray, slate, or blue color results from the presence of dermal melanocytes or phagocytized melanin in the dermis.

Source: Fitzpatrick, T. B., Eisen, A. Z., Wolff, K., Freedberg, I. M., and Austen, K. F.: Dermatology in General Medicine. 2nd ed. New York, McGraw-Hill Book Company, 1979.

of melanocytes also decreases in the skin with age. Although graying of hair ordinarily begins in the fourth or early part of the fifth decade, "premature" graying may occur in the early part of the second decade. Premature graying occurs in over one third of patients with vitiligo.

Failure of replication of melanocytes apparently occurs in the disorder *vitiligo* leading to their absence. Vitiligo is a common, acquired, patterned, idiopathic hypomelanosis (Fig. 10) that is often familial and is characterized by pale white macules that enlarge over time. The general health is usually not impaired but the disfigurement, especially in pigmented persons, can be socially catastrophic, notably in India, Africa, and the Middle Eastern countries.

Vitiligo is associated with thyroid disease (Graves' disease, thyroiditis, toxic goiter) (2 to 30 per cent), Addison's disease (2 per cent), pernicious anemia (10 per cent), diabetes mellitus (1 to 7 per cent), and alopecia areata (16 per cent). There are three hypotheses for the occurrence of vitiligo in this melange of medical disorders: the immune hypothesis, the neural hypothesis, and the "self-destruct" hypothesis.

The immune hypothesis proposes an aberration of

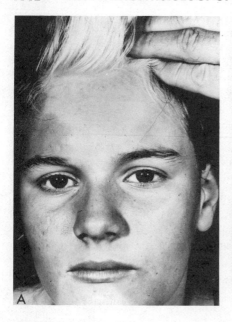

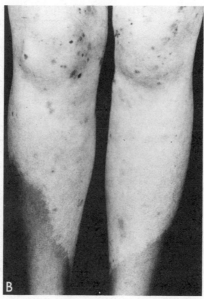

Figure 9. Piebaldism. *A,* There is a striking triangular hypomelanosis involving both the skin and the hair; the eye color is normal, and there is no iris translucence. *B,* The hypomelanosis on the legs appears as white as vitiligo, but, in contrast with vitiligo, there are islands of normally pigmented skin in the large areas of hypomelanosis. (From Fitzpatrick, T. B., Arndt, K. A., Clark, W. H., Jr., Eisen, A. Z., Van Scott, E. J., and Vaughan, J. H. (eds.): Dermatology in General Medicine. New York, McGraw-Hill Book Co., 1971.)

immune surveillance that results in melanocyte destruction or dysfunction, or both. The primary event could be an injury to melanocytes with release of antigen and subsequent autoimmunization. Antimelanocyte antibodies have been isolated in two patients with vitiligo and multiglandular deficiencies.

The neural hypothesis postulates a neurochemical mediator that destroys melanocytes. This is suggested by the occasional patient whose vitiligo occurs in a quasi-dermatomal distribution, or vitiligo following peripheral nerve injury, or vitiligo with multiple sclerosis and Horner's syndome.

The "self-destruct" hypothesis postulates the excessive accumulation of an intermediate in melanin metabolism (tyrosine or dopa, or another intermediate) that causes destruction of melanocytes.

None of these hypotheses is entirely satisfactory. The most reasonable hypothesis is that any etiologic factor leading to melanocyte destruction releases an

antigen that could then produce antibodies to melanocytes. One phenomenon that supports an immune basis for vitiligo is the repigmentation effect of topical corticosteroids, which could act as local immunosuppressive agents. The positive responses of vitiligo to prolonged therapy with orally administered psoralens followed by exposure to long-wave ultraviolet (PUVA) photochemotherapy also suggest an immune hypothesis, as PUVA has a topical immunosuppressive effect, probably by the reduction of the T lymphocytes. PUVA, however, also induces mitosis in melanocytes, and it increases cyclic AMP in melanocytes. Cyclic AMP, in turn, increases melanosome and tyrosinase activity in melanocytes.

Steps 4 to 8 (tyrosinase synthesis, melanosome matrix synthesis, tyrosinase transport, melanosome formation, and melanosome melanization) in Figure 8 are altered in various pigment disorders as a group or singly—in other words, some pigment disorders affect more than one of these steps. For example, in the genetic disorder *tuberous sclerosis,* there is reduced melanosome size (Step 7) and reduced melanosome melanization (Step 8), while in other disorders, such as the genetic disorder *neurofibromatosis,* melanocytes contain melanosomes that are very large (five times the normal size), therefore involving only Step 7.

Tyrosinase Synthesis—Step 4. In the familiar disorder *albinism,* a genetic trait affecting humans and other mammals as well as fish, reptiles, and birds, there is a dilution of skin, hair (or feather), and eye color based on a failure of synthesis of tyrosinase. In humans, albinism occurs as six different types in which a congenital absence or dilution of skin, hair, and eye color is noted, and also disturbing eye defects: decreased visual acuity, nystagmus, and photophobia. The six types of albinism are distinguished from one another by clinical and biochemical criteria. In the classic type of albinism in mice, an autosomal recessive trait, there is a total absence of functioning tyrosinase in the skin, hair, and eye pigment cells. In the different types of human albinism, tyrosinase activity and vary-

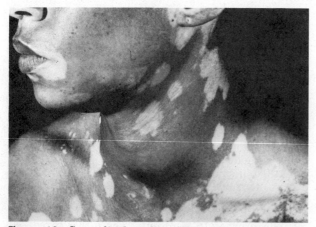

Figure 10. Generalized vitiligo. (From Fitzpatrick, T. B., Arndt, K. A., Clark, W. H., Jr., Eisen, A. Z., Van Scott, E. J., and Vaughan, J. H. (eds.): Dermatology in General Medicine. New York, McGraw-Hill Book Co., 1971.)

ing amounts of melanin are present. There are biochemical as well as clinical differences in the skin, eye, and hair color, and there is a variation from no tyrosinase activity to moderate activity. It is thus possible to classify albinism as *tyrosinase-negative* (TY-NEG) or *tyrosinase-positive* (TY-POS) albinism.

As melanocytes and melanosomes are present in albinism, the decreased pigmentation results from a reduction of tyrosinase (Step 4). The absence of detectable tyrosinase, so-called TY-NEG albinism, suggests that either the enzyme tyrosinase is completely absent or, if present, is functionally inactive. The presence of small amounts of tyrosinase could indicate different "doses" of enzyme. Human oculocutaneous albinism is apparently a deficiency in tyrosinase, whereas the other biologic processes—melanosome matrix synthesis, tyrosinase transport, and melanosome formation—are not altered.

The reduction in melanin in the epidermis leads to a failure of the epidermis to filter the carcinogenic solar ultraviolet radiation (UV-B); albinos living near the equator develop carcinomas and connective tissue degeneration ("wrinkling") at an early age (10 to 12 years).

Melanosome Matrix Synthesis—Step 5, and Tyrosinase Transport—Step 6. Vitiligo-like leukoderma may occur in patients with malignant melanoma, characterized by the appearance of circumscribed hypomelanosis that differs from that in idiopathic vitiligo in distribution pattern and color ("off-white") of the lesions. The pathogenesis of the leukoderma is believed to be a marked reduction of melanocytes, possibly on an immunologic basis. The residual melanocytes in the leukodermic macules are larger in size than normal melanocytes and contain large amounts of tyrosinase on the smooth and rough endoplasmic reticulum, but have virtually no melanosomes. This suggests a defect in the formation of the melanosome matrix and/or tyrosinase transport (see Fig. 8).

Melanosome Formation—Step 7. The normal melanosome in skin is a highly structured ellipsoidal organelle that contains filamentous, sheetlike structures as well as varying amounts of melanin and is surrounded by a unit membrane. Abnormally large spherical melanosomes are observed very frequently in the so-called *café-au-lait macules* that occur in the autosomal dominant trait *neurofibromatosis*, or von Recklinghausen's disease. These large melanin macroglobules, whose long and short axes are at least ten times larger than those of melanosomes, have characteristics that indicate that they are formed within melanocytes by a merger of autophagosomes and lysosomes (Fig. 11).

Melanosome Melanization—Step 8. Another type of hypomelanosis with decreased melanization occurs in the serious genetic disorder *tuberous sclerosis*, an autosomal dominant trait often associated with mental retardation and seizures. In over 90 per cent of the infants born with this disorder there are four to more than 100 hypomelanotic macules that are usually larger than 1.0 cm. These macules generally have a characteristic shape that simulates the outline of an American mountain-ash leaf—this important diagnostic sign is familiarly known as the "ash leaf spot." The melanosomes in the white macules are reduced in size, and the melanin content is markedly reduced, suggesting a lower concentration of tyrosinase, or possibly the presence of an inhibitor of melanogenesis.

Melanosome Transfer—Step 9. A functioning epidermal melanin unit implies a melanocyte capable of transferring melanosomes to keratinocytes. This requires not only melanocytes with adequate dendrites but also "receptive" keratinocytes. If there are pathologic alterations in melanocyte morphology, such as inadequate dendrites, or if there are pathologic changes in the keratinocytes that do not accept melanosomes after they leave the melanocyte dendrite, a reduction of melanin pigmentation will occur. As emphasized earlier, clinically visible melanin pigmenta-

Figure 11. Melanin macroglobules (MMs) in a melanocyte of the café-au-lait pigmented macule in a patient with neurofibromatosis. (a) Low-power view of the (MMs). Compare the difference in the size of the normal melanosomes (NMs) (shown in cross section) and the MM which is spherical. × 6,000. (b) High-power view of the MM, which is surrounded by a membrane. Between the electron-dense inner core and the outer membrane, there is a region in which vesiculoglobular bodies are aggregated. × 55,000. (From Jimbow, K., Quevedo, W. C., Jr., Fitzpatrick, T. B., and Szabo, G.: Some aspects of melanin biology: 1950–1975. J Invest Dermatol 67:72, 1976.)

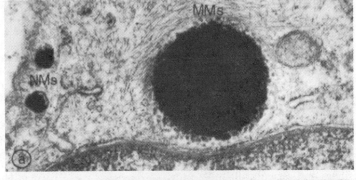
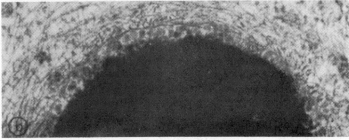

tion of the skin or hair requries the presence of melanized melanosomes in keratinocytes. Even if the melanocyte contains myriads of melanized melanosomes, clinical pigmentation will not be evident. A syndrome has been described in two children with dilution of pigmentation and immunodeficiency. In the skin of these children the melanocytes were "stuffed with nonaggregated Stage IV melanosomes" and the keratinocytes were "hypopigmented," interpreted as reflecting a defect in melanosome transfer. The immunodeficiency was of an unusual type in which there were normal numbers of circulating T and B lymphocytes, but the skin reactivity to DNCB and PHA, skin graft rejection, and antibody formation were markedly impaired.

Melanosome Degradation—Step 10. As discussed above, melanosomes are present in melanocytes of all races as a single organelle surrounded by a unit membrane. When melanosomes are transferred, they may remain isolated organelles (nonaggregated), or a few or several melanosomes may become surrounded by a limiting membrane (aggregated). Lysosomal enzymes progressively degradate the protein and the lipid moiety of the melanosome, but not the melanin polymer, which is apparently nonbiodegradable. Melanosome degradation can occur in the melanocytes in skin that has been exposed to ultraviolet radiation and in the malignant melanocytes that occur in primary melanoma of the skin.

THE DERMIS: CELLULAR, CONNECTIVE TISSUE, AND VASCULAR COMPONENTS AS THE SITE OF IMMUNOPATHOLOGIC REACTIONS AFFECTING THE SKIN

The dermis, which may constitute up to 20 per cent of body weight, is composed of connective tissue containing fibrous proteins—collagen, elastin, and reticulin and ground substance. The dermis also contains the pilosebaceous unit, eccrine sweat glands, blood vessels, lymphatics, and nerves. A major function of the dermis is protection of the body from mechanical injury. It maintains an interaction with the epidermis during embryogenesis, morphogenesis, and wound repair. The dermis is stratified and its connective tissue layers are oriented in such a manner that it becomes a mobile tissue capable of extension and relaxation, thus providing the dermis with the capacity to adapt to body movement.

Two major divisions can be recognized—the superficial portion, or papillary dermis, and a deeper portion, or reticular dermis (Fig. 2A). In the papillary layer, a few thin collagen fibers form a loose three-dimensional network. The reticular dermis contains denser and thick collagen fibers between which are the elastic fibers and reticular fibers.

Collagen is the major constituent of the dermis, apart from water, and is embedded in ground substance composed mainly of glycosaminoglycans. The structure and formation of collagen are described in Section IX, to which the reader is referred.

The *elastic fibers* are highly branching structures whose presence is responsible for the elasticity of connective tissues. In normal human skin, the elastic tissue proteins represent only a small fraction of the total dermal proteins. Elastic fibers consist of amorphous and fibrillar components. The major component, which has an amorphous appearance without periodic structures, represents biochemically the elastin. A complete discussion of elastin and the disorders associated with its formation is contained in Section IX. The two inherited dermatologic conditions demonstrating derangement of elastic fibers are pseudoxanthoma elasticum and cutis laxa. In pseudoxanthoma elasticum, the amorphous elastin component of the fibers has been replaced by bundles of granular material. In cutis laxa, there is degeneration of the dermal elastic fibers, which are deficient in elastin with normal elastic microfilaments. In some patients there may be decreased cross-linking of elastin, leading to connective tissue weakness.

The *ground substance* is the amorphous material that, together with collagen and elastin fibers, makes up the matrix of the dermis and subcutaneous connective tissue. This ground substance is composed primarily of proteoglycans and also contains water, salt, and glycoproteins similar to those of plasma. In the ground substance of skin these acidic proteoglycans are chiefly hyaluronic acid, dermatan sulfate, and chondroitin-6-sulfate. Ground substance is discussed in more detail in Section IX. The site of synthesis of hyaluronic acid and dermatan sulfate is the fibroblast. In human skin there is a general decrease with age in acidic proteoglycan content relative to weight and collagen content. Sex hormones have also been noted to affect the acid proteoglycan content of the skin of experimental animals. For example, testosterone administration is followed by increases in hyaluronic acid, while corticosteroid administration has resulted in both increases and decreases in various acidic proteoglycans. There are reports of changes in the amounts of skin acidic proteoglycans in various diseases, notably pseudoxanthoma elasticum, systemic lupus erythematosus, and scleroderma. Hypothyroid animals accumulate hyaluronic acid, and diabetes is associated with decreased levels of hyaluronic acid.

CELLS OF THE DERMIS

The normal dermis contains a variety of cell types, including mast cells, fibroblasts, monocyte-macrophages, and lymphocytes. None of the three classes of polymorphonuclear leukocytes—that is, neutrophils, eosinophils, or basophils—is present in normal skin.

Mast cells (Fig. 12), which are especially prominent in skin are described in Section III. Human skin mast cells have the distinguishing features of long villous extensions of the plasma membrane and prominent microfilaments. Upon activation by a variety of mechanisms, exocytosis of granules occurs that involves fusion between the cell membrane and the membranes of the granules. Continuity between cell exterior and the granules is thus established, which allows the release of certain granule contents while the cell membrane and cytoplasm remain intact. The human mast cell contains substances with vasoactive and smooth muscle–contracting ability such as histamine, prostaglandin D_2, and the sulfidopeptide leukotrienes; a variety of chemotactic factors for eosinophilic and neutrophilic polymorphonuclear leukocytes; enzymes, such as neutral proteases and acid hydrolases; and the acidic proteoglycan heparin (Table 6).

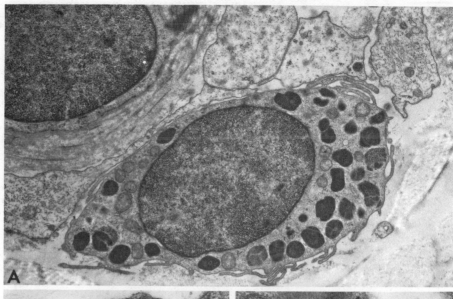

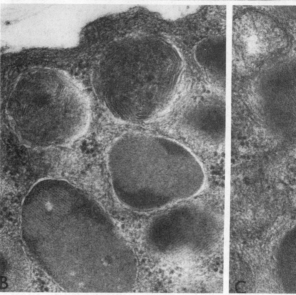

Figure 12. Electron micrographs of a mast cell in normal human skin. *A* shows a mast cell, revealing characteristic granules (dark) and mitochondria (pale) in cytoplasm and microvilli at cell surface. × 11,700. *B* and *C* reveal details of mast cell granules. × 75,000. (From Fitzpatrick, T. B., Arndt, K. A., Clark, W. H., Jr., Eisen, A. Z., Van Scott, E. J., and Vaughan, J. H. (eds.): Dermatology in General Medicine. New York, McGraw-Hill Book Co., 1971.)

Antigen-induced release of histamine after the passive sensitization with IgE-rich serum has been demonstrated in human skin slices. Disodium cromoglycate, an agent that inhibits histamine release from lung and rodent skin mast cells, fails to suppress passive transfer reactions in human skin and the antigen-induced release of histamine from skin slices. These data suggest that human cutaneous mast cells may possess specific biochemical and functional differences from mast cells in other tissues. Mast cells participate in various forms of cutaneous inflammation. The activation of human skin mast cells by IgE-dependent mechanisms is based upon the passive transfer phenomenon in vivo. Mast cells may also be activated secondary to the formation of immune complexes, with activation of the classic complement system and subsequent elaboration of the anaphylatoxins C3a and C5a. When the latter materials are injected into the skin, erythema, urticaria, and pruritus result. Mast cell degranulation has been noted in urticaria/angioedema, in certain forms of necrotizing vasculitis, and in cellular-type hypersensitivity reactions in skin.

The skin contains a population of lymphocytes that has the capacity to produce a group of biologically active molecules (lymphokines) and also to participate in cell-mediated or delayed-type hypersensitivity reactions. This class of response includes contact dermatitis, resistance to infection with viruses and other microorganisms, resistance to tumors, and allograft rejection.

The skin contains a resident number of macrophages in the dermis surrounding blood vessels. In addition, dendritic cells known as Langerhans' cells are located in the dermis and especially in the epidermis. Their membrane contains receptors for the Fc portion of IgG, C3b, and HLADr. The Langerhans' cells represent the

TABLE 6. HUMAN MAST CELL MEDIATORS

MEDIATOR	FUNCTION
Vasoactive and Smooth Muscle Contracting Substances	
Histamine	H1: Contracts smooth muscle, increases venular permeability, enhances chemotaxis of neutrophils and eosinophils
	H2: Stimulates suppressor T lymphocytes, increases venular permeability, inhibits chemotaxis of neutrophils and eosinophils, augments gastric acid secretion, stimulates cardiac effects
Prostaglandin D2	Contracts smooth muscle, vasodilation, chemokinesis of neutrophils
Leukotrienes C4, D4, and E4	Contract smooth muscle, increase vascular permeability
Chemotactic Factors	
Eosinophil chemotactic factor of anaphylaxis (ECF-A)	Attracts and deactivates eosinophils and secondarily neutrophils
Eosinophil chemotactic oligopeptides	Attracts and deactivates eosinophils and secondarily neutrophils
Neutrophil chemotactic factor	Attracts and deactivates neutrophils
Enzymes	
Tryptase	Neutral protease
Arylsulfatases	Hydrolysis of sulfate esters
N-Acetyl-β-D-glucosaminidase	Cleavage of glucosamine residues
β-Glucuronidase	Cleavage of glucuronide residues
Structural Component	
Heparin	Anticoagulant, antithrombin-III interaction, inhibits complement activation

sentinel cells in skin for delayed-type hypersensitivity reactions and are functionally similar to macrophages in their interactions with antigens.

The skin also contains fibroblasts that produce collagen, elastin, and ground substance.

Cutaneous Microvasculature

Skin is pervaded by a continuous three-dimensional network of blood vessels composed of several plexuses parallel to the skin surface at different levels and linked by vertically oriented communicating vessels. No vessels pass the dermoepidermal junction.

Medium-size arteries enter the subcutaneous fat and branch in the lower reticular dermis to form a deep arterial plexus that is horizontal to the long axis of the epidermis (Fig. 3A). From this plexus vertical branches (ART) of diminishing caliber form arcades of small arteries and arterioles (SM ART/A) that extend to the superficial reticular dermis and, in turn, branch into the horizontally oriented superficial arteriolar plexus (SAP). Afferent vessels arise from this plexus and ascend vertically into the dermal papillae, where they form loops that then descend to the lower papillary and upper reticular dermis. The efferent limb of the superficial capillary venule (SCV) drains into the horizontally disposed superficial arteriolar plexus. Larger vertically oriented venules and small veins (VSM/VN) drain from the superficial venular plexuses in a fashion parallel to the arteriolar system, with medium-size veins (VN) exiting from the lower dermis into the fat. Cutaneous appendages are enveloped by a plexus of small venules that drain into small veins. The venular portion of the cutaneous microvasculature is the most permeable and is the predominant site of dilatation and leakage in urticaria and of inflammation in most forms of necrotizing vasculitis in the skin. Necrotizing venulitis is most frequently recognized as a raised, solid, purpuric elevation of the skin

(*palpable purpura*). Edema; infiltration with neutrophilic leukocytes; participation of lymphocytes and mast cells; venular endothelial cell changes, including necrosis; and fibrin deposition characterize these lesions.

Multiple microcirculatory units arise from the interconnecting networks of arterioles and venules that supply the glands and appendages. In various parts of the body the skin shows differences in form, number, and distribution of blood vessels; for example, the microcirculation of the scalp and palms differs from that of the forearms. In addition, multiple arteriovenous anastomoses provide for a direct by-pass of the normal arterial-capillary-venous circuit and thus allow the blood to flow through preferential channels that shorten the distance between artery and vein. These arteriovenous anastomoses, which are particularly numerous in the digits, have a tendency to close if the blood pressure does not exceed a critical value. The opening of these shunts excludes the capillary bed and permits the dermal vasculature to meet various thermal regulatory requirements.

The vasculature of skin is developed beyond the degree necessary for the nutrition of this organ. The excess of blood vessels aids in temperature control and regulation of blood pressure. The amount of blood normally circulating through the digits is 20 to 30 times the minimum required for oxygenation of the tissue, and in vasodilatation it may rise to over 100 times the minimum value.

Immunopathologic Reactions

The dermis, with its cells, blood vessels, and nerves, constitutes a primary site of inflammatory and immunologic reactions in the skin. These processes involve complex biologic interactions that participate in host defense against foreign substances. Immunologically induced inflammatory responses may be acute, subacute, or chronic and may involve immediate-type hypersensitivity, immune complex–mediated reactions, or cellular-type hypersensitivity, singly or in combination. A variety of effector systems derived from cells and plasma may be involved. The effects of these systems reflect the biologic products of mast cells and lymphocytes; of the membrane-derived arachidonic acid–prostaglandin sequence; of the complement reaction products; and of the Hageman factor-dependent pathways of coagulation, fibrinolysis, and kinin generation.

SKIN APPENDAGES: SEBACEOUS GLANDS

While sweat glands have an important role in temperature regulation, sebaceous glands have no known function and are of importance in humans only as the site of a very common disfiguring disorder of young adults, *acne.*

Sebaceous glands produce a complex lipid mixture, *sebum,* that is emptied through a small duct into the neck of the hair follicle. They are largest on the face, scalp, and scrotum, but are present in all areas of the skin except on the palms, soles, and the dorsa of the feet.

Sebaceous glands open to the skin surface by a widely dilated follicular orifice (the "pore," most easily observed on the nose). A vellus hair is always present in the follicle. A short duct leads from the huge collection of acinar glands to the large hair follicle duct (Fig. 13). The sebaceous cells are derived from and have ultrastructural similarities to epidermal cells, except that they gradually accumulate lipid droplets that ultimately fill the cytoplasm of the cell (Fig. 13). Whole sebaceous cells move out of the gland, and thus the secretory product is actually a whole cell without a nucleus and contains membrane-enclosed masses of lipid droplets. The sebaceous gland is thus a *holocrine* gland in which the differentiated sebaceous cells are pushed forward by pressure of cell replication and emptied through the short duct into the large hair follicular duct. The cells finally rupture and the lipid droplets and sebum (from Latin *sebum,* tallow, grease) are a mixture of free fatty acids, triglycerides, diglycerides, monoglycerides, sterol esters, sterols, and squalene. Squalene and wax esters are unique products of sebaceous glands.

Sebaceous cell proliferation (and therefore sebum production) is uniquely responsive to *direct* hormonal stimulation by androgen. Newborns may have enlarged sebaceous glands and even acne because of androgen stimulation in utero. The size and development of sebaceous glands can be clearly correlated with early puberty and the secretion of sex steroids. Topical androgen administration can cause enlargement of sebaceous glands at the site of application of the scalp of prepubertal persons. Estrogens have the opposite effect, causing a decrease in the size of the gland and in the production of sebum secretion, but this not a direct effect. The activity of sebaceous glands varies with age and sex: low in children, higher in adults (more in men than women), and decreasing in males over the age of 50 but only slightly decreasing in women. These effects are related to changes in gonadal and adrenal function. In women, adrenal and

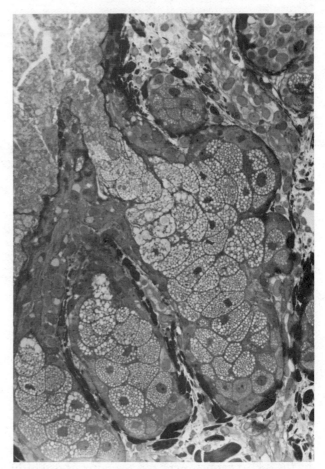

Figure 13. Sebaceous gland from skin of human face. Three acini are shown, and the duct of one of these is seen to open into the follicle at upper left. Observe the character of peripheral acinar cells, and compare with more centrally disposed lipid-containing cells. × 450. (From Fitzpatrick, T. B., Arndt, K. A., Clark, W. H., Jr., Eisen, A. Z., Van Scott, E. J., and Vaughan, J. H. (eds.): Dermatology in General Medicine. New York, McGraw-Hill Book Co., 1971.)

ovarian androgens maintain sebaceous activity, but in males testicular androgen is the principal, although not the only, stimulus for sebaceous activity. Orchiectomy causes a marked fall in sebum production. In virilizing syndromes (malignant adrenal tumors, ovarian arrhenoblastoma, and Stein-Leventhal syndrome), increased androgens of ovarian or adrenal origin can cause typical acne vulgaris, marked seborrhea of the face, as well as clitoral enlargement, hypertrophy of the penis, male-pattern alopecia, and hirsutism.

THE PATHOGENESIS OF ACNE

Acne is not solely related to sebaceous gland activity, and there is considerable variation in sebum secretion in patients with acne. Sebaceous gland activity, however, is the major factor in acne; when the gland is suppressed by estrogens acne can be controlled. Comedones can be produced by sebum, and sebum causes inflammation when injected into the skin, probably because it contains free fatty acids; these cause severe inflammation when injected into the skin.

Why do only certain persons develop acne? Possibly

the sebum of acne patients is different, but no consistent pattern has been shown. What is the role of infection, inasmuch as oral and topical antibiotics are effective in controlling acne? The predominant organism in the follicular duct is the anaerobic, pleomorphic diphtheroid *Propionibacterium acnes*. There is a marked increase in the number of *P. acnes* in children aged 11 to 15 *with acne,* but virtually no *P. acnes* in children without acne. Similar differences are found in persons aged 16 to 20. Older persons, however, have the same numbers of *P. acnes* organisms, whether they have acne or not. Injection of *P. acnes* causes rupture of acne cysts and severe inflammation; very little inflammation results when nonviable *P. acnes* organisms are similarly injected into the cysts. *P. acnes* contains lipases, and these enzymes can result in lipolytic activity producing free fatty acids. The path of *P. acnes* lipase (free fatty acids) inflammation is a highly possible mechanism for the production of acne. In certain types of acne, topical antibiotics, especially clindamycin, erythromycin, and tetracycline, have been shown to be efficacious.

As mentioned above, orally administered estrogen inhibits the sebaceous glands and is therefore very effective in the control of acne. Serious side effects, however, preclude its use in males (gynecomastia, inhibition of spermatogenesis, impotence, and so on).

For years it has been almost an article of dogma that diet, especially chocolate or iodine-containing foods, can cause exacerbations of acne. Controlled studies have almost eliminated any possibility of a dietary factor in the pathogenesis of acne.

An enigma in the pathogenesis of acne is that almost all patients undergo a spontaneous remission—usually by the early twenties. Acne can begin from age 8 to 20 and usually persists for several years. The cause of spontaneous remission is unknown. At the time of remission, the sebaceous glands are still active, the *P. acnes* organisms are still present, and yet the disease completely disappears! By unknown mechanisms, remissions or exacerbations may occur during the same age span, from 8 to 20 years. For example, the typical premenstrual flare of acne cannot be explained by increased sebum production, as there is no change in sebum production during the luteal phase of the menstrual cycle. Also, for no known reason, a remission commonly occurs in northern latitudes during the summer. This may be the effect of a combination of factors: less emotional stress, for instance, or more exposure to sunlight.

Acne is one of the most serious problems of adolescence because of the marked disfigurement that it can produce at a time when acceptance by peers is a chief concern and when young adults are undergoing profound psychological adjustments in their schools and communities. Until recent years there was no method for even partial control. New agents such as a vitamin A derivative, 13-*cis*-retinoic acid, are now available and are powerful new oral agents in the control of severe forms of *cystic acne.*

SKIN APPENDAGES: SWEAT GLANDS AND THERMOREGULATION

Humans possess two to four million *eccrine sweat glands* distributed over nearly the entire surface of the body. In adults these glands are most numerous on the sole of the foot and least abundant over the back. Eccrine sweat glands produce a hypotonic skin surface fluid, thus serving as an excretory organ for water, electrolytes, heavy metals, organic compounds, and macromolecules. During conditions in which the rate of sweating reaches several liters a day, ductal reabsorption assumes a role in maintaining body homeostasis.

The eccrine sweat glands are of the merocrine type; that is, they achieve secretion without damage to the cell's cytoplasm. The eccrine sweat gland consists of two segments: a secretory coil and a duct. The secretory coil is composed of three cell types: clear secretory, dark mucoid, and myoepithelial. The clear cell is probably responsible for the secretion of water and electrolytes and the dark cell for the mucosubstance in sweat. The myoepithelial cells lie on the basement membrane and contain substantial numbers of myofilaments but are currently thought to have a minimal role in sweat expulsion.

Control of sweating is located in the hypothalamus, which regulates body temperature. Afferent stimuli that influence the hypothalamic sweat center are neuromuscular drive and temperature of the body core, skin, muscles, and subdermal areas. Efferent impulses descend through the brain stem, spinal cord, and peripheral nerves. The nerves surrounding the sweat glands are composed of nonmyelinated class C fibers of the sympathetic system; physiologically, however, the gland responds to parasympathetic or cholinergic stimuli. Since eccrine sweat glands respond to the intradermal injection of acetylcholine and to a minimal degree to epinephrine, and are inhibited by the prior administration of atropine, it is concluded that only cholinergic fibers control eccrine sweat secretion. Glands over the entire skin surface respond predominantly to thermal stimuli and also to emotional stress, but emotionally induced sweating is usually restricted to the forehead, axillae, palms, and soles.

In studies of isolated eccrine sweat glands, predominantly beta-adrenergic (and to a lesser extent alpha-adrenergic agents) and also calcium ionophore, prostaglandin E_1, and theophylline stimulate sweat secretion. However, the cellular levels of cyclic AMP do not increase after stimulation with acetylcholine.

The sweat rate varies from one body area to another according to such factors as sweat gland density, age, water intake, skin temperature, vascular supply, and acclimatization. An ultrafiltrate of plasma-like isotonic precursor fluid is secreted by the secretory coil. As this precursor fluid flows through the duct, a portion of the sodium and chloride is reabsorbed in excess of water by the duct to produce hyposmotic skin surface sweat. Sweat sodium and chloride levels are low at lower sweat rates but increase with an increase in secretory rate. The concentrations never reach the isotonic level unless there is a defect as in cystic fibrosis. The potassium content is higher than that of plasma. The sweat also contains calcium, magnesium, iodide, zinc, cobalt, lead, manganese, molybdenum, tin, and mercury. Organic compounds found in sweat include lactate, urea, ammonia, amino acids, glycoproteins, and acidic glycosaminoglycans. IgG is the major immunoglobulin in sweat, although IgA and IgD are present. Albumin, transferrin, ceruloplasmin, and orosomucoid have been detected.

Humans are capable of maintaining a relatively constant core body temperature despite great variations in both skin and environmental temperature. The surface temperature varies over different parts of the skin but normally lies between that of the body core and that of the surroundings. It may fluctuate between 20° C and 40° C without damage. It is through changes in skin temperature that environmental temperatures are sensed by the body. Certain cells within the brain and possibly elsewhere are capable of responding directly to signals from the skin's thermoreceptors. These thermoreceptors are distributed unevenly over the skin in a spotty fashion, and are of two kinds—those that respond to increasing temperature and those that respond to decreasing temperature. The skin influences the basal metabolic rate only at hypothalamic temperatures below 37° C. Sweating does not occur unless hypothalamic temperature exceeds 37° C regardless of skin temperature. At hypothalamic temperatures in excess of 37° C, increasing the skin temperature increases sweating. Skin temperatures in excess of 31° C prevent increased heat production, whereas a skin temperature less than 29° C blocks sweating. Heat reaching the skin surface is transferred to the environment by radiation, conduction, convection, and/or evaporation. Heat loss to the environment depends primarily on skin temperature and skin area. Human skin can radiate and absorb heat by infrared radiation with great efficiency; but, except when a large area of bare skin comes in contact with a good conductor and low temperature, conduction does not play a predominant role in thermoregulation. Rapid evaporation of sweat can lower skin temperature. Heat regulation is the primary function of the skin's rich circulation.

There is a congenital absence of eccrine sweat glands in patients with hereditary anhidrotic ectodermal dysplasia.

SKIN APPENDAGES: APOCRINE GLANDS

Apocrine glands have a duct that opens into a hair follicle. In humans the glands are confined to the regions of the axilla and perineum and do not become functional until puberty. It is assumed that their development, but not their maintenance, depends on sex hormones. The apocrine glands of many species produce pheromones. Since the apocrine glands of humans do not begin to function until puberty and are odor producing, it has been suggested that they have some sexual function.

The apocrine sweat of humans has been described as milky and viscid and without odor when secreted. Studies in humans are limited, since apocrine sweat gland secretion is mixed with sebum. The secretion is pulsatile. The apocrine sweat glands of humans respond to stimuli only after puberty. They can be stimulated by epinephrine or norepinephrine; the response cannot be abolished by denervation. Drugs that affect adrenergic systems also have an effect on apocrine sweat glands.

SKIN APPENDAGES: HAIR

Hair performs no vital function in humans, not even in thermoregulation; however, the psychological functions are inestimable. Physiologically, body hair prob-

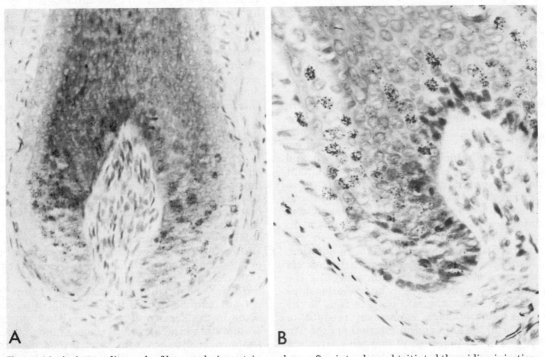

Figure 14. *A*, Autoradiograph of human hair matrix one hour after intradermal tritiated thymidine injection. Numerous labeled cells are found in the lower half of the hair matrix. *B*, Forty-eight hours later, cells have moved distad above the dermal papilla. (From Fitzpatrick, T. B., Arndt, K. A., Clark, W. H., Jr., Eisen, A. Z., Van Scott, E. J., and Vaughan, J. H. (eds.): Dermatology in General Medicine. New York, McGraw-Hill Book Co., 1971.)

ably remains as an apparatus for odor dissemination in social or sexual communication.

Hair is a cylinder of keratinized cells (Fig. 14). Its bulk is formed by the cortex, which often surrounds a medulla and is itself surrounded by a cuticle. Hair is formed within an inner root sheath by the cell matrix, the outer surface of the dermal papilla. The inner root sheath undergoes keratinization and is lost as the hair emerges.

Hair can be divided into *vellus,* which is soft, without a medulla, and seldom more than two cm in length, and *terminal* hair, which is longer, coarser, and often contains a medulla. Vellus hair is replaced by terminal hair at puberty.

Both the form of scalp hair and the distribution of body hair differ between human groups. Scalp hair has the roundest cross-section and is usually straight in Mongoloids, more elliptic and slender in Caucasoids, and flat and curled in Negroids. Mongoloids have less pubic, axillary, beard, and body hair than Caucasoids. Only minor differences in body hair distribution between Caucasoids and Negroids can be detected.

The activity of hair follicles is cyclic. The active, or *anagen,* hair shows a lightening of pigment at the base of its shaft with a decrease and transfer of melanin. The distal region of the hair bulb expands to form a club, becoming the *catagen* hair, characterized by a thick and corrugated vitreous membrane that forms a portion of the connective tissue sheath of the follicle. The resting hair is known as the *telogen* hair. In the human scalp at any one time less than one per cent of the follicles are in catagen and 13 per cent are in telogen. Anagen may last three or more years. About 100 hairs are normally shed each day.

SKIN CANCER

PATHOGENESIS OF SKIN CANCER AND OF SKIN RESPONSES TO SYSTEMIC CANCER

Epithelial cancers are the most common cancers in humans. White persons who are susceptible and who are repeatedly exposed to carcinogenic solar ultraviolet radiation will *all* develop skin cancers if they live long enough (Fig. 15). Epithelial cancers (basal cell and squamous cell) and cancer of melanocytes (malignant melanoma) are so readily visible and the tissue so accessible that it is possible to study the natural history of spontaneous skin cancers in humans, and experimentally induced skin cancers in animals. In some human cancers, both the precursor lesion and the cancer are visible in the same lesion. In addition, the skin exhibits a number of responses to cancers arising in organs other than the skin, reflecting the complex immunologic and metabolic interrelationships of malignant neoplasms; the skin may, in fact, be the target of the same etiologic agent that produces a primary cancer in the skin and in internal organs. An example of this is the ingestion of inorganic trivalent arsenic, a quite common medical treatment in the early part of this century, that can cause a primary squamous cell carcinoma in the skin (Fig. 15) and a primary bronchiogenic squamous cell carcinoma of the lung.

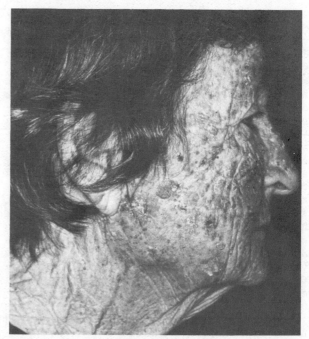

Figure 15. Multiple squamous cell carcinomas arising in solar keratoses. (From Fitzpatrick, T. B., Arndt, K. A., Clark, W. H., Jr., Eisen, A. Z., Van Scott, E. J., and Vaughan, J. H. (eds.): Dermatology in General Medicine. New York, McGraw-Hill Book Co., 1971.)

Ultraviolet and Skin Cancer

Of the various etiologic agents that cause skin cancer in humans, ultraviolet radiant energy is a useful model for the study of the pathogenesis of skin cancer. Ultraviolet light is presumed to be carcinogenic by virtue of its action on DNA. UV-B (290 to 310 nm) can induce thymine dimers in skin; the peak action spectrum of this effect is 290 nm. Excision repair of thymine dimers is an essential step before replication begins.

Persons who are homozygous for the autosomal recessive trait xeroderma pigmentosum (XP) are extraordinarily susceptible to the development of sun-induced skin cancer (basal cell and squamous cell carcinoma and malignant melanoma). The cells of these individuals are defective in excision repair (one of the several molecular mechanisms that repair ultraviolet damage to DNA). Evidence that there is a correlation between the capacity of an agent to produce mutations in DNA and its ability to produce cancer has been obtained for the most part from the study of a few rare genetic diseases such as XP. This entity is discussed later in this chapter.

High-Risk Population for Development of UV-Induced Skin Cancer. Even heterozygotes (carriers) of XP genes appear to have an increased incidence of skin cancer. This would suggest that the increased incidence of epithelial skin cancers in certain "normal" persons may be related to DNA repair processes that occur in the keratinocytes. There is a high incidence of nonfatal skin cancers in pale-skinned persons who sunburn easily and tan poorly, regardless of their phenotype (for example, they may have black hair and brown eyes). Possibly these persons have a defect in DNA repair.

The fatal skin cancer, malignant melanoma, may

also be related to an increased susceptibility (fair skin, easy burning, and poor tanning) to sunlight exposure. Malignant melanoma, which affects the young and the middle-aged, is the leading cause of death among diseases arising in the skin and will be discussed later. Nonwhite persons have very few melanomas or non-melanoma skin cancers (basal cell and squamous cell cancer). Also, nonwhite persons have virtually no sun-induced pathologic changes such as actinic keratoses, actinic dermal degeneration, or other consequences of chronic insolation that plague about 30 per cent of the white population. This susceptible 30 per cent of white people (living in northern Europe, the United Kingdom, North America, South Africa, and Australia) have *white* skin, while the 500 million people living in the Middle East, although classified as "white," have constitutively a *tan,* not white, skin. The curious fact is that even these susceptible white people are not alike in their reactions to sun exposure or in their potential risk for developing sun-induced skin disorders. Among the white population, there is a wide variation in the constitutive or genetic melanin pigmentation and in the facultative tanning responses.

Sun-Reactive Skin Types. How do we identify this population at high risk for the development of sun-induced skin changes, including skin cancer? A simple working classification has been proposed that is based, not on the phenotype (that is, hair and eye color), but on the response to an *initial* sun exposure of three minimal erythema doses (MEDs)—about one hour in northern latitudes in the summer. We need ask only two questions about the response to three MED exposures:

How much *painful* sunburn do you have after 24 hours?
How much tan will you develop in 7 days?

There are two groups of the white population who have a clear-cut answer (Fig. 16). One group will reply, a painful burn at 24 hours and no tan at 7 days. This is termed Type I sun-reactive skin type. Another group will respond: no burn at 24 hours and a dark tan at 7 days. This group is called Type IV. One of the two subgroups of Type I and IV will answer: a painful burn at 24 hours (the same as Type I response) and a light tan at 7 days; this group is termed Type II. Another subgroup will testify to a slightly tender burn at 24

hours and a good tan at 7 days; this is Type III and is the largest group, with a life style of repeated and prolonged sun exposure. Types I and II are at high risk for sun-induced skin damage; Type IV persons have a low risk for sun-induced skin damage; Type III persons at moderate risk.

Of the three factors affecting melanin pigmentation in humans—genes, light, and hormones—only genes and sunlight are major determinants of pigmentation in the normal population. Genes set the level of tyrosinase production and determine the rate of synthesis, the number and size of melanosomes within the melanocyte itself, and also control the manner of melanosome degradation in keratinocytes. After three MEDs of sun exposure, persons with skin Types I and II develop a few melanized melanosomes, and these are, in fact, rapidly degraded in keratinocytes so that a melanin filter never develops in the stratum corneum, and the epidermis is virtually devoid of melanin. In Type IV skin, after three MEDs, there is a high level of tyrosinase and large numbers of heavily melanized melanosomes; the stratum corneum contains myriads of ultraviolet melanin particles, and the epidermis is heavily populated with bundles of aggregated melanosomes. The Type IV skin in response to sun exposure creates its own density filter that absorbs UV-B and thus prevents damage to the nucleus by photons.

Melanoma and Sunlight Exposure: The Paradox of Site of Origin. There appear to be persons at risk for developing melanoma based on genetic control of their melanocytes to supply protective-shielding melanin pigment. Patients with melanoma are reported to be more likely to give a history of developing painful sunburn and poor or no tanning than are control groups. Melanoma can no longer be considered a rare disease. In the United States alone, for example, there were 17,400 (in 1983) new cases and this figure is increasing by 5 to 10 per cent each year. Based on the current survival rates, this means that approximately 5200 of these new patients will die within five years.

There is a heavy density of primary melanomas on totally exposed (face) and intermittently exposed (trunk) areas and a low density of melanomas on the totally unexposed areas (covered parts of the breasts in females, bathing trunk areas of males and panty areas of females). Also, there is a striking disparity in the number of melanomas on the lower legs of females

Figure 16. Sun-reactive skin types. Based on exposure of white skin to three minimal erythema doses. Peak erythema and pigment reactions (0 to 4 intensity) noted at 24 hours and 7 days respectively.

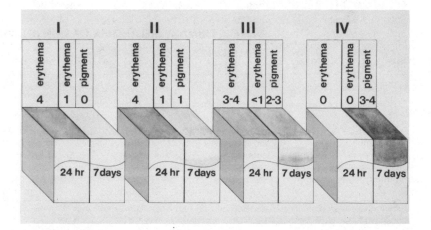

and males. The increased number of melanomas on the lower legs in females might be related to the incremental exposure of the skin surfaces below the knee.

Types of Melanoma. Malignant melanoma arising in the skin is not one but three different specific types of cancer of pigment cells (Table 7). The differences are related to the age of onset, the clinical appearance, the cellular pattern (histology), the rate and manner of growth in the skin, and the survival rate. There are discrepancies in the incidence of the three types, as seen in various hospitals; superficial spreading is reported to be as high as 80 per cent in general hospitals and as low as 10 per cent in specialized cancer hospitals. Because two of the three types of melanoma may be present as an identifiable cancer for several years before invading deeply in the skin, it is possible to remove these early lesions surgically and cure the disease before deep invasion occurs. This, of course, depends on early detection of primary melanoma by the patient or physician, which in turn depends on an intensive program of public education, even as simple a program as the one in the following paragraph:

Examination of the human body for early stages of superficial spreading melanomas, the most common type, is very easy. One has only to look at moles carefully, noting whether (a) the mole's edges are rough and contain a notch or (b) the color is speckled and contains red, white, or, particularly, blue. If either of these conditions is found, examination by a specialist is imperative (very few moles with either of these characteristics are noncancerous). An important acquired "mole" can be considered a precursor lesion of malignant melanoma. This is called the dysplastic nevus, a unique type of melanocytic nevus that has the physical characteristics of early primary melanoma just enumerated previously: variegation of color (varying shades of brown, red, and flesh tones) and irregular borders. These lesions (dysplastic nevi) occur in 1 to 2 per cent of the general population but have a high incidence in patients with malignant melanoma of the skin; e.g., 30 per cent of patients with sporadic melanoma have one or more dysplastic nevi, and in patients with familial malignant melanoma 94 per cent arise in contiguity to a dysplastic nevus.

The conjecture that sunlight is a major or contributing cause of melanoma or nonmelanoma* skin cancer

---

*The term nonmelanoma skin cancer includes basal cell and squamous cell cancers.

is supported by the following data: (1) the difference in incidence of mortality with different latitudes can be generally equated with differences in solar exposure (UV-B flux); (2) the anatomic sites of skin cancer are directly related to different degrees of protection by clothing; (3) the incidence or mortality is inversely related to the degree of pigmentation of the skin; that is, black people have a much lower incidence than white Caucasians and have lesions located mainly on the foot, while malignant melanoma occurs more frequently in persons with fair complexions who tan poorly; (4) the changes in incidence or mortality over a period of time are related to changes in exposure. In the following discussion, these pieces of evidence will be compared with reference to nonmelanoma and melanoma skin cancer.

Nonmelanoma Skin Cancer

The incidence of nonmelanoma skin cancer (over 400,000 new cases in the United States each year) is directly dependent on latitude and intensity of UV-B flux. Nonmelanoma skin cancer occurs on sites of the body receiving maximal exposure to sunlight. Over 90 per cent of basal cell carcinomas occur on the face and neck. Squamous cell carcinomas have been shown to occur almost exclusively on the head and neck. Nonmelanoma cancers also occur more frequently in persons with outdoor occupations who receive extensive solar exposure (for example, sailors and farmers). Pigmented peoples rarely develop nonmelanoma skin cancer and then most frequently in sites that do not receive maximum solar exposure. Albino blacks in Nigeria have a high incidence of nonmelanoma skin cancer. These facts suggest that sunlight exposure is the principal etiologic agent in nonmelanoma skin cancer.

Malignant Melanoma

Latitude also strongly influences the incidence of malignant melanoma. A higher incidence is seen in fair-skinned individuals and a lower incidence in pigmented peoples. The relationship of solar exposure to anatomic sites of tumor development is more complex for melanoma than for nonmelanoma, since melanoma does not appear most frequently in the maximally exposed sites. The remarkable increase in incidence since World War II is probably related to changes in exposure behavior. Melanoma is rare in blacks. The

---

TABLE 7. PRIMARY MELANOMA OF SKIN (IN WHITE PERSONS)

TYPE OF MELANOMA	MEDIAN AGE (yr)	SPECIFIC SITES*	RATE OF DEVELOPMENT	APPEARANCE
Lentigo maligna melanoma	70	Face, neck, and hands	Slow: 5–20 years	Predominantly flat (macule) 2–20 cm in size, with *irregular* borders and with raised portions throughout
Superficial spreading melanoma	56	Face, neck, upper trunk, and lower legs (in females)	Moderately slow: 1–7 years	Elevated lesion (papule or plaque) with *irregular* borders; the brown or black color is speckled or blue, white, and red, or both
Nodular	49		Rapid: months	Isolated, small (3.0 cm) nodule with *smooth* borders; color uniform blue-black

*All three types occur either on the exposed parts of the face, neck, and hands or on the relatively exposed areas of the chest, back, and legs. Only a few lesions are seen on covered areas such as the breasts of females, bathing trunk areas of males, and bathing suit areas of females.

age-adjusted rate in 1982 for whites was 9.0 per 100,000 while for blacks the rate was 0.9 per 100,000. Both males and females have a predominance of melanomas on the upper back and, in addition, females show a high incidence on the lower legs.

Skin Cancer from Agents Other Than Ultraviolet Light

Very low doses of mutagenic agents (x-ray, chemicals, and ultraviolet) can elicit an error-prone postreplication repair process. These agents apparently induce an enzymatic pathway that can replicate DNA, resulting in a marked increase of mutations. A variety of occupational cancers have arisen from exposure to soot (observed in 1775), arsenic, coal tar, shale oil, creosote oil, and petroleum lubricating oil.

Most investigators now propose a two-, three-, or multiple-stage concept of the pathogenesis of cancer. Initiation, promotion, and progression have been postulated as the three stages of cancer growth. By epidemiologic evidence, arsenic has been shown to be carcinogenic. There is increased incidence of carcinoma in those regions in the world where there is a high content of arsenic in the drinking water, or where there is occupational exposure to the chemical.

X-rays and gamma rays are established causes of skin cancer in humans receiving more than 1000 rads to the skin. Various carcinogenic aromatic hydrocarbons, viruses, and rare metals have been used in the experimental induction of skin cancer in rodents. Only a few of these, however, are relevant to humans. The enhancement of ultraviolet carcinogenesis by a number of chemicals (coal tar, 8-methoxypsoralen, and phenanthrene hydrocarbons) has been demonstrated in recent years.

Mechanisms of Skin Alterations in Patients with Systemic Cancer (Table 8)

The skin changes that occur in the presence of some malignancies are believed to be based on immunologic mechanisms (dermatomyositis), the production of metabolic substances by tumors (carcinoid), and functional disturbances in other systems induced by nonendocrine malignancies (obstructive jaundice). In addition, the skin may contain metastatic cancer or may be involved simultaneously with an internal organ by exposure to a carcinogen (arsenic). Finally, the skin may exhibit quite specific and diagnostic alterations.

Dermatomyositis. Dermatomyositis not only affects upper trunk muscles, which leads eventually to severe muscle degeneration, but the skin develops a striking erythematous, telangiectatic, macular, and papular eruption usually occurring on the upper chest, arms, knuckles, and digits. The cancer may precede or follow the onset of dermatomyositis. Only adult dermatomyositis has been linked to an underlying cancer; the

---

TABLE 8. CLASSIFICATION OF SKIN SIGNS OF INTERNAL MALIGNANCY

Skin infiltration by an internal malignancy:
  Metastatic, lymphatic, hematogenous, or by surgical implantation:
    Carcinoma
    Leukemia
  Metastatic, intraepidermal:
    Paget's disease of the breast
    Extramammary Paget's disease
  Autochthonous or metastatic (?):
    Lymphoma
    Malignant histiocytosis

Skin changes due to exposure to a carcinogen that also induces internal malignancy:
  Arsenical keratoses
  Bowen's disease

Skin malignancies associated with increased risk of separate primary internal malignancy:
  Bowen's disease
  Kaposi's sarcoma

Skin changes due to metabolic products of malignancies:
  Malignant carcinoid syndrome
  Addisonian hyperpigmentation with Cushing's syndrome, from carcinomas producing MSH- and ACTH-like peptides
  Generalized dermal melanosis (slate-gray), from malignant melanoma
  Nodular fat necrosis, due to lipases from pancreatic carcinoma
  Raynaud's syndrome with cryoproteinemia, from multiple myeloma
  Amyloidosis, from multiple myeloma
  Necrolytic migrating erythema, from functioning glucagonoma

Skin changes due to functional disturbances in other systems induced by nonendocrine malignancies:
  Jaundice, obstructive
  Addisonian hyperpigmentation, from adrenal infiltration by a tumor
  Purpura, thrombocytopenic
  Pallor, from anemia
  Herpes zoster
  Herpes simplex, severe, protracted
  Pyoderma, recurrent
  Delayed hypersensitivity, exaggerated response to mosquito bites

Skin changes, idiopathic:
  Changes frequently related to internal malignancy:
    Dermatomyositis, adult-onset
    Acanthosis nigricans
    Thrombophlebitis, migratory
    Ichthyosis, adult-onset
    Alopecia mucinosa, adult
    Pachydermoperiostosis, acquired
    Hypertrichosis lanugosa, acquired "malignant down"
    Erythema gyratum repens
  Changes occasionally related to internal malignancy:
    Pruritus, without causative skin lesions
    Clubbing, with and without hypertrophic osteoarthropathy
    Erythroderma
    Normolipemic xanthomatosis
    Erythema multiforme
    Urticaria and erythema annulare centrifugum
    Pyoderma gangrenosum, atypical
    Bullous disease and dermatitis herpetiformis
    Dermatoses, bizarre

Heritable diseases with skin manifestations and the propensity to develop internal malignancy

Source: Fitzpatrick, T. B., Eisen, A. Z., Wolff, K., Freedberg, I. M., and Austin, K. F. (eds.): Dermatology in General Medicine. 2nd ed. New York, McGraw-Hill Book Company, 1979.

association is present in less than 25 per cent of patients with dermatomyositis. There is no satisfactory hypothesis to explain the skin and muscle findings except the observation that the inflammation is a hypersensitivity response to a tumor antigen. Hypersensitivity to an extract of tumor tissue was demonstrated in two instances. Passive transfer of the cutaneous hypersensitivity by serum to a normal host was successful. These results and others have led to the proposal that the combined skin and muscle response are related to antibodies cross-reacting to a common antigen produced by the tumor.

Acanthosis Nigricans. This rare disorder is a striking example of skin response to malignancy. "Nigricans" (from the Latin *nigricare,* to turn black) refers to the hypermelanosis, a dark brown pigmentation of the body folds, especially the axillae, the umbilicus, and the inguinal area. Not only are the areas dark brown but there is "acanthosis"—that is, a diffuse, "velvety" hyperplasia of the epidermis with accentuation of the skin lines. A cancer is present in almost 100 per cent of adult patients with acanthosis nigricans. Two thirds are associated with primary cancer of the stomach, but acanthosis nigricans may also be associated with primary cancers of the pancreas, colon, rectum, uterus, ovary, prostate, esophagus, breast, and lung. The cancer and the skin change run parallel, once established; the skin findings regress as the tumor is removed or treated with chemotherapy. It has been postulated that a humoral agent (not melanocyte-stimulating hormone) produced by the tumor is responsible for the dual epidermal response of increased melanogenesis and keratinocytic hyperplasia. This notion has not as yet been proved.

Nodular Fat Necrosis Due to Lipases from Pancreatic Carcinoma. Here the pancreatic acinous adenocarcinoma releases the enzyme lipase, which is reflected in the very high serum lipase levels, along with high serum amylase. This lipolytic enzyme acts on the fat cells in the panniculus adiposus to produce a lobular panniculitis characterized by fat necrosis and by intensely basophilic crystals of calcium soaps. These localized sites of panniculitis appear clinically as painful, violaceous or red, subcutaneous nodules on the legs, especially on the ankles. Distinctive from erythema nodosum, which never ulcerates, are the large nodose lesions sometimes present from pancreatitis; these may undergo abscess-like change and spontaneously rupture, exuding an oily, viscous material.

Glucagonoma Syndrome. The glucagonoma syndrome is composed of skin eruption, weight loss, anemia, and sometimes hyperglycemia and stomatitis. It results from a functioning islet cell tumor of the pancreas that is usually malignant and that secretes large amounts of glucagon. Glucagon is a polypeptide hormone with a molecular weight of 3485 secreted by the alpha cells of the islets of Langerhans. In glucagonoma syndrome there may be a tenfold or greater increase in the plasma concentration of glucagon that decreases following removal of the pancreatic neoplasm; in addition, the skin eruption disappears within hours after surgical excision of the tumor.

The skin alterations in glucagonoma syndrome have been termed "necrolytic migrating erythema," which described the arciform and polycyclic erythematous scaling papules and plaques, often with vesicles, bul-

lae, and necrosis and a tendency to heal centrally. The eruption most often occurs around the mouth, on the lower abdomen, and in the groin and anogenital area. The eruption present in the glucagonoma syndrome is commonly misdiagnosed, sometimes for years, as mucocutaneous moniliasis or atypical psoriasis.

MECHANISM OF REACTIONS UNIQUE TO HUMANS

PRURITUS

Pruritus is one of the most miserable sensations that humans can experience. More troublesome than pain, which can usually be controlled with analgesics, pruritus is difficult to modify significantly by any pharmacologic agent. The management of severe pruritus is one of the most urgent problems in pharmacology. Any normal person, on adequate stimulation, can experience the itch sensation. Therefore, itch is an exaggerated normal sensation; normal persons experience transient pruritus of short duration that may not enter consciousness. Pathologic pruritus is of such severity and tormenting persistence that it can lead to loss of sleep, and even suicide.

Pathologic itching sensations are mediated by Class C fibers: thin, unmyelinated, very slowly conducting (1 m/sec) fibers. Itch-mediating bundles enter the posterior lateral ventral nucleus of the thalamus and proceed through the internal capsule to the secondary area of the posterior central gyrus of the cortex.

Pruritus is defined as "an unpleasant sensation that provokes the desire to scratch." Any area of skin can itch, but certain areas have an increased susceptibility to itch, such as the anogenital region, ear canals, eyelids, and nostrils.

Pruritus requires an intact epidermis, and while a denuded skin can still perceive pain (for example, a leg ulcer), itching is not possible unless the skin is intact.

The itch sensation is presumed to result from the release of mediators following damage to cells. The mediators for itching have not yet been isolated. One interesting, but as yet unconfirmed, hypothesis is that itching is related to the release of endopeptidases. A number of mediators can provoke itching, including kallikrein and histamine. Substance P appears to evoke itching through histamine, and prostaglandins of the E series potentiate itch due to other factors. Experimental evidence has shown that the itch threshold is lower at night, or with increased stress, or with vasodilatation, or decreased skin hydration, or with a present or previous dermatosis, and, finally, in the area immediately surrounding a central itch focus.

Many skin disorders are associated with severe pruritus; these include scabies, atopic eczematous dermatitis, miliaria (heat rash), and pediculosis. More important for the patient are those medical disorders that are associated with severe generalized pruritus in the absence of direct involvement of the skin (see Table 9). For example, severe itching is associated with obstructive biliary disease (primary biliary cirrhosis, extrahepatic biliary obstruction, and intrahepatic cholestasis of pregnancy). In these conditions there is an elevation of bilirubin in the serum and extracellular compartment of the dermis, which leads to jaundice.

TABLE 9. CONDITIONS WITH GENERALIZED PRURITUS WITHOUT DIAGNOSTIC SKIN LESIONS

Psychogenic States
Transitory: periods of
emotional stress
Persistent: delusions of
parasitosis

Malignant Neoplasms
Lymphoma and leukemia
Abdominal cancer*
CNS tumors*
Multiple myeloma*

Infestations
Pediculosis corporis
Scabies†
Hookworm
(ancylostomiasis)
Onchocerciasis

Hepatic Disease
Obstructive biliary disease
Pregnancy (intrahepatic
cholestasis)

**Metabolic and Endocrine
Conditions**
Hyperthyroidism
Diabetes mellitus*
Carcinoid syndrome

Drug Ingestion
Opium derivatives
Subclinical drug sensitivities

Renal Disease
Chronic renal failure

Hematologic Disease
Polycythemia vera‡

Miscellaneous Conditions
Dry skin§
"Senile" pruritus§

---

*Not definitely proved.
†Diagnostic lesions may be present.
‡Especially after a bath.
§Unexplained intense pruritus in patients over 65 years without obvious
"dry skin" and with no apparent emotional stress.
  Source: Fitzpatrick, T. B., Eisen, A. Z., Wolff, K., Freedberg, I. M., and
Austen, K. F. (eds.): Dermatology in General Medicine. 2nd ed. New York,
McGraw-Hill Book Co., 1979.

Bile acids have been identified in the skin, and itching can be produced by application of bile acids to cellophane-stripped skin, possibly through the release of proteolytic enzymes contained in lysosomes, which have a detergent effect on the lipid cell membrane.

By using a nonabsorbable anion-exchange resin, cholestyramine, it is possible to lower the bile acid concentration and thereby stop the pruritus. For some unknown reason, the severe pruritus that occurs in patients on hemodialysis can be markedly decreased by exposing the skin to total-body irradiation with ultraviolet light (UV-B, 290 to 320 nm).

PHOTOSENSITIVITY

The warm, relaxing rays of the sun are not beneficial to the skin, but actually noxious, producing in humans a diverse variety of deleterious effects ranging from an acute sunburn to crippling photosensitivity and even fatal skin cancer. Sunlight occupies almost a divine position in our society. Millions of dollars and countless hours are spent by people seeking the sun. Man is truly phototropic—turning to the sun at every opportunity.

Sunlight comprises infrared radiation (60 per cent), visible radiation (37 per cent), and ultraviolet radiation (3 per cent). Visible light, in turn, is composed of a spectrum of colors from red (700 nm) at one end to violet (400 nm) at the other end.

Most of the ultraviolet radiation emitted by the sun is absorbed by ozone (O_3) in the stratosphere; the portion that reaches the earth's surface covers a range of 286 to 400 nm. Ultraviolet radiation evoking the biologic effects on the skin is arbitrarily divided into three regions: (1) Ultraviolet A (or UV-A) extends from 400 to 320 nm and evokes biologic response in normal skin. (2) Ultraviolet B (or UV-B) includes wavelengths from 320 to 286 nm, the latter being the shortest wavelengths to reach the earth's surface. UV-B is also called the "sunburn" spectrum, because exposure to the 290 to 320 nm radiation results in acute vascular response (erythema or "sunburn") in some white people on short exposures in the summer at all latitudes, and at all seasons in geographic regions near the equator. (3) Ultraviolet C (UV-C) does not reach the earth's surface, being absorbed by ozone in the stratosphere. UV-C is highly toxic to life and artificially produced UV-C is, in fact, a germicidal agent, used in surgical operating rooms and anywhere that a sterile environment is necessary. While quartz transmits UV-A, UV-B, and UV-C, ordinary window glass transmits only UV-A; this is why it is not possible to obtain a sunburn while sitting behind a window glass.

Types of Reactions to Sunlight Exposure

The photosensitivity reactions of the skin to sunlight exposure (UV-A, UV-B, and visible wavelengths) depend on the amount of exposure and the skin type (see below). Pathologic responses can also be related to (1) light per se, (2) light in combination with an exogenous agent (e.g., drugs or chemicals), (3) light in combination with an endogenously produced metabolite (e.g., photosensitizing porphyrins), and (4) light causing an abnormal response by its action on skin that has an inherent pathologic alteration (e.g., defective DNA repair in xeroderma pigmentosum) (Table 10). Finally, individuals may develop pruritic rashes following sun exposure for no known reason.

The following classification divides light-induced disorders into eight categories (Table 11).

Category I—Physiologic Phototoxicity (Sunburn)

Definition. Excessive sun exposure in normal persons.

Sunburn occurs when white persons exceed their normal skin tolerance, which is 15 to 20 minutes in northern latitudes in summer, but which varies with the skin type. Skin types I and II will exceed their tolerance in 12 to 20 minutes of noon exposure in northern latitudes in the summer, while persons with skin type IV may not exceed their tolerance even after 45 minutes of sun exposure.

The mechanism of the sunburn delayed erythema response is not entirely known, but there is evidence to implicate prostaglandins (PG) as indomethacin blocks PG synthesis from arachidonic acid and also prevents the erythema response. Histamine is not involved in the delayed sunburn response. Whether other mediators such as kinins are involved in the sunburn erythema is not known.

Sun Reactive Skin Types. Normal persons who go out in the sun do not all have the same skin reaction. Individuals are predisposed to sunburn based on a congenital partial or total deficiency of melanin follow-

TABLE 10. DISEASES* INDUCED OR EXACERBATED BY LIGHT†

COFACTOR IN PATHOGENESIS	LIGHT ALONE	LIGHT + EXOGENOUS AGENT	LIGHT + METABOLITE	LIGHT + PREEXISTING DISEASE
Genetic	Ephelides (freckles)		Porphyrias: Erythropoietic porphyria Erythropoietic protoporphyria Variegate porphyria (mixed porphyria) Hereditary coproporphyria Porphyria cutanea tarda	Xeroderma pigmentosum Oculocutaneous albinism
Chemical or drug		"Phototoxic" reactions Phytophotodermatitis Lupus erythematosus, hydralazine, and procainamide	Porphyria cutanea tarda from hexachlorobenzene, estrogens, stilbestrol, and alcohol	
Chemical (drug) and immunologic		"Photoallergic" reactions		
Nutritional and metabolic				Pellagra Malignant carcinoid
Infectious agent				Herpes simplex
Not defined	Acute solar skin damage (sunburn) Connective tissue degeneration (wrinkling) Telangiectasia Solar keratoses and solar lentigo Basal cell carcinoma Squamous cell carcinoma Malignant melanoma Polymorphous photodermatosis Solar urticaria			

*Excludes some rare disorders caused or exacerbated by light exposure.
†All responses are caused by UV-B, UV-A, and visible light.

TABLE 11. CATEGORIES OF REACTIONS TO SUNLIGHT EXPOSURE

PHOTOTOXIC[1]	Acute[3]	Chronic[4]
	Category I—Physiologic phototoxicity (sunburn)	Category VI—Dermatoheliosis (telangiectasia, lentigo, keratoses, wrinkling)
	Category II—Chemical phototoxicity (e.g., tetracycline)	Category VII—Dermatoheliosis with multiple skin cancers resulting from a heritable defect in DNA repair (xeroderma pigmentosum)
	Category III—Metabolic phototoxicity (e.g., erythropoietic protoporphyria)	
PHOTOIMMUNOLOGIC[2]		
	Category IV—Chemical photoallergy (e.g., oral or topical drugs or chemicals)	
IDIOPATHIC PHOTOIMMUNOLOGIC-TYPE REACTIONS[2]		
	Category V—Acute idiopathic photoimmunologic reactions (e.g., polymorphous light eruption)	Category VIII—Chronic idiopathic photoimmunologic-type reactions (e.g., actinic reticuloid)

1—Morphology—Sunburn: confluent erythema, edema, vesicles.
2—Morphology—"Rashes": discrete papules, plaques, wheals.
3—Occurring within minutes to hours following exposure.
4—Following repeated exposures over years.

ing exposure (i.e., tan). This individual reactivity can be easily ascertained by history of the person's response to a short, single exposure of untanned skin: the degree of sunburn response and the "tan" that can be developed. Swarthy-skinned or black people have little or no response to sun exposure except to develop an immediate, short-lived tan (so-called immediate pigment darkening). Fair-skinned white persons react differently depending on their skin type. The different skin types have been discussed earlier in this chapter.

Prolonged and repeated exposure to sunlight leads to actinic changes and premature aging of the skin which we have termed dermatoheliosis. These changes, limited to the areas that are habitually exposed, occur in persons who are genetically deficient in melanin pigmentation responses, i.e., types I and II sun-reactive skin types. So-called sailor's skin and farmer's skin, which can also be called beach bum's skin, is markedly wrinkled, contains telangiectases, has a loss of elasticity, and develops punctate warty lesions known as actinic keratoses. The connective tissue of the dermis becomes markedly altered, the fibers become hypertrophied, curled, fragmented, and degenerated; decrease in insoluble collagen occurs, and there is a real or apparent increase in elastin and ground substance. The mechanism of age-dependent changes in cells and tissues may be due to intramolecular and intermolecular cross-linking reactions.

Category II—Chemical Phototoxicity

Definition. Normal sun exposure in persons who have ingested certain chemicals (i.e., tetracycline or its derivatives).

Phototoxicity is a dose-related response and occurs in all persons after exposure of normal skin containing a phototoxic chemical to an appropriate wavelength. Phototoxicity occurs only when both the chemical and the appropriate wavelength are present. Certain phototoxic chemicals appear to act by selective localization in the cell membrane (e.g., anthracene); others, such as psoralens, attach to DNA; and some chemicals appear to concentrate on lysosomes and, on exposure to ultraviolet radiation, cause destruction of lysosomes.

Category III—Metabolic Phototoxicity

Definition. Normal sun exposure in persons with an inherited metabolic disease (e.g., erythropoietic protoporphyria).

A dark-haired girl of six years cried every summer and had to stay indoors because when she played outside for more than even a few minutes, she would begin to feel an uncomfortable pruritus, her skin would become warm, and her hands would begin to swell. A few hours later she would be very uncomfortable because of swollen hands, swelling and painful blisters on the nose, and severe red "sunburn." After one or two such episodes, the child's mother could not convince her to go outside at all, and she remained in the house in a darkened room. Her father had the same problem and was forced to work inside and restrict his outdoor activities. Within six weeks after taking 180 mg beta-carotene daily, both the child and the father could assume a nearly normal life out of doors with no necessity to avoid the sun. This is a vignette of erythropoietic protoporphyria, an autosomal dominant trait, in which moderate to severe photosensitivity occurs. In this disorder there is elevated protoporphyrin in the skin because of a deficiency of the enzyme, ferrochelatase, which catalyzes the conversion of protoporphyrin to heme. Protoporphyrin absorbs the visible light and generates singlet oxygen which, being highly reactive, damages the cell membrane. Beta-carotene is capable of effectively quenching singlet oxygen, and thus the damaging effect does not occur.

Category IV—Chemical Photoallergy

Definition. Normal sun exposure that produces rashes in certain persons taking drugs (e.g., oral diazide derivatives).

A rash (urticarial wheals, eczema-like eruptions, or mobilliform eruptions) may occur in white or black persons taking sulfonamide-type drugs, especially thiazide diuretics, or phenothiazines. These are called "photoallergic" reactions. "Photoallergy" is a response to chemicals and radiation, but by an immune mechanism, in contrast to "phototoxicity."

This reaction does not occur in all persons, is not dose-related, and very small amounts of drug can elicit the response. Photoallergy was first described in patients who develop rashes while receiving sulfanilamide. Ultraviolet radiation alters the sulfanilamide in the skin, producing a new product, p-hydroxyaminobenzene-sulfonamide. Applied to the skin, this new allergen can evoke a response *without* ultraviolet irradiation; in other words, the allergen produces contact sensitization.

Category V—Acute Idiopathic Photoimmunologic Reactions (e.g., polymorphous light eruption)

Definition. Normal sun exposure that produces rashes in "normal" persons not taking photosensitizing drugs.

Rashes from the sun can occur without any apparent cause. These eruptions may consist of hives (solar urticaria) or of a variety of rashes—eczema-like or bumpy, itching tiny blisters, or large, red, nonitchy, raised areas—these are collectively known as *polymorphous light eruptions* (called PMLE). Like normal sunburn, PMLE is often not associated with any symptoms during the actual exposure and the eruption is usually delayed in appearing on the skin, becoming evident several hours after exposure. PMLE can be controlled with certain topical sunscreens that filter UV-B *and* UV-A, or, if these fail, by PUVA (see pp. 1312 and 1329) or, finally, by orally administered antimalarial drugs such as hydroxychloroquine or atabrine.

Category VI—Dermatoheliosis (telangiectasia, keratosis, solar lentigo, wrinkling)

Definition. The effects of repeated exposures to the sun on normal skin. These effects occur following the first exposures in early life and are cumulative and irreversible.

The magnitude and variety of the effects depend on the natural defense mechanisms (constitutive pigmentation and facultative tanning) and on whether or not susceptible persons use effective topical sun-protective agents throughout life. The dermatoheliosis syndrome is a polymorphic response to sunlight exposure of various components of the skin: (1) the *vascular system* of the dermis, with acute transient mediator-induced vasodilatation (sunburn erythema) or permanent dilatation of vessels (telangiectasia); (2) the *keratinocytes* of the epidermis leading to localized atypical keratinocytic hyperplasia (solar keratosis); (3) the *melanocytes* of the epidermis leading to macular pigmented lesions with sharply irregular borders and variegated brown color (freckles) and to isolated, smooth-bordered, uniformly brown macules (solar lentigo); and (4) the *connective tissue components* of the dermis, collagen and elastic tissue, leading to wrinkling, roughening, and yellowing of the skin.

Dermatoheliosis, which is analogous to pneumoconiosis, is a preventable environmental hazard that can potentially affect the health of approximately 25 per cent of the population of the United States. Persons at risk need to be identified at an early age and need to be made aware of the noxious long-term effects of the sun: (1) avoiding exposure during the peak flux of UV-B in the middle hours of the day, and (2) using substantive and effective topical sunscreens in a daily program of self-protection.

Category VII—Chronic Idiopathic Photoimmunologic Reactions (e.g., photosensitive eczema or actinic reticuloid)

Definition. Photosensitive eczema and actinic reticuloid, both of unknown etiology and insidious onset, are chronic persistent "rashes" or "dermatitis" that affect middle-aged or older men.

Photosensitive eczema (PSE) can be separated from actinic reticuloid on the basis of clinical, histologic, and photobiologic findings. PSE is not an erythroderma but essentially a chronic eczema (erythemato-papulo-vesicular or erythemato-squamous) that may resemble or be indistinguishable from actinic reticuloid. The pathology is that of a chronic eczema. Patch tests (with irradiation) may be positive, especially to rubber. The photobiologic responses are almost entirely in the 300 nm region.

Actinic reticuloid is a curious disorder resembling the early stages of *photosensitive eczema* that presents initially as an eczematous eruption. Later, however, and in contrast to photosensitive eczema, the skin becomes markedly thickened and lichenified, and episodes of an almost universal erythroderma are an important and common clinical feature. Monochromatic irradiation in actinic reticuloid reveals a wide spectrum of abnormal response from 300 to 360 nm (and frequently extending to 400 nm and even to 600 nm). The nature of the dermal infiltrate suggests a cell-mediated rather than an immunoglobulin (IgE) reaction. The course of actinic reticuloid is relentless, but no true transition to lymphoma has ever been reported.

Category VIII—Heritable Dermatoheliosis and Multiple Skin Cancers

Definition. Normal sun exposure in persons with an inherited defect in DNA repair (xeroderma pigmentosa).

DNA is one of the principal targets of UV-B. Intense exposure leads to inhibition of cell division and even to cell death. Sublethal damage is repaired, but if the repair is not accurate there is a mutation and possibly a carcinoma. Ultraviolet causes base alterations and chain breaks. The most frequent base alteration is the formation of pyrimidine dimers, a covalent linkage of two pyrimidine residues to form a cyclobutane ring. Thymine-thymine dimers are most frequently encountered from exposure to UV-B irradiation. Repair of UV-damaged DNA occurs by three enzyme repair processes: excision repair, photoreactivation repair, and postreplication (recombination) repair. In excision repair there is a recognition and removal from single strands of DNA of a dimer and then a synthesis and rejoining of a new sequence of bases of DNA (so-called cut and patch). The photoreactivation system involves a split of the dimer following exposure to 300 to 500 nm by the action of a photoreactivating enzyme. The role of photoreactivation in humans is not known, although the photoreactivating enzyme has been demonstrated. In postreplication repair, the damaged segment of DNA is bypassed by the normal repair replication. The gap that remains in the daughter segment opposite the damaged segment is filled by a segment of normal parental segment (recombination). This parent dimer is removed by excision repair. Repair replication is error-prone and can, therefore, lead to mutation.

Xeroderma pigmentosum (XP), an autosomal recessive trait, is a defect in excision repair of dimers and of postreplication repair. In XP there is a high incidence of sun-induced skin cancers, including basal cell and squamous cell carcinomas, malignant melanomas, and sarcomas. XP patients have a striking, freckle-like pigmentation, depigmentation, and telangiectasia limited to areas exposed to the sun. In some types of XP there are associated neurologic disorders (mental retardation, ataxia, choreoathetosis, and spasticity). The skin changes are limited to the sun-exposed areas, develop in early childhood, and may begin in infancy.

Mechanism of Action of Light in Phototherapy, and Photoprotection

Light alone or light combined with certain photoactive chemicals has been used as a therapeutic modality, with only little success until recently. Certain diseases improve following exposure to the sun; these include common and disfiguring diseases such as psoriasis, eczema, and acne. These same diseases respond quite well to artificial UV-B irradiation, although its mechanism of action is not known. In psoriasis it is presumed that ultraviolet inhibits DNA synthesis. UV-B also appears to improve the severe pruritus that occurs in patients on chronic hemodialysis, but the mode of action is not yet understood.

Visible light (with a maximum efficacy at 410 to 460 nm) is effective in treating premature infants with hyperbilirubinemia. Bilirubin is toxic to neurons and causes a bilirubin encephalopathy, especially in premature infants. Phototherapy acts by preventing increased bilirubin concentrations, presumably by a photodecomposition of bilirubin, but also by an unexplained enhancement of excretion of the unconjugated bilirubin during and after phototherapy. When the interaction of drugs and light produces biologic changes in the skin, the effects are usually considered deleterious and are often referred to as phototoxic or photoallergic reactions. The term photochemotherapy describes quite the opposite effect on the skin: the combination of drug and light produces a beneficial effect. Photochemotherapy can be considered an example of the pharmacologic phenomenon of potentiation: the combined action of two agents is greater than the sum of their individual actions. Oral psoralen photochemotherapy involves the ingestion of psoralens (P) followed, at a specified interval, by exposure of the skin to long-wave ultraviolet light (UV-A), abbreviated PUVA. PUVA inhibits DNA synthesis and leads to improvement of diseases associated with cellular proliferation in the epidermis (psoriasis) and in the dermis (mycosis fungoides) and a large variety of other skin diseases (lichen planus, polymorphous light eruption, disabling chronic light diseases, vitiligo). The compound most effective in oral psoralen photochemotherapy of psoriasis is methoxsalen or 8-methoxypsoralen. The light system must deliver UV-A uniformly to the entire body surface without significant UV-B.

Topical sunburn prevention is accomplished by application of UV-B–absorbing chemicals in alcoholic solutions, in oil-in-water emulsions, or in acid, cinnamates, and benzophenones. The aim of photoprotection of normal and abnormal skin is to reduce the penetration of ultraviolet radiation into the epidermis. There are very effective preparations that prevent sunburn from UV-B, even type I and type II persons. UV-A sunscreens are currently available but are not as effective as UV-B sunscreens; nevertheless, most sunscreens now contain both UV-A and UV-B filters. The effectiveness and substantivity of sunscreens depend not only on the concentration of the absorbing chemical but equally on the selection of the vehicle.

REFERENCES

Anderson, R., Coons, R. L., and Smith, D. E.: The effect of oral and topical tetracycline on acne severity and on surface lipid composition. J Invest Dermatol 66:172, 1976.

Bergstresser, P. E., and Taylor, J. R.: Epidermal turnover time—a new examination. Br J Dermatol 96:503, 1977.

Braverman, I. M., and Yen, A.: Ultrastructure of the human dermal microcirculation. II. The capillary loops of the dermal papillae. J Invest Dermatol 68:44, 1977.

Briggaman, R. A.: Biochemical composition of the epidermal-dermal junction and the basement membrane. J Invest Dermatol 78:1, 1982.

Clark, W. H., Jr., et al.: Origin of familial malignant melanomas from heritable melanocytic lesions: The B-K mole syndrome. Arch Dermatol 114:732, 1978.

Cleaver, J.: Xeroderma pigmentosum. In Stanbury, J. B., Wyngaarden, J. B., Fredrickson, D. S., Goldstein, J. L., and Brown, M. S. (eds.): The Metabolic Basis of Inherited Disease. 5th ed. New York, McGraw-Hill Book Co., 1983.

Cooke, A., and Johnson, B. E.: Dose response, wave-length dependence and rate of excision of ultraviolet radiation–induced pyrimidine dimers in mouse skin DNA. Biochim Biophys Acta 577:24, 1978.

Elder, D. E., et al.: Dysplastic nevus syndrome: A phenotypic of sporadic cutaneous melanoma. Cancer 46:1787, 1980.

Elias, P. M., and Friend, D. S.: The permeability barrier in mammalian epidermis. J Cell Biol 65:180, 1975.

Fitzpatrick, T. B., Sober, A. J., Pearson, B. J., and Lew, R.:

Cutaneous carcinogenic effects of sunlight in humans. In Castellani, A. (ed.): Research in Photobiology. New York/London, Plenum Press, 1978.

Fitzpatrick, T. B., Pathak, M. A., and Parrish, J. A.: Protection of human skin against the effects of the sunburn ultraviolet (290–320 nm). In Pathak, M. A., Harber, L. C., Seiji, M., and Kukita, A. (eds.); and Fitzpatrick, T. B. (consulting ed.): Sunlight and Man: Normal and Abnormal Photobiologic Responses. Tokyo, University of Tokyo Press, 1974, p. 751.

Fitzpatrick, T. B., et al.: Heritable melanin deficiency syndromes. Diagnosis and prophylactic treatment with sunprotective agents. In Update: Dermatology in General Medicine. New York, McGraw-Hill Book Co., 1983, p. 46.

Fuchs, E., and Green, H.: Changes in keratin gene expression during terminal differentiation of the keratinocyte. Cell 19:1033, 1980.

Greaves, M. W., Yamamoto, S., and Fairley, V. M.: IgE-mediated hypersensitivity in human skin studied using a new in vitro method. Immunology 23:239, 1972.

Harrison, G. A.: Differences in human pigmentation: Measurement, geographic variation, and causes. J Invest Dermatol 60:418, 1973.

Hertz, K.: Autoimmune vitiligo: Detection of antibodies to melanin producing cells. N Engl J Med 297:634, 1977.

Higgins, J. C., and Eady, R. A. J.: Human dermal microvasculature. I. Its segmental differentiation. Light and electron microscopic study. Br. J Dermatol 104:117, 1981.

Jimbow, K., Fitzpatrick, T. B., Szabo, G., and Hori, Y.: Congenital circumscribed hypomelanosis: A characterization based on electron microscopic study of tuberous sclerosis, nevus depigmentosus and piebaldism. J Invest Dermatol 64:30, 1975.

Lampe, M. A., Williams, M. L., and Elias, P. M.: Human epidermal lipids: Characterization and modulations during differentiation. J Lipid Res 24:131, 1983.

Lavker, R. M., and Sun, T.-T.: Heterogeneity in basal keratinocytes: Morphological and functional correlations. Science 215:1239, 1982.

Lerner, A. B.: Neural control of pigment cells. In Kawamura, T., Fitzpatrick, T. B., and Seiji, M. (eds.): The Biology of Normal and Abnormal Melanocytes. Tokyo, University Park Press, 1971, p. 3.

Leyden, J. J., McGinley, K. J., Mills, O. H., and Kligman, A. M.: Propionibacterium levels in patients with and without acne vulgaris. J Invest Dermatol 65:382, 1975.

Marx, J. F.: DNA repair. New clues to carcinogenesis. Science 200:518, 1978.

Nakagawa, H., Hori, Y., Sato, S., Fitzpatrick, T. B., and Murtuza, R. L.: The nature and origin of the melanin macroglobule. J Invest Dermatol 83:134, 1984.

Ortonne, J.-P., Mosher, D. B., and Fitzpatrick, T. B.: Vitiligo and Other Hypomelanoses of Hair and Skin. New York, Plenum Medical Books, 1983.

Pathak, M. A., Kramer, D. M., and Gungerick, U.: Formation of thymine dimers in mammalian skin by ultraviolet radiation in vivo. Photochem Photobiol 15:177, 1972.

Peck, G. L.: Prolonged remission of cystic and conglobate acne with 13 cis retinoic acid. N Engl J Med 300:329, 1979.

Pochi, P. E., Strauss, J. S., and Downing, D. T.: Skin surface lipid composition, acne, pubertal development and urinary excretion of testosterone and 17-ketosteroids in children. J Invest Dermatol 69:485, 1977.

Snyder, D. S., and Eaglstein, W. H.: Intradermal anti-prostaglandin agents and sunburn. J Invest Dermatol 62:47, 1974.

Soter, N. A., Lewis, R. A., Corey, E. J., and Austen, K. F.: Local effects of synthetic leukotrienes (LTC$_4$, LTD$_4$, LTE$_4$, and LTB$_4$) in human skin. J Invest Dermatol 80:115, 1983.

Soter, N. A.: Physical urticaria/angioedema as an experimental model of acute and chronic inflammation in human skin. Springer Semin Immunopathol 4:73, 1981.

Soter, N. A., Mihm, M. C., Jr., Gigli, I., Dvorak, H. F., and Austen, K. F.: Two distinct cellular patterns in cutaneous necrotizing angiitis. J Invest Dermatol 66:344, 1976.

Soter, N. A., Mihm, M. C., Jr., Dvorak, H. F., and Austen, K. F.: Cutaneous necrotizing venulitis: A sequential analysis of the morphologic alterations occurring after mast cell degranulation in a patient with a unique syndrome. Clin Exp Immunol 32:46, 1978.

Stanley, J. R., Hawley-Nelson, P., Yaar, M., Martin, G. R., and Katz, S. I.: Laminin and bullous pemphigoid antigen are distinct basement membrane proteins synthesized by epidermal cells. J Invest Dermatol 82:456, 1982.

Sun, T.-T., Eichner, R., Schermer, A., Cooper, D., Nelson, W., and Weiss, R. A.: Classification, expression and possible mechanisms of evolution of mammalian epithelial keratins: A unifying model. In Levine, A., Topp, W., VandeWoude, G., and Watson, J. D. (eds.): The Cancer Cell. Vol. I, The Transformed Phenotype. New York, Cold Spring Harbor Lab., 1984, p. 169.

Sun, T.-T., Shih, C., and Green, H.: Keratin cytoskeletons in epithelial cells of internal organs. Proc Natl Acad Sci USA 76:2813, 1979.

Uitto, J.: Biochemistry of the elastic fibers in normal connective tissues and its alterations in disease. J Invest Dermatol 72:1, 1979.

Urbach, F., Epstein, J. H., and Forbes, P. D.: Ultraviolet carcinogenesis: Experimental, global and genetic aspects. In Pathak, M. A., Harber, L. C., Seiji, M., and Kukita, A. (eds.), and Fitzpatrick, T. B. (consulting ed.): Sunlight and Man: Normal and Abnormal Photobiologic Responses. Tokyo, University of Tokyo Press, 1974, p. 259.

Voorhees, J. J., and Marcelo, C.: Molecular mechanisms and the cyclic nucleotide cascade in psoriasis. In Farber, E. M., and Cox, A. V. (eds.): Psoriasis: Proceedings of the Second International Symposium. New York, Yorke Medical Books, 1977, p. 91.

Williams, M. L., and Elias, P. M.: Elevated n-alkanes in congenital ichthyosiform erythroderma. J Clin Invest 74:296, 1984.

Witkop, C., Jr., Quevedo, W. C., Jr., and Fitzpatrick, T. B.: Albinism. In Stanbury, J. B., Wyngaarden, J. B., Fredrickson, D. S., Goldstein, J. L., and Brown, M. S. (eds.): The Metabolic Basis of Inherited Disease. 5th ed. New York, McGraw-Hill Book Co., 1983.

INDEX

Note: The expression "vs." has been used to denote "differential diagnosis." Italics indicate illustrations and t indicates tables.